HANDBOOK *of* NUTRITION *and* FOOD

HANDBOOK *of* NUTRITION *and* FOOD

Edited by

CAROLYN D. BERDANIER

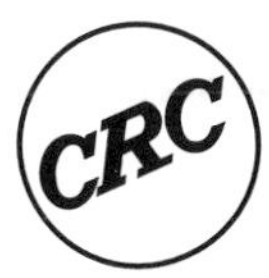

CRC PRESS

Boca Raton London New York Washington, D.C.

Library of Congress Cataloging-in-Publication Data

CRC handbook of nutrition and food / edited by Carolyn D. Berdanier … [et al.].
p. cm.
Includes bibliographical references and index.
ISBN 0-8493-2705-9
1. Nutrition—Handbooks, manuals, etc. I. Title: Handbook of nutrition and food. II. Berdanier, Carolyn D.

QP141 .C774 2001
612.3'9—dc21 2001035595
CIP

Direct all inquiries to CRC Press LLC, 2000 N.W. Corporate Blvd., Boca Raton, Florida 33431.

International Standard Book Number 0-8493-2705-9
Library of Congress Card Number 2001035595
Printed in the United States of America 2 3 4 5 6 7 8 9 0
Printed on acid-free paper

Part VI Modified Diets

Part VII Clinical Nutrition

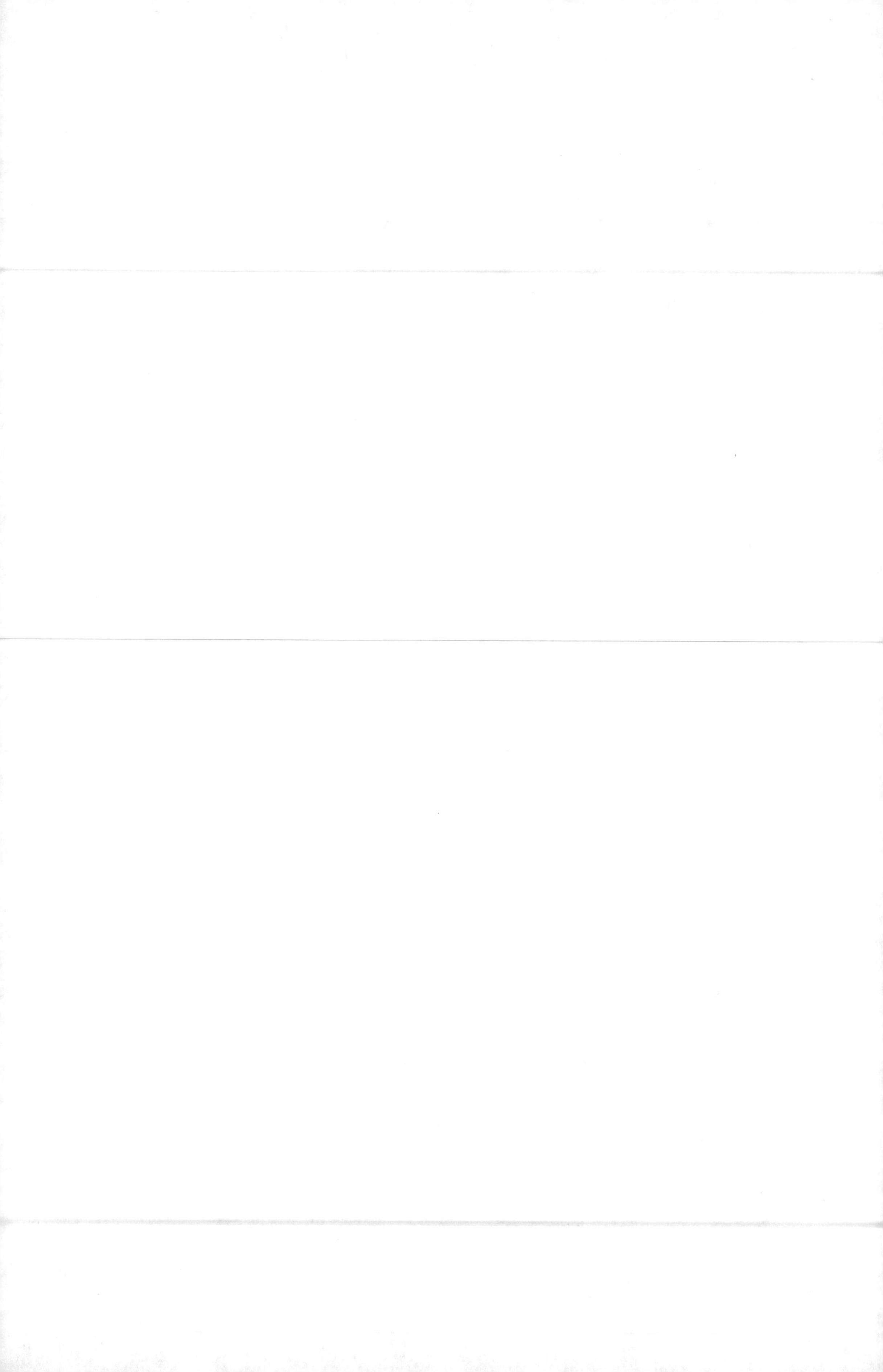

Part I

Food

1

Food Constituents

Carolyn D. Berdanier

Animals, including man, consume food to obtain the nutrients they need. Throughout the world there are differences in food consumption related to socioeconomic conditions, food availability, and cultural dictates. If a variety of fresh and cooked foods is consumed in sufficient quantities to meet the energy needs of the consumer, then the needs for protein and the micronutrients should be met. Having this in mind, it is surprising to learn that some people are poorly nourished, and indeed may develop one or more nutrition-related diseases. The early years of nutrition research focused on diseases related to inadequate vitamin and mineral intake. An important component of this research was the determination of the vitamin and mineral content of a vast variety of foods. The composition of these foods has been compiled by the USDA, and Table 1.1 provides web addresses to access these data sets. Several data sets that may not be available on the web can be found in this section. Table 1.2 provides the sugar content of selected foods in 100 g portions. This may be a very large serving size or a very small one, depending on the food in question. However, using a standard portion allows one to compare the sugar content of a variety of foods. Those that are very rich sources, i.e., honey or table sugar (sucrose), of course will have a very high value, yet one would not consume this much in a single food under most circumstances. Usually, one would select a portion size compatible with the need for sweetness in the particular food product. For example, one might add a teaspoon of table sugar to a cup of coffee. That teaspoon of sugar might weigh 8 grams.Table 1.3 provides information on the tagatose content of food. Tagatose is a new food additive used to reduce the amount of sugar in a food. It has a sweet taste, yet does not have the same energy value as sucrose. Other sugar substitutes are also used in the preparation of reduced-energy foods; however, data on their quantitative occurrence is not as readily available because of the proprietary interests of food producers. A list of sweeteners added to foods is provided in Table 1.5. Following this table is a list of the types of food additives that change the properties of food (Table 1.6). This table describes compounds that increase the shelf life of a class of foods, or additives that change the texture of a food. The specific attributes of individual food additives are described in Table 1.7. This table provides information on how these additives function in particular food products. Table 1.8 is a list of mycotoxins and bacterial toxins that can occur in food. The reader should also review Section 52 for an extensive description of foodborne illness. Table 1.9 provides a list of antinutrients sometimes found in food, and Table 1.10 is a list of toxic substances that can be present in food. Some of these toxic substances are added inadvertently by the food processing methods, but some occur naturally. If consumed in minute quantities, some of these toxic materials are without significant effect, yet other compounds (e.g., arsenic), even in minute amounts, could accumulate and become lethal.

0-8493-2705-9/01/$0.00+$1.50

Tables 1.11, 1.12, and 1.14 overlap to some extent. All contain information about plants. Some of these plants can have both a food and a non-food use. Non-food use is defined as a use that may have a real or imagined pharmacologic (drug/herbal) effect. The reader should use this information with considerable caution. Plants can differ from variety to variety, and indeed from one growing condition to another in the content of certain of their herbal or nutritive ingredients. Over-the-counter herbal preparations can also vary. There is little regulation of these preparations and few safeguards exist to protect the consumer with respect to biopotency. Furthermore, the consumer should be aware of the fact that some of these herbal remedies may interact with prescribed drugs, either nullifying the drug effect or, worse, interacting to cause an unwarranted or even lethal effect. Consumers of plants used for herbal remedies should consult their pharmacists and physicians about these potentially dangerous uses.

The next six tables provide information about the micronutrients. Table 1.14 gives vitamin terminology. Table 1.15 is a list of compounds that have vitamin A activity. Table 1.16 gives the structures and characteristics of the vitamins. The use of vitamin supplements as well as descriptions of vitamin deficiency is covered in Sections 43, 61, and 62. Table 1.17 summarizes vitamin deficiencies and needs. Table 1.18 summarizes the essential minerals and their functions. A more detailed description of the minerals is provided in Section 57. Table 1.19 lists the essential fatty acids, and Table 1.20 gives the common and technical names for fatty acids. It should be noted that felines require arachidonic acid as well as linoleic and linolenic acid in their diets. Other mammals only require linoleic and linolenic acids.

TABLE 1.1

Web Addresses for Information on the Composition of Food

Data Set	Web Address
Composition of foods, raw, processed, prepared; 6200 foods, 82 nutrients	http://www.nal.usda.gov/fnic/foodcomp/Data/
Daidzein, genisten, glycitein, isoflavone content of 128 foods	Use above address, click on this file to open
Carotenoid content of 215 foods	Use above address, click on this file to open
Trans fatty acid content of 214 foods	Use above address, click on this file to open
Sugar content of 500+ foods	Use above address, click on this file to open
Nutritive value of food in common household units; more than 900 items are in this list	Use above address, click on Nutritive Value of Foods (HG-72) to open
Vitamin K	Use above address, click on vitamin K to open
List of key foods (foods that contribute up to 75% of any one nutrient)	Use above address, click on Key Foods to open
Nutrient retention factors: calculations of retention of specific micronutrients	Use above address, click on Nutrient Retention Factors, Release 4 (1998)
Primary nutrient datasets (results of USDA surveys)	Use above address, click on Primary Nutrient for USDA Nationwide Food Surveys Dataset
Selenium and vitamin D (provisional values)	Use above address, click on selenium and vitamin D to open
Food composition (foods from India)	www.unu.edu/unupress/unupbooks/80633e/80633Eoi.htm
European foods	Cost99/EUROFOODS:Inventory of European Food Composition food.ethz.ch/cost99db-inventory.htm
Foods in developing countries	www.fao.org/DOCREP/W0073e/woo73eO6.htm
Other food data	www.arborcom.com/frame/foodc.htm
Soy foods (beneficial compounds)	See above, isoflavone, etc.
Individual amino acids and fatty acids	http://www.infinite faculty.org/sci/cr/crs/1994

Note: Most of these databases can be accessed as subdirectories of: http://www.Nal.USDA.gov/foodcomp/data/. A printed format can be obtained from the Superintendent of Documents, U.S. Printing Office, Washington D.C. 20402. Request USDA Handbooks 8 through 16. A CD-ROM can also be obtained. None of these are free.

TABLE 1.2

Sugar Content of Selected Foods, 100 Grams, Edible Portion[1]

Food Item	Moisture (%)	Monosaccharides (in grams)			Disaccharides (in grams)			Other Sugars	Total Sugars
		Galactose	Glucose	Fructose	Lactose	Sucrose	Maltose		
Dairy Products									
Cheese									
Brie	47.7	—	1.0	0.3	0.2	0.1	TR	—	1.6
Edam	41.1	—	0.1	—	—	0.1	—	—	0.2
Mozzarella	47.0	—	1.1	—	TR	—	—	—	1.1
Ice cream									
Chocolate	53.7	—	—	—	3.7	14.9	TR	—	18.6
Strawberry	56.9	—	1.5	0.8	4.1	8.5	TR	—	14.9
Vanilla	60.5	—	—	—	5.1	8.9	TR	—	14.0
Ice milk, vanilla	59.3	—	1.6	0.8	5.8	6.5	TR	—	14.7
Yogurt									
Plain	86.0	—	0.3	—	3.0	—	—	—	3.3
Strawberry	72.5	—	2.3	2.1	3.2	7.3	—	—	14.9

TABLE 1.2 *(Continued)*

Sugar Content of Selected Foods, 100 Grams, Edible Portion[1]

Food Item	Moisture (%)	Monosaccharides (in grams)			Disaccharides (in grams)			Other Sugars	Total Sugars
		Galactose	Glucose	Fructose	Lactose	Sucrose	Maltose		
Grains and Baked Products									
Bread									
Banana	32.9	—	TR	0.1	—	25.8	—	—	25.9
Hamburger buns	34.7	—	1.7	1.3	0.2	—	0.2	—	3.4
Pita	20.5	—	0.1	0.2	—	—	1.0	—	1.3
Pumpernickel	37.1	—	0.6	0.1	—	—	1.0	—	1.7
Raisin	31.5	—	7.3	6.6	—	TR	TR	—	13.9
Rye	36.5	—	0.6	0.4	—	0.6	—	—	1.6
White	36.3	—	1.8	1.2	—	0.4	0.2	—	3.6
Whole wheat	39.3	—	0.7	0.6	—	—	0.6	—	1.9
Cake									
Angel food	34.8	—	—	—	—	33.7	—	—	33.7
Sponge	21.1	—	TR	—	—	23.6	—	—	23.6
Yellow	33.9	—	TR	—	—	25.8	—	—	25.8
Cheesecake, plain	38.2	—	TR	—	0.1	7.0	—	—	7.1
Chocolate chip cookies	3.7	—	TR	TR	—	18.7	—	—	18.7
Corn flakes	1.7	—	2.2	2.1	—	2.9	—	—	7.2
Crude wheat germ	9.6	—	0.9	TR	—	6.9	—	—	7.8
Donuts									
Cake type	20.8	—	0.9	0.1	TR	8.6	TR	—	9.6
Yeast type	26.3	—	1.4	1.4	1.0	—	1.4	—	5.2
Flour									
Rye	11.0	—	0.2	0.1	—	0.6	—	—	0.9
White	10.5	—	TR	TR	—	0.1	TR	—	0.1
Whole wheat	9.3	—	TR	TR	—	0.4	—	—	0.4
Graham crackers	5.6	—	1.9	1.2	—	12.6	—	—	5.7
Pasta									
Egg noodles, raw	8.8	—	—	—	—	0.1	0.8	—	0.9
Egg noodles, cooked	67.0	—	0.1	—	—	TR	0.2	—	0.3
Spaghetti, raw	9.8	—	TR	—	—	0.1	0.4	—	0.5
Spaghetti, cooked	62.7	—	0.1	—	—	—	0.2	—	0.3
Rice									
Parboiled, raw	9.8	—	TR	—	—	0.1	—	—	0.1
Parboiled, cooked	72.8	—	0.1	TR	—	0.1	—	—	0.2
Tortillas									
Flour	18.5	—	—	TR	—	0.1	0.5	—	0.6
Corn	49.6	—	—	TR	—	0.5	—	—	0.5
Fruits and Fruit Juices									
Apples									
Delicious, golden	84.5	—	1.8	6.4	—	1.8	—	—	10.0

TABLE 1.2 *(Continued)*

Sugar Content of Selected Foods, 100 Grams, Edible Portion[1]

Food Item	Moisture (%)	Monosaccharides (in grams)			Disaccharides (in grams)			Other Sugars	Total Sugars
		Galactose	Glucose	Fructose	Lactose	Sucrose	Maltose		
Delicious, red	84.9	—	2.4	6.2	—	2.0	—	—	10.6
Winesap	84.7	—	3.5	6.7	—	3.6	—	—	13.8
Apricot nectar	84.6	—	6.3	4.6	—	2.0	—	—	12.9
Cantaloupe	90.0	—	1.1	1.3	—	5.9	—	—	8.3
Dried apricots	26.5	—	13.1	7.6	—	5.8	—	—	26.5
Dried peaches	22.6	—	9.9	11.4	—	17.6	—	—	38.9
Dried pears	33.1	—	8.9	23.0	—	—	—	—	31.9
Dried prunes	3.8	—	19.5	10.6	—	—	—	—	30.1
Grapes, Thompson, seedless	74.9	—	7.9	7.8	—	1.1	—	—	16.8
Grapefruit, white, seedless	87.7	—	2.0	1.9	—	2.5	—	—	6.4
Kiwi	83.1	—	3.5	3.9	—	0.9	—	—	8.3
Orange juice, canned	87.7	—	2.4	2.6	—	2.8	—	—	7.8
Peaches	87.5	—	0.9	0.9	—	—	—	—	1.8
Pears, Bartlett	83.6	—	4.4	6.7	—	0.9	—	—	12.0
Persimmon	78.9	—	5.4	5.6	—	1.5	—	—	12.5
Plums	89.1	—	3.1	2.6	—	2.7	—	—	8.4
Strawberries									
Fresh, raw	91.7	—	1.6	1.8	—	0.2	—	—	3.6
Frozen with sugar added	71.2	—	5.8	5.1	—	16.3	—	—	27.2
Frozen without sugar added	90.4	—	1.9	1.8	—	—	—	—	3.7
Tangelos	86.5	—	1.5	1.6	—	4.0	—	—	7.1
Tangerines	82.3	—	2.2	2.6	—	6.7	—	—	11.5
Watermelon	91.1	—	1.6	3.4	—	3.7	—	—	8.7
Vegetable Products									
Broccoli									
Raw	90.9	—	0.4	0.4	—	0.1	—	—	0.9
Cooked	90.7	—	0.4	0.3	—	0.1	—	—	0.8
Cabbage									
Raw	92.7	—	1.5	1.1	—	TR	TR	—	2.6
Cooked	93.8	—	1.0	0.7	—	0.1	—	—	1.8
Carrots									
Raw	88.3	—	0.6	0.5	—	3.1	—	—	4.2
Cooked	90.1	—	0.3	0.3	—	1.6	—	—	2.2
Mushrooms, raw	93.2	—	2.6	TR	—	—	—	—	2.6
Spinach									
Raw	93.5	—	0.1	TR	—	TR	—	—	0.1
Cooked	93.2	—	0.1	TR	—	TR	—	—	0.1
Sprouts									
Alfalfa, raw	92.3	—	0.1	0.1	—	TR	—	—	0.2
Mung bean, raw	91.0	—	1.0	0.5	—	0.2	—	—	1.7
Sweet potatoes									
Raw	73.4	—	0.9	0.7	—	3.5	—	—	5.1
Cooked	82.1	—	0.7	0.8	—	2.4	2.6	—	6.5

TABLE 1.2 *(Continued)*

Sugar Content of Selected Foods, 100 Grams, Edible Portion[1]

Food Item	Moisture (%)	Monosaccharides (in grams) Galactose	Glucose	Fructose	Disaccharides (in grams) Lactose	Sucrose	Maltose	Other Sugars	Total Sugars
Beverages									
Beer									
Light	97.9	—	TR	TR	—	—	TR	—	TR
Regular	96.1	—	TR	—	—	—	—	—	TR
Sherry									
Dry	72.2	—	0.6	0.5	—	TR	TR	—	1.1
Medium	71.7	—	1.6	1.3	—	—	—	—	2.9
Sweet	70.8	—	0.9	5.2	—	—	—	—	6.1
Wine									
Port, dessert	69.0	—	4.3	5.1	—	TR	—	—	9.4
Red, dry	85.1	—	0.4	0.3	—	0.1	—	—	0.8
Rose, dry	84.2	—	1.4	1.4	—	—	—	—	2.8
White, dry	86.5	—	0.6	0.6	—	—	0.1	—	1.3
Vermouth, dry	72.8	—	0.6	0.5	—	—	—	—	1.1
Sweets									
Honey	7.8	—	38.7	45.2	—	TR	TR	—	83.9
Maple syrup	32.7	—	TR	TR	—	55.4	—	—	55.4
Milk chocolate, plain	1.4	—	—	—	6.6	46.4	—	—	53.0
Molasses	17.4	—	15.7	14.8	—	24.5	—	—	55.9
Molasses, blackstrap	23.0	—	—	9.8	—	42.5	—	—	52.3
Nuts and Seeds									
Coconut, dried, sweetened	10.6	—	0.4	0.2	—	3.9	—	—	4.5
Sesame seeds									
Dehulled	4.1	—	0.1	—	—	0.1	—	—	0.2
Whole	5.4	—	TR	—	—	0.3	—	—	0.3
Sunflower nuts, dried roasted	1.4	—	1.5	—	—	1.5	—	—	3.0
Legumes									
Baked beans									
In tomato sauce	73.8	—	0.6	0.5	—	4.2	—	0.3	5.6
With pork	69.0	—	1.4	1.0	—	4.2	—	0.3	6.9
Black-eyed peas	75.9	—	—	0.2	—	0.3	—	—	0.5
Chickpeas	65.0	—	—	0.2	—	0.2	—	—	0.4

Note: Dash denotes lack of data for sugar that may be present; (0.0) denotes lack of data for sugar thought not to be present; TR denotes trace.

[1] See also http://www.nal.usda./goo/fnic/foodcomp/data/sugar.

TABLE 1.3
Tocopherols and Tocotrienols in Selected Food Products (mg/100 g)

Product	α-T	α-T3	β-T	β-T3	γ-T	γ-T3	δ-T	δ-T3	Total	α Tocopherol Equivalents
Breakfast Cereals										
Fortified										
Total	104.50				ND		ND		104.50	104.50
King Vitamin	35.10				ND		ND		35.10	35.10
Non-Fortified										
Post Natural Raisin Bran	1.50				ND		ND		1.50	1.50
Kellogg's	1.30				ND		ND		1.30	1.30
Cheese										
American										
Low fat Weight Watchers	1.50				ND		ND		1.50	1.50
Borden Lite Line	0.10				ND		ND		0.10	0.10
Processed										
Kraft	0.40				ND		ND		0.40	0.40
American processed										
Kroger	0.40				ND		ND		0.40	0.40
Cheddar										
Kraft	0.30				ND		ND		0.30	0.30
Kroger	0.20				ND		ND		0.20	0.20
Munster										
Sargento	0.50				ND		ND		0.50	0.50
Kroger	0.30				ND		ND		0.30	0.30
Swiss										
Kraft	0.60				ND		ND		0.60	0.60
Beatrice City Line Old World	0.40				ND		ND		0.40	0.40
Chips										
Potato										
Lay's	1.30				4.60		1.30		7.20	1.80
Wise	7.40				1.20		0.10		8.70	7.52
Tortilla										
Tostitos	1.10				2.40		0.50		4.00	1.36
Tostados	1.50				1.00		0.30		2.80	1.61
										0.00

TABLE 1.3 *(Continued)*

Tocopherols and Tocotrienols in Selected Food Products (mg/100 g)

Product	α-T	α-T3	β-T	β-T3	γ-T	γ-T3	δ-T	δ-T3	Total	α Tocopherol Equivalents
Fish										
Salmon, waterpack										
Chicken of the Sea	0.70				ND		ND		0.70	0.70
Black Top	0.60				ND		ND		0.60	0.60
Sardines, in tomato sauce										
Spirit of Norway	3.60				0.20		0.10		3.90	3.62
Orleans	3.90				ND		0.10		4.00	3.90
Tuna, canned in oil										0.00
Starkist	1.00				4.80		1.90		7.70	1.54
Chicken of the Sea	0.98				2.60		1.10		4.68	1.27
Fruits and Fruit Juices										
Grape juice, bottled										
Welch's	ND				ND		ND		0.00	0.00
Seneca	ND				ND		ND		0.00	0.00
Orange juice										
Fresh Tropicana	0.20				ND		ND		0.20	0.20
Frozen Minute Maid	0.20				0.10		ND		0.30	0.21
Plums										0.00
Variety 1	0.70				0.10		ND		0.80	0.71
Variety 2	0.50				0.04		ND		0.54	0.50
Milk chocolate, plain	0.50				2.00		ND		2.50	0.70
Nuts										
Brazil nuts										
Health food store	6.60				2.10		1.60		10.30	6.86
Dekalb Farmers Market	11.00				5.10		2.60		18.70	11.59
English walnuts										
Diamond	1.40				9.20		0.60		11.20	2.34
Kroger					6.70		0.50		7.20	0.69
Hazelnuts										
Health food store	21.50				0.10		0.01		21.61	21.51
Dekalb Farmers Market	16.80				0.70		ND		17.50	16.87

Oils					
Margarine, stick					
Mazzola	8.40	24.40	0.40	33.20	10.85
Fleischman	7.90	23.10	0.60	31.60	10.23
Mayonnaise					
Kraft	1.30	6.60	1.00	8.90	1.99
Hellman	1.60	9.80	1.90	13.30	2.64
Shortenings, Crisco	5.60	25.20	5.40	36.20	8.28
Vegetable oil					0.00
Crisco	2.90	33.30	7.00	43.20	6.44
Wesson	2.80	18.30	3.00	24.10	4.72
Protein Diet Powder					
Slimfast	26.50	ND	ND	26.50	26.50
Herbalife	24.60	ND	ND	24.60	24.60
Salad Dressings					
Bleu Cheese					
Marie's	4.70	57.50	25.40	87.60	11.21
Kraft	2.80	49.00	14.40	66.20	8.13
French					
Wishbone	3.00	66.90	27.70	97.60	10.52
Kraft	3.10	61.90	18.20	83.20	9.84
Italian					
Wishbone	4.40	60.60	30.00	95.00	11.36
Kraft	4.00	62.70	17.80	84.50	10.80
Tea					
Tea leaves from tea bags					
Tetley	2.40	0.60	ND	3.00	2.46
Lipton	12.30	3.20	ND	15.50	12.62
Tea brewed from tea bags					
Tetley	ND	ND	ND	0.00	0.00
Lipton	ND	ND	ND	0.00	0.00
Tomato Products					
Barbecue sauce					
Kraft	1.00	0.80	0.10	1.90	1.08

TABLE 1.3 *(Continued)*

Tocopherols and Tocotrienols in Selected Food Products (mg/100 g)

Product	α-T	α-T3	β-T	β-T3	γ-T	γ-T3	δ-T	δ-T3	Total	α Tocopherol Equivalents
Heinz	1.10				0.40		0.10		1.60	1.14
Catsup										
Heinz	1.10				0.10		ND		1.20	1.11
Hunt's	1.80				0.20		ND		2.00	1.82
Tomato chili sauce										
Del Monte	2.70				0.20		ND		2.90	2.72
Heinz	3.20				0.30		ND		3.50	3.23
Tomato paste										
Hunt's	4.10				0.30		ND		4.40	4.13
Contadina	4.50				0.70		ND		5.20	4.57
Tomato sauce										
Hunt's	1.40				0.10		ND		1.50	1.41
Progresso	1.50				0.20		ND		1.70	1.52
Tomato soup										
Campbell's	0.70				0.30		0.10		1.10	0.73
Kroger	0.60				0.10		ND		0.70	0.61
Tomatoes, stewed										
Del Monte	0.90				0.20		ND		1.10	0.92
Stokely's	0.70				0.20		ND		0.90	0.72
Vegetables										
Asparagus										
Sample 1	1.00				0.10		ND		1.10	1.01
Sample 2	1.30				0.10		ND		1.40	1.31
Cabbage										
Sample 1	0.12				ND		ND		0.12	0.12
Sample 2	0.09				ND		ND		0.09	0.09
Cucumbers										
Sample 1	0.04				0.02		ND		0.06	0.04
Sample 2	0.09				0.02		ND		0.11	0.09
Turnip greens										
Sample 1	2.90				0.10		ND		3.00	2.91
Sample 2	2.80				0.20		ND		3.00	2.82

Note: ND, not detectable.

TABLE 1.4

Occurrence of D-Tagatose in Foods[1]

Food	Result (mg/kg)	Sample Preparation	Apparatus
Sterilized cow's milk	2 to 3000	Extracted with methanol; prepared trimethylsilyl (TMS) derivatives	Gas chromatography (GC), fused silica capillary column (18m × 0.22mm) coated with AT-1000; carrier gas-N_2; flame ionization detector (FID)
Hot cocoa (processed with alkali) prepared with milk	140	Extracted with deionized (DI) water	High performance liquid chromatography (HPLC); used Bio-Rad Aminex® HPX-87C column (300 mm × 7.8 mm) heated to 85° C; mobile phase-DI water; flow rate-0.6 mL/min; refractive index (RI) detector
Hot cocoa prepared with milk	190	Extracted with DI water	HPLC; Bio-Rad Aminex® HPX-87C column heated to 85°C; mobile phase-DI water; flow rate-0.6 mL/min; RI detector
Powdered cow's milk	800	Extracted three times with distilled water for 3h at 60°C; column chromatography to remove organic acids and bases; fractionation by partition chromatography	Paper partition chromatography, descending method on Whatman no.1 paper; used three solvent systems
Similac® infant formula	4	Extracted with 90% ethanol; prepared TMS derivatives	GC; DB-5 fused-silica capillary column (15 m × 0.53 mm, 1.5 μm film thickness); carrier gas-He; FID detector
Enfamil® infant formula	23	Extracted with 90% aqueous ethanol; prepared TMS derivatives	GC; DB-17 fused-silica capillary column (15 m × 0.53 mm,1 μm film thickness); carrier gas-He; FID detector
Parmesan cheese	10	Extracted with 80% aqueous methanol; prepared TMS derivatives	GC; DB-5 fused silica capillary column (30 m, 0.25 μm film thickness); carrier gas-He; FID detector
Gjetost cheese	15	Extracted with 80% aqueous methanol; prepared TMS derivatives	GC; DB-5 fused silica capillary column (30 m, 0.25 μm film thickness); carrier gas-He; FID detector
Cheddar cheese	2	Extracted with 80% aqueous methanol; prepared TMS derivatives	GC; DB-5 fused silica capillary column (30 m, 0.25 μm film thickness); carrier gas-He; FID detector
Roquefort cheese	20	Extracted with 80% aqueous methanol; prepared TMS derivatives	GC; DB-5 fused silica capillary column (30 m, 0.25 μm film thickness); carrier gas-He; FID detector
Feta cheese	17	Extracted with 80% aqueous methanol; prepared TMS derivatives	GC; DB-5 fused silica capillary column (30 m, 0.25 μm film thickness); carrier gas-He; FID detector

TABLE 1.4 *(Continued)*

Occurrence of D-Tagatose in Foods[1]

Food	Result (mg/kg)	Sample Preparation	Apparatus
Ultra high temperature milk	~5	Dried under vacuum; water was added, then volatile derivatives extracted with isooctane	GC; Rescom type OV1 capillary column (25 m × 0.25 mm, 0.1 or 0.25 μm film thickness); carrier gas-H 2; FID detector
BA Nature® Yogurt	29	Extracted with DI water; passed through a strong cation exchange column followed by an amine column	HPLC; Bio-Rad Aminex® HPX-87C column heated to 85°C; mobile phase-DI water; flow rate-0.6 mL/min; RI detector
Cephulac®, an orally-ingested medication for treatment of portal-systemic encephalopathy	6500	Deionized with Amberlite IR-120 (H) and Duolite A-561 (free base); diluted to 20 mg/mL with a 50:50 mixture of acetonitrile and water	HPLC; Waters Carbohydrate Analysis Column (300 mm × 3.9 mm); mobile phase-water: acetonitrile, 77:23 (w/w); flow rate-2 mL/min; RI detector
Chronulac®, an orally ingested laxative	6500	Deionized with Amberlite IR-120 (H) and Duolite A-561 (free base); diluted to 20 mg/mL with a 50:50 mixture of acetonitrile and water	HPLC; Waters Carbohydrate Analysis Column (300 mm × 3.9 mm); mobile phase-water: acetonitrile, 77:23 (w/w); flow rate-2 mL/min; RI detector

[1] This table was prepared by Lee Zehner, Beltsville, MD.

TABLE 1.5

Sweetening Agents, Sugar Substitutes

Name	Sweetness	Classification	Uses	Comments
Acesulfame-K (sold under brand Sunette)	130	Nonnutritive; artificial	Tabletop sweetener, chewing gum, dry beverage mixes, puddings	This is actually the potassium salt of the 6-methyl derivative of a group of chemicals called oxathiazinone dioxides; approved by the FDA in 1988
Aspartame	180	Nutritive; artificial	In most diet sodas; also used in cold cereals, drink mixes, gelatin, puddings, toppings, dairy products, and at the table by the consumer; not used in cooking due to lack of stability when heated	Composed of the two naturally occurring amino acids, aspartic acid and phenylalanine; sweeter than sugar, therefore less required, hence fewer calories
Cyclamate	30	Nonnutritive; artificial	Tabletop sweetener and in drugs in Canada and 40 other countries	Discovered in 1937; FDA banned all cyclamate-containing beverages in 1969 and all cyclamate-containing foods in 1970 Cyclamate safety is now being reevaluated by the FDA
Dulcin (4-ethoxy-phenyl-urea)	250	Nonnutritive; artificial	None	Not approved for food use in the U.S.; used in some European countries; also called Sucrol and Valzin
Fructose (levulose)	1.7	Nutritive; natural	Beverages, baking, canned goods; anywhere invert sugar or honey may be used	A carbohydrate; a monosaccharide; naturally occurs in fruits; makes up about 50% of the sugar in honey; commercially found in high-fructose syrups and invert sugars; contributes sweetness and prevents crystallization
Glucose (dextrose)	0.7	Nutritive; natural	Primarily in the confection, wine, and canning industries; and in intravenous solutions	Acts synergistically with other sweeteners
Glycine	0.8	Nutritive; natural	Permissible to use to modify taste of some foods	A sweet-tasting amino acid; tryptophan is also a sweet-tasting amino acid
Mannitol	0.7	Nutritive; natural	Candies, chewing gums, confections, and baked goods; dietetic foods	A sugar alcohol or polyhydric alcohol (polyol); occurs naturally in pineapples, olives, asparagus, and carrots; commercially prepared by the hydrogenation of mannose or glucose; slowly and incompletely absorbed from the intestines; only slightly metabolized, most excreted unchanged in the urine; may cause diarrhea

TABLE 1.5 *(Continued)*

Sweetening Agents, Sugar Substitutes

Name	Sweetness[1]	Classification	Uses	Comments
Miraculin	—	Nutritive; natural	None	Actually a taste-modifying protein rather than a sweetener; after exposing tongue to miraculin, sour lemon tastes like sweetened lemon; responsible for the taste-changing properties of mircale fruit, red berries of *Synsepalum dulcificum*, a native plant of West Africa; first described in 1852; one attempt made to commercialize by a U.S. firm but FDA denied approval and marketing was stopped
Monellin	3000	Nutritive; natural	None; only a potential low-calorie sweetener	Extract of the pulp of the light red berries of the tropical plant *Dioscoreophyllum cumminsii;* also called Serendipity Berry; first protein found to elicit a sweet taste in man; first extracted in 1969; potential use limited by lack of stability; taste sensation is slow and lingering; everything tastes sweet after monellin.
Neohesperidin dihydrochalone (Neo DHC, NDHC)	1250	Nonnutritive; artificial	None approved; potential for chewing gum, mouthwash, and toothpaste	Formed from naringen isolated from citrus fruit; slow to elicit the taste sensation; lingering licorice-like aftertaste; animal studies indicate not toxic
P-4000 (5-nitro-2-propoxyaniline)	4100	Nonnutritive; artificial	None approved	Derivative of nitroaniline; used as a sweetener in some European countries but banned in the U.S. due to toxic effects on rats; no bitter aftertaste; major drawback of P-4000 is powerful local anesthetic effect on the tongue and mouth; used in the Netherlands during German occupation and Berlin blockade
Phyllodulcin	250	Natural	None approved	Isolated from *Hydrangea macrophylla Seringe* in 1916; displays a lagging onset of sweetness with licorice aftertaste; not well studied; possible market for hard candies, chewing gums, and oral hygiene products
Saccharin (0 benzo-sulfimide)	500	Nonnutritive; artificial	Used in beverages, as a tabletop sweetener, and in cosmetics, toothpaste, and cough syrup; used as a sweetener by diabetics	Both sodium and calcium salts of saccharin used; passes through body unchanged; excreted in urine; originally a generally recognized as safe (GRAS) additive Subsequently, saccharin was classed as a carcinogen based on experiments with rats; however, recent experiments indicate that saccharin causes cancer in rats, but not in mice and people

Sorbitol	0.6	Nutritive; natural	Chewing gum, dairy products, meat products, icing, toppings, and beverages	A sugar alcohol or polyhydric alcohol (polyol); occurs naturally in many fruits commercially prepared by the hydrogenation of glucose; many unique properties besides sweetness; on the FDA list of GRAS food additives; the most widely used sugar alcohol; slow intestinal absorption; consumption of large amounts may cause diarrhea
SRI Oxime V (Perilla sugar)	450	Nonnutritive; artificial	None approved	Derived from extract of Perilla namkinensis; clean taste; needs research; used as sweetening agent in Japan
Stevioside	300	Nutritive; natural	None approved	Isolated from the leaves of the wild shrub *Stevia rebaudiana Bertoni;* used by the people of Paraguay to sweeten drinks; limited evidence suggests nontoxic to humans Rebaudioside A is isolated from the same plant and is said to taste superior to stevioside; its chemical structure is very similar to stevioside and it is 190 times sweeter than sugar
Sucrose (brown sugar, liquid sugar, sugar, table sugar, white sugar	1.0	Nutritive; natural	Many beverages and processed foods; home use in a wide variety of foods	The chemical combination of the sugars fructose and glucose; one of the oldest sweetening agents; most popular and most available sweetening agent; occurs naturally in many fruits; commercially extracted from sugar cane and sugar beets
Thaumatins	1600	Nutritive; natural	None	Source of sweetness of the tropical fruit from the plant *Thaumatococcus daniellii;* enjoyed by inhabitants of western Africa; doubtful commercial applications
Xylitol (Also see XYLITOL)	0.8	Nutritive; natural	Chewing gums and dietetic foods	A sugar alcohol or polyhydric alcohol (polyol); occurs naturally in some fruits and vegetables; produced in the body; commercial production from plant parts (oat hulls, corncobs, and birch wood chips) containing xylans — long chains of the sugar xylose; possible diarrhea; one British study suggests xylitol causes cancer in animals

Adapted from Ensminger et al. *Foods and Nutrition Encyclopedia*, 2nd ed., CRC Press, Boca Raton, 1994, pp. 2082–2087.

TABLE 1.6

Terms used to Describe the Functions of Food Additives

Term	Function
Anticaking agents and free-flow agents	Substances added to finely powdered or crystalline food products to prevent caking
Antimicrobial agents	Substances used to preserve food by preventing growth of microorganisms and subsequent spoilage, including fungicides, mold and yeast inhibitors, and bacteriocides
Antioxidants	Substances used to preserve food by retarding deterioration, rancidity, or discoloration due to oxidation
Colors and coloring adjuncts	Substances used to impart, preserve, or enhance the color or shading of a food, including color stabilizers, color fixatives, color-retention agents
Curing and pickling agents	Substances imparting a unique flavor and/or color to a food, usually producing an increase in shelf life stability
Dough strengtheners	Substances used to modify starch and gluten, thereby producing a more stable dough
Drying agents	Substances with moisture-absorbing ability, used to maintain an environment of low moisture
Emulsifiers and emulsifier salts	Substances which modify surface tension of two (or more) immiscible solutions to establish a uniform dispersion of components; called an emulsion
Enzymes	Substances used to improve food processing and the quality of the finished food
Firming agents	Substances added to precipitate residual pectin, thus strengthening the supporting tissue and preventing its collapse during processing
Flavor enhancers	Substances added to supplement, enhance, or modify the original taste and/or aroma of a food without imparting a characteristic taste or aroma of its own
Flavoring agents and adjuvants	Substances added to impart or help impart a taste or aroma in food
Flour treating agents	Substances added to milled flour, at the mill, to improve its color and/or baking qualities, including bleaching and maturing agents
Formulation aids	Substances used to promote or produce a desired physical state or texture in food, including carriers, binders, fillers, plasticizers, film-formers, and tableting aids
Fumigants	Volatile substances used for controlling insects or pests
Humectants	Hygroscopic substances incorporated in food to promote retention of moisture, including moisture-retention agents and antidusting agents
Leavening agents	Substances used to produce or stimulate production of carbon dioxide in baked goods to impart a light texture, including yeast, yeast foods, and calcium salts
Lubricants and release agents	Substances added to food contact surfaces to prevent ingredients and finished products from sticking to them
Nonnutritive sweeteners	Substances having less than 2% of the caloric value of sucrose per equivalent unit of sweetening capacity
Nutrient supplements	Substances which are necessary for the body's nutritional and metabolic processes
Nutritive sweeteners	Substances having greater than 2% equivalent unit of sweetening capacity
Oxidizing and reducing agents	Substances which chemically oxidize or reduce another food ingredient, thereby producing a more stable product
pH control agents	Substances added to change or maintain active acidity or alkalinity, including buffers, acids, alkalis, and neutralizing agents
Processing aids	Substances used as manufacturing aids to enhance the appeal or utility of a food or food component, including clarifying agents, clouding agents, catalysts, flocculents, filter aids, and crystallization inhibitors

TABLE 1.6 *(Continued)*

Terms used to Describe the Functions of Food Additives

Term	Function
Propellants, aerating agents, and gases	Gases used to supply force to expel a product, or used to reduce the amount of oxygen in contact with the food in packaging
Sequestrants	Substances which combine with polyvalent metal ions to form a soluble metal complex, to improve the quality and stability of products
Solvents and vehicles	Substances used to extract or dissolve another substance
Stabilizers and thickeners	Substances used to produce viscous solutions or dispersions, to impart body, improve consistency, or stabilize emulsions, including suspending and bodying agents, setting agents, gelling agents, and bulking agents
Surface-active agents	Substances used to modify surface properties of liquid food components for a variety of effects, other than emulsifiers but including solubilizing agents, dispersants, detergents, wetting agents, rehydration enhancers, whipping agents, foaming agents, and defoaming agents
Surface-finishing agents	Substances used to increase palatability, preserve gloss, and inhibit discoloration of foods, including glazes, polishes, waxes, and protective coatings
Synergists	Substances used to act or react with another food ingredient to produce a total effect different or greater than the sum of the effects produced by the individual ingredients
Texturizers	Substances which affect the appearance or feel of the food

Taken from Ensminger, et al. *Foods and Nutrition Encyclopedia*, 2nd ed., CRC Press, Boca Raton, 1994, p. 11.

TABLE 1.7

Specific Food Additives and Their Functions

Name	Function[1]	Food Use and Comments[2]
Acetic acid	pH control, preservative	Acid of vinegar is acetic acid; miscellaneous and/or general purposes; many food uses; GRAS additive
Adipic acid	pH control	Buffer and neutralizing agent; use in confectionery; GRAS additive
Ammonium alginate	Stabilizer and thickener, texturizer	Extracted from seaweed; widespread food use; GRAS additive
Annatto	Color	Extracted from seeds of *Bixa crellana*; butter, cheese, margarine, shortening, and sausage casings; coloring foods in general
Arabinogalactan	Stabilizer and thickener, texturizer	Extracted from Western larch; widespread food use; bodying agent in essential oils, nonnutritive sweeteners, flavor bases, nonstandardized dressings, and pudding mixes
Ascorbic acid (Vitamin C)	Nutrient, antioxidant, preservative	Widespread use in foods to prevent rancidity, browning; used in meat curing; GRAS additive
Aspartame	Sweetener; sugar substitute	Soft drinks, chewing gum, powdered beverages, whipped toppings, puddings, gelatin; tabletop sweetener
Azodicarbonamide	Flour treating agent	Aging and bleaching ingredient in cereal flour
Benzoic acid	Preservative	Occurs in nature in free and combined forms; widespread food use; GRAS additive
Benzoyl peroxide	Flour treating agent	Bleaching agent in flour; may be used in some cheeses
Beta-apo-8′ carotenal	Color	Natural food color; general use not to exceed 30 mg/lb or pt of food

TABLE 1.7 *(Continued)*

Specific Food Additives and Their Functions

Name	Function[1]	Food Use and Comments[2]
BHA (butylated hydroxyanisole)	Antioxidant, preservative	Fats, oils, dry yeast, beverages, breakfast cereals, dry mixes, shortening, potato flakes, chewing gum, sausage; often used in combination with BHT; GRAS additive
BHT (butylated hydroxytoluene)	Antioxidant, preservative	Rice, fats, oils, potato granules, breakfast cereals, potato flakes, shortening, chewing gum, sausage; often used in combination with BHA; GRAS additive
Biotin	Nutrient	Rich natural sources are liver, kidney, pancreas, yeast, milk; vitamin supplement; GRAS additive
Calcium alginate	Stabilizer and thickener, texturizer	Extracted from seaweed; widespread food use; GRAS additive
Calcium carbonate	Nutrient	Mineral supplement; general purpose additive; GRAS additive
Calcium lactate	Preservative	General purpose and/or miscellaneous use; GRAS additive
Calcium phosphate	Leavening agent, sequestrant, nutrient	General purpose and/or miscellaneous use; mineral supplement; GRAS additive
Calcium propionate	Preservative	Bakery products, alone or with sodium propionate; inhibits mold and other microorganisms; GRAS additive
Calcium silicate	Anticaking agent	Used in baking powder and salt; GRAS additive
Canthaxanthin	Color	Widely distributed in nature; color for foods; more red than carotene
Caramel	Color	Miscellaneous and/or general purpose use in foods for color; GRAS additive
Carob bean gum	Stabilizer and thickener	Extracted from bean of carob tree (Locust bean); numerous foods, e.g., confections, syrups, cheese spreads, frozen desserts, and salad dressings; GRAS additive
Carrageenan	Emulsifier, stabilizer, and thickener	Extracted from seaweed; a variety of foods, primarily those with a water or milk base
Cellulose	Emulsifier, stabilizer, and thickener	Component of all plants; inert bulking agent in foods; may be used to reduce energy content of food; used in foods which are liquid and foam systems
Citric acid	Preservative, antioxidant, pH control agent, sequestrant	Widely distributed in nature in both plants and animals; miscellaneous and/or general purpose food use; used in lard, shortening, sausage, margarine, chili con carne, cured meats, and freeze-dried meats; GRAS additive
Citrus Red No. 2	Color	Coloring skins of oranges
Cochineal	Color	Derived from the dried female insect, *Coccus cacti;* raised in West Indies, Canary Islands, southern Spain, and Algiers; 70,000 insects to 1 lb.; provides red color for meat products and beverages
Corn endosperm oil	Color	Source of xanthophyll for yellow color; used in chicken feed to color yolks of eggs and chicken skin
Cornstarch	Anticaking agent, drying agent, formulation aid, processing aid, surface-finishing agent	Digestible polysaccharide used in many foods, often in a modified form; these include baking powder, baby foods, soups, sauces, pie fillings, imitation jellies, custards, and candies
Corn syrup	Flavoring agent, humectant, nutritive sweetener, preservative	Derived from hydrolysis of cornstarch; employed in numerous foods, e.g., baby foods, bakery products, toppings, meat products, beverages, condiments, and confections; GRAS additive

TABLE 1.7 *(Continued)*

Specific Food Additives and Their Functions

Name	Function[1]	Food Use and Comments[2]
Dextrose (glucose)	Flavoring agent, humectant, nutritive sweetener, synergist	Derived from cornstarch; major users of dextrose are confection, wine, and canning industries; used to flavor meat products; used in production of caramel; variety of other uses
Diglycerides	Emulsifiers	Uses include frozen desserts, lard, shortening, and margarine; GRAS additive
Dioctyl sodium sulfosuccinate	Emulsifier, processing aid, surface active agent	Employed in gelatin dessert, dry beverages, fruit juice drinks, and noncarbonated beverages with cocoa fat; used in production of cane sugar and in canning
Disodium guanylate	Flavor enhancer	Derived from dried fish or seaweed
Disodium inosinate	Flavor adjuvant	Derived from seaweed or dried fish; sodium guanylate is a byproduct
EDTA (ethylenediamine-tetraacetic acid)	Antioxidant, sequestrant	Calcium disodium and disodium salt of EDTA employed in a variety of foods including soft drinks, alcoholic beverages, dressings, canned vegetables, margarine, pickles, sandwich spreads, and sausage
FD&C colors: Blue No. 1 Red No. 40 Yellow No. 5	Color	Coloring foods in general, including dietary supplements
Gelatin	Stabilizer and thickener, texturizer	Derived from collagen by boiling skin, tendons, ligaments, bones, etc. with water; employed in many foods including confectionery, jellies, and ice cream; GRAS additive
Glycerine (glycerol)	Humectant	Miscellaneous and general purpose additive; GRAS additive
Grape skin extract	Color	Colorings for carbonated drinks, beverage bases, and alcoholic beverages
Guar gum	Stabilizer and thickener, texturizer	Extracted from seeds of the guar plant of India and Pakistan; employed in such foods as cheese, salad dressings, ice cream, and soups
Gum arabic	Stabilizer and thickener, texturizer	Gummy exudate of Acacia plants; used in variety of foods; GRAS additive
Gum ghatti	Stabilizer and thickener, texturizer	Gummy exudate of plant growing in India and Ceylon; a variety of food uses; GRAS additive
Hydrogen peroxide	Bleaching agent	Modification of starch and bleaching tripe; GRAS bleaching agent
Hydrolyzed vegetable (plant) protein	Flavor enhancer	Used to flavor various meat products
Invert sugar	Humectant, nutritive sweetener	Main use in confectionery and brewing industry
Iron	Nutrient	Dietary supplements and food; GRAS additive
Iron-Ammonium citrate	Anticaking agent	Used in salt
Karraya gum	Stabilizer and thickener	Derived from dried extract of *Sterculia urens* found primarily in India; variety of food uses; a substitute for tragacanth gum; GRAS additive
Lactic acid	Preservative, pH control	Normal product of human metabolism; numerous uses in foods and beverages; a miscellaneous general purpose additive; GRAS additive
Lecithin (phosphatidyl-choline)	Emulsifier, surface active agent	Normal tissue component of the body; edible and digestible additive naturally occurring in eggs; commercially derived from soybeans; margarine, chocolate, and wide variety of other food uses; GRAS additive

TABLE 1.7 *(Continued)*

Specific Food Additives and Their Functions

Name	Function[1]	Food Use and Comments[2]
Mannitol	Anticaking, nutritive sweetener, stabilizer and thickener, texturizer	Special dietary foods; GRAS additive; supplies 1/2 the energy of glucose; classified as a sugar alcohol or polyol
Methylparaben	Preservative	Food and beverages; GRAS additive
Modified food starch	Drying agent, formulation aid, processing aid, surface finishing agent	Digestible polysaccharide used in many foods and stages of food processing; examples include baking powder, puddings, pie fillings, baby foods, soups, sauces, candies, etc.
Monoglycerides	Emulsifiers	Widely used in foods such as frozen desserts, lard, shortening, and margarine; GRAS additive
MSG (monosodium glutamate)	Flavor enhancer	Enhances the flavor of a variety of foods including various meat products; possible association with the Chinese restaurant syndrome
Papain	Texturizer	Miscellaneous and/or general purpose additive; GRAS additive; achieves results through enzymatic action; used as meat tenderizer
Paprika	Color, flavoring agent	Provides coloring and/or flavor to foods; GRAS additive
Pectin	Stabilizer and thickener, texturizer	Richest source of pectin is lemon and orange rind; present in cell walls of all plant tissues; used to prepare jellies and jams; GRAS additive
Phosphoric acid	pH control	Miscellaneous and/or general purpose additive; used to increase effectiveness of antioxidants in lard and shortening; GRAS additive
Polyphosphates	Nutrient, flavor improver, sequestrant, pH control	Numerous food uses; most polyphosphates and their sodium, calcium, potassium, and ammonium salts; GRAS additive
Polysorbates	Emulsifiers, surface active agent	Polysorbates designated by numbers such as 60, 65, and 80; variety of food uses including baking mixes, frozen custards, pickles, sherbets, ice creams, and shortenings
Potassium alginate	Stabilizer and thickener, texturizer	Extracted from seaweed; wide usage; GRAS additive
Potassium bromate	Flour treating agent	Employed in flour, whole wheat flour, fermented malt beverages, and to treat malt
Potassium iodide	Nutrient	Added to table salt or used in mineral preparations as a source of dietary iodine
Potassium nitrite	Curing and pickling agent	To fix color in cured products such as meats
Potassium sorbate	Preservative	Inhibits mold and yeast growth in foods such as wines, sausage casings, and margarine; GRAS additive
Propionic acid	Preservative	Mold inhibitor in breads and general fungicide; GRAS additive; used in manufacture of fruit flavors
Propyl gallate	Antioxidant, preservative	Used in products containing oil or fat; employed in chewing gum; used to retard rancidity in frozen fresh pork sausage
Propylene glycol	Emulsifier, humectant, stabilizer and thickener, texturizer	Miscellaneous and/or general purpose additive; uses include salad dressings, ice cream, ice milk, custards, and a variety of other foods; GRAS additive
Propylparaben	Preservative	Fungicide; controls mold in sausage casings; GRAS additive
Saccharin	Nonnutritive sweetener	Special dietary foods and a variety of beverages; baked products; tabletop sweeteners
Saffron	Color, flavoring agent	Derived from plant of western Asia and southern Europe; all foods except those where standards forbid; to color sausage casings, margarine, or product branding inks

TABLE 1.7 *(Continued)*

Specific Food Additives and Their Functions

Name	Function[1]	Food Use and Comments[2]
Silicon dioxide	Anticaking agent	Used in feed or feed components, beer production, production of special dietary foods, and ink diluent for marking fruits and vegetables
Sodium acetate	pH control, preservative	Miscellaneous and/or general purpose use; meat preservation; GRAS additive
Sodium alginate	Stabilizer and thickener, texturizer	Extracted from seaweed; widespread food use; GRAS additive
Sodium aluminum sulfate	Leavening agent	Baking powders, confectionery; sugar refining
Sodium benzoate	Preservative	Variety of food products; margarine to retard flavor reversion; GRAS additive
Sodium bicarbonate	Leavening agent, pH control	Miscellaneous and/or general purpose uses; separation of fatty acids and glycerol in rendered fats; neutralize excess and clean vegetables in rendered fats, soups, and curing pickles; GRAS additive
Sodium chloride (salt)	Flavor enhancer, formulation acid, preservation	Used widely in many foods; GRAS additive
Sodium citrate	pH control, curing and pickling agent, sequestrant	Evaporated milk; miscellaneous and/or general purpose food use; accelerate color fixing in cured meats; GRAS additive
Sodium diacetate	Preservative, sequestrant	An inhibitor of molds and rope-forming bacteria in baked products; GRAS additive
Sodium nitrate (Chile saltpeter)	Curing and pickling agent, preservative	Used with or without sodium nitrite in smoked, cured fish, cured meat products
Sodium nitrite	Curing and pickling agent, preservative	May be used with sodium nitrate in smoked or cured fish, cured meat products, and pet foods
Sodium propionate	Preservative	A fungicide and mold preventative in bakery products; GRAS additive
Sorbic acid	Preservative	Fungistatic agent for foods, especially cheeses; other uses include baked goods, beverages, dried fruits, fish, jams, jellies, meats, pickled products, and wines; GRAS additive
Sorbitan monostearate	Emulsifier, stabilizer and thickener	Widespread food usage such as whipped toppings, cakes, cake mixes, confectionery, icings, and shortenings; also many nonfood uses
Sorbitol	Humectant, nutritive sweetener, stabilizer and thickener, sequestrant	A sugar alcohol or polyol; used in chewing gum, meat products, icings, dairy products, beverages, and pet foods
Sucrose	Nutritive sweetener, preservative	The most widely used additive; used in beverages, baked goods, candies, jams and jellies, and other processed foods
Tagetes (Aztec marigold)	Color	Source is flower petals of Aztec marigold; used to enhance yellow color of chicken skin and eggs, incorporated in chicken feed
Tartaric acid	pH control	Occurs free in many fruits, free or combined with calcium, magnesium, or potassium; used in the soft drink industry, confectionery products, bakery products, and gelatin desserts
Titanium dioxide	Color	For coloring foods generally, except standardized foods; used for coloring ingested and applied drugs
Tocopherols (vitamin E)	Antioxidant, nutrient	To retard rancidity in foods containing fat; used in dietary supplements; GRAS additive
Tragacanth gum	Stabilizer and thickener, texturizer	Derived from the plant *Astragalus gummifier* or other Asiatic species of *Astragalus*; general purpose additive

TABLE 1.7 *(Continued)*

Specific Food Additives and Their Functions

Name	Function[1]	Food Use and Comments[2]
Turmeric	Color	Derived from rhizome of *Curcuma longa;* used to color sausage casings, margarine or shortening, and ink for branding or marking products
Vanilla	Flavoring agent	Used in various bakery products, confectionery, and beverages; natural flavoring extracted from cured, full grown unripe fruit of *Vanilla panifolia;* GRAS additive
Vanillin	Flavoring agent and adjuvant	Widespread confectionery, beverage and food use; synthetic form of vanilla; GRAS additive
Yellow prussiate of soda	Anticaking agent	Employed in salt

[1] Function refers to those defined in Table 1.3.
[2] Adapted from Ensinger et al., *Food and Nutrition Encyclopedia,* 2nd ed., CRC Press, Boca Raton, 1994, pp. 13-18.

TABLE 1.8

Mycotoxins/Bacterial Toxins in Foods

Toxins from Bacteria

Staphylococcus aureus: α exotoxin (lethal, dermonecrotic, hemolytic, leucolytic)
β exotoxin (hemolytic)
γ exotoxin (hemolytic)
δ exotoxin (dermonecrotic, hemolytic)
leucocidin (leucolytic)
exfoliative toxin
enterotoxin

Clostridium botulinum (four strains): Toxins are lettered as A,B, Cα (1,2,D), Cβ, D(C_1 and D), E, F, G. All of the toxics are proteolytic and produce NH_3, H_2S, CO_2, and volatile amines. The toxins are hemolytic and neurotoxic

Escherichi coli (several serotypes): Induce diarrhea, vomiting; produce toxins that are heat labile

Bacillus cereus (several types): Produces heat labile enterotoxins that induce vomiting and diarrhea

Mycotoxins Produced by Fungi

Aspergillus flavis
Claviceps purpura
Fusarium graminearum
Aspergillus ochraceus
Aspergillus parasiticus
Penicillium viridicatum

TABLE 1.9

Antinutrients in Food

Type of Factor(s)	Effect of Factor(s)	Legumes Containing the Factor(s)
Antivitamin factors	Interfere with the actions of certain vitamins	
Antivitamin A	Lipoxidase oxidizes and destroys carotene (provitamin A)	Soybeans
Antivitamin B_{12}	Increases requirement for Vitamin B_{12}	Soybeans
Antivitamin D	Causes rickets unless extra vitamin D is provided	Soybeans
Antivitamin E	Damage to the liver and muscles	Alfalfa, Common beans (*Phaseolus vulgaris*), Peas (*Pisum sativum*)

TABLE 1.9 *(Continued)*

Antinutrients in Food

Type of Factor(s)	Effect of Factor(s)	Legumes Containing the Factor(s)
Cyanide-releasing glucosides	Releases hydrocyanic acid. The poison may also be released by an enzyme in *E. coli*, a normal inhabitant of the human intestine	All legumes contain at least small amounts of these factors; however, certain varieties of lima beans (*Phaseolus lunatus*) may contain much larger amounts
Favism factor	Causes the breakdown of red blood cells in susceptible individuals	Fava beans (*Vicia faba*)
Gas-generating carbohydrates	Certain indigestible carbohydrates are acted upon by gas-producing bacteria in the lower intestine	Many species of mature dry legume seeds, but not peanuts; the immature (green) seeds contain much lower amounts
Goitrogens	Interfere with the utilization of iodine by the thyroid gland	Peanuts and soybeans
Inhibitors of trypsin	The inhibitor(s) binds with the digestive enzyme trypsin	All legumes contain trypsin inhibitors; these inhibitors are destroyed by heat
Lathyrogenic neurotoxins	Consumption of large quantities of lathyrogenic legumes for long periods (several months) results in severe neurological disorders	Lathyrus pea (*L. sativus*) which is grown mainly in India Common vetch (*Vicia sativa*) may also be lathyrogenic
Metal binders	Bind copper, iron, manganese, and zinc	Soybeans, Peas (*Pisum sativum*)
Red blood cell clumping agents (hemagglutinins)	The agents cause the red blood cells to clump together	Occurs in all legumes to some extent

Adapted from Ensminger et al., *Food and Nutrition Encyclopedia,* 2nd ed., CRC Press, Boca Raton, 1994, pp. 1284–1285.

Type A antinutritives. Substances primarily interfering with the digestion of proteins or the absorption and utilization of amino acids. Also known as antiproteins. People depending on vegetables for their protein supply, as in less developed countries, are in danger of impairment by this type of antinutritives. The most important type A antinutritives are protease inhibitors and lectins.

Protease inhibitors, occurring in many plant and animal tissues, are proteins which inhibit proteolytic enzymes by binding to the active sites of the enzymes. Proteolytic enzyme inhibitors were first found in avian eggs around the turn of the century. They were later identified as ovomucoid and ovoinhibitor, both of which inactivate trypsin. Chymotrypsin inhibitors also are found in avian egg whites. Other sources of trypsin and/or chymotrypsin inhibitors are soybeans and other legumes and pulses, vegetables, milk and colostrum, wheat and other cereal grains, guar gum, and white and sweet potatoes. The protease inhibitors of kidney beans, soybeans, and potatoes can additionally inhibit elastase, a pancreatic enzyme acting on elastin, an insoluble protein in meat. Animals given food containing active inhibitors show growth depression. This appears to be due to interference in trypsin and chymotrypsin activities and to excessive stimulation of the secretory exocrine pancreatic cells, which become hypertrophic. Valuable proteins may be lost to the feces in this case. *In vitro* experiments with human proteolytic enzymes have been shown that trypsin inhibitors from bovine colostrum, lima beans, soybeans, kidney beans, and quail ovomucoid were active against human trypsin, whereas trypsin inhibitors originating from bovine and porcine pancrease, potatoes, chicken ovomucoid, and chicken ovoinhibitor were not. The soybean and lima bean trypsin inhibitors are also active against human chymotrypsin. Many protease inhibitors are heat labile, especially with moist heat.

Relatively heat resistant protease inhibitors include the antitryptic factor in milk, the alcohol-precipitable and nondialyzable trypsin inhibitor in alfalfa, the chymotrypsin inhibitor in potato, the kidney bean inhibitor, and the trypsin inhibitor in lima beans.

Lectin is the general term for plant proteins that have highly specific binding sites for carbohydrates. They are widely distributed among various sources such as soybeans, peanuts, jack beans, mung beans, lima beans, kidney beans, fava beans, vetch, yellow wax beans, hyacinth beans, lentils, peas, potatoes, bananas, mangoes and wheat germ. Most plant lectins are glycoproteins, except concanavalin A from jack beans, which is carbohydrate-free. The most toxic lectins in food include ricin in castor bean (oral toxic dose in man: 150-200 mg; intravenous toxic dose: 20 mg), and the lectins of kidney bean and hyacinth bean. The mode of action of lectins may be related to their ability to bind to specific cell receptors in a way comparable to that of antibodies. Because they are able to agglutinate red blood cells, they are also known as hemaglutinins. The binding of bean lectin on rat intestinal mucosal cells has been demonstrated *in vitro*, and it has been suggested that this action is responsible for the oral toxicity of the lectins. Such bindings may disturb the intestines' absorptive capacity for nutrients and other essential compounds. The lectins, being proteins, can easily be inactivated by moist heat. Germination decreases the hemaglutinating activity in varieties of peas and species of beans.

Type B antinutritives. Substances interfering with the absorption or metabolic utilization of minerals are also known as antiminerals. Although they are toxic per se, the amounts present in foods seldom cause acute intoxication under normal food consumption. However, they may harm the organism under suboptimum nutriture. The most important type B antinutritives are phytic acid, oxalates, and glucosinolates.

Phytic acid, or myoinositol hexaphosphate, is a naturally occurring strong acid which binds to many types of bivalent and trivalent heavy metal ions, forming insoluble salts. Consequently, phytic acid reduces the availability of many minerals and essential trace elements. The degree of insolubility of these salts appears to depend on the nature of the metal, the pH of the solution, and for certain metals, on the presence of another metal. Synergism between two metallic ions in the formation of phytate complexes has also been observed. For instance, zinc-calcium phytate precipitates maximally at pH 6, which is also the pH of the duodenum, where mainly calcium and trace metals are absorbed. Phytates occur in a wide variety of foods, such as cereals (e.g. wheat, rye, maize, rice, barley), legumes and vegetables (e.g. bean, soybean, lentil, pea, vetch); nuts and seeds (e.g. walnut, hazelnut, almond, peanut, cocoa bean), and spices and flavoring agents (e.g. caraway, coriander, cumin, mustard, nutmeg). From several experiments in animals and man it has been observed that phytates exert negative effects on the availability of calcium, iron, magnesium, zinc, and other trace essential elements. These effects may be minimized considerably, if not eliminated, by increased intake of essential minerals. In the case of calcium, intake of cholecalciferol must also be adequate, since the activity of phytates on calcium absorption is enhanced when this vitamin is inadequate or limiting. In many foodstuffs the phytic acid level can be reduced by phytase, an enzyme occurring in plants, that catalyzes the dephosphorylation of phytic acid.

Oxalic acid is a strong acid which forms water soluble Na^+ and K^+ salts, but less soluble salts with alkaline earth and other bivalent metals. Calcium oxalate is particularly insoluble at neutral or alkaline pH, whereas it readily dissolves in acid medium. Oxalates mainly exert effects on the absorption of calcium. These effects must be considered in terms of the oxalate/calcium ratio (in milliequivalent/milliequivalent): foods having a ratio greater than 1 may have negative effects on calcium availability, whereas foods with a ratio of 1 or below do not. Examples of foodstuffs having a ratio greater than 1 are: rhubarb (8.5), spinach (4.3), beet (2.5 to 5.1), cocoa (2.6), coffee (3.9), tea (1.1), and potato (1.6). Harmful oxalates in food may be removed by soaking in water. Consumption of calcium-rich foods (e.g. dairy products and seafood), as well as augmented cholecalciferol intake, are recommended when large amounts of high oxalate food are consumed.

A variety of plants contain a third group of type B antinutritives, the glucosinolates, also known as thioglucosides. Many glucosinolates are goitrogenic. They have a general structure, and yield on hydrolysis the active or actual goitrogens, such as thiocyanates, isothiocyanates, cyclic sulfur compounds, and nitriles. Three types of goiter can be identified: 1) cabbage goiter, 2) brassica seed goiter, and 3) legume goiter. Cabbage goiter, also known as struma, is induced by excessive consumption of cabbage. It seems that cabbage goitrogens inhibit iodine uptake by directly affecting the thyroid gland. Cabbage goiter can be treated by iodine supplementation. Brassica seed goiter can result from the consumption of the seeds of Brassica plants (e.g. rutabaga, turnip, cabbage, rape) which contain goitrogens that prevent thyroxine synthesis. This type of goiter can only be treated by administration of the thyroid hormone. Legume goiter is induced by goitrogens in legumes like soybeans and peanuts. It differs from cabbage goiter in that the thyroid gland does not lose its activity for iodine. Inhibition of the intestinal absorption of iodine or the reabsorption of thyroxine has been shown in this case. Legume goiter can be treated by iodine therapy. Glucosinolates which have been shown to induce goiter, at least in experimental animals, are found in several foods and feedstuffs: broccoli (buds), brussels sprouts (head), cabbage (head), cauliflower (buds), garden cress (leaves), horseradish (roots), kale (leaves), kohlrabi (head), black and white mustard (seed), radish (root), rape (seed), rutabaga (root), and turnips (root and seed). One of the most potent glucosinolates is progoitrin from the seeds of Brassica plants and the roots of rutabaga. Hydrolysis of this compound yields 1-cyano-2-hydroxy-3-butene, 1-cyano-2-hydroxy-3,4-butylepisulfide, 2-hydroxy-3,4-butenylisothiocyanate, and (*S*)-5-vinyl-oxazolidone-2-thione, also known as goitrin. The latter product interferes, together with its R-enantiomer, in the iodination of thyroxine precursors, so that the resulting goiter cannot be treated by iodine therapy.

Type C antinutritives. Naturally occurring substances which can decompose vitamins, form unabsorbable complexes with them, or interfere with their digestive or metabolic utilization. Also known as antivitamins. The most important type C antinutritives are ascorbic acid oxidase, antithiamine factors, and antipyridoxine factors.

Ascorbic acid oxidase is a copper-containing enzyme that catalyzes the oxidation of free ascorbic acid to diketogluconic acid, oxalic acid, and other oxidation products. It has been reported to occur in many fruits (e.g. peaches, bananas) and vegetables (e.g. cucumbers, pumpkins, lettuce, cress, cauliflowers, spinach, green beans, green peas, carrots, potatoes, tomatoes, beets, kohlrabi). The enzyme is active between pH 4 and 7 (optimum pH 5.6 to 6.0); its optimum temperature is 38°C. The enzyme is released when plant cells are broken. Therefore, if fruits and vegetables are cut, the vitamin C content decreases gradually. Ascorbic acid oxidase can be inhibited effectively at pH 2 or by blanching at around 100°C. Ascorbic acid can also be protected against ascorbic acid oxidase by substances of plant origin. Flavonoids, such as the flavonoles quercetin and kempferol, present in fruits and vegetables, strongly inhibit the enzyme.

A second group of type C antinutritives are the antithiamine factors, which interact with thiamine, also known as vitamin B_1. Antithiamine factors can be grouped as thiaminases, catechols, and tannins. Thiaminases, which are enzymes that split thiamine at the methylene linkage, are found in many freshwater and saltwater fish species, and in certain species of crab and clam. They contain a nonprotein coenzyme structurally related to hemin. This coenzyme is the actual antithiamine factor. Thiaminases in fish and other sources can be destroyed by cooking. Antithiamine factors of plant origin include catechols and tannins. The most well known ortho-catechol is found in bracken fern. In fact, there are two types of heat-stable antithiamine factors in this fern, one of which has been identified as caffeic acid, which can also by hydrolyzed from chlorogenic acid (found in green coffee beans) by intestinal bacteria. Other ortho-catechols, such as methylsinapate occurring in mustard seed and rapeseed, also have antithiamine activity. The mechanism of thiamine inactivation by these compounds requires oxygen and is dependent on temperature and pH. The reaction appears to proceed in two phases: a rapid initial phase, which is reversible by addition of reducing agents (e.g. ascorbic acid), and a slower subsequent phase, which is irreversible. Tannins, occurring in a variety of plants, including tea, similarly possess antithiamine activity. Thiamine is one of the vitamins likely to be deficient in the diet. Thus, persistent consumption of antithiamine factors and the possible presence of thiaminase-producing bacteria in the gastrointestinal tract may compromise the already marginal thiamine intake.

A variety of plants and mushrooms contain pyridoxine (a form of vitamin B_6) antagonists. These antipyridoxine factors have been identified as hydrazine derivatives. Linseed contains the water-soluble and heat-labile antipyridoxine factor linatine (γ-glutamyl-1-amino-D-proline). Hydrolysis of linatine yields the actual antipyridoxine factor 1-amino-proline. Antipyridoxine factors have also been found in wild mushrooms, the common commercial edible mushroom, and the Japanese mushroom shiitake. Commercial and shiitake mushrooms contain agaritine. Hydrolysis of agaritine by γ-glutamyl transferase, which is endogenous to the mushroom, yields the active agent 4-hydroxymethylphenylhydrazine. Disruption of the cells of the mushroom can accelerate hydrolysis; careful handling of the mushrooms and immediate blanching after cleaning and cutting can prevent hydrolysis. The mechanism underlying the antipyridoxine activity is believed to be condensation of the hydrazines with the carbonyl compounds pyridoxal and pyridoxal phosphate (the active form of the vitamin), resulting in the formation of inactive hydrazones.

TABLE 1.10

Toxic Substances in Food (Toxic if Consumed in Excess)

Poison (Toxin)	Source	Symptoms and Signs	Distribution; Magnitude	Prevention; Treatment	Remarks
Aflatoxins (See Table 1.8).					
Aluminum (Al)	Food additives, mainly presented in such items as baking powder, pickles, and processed cheeses. Aluminum-containing antacids.	Abnormally large intakes of aluminum irritate the digestive tract. Also, unusual conditions have sometimes resulted in the absorption of sufficient aluminum from antacids to cause brain damage. Aluminum may form non-absorbable complexes with essential trace elements, thereby creating deficiencies of these elements.	**Distribution**: Aluminum is widely used throughout the world. **Magnitude**: The U.S. uses more aluminum than any other mineral except iron. However, known cases of aluminum toxicity are rare.	**Prevention**: Based on the evidence presented, no preventative measures are recommended.	Aluminum toxicity has been reported in patients receiving renal dialysis.
Arsenic (As)	Consuming contaminated foods and beverages. Arsenical insecticides used in vineyards exposing the workers (1) when spraying or (2) by inhaling contaminated dusts and plant debris. Arsenic in the air from three major sources; smelting of metals, burning of coal, and use of arsenical pesticides.	Burning pains in the throat or stomach, cardiac abnormalities, and the odor of garlic on the breath. Other symptoms may be diarrhea and extreme thirst along with a choking sensation. Small doses of arsenic taken into the body over a long period of time may produce hyperkeratosis (irregularities in pigmentation, especially on the trunk); arterial insufficiency; and cancer. There is strong evidence that inorganic arsenic is a skin and lung carcinogen in man.	**Distribution**: Arsenic is widely distributed, but the amount of the element consumed by man in food and water, or breathed, is very small and not harmful. **Magnitude**: Cases of arsenic toxicity in man are infrequent. Two noteworthy episodes occurred in Japan in 1955. One involved tainted powdered milk; the other contaminated soy sauce. The toxic milk caused 12,131 cases of infant poisoning, with 130 deaths. The soy sauce poisoned 220 people.	**Treatment**: Induce vomiting, followed by an antidote of egg whites in water or milk. Afterward, give strong coffee or tea, followed by Epsom salts in water or castor oil.	Arsenic is known to partially protect against selenium poisoning. The highest residues of arsenic are generally in the hair and nails. Arsenic in soils may sharply decrease crop growth and yields, but it is not a hazard to people or livestock that eat plants grown in these fields.

TABLE 1.10 *(Continued)*

Toxic Substances in Food (Toxic if Consumed in Excess)

Poison (Toxin)	Source	Symptoms and Signs	Distribution; Magnitude	Prevention; Treatment	Remarks
Chromium (Cr)	Food, water, and air contaminated by chromium compounds in industrialized areas.	Inorganic chromium salt reduces the absorption of zinc; hence, zinc deficiency symptoms may become evident in chronic chromium toxicity.	**Distribution**: Chromium toxicity is not common. **Magnitude**: Chromium toxicity is not very common.	**Prevention**: It is unlikely that people will get too much chromium because (1) only minute amounts of the element are present in most foods, (2) the body utilizes chromium poorly, and (3) the toxic dose is about 10,000 times the lowest effective medical dose.	
Copper (Cu)	Diets with excess copper, but low in other minerals that counteract its effects. Acid foods or beverages (vinegar, carbonated beverages, or citrus juices) that have been in prolonged contact with copper metal may cause acute gastrointestinal disturbances.	**Acute copper toxicity**: Characterized by headache, dizziness, metallic taste, excessive salivation, nausea, vomiting, stomachache, diarrhea, and weakness. If the disease is allowed to get worse, there may also be racing of the heart, high blood pressure, jaundice, hemolytic anemia, dark-pigmented urine, kidney disorders, and even death. **Chronic copper toxicity**: May be contributory to iron-deficiency anemia, mental illness following childbirth (postpartum psychosis), certain types of schizophrenia, and perhaps heart attacks.	**Distribution**: Copper toxicity may occur wherever there is excess copper intake, especially when accompanied by low iron, molybdenum, sulfur, zinc, and vitamin C. **Magnitude**: The incidence of copper toxicity is extremely rare in man. Its occurrence in significant form is almost always limited to (1) suicide attempted by ingesting large quantities of copper salt, or (2) a genetic defect in copper metabolism inherited as an autosomal recessive, known as Wilson's disease.	**Prevention**: Avoid foods and beverages that have been in prolonged contact with copper metal. Administration of copper chelating agents to remove excess copper.	Copper is essential to human life and health, but like all heavy metals, it may be toxic in excess.

Ergot	Rye, wheat, barley, oats and triticale carry this mycotoxin. Ergot replaces the seed in the heads of cereal grains, in which it appears as a purplish-black, hard, banana-shaped, dense mass from 1/4-3/4 in. (6-9 mm) long.	When a large amount of ergot is consumed in a short period, convulsive ergotism is observed. The symptoms include itching, numbness, severe muscle cramps, sustained spasms and convulsions, and extreme pain. When smaller amounts of ergot are consumed over an extended period, ergotism is characterized by gangrene of the fingertips and toes, caused by blood vessel and muscle contraction stopping blood circulation in the extremities. These symptoms include cramps, swelling, inflammation, alternating burning and freezing sensations ("St. Anthony's fire") and numbness; eventually the hands and feet may turn black, shrink, and fall off. Ergotism is a cumulative poison, depending on the amount of ergot eaten and the length of time over which it is eaten.	**Distribution**: Ergot is found throughout the world wherever rye, wheat, barley, oats, or triticale are grown. **Magnitude**: There is considerable ergot, especially in rye. But, normally, screening grains before processing alleviates ergotism in people.	**Prevention**: Consists of an ergot-free diet. Ergot in food and feed grains may be removed by screening the grains before processing. In the U.S., wheat and rye containing more than 0.3% ergot are classed as "ergoty." In Canada, government regulations prohibit more than 0.1% ergot in feeds. **Treatment**: An ergot-free diet; good nursing; treatment by a doctor.	Six different alkaloids are involved in ergot poisoning. Ergot is used to aid the uterus to contract after childbirth, to prevent loss of blood. Also, another ergot drug (ergotamine) is widely used in the treatment of migraine headaches.

TABLE 1.10 *(Continued)*

Toxic Substances in Food (Toxic if Consumed in Excess)

Poison (Toxin)	Source	Symptoms and Signs	Distribution; Magnitude	Prevention; Treatment	Remarks
Fluorine (F) (fluorosis)	Ingesting excessive quantities of fluorine through either the food or water, or a combination of these. Except in certain industrial exposures, the intake of fluoride inhaled from the air is only a small fraction of the total fluoride intake in man. Pesticides containing fluorides, including those used to control insects, weeds, and rodents. Although water is the principal source of fluoride in an average human diet in the U.S., fluoride is frequently contained in toothpaste, tooth powder, chewing gums, mouthwashes, vitamin supplements, and mineral supplements.	**Acute fluoride poisoning**: Abdominal pain, diarrhea, vomiting, excessive salivation, thirst, perspiration, and painful spasms of the limbs. **Chronic fluoride poisoning**: Abnormal teeth (especially mottled enamel) during the first 8 years of life; brittle bones. Other effects, predicted from animal studies, may include loss of body weight and altered structure and function of the thyroid gland and kidneys. Water containing 3-10 ppm of fluoride may cause mottling of the teeth. An average daily intake of 20-80 mg of fluoride over a period of 10-20 years will result in crippling fluorosis.	**Distribution**: The water in parts of Arkansas, California, South Carolina, and Texas contains excess fluorine. Occasionally, throughout the U.S., high-fluorine phosphates are used in mineral mixtures. **Magnitude**: Generally speaking, fluorosis is limited to high-fluorine areas. Only a few instances of health effects in man have been attributed to airborne fluoride, and they occurred in persons living in the vicinity of fluoride-emitting industries.	**Prevention**: Avoid the use of food and water containing excessive fluorine. **Treatment**: Any damage may be permanent, but people who have not developed severe symptoms may be helped to some extent if the source of excess fluorine is eliminated. High dietary levels of calcium and magnesium may reduce the absorption and utilization of fluoride.	Fluorine is a cumulative poison. The total fluoride in the human body averages 2.57 g. Susceptibility to fluoride toxicity is increased by deficiencies of calcium, vitamin C, and protein. Virtually all foods contain trace amounts of fluoride.

Lead (Pb)	Consuming food or medicinal products (including health food products) contaminated with lead. Inhaling the poison as a dust by workers in such industries as painting, lead mining, and refining. Inhaling airborne lead discharged into the air from auto exhaust fumes. Consuming food crops contaminated by lead being deposited on the leaves and other edible portions of the plant by direct fallout. Consuming food or water contaminated by contact with lead pipes or utensils. Old houses in which the interiors were painted with leaded paints prior to 1945, with the chipped wall paint eaten by children. Such miscellaneous sources as illicitly distilled whiskey, improperly lead-glazed earthenware, old battery casings used as fuel, and toys containing lead.	Symptoms develop rapidly in young children, but slowly in mature people. **Acute lead poisoning**: Colic, cramps, diarrhea or constipation, leg cramps, and drowsiness. The most severe form of lead poisoning, encountered in infants and in heavy drinkers of illicitly distilled whiskey, is characterized by profound disturbances of the central nervous system and permanent damage to the brain; damage to the kidneys; and shortened life span of the erthrocytes. **Chronic lead poisoning**: Colic, constipation, lead palsy especially in the forearm and fingers, the symptoms of chronic nephritis, and sometimes mental depression, convulsions, and a blue line at the edge of the gums.	**Distribution**: Predominantly among children who may eat chips of lead-containing paints, peeled off from painted wood. **Magnitude**: The Centers for Disease Control, Atlanta, GA, estimates that (1) lead poisoning claims the lives of 200 children each year, and (2) 400,000-600,000 children have elevated lead levels in the blood. Lead poisoning has been reduced significantly with the use of lead-free paint.	**Prevention**: Avoid inhaling or consuming lead. **Treatment**: **Acute lead poisoning**: An emetic (induce vomiting), followed by drinking plenty of milk and 1/2 oz (14 g) of Epsom salts in 1/2 glass of water. **Chronic lead poisoning**: Remove the source of lead. Sometimes treated by administration of magnesium or lead sulphate solution as a laxative and antidote on the lead in the digestive system, followed by potassium iodide which cleanses the tracts. Currently, treatment of lead poisoning makes use of chemicals that bind the metal in the body and help in its removal.	Lead is a cumulative poison. When incorporated in the soil, nearly all the lead is converted into forms that are not available to plants. Any lead taken up by plant roots tends to stay in the roots, rather than move up to the top of the plant. Lead poisoning can be diagnosed positively by analyzing the blood tissue for lead content; clinical signs of lead poisoning usually are manifested at blood lead concentrations above 80 µg/100 grams.

TABLE 1.10 *(Continued)*

Toxic Substances in Food (Toxic if Consumed in Excess)

Poison (Toxin)	Source	Symptoms and Signs	Distribution; Magnitude	Prevention; Treatment	Remarks
Mercury (Hg)	Mercury is discharged into air and water from industrial operations and is used in herbicide and fungicide treatments. Mercury poisoning has occurred where mercury from industrial plants has been discharged into water, then accumulated as methylmercury in fish and shellfish. Accidental consumption of seed grains treated with fungicides that contain mercury, used for the control of fungus diseases of oats, wheat, barley, and flax.	The toxic effects of organic and inorganic compounds of mercury are dissimilar. The organic compounds of mercury, such as the various fungicides (1) affect the central nervous system, and (2) are not corrosive. The inorganic compounds of mercury include mainly mercuric chloride, a disinfectant; mercurous chloride (calomel), a cathartic; and elemental mercury. Commonly the toxic symptoms are corrosive gastrointestinal effects, such as vomiting, bloody diarrhea, and necrosis of the alimentary mucosa.	**Distribution**: Wherever mercury is produced in industrial operations or used in herbicide or fungicide treatments. **Magnitude**: Limited. But about 1200 cases of mercury poisoning identified in Japan in the 1950s were traced to the consumption of fish and shellfish from Japan's Minamata Bay contaminated with methylmercury. Some of the offspring of exposed mothers were born with birth defects, and many victims suffered central nervous system damage. Another outbreak of mercury toxicity occurred in Iraq, where more than 6000 people were hospitalized after eating bread made from wheat that had been treated with methylmercury.	Control mercury pollution from industrial operations.	Mercury is a cumulative poison. FDA prohibits use of mercury-treated grain for food or feed. Grain crops produced from mercury-treated seed and crops produced on soils treated with mercury herbicides have not been found to contain harmful concentrations of this element.

Polychlorinated biphenyls (PCBs), industrial chemicals; chlorinated hydrocarbons which may cause cancer when taken into the food supply.	Sources of contamination to man include: 1. Contaminated foods 2. Mammals or birds that have fed on contaminated foods of fish. 3. Residues on foods that have been wrapped in papers and plastics containing PCBs. 4. Milk from cows that have been fed silage from silos coated with PCB-containing paint; and eggs from layers fed feeds contaminated with PCBs.	Clinical effects on people are: an eruption of the skin resembling acne, visual disturbances, jaundice, numbness, and spasms. Newborn infants from mothers who have been poisoned show discoloration of the skin which regresses after 2-5 months. PCBs are fat soluble.	**Distribution**: PCBs are widespread. Their use by industry is declining.		Although the production of PCBs was halted in 1977 and the importing of PCBs was banned January 1, 1979, the chemicals had been widely used for 40 years, and they are exceptionally long-lived. PCBs have been widely used in dielectric fluids in capacitors and transformers, hydraulic fluids, and heat transfer fluids. Also, they have more than 50 minor uses including plasticizers and solvents in adhesives, printing ink, sealants, moisture retardants, paints, and pesticide carriers. PCB will cause cancer in laboratory animals (rats, mice, and rhesus monkeys). It is not known if it will cause cancer in humans. More study is needed to gauge its effects on the ecological food chain and on human health. When fed Coho salmon from Lake Michigan with 10-15 ppm PCB, mink in Wisconsin stopped reproducing or their kits died.

TABLE 1.10 *(Continued)*

Toxic Substances in Food (Toxic if Consumed in Excess)

Poison (Toxin)	Source	Symptoms and Signs	Distribution; Magnitude	Prevention; Treatment	Remarks
Salt (NaCl-sodium chloride) poisoning	Consumption of high-salt food and beverages.	Salt may be toxic (1) when it is fed to infants or others whose kidneys cannot excrete the excess in the urine, or (2) when the body is adapted to a chronic low-salt diet.	**Distribution**: Salt is used all over the world. Hence, the potential for salt poisoning exists everywhere. **Magnitude**: Salt poisoning is relatively rare.	**Treatment**: Drink large quantities of fresh water.	Even normal salt concentration may be toxic if water intake is low.
Selenium (Se)	Consumption of high levels in food or drinking water. Presence of malnutrition, parasitic infestation, or other factors which make people highly susceptible to selenium toxicity.	Abnormalities in the hair, nails, and skin. Children in a high-selenium area of Venezuela showed loss of hair, discolored skin, and chronic digestive disturbances. Normally, people who have consumed large excesses of selenium excrete it as trimethyl selenide in the urine, and/or as dimethyl selenide on the breath. The latter substance has an odor resembling garlic.	**Distribution**: In certain regions of western U.S., especially in South Dakota, Montana, Wyoming, Nebraska, Kansas, and perhaps areas in other states in the Great Plains and Rocky Mountains. Also, in Canada. **Magnitude**: Selenium toxicity in people is relatively rare.	**Treatment**: Selenium toxicity may be counteracted by arsenic or copper, but such treatment should be carefully monitored.	Confirmed cases of selenium poisoning in people are rare because (1) only traces are present in most foods, (2) foods generally come from a wide area, and (3) the metabolic processes normally convert excess selenium into harmless substances which are excreted in the urine or breath.
Tin (Sn)	From acid fruits and vegetables canned in tin cans. The acids in such foods as citrus fruits and tomato products can leach tin from the inside of the can. Then the tin is ingested with the canned food. In the digestive tract tin goes through a methylation process in which nontoxic tin is converted to methylated tin, which is toxic.	Methylated tin is a neurotoxin — a toxin that attacks the central nervous system, the symptoms of which are numbness of the fingers and lips followed by a loss of speech and hearing. Eventually, the afflicted person becomes spastic, then coma and death follow.	**Distribution**: Worldwide. **Magnitude**: The use of tin in advanced industrial societies has increased 14-fold over the last 10 years.	**Prevention**: Tin cans are rare. Many tin cans are coated on the inside with enamel or other materials. Most cans are steel.	Currently, not much is known about the amount of tin in the human diet.

Adapted from Ensminger et al. *Foods & Nutrition Encyclopedia,* 2nd ed., CRC Press, Boca Raton, 1994, pp. 1790-1803.

TABLE 1.11
Edible Weeds

Common Name	Scientific Name	Use
Maple tree	*Acer* (many varieties)	Sap can be collected and reduced by evaporation into syrup.
Sweetflag	*Acorus calamus*	Rootstocks or stems are edible with a sweet taste. Young shoots can be used as salad.
Quackgrass	*Agropyron repens* L. (has many other names)	Rootstocks can be chewed or scorched to use as coffee substitute; seeds can be used for breadstuffs and for beer.
Waterplantain	*Alisma* spp.	Root is starchy and edible; should be dried to reduce acrid taste. Three varieties of this plant can be toxic.
Garlic mustard	*Alliaria petiolata*	Leaf, stem, flower, and fruit are spicy and hot. If cooked, some of this spiciness is lost. Several plants that resemble this one are not edible.
Wild garlic	*Allium vineale* L.	Used as an herbal seasoning; there are similar plants that are not garlic in aroma; they can be toxic.
Pigweed	*Amaranthus* spp.	Leaves from a young plant can be eaten raw as salad or boiled like spinach.
Serviceberry	*Amelanchier* spp.	Berries are rich and sweet; pits and leaves contain cyanide; also called shadbush or juneberry.
Hog peanut	*Amphicarpaea bracteata*	Fleshy seedpods found underground are edible.
Ground nut	*Apios americana* *Medik*	Root can be eaten raw or cooked. Seeds can also be used. Europeans use the term ground nut to refer to peanuts. This is not the same plant.
Common burdock	*Arctium minus*	Young leaves can be eaten as salad; roots are carrot-like in shape and can be cooked (boiled) and eaten. A little baking soda added to the cooking water improves tenderness and flavor. Scorched roots can be used as a coffee substitute.
Giant reed	*Arundo donax* L.	Young shoots and rootstalks are sometimes sweet enough to be used as a substitute for sugar cane. Infusions of the root stocks can have some herbal properties; local weak anesthetic and in some instances either a hypotensive agent or hypertensive agent (depends on dose).
Milkweed	*Asclepias syriaca* L.	Young shoots, flower buds boiled with at least two changes of water. The plant contains cardiac glycosides and can be toxic.
Pawpaw	*Asimina triloba* L.	The aromatic fruits are quite tasty. Seeds and bark have pesticide properties and should be handled with caution.
Wild oat	*Avena Fatua* L.	Seeds are similar to cultivated oats. Useful when dried and ground as a cereal. Seeds can be scorched and used as a coffee substitute.
Wintercress/Yellow rocket	*Barbarea* spp. (*B. vcma; B. vulgaris*)	Young leaves and stems can be used as a salad.
Birches	*Betula* spp. (*Betulacea*)	Spring sap can be reduced to a syrup; bark can be boiled for tea.
Mustard; black or yellow	*Brassica nigra*	Seeds used to prepare mustard; leaves can be boiled for consumption, as can young stalks.
Bromegrass	*Bromus japonicus*	Seeds can be dried, ground, and used as cereal.
Shepherd's purse	*Capsella bursa-pastoris*	Seeds are used as a spicy pot herb. Tender young shoots can be eaten raw. Has a peppery taste.
Bittercress	*Cardamme bulbosa*	Roots can be ground for a horseradish substitute; leaves and stems can be added to salad. The roots of some species (*C. bulbosa*) can be toxic.

TABLE 1.11 *(Continued)*

Edible Weeds

Common Name	Scientific Name	Use
Hornbeam	*Carpus caroliniana*	Nuts are edible.
Hickory	*Carya* spp.	Nuts are edible.
Chestnut	*Castanea* spp.	Nuts are edible but are covered by a prickly coat. Roasting improves flavor and texture.
Sandbur	*Cenchrus* spp.	Seeds and burrs can be used as cereal grains.
Lambsquarter	*Chenopodium album* L.	Leaves can be eaten raw or cooked as spinach. The Mexican version (*Mexicantea, C. ambrosioides*) is toxic.
Oxeye daisy	*Chrysanthemum leucanthemum*	Leaves and flowers can be eaten raw or cooked.
Chicory	*Cichorium intybus* L.	Leaves are good salad ingredients.
Thistles	*Cirsium* spp.	The taproot is chewy but tasty.
Wandering jew	*Commelina communis*	Leaves can be used as potherbs; flowering shoots can be eaten raw.
Hawthorn	*Crataegus* spp.	Berries are edible, thorns can be a problem when gathering the berries. Some species contain heart stimulants.
Wild chervil	*Cryototaenia canadensis*	Roots can be boiled, with a taste like parsnips; young leaves and stems can be eaten as salad; has an herb use in stews and soups.
Nutgrass	*Cyperus* spp.	Tubers can be eaten or ground up to make a beverage called "chufa" or "horchata."
Queen Anne's lace, also called wild carrot	*Daucus carota* L.	Root can be eaten after boiling; however, because it looks like poisonous hemlock, one should be cautious.
Crabgrass	*Digitaria snaguinalis* L.	Seeds can be dried and ground for use as a cereal.
Persimmon	*Diospyros virginiana* L.	Fruits when ripe are very sweet.
Barnyard grass	*Echinochloa crusgalli* L.	Seeds can be dried and used as cereal.
Russian olive	*Elaegnus angustifolia* L.	Fruits are edible though astringent.
American burnweed	*Erechtites hieracifolia*	Leaves can be eaten raw as salad or cooked.
Redstem filaree	*Erodium cicutarium*	Tender leaves are eaten as salad; can also be used as potherb.
Wild strawberry	*Fragaria virginiana*	Fruits are small but delicious.
Catchweed bedstraw	*Galium aparine*	Young shoots are good potherbs; leaves and stems can be steamed and eaten as vegetable.
Wintergreen	*Gaultheria procumbens* L.	Berries, foliage, and bark can be used to make tea. Berries can be eaten raw.
Huckleberry	*Gaylussacia baccata*	Berries can be eaten raw or cooked.
Honey locust	*Gleditsia triacanthos*	The pulp around the seeds can be used as a sweetener. (Tender green pods can also be cooked and eaten as a vegetable.) The tree is similar in appearance to the Kentucky coffee tree, and the pods of this tree cannot be eaten.
Jerusalem artichoke	*Helianthus tuberosus*	The tubers are crisp and can be used in place of chinese chestnuts in salads; can also be cooked and mashed.
Daylily	*Hemerocallis fulva* L.	Flower buds can be used in salads. Tubers can be cooked and eaten. Can cause diarrhea in sensitive people.
Foxtail barley	*Hordeum jubatum*	Seeds can be dried and used as cereal.
Touch-me-not	*Impatients* spp.	Leaves can be used for an herbal tea; leaves can be eaten as salad; pods are also edible.
Burning bush	*Kochia scoparia*	Young shoots can be used as a potherb; seeds can be dried and used as cereal.
Prickly lettuce	*Lactuca scariola* L.	Young leaves can be used as salad, however may have a bitter taste.

TABLE 1.11 *(Continued)*

Edible Weeds

Common Name	Scientific Name	Use
Virginia peppergrass	*Lepidium virginicum*	Has a pungent mustard-like taste; used as a potherb.
Bugleweed	*Lycorise* spp.	Roots can be eaten raw or cooked.
Common mallow	*Malva neglecta*	Boiled leaves have a slimy consistency much like okra. Flower buds can be pickled; leaves can be used as a thickener for soup.
Black medic	*Medicago lupulina*	Sprouts can be added to salads for texture; leaves can be used as a potherb.
Mulberry	*Mortis* spp.	Berries can be eaten out of hand.
Watercress	*Nasturtium officinale* R.	Leaves can be eaten raw or used as a potherb.
American lotus	*Nelumbo lutea*	Entire plant is edible.
Yellow water lily	*Nuphar luteum* L.	Tubers when cooked are a starch substitute.
Fragrant water lily	*Nymphaea odorata*	Flower buds and young leaves can be boiled and eaten; seeds can be dried and used as cereal.
Evening primrose	*Oenothera biennis* L.	Seeds are a source of γ linolenic acid; tap roots can be eaten raw or cooked.
Wood sorrel	*Oxalis* spp.	Leaves can be eaten cooked or raw; seed pods can also be eaten.
Perilla mint	*Perilla frutescens* L.	Leaves can be eaten cooked or raw.
Common reed	*Phragmites communis*	Young shoots are edible. Plant is similar to the poisonous Arundo, so the forager should be very careful to correctly identify the plant.
Ground cherry (Chinese lanterns)	*Physalis heterophylla*	Berries can be eaten cooked or raw.
Pokeweed	*Phytolacca americana* L.	Young shoots can be used as a potherb; berries and roots may be poisonous.
Plantain	*Plantago major* L.	Leaves can be used in salads.
Mayapple	*Podophyllum peltatum*	Fruits are edible raw or cooked, rest of the plant may be poisonous.
Japanese knotweed	*Polygonum cuspidatum*	Young sprouts can be cooked and eaten like asparagus.
Purslane	*Portulaca oleracea* L.	Young leaves can be used as a potherb or salad ingredient.
Healall	*Prunella vulgaris* L.	Boiled and used as a potherb.
Wild cherry	*Prunus serotina*	Fruits are edible.
Kudzu	*Pueraria lobata*	Roots and leaves are edible.
Rock chestnut oak	*Quercus prinus* L.	Nuts (acorns) are edible.
Sumac	*Rhus glabra* L.	Berries are edible as are the roots; however, some people are allergic to all parts of the plant and will develop skin rash.
Multiflora rose	*Rosa multifora*	The hips are edible in small quantities.
Raspberry, blackberry	*Rubus* spp.	Fruits are eaten raw or used to make juice or jam.
Red sorrel	*Rumex acetosella* L.	Leaves can be eaten as salad or cooked in water. The leaves contain a lot of oxalic acid, so small quantities would be preferred.
Arrowhead	*Sagittaria latifolia Willd*	Roots can be eaten raw or cooked. Plants resemble the poisonous Jack-in-the-pulpit plant so gatherers should beware.
Elderberry	*Sambucus canadensis*	Fruits can be eaten raw or cooked.
Hardstem bulrush	*Scrpus acutus Muhl*	Roots can be boiled and eaten.
Foxtail grass	*Setaria* spp.	Seed grains can be dried and used as cereal.
Tumble mustard	*Sisymbrium altissimum* L.	All parts of the plant are edible but have a strong mustard flavor; better used as a potherb.
Roundleaf cabriar	*Smilax rotundiflora* L.	Young tender shoots can be eaten raw. Young leaves can be eaten as salad; roots can be used for tea.

TABLE 1.11 *(Continued)*

Edible Weeds

Common Name	Scientific Name	Use
Sowthistle	*Sonchus oleraceus* L.	Leaves are prickly and bitter but can be used as a potherb.
Johnson grass	*Sorghum halepense* L.	Young shoots can be eaten raw; seeds can be dried and used as cereal; mature stalks can be ground and the liquid extracted for use as syrup.
Chickweed	*Stellaria media* L.	Leaves can be eaten raw or cooked.
Dandelion	*Taraxacum officinale*	All parts of the plant are edible.
Stinkweed	*Thlaspi arvense* L.	All parts of the plant are edible after cooking.
Westem salsify	*Tragopogon dubius Scopoli*	Roots can be eaten after boiling; leaves, flowers, and stems can be eaten raw.
Red clover	*Trifolium pratense* L.	Flowers can be boiled to make a broth; powdered leaves and flowers can be used as seasoning.
Coltsfoot	*Tussilago farfara* L.	Can be used as a potherb in small amounts.
Cattail	*Typha* spp.	Roots, stalks, and spears are edible.
Stinging nettle	*Urtica dioica* L.	Can be eaten cooked or used as a potherb.
Bellwort	*Uvularia perfoliata* L.	Young shoots can be cooked and eaten; leaves are bitter.
Blueberry, gooseberry	*Vaccinium, stamineun*	Berries can be eaten raw or used to make juice, jam, or jelly.
Violet	*Viola papilionacea Purish*	Flowers are edible.
Wild grapes	*Vitis* spp.	Fruits can be eaten raw or cooked.
Spanish bayonnet	*Yucca filimentosa* L.	Flower buds can be eaten raw.

1 Persons using this list should be aware that individuals may differ in their responses to these plants. For some consumers allergic reactions may be elicited. For others, there may be chemicals in the plants that elicit an undesirable physiological effect. Still other plants, especially the water plants, may harbor parasites that may be injurious. The serious forager should consult a plant taxonomist to be sure that the plant gathered is an edible plant. There are may similar plants that may in fact be poisonous, while others are safe to consume.

2 Weeds are plants that grow in places where we humans do not want them to grow. As such, we may not recognize them as food. The above plants contain edible portions. Not all parts of these plants may be useful as human food. Some varieties, in fact, may contain toxic chemicals that if consumed in large quantities may cause problems. A number of the plants have been identified based on their use by native Americans. These plants can have many different names as common names. This list is an abstract provided by James A. Duke in *Handbook of Edible Weeds,* CRC Press, Boca Raton, 1992, 246 pages.

TABLE 1.12

Toxic Plants

Common and Scientific Name	Description; Toxic Parts	Geographical Distribution	Poisoning; Symptoms	Remarks
Baneberry *Actaea* sp.	**Description**: Perennial growing to 3 ft (1 m) tall from a thick root; compound leaves; small, white flowers; white or red berries with several seeds borne in short, terminal clusters. **Toxic parts**: All parts, but primarily roots and berries.	Native woodlands of North America from Canada south to Georgia, Alabama, Louisiana, Oklahoma, and the northern Rockies; red-fruited western baneberry from Alaska to central California, Arizona, Montana, and South Dakota.	**Poisoning**: Attributed to a glycoside or essential oil which causes severe inflammation of the digestive tract. **Symptoms**: Acute stomach cramps, headache, increased pulse, vomiting, delirium, dizziness, and circulatory failure.	As few as 6 berries can cause symptoms persisting for hours. Treatment may be a gastric lavage or vomiting. Bright red berries attract children.
Buckeye; Horsechestnut *Aesculus* sp.	**Description**: Shrub or tree; deciduous, opposite, palmately, divided leaves with 5-9 leaflets on a long stalk; red, yellow, or white flowers; 2- to 3-valved, capsule fruit; with thick, leathery husk enclosing 1-6 brown shiny seeds. **Toxic parts**: Leaves, twigs, flowers, and seeds.	Various species throughout the United States and Canada; some cultivated as ornamentals, others growing wild.	**Poisoning**: Toxic parts contain the glycoside, esculin. **Symptoms**: Nervous twitching of muscles, weakness, lack of coordination, dilated pupils, nausea, vomiting, diarrhea, depression, paralysis, and stupor.	By making a "tea" from the leaves and twigs or by eating the seeds, children have been poisoned. Honey collected from the buckeye flower may also cause poisoning. Roots, branches, and fruits have been used to stupefy fish in ponds. Treatment usually is a gastric lavage or vomiting.
Buttercup *Ranunculus* sp.	**Description**: Annual or perennial herb growing to 16–32 in. (41–81 cm) high; leaves alternate entire to compound, and largely basal; yellow flowers borne singly or in clusters on ends of seed stalks; small fruits, 1-seeded pods. **Toxic parts**: Entire plant.	Widely distributed in woods, meadows, pastures, and along streams throughout temperate and cold locations.	**Poisoning**: The alkaloid protoanemonin, which can injure the digestive system and ulcerate the skin. **Symptoms**: Burning sensation of the mouth, nervousness, nausea, vomiting, low blood pressure, weak pulse, depression, and convulsions.	Sap and leaves may cause dermatitis. Cows poisoned by buttercups produce bitter milk or milk with a reddish color.

TABLE 1.12 *(Continued)*

Toxic Plants

Common and Scientific Name	Description; Toxic Parts	Geographical Distribution	Poisoning; Symptoms	Remarks
Castor bean *Ricinus communis*	**Description**: Shrublike herb 4-12 ft. (1.2-3.7 m) tall; simple, alternate, long-stalked leaves with 5 to 11 long lobes which are toothed on margins; fruits oval, green, or red, and covered with spines; 3 elliptical, glossy, black, white, or mottled seeds per capsule. **Toxic parts**: Entire plant, especially the seeds.	Cultivated as an ornamental or oilseed crop primarily in the southern part of the United States and Hawaii.	**Poisoning**: Seeds, pressed cake, and leaves poisonous when chewed; contain the phytotoxin, ricin. **Symptoms**: Burning of the mouth and throat, nausea, vomiting, severe stomach pains, bloody diarrhea, excessive thirst, prostration, dullness of vision, and convulsions; kidney failure and death 1–12 days later.	Fatal dose for a child is 1-3 seeds, and for an adult 2-8 seeds. The oil extracted from the seeds is an important commercial product. It is not poisonous and it is used as a medicine (castor oil), for soap, and as a lubricant.
Chinaberry *Melia azedarach*	**Description**: Deciduous tree 20–40 ft (6–12 m) tall; twice, pinnately divided leaves and toothed or lobed leaflets, purple flowers borne in clusters; yellow, wrinkled, rounded berries which persist throughout the winter. **Toxic parts**: Berries, bark, flowers, and leaves.	A native of Asia introduced as an ornamental in the United States; common in the southern United States and lower altitudes in Hawaii; has become naturalized in old fields, pastures, around buildings, and along fence rows.	**Poisoning**: Most result from eating pulp of berries; toxic principle is a resinoid with narcotic effects. **Symptoms**: Nausea, vomiting, diarrhea, irregular breathing, and respiratory distress.	Six to eight berries can cause the death of a child. The berries have been used to make insecticide and flea powder.
Death camas *Zigadenus paniculatus*	**Description**: Perennial herb resembling wild onions but the onion odor lacking; long, slender leaves with parallel veins; pale yellow to pink flowers in clusters on slender seedstalks; fruit a 3-celled capsule. **Toxic parts**: Entire plant, especially the bulb.	Various species occur throughout the United States and Canada; all are more or less poisonous.	**Poisoning**: Due to the alkaloids zygadenine, veratrine, and others. **Symptoms**: Excessive salivation, muscular weakness, slow heart rate, low blood pressure, subnormal temperature, nausea, vomiting, diarrhea, prostration, coma, and sometimes death.	The members of Lewis and Clark Expedition made flour from the bulbs and suffered the symptoms of poisoning. Later some pioneers were killed when they mistook death camas for wild onions or garlic.

Dogbane (Indian hemp) *Apocynum cannabinum*	**Description**: Perennial herbs with milky juice and somewhat woody stems; simple, smooth, and oppositely paired leaves; bell-shaped, small, white to pink flowers borne in clusters at ends of axillary stems; paired, long, slender seed pods. **Toxic parts**: Entire plant.	Various species growing throughout North America in fields and forests, and along streams and roadsides.	**Poisoning**: Only suspect since it contains the toxic glycoside, cymarin and is poisonous to animals. **Symptoms**: In animals, increased temperature and pulse, cold extremities, dilation of the pupils, discoloration of the mouth and nose, sore mouth, sweating, loss of appetite, and death.	Compounds extracted from roots of dogbane have been used to make a heart stimulant.
Foxglove *Digitalis purpurea*	**Description**: Biennial herb with alternate, simple, toothed leaves; terminal, showy raceme of flowers, purple, pink, rose, yellow, or white; dry capsule fruit. **Toxic parts**: Entire plant, especially leaves, flowers, and seeds.	Native of Europe commonly planted in gardens of the United States; naturalized and abundant in some parts of the western United States.	**Poisoning**: Due to digitalis component. **Symptoms**: Nausea, vomiting, dizziness, irregular heartbeat, tremors, convulsions, and possibly death.	Foxglove has long been known as a source of digitalis and steroid glycosides. It is an important medicinal plant when used correctly.
Henbane *Hyoscyamus niger*	**Description**: Erect annual or biennial herb with coarse, hairy stems 1–5 ft (30–152 cm) high; simple, oblong, alternate leaves with a few, coarse teeth, not stalked; greenish-yellow or yellowish with purple vein flowers; fruit a rounded capsule. **Toxic parts**: Entire plant.	Along roads, in waste places across southern Canada and northern United States, particularly common in the Rocky Mountains.	**Poisoning**: Caused by the alkaloids, hyoscyamine hyoscine, and atropine. **Symptoms**: Increased salivation, headache, nausea, rapid pulse, convulsions, coma, and death.	A gastric lavage of 4% tannic acid solution may be used to treat the poisoning.
Iris (Rock Mountain Iris) *Iris missouriensis*	**Description**: Lilylike perennial plants often in dense patches; long, narrow leaves; flowers blue-purple; fruit a 3-celled capsule. **Toxic parts**: Leaves, but especially the root stalk.	Wet land of meadows, marshes, and along streams from North Dakota to British Columbia, Canada; south to New Mexico, Arizona, and California; scattered over entire Rocky Mountain area; cultivated species also common.	**Poisoning**: An irritating resinous substance, irisin. **Symptoms**: Burning, congestion, and severe pain in the digestive tract; nausea and diarrhea.	Rootstalks have such an acrid taste that they are unlikely to be eaten.

TABLE 1.12 *(Continued)*
Toxic Plants

Common and Scientific Name	Description; Toxic Parts	Geographical Distribution	Poisoning; Symptoms	Remarks
Jasmine *Geisemium sempervirens*	**Description**: A woody, trailing, or climbing evergreen vine; opposite, simple, lance-shaped, glossy leaves; fragrant, yellow flowers; flattened 2-celled, beaked capsule fruits. **Toxic parts**: Entire plant, but especially the root and flowers.	Native to the southeastern United States; commonly grown in the Southwest as an ornamental.	**Poisoning**: Alkaloids, geisemine, gelseminine, and gelsemoidine found throughout the plant. **Symptoms**: Profuse sweating, muscular weakness, convulsions, respiratory depression, paralysis, and death possible.	Jasmine has been used as a medicinal herb, but overdoses are dangerous. Children have been poisoned by chewing on the leaves.
Jimmyweed (Rayless goldenrod) *Haplopappus heterophyllus*	**Description**: Small, bushy, half-shrub with erect stems arising from the woody crown to a height of 2–4 ft (61–122 cm); narrow, alternate, sticky leaves; clusters of small, yellow flower heads at tips of stems. **Toxic parts**: Entire plant.	Common in fields or ranges around watering sites and along streams from Kansas, Oklahoma, and Texas to Colorado, New Mexico, and Arizona.	**Poisoning**: Contains the higher alcohol, tremetol, which accumulates in the milk of cows and causes human poisoning known as "milk sickness."	Other species of Haplopappus probably are equally dangerous. White snakeroot also contains tremetol, and causes "milk sickness."
Jimsonwood (Thornapple) *Datura stramonium*	**Description**: Coarse, weedy plant with stout stems and foul-smelling foliage; large, oval leaves with wavy margins; fragrant, large, tubular, white to purple flowers; round, nodding or erect prickly capsule. **Toxic parts**: Entire plant, particularly the seeds and leaves.	Naturalized throughout North America; common weed of fields, gardens, roadsides, and pastures.	**Poisoning**: Due to the alkaloids hyoscyamine, atropine, and hyoscine (scopolamine). **Symptoms**: Dry mouth, thirst, red skin, disturbed vision, pupil dilation, nausea, vomiting, headache, hallucination, rapid pulse, delirium, incoherent speech, convulsion, high blood pressure, coma, and possibly death.	Sleeping near the fragrant flowers can cause headache, nausea, dizziness, and weakness. Children pretending the flowers were trumpets have been poisoned.

Lantana (Red Sage) *Lantana camara*	**Description**: Perennial shrub with square twigs and a few spines; simple, opposite or whorled oval-shaped leaves with tooth margins; white, yellow, orange, red, or blue flowers occurring in flat-topped clusters; berry-like fruit with a hard, blue-black seed. **Toxic parts**: All parts, especially the green berries.	Native of the dry woods in the southeastern United States; cultivated as an ornamental shrub in pots in the northern United States and Canada; or a lawn shrub in the southeastern coastal plains, Texas, California, and Hawaii.	**Poisoning**: Fruit contains high levels of an alkaloid, lantanin or lantadene A. **Symptoms**: Stomach and intestinal irritation, vomiting, bloody diarrhea, muscular weakness, jaundice, and circulatory collapse; death possible but not common.	In Florida, these plants are considered a major cause of human poisoning. The foliage of lantana may also cause dermatitis.
Larkspur *Delphinium* sp.	**Description**: Annual or perennial herb 2–4 ft (61–122 cm) high; finely, palmately divided leaves on long stalks; white, pink, rose, blue, or purple flowers each with a spur; fruit a many-seeded, 3-celled capsule. **Toxic parts**: Entire plant.	Native of rich or dry forest and meadows throughout the United States but common in the West; frequently cultivated in flower gardens.	**Poisoning**: Contains the alkaloids delphinine, delphineidine, ajacine, and others. **Symptoms**: Burning sensation in the mouth and skin, low blood pressure, nervousness, weakness, prickling of the skin, nausea, vomiting, depression, convulsions, and death within 6 hours if eaten in large quantities.	Poisoning potential of larkspur decreases as it ages, but alkaloids still concentrated in the seeds. Seeds are used in some commercial lice remedies.
Laurel (Mountain laurel) *Kalmia latifolia*	**Description**: Large evergreen shrubs growing to 35 ft (11 m) tall; alternate leaves dark green on top and bright green underneath; white to rose flowers in terminal clusters; fruit in a dry capsule. **Toxic parts**: Leaves, twigs, flowers, and pollen grains.	Found in moist woods and along streams in eastern Canada southward in the Appalachian Mountains and Piedmont, and sometimes in the eastern coastal plain.	**Poisoning**: Contains the toxic resinoid, andromedotoxin. **Symptoms**: Increased salivation, watering of eyes and nose, loss of energy, slow pulse, vomiting, low blood pressure, lack of coordination, convulsions, and progressive paralysis until eventual death.	The Mountain laurel is the state flower of Connecticut and Pennsylvania. By making "tea" from the leaves or by sucking on the flowers, children have been poisoned.

TABLE 1.12 *(Continued)*

Toxic Plants

Common and Scientific Name	Description; Toxic Parts	Geographical Distribution	Poisoning; Symptoms	Remarks
Locoweed (Crazyweed) *Oxtropis* sp.	**Description:** Perennial herb with erect or spreading stems; pealike flowers and stems — only smaller.	Common throughout the southwestern United States.	**Poisoning**: Contains alkaloidlike substances — a serious threat to livestock. **Symptoms**: In animals, loss of weight, irregular gait, loss of sense of direction, nervousness, weakness, and loss of muscular control.	Locoweeds are seldom eaten by humans, hence they are not a serious problem. There are more than 100 species of locoweeds.
Lupine (Bluebonnet) *Lupinus* sp.	**Description**: Annual or perennial herbs; digitately divided, alternate leaves; pear-shaped blue, white, red, or yellow flowers borne in clusters at ends of stems; seeds in flattened pods. **Toxic parts**: Entire plant, particularly the seeds.	Wide distribution but most common in western North America; many cultivated as ornamentals.	**Poisoning**: Contains lupinine and related toxic alkaloids. **Symptoms**: Weak pulse, slowed respiration, convulsions, and paralysis.	Rarely have cultivated varieties poisoned children. Not all lupines are poisonous.
Marijuana (hashish, Mary Jane, pot, grass)	**Description**: A tall coarse, annual herb; palmately divided and long stalked leaves; small, green flowers clustered in the leaf axils. **Toxic parts**: Entire plant, especially the leaves, flowers, sap and resinous secretions.	Widely naturalized weed in temperate North America; cultivated in warmer areas.	**Poisoning**: Various narcotic resins but mainly tetrahydrocannabinol (THC) and related compounds. **Symptoms**: Exhilaration, hallucinations, delusions, mental confusion, dilated pupils, blurred vision, poor coordination, weakness, and stupor; coma and death in large doses.	Poisoning results form drinking the extract, chewing the plant parts, or smoking a so-called "reefer" (joint). The hallucinogenic and narcotic effects of marijuana have been known for more than 2000 years. Laws in the United States and Canada restrict the possession of living or dried parts of marijuana.

Mescal bean (Frijolito) *Sophora secundiflora*	**Description**: Evergreen shrub or small tree growing to 40 ft (12 m) tall; stalked, alternate leaves 4–6 in. (10–15 cm) long, which are pinnately divided and shiny, yellow-green above and silky below when young; violet-blue, pealike flowers; bright red seeds. **Toxic parts**: Entire plant, particularly the seed.	Native to southwestern Texas and southern New Mexico; cultivated as ornamentals in the southwestern United States.	**Poisoning**: Contains cytisine and other poisonous alkaloids. **Symptoms**: Nausea, vomiting, diarrhea, excitement, delirium, hallucinations, coma, and death; deep sleep lasting 2–3 days in nonlethal doses.	One seed, if sufficiently chewed, is enough to cause the death of a young child. The Indians of Mexico and the Southwest have used the seeds in medicine as a narcotic and as a hallucinatory drug. Necklaces have been made from the seeds.
Mistletoe *Phoradendron serotinum*	**Description**: Parasitic evergreen plants that grow on trees and shrubs; oblong, simple, opposite leaves, which are leathery; small, white berries. **Toxic parts**: All parts, especially the berries.	Common on the branches of various trees from New Jersey and southern Indiana southward to Florida and Texas; other species throughout North America.	**Poisoning**: Contains the toxic amines, beta-phenylethylamine and tyrosamine. **Symptoms**: Gastrointestinal pain, diarrhea, slow pulse, and collapse; possibly nausea, vomiting, nervousness, difficult breathing, delirium, pupil dilation, and abortion; in sufficient amounts, death within a few hours.	Mistletoe is a favorite Christmas decoration. It is the state flower of Oklahoma. Poisonings have occurred when people eat the berries or make "tea" from the berries. Indians chewed the leaves to relieve toothache.
Monkshood (Wolfsbane) *Aconitum columbianum*	**Description**: Perennial herb about 2–5 ft (61–152 cm) high; alternate, petioled leaves which are palmately divided into segments with pointed tips; generally dark blue flowers with a prominent hood; seed in a short-beaked capsule. **Toxic parts**: Entire plant, especially roots and seeds.	Rich, moist soil in meadows and along streams from western Canada south to California and New Mexico.	**Poisoning**: Due to several alkaloids, including aconine and aconitine. **Symptoms**: Burning sensation of the mouth and skin; nausea, vomiting, diarrhea, muscular weakness, and spasms, weak, irregular pulse, paralysis of respiration, dimmed vision, convulsions, and death within a few hours.	Small amounts can be lethal. Death in humans reported from eating the plant or extracts made from it. It has been mistaken for horseradish.

TABLE 1.12 *(Continued)*

Toxic Plants

Common and Scientific Name	Description; Toxic Parts	Geographical Distribution	Poisoning; Symptoms	Remarks
Mushrooms (toadstools) *Amanita muscaria, Amantia verna, Chlorophyllum molybdites*	**Description**: Common types with central stalk, and cap; flat plates (gills) underneath cap; some with deeply ridged, cylindrical top rather than cap. **Toxic parts**: Entire fungus.	Various types throughout North America.	**Poisoning**: Depending on type of mushroom; complex polypeptides such as amanitin and possibly phalloidin; a toxic protein in some; the poisons ibotenic acid, muscimol, and related compounds in others. **Symptoms**: Vary with type of mushroom but include deathlike sleep, manic behavior, delirium, seeing colored visions, feeling of elation, explosive diarrhea, vomiting, severe headache, loss of muscular coordination, abdominal cramps, and coma and death from some types; permanent liver, kidney, and heart damage from other types.	Wild mushrooms are extremely difficult to identify and are best avoided. There is no simple rule of thumb for distinguishing between poisonous and nonpoisonous mushrooms — only myths and nonsense. Only one or two bites are necessary for death from some species. During the month of December 1981, three people were killed, and two hospitalized in California after eating poisonous mushrooms.
Nightshade *Solanum nigrum, Solanum eleagnifolium*	**Description**: Annual herbs or shrublike plants with simple alternate leaves; small, white, blue or violet flowers; black berries or yellow to yellow-orange berries depending on species. **Toxic parts**: Prinarily the unripe berries.	Throughout the United States and southern Canada in waste places, old fields, ditches, roadsides, fence rows, or edges of woods.	**Poisoning**: Contains the alkaloid solanine; possibly saponin, atropine, and perhaps high levels of nitrate. **Symptoms**: Headache, stomach pain, vomiting, diarrhea, dilated pupils, subnormal temperature, shock, circulatory and respiratory depression, possible death.	Some individuals use the completely ripe berries in pies and jellies. Young shoots and leaves of the plant have been cooked and eaten like spinach.

Oleander *Nerium oleander*	**Description**: An evergreen shrub or small tree growing to 25 ft (8 m) tall; short-stalked, narrow, leathery leaves, opposite or in whorls of 3; white to pink to red flowers at tips of twigs. **Toxic parts**: Entire plant, especially the leaves.	A native of southern Europe but commonly cultivated in the southern United States and California.	**Poisoning**: Contains the poisonous glycosides oleandrin and nerioside, which act similar to digitalis. **Symptoms**: Nausea, severe vomiting, stomach pain, bloody diarrhea, cold feet and hands, irregular heartbeat, dilation of pupils, drowsiness, unconsciousness, paralysis of respiration, convulsions, coma, death within a day.	One leaf of an oleander is said to contain enough poison to kill an adult. In Florida, severe poisoning resulted when oleander branches were used as skewers. Honey made from oleander flower nectar is poisonous.
Peyote (Mescal buttons) *Lophophora williamsii*	**Description**: Hemispherical, spineless member of the cactus family growing from carrot-shaped roots; low, rounded sections with a tuft of yellow-white hairs on top; flower from the center of the plant, white to rose-pink; pink berry when ripe; black seeds. **Toxic parts**: Entire plant, especially the buttons.	Native to southern Texas and northern Mexico; cultivated in other areas.	**Poisoning**: Contains mescaline, lophophorine and other alkaloids. **Symptoms**: Illusions and hallucinations with vivid color, anxiety, muscular tremors and twitching, vomiting, diarrhea, blurred vision, wakefulness, forgetfulness, muscular relaxation, dizziness.	The effects of chewing fresh or dried "buttons" of peyote are similar to those produced by LSD, only milder. In some states, peyote is recognized as a drug. Peyote has long been used by the Indians and Mexicans in religious ceremonies.
Poison hemlock (poison parsley) *Conium maculatum*	**Description**: Biennial herb with a hairless purple-spotted or lined, hollow stem growing up to 8 ft (2.4 m) tall; turniplike, long, solid taproot; large, alternate, pinnately divided leaves; small, white flowers in umbrella-shaped clusters, dry; ribbed, 2-part capsule fruit. **Toxic parts**: Entire plant, primarily seeds and root.	A native of Eurasia, now a weed in meadows, and along roads and ditches throughout the United States and southern Canada where moisture is sufficient.	**Poisoning**: The poisonous alkaloid coniine and other related alkaloids. **Symptoms**: Burning sensation in the mouth and throat, nervousness, dyscoordination, dilated pupils, muscular weakness, weakened and slowed heartbeat, convulsions, coma, death.	Poisoning occurs when the leaves are mistaken for parsley, the roots for turnips, or the seeds for anise. Toxic quantities seldom consumed because the plant has such an unpleasant odor and taste. Assumed by some to be the poison drunk by Socrates.

TABLE 1.12 *(Continued)*

Toxic Plants

Common and Scientific Name	Description; Toxic Parts	Geographical Distribution	Poisoning; Symptoms	Remarks
Poison ivy (poison oak) *Toxicondendron radicans*	**Description**: A trailing or climbing vine, shrub, or small tree; alternate leaves with 3 leaflets; flowers and fruits hanging in clusters; white to yellowish fruit (drupes). **Toxic parts**: Roots, stems, leaves, pollen, flowers, and fruits.	An extremely variable native weed throughout southern Canada and the United States with the exception of the west coast; found on flood plains, along lake shores, edges of woods, stream banks, fences, and around buildings.	**Poisoning**: Skin irritation due to an oil-resin containing urushiol. **Symptoms**: Contact with skin causes itching, burning, redness, and small blisters; severe gastric disturbance and even death by eating leaves or fruit.	Almost half of all persons are allergic to poison ivy. Skin irritation may also result from indirect contact such as animals (including dogs and cats), clothing, tools, or sports equipment.
Pokeweed (Pokeberry) *Phytolacca americana*	**Description**: Shrublike herb with a large fleshy taproot; large, entire, oblong leaves which are pointed; white to purplish flowers in clusters at ends of branches; mature fruit a dark purple berry with red juice. **Toxic parts**: Rootstalk, leaves, and stems.	Native to the eastern United States and southeastern Canada.	**Poisoning**: Highest concentration of poison mainly in roots; contains the bitter glycoside, saponin and glycoprotein. **Symptoms**: Burning and bitter taste in mouth, stomach cramps, nausea, vomiting, diarrhea, drowsiness, slowed breathing, weakness, tremors, convulsions, spasms, coma and death if eaten in large amounts.	Young tender leaves and stems of pokeweed are often cooked as greens. Cooked berries are used for pies without harm. It is one of the most dangerous poisonous plants because people prepare it improperly.
Poppy (common poppy) *Papaver somniferum*	**Description**: An erect annual herb with milky juice, simple, coarsely toothed, or lobed leaves; showy red, white, pink, or purple flowers; fruit an oval, crowned capsule; tiny seeds in capsule. **Toxic parts**: Unripe fruits or their juice.	Introduced from Eurasia and widely grown in the United States until cultivation without a license became unlawful.	**Poisoning**: Crude resin from unripe seed capsule source of narcotic opium alkaloids. **Symptoms**: From unripe fruit, stupor, coma, shallow and slow breathing, depression of the central nervous system; possibly nausea and severe retching (straining to vomit).	The use of poppy extracts is a double edged sword — addictive narcotics and valuable medicines. Poppy seeds used as toppings on breads are harmless.

Rhododendron, azaleas *Rhododendron sp.*	**Description**: Usually evergreen shrubs; mostly entire, simple, leathery leaves in whorls or alternate; snowy white to pink flowers in terminal clusters; fruit a wood capsule. **Toxic part**: Entire plant.	Throughout the temperate parts of the United States as a native and as an introduced ornamental.	**Poisoning**: Contains the toxic resinoid, andromedotoxin. **Symptoms**: Watering eyes and mouth, nasal discharge, nausea, severe abdominal pain, vomiting, convulsions, lowered blood pressure, lack of coordination and loss of energy; progressive paralysis of arms and legs until death, in severe cases.	Cases of poisoning are rare in this country but rhododentrons should be suspected of possible danger.
Rosary pea (precatory pea) *Abrus precatorius*	**Description**: A twining, more or less woody perennial vine; alternate and divided leaves with small leaflets; red to purple or white flowers; fruit a short pod containing ovoid seeds which are glossy, bright scarlet over 3/4 of their surface, and jet black over the remaining 1/4. **Toxic parts**: Seeds.	Native to the tropics, but naturalized in Florida and the Keys.	**Poisoning**: Contains the phytotoxin abrin and tetanic glycoside, abric acid. **Symptoms**: Severe stomach pain, in 1-3 days, nausea, vomiting, severe diarrhea, weakness, cold sweat, drowsiness, weak, fast pulse, coma, circulatory collapse, death.	The beans are made into rosaries, necklaces, bracelets, leis, and various toys which receive wide distribution. Seeds must be chewed and swallowed to cause poisoning. Whole seeds pass through the digestive tract without causing symptoms. One thoroughly chewed seed is said to be potent enough to kill an adult or child.
Snow-on-the-mountain *Euphorbia marginata*	**Description**: A tall annual herb, browing up to 4 ft (122 cm) high; smooth, lance-shaped leaves with conspicuously white margins; whorls of white petal-like leaves border flowers; fruit a 3-celled, 3-lobed capsule. **Toxic parts**: Leaves, stems, milky sap.	Native to the western, dry plains and valleys from Montana to Mexico; sometimes escapes in the eastern United States.	**Poisoning**: Toxins causing dermatitis and severe irritation of the digestive tract. **Symptoms**: Blistering of the skin, nausea, abdominal pain, fainting, diarrhea, possibly death in severe cases.	Milky juice of this plant is very caustic. Outwardly resembles a poinsettia.

TABLE 1.12 *(Continued)*

Toxic Plants

Common and Scientific Name	Description; Toxic Parts	Geographical Distribution	Poisoning; Symptoms	Remarks
Skunkcabbage *Veratrum californicum*	**Description**: Tall, broadleaved herbs of the lily family, growing to 6 ft (183 cm) high; large, alternate pleated, clasping, and parallel-veined leaves; numerous whitish to greenish flowers in large terminal clusters; 3-lobed, capsule fruit. **Toxic parts**: Entire plant.	Various species throughout North America in wet meadows, forests, and along streams.	**Poisoning**: Contains such alkaloids as veradridene and veratrine. **Symptoms**: Nausea, vomiting, diarrhea, stomach pains, lowered blood pressure, slow pulse, reduced body temperature, shallow breathing, salivation, weakness, nervousness, convulsions, paralysis, possibly death.	These plants have been used for centuries as a source of drugs and as a source of insecticide. Since the leaves resemble cabbage, they are often collected as an edible wild plant, but with unpleasant results.
Tansy *Tanacetum vulgare*	**Description**: Tall, aromatic herb with simple stems to 3 ft (91 cm) high; alternate, pinnately divided, narrow leaves, flower heads in flat-topped clusters with numerous small, yellow flowers. **Toxic parts**: Leaves, stems, and flowers.	Introduced from Eurasia; widely naturalized in North America; sometimes found escarped along roadsides, in pastures, or other wet places; grown for medicinal purposes.	**Poisoning**: Contains an oil, tanacetin, or oil of tansy. **Symptoms**: Nausea, vomiting, diarrhea, convulsions, violent spasms, dilated pupils, rapid and feeble pulse, possibly death.	Tanys and oil of tansy are employed as an herbal remedy for nervousness, intestinal worms, to promote menstruation, and to induce abortion. Some poisonings have resulted from the use of tansy as a home remedy.

Waterhemlock *Cicuta sp.*	**Description**: A perennial with parsleylike leaves; hollow, jointed stems and hollow, pithy roots; flowers in umbrella clusters; stems streaked with purple ridges; 2-6 ft (61-183 cm) high. **Toxic parts**: Entire plant, primarily the roots and young growth.	Wet meadows, pastures, and flood plains of western and eastern United States, generally absent in the plains states.	**Poisoning**: Contains the toxic resinlike higher alcohol, cicutoxin. **Symptoms**: Frothing at the mouth, spasms, dilated pupils, diarrhea, convulsions, vomiting, delirium, respiratory failure, paralysis, and death.	One mouthful of the waterhemlock root is reported to contain sufficient poison to kill a man. Children making whistles and peashooters from the hollow stems have been poisoned. The waterhemlock is often mistaken for the edible wild artichoke or parsnip. However, it is considered to be one of the poisonous plants of the North Temperate Zone.
White snakeroot *Eupatorium rogosum*	Description: Erect perrenial with stems 1-5 ft (30-152 cm) tall; opposite oval leaves with pointed tips and sharply toothed edges, and dull on the upper surface but shiny on the lower surface; showy, snow white flowers in terminal clusters. Toxic parts: Entire plant.	From eastern Canada to Saskatchewan and south to Texas, Louisiana, Georgia, and Virginia.	Poisoning: Contains the higher alcohol, tremetol and some glycosides. Symptoms: Weakness, nausea, loss of appetite, vomiting, tremors, labored breathing, constipation, dizziness, delirium, convulsions, coma, and death.	Recovery from a nonlethal dose is a slow process, due to liver and kidney damage. Poison may be in the milk of cows that have eaten white snakeroot — "milk sickness."

Taken from Ensminger et al., *Foods and Nutrition Encyclopedia,* 2nd ed., CRC Press, Boca Raton, 1994, pp. 1776-1785.

TABLE 1.13

Plants Used as Herbal Remedies[1]

Common and Scientific Name	Description	Production	Part(s) of Plant Used	Reported Uses
Agrimony *Agrimonia gryposepala*	Small yellow flowers on a long spike; leaves hairy and at least 5 in. (13 cm) long, narrow and pointed; leaf edges toothed; a perennial.	Needs good soil and sunshine; grows in New England and Middle Atlantic states.	Whole plant including roots	A tonic, alterative, diuretic, and astringent; infusions from the leaves for sore throats; treatment of kidney and bladder stones; root for jaundice.
Aletris root (whitetube stargrass) *Aletris farinosa*	Grasslike leaves in a flat rosette around a spike-like stem; white to yellow tubular flowers along stem.	Moist locations in woods, meadows, or bogs; New England to Michigan and Wisconsin; south to Florida and west to Texas.	Leaves, roots	Poultice of leaves for sore breast; liquid from boiled roots for stomach pains, tonic, sedative, and diuretic.
Alfalfa *Medicago sativa*	Very leafy plant growing 1–2 ft (30–61 cm) high; small green leaves; bluish-purple flowers; deep roots.	A legume cultivated widely in the United States.	Leaves	Powdered and mixed with cider vinegar as a tonic; infusions for a tasty drink; leaves may also be used green.
Aloe vera *Aloe barbadensis*	A succulent plant with leathery sword-shaped leaves, 6–24 in. (15–61 cm) long.	A semidesert plant which grows in Mexico and Hawaii; temperature must remain above 50°F (10°C); can be a house plant.	Mucilaginous juice of the leaves	Effective on small cuts and sunburn; speeds healing; manufactured product for variety of cosmetic purposes.
Angelica *Angelica atropurpurea*	Shrub growing to 8 ft (2.4 m) high; stem purplish with 3 toothed leaflets at tip of each leaf stem; white or greenish flowers in clusters at end of each stalk.	Grows in rich low soil near streams and swamps and in gardens; from New England west to Ohio, Indiana, Illinois, and Wisconsin; south to Delaware, Maryland, West Virginia, and Kentucky.	Roots, seeds	Small amount of dried root or seeds for relief of flatulence; roots for the induction of vomiting and perspiration; roots for treatment of toothache, bronchitis, rheumatism, gout, fever, and to increase menstrual flow.
Anise (Anise seed) *Pimpinella anisum*	Annual plant, 1–2 ft (30–61 cm) high; belongs to carrot family; small white flowers on long hairy stalk; lower leaves egg-shaped; upper leaves feathery.	Grown all over the world; grows wild in countries around the Mediterranean; much is imported to United States.	Seed	As a hot tea to relieve flatulence or for colic.

TABLE 1.13 *(Continued)*

Plants Used as Herbal Remedies[1]

Common and Scientific Name	Description	Production	Part(s) of Plant Used	Reported Uses
Asafetida *Ferula* sp.	A coarse plant growing to 7 ft (2.1 m) high with numerous stem leaves; pale green-yellow flowers; flowers and seeds borne in clusters on stalks; large fleshly root; tenacious odor.	Indigenous to Afghanistan, but some species grow in other Asiatic countries.	Gummy resin from the root	As an antispasmodic; to ward off colds and flu by wearing in a bag around the neck.
Bayberry (Southern wax myrtle) *Myrica cerifera*	Perennial shrub growing to 30 ft (9.2 m) high; waxy branchlets; narrow evergreen leaves tapering at both ends; yellowish flowers; fruits are grayish berries.	Grows in coastal regions from New Jersey, Delaware and Maryland to Florida, Alabama, Mississippi, and Arkansas.	Root bark, leaves, stems	Decoction of root bark to treat uterine hemorrhage, jaundice, dysentery, and cankers; leaves and stems boiled and used to treat fevers; decoction of boiled leaves for intestinal worms.
Bearberry *Arctostaphylos uva-ursi*	Creeping evergreen shrub with stems up to 6 in. (15 cm) high; reddish bark; bright green leaves, 1 in. (3 cm) long; white flowers with red markings, in clusters; smooth red fruits.	Grows in well-drained soils at higher altitudes; from Oregon, Washington, and California, to Colorado and New Mexico.	Leaves	As a diuretic; also boiled infusions used as a drink to treat sprains, stomach pains, and urinary problems; poison oak inflammations treated with leaf decoction by pioneers.
Blackberry (brambleberry, dewberry, raspberry) *Rubus*	Shrubby or viny thorny perennial; numerous species; large white flowers; red or black fruit.	Grows wild or in gardens throughout the United States; wild in old fields, waste areas, forest borders, and pastures.	Roots, root bark, leaves, fruit	Infusion made from roots used to dry up runny noses; infusion from root bark to treat dysentery; fruit used to treat dysentery in children; leaves also used in similar manner.
Black cohosh *Cimicifuga racemosa*	Perennial shrub growing to 9 ft (2.7 m) or more in height; leaf has 2 to 5 leaflets; plant topped with spike of slender candlelike, white or yellowish flowers; rhizome gnarled and twisted.	Grows throughout eastern United States; commercial supply from Blue Ridge Mountains.	Rhizomes, roots	Infusion and decoctions used to treat sore throat, rheumatism, kidney trouble, and general malaise; also used for "women's ailments" and malaria.

TABLE 1.13 *(Continued)*

Plants Used as Herbal Remedies[1]

Common and Scientific Name	Description	Production	Part(s) of Plant Used	Reported Uses
Black Walnut *Juglans nigra*	A tree growing up to 120 ft (36.6 m) high; leaflets alternate 12–23 per stem, finely toothed and about 3–3.5 in. (8–9 cm) long; nut occurs singly or in clusters with fleshy, aromatic husk.	Native to a large section of the rich woods of eastern and midwestern United States.	Bark, nut husk, leaves	Inner bark used as mild laxative; husk of nut used for treating intestinal worms, ulcers, syphilis, and fungus infections; leaf infusion for bedbugs.
Blessed thistle *Cnicus benedictus*	Annual plant growing to 2 ft (61 cm) high; spiny tooth, lobed leaves; many flowered yellow heads.	Grows along roadsides and in waste places in eastern and parts of southwestern United States.	Leaves and flowering tops in full bloom, seeds	Infusions from leaves and tops for cancer treatment, to induce sweating, as a diuretic, to reduce fever, and for inflammations of the respiratory system; infusion of tops as Indian contraceptive; seeds induce vomiting.
Boneset *Eupatorium perfoliatum*	Perennial bush growing to 5 ft (1.5 m) in height; heavy stems with leaves opposite; purplish to white flowers borne in flat heads.	Commonly found in wet areas such as swamps, rich woods, marshes, and pastures; grows from Canada to Florida and west to Texas and Nebraska.	Leaves, flowering tops	Infusions made from leaves used for laxative and treatment of coughs and chest illnesses — a cold remedy; Negro slaves and Indians used it to treat malaria.
Borage *Borago officinalis*	Entire plant not over 1 ft (30 cm) high; nodding heads of starlike flowers grow from clusters of hairy obovate leaves.	Introduced in United States from Europe; occasionally grows in waste areas in northern states; cultivated widely in gardens.	Leaves	Most often used as an infusion to increase sweating, as a diuretic, or to soothe intestinal tract; can be applied to swellings and inflamed areas for relief.
Buchu *Rutaceae*	Low shrubs with angular branches and small leaves growing in opposition; flowers from white to pink.	Grown in rich soil in warm climate of South Africa.	Dried leaves	Prepared as tincture or infusion; used for genito-urinary diseases, indigestion, edema, and early stages of diabetes.
Buckthorn *Rhamnus purshiana*	Deciduous tree growing to 25 ft (7.6 m) high; leaves 2–6 in. (5–15 cm) long; flowers small greenish yellow; fruit globular and black, about 1/4 in. (6 mm) across.	Grows usually with conifers along canyon walls, rich bottom lands, and mountain ridges in western United States.	Bark, fruit	Bark used as a laxative and tonic; fruit (berries) used as a laxative.

TABLE 1.13 *(Continued)*

Plants Used as Herbal Remedies[1]

Common and Scientific Name	Description	Production	Part(s) of Plant Used	Reported Uses
Burdock *Arctium minus*	Biennial or perennial growing 5–8 ft (1.5–2.4 m) high; large leaves resembling rhubarb; tube-shaped white and pink to purple flowers in heads; brown bristled burrs contain seeds.	Grows in wastelands, fields, and pastures throughout the United States.	Root	Infusion of roots for coughs, asthma, and to stimulate menstruation; tincture of root for rheumatism and stomachache.
Calamus (Sweet flag) *Acorus calamus*	Perennial growing 3–5 ft (1.0–1.5 m) high; long narrow leaves with sharp edges; aromatic leaves; flower stalk 2–3 in. (3–8 cm) long and clublike; greenish-yellow flowers.	Grows in swamps, edges of streams and ponds from New England west to Oregon and Montana, and from Texas east to Florida and north.	Rhizomes	Root chewed to clear phlegm (mucous) and ease stomach gas; infusions to treat stomach distress; considered useful as tonic and stimulant.
Catnip *Nepeta cataria*	Perennial growing to 3 ft (1 m) in height; stem downy and whitish; leaves heart-shaped opposite coarsely toothed and 2–3 in. (3–8 cm) long; tubular whitish with purplish marked flowers in compact spikes.	Grows wild along fences, roadsides, waste places, and streams in Virginia, Tennessee, West Virginia, Georgia, New England, Illinois, Indiana, Ohio, New Mexico, Colorado, Arizona, Utah, and California; readily cultivated in gardens.	Entire plant	Infusions for treating colds, nervous disorders, stomach ailments, infant colic, and hives; smoke relieves respiratory ailments; poultice to reduce swellings.
Celery *Apium graveolens*	A biennial producing flower stalk second year; terminal leaflet at end of stem; fruit brown and round.	Cultivated in California, Florida, Michigan, New York, and Washington.	Seeds	As an infusion to relieve rheumatism and flatulence (gas); to act as a diuretic; to act as a tonic and stimulant; oil from seeds used similarly.

TABLE 1.13 *(Continued)*
Plants Used as Herbal Remedies[1]

Common and Scientific Name	Description	Production	Part(s) of Plant Used	Reported Uses
Chamomile *Anthemis nobilis*	Low growing, pleasantly strong-scented, downy, and matlike perennial; daisylike flowers with white petals and yellow center.	Cultivated in gardens; some wild growing which escaped from gardens.	Leaves, flowers	Powdered and mixed with boiling water to stimulate stomach, to remedy nervousness in women, and stimulate menstrual flow, also a tonic; flowers for poultice to relieve pain; chamomile tea known as soothing, sedative, completely harmless.
Chaparral *Croton corynbulosus*	Shrubby perennial plant of the Spurge family.	Grows in dry rock areas from Texas west.	Flowering tips	Infusions act as laxative; some claims as cancer treatment.
Chickweed *Stellaria media*	Annual growing 12–15 in. (30–38 cm) high; stems matted to somewhat upright; upper leaves vary but lower leaves ovate; white, small individual flowers.	Grows in shaded areas, meadows, wasteland, cultivated land, thickets, gardens, and damp woods in Virginia to South Carolina and southeast.	Entire plant in full bloom	Poultice made to treat sores, ulcers, infections, and hemorrhoids.
Chicory *Cichorium intybus*	Easily confused with its close relative the dandelion; in bloom bears blue or soft pink blooms not resembling dandelion.	Introduced from Europe, now common wild plant in United States; some grown in gardens.	Roots, leaves	No great medicinal value; some mention of diuretic, laxative, and tonic use; mainly added to give coffee distinctive flavor.
Cinnamon *Cinnamomum zeylanicum*	An evergreen bush or tree growing to 30 ft (9 m) high.	A native plant of Sri Lanka, India, and Malaysia; tree kept pruned to a shrub; bark of lower branches peeled and dried.	Bark	Treatment for flatulence, diarrhea, vomiting, and nausea.
Cleaver's herb (Catchweed bedstraw) *Galium aparine*	Annual plant; weak reclining bristled stem with hairy joints; leaves in whorls of 8; white flowers in broad, flat cluster; bristled fruit.	Grows in rich woods, thickets, seashores, waste areas, and shady areas from Canada to Florida and west to Texas.	Entire plant during flowering	To increase urine formation; to stimulate appetite; to reduce fever; to remedy vitamin C deficiency.

TABLE 1.13 *(Continued)*

Plants Used as Herbal Remedies[1]

Common and Scientific Name	Description	Production	Part(s) of Plant Used	Reported Uses
Cloves *Syzygium aromaticum*	Dried flower bud of a tropical tree which is a 30-ft (9 m) high red flowered evergreen.	Tree native to Molucca, but widely cultivated in tropics; flower bud picked before flower opens and dried.	Flower bud	To promote salivation and gastric secretion; to relieve pain in stomach and intestines; applied externally to relieve rheumatism, lumbago, toothache, muscle cramps, and neuralgia; clove oil used, too; infusions with clove powder relieves nausea and vomiting.
Colt's foot (Canada wild ginger) *Asarum canadense*	Low growing stemless perennial; heart-shaped leaves; flowers near root are brown and bell-shaped.	Found in moist woods from Maine to Georgia and west to Ohio.	Roots, leaves	Infusion of root to relieve flatulence; powdered root to relieve flatulence; induce sweating, and to relieve aching head and eyes; leaves substitute for ginger.
Comfrey *Symphytum officinale*	A perennial which reaches about 2 ft (61 cm) in height; leaves are large and broad at base but lancelike at terminal; fine hair on leaves; tail-shaped head of white to purple flowers at terminal.	Prefers a moist environment; a European plant now naturalized in the United States.	Roots, leaves	Numerous uses including treatments for pneumonia, coughs, diarrhea, calcium deficiency, colds, sores, ulcers, arthritis, gallstones, tonsils, cuts and wounds, headaches, hemorrhoids, gout, burns, kidney stones, anemia, and tuberculosis; used as a poultice, infusion, powder, or in capsule form.
Dandelion *Taraxacum officinale*	Biennial growing 2–12 in. (5–30 cm) high; leaves deeply serrated forming a basal rosette in spring; yellow flower but turns to gray upon maturing.	Weed throughout the United States; the bane of lawns.	Flowers, roots, green leaves	Root uses include diuretic, laxative, tonic, and to stimulate appetite; infusion from flower for heart troubles; paste of green leaves for bruises.
Echinacea (Purple echinacea) *Echinacea purpurea*	Perennial from 2–5 ft (0.6–1.5 m) high; alternate lance-shaped leaves; leaf margins toothed; top leaves lack stems; purple to white flower.	Grows wild on road banks, prairies, and dry, open woods in Ohio to Iowa, south to Oklahoma, Georgia, and Alabama.	Roots	Treatment of ulcers and boils, syphilis, snakebites, skin diseases, and blood poisoning; used as powder and in capsules.

TABLE 1.13 *(Continued)*

Plants Used as Herbal Remedies[1]

Common and Scientific Name	Description	Production	Part(s) of Plant Used	Reported Uses
Eucalyptus *Eucalyptus globulus*	Tall, fragrant tree growing up to 300 ft (92 m) high; reddish-brown stringy bark.	Native to Australia but grown in other semitropical and warm temperate regions.	Leaves and oil distilled from leaves	Antiseptic value; inhaled freely for sore throat; asthma relief; local application to ulcers; used on open wounds.
Eyebright (Indian tobacco) *Lobelia inflata*	Branching annual growing to 3 ft (1 m) high with leaves 1–3 in. (3–8 cm) long; small violet to pinkish-white flowers in axils of leaves; seed capsules at base of flower containing many tiny brown seeds.	Roadside weed of eastern United States, west to Kansas.	Entire plant in full bloom or when seeds are formed	Treatment of whooping cough, asthma, epilepsy, pneumonia, hysteria, and convulsion; alkaloid extracted for use in antismoking preparations.
Fenugreek *Trigonella foenum-graceum*	Annual plant similar to clover in size.	Native to the Mediterranean regions and northern India; widely cultivated; easily grown in home gardens.	Seed	Poultice for wounds; gargle for sore throat.
Flax (Linseed) *Linum usitatissimum*	Herbaceous annual; slender upright plant with narrow leaves and blue flowers; grows to about 2 ft (61 cm) high.	Originated in Mediterranean region; cultivated widely for fiber and oil.	Seed	Ground flaxseed mixed with boiling water for poultice on burns, boils, carbuncles, and sores; internally as a laxative.
Garlic *Allium sativum*	Annual plant growing to 12 in. (30 cm) high; long, linear, narrow leaves; bulb composed of several bulblets.	Throughout the United States under cultivation; some wild.	Entire plant when in bloom; bulbs	Fresh poultice of the mashed plant for treating snake bite, hornet stings, and scorpion stings; eaten to expel worms, treat colds, coughs, hoarseness, and asthma; bulb expressed against the gum for toothache.
Gentian (Sampson snakeroot) *Gentiana villosa*	Perennial with stems growing 8–10 in. (20–25 cm) high; opposite ovate, lance-shaped leaves; pale blue flowers.	Grows wild in swampy areas Florida west to Louisiana, north to New Jersey, Pennsylvania, Ohio, and Indiana.	Rhizomes and roots	Treatment of indigestion, gout, and rheumatism; induction of vomiting; aid to digestion; a tonic.
Ginger *Zingiber officinale*	Perennial plant; forms irregular-shaped rhizomes at shallow depth.	Native to southeastern Asia; now grown all over tropics.	Rhizome	An expectorant; treatment of flatulence, colds, and sore throats.

TABLE 1.13 *(Continued)*

Plants Used as Herbal Remedies[1]

Common and Scientific Name	Description	Production	Part(s) of Plant Used	Reported Uses
Ginseng *Panax quinquefolia*	Hollow stems solid at nodes; leaves alternate; root often resembles shape of a man; small, inconspicuous flowers; vivid, shiny, scarlet berries.	Grows in eastern Asia, Korea, China, and Japan; some grown in United States.	Root	As a tonic and stimulant; treatment of convulsions, dizziness, vomiting, colds, fevers, headaches, and rheumatism.
Goldenrod *Solidago odora*	Grows 18–36 in. (46–91 cm) high with narrow leaves scented like anise; inconspicuous head with 6–8 flowers.	Grows throughout the United States.	Leaves	Infusions from dried leaves as aromatic stimulant and a diuretic.
Goldenseal *Hydrastis canadensis*	Perennial growing to about 1 ft (30 cm) high; one stem with 5–7 lobed leaves near top; several single leafstalks topped with petalless flowers; raspberrylike fruit but inedible.	Grows in rich, shady woods of southeastern and midwestern United States; grown under cultivation in Washington.	Roots, leaves, stalks	Root infusion as an appetite stimulant and tonic; root powder for open cuts and wounds; chewing root for mouth sores; leaf infusion for liver and stomach ailments.
Guarana *Paullinia cupana*	Climbing shrub of the soapberry family; yellow flowers; pear-shaped fruit; seed in 3-sided, 3-celled capsules.	Grows in South America, particularly Brazil and Uruguay.	Seeds	Stimulant; seeds high in caffeine.
Hawthorn *Crataegus oxycantha*	Hardy shrub or tree depending upon growth conditions; small, berry fruit; cup-shaped flowers with 5 parts; thorny stems.	Originally grown throughout England as hedges; also grows wild; some introduced in the United States.	Berry	Tonic for heart ailments such as angina pectoris, valve defects, rapid and feeble heart beat, and hypertrophied heart; reverses arteriosclerosis.
Hop *Humulus lupulus*	Twining, perennial growing 20 ft (6 m) or more; 3 smooth-lobed leaves 4–5 in. (10–13 cm) long; membranous, conelike fruit.	Grows throughout the United States; often a cultivated crop.	Fruit (hops)	Straight hops or powder used; hot poultice of hops for boils and inflammations; treatment of fever, worms, and rheumatism; as a diuretic; as a sedative.

TABLE 1.13 *(Continued)*

Plants Used as Herbal Remedies[1]

Common and Scientific Name	Description	Production	Part(s) of Plant Used	Reported Uses
Horehound (White horehound) *Marrubium vulgare*	Shrub growing to 3 ft (1 m) in height; fuzzy ovate-round leaves which are whitish above and gray below; foliage aromatic when crushed.	Grows wild throughout most of United States in pastures, old fields, and waste places, except in arid southwest.	Leaves and small stems; bark	Decoctions to treat coughs, colds, asthma, and hoarseness; other uses include treatment for diarrhea,menstrual irregularity, and kidney ailments.
Huckleberry (Sparkleberry) *Vaccinium arboreum*	Shrub or tree growing to 25 ft (7.6 m) high; leathery; shiny, thick leaves; white flowers; black berries; other species.	Grows wild in woods, clearings, sandy and dry woods in Virginia, Georgia, Florida, Mississippi, Indiana, Illinois, Missouri, Texas, and Oklahoma.	Leaves, root bark, berries	Decoctions of leaves and root bark to treat sore throat and diarrhea; drink from berry for treating chronic dysentery.
Hyssop *Hyssopus officinalis*	Hardy, fragrant, bushy plants belonging to the mint family; stem woody; leaves hairy, pointed, and about 1/2 in. (20 mm) long; blue flowers in tufts.	Grows in various parts of Europe including the Middle East; some grown in United States.	Leaves	Infusions for colds, coughs, tuberculosis, and asthma; an aromatic stimulant; healing agent for cuts and bruises.
Juniper (Commonjuniper) *Juniperus communis*	Small evergreen shrub growing 12–30 ft (3.7–9.2 m) high; bark of trunk reddish-brown and tends to shred; needles straight and at right angles to branchlets; dark, purple, fleshy berrylike fruit.	Widely distributed from New Mexico to Dakotas and east; dry areas.	Fruit (berries)	Used as a diuretic, to induce menstruation, to relieve gas, and to treat snake bites and intestinal worms.
Lemon balm *Melissa officinalis*	Persistent perennial growing to 1 ft (30 cm) high; light green, serrated leaves; lemon smell and taste to crushed leaves.	Wild in much of the United States; grown in gardens.	Leaves	Infusion used as a carminative, diaphoretic, or febrifuge.
Licorice (Wild licorice) *Glycyrrhiza lepidota*	Erect perennial growing to 3 ft (1 m) high; pale yellow to white flowers at end of flower stalks; brown seed pods resemble cockleburs.	Grows wild on prairies, lake shores, and railroad right-of-ways throughout much of the United States.	Root **Caution:** Licorice raises the blood pressure of some people dangerously high, due to the retention of sodium.	Root extract to help bring out phlegm (mucus); treatment of stomach ulcers, rheumatism, and arthritis; root decoctions for inducing menstrual flow, treating fevers, and expulsion of afterbirth.

TABLE 1.13 *(Continued)*

Plants Used as Herbal Remedies[1]

Common and Scientific Name	Description	Production	Part(s) of Plant Used	Reported Uses
Marshmallow *Althaea officinalis*	Stems erect and 3–4 ft (0.9–1.2 m) high with only a few lateral branches; roundish, ovate-cordate leaves 2–3 in. (5–8 cm) long and irregularly toothed at margin; cup-shaped, pale-colored flowers.	Introduced into United States from Europe; now found on banks of tidal rivers and brackish streams; grew wild in salt marshes, damp meadows, by ditches, by the sea, and banks of tidal rivers from Denmark south.	Root	Primarily a demulcent and emollient; used in cough remedies; good poultice made from crushed roots.
Motherwort *Leonurus cardiaca*	Perennial growing 5–6 ft (1.5–1.8 m) high; lobed, dented leaves, 5 in. (13 cm) long; very fuzzy white to pink flowers.	Grows wild in pastures, waste places, and road-sides from northeastern states west to Montana and Texas, south to North Carolina and Tennessee.	Entire plant above ground	Used as a stimulant, tonic, and diuretic; Europeans used for asthma and heart palpitation; usually taken as an infusion.
Mullien (Aaron's rod) *Verbascum thapsus*	At base a rosette of woody, lance-shaped, oblong leaves with a diameter of up to 2 ft (61 cm); yellow flowers along a clublike spike arising from the rosette to a height of up to 7 ft (2.1 m).	Grows wild throughout the United States in dry fields, meadows, pastures, rocky or gravelly banks, burned areas, etc.	Leaves, roots, flowers	Infusions of leaves to treat colds and dysentery; dried leaves and flowers serve as a demulcent and emollient; leaves smoked for asthma relief; boiled roots for croup; oil from flowers for earache; local applications of leaves for hemorrhoids, inflammations, and sunburn.
Nutmeg *Muristica fragrans*	Evergreen tree growing to about 25 ft (7.6 m) high; grayish-brown, smooth bark; fruit resembles yellow plum, the seed of which is known as nutmeg.	Native to Spice Islands of Indonesia; now cultivated in other tropical areas.	Seed	For the treatment of nausea and vomiting; grated and mixed with lard for hemorrhoid ointment.
Papaya *Carica papaya*	Small tree seldom above 20 ft (6.1 m) high; soft, spongy wood; leaves as large as 2 ft (61 cm) in diameter and deeply cut into 7 lobes; fruit oblong and dingy green-yellow.	Originated in South American tropics; now cultivated in tropical climates.	Leaves	Dressing for wounds, and aid for digestion; contains proteolytic enzyme, papain, used as a meat tenderizer.

TABLE 1.13 *(Continued)*

Plants Used as Herbal Remedies[1]

Common and Scientific Name	Description	Production	Part(s) of Plant Used	Reported Uses
Parsley *Petroselinum crispum*	Biennial which is usually grown as an annual; finely divided, often curled, fragrant leaves.	Originated in the Mediterranean area; now grown worldwide.	Leaves, seeds, roots	As diuretic with aromatic and stimulating properties.
Passion flower (Maypop passion-flower) *Passiflora incarnata*	Perennial vine growing to 30 ft (9.2 m) in length; alternate leaves composed of 3–5 finely toothed lobes; showy, vivid, purple, flesh-colored flowers; smooth, yellow ovate fruit 2–3 in. (5–8 cm) long.	Grows wild in West Indies and southern United States; cultivated in many areas.	Flowering and fruiting tops	Crushed parts for poultice to treat bruises and injuries; other uses include treatment of nervousness, insomnia, fevers, and asthma.
Peppermint *Mentha piperita*	Perennial growing to about 3.5 ft (1 m) high; dark, green, toothed leaves; purplish flowers in spike-like groups.	Originated in temperate regions of the Old World where most is still grown; grows in shady damp areas in many areas of the United States; grown in gardens.	Flowering tops, leaves	Infusions for relief of flatulence, nausea, headache, and heartburn; fresh leaves rubbed into skin to relieve local pain; extracted oil contains medicinal properties.
Plantain *Plantago* sp.	Low perennial with broad leaves; flowers on erect spikes.	Grows wild throughout the United States in poor soils, fields, lawns, and edges of woods.	Leaves, seeds, root	Infusion of leaves for a tonic; seeds for laxative; soaking seeds provides sticky gum for lotions; fresh, crushed leaves to reduce swelling of bruised body parts; fresh, boiled roots applied to sore nipples.
Pleurisy root (Butterfly milkweed) *Asclepias tuberosa*	Leafy perennial growing to 3 ft (1 m) high; alternate leaves which are 2–6 in. (5–15 cm) long and narrow; bright orange flowers in a cluster; root spindle-shaped with knotty crown.	Grows in sandy, dry soils; pastures, roadsides, and gardens; south to Florida and west to Texas and Arizona.	Root	Small doses of dried root as a diaphoretic, diuretic, expectorant, and alternative; ground roots fresh or dried for poultice to treat sores.

TABLE 1.13 *(Continued)*

Plants Used as Herbal Remedies[1]

Common and Scientific Name	Description	Production	Part(s) of Plant Used	Reported Uses
Queens delight *Stillingia sylvatica*	Perennial growing to 3 ft (1 m) high; contains milky juice; leathery, fleshy, stemless leaves; yellow flowers.	Grows wild in dry woods, sandy soils, and old fields; Virginia to Florida, Kansas, and Texas, north to Oklahoma.	Root	Treatment of infectious diseases.
Red clover *Trifolium pratense*	Biennial or perennial legume less than 2 ft (61 cm) high; 3 oval-shaped leaflets form leaf; flowers globe-shaped and rose to purple colored.	Throughout United States; some wild, some cultivated.	Entire plant in full bloom	Infusions to treat whooping cough; component of salves for sores and ulcers; flowers as sedative; to relieve gastric distress and improve the appetite.
Rosemary *Rosmarinus officinalis*	Low-growing perennial evergreen shrub; leaves about 1 in. (3 cm) in height; orange-yellow flowers; white, shiny seeds.	Native to Mediterranean region; now cultivated in most of Europe and the Americas.	Leaves	Used as a tonic, astringent, diaphoretic, stimulant, carminative, and nervine.
Saffron (Safflower) *Carthamus tinctorius*	Annual with alternate spring leaves; grows to 3 ft (1 m) in height; orange-yellow flowers; white, shiny seeds.	Wild in Afghanistan; cultivated in the United States, primarily in California.	Flowers, seeds, entire plant in bloom	Paste of flowers and water applied to boils; flowers soaked in water to make a drink to reduce fever, as a laxative, to induce perspiration, to stimulate menstrual flow, and to dry up skin symptoms of measles.
Sage (Garden sage) *Salvia officinalis*	Fuzzy perennial belonging to the mint family; leaves with toothed edges; terminal spikes bearing blue or white flowers in whorls.	Originated in the Mediterranean area where it grows wild and is cultivated; grown throughout the United States, some wild.	Leaves	Treatment for wounds and cuts, sores, coughs, colds, and sore throat; infusions used as a laxative and to relieve flatulence; major use for treatment of dyspepsia.
Sarsaparilla *Smilax* sp.	Climbing evergreen shrub with prickly stems; leaves round to oblong; small, globular berry for fruit.	Grown in tropical areas of Central and South America and in Japan and China.	Root	Primarily an alterative for colds and fevers; to relieve flatulence; best used as an infusion.

TABLE 1.13 *(Continued)*

Plants Used as Herbal Remedies[1]

Common and Scientific Name	Description	Production	Part(s) of Plant Used	Reported Uses
Sassafras *Sassafras album*	Tree growing to 40 ft (12.2 m) high; leaves may be 3-lobed, 2-lobed, mitten-shaped, or unlobed; yellowish-green flowers in clusters; pea-sized, 1-seeded berries in fall.	Originated in New World; grows in New England, New York, Ohio, Illinois, and Michigan, south to Florida and Texas; grows along roadsides, in woods, along fences, and in fields.	Root bark	Sassafras was formerly used for medical purposes, but the use of the roots was banned by the FDA because of their carcinogenic qualities.
Saw palmetto *Serenoa serrulata*	Low-growing fan palm; whitish bloom covers sawtoothed, green leaves; flowers in branching clusters; fruit varies in size and shape.	Grows in warm, swampy, low areas near the coast.	Fruit (berries)	To improve digestion; to treat respiratory infections; as a tonic and as a sedative.
Senna (Wild senna) *Cassia marilandica*	Perennial growing to 6 ft (1.8 m) in height; alternate leaves with leaflets in pairs of 5–10; bright yellow flowers.	Grows along roadsides and in thickets from Pennsylvania to Kansas and Iowa, south to Texas and Florida.	Leaves	Infusions primarily employed as a laxative.
Skullcap *Scutellaria lateriflora*	Perennial growing 1–2 ft (30–61 cm) high; toothed, lance-shaped leaves; blue or whitish flowers.	Native to most sections of the United States; prefers moist woods, damp areas, meadows, and swampy areas.	Entire plant in bloom	Powdered plant primarily a nervine.
Spearmint *Mentha spicata*	Perennial resembling other mints; grows to 3 ft (1 m) in height; pink or white flowers borne in long spikes.	Throughout the United States in damp places; cultivated in Michigan, Indiana, and California.	Above ground parts	Primarily a carminative; administered as an infusion through extracted oils.
Tansy *Tanacetum vulgare*	Perennial growing to 3 ft (1 m) in height; pungent fernlike foliage with tops of composite heads of buttonlike flowers.	Grown or escaped into the wild in much of the United States.	Leaves and flowering tops	Infusions used as stomachic, emmenagogue, or to expel intestinal worms; extracted oil induced abortion often with fat results; poultice for sprains and bruises.

TABLE 1.13 *(Continued)*

Plants Used as Herbal Remedies[1]

Common and Scientific Name	Description	Production	Part(s) of Plant Used	Reported Uses
Valerian *Valeriana officinalis*	Coarse perennial growing to 5 ft (1.5 m) high; fragrant, pinkish-white flowers opposite pinnate leaves.	Native to Europe and Northern Asia; cultivated in the United States.	Root	As a calmative and as a carminative.
Witch hazel *Hamamelis virginiana*	Crooked tree or shrub 8–15 ft (2.4–4.6 m) in height; roundish to oval leaves; yellow, threadlike flowers; fruits in clusters along the stem eject shiny, black seeds.	Found in damp woods of North America from Nova Scotia to Florida and west to Minnesota and Texas.	Leaves, bark, twigs	Twigs, leaves, and bark basis for witch hazel extract which is included in many lotions for bruises, sprains, and shaving; bark sometimes applied to tumors and skin inflammations; some preparations for treating hemorrhoids.
Yerba santa *Eriodictyon californicum*	Evergreen shrub with lance-shaped leaves.	Part of flora of the west coast of the United States.	Leaves	As an expectorant; recommended for asthma and hay fever.

Adapted from Ensminger et al., *Foods and Nutrition Encyclopedia,* 2nd ed., CRC Press, Boca Raton, 1994, pp. 1430–1441.

[1] Herbal remedies can vary widely in potency. Some may be toxic. These remedies should not be used without the advice of a physician.

TABLE 1.14

Vitamin Terminology

Vitamins were named according to a) their function; b) their location; c) the order in which they were discovered; or d) combinations of a, b, or c. Some of these names became obsolete as their proposed functions or their isolated structures were found to duplicate already named and described vitamins. Obsolescence also occurred as research showed that certain of these compounds were not needed dietary factors but were synthesized by the body in needed amounts.

Name	Comment
Vitamin A	A number of compounds have vitamin A activity but differ in biopotency. All trans retinol is the standard, and the activity of other compounds can be stated as retinol equivalents. This includes the aldehyde (retinal), acid (retinoic acid), and provitamin (carotene) forms.
Vitamin B	Although orginally thought to be a single compound, researchers found that eight major compounds comprised this "vitamin."
Vitamin B complex	A group of vitamins; includes thiamin, riboflavin, niacin, pyridoxine (3 forms), pantothenic acid, biotin, cyanocobalamin (B_{12}), folacin.
Vitamin B_1	Aneurin; antineuritic factor. Obsolete synonym for thiamin.
Vitamin B_2	Lactoflavin, Ovoflavin. Obsolete synonyms for riboflavin.
Vitamin B_3	Antipellagra factor. Obsolete synonym for niacin.
Vitamin B_4	Not proven to have vitamin activity; thought to be a mixture of arginine, glycine, riboflavin, and pyridoxine.
Vitamin B_5	Probably identical to niacin.
Vitamin B_6	Synonym for pyridoxine, pyridoxal, pyridoxamine.
Vitamin B_7	Not proven to have vitamin activity;[1] sometimes referred to as Vitamin I, a factor which improves food digestibility in pigeons.

TABLE 1.14 *(Continued)*
Vitamin Terminology

Name	Comment
Vitamin B_8	Not proven to have vitamin activity;[1] found to be adenylic acid.
Vitamin B_{10}, B_{11}	An unrefined mixture of folacin and cyanocobalamin; obsolete term.
Vitamin B_{12}	Cyanocobalamin; B_{12a} is aquacobalamin; B_{12b} is hydroxocobalamin; B_{12c} is nitritocobalamin.
Vitamin B_{13}	Orotic acid; a metabolite of pyrimidine metabolism; not considered a vitamin.[1]
Vitamin B_{15}	Synonym for "pangamic acid" a compound of no known biologic value; not a vitamin.[1]
Vitamin B_{17}	Synonym for laetrile; a cyanogenic glycoside of no known biologic value; not a vitamin.[1]
Vitamin B_c	Obsolete term for pteroylglutamic acid; a component of folacin.
Vitamin B_p	A compound which prevents perosis in chicks, can be replaced by choline and manganese.
Vitamin B_f	Shown to be carnitine.
Vitamin B_x	Probably a mixture of pantothenic acid and p-aminobenzoic acid.
Vitamin C	Synonym for ascorbic acid.
Vitamin C_2	Unrecognized, unconfirmed compound purported to have antipneumonia activity; also called vitamin J.
Vitamin D	Antirachitic factor; a group of sterols (the calciferols) that serve to enhance bone calcification.
Vitamin D_2	Ergocalciferol; one of the D vitamins from plant sources.
Vitamin D_3	Cholecalciferol; one of the D vitamins from animal sources.
Vitamin E	A group of tocopherols that have an important function in the antioxidant system; suppresses free radical formation.
Vitamin F	Obsolete term for the essential fatty acids (linoleic and linolenic acids).
Vitamin G	Obsolete term for riboflavin before riboflavin and niacin were recognized as separate vitamins.
Vitamin H	Obsolete term for biotin.
Vitamin I	Obsolete term for a mixture of B vitamins.
Vitamin K	A group of fat soluble compounds that function in the post translational carboxylation of the glutamic acid residues of prothrombin.
Vitamin K_1	Phylloquinone; vitamin K of plant origin.
Vitamin K_2	Menaquinone; vitamin K of animal origin.
Vitamin K_3	Menadione; synthetic vitamin K.
Vitamin L_1	Unrecognized factor which may be related to anthranitic acid and which has been proposed to be important for lactation; not proven to have vitamin activity.[1]
Vitamin L_2	See above.
Vitamin M	Obsolete term for pteroylglutamic acid (folacin).
Vitamin N	Obsolete term used to designate an anticancer compound mixture; undefined and unrecognized.
Vitamin P	Not a vitamin;[1] but is a metabolite of citrin.
Vitamin Q	Not a vitamin;[1] but is probably a synonym for coenzyme Q.
Vitamin R	Obsolete term for folacin.
Vitamin S	Not a vitamin;[1] but does act to enhance chick growth; related to the peptide "streptogenin" and also to biotin.
Vitamin T	Not a vitamin;[1] reported to improve protein utilization in rats; an extract from termites.
Vitamin U	Not a vitamin;[1] an extract from cabbage that has been reported to suppress gastric acid production; may be important to folacin activity.
Vitamin V	Not a vitamin.[1]
Bioflavinoids	Not a vitamin.[1]
Carnitine	Not a vitamin;[1] except in preterm infants and in severely traumatized persons.
Choline	Can be synthesized by the body but some conditions interfere with adequate synthesis.
Citrovorum factor	Synonym for folacin; a B vitamin.
Extrinsic factor	Obsolete term for vitamin B_{12}, cyanocobalamin.
Factors U, R, X	Obsolete terms for folacin.
Filtrate factor	Obsolete term for riboflavin.
Flavin	A general term for the riboflavin containing coenzymes, FMN, and FAD.
Hepatoflavin	Obsolete term for riboflavin.
Intrinsic factor	Not a vitamin;[1] an endogenous factor needed for vitamin B_{12}, cyanocobalamin, absorption.

TABLE 1.14 *(Continued)*

Vitamin Terminology

Name	Comment
LLD factor	Obsolete term for vitamin B_{12}, cyanocobalamin.
Lipoic acid	Not a vitamin,[1] but does serve as a cofactor in oxidative decarboxylation.
Myoinositol	Sometimes a vitamin when endogenous synthesis is inadequate.
Norite eluate	Not a vitamin.[1]
P-P factor	Obsolete term for niacin.
Pyrroloquinoline quinone	Not a vitamin;[1] component of metallo-oxido-reductases.
Rhizopterin	Obsolete term for folacin.
SLR factor	Obsolete term for folacin.
Streptogenin	Not a vitamin.[1]
Wills factor	Obsolete term for folacin.
Zoopherin	Obsolete term for vitamin B_{12}, cyanocobalamin.

[1] A vitamin is an organic compound required in small amounts for the maintenance of normal biochemical and physiological function of the body. These compounds must be present in food and if absent, well defined symptoms of deficiency will develop. An essential nutrient such as a vitamin cannot be synthesized in amounts sufficient to meet needs.

TABLE 1.15

Nomenclature of Compounds with Vitamin A Activity

Recommended Name	Synonyms
Retinol	Vitamin A alcohol
Retinal	Vitamin A aldehyde, retinene, retinaldehyde
Retinoic acid	Vitamin A acid
3-dehydroretinol	Vitamin A_2 (alcohol)
3-Dehydroretinal	Vitamin A_2 aldehyde, retinene$_2$
3-Dehydroretinoic acid	Vitamin A_2 acid
Anhydroretinol	Anhydrovitamin A
Retro retinol	Rehydrovitamin A
5,6-Epoxyretinol	5,6-Epoxyvitamin A alcohol
Retinyl palmitate	Vitamin A palmitate
Retinyl acetate	Vitamin A acetate
Retinyl β-glucuronide	Vitamin A acid β-glucuronide
11-*cis*-retinaldehyde	11-*cis* or neo β vitamin A aldehyde
4-Ketoretinol	4-Keto vitamin A alcohol
Retinyl phosphate	Vitamin A phosphate
β-Carotene	Provitamin A
α-Carotene	Provitamin A
γ-Carotene	Provitamin A

TABLE 1.16

Chemical and Physical Properties of Vitamins

Generic Name	Compound Name	Structure	Molecular wt.	Absorption (nm)	Solubility	Melting pt.	Biopotency	Stability
Vitamin A	all *trans* 3 dehydroretinol	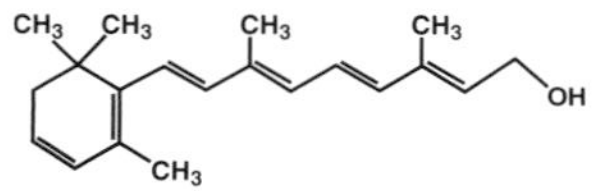	286.4	325	Ether, ethanol, chloroform benzene acetone hexane	62–64	30	unstable to UV light, oxygen, acids, metal
	all *trans* retinol	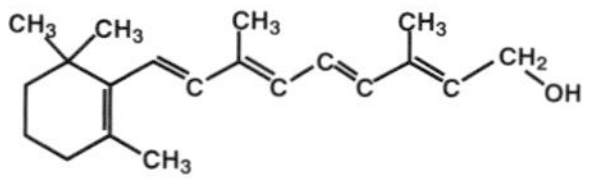	286.4	325		63–64	100	
	13-*cis* retinol	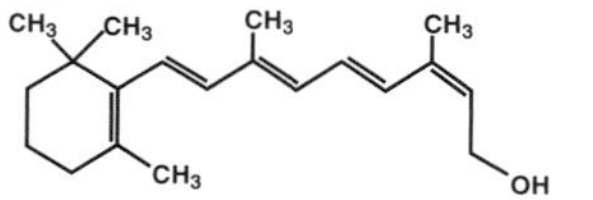	286.4				23–75	
	all *trans* retinal	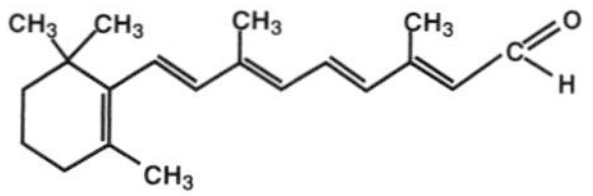	284.4				100	
	11-*cis* retinal	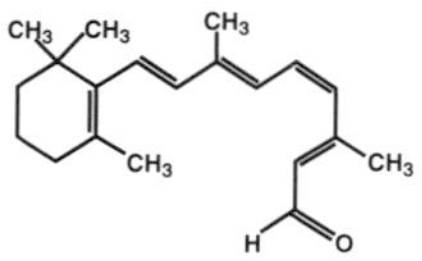	284.4	373		61–64		
	13-*cis*-retinoic acid	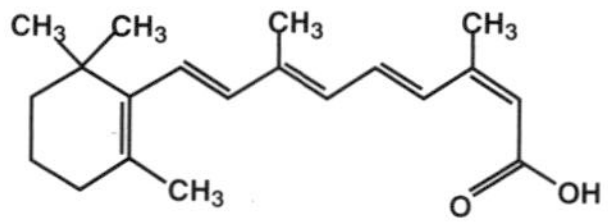	300.4	351			180–182	
	all *trans* retinoic acid	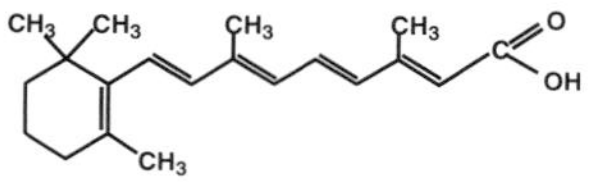	300.4	351				
	all *trans* retinyl phosphate	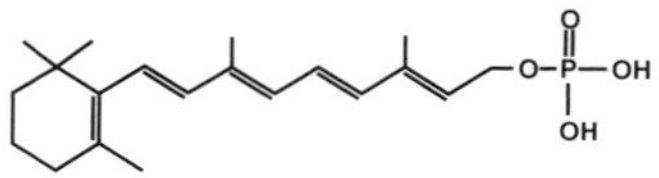	364			10–100		

Provitamin A	α carotene	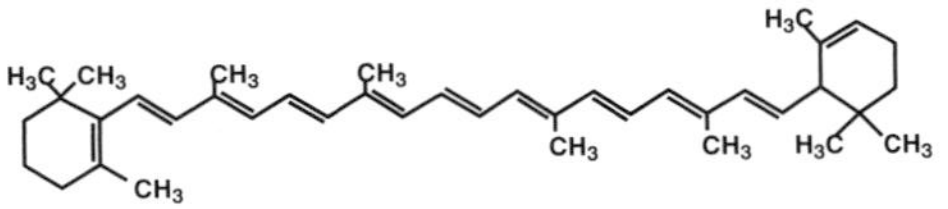 536.9		Ether, benzene	187.5	26	
	β carotene	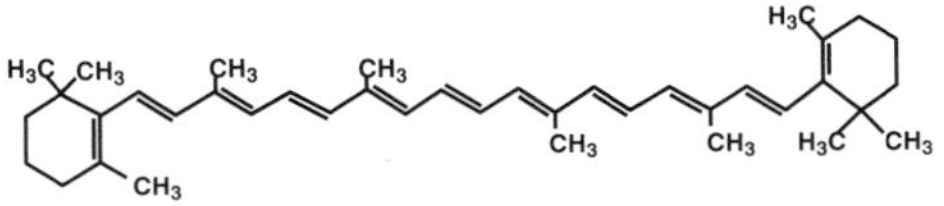 536.9			184	50	
	γ carotene	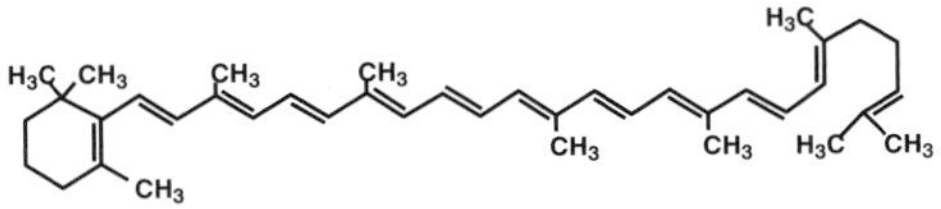 536.9		Ethanol Acetone	178	21	
	cryptoxanthin (β-carotene-3-ol)	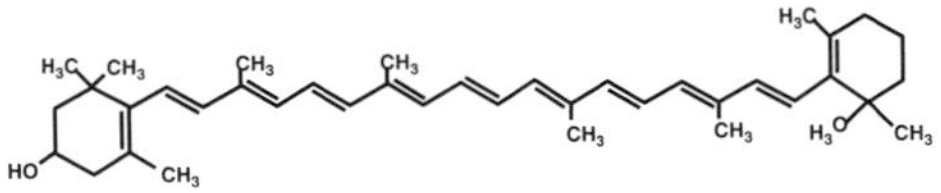 552.9			169	28	
Vitamin D_2	Ergocalciferol	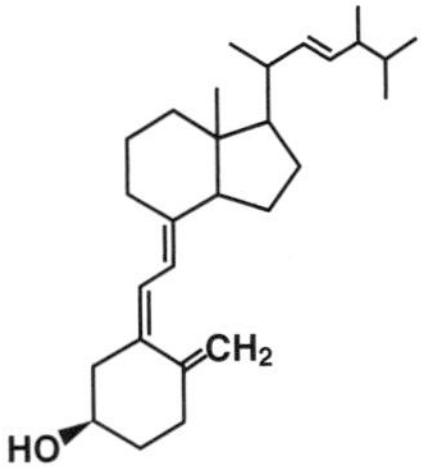 396.67	264	Alcohol Ether Acetone	115–118	100	Unstable to UV light, oxygen, iodine, heat, mild acid
	25-OH-Vitamin D_3	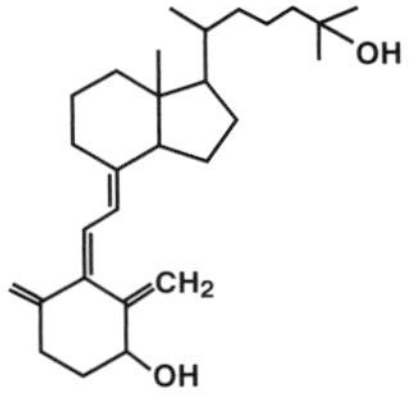 411.67	265		84–85	200–500	

TABLE 1.16 *(Continued)*
Chemical and Physical Properties of Vitamins

Generic Name	Compound Name	Structure	Molecular wt.	Absorption (nm)	Solubility	Melting pt.	Biopotency	Stability
Vitamin D_3	Cholecalciferol	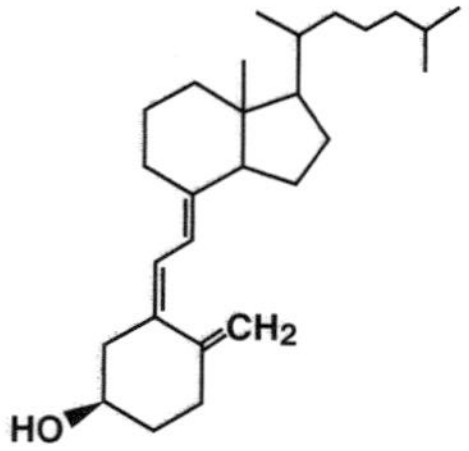	396.67	265	|	84–85	100	
	1,25-$(OH)_2$ vitamin D_3	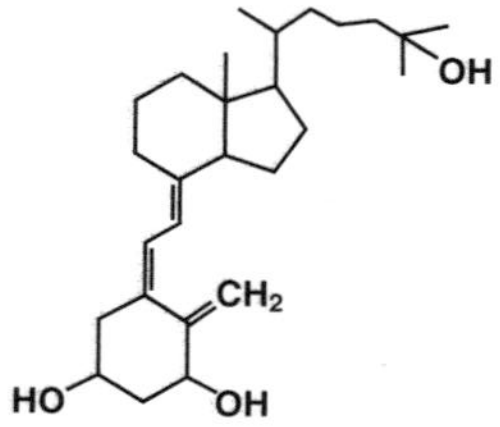	426.67	265	↓	84–85	500–1000	
Vitamin E	Tocopherols	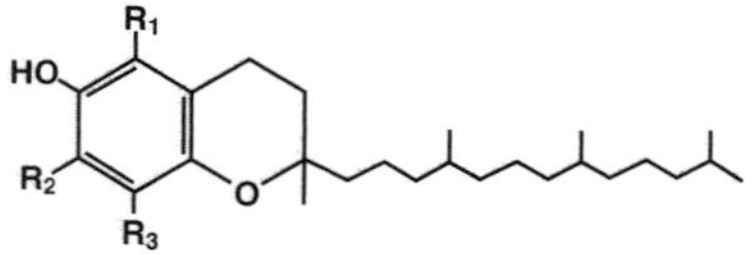						Unstable to oxygen, light, metal, salts

			R_1	R_2	R_3						
	Tocotrienols	HO, R_1, R_2, R_3, O									
	tocol or tocotrierol	α	CH_3	CH_3	CH_3	430.7	294	Alcohol,	2.5–3.5	1.49	Unstable to O_2,
	tocol or tocotrierol	β	CH_3	H	CH_3	416.7		ether,		0.12	light, metals,
	tocol or tocotrierol	γ	H	CH_3	CH_3	416.7	298	acetone		0.05	salts
	tocol or tocotrierol	δ	H	H	CH_3	416.7		↓		0.32	
										0.05	
Vitamin K	Phylloquinone	CH_3, O, 3, CH_3, CH_3, H, n(1-6) repeats			n=1	325	240–270	Alcohol,	0°C	5	Unstable to light
					n=2	396		ether,		10	and alkali, stable
					n=3	450.7		acetone,	−20	30	to heat
					n=4			benzene		100	
					n=5					80	
					n=6					50	
	Menaquinone	3-(preny1)$_n$ preny1$_{n-1}$; CH_3, O, 2, CH_3, CH_3, H, n(2-7) repeats			n=2					15	
					n=3					40	
					n=4	448.7	243–328	↓	54	100	
					n=5					120	
					n=6					100	
					n=7					70	

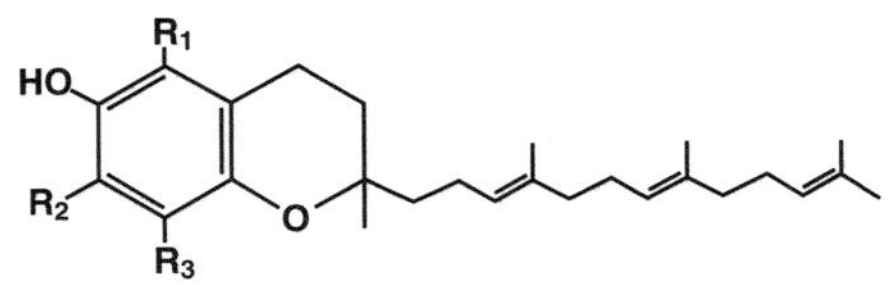

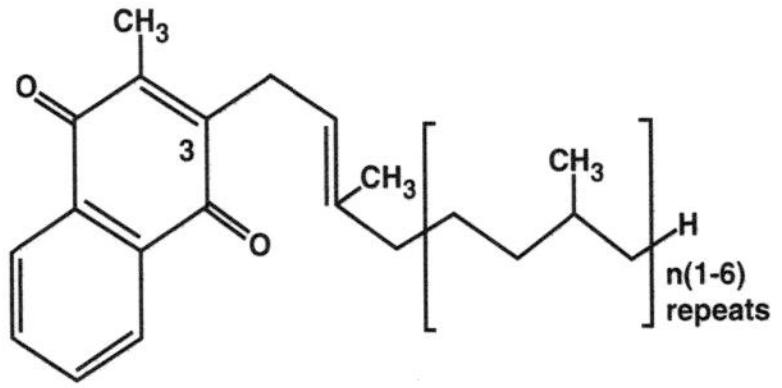

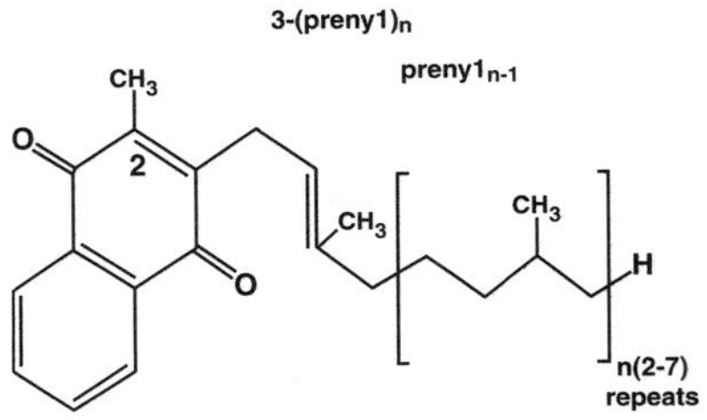

TABLE 1.16 *(Continued)*

Chemical and Physical Properties of Vitamins

Generic Name	Compound Name	Structure	Molecular wt.	Absorption (nm)	Solubility	Melting pt.	Biopotency	Stability
	Menadione	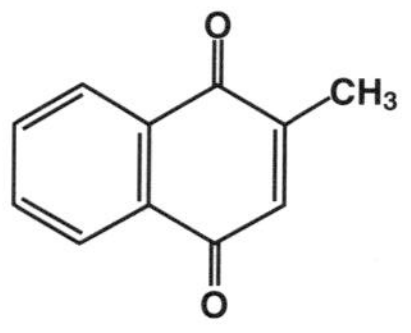	172.2		↓		40–150	
Vitamin C	Ascorbic acid	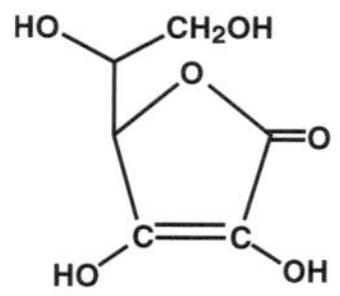	176.14	245	Water	190–192	100	Unstable to heat and alkali
	Dehydroascorbic acid	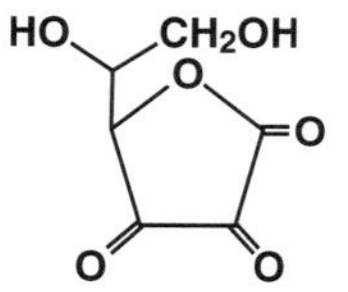	174.14	245	Water	190–192	80	↓
Vitamin B_1	Thiamin	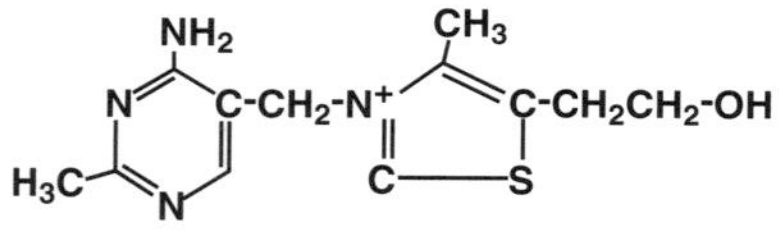	337.27	—	Water	177	100	

Vitamin B_2	Riboflavin	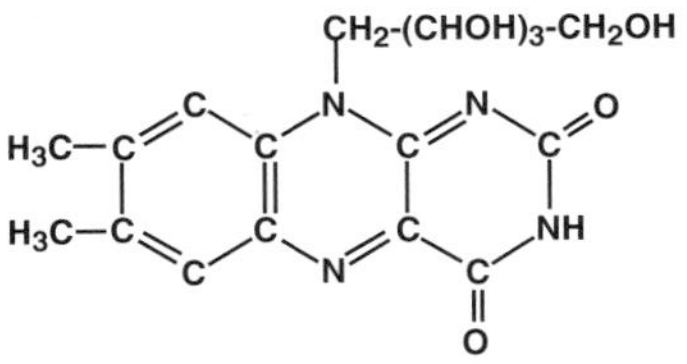	376.4	220, 225, 266, 371, 444, 475	Water	278	100	Unstable to UV light and heat
Vitamin B_3	Niacin Nicotinic acid	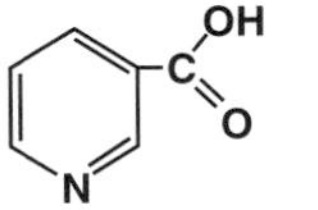	123.1	263	Water	237	100	
	Nicotinamide	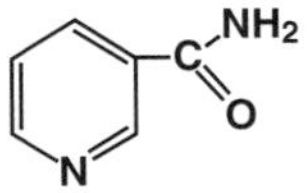	122.1	263	Water	128–131	100	
Vitamin B_6	Pyridoxal	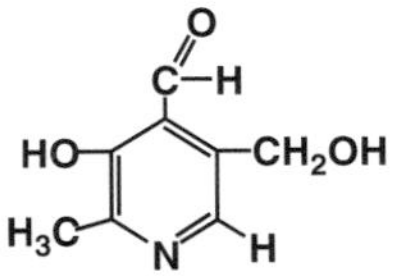	167.2	293	Water	165	100	
	Pyridoxamine	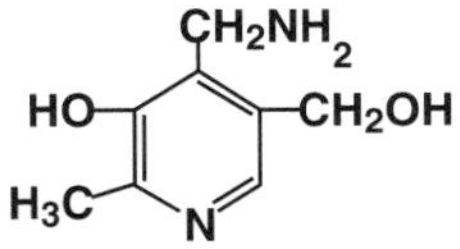	205.6	255, 326	Water	160	100	
	Pyridoxine	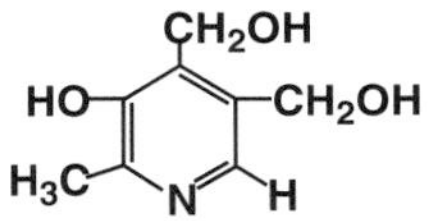	169.18	—	Water	160	100	

TABLE 1.16 *(Continued)*

Chemical and Physical Properties of Vitamins

Generic Name	Compound Name	Structure	Molecular wt.	Absorption (nm)	Solubility	Melting pt.	Biopotency	Stability
	Biotin	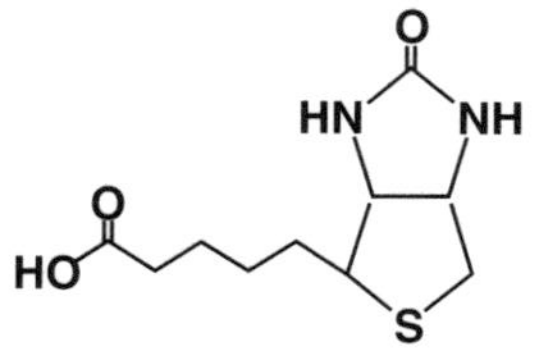	244.3	—	Water	167	100	Unstable to acid and alkaline conditions
	Pantothenic acid	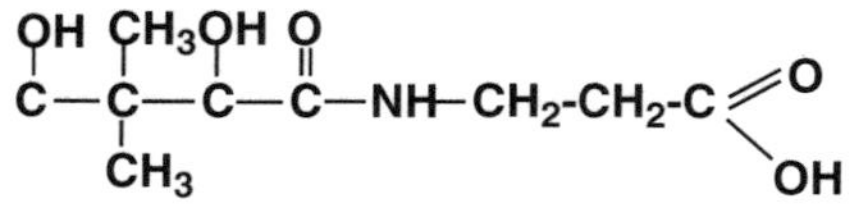	219.2	—	Water	—	100	Unstable to heat
		as calcium salt	476.5	—	Water	195	100	
	Folate Folacin (pteroylmonoglutamic acid)	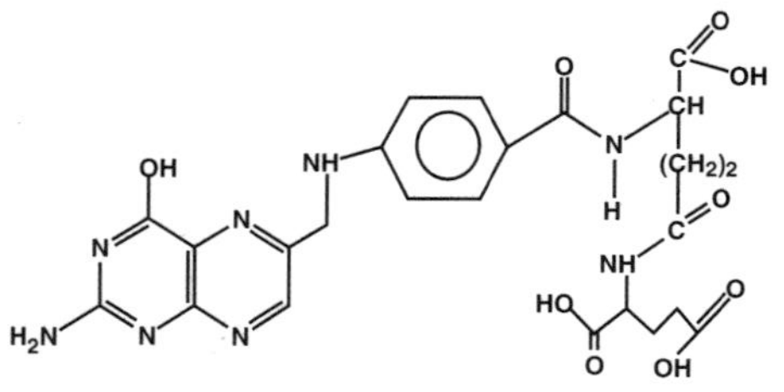	441	256, 283, 368	Water	250	100	Unstable to light, acid, alkaline, reducing agents, heat

Vitamin B_{12}	Cyanocobalamin	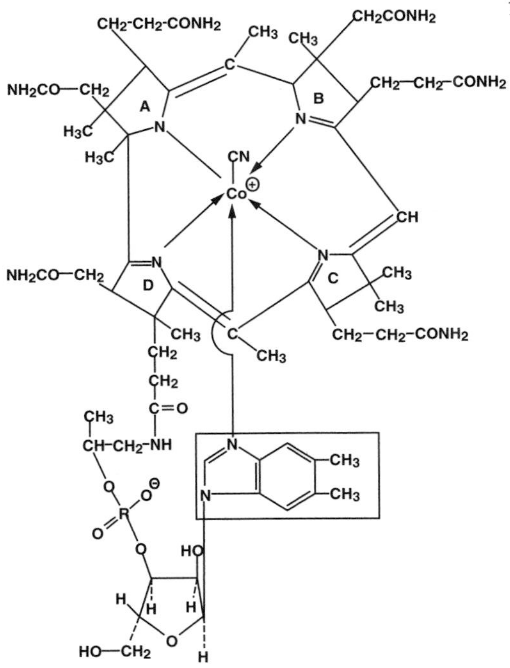	1355.4	278, 361, 550	Water	>300	100	Unstable to light

TABLE 1.17

Summary of Vitamin Deficiency Signs and Need[1]

Functions	Deficiency and Toxicity Symptoms	Sources	Comments
Fat-Soluble Vitamins			
Vitamin A Helps maintain normal vision in dim light — prevents night blindness and xerophthalmia. Essential for body growth. Necessary for normal bone growth and normal tooth development. Acts as a coenzyme in glycoprotein synthesis; functions like steroid hormones, with a role in the cell nuclei, leading to tissue differentiation. Necessary for (1) thyroxine formation and prevention of goiter; (2) protein synthesis; and (3) synthesis of corticosterone from cholesterol, and the normal synthesis of glycogen.	**Deficiency symptoms**: Night blindness (nyctalopia) xerosis, and xerophthalmia. Stunted bone growth, abnormal bone shape, and paralysis. Unsound teeth, characterized by abnormal enamel, pits, and decay. Rough, dry, scaly skin — a condition known as follicular hyperkeratosis (it looks like "gooseflesh"); increased sinus, sore throat, and abscesses in ears, mouth, or salivary glands; increased diarrhea and kidney and bladder stones. Reproductive disorders, including poor conception, abnormal embryonic growth, placental injury, and death of the fetus. **Toxicity**: Characterized by loss of appetite, headache, blurred vision, excessive irritability, loss of hair, dryness and flaking of skin (with itching), swelling over the long bones, drowsiness, diarrhea, nausea, and enlargement of the liver and spleen.	Liver, carrots, dark-green leafy vegetables. Yellow vegetables: pumpkins, sweet potatoes, squash (winter). Yellow fruits: apricots, peaches. Some seafoods (crab, halibut, oysters, salmon, swordfish); milk and milk products, eggs. **Supplemental sources**: Synthetic vitamin A, cod and other fish liver oils.	The forms of vitamin A are alcohol (retinol), ester (retinyl palmitate), aldehyde (retinal or retinene), and acid (retinoic acid). Retinol, retinyl palmitate, and retinal are readily converted from one form to other forms. Retinoic acid fulfills some of the functions of vitamin A, but it does not function in the visual cycle. β carotene found in vegetables serves as a vitamin A precursor.

Vitamin D Increases calcium absorption from the small intestine. Promotes growth and mineralization of bones. Promotes sound teeth. Increases absorption of phosphorus through the intestinal wall; increases resorption of phosphates from the kidney tubules. Maintains normal level of citrate in the blood. Protects against the loss of amino acids through the kidneys.	**Deficiency symptoms**: Rickets in infants and children, characterized by enlarged joints, bowed legs, knocked knees, outward projection of the sternum (pigeon breast), a row of beadlike projections on each side of the chest at the juncture of the rib bones and joining (costal) cartilage (called rachitic rosary), bulging forehead, pot belly; delayed eruption of temporary teeth and unsound permanent teeth. Osteomalacia in adults, in which the bones soften, become distorted, and fracture easily. Tetany, characterized by muscle twitching, convulsions, and low serum calcium. **Toxicity**: Excessive vitamin D may cause hypercalcemia (increased intestinal absorption, leading to elevated blood calcium levels), characterized by loss of appetite, excessive thirst, nausea, vomiting, irritability, weakness, constipation alternating with bouts of diarrhea, retarded growth in infants and children, and weight loss in adults.	**D-fortified foods**: Milk (400 IU/qt) and infant formulas. Other foods to which vitamin D is often added include: breakfast and infant cereals, breads, margarines, milk flavorings, fruit and chocolate beverages, and cocoa. **Supplemental sources**: Fish liver oils (from cod, halibut, or swordfish); irradiated ergosterol or 7-dehydro-cholesterol such as viosterol. Exposure to sunlight or sunlamp converts the vitamin D precursor to active vitamin D.	Vitamin D includes both D_2 (ergocalciferol, calciferol, or viosterol) and D_3 (cholecalciferol). Vitamin D is unique among vitamins because it can be formed in the body and in certain foods by exposure to ultraviolet rays, and the active compound of vitamin D (1, 25-$(OH)_2$-D_3) functions as a hormone.

TABLE 1.17 *(Continued)*

Summary of Vitamin Deficiency Signs and Need[1]

Functions	Deficiency and Toxicity Symptoms	Sources	Comments
Vitamin E (Tocopherols) An antioxidant which protects body cells from free radicals formed from the unsaturated fatty acids. Maintains the integrity of red blood cells by its action as a suppressor of free radicals. An agent essential to cellular respiration, primarily in heart and skeletal muscle tissues.	**Deficiency symptoms**: Newborn infants (especially the premature). Anemia caused by shortened life span of red blood cells, edema, skin lesions, and blood abnormalities. Patients unable to absorb fat have low blood and tissue tocopherol levels, decreased red blood cell life span, and increased urinary excretion of creatine. **Toxicity**: Relatively nontoxic. Some persons consuming daily doses of more than 300 IU of vitamin E have complained of nausea and intestinal distress. Excess intake of vitamin E appears to be excreted in the feces.	Vegetable oils (except coconut oil), alfalfa seeds, margarine, nuts (almonds, Brazil nuts, filberts, peanuts, pecans), sunflower seed kernels. **Good sources**: Asparagus, avocados, beef and organ meats, blackberries, butter, eggs, green leafy vegetables, oatmeal, potato chips, rye, seafoods (lobster, salmon, shrimp, tuna), tomatoes. **Supplemental sources**: Synthetic di-alpha-tocopherol acetate, wheat germ, wheat germ oil.	There are 8 tocopherols and tocotrienols, of which α-tocopherol has the greatest vitamin E activity.
Vitamin K Essential for the synthesis in the liver of four bloodclotting proteins: 1. Factor II, prothrombin 2. Factor VII, proconvertin 3. Factor IX, Christmas factor 4. Factor X, Stuart-Power. Its action is on the post translational carboxylation of glutamic acid residues.	**Deficiency symptoms**: 1. Delayed blood clotting 2. Hemorrhagic disease of newborn Vitamin K deficiency symptoms are likely in: 1. Newborn infants 2. Infants born to mothers receiving anticoagulants 3. Obstructive jaundice (lack of bile) 4. Fat absorption defects (celiac disease, sprue) 5. Anticoagulant therapy or toxicity **Toxicity**: The natural forms of vitamin K_1 and K_2 have not produced toxicity even when given in large amounts. However, synthetic menadione and its various derivatives have produced toxic symptoms in rats and jaundice in human infants when given in amounts of more than 5 mg daily.	Vitamin K is fairly widely distributed in foods and is available synthetically.	Two forms: K_1 (phylloquinone, or phytylmenaquinone), and K_2 (menaquinones), multiprenyl-menaquinones. Vitamin K is synthesized by bacteria in the intestinal tracts of human beings and other species. There are several synthetic compounds, the best known of which is menadione, formerly known as K_3.

Water-Soluble Vitamins

Biotin Functions as a coenzyme mainly in decarboxylation-carboxylation and in deamination reactions.	**Deficiency symptoms**: The deficiency symptoms in man include a dry, scaly dermatitis, loss of appetite, nausea, vomiting, muscle pains, glossitis (inflammation of the tongue), pallor of skin, mental depression, decrease in hemoglobin and red blood cells, high cholesterol level, and a low excretion of biotin, all of which respond to biotin administration. **Toxicity**: There are no known toxic effects.	**Rich sources**: Cheese (processed), kidney, liver, soybean flour. **Good sources**: Cauliflower, chocolate, eggs, mushrooms, nuts, peanut butter, sardine and salmon, wheat bran. Supplemental sources — Synthetic biotin, yeast (brewers' torula), alfalfa leaf meal (dehydrated). Considerable biotin is synthesized by the microorganisms in the intestinal tract.	Avidin, found in raw egg white, binds biotin, making it unavailable. Avidin is destroyed by cooking.
Choline 1. As part of the neurotransmitter acetyl choline, transmits nerve impulses. 2. Is essential for one of the membrane phospholipids (phosphatidylcholine) 3. Serves as a methyl donor.	**Deficiency symptoms**: Poor growth and fatty livers are the deficiency symptoms in most species except chickens and turkeys. Chickens and turkeys develop slipped tendons (perosis). In young rats, choline deficiency produces hemorrhagic lesions in the kidneys and other organs. **Toxicity**: No toxic effects have been observed.	**Rich sources**: Egg yolk, eggs, liver (beef, pork, lamb). **Good sources**: Soybeans, potatoes (dehydrated), cabbage, wheat bran, navy beans, alfalfa leaf meal, dried buttermilk and dried skimmed milk, rice polish, rice bran, whole grains (barley, corn, oats, rice, sorghum, wheat), hominy, turnips, wheat flour, blackstrap molasses. **Supplemental sources**: Yeast (brewers', torula), wheat germ, soybean lecithin, egg yolk lecithin, and synthetic choline and choline derivatives.	The classification of choline as a vitamin is debated because it does not meet all the criteria for vitamins, especially those of the B vitamins. The body manufactures choline from methionine, with the aid of folacin and vitamin B_{12}.

TABLE 1.17 *(Continued)*

Summary of Vitamin Deficiency Signs and Need[1]

Functions	Deficiency and Toxicity Symptoms	Sources	Comments
Folacin/Folate (Folic Acid) Folacin coenzymes are responsible for the following important functions: 1. The formation of purines and pyrimidines which, in turn, are needed for the synthesis of the nucleic acids DNA and RNA. 2. The formation of heme, the iron-containing protein in hemoglobin. 3. The interconversion of the three-carbon amino acid serine from the two-carbon amino acid glycine. 4. The formation of the amino acids tyrosine from phenylalanine and glutamic acid from histidine. 5. The formation of the amino acid methionine from homocysteine. 6. The synthesis of choline from ethanolamine. 7. The conversion of nicotinamide to N-methylnicotinamide, one of the metabolites of niacin that is excreted in the urine.	**Deficiency symptoms**: Megaloblastic anemia (of infancy), also called macrocyticanemia (of pregnancy), in which the red blood cells are larger and fewer than normal, and also immature. The anemia is due to inadequate formation of nucl-proteins, causing failure of the megaloblasts (young red blood cells) in the one marrow to mature. The hemoglobin level is low because of the reduced number of red blood cells and the white blood cell, blood platelet, and serum folate levels are low. Other symptoms include a sore, red, smooth red tongue (glossitis), disturbances of the digestive tract (diarrhea), and poor growth. **Toxicity**: Normally, no toxicity.	**Rich sources**: Liver and kidney. **Good sources**: Avocados, beans, beets, celery, chickpeas, eggs, fish, green leafy vegetables (such as asparagus, broccoli, Brussels sprouts, cabbage, cauliflower, endive, lettuce, parsley, spinach, turnip greens), nuts, oranges, orange juice, soybeans, and whole wheat products. **Supplemental sources**: Yeast, wheat germ, and commercially synthesized folic acid (pteroyl-glutamic acid, or PGA).	There is no single vitamin compound with the name folacin; rather, the term folacin is used to designate folic acid and a group of closely related substances which are essential for all vertebrates, including man. Ascorbic acid, vitamin B_{12}, and vitamin B_6 are essential for the activity of the folacin coenzymes. Folacin deficiencies are thought to be a health problem in the U.S. and throughout the world. Infants, adolescents, and pregnant women are particularly vulnerable. The folacin requirement is increased by tropical sprue, certain genetic disturbances, cancer, parasitic infection, alcoholism, and oral contraceptives. Raw vegetables stored at room temperature for 2–3 days lose as much as 50–70% of their folate content. Between 50 and 95% of food folate is destroyed in cooking. Intestinal synthesis provides some folacin.

Niacin
(Nicotinic acid; nicotinamide) is a constituent of two important coenzymes in the body; nicotinamide adenine and dinucleotide (NAD) and nicotinamide adenine dinucleotide phosphate (NADP). These coenzymes function as reducing equivalent (H^+) acceptors or donors.

Deficiency symptoms: A deficiency of niacin results in pellagra, the symptoms of which are: dermatitis, particularly of areas of skin which are exposed to light or injury; inflammation of mucous membranes, including the entire gastrointestinal tract, which results in a red, swollen, sore tongue and mouth, diarrhea, and rectal irritation; and psychic changes, such as irritability, anxiety, depression, and in advanced cases, delirium, hallucinations, confusion, disorientation, and stupor.
Toxicity: Only large doses of niacin, sometimes given to individuals with mental illness, are known to be toxic. However, ingestion of large amounts may result in vascular dilation, or "flushing" of the skin, itching, liver damage, elevated blood glucose, elevated blood enzymes, and/or peptic ulcer.

Generally speaking, niacin is found in animal tissues as nicotinamide and in plant tissues as nicotinic acid. Both forms are of equal niacin activity.
Rich sources: Liver, kidney, lean meats, poultry, fish, rabbit, corn flakes (enriched), nuts, peanut butter, milk, cheese, and eggs, although low in niacin content, are good antipellagra foods, because their niacin is in available form.
Enriched cereal flours and products are good sources of niacin.
Supplemental sources: Both synthetic nicotinamide and nicotinic acid are commercially available. For pharmaceutical use, nicotinamide is usually used; for food nutrification, nicotinic acid is usually used. Also, yeast is a rich natural source of niacin.

An average mixed diet in the U.S. provides about 1% protein as tryptophan. Thus, a diet supplying 60 g of protein contains about 600 mg of tryptophan, which will yield about 10 mg of niacin (on the average, 1 mg of niacin is derived from each 60 mg of dietary tryptophan).
Niacin is the most stable of the B-complex vitamins. Cooking losses of a mixed diet usually do not amount to more than 15–25%.

Pantothenic acid
(Vitamin B_3) Pantothenic acid functions as part of two enzymes — coenzyme A (CoA) and acyl carrier protein (ACP).
CoA functions in the following important reactions:
1. The formation of acetyl-choline, a substance of importance in transmitting nerve impulses.
2. The synthesis of porphyrin, a precursor of heme, of importance in hemoglobin synthesis.
3. The synthesis of cholesterol and other sterols.
4. The steroid hormones formed by the adrenal and sex glands.
5. The maintenance of normal blood sugar, and the formation of antibodies.
6. The excretion of sulfonamide drugs.

ACP, along with CoA, required by the cells in the synthesis of fatty acids.

Deficiency symptoms:
The symptoms: irritableness and restlessness; loss of appetite, indigestion, abdominal pains, nausea; headache; sullenness, mental depression; fatigue, weakness; numbness and tingling of hands and feet, muscle cramps in the arms and legs; burning sensation in the feet; insomnia; respiratory infections; rapid pulse; and a staggering gait. Also, in these subjects there was increased reaction to stress; increased sensitivity to insulin, resulting in low blood sugar levels; increased sedimentation rate for erythrocytes; decreased gastric secretions; and marked decrease in antibody production.
Toxicity: Pantothenic acid is relatively nontoxic. However, doses of 10 to 20 g per day may result in occasional diarrhea and water retention.

Organ meat (liver, kidney, and heart), cottonseed flour, wheat bran, rice bran, rice polish, nuts, mushrooms, soybean flour, salmon, bleu cheese, eggs, buckwheat flour, brown rice, lobster, sunflower seeds.
Supplemental sources: Synthetic calcium pantothenate is widely used as a vitamin supplementation. Yeast is a rich natural supplement.
Intestinal bacteria synthesize pantothenic acid, but the amount and availability is unknown.

Coenzyme A, of which pantothenic acid is a part, is one of the most important substances in body metabolism. It functions in acetyl group transfer and thus is important to fatty acid synthesis and degradation.

TABLE 1.17 *(Continued)*

Summary of Vitamin Deficiency Signs and Need[1]

Functions	Deficiency and Toxicity Symptoms	Sources	Comments
Riboflavin (Vitamin B_2) Riboflavin fu as an integral part of the coenzymes FAD and FMN. These coenzymes accept or donate reducing equivalents.	**Deficiency symptoms**: Unlike all the other vitamins, riboflavin deficiency is not the cause of any severe or major disease of man. Rather, riboflavin often contributes to other disorders and disabilities such as beriberi, pellagra, scurvy, keratomalacia, and nutritional megaloblastic anemia. Riboflavin deficiency symptoms are: sores at the angles of the mouth (angular stomatitis); sore swollen, and chapped lips (cheilosis); swollen, fissured, and painful tongue (glossitis); redness and congestion at the edges of the cornea of the eye; and oily, crusty, scaly skin (seborrheic dermatitis). **Toxicity**: There is no known toxicity of riboflavin.	**Rich sources**: Organ meats (liver, kidney, heart). **Good sources**: Corn flakes (enriched), almonds, cheese, eggs, lean meat (beef, pork, lamb), mushrooms (raw), wheat flour (enriched), turnip greens, wheat bran, soybean flour, bacon, cornmeal (enriched). **Supplemental sources**: Yeast (brewers', torula). Riboflavin is the only vitamin present in significant amounts in beer.	Riboflavin is destroyed by light, and by heat in an alkaline solution.
Thiamin (Vitamin B_1) As a coenzyme in transketolation (Keto-carrying). In direct functions in the body, including (1) maintenance of normal appetite (2) the tone of the muscles (3) a healthy mental attitude	**Deficiency symptoms**: Moderate thiamin deficiency symptoms include fatigue; apathy (lack of interest); loss of appetite; nausea; moodiness; irritability; depression; retarded growth; a sensation of numbness in the legs; and abnormalities of the electrocardiogram. Severe thiamin deficiency of long duration culminates in beriberi, the symptoms of which are polyneuritis (inflammation of the nerves), emaciation and/or edema, and disturbances of heart function. **Toxicity**: None.	Thiamin is found in a large variety of animal and vegetable products but is abundant in few. **Rich sources**: Lean pork, sunflower seed, corn flakes (enriched), peanuts, safflower flour, soybean flour. **Good sources**: Wheat bran, kidney, wheat flour (enriched), rye flour, nuts (except peanuts, which are a rich source), whole wheat flour, cornmeal (enriched), rice (enriched), white bread (enriched), soybean sprouts. **Supplemental sources**: Thiamin hydrochloride, thiamin mononitrate, yeast (brewers', torula), rice bran, wheat germ, and rice polish. Enriched flour (bread) and cereal has been of special significance in improving the dietary level of thiamin in the U.S.	

Vitamin B_6 (Pyridoxine; pyridoxal; pyridoxamine) Vitamin B_6 functions as a coenzyme (pyridoxal phosphate) a. Transamination b. Decarboxylation c. Transsulfuration d. Tryptophan conversion to nicotinic acid e. Absorption of amino acids f. The conversion of glycogen to glucose-1-phosphate g. The conversion of linoleic acid to arachidonic acid	**Deficiency symptoms**: In adults: greasy scaliness (seborrheic dermatitis) in the skin around the eyes, nose, and mouth, which subsequently spread to other parts of the body; a smooth, red tongue; loss of weight; muscular weakness; irritability; mental depression. In infants, the deficiency symptoms are irritability, muscular twitchings, and convulsions. **Toxicity**: B_6 is relatively nontoxic, but large doses may result in sleepiness and be habit-forming when taken over an extended period.	Rice bran, wheat bran, sunflower seeds, avocados, bananas, corn, fish, kidney, lean meat, liver, nuts, poultry, rice (brown), soybeans, whole grain. **Supplemental sources**: Pyridoxine hydrochloride is the most commonly available synthetic form, and yeast (torula, brewers'), rice polish, and wheat germ are used as natural source supplements.	In rats, the three forms of vitamin B_6 have equal activity; and it is assumed that the same applies to man. Processing or cooking foods may destroy up to 50% of the B_6. Because vitamin B_6 is limited in many foods, supplemental B_6 with synthetic pyridoxine hydrochloride may be indicated, especially for infants and during pregnancy and lactation.
Vitamin B_{12} (Cobalamins) 1. Synthesis or transfer of single carbon units. 2. Biosynthesis of methyl groups (-CH3), and in reduction reactions such as the conversion of disulfide (S-S) to the sulfhydryl group (-SH).	**Deficiency symptoms**: Vitamin B_{12} deficiency in man may occur as a result of (1) dietary lack, which sometimes occurs among vegetarians who consume no animal food; or (2) deficiency of intrinsic factor due to total or partial removal of the stomach by surgery, or infestation with parasites such as the fish tapeworm. The common symptoms of a dietary deficiency of vitamin B_{12} are: sore tongue, weakness, loss of weight, back pains, tingling of the extremities, apathy, and mental and other nervous abnormalities. Anemia is rarely seen in dietary deficiency of B_{12}. In pernicious anemia, the characteristic symptoms are: abnormally large red blood cells, lemon-yellow pallor, anorexia, prolonged bleeding time, abdominal discomfort, loss of weight, glossitis, an unsteady gait, and neurological disturbances, including stiffness of the limbs, irritability, and mental depression. Without treatment death follows. **Toxicity**: No toxic effects of vitamin B_{12} are known.	Liver and other organ meats — kidney, heart, muscle meats, fish, shellfish, eggs, and cheese. **Supplemental sources**: Cobalamin, of which there are at least three active forms, produced by microbial growth; available at the corner drugstore. Some B_{12} is synthesized in the intestinal tract of human beings. However, little of it may be absorbed.	Plants cannot manufacture vitamin B_{12}. Vitamin B_{12} is the largest and the most complex of all vitamin molecules. Vitamin B_{12} is the only vitamin that requires a specific gastrointestinal factor for its absorption (intrinsic factor); and (2) that the absorption of vitamin B_{12} in the small intestine requires about 3 hours.

TABLE 1.17 *(Continued)*

Summary of Vitamin Deficiency Signs and Need

Functions	Deficiency and Toxicity Symptoms	Sources	Comments
Vitamin C (Ascorbic acid) Formation and maintenance of collagen, the substance that binds body cells together. Metabolism of the amino acids tyrosine and tryptophan. Absorption and movement of iron. Metabolism of fats and lipids, and cholesterol control. Sound teeth and bones. Strong capillary walls and healthy blood vessels. Metabolism of folic acid.	**Deficiency symptoms**: Early symptoms, called latent scurvy: loss in weight, listlessness, fatigue, fleeting pains in the joints and muscles, irritability, shortness of breath, sore and bleeding gums, small hemorrhages under the skin, bones that fracture easily, and poor wound healing. Scurvy: Swollen, bleeding and ulcerated gums; loose teeth; malformed and weak bones, fragility of the capillaries with resulting hemorrhages throughout the body; large bruises; big joints, such as the knees and hips, due to bleeding into the joint cavity; anemia; degeneration of muscle fibers; including those of the heart; and tendency of old wounds to become red and break open. Sudden death from severe internal hemorrhage and heart failure. **Toxicity**: Adverse effects reported of intakes in excess of 8 g per day (more than 100 times the recommended allowance) include: nausea, abdominal cramps, and diarrhea; absorption of excessive amounts of iron; destruction of red blood cells; increased mobilization of bone minerals; interference with anticoagulant therapy; formation of kidney and bladder stones; inactivation of vitamin B_{12}; rise in plasma cholesterol; and possible dependence upon large doses of vitamin C.	Natural sources of vitamin C occur primarily in fruits (especially citrus fruits) and leafy vegetables: acerola cherry, *camu-camu*, and rose hips, raw, frozen, or canned citrus fruit or juice: oranges, grapefruit, lemons, and limes. Guavas, peppers (green, hot), black currants, parsley, turnip greens, poke greens, and mustard greens. **Good sources**: Green leafy vegetables: broccoli, Brussels sprouts, cabbage (red), cauliflower, collards, kale, lamb's-quarter, spinach, Swiss chard, and watercress. Also, cantaloupe, papaya, strawberries, and tomatoes and tomato juice (fresh or canned). **Supplemental sources**: Vitamin C (ascorbic acid) is available wherever vitamins are sold.	All animal species appear to require vitamin C, but dietary need is limited to humans, guinea pigs, monkeys, fruit bats, birds, certain fish, and certain reptiles. Of all the vitamins, ascorbic acid is the most unstable. It is easily destroyed during storage, processing, and cooking; it is water soluble, easily oxidized, and attacked by enzymes.

[1] See also Section 64.

TABLE 1.18

Essential Minerals and Their Functions

Function	Deficiencies and Toxicity Symptoms	Sources	Comments
Macrominerals			
Calcium (Ca) The primary function of calcium is to build the bones and teeth and to maintain the bones. Other functions are: 1. Blood clotting. 2. Muscle contraction and relaxation, especially the heartbeat. 3. Nerve transmission. 4. Cell wall permeability. 5. Enzyme activation. 6. Secretion of a number of hormones and hormone-releasing factors.	**Deficiency symptoms:** 1. Stunting of growth. 2. Poor quality bones and teeth. 3. Malformation of bones — rickets. The clinical manifestations of calcium related diseases are: 1. Rickets in children. 2. Osteomalacia, the adult counterpart of rickets. 3. Osteoporosis, a condition of too little bone, resulting when bone resorption exceeds bone formation. 4. Hypercalcemia, characterized by high serum calcium. 5. Tetany, characterized by muscle spasms and muscle pain. 6. Kidney stones. **Toxicity**: Normally, the small intestine prevents excess calcium from being absorbed. However, a breakdown of this control may raise the level of calcium in the blood and lead to calcification of the kidneys and other internal organs. High calcium intake may cause excess secretion of calcitonin and very dense bones.	Cheeses, wheat-soy flour, blackstrap molasses, milk, and milk products.	Calcium is the most abundant mineral in the body. It comprises about 40% of the total minerals present; 99% of it is in the bones and teeth. Generally, nutritionists recommend a calcium–phosphorus ratio of 1.5:1 in infancy, decreasing to 1:1 at 1 year of age and remaining at 1:1 throughout the rest of life; although they consider ratios between 2:1 and 1:2 as satisfactory.

TABLE 1.18 *(Continued)*

Essential Minerals and Their Functions

Function	Deficiencies and Toxicity Symptoms	Sources	Comments
Phosphorus (P) Essential for bone formation and maintenance. Important in the development of teeth. Essential for normal milk secretion. Important in building muscle tissue. As a component of nucleic acids (RNA and DNA), which are important in genetic transmission and control of cellular metabolism. Maintenance in many metabolic functions, especially: 1. Energy utilization 2. Phospholipid formation 3. Amino acid metabolism; protein formation 4. Enzyme systems	**Deficiency symptoms**: General weakness, loss of appetite, muscle weakness, bone pain, and loss of calcium. Severe and prolonged deficiencies of phosphorus may be manifested by rickets, osteomalacia, and other phosphorus related diseases. **Toxicity**: There is no known phosphorus toxicity per se. However, excess phosphate consumption may cause hypocalcemia (a deficiency of calcium in the blood).	Cocoa powder, cottonseed flour, fish flour, peanut flour, pumpkin and squash seeds, rice bran, rice polish, soybean flour, sunflower seeds, wheat, and bran.	Phosphorus comprises about 1/4 the total mineral matter in the body. Eighty percent of the phosphorus is in the bones and teeth in inorganic combination with calcium. Normally, 70% of the ingested phosphorus is absorbed. Generally, nutritionists recommend a calcium–phosphorus ratio of 1.5:1 in infancy, decreasing to 1:1 at 1 year of age, and remaining at 1:1 throughout the rest of life, although they consider ratios between 2:1 and 1:2 as satisfactory.
Sodium (Na) Helps to maintain the balance of water, acids, and bases in the fluid outside the cells. As a constituent of pancreatic juice, bile, sweat, and tears. Associated with muscle contraction and nerve functions. Plays a specific role in the absorption of carbohydrates.	**Deficiency symptoms**: Reduced growth, loss of appetite, loss of body weight due to loss of water, reduced milk production of lactating mothers, muscle cramps, nausea, diarrhea, and headache. Excess perspiration and salt depletion may be accompanied by heat exhaustion. **Toxicity**: Salt may be toxic when (1) a high intake is accompanied by a restriction of water, (2) when the body is adapted to a chronic low salt diet, or (3) when it is fed to infants or others whose kidneys cannot excrete the excess in the urine.	Table salt, processed meat products, and pickled/cured products.	Deficiencies of sodium may occur when there has been heavy, prolonged sweating, diarrhea, vomiting, or adrenal cortical insufficiency. In such cases, extra salt should be taken.

Chlorine (Cl) Plays a major role in the regulation of osmotic pressure, water balance, and acid-base balance. Required for the production of hydrochloric acid in the stomach; this acid is necessary for the proper absorption of Vitamin B_{12} and iron, for the activation of the enzyme that breaks down starch, and for suppressing the growth of microorganisms that enter the stomach with food and drink.	**Deficiency symptoms**: Severe deficiencies may result in alkalosis (an excess of alkali in the blood), characterized by slow and shallow breathing, listlessness, muscle cramps, loss of appetite, and, occasionally, by convulsions. Deficiencies of chloride may develop from prolonged and severe vomiting, diarrhea, pumping of the stomach, injudicious use of diuretic drugs. **Toxicity**: An excess of chlorine ions is unlikely when the kidneys are functioning properly.	Table salt (sodium chloride) and foods that contain salt.	Persons whose sodium intake is severely restricted (owing to diseases of the heart, kidney, or liver) may need an alternative source of chloride; a number of chloride-containing salt substitutes are available for this purpose.
Magnesium (Mg) Constituent of bones and teeth. Essential element of cellular metabolism, often as an activator of enzymes involved in phosphorylated compounds and of high energy phosphate transfer of ADP and ATP. Involved in activating certain peptidases in protein digestion. Relaxes nerve impulse, functioning antagon-istically to calcium which is stimulatory.	**Deficiency symptoms**: A deficiency of magnesium is characterized by (1) muscle spasms (tremor, twitching) and rapid heartbeat; (2) confusion, hallucinations, and disorientation; and (3) lack of appetite, listlessness, nausea, and vomiting. **Toxicity**: Magnesium toxicity is characterized by slowed breathing, coma, and sometimes death.	**Rich sources**: Coffee (instant), cocoa powder, cottonseed flour, peanut flour, sesame seeds, soybean flour, spices, wheat bran, and wheat germ.	Overuse of such substances as "milk of magnesia" (magnesium hydroxide) or "Epsom salts" (magnesium sulfate) may lead to deficiencies of other minerals or even to toxicity.

TABLE 1.18 *(Continued)*

Essential Minerals and Their Functions

Function	Deficiencies and Toxicity Symptoms	Sources	Comments
Potassium (K) Involved in the maintenance of proper acid-base balance and the transfer of nutrients in and out of individual cells. Relaxes the heart muscle — action opposite to that of calcium which is stimulatory. Required for the secretion of insulin by the pancreas in enzyme reactions involving the phosphorylation.	**Deficiency symptoms**: Potassium deficiency may cause rapid and irregular heartbeats and abnormal electrocardiograms; muscle weakness, irritability, and occasionally paralysis; and nausea, vomiting, diarrhea, and swollen abdomen. Extreme and prolonged deficiency of potassium may cause hypokalemia, culminating in the heart muscles stopping. **Toxicity**: Acute toxicity from potassium (known as hyperpotassemia or hyperkalemia) can result when kidneys are not functioning properly. The condition may prove fatal due to cardiac arrest.	Dehydrated fruits, molasses, potato flour, rice bran, seaweed, soybean flour, spices, sunflower seeds, and wheat bran.	Potassium is the third most abundant element in the body, after calcium and phosphorus, and it is present in twice the concentration of sodium
Cobalt (Co) The only known function of cobalt is that of an integral part of Vitamin B_{12}, an essential factor in the formation of red blood cells.	A cobalt deficiency as such has never been produced in humans. The signs and symptoms that are sometimes attributed to cobalt deficiency are actually due to lack of Vitamin B_{12}, characterized by pernicious anemia, poor growth, and occasionally neurological disorders.	Cobalt is present in many foods.	Cobalt is an essential constituent of Vitamin B_{12} and must be ingested in the form of vitamin molecule inasmuch as humans synthesize little of the vitamin. (A small amount of Vitamin B_{12} is synthesized in the human colon by *E. coli*, but absorption is very limited.)

Copper (Cu) Facilitating the absorption of iron from the intestinal tract and releasing it from storage in the liver and the reticuloendothelial system. Essential for the formation of hemoglobin, although it is not a part of hemoglobin as such. Constituent of several enzyme systems. Development and maintenance of the vascular and skeletal structures (blood vessels, tendons, and bones). Structure and function of the central nervous system. Required for normal pigmentation of hair. Component of important copper-containing proteins. Reproduction (fertility).	**Deficiency symptoms**: Deficiency is most apt to occur in malnourished children and in premature infants fed exclusively on modified cow's milk and in infants breast fed for an extended period of time. Deficiency leads to a variety of abnormalities, including anemia, skeletal defects, demyelination and degeneration of the nervous system, defects in pigmentation and structure of the hair, reproductive failure, and pronounced cardiovascular lesions. **Toxicity**: Copper is relatively nontoxic to monogastric species, including man. The recommended copper intake for adults is in the range of 2–3 mg/day. Daily intakes of more than 20–30 mg over extended periods would be expected to be unsafe.	Black pepper, blackstrap molasses, Brazil nuts, cocoa, liver, and oysters (raw).	Most cases of copper poisoning result from drinking water or beverages that have been stored in copper tanks and/or pass through copper pipes. Dietary excesses of calcium, iron, cadmium, zinc, lead, silver, and molybdenum plus sulfur reduce the utilization of copper.
Fluorine (F) Constitutes 0.02–0.05% of the bones and teeth. Necessary for sound bones and teeth. Assists in the prevention of dental caries.	**Deficiency symptoms**: Excess dental caries. Also, there is indication that a deficiency of fluorine results in osteoporosis in the aged. **Toxicity**: Deformed teeth and bones, and softening, mottling, and irregular wear of the teeth.	Fluorine is found in many foods, but seafoods and dry tea are the richest food sources. Fluoridation of water supplies to bring the concentration of fluoride to 1 ppm.	Large amounts of dietary calcium, aluminum, and fat will lower the absorption of fluorine. Fluoridation of water supplies (1 ppm) is the simplest and most effective method of providing added protection against dental caries.

TABLE 1.18 *(Continued)*

Essential Minerals and Their Functions

Function	Deficiencies and Toxicity Symptoms	Sources	Comments
Iodine (I) The sole function of iodine is making the iodine-containing thyroid hormones.	**Deficiency symptoms**: Iodine deficiency is characterized by goiter (an enlargement of the thyroid gland at the base of the neck), coarse hair, obesity, and high blood cholesterol. Iodine-deficient mothers may give birth to infants with a type of dwarfism known as cretinism, a disorder characterized by malfunctioning of the thyroid gland, goiter, mental retardation, and stunted growth. A similar disorder of the thyroid gland, known as myxedema, may develop in adults. **Toxicity**: Long-term intake of large excesses of iodine may disturb the utilization of iodine by the thyroid gland and result in goiter.	Among natural foods the best sources of iodine are kelp, seafoods, and vegetables grown in iodine-rich soils and iodized salt. Stabilized iodized salt contains 0.01% potassium iodide (0.0076% I), or 76 mcg of iodine per gram.	Certain foods (especially plants of the cabbage family) contain goitrogens, which interfere with the use of thyroxine and may produce goiter. Fortunately, goitrogenic action is prevented by cooking.
Iron (Fe) Iron (heme) combines with protein (globin) to make hemoglobin, the iron-containing compound in red blood cells which transports oxygen. Iron is also a component of enzymes which are involved in energy metabolism.	**Deficiency symptoms**: Iron-deficiency (nutritional) anemia, the symptoms of which are paleness of skin and mucous membranes, fatigue, dizziness, sensitivity to cold, shortness of breath, rapid heartbeats, and tingling of the fingers and toes. An excess of iron in the diet can tie up phosphorus in an insoluble iron-phosphate complex, thereby creating a deficiency of phosphorus.	Red meat, egg yolk, and dark green, leafy vegetables.	About 70% of the iron is present in the hemoglobin, the pigment of the red blood cells. The other 30% is present as a reserve store in the liver, spleen, and bone marrow.

Manganese (Mn) Formation of bone and the growth of other connective tissues. Blood clotting. Insulin action. Cholesterol synthesis. Activator of various enzymes in the metabolism of carbohydrates, fats, proteins, and nucleic acids.	**Deficiency symptoms**: No clear deficiency disease in man has been reported. **Toxicity**: Toxicity in man as a consequence of dietary intake has not been observed. However, it has occurred in workers (miners and others) exposed to high concentrations of manganese dust in the air. The symptoms resemble those found in Parkinson's and Wilson's disease.	Rice (brown), rice bran and polish, walnuts, wheat bran, and wheat germ.	In average diets, only about 45% of the ingested magnesium is absorbed. The manganese content of plants is dependent on soil content.
Molybdenum (Mo) As a component of three different enzyme systems which are involved in the metabolism of carbohydrates, fats, proteins, sulfur-containing amino acids, nucleic acids (DNA and RNA), and iron.	**Deficiency symptoms**: Naturally occurring deficiency in man is not known. Molybdenum-deficient animals are especially susceptible to the toxic effects of bisulfite, characterized by breathing difficulties and neurological disorders. Severe molybdenum toxicity in animals (molybdenosis), particularly cattle, occurs throughout the world wherever pastures are grown on high-molybdenum soils. The symptoms include diarrhea, loss of weight, decreased production, fading of hair color, and other symptoms of copper deficiency.	The concentration of molybdenum in food varies considerably, depending on the soil in which it is grown. Most of the dietary molybdenum intake is derived from organ meats, whole grains, leafy vegetables, legumes, and yeast.	The utilization of molybdenum is reduced by excess copper, sulfate, and tungsten. In cattle, a relationship exists between molybdenum, copper, and sulfur. Excess molybdenum will cause copper deficiency. However, when the sulfate content of the diet is increased, the symptoms of toxicity are avoided inasmuch as the excretion of molybdenum is increased.

TABLE 1.18 *(Continued)*

Essential Minerals and Their Functions

Function	Deficiencies and Toxicity Symptoms	Sources	Comments
Selenium (Se) Component of the enzyme glutathione peroxidase, the metabolic role of which is to protect against oxidation of polyunsaturated fatty acids and resultant tissue damage.	**Deficiency symptoms**: There are no clear-cut deficiencies of selenium, because this mineral is so closely related to vitamin E that it is difficult to distinguish deficiency due to selenium alone. **Toxicity**: Poisonous effects of selenium are manifested by (1) abnormalities of the hair, nails, and skin; (2) garlic odor on the breath; (3) intensification of selenium toxicity by arsenic or mercury; and (4) higher than normal rates of dental caries.	The selenium content of plant and animal products is affected by the selenium content of the soil and animal feed, respectively. Brazil nuts, butter, flour, fish, lobster, and smelt.	The high selenium areas are in Great Plains and the Rocky Mountain states — especially in parts of the Dakotas and Wyoming.
Zinc (Zn) Needed for normal skin, bones, and hair. A component of several different enzyme systems which are involved in digestion and respiration. Required for the transfer of carbon dioxide in red blood cells, for proper calcification of bones, for the synthesis and metabolism of proteins and nucleic acids, for the development and functioning of reproductive organs, for wound and burn healing, for the functioning of insulin, and for normal taste acuity.	**Deficiency symptoms**: Loss of appetite, stunted growth in children, skin changes, small sex glands in boys, loss of taste sensitivity, lightened pigment in hair, white spots on the fingernails, and delayed healing of wounds. In the Middle East, pronounced zinc deficiency in man has resulted in hypogonadism and dwarfism. In pregnant animals, experimental zinc deficiency has resulted in malformation and behavioral disturbances in offspring. **Toxicity**: Ingestion of excess soluble salts may cause nausea, vomiting, and purging.	Beef, liver, oysters, spices, and wheat bran.	The biological availability of zinc in different foods varies widely; meats and seafoods are much better sources of available zinc than vegetables. Zinc availability is adversely affected by phytates (found in whole grains and beans), high calcium, oxalates (in rhubarb and spinach), high fiber, copper (from drinking water conveyed in copper piping), and EDTA (an additive used in certain canned foods).

Adapted from Ensminger, et al. *Foods & Nutrition Encyclopedia,* 2nd ed., CRC Press, Boca Raton, 1994, pp. 1511–1521.

TABLE 1.19

Essential Fatty Acids

Structure	Name
H H H H $CH_3CH_2CH_2CH_2C{=}C{-}CH_2{-}C{=}CCH_2CH_2CH_2CH_2CH_2CH_2CH_2COOH$ 18 12 9	linoleic acid [18:2, (9, 12)]
H H H H H H $CH_3CH_2CH_2CH_2CH_2C{=}C{-}CH_2{-}C{=}C{-}CH_2{-}C{=}CCH_2CH_2CH_2CH_2COOH$ 18 12 9 6 1	γ linolenic acid [18:3, (6, 9, 12)]
H H H H H H $CH_3CH_2C{=}C{-}CH_2{-}C{=}C{-}CH_2{-}C{=}C{-}(CH_2)_7COOH$ 18 15 12 9	linolenic acid [18:3 (9, 12, 15)]

TABLE 1.20

Structure and Names of Fatty Acids Found in Food

Structure	# Carbons: Double Bonds	Systematic Name	Trivial Name	Source
Saturated Fatty Acids				
$CH_3(CH_2)_2COOH$	4:0	*n*-Butanoic	Butyric	Butter
$CH_3(CH_2)_4COOH$	6:0	*n*-Hexanoic	Caproic	Butter
$CH_3(CH_2)_6COOH$	8:0	*n*-Octanoic	Caprylic	Coconut oil
$CH_3(CH_2)_8COOH$	10:0	*n*-Decanoic	Capric	Palm oil
$CH_3(CH_2)_{10}COOH$	12:0	*n*-Dodecanoic	Lauric	Coconut oil, nutmeg, butter
$CH_3(CH_2)_{12}COOH$	14:0	*n*-Tetradecanoic	Myristic	Coconut oil
$CH_3(CH_2)_{14}COOH$	16:0	*n*-Hexadecanoic	Palmitic	Most fats and oils
$CH_3(CH_2)_{16}COOH$	18:0	*n*-Octadecanoic	Stearic	Most fats and oils
$CH_3(CH_2)_{18}COOH$	20:0	*n*-Eicosanoic	Arachidic	Peanut oil, lard
Unsaturated Fatty Acids				
$CH_3(CH_2)_5CH{=}CH(CH_2)_7COOH$	16:1	9-Hexadecenoic	Palmitoleic	Butter and seed oils
$CH_3(CH_2)_7CH{=}CH(CH_2)_7COOH$	18:1	9-Octadecenoic	Oleic	Most fats and oils
$CH_3(CH_2)_5CH{=}CH(CH_2)_9COOH$	20:1	11-Octadecenoic	*trans*-Vaccenic	Hydrogenated vegetable oils
$CH_3(CH_2)_4CH{=}CHCH_2CH{=}CH(CH_2)_7COOH$	18:2	9,12-Octadecadienoic	Linoleic	Linseed oil, corn oil, cottonseed oil
$CH_3CH_2(CH{=}CHCH_2)_3(CH_2)_7COOH$	18:3	9,12,15-Octadecatrienoic	Linolenic	Soybean oil, marine oils
$CH_3(CH_2)_4(CH{=}CHCH2)_4(CH_2)_2COOH$	20:4	5,8,11,14-Eicosatetraenoic	Arachidonic	Cottonseed oil

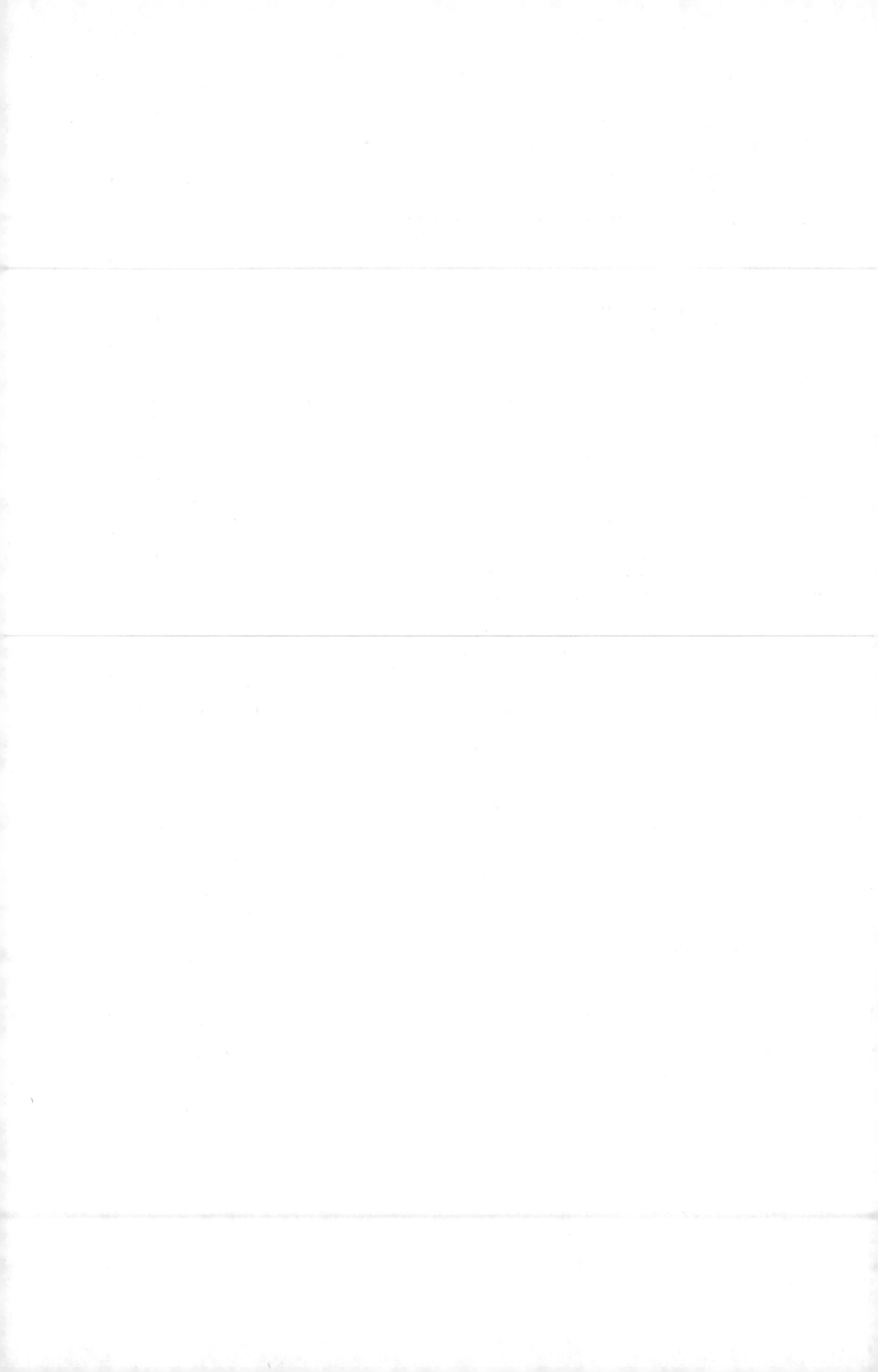

Part II

Metabolism

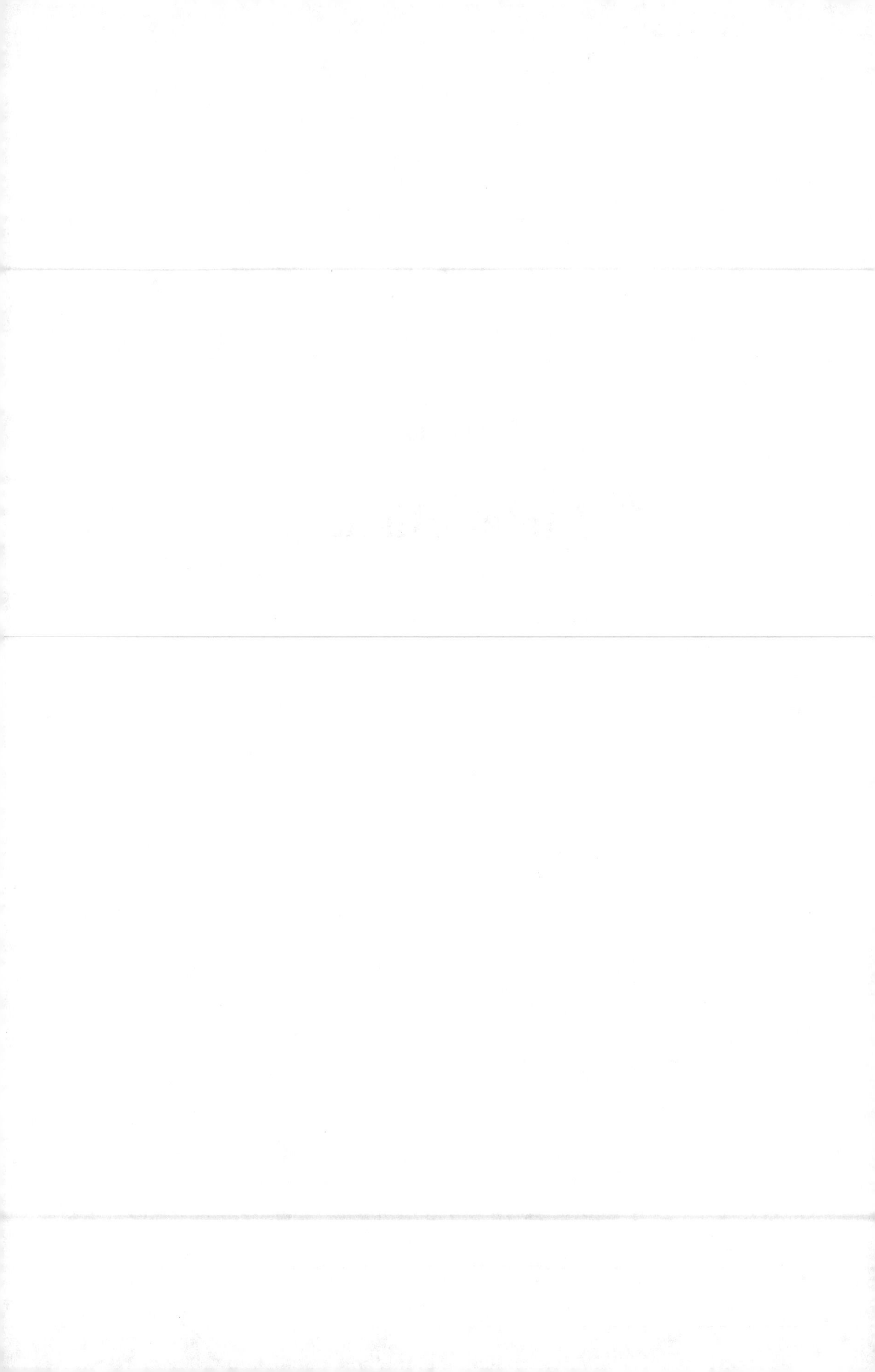

2

Metabolic Maps

Carolyn D. Berdanier

The individual reactions of metabolisms have been studied extensively. The details of their regulation within a given pathway has likewise received considerable attention. The entire map can be obtained from Boehringer Manheim (BM) at minimal cost. (Boehringer Mannheim, PO Box 31 01 20, D-6800 Mannheim 31 Germany.) The maps come complete with citations of the works that provided the critical information for these maps as well as notations on species differences and differences between mammals, plants, and microorganisms.

The maps that follow are general and lack the detail found in the BM maps. They are provided to give the user an idea of where in metabolism the use of the various macronutrients occur. They also provide some details about intermediary metabolism.

0-8493-2705-9/01/$0.00+$1.50

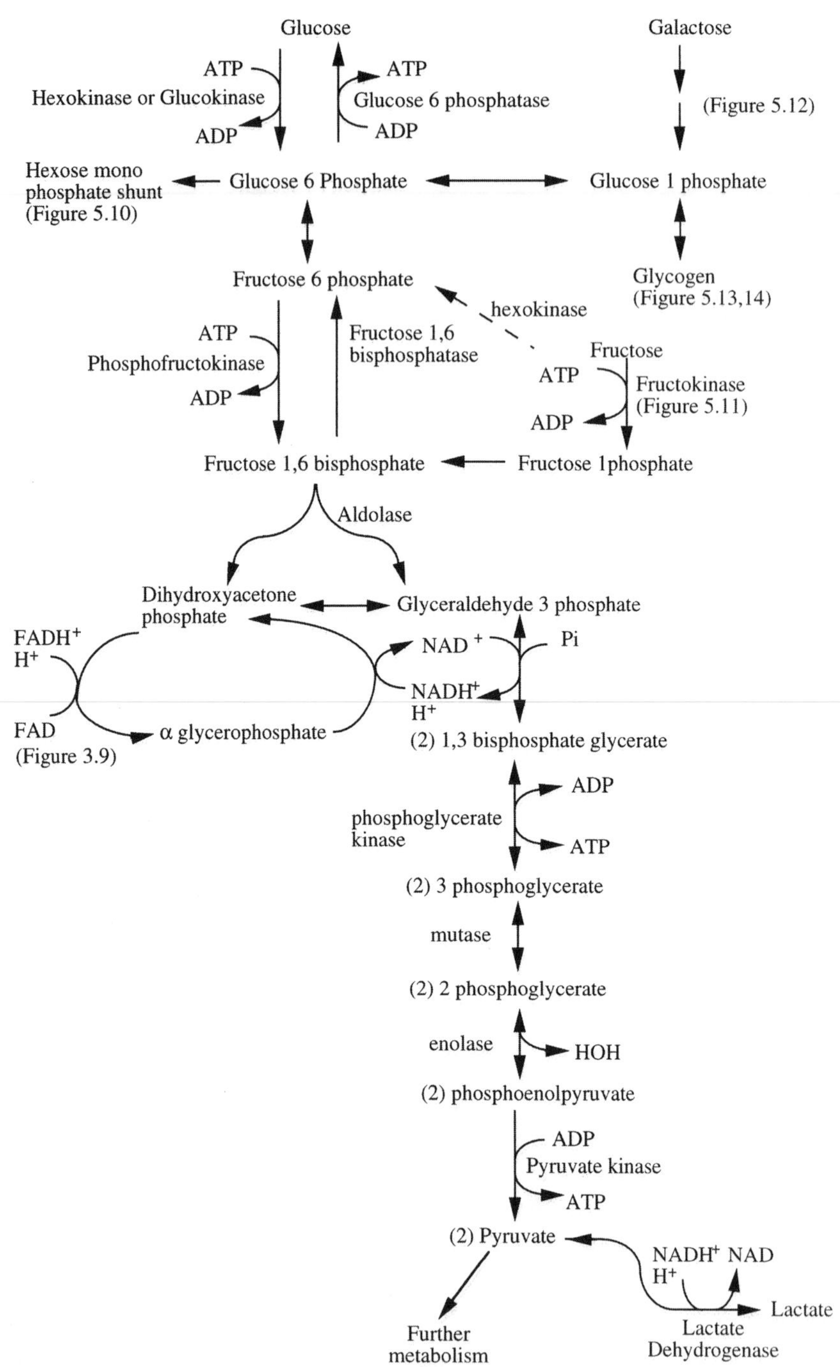

FIGURE 2.1
The glycolytic pathway.

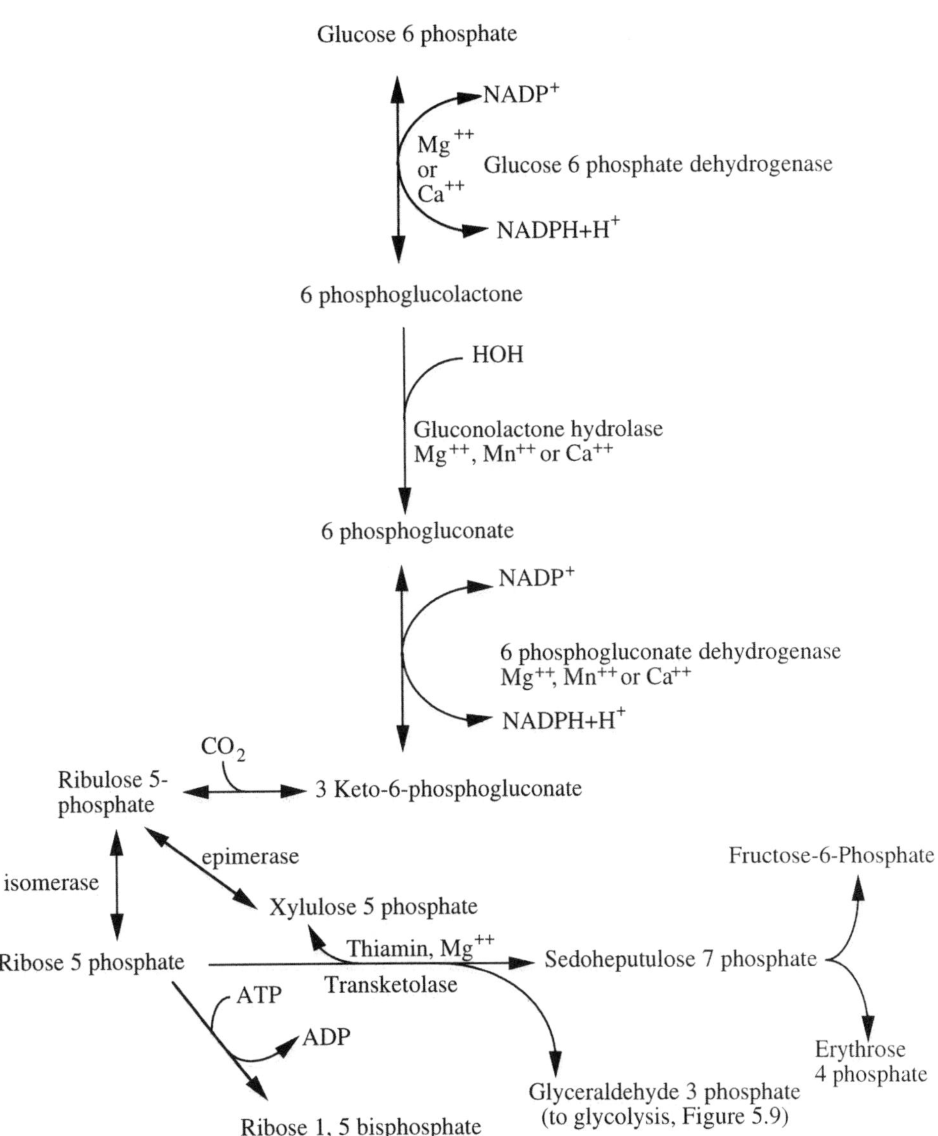

FIGURE 2.2
Reaction sequence of the hexose monophosphate shunt commonly referred to as the "shunt."

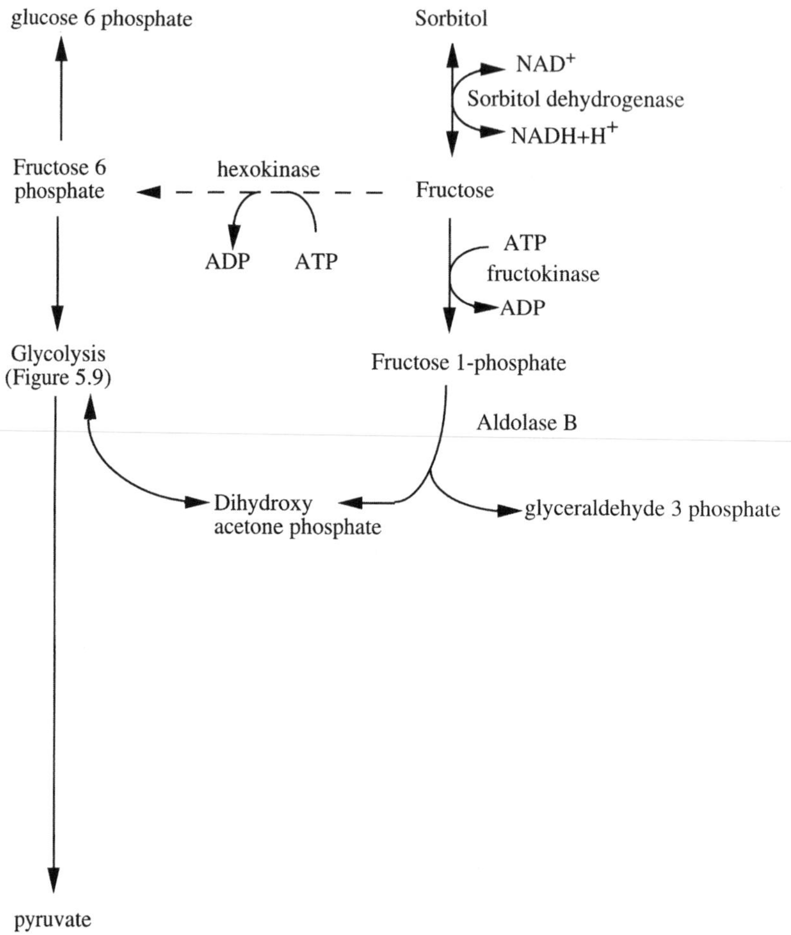

FIGURE 2.3
Metabolism of fructose.

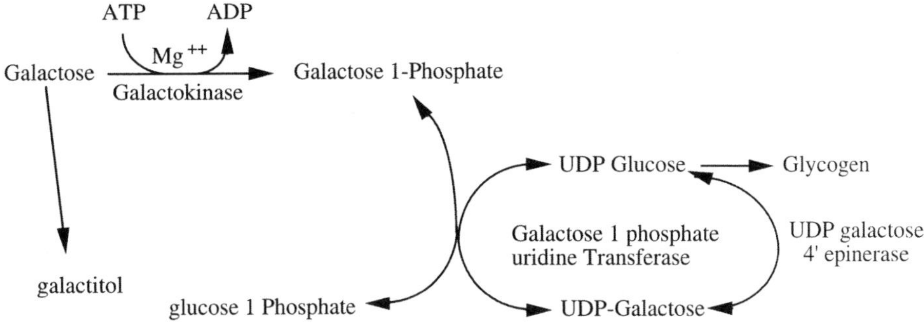

FIGURE 2.4
Conversion of galactose to glucose.

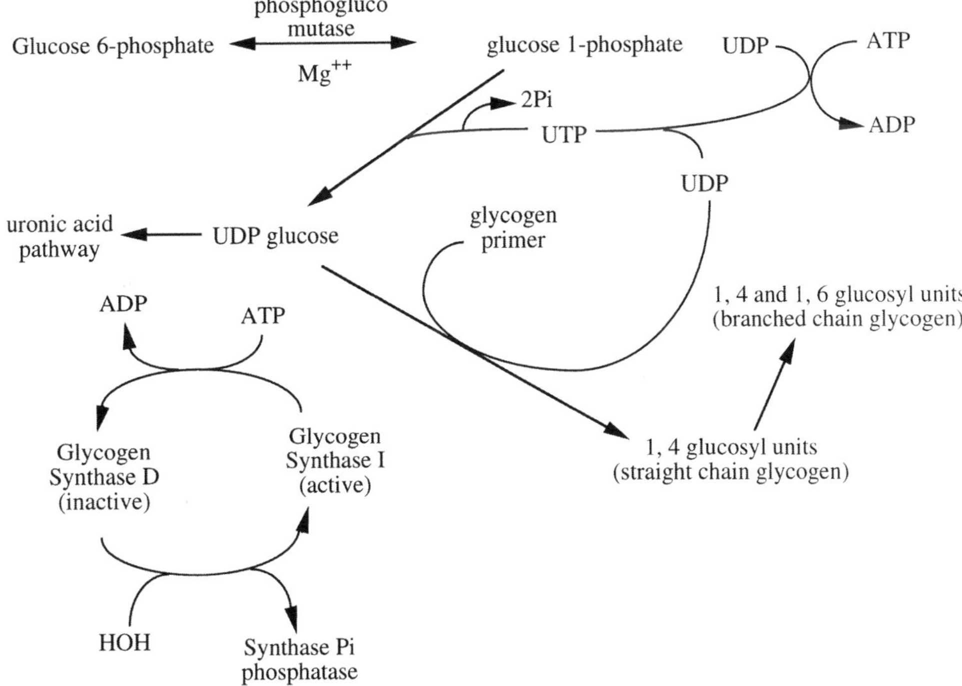

FIGURE 2.5
Glycogen synthesis (glycogenesis).

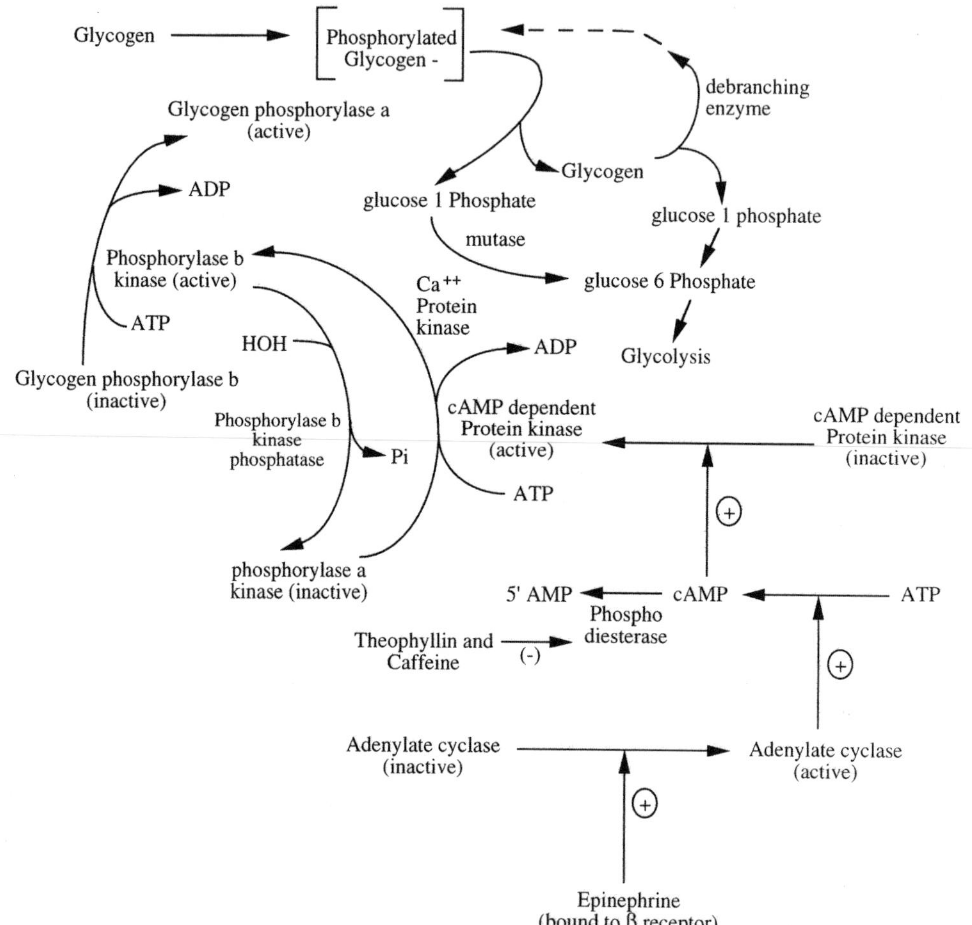

FIGURE 2.6
Stepwise release of glucose molecules from the glycogen molecule.

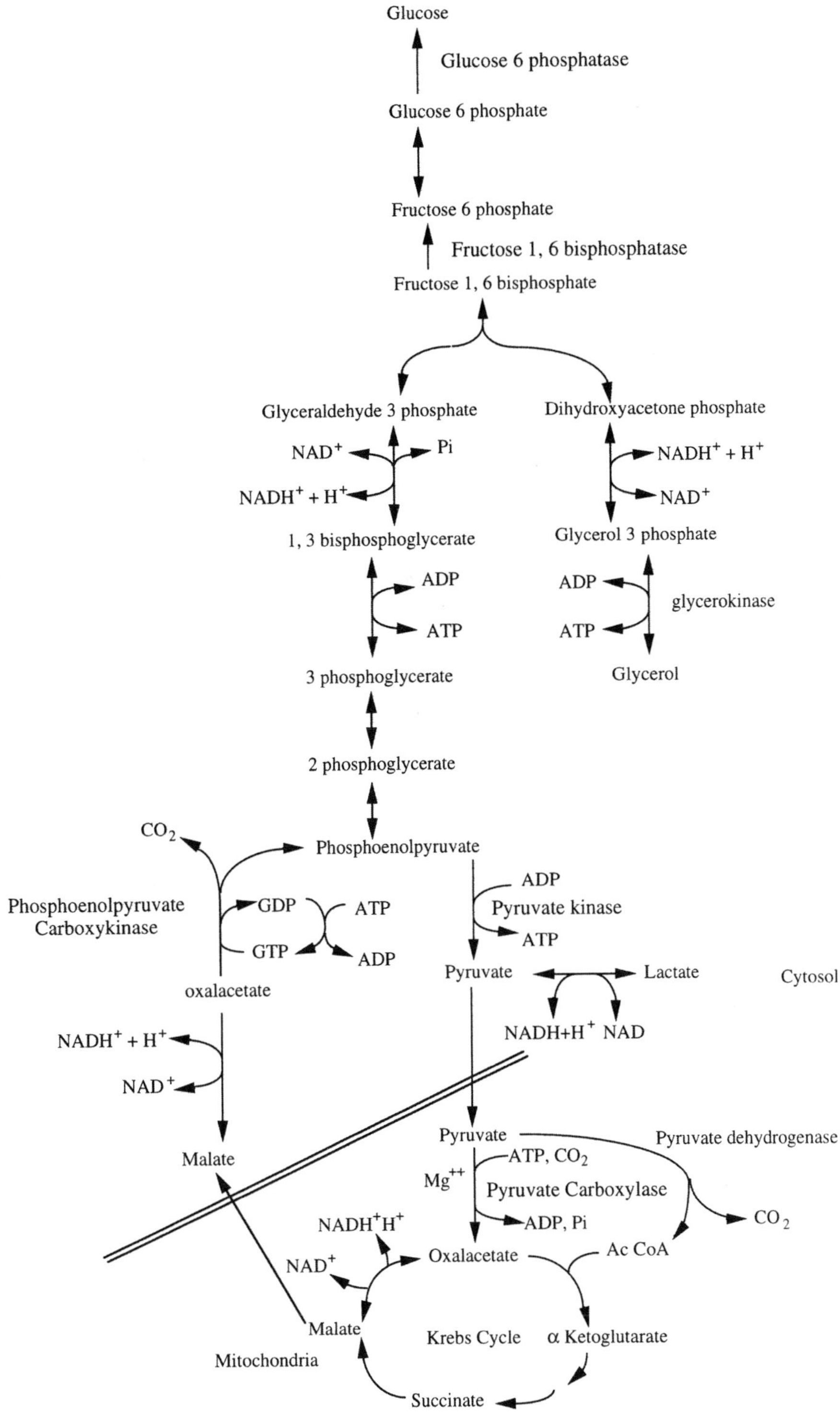

FIGURE 2.7
Pathway for gluconeogenesis.

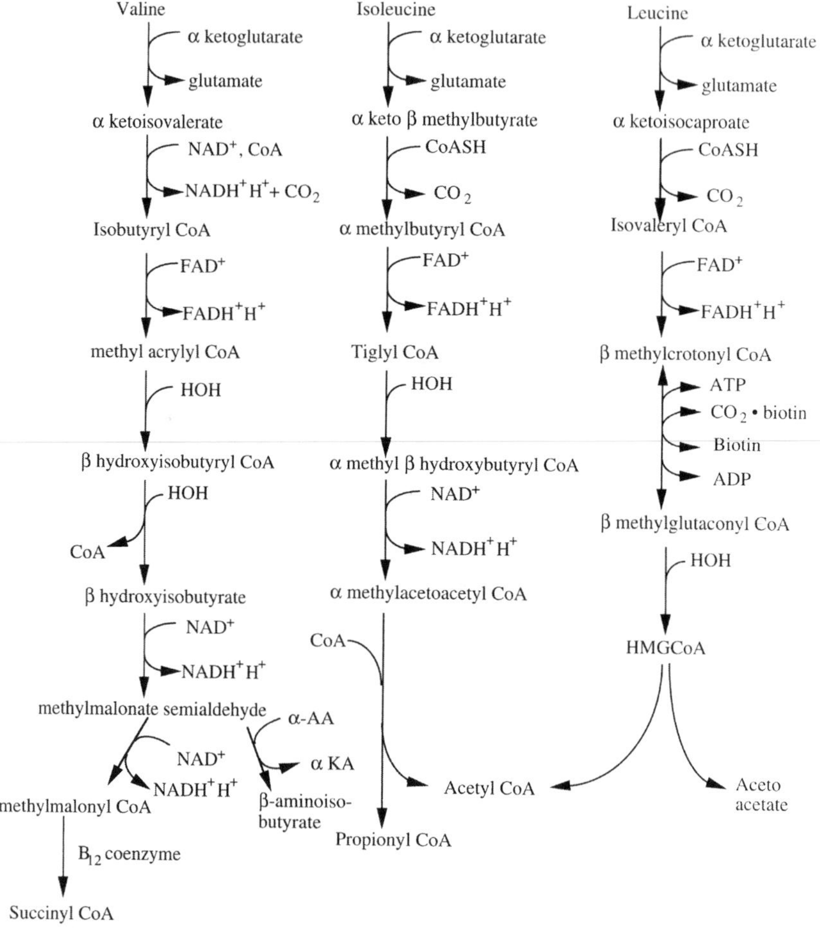

FIGURE 2.8
Catabolism of branched chain amino acids showing their use in the production of metabolites that are either lipid precursors or metabolites than can be oxidized via the Krebs cycle.

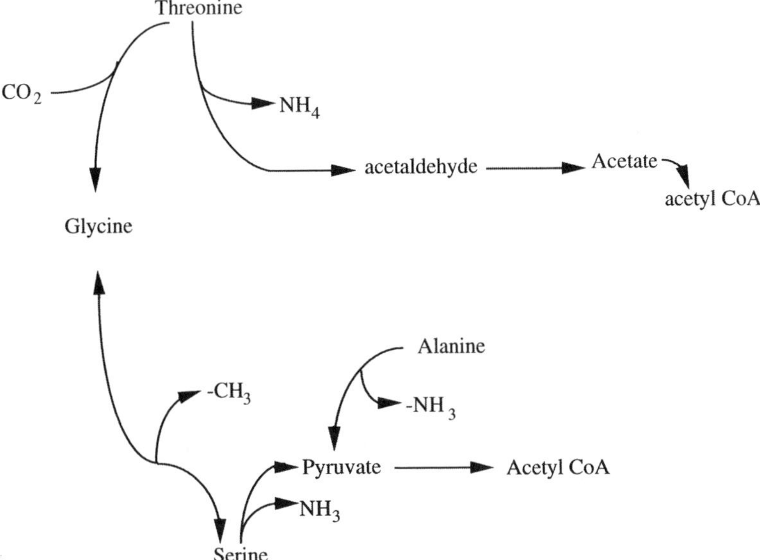

FIGURE 2.9
Catabolism of threonine showing its relationship to that of serine and glycine.

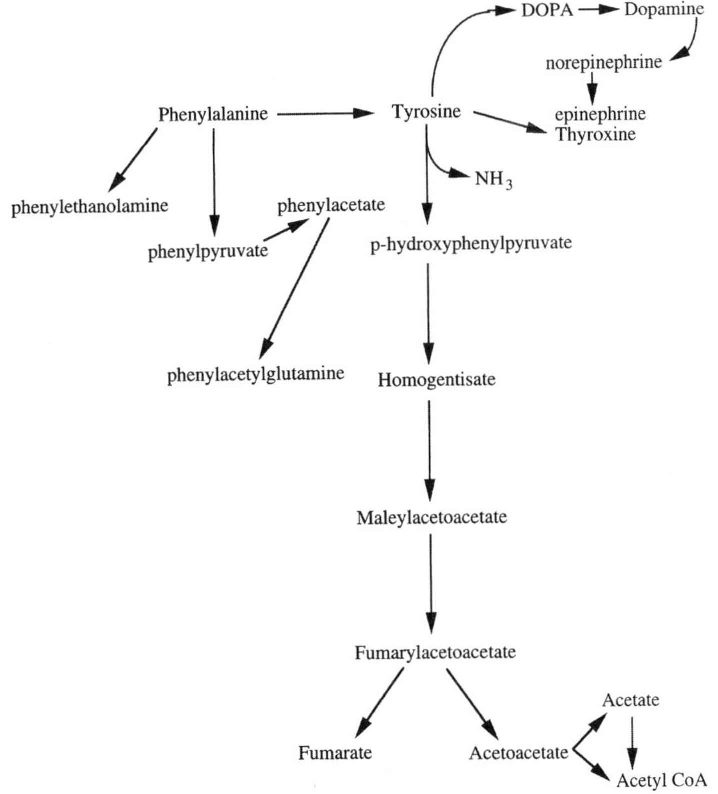

FIGURE 2.10
Phenylalanine and tyrosine catabolism. This pathway has a number of mutations that result in a variety of genetic disease.

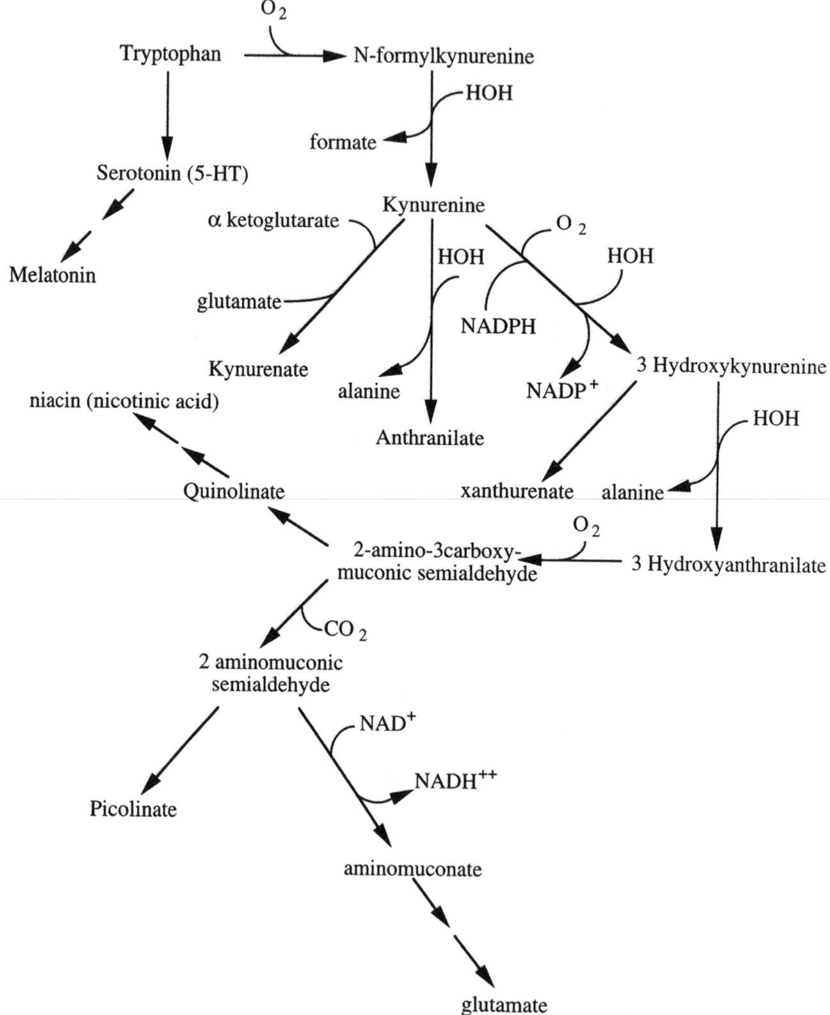

FIGURE 2.11
Catabolism of tryptophan showing conversion to the vitamin niacin. This conversion is not very efficient. Tryptophan catabolism also results in picolinate, which is believed by some to play a role in trace-mineral conservation.

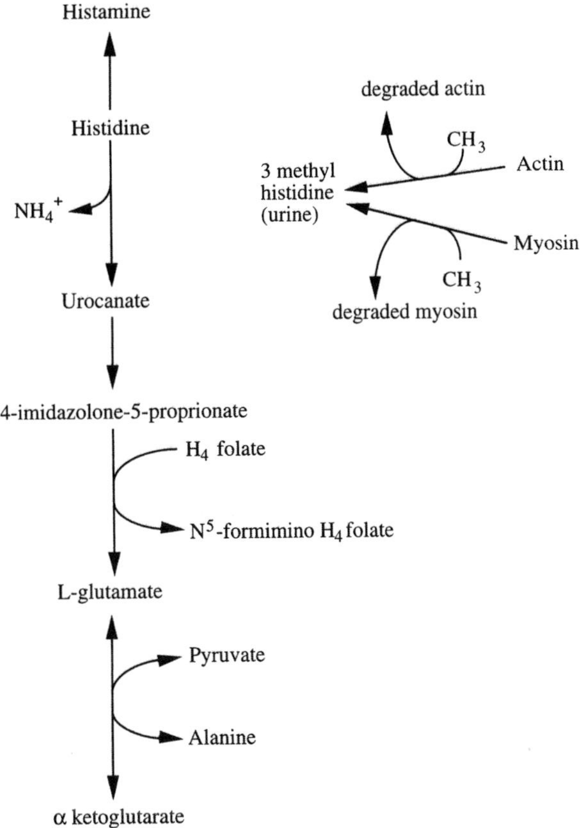

FIGURE 2.12
Catabolism of histidine. Note that 3-methyl histidine is not part of the pathway. This metabolite is formed in the muscle when the contractile proteins actin and myosin are methylated.

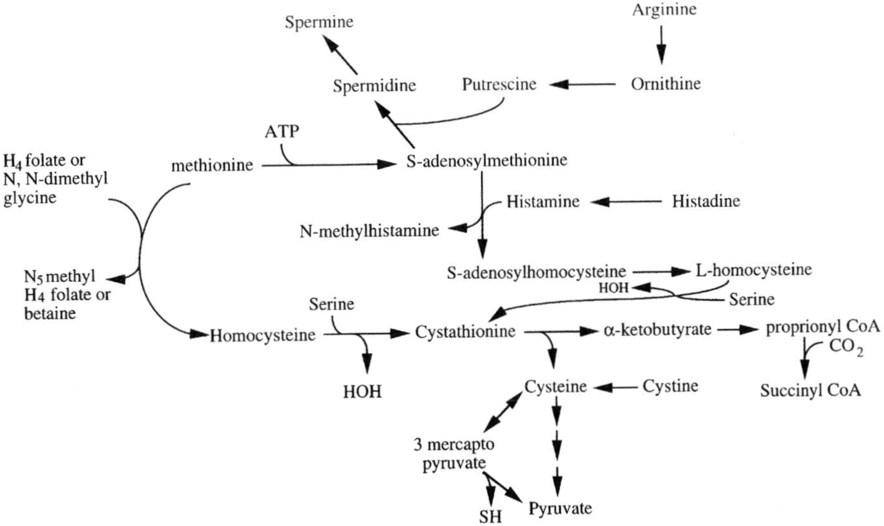

FIGURE 2.13
Conservation of SH groups via methionine–cysteine interconversion. Spermine, putrescine, and spermidine are polyamines that are important in cell and tissue growth.

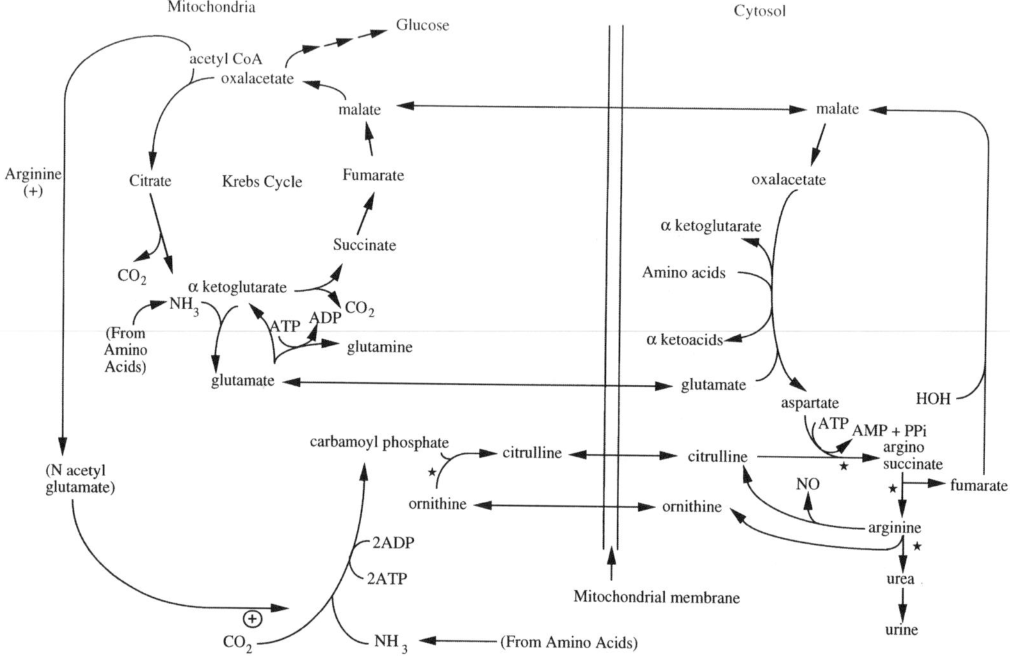

FIGURE 2.14
The urea cycle. Locations of mutations in the urea cycle enzymes are indicated with a star. Persons with these mutations have very short lives, with evidence of mental retardation, seizures, coma, and early death due to the toxic effects of ammonia accumulation. Rate controlling steps are indicated with a circled cross.

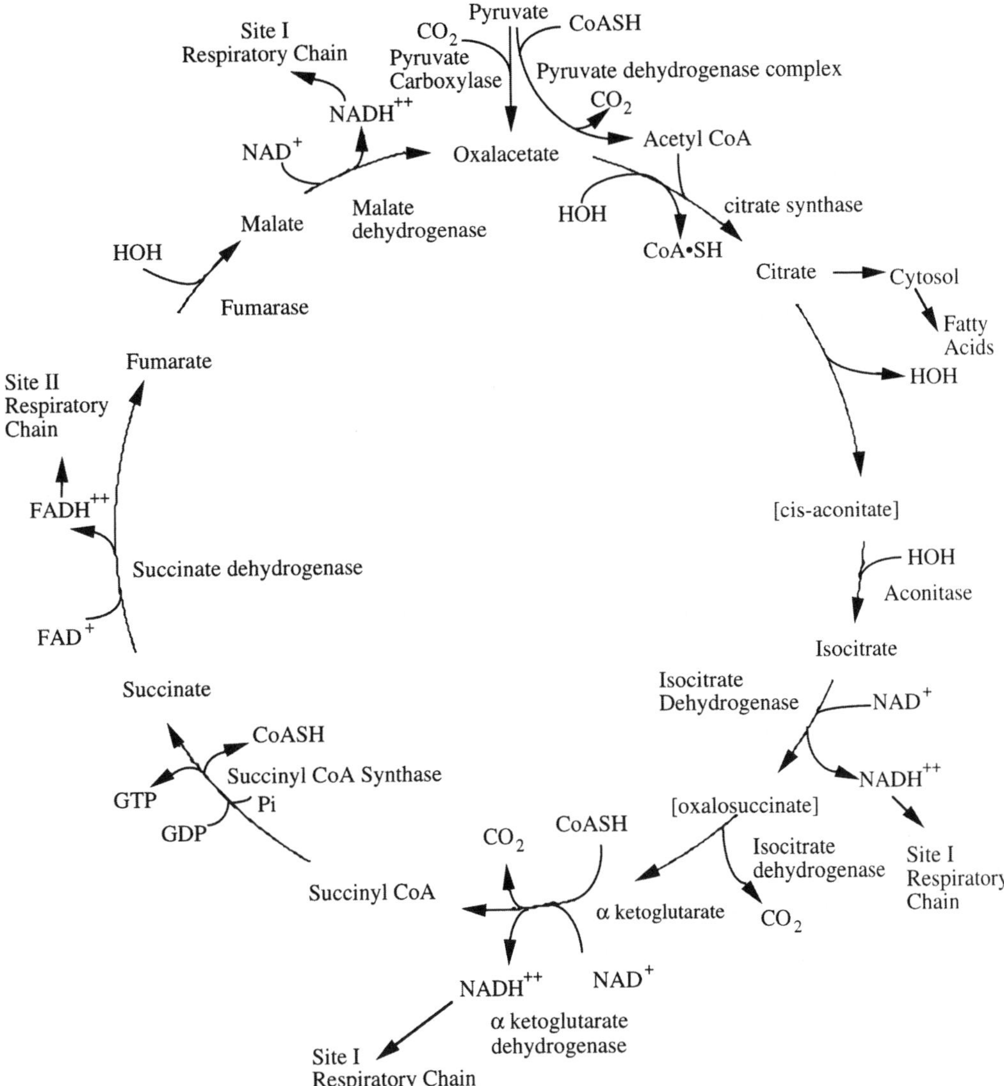

FIGURE 2.15
Krebs citric acid cycle in the mitochondria. This cycle is also called the tricarboxylate cycle (TCA).

ATP
ATP
ATP
F_1F_0 ATPase
F_1F_0 ATPase
F_1F_0 ATPase
NADH+H+
FAD
FMN
CoQH2
Fe+++
Fe++
Fe+++
Fe++
1/2 O2
SITE I
SITE II
Cytochrome b
Cytochrome C1
Cytochrome C
Cytochrome aa3
NAD+
FMNH2
CoQ
Fe++
Fe+++
Fe++
Fe+++
ADP, Pi
FADH+H+
ADP, Pi
Krebs Cycle
FADH++
HOH
Pyruvate
Fatty Acid Oxidation
2H+

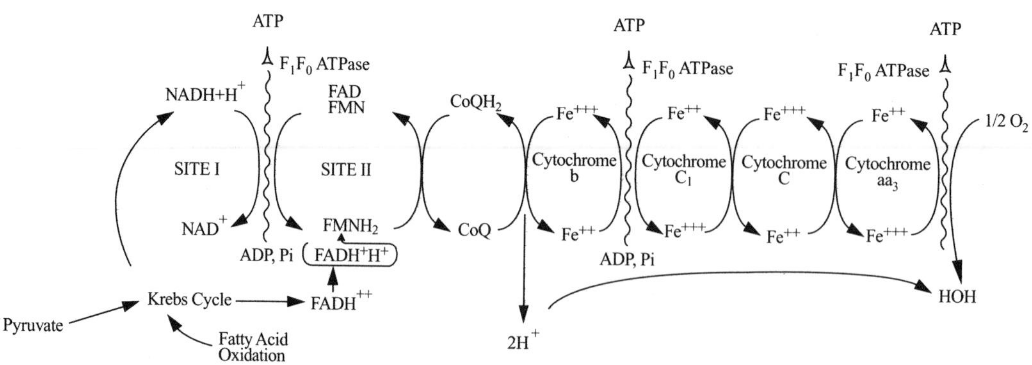

FIGURE 2.16
The respiratory chain showing the points where sufficient energy has been generated to support the synthesis of 1 molecule of ATP from ADP and Pi. Each of the segments generates a proton gradient. This energy is captured by the F_0 portion of the ATPase and transmitted to the F_1 portion of the ATPase. If uncouplers are present, the proton gradient is dissipated and all of the energy is released as heat.

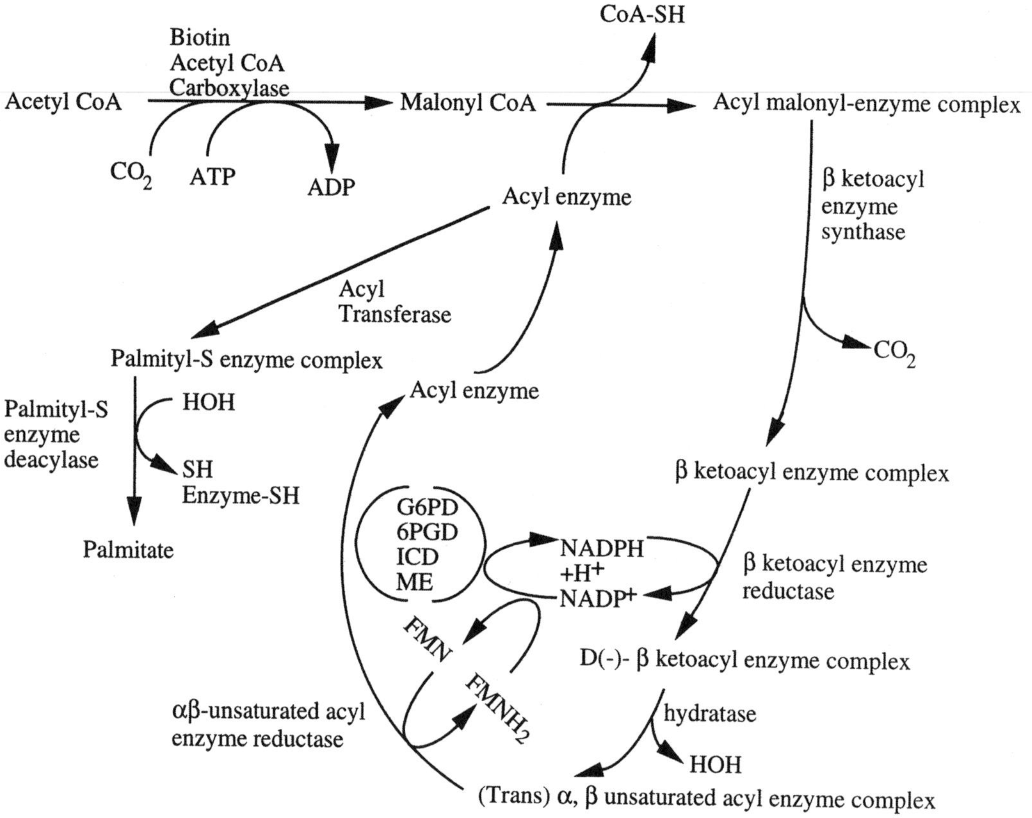

CoA-SH
Biotin
Acetyl CoA
Carboxylase
Acetyl CoA
Malonyl CoA
Acyl malonyl-enzyme complex
CO2
ATP
ADP
Acyl enzyme
β ketoacyl
enzyme
synthase
Acyl
Transferase
CO2
Palmityl-S enzyme complex
Acyl enzyme
Palmityl-S
enzyme
deacylase
HOH
SH
Enzyme-SH
β ketoacyl enzyme complex
Palmitate
G6PD
6PGD
ICD
ME
NADPH
+H+
NADP+
β ketoacyl enzyme
reductase
FMN
FMNH2
D(-)- β ketoacyl enzyme complex
αβ-unsaturated acyl
enzyme reductase
hydratase
HOH
(Trans) α, β unsaturated acyl enzyme complex

FIGURE 2.17
Fatty acid synthesis.

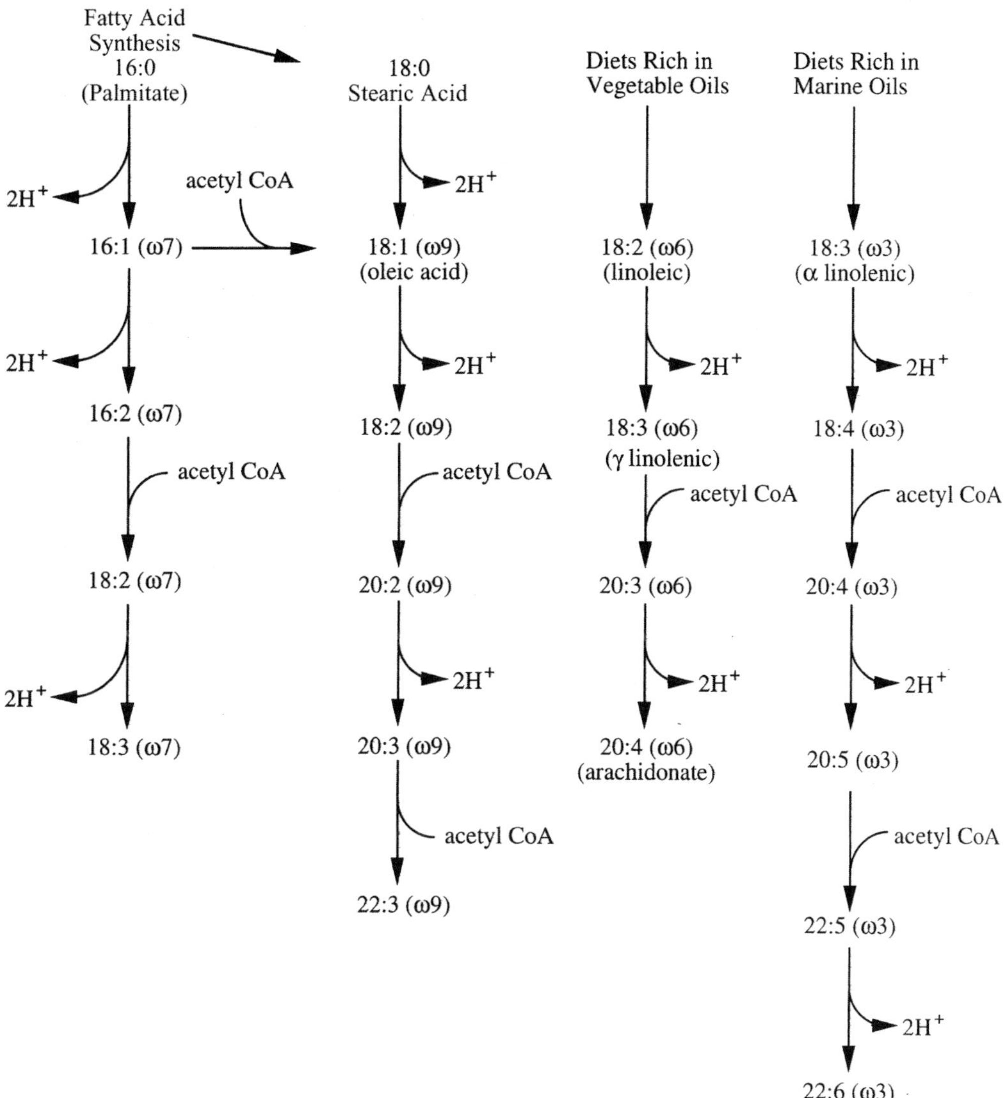

FIGURE 2.18
Pathways for synthesis of long-chain polyunsaturated fatty acids (PUFA) through elongation and desaturation. Not all of these reactions occur in all species. The ω symbol is the same as the n symbol. Thus, 18:2ω6, linoleic acid, could also be written 18:2n6.

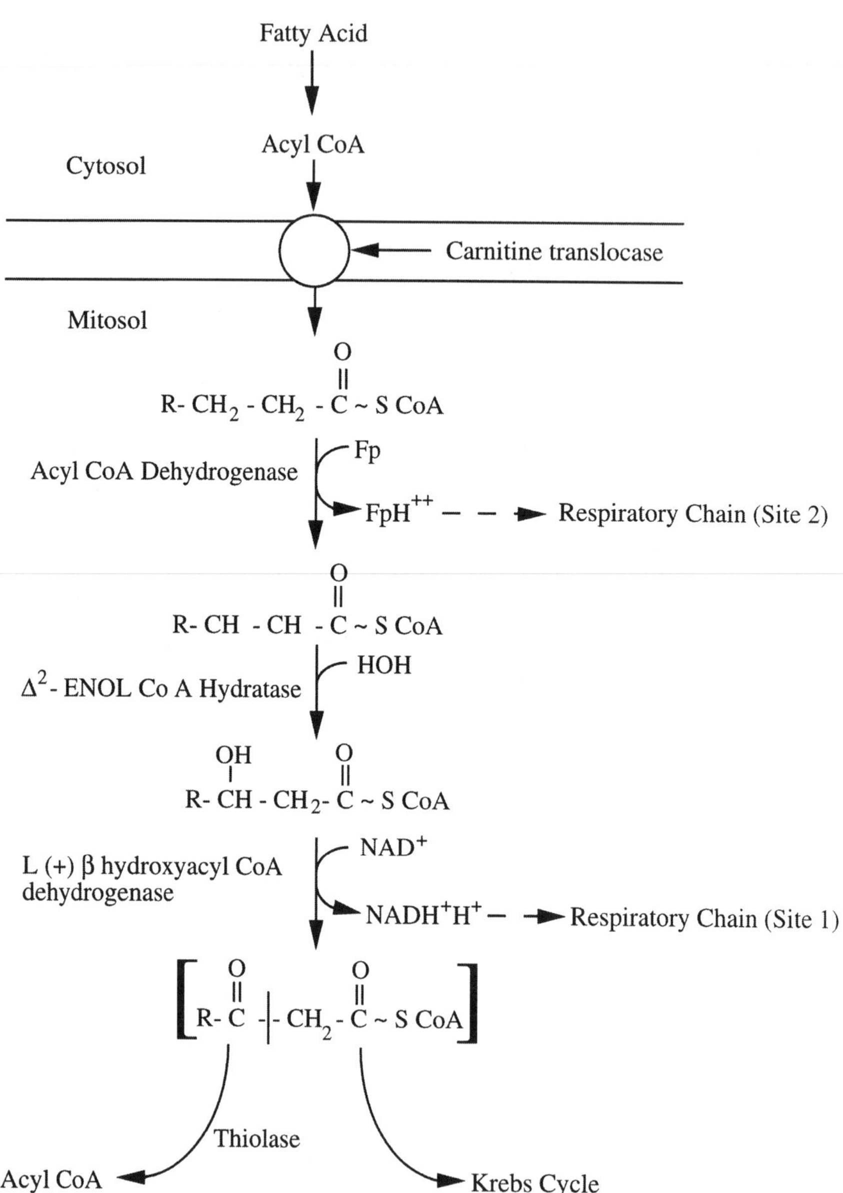

FIGURE 2.19
Pathway for β oxidation of fatty acids in the mitochondria.

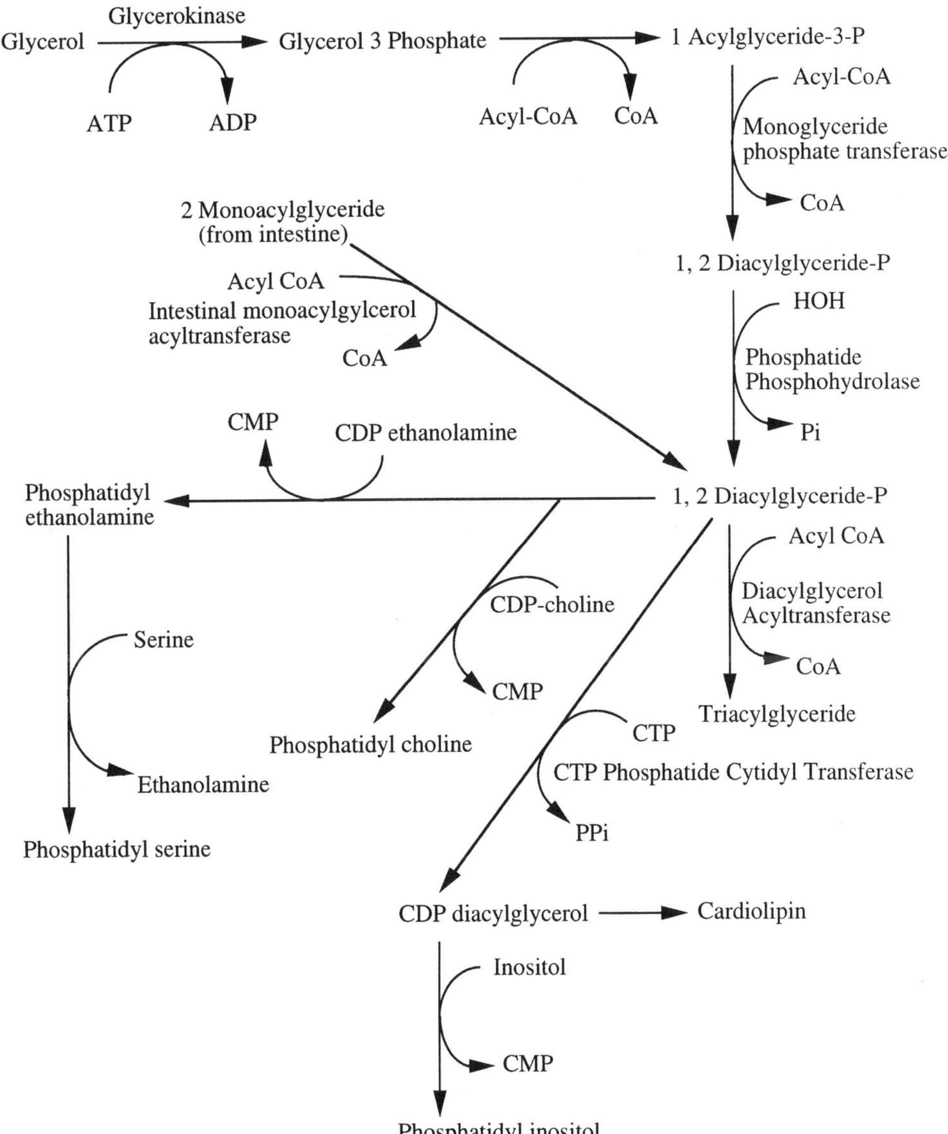

FIGURE 2.20
Pathways for the synthesis of triacylglycerides and phospholipids.

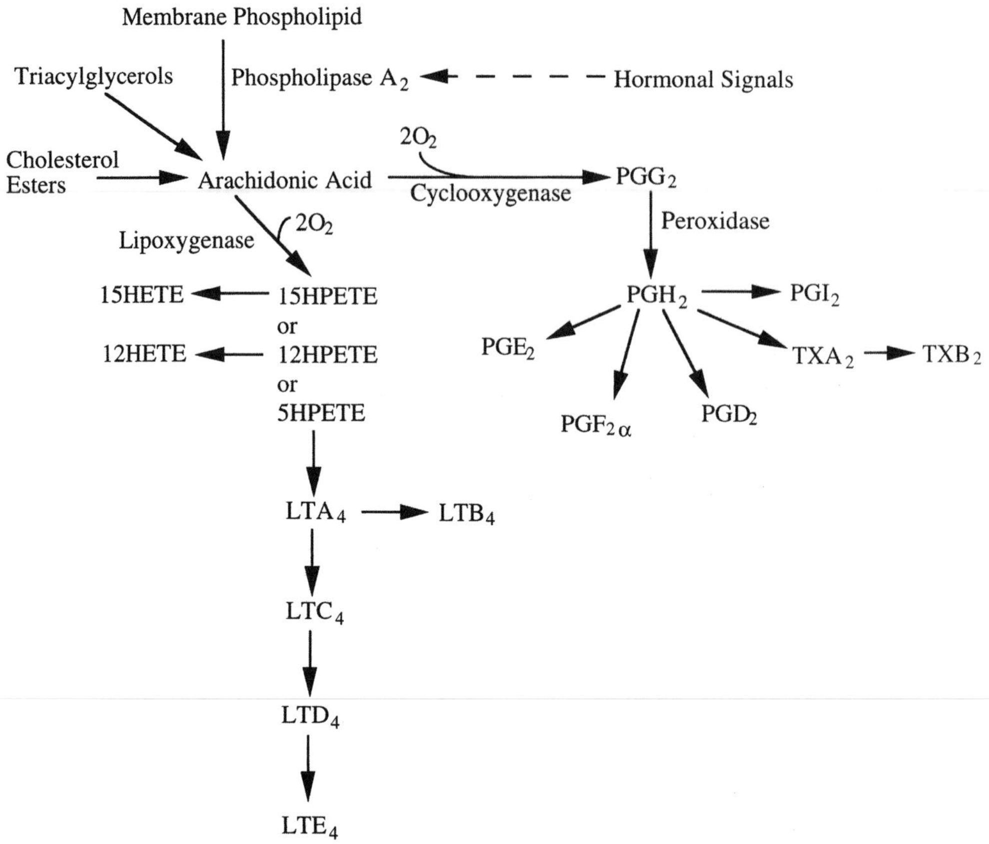

Membrane Phospholipid
Triacylglycerols
Phospholipase A2
Hormonal Signals
Cholesterol Esters
Arachidonic Acid
2O2
Cyclooxygenase
PGG2
Peroxidase
Lipoxygenase
2O2
15HETE
15HPETE
or
12HETE
12HPETE
or
5HPETE
PGH2
PGI2
PGE2
TXA2
TXB2
PGF2α
PGD2
LTA4
LTB4
LTC4
LTD4
LTE4

FIGURE 2.21
Eicosanoid synthesis from arachidonic acid.

CoA
HMG CoA reductase
Acetyl CoA + Acetoacyl CoA
HMG CoA
Mevalonate
HOH
2NADPH+H+
2NADP+
3ATP
3ADP
Lanosterol
Squalene 2,3 Epoxide
Squalene
Farnesyl Phosphate
Farnesyl Phosphate
Cholesterol
Cholesterol Esters
Fatty Acids

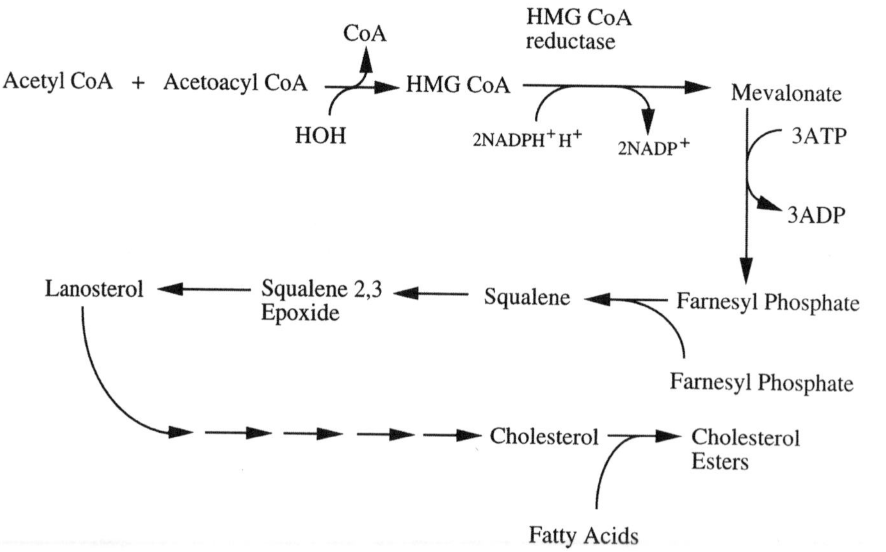

FIGURE 2.22
Cholesterol biosynthesis.

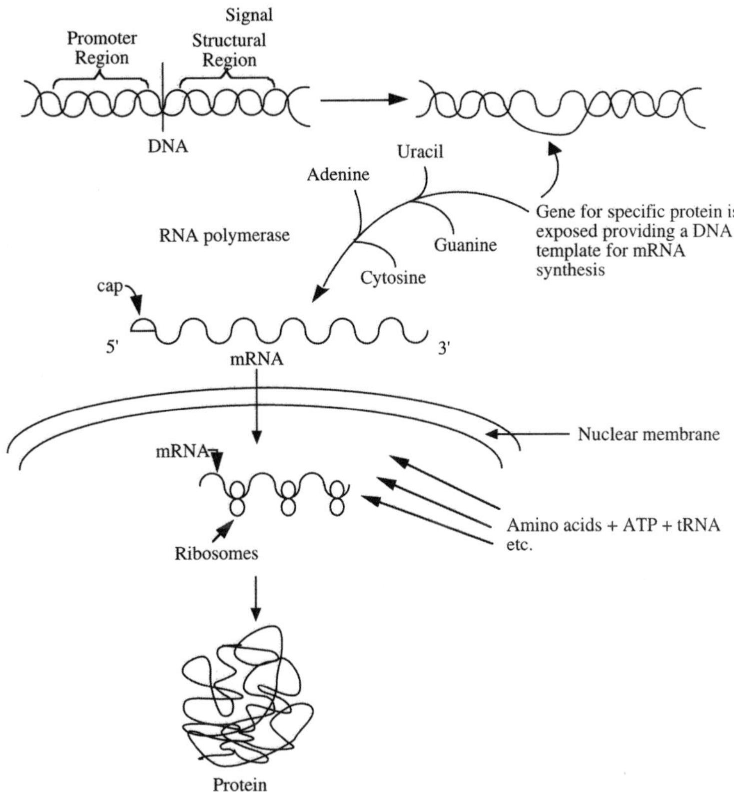

FIGURE 2.23
Overview of protein synthesis. Signals are transmitted to the nucleus that stimulate the exposure of a gene for a specific protein. A specific messenger RNA is synthesized. The mRNA moves out into the cytosol and attaches to the ribosome, whereupon tRNAs attached to amino acids dock at appropriate complementary bases and the amino acids are joined together to make protein.

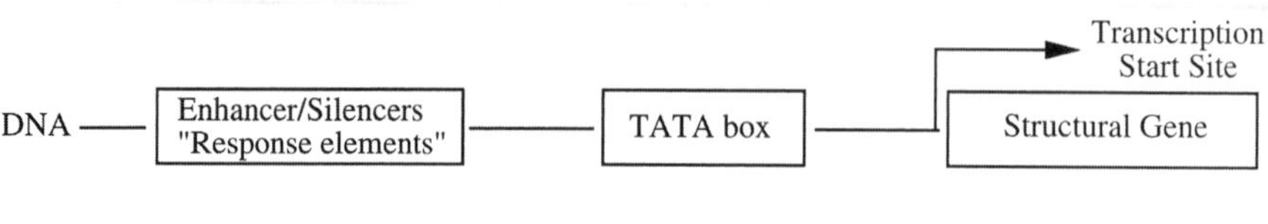

FIGURE 2.24
Detailed structure of the components of a gene that is to be transcribed.

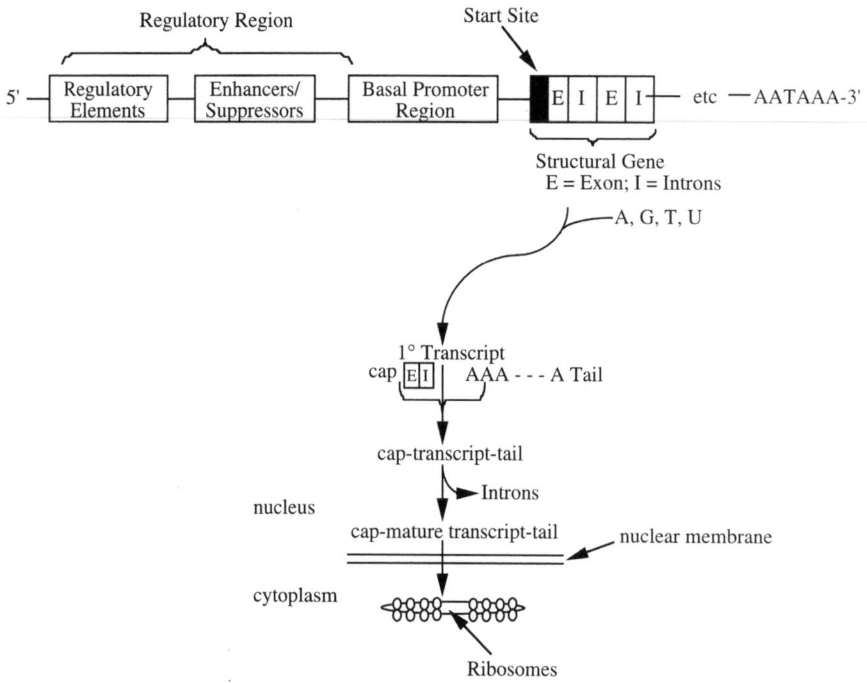

FIGURE 2.25
Synthesis of messenger RNA and its migration to the ribosomes in the cytoplasm.

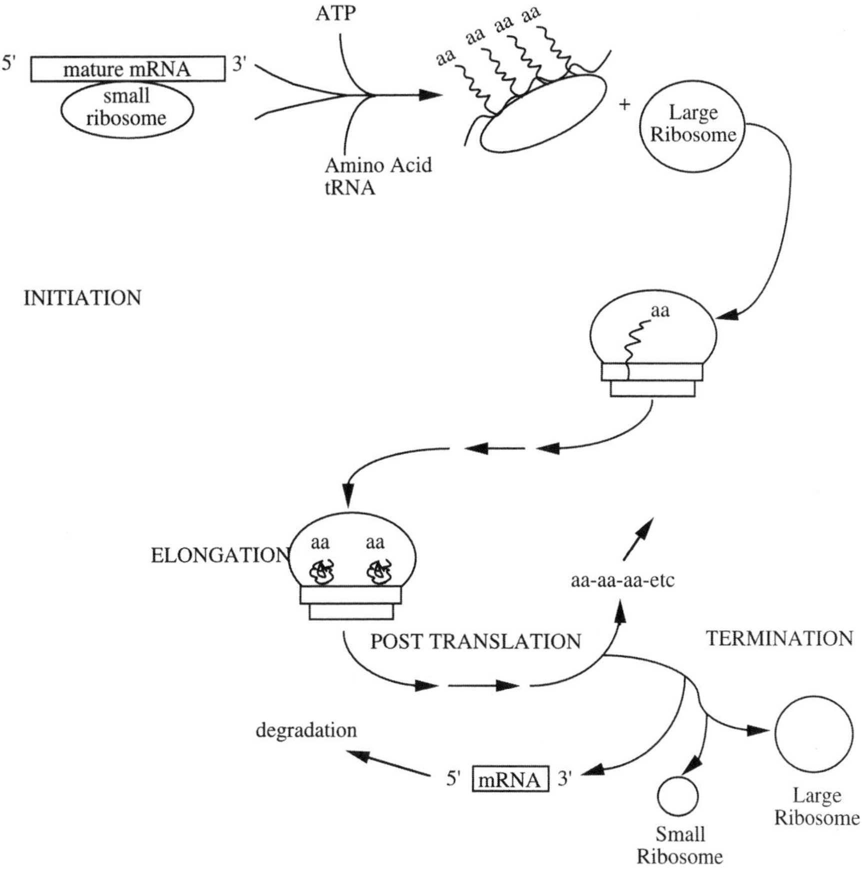

FIGURE 2.26
Overview of translation involving mRNA, tRNA-amino acids, and small and large ribosomal units.

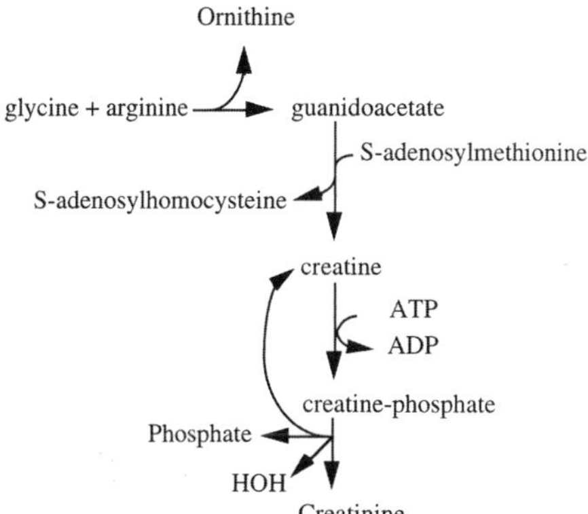

FIGURE 2.27
Synthesis of creatine and creatinine.

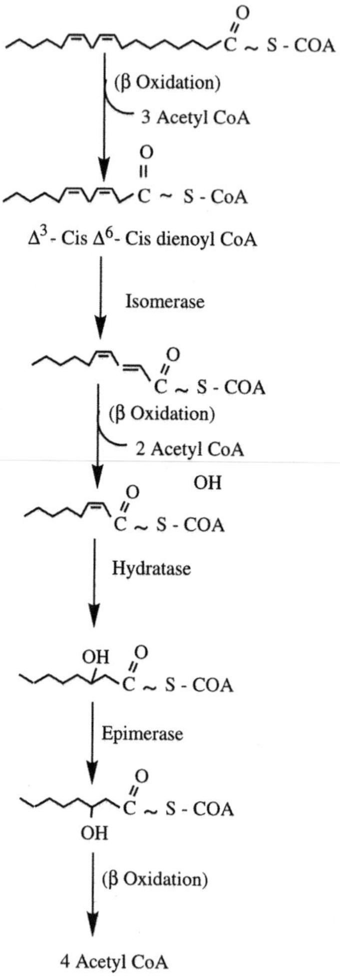

C ~ S - COA

(β Oxidation)

3 Acetyl CoA

C ~ S - CoA

Δ^3- Cis Δ^6- Cis dienoyl CoA

Isomerase

C ~ S - COA

(β Oxidation)

2 Acetyl CoA

OH

C ~ S - COA

Hydratase

OH

C ~ S - COA

Epimerase

C ~ S - COA

OH

(β Oxidation)

4 Acetyl CoA

FIGURE 2.28
Modification of β oxidation for unsaturated fatty acid.

3

Tables of Clinical Significance

Carolyn D. Berdanier

In this section can be found a variety of tables with importance to the clinician and nutrition scientist. There are no discussions of these tables because sections later in the book address key issues related to them. Rather, these tables represent a quick look at topics essential to an understanding of the health-related, nutrition-related human conditions.

TABLE 3.1

Proteins Involved in Lipid Transport

Protein	Function
apo A-II	Transport protein in HDL
apo B-48	Transport protein for chylomicrons; synthesized in the enterocyte in the human.
High density lipoprotein binding protein (HDLBP)	Binds HDL and functions in the removal of excess cellular cholesterol
apo D	Transport protein similar to retinol-binding protein
apo (a)	Abnormal transport protein for LDL
apo A-I	Transport protein for chylomicrons and HDL; synthesized in the liver and its synthesis is induced by retinoic acid
apo C-III	Transport protein for VLDL
apo A-IV	Transport protein for chylomicrons
CETP	Participates in the transport of cholesterol from peripheral tissue to liver; reduces HDL size
LCAT	Synthesized in the liver and is secreted into the plasma where it resides on the HDL. Participates in the reverse transport of cholesterol from peripheral tissues to the liver; esterifies the HDL cholesterol.
apo E	Mediates high affinity binding of LDL's to LDL receptor and the putative chylomicron receptor. Required for clearance of chylomicron remnant. Synthesized primarily in the liver.
apo C-I	Transport protein for VLDL
apo C-II	Chylomicron transport protein required cofactor for LPL activity
Apo B-100	Synthesized in the liver and is secreted into the circulation as part of the VLDL. Also serves as the ligand for the LDL receptor mediated hepatic endocytosis.
Lipoprotein lipase	Catalyzes the hydrolysis of plasma triglycerides into free fatty acids
Hepatic lipase	Catalyzes the hydrolysis of triglycerides and phospholipids of the LDL and HDL. It is bound to the surfaces of both hepatic and non hepatic tissues.

0-8493-2705-9/01/$0.00+$1.50

TABLE 3.2

Inherited Disorders of Carbohydrate Metabolism

	Disease	Mutation	Characteristics
Digestion	Lactose intolerance	Lactase	Chronic or intermittent diarrhea, flatulence, nausea, vomiting, growth failure in young children
	Sucrose intolerance	Sucrase	Diarrhea, flatulence, nausea, poor growth in infants
Intestinal transport	Glucose-galactose intolerance	Glucose-galactose carrier	Diarrhea, growth failure in infants, stools contain large quantities of glucose and lactic acid
Interconversion of sugars	Galactosemia	Galactose-1-P-uridyl transferase	Increased cellular content of galactose 1-phosphate, eye cataracts, mental retardation, increased cellular levels of galactitol; three mutations have been reported
		Galactokinase	Cataracts, cellular accumulation of galactose and galactitrol; two mutations have been reported
		Galactoepimerase	No severe symptoms; two mutations have been reported
	Fructosemia	Fructokinase	Fructosuria, fructosemia
		Fructose-1-P-aldolase	Hypoglycemia, vomiting after fructose load, fructosemia, fructosuria; in children: poor growth, jaundice, hyperbilirubinemia, albuminuria, amino-aciduria
		Fructose-1,6-diphosphatase	Hypoglycemia, hepatomegaly, poor muscle tone, increased blood lactate levels
	Pentosuria	NADP-lined xylitol dehydrogenase	Elevated levels of xylose in urine
Glucose catabolism	Hemolytic anemia	Glucose-6-phosphate dehydrogenase	Low erythrocyte levels of NADPH, hemolysis of the erythrocyte
		Pyruvate kinase	Nonspherocytic anemia, accumulation of phosphorylated glucose metabolites in the cell, jaundice in newborn
	Type VII glycogenosis	Phosphofructokinase	Intolerance to exercise, elevated muscle glycogen levels, accumulation of hexose monophosphates in muscle
Gluconeogenesis	Von Gierke's disease (Type I glycogenosis)	Glucose-6-phosphatase	Hypoglycemia, hyperlipemia, brain damage in some patients, excess liver glycogen levels, shortened lifespan, increased glycerol utilization
Glycogen synthesis	Amylopectinosis (Type IV glycogenosis)	Branching enzyme Liver amylo (1,4→1,6)-transglucosidase	Tissue accumulation of long-chain glycogen that is poorly branched, intolerance to exercise
Glycogenolysis	Pompe's disease (Type II glycogenosis)	Lysosomal a-1,4-glucosidase (acid maltase)	Generalized glycogen excess in viscera, muscles, and nervous system, extreme muscular weakness, hepatomegaly, enlarged heart
	Forbe's disease (Type III glycogenosis)	Amylo-1,6-glucosidase (debrancing enzyme)	Tissue accumulation of highly branched, short-chain glycogen, hypoglycemia, acidosis, muscular weakness, enlarged heart

TABLE 3.2 *(Continued)*

Inherited Disorders of Carbohydrate Metabolism

Disease	Mutation	Characteristics
McArdle's disease (Type V glycogenosis)	Muscle phosphorylase	Intolerance to exercise
Her's disease (Type VI glycogenosis)	Liver phosphorylase	Hepatomegaly, increased liver glycogen content, elevated serum lipids, growth retardation
(Type IX glycogenosis)	Phosphorylase kinase	Hepatomegaly, increased liver glycogen levels, decreasd phosphorylase activity in hepatocytes and leukocytes, elevated blood lipids, hypoglycemia after prolonged fasting, increased gluconeogenesis

TABLE 3.3

Genetic Diseases in Lipid Metabolism

Disease	Mutation	Characteristics
Tay-Sachs disease	Hexosaminidase A deficiency	Early death, CNS degeneration, ganglioside GM2 accumulates
Gaucher's disease	Glucocerebrosidase deficiency	Enlarged liver and spleen; erosion of long bones and pelvis; mental retardation; glucocerebroside accumulates
Fabry's disease	α Galactosidase A deficiency	Skin rash, kidney failure, pain in legs and feet, ceramide trihexoside accumulates
Niemann-Pick disease	Sphingomyelinase deficiency	Enlarged liver and spleen, mental retardation, sphingomyelin accumulates
Krabbe's disease (globoid leukodystrophy)	Galactocerebroside deficiency	Mental retardation, absence of myelin
Metachromatic leukodystrophy	Arylsulfatase A deficiency	Mental retardation, sulfatides accumulate
Generalized gangliosidosis	Gmi,Gandioside: β galactosidase deficiency	Mental retardation, enlarged liver
Sandhoff-Jatzkewitz disease	Hexosaminidase A and B deficiency	Same as Tay-Sachs but develops quicker
Fucosidosis	α-L-Fucosidase	Cerebral degeneration, spastic muscles, thick skin
Acetyl CoA carboxylase deficiency	Acetyl CoA carboxylase deficiency	No de novo fatty acid synthesis
Hypercholesterolemia	LDL receptor deficiency	Premature atherosclerosis and death from CVD
Refsum's disease	α hydroxylating enzyme	Neurological problems: deafness, blindness, cerebellar ataxia, phytanic acid accumulates

TABLE 3.4

Genetic Mutations in Enzymes of Amino Acid Metabolism

Disease	Mutation	Characteristics
Maple syrup urine disease	Branched chain keto acid dehydrogenase (Several variants)	Elevated levels of α ketoacids and their metabolites in blood and urine; mental retardation, ketoacidosis, early death
Methylmalonuria	Methylmalonyl CoA mutase (Several variants) Inability to use vitamin B_{12}	High blood levels of methylmalonate; pernicious anemia, early death
Nonketotic hyperglycinemia	Glycine cleavage enzyme	Severe mental retardation, early death, high blood glycine levels
Hypermethioninemia	Methionine adenosyltransferase ($\uparrow$ Km not deficiency per se)	Accumulation of methionine in blood (condition is benign)
Homocysteinemia	Cystathionine synthase	Elevated blood levels of methionine, homocysteine; abnormal collagen (no cross linking); dislocated lenses and other ocular malformations; osteoporosis; mental retardation, thromboembolism and vascular occlusions; short lifespan
Cystathioninuria	Cystathionase	Elevated levels of cystathionine in urine (condition is benign)
Phenylketonuria	Phenylalanine hydroxylase (several variants)	Increased levels of phenylalanine and deaminated metabolites in blood and urine; mental retardation; decreased neurotransmitter synthesis; shortened lifespan
Tyrosinemia	Tyrosine transaminase	Eye and skin lesions, mental retardation
	Fumarylacetoacetate hydrolase	Liver failure, renal failure
	p-hydroxylphenylpyruvate oxidase	Increased need for ascorbic acid
Albinism	Tyrosinase	Lack of melanin (skin pigment) formation; increased sensitivity to sunlight; lack of eye pigment
Alcaptonuria	Homogentisate oxidase	Elevated urine levels of homogentisate; slow deposits of homogentisate in bones, connective tissue and internal organs resulting in gradual darkening of these structures. Increased susceptibility to arthritis
Histidenemia	Histidase	Elevated levels of histidine in blood and urine. Can give false positive result in test for phenylketonuria. Elevated urocanase levels in sweat. Decreased histamine formation.

TABLE 3.5

Mutations that Phenotype as Obesity

Genotype	Species	Phenotype
Estrogen receptor β		
Codons 238-244 — 21 bp deletion	human	obesity[1]
846G to A	human	obesity[1]
1421T to C	human	obesity[1]
1730A to G	human	obesity[1]
POMC (Proopiomelanocortin gene)		
codon 73-74 (btwn. 6997 and 6998)	human	extreme childhood and adolescent obesity[2]
within codon 176 (btwn. 7304 and 7305)	human	extreme childhood and adolescent obesity[2]
G7316T	human	extreme childhood and adolescent obesity[2]
G7341G	human	extreme childhood and adolescent obesity[2]
C6982T	human	extreme childhood and adolescent obesity[2]
C7111G	human	extreme childhood and adolescent obesity[2]
LEP (Leptin gene)		
G144A substitution in codon 48	human	extreme obesity and very low serum leptin levels[3]
G328A substitution in codon 110	human	extreme obesity and very low serum leptin levels[3]
c'some 6-10.5	mouse	obesity[4]
c'some 7-q32	human	obesity[4]
LEPR (Leptin receptor)		
c'some 4-46.7	mouse	obesity[4]
c'some 1-p31	human	obesity[4]
UCP1 (Uncoupling protein)		
Arg/Trp 40	human	juvenile onset obesity[5]
Ala/Thr 64	human	juvenile onset obesity[5]
Val/Met 137	human	juvenile onset obesity[5]
Met/Leu 229	human	juvenile onset obesity[5]
Lys/Asn 257	human	juvenile onset obesity[5]
UCP2 (11q13)	human	obesity[4]
UCP3 (11q13)	human	obesity[4]
MC3R (20q13)	human	obesity[4]
NPYR5 (4q31-q32)	human	obesity[4]
MSTN (2q32.1)	human	obesity[4]
Chromosome 2p12-13	human	Alstrom Syndrome (retinal pigment degeneration, neurogenic deafness, infantile obesity, hyperlipidemia, NIDDM[6]
fa mutation		
269Gln to Pro	Zucker rat	Obesity: Severe insulin resistance, hyperinsulinemia, hyperglycemia, hyperlipidemia, hypercortisolemia[7]
Ob-Rb (269Gln to Pro)	Zucker rat	Obesity: Decreased cell-surface expression and decreased leptin binding affinity[7]
C57 BLKS/J-Lepr^{db}/Lepr^{db}	mouse	hyperphagia, obesity, hyperinsulinemia, hyperglycemia[8]
Gsalpha		
R258W	human	Albright hereditary osteodystrophy: skeletal abnormalities and obesity[9]
R258A	human	Albright hereditary osteodystrophy: skeletal abnormalities and obesity[9]
PPARg2		
Pro115Gln	human	extreme obesity[10]
CPE (carboxypeptidase E)	mouse	hyperproinsulinemia, late onset obesity, diabetes[11]
IRS 1 (insulin receptor substrate) S13 and 972	human	NIDDM and obesity[12]
Beta3 AR 64 (Beta 3 adrenergic receptor)	human	NIDDM and obesity[12]
OB D75514 — D7S530	human	NIDDM, obesity, hypertension, and insulin resistance[13]

TABLE 3.5 *(Continued)*

Mutations that Phenotype as Obesity

Genotype	Species	Phenotype
Insulin receptor gene		
Ile1153Met	human	obesity, insulin resistance, hypoandrogenism, acanthosis nigricans[14]
ASIP (agouti signaling protein)		
2-88.8	mouse	obesity[4]
20q11.2-q12	human	obesity[4]
TUB (tubby)		
c'some 7-51.45	mouse	obesity[4]
c'some 11p15.4-p15.5	human	obesity[4]
TNFA (tumor necrosis factor)		
c'some 17-19.1	mouse	obesity[4]
c'some 6p21.3	human	obesity[4]
4p16.3 (autosomal dominant)	human	obesity — Achondroplasia[15]
20q11 (autosomal dominant)	human	obesity — Posterior Polymorphous Corneal Dystrophy[15]
15q11.2-q12(autosomal dominant)	human	obesity — Prader-Willi Syndrome[15]
12q23-q24.1(autosomal dominant)	human	obesity — Schinzel Syndrome[15]
11q13 (autosomal recessive)	human	obesity — BBS 1 (Bardet-Biedl Syn)[15]
16q21 (autosomal recessive)	human	obesity — BBS2[15]
3p13-p12 (autosomal recessive)	human	obesity — BBS3[15]
15q22.3-q23(autosomal recessive)	human	obesity — BBS4[15]
8q22-q23(autosomal recessive)	human	obesity — Cohen Syndrome (CHS1)[15]
Xq26-q27 (X linked)	human	obesity — Borjeson-Forssman-Lehman[15]
Xq21 **(X linked)**	human	obesity[15]
Xq21.1-q22 **(X linked)**	human	obesity — Wilson-Turner Syndrome[15]
Xq26 **(X linked)**	human	obesity — Simpson-Golabi Behmel [15]
HSD3B1 (1p13.1)	human	obesity[15]
ATP1A2 (1q21-q23)	human	obesity[15]
ACP1 (2p25)	human	obesity[15]
APOB (2p24-p23)	human	obesity[15]
APOD (3q27-qter)	human	obesity[15]
UCP (4q28-q31)	human	obesity[15]
TNFir24 (6p21.3)	human	obesity[15]
LPL (8p22)	human	obesity[15]
ADRB3 (8p12-p11.1)	human	obesity[15]
SUR (11p15.1)	human	obesity[15]
DRD2 (11q22.2-q22.3)	human	obesity[15]
APOA4 (11q23-qter)	human	obesity[15]
LDLR (19p13.2)	human	obesity[15]

1.Rosenkranz, K, Hinney, A, Ziegler, A, et al. *J Clin Endocrinol Metab* 83: 4524; 1998.
2. Hinney, A, Becker, I, Heibut, O, et al. *J Endocrinol Metab* 83: 3737; 1998.
3. Karvonen, MK, Pesonen, U, Heinonen, P, et al. *J Endocrinol Metab* 83: 3239; 1998.
4. Comuzzie, AG, Allison, DB, *Science* 280: 1374; 1998.
5. Urhammer, SA, Fridberg, M, Sorensen, TI, et al., *J Clin Endocrinol Metab* 82: 4069; 1997.
6. Macari, F, Lautier, C, Girardet, A, *Hum Genet* 103: 658; 1998.
7. da Silva, BA, Bjorbaek, C, Uotani, S, Flier, JS, *Endocrinology* 139: 3681; 1998.
8. Igel, M, Becker, W, Herberg, L, Joost, HG, *Endocrinology* 138: 4234; 1997.
9. Warner, DR, Weng, G, Yu, S, et al. *J Biol Chem* 273: 23976; 1998.
10. Ristow, M, Muller-Wieland, D, Pfeiffer, A, et al. *N Eng J Med* 339: 953; 1998.
11. Utsunomiya, N, Ohagi, S, Sanke, T, et al. *Diabetologia* 41: 701; 1998.
12. Zhang, Y, Wat, N, Stratton, IM, et al. *Diabetologia* 39: 1505; 1996.
13. Hani, EH, Boutin, P, Durand, E, et al. *Diabetologia* 41: 1511; 1998.
14. Cama, A, Sierra, ML, Ottini, L, *J Clin Endocrinol Metab* 73: 894; 1991.
15. Perusse, L, Chagnon, YC, Dionne, FT, Bouchard, C, *Obesity Res* 5: 1225; 1996.

TABLE 3.6

Mutations that Phenotype as Heart Disease

Genotype	Species	Phenotype
LPL gene		
G188E (exon 5)	human	High plasma TG — heart disease[1]
P207L (exon 5)	human	High plasma TG — heart disease[1]
D250N (exon 6)	human	High plasma TG — heart disease[1]
Homocysteine gene		
373C/T = R125W(autosomal recessive)	human	Homocystinuria[2]
456C/G = I152M (autosomal recessive)	human	Homocystinuria[2]
494G/A = C165Y(autosomal recessive)	human	Homocystinuria[2]
539T/C = V180A(autosomal recessive)	human	Homocystinuria[2]
833T/C = I278T(autosomal recessive)	human	Homocystinuria[2]
1105C/T = R369C(autosomal recessive)	human	Homocystinuria[2]
1111G/A = V137M(autosomal recessive)	human	Homocystinuria[2]
1301 C/A = T434N(autosomal recessive)	human	Homocystinuria[2]
1330 G/A = D444N(autosomal recessive)	human	Homocystinuria[2]
1471 C/T = R491C(autosomal recessive)	human	Homocystinuria[2]
MTHR gene		
792+1G to A/?	human	Hyperhomocysteinemia/Hypomethioninemia[3]
G458T/G458T	human	Hyperhomocysteinemia/Hypomethioninemia[3]
C692T/C692T	human	Hyperhomocysteinemia/Hypomethioninemia[3]
C559T/C559T	human	Hyperhomocysteinemia/Hypomethioninemia[3]
249-IG to T/G164C	human	Hyperhomocysteinemia/Hypomethioninemia[3]
G428A/?	human	Hyperhomocysteinemia/Hypomethioninemia[3]
C985T/C985T	human	Hyperhomocysteinemia/Hypomethioninemia[3]
G167A/C1015T	human	Hyperhomocysteinemia/Hypomethioninemia[3]
C559T/C559T	human	Hyperhomocysteinemia/Hypomethioninemia[3]
C764T/C764T	human	Hyperhomocysteinemia/Hypomethioninemia[3]
G167A/C1081T	human	Hyperhomocysteinemia/Hypomethioninemia[3]
T980C/C1141T	human	Hyperhomocysteinemia/Hypomethioninemia[3]
C559T/N	human	Hyperhomocysteinemia/Hypomethioninemia[3]
833T to C = I278T	human	Mild hyperhomocysteinuria[2]
677C to T (A to V)	human	Mild hyperhomocysteinuria[2]
4p16.1 (btwn. D4S2957 and D4S827)	human	Ellis van Creveld Syn (cardiac malformations)[4]
9q31		
TD1 = G1764del to Stop (autosomal recessive)	human	Tangier disease — premature CAD[5]
TD2 = 3' del (autosomal recessive)	human	Tangier disease — premature CAD[5]
TD3 = N875S (autosomal recessive)	human	Tangier disease — premature CAD[5]
TD4 = A877V (autosomal recessive)	human	Tangier disease — premature CAD[5]
TD5 = W530S (autosomal recessive)	human	Tangier disease — premature CAD[5]
LDLR gene		
Missense C240 to F (Cys to Phe) Exon 5	human	Hypercholesterolemia/Premature CVD[6]
Missense G5218 to D (Gly to Asp) Exon 11	human	Hypercholesterolemia/Premature CVD[6]
Nonsense C122 to X (Cys to stop) Exon 4A	human	Hypercholesterolemia/Premature CVD[6]
Nonsense C122 to X (Cys to stop) Exon 4A	human	Hypercholesterolemia/Premature CVD[6]
Missense E187 to K (Glu to Lys) Exon 4B	human	Hypercholesterolemia/Premature CVD[6]
Missense C356 to Y (Cys to Tyr) Exon 8	human	Hypercholesterolemia/Premature CVD[6]
Nonsense C122 to X (Cys to stop) Exon 4A	human	Hypercholesterolemia/Premature CVD[6]
Nonsense C122 to X (Cys to stop) Exon 4A	human	Hypercholesterolemia/Premature CVD[6]
Missense w66 to G (Trp to Gly) Exon 3	human	Hypercholesterolemia/Premature CVD[6]
Missense W66 to G (Trp to Gly) Exon3	human	Hypercholesterolemia/Premature CVD[6]
Missense 187E to K (Glu to Lys) Exon 4B	human	Hypercholesterolemia/Premature CVD[6]
Missense W66 to G (Trp to Gly) exon 3	human	Hypercholesterolemia/Premature CVD[6]
Insertion 785insG (frameshift) Exon 17	human	Hypercholesterolemia/Premature CVD[6]
Missense W66 to G (Trp to Gly) Exon 3	human	Hypercholesterolemia/Premature CVD[6]
Deletion 165delG (frameshift) Exon 4A	human	Hypercholesterolemia/Premature CVD[6]
Missense D245 to E (Asp to Glu) Exon 5	human	Hypercholesterolemia/Premature CVD[6]

TABLE 3.6 *(Continued)*

Mutations that Phenotype as Heart Disease

Genotype	Species	Phenotype
C-45T in promoter	human	Hypercholesterolemia/Premature CAD[7]
Trp66Gly	human	Hypercholesterolemia/Premature CAD[7]
Cys68Tyr	human	Hypercholesterolemia/Premature CAD[7]
Cys88Tyr	human	Hypercholesterolemia/Premature CAD[7]
Glu387Lys	human	Hypercholesterolemia/Premature CAD[7]
Ala519Thr	human	Hypercholesterolemia/Premature CAD[7]
Ala585Ser	human	Hypercholesterolemia/Premature CAD[7]
Pro587Arg	human	Hypercholesterolemia/Premature CAD[7]
Phe598Leu	human	Hypercholesterolemia/Premature CAD[7]
Trp599Arg	human	Hypercholesterolemia/Premature CAD[7]
Arg723Gln	human	Hypercholesterolemia/Premature CAD[7]
Cys660stop	human	Hypercholesterolemia[8]
Asp206Glu	human	Hypercholesterolemia[8]
Val208Met	human	Hypercholesterolemia[8]
DelGly197	human	Hypercholesterolemia[8]
Glu80toLys	human	Hypercholesterolemia[8]
Asp206toGlu	human	Hypercholesterolemia[8]
Tyr807Lys	human	Hypercholesterolemia[8]
Glu207Lys	human	Hypercholesterolemia[8]
Pro664Leu	human	Hypercholesterolemia[8]
CBS gene		
G919 to A	human	Homocystinuria[9]
Elastin Gene		
7q11.23	human	Williams Syn (Supravalvular aortic stenosis)[10]
11p15.5	human	Long QT Syn (congenital heart & vascular disease)[10]
7q35-36	human	Long QT Syn (congenital heart & vascular disease)[10]
3p21-24	human	Long QT Syn (congenital heart & vascular disease)[10]
Paraoxonase gene		
Leu 54 to Met	human	CVD[11]
Troponin T gene		
Ile79Asn	human	Hypertrophic cardiomyopathy[12]
Arg92Gln	human	Hypertrophic cardiomyopathy[12]
Phe110Ile	human	Hypertrophic cardiomyopathy[12]
Glu163Lys	human	Hypertrophic cardiomyopathy[12]
Glu244Asp	human	Hypertrophic cardiomyopathy[12]
Arg278Cys	human	Hypertrophic cardiomyopathy[12]
Alpha Tropomyosin gene		
Asp175Asn	human	Hypertrophic cardiomyopathy[12]
Myosin gene		
Arg403Gln	human	Hypertrophic cardiomyopathy[12]
Arg453Gln	human	Hypertrophic cardiomyopathy[12]
Arg719Trp	human	Hypertrophic cardiomyopathy[12]
Val606Met	human	Hypertrophic cardiomyopathy[12]
Phe513Cys	human	Hypertrophic cardiomyopathy[12]
Leu908Val	human	Hypertrophic cardiomyopathy[12]
ApoB gene		
Arg3500 to Gln	human	hypercholesterolemia/peripheral vascular disease[13]
arg3531 to Cys	human	hypercholesterolemia/peripheral vascular disease[13]
Glu to Lys 4154	human	CAD[14]
Arg to Glu 3611	human	CAD[14]

TABLE 3.6 *(Continued)*

Mutations that Phenotype as Heart Disease

Genotype	Species	Phenotype
11 βHSD		
R208C	human	hypertension[15]
R213C	human	hypertension[15]
L250P	human	hypertension[15]
L251S	human	hypertension[15]
R337H	human	hypertension[15]
Y338	human	hypertension[15]
hBENaC		
C to T at Arg 564 (autosomal dominant)	human	Liddle's Syn (hypertension)[16]
Bradykinin receptor (14q32)		
845C/T	human	CVD[17]
704C/T	human	CVD[17]
649insG	human	CVD[17]
640T/C	human	CVD[17]
536T/C	human	CVD[17]
412C/G	human	CVD[17]
143C/T	human	CVD[17]
78C/T	human	CVD[17]
Transcription factor NKX2-5		
Thr178Met	human	Congenital heart disease[18]
Gln170ter	human	Congenital heart disease[18]
Gln198ter	human	Congenital heart disease[18]

1. Julien, P, Vohl, MC, Gaudet, D, et al. *Diabetes* 46: 2063; 1997.
2. Kluijtmans, LA, van den Heuvel, LP, Boers, GH, et al. *Am J Hum Genet* 58: 35; 1996.
3. Goyette, P, Christensen, B, Rosenblatt, DS, Rozen, R. *Am J Hum Genet* 59: 1268; 1996.
4. Howard, TD, Guttmacher, AE, McKinnon, W, et al. *Am J Hum Genet* 61: 1405; 1997.
5. Bodzioch, 1999.
6. Eckstrom, U, Abrahamsoon, M, Wallmark, A, et al. *Eur J Clin Invest* 28: 740; 1998.
7. Sun, XM, Patel, DD, Knight, BL, Soutar, AK. *Atherosclerosis* 136: 175; 1998.
8. Soutar, AK, *J Intern Med* 231: 633; 1992.
9. Folsom, AR, Nieto, FJ, McGovern, PG, et al. *J Clin Invest* 98(3): 204; 1998.
10. Keating, MT, *Circulation* 92: 142; 1995.
11. Garin, MC, James, RW, Dussoix, P, et al. *J Clin Invest* 99: 62; 1997.
12. Watkins, H, McKenna, WJ, Thierfelder, HJ, et al. *N Eng J Med* 332: 1058; 1995.
13. Pullinger, CR, Hennessy, LK, Chatterton, JE, et al. *J Clin Invest* 95: 1225; 1995.
14. Genest, JJ, Ordovas, JM, McNamara, JR, et al. *Atherosclerosis* 82: 7; 1990.
15. Mune, T, Rogerson, RM, Nikkila, H, et al. *Nat Genet* 10: 394; 1995.
16. Shimkets, RA, Warnock, DG, Bositis, CM. *Cell* 79: 407; 1994.
17. Erdmann, J, Hegemann, N, Weidemann, A, et al. *Am J Med Genet* 80: 521; 1998.
18. Schott, JJ, Benson, DW, Basson, CT, et al. *Science* 281: 108; 1998.

TABLE 3.7

Mutations that Phenotype as Diabetes

Genotype	Species	Phenotype
PC1 (prohormone convertase 1)		
Gly483Arg	human	Extreme childhood obesity, abnormal glucose homeostasis[1]
PC2 (prohormone convertase 2)	mouse	NIDDM: elevation of proinsulin level and/or proinsulin/insulin ratio[2]
PC3 (prohormone convertase 3)	mouse	NIDDM: elevation of proinsulin level and/or proinsulin/insulin ratio[2]

TABLE 3.7 *(Continued)*
Mutations that Phenotype as Diabetes

Genotype	Species	Phenotype
GCK (glucokinase)		NIDDM: low prevalence of micro-and macrovascular complications of diabetes[3]
A53S	human	MODY[4]
G80A	human	MODY[4]
H137R	human	MODY[4]
T168P	human	MODY[4]
M210T	human	MODY[4]
C213R	human	MODY[4]
V226M	human	MODY[4]
S336L	human	MODY[4]
V367M	human	MODY[4]
E248X	human	MODY[4]
S360X	human	MODY[4]
V401del1	human	MODY[4]
L1221G to T	human	MODY[4]
K161+2del10	human	MODY[4]
R186X	human	MODY[4]
G261R	human	MODY[4]
G279T	human	MODY[5]
Ala188Thr (autosomal dominant)	human	NIDDM[6]
7p (alleles z+4, z+2, Z22) (autosomal dominant)	human	NIDDM[7]
IRS 1 (insulin receptor substrate)		
S13 and 972	human	NIDDM and obesity[8]
Beta3 AR 64 (Beta 3 adrenergic receptor)	human	NIDDM and obesity[8]
OB D75514 — D7S530	human	NIDDM, obesity, hypertension, and insulin resistance[9]
Insulin receptor gene		
Codon 897 — nonsense mutation	human	Leprechaun/Minn 1:Leprechaunism-intrauterine growth retardation, extreme insulin resistance Death usually occurs before age 1.[10]
Glu460Lys	human	Leprechaun/Ark-1 Leprechaunism — intrauterine growth retardation, extreme insulin resistance Death usually occurs before age 1[10]
Leu233Pro	human	insulin resistance/NIDDM[10]
Phe382Val	human	insulin resistance/NIDDM[10]
Lys460Glu	human	insulin resistance/NIDDM[10]
Gln672stop	human	insulin resistance/NIDDM[10]
Arg735Ser	human	insulin resistance/NIDDM[10]
Arg897stop	human	insulin resistance/NIDDM[10]
Gly1008Val	human	insulin resistance/NIDDM[10]
Trp1200Ser	human	insulin resistance/NIDDM[10]
Val382Ser	human	Rabson-Mendenhall Syndrome — insulin resistance (NIDDM), abnormalities of teeth, nails, and pineal hyperplasia[10]
Amber133/Ser462	human	NIDDM, acanthosis nigricans, hypoandrogenism[11]
Ser735	human	NIDDM, acanthosis nigricans, hypoandrogenism[11]
Thr1134Ala	human	NIDDM, acanthosis nigricans, hypoandrogenism[11]
Arg209His	human	Leprechaun/Winnipeg — leprechaunism, extreme insulin resistance (NIDDM)[12]

TABLE 3.7 *(Continued)*

Mutations that Phenotype as Diabetes

Genotype	Species	Phenotype
Asn15Lys	human	Rabson-Mendenhall Syndrome — insulin resistance (NIDDM), abnormalities of teeth, nails, and pineal hyperplasia[12]
Asn462Ser	human	NIDDM — extreme insulin resistance, acanthosis nigricans, Hyperandrogenism[12]
Trp133stop	human	NIDDM[12]
His209Arg	human	NIDDM[12]
Arg1000stop	human	NIDDM[12]
Gly996Val	human	NIDDM and acanthosis nigricans[13]
Glu 1135/WT	human	type A extreme insulin resistance[14]
Ile 1153	human	type A extreme insulin resistance[14]
Del exon 3/WT	human	type A extreme insulin resistance[14]
Del codon 1109/WT	human	type A extreme insulin resistance[14]
Glu993/Opal 1000	human	type A extreme insulin resistance[14]
Leu 1178/WT	human	type A extreme insulin resistance[14]
Ser 1200	human	type A extreme insulin resistance[14]
Lys15/Opal 1000	human	type A extreme insulin resistance[14]
AG to GG (intron4)	human	type A extreme insulin resistance[14]
Glu460/Amber 672	human	type A extreme insulin resistance[14]
Pro223	human	type A extreme insulin resistance[14]
Arg31	human	type A extreme insulin resistance[14]
Opal897	human	type A extreme insulin resistance[14]
Del codon 1109/Met910	human	type A extreme insulin resistance[14]
Ala28/Arg366	human	type A extreme insulin resistance[14]
KIR6.2		
E23R	human	NIDDM[15]
L270V	human	NIDDM[15]
I337V	human	NIDDM[15]
20q12-q13.1	human	MODY 1[16]
7p15-p13	human	MODY 2[16]
12q24.2	human	MODY 3[16]
13q12.1	human	MODY 4[16]
17cen-q21.3	human	MODY 5[16]
HNF1 alpha		
G31D	human	NIDDM- defective insulin secretion[17]
R159W	human	NIDDM- defective insulin secretion[17]
A161T	human	NIDDM- defective insulin secretion[17]
R200W	human	NIDDM- defective insulin secretion[17]
R271W	human	NIDDM- defective insulin secretion[17]
IVS5nt+2T to A	human	NIDDM- defective insulin secretion[17]
P379fsdelT	human	NIDDM- defective insulin secretion[17]
G292fsdelG	human	MODY[18]
Y122C	human	MODY[18]
R159Q	human	MODY[18]
S142F	human	MODY[18]
R55G56fsdelGACGG	human	MODY[18]
Q7X	human	MODY[18]
R171X	human	MODY[18]
P291fsdelC	human	MODY[18]
A443fsddCA	human	MODY[19]
P129T	human	MODY[19]

TABLE 3.7 *(Continued)*
Mutations that Phenotype as Diabetes

Genotype	Species	Phenotype
R131W	human	MODY[19]
R159W	human	MODY[19]
P519L	human	MODY[19]
T620I	human	MODY[19]
I128N	human	MODY[20]
H143Y	human	MODY[20]
P447L	human	MODY[20]
A559fsinsA	human	MODY[20]
CD38 gene		
Arg140Trp	human	Type II diabetes mellitus[21]
Insulin gene		
ValA3Leu (autosomal dominant)	human	mild diabetes or glucose intolerance[22]
PheB24Ser (autosomal dominant)	human	mild diabetes or glucose intolerance[22]
PheB25Leu (autosomal dominant)	human	mild diabetes or glucose intolerance[22]
His 65 (autosomal dominant)	human	mild diabetes or glucose intolerance[22]
Xaa 65 (autosomal dominant)	human	mild diabetes or glucose intolerance[23]
AspB10 (autosomal dominant)	human	mild diabetes or glucose intolerance[23]
mGPDH gene		
ACA:Thr243-ACG:Thr243	human	NIDDM[24]
CAT: His264-CGT: Arg264	human	NIDDM[24]
GCA:Ala305-GCC:Ala305	human	NIDDM[24]
GCA:Ala306-TCA:Ser306	human	NIDDM[24]
4p16 between D4S432 and D4S431	human	Wolfram Syn (DM, DI, optic atrophy, deafness)[25]
Mitochondrial DNA mutations(phenotype depends on % mutation in the heteroplasmic individual) [26,27]		
tRNA $^{Leu\ (UUR)}$		
A3423G,A3252G,C3256T, T3271C, T3290C, T3291C	human	NIDDM and deafness
ND 1		
G3316A, A3348G, T3394C, T3396C, G3423T,A3434G, G3438A, A3447G, A3480G G3483A, T4216	human	Diabetes with varying degrees of severity; CNS, Muscle, heart, and kidney involvement
ND2		
A4917	human	same as above
tRNA^{cys}		
C5780A	human	same as above
tRNA^{ser}		
C7476T	human	same as above
COX II		
A8245G,G8251A	human	same as above
tRNA^{lys}		
A8344G	human	same as above
ATPase 6,8 (genes overlap on the mt genome)		
T8993G or C, A8860G,G8894A	human	same as above
G8204A, C8289T	rat	same as above but milder
ND3		
C10398T, T11778C	human	same as above
ND4		
T11778C	human	same as above
tRNA ^{glu}		
T14709C	human	same as above

TABLE 3.7 *(Continued)*

Mutations that Phenotype as Diabetes

Genotype	Species	Phenotype
TRNAthr		
C15904T, A15924G, G15927A	human	same as above
G15928A		
D-loop		
C16069T,T16093C,C16126T	human	same as above

1. Jackson, RS, Creemers, JW, Ohagi, S, et al. *Nat Genet* 16: 303; 1997.
2. Utsunomiya, N, Ohagi, S, Sanke, T, et al. *Diabetologia* 41: 701; 1998.
3. Froguel, P, Vaxillaire, M, Velho, G. *Diabetes Rev* 5: 123; 1997.
4. Velho, G, Blanche, H, Vaxillaire, M, et al. *Diabetologia* 40 : 217; 1997.
5. Vionnet, N, Stoffel, M, Takeda, J, et al. *Nature* 356: 721; 1992.
6. Shimada, F, Makino, H, Hashimoto, H. *Diabetologia* 36: 433; 1993.
7. Hattersley, AT, Turner, RC, Permutt, MA. *Lancet* 339:1307; 1993.
8. Zhang, Y, Wat, N, Stratton, IM, et al. *Diabetologia* 39: 1505; 1996.
9. Shitani, M, Ikegami, H, Yamato, E, et al. *Diabetologia* 39: 1398; 1996.
10. Taylor, SI, Kadowaki, H, Accili, D, et al. *Diab Care* 13: 257; 1990.
11. Cama, A, Sierra, ML, Ottini, L. *J Clin Endocrinol Metab* 73: 894; 1991.
12. Kadowaki, T, Kadowaki, H, Rechler, MM. *J Clin Invest* 86: 254; 1990.
13. Odawara, M, Kadowaki, T, Yamamoto, R. *Science* 245: 66; 1989.
14. Taylor, SI, Cama, A, Accili, D, et al. *Endocr Rev* 13: 566; 1992.
15. Hani, EH, Boutin, P, Durand, E, et al. *Diabetologia* 41: 1511; 1998.
16. Chevre, JC, Hani, EH, Boutin, P, et al. *Diabetologia* 41: 1017; 1998.
17. Velho, G, Froguel, P, *Endocrinology* 138: 233; 1998.
18. Vaxillaire, M, Rouard, M, Yamagata, K, et al. *Hum Mol Genet* 6: 583; 1997.
19. Frayling, TM, Bulamn, MP, Ellard, S, et al. *Diabetes* 46: 720; 1997.
20. Hansen, T, Eiberg, H, Rouard, M, et al. *Diabetes* 46: 726; 1997.
21. Yagui, K, Shimada, F, Mimura, M, et al. *Diabetologia* 41: 1024; 1998.
22. Steiner, DF, Tager, HS, Chan, SJ, et al. *Diabetes Care* 13: 600; 1990.
23. DeFronzo, RA, *Diabetes Rev* 5; 177; 1997.
24. Strom, TM, Hortnagel, K, Hofmann, S, et al. *Hum Mol Genet* 7: 2021; 1998.
25. van den Ouweland, JMW, Lemkes, HHPJ, Ruitenbeek, W, et al. *Nat Genet* 1: 368; 1992.
26. Mathews, CE, Berdanier, CD. *Proc Soc Exp Biol Med* 219: 97; 1998.

TABLE 3.8

Normal Values for Micronutrients in Blood

Ascorbic acid, plasma	0.6–1.6 mg/dl	Phosphorus	3.4–4.5 mg/dl
Calcium, serum	4.5–5.3 meq/l	Potassium	3.5–5.0 meq/l
β-Carotene, serum	40–200 μg/dl	Riboflavin, red cell	>14.9 μg/dl cells
Chloride, serum	95–103 meq/l	Folate, plasma	>6 ng/ml
Lead, whole blood	0–50 μg/dl	Pantothenic acid, plasma	≥6 μg/dl
Magnesium, serum	1.5–2.5 meq/l	Pantothenic acid, whole blood	≥80 μg/dl
Sodium, plasma	136–142 meq/l	Biotin, whole blood	>25 ng/ml
Sulfate, serum	0.2–1.3 meq/l	B_{12}, plasma	>150 pg/ml
Vitamin A, serum	15–60 μg/dl	Vitamin D 25(OH)–D_3, plasma	>10 ng/ml
Retinol, plasma	>20 μg/dl	α-Tocopherol, plasma	>0.80 mg/dl

Note: For more information on blood analysis see: NHANES Manual for Nutrition Assessment, CDC, Atlanta, GA (contact Elaine Gunter); ICNND Manual for Nutrition Surveys, 2nd ed., 1963, U.S. Government Printing Office, Washington, D.C.; Sauberlich et al., 1974, *Laboratory Tests for the Assessment of Nutritional Status,* CRC Press, Boca Raton, FL.

TABLE 3.9

Normal Clinical Values for Constituents of Blood

	Common Units or SI Units
Ammonia	22-39 umol/L
Calcium	8.5-10.5 mg/dl or 2.25-2.65 mmol/L
Carbon dioxide	24-30 meq/l or 24-29 mmol/L
Chloride	100-106 meq/L or mmol/L
Copper	100-200 µg/dl or 16-31 µmol/L
Iron	50-150 µg/dl or 11.6-31.3 µmol/L
Lead	50 µg/dl or less
Magnesium	1.5-2.0 meq/L or 0.75-1.25 mmol/L
P CO_2	35-40 mm Hg
pH	7.35-7.45
Phosphorus	3.0-4.5 mg/dl or 1-1.5 mmol/L
PO_2	75-100 mm Hg
Potassium	3.5-5.0 meq/L or 2.5-5.0 mmol/L
Sodium	135-145 meq/L or 135-145 mmol/L
Acetoaetate	less than 2 mmol
Ascorbic adic	0.4-15 mg/dl or 23-85 µmol/L
Bilirubin	0.4-0.6 mg/dl or 1.71-6.84 µmol/L
Carotinoids	0.8-4.0 µg/ml
Creatinine	0.6-1.5 mg/dl or 60-130 µmol/L
Lactic acid	0.6-1.8 meq/L or 0.44-1.28 µmol/L
Cholesterol	120-220 mg/dl or 3.9-7.3 mmol/L
Triglycerides	40-150 mg/dl or 6-18 mmol/L
Pyruvic acid	0-0.11 meq/L or 79.8-228 µmol/L
Urea nitrogen	8-25 mg/dl or 2.86-7.14 mmol/L
Uric acid	3.0-7.0 mg/dl or 0.18-0.29 mmol/L
Albumin	3.5-5.0 g/dl
Insulin	6-20 µU/dl
Glucose	70-100 mg/dl or 4-6 mmol/L

TABLE 3.10

Normal Values for Micronutrients in Urine

Calcium, mg/24 hr	100–250
Chloride, meq/24 hr	110–250
Copper, µg/24 hr	0–100
Lead, µg/24 hr	< 100
Phosphorus, g/24 hr	0.9–1.3
Potassium, meq/24 hr	25–100
Sodium, meq/24 hr	130–260
Zinc, mg/24 hr	0.15–1.2
Creatinine, mg/kg bodyweight	15–25
Riboflavin, µg/g creatinine	> 80
Niacin metabolite,[a] µg/g creatinine	> 1.6
Pyridoxine, µg/g creatinine	≥ 20
Biotin, µg/24 hr	> 25
Pantothenic acid, mg/24 hr	≥ 1
Folate, FIGLU[b] after histidine load	< 5 mg/8 hr
B_{12}, methylmalonic acid after a valine load	≤ 2 mg/24 hr

Note: For more information on urine analyses see: ICNNO, 1963, *Manual for Nutrition Surveys*, 2nd ed., U.S. Government Printing Office, Washington, D.C.; Sauberlich et al., 1974, *Laboratory Tests for the Assessment of Nutritional Status*, CRC Press, Boca Raton, FL; NHANES Manual for Nutrition Assessment, CDC, Atlanta, GA; Gibson, R.S., 1990. *Principles of Nutrition Assessment*, Oxford University Press, New York.

[a] N^1-methylnicotinamide.

[b] Formiminoglutamic acid.

TABLE 3.11

Normal Clinical Values for Constituents of Human Urine

Constituent	Content
Aldosterone	2–26 μg/24 hr; 5.5–72 nmol/d
Catecholamines (total)	< 100 μg/24 hr
Epinephrine	< 10 μg/24 hr; <100 nmol/d
Norepinephrine	< 100 μg/24 hr; <590 nmol/d
Cortisol, free	20–100 μg/24 hr; 0.55–2.76 μmol/d
11,17-Hydroxycorticoids	men: 4–12 μg/24 hr; women, 4–8 μg/24 hr
17-Ketosteroids	<8 yrs: 0–2 mg/24 hr; 9–20 yrs: 2–20 mg/24
Metanephrine	< 1.3 mg/24 hr; 6.6 umol/d
Vanillylmandilic acid	< 7 mg/24 hr; < 35 μmol/d
Lead	< 80 μg/24 hr; 0.4 μmol/d
Sodium	190 mmol/l
Potassium	70 mol/l
Chloride	200 mmol/l
Phosphate (PO_4)	35 mmol/l
Phosphorus	22.5 mmol/g creatinine/l urine
Sulfate (SO_4)	21–34 mmol/l
Calcium	204 ± 73 mg/24 hr; 1.25–12.5 mmol/24 hr
Iodine	>50 μg/g creatinine
Chromium	3.27–3.85 nmol/l
Manganese	7–10.6 nmol/24 hr
Urea	330–580 mmol/l (depends on diet)
Uric acid	0.4–5.8 mmol/l
Amino nitrogen	19–31 mmol/l (depends on diet)
Ammonia	29–72 mmol/l (depends on diet)
Creatinine	9.5–28.5 mmol/l
Porphyrins	
D aminolevulinic acid	1.5–7.5 mg/24 hr; 11–57 umol/d
Coproporphyrin	< 230 μg/24 hr; < 350 nmol/d
Uroporphyrin	< 50 μg/24 hr; < 60 nmol/d
Porphobilinogen	< 2 mg/24 hr; 8.8 μmol/d
Urobilinogen	< 2.5 mg/24 hr; 70–470 μmol/d
Vitamins (well nourished adult subjects)	
Riboflavin	> 120 μg/24 hr
Niacin	> 66 μg/g creatinine
B_6	> 20 μg/g creatinine
Methylmalonic acid (B_{12} deficient)	>5.0 ug/mg creatinine
Gla:creatinine (K deficient)	Men: 3.16 ± 0.06; women 3.83±0.08
Specific gravity of urine	1.003–1.030
pH	5.5–7.0

Note: Values were from: Sauberlich, HE *Assessment of Nutritional Status*, 2nd Edition CRC Press, Boca Raton, 1999; Banks, P, Bartley, W, Birt, LM, *The Biochemistry of Tissues* 2nd Edition John Wiley 1976; and Murray, RK, Granner, DK, Mayes, PA, Rodwell, *VW Harper's Biochemistry* 24th Edition Appleton & Lange, 1996.

TABLE 3.12

Retinol Binding Proteins

Acronym	Protein	Molecular Weight	Location	Function
RBP	Retinol binding protein	21,000	Plasma	Transports all-*trans* retinol from intestinal absorption site to target tissues
CRBP	Cellular retinol binding protein	14,600	Cells of target tissue	Transports all-*trans* retinol from plasma membrane to organelles within the cell
CRBP II	Cellular retinol binding protein Type II	16,000	Absorptive cells of small intestine	Transports all-*trans* retinol from absorptive sites on plasma membrane of mucosal cells
CRABP	Cellular retinoic acid binding protein	14,600	Cells of target tissue	Transports all-*trans* retinoic acid to the nucleus
CRALBP	Cellular retinal binding protein	33,000	Specific cells in the eye	Transports 11-*cis* retinal and 11-*cis* retinol as part of the visual cycle
IRBP	Interphotoreceptor or interstitial retinol binding protein	144,000	Retina	Transports all-*trans* retinol and 11-*cis* retinal in the retina extracellular space
RAR	Nuclear retinoic acid receptor, 3 main forms (α, β, γ)		All cells α-liver β-brain γ-liver, kidney, lung	Binds retinoic acid and regions of DNA having the GGTCA sequence
RXR	Nuclear retinoic acid receptors, multiple forms			

TABLE 3.13

Drugs that Alter Nutritional State

Drug	Effect
Spironolactone	Increases need for vitamin A
Thiazides	Increases potassium excretion
Cholestyramine	Increases fecal excretion of cholesterol, vitamin A, B_{12}, folacin
Colestipol	Increases fecal excretion of bile acids, cholesterol, Vitamin A, K, & D
Phenolphthalein	Increases fecal excretion of ingesta (laxative effect) also affects availability of vitamins A, D, K and increases potassium loss
Phenytoin, dilantin	Impairs use of folate
Coumarin, dicoumarol	Interferes with vitamin K in its role in coagulation
Cyclosporin	Interferes with vitamin K metabolism
Isoniazid	Increases need for niacin and B_6
Sulfasalazine	Increases need for folacin
p-aminosalicylic acid	Increases need for vitamin B_{12}
Neomycin	Increases need for vitamin B_{12}
Tetracycline	Interferes with uptake of calcium, magnesium, iron, and zinc
EDTA	Binds divalent ions in the intestine thus decreasing availability
Phenylbutazone	Increases niacin need
Penicillamine	Binds copper and B_6 thus increasing need
Thiosemicarbazide	Binds vitamin B_6
L-DOPA	Increases need for vitamin B_6
Hydralazine	Increases need for vitamin B_6
Pyrimethane	Increases need for folacin
Methotrexate	Increases need for folacin
Theophylline	Increases protein turnover, increases calcium mobilization in cells
Ametine	Interferes with vitamin B_{12}
Aluminum hydroxide	Reduces folate availability as well as phosphate use
Magnesium hydroxide	Counteracts phosphate in intestine
Sodium bicarbonate	Reduces folate availability
Ethanol	Drives up need for niacin, riboflavin, B_6 and folacin
Mineral oil	Impairs absorption of vitamin A & β carotene
Azulfidine	Impairs absorption of folacin, B_{12} and fat soluble vitamins
Oral contraceptives	Increases folacin turnover
Amphetamine	Anorexia
Phenethylamine & related compounds	Anorexia
Colchicine	Promotes peristalsis thus reducing the absorption of all nutrients
Biguanides	Promotes glucose use; decreases absorption of B_{12}

Note: The information in this table provided by the *Physicians' Desk Reference*; *The Merck Index*; Sauberlich, HE, *Assessment of Nutritional Status*, 2nd ed., CRC Press, 1999; and Murray, RK, Granner, DK, Mayes, PA, Rodwell, VW, *Harper's Biochemistry* 24 ed. Appleton & Lange, Stamford, CN, 1997.

TABLE 3.14

Drugs that May Have Anti-Obesity Properties

Drug	Example	Effect
a) Anti Nutrition Drugs		
1. Gastric emptying inhibitors	(--) threochlorocitric acid	Delays gastric emptying, induces satiety
2. Glucosidase inhibitors	Acarbose, miglitol	Inhibits carbohydrate digestion
3. Inhibitors of lipid uptake	Cholestyramine	Binds bile acids, disrupts micelle formation
4. Pseudonutrients	Olestra	Fat substitute with less energy
	Artificial sweeteners	Sugar substitute, no energy
	Bulking agents, fibers	Induce satiety at lower energy intake
5. Lipase inhibitor	Xenecal	Inhibits hydrolysis of triacylglycides
b) Drugs that Affect Nutrient Partitioning		
1. Growth hormone		Stimulates protein synthesis
2. Testosterone		Stimulates protein synthesis in males only
3. α_2 adrenergic antagonists		Enhances lipolysis
4. Thermogenic drugs		
β_2 and β_3 adrenergic	BRL-26830A, terbutaline	Stimulates protein synthesis and lipolysis; can have serious side effects
Dinitrophenol		Metabolic poison; not recommended
c) Appetite Suppressors		
1. β phenethylamine derivatives	Fastin, Dexatrim	Interferes with hunger signaling via norepinephrine
2. Serotonergic agents	Fenfluramine, fluoxetine	Increases serotonin release and signals satiety
3. Amine reuptake inhibitor	Sibutramine	Blocks reuptake of norepinephrine and 5-HT and suppresses appetite

TABLE 3.15
Micronutrient Interactions

	Calcium	Phosphorus	Potassium	Sodium	Magnesium	Zinc	Iron	Copper	Iodine	Fluorine	Vitamin A	Vitamin D	Vitamin E	B_{12}	Vitamin K	Riboflavin	Niacin	Thiamin	Ascorbic acid	B_6	Folacin
Calcium	X	↑a	↓a	↓a↑m	↑m↓a						↑a	↑a, m							↑m		
Phosphorus	↑a	X	↑m	↑m	↓a							↑a				↑m	↑m	↑m			
Potassium	↑↓m	↑a	X	↑a	↓a, ↑m							↑a								↑↓m	
Sodium	↑↓m	↑a		X	↓a, ↑m							↑m								↑↓m	
Magnesium	↓a	↑m		↓a, ↑m	X				↑m			↑a						↑m	↑m	↑m	
Zinc						X		↓a, ↑m			↑m	↑a	↑m				↑m			↑m	
Iron	↑m	↓a				↓a	X	↓a, ↑m						↑m		↑m	↑m		↑a	↓a	↑m
Copper						↓a	↓a, ↑m	X			↑m					↑m				↑m	
Iodine									X			↓a		↑a			↑m		↑m		
Fluorine	↓a									X											
Cobalt							↓a														
Chromium						↓a															
Manganese					↓a		↓a														
Molybdenum							↑m	↓a													
Selenium								↑m													

Note: ↑ increase; ↓ decrease; a, absorption; m, metabolism.

TABLE 3.16

Preferred Ligand Binding Groups for Metal Ions

Metal	Ligand Groups
K^+	Singly charged oxygen donors or neutral oxygen ligands
Mg^{2+}	Carboxylase, phosphate, nitrogen donors
Ca^{2+}	$=Mg^{2+}$, but less affinity for nitrogen donors, phosphate, and other multidentate anions
Mn^{2+}	Similar to Mg^{2+}
Fe^{2+}	–SH, NH_2 > carboxylates
Fe^{3+}	Carboxylate, tyrosine, $-NH_2$, porphyrin (four 'hard' nitrogen donors)
Co^{3+}	Similar to Fe^{3+}
Cu^+	–SH (cysteine)
Cu^{2+}	Amines >> carboxylates
Zn^{2+}	Imidazole, cysteine
Mo^{2+}	–SH
Cd^{2+}	–SH

TABLE 3.17

Food Components That Affect Calcium Absorption

Component	Effect
Alcohol	↓
Ascorbic acid	↓↑
Cellulose	↓
Fat[a]	↑↓
Fiber	↓
Lactose	↑
Medium-chain triglycerides	↑
Oxalates	↓
Pectin	↑↓
Phytate	↓
Protein[b]	↑↓
Sodium alginate	↓
Uronic acid	↓

[a] In cases of steatorrhea, calcium absorption is reduced.
[b] Certain proteins, e.g., those in milk, enhance calcium availability while others, e.g., those in plants, reduce it.

TABLE 3.18

Calcium Binding Proteins

Protein	Function
α-Laçtalbumin	Carries calcium in milk
Casein	Carries calcium in milk
Calmodulin	Serves as major intracellular calcium receptor; activates cyclic nucleotidephosphodiesterase
Calbindin D_{9k} and D_{28k}	Facilitates intracellular Ca^{2+} translocation
Osteocalcin	Essential for calcium deposition in bone
$Ca^{2+}Mg^{2+}$ ATPase	Essential to movement of calcium across membranes
Prothrombin	Essential to blood clot formation
Calcitonin	Inhibits osteoclast-mediated bone resorption Regulates blood calcium levels by preventing hypercalcemia
Parathyroid hormone	Stimulates calcitonin synthesis, bone Ca resorption, renal Ca conservation
Albumin	Carries calcium in the blood
Globulin	Carries calcium in the blood
Osteopontin	Essential for calcium mobilization from bone
Troponin C	Muscle contraction
Alkaline phosphatase	Mineralization of bone
Sialoprotein	Embryonic bone growth
GLA-rich clotting proteins	Binds calcium in the coagulation cascade (see vitamin K)
Villin, gelsolin	Cytoskeleton stabilization

TABLE 3.19

The Body Content of Iron

Types of Iron	Male (70 kg)	Female (60 kg)
Essential Iron	3.100 g	2.100 g
Hemoglobin	2.700	1.800
Myoglobin, cytochromes, and other enzymes	0.400	0.300
Storage and transport iron	0.900	0.500
Ferritin, Hemosiderin	0.897	0.407
Transferrin	0.003	0.003
Total iron	4.000	2.600

TABLE 3.20

Body Mass Index Calculated as Body Mass Index = Body Weight/Height.[2] BMI for a given height

wt/lb	wt/kg													
Height		56	57	58	59	60	61	62	63	64	65	66	67	68
		142.2	144.8	147.3	149.9	152.4	154.9	157.5	160.0	162.6	165.1	167.6	170.2	172.7
100	45.5	22.5	21.7	20.9	20.2	19.6	18.9	18.3	17.8	17.2	16.7	16.2	15.7	15.2
110	50.0	24.7	23.8	23.0	22.3	21.5	20.8	20.2	19.5	18.9	18.3	17.8	17.3	16.8
120	54.5	27.0	26.0	25.1	24.3	23.5	22.7	22.0	21.3	20.6	20.0	19.4	18.8	18.3
130	59.1	29.2	28.2	27.2	26.3	25.4	24.6	23.8	23.1	22.4	21.7	21.0	20.4	19.8
140	63.6	31.5	30.4	29.3	28.3	27.4	26.5	25.7	24.9	24.1	23.3	22.7	22.0	21.3
150	68.2	33.7	32.5	31.4	30.3	29.4	28.4	27.5	26.6	25.8	25.0	24.3	23.5	22.9
160	72.7	36.0	34.7	33.5	32.4	31.3	30.3	29.3	28.4	27.5	26.7	25.9	25.1	24.4
170	77.3	38.2	36.9	35.6	34.4	33.3	32.2	31.2	30.2	29.2	28.3	27.5	26.7	25.9
180	81.8	40.5	39.0	37.7	36.4	35.2	34.1	33.0	32.0	30.9	30.0	29.1	28.2	27.4
190	86.4	42.7	41.2	39.8	38.4	37.2	36.0	34.8	33.7	32.7	31.7	30.7	29.8	29.0
200	90.9	45.0	43.4	41.9	40.5	39.1	37.9	36.6	35.5	34.4	33.4	32.4	31.4	30.5
210	95.5	47.2	45.5	44.0	42.5	41.1	29.8	38.5	37.3	36.1	35.0	34.0	33.0	32.0
220	100.0	49.5	47.7	46.1	44.5	43.1	41.7	40.3	39.1	37.8	36.7	35.6	34.5	33.5
230	104.5	51.7	49.9	48.2	46.5	45.0	43.6	42.1	40.8	39.5	38.4	37.2	36.1	35.1
240	109.1	53.9	42.0	50.3	48.5	47.0	45.5	44.0	42.6	41.3	40.0	38.8	37.7	36.6
250	113.6	56.2	54.2	52.4	50.6	48.9	47.4	45.8	44.4	43.0	41.7	40.5	39.2	38.1
260	118.2	58.4	56.4	54.5	52.6	50.9	49.3	47.6	46.2	44.7	43.4	42.1	40.8	39.6
270	122.7	60.7	58.5	56.6	54.6	52.8	51.1	49.5	47.9	46.4	45.0	43.7	42.4	41.1
280	127.3	62.9	60.7	58.7	56.6	54.8	53.0	51.3	49.7	48.1	46.7	45.3	43.9	43.7
290	131.8	65.2	62.9	60.8	58.7	56.8	54.9	53.1	51.5	49.9	48.4	46.9	45.5	44.2
300	136.4	67.4	65.0	62.8	60.7	58.7	56.8	55.0	53.3	51.6	50.0	48.5	47.1	45.7
310	140.9	69.7	67.2	64.9	62.7	60.7	58.7	56.8	55.0	53.3	51.7	50.2	48.6	47.2
320	145.5	71.9	69.4	67.0	64.7	62.6	60.6	58.6	56.8	55.0	53.4	51.8	50.2	48.8
330	150.0	74.2	71.5	69.1	66.8	64.6	62.5	60.5	58.6	56.7	55.0	53.4	51.8	50.3
340	154.5	76.4	73.7	71.2	68.8	66.5	64.4	62.3	60.4	58.5	56.7	55.0	53.4	51.8
350	159.1	78.7	75.9	73.3	70.8	68.5	66.3	64.1	62.1	60.2	58.4	56.6	54.9	53.3
360	163.6	80.9	78.0	75.4	72.8	70.5	68.2	66.0	63.9	61.9	60.0	58.3	56.5	54.9
370	168.2	83.2	80.2	77.5	74.8	72.4	70.1	67.8	65.7	63.6	61.7	59.9	58.1	56.4
380	172.7	85.4	82.4	79.6	76.9	74.4	72.0	69.6	67.5	65.3	63.4	61.5	59.6	57.9
390	177.3	87.7	84.5	81.7	78.9	76.3	73.9	71.5	69.2	67.1	65.0	63.1	61.2	59.4
400	181.8	89.9	86.7	83.8	80.9	78.3	75.8	73.3	71.0	68.8	66.7	64.7	62.8	61.0

and weight is where the horizontal line intersects the vertical line.

69	70	71	72	73	74	75	76	77	78	79	80	81	82	83	84
175.3	177.8	180.3	182.9	185.4	188.0	190.5	193.0	195.6	198.1	200.7	203.2	205.7	208.3	210.8	213.4
14.8	14.4	14.0	13.6	13.2	12.9	12.5	12.2	11.9	11.6	11.3	11.0	10.7	10.5	10.2	10.0
16.3	15.8	15.4	14.9	14.5	14.1	13.8	13.4	13.1	12.7	12.4	12.1	11.8	11.5	11.3	11.0
17.7	17.3	16.8	16.3	15.9	15.4	15.0	14.6	14.3	13.9	13.5	13.2	12.9	12.6	12.3	12.0
19.2	18.7	18.2	17.7	17.2	16.7	16.3	15.9	15.4	15.1	14.7	14.3	14.0	13.6	13.3	13.0
20.7	20.1	19.6	19.0	18.5	18.0	17.5	17.1	16.6	16.2	15.8	15.4	15.0	14.7	14.3	14.0
22.2	21.6	21.0	20.4	19.8	19.3	18.8	18.3	17.8	17.4	16.9	16.5	16.1	15.7	15.3	15.0
23.7	23.0	22.4	21.7	21.2	20.6	20.0	19.5	19.0	18.5	18.1	17.6	17.2	16.8	16.4	16.0
25.1	24.4	23.8	23.1	22.5	21.9	21.3	20.7	20.2	19.7	19.2	18.7	18.3	17.8	17.4	17.0
26.6	25.9	25.2	24.5	23.8	23.1	22.5	22.0	21.4	20.8	20.3	19.8	19.3	18.9	18.4	18.0
28.1	27.3	26.6	25.8	25.1	24.4	23.8	23.2	22.6	22.0	21.4	20.9	20.4	19.9	19.4	19.0
29.6	28.8	28.0	27.2	26.4	25.7	25.1	24.4	23.8	23.2	22.6	22.0	21.5	21.0	20.5	20.0
31.1	30.2	29.4	28.5	27.8	27.0	26.3	25.6	24.9	24.3	23.7	23.1	22.6	22.0	21.5	21.0
32.5	31.6	30.8	29.9	29.1	28.3	27.6	26.8	26.1	25.5	24.8	24.2	23.6	23.0	22.5	22.0
34.0	33.1	32.2	31.3	30.4	29.6	28.8	28.1	27.3	26.6	26.0	25.3	24.7	24.1	23.5	23.0
35.5	34.5	33.6	32.6	31.7	30.9	30.1	29.3	28.5	27.8	27.1	26.4	25.8	25.1	24.5	24.0
37.0	35.9	35.0	34.0	33.1	32.2	31.3	30.5	29.7	29.0	28.2	27.5	26.9	26.2	25.6	25.0
38.5	37.4	36.4	35.3	34.4	33.4	32.6	31.7	30.9	30.1	29.3	28.6	27.9	27.2	26.6	26.0
39.9	38.8	37.8	36.7	35.7	34.7	33.8	32.9	32.1	31.3	30.5	29.7	39.0	28.3	27.6	26.9
41.4	40.3	39.2	38.0	37.0	36.0	35.1	34.2	33.3	32.4	31.6	30.8	30.1	29.3	28.6	27.9
42.9	41.7	40.5	39.4	38.3	37.3	36.3	35.4	34.5	33.6	32.7	31.9	31.2	30.4	29.7	28.9
44.4	43.1	41.9	40.8	39.7	38.6	37.6	36.6	35.6	34.7	33.9	33.0	32.2	31.4	30.7	29.9
45.9	44.6	43.3	42.1	41.0	39.9	38.8	37.8	36.8	35.9	35.0	34.1	33.3	32.5	31.7	30.9
47.3	46.0	44.7	43.5	42.3	41.2	40.1	39.0	38.0	37.1	36.1	35.2	34.4	33.5	32.7	31.9
48.8	47.4	46.1	44.8	43.6	42.4	41.3	40.3	39.2	38.2	37.2	36.3	35.5	34.6	33.8	32.9
50.3	48.9	47.5	46.2	45.0	43.7	52.6	41.5	40.4	39.4	38.4	37.4	36.5	35.6	34.8	33.9
51.8	50.3	48.9	47.6	46.3	45.0	43.8	42.7	41.6	40.5	39.5	38.5	37.6	36.7	35.8	34.9
53.2	51.8	50.3	48.9	47.6	46.3	45.1	43.9	42.8	41.7	40.6	39.6	38.7	37.7	36.8	35.9
54.7	53.2	51.7	50.3	48.9	47.6	46.3	45.2	44.0	42.9	41.8	40.7	39.7	38.8	37.8	36.9
56.2	54.6	53.1	51.6	50.3	48.9	47.6	46.4	45.1	44.0	42.9	41.8	40.8	39.8	38.9	37.9
57.7	56.1	54.5	53.0	51.6	50.2	48.8	47.6	46.3	45.2	44.0	42.9	41.9	40.9	39.9	38.9
59.2	57.5	55.9	54.4	52.9	51.4	50.1	48.8	47.5	46.3	45.1	44.0	43.0	41.9	40.9	39.9

TABLE 3.21

Standard International Units (SI Units) for Reporting Clinical Data

Physical Quantity	Base Units	SI Symbol
I. Base Units		
Length	Meter	m
Mass	Kilogram	kg
Time	Second	s
Amount	Moles	mol
Thermodynamic Temperature	Kelvin	K
Electric Current	Ampere	A
Luminous Intensity	Candela	cd
II. Derived Units		
Area	Square Meter	m^2
Volume	Cubic Meter	m^3
Force	Newton (N)	$kg \cdot m \cdot s^{-2}$
Pressure	Pascal (Pa)	$kg \cdot m^{-2} \cdot s^{-2}$ (N/m^2)
Work, Energy	Joule (J)	$kg \cdot m^2 \cdot s^{-2}$ $(N \cdot m)$
Mass Density	Kilogram per cubic meter	kg/m^3
Frequency	Hertz (Hz)	s^{-1}

TABLE 3.22

Conversion Factors for Values in Clinical Chemistry (SI Units)

Component	Present Reference Intervals (examples)	Present Unit	Conversion Factor	SI Reference Intervals	SI Unit Symbol	Significant Digits	Suggested Minimum Increment
acetaminophen (P) - toxic	>5.0	mg/dL	66.16	>330	µmol/L	XXO	10 µmol/L
acetoacetate (S)	0.3-3.0	mg/dL	97.95	30-300	µmol/L	XXO	10 µmol/L
acetone (B,S)	0	mg/dL	172.2	0	µmol/L	XXO	10 µmol/L
acid phosphatase (S)	0-5.5	U/L	16.67	0-90	nkat/L	XX	2 nkat/L
adrenocorticotropin [ACTH] (P)	20-100	pg/mL	0.2202	4-22	pmol/L	XX	1 pmol/L
alanine aminotransferase [ALT] (S)	0-35	U/L	0.01667	0-0.58	µkat/L	X.XX	0.02 µkat/L
albumin (S)	4.0-6.0	g/dL	10.0	40-60	g/L	XX	1 g/L
aldolase (S)	0-6	U/L	16.67	0-100	nkat/L	XXO	20 nkat/L
aldosterone (S)							
normal salt diet	8.1-15.5	ng/dL	27.74	220-430	pmol/L	XXO	10 pmol/L
restricted salt diet	20.8-44.4	ng/dL	27.74	580-1240	pmol/L	XXO	10 pmol/L
aldosterone (U) - sodium excretion							
=25 mmol/d	18-85	µg/24 h	2.774	50-235	nmol/d	XXX	5 nmol/d
=75-125 mmol/d	5-26	µg/24 h	2.774	15-70	nmol/d	XXX	5 nmol/d
=200 mmol/d	1.5-12.5	µg/24 h	2.774	5-35	nmol/d	XXX	5 nmol/d
alkaline phosphatase (S)	0-120	U/L	0.01667	0.5-2.0	µkat/L	X.X	0.1 µkat/L
$alpha_1$-antitrypsin (S)	150-350	mg/dL	0.01	1.5-3.5	g/L	X.X	0.1 g/L
alpha-fetoprotein (S)	0-20	ng/mL	1.00	0-20	µg/L	XX	1 µg/L
alpha-fetoprotein (Amf)	Depends on gestation	mg/dL	10	Depends on gestation	mg/L	XX	1 mg/L
$alpha_2$-macroglobulin (S)	145-410	mg/dL	0.01	1.5-4.1	g/L	X.X	1 mg/L
aluminum (S)	0-15	µg/L	37.06	0-560	nmol/L	XXO	10 nmol/L
amino acid fractionation (P)							
alanine	2.2-4.5	mg/dL	112.2	245-500	µmol/L	XXX	5 µmol/L
alpha aminobutyric acid	0.1-0.2	mg/dL	96.97	10-20	µmol/L	XXX	5 µmol/L
arginine	0.5-2.5	mg/dL	57.40	30-145	µmol/L	XXX	5 µmol/L
asparagine	0.5-0.6	mg/dL	75.69	35-45	µmol/L	XXX	5 µmol/L
citrulline	0.2-1.0	mg/dL	75.13	0-20	µmol/L	XXX	5 µmol/L

TABLE 3.22 *(Continued)*

Conversion Factors for Values in Clinical Chemistry (SI Units)

Component	Present Reference Intervals (examples)	Present Unit	Conversion Factor	SI Reference Intervals	SI Unit Symbol	Significant Digits	Suggested Minimum Increment
cystine	0.2-2.2	mg/dL	57.08	15-55	µmol/L	XXX	5 µmol/L
glutamic acid	0.2-2.8	mg/dL	67.97	15-190	µmol/L	XXX	5 µmol/L
glutamine	6.1-10.2	mg/dL	68.42	420-700	µmol/L	XXX	5 µmol/L
glycine	0.9-4.2	mg/dL	133.2	120-560	µmol/L	XXX	5 µmol/L
histidine	0.5-1.7	mg/dL	64.45	30-110	µmol/L	XXX	5 µmol/L
hydroxyproline	0-trace	mg/dL	76.26	0-trace	µmol/L	XXX	5 µmol/L
isoleucine	0.5-1.3	mg/dL	76.24	40-100	µmol/L	XXX	5 µmol/L
leucine	1.2-3.5	mg/dL	76.24	75-175	µmol/L	XXX	5 µmol/L
lysine	1.2-3.5	mg/dL	68.40	80-240	µmol/L	XXX	5 µmol/L
methionine	0.1-0.6	mg/dL	67.02	5-40	µmol/L	XXX	5 µmol/L
ornithine	0.4-1.4	mg/dL	75.67	30-400	µmol/L	XXX	5 µmol/L
phenylalanine	0.6-1.5	mg/dL	60.54	35-90	µmol/L	XXX	5 µmol/L
proline	1.2-3.9	mg/dL	86.86	105-340	µmol/L	XXX	5 µmol/L
serine	0.8-1.8	mg/dL	95.16	75-170	µmol/L	XXX	5 µmol/L
taurine	0.9-2.5	mg/dL	79.91	25-170	µmol/L	XXX	5 µmol/L
threonine	0.9-2.5	mg/dL	83.95	75-210	µmol/L	XXX	5 µmol/L
tryptophan	0.5-2.5	mg/dL	48.97	25-125	µmol/L	XXX	5 µmol/L
tyrosine	0.4-1.6	mg/dL	55.19	20-90	µmol/L	XXX	5 µmol/L
valine	1.7-3.7	mg/dL	85.36	145-315	µmol/L	XXX	5 µmol/L
amino acid nitrogen (P)	4.0-6.0	mg/dL	0.7139	2.9-4.3	mmol/L	X.X	0.1 mmol/L
amino acid nitrogen (U)	50-200	mg/24 h	0.07139	3.6-14.3	mmol/d	X.X	0.1 mmol/d
delta-aminolevulinate [as levulinic acid] (U)	1.0-7.0	mg/24 h	7.626	8-53	µmol/d	XX	1 µmol/d
amitriptyline (P,S) therapeutic	50-200	ng/mL	3.605	180-270	µmol/L	XO	10 nmol/L
ammonia (vP)							
as ammonia [NH_3]	10-80	µg/dL	0.5872	5-50	µmol/L	XXX	5 µmol/L
as ammonium ion [NH_4+]	10-85	µg/dL	0.5543	5-50	µmol/L	XXX	5 µmol/L
as nitrogen [N]	10-65	µg/dL	0.7139	5-50	µmol/L	XXX	5 µmol/L
amylase (S)	0-130	U/L	0.01667	0-2.17	µkat/L	XXX	0.01 µkat/L
androstenedione (S)							
male > 18 years	0.2-3.0	mg/L	3.492	0.5-10.5	nmol/L	XX.X	0.5 nmol/L
female > 18 years	0.8-3.0	mg/L	3.492	3.0-10.5	nmol/L	XX.X	0.5 nmol/L

angiotensin converting enzyme (S)	<40	nmol/mL/min	16.67	<670	nkat/L	XXO	10 nkat/L
arsenic (H) [as As]	<1	µg/g (ppm)	13.35	<13	nmol/g	XX.X	0.5 nmol/g
arsenic (U) [as As]	0-5	µg/24 h	13.35	0-67	nmol/d	XX	1nmol/d
[as As_2O_3]	<25	µg/dL	0.05055	<1.3	µmol/L	XX.X	0.1 µmol/L
ascorbate (P) [as ascorbic acid]	0.6-2.0	µg/dL	56.78	30-110	µmol/L	XO	10 µmol/L
aspartate amino-transferase [AST] (S)	0-35	U/L	0.0167	0-0.58	µkat/L	O.XX	0.01 µkat/L
barbiturate (S) overdose total expressed as:	Depends on						
phenobarbital	composition of						
sodium phenobarbital	mixture.						
barbitone	Usually not	mg/dL	43.06	. . .	µmol/L	XX	5 µmol/L
	known.	mg/dL	39.34		µmol/L	XX	5 µmol/L
		mg/dL	54.29		µmol/L	XX	5 µmol/L
barbiturate (S) therapeutic							
see phenobarbital							
see pentobarbital	. . .	. . .	. . .	. . .	. . .	. . .	. . .
see thiopental							
bile acids, total (S)							
[as chenodeoxycholic acid]	Trace-3.3	µg/mL	2.547	Trace-8.4	µmol/L	X.X	0.2 µmol/L
cholic acid	Trace-1.0	µg/mL	2.448	Trace-2.4	µmol/L	X.X	0.2 µmol/L
chenodeoxycholic acid	Trace-1.3	µg/mL	2.547	Trace-3.4	µmol/L	X.X	0.2 µmol/L
deoxycholic acid	Trace-1.0	µg/mL	2.547	Trace-2.6	µmol/L	X.X	0.2 µmol/L
lithocholic acid	Trace	µg/mL	2.656	Trace	µmol/L	X.X	0.2 µmol/L
bile acids (Df) [after cholcystokinin stimulation]							
total as chenodeoxycholic acid	14.0-58.0	mg/mL	2.547	35.0-148	mmol/L	XX.X	0.2 mmol/L
cholic acid	2.4-33.0	mg/mL	2.448	6.8-81.0	mmol/L	XX.X	0.2 mmol/L
chenodeoxycholic acid	4.0-24.0	mg/mL	2.547	10.0-61.4	mmol/L	XX.X	0.2 mmol/L
deoxycholic acid	0.8-6.9	mg/mL	2.547	2.0-18.0	mmol/L	XX.X	0.2 mmol/L
lithocholic acid	0.3-0.8	mg/mL	2.656	0.8-2.0	mmol/L	XX.X	0.2 mmol/L
bilirubin, total (S)	0.1-1.0	mg/dL	17.10	2-18	µmol/L	XX	2 µmol/L
bilirubin, conjugated (S)	0-0.2	mg/dL	17.10	0-4	µmol/L	XX	2 µmol/L
bromide (S), toxic							
as bromide ion	>120	mg/dL	0.1252	>15	mmol/L	XX	1 mmol/L
as sodium bromide	>150	mg/dL	0.09719	>15	mmol/L	XX	1 mmol/L
	>15	mEq/L	1.00	>15	mmol/L	XX	1 mmol/L
cadmium (S)	<3	mg/dL	0.08897	<0.3	µmol/L	X.X	0.1 µmol/L
calcitonin (S)	<100	pg/mL	1.00	<100	ng/L	XXX	10 ng/L

TABLE 3.22 *(Continued)*

Conversion Factors for Values in Clinical Chemistry (SI Units)

Component	Present Reference Intervals (examples)	Present Unit	Conversion Factor	SI Reference Intervals	SI Unit Symbol	Significant Digits	Suggested Minimum Increment
calcium (S)							
male	8.8-10.3	mg/dL	0.2495	2.20-2.58	mmol/L	X.XX	0.02 mmol/L
female <50 y	8.8-10.0	mg/dL	0.2495	2.20-2.50	mmol/L	X.XX	0.02 mmol/L
female >50 y	8.8-10.2	mg/dL	0.2495	2.20-2.56	mmol/L	X.XX	0.02 mmol/L
	4.4-5.1	mEq/L	0.500	2.20-2.56	mmol/L	X.XX	0.02 mmol/L
calcium ion (S)	2.00-2.30	mEq/L	0.500	1.00-1.15	mmol/L	X.XX	0.01 mmol/L
calcium (U), normal diet	<250	mg/24 h	0.02495	<6.2	mmol/d	X.X	0.1 mmol/d
carbamazepine (P)							
- therapeutic	4.0-10.0	mg/L	4.233	17-42	µmol/L	XX	1 µmol/L
carbon dioxide content (B, P, S) [bicarbonate + CO_2]	22-28	mEq/L	1.00	22-28	mmol/L	X	1 mmol/L
carbon monoxide (B) [proportion of Hb which is COHb]	<15	%	0.01	<0.15	1	0.XX	0.01
beta carotenes (S)	50-250	mg/dL	0.01863	0.9-4.6	µmol/L	X.X	0.1 µmol/L
catecholamines, total (U) [as norepinephrine]	<120	mg/24 h	5.911	<675	nmol/d	XXO	10 mg/d
ceruloplasmin (S)	20-35	mg/dL	10.0	200-350	mg/L	XXO	10 mg/L
Chlordiazepoxide (P)							
- therapeutic	0.5-5.0	mg/L	3.336	2-17	µmol/L	XX	1 µmol/L
- toxic	>10.0	mg/L	3.336	>33	µmol/L	XX	1 µmol/L
chloride (S)	95-105	mEq/L	1.00	95105	mmol/L	XXX	1 mmol/L
chlorimipramine (P) [includes desmethyl metabolite}	50-400	ng/mL	3.176	150-1270	nmol/L	XXO	10 nmol/L
chlorpromazine (P)	50-300	ng/mL	3.136	150-950	nmol/L	XXO	10 nmol/L
chlorpropamide (P)							
-therapeutic	75-250	mg/L	3.613	270-900	mmol/L	XXO	10 mmol/L
cholestanol (P) [as a fraction of total cholesterol]	1-3	%	0.01	0.01-0.03	1	0.XX	0.01
cholesterol (P)							
- <29 years	<200	mg/dL	0.02586	<5.20	mol/L	X.XX	0.05 mmol/L

- 30-39 years	<225	mg/dL	0.02586	<5.85	mmol/L	X.XX	0.05 mmol/L
- 40-49 years	<245	mg/dL	0.02586	<6.35	mmol/L	X.XX	0.05 mmol/L
- >50 years	<265	mg/dL	0.02586	<6.85	mmol/L	X.XX	0.05 mmol/L
cholesterol esters (P) [as a fraction of total cholesterol]	60-75	%	0.01	0.60-0.75	1	0.XX	0.01
cholinesterase (S)	620-1370	U/L	0.01667	10.3-22.8	mkat/L	XX.X	0.1 mkat/L
chorionic gonadotropin (P) [beta HCG]	0 if not pregnant	mIU/mL	1.00	0 if not pregnant	IU/L	XX	1 IU/L
citrate (B) [as citric acid]	1.2-3.0	mg/dL	52.05	60-160	μmol/L	XXX	5 μmol/L
complement, C3 (S)	70-160	mg/dL	0.01	0.7-1.6	g/L	X.X	0.1 g/L
complement, C4 (S)	20-40	mg/dL	0.01	0.2-0.4	g/L	X.X	0.1 g/L
copper (S)	70-140	μg/dL	0.1574	11.0-22.0	μmol/L	XX.X	0.2.μmol/L
copper (U)	<40	μg/24 h	0.01574	<0.6	μmol/d	X.X	0.2 μmol/L
coproporphyrins (U)	<200	μg/24 h	1.527	<300	nmol/d	XXO	10 nmol/d
cortisol (S)							
-800 h	4-19	μg/dL	27.59	110-520	nmol/L	XXO	10 nmol/L
-1600 h	2-15	μg/dL	27.59	50-410	nmol/L	XXO	10 nmol/L
-2400 h	5	μg/dL	7.59	140	nmol/L	XXO	10 nmol/L
cortisol, free (U)	10-110	μg/24 h	2.759	30-300	nmol/d	XXO	10 nmol/d
creatine (S)							
-male	0.17-0.50	μg/dL	76.25	10-40	mmol/L	XO	10 mmol/L
-female	0.35-0.93	μg/dL	76.25	30-70	mmol/L	XO	10 mmol/L
creatine (U)							
-male	0-40	mg/24 h	7.625	0-300	μmol/d	XXO	10 μmol/d
-female	0-80	mg/24 h	7.625	0-600	μmol/d	XXO	10 μmol/d
creatine kinase [CK] (S)							
creatine kinase isoenzymes (S)	0-130	U/L	0.01667	0-2.16	μkat/L	X.XX	0.01 μkat/L
-MB fraction	>5 in myocardial infarction	%	0.01	>0.05	1	O.XX	0.01
creatinine (S)	0.6-1.2	mg/dL	88.40	50-110	μmol/L	XXO	10 μmol/L
creatinine (U)	Variable	g/24 h	8.840	Variable	mmol/d	XX.X	0.1 mmol/d
creatinine clearance (S, U)	75-125	mL/min	0.01667	1.24-2.08	mL/s	X.XX	0.02 mL/s

$$\text{creatinine clearance corrected for body} = \frac{\text{mmol / L (urine creatinine)}}{\text{mmol / L (serum creatinine)}} \times \text{mL / s} \times \frac{1.73}{A}$$

[where A is the body surface area in square meters (m^2)]

cyanide (B) - lethal	>0.10	mg/dL	384.3	>40	μmol/L	XXX	5 μmol/L
cyanocobalamin (S)							

TABLE 3.22 *(Continued)*

Conversion Factors for Values in Clinical Chemistry (SI Units)

Component	Present Reference Intervals (examples)	Present Unit	Conversion Factor	SI Reference Intervals	SI Unit Symbol	Significant Digits	Suggested Minimum Increment
[vitamin B_{12}]	200-100	pg/mL	0.7378	150-750	pmol/L	XXO	10 pmol/L
cyclic AMP (S)	2.6-6.6	μg/L	3.038	8-20	nmol/L	XXX	1 nmol/L
cyclic AMP (U)							
-total urinary	2.9-5.6	μmol/g creatinine	113.1	330-630	nmol/mmol creatinine	XXO	10nmol/mmol creatinine
-renal tubular	<2.5	μmol/g creatinine	113.1	<280	nmol/mmol creatinine	XXO	10nmol/mmol creatinine
cyclic GMP (S)	0.6-3.5	μg/L	2.897	1.7-10.1	nmol/L	XX.X	0.1 nmol/L
cyclic GMP (U)	0.3-1.8	μmol/g creatinine	113.1	30-200	nmol/mmol creatinine	XXO	10nmol/mmol creatinine
cystine (U)	10-100	mg/24 h	4.161	40-420	mmol/d	XXO	10 mmol/d
dehydroepiandrosterone (P,S)							
[DHEA]- 1-4 years	0.2-0.4	μg/L	3.467	0.6-1.4	nmol/L	XX.X	0.2 nmol/L
4-8 years	0.1-1.9	μg/L	3.467	0.4-6.6	nmol/L	XX.X	0.2 nmol/L
8-10 years	0.2-2.9	μg/L	3.467	0.6-10.0	nmol/L	XX.X	0.2 nmol/L
10-12 years	0.5-9.2	μg/L	3.467	1.8-31.8	nmol/L	XX.X	0.2 nmol/L
12-14 years	0.9-20.0	μg/L	3.467	3.2-69.4	nmol/L	XX.X	0.2 nmol/L
14-16 years	2.5-20.0	μg/L	3.467	8.6-69.4	nmol/L	XX.X	0.2 nmol/L
premenopausal female	2.0-15.0	μg/L	3.467	7.0-52.0	nmol/L	XX.X	0.2 nmol/L
male	0.8-10.0	μg/L	3.467	2.8-34.6	nmol/L	XX.X	0.2 nmol/L
dehydroepiandrosterone (U)	See Steroids	Fractionation	. . .	. . .	. . .	. . .	. . .
dehydroepiandrosterone sulphate [DHEA-S] (P, S)							
newborn	1670-3640	ng/mL	0.002714	4.5-9.9	μmol/L	XX.X	μmol/L
pre-pubertal children	100-600	ng/mL	0.002714	0.3-1.6	μmol/L	XX.X	μmol/L
male	2000-3500	ng/mL	0.002714	5.4-9.1	μmol/L	XX.X	μmol/L
female (premenopausal)	820-3380	ng/mL	0.002714	2.2-9.2	μmol/L	XX.X	μmol/L
female (post-menopausal)	110-610	ng/mL	0.002714	0.3-1.7	μmol/L	XX.X	μmol/L
pregnancy [term]	0-1170	ng/mL	0.002714	0.6-3.2	μmol/L	XX.X	μmol/L
11-deoxycortisol (S)	0-2	μg/dL	28.86	0-60	nmol/L	XXO	10 nmol/L
desipramine (P)							
-therapeutic	50-200	ng/mL	3.754	170-700	nmol/L	XXO	10 nmol/L

diazepam (P)							
-therapeutic	0.10-0.25	mg/L	3512	350-900	nmol/L	XXO	10 nmol/L
-toxic	>1.0	mg/L	3512	>3510	nmol/L	XXO	10 nmol/L
dicoumarol (P)							
-therapeutic	8-30	mg/L	2.974	25-90	μmol/L	XX	5 μmol/L
digoxin (P)							
-therapeutic	0.5-2.2	ng/mL	1.281	0.6-2.8	nmol/L	X.X	0.1 nmol/L
	0.5-2.2	μg/L	1.281	0.6-2.8	nmol/L	X.X	0.1 nmol/L
-toxic	>2.5	ng/mL	1.281	>3.2	nmol/L	X.X	0.1 nmol/L
dimethadione (P)							
-therapeutic	<1.00	g/L	7.745	<7.7	mmol/L	X.X	0.1 mmol/L
disopyramide (P)							
-therapeutic	2.0-6.0	mg/L	2.946	6-18	μmol/L	XX	1 μmol/L
doxepin (P)							
-therapeutic	50-200	n/mL	3.579	180-720	nmol/L	XO	10 nmol/L
electrophoresis, protein (S)							
albumin	60-65	%	0.01	0.60-0.65	1	O.XX	0.01
$alpha_1$-globulin	1.7-5.0	%	0.01	0.02-0.05	1	O.XX	0.01
$alpha_2$-globulin	6.7-12.5	%	0.01	0.07-0.13	1	O.XX	0.01
beta-globulin	8.3-16.3	%	0.01	0.08-0.16	1	O.XX	0.01
gamma-globulin	10.7-20.0	%	0.01	0.11-0.20	1	O.XX	0.01
albumin	3.6-5.2	g/dL	10.0	36-52	g/L	XX	1 g/L
$alpha_1$-globulin	0.1-0.4	g/dL	10.0	1-4	g/L	XX	1 g/L
$alpha_2$-globulin	0.4-1.0	g/dL	10.0	4-10	g/L	XX	1 g/L
beta-globulin	0.5-1.2	g/dL	10.0	5-12	g/L	XX	1 g/L
gamma-globulin	0.6-1.6	g/dL	10.0	6-16	g/L	XX	1 g/L
epinephrine (P)	31-95 (at rest for 15 min)	pg/mL	5.458	170-520	pmol/L	XXO	10 pmol/L
epinephrine (U)	<10	μg/24 h	5.458	<55	nmol/d	XX	5 nmol/d
estradiol (S)							
male >18 yrs	15-40	pg/mL	3.671	55-150	pmol/L	XX	1 pmol/L
estriol (U)							
[non pregnant]							
onset of menstruation	4-25	μg/24 h	3.468	15-85	nmol/d	XXX	5 nmol/d
ovulation peak	28-99	μg/24 h	3.468	95-345	nmol/d	XXX	5 nmol/d
luteal peak	22-105	μg/24 h	3.468	75-365	nmol/d	XXX	5 nmol/d
menopausal woman	1.4-19.6	μg/24 h	3.468	5-70	nmol/d	XXX	5 nmol/d
male	5-18	μg/24 h	3.468	15-60	nmol/d	XXX	5 nmol/d

TABLE 3.22 *(Continued)*

Conversion Factors for Values in Clinical Chemistry (SI Units)

Component	Present Reference Intervals (examples)	Present Unit	Conversion Factor	SI Reference Intervals	SI Unit Symbol	Significant Digits	Suggested Minimum Increment
estrogens (S) [as estradiol]							
female	20-300	pg/mL	3.671	70-1100	pmol/L	XXXO	10 pmol/L
peak production	200-800	pg/mL	3.671	750-2900	pmol/L	XXXO	10 pmol/L
male	<50	pg/mL	3.671	<180	pmol/L	XXO	10 pmol/L
estrogens, placental (U) [as estriol]	Depends on period of gestation	mg/24 h	3.468	Depends on period of gestation	µmol/d	XXX	1 µmol/d
estrogen receptors (T)							
negative	0-3	fmol estradiol bound/mg cytosol protein	1.00	0-3	fmol estradiol/mg cytosol protein	XXX	1 fmol/mg protein
doubtful	4-10	fmol estradiol bound/mg cytosol protein	1.00	4-10	fmol estradiol/mg cytosol protein	XXX	1 fmol/mg protein
positive	>10	fmol estradiol bound/mg cytosol protein	1.00	>10	fmol estradiol/mg cytosol protein	XXX	1 fmol/mg protein
estrone (P, S)							
- female 1-10 days of cycle	43-180	pg/mL	3.699	160-665	pmol/L	XXX	5 pmol/L
-female 11-20 days of cycle	75-196	pg/mL	3.699	275-725	pmol/L	XXX	5 pmol/L
-female 20-39 days of cycle	131-201	pg/mL	3.699	485-745	pmol/L	XXX	5 pmol/L
-male	29-75	pg/mL	3.699	105-275	pmol/L	XXX	5 pmol/L
estrone (U) female	2-25	µg/24 h	3.699	5-90	nmol/d	XXX	5 nmol/d
ethanol (P)							
legal limit [driving]	<80	mg/dL	0.2171	<17	mmol/L	XX	1 nmol/L
-toxic	>100	mg/dL	0.2171	>22	mmol/L	XX	1 mmol/L
ethchlorvynol (P) toxic	>40	mg/L	6.915	>280	µmol/L	XXO	10 µmol/L
ethosuximide (P)							
therapeutic	40-110	mg/L	7.084	280-780	µmol/L	XXO	10 µmol/L
ethylene glycol (P)							
toxic	>30	mg/dL	0.1611	>5	mmol/L	XX	1 mmol/L

fat (F)							
[as stearic acid]	2.0-6.0	g/24 h	3.515	7-21	mmol/d	XXX	1 mmol/d
fatty acids, non-							
esterified (P)	8-20	mg/dL	10.00	80-200	mg/L	XXO	10 mg/L
ferritin (S)	18-300	ng/mL	1.00	18-300	µg/L	XXO	10 µg/L
fibrinogen (P)	200-400	mg/dL	0.01	2.0-4.0	g/L	X.X	0.1 g/L
fluoride (U)	<1.0	mg/24 h	52.63	<50	µmol/d	XXO	10 µmol/d
folate (S) [as pteroylglutamic acid]	2-10	ng/mL	2.266	4-22	nmol/L	XX	2 nmol/L
		µg/dL	22.66		nmol/L		2 nmol/L
folate (Erc)	140-960	ng/mL	2.266	550-2200	nmol/L	XXO	10 nmol/L
follicle stimulating hormone							
[FSH] (P)							
female	2.0-15.0	mIU/mL	1.00	2-15	IU/L	XX	1 IU/L
peak production	20-50	mIU/mL	1.00	20-50	IU/L	XX	1 IU/L
male	1.0-10.0	mIU/mL	1.00	1-10	IU/L	XX	1 IU/L
follicle stimulating hormone [FSH] (U)							
follicular phase	2-15	IU/24 h	1.00	2-15	IU/d	XXX	1 IU/d
midcycle	8-40	IU/24 h	1.00	8-40	IU/d	XXX	1 IU/d
luteal phase	2-10	IU/24 h	1.00	2-10	IU/d	XXX	1 IU/d
menopausal women	35-100	IU/24 h	1.00	35-100	IU/d	XXX	1 IU/d
male	2-15	IU/24 h	1.00	2-15	IU/d	XXX	1 IU/d
fructose (P)	<10	mg/dL	0.05551	<0.6	mmol/L	X.XX	0.1 mmol/L
galactose (P) [children]	<20	mg/dL	0.05551	<1.1	mmol/L	X.XX	0.1 mmol/L
gases (aB)							
pO_2	75-105	mm Hg (= Torr)	0.1333	10.0-14.0	kPa	XX.X	0.1 kPa
pCO_2	33-44	mm Hg (= Torr)	0.1333	4.4-5.9	kPa	X.X	0.1 kPa
gamma-glutamyltransferase [GGT] (S)	0-30	U/L	0.01667	0-0.50	µkat/L	X.XX	0.01 µkat/L
gastrin (S)	0-180	pg/mL	1	0-180	ng/L	XXO	10 ng/L
globulins (S) [see immunoglobulins]	...	...	...	...	...	...	...
glucagon (S)	50-100	pg/mL	1	50-100	ng/L	XXO	10 ng/L
glucose (P) fasting	70110	mg/dL	0.05551	3.9-6.1	mmol/L	XX.X	0.1 mmol/L
glucose (Sf)	50-80	mg/dL	0.05551	2.8-4.4	mmol/L	XX.X	0.1 mmol/L
glutethimide (P)							
-therapeutic	<10	mg/L	4.603	<46	µmol/L	XX	1 µmol/L
-toxic	>20	mg/L	4.603	>92	µmol/L	XX	1 µmol/L
glycerol, free (S)	<1.5	mg/dL	0.1086	<0.16	mmol/L	X.XX	0.01 mmol/L
gold (S) therapeutic	300-800	µg/dL	0.05077	15.0-40.0	µmol/L	XX.X	0.1 µmol/L
gold (U)	<500	µg/24 h	0.005077	<2.5	µmol/d	X.X	0.1 µmol/d

TABLE 3.22 *(Continued)*

Conversion Factors for Values in Clinical Chemistry (SI Units)

Component	Present Reference Intervals (examples)	Present Unit	Conversion Factor	SI Reference Intervals	SI Unit Symbol	Significant Digits	Suggested Minimum Increment
palmitic acid (Amf)	Depends on gestation	mmol/L	1000	Depends on gestation	µmol/L	XXX	5 µmol/L
pentobarbital (P)	20-40	mg/L	4.419	90-170	µmol/L	XX	5 µmol/L
phenobarbital (P)							
-therapeutic	2-5	mg/L	43.06	85-215	µmol/L	XXX	5 µmol/L
phensuximide (P)	4-8	mg/L	5.285	20-40	µmol/L	XX	5 µmol/L
phenylbutazone (P)							
-therapeutic	<100	mg/L	3.243	<320	µmol/L	XXO	10 µmol/L
phenytoin (P)							
-therapeutic	10-20	mg/L	3.964	40-80	µmol/L	XX	5 µmol/L
-toxic	>30	mg/L	3.964	>12	µmol/L	XX	5 µmol/L
phosphate (S) [as phosphorus, inorganic]	2.5-5.0	mg/dL	0.3229	0.80-1.60	mmol/L	X.XX	0.05 mmol/L
phosphate (U) [as phosphorus, inorganic]	Diet dependent	g/24 h	32.29	Diet dependent	mmol/d	XXX	1 mmol/d
phospholipid phosphorus, total (P)	5-12	mg/dL	0.3229	1.60-3.90	mmol/L	X.XX	0.05 mmol/L
phospholipid phosphorus, total (Erc)	1.2-12	mg/dL	0.3229	0.40-3.90	mmol/L	X.XX	0.05 mmol/L
phospholipids (P)							
substance fraction of total phospholipid							
phosphatidyl choline	65-70	%/total	0.01	0.65-0.70	1	O.XX	0.01
phosphatidyl ethanolamine	4-5	%/total	0.01	0.04-0.05	1	O.XX	0.01
sphingomyelin	15-20	%/total	0.01	0.15-0.20	1	O.XX	0.01
lysophosphatidyl choline	3-5	%/total	0.01	0.03-0.05	1	O.XX	0.01
phospholipids (Erc)							
substance fraction of total phospholipid							
phosphatidyl choline	28-33	%/total	0.01	0.28-0.33	1	O.XX	0.01
phosphatidyl ethanolamine	24-31	%/total	0.01	0.24-0.31	1	O.XX	0.01
sphingomyelin	22-29	%/total	0.01	0.22-0.29	1	O.XX	0.01

phosphatidyl serine + phosphatidyl inositol	12-20	%/total	0.01	0.12-0.20	1	O.XX	0.01
lysophosphatidyl choline	1-2	%/total	0.01	0.01-0.02	1	O.XX	0.01
phytanic acid (P)	Trace-0.3	mg/dL	32.00	<10	µmol/L	XX	5 µmol/L
[human] placental lactogen (SO [HPL]	>4.0 after 30 wk gestation	µg/mL	46.30	>180	nmol/L	XXO	10 nmol/L
porphobilinogen (U)	0.0-2.0	mg/24 h	4.420	0-9.0	µmol/d	X.X	0.5 µmol/d
porphyrins							
coproporphyrin (U)	45-180	µg/24 h	1.527	68-276	nmol/d	XXX	2 nmol/d
protoporphyrin (Erc)	15-50	µg/dL	0.0177	0.28-0.90	µmol/L	X.XX	0.02 µmol/L
uroporphyrin (U)	5-20	µg/24 h	1.204	6-24	nmol/d	XX	2 nmol/d
uroporphyrinogen synthetase (Erc)	22-42	mmol/mL/h	0.2778	6.0-11.8	mmol/ (L.s)	X.X	0.2 mmol/(L.s)
potassium ion (S)	3.5-5.0	mEq/L	1.00	3.5-5.0	mmol/L	X.X	0.1 mmol/L
		mg/dL	0.2558		mmol/L	X.X	0.1 mmol/L
potassium ion (U) [diet dependent]	25-100	mEq/24 h	1.00	25-100	mmol/d	XX	1 mmol/d
pregnaediol (U)							
-normal	1.0-6.0	mg/24 h	3.120	3.0-18.5	µmol/d	XX.X	0.5 µmol/d
-pregnancy	Depends on gestation						
pregnanetriol (U)	0.5-2.0	mg/24 h	2.972	1.5-6.0	µmol/d	XX.X	0.5 µmol/d
primidone (P)							
-therapeutic	6.0-10.0	mg/L	4.582	25-46	µmol/L	XX	1 µmol/L
-toxic	>10.0	mg/L	4.582	>46	µmol/L	XX	1 µmol/L
procainamide (P)							
-therapeutic	4.0-8.0	mg/L	4.249	17-34	µmol/L	XX	1 µmol/L
-toxic	>12.0	mg/L	4.249	>50	µmol/L	XX	1 µmol/L
N-acetyl procainamide (P)							
-therapeutic	4.0-8.0	mg/L	3.606	14-29	µmol/L	XX	1 µmol/L
progesterone (P)							
follicular phase	<2	ng/mL	3.180	<6	nmol/L	XX	2 nmol/L
luteal phase	2-20	ng/mL	3.180	6-64	nmol/L	XX	2 nmol/L
progesterone receptors (T)							
negative	0-3	fmol progesterone bound/mg cytosol protein	1.00	0-3	fmol progesterone bound/mg cytosol protein	XX	1 fmol/mg protein

TABLE 3.22 *(Continued)*

Conversion Factors for Values in Clinical Chemistry (SI Units)

Component	Present Reference Intervals (examples)	Present Unit	Conversion Factor	SI Reference Intervals	SI Unit Symbol	Significant Digits	Suggested Minimum Increment
doubtful	4-10	fmol progesterone bound/mg cytosol protein	1.00	4-10	fmol progesterone bound/mg cytosol protein	XX	1 fmol/mg protein
positive	>10	fmol progesterone bound/mg cytosol protein	1.00	>10	fmol progesterone bound/mg cytosol protein	XX	1 fmol/mg protein
prolactin (P)	<20	ng/mL	1.00	<20	μg/L	XX	1 μg/L
propoxyphene (P) toxic	>2.0	mg/L	2.946	>5.9	μmol/L	X.X	0.1 μmol/L
propranolol (P)							
[Inderal] therapeutic	50-200	ng/mL	3.856	190-770	nmol/L	XXO	10 nmol/L
protein, total (S)	6.0-8.0	g/dL	10.0	60-80	g/L	XX	1 g/L
protein, total (Sf)	<40	mg/dL	0.01	<0.40	g/L	X.XX	0.1 g/L
protein, total (U)	<150	mg/24 h	0.001	<0.15	g/d	X.XX	0.01 g/d
protryptyline (P)	100-300	ng/mL	3.797	380-1140	nmol/L	XXO	10 nmol/L
pyruvate (B) [as pyruvic acid]	0.30-0.90	mg/dL	113.6	35-100	μmol/L	XXX	1 μmol/L
quinidine (P)							
-therapeutic	1.5-3.0	mg/L	3.082	4.6-9.2	μmol/L	X.X	0.1 μmol/L
-toxic	>6.0	mg/L	3.082	>18.5	μmol/L	X.X	0.1 μmol/L
renin (P)							
normal sodium diet	1.1-4.1	ng/mL/h	0.2778	0.30-1.14	ng/(L.s)	X.XX	0.2 ng/(L.s)
restricted sodium diet	6.2-12.4	ng/mL/h	0.2778	1.72-3.44	ng/(L.s)	X.XX	0.02 ng/(L.s)
salicylate (S) [salicylic acid]							
toxic	>20	mg/dL	0.07240	>1.45	mmol/L	X.XX	0.05 mmol/L
serotonin (B) [5 hydroxytryptamine]	8-21	μg/dL	0.05675	0.45-1.20	μmol/L	X.XX	0.05 μmol/L
sodium ion (S)	135-147	mEq/L	1.00	135-147	mmol/L	XXX	1 mmol/L

sodium ion (U)	Diet dependent	mEq/24 h	1.00	Diet dependent	mmol/d	XXX	2 mmol/d
steroids							
17-hydroxy-corticosteroids (U) [as cortisol]							
-female	2.0-8.0	mg/24 h	2.759	5-25	µmol/d	XX	1 µmol/d
-male	3.0-10.0	mg/24 h	2.759	10-30	µmol/d	XX	1 µmol/d
17-ketogenic steroids (U) [as dehydroepiandrosterone]							
-female	7.0-12.0	mg/24 h	3.467	25-40	µmol/d	XX	1 µmol/d
-male	9.0-17.0	mg/24 h	3.467	30-60	µmol/d	XX	1 µmol/d
17-ketosteroids (U) [as dehydroepiandrosterone]							
-female	6.0-17.0	mg/24 h	3.467	20-60	µmol/d	XX	1 µmol/d
-male	6.0-20.0	mg/24 h	3.467	20-70	µmol/d	XX	1 µmol/d
ketosteroid fractions (U) androsterone							
-female	0.5-2.0	mg/24 h	3.443	1-10	µmol/d	XX	1 µmol/d
-male	2.0-5.0	mg/24 h	3.443	7-17	µmol/d	XX	1 µmol/d
dehydroepiandrosterone							
-female	0.2-1.8	mg/24 h	3.467	1-6	µmol/d	XX	1 µmol/d
-male	0.2-2.0	mg/24 h	3.467	1-7	µmol/d	XX	1 µmol/d
etiocholanolone							
-female	0.8-4.0	mg/24 h	3.443	2-14	µmol/d	XX	1 µmol/d
-male	1.4-5.0	mg/24 h	3.443	4-17	µmol/d	XX	1 µmol/d
sulfonamides (B) [as sulfanilamide]							
-therapeutic	10.0-15.0	mg/dL	58.07	580-870	µmol/L	XXO	10 µmol/L
testosterone (P)							
-female	0.6	ng/mL	3.467	2.0	nmol/L	XX.X	0.5 nmol/L
-male	4.6-8.0	ng/mL	3.467	14.0-28.0	nmol/L	XX.X	0.5 nmol/L
theophylline (P)							
-therapeutic	10.0-20.0	mg/L	5.550	55-110	µmol/L	XX	1 µmol/L
thiocyanate (P) (nitroprusside toxicity)	10.0	mg/dL	0.1722	1.7	mmol/L	X.XX	0.1 mmol/L
thiopental (P)	individual	mg/L	4.126	individual	µmol/L	XX	5 µmol/L
thyroid tests:							
thyroid stimulating hormone [TSH] (S)	2-11	µU/mL	1.00	2-11	mU/L	XX	1 mU/L
thyroxine [T_4] (S)	4.0-11.0	µg/dL	12.87	51-142	nmol/L	XXX	1 nmol/L

TABLE 3.22 *(Continued)*

Conversion Factors for Values in Clinical Chemistry (SI Units)

Component	Present Reference Intervals (examples)	Present Unit	Conversion Factor	SI Reference Intervals	SI Unit Symbol	Significant Digits	Suggested Minimum Increment
thyroxine binding globulin [TGB] (S) [as thyroxine]	12.0-28.0	μg/dL	12.87	150-360	nmol/L	XXO	1 nmol/L
thyroxine, free (S)	0.8-2.8	ng/dL	12.87	10-36	pmol/L	XX	1 pmol/L
triiodothyronine [T_3] (S)	75-220	ng/dL	0.01536	1.2-3.4	nmol/L	X.X	0.1 nmol/L
T_3 uptake (S)	25-35	%	0.01	0.25-0.35	1	O.XX	0.01
tolbuamide (P)							
-therapeutic	50-120	mg/L	3.699	180-450	mmol/L	XXO	10 mmol/L
transferrin (S)	170-370	mg/dL	0.01	1.70-3.70	g/L	X.XX	0.01 g/L
triglycerides (P) [as triolein]	<160	mg/dL	0.01129	<1.80	mmol/L	X.XX	0.02 mmol/L
trimethadione (P)							
- therapeutic	<50	mg/L	6.986	<350	μmol/L	XXO	10 μmol/L
trimipramine (P)							
-therapeutic	50-200	ng/mL	3.397	170-680	nmol/L	XXO	10 nmol/L
urate (S) [as uric acid]	2.0-7.0	mg/dL	59.48	120-420	μmol/L	XXO	10 μmol/L
urate (U) [as uric acid]	Diet dependent	g/24 h	5.948	Diet dependent	mmol/d	XX	1 mmol/d
urea nitrogen (S)	8-18	mg/dL	0.3570	3.0-6.5	mmol/L UREA	X.X	0.5 mmol/L
urea nitrogen (U)	2.0-20.0 diet dependent	g/24 h	35.700	450-700	mmol/d UREA	XXO	10 mol/d
urobilinogen (U)	0.0-4.0	mg/24 h	1.693	0.0-6.8	μmol/d	X.X	0.1 μmol/d
valproic acid (P)							
-therapeutic	50-100	mg/L	6.934	350-700	μmol/L	XO	10 μmol/L
vanillylmandelic acid [VMA] (U)*	<6.8	mg/24 h	5.046	<35	μmol/d	XX	1 μmol/d

vitamin A [retinol] (P,S)	10-50	μg/dL	0.03491	0.35-1.75	μmol/L	X.XX	0.05 μmol/L
vitamin B_1 [thiamine hydrochloride] (U)	60-500	mg/24 h	0.002965	0.18-1.48	μmol/d	ZX.XX	0.01 μmol/d
vitamin B_2 [riboflavin] (S)	2.6-3.7	μg/dL	26.57	70-100	nmol/L	XXX	5 nmol/L
vitamin B_6 [pyridoxal] (B)	20-90	ng/mL	5.982	120-540	nmol/L	XXX	5 nmol/L
vitamin B_{12} (P,S) [cyanocobalamin]	200-1000	pg/mL	0.7378	150-750	pmol/L	XO	10 pmol/L
vitamin C [see ascorbate] (B,P,S)	...	...	...	...	...	...	...
vitamin D_3 [cholecalciferol] (P)	24-40	mg/mL	2.599	60-105	nmol/L	XXX	5 nmol/L
25 OH-cholecacliferol	18-36	ng/mL	.496	45-90	nmol/L	XXX	5 mmol/L
vitamin E [alpha-tocopherol] (P,S)	0.78-1.25	mg/dL	23.22	18-29	μmol/L	XX	1 μmol/L
warfarin (P)							
-therapeutic	1.0-3.0	mg/L	3.243	3.3-9.8	μmol/L	XX.X	0.1 μmol/L
xanthine (U)							
-hypoxanthine	5-30	mg/24	6.574	30-200	μmol/d	XXO	10 μmol/d
		hmg/24 h	7.347		μmol/d	XXO	10 μmol/d
D-xylose (B) [25 g dose]	30-40 (30-60 min)	mg/dL	0.06661	.0-2.7 (30-60 min)	mmol/L	X.X	0.1 mmol/L
D-xylose excretion (U) [25 g dose]	21-31	%	0.01	0.21-0.31 (excreted in 5 h)	1	0.XX	0.01
zinc (S)	75-120	μg/dL	0.1530	11.5-18.5	μmol/L	XX.X	0.1 μmol/L
zinc (U)	150-1200	μg/24 h	0.01530	2.3-18.3	μmol/d	XX.X	0.1 μmol/d

TABLE 3.23

Small Animal Analogs of Human Degenerative Diseases*

Type 1 Diabetes Mellitus (IDDM)

Streptozotocin or alloxan treated animals of most species
Pancreatectomy will also produce IDDM
BB rat, NOD mouse (Both of these develop diabetes as an autoimmune disease and both mimic Type I diabetes mellitus as found in humans.)
db/db mouse
FAT mouse
NZO mouse
TUBBY mouse
Adipose mouse
Chinese hampster (*Cricetulus griseus*)
South African hamster (*Mystromys alb*)
Tuco-Tuco (*Clenomys tabarum*)

Type 2 Diabetes Mellitus

ob/ob mouse
KK, yellow KK mouse
A^{vy}, A^{y} yellow mouse
P, PB 13/Ld mouse
db PAS mouse
BHE/Cdb rat
Zucker diabetic rat
SHR/N-cp rat
Spiny mouse
HUS rat
LA/N-cp rat
Wistar Kyoto rat

Obesity

Zucker rat
db/db mouse
SHR/N-cp rat
LA/N-cp rat
ob/ob mouse
Ventral hypothalamus lesioned animals
Osborne-Mendel rats fed high fat diets

Hypertension

SHR rats
JCR:LA rats
WKY rats
Transgenic rats

Gallstones

(The rat does not have a gall bladder nor does it have stones.)
Gerbil fed a cholesterol-rich, cholic acid-rich diet
Hamster, prairie dog, squirrel monkey, or tree shrew fed a cholesterol-rich diet

Lipemia

Zucker fatty rat
BHE/Cdb rat
NZW mouse
Transgenic mice given gene for atherosclerosis

Atherosclerosis

Transgenic mice given gene for atherosclerosis
NZW mouse
JCR:LA cp/cp rat

* There are several compilations of animal models for human disease. See the series of books edited by Shafrir having the general title *Lessons from Animal Diabetes* published by Smith Gordon, London. See also the NIH Guide for Animal Resources, updated annually, and the Jackson Laboratory catalog, Bar Harbor, Maine.

TABLE 3.24

Composition of the AIN-93 Maintenance (M) and Growth (G) Diets

Ingredient	AIN-93M (g/kg)	AIN-93G (g/kg)
Casein	140	200
Cornstarch	465.692	397.486
Dextrose	155	132
Sucrose	100	100
Cellulose	50	50
Soybean oil	40	70
Mineral mix	35	35
Vitamin mix	10	10
L-cystine	1.8	3
Choline bitartrate	2.5	2.5
t-Butylhydroquinone	0.008	0.014
Energy	~3.8 kcal or ~16 kJ/g	~3.9 kcal or ~16.4 kJ/g

From: *Journal of Nutrition* 123:1941-44, 1993.

Part III

Comparative Nutrition

4

Animal Needs and Uses (Comparative Nutrition)

William P. Flatt

Overview — Nutritional Requirements for Different Species

The nutritional requirements for different species of animals, including mammals, birds and fish, vary markedly. Many factors influence the requirements for specific nutrients. Within species, some of the factors affecting nutritional requirements are age, gender, stage of maturity, level of activity (work), body size, type and level of production (i.e. lean or adipose body tissue, milk, eggs, wool, bone growth, etc.), environment, physiological function (i.e. maintenance, pregnancy, lactation), health, and endocrinological factors. Between and among species, the type of gastrointestinal tract greatly influences the nutritional requirements of the animal, and the type of food it may eat to provide the nutrients. For example, ruminants (cattle, sheep, goats, and deer), as a result of microbial fermentation in the upper gastrointestinal tract, have quite different nutritional requirements than nonruminants (humans, swine, dogs, cats, non-human primates). Ruminants, and other herbivores that have extensive microbial fermentation in the large intestine and cecum, may utilize cellulose, hemicellulose, and other high fiber diets that nonruminants cannot digest. This adaptation also results in differences in the requirements for dietary sources of some of the B vitamins and amino acids.

Some species store bile from the liver in the gallbladder (humans, swine, cattle, sheep, chickens), whereas others (rats, horses, deer, elk, moose, camels) have no reservoir to store bile, and this in turn may affect lipid digestion. Another species difference is in nitrogen utilization. For example, mammals excrete excess nitrogen resulting from protein metabolism as urea, whereas birds excrete uric acid. Many different species of animals have been used extensively as research models to obtain data on the nutrient requirements of humans, and to learn the mode of action of various dietary additives. The researcher must be aware of differences in the nutritional requirements of different species, or erroneous conclusions could be drawn. For example, vitamin C is required for humans, guinea pigs, and monkeys but not for swine and rats, which are frequently used as animal models.

It is essential for livestock, poultry, and aquatic food producers as well as veterinarians, animal caretakers, biomedical research scientists, and others involved in caring for and feeding animals to know what nutrients are required and the amounts of each, the effects of different factors on the efficiency of nutrient utilization, and how best to provide feeds

0-8493-2705-9/01/$0.00+$1.50

with the proper proportions of these nutrients to the animals. Because of the economic importance of this knowledge, scientists throughout the world have conducted research with different species of animals, birds, and fish, and feeding standards based on this research have been developed to formulate diets and rations for domestic livestock, poultry, companion animals, laboratory animals, and other species.

During the past century, scientists from many nations have conducted research on the specific nutritional requirements of numerous species of animals, but there are so many interactions among nutrients — and so many factors that influence nutrient utilization by different species — that tables or formulae for calculating nutritional requirements must be modified periodically. The data presented in this section are based on research summarized by groups of scientists who are most knowledgeable about the nutritional research that has been conducted anywhere in the world on that particular species. In the United States, the National Academy of Sciences, National Research Council (NRC), Board on Agriculture, Committee on Animal Nutrition has been responsible for appointing committees of expert animal scientists to publish periodical reports that summarize the most up-to-date information on nutritional requirements of various species. The nutrient composition of feeds usually consumed by these animals is also included in each of the publications, because the feed evaluation system used to express the nutritional value of feeds determines the manner in which the nutritional requirements of the animal are expressed. Specific information on each species may be obtained by obtaining the most recent NRC publication on that species.

The health and wellbeing of animals are affected markedly by their nutritional status. It is important to know how to properly provide feed that contains the nutrients animals need to meet their nutritional requirements. This applies to companion animals such as dogs, cats, birds, and fish as well as recreational animals such as horses, ponies, donkeys, and camels. The efficient and economical production of food and fiber by domestic livestock and poultry requires good management practices, and especially balanced rations that contain adequate supplies of protein, minerals, vitamins, and energy. In most, if not all, animal production systems a limited energy supply more frequently retards growth and limits production than a deficiency of any other nutrient. Crampton (1956)[1] stated that "the basic need of animals fed normal rations is for energy, and this demand is the basis for most, and perhaps all, of the other nutrient requirements."

The National Research Council, Board on Agriculture, Committee on Animal Nutrition subcommittees prepare reports periodically published by the National Academy Press, 2101 Constitution Avenue NW, Washington, D.C. 20055. The most recent publications (dairy cattle, horses, beef cattle, and swine) have included computer disks with tables of nutrient requirements and feed composition. The full text, including tables, for *Nutrient Requirements of Swine,* 10th Revised Edition, 1998, and may be accessed on the web site of the National Academy Press (http://books.nap.edu).

The most recent National Academy Press series of publications on Nutrient Requirements of Domestic Animals is summarized in Table 4.1. The pages of the tables of nutrient requirements of each species are included, but in order to use this information most effectively, the tables of nutrient composition of most commonly used feed ingredients are needed. The feed composition tables are included in each of these publications. The 1999 *Feedstuffs* Reference Issue (Volume 71, Number 31, July 30, 1999, pages 40-84) has tables based on the NRC publications for swine, beef cattle, dairy cattle, chickens and turkeys, horses, and pets (dogs and cats). There are numerous publications, including animal nutrition textbooks, that have used the tables of nutrient requirements of various species of livestock as well as the tables of nutrient composition. One recent example is *Livestock Feeds and Feeding, 4th Edition,* 1998, by Richard O. Kellems and D.C. Church, Prentice Hall, New Jersey. The species included in this text are: beef cattle, dairy cattle, sheep, goats, swine, poultry, horses, dogs and cats, and rabbits (pages 485–552). Tables of the composition of feedstuffs commonly fed to livestock are on pages 468–484.

Sources of Information for the Nutrient Requirements of Various Species

Nutrient Requirements of Domestic Animals: A Series. Subcommittees of the Committee on Animal Nutrition, Board on Agriculture, National Research Council. National Academy Press. Washington, D.C.

Publications with details, including complete text of most of the current publications are on the computer web site (URL) at http://books.nap.edu. To locate each publication type "Nutrient Requirements" in the box labeled SEARCH ALL TITLES. Tables with specific information on the nutrient requirements of each species as well as the composition of diet ingredients (feedstuffs) may be accessed by clicking on OPEN BOOK Searchable READ.

Companion Animals (Cats and Dogs)

Cats

Nutrient Requirements of Cats, Revised Edition, 1986, 88 pp. 8.5 X 11, 1986 ISBN 0-309-03682-8 (SF 447.6 .N88 1986).

Subcommittee on Cat Nutrition

Quinton R. Rogers, Chairman, University of California, Davis

David H. Baker, University of Illinois

Kenneth C. Hayes, Brandeis University

Peter T. Kendall, Pedigree Foods

James C. Morris, University of California, Davis

Dogs

Nutrient Requirements of Dogs, Revised 1985, 79 pp. ISBN 0-309-03496-5 (S 95 .N28 1985).

Subcommittee on Dog Nutrition

Ben E. Sheffy, Chairman, Cornell University

Kenneth C. Hayes, Brandeis University

Joseph J. Knapka, National Institutes of Health

John A. Milner, University of Illinois at Urbana-Champaign

James G. Morris, University of California, Davis

Dale R. Romsos, Michigan State University

Mink and Foxes

Nutrient Requirements of Mink and Foxes, Second Revised Edition, 1982 (BOA) 72 pp. ISBN 0-309-03325-X.

Subcommittee on Furbearer Nutrition, 1982
Hugh Travis, Chairman, USDA, SEA, Cornell University
E.V. Evans, University of Guelph, Ontario
Gunnar Joergensen, National Institute of Animal Science, Denmark
Richard J. Aulerich, Michigan State University
William L. Leoschke, Valparaiso University, Indiana
James E. Oldfield, Oregon State University

Rabbits

Nutrient Requirements of Rabbits, Second Revised Edition, 1977.

Subcommittee on Rabbit Nutrition, 1977
Arrington Lewis, Chairman
Peter R. Cheeke
Francois Lebas
Sedgwick E. Smith, Cornell University

Laboratory Animals

Rat, mouse, guinea pigs, hamster, gerbils, voles

Nutrient Requirements of Laboratory Animals, Fourth Revised Edition, 1995 (BOA), Nutrient Requirements of Domestic Animals, National Research Council, National Academy Press, Washington, D.C. 1995. 173 pp. ISBN 0-309-05126-6 (SF 406.2 .N88 1995).

Subcommittee on Laboratory Animal Nutrition
Norlin J. Benevenga, Chair, University of Wisconsin, Madison
Christopher Calvert, University of California, Davis
Curtis D. Eckhert, University of California, Los Angeles
Janet L. Greger, University of Wisconsin, Madison
Carl L. Keen, University of California, Davis
Joseph J. Knapka, National Institutes of Health, Bethesda, Maryland
Hulda Magalhaes, Bucknell University
Olav T. Oftedal, National Zoological Park, Washington, D.C.
Philip G. Reeves, Agricultural Research Service, U.S. Department of Agriculture, Grand Forks, North Dakota
Helen Anderson Shaw, University of North Carolina, Greensboro
John Edgar Smith, Pennsylvania State University, University Park
Robert D. Steele, University of Wisconsin

Fish

Nutrient Requirements of Fish (BOA) 128 pp., ISBN-04891-5, 1993 (SH 156 .N86 1993).

Subcommittee on Fish Nutrition

Richard T. Lovell, Chair, Auburn University

C. Young Cho, University of Guelph and Fisheries Branch, Ontario

Ministry of Natural Resources, Canada

Colin B. Cowey, University of Guelph, Canada

Konrad Dabrowski, The Ohio State University

Steven Hughes, U.S. Fish and Wildlife Service, Monell Chemical

Senses Center, Philadelphia, Pennsylvania

Santosh Lall, Nova Scotia Department of Fisheries and Ocean, Canada

Takeshi Murai, National Institute of Fisheries Science, Tokyo, Japan

Robert P. Wilson, Mississippi State University

Avian Species

Poultry (chickens, turkeys, geese, ducks, pheasants, Japanese quail, bobwhite quail)

Nutrient Requirements of Poultry, Ninth Revised Edition, 1994 (BOA) 176 pp., ISBN 0-309-04892-3.

Subcommittee on Poultry Nutrition

Jerry L. Sell, Chair, Iowa State University

F. Howard Kratzer, University of California, Davis

J. David Latshaw, The Ohio State University

Steven L. Leeson, University of Guelph

Edwin T. Moran, Auburn University

Carl M. Parsons, University of Illinois

Park W. Waldroup, University of Arkansas

Domestic Livestock

Nonruminant Species

Swine

Nutrient Requirements of Swine, Tenth Revised Edition, 1998 (BOA) 210 pp., ISBN 0-309-05993-3, Computer laser optical disc (4 3/4 in.).

Subcommittee on Swine Nutrition

Gary L. Cromwell, Chair, University of Kentucky

David H. Baker, University of Illinois

Richard C. Ewan, Iowa State University

E.T. Kornegay, Virginia Polytechnic Institute and State University

Austin J. Lewis, University of Nebraska

James E. Pettigrew, Pettigrew Consulting International, Louisiana, Missouri

Norman C. Steele, U.S.D.A., A.R.S., Beltsville, Maryland

Philip A. Thacker, University of Saskatchewan, Canada

Horses

Nutrient Requirements of Horses, Fifth Revised Edition, 1989 (BOA) 112 pp., ISBN 03989-4.

Subcommittee on Horse Nutrition

Edgar, A. Ott, Chairman, University of Florida, Gainesville

John P. Baker, Uniiversity of Kentucky

Harold F. Hintz, Cornell University

Gary D. Potter, Texas A & M University

Howard D. Stowe, Michigan State University

Duane E. Ullrey, Michigan State University

Ruminant Species

Beef cattle

Nutrient Requirements of Beef Cattle, Seventh Revised Edition, 1996 (BOA) Note: The 7th Revised Edition Update 2000 was released and is on the web site. 242 pp., ISBN 0-309-05426-5, 1 computer disk (3 1/2 in.).

Subcommittee on Beef Cattle Nutrition, 1996

Jock G. Buchanan-Smith, Chair, University of Guelph, Canada

Larry L. Berger, University of Illinois

Calvin L. Ferrell, U.S.D.A., A.R.S., Clay Center, Nebraska

Danny G. Fox, Cornell University

Michael L. Galyean, Clayton Livestock Research Center, Clayton, New Mexico

David P. Hutcheson, Animal Agricultural Consulting, Inc., Amarillo, Texas

Terry J. Klopfenstein, University of Nebraska

Jerry W. Spears, North Carolina State University

Dairy cattle

Nutrient Requirements of Dairy Cattle, Sixth Revised Edition, Update l989 (BOA) 168 pp., ISBN 0-309-03826-X.

Subcommittee on Dairy Cattle Nutrition

Roger W. Hemken, Chairman, University of Kentucky

Clarence B. Ammerman, University of Florida

Donald L. Bath, University of California, Davis

Jimmy H. Clark, University of Illinois

Neal A. Jorgersen, University of Wisconsin

Paul W. Moe, U.S. Department of Agriculture, Beltsville, Maryland

Lawrence D. Muller, Pennsylvania State University

Dale R. Waldo, U.S. Department of Agriculture, Beltsville, Maryland

Sheep

Nutrient Requirements of Sheep, Sixth Revised Edition, 1985 (BOA) 112 pp., ISBN 0-309-03596-1.

Subcommittee on Sheep Nutrition

Robert M. Jordan, Chairman, University of Minnesota

Millard C. Calhoun, Texas Agricultural Experiment Station, San Angelo

Donald G. Ely, University of Kentucky

David P. Heaney, Research Branch, Agriculture Canada, Ottawa

Frank C. Hinds, University of Wyoming

Donald E. Johnson, Colorado State University

Goats

Nutrient Requirements of Goats: Angora, Dairy, and Meat Goats in Temperate and Tropical Countries (BOA) 84 pp., ISBN 0-309-03185-0 (SF 95. N28 no. 15).

Subcommittee on Goat Nutrition

George F.W. Haenlein, Chairman, University of Delaware, Newark

Canagasaby Devendra, Maylasian Agricultural Research and Development Institute, Serdang, Maylasia

James E. Huston, Texas A&M University, San Angelo

O.P.S. Sengar, Raja Balwant Singh College, Bichpuri (Agra), India

Maurice Shelton, Texas A&M University, San Angelo

S.N. Singh, Raja Balwant Singh College, Bichpuri (Agra), India

Nonhuman Primates

Nutrient Requirements of Nonhuman Primates 1978 ix, 83 p.: ill. :28 cm. 1978 ISBN 0-309-02786-1 (SF 95 .N28 1978).

Panel on Nonhuman Primates

George R. Kerr, Chairman, University of Texas School of Public Health

Coy D. Fitch, St. Louis University

Ronald D. Hunt, New England Regional Primate Center

Nutrient Requirement Table 1 pages 18-19.

Nutrient Requirements of Nonhuman Primates: Second Revised Edition, 2000, 300 pages (not yet available).

TABLE 4.1

Web Addresses for Tables of Nutrient Requirements for a Variety of Animals

National Academy Press. Washington, D.C. List of publications with tables of nutrient requirements of each species. http://books.nap.edu. To obtain complete text, including tables, fill in the box labeled SEARCH ALL TITLES with "Nutrient Requirements" and all the following publications with hyperlinks will appear at URL http://books.nap.edu/catalog/910.html.

Nutrient Requirements of Cats, Revised Edition, 1986 (SF 447.6 .N88 1986) Nutrient Requirement Tables, pages 41-44. (http://www.nap.edu/openbook/0309036828/html)

Nutrient Requirements of Dogs, Revised 1985 (S 95 .N28 1985) Nutrient Requirement Tables, pages 44-45. (http://www.nap.edu/openbook/0309034965/html/44.html)

Nutrient Requirements of Mink and Foxes, Second Revised Edition, 1982 (SF 95 .N28 1982) Nutrient Requirement Tables, pages 33-36. (http://www.nap.edu/openbook/030903325X/html/33.html)

Nutrient Requirements of Rabbits, Second Revised Edition, 1977 (SF 95 .N32 1977) Nutrient Requirement Tables, pages 14-15. (http://www.nap.edu/openbook/0309026075/html/14.html)

Nutrient Requirements of Laboratory Animals, Fourth Revised Edition, 1995 (SF 406.2 .N88 1995) Nutrient Requirement Tables for Rats, page 13; Mice, page 82; Guinea Pigs, page 104-105; (Hamsters, Gerbils, and Voles — text rather than tables) (http://www.nap.edu/openbook/0309051266/html/11.html)

Nutrient Requirements of Fish, 1993 (SH 156 .N86 1993) Nutrient Requirements Table, pages 62-63. (http://www.nap.edu/openbook/0309048915/html/62.html)

Nutrient Requirements of Poultry, Ninth Revised Edition, 1994 (SF 95 .N28 1994) Nutrient Requirement Tables for Chickens, pages 19-34 for Tables 2-1 through 2-8; for Turkeys, pages 35-39, Tables 3-1 through 3-3; for Geese pages 40-41; for Ducks, pages 42-43; for Ring-Necked Pheasants, page 44; for Japanese Quail, page 45; for Bobwhite Quail, page 45. (http://www.nap.edu/openbook/0309048923/html/19.html)

Nutrient Requirements of Swine, 10th Revised Edition, 1998 (SF 396.5 .N87 1998). Nutrient Requirement Tables, pages 110-123. Computer laser optical disc (4 3/4 in.). (http://www.nap.edu/openbook/0309059933/html/110.html)

Nutrient Requirements of Horses, Fifth Revised Edition, 1989 (SF 285.5 .N37 1989). Nutrient Requirement Tables, pages 39-48. Computer disk (5 1/4 in.). (http://www.nap.edu/openbook/0309039894/html/39.html)

Nutrient Requirements of Beef Cattle, Seventh Revised Edition, 1996 (SF 203 .N88 1996) Nutrient Requirement Tables, pages 102-112. Prediction Equations and Computer Models, pages 113-131. Computer disk (3 1/2 in.). (http://www.nap.edu/openbook/0309069343/html/102.html)

Nutrient Requirements of Beef Cattle, Seventh Revised Edition: Update 2000, NRC Model Application software available on line at http://stills.nap.edu/readingroom/books/beefmodel/

Nutrient Requirements of Dairy Cattle, Sixth Revised Edition, Update 1989 (SF 203 .N34 1988) Nutrient Requirement Tables, pages 78-88. Computer disk (5 1/4 in.). (http://www.nap.edu/openbook/030903826X/html/78.html)

Nutrient Requirements of Sheep, Sixth Revised Edition, 1985 (SF 376 .N85 1985) Nutrient Requirement Tables, pages 45-53. (http://www.nap.edu/openbook/0309035961/html/45.html)

Nutrient Requirements of Goats: Angora, Dairy, and Meat Goats in Temperate and Tropical Countries, 1981 (S 95 .N28 1981) Nutrient Requirement Tables, pages 10-12. (http://www.nap.edu/openbook/0309031850/html/10.html)

Nutrient Requirements of Nonhuman Primates 1978 (SF 95 .N28 1978) Nutrient Requirement Table 1 pages 18-19. Print-On-Demand. (http://books.nap.edu/catalog/34.html)

Nutrient Requirements of Nonhuman Primates: Second Revised Edition, 2000 300 pages In press, not yet available.

TABLE 4.2

Publications Providing Information on the Nutrient Needs of Specific Animals

A. Nutrient requirements of companion animals (cats and dogs), rabbits, mink and foxes, and laboratory animals (rats, mice, guinea pigs, hamsters, gerbils, and voles) and rabbits, mink, and foxes. Tables of nutrient requirements from *Nutrient Requirements of Domestic Animals: A Series.* National Research Council, National Academy Press (http://books.nap.edu)

Species	NRC Publication	Year last revised	Pages of Tables	Computer disk	NAP Web site of Tables
Companion Animals					
Cats	*Nutrient Requirements of Cats*	1986	41–44	No	Yes
Dogs	*Nutrient Requirements of Dogs*	1985	44–45	No	Yes
Laboratory Animals					
	Nutrient Requirements of Laboratory Animals	1995	13–105	No	Yes
Rats	*Nutrient Requirements of Laboratory Animals*	1995	13	No	Yes
Mice	*Nutrient Requirements of Laboratory Animals*		82	No	Yes
Guinea pigs	*Nutrient Requirements of Laboratory Animals*		104–105	No	Yes
Hamsters	*Nutrient Requirements of Laboratory Animals*		Text	No	Yes
Gerbils	*Nutrient Requirements of Laboratory Animals*		Text	No	Yes
Voles	*Nutrient Requirements of Laboratory Animals*		Text	No	Yes
Other Small Animals					
Rabbits	*Nutrient Requirements of Rabbits*	1977	14–15	No	Yes
Mink	*Nutrient Requirements of Mink and Foxes*	1982	33–34	No	Yes
Foxes	*Nutrient Requirements of Mink and Foxes*	1982	35–36	No	Yes

B. Nutrient requirements of poultry (chickens, turkeys, geese, ducks, ring-necked pheasants, Japanese quail and bobwhite quail), fish, nonhuman primates, horses and swine. Tables of nutrient requirements from *Nutrient Requirements of Domestic Animals: A Series.* National Research Council, National Academy Press (http://books.nap.edu)

Species	NRC Publication	Year last revised	Pages of Tables	Computer disk	NAP Web site of Tables
Avian Species					
	Nutrient Requirements of Poultry	1994	19–45	No	Yes
Chickens	*Nutrient Requirements of Poultry*	1994	19–34	No	Yes
Turkeys	*Nutrient Requirements of Poultry*	1994	35–39	No	Yes
Geese	*Nutrient Requirements of Poultry*	1994	40–41	No	Yes
Ducks	*Nutrient Requirements of Poultry*	1994	42–43	No	Yes
Ring-necked pheasants	*Nutrient Requirements of Poultry*	1994	44	No	Yes
Japanese quail	*Nutrient Requirements of Poultry*	1994	45	No	Yes
Bobwhite quail	*Nutrient Requirements of Poultry*	1994	45	No	Yes

B. Nutrient requirements of poultry (chickens, turkeys, geese, ducks, ring-necked pheasants, Japanese quail and bobwhite quail), fish, nonhuman primates, horses and swine. Tables of nutrient requirements from *Nutrient Requirements of Domestic Animals: A Series.* National Research Council, National Academy Press (http://books.nap.edu)

Species	NRC Publication	Year last revised	Pages of Tables	Computer disk	NAP Web site of Tables
Other Species					
Fish	*Nutrient Requirements of Fish*	1993	62–63	No	Yes
Nonhuman Primates	*Nutrient Requirements of Nonhuman Primates*	1978 (2000 in press)	18–19	No	No (Yes, soon for 2000)
Horses	*Nutrient Requirements of Horses*	1989	39–48	Yes (5 1/4 in.)	Yes
Swine	*Nutrient Requirements of Swine*	1998	110–123	Yes (Laser optical disk, 4 3/4 in.	Yes

C. Nutrient requirements of ruminants (beef cattle, dairy cattle, sheep and goats). Tables of nutrient requirements from *Nutrient Requirements of Domestic Animals: A Series.* National Research Council, National Academy Press (http://books.nap.edu)

Species	NRC Publication	Year last revised	Pages of Tables	Computer disk	NAP Web site of Tables
Ruminant Species					
Beef Cattle	*Nutrient Requirements of Beef Cattle*	2000	102–112	Yes (3 1/2 in.)	Yes
Dairy Cattle	*Nutrient Requirements of Dairy Cattle*	1989	78–88	Yes (5 1/4 in.)	Yes
Sheep	*Nutrient Requirements of Sheep*	1985	45–53	No	Yes
Goats	*Nutrient Requirements of Goats: Angora, Dairy and Meat Goats in Temperate and Tropical Countries*	1981	10–12	No	Yes

References

1. Crampton, EW. 1956. *Applied Animal Nutrition. The Use of Feedstuffs in the Formulation of Livestock Rations.* W.H. Freeman and Co., San Francisco, CA.

Part IV

Human Nutrient Needs in the Life Cycle

5

Nutrition during Pregnancy and Lactation

Kathryn M. Kolasa and David G. Weismiller

Recommendations for Women before Pregnancy

It seems logical that the nutritional status of a woman prior to pregnancy as well as maternal nutrition should affect fetal development and subsequent pregnancy outcome. However, many confounding variables are common to the investigation of maternal nutrition and fetal development.[1] This section briefly summarizes recommendations for maternal nutrition.[2-7] It also includes comments about lactation, since maternal diet plays a central role in the transfer of nutriments to the infant. Table 5.1 includes special recommendations for women during childbearing years. Suggestions for counseling and treatment during a preconception care office visit are given in Table 5.2.

Risk Factors for Prenatal Nutrition Risk and Indications for Referral

Table 5.2 includes nutrition assessment, counseling, and treatment strategies for women seeking care in both the prenatal and postnatal stages. Fetal growth is affected by the

TABLE 5.1

Special Recommendations for Women before Pregnancy

Maintain a healthy weight.
Engage in physical activity regularly.
If you need to gain or lose weight, do so gradually (no more than 1–2 pounds/week).
If trying to become pregnant and ordinarily drink alcoholic beverages, stop drinking or cut back on the amount you drink.
If you smoke, quit or cut back to improve health.
To minimize risk of having an infant with a neural tube defect, eat a highly fortified breakfast cereal that provides 100% of the Daily Value (DV) for folate or take a vitamin supplement that provides 400 μg/day of folic acid. Folic acid, the synthetic form of folate, is obtained only from fortified foods or vitamin supplements. It is not yet known whether naturally occurring folate is as effective as folic acid in the prevention of neural tube defects.

0-8493-2705-9/01/$0.00+$1.50

TABLE 5.2

Nutritional Care at Preconception, Prenatal, and Postnatal Visits

Visit	Assessment	Counseling/Treatment
Preconception care	Determine BMI	If <18 or >25, counsel on appropriate weight
	Evaluate diet/supplement intake	Develop a concrete plan for eating enough food to achieve/maintain a healthy weight Begin prenatal vitamin/mineral supplement Prescribe calcium supplement if intake <1000 mg Prescribe synthetic folic acid supplement of 400 µg per day
	Botanical use	Discontinue those with known or potential toxicities
	Evaluate for anemia	Hgb <12 g/dl, start therapeutic regimen of approximately 60–120 mg/day of ferrous iron; give multivitamin/mineral supplement that contains ~15 mg of zinc and ~2 mg of copper When anemia has resolved, discontinue high-dose iron
	Use of harmful substances	Reinforcement for any constructive steps already taken; provide assistance with quitting, and refer for further evaluation
Prenatal	Evaluate diet	Utilize dietary intake questionnaire, e.g. Diet Score, food frequency questionnaires
	Optimal weight gain during pregnancy	BMI <19.8 28–40 lbs 19.8–26.0 25–35 lbs 26.1–29.0 15–25 lbs >29 ~15 lbs
	Rate of weight gain	First trimester 1 1/2–5 lbs Second and third trimester 1/2–2 lbs/week
	Poor weight gain < 2 lbs/month < 10 lbs by mid-pregnancy	Intensive assessment and counseling
	Nutritional needs/barriers	If patient is economically unable to meet nutritional needs — referral to federal food and nutrition programs (WIC) Increase knowledge with dietary counseling
	Vitamin/mineral supplementation	No requirement for routine supplementation except folate (400 µg/day) and iron (30–60 mg elemental iron/day) Dietary supplements should be given if the adequacy of a patient's diet is questionable or if she is at high nutritional risk Excessive vitamin and mineral intake (more than twice the RDA) should be avoided
	Prophylaxis for iron deficiency	Supplement of ferrous iron — 30 mg elemental iron daily
	Iron deficiency anemia	60–120 mg elemental iron daily
	Evaluate use of alcohol, tobacco, drugs	Effects of substance use/abuse on perinatal outcomes Abstinence from alcoholic beverages
	Caffeine intake	Consumption of 2–3 servings of caffeinated beverages is unlikely to have adverse effects; in general, caffeinated beverages provide few essential nutrients and often crowd out better sources of nutrients
	Lactose intolerance	May result in insufficient calcium intake Supplemental calcium necessary if insufficient calcium consumed from food sources
	Gestational diabetes mellitus	Referral for nutrition assessment and counseling
	Nausea/emesis	Eat crackers before getting out of bed in the morning; eat frequent small meals; eat low-fat, bland foods; eat ginger (soda, tea, or ginger snaps); suck on hard candy; eat salty/tart foods combined (e.g., potato chips with lemonade); supplement with vitamin B_6 (25 mg three times daily); wear Sea Band® (an elastic band worn on wrists to counter nausea caused by sea-sickness)

TABLE 5.2 *(Continued)*

Nutritional Care at Preconception, Prenatal, and Postnatal Visits

Visit	Assessment	Counseling/Treatment
	Hyperemesis gravidarum	Doxylamine (Unisom), 12.5–25 mg three times daily; ginger in any form (tea, soda, tablets [250-mg capsule, 4 times daily for 4–5 days]); emetrol, 5–10 mL in the morning and every 3–4 hours as needed; anti-emetic/anti-nausea medications (e.g., trimethobenzamine [Tebamide, Tigan, Trimazide], 200 mg suppository three times daily, or promethazine, 12.5–25 mg orally, rectally, or intravenously every 4–6 hours)
	Constipation	Foods high in dietary fiber, including cereals, bread, fruits, and vegetables; adequate fluids; moderate exercise; soluble fiber (e.g., Metamucil, Citrucel); docusate; change brand of iron supplement
Postpartum	Diet	Utilize dietary intake questionnaire Dietary guidelines are similar to those established during pregnancy Balanced, nutritious diet will ensure both the quality and quantity of milk produced without depletion of maternal stores
	Caloric requirement	Minimal caloric requirement for adequate milk production in a woman of average size is 1800 kcal/day
	Vitamin/mineral supplement	Not needed routinely; mothers at nutritional risk should be given a multivitamin supplement with particular emphasis on calcium and vitamins B_{12} and D
	Weight retention	There is no relationship between BMI or total weight gain and weight retention Aging, rather than parity, is the major determinant of increases in a woman's weight over time
	Residual postpartum weight retention	Special attention to lifestyle, including exercise and eating habits

quality and quantity of the maternal diet, the ability of the mother to digest and absorb nutrients, maternal cardiorespiratory function, uterine blood flow, placental transfer, placental blood flow, and appropriate distribution and handling of nutrients and oxygen by the fetus. Factors that put women at nutritional risk for pregnancy are listed in Table 5.3.[5,8-10] Patients at high nutritional risk should be provided professional nutritional counseling and/or referral to a nutrition intervention program. (Table 5.4). The Women, Infants, and Children (WIC) Program is a food prescription program designed and proven to reduce poor pregnancy outcomes (Table 5.5).

Weight Gain and Pregnancy

Pregnancy Weight Goals

There is a lack of consistent findings concerning relationships of birth interval, parity, prepregnancy weight or body mass index (BMI), height, and physical activity to maternal weight or weight gain.[11-24] The Cochrane Pregnancy and Childbirth Group[25] summarized the findings on the effects of advising pregnant women to increase their energy and protein intakes, on gestational weight gain, and on the outcome of pregnancy. They found that nutritional advice appears to be effective in increasing pregnant women's energy and

TABLE 5.3

Risk Factors for Prenatal Nutritional Risk

Risk Factor	Low Risk	High Risk
Is patient pre- or adolescent or less than 3 yrs post menarche?	No	Yes
Is patient economically disadvantaged or have limited income for food?	No	Yes
Does patient have history of anemia or is anemic (hematocrit <32 mg/% during pregnancy)?	No	Yes
Is patient's BMI <19.8 or >26.1?	No	Yes
Does patient have history of fad dieting, or restrictive eating?	No	Yes
Does patient have illness or medication that will interfere with absorption; is she HIV+ ?	No	Yes
Does patient use tobacco, alcohol, or drugs?	No	Yes
Does patient practice pica (consume ice, starch, clay, or other substances in large amounts)?	No	Yes
Does patient experience nausea and/or vomiting?	No	Yes
Is patient lactose intolerant?	No	Yes
Is weight gain 0.8–1.0 lb/wk?	No	Yes
Does patient stay within the weight gain range recommended for her prepregnancy BMI?	Yes	No
Weight gain less than 15 lbs or more than 45 lbs?	No	Yes

TABLE 5.4

Indications for a Referral of Pregnant Patients for Nutrition Assessment and Counseling

Patient has interest in and desire to see a nutritionist
Patient has inappropriate weight gain
Patient has gestational diabetes
Patient has chronic condition managed with diet (e.g., diabetes, hyperlipidemia)
Patient has history of anemia
Patient has inadequate or inappropriate food supply
Patient has history of prepregnancy anorexia or bulimia
Patient has significant discomforts of pregnancy (e.g., heartburn, nausea, vomiting)
Patient has preeclampsia
Patient has multiple gestation
Patient is adolescent
Patient is vegetarian
Patient is interested in or undecided about breastfeeding

TABLE 5.5

Characteristics of Women, Infants, and Children (WIC) Program

Target Audience	Pregnant women Breastfeeding women Non-breastfeeding mothers of infants <6 months old Infants <1 y/o Children <5 y/o
Purpose	Provide nutritious foods, health checks, referrals, nutrition education, and counseling
Eligibility Criteria	Low income: <185% U.S. federal poverty level for women and children
Food	Nutrient rich, high in protein, calcium, iron and vitamins A & C Limited brand names Patient-purchased food and infant formula from local supermarkets
Nutrition Education	Individual and group Specific to risk
Health Checks	Height, weight, and anemia testing for women, infants and children Height, weight, and anemia testing for women and children 1 yr old test for lead

TABLE 5.6

Pregnancy Weight Goals

Optimal Weight Gain (pounds)	Characteristic
25–35	Most women and normal pregnancy Prepregnancy BMI 19.8–26.0 or 100% prepregnancy ideal body weight
28–40	Women at higher risk for low birth weight babies including adolescents and African American women Prepregnancy BMI <19.8 (underweight) or 90% ideal body weight Twin pregnancy
15–25	Prepregnant BMI >26.1 (overweight or obese) or >120% ideal body weight
15	Prepregnant BMI >29 or >135% ideal body weight

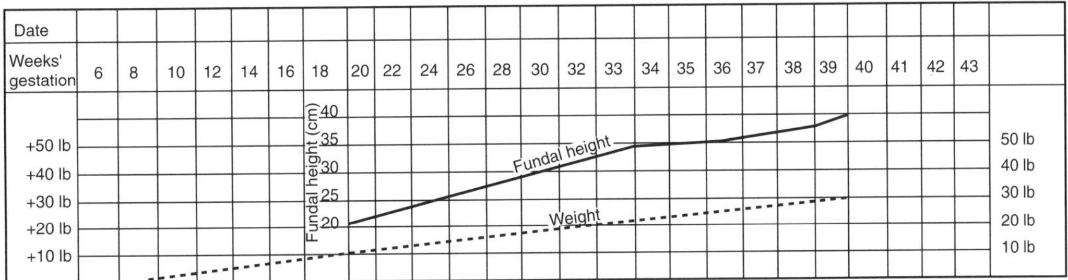

FIGURE 5.1
Graph for tracking weight and fundal height. (From Kolasa, K.M. and Weismiller, D.G., Nutrition during pregnancy, *Am Fam Phys*, 56(1): 206, July 1995. With permission.)

protein intakes but the implications for fetal, infant, or maternal health cannot be judged from the available trials.[26]

Some researchers question the recommendation that African American women gain more weight than caucasian women, suggesting that the data only show questionable benefit in reducing risks for low birth weight babies. Obese women have a greater risk of pregnancy complications, especially gestational diabetes, hypertensive disorders, cesarean deliveries, and postoperative morbidity. Infants of obese women may be at greater risk for macrosomia and perinatal death.[21,25]

The recommendations in Table 5.6 were established by the National Academy of Sciences of the National Institute of Medicine in 1990.[16] They were reviewed and left unchanged by the Maternal Weight Gain Expert Group in 1996.[24] Weight gain goals are determined to provide optimal risk reduction for delivering a low birth weight baby while avoiding adverse effects on the mother's health. The recommendations vary based on prepregnancy weight, age, and ethnicity. The weight gain expected is essentially linear, as demonstrated in Figure 5.1.[4]

Women with prepregnant body mass index (BMI) >35 are at increased risk for gestational diabetes, preeclampsia, placenta abrupta, cesarean delivery, and endometriosis.

Rate of Weight Gain

In 1996, the Maternal and Weight Gain Expert Group[24] suggested a weight gain of 1.5 pounds/week for normal weight women during the second half of a twin pregnancy.

TABLE 5.7

Rate of Weight Gain (Pounds)

Timing (trimester)	Appropriate	Inadequate	Excessive
1st	3–5 Total	Less	More
2nd, 3rd	1/wk	Less than 2 lbs in a single month for normal wt women or less than 1 lb in obese	More than 6.5 in a single month

TABLE 5.8

Weight Gain Distribution during Pregnancy (Pounds)

Source	Pounds
Amniotic fluid	2–2.6
Baby	7–8.5
Fat/breast tissue stores for breastfeeding	1–4
Increased blood volume	4–5
Increased weight of uterus	2
Maternal fat stores	4–7
Placenta	0.7–1.0
Tissue fluid	3–5
Total	25–35

Weight gain is the single most reliable indicator of pregnancy outcome.[11,23] Weight status should be routinely assessed for amount and rate. Figure 5.1 depicts an example of a graph for tracking weight. Weight charts should be shown to women and their support partners. Table 5.7 gives recommended weight gains. The optimal weight for a newborn infant of 39 to 41 weeks gestation is 6.6 to 8.8 pounds.[9]

Women with inadequate weight gain should eat more frequently, be referred to a dietitian for nutrient assessment and counseling, choose more nutrient-dense foods, avoid alcohol and tobacco use, limit activity, and avoid caffeine or other appetite depressants. Women with excessive gain should reduce portion sizes, limit intake of sweets and foods high in fat, increase activity, and be evaluated by a registered dietitian.

Weight Gain Distribution during Pregnancy

Weight gain by pregnant women consists of water, protein, and fat. Measurements of maternal water gain may predict birth weight better than measurements of composite weight gain. The total amount of weight gained, the composition of gain, and the rate of energy metabolism all differ among healthy pregnant women. Table 5.8 is a typical teaching tool about weight gain distribution.

Nutrition Snacks

Pregnant women may need suggestions for healthy snacks. Table 5.9 includes snacks of about 100 calories.

Dietary Requirements for Pregnancy and Lactation

Dietary Reference Intake (DRI)

Dietary Reference Intakes are the levels of intake of essential nutrients considered adequate to meet or exceed known nutritional needs of practically all healthy people. Table 5.10

TABLE 5.9

Nutritious Snacks of 100 kcalories or Less

Food Item	Serving Size
Applesauce	2/3 cup
Bagel	1/2
Carrot, raw	1 cup or 1 large
Cheese, low-fat	1 oz.
Cottage cheese, low-fat	1/3 cup
Entenmann's® fat-free cakes/pastries	1 small slice
Figs, low-fat or other Newton® cookies	1-1/2 tsp
fruit, dried (like apricots, raisins, prunes)	4 tsp.
Fruit, fresh	1 medium
Graham crackers	2
Grits	1 package
Milk, skim	1 cup
Pretzels	15
Pudding made w/skim milk	1/3 cup
Rice cakes, flavored	2
Tortilla chips, baked, low-fat and w/salsa	12
Tuna	1/2 cup
Yogurt, frozen	1/2 cup
Yogurt, low-fat	1/2 cup

includes the Recommended Dietary Allowances (RDA) and Adequate Intakes (AI) as available in 1999 for pregnancy and lactation.[27,28] These levels are set by the Food and Nutrition Board of the National Academy of Sciences.

Nutrient needs that are increased during pregnancy and/or lactation include protein, folate, vitamins A, B6, C, and D, calcium, iron, and zinc.[18,29-34] Energy needs are also increased by 300 kcal/day at the second trimester of pregnancy and by 850 kcal/day during lactation to produce adequate breast milk supply. During lactation 500 calories should be consumed as nutrient-dense foods, with the remaining 350 calories coming from maternal fat stores accumulated during pregnancy.[35]

The Food Guide Pyramid Servings

The Food Guide Pyramid (Table 5.11) provides guidelines for the number of servings from each food group that should be eaten daily during pregnancy and lactation. Pregnant women should drink 8 to 10 glasses of water each day.

Dietary Assessment of the Pregnant Woman

Individualized nutrition assessment and planning is important because of the strong associations between extremes in prepregnancy BMI, extremes in weight gain, and adverse pregnancy outcomes.[3,4,7,36,37]

Behavior Change Tool

Assessment relies on the woman's medical record, history, and physical examination. Nutritional factors of importance include previous nutritional challenges, eating disorders, pica, fad dieting, strict vegetarian diet, medications, and quantity and quality of current diet. The Institute of Medicine provides a sample dietary history tool (Table 5.12).[3]

TABLE 5.10

Food and Nutrition Board, National Academy of Sciences — National Research Council Recommended Dietary Allowances,[a] revised 1989 (abridged) and Dietary Reference Intakes (DRI)

Designed for the maintenance of good nutrition of practically all healthy people in the United States

Category	Condition	Protein (g)	Vitamin A (μg RE)[b]	Vitamin E (mg α-TE)[c]	Vitamin K (μg)	Vitamin C (mg)	Iron (mg)	Zinc (mg)	Iodine (μg)	Selenium (μg)
Pregnant		60	800	10	65	70	30	15	175	65
Lactating	1st 6 months	65	1300	12	65	95	15	19	200	75
	2nd 6 months	62	1200	11	65	90	15	16	200	75

Note: *Dietary Reference Intakes for Calcium, Phosphorus, Magnesium, Vitamin D, and Fluoride* [1997] and *Dietary Reference Intakes for Thiamin, Riboflavin, Niacin, Vitamin B_6, Folate, Vitamin B_{12}, Pantothenic Acid, Biotin, and Choline* [1998].

[a] The allowances, expressed as average daily intakes over time, are intended to provide for individual variations among most normal persons as they live in the U.S. under usual environmental stresses. Diets should be based on a variety of common foods in order to provide other nutrients for which human requirements have been less well defined.

[b] Retinol equivalents. 1 retinol equivalent = 1 μg retinol or 6 μg β-carotene.

[c] α-Tocopherol equivalents. 1 mg d-α tocopherol = α-TE.

TABLE 5.10 *(Continued)*

Food and Nutrition Board, Institute of Medicine — National Academy of Sciences

Dietary Reference Intakes: Recommended Intakes For Individuals

Life-Stage Group	Calcium (mg/d)	Phosphorus (mg/d)	Magnesium (mg/d)	Vitamin D (μg/d)[a,b]	Fluoride (mg/d)	Thiamin (mg/d)	Riboflavin (mg/d)	Niacin (mg/d)[c]	Vitamin B_6 (mg/d)	Folate (μg/d)[d]	Vitamin B_{12} (μg/d)	Pantothenic Acid (mg/d)	Biotin (μg/d)	Choline[c] (mg/d)
Pregnancy														
≤ 18 yr	1300*	**1250**	**400**	5*	3*	**1.4**	**1.4**	**18**	**1.9**	**600**[h]	**2.6**	6*	30*	450*
19-30 yr	1000*	**700**	**350**	5*	3*	**1.4**	**1.4**	**18**	**1.9**	**600**[h]	**2.6**	6*	30*	450*
31-50 yr	1000*	**700**	**360**	5*	3*	**1.4**	**1.4**	**18**	**1.9**	**600**[h]	**2.6**	6*	30*	450*
Lactation														
≤ 18 yr	1300*	**1250**	**360**	5*	3*	**1.5**	**1.6**	**17**	**2.0**	**500**	**2.8**	7*	35*	550*
19-30 yr	1000*	**700**	**310**	5*	3*	**1.5**	**1.6**	**17**	**2.0**	**500**	**2.8**	7*	35*	550*
31-50 yr	1000*	**700**	**320**	5*	3*	**1.5**	**1.6**	**17**	**2.0**	**500**	**2.8**	7*	35*	550*

Note: This table presents Recommended Dietary Allowances (RDAs) in bold type and Adequate Intakes (AIs) in ordinary type followed by an asterisk (*).

[a] As cholecalciferol. 1μg cholecalciferol = 40 IU vitamin D.

[b] In the absence of adequate exposure to sunlight.

[c] As niacin equivalents (NE). 1 mg of niacin = 60 mg of tryptophan; 0-6 months = preformed niacin (not NE).

[d] As dietary folate equivalents (DFE). 1 DFE = 1μg food folate = 0.6 μg of folic acid (from fortified food or supplement) consumed with food = 0.5 μg of synthetic (supplemental) folic acid taken on an empty stomach.

[e] In view of evidence linking folate intake with neural tube defects in the fetus, it is recommended that all women capable of becoming pregnant consume 400 μg of synthetic folic acid from fortified foods and/or supplements in addition to intake of food folate from a varied diet.

[f] It is assumed that women will continue consuming 400 μg of folic acid until their pregnancy is confirmed and they enter prenatal care, which ordinarily occurs after the end of the periconceptional period — the critical time for formation of the neural tube.

TABLE 5.11

Food Guide Pyramid Servings

Food Group	Serving Size	Number of Servings: During Adolescent Pregnancy	During Pregnancy	During Pregnancy
Milk/dairy	1 milk, cottage cheese, or yogurt; 1 oz. cheese	5	4	4
Protein-rich	3 oz. meat, fish, or poultry; 1 dried beans	4	3–4	3–4
Breads/cereals, rice/pasta	1/2 cooked rice, cereal, or pasta; 1 slice bread; 4 crackers	9–11	6–11	6–11
Fruits	1 small piece fresh fruit; 1/2 canned fruit; 1/3 fruit juice	2–4	2–4	2–4
Vegetables	1/2 fresh, cooked, or canned	3–5	3–5	3–5
Fats/oils/sweets	1 tsp margarine, mayonnaise, salad dressing or gravy	use in moderation	use sparingly	use sparingly

TABLE 5.12

Behavior Change Dietary Assessment Tool

What you eat and some of the lifestyle choices you make can affect your nutrition and health now and in the future. Your nutrition can also have an important effect on your baby's health. Please answer these questions by circling the answers that apply to you.

Eating Behavior

1. Are you frequently bothered by any of the following? (circle all that apply)
   Nausea Vomiting Heartburn Constipation
2. Do you skip meals at least 3 times a week? No Yes
3. Do you try to limit the amount or kind of food you eat to control your weight? No Yes
4. Are you on a special diet now? No Yes
5. Do you avoid any foods for health or religious reasons? No Yes

Food Sources

6. Do you have a working stove? No Yes
   Do you have a working refrigerator? No Yes
7. Do you sometimes run out of food before you are able to buy more? No Yes
8. Can you afford to eat the way you should? No Yes
9. Are you receiving any food assistance now? (circle all that apply)
   Food stamps School breakfast School lunch
   Donated food Commodity Supplemental Food Program
   Food from a food pantry, soup kitchen, or food banks
10. Do you feel you need help in obtaining food? No Yes

Food and Drink

11. Which of these did you drink yesterday? (circle all that apply)
    Soft drinks Coffee Tea Fruit drink
    Orange juice Grapefruit juice Other juices Milk
    Kool-Aid® Beer Wine Alcoholic drinks
    Water Other beverages (list) ____________________
12. Which of these foods did you eat yesterday (circle all that apply):
    Cheese Pizza Macaroni and cheese
    Yogurt Cereal with milk

13. Other foods made with cheese (such as tacos, enchiladas, lasagna, cheeseburgers)

Corn	Potatoes	Sweet potatoes	Green salad	
Carrots	Collard greens	Spinach	Turnip greens	
Broccoli	Green beans	Green peas	Other vegetables	
Apples	Bananas	Berries	Grapefruit	
Melon	Oranges	Peaches	Other fruit	
Meat	Fish	Chicken	Eggs	
Peanut butter	Nuts	Seeds	Dried beans	
Cold cuts	Hot dog	Bacon	Sausage	
Cake	Cookies	Doughnut	Pastry	
Chips	French fries	Deep fried foods, such as fried chicken or egg rolls		
Bread	Rolls	Rice	Cereal	
Noodles	Spaghetti	Tortillas		

Were any of these whole grain? No Yes

13. Is the way you ate yesterday the way you usually eat? No Yes

Lifestyle

14. Do you exercise for at least 30 minutes on a regular basis — 3 times a week or more? No Yes
15. Do you ever smoke cigarettes or use smokeless tobacco? No Yes
16. Do you ever drink beer, wine, liquor, or any other alcoholic beverages? No Yes
17. Which of these do you take? (circle all that apply)
    Prescribed drugs or medications
    Any over the counter products (such as aspirin, acetaminophen, antacids, or vitamins)
    Street drugs (such as marijuana, speed, downers, crack, or heroin)

From: Institute of Medicine, 1992.

Systematic assessment of the diet is preferable to questions like "How are you eating?" The 24-hour dietary recall method is commonly used to recall the types and amounts of foods and beverages consumed during the previous day. The food frequency questionnaire has been demonstrated to detect pregnancy-related changes in diet.

Nutritional Risk Tool

Table 5.13 is an example of a more quantitative method for assessing the diet.[37] The mother's usual intake is determined for each of the food groups (meats and alternatives, dairy, bread and cereal, fruits and vegetables) and the score is tallied. A patient with fewer than 80 points is at nutritional risk. The evaluator should determine whether the patient has problems such as nausea/vomiting, lactose intolerance, constipation, or cravings for non-food items. Women with a score of fewer than 50 points should be referred to a registered dietitian for counseling.

Complications of Pregnancy that May Impact Nutritional Status

A number of complications of pregnancy may impact nutritional status. Some of these include nausea and vomiting, constipation, caffeine intake, and alcohol intake.

Nausea and Vomiting

About 70% of pregnant women report nausea during the first 14–16 weeks of pregnancy, and 37–58% experience vomiting. The etiology is unknown. The remedies include diet, fluids, and reassurance.[38,39] Table 5.14 is a collection of remedies.

TABLE 5.13

Nutritional Risk Score (Massachusetts Department of Health)

Foods Usually Eaten	Amount
Meat or alternates	
meats, fish, poultry (fresh or processed), liver, eggs, nuts, peanut butter, legumes	_______ servings
1 oz = 5 points	_______ oz. meat, fish, cheese[a]
maximum score = 40 points	_______ oz. alternate
Milk (type) 1 unit = 5 points	_______ fluid
1 unit = 8 fl oz.	_______ cups
Cheese[b] (type) ____________	_______ oz.
maximum score = 15 points	
Bread and cereal[c] whole grain, enriched, other maximum score = 15 points	_______ servings
Fruits and vegetables	
citrus and/or vitamin C-rich vegetables	_______ servings
green and yellow vegetables	_______ servings
all other, including potato	_______ servings
	Total fruits
vitamin A / vitamin C	
1 unit = 5 points / 1 unit = 5 points	
2 units = 15 points / 2 units = 15 points	_______ servings
Supplements[d] (type)	_______ amount
Other foods and beverages	
total score: more than 80 = no risk, less, less than 80 = risk, less than 50 = high risk	

[a] Cheese in excess of the 3 units scored in milk; 1 oz. cheese equals 1 unit
[b] Maximum of 3 oz. scored
[c] Unit = 1 slice of bread or 1 oz cereal. Less than 3 units = 0, 3 units = 5 points, 4 units = 10 points, 5 units = 15 points
[d] Not given a score

From *JADA*: 86(10), 1986, with permission.

TABLE 5.14

Nonpharmacological Remedies for Nausea and Vomiting

Eat small, frequent meals
Eat dry foods/cold foods
Take dietary supplements after meals
Suck on candy
Switch brands of iron supplements
Eat combinations of foods that are salty and tart
Eat vitamin B6-rich foods
Try seabands or accupressure bands
Avoid beverages with meat
Avoid caffeine
Avoid spicy, acidic foods, strong odors
Sniff lemon
Drink ginger root tea, ginger ale; eat ginger snaps; take ginger tablets (250 mg tablets 4x daily for 4–5 days)
Drink plenty of fluids to avoid dehydration

TABLE 5.15

Hyperemesis Gravidurum

Medication	Dosage
Vitamin B_6	25 mg tid
Doxylamine	12.5–25 mg tid
Emetrol	5–10 cc in the morning and every 3–4 hrs as needed
Anti-emetic/anti-nausea medications, e.g., trimethobenyamine (Tigan)	200 mg suppository q 8 prn
Promethazine	12.5–25 mg po. Pr or iv q 4-6

Hyperemesis Gravidarum

Vomiting that produces weight loss, dehydration, acidosis from starvation, alkalosis from loss of hydrochloric acid in vomitus, and/or hypokalemia may be treated pharmacologically. Management is to correct dehydration, fluid and electrolyte deficits, acidosis, and alkalosis. Table 5.15 includes some pharmacological approaches.

Constipation

Constipation is extremely common in pregnancy due to decreased motility of the gastrointestinal (GI) tract. Constipation can be exacerbated by iron supplementation. Constipation is often related to low dietary fiber intake and low fluid intake. Table 5.16 includes foods rich in dietary fiber. The recommended intake is 20 to 30 grams of dietary fiber daily.

Caffeine during Pregnancy and Lactation

The literature is mixed on the effects of caffeine during pregnancy. The official FDA position advises pregnant women to avoid caffeine or consume it sparingly. Most experts agree that caffeine should be limited to less than two servings per day. Caffeine is known to decrease availability of calcium, iron, and zinc. It is not known to exert effects on the fetus. The relationship of caffeine to spontaneous abortion remains controversial. A recent report suggests that risk increases with the consumption in the range of 6 to 18 cups of coffee per day.[40]

Caffeine does pass into breast milk, and therefore consumption during lactation should be limited. Table 5.17 lists caffeine values for popular beverages.

Some suggestions for reducing caffeine consumption include: 1) switching to decaffeinated coffee or soft drinks; 2) cutting down on caffeinated beverages; 3) mixing caffeinated and decaffeinated coffee grounds together before making coffee; or 4) limiting consumption of caffeinated beverages to a preselected number and then switching to decaffeinated beverages over time.

Alcohol

Consumption of alcohol during pregnancy and lactation is controversial.

Pregnancy

A safe lower limit of alcohol during pregnancy is not known. Therefore, the only sure way to avoid the possible harmful effects of alcohol on the fetus is to abstain. Binge

TABLE 5.16

Dietary Sources of Fiber

Serving Size	Food	Grams of Fiber
Breads, Cereals, Pastas		
3 cups	Air-popped popcorn	4
1 medium	Bran muffin	3
2/3 cup	Brown rice	3
1 slice	Whole wheat bread	3
1/2 cup	Cooked legumes	5
1/2 cup	Baked beans	10
1/2 cup	Great northern beans	7
1/2 cup	Lima beans	7
Fruits		
1 cup	Raisins	6
3	Dried prunes	5
1 medium	Pear with skin	4
1 medium	Apple with skin	3
1 cup	Strawberries	3
1 medium	Banana	3
1 medium	Orange	3
Vegetables		
1/2 cup	Cooked frozen peas	4
1 medium	Baked potato w/ skin	4
1/2 cup	Brussels sprouts	3
1/2 cup	Cooked broccoli tops	3
1/2 cup	Cooked carrots	3
1/2 cup	Cooked corn	3

drinking or excessive drinking during pregnancy results in fetal alcohol syndrome. However, even small amounts of alcohol can temporarily alter fetal function. Adverse outcomes have not been found with daily consumption of fewer than two standard drinks. The danger from light drinking should not be overstated. This may cause undue stress in some patients who had a few drinks before realizing they were pregnant (see Table 5.18).

Lactation

Alcohol does not increase milk volume. Chronic consumption can inhibit milk ejection reflex. The American Academy of Pediatrics does, however, consider minimal alcohol (no more than 2 to 2.5 oz liquor, 8 oz wine, or 2 cans of beer on any day) compatible with lactation.

Hypertension

In 1999 the National High Blood Pressure Education Committee issued an advisory on diagnoses and treatment of high blood pressure.[41] Using evidence-based medicine and consensus, this report updates contemporary approaches to hypertension control during pregnancy by expanding on recommendations made in the *Sixth Report of the Joint National Committee on Prevention, Detection, Evaluation, and Treatment of High Blood Pressure (JNC VI).*

TABLE 5.17

Caffeine Audit

Approximate the caffeine you consume by filling in the table. Recall caffeine consumption during the past 24 hours and record in column A, the number of servings or doses for each listed item. Then multiply the column A value by its corresponding column B value and record the product in column C. Add all values in column C to estimate your intake.

Sources of Caffeine	Column A Number of Servings per Day		Column B Amount of Caffeine per Serving (mg)		Column C Total Caffeine (mg)
Coffee (6 oz.)					
Automatic drip	________	×	180	=	________
Automatic perk	________	×	135	=	________
Instant	________	×	125	=	________
Decaffeinated	________	×	5	=	________
Soft Drinks (12 oz.)					
Regular colas	________	×	37	=	________
Diet colas	________	×	50	=	________
Cocoa Products					
Chocolate candy (2 oz.)	________	×	45	=	________
Baking chocolate (1 oz.)	________	×	30	=	________
Milk chocolate (2 oz.)	________	×	10	=	________
South American cocoa (6 oz.)	________	×	40	=	________
Drugs (one tablet or capsule)					
Dexatrim (not caffeine free)	________	×	200	=	________
NoDoz	________	×	100	=	________
Anacin	________	×	35	=	________
Midol	________	×	30	=	________
Coricidin	________	×	30	=	________
Tea (6 oz.)					
Iced tea	________	×	36	=	________
Hot tea (moderate steeping time)	________	×	65	=	________
Total				=	________

The recommendations to use K5 for determining diastolic pressure and to eliminate edema as a criterion for diagnosing preeclampsia are discussed. In addition, the use of blood pressure increases of 30 mm Hg systolic or 15 mm Hg diastolic as a diagnostic criterion has not been recommended, as available evidence shows that women in this group are not likely to suffer increased adverse outcomes. Management considerations are made between chronic hypertension present before pregnancy and hypertension occurring as part of the pregnancy-specific condition preeclampsia, as well as management considerations in women with comorbid conditions. A discussion of the pharmacologic treatment of hypertension in pregnancy includes recommendations for specific agents. The use of low-dose aspirin, calcium, or other dietary supplements in the prevention of preeclampsia is described, and expanded sections on counseling women for future pregnancies and recommendations for future research are included.[14]

TABLE 5.18

Effects of Alcohol, Tobacco, and Drug Use on Nutritional Status and Pregnancy Outcomes and Lactation

Effect	Cause
Increased nutrient requirements/impaired nutrient absorption	Smokers have reduced vitamin C levels
	Drinkers have reduced serum folate, vitamin C levels
Impaired growth of the fetus/stunted growth of child	Drinkers (1–2 alcoholic beverages/day) associated with LBW, and slow weight gain and failure to thrive
	Smokers
Infant sleep disruption/increased arousal	Consumption of one drink/day in first trimester
Delayed development/mental retardation	Drinkers have children who are more at risk for hyperactivity, poor attention span, language dysfunction
Reduced fertility	Chronic drinking and smoking associated with lower fertility in men and women
Transfer to baby during lactation disrupted sleep pattern of infant	Alcohol found in breast milk about 30 min after consumption; if woman chooses to drink during lactation, limit to 1.5 oz distilled spirits, 5 oz wine, or 12 oz beer, and consume after breastfeeding

Vitamin and Mineral Requirements, Food Sources, and Supplementation

In the United States, vitamin and mineral supplementation is common among pregnant women. During pregnancy, maternal requirements for all nutrients increase. For some nutrients, the evidence indicates a direct link between chronic maternal deficiency and poor outcome for the mother and infant. Excessive intake (usually defined as more than twice the RDA) of some nutrients may be harmful to the fetus, especially very early in the pregnancy.[16,26]

Supplementation is recommended only after assessment of dietary practices of pregnant women. The Institute of Medicine does not recommend routine use of prenatal vitamins; however, many physicians prescribe them because of the marginal nutritional status of their patients or because it is difficult to be completely sure of their patients' nutritional status.[3] Prenatal vitamins and minerals are indicated for high risk populations and those with an obstetric history of high parity, previous delivery of a low-birth-weight infant, a short interval between births, and smokers, drug or alcohol abusers, and those with multiple pregnancies.

Prenatal Vitamins

Indications for vitamin and mineral supplementation are in shown Table 5.19, which lists nutrient dose and indication for use. The contents of typical prenatal vitamin-mineral supplements are shown in Table 5.20, which includes usual formation of an over-the-counter (OTC) and a prescription supplement recommended to pregnant women.

Vitamin A

Most pregnant women do not need supplemental vitamin A, the teratogenic threshold of which may be lower than previously thought. Vitamin A is essential for embryogenesis,

TABLE 5.19

Indications for Vitamin and Mineral Supplementation

Indication	Nutrient	Dose
Inadequate diet; during first two trimesters for women at risk for preterm labor or low birth weight baby	Prenatal Supplements	Read label
Up to 1200 mg/day if dairy or fortified foods not consumed	Calcium	250–300 mg
For women receiving supplemental iron	Copper	2 mg
For all women of child bearing age	Folate	400 ug
Inadequate diet; anemia	Iron[a]	30–60 mg elemental
Inadequate diet	Vitamin B_6	2 mg
Inadequate diet	Vitamin C	50 mg
Inadequate diet; no exposure to sunlight	Vitamin D	10 µg
For women receiving supplemental iron	Zinc	15 mg

[a] Supplements containing high levels of folate or iron negatively affect zinc metabolism. Supplementary forms of folic acid are better absorbed than folate occurring in food.

TABLE 5.20

Prenatal Vitamin Mineral Supplements

	Flintstones Complete Chewables	Prenatal Vitamin (PreCare®)
Vitamin A	5000 IU	—
Vitamin C	60 mg	50 mg
Vitamin D	400 IU	6 µg
Thiamin	1.5 mg	—
Riboflavin	1.7 mg	—
Niacin	20 mg	—
B_6	2 mg	2 mg
Folic acid	400 µg	1 mg
B_{12}	6 µg	—
Biotin	40 µg	—
Pantothenic acid	10 mg	—
Calcium (as carbonate)	100 mg	250 mg
Iron	18 mg	40 mg
Phosphorus	100 mg	—
Iodine	150 µg	—
Magnesium	20 mg	50 mg
Zinc	15 mg	15 mg
Copper	2 mg	2 mg
Vitamin E	—	3.5 mg

growth, and epithelial differentiation. Case reports have suggested an association between high doses of vitamin A (> 25,000 IU) during pregnancy and birth defects. The American College of Obstetricians and Gynecologists established 10,000 IU as the cutoff for supplemental vitamin A (retinol) prior to or during pregnancy.[2]

Calcium and Magnesium

About 99% of calcium in pregnant women and their fetus is located in their bones and teeth. Pregnancy and lactation are associated with increased bone turnover to meet fat needs. If dietary deficiencies occur, maternal bone will supply the calcium to the fetus. Calcium supplementation during pregnancy has been shown to lead to an important reduction in systolic and diastolic blood pressure.[29,31] Controlled clinical trials to test the hypothesis that calcium supplements during pregnancy reduce the incidence of pregnancy-induced hypertension have had mixed results. Therefore there is no support for routine supplementation with 2000 mg/day for all pregnant women. In pregnant women who have diets deficient in calcium, prepregnancy hypertension, history of preeclampsia, or chronic use of heparin and steroids, supplemental calcium is recommended.[42]

The fetus absorbs 6 mg of magnesium each day. Maternal magnesium levels remain constant during pregnancy despite reported inadequate intakes. Magnesium supplementation has been associated with fewer hospitalizations, fewer preterm births, and more perinatal hemorrhages compared with placebo-supplemented women. Thus, further study is needed before routine supplementation is recommended.

Folate

The available data from controlled trials provide clear evidence of an improvement in hematological indices in women receiving routine iron and folate supplementation in pregnancy.[30] No conclusions can be drawn in terms of any beneficial or harmful effects on clinical outcomes for mother and baby. However, the Cochrane Pregnancy and Childbirth Group concludes that there is no evidence to advise against a policy of routine iron and folate supplementation in pregnancy.[25] Both folate intake from food and synthetic folic acid should be included in assessing and planning diet. The literature contains a variety of recommendations. The DRI is higher than can usually be obtained from food. The current recommendation during pregnancy is 600 µg/day of folic acid per day. It is well established that periconceptional use of folic acid supplementation reduces the risk of first occurrence and recurrence of neural tube defect (NTD)-affected pregnancies. The Center for Disease Control (CDC) recommends supplementation with 400 µg/day. Research is needed to determine effective strategies for disseminating information about the protective effects of folate.[26]

Iron

Additional iron is needed by most pregnant women in the U.S. A substantial amount of iron is required, given the amount of erythropoiesis. For example, a term infant contains an average of 225 mg of iron, the placenta and cord contain 50 mg of iron through the pregnancy, and the maternal red blood count volume increases 500 mL. Although maternal absorption of iron from the GI tract is increased by about 15%, it remains difficult to meet the increased iron need through diet alone. Iron absorption is increased in the presence of ascorbic acid. Adverse pregnancy outcomes are associated with hemoglobin levels below 10.4 g/dL or above 13.2 g/dL. Clinical diagnosis of anemia is made based on hemoglobin below 10.5 g/dL, a low MCV, and serum ferritin level below 12 µg/dL. Supplementation of 30 to 60 mg per day of elemental iron is usually prescribed, although the benefit of routine iron supplementation for healthy, well nourished women during pregnancy is unproven.[26,32] Common side effects include stomach upset, nausea, and constipation. These effects may be relieved by reducing the dosage or switching the brand of iron supplement. Some, but not all, sustained release preparations have been clinically shown to be associated with fewer discomforts. The safety of iron supplementation at dosages greater than 100 mg per day has been questioned. Researchers suggest that excess iron may lead to zinc depletion, which is associated with intrauterine growth retardation.

Zinc

The prevalence and effects of mild zinc deficiency in pregnancy are poorly defined. However, there have been a few case reports of severe human zinc deficiency in pregnancy that led to major obstetric complications and congenital malformations in the fetus. Supplementation studies have yielded mixed results. Iron appears to depress plasma zinc in pregnant women; therefore, zinc supplementation is recommended when >30 mg supplemental iron is taken.[43] Higher birth weights in infants of women with low prepregnancy weight (BMI <26) and low plasma zinc levels have been reported in women who received 25 mg zinc daily.

Vitamin B_6

The value of supplementation with Vitamin B_6 in pregnancy is controversial. However, it is included in most prenatal vitamins.

Vitamin C

Taking iron tablets along with a source of vitamin C facilitates iron absorption.

Vitamin D

Vitamin D is critical in the absorption, distribution, and storage of calcium. Relatively few foods are good sources of vitamin D.

Food Sources of Selected Nutrients

There are a variety of published recommendations for calcium in pregnancy and lactation. The optimal calcium intake recommended by the National Institutes of Health is 1200 mg per day. This is difficult to meet with a diet containing little dairy or calcium-fortified foods. The recommended daily intake (RDI) for pregnancy and lactation varies based on age from 1000 to 1300 mg/day. The usual calcium intake in the U.S. averages less than 700 mg per day. The benefit of meeting calcium needs has been demonstrated in reducing pregnancy induced hypertension. However, no benefit in reducing preeclampsia is seen with supplementing greater than 1200 mg calcium daily. Table 5.21 lists common dietary

TABLE 5.21

Dietary Sources of Calcium (DRI = 1000–1300 mg/d)

Food Item	Serving Size
Good: > 200 mg	
Broccoli/greens	2 cups
Calcium fortified foods (juice, cereal)	varies, read label
Canned salmon w/bones	3 oz.
Canned sardines w/bones	3 oz.
Cheese (cheddar, edam, Monterey jack, mozzarella, Parmesan, provolone, ricotta)	1 oz.
Ice cream	1 cup
Ice milk	1 cup
Milk (skim, 2%, whole, buttermilk)	1 cup
Yogurt	6-8 oz.

TABLE 5.22

Dietary Sources of Folate (DRI = 500–600 μg/d of dietary folate equivalents (DFE)

Food Item	Serving Size
Excellent >100 μg	
Asparagus	1/2 cup
Baked beans	1 cup
Bean burritos	2
Black-eyed peas	1 cup
Fortified grain and cereal products	varies, read label
Kidney beans	1 cup
Lentils	1 cup
Liver and other organ meats:	
beef	3.5 oz.
chicken	3.5 oz.
Orange Juice	1 cup
Peanuts	4 oz.
Spinach	1/2 cup
Good: 15–99 μg	
Almonds	4 oz.
Bread, fortified	1 slice
Beets	1/2 cup
Broccoli, cooked	1/2 cup
Cantaloupe/Honeydew melon	1 cup
Cauliflower	1/2 cup
Egg	1
French fries	large order
Lettuce (romaine)	1/2 cup
Orange	1 med
Turnip greens	1/2 cup

sources of calcium. Table 5.22 lists common food sources of folate, Table 5.23 includes common dietary sources of iron, and Table 5.24 includes common dietary sources.

Physical Activity during Pregnancy

Several factors influence physical activity during pregnancy, including prepregnancy exercise levels, current exercise levels, personal preferences, risk, limitations, and contraindications.[13] Tables 5.25 through 5.29 include guidelines for physical activity.

Postpartum Weight Loss

While a great deal of attention is given to counseling women about appropriate weight gain for pregnancy, clinicians have typically given less assistance in achieving postpartum weight loss. Researchers are beginning to link failure to return to prepregnancy weight

TABLE 5.23

Dietary Sources of Iron (DRI = 15–30 mg/d)

Food Item	Serving Size
Excellent >4 mg	
Beef liver	3 oz.
Clams	1/2 cup
Figs (dried)	10
Iron-fortified infant cereal	1/2 cup
Iron-fortified infant cereal	3 Tsp
Kidney beans	1 cup
Molasses (blackstrap)	3 Tbsp
Peaches (dried)	10 halves
Pinto beans	1 cup
Ready-to-eat, fortified cereals (like Product 19®, Total ®)	3/4 cup
Sunflower seeds (dried, hulled)	2/3 cup
Good: 2–4 mg	
Beef	3 oz.
Egg yolks	3
Iron-fortified infant formula	4 oz.
Lamb	3 oz.
Lima beans	1/2 cup
Oysters	3 oz.
Peas	1 cup
Pork	3 oz.
Prune juice	1 cup
Raisins	2/3 cup
Soybeans	1/2 cup

TABLE 5.24

Dietary Sources of Zinc (DRI = 15–19 mg/d)

Food Item	Serving Size	mg/Serving
Excellent: >4 mg		
Beef (lean, cooked)	3 oz.	5.1
Calves' liver (cooked)	3 oz.	5.3
Lamb (lean, cooked)	3 oz.	4.0
Oysters, Atlantic	3 oz.	63.0
Oysters, Pacific	3 oz.	7.6
Good: 0.9–3.4 mg		
Black-eyed peas (cooked)	1/2 cup	3.4
Chicken	3 oz.	2.4
Crabmeat	1/2 cup	3.4
Green peas (cooked)	1/2 cup	0.9
Lima beans (cooked)	3 oz.	0.9
Milk (whole)	1 cup	0.9
Pork loin (cooked)	3 oz.	2.6
Potato (baked with skin)	1 medium	1.0
Shrimp	1/2 cup	1.4
Tuna (oil-packed, drained)	3 oz.	0.9
Whitefish	3 oz.	0.9
Yogurt (plain)	1 cup	1.1

TABLE 5.25

Benefits of Physical Activity during Pregnancy

Improvement in circulation
Improved posture
Improved or maintained cardiovascular fitness
Reduced risk of cesarean section, decreased labor time, decreased use of epidural and forceps
Positive effects on mood, energy level
Release of tension and reduction of stress
Prevention of injury

TABLE 5.26

Contraindications to Physical Activity

Active myocardial disease, congestive heart failure, rheumatic heart disease
Thrombophlebitis
Risk of premature labor; incompetent cervix; uterine bleeding; ruptured membranes
Intrauterine growth retardation
Severe hypertensive disease
Suspected fetal distress

TABLE 5.27

Warning Signs to Stop Physical Activity

Vaginal bleeding
Uterine contractions
Nausea, vomiting
Dizziness or faintness
Difficulty walking
Decreased fetal activity
Palpitations or rapid heart rate
Numbness in any part of the body
Problems with vision

TABLE 5.28

Guidelines for Physical Activity

Activity	Guideline
Intensity	Reduce the intensity of exercise by 25%
Heart rate	Not to exceed 140 beats per minute
Temperature	Not to go above 101 degrees
Time	Moderate activity should not exceed 30 minutes; intersperse with low-intensity exercise and rest periods
Position	Avoid lying on back for more than 5 minutes after entering the 2nd trimester
Frequency	Exercise should be performed consistently at least three times per week and include a warm-up and a cool-down period

TABLE 5.29

Guidelines for Recreational Activity

Activity	Guideline
General conditioning exercises	Kegel, breathing, calf pumping, abdominal, bridging, lower trunk rotation, tail wagging
Jogging	May be continued moderately, however should not be started as a new activity after pregnancy; watch out for joint pain and decrease overall distance — recommendation is 2 miles or less per day
Aerobics	Avoid high impact or step aerobics; as for jogging, look out for joint pain or signs of over exertion; avoid exercises that involve lying on the back for more than 5 minutes
Bicycling	In the third trimester it may be necessary to switch to a stationary bike due to problems with balance
Weight lifting	Can be continued during pregnancy — use light weights and moderate repetitions; avoid heavy resistance
Avoid during pregnancy	Downhill skiing, gymnastics, horseback riding, scuba diving, any contact sports

TABLE 5.30

Strategies for Postpartum Weight Loss

Encourage a healthy diet based on current dietary guidelines
Make energy intake less than energy expenditure
Reduce portion size but do not restrict kcalories to less than 1800 per day
Determine foods high in fats and calories and substitute with fruits, vegetables, lean meats and fish, skinless poultry
Avoid cooking in oil, butter, margarine
Drink 8–10 glasses fluid per day
Discuss feasible physical activity
Monitor women who
Restrict intake to less than 1800 kcalories per day
Are vegans (avoid all animal products including dairy, eggs, and meats)
Avoid foods enriched with Vitamin D and have limited exposure to sunlight

with increased risks for chronic disease later in life. Table 5.30 includes currently recommended strategies for post partum weight loss.

Nutrition and Lactation

The RDA and AI for lactation are listed in Table 5.10. Suggestions for maternal nutrition to meet the increased energy and nutrient needs are listed in Table 5.31. Until relatively recently, breastfeeding has been considered too imprecise to study. A wealth of information is being developed about lactation and breast milk.[50] Table 5.32 lists some of the benefits of unrestricted nursing for the infant. Many women and their clinicians still are concerned about ways to identify whether an infant is obtaining enough nutriture. Table 5.33 lists signs of insufficient milk intake. The social history of infant feeding from the late 1800s to the 1950s in the U.S. shows a transition from breastfeeding to scientific feeding of infants. As a result of that, much cultural knowledge and support for breastfeeding had been lost. Guidebooks are important for women and clinicians.[46-50] Tables 5.34 and 5.35 include common concerns and recommended actions to support breastfeeding.

TABLE 5.31

Maternal Nutrition during Breastfeeding

Encourage a healthy diet based on current dietary guidelines
Reinforce that milk quality is generally not affected by the mother's diet
Suggest eating meals and snacks that are easy to prepare
Provide patient with information on normal postpartum weight loss in a breastfeeding woman
Drink enough fluids to keep from getting thirsty
Eat at least 1800 kcalories per day
Use appetite as a guide to amount of food eaten in first six weeks
Keep intake of coffee, cola, or other sources of caffeine to 2 servings or less per day. Caffeine accumulates in the infant and use should be discontinued if infant becomes wakeful, hyperactive, or has disturbed sleep patterns. This reaction is intensified with a smoking mother.

TABLE 5.32

Benefits of Frequent, Early, Unrestricted Nursing

Provides colostrum that the baby needs
Helps decrease newborn jaundice because of the laxative effect of colostrum
Provides a period of practice time before milk volume increases
Stimulates uterine contractions, lessening chances of maternal postpartum hemorrhage
Prevents infant hypoglycemia

TABLE 5.33

Signs of Insufficient Milk Intake in the Newborn

Failure to regain birth weight by 2 weeks of age
Weight gain of less than 7 oz per week after regaining birth weight and less than 4 lbs in 4 months
Fewer than 3–4 stools per day after day 5
Fewer than 6 urinations per day after day 5. (During the first 5 days wet and soiled diapers should increase in number each day.)

TABLE 5.34

Breastfeeding Tips: Common Concerns about the Infant

Concern	Recommended Action
Jaundice	Continue to breastfeed at least every 2 hours around the clock. If breastfeeding is stopped, pump breasts to maintain milk supply. Avoid water or formula feedings.
Latch-on	Latch-on is necessary for baby to begin sucking at the breast. Poor latch-on is a major cause of sore nipples. Baby's mouth should be at nipple level. Support the breast by placing the thumb on the top and four fingers underneath. Tickle baby's bottom lip with nipple until baby opens mouth very wide. Center nipple quickly and bring baby very close. Baby's nose and chin should be touching breast.
Leaking	Leaking is a sign of normal letdown in the early weeks of breastfeeding. Use breast pads in bra between feedings. Avoid pads with plastic lining. During sexual activity, leaking may occur; breastfeed your baby first.
Duration of breastfeeding: how long and how often?	Frequent (every 2–3 hours) and unrestricted breastfeeding for the first weeks. Baby should empty one breast, be burped, and offered the second breast. Watch baby for signs that he is full, like falling asleep, losing interest in feeding, or stopping breastfeeding.
Early first feeding	Put baby to breast soon after delivery, if possible within the first 2 hours. Cuddling, licking, and brief sucking are good signs that baby is learning to breastfeed. Offer your breast often to let your baby practice. Ask a supportive nurse for help.
Extra feedings	Healthy breastfed newborns do not need formula, water, or juice. Breastfeed at least every 2–3 hours during the first month. Older breastfed babies will be ready for solid foods and juices between 4-6 months of age.

TABLE 5.35
Breastfeeding Tips: Common Discomforts That Lead to Breastfeeding Termination

Concern	Recommended Action
Hospital survival skills	"Rooming-in" with your baby is your right as a consumer. Keep your baby with you as much as possible so you can breastfeed often. Do not give bottles of formula or water. Do not limit feeding time at breast. Ask a supportive nurse for help. Do not accept formula gift packs.
Mastitis	Mastitis is a swollen, inflamed, or infected area in the breast. Watch for flu-like symptoms such as fever above 101°F, chills and muscle aches, and a reddened, hot, tender, or swollen area in the breast. Rest, breastfeed often, and drink more fluids. Avoid tight bra or clothing. Apply warm water soaks, heating pad. Massage affected area. Antibiotics may be needed. No reason to stop breastfeeding.
Myths and misconceptions	Breast sagging is not a result of breastfeeding. Breast size does not affect ability to breastfeed. Drinking beer, manzanilla tea, or large amounts of fluids does not make more milk.
Nipples, flat or inverted (before birth)	Flat or inverted nipples retract or move in toward the breast. Breast shells (milk cups) may be worn during the last month of pregnancy to help minimize inverted nipples. Gradually increase time of use from a few hours to 8–10 hours/day. Do not wear while sleeping. Air-dry nipples if leaking occurs. Breast shells should not be used by women at risk for preterm labor.
Nipples, flat or inverted (after birth)	Begin breastfeeding as soon as possible after birth. Breastfeed frequently to avoid engorgement. Use nipple rolling or stretching before each breastfeeding. Pump breast for a short period before breastfeeding, or apply ice wrapped in a cloth and placed on the nipple before feeding. Breast shells (milk cups) may be used between feedings. Remove the breast shell just before placing baby at breast.
Engorgement	Engorgement may occur when milk first comes in or when feedings are missed or delayed. Use warm compresses or shower before feedings. Hand-express to soften areola, making it easier for baby to latch on. Breastfeed every 1–2 hours for 10–20 minutes per breast. Apply ice to breast and under arm after feeding until swelling decreases. Gentle breast massage toward nipple. Take non-aspirin pain reliever.
Breast care	Nipple pulling, tugging, or rolling during pregnancy is not necessary to prepare for breastfeeding. Avoid soaps or lotions to the nipples. Air dry nipples after breastfeeding.
Breast creams	Vitamin E, breast creams, or ointments are not recommended. No evidence exists that they heal the nipple. May make soreness worse by keeping the nipple moist. Use pure lanolin. Can massage drops of breast milk on nipples.
Breast surgery	Any type of breast surgery may interfere with milk supply.
Cesarean section	Breastfeed baby as soon as possible after delivery, preferably in the recovery room. Hold baby in a comfortable position. Use pillows across abdomen to protect the incision and support baby.

Resource Materials

American College of Obstetricians and Gynecologists, Office of Public Information, 409 12th Street SW, Washington, DC 20024-2188; 202-638-5577.

Best Start Social Marketing. 3500 E. Fletcher Avenue, Suite 519, Tampa, FL 33613; 1-800-277-4975. Best Start is a not-for-profit corporation. One of its largest social marketing projects was developed in 1997 for USDA as part of the WIC National Breastfeeding Promotion Project. A wide variety of campaign and professional materials is available. Beststart@mindspring.com; Also see http://www.opc.on.ca/beststart/info_sheets/feed.html

Erick M. *No More Morning Sickness. A Survival Guide for Pregnant Women,* Plume Book, NJ. 1-800-245-6476.

Food and Nutrition Information Center, National Agricultural Library, ARS, USDA, Beltsville, MD 20705-2351. 301-504-5719.
http://www.nal.usda.gov/fnic

La Leche League International, 1400 N Meacham Rd, PO Box 4079, Schaumburg IL 60168-4079.
http://www.lalecheleague.org

Lopes GL. *Gestational Diabetes and You.* NCES, Inc. 1995. 913-782-4385.

March of Dimes Birth Defects Foundation Resource Center, 1275 Mamoroneck Ave, White Plains, NY 10605.
http://modimes.org

National Maternal and Child Health Clearinghouse, 2070 Chain Bridge Road, Suite 450, Vienna, VA 22182-2536. 703-356-1964; fax: 703-821-2098.
e-mail: nmchc@circsol.com; Web site: http://www.circsol.com/mch.

National Center for Nutrition and Dietetics, The American Dietetic Association, 216 W Jackson Blvd, Suite 800, Chicago, IL 60606-6995.
http://www.eatright.org

USDA. Is Someone You Know At Risk for Foodborne Illness? Food Safety and Inspection Service, April 1990.
http://www.fightbac.org

References

1. Am Coll OB-GYN. ACOG Technical Bulletin No. 205, May, 1995.
2. Am Acad Ped. Am Coll OB-GYN. Chapter 11, pages 279-284. In *Guidelines for Perinatal Care,* 1997.
3. Institute of Medicine, Subcommittee for a Clinical Application Guide. *Nutrition During Pregnancy and Lactation: An Implementation Guide,* National Academy Press, Washington, DC, 1992.
4. Kolasa KM, Weismiller D. *AFP* 56:205; 1997.
5. Newton E. Maternal nutrition. In *Management of High Risk Pregnancy.* (Queen, JT, Ed) Blackwell Science, 4th ed. 1999.
6. Peshicka D, Riley J, Thomson C. *Obstetrics/Gynecology Nutrition Handbook.* Chapman and Hall, New York, NY 10003, 1996.
7. Suitor CW. Update for Nutrition during Pregnancy and Lactation: An Implementation Guide. National Center for Education in Maternal and Child Health. Maternal and Child Health Bureau, Health Resources and Services Administration, Public Health Service, U.S. Department of Health and Human Services.
8. Homan RK, Korenbrot CC. *Medical Care* 36: 190; 1998.
9. Luke B. *Clin Obstet Gynecol* 37: 538; 1994.
10. Matthews F, Yudkin P, Neil A. *Brit Med J* 319: 339; 1999.
11. Abrams B, Carmichael S, Selvin S. *Obstet Gynecol* 86: 170; 1995.
12. Ananth CV, Vintzileos AM, Shen-Schwarz S, et al. *Obstet Gynecol* 91: 917; 1998.
13. Boardley DJ, Sargent RG, Coker AL, et al. *Obstet Gynecol* 86: 834; 1995.
14. Cattingius S, Bergstrom R, Lipworth L, Kramer M. 338: 147; 1998.
15. Cogswell ME, Serdula MK, Hungerford DW, Yip R. *Am J Ob-Gyn* 172: 705; 1995.
16. Keppel KG, Taffel SM. *AJPHA* 83: 1100; 1993.
17. King JC, Butte NF, Bronstein MN, et al. *Am J Clin Nutr* 59(suppl): 439S; 1994.
18. Luke B, Hediger ML, Scholl TO. *J Mat Fetal Med* 5: 168; 1996.
19. Parker JD, Abrams B. *Obstet Gynecol* 79: 664; 1992.
20. Schieve LA, Cogswell ME, Scanlon KS. *Obstet Gynecol* 91: 878; 1998.
21. Scholl TO, Hedinger ML, Schall JI, et al. *Obstet Gynecol* 86: 423; 1995.
22. Siega-Riz AM, Adair LS, Hobel CJ. *Nutrition* 126: 146; 1996.
23. Taffel SM, Keppel KG, Jones GK. *Ann NY Acad Sci* 678: 293; 1993.
24. Suitor CW. Maternal Weight Gain: A Report of an Expert Work Group, National Center for Education in Maternal and Child Health, Arlington, VA, 1997.

25. Cochrane Pregnancy and Childbirth Group. Cochrane Database of Systematic Reviews. Issue 3, 1999.
26. Institute of Medicine, Food and Nutrition Board. *Dietary Reference Intakes for Thiamin, Riboflavin, Niacin, Vitamin B6, Folate, Vitamin B12, Pantothenic Acid, Biotin, and Choline.* National Academy Press, Washington, DC, 1998.
27. Institute of Medicine, Food and Nutrition Board, *Dietary References Intakes for Calcium, Phosphorus, Magnesium, Vitamin D, and Fluoride.* National Academy Press, Washington, DC, 1997.
28. Allen L. *Am J Clin Nutr* 67: 591; 1998.
29. Kloeblen AS. *J Am Diet A* 99: 33; 1999.
30. Levine RJ, Hauth JC, Curet LB, et al. *N Engl J Med* 337: 69; 1997.
31. Long PJ. *J Nurse Midwifery* 40: 36; 1995.
32. Matthews F. *Nutr Res Rev* 9: 175; 1996.
33. Rose NC, Mennuti MT. *Clin Obstet Gynecol* 37: 605; 1998.
34. Brown JE, Buzzard M, Jacobs DR, et al. *JADA* 96: 262; 1996.
35. Kennedy E. *JADA* 86: 1372; 1986.
36. Erick M. *Nutrition Rev* 53: 289; 1995.
37. Stainton MC, Neff EJA. *Health Care for Women International* 15: 563; 1994.
38. Klebanoff MA, Levine RJ, DerSimonian R, et al. *N Engl J Med* 341: 1639; 1999.
39. Bucher HC, Guyatt GH, Cook RJ, et al. *JAMA* 275: 1113 1996.
40. Goldenberg RL, Tamura T, Neggers Y, et al. *JAMA* 274: 463; 1995.
41. Institute of Medicine, Subcommittee on Nutrition During Lactation. *Nutrition During Lactation.* National Academy Press: Washington, DC, 1991.
42. National Academy of Sciences, Institute of Medicine, Food and Nutrition Board, Committee on Nutritional Status During Pregnancy and Lactation. *Nutrition Services in Perinatal Care* (2nd ed.). National Academy Press, Washington, DC, 1992.
43. Lawrence, RA . Maternal and Child Health Technical Information Bulletin. National Center for Education in Material and Child Health, Arlington, VA, 1997.
44. Lawrence RA and Lawrence RM. *Breastfeeding: A Guide for the Medical Profession.* C.V. Mosby, St. Louis, MO, 1998.
45. Mohrbacher N and Stock J. *The Breastfeeding Answer Book.* La Leche League International. Schaumburg, IL, 1997.
46. Am Acad Ped. Work Group on Breastfeeding. *Pediatrics* 100: 1035; 1997.
47. Riordan J and Auerbach KG. *Pocket Guide to Breastfeeding and Human Lactation,* Jones and Bartlett, Boston, MA, 1997.
48. Prentice A. *N Engl J Med* 337: 558; 1997.

6

Feeding the Premature Infant

Jatinder Bhatia, Colleen Bucher, and Chantrapa Bunyapen

Nutritional management of the premature infant has become an integral part of the medical care provided to these infants. With the ever increasing survival of low-birth-weight and very-low-birth-weight infants, understanding the principles of nutritional therapy becomes all the more important. It is estimated that there are four million births in the United States every year; with an estimated prematurity rate of 9%, the number of infants requiring such management is enormous. This section focuses on nutritional goals, nutrient requirements, and enteral and parenteral routes of nutritional therapy.

Nutritional Goals for the Premature Infant

Prematurity is defined as an infant with a gestational age of less than 38 weeks born before completion of 37 weeks gestation. A post-term infant is one whose birth occurs from the beginning of the first day of week 43 (>42 weeks). Classifying infants as preterm, term, or post-term assists in establishing the level of risk for neonatal morbidity, nutritional needs, and long-term sequelae. Assessment of gestational age is based on maternal dates, obstetric dating by ultrasonography, and physical examination.[1] Ultrasonography has improved the ability to estimate gestational age. Estimation by physical exam relies on the predictable changes in the pattern of physical and neurological changes that occur with advancing gestation and form the basis of the examinations for the estimation of gestational age. The Ballard exam may overestimate the age of premature infants and, on the other hand, may underestimate that of post-term infants.[2] Because of the error in gestational age assessment, particularly in very-low-birth-weight infants, a New Ballard Score is currently used.[3] This modified examination is particularly suited for the very small premature infant, and the estimated gestational age is accurate to within one week. Items of neuromuscular maturity and physical maturity are scored from –1 to 5, a total score obtained, and gestational age estimated based on maturity rating score.

Infants are considered low birth-weight if birth weight is less than 2500 g regardless of gestational age. Very-low-birth-weight defines infants with weight less than 1500 g, with an additional classification of extremely low-birth-weight describing infants less than 1000 g.

Crown–heel length performed by two examiners is measured by achieving full extension of the infant on a measuring board with a fixed headpiece and movable footpiece. The

0-8493-2705-9/01/$0.00+$1.50

infant needs to be supine, head held in the Frankfurt plane vertical, legs extended, and ankles flexed, and the movable footpiece is brought to rest firmly against the infant's heels. An average of two measurements documents the length. If crown–heel length cannot be measured due to limb anomalies or if there is a discrepancy between weight and length, a crown–rump length is sometimes measured.

Head circumference measured with a non-stretchable tape is the largest of three measurements around the head, with the tape held snugly above the ears.

Weight, length, and head circumference are then plotted on standard curves to classify an infant as appropriate, small, or large for gestational age for each measurement. Most measurements[6] define appropriate for age as measurements that fall within the 10th to 90th percentiles, ideally based on charts constructed for similar race and height above sea level. Infants who are appropriate for age on the three measures are at the lowest risk, within that gestational age grouping, for problems associated with neonatal morbidity and mortality. An example of growth curves commonly used in neonatal nurseries is depicted in Figure 6.1.

Growth and Nutrient Requirements

Estimation of nutrient requirements in premature infants is based on the goals for growth of this cohort of infants. The common goal has been to achieve growth similar to that of the "reference fetus."[4,5] These growth standards serve as a reference to judge the adequacy of growth; however, postnatal changes in energy requirements as well as environmental stresses are likely to be different, and the ideal growth of these infants remains to be defined. An alternative approach may be to achieve the best possible growth without adverse metabolic consequences.

Nutrient requirements for preterm infants have been estimated by various methods, including the factorial method based on the reference fetus, nitrogen balance studies, and turnover studies, or based on nutrient values in the serum. For example, Figure 6.2 depicts the composition of weight gain in normal human fetuses.[4] This reference fetus (Table 6.1) has not only served as a basis for calculation of nutrient needs, but also as a measure of sufficiency of particular nutrients, as discussed above. The factorial approach is based on the assumption that the requirement for a nutrient is the sum of losses (fecal, urine, dermal, and other, if any) and the amount required for growth, i.e., incorporation into new tissues. An example of such an approach to calculate protein requirements of preterm infants is that of Ziegler.[6] Advisable intakes of protein are obtained by adding 8–10% of the estimated requirement.

Provision of Nutrients

Energy Needs

Energy needs are based on basal metabolic rate, cost of growth, and losses in stool and urine. The factorial method cannot be used to estimate energy requirements. It is generally recognized that preterm infants have higher energy requirements compared to their term counterparts.[7] To gain the predicted growth in weight for premature infants

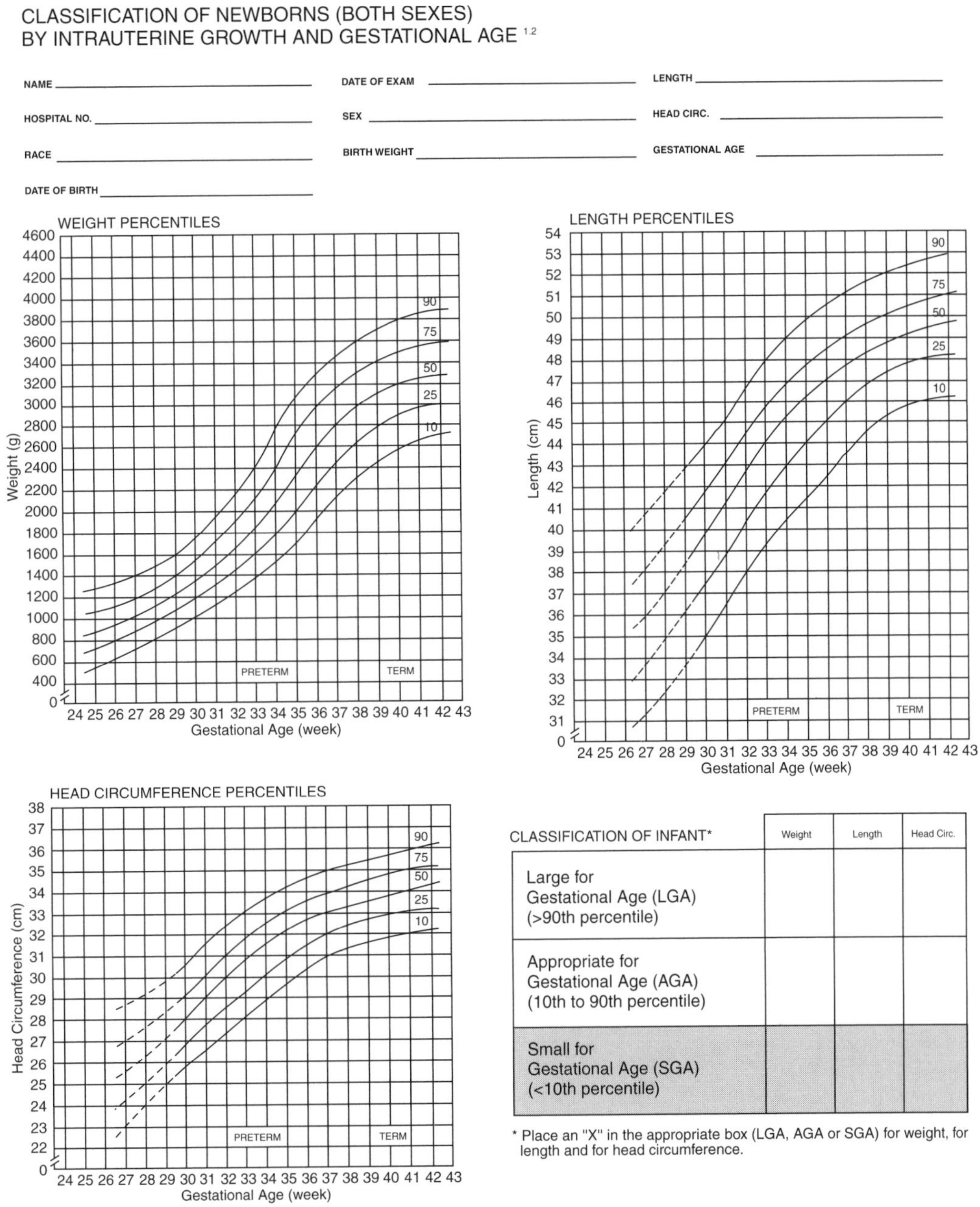
CLASSIFICATION OF NEWBORNS (BOTH SEXES)
BY INTRAUTERINE GROWTH AND GESTATIONAL AGE 1,2
NAME
DATE OF EXAM
LENGTH
HOSPITAL NO.
SEX
HEAD CIRC.
RACE
BIRTH WEIGHT
GESTATIONAL AGE
DATE OF BIRTH
WEIGHT PERCENTILES
Weight (g)
Gestational Age (week)
90
75
50
25
10
PRETERM
TERM
LENGTH PERCENTILES
Length (cm)
HEAD CIRCUMFERENCE PERCENTILES
Head Circumference (cm)
CLASSIFICATION OF INFANT*
Weight
Length
Head Circ.
Large for Gestational Age (LGA) (>90th percentile)
Appropriate for Gestational Age (AGA) (10th to 90th percentile)
Small for Gestational Age (SGA) (<10th percentile)
* Place an "X" in the appropriate box (LGA, AGA or SGA) for weight, for length and for head circumference.

FIGURE 6.1
Classification of newborns by intrauterine growth and gestational age.

(10 to 15g/kg/d), it is estimated that premature infants would need 110 to 130 kcal/kg/d. Energy requirements must take into account the route of administration, enteral vs. parenteral, since 90 to 95 kcal/kg/d may satisfy energy requirements by the parenteral route. Disease states such as sepsis, chronic lung disease,[8,9] and concomitant use of corticosteroids will increase energy needs. The mainstay of energy support should be balanced between carbohydrates, fat, and amino acids.

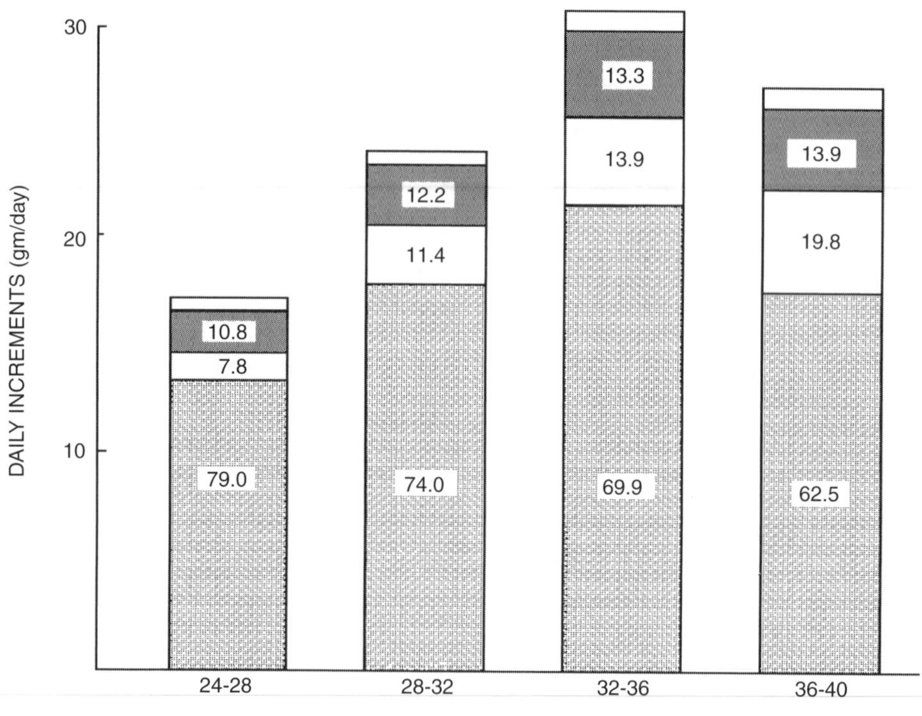

FIGURE 6.2
Average composition of weight gain of the reference fetus; numbers indicate percentages of gained accounted for by components. From Ziegler E.E., O'Donnell A.M., Nelson S.E., Fomon S.J. *Growth* 40: 329; 1976. With permission.

TABLE 6.1
Daily Increments of Body Weight and Body Composition of the Reference Fetus

Age Interval (Weeks)	Weight (g)	Protein (g)	Lipid (g)	Ca (mg)	P (mg)	Mg (mg)	Na (mEq)	K (mEq)	Cl (mEq)
24–25	11.4	1.25	0.5	61	39	1.8	0.9	0.5	0.8
25–26	15.7	1.67	1.2	84	54	2.4	1.3	0.6	1.0
26–27	18.6	2.00	1.6	101	65	2.8	1.5	0.8	1.1
27–28	21.4	2.37	2.0	119	76	3.3	1.7	0.9	1.3
28–29	22.6	2.59	2.3	129	83	3.5	1.7	0.9	1.3
29–30	23.1	2.76	2.6	138	89	3.7	1.7	1.0	1.3
30–31	24.3	3.00	2.9	152	97	4.0	1.8	1.0	1.3
31–32	25.7	3.28	3.2	171	109	4.4	1.8	1.1	1.3
32–33	27.1	3.55	3.5	193	123	4.8	1.9	1.1	1.3
33–34	30.0	3.97	4.0	228	144	5.5	2.1	1.2	1.4
34–35	31.4	4.23	4.4	258	162	6.0	2.2	1.3	1.4
35–36	34.3	4.62	5.1	301	189	6.9	2.4	1.4	1.4
36–37	35.7	4.83	5.6	341	212	7.5	2.5	1.5	1.4
37–38	31.4	4.34	5.6	344	211	7.1	2.1	1.3	1.1
38–39	24.3	3.44	5.4	325	197	6.1	1.6	1.0	0.7
39–40	17.1	2.50	5.0	302	179	5.0	1.0	0.6	0.3

From Ziegler E.E., O'Donnell A.M., Nelson S.E., Fomon S.J. *Growth* 40: 329; 1976. With permission.

Amino Acid Needs

The factorial approach is commonly used to estimate protein requirements. The protein need will be greater if catch-up growth is also to be produced. It is generally accepted that the newborn infant will lose up to 10% of his/her body weight. In sick premature infants where nutrition cannot be provided or is not tolerated, the amount of catch-up may be greater. Several studies suggest that endogenous protein losses in the absence of exogenous protein intake are at least 1 g/kg/d.[10,11] When fed in the conventional manner, premature infants run the risk of under-nutrition. Therefore, strategies to optimize amino acid intakes to include provision for catch-up growth need to be developed, since early initiation of parenteral nutrition results in positive nitrogen balance and has been shown to be safe.[11,12-14]

Cysteine and tyrosine are provided as cysteine hydrochloride (40 mg/g/amino acid, not to exceed 100 mg/kg/d) and N-acetyl-L-tyrosine (0.24 g%);[15] it has been demonstrated that infants receiving cysteine retain significantly more nitrogen that do infants receiving an isonitrogenous amino acid intake without cysteine.[11]

It is generally accepted that infants receiving 80 to 90 kcal/kg/d from parenteral nutrition with an adequate amino acid intake should gain weight similar to the intrauterine rate.[16] Most of this energy intake is provided by glucose and lipids. However, premature and sick infants may not tolerate increasing glucose concentrations/delivery without concomitant hyperglycemia, making the goal of achieving adequate energy intake difficult in the first week of life.

Lipid Needs

Lipid emulsions are used in conjunction with glucose and amino acid solutions. Generally, lipids are started at 0.5 g/kg/d intravenously, increasing by 0.5 g/kg to a maximum of 3.0 g/kg/d. Infusion rates are maintained between 0.15 to 0.25 g/kg/h in order to avoid hypertriglyceridemia (triglycerides > 175 mg/dL). Essential fatty acid deficiency may be prevented by lipid intakes as low as 0.5 to 1.0 g/kg/d.

Fat particle size is between 0.4 and 0.5μ in diameter, similar to that of endogenous chylomicrons. Clearance of lipids by premature infants may be limited, thereby requiring frequent assessment of tolerance. Emulsions of 20% are preferred due to lower total phospholid and liposome content per gram of triglyceride.[17,18]

Parenteral Nutrition

It is common practice to provide initial nutrient requirements, especially in a sick neonate, by the parenteral route. A typical parenteral regimen is depicted in Table 6.2. Commonly available lipid products are listed in Table 6.3. Currently, two amino acid formulations are available in the U.S. specifically designed for preterm infants: Trophamine® and Aminosyn-PF®. These amino acid formulations were designed to result in a plasma amino acid profile similar to that of a 30-day-old breastfed infant.[19] It is generally recommended that parenteral nutrition be started within the first two days of life in preterm infants and advanced in a systematic fashion to achieve 3.0–4.0 g/kg/d of amino acids, 90–100 kcal/kg/d of energy. Most preterm infants do not achieve these intakes until well into the second week of life because of issues such as glucose and lipid intolerance.

Mineral Requirements

Mineral requirements have also been estimated based on body composition and the reference fetus.[4,5] From a practical standpoint, daily needs for sodium, potassium, and

TABLE 6.2

Parenteral Nutrition Regimen

Component		Amount/kg/d
Amino acids (g)		3–4
Glucose (g)		15–25
Lipid (g)		0.5–3.0
Sodium (mEq)[1]		2–5
Potassium (mEq)[2]		2–4
Calcium (mg)		80–100
Magnesium (mg)		3–6
Chloride (mEq)		2–3
Phosphorus (mg)[2]		40–60
Zinc (μg)		200–400
Copper (μg)		20
Iron (μg)		100–200
Other trace minerals[3]		
Vitamins[4]		
Total Volume		120–150 mL
Nutrient	**<14 d**	**>14 d**
Manganese (μg)	0.0–0.75	1.0
Chromium (μg)	0.0–0.05	0.2
Selenium (μg)	0.0–1.3	2.0
Iodide (μg)	0.0–1.0	1.0
Molybdenum (μg)	0	0.25
C (mg)		80
A (mg)		0.7
D (μg)		10 (= 400 μ)
B_1 (mg)		1.2
B_2 (mg)		1.4
B_6 (mg)		1
Niacin (mg)		17

[1] Sodium requirements may vary between infants and within the same infant, and should be tailored to serum values.

[2] Phosphorus intakes are maintained in a ratio of 1:2 to 1:2.6 with calcium (mEq:mM) and may be limiting in parenteral nutrition because of insolubility; in general, the more acidic the TPN, the more calcium and phosphorus can be dissolved in the solution without precipitation. Care must be taken to avoid hyperphosphatemia with its resultant hypocalcemia.

[3] amount/kg/d.

[4] Provided as MVI-Pediatric®; each 5 mL provides (MVI is to be provided in amounts not exceeding 2.0 ml/kg/d).

chloride are based on serum measurements, while calcium and phosphorus needs are based on the factorial method.[4,5] Requirements are listed in Table 6.2. In general, the preterm infant has higher requirements of most minerals than term infants. During total parenteral nutrition, requirements for calcium and phosphorus may not be met because of the insolubility of calcium salts. Human milk may not provide adequate amounts of sodium, and hyponatremia has been reported.[20] Calcium and phosphorus needs of preterm infants cannot be met by human milk from mothers delivering preterm or term infants, and will need to be supplemented.[21] Since calcium transfer across the placenta occurs in the third trimester, the very premature infant is relatively osteopenic, and prolonged

TABLE 6.3

Fatty Acid Composition of Commonly Used Lipid Emulsions

	Intralipid® 20%	Liposyn III® 20%
Oils %	—	—
Safflower	0	0
Soybean	20	20
Fatty acid content (%)	—	—
Linoleic	50	54.5
Oleic	26	22.4
Palmitic	10	10.5
Linolenic	9	8.3
Stearic	3.5	4.2
Egg yolk phospholipid %	1.2	1.2
Glycerine %	2.25	2.5
kcal/mL	2	2
mOsm/L	260	292

parenteral nutrition and/or unfortified human milk feedings puts the infant at great risk for metabolic bone disease.

Iron is accumulated in the fetus in the third trimester with an iron content of 75 mg/kg at term. Small-for-gestational-age infants, preterm infants, and infants of diabetic mothers have low iron stores at birth. Coupled with the need for frequent blood sampling, the premature infant is at great risk for the development of iron deficiency anemia, and the exact time for supplementation remains controversial. However, given that the criteria for blood transfusion have become more stringent,[21] iron should be supplemented as early as two weeks. If recombinant erythropoietin is used to stimulate endogenous iron production,[22] iron requirements may be 6.0 mg/kg/d or higher.

Nutrient Delivery

Delivery of enteral nutrients is based on gestational age. In general, infants of 33 weeks gestation and beyond can be fed orally soon after birth. However, if medical or surgical illness precludes enteral feedings, parenteral nutrition is indicated. Parenteral nutrition can be considered as total (where all nutrients are delivered, for example in an infant with a surgical condition precluding enteral nutrition: gastroschisis) or supplemental (to complement enteral nutrition). It can be further described as peripheral parenteral nutrition (provided by a peripheral intravenous line) or central (where the tip of the catheter is in a central location or deep vein). The latter should be the route if long-term parenteral nutrition (for example, greater than 2 weeks) is anticipated, since it allows for higher glucose delivery compared to the peripheral vein (>12.5% dextrose in water). A typical nutrition plan for a very-low-birth weight infant is depicted in Table 6.4, and indications for parenteral nutrition are listed in Table 6.5.

The metabolic complications (Table 6.6) can be avoided by careful assessment of tolerance to the macronutrients as nutrition delivery is advanced. Premature infants do not tolerate high concentrations of glucose or rapid advances in glucose delivery; similarly, rates of fat infusion of greater than 2.0 g/kg/d may result in hypertriglyceridemia, particularly in the small or ill preterm infant (triglycerides >175 mg/dL). A suggested regimen of monitoring parenteral nutrition is depicted in Table 6.7. A multidisciplinary approach with physicians, pharmacists, nutritionists, and nursing staff who are knowledgeable in parenteral nutrition and monitoring should be implemented for the care of such infants. Early recognition of metabolic effects (pharmacist/nutritionist) or catheter-related effects

TABLE 6.4

Initiation and Advancement of Parenteral and Minimal Enteral Feedings in an Infant with a Birthweight of <1000 g

Age, d	Parenteral Amino Acid [g/kg]	Glucose	Lipids [g/kg]	Electrolytes	Enteral mL/h
1	0.0	D_5W	0.0	0.0	0.0
2	1.0	D_5W	0.5	Add if Na <130 mEq/l	0.25
3	1.5	Increments of 2.5%	1.0[a]	Standard	0.25
4	2.0	Increase as tolerated	1.5[a]	Standard	0.5
5	2.5	Increase as tolerated	2.0[a]	Standard	0.5
6	3.0	Increase as tolerated	2.5[a]	Standard	0.75
7	3.0 or higher[b]	Same or higher	3.0[a]	Standard	0.75

[a] Monitor triglycerides to assess lipid tolerance.

[b] Optional; infants requiring catch up growth, on corticosteroids or demonstrating low BUN despite adequate protein intakes may need higher amino acid intakes at later stages.

TABLE 6.5

Parenteral Nutrition is Indicated in the Following Conditions

Condition	Indication
Medical	Inadequate enteral nutrition
	Necrotizing enterocolitis
	Feeding intolerance/difficulty
	Ileus
Surgical	Omphalocele
	Gastroschisis
	Tracheo-esophageal fistula
	Atresias of the intestine (duodenal/jejunal/ileal)
	Diaphragmatic hernia
	Hirschsprung's disease

TABLE 6.6

Complications of Parenteral Nutrition

Type	Complication
Metabolic	Hypo- or hyperglycemia
	Electrolyte imbalance
	Metabolic bone disease
	Hepatic dysfunction
Infectious	Bacterial sepsis
	Fungal sepsis
Mechanical	Extravasation
	Thrombosis
	Pericardial effusion
	Diaphragmatic palsy

(nursing) could help to minimize the potential complications of parenteral nutrition. The most common metabolic complications observed are hepatic dysfunction and metabolic bone disease.

Hepatic dysfunction is defined as an increase in serum bile acids followed by an increase in direct bilirubin, alkaline phosphatase, and gamma-glutamyl transferase. The hepatocellular enzymes, ALT and AST, are late to increase, and are often seen in the more severe cases. Gamma-glutamyl transferase is probably the most sensitive but least specific

TABLE 6.7

Suggested Monitoring during Parenteral Nutrition

Component	Initial	Later
Weight	Daily	Daily
Length	Weekly	Weekly
Head circumference	Weekly	Weekly
Na, K, Cl, CO_2	Daily until stable	Weekly
Glucose	Daily	PRN
Triglycerides	With every lipid change	Weekly or biweekly
Ca, PO_4	Daily until stable	Weekly or biweekly
Alkaline phosphatase	Initial	Weekly or biweekly
Bilirubin	Initial	Weekly or biweekly
Mg	Initial	Weekly or biweekly
Ammonia	PRN	PRN
Gamma GT	Initial	Weekly or biweekly
ALT/AST	Initial	Weekly or biweekly
Complete blood count	Initial	Weekly or PRN

indicator, whereas elevation in direct bilrubin is the most specific and least sensitive indicator of hepatic dysfunction. The etiology is multi-factorial,[23-25] but the incidence appears to be declining as a result of both specialized amino acid solutions and early provision of enteral nutrients.

Premature infants are at high risk for the development of metabolic bone disease most commonly due to inadequate intakes of calcium and phosphorus during parenteral nutrition. Infants born before 32 weeks of gestation have some degree of hypomineralization which is worsened during the subsequent period of hospitalization, especially coupled with inadequate intakes of calcium and phosphorus. In general, both calcium and phosphorus levels are maintained in serum, while the bones appear more osteopenic on radiographs, and ultimately hypophosphatemia with increasing alkaline phosphatase is observed. Rising alkaline phosphatase in the absence of elevated liver enzymes is a strong indicator of metabolic bone disease. Incidence of rickets (metabolic bone disease) is inversely proportional to birth-weight, and has been reported to be as high as 50–60% in very-low-birth-weight infants.[26] Diagnosis is made by routine radiographs which in the initial stages would demonstrate bone undermineralization, especially in the ribs and scapula, subsequently showing the classic forms of rickets in the wrists and long bones. Strategies to increase calcium and phosphorus delivery should be considered. Unfortunately, the very small preterm infant is more often at risk for these complications, given the duration of parenteral nutrition and the coexistence of hepatic dysfunction.

Enteral Nutrition

Even if enteral nutrition is started in the first days after birth, it is suggested that supplemental parenteral nutrition be started because immaturity, feeding intolerance, and GI motility may affect the rate of advancement of enteral nutrition. Further, intakes are also dictated by the feedings used: human milk or formula. Composition of formulas available in the U.S. is depicted in Table 6.8. Composition of human milk (Table 6.9), especially from a mother delivering a preterm infant, is different from that of mothers delivering at term; further, differences between and within the same woman makes the average content difficult to estimate. The route of enteral nutrition is dictated not only by the gestational age of the infant, but also the coexistence of medical or surgical morbidity. Routes and types of delivery are depicted in Table 6.10.

TABLE 6.8

Composition of Formulas Commonly Used in Premature Infants

Nutrients per 100 Calories	Enfamil® Premature Formula 24 with Iron	Similac® Special Care® 24 with Iron	Enfamil 22™ with Iron	Similac® NeoCare™ 22 with Iron
Protein, g	3	2.71	2.8	2.6
Whey:casein	60:40	60:40	60:40	50:50
Fat, g	5.1	5.43	5.3	5.5
Source	MCT, soy, coconut oils	MCT, soy, coconut oils	High oleic sunflower, soy, MCT, coconut oils	Soy, MCT, coconut oils**
Carbohydrate, g	11.1	10.6	10.7	10.3
Source	Corn syrup, solids, lactose	Corn syrup, solids, lactose	Corn syrup solids,* lactose	Corn syrup solids, lactose
Water, g	108	109	120	120
Lineoleic acid, mg	1060	700	950	750
Vitamin A, IU	1250	1250	450	460
Vitamin D, IU	270	150	80	70
Vitamin E, IU	603	4	4	3.6
Vitamin K, mcg	8	12	8	11
Thiamin (B_1), mcg	200	250	200	220
Riboflavin (B_2), mcg	300	620	200	150
Vitamin B_6, mcg	150	250	100	100
Vitamin B_{12}, mcg	0.25	0.55	0.3	0.4
Niacin, mcg	4000	5000	2000	1950
Folic acid, mcg	35	37	26	25
Pantothenic acid, mcg	1200	1900	850	800
Biotin, mcg	4	37	6	9
Vitamin C, mg	20	37	16	15
Choline, mg	12	10	15	16
Inositol, mg	17	5.5	30	6
Calcium, mg	165	180	120	105
Phosphorus, mg	83	100	66	62
Calcium: phosphorus	2:1	1.8:1	1.8:1	1.7:1
Magnesium, mg	6.8	12	8	9
Iron, mg	108	1.8	1.8	1.8
Zinc, mg	105	1.5	1.25	1.2
Manganese, mcg	603	12	15	10
Copper, mcg	125	250	120	120
Iodine, mcg	25	6	15	15
Selenium, mcg	1.8	1.8	2.3	2.3
Sodium, mg	39	43	35	33
Potassium, mg	103	129	105	142
Chloride, mg	85	81	78	75
Osmolality, m0sm/kg water	310	280	260	250

* Powder form only. Ready-to-use form contains maltodextrin.
** Ready to feed.

TABLE 6.9

Composition of Human Milk

		Human milk (2 wks postpartum)	
		Term	Preterm
Volume (ml)		147–161	139–150
Water (ml)		133–145	125–135
Protein			
Content (gm)		1.8–2.5	2.4–3.1
% of energy		7–11	9.6–12
Whey/casein ratio		80:20	80 : 20
Lipid			
Content (gm)		4.4–6	4.9–6.3
% of energy		44–56	42–55
Composition			
Saturated (%)		43	41–47
Monosaturated (%)		42	39–40
Polyunsaturated (%)		15	12–14
Carbohydrate			
Content (gm)		9–10.6	8–9.8
% of energy		38–44	31–38
Lactose (%)		100	100
Minerals and Trace Elements			
Calcium	(mg)	39–42	31–40
	(mmol)	0.9–1	0.7–1
Chloride	(mg)	69–76	76–127
	(mmol)	1.9–2.1	2.1–3.6
Copper (mg)		37–85	107–111
Iodine	(μg)	16	—
	(mmol)		
Iron (mg)		0.04–0.12	0.13–0.14
Magnesium	(mg)	3.9–4.5	4.3–4.7
	(mmol)	0.16–0.18	0.17–0.2
Manganese (μg)		0.9	—
Phosphorus	(mg)	22–25	20–23
	(mmol)	0.7–0.9	0.6–0.7
Potassium	(mg)	90–91	81–93
	(mmol)	2.2–2.4	2.1–2.4
Sodium	(mg)	37–43	44–77
	(mmol)	1.6–1.9	1.9–3.3
Zinc (mg)		0.18–0.50	0.61–0.69
Vitamins			
Fat-soluble			
Vitamin A (IU)		155–333	72–357
Vitamin D (IU)		0.7–3.3	0.7–12
Vitamin E (IU)		0.45–0.75	0.42–1.42
Vitamin K (μg)		0.29–3	0.29–3

TABLE 6.9 *(Continued)*

Composition of Human Milk

	Human milk (2 wks postpartum)	
	Term	Preterm
Water-soluble		
Vitamin B_6 (μg)	15–119	9–129
Vitamin B_{12} (μg)	0.01–1.2	0.01–0.07
Vitamin C (mg)	6.6–7.8	6.3–7.4
Biotin (μg)	0.01–1.2	0.01–1.2
Folic Acid (μg)	7.5–9	5–8.6
Niacin (mg)	0.2–0.25	0.24–0.3
Pantothenic acid (mg)	0.26	0.33
Riboflavin (μg)	15–104	14–79
Thiamin (μg)	3–31	1.4–31
Other		
Carnitine (mg)	1.04	—
Choline (mg)	13.4	10–13
Inositol (mg)	22.2–83.5	21.3

TABLE 6.10

Routes of Feeding Preterm Infants

Route	<34 weeks	>34 weeks
Per os	No	Yes
Continuous gastric	<1250 g	Failure to tolerate bolus gastric, significant GER
Bolus gastric (every 3 h)	>1250 g; infants <1250 g not tolerating continuous	Failure to tolerate per os
Transpyloric, continuous	Failure to tolerate gastric feeds, gastric distention due to positive pressure, poor gastric emptying	Same as <34 weeks

Motor responses to feedings are similar whether feedings are provided by the gastric or transpyloric route.[27] However, when feeds are provided slowly over 120 min as compared to 15 min, gastric emptying is better, suggesting that in the smaller premature infant, slow infusions may be better tolerated.[28,29]

Oral Feeding

Term and preterm infants greater than 33 to 34 weeks gestation may be fed soon after birth by the oral route. This should be attempted in the delivery room in healthy infants or initiated soon after birth. Human milk feedings (i.e., breast feeding) should be encouraged, and all steps should be taken by the medical team and hospital staff to encourage breast feeding once the decision is made.[30] If breast feeding is precluded due to craniofacial anomalies such as cleft lip or palate, feeding devices are available and speech and/or feeding teams may need to be involved. Lactation consultation should be sought for mothers who have difficulty in either initiation or maintenance of breast feeding. Hospitals should avoid supplementing breastfed infants and the use of pacifiers.[30]

Most mothers delivering preterm infants have not made a decision about breast feeding, and should be counseled appropriately. All delivery sites should have facilities to pump breast milk if actual breastfeeding is not possible and the mother wishes to breastfeed. Teaching should include appropriate techniques for pumping and storing milk.

Nutrient Delivery

For infants born after 33 to 34 weeks of gestation, enteral feedings may be started *per os*. Although it is recognized that infants at this gestational age can coordinate their suck, swallow, and respiratory activities, thus enabling feedings, not all infants respond in such a fashion and careful assessment is warranted. In the event that nipple feedings are not achieved, the infant may be fed by the gastric route.

In general, the alternatives to feedings by mouth are gastric and transpyloric. Gastric feedings can be further described as bolus or continuous, where the feedings are either provided intermittently every 2 to 3 hours, or by a pump continuously. Transpyloric feeds are provided continuously, with the tip of the feeding tube in the second part of the duodenum. General indications for the latter include failure to tolerate gastric feeding due to delayed gastric emptying, gastric distention due to positive pressure ventilation, or gastroesophageal reflux. Feedings can also be planned based on birth-weight. In general, infants below 1250 g are fed by the continuous gastric method, whereas bigger infants are fed by the intermittent method.

Special Considerations

Essential Fatty Acids

Vegetable oils contain the precursor essential fatty acids linoleic acid (18:2w-6) and in most cases alpha linolenic acid (18:3w-3). Linoleic and linolenic acids serve as precursors for the synthesis of long-chain polyunsaturated fatty acids (LC-PUFA) including arachdonic (20:4w-6), eicosopentaenoic (20:5w-3), and docosahexaenoic (22:6w-3) acids. Human milk lipids contain preformed LC-PUFA; LC-PUFA are essential components of membrane systems and are incorporated in membrane-rich tissues such as the brain during early growth.[31,32] Some of the LC-PUFA serve as precursors for prostaglandins, prostacyclin, thromboxanes, and leukotrienes. The fetus and the fully breastfed infant do not depend on active synthesis of LC-PUFA, since the placenta and human milk provide LC-PUFA in amounts considered appropriate.[33-36] Premature infants fed formulas without LC-PUFA develop depletion of LC-PUFA in plasma and red cell membranes, indicating limited endogenous LC-PUFA synthesis.[37] Recent studies by Carlson et al. demonstrate that preterm infants have high cord blood phosphatidlyethalonamine (PE), phosphatidlycholine (PC), docosahexanoic acid (DHA), and arachadonic acid (AA), but that these levels decline rapidly.[38] Further, PE, PC, DHA, and PC AA declined in formula-fed infants, but were maintained in human milk-fed infants;[38] at the end of the six-week study period, although PE, PC DHA, and AA were significantly higher in human milk-fed than formula-fed infants, these levels did not reach cord blood levels.[38] These declines in erythrocyte PE DHA could be prevented with supplementation of DHA.[39] However, supplementation with DHA (0.5% total fatty acids) resulted in decreased AA concentrations compared to feeding with 0.2% DHA, suggesting adverse effects on AA synthesis at the higher concentration.[40] Similar effects on AA were observed in premature infants fed formulas with similar linoleic acid content (16%) but different alpha-linolenic acid contents (1 vs. 3.2%); high alpha-linolenic acid-supplemented infants had lower AA and despite a higher DHA content, rate of weight gain was significantly less than the lower-supplemented infants throughout the study.[41] There were no demonstrable effects on visual evoked potential or latency at 56 weeks between the two groups of infants, although mean latency in both groups was higher and mean amplitude lower than in age-matched breastfed term infants or in term infants fed similar formulas. Higher visual acuity in DHA-supplemented infants has been reported at 2 and 4 months[42-44] but not at 6, 9, and 12 months. Further studies are required before the optimal dose of DHA can be determined on growth and longer term followup of premature infants.

Carnitine

Current parenteral nutrition regimens do not contain carnitine. Low plasma concentrations of carnitine and its decline with postnatal age has been demonstrated in infants receiving carnitine-free nutrition.[45,46] Although fatty acid metabolism has not been shown to be impaired in short-term parenteral nutrition, carnitine is an accepted additive for infants requiring parenteral nutrition for longer periods.[47-49] Carnitine is provided at doses of 8.0 to 20 mg/kg/d.

Glutamine

Glutamine is the most abundant amino acid in the human body and is the most important "nitrogen shuttle," accounting for 30 to 35% of all amino acid nitrogen transported in the blood.[50] Glutamine concentrations in blood and tissue fall following starvation, surgery, infection, and trauma.[51,52] In addition, glutamine plays an important role in protein and energy metabolism, nucleotide synthesis, and lymphocyte function.[53] Glutamine is known to be an important fuel for small intestinal enterocytes;[54] however, an absolute need of glutamine for gut growth has not been demonstrated with either detrimental or negligible effects reported in the literature.[55-57] Nonetheless, absence of glutamine in the diet has been shown to cause villous atrophy, fall in lumina propria lymphocyte populations, and increased bacterial translocation.[58-62] While optimal intakes of glutamine for premature infants is not known, enteral supplementation with glutamine has been shown to decrease feeding intolerance,[63] and there is a possible decrease in hospital costs[64] with glutamine supplemented up to 0.3 g/kg/d. Further studies on optimal supplementation of glutamine, enterally and parenterally, in preterm infants are required.

Summary

Despite the many questions that remain regarding optimal nutritional management of the neonate, it is nonetheless important to develop rational protocols for the management of nutritional issues that arise. This chapter has provided some guidelines and the framework from which these guidelines arose. There are numerous different approaches to feeding a neonate. The ultimate goal should be to optimize nutrition, and hence growth and ultimately development in this ever-increasing population of small premature infants.

References

1. Ballard J. L., Novak K. K., Driver, M. *J Pediatr* 95: 769; 1979.

2. Alexander G. R., de Caunes F., Hulsey T. C., Thompkins M. E., Allen M. *Am J Obstet Gynecol* 166: 891; 1992.
3. Ballard J. L., Khoury J. C., Wedig K., Wang L., Wilers-Walsman B. L., Lipp R. *J Pediatr* 119: 417; 1991.
4. Ziegler E. E., O'Donnell A. M., Nelson S. E., Fomon S. J. *Growth* 40: 329; 1976.
5. Widdowson, E. M., Spray, C. M. *Arch Dis Child* 26: 205; 1951.
6. Ziegler E.E. *Energy and Protein Needs during Infancy,* Academic Press, Florida, 1996.
7. Weinstein M. R. Oh W. *J Pediatr* 99: 958; 1981.
8. Billeaud C., Piedboeuf B., Chessex P. *J Pediatr* 120: 461; 1992.
9. Kashyap S., Hierd W. C. NCR [ed]: *Protein Metabolism During Infancy, Nestle Nutrition Workshop Series,* Raven Press, New York, 33: 133; 1994.
10. Rivera A. Jr., Bell E. F., Stegink L. D., Ziegler E. E. *J Pediatr* 115: 465; 1989.
11. Kashyap S., Abildskov A., Heird W.C. *Pediatr Res* 31: 290A; 1992.
12. Saini J., MacMahon P., Morgan J. B., Kovar I. Z. *Arch Dis Child* 64: 1362; 1989.
13. Van Lingen R.A., van Goudoever J. B., Luijendijk I. H., et al. *Clin Sci* 82:199; 1992.
14. van Goudoever J. B., Sucklers E. J., Timmerman M., et al. *J Parent Enteral Nutr* 18: 404; 1994.
15. Zlotkin S. H., Bryan M. H., Anderson G. H. *J Pediatr* 99: 115; 1981.
16. Haumont D., Deckelbaum R. J., Richelle M., et al. *J Pediatr* 115: 787; 1989.
17. Brans Y. W., Andrews D. S., Carrillo D. W., et al. *Am J Dis Child* 142: 145; 1988.
18. Wu P. Y., Edwards N., Storm M. C. *J Pediatr* 109: 347; 1986.
19. Schanler R. J. *Clin Perinatol* 22: 207; 1995.
20. Schanler R. J., Garza C. *J Pediatr* 112: 452; 1988.
21. Widness J. A., Seward, V. J., Kromer, I. J., et al. *J Pediatr* 129: 680; 1996.
22. Shannon K. M., Keith J. F., Mentzer W. C., et al. *Pediatrics* 95: 1; 1995.
23. Grant J. P., Cox C. E., Kleinman L. M. et al., *Surg Gynecol Obstet* 145: 573; 1977.
24. Balistreri W. F., Bove K. E. *Prog Liver Dis* 9: 567; 1990.
25. Bhatia J., Moslen M. T., Haque A. K. *Pediatr Res* 33: 487; 1993.
26. Greer F. R. *Ann Rev Nutr* 14: 169; 1994.
27. Koenig W. J., Amarnath R. P., Hench V., Berseth C. L. *Pediatrics* 95: 203; 1995.
28. Berseth C. L. *J Pediatr* 117: 777; 1990.
29. Berseth C. L., Ittmann P. I. *J Pediatr Gastroenterol Nutr* 14: 182; 1992.
30. American Academy of Pediatrics. Work Group on Breastfeeding. *Pediatrics* 100: 1035; 1997.
31. Clandinin M. T., Chappell J. E., Leong S., et al. *Human Dev* 4: 121; 1980.
32. Martinez M., Ballabriga A. *Lipids* 22: 133; 1987.
33. Koletzko B., Thiel I., Springer S. *Eur J Clin Nutr* 46: S45; 1992.
34. Jensen R. G., *The Lipids of Human Milk,* CRC Press, Boca Raton, 1995.
35. Sanders T. A., Naismith D. J. *Br J Nutr* 41: 619; 1979.
36. Putnam J. C., Carlson S. E., DeVoe P. W., Barness L. A. *Am J Clin Nutr* 36: 106; 1982.
37. Koletzko B., Schmidt E., Bremer H. J., et al. *Eur J Pediatr* 148: 669; 1989.
38. Carlson S. E., Rhodes P. G., Ferguson M. G. *Am J Clin Nutr* 44: 798; 1986.
39. Carlson S. E., Rhodes P. G., Rao V. S., Goldgar D. E. *Pediatr Res* 21: 507; 1987.
40. Liu C. C., Carlson S. E., Rhodes P. G., et al. *Pediatr Res* 22: 292; 1987.
41. Jensen C. L., Chen H. M., Prager T. C., et al. *Pediatr Res* 37: 311A, 1995.
42. Uauy R. D., Birch D. G., Birch E. E. et al., *Pediatr Res* 28: 485; 1990.
43. Carlson S. E., Werkman S. H., Tolley E. A. *Am J Clin Nutr* 63: 687; 1996.
44. Carlson S. E., Werkman S. H., Rhodes P. G., Tolley E. *Am J Clin Nutr* 58: 35; 1993.
45. Penn D., Schmidt-Sommerfeld E., Pascu F. *Early Hum Develop* 4: 23; 1979.
46. Shenai J. P., Borum P. R. *Pediatr Res* 18: 679; 1984.
47. Orzali A., Donzelli F., Enzi G., Rubaltelli F. *Biol Neonate* 43: 186; 1983.
48. Orzali A., Maetzke G., Donzelli F., Rubaltelli F. F. *J Pediatr* 104: 436; 1984.
49. Schmidt-Sommerfeld E., Penn D., Wolf H. *J Pediatr* 102: 931; 1983.
50. Souba W. W. *J Parent Enteral Nutr* 11: 569; 1987.
51. Askanazi J., Carpentier Y. A., Michelsen C. B., et al. *Ann Surg* 192: 78; 1980.
52. Roth E., Funovics J., Muhlbacher F., et al. *Clin Nutr* 1:25; 1982.
53. Neu J., Shenoy V., Chakrabarti R. *FASEB J* 10: 829; 1996.

54. Souba W. W., Herskowitz, K., Salloum, R. M., et al. *J Parent Enteral Nutr* 14: 45S; 1990.
55. Bark T., Svenberg T., Theodorsson E., et al. *Clin Nutr* 13:79; 1994.
56. Burrin D. G., Shulam R. J., Storm M. C., Reeds P. J. *J Parent Enteral Nutr* 15: 262; 1991.
57. Vanderhoof J. A., Blackwood D. J., Mohammadpour H., Park, J. H. *J Am Coll Nutr* 11: 223; 1992.
58. Hwang T. L., O'Dwyer S. T., Smith R. J., et al. *Surg Forum* 38: 56; 1987.
59. Grant J. *J Surg* 44: 506; 1988.
60. Burke D. J., Alverdy J. C., Aoys E., Moss G. S. *Arch Surg,* 124: 1396; 1989.
61. Alverdy J. C., Aoys E., Weiss-Carrington P., Burke D. A. *J Surg Res* 52: 34; 1992.
62. Neu J., Roig J. C., Meetze W. H., et al. *J Pediatr* 131: 691; 1997.
63. Dallas M. J., Bowling D., Roig J. C., et al. *J Parent Enteral Nutr* 22: 352; 1998.

7

Feeding the Term Infant

Jatinder Bhatia, Colleen Bucher, and Chantrapa Bunyapen

Growth, particularly in weight, length, and additional anthropometric measurements, remains a measure of adequacy of nutritional regimens for the growing infant and child. Infant feeding decisions have an impact on lifelong medical illnesses, growth, and developmental abilities well beyond infancy. This section will review normal growth and requirements in healthy term infants.

Growth

The average weight of a healthy term infant is 3.5 kg. With an anticipated loss of 10% in body weight in the first week of life, birth weight is regained by two weeks of age in both breast-fed and formula-fed infants, with the formula-fed infants demonstrating a tendency to regain birth weight sooner than their breast-fed counterparts.

Body weight should be measured with an electronic scale or a beam balance without detachable weights, with the balances capable of weighing to the nearest 10 g. Even with the use of electronic scales, balances should be tared with calibrated weights at least two times a year. Mean weight and selected centiles for weight are summarized in Table 7.1. In clinical practice, however, weight and other anthropometric measurements including length, head circumference, and weight for length are plotted on growth charts (Figures 7.1 and 7.2) adapted from Hamill et al.[1] The plotting of growth on these charts will suffice for monitoring of normal infants; however, a different and more sensitive approach will be needed for infants with faltering growth. The "reference data" provided by Fomon[2] combine data from the University of Iowa and the Fels Longitudinal Study, the latter data used in the growth charts.

Length

Length should be measured by two examiners using a calibrated length board with a fixed headpiece and a movable foot board. The head is held by one examiner with the Frankfort plane (defined as a line that passes through the left porion, the right porion, and the orbits)

0-8493-2705-9/01/$0.00+$1.50

TABLE 7.1

Mean Body Weight and Selected Centiles for Males and Females, 0–12 Months of Age

Age	Mean	5th centile (g)	50th centile (g)	95th centile (g)
Mean body weight and selected centiles for males, 0–12 months of age				
Birth	3350	2685	3530	4225
1 mo	4445	3640	4448	5238
2 mo	5519	4574	5491	6475
3 mo	6326	5321	6323	7393
6 mo	7927	6670	7877	9146
9 mo	9087	7785	9008	10,448
12 mo	10,059	8606	9978	11,676
Mean body weight and selected centiles for females, 0–12 months of age				
Birth	3367	2750	3345	4095
1 mo	4160	3548	4123	4885
2 mo	5049	4301	5009	5878
3 mo	5763	4837	5729	6712
6 mo	7288	6063	7239	8547
9 mo	8449	7072	8373	9723
12 mo	9425	7942	9362	10,863

Modified from Fomon S.J. and Nelson S.E. In *Nutrition of Normal Infants,* CV Mosby, 1993, 36, p. 155.

in the vertical position, and gentle traction is placed to bring the head into contact with the headpiece. A second examiner holds the infant's feet with the toes pointing upwards, and while applying gentle traction, brings the footpiece to rest firmly against the infant's heels. Measurements agreeing to within 0.4 cm are considered adequate, and the importance of length measurements is underscored, particularly when serial measurements are made in a longitudinal fashion. It is generally agreed that faltering in length as well as weight suggests growth faltering of a longer duration than when weight alone is affected.

Head Circumference

Head circumference is measured by a narrow flexible steel or paper tape applied to the head above the supraorbital ridges and encircling the most prominent parts of the forehead and the occiput. The maximum of three measurements should be used as the maximal circumference. Weight-for-length measurements (Figures 7.1 and 7.2) are also available and are useful in defining obesity as well as leanness.

A variety of other measures to define growth include skin fold thickness, limb length and circumference, and body mass index. The latter, body mass index, is calculated by dividing weight in kilograms by length in meters squared, replacing weight for length in older children. In any case, accurate measurements are essential to the interpretation of growth charts.

Normal growth is a strong indicator of nutritional sufficiency and overall health of an infant. Since infancy is a period of rapid growth, particularly early infancy, identifying growth failure is important and requires prompt medical attention. As we understand more about the complex interactions between genetic, immunologic, metabolic, physiologic, and psychologic factors and their effects on long-term outcomes of infant feeding decisions, defining appropriate growth becomes a very important issue for health care providers of children.

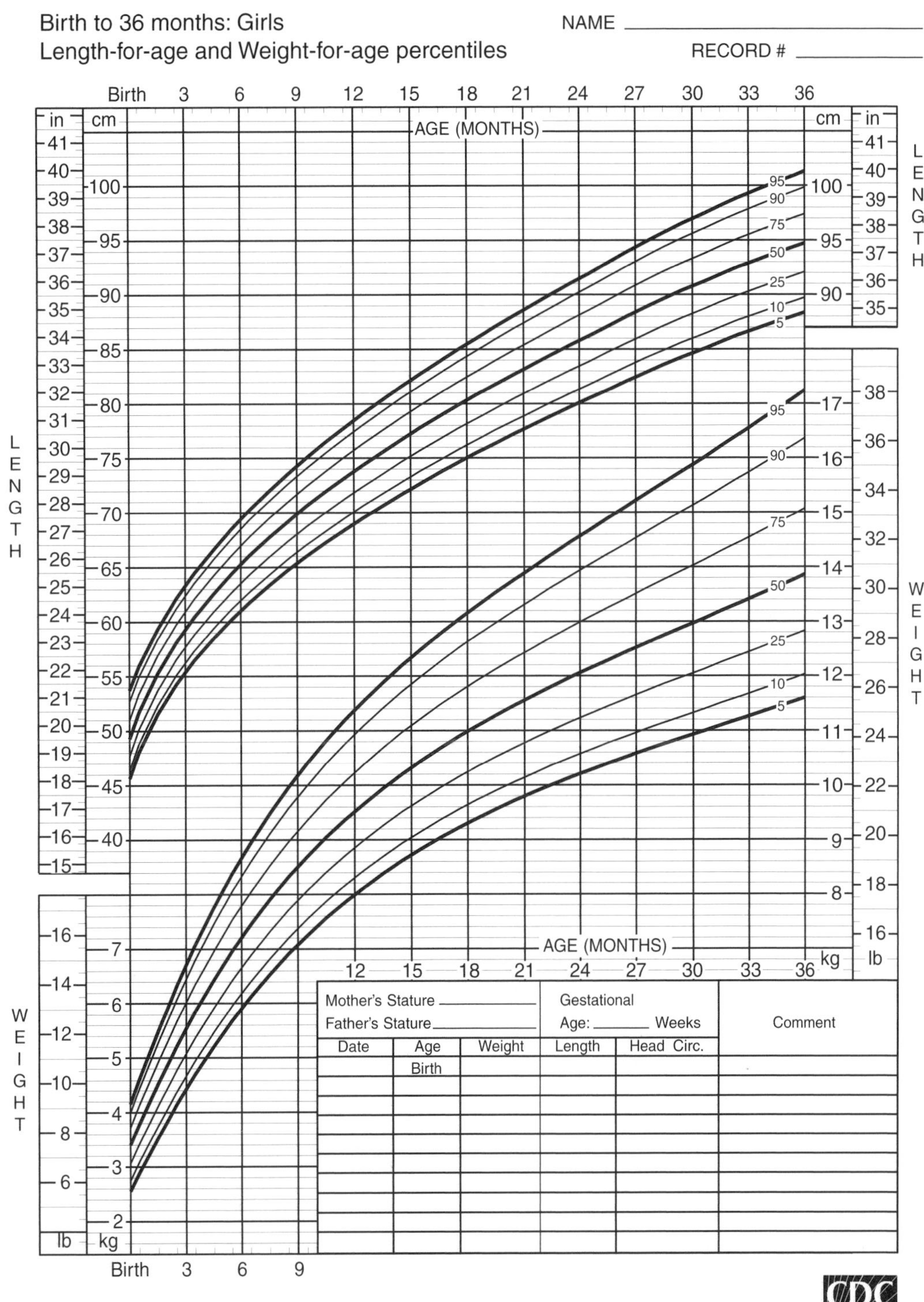

FIGURE 7.1
Girls: birth to 36 months: physical growth NCHS percentiles.

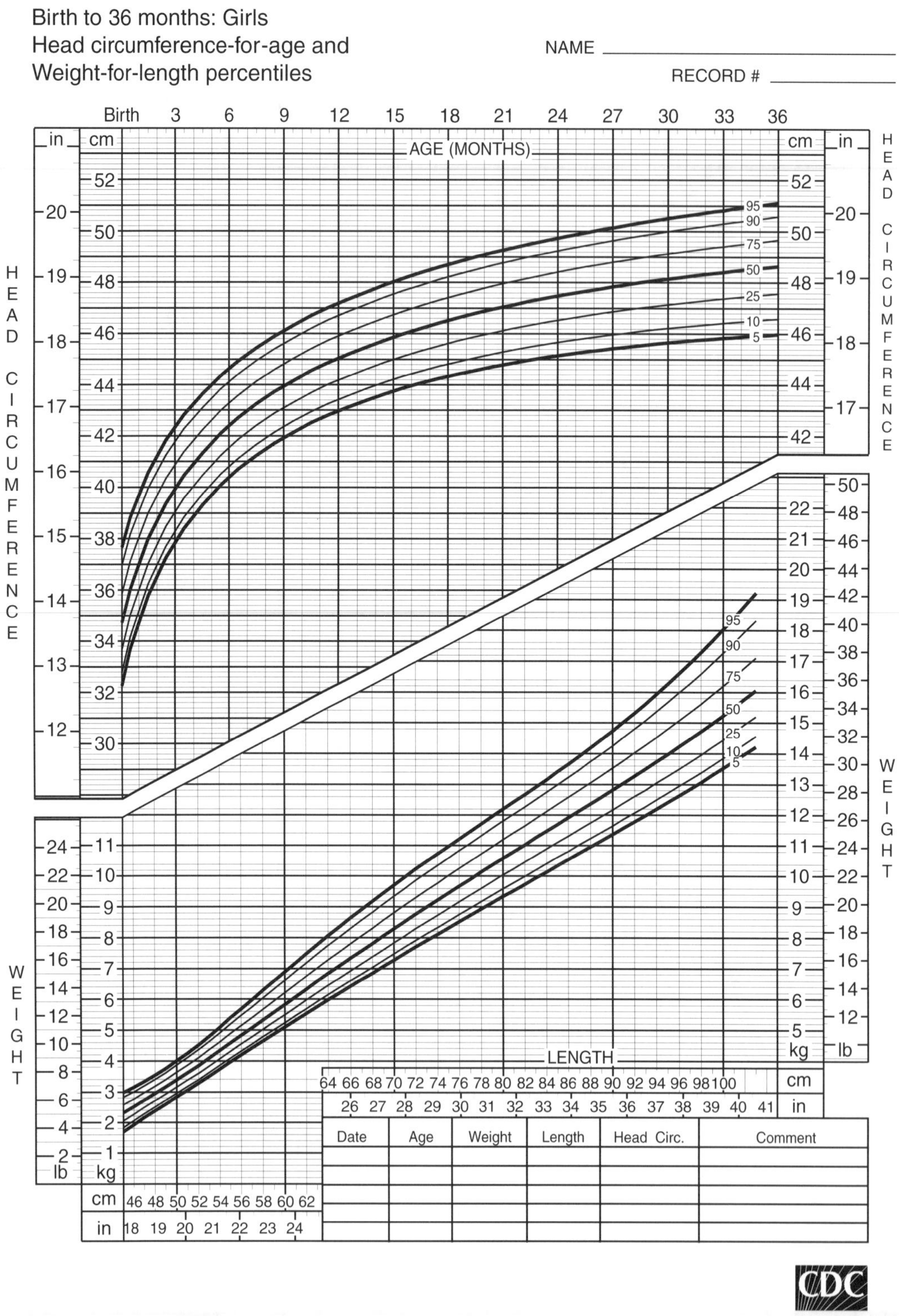

Birth to 36 months: Girls
Head circumference-for-age and
Weight-for-length percentiles

NAME ______________________

RECORD # __________

AGE (MONTHS)

Birth 3 6 9 12 15 18 21 24 27 30 33 36

HEAD CIRCUMFERENCE

in: 12 13 14 15 16 17 18 19 20

cm: 30 32 34 36 38 40 42 44 46 48 50 52

Percentiles: 95 90 75 50 25 10 5

WEIGHT

kg: 1 2 3 4 5 6 7 8 9 10 11 12 13 14 15 16 17 18 19 20 21 22

lb: 2 4 6 8 10 12 14 16 18 20 22 24 26 28 30 32 34 36 38 40 42 44 46 48 50

LENGTH

cm: 46 48 50 52 54 56 58 60 62 64 66 68 70 72 74 76 78 80 82 84 86 88 90 92 94 96 98 100

in: 18 19 20 21 22 23 24 26 27 28 29 30 31 32 33 34 35 36 37 38 39 40 41

Date	Age	Weight	Length	Head Circ.	Comment

FIGURE 7.1
Continued.

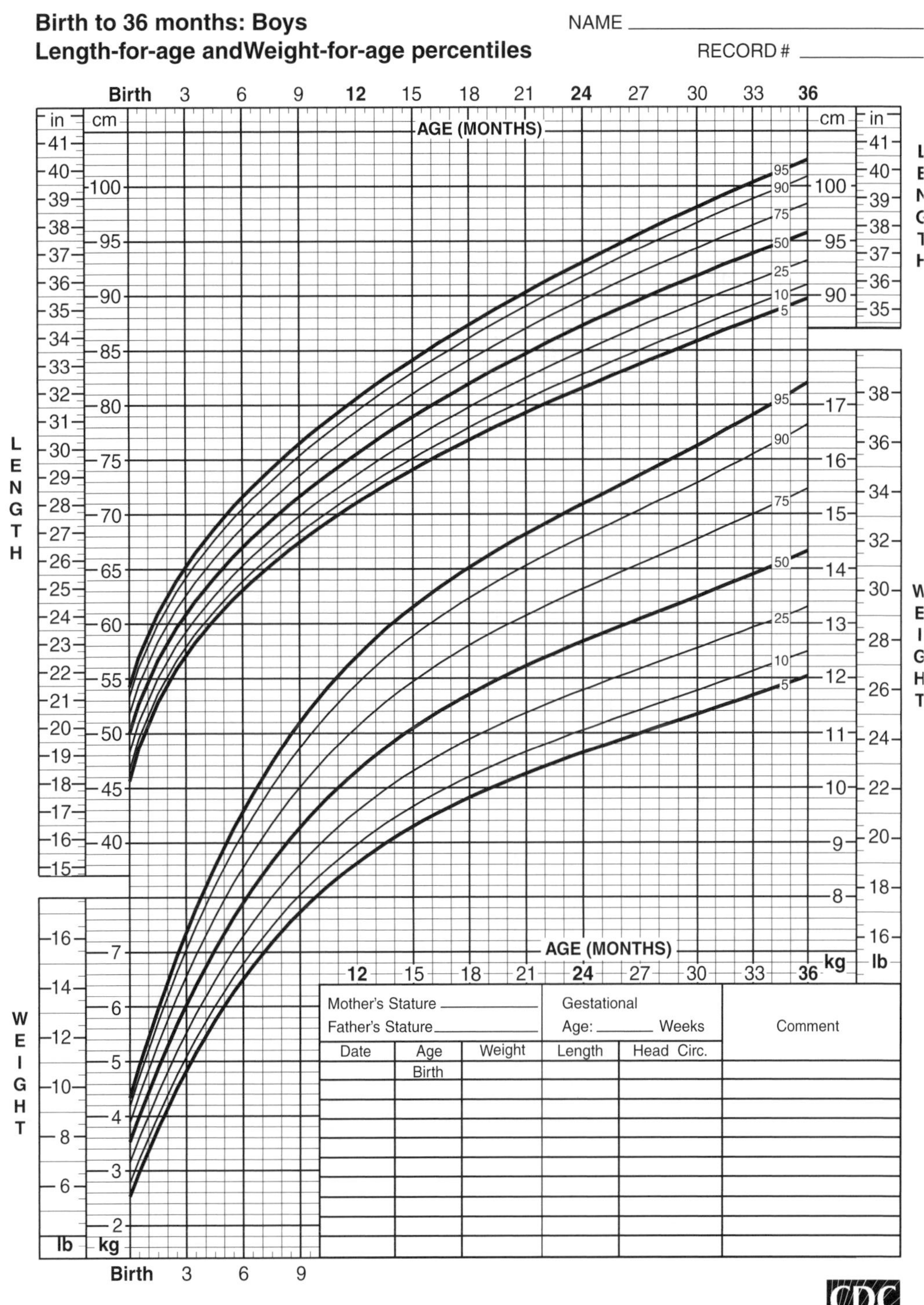

FIGURE 7.2
Boys: birth to 36 months: physical growth NHS percentiles.

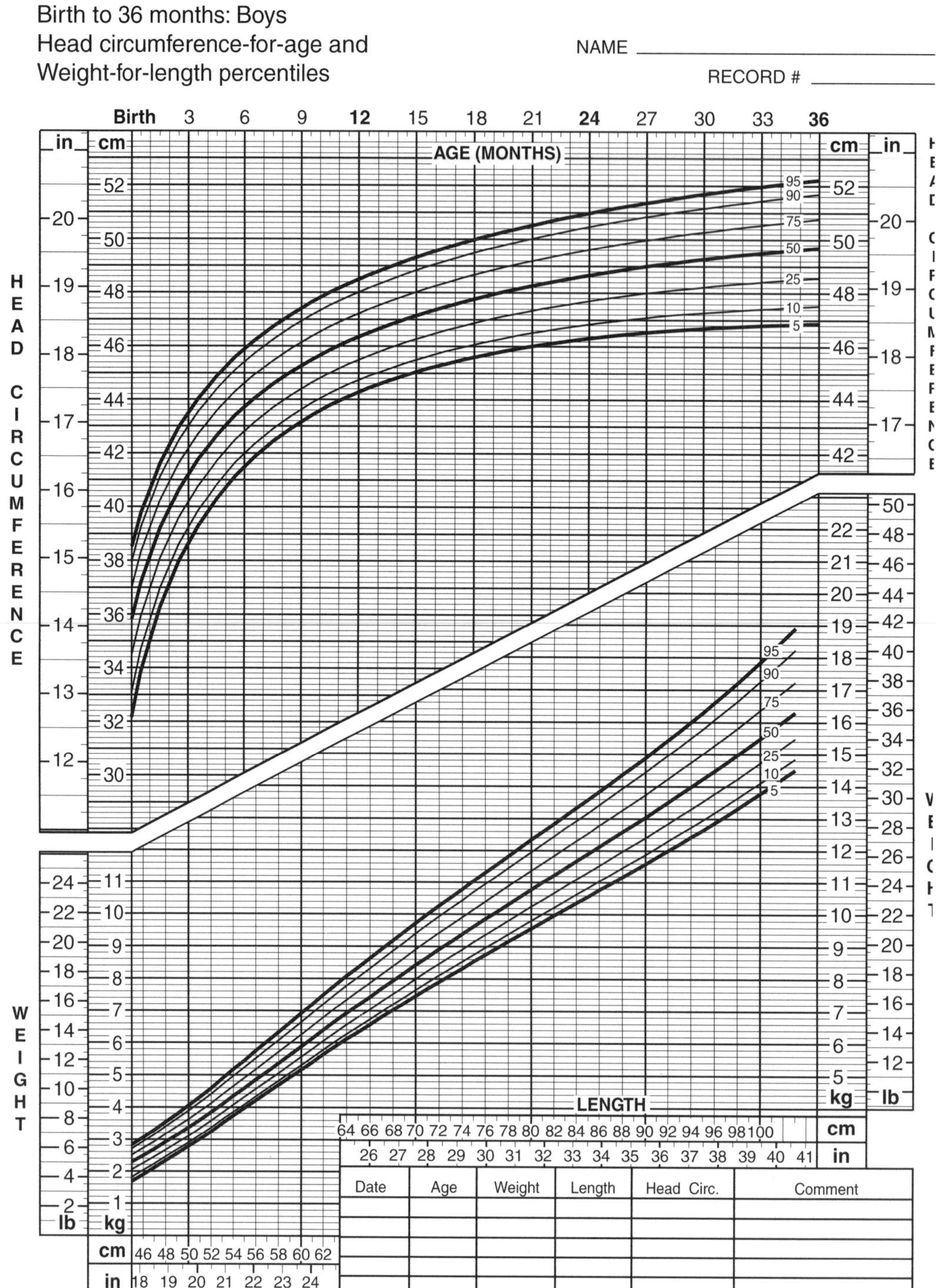

FIGURE 7.2
Continued.

Energy

Energy requirements during infancy may be partitioned into basal metabolism, thermic effect of feeding, thermoregulation, physical activity, and growth. The energy requirements for growth relative to maintenance, except in early infancy, are small, and satisfactory growth can be considered a sensitive indicator that energy requirements are being met. Energy balance may be defined as gross energy intake = energy excreted + energy expended + energy stored. Gross energy intake, measured by the heat of combustion, is greater than energy available when fed because most foods are not completely digested, and protein oxidation is incomplete. Fat absorption varies widely among infants fed various formulas, particularly in infancy. Urea and other nitrogenous compounds are excreted in the urine. Gross intake is calculated as 5.7 kcal/g, 9.4 kcal/g, and 4.1 kcal/g obtained from protein, fat, and carbohydrate, respectively, and therefore it varies given the type of diet fed. The term "digestible energy" refers to gross energy intake minus energy excreted in the feces. Metabolizable energy is defined as digestible energy minus energy lost in urine. The metabolizable energy values for protein, fat, and carbohydrate are close to 4, 9, and 4 kcal/g, respectively. Losses of energy, other than feces and urine, are negligible and are ignored for practical purposes.

The energy intake of normal infants per unit body weight is much greater than in adult counterparts. Energy requirements for term infants have been estimated by various groups and vary from 100–116 kcal/kg/d from 0–3 months and decline to about 100 kcal/kg/d by the end of the first year.[3-7] These recommendations are based on the median intake of thriving infants; the intakes of breast-fed infants are lower than that of formula-fed infants, with an average of 3–4% lower in the first three months, and 6–7% from three to six months. As new, more precise estimates of energy expenditure become available, these recommendations are apt to change, given that current recommendations are higher than the "gold" standard — the breast-fed infant. Energy intakes of infants from 6 to 12 months of age have been reported to be between 91 and 100 kcal/kg/d.[8-10]

Protein

Intakes of protein and essential amino acids are generally sufficient in developed countries, in contrast to developing countries where protein and protein-energy malnutrition are still a frequent occurrence. In appropriately fed infants, protein is not a limiting dietary component in infancy and is clearly essential for normal growth and development. For the human infant, histidine, isoleucine, leucine, lysine, methionine, phenylalanine, threonine, tryptophan, and valine are considered essential amino acids. The data for cysteine are conflicting[11,12] for the term infant, although the data are clear for the preterm infant. Conditionally essential amino acids are those that become essential under certain circumstances, since they may be produced in inadequate amounts endogenously. An example of this is taurine, which is now added to formulas based on reports of greater concentrations of taurine in the plasma and urine of preterm[13,14] and term[15] infants. The concern about taurine depletion stems from the observations of growth retardation, abnormal retinal findings, and impaired bile acid metabolism in taurine-deficient animals and humans.

Recommended dietary intakes of protein are summarized in Table 7.2. In contrast, intakes recommended by WHO[16] are 2.25, 1.86, 1.65, and 1.48 g/100 kcal from 1–2, 3–6,

TABLE 7.2

Recommended Dietary Intakes of Protein

Age Interval (mo)	Recommended Dietary Intake ($g \cdot kg^{-1} \cdot d^{-1}$)	(g/100 kcal)
0 to 1	2.6	2.2
1 to 2	2.2	2.0
2 to 3	1.8	1.8
3 to 4	1.5	1.6
4 to 5	1.4	1.6
5 to 6	1.4	1.6
6 to 9	1.4	1.5
9 to 12	1.3	1.5

Reproduced with permission from Fomon, S. J. *Pediatric Research* 30, 391, 1991.

6–9, and 9–12 months, respectively. Both of these recommendations are generally higher than the intakes observed in human milk-fed infants.

Fat

The importance of dietary fat is underscored by the fact that 35% of the weight gain of an infant in early infancy is accounted for by fat.[17] Most of the dietary fat is in the form of triglyceride formed by three fatty acids esterified to a glycerol backbone. In the body, triglycerides are the main form of storage and transport of fatty acids. Phospholipids and cholesterol are indispensable components of the lipid bi-layer of all cell membranes, and the amount of different phospholipids and cholesterol, as well as the fatty acid pattern of incorporated phospholipids, modulate membrane fluidity, permeability, enzyme and receptor activity, and signal transduction. Cholesterol is required for the synthesis of steroids and bile acids, although the majority of the cholesterol pool in tissue and plasma is derived from endogenous synthesis; dietary cholesterol contributes to the pool, and diet modifies liver synthesis.[18] Fatty acids (4-26 carbon atoms) are either saturated (no double bonds in the carbon chain), mono-unsaturated (one double bond) or polyunsaturated (two or more double bonds). Double bonds occur in two isomeric forms: cis and trans; unsaturated fatty acids are folded at the site of each double bond, cis, and trans-fatty acids have straight carbon chains.

Human milk contains approximately 4% lipids, but the reported variation is between 3.1 and 5.2%,[19,20] with 99% of the fat present in the form of triglycerides and the rest in the form of diglycerides, monoglycerides, free fatty acids, phospholipids, and cholesterol. The fat content of human milk increases with duration of lactation.[19,21] During this period, the average size of the fat globules increases, and the ratio of phospholipids and cholesterol to triglycerides decreases.[22] The concentration of fat in human milk remains similar regardless of maternal diet or nutritional status, although poor nutrition has been shown to decrease fat content.[23] Fatty acid content of human milk has been reported by numerous investigators and demonstrates a wide range, as summarized by Fomon.[2] Fatty acid content of human milk is also altered by dietary manipulation.[24-27] Human milk fat provides the essential fatty acids linoleic and α-linolenic acids, along with the long-chain polyunsaturated fatty acids such as arachidonic and docosahexaenoic acids. The decrease of milk phospholipid content during the first few weeks after birth is accompanied by a decrease in arachidonic and docosahexaenoic acids.[28] Fat content of human milk and commonly used formulas is summarized in Table 7.3.

TABLE 7.3

Nutritional Composition of Human Milk and Commonly Used Formulas

	Kilocalories/ oz.	Protein		Fat		Carbohydrate		Na mEq/dl	K mEq/dl	Phosphorus mg/dl	Calcium mg/dl	Osmolality mOsm/kg water
		Source	gm/dl	Source	gm/dl	Source	gm/dl					
Mature human milk	20	Human milk	1.0	Human milk	4.4	Lactose	6.9	0.7	1.3	14	32	300
Enfamil (Mead Johnson)	20	Whey, nonfat milk	1.5	Palm olein, soy coconut, high-oleic sunflower oils	3.6	Lactose	7.3	0.8	1.9	36	53	300
Enfamil AR (Mead Johnson)	20	Nonfat milk	1.7	Palm olein, soy coconut, sunflower oils	3.5	Lactose, rice starch maltodextrin	7.4	1.2	1.9	36	53	240
Good Start (Nestle/ Carnation)	20	Enzymatically hydrolyzed reduced mineral whey	1.6	Palm olein, soybean, coconut, high-oleic safflower oils	3.4	Lactose, maltodextrin	7.4	0.7	1.7	24	43	265
Lactofree (Mead Johnson)	20	Milk protein isolate	1.4	Palm olein, soy coconut, high-oleic sunflower oils	3.6	Corn syrup solids	7.4	0.9	1.9	37	55	200
Similac Improved (Ross)	20	Nonfat milk, whey	1.4	High-oleic safflower, coconut, soy oils	3.7	Lactose	7.3	0.7	1.8	28	53	300
Similac Lactose Free (Ross)	20	Milk protein isolate	1.4	Soy, coconut oils	3.6	Corn syrup solids, sucrose	7.2	0.8	1.8	38	57	230
Similac PM/ 60/40 (Ross)	20	Whey, sodium caseinate	1.5	Soy, corn, coconut oils	3.8	Lactose	6.9	0.7	1.5	19	38	280
Alsoy (Nestle/ Carnation)	20	Soy protein isolate with L-methionine	1.9	Palm olein, soy, coconut, high-oleic safflower oils	3.3	Corn maltodextrin, sucrose	7.5	0.9	2.0	41	71	200

TABLE 7.3 *(Continued)*

Nutritional Composition of Human Milk and Commonly Used Formulas

	Kilocalories/ oz.	Protein		Fat		Carbohydrate		Na mEq/dl	K mEq/dl	Phosphorus mg/dl	Calcium mg/dl	Osmolality mOsm/kg water
		Source	gm/dl	Source	gm/dl	Source	gm/dl					
Babysoy (pwd) (Wyeth Nutritionals, Inc.)	20	Soy protein isolate with L-methionine	2.1	Oleo, coconut, high-oleic (saff. or sun.), soybean oils	3.6	Corn syrup solids, sucrose	6.9	0.9	1.8	42	60	228
Isomil (Ross)	20	Soy protein isolate with L-methionine	1.7	High-oleic safflower, coconut, soy oils	3.7	Corn syrup, sucrose	7.0	1.3	1.9	51	71	230
Isomil DF (Ross)	20	Soy protein isolate with L-methionine	1.8	Soy, coconut oils	3.7	Corn syrup, sucrose, soy fiber	6.8	1.3	1.9	51	71	240
ProSobee (Mead Johnson)	20	Soy protein isolate with L-methionine	1.7	Palm olein, soy, coconut, high-oleic sunflower oils	3.7	Corn syrup solids	7.3	1.0	2.1	56	71	200
Alimentum (Ross)	20	Casein hydrolysate with added amino acids	1.9	MCT 33%, safflower, soy oils	3.7	Sucrose, modified tapioca starch	6.9	1.3	2.0	51	71	370
Nutramigen (Mead Johnson)	20	Casein hydrolysate with added amino acids	1.9	Palm olein, soy, coconut, high-oleic sunflower oils	3.4	Corn syrup solids, modified corn starch	7.5	1.4	1.9	43	64	320
Pregestimil Powder (Mead Johnson)	20	Casein hydrolysate with added amino acids	1.9	MCT (55%), corn, soy, high-oleic oils	3.8	Corn syrup solids, dextrose, modified corn starch	6.9	1.4	1.9	51	78	340

Pregestimil Liquid (Mead Johnson)	20	Casein hydrolysate with added amino acids	1.9	MCT (55%), soy, high-oleic safflower oils	3.8	Corn syrup solids, modified corn starch	6.9	1.4	1.9	51	78	280
Neocate (SHS)	20	L-amino acids	2.1	Hybrid safflower, refined vegetable oils, (coconut, soy)	3.0	Corn syrup solids	7.8	1.1	2.7	62	82	342
Follow-Up (Nestle/Carnation)	20	Nonfat milk	1.8	Palm olein, soy, coconut, high-oleic safflower oils	2.8	Corn syrup solids, lactose	8.9	1.2	2.3	61	91	326
Follow-Up Soy (Nestle/Carnation)	20	Soy protein isolate with L-methionine	2.1	Palm olein, soy, coconut, high-oleic safflower oils	3.0	Corn maltodextrin, sucrose	8.1	1.2	2.0	61	91	200
Whole cow's milk	20	Cow's milk	3.3	Cow's milk	3.7	Lactose	4.7	2.1	3.9	93	119	288
Next Step (Mead Johnson)	20	Nonfat milk	1.8	Palm olein, soy, coconut, high-oleic sunflower oils	3.4	Lactose, corn syrup solids	7.5	1.2	2.3	57	81	270
Next Step Soy (Mead Johnson)	20	Soy protein isolate with L-methionine	2.2	Palm olein, soy, coconut, high-oleic sunflower oils	3.0	Corn syrup solids, sucrose	8.0	1.3	2.6	61	78	260

Essential Fatty Acid Metabolism

Human milk lipids contain preformed long-chain polyunsaturated fatty acids (LC-PUFA) in considerable amounts, whereas vegetable oils (with the exception of coconut oil) are also rich in PUFA. The latter has a higher percentage of medium- and short-chain fatty acids.

For the healthy full term infant, the concerns of the premature infant may not apply given the larger body stores of LC-PUFA at birth and the lower requirements compared to the preterm infant because of slower growth. However, nutritional requirements for PUFAs are not clearly defined for infants, and the issue is complicated by the fact that linoleic acid (18:2n-6) and α-linolenic acid (18:3n-3) can be converted to both 20 and 22 carbon length long-chain PUFAs with significant biological activities. The absence of linoleic acid in the diet results in growth retardation and dermatologic manifestations. Intakes of linoleic acid, as low as 0.6% of daily energy intake, can obviate essential fatty acid deficiency as defined by the triene to tetraene ratio, and current recommendations[29] specify the minimum level of 0.3g/100 kcal in infant formulas.

Fully breastfed infants have a dietary lipid intake of approximately 50% of their energy intake (3.1 to 5.2g/dL, see earlier discussion), whereas formulas contain between 3.4 and 3.8 g/dL. Although the importance of limiting the dietary intake of saturated and total fats to prevent cardiovascular disease, obesity, and diabetes is well recognized, adverse effects of limiting fat on weight gain and growth[30,31] should be balanced against providing increased amounts of fat.

Carbohydrate

Carbohydrates generally account for 35 to 42% of the energy intake of breast- or formula-fed infants, and the usual carbohydrates in infants' diets are listed in Table 7.4. Carbohydrates may be classified as monosaccharides, oligosaccharides, and polysaccharides. *Monosaccharides* can be further defined as aldoses (glucose, galactose, xylose, for example) or ketoses (fructose). *Oligosaccharides* are consumed in the diet mainly in milk with lactose, maltose and sucrose being the main sugars present. *Polysaccharides* are starches, starch hydrolysates, glycogen, or components of fiber. The major carbohydrate in human milk is lactose, although small amounts of glucose and other oligosaccharides are also present. Carbohydrate content of human milk and various formulas is listed in Table 7.3. Carbohydrate malabsorption, apart from genetic causes, is unusual. When the colonic capacity to ferment carbohydrate is exceeded by the unabsorbed load, symptoms of carbohydrate intolerance, usually in the form of diarrhea, occur. The diarrhea improves when dietary carbohydrates are reduced or eliminated from the diet, making the diagnosis of carbohydrate intolerance. Normally, electrolytes in the distal gastrointestinal tract and unabsorbed

TABLE 7.4

Usual Carbohydrates and Related Enzymes

Carbohydrate	Enzyme
Lactose	Lactase
Sucrose	Sucrase-isomaltase
Isomaltose	Sucrase-isomaltase
Maltose	Maltase-glucoamylase
Amylose	α-Amylase
Amylopectin	β-Amylase

TABLE 7.5

Commonly Used Formulas and Their Indications

Commonly Used Formulas and Their Indications				
Formula	**Carbohydrate**	**Protein**	**Fat**	**Indication**
Bovine milk-based	Lactose	Bovine whey and casein	Vegetable, animal	Normal function
Soy-protein-based	Sucrose, glucose	Soy	Soy	Lactose intolerance
Hydrolyzed protein	Sucrose, glucose	Hydrolyzed whey or casein	Medium chain triglycerides	Cow milk and soy protein hypersensitivity; pancreatic insufficiency
Casein-based (modular)	Modified tapioca starch, added carbohydrate	Casein hydrolysate with added amino acids	MCT oil, corn oil	Lactase, sucrase and maltase deficiency, impaired glucose transport
Elemental	Lactose- and sucrose-free, corn syrup solids, modified corn starch	Hydrolyzed casein	Vegetable	Cow milk allergy
"Metabolic"	Depends on condition	Corn syrup solids/ sucrose	Corn oil/ coconut oil	Specific metabolic disorders

carbohydrates (fermented to volatile fatty acids) are rapidly absorbed. Inadequate colonic salvage results in diarrhea. In young infants and children with disorders of carbohydrate metabolism, the ultimate goal of carbohydrate digestion and absorption is to render all available carbohydrates into smaller compounds that the body can use; chiefly, glucose and fructose. *Lactase deficiency* is exceedingly rare in newborn infants. Infants usually develop diet-induced diarrhea following introduction of lactose-containing milk. The disease, thought to be autosomal recessive, is treated with the elimination or limitation of lactose in the diet. More commonly, a transient lactose intolerance can occur after acute or repeated bouts of diarrhea. *Sucrase-Isomaltase deficiency* is a rare disease that does not appear until diets containing sucrose, dextrin, or starch are begun. Bouts of diarrhea may be observed in infants with this deficiency, and management includes eliminating sucrose and limiting starch in the diet. Older affected children and adults usually tolerate normal quantities of carbohydrates. *Glucose-Galactose deficiency* manifests itself with diet-induced diarrhea soon after birth and responds to withdrawal of these carbohydrates from the diet. The defect appears to be a specific absence of glucose and galactose transport mechanisms, whereas amino acid transport is normal. Fructose transport is normal, and these infants respond to a diet containing fructose with relief from diarrhea. With age, variable amounts of starch and milk may be tolerated. Commonly used formulas for various forms of intolerance are listed in Table 7.5.[32]

Iron

Iron deficiency is the most common nutritional deficiency in the U.S. and worldwide, with young children the most susceptible. The increased susceptibility comes from an increased iron requirement for the rapid growth during this period and inadequate amounts of iron in the diet unless adequately supplemented.[33] According to the third National Health and Nutrition Examination Survey (NHANES, 1991), ~5% of children between one and two

TABLE 7.6

Stages of Iron Deficiency

Iron Nutritional Status	Indices
Adequate stores	Normal
Decreased stores	Decreased ferritin (10–20 ng/mL), transferrin normal, erythrocyte protoporphyrin normal, MCV normal, hemoglobin normal, transferrin receptor normal
Iron deficiency	Decreased ferritin, transferrin saturation decreased, erythrocyte protoporphyrin increased, MCV normal, hemoglobin normal, transferrin receptor increased
Iron deficiency anemia	Decreased ferritin, transferrin saturation decreased, erythrocyte protoporphyrin increased, MCV decreased, hemoglobin decreased, transferrin receptor increased

years of age had evidence of iron deficiency, and about half were also anemic. However, between the two previously published studies, NHANES II and I, prevalence of iron deficiency was observed to be decreasing.[34] Stages of iron nutritional status are listed in Table 7.6.

One should distinguish between anemia and iron deficiency anemia, since the latter occurs when hemoglobin concentration falls below the 90 to 95% range for the same age and sex.[34] A diagnosis of iron deficiency is made when the anemia is accompanied by evidence of iron deficiency or when there is a rise in hemoglobin following treatment with iron. In this regard, serum transferrin receptor may offer an advantage for screening for iron deficiency, since it rises with iron deficiency and is not affected by infection or acute liver disease.[35]

Iron deficiency peaks between six and nine months of age and is a consequence of multiple factors: rapid growth, depleted stores, low iron content of the diet, and early feeding of cow's milk.[36,37] Since a milk-based diet is the predominant source of energy, at least in the first six months of life, the iron content and its bioavailability are strong predictors of iron nutritional status.[38] The estimated requirement of absorbed iron from birth to one year is 0.55 to 0.75 mg/d, thereby underscoring the need for adequate iron in the diet to meet these needs. Iron concentration in human milk is low (0.3 to 0.5 mg/L), and although well absorbed, iron content declines between 14 and 183 days of age.[39] Therefore, even given the better absorption as milk intake increases and iron content decreases, it is easy to see that the amount of absorbed iron will be inadequate to meet the estimated requirements. Therefore, breastfed infants who do not receive iron supplements or iron from other sources are at risk of becoming iron deficient between 6 and 12 months of age.[40] Iron-fortified cow's milk or soy-based formulas are effective in preventing iron deficiency, and the decline in iron deficiency anemia over the past few decades has been attributed to their use.[34] Systemic manifestations of iron deficiency anemia include behavioral and cognitive abnormalities expressed as lower scores on tests of psychomotor development. These effects have to be interpreted keeping the confounding variables of poor nutrition, environment, and poor socioeconomic background that often coexist. The studies suggest that infants with iron deficiency anemia, but not iron deficiency without anemia, have impaired performance of mental and psychomotor development.[41-45] These deficiencies do not improve with iron therapy, and follow-up studies at five to six years of age still demonstrate poorer scores in the children who were previously anemic.[43,44] Strategies to prevent iron deficiency could include the feeding of iron-fortified formulas, avoidance of non-iron fortified milks and cow's milk (the latter, at least, till beyond 12 months of age), the feeding of meats and iron-fortified foods, and, if needed, medicinal iron supplementation in the form of ferrous sulfate.

TABLE 7.7

Unique Constituents of Breast Milk

	Unique Constituents of Breast Milk
Docosahexanoic acid	Necessary for growth and development of the brain and retina and for myelinization of nervous tissue
Cholesterol	Enhances myelinization of nervous tissue
Taurine	Second most abundant amino acid in human milk, important for bile acid conjugation
Choline	May enhance memory
Enzymes	Numerous enzymes such as lipases that are important in digestion and absorption of fat
Lactoferrin	Prevents iron from being available to bacteria
Inositol	Enhances synthesis and secretion of surfactant in immature lung tissue
Poly- and Oligosaccharides	Inhibit bacterial binding to mucosal surfaces
Protein (such as α-lactalbumin)	Supply amino acids to the infant, help synthesize lactose in the mammary gland, and bind calcium and zinc
Bifidobacterium species	Predominant bacterial flora in the gastrointestinal tract of breastfed infants, creates unfavorable pH conditions for the growth of enteric pathogens
Macrophages	Macrophages in human colostrum have high concentrations of slgA which is released during phagocytosis
Epidermal growth factor	Promotes cell proliferation in the gastrointestinal mucosa

Breastfeeding

The benefits of breastfeeding to the infant, mother, family, and society are numerous and impressive, but they must be put into context when making individual decisions about breast feeding. These include ready availability, possible enhancement of intestinal development, resistance to infection, and bonding between mother and infant. It is the preferred feeding method for the normal infant. Breast milk, in addition to providing the required nutrients for the healthy infant, has unique constituents, as listed in Table 7.7.

Protein

Approximately 20% of the total nitrogen in human milk is in the form of non-protein nitrogen compounds such as free amino acids, and urea, which is considerably greater than the 5% found in bovine milk,[46] although there remains a debate about their contribution to nitrogen utilization.[47] The quality of the protein differs from that of bovine milk as well, with the whey-to-casein protein ratios being 70:30 and 18:82 in human and bovine milk, respectively. These differences in whey-to-casein ratio are reflected in the plasma amino acid profile of infants and are readily observed within the first three days of age.[48] Further, plasma amino acid patterns in human milk-fed infants has been used as a reference in infant nutrition.[49,50] In addition, specific human whey proteins — lactoferrin, lysozyme, and slgA — are involved in host defense.[51,52]

Lipids

Lipids in human milk provide 40 to 50% of the energy content and are vehicles for fat soluble vitamins. The total fat content varies from 2% in colostrum to 2.5–3.0% in transitional milk, and 3.5–4.5% in mature human milk.[19] Cholesterol, phospholipids, and essential fatty acids are highest in colostrum, and more than 98% of human milk fat comes from 11 major fatty acids of 10-20 carbon length. Human milk lipids can inactivate enveloped viruses including herpes simplex I, measles, and cytomegalovirus, to name a few. Monoglycerides also exert antiviral activity.

Fat content of human milk is variable, with the fat content rising throughout lactation but with changes apparent within the course of one day, within feeds and between women.[53] The effects of these differences in thriving infants is not clear, even given that hind milk has a higher fat content than fore milk. Human milk lipids provide preformed LC-PUFAs in amounts sufficient to meet nutrient needs. In term infants, plasma concentrations of essential fatty acids (arachidonic acid) at two and four weeks of age were significantly lower in infants fed formula without LC-PUFA compared to breastfed infants. Docosahexanoic acid concentrations were similarly lower at four and eight weeks of age. Neuringer and colleagues showed that visual acuity and learning abilities correlate well with the amount of DHA in the retina and brain phospholipids.[54]

Nucleotides

Nucleotides represent 2 to 5% of the non-protein nitrogen in human milk.[55] Nucleotides participate in many biological functions such as forming the basis of genetic information (DNA, RNA) and storing energy (AMP, GMP), and they play roles in immunity as well as cellular activities. Although they can be produced by the liver, the body's requirements vary considerably, especially during infancy.[56] The effect of nucleotides on immune function is not well understood, but infants fed breast milk or nucleotide-supplemented formula have been shown to exhibit increased natural killer cell activity compared to infants fed unsupplemented formula.[57] Infants fed nucleotide formulas had enhanced Haemophilus influenza type B and diphtheria humoral responses compared to non-supplemented infants.[58] Feeding of human milk resulted in significantly higher neutralizing antibody titers to polio virus at six months of age than were found in control or formula-fed cohorts. These data suggest that dietary factors play a role in the antibody response to immunization, and more studies are needed to better understand the mechanisms involved.

Infection

There are several enzymes present in human milk that appear to be important in the prevention of infection. These include glutathione peroxidase, alkaline phosphatase, and xanthine oxidase. In addition, other anti-inflammatory agents such as catalase, lactoferrin, immunoglobulins, and lysozyme are also present in human milk. The antimicrobial activities of these are generally found at mucosal surfaces, such as the gastrointestinal, urinary, and respiratory tracts. Specific factors, such as lactoferrin, lysozyme, and slgA, resist proteolytic degradation and can line the mucosal surfaces, preventing microbial attachment and inhibiting microbial activity. Each of the mammary immune systems is active against a variety of antigens. Prospective studies in developing countries indicate that breast milk feeding reduces the incidence or severity of diarrhea,[59] lower respiratory tract infection,[60] otitis media,[61] bacteremia,[62] bacterial meningitis,[63] botulism,[64] urinary tract infection,[65] and necrotizing enterocolitis.[66]

Hyperbilirubinemia is more common in breast-fed than formula-fed infants. This is usually transient, and discontinuation of breast feeding is not recommended unless bilirubin values reach excessively high levels or the jaundice persists. Usually, switching to a formula for one to two days is therapeutic and diagnostic, and breastfeeding can be safely resumed. Other causes of jaundice should be sought before making a firm diagnosis of breast-milk jaundice.

Certain chemicals, drugs, foreign proteins, and viruses may be present in human milk.[67] However, the risk–benefit ratio of artificial milk needs to be weighed, especially if the water sources for mixing the milk are contaminated. Breastfeeding is currently contraindicated in disease states such as active herpes, tuberculosis, and AIDS.

Formula Feeding

A variety of formulas are available for feeding infants (Table 7.3). The most commonly used formulas are from bovine milk, and nutrient specifications for infant formulas are available.[68] Commercially available formulas are recommended when breast feeding is not chosen. Cow's milk is not recommended in the first year of life due to its nutritional limitations and inappropriate nutrient concentrations. Cow's milk has higher concentrations of protein and phosphorus, a lower calcium-to-phosphorus ratio, limited iron, less essential fatty acids, vitamin C, and zinc than human milk. Increased renal solute load due to cow's milk and increased occult blood loss via the gastrointestinal tract leading to iron deficiency and anemia in infants fed cow's milk unsupplemented by other nutrients are additional reasons to discourage the feeding of cow's milk in early infancy.

Soy Protein-Based Formulas

The Committee on Nutrition of the American Academy of Pediatrics reviewed the indications of soy protein-based formulas.[69] Some of the conclusions include:

1. Isolated soy protein-based formulas are safe and effective alternatives to provide appropriate nutrition if breast milk or cow milk-based formulas do not meet the nutritional needs in term infants. However, no advantage is provided over cow's milk protein-based formulas as a supplement for breast feeding.
2. Soy protein-based formulas are appropriate for use in infants with galactosemia and hereditary lactase deficiency.
3. There is no proven value of the routine use of soy-protein based formula in the prevention or management of infantile colic.
4. There is no proven value of the routine use of soy protein-based formula in the prevention of atopic disease in healthy or at-risk infants.
5. Infants with documented cow milk protein-induced enteropathy or enterocolitis should not be given soy protein-based formula routinely.

The nutritional needs of infants zero to six months can be met by breast milk or infant formulas. Although both groups of infants need to have health surveillance including growth and development, breastfed infants need to be followed closely over the first few weeks to assure appropriate feeding practices and resultant growth. Appropriate counseling for common breast feeding problems needs to be provided, and community support groups can be involved if needed. Beyond six months, recommendations for infant feeding are variable, and the recommendations are largely based on extrapolation from data on younger infants. Nutritional composition of "follow-up" formulas is specified with minimum lower limits for energy (60 kcal/dL), higher minimum limits for protein (2.25 to 3.0 g/100 kcal) and lower minimum limits for fat (3.0 to 4.0 g/100 kcal) compared to formulas for younger infants. Nonetheless, iron-fortified formulas designed for younger infants may be safely fed from 6 to 12 months. Infants by this age are physiologically and developmentally ready to accept a variety of dietary items, and feeding practices vary based on ethnic, cultural, and economic reasons. As stated earlier, feeding of bovine milk is discouraged during this period, although a substantial number of infants are indeed fed bovine milk.[70] In addition, there are concerns about the substitution of low-fat or skimmed milks during this period because of higher intakes of protein and sodium and lower intakes of iron and essential fatty acids. However, if infants are being fed non-milk foods, the actual intake of energy may not be lower than of infants fed bovine milk or formula.[71]

Weaning

The transition from suckling to eating of non-milk foods occurs during the first year of life based on cultural beliefs and practices, physicians beliefs, mothers' perceptions of their infants' needs, and economic realities. Complementary foods are introduced from before three months to by six months of age, and a variety of foods are offered.[72-74] In the U.S., the total transition to beikost usually occurs by the end of the first year of life and continues during the second year.

The weaning process can be considered in three ways. First, it could be the weaning from breast feeding to other milks which may replace breast feeding partially or completely. In the second form, weaning could be considered the transition from liquid to non-liquid diet. Health concerns may arise during this period if the added foods are too nutrient dense (protein or energy) or nutrient-deficient (iron, protein), thus altering the protein:energy ratio or causing deficiency of specific nutrients. The third aspect of weaning may be the transition from human milk or formula to bovine milk in addition to the provision of beikost. Since weaning typically occurs during a period of rapid growth, attention to both nutritional and developmental issues during this period is warranted. Complementary foods, in addition to providing the required nutrients, are also important in establishing lifelong patterns of eating.

Failure to Thrive

Growth, as assessed by weight, length (and subsequently height) and head circumference, is an important part of anticipatory guidance provided in well child care. These anthropometric measurements, especially weight, can be used to detect inadequate attained growth or reduced growth velocity. The average birth weight of a full term infant is 3300 to 3500 g; after a weight loss of ~10%, infants should regain their birth weight by two weeks, with formula-fed infants tending to regain their birth weight a little sooner than their breastfed counterparts. On an average, infants gain about 1 kg per month for the first three months, 1/2 kilogram per month for the next three months, 1/3 kilogram per month from 6 to 9 months and 1/4 kilogram per month from 9 to 12 months. Full term infants double their weight by 4 months and triple their weight by 12 months, while doubling their length during the same period. Both weight and length gain are slower in the second year of life, underscoring the anticipatory nutritional guidance needed during that period. Growth faltering, or failure to thrive, a descriptive term, is then identified by the following criteria: (1) weight less than 80 to 85% of the 50th percentile on the National Center for Health Statistics (NCHS) growth charts, (2) weight for age less than the 3 to 5 percentile on the NCHS growth charts, (3) drop in weight that crosses two or more percentile categories on standard growth charts from previously established pattern of adequate growth, and (4) a Z-score of –2 SD below the normal 50th percentile. If growth velocity is used, a decrement of 2 SD over a 90-day period and loss of >1 SD Z score over 90 days is used as a measure of growth faltering.

Since decline in rate of weight gain or growth velocity is more sensitive than decline in length or head circumference, serial measurements of weight are an important part of the anticipatory guidance given during well child checks, and provide an early warning of growth faltering.[75,76] The Body Mass Index (BMI), calculated by dividing weight in kilograms by length/height in meters squared, has largely replaced weight for stature. It should be recognized that there are growth differences between breast and formula-fed infants. As reported by Nelson et al.,[77] mean gains in both weight (g/d) and length (cm/d) were greater in formula-fed males and females than their breastfed counterparts from 8–122 days of age. Since the NCHS growth charts were made from data that was cross-sectional and the infants were fed formulas, attention to growth faltering in the breastfed infant requires both understanding of the growth of breastfed infants and the early recognition of decrease in weight or growth velocity.[78] There are numerous organic and non-organic causes of growth failure or faltering which need to be addressed during such an evaluation. It is important to realize that failure to thrive or malnutrition may occur in hospitalized infants and children, as well, and efforts to recognize and nourish these infants and children should be made.

Summary

In summary, the period of infancy is one of rapid changes in growth and attainment of developmental milestones. This period imposes unique nutritional needs and challenges for the health care provider. Understanding nutritional needs, ways of meeting these needs (Table 7.8), deviations in growth and their causes, and providing nutrition in age-appro-

TABLE 7.8

Recommendations for Feeding Healthy Full-Term Infants

Breastfeeding is strongly recommended.
Infant formulas that meet AAP guidelines are recommended when breastfeeding is not chosen or breast milk is not available.
Breast milk or infant formula is the preferred feeding in the first year of life.
Adequate intakes of human milk or formula meet all nutrient requirements for the first 6 months of life (exception may be vitamin D in dark-skinned, sun deprived breast fed infants). Infant formula or "follow-up" formula may be fed in the second 6 months of life.
Introduction of complementary foods should be based on growth, developmental, cultural, social, psychological and economic considerations. As a general rule, when an infant is consuming 32 ounces of milk per day and appears to want more, supplemental feedings may be indicated. This usually occurs between 4 and 6 months of age.

priate, culturally and ethnically sensitive ways while addressing economic issues is the task of the health care team. Ideally, the infant's nutritional need (expressed as hunger), developmental progress (as observed in attainment of feeding skills), and mother's and care provider's beliefs within the context of the family will guide the infant's feeding experience and transition to the next phase in life.

Acknowledgment

The authors thank Tina Corbin for her tireless secretarial support in the preparation of this manuscript.

References

1. Hamill P. V., Drizd T. A., Johnson C. L., et al. *Am J Clin Nutr* 32: 607; 1979.
2. Fomon S. J., Nelson S. E. Size and growth: In *Nutrition of Normal Infants,* CV Mosby, 1993, 36, p. 155.
3. Butte N. F. *Eur J Clin Nutr* 50: 24S; 1996.
4. Health and Welfare Canada. Nutrition Recommendations. The report of the scientific review committee, Ottawa, Canada: Supply and Services, 1990.
5. Dewey K. G., Lonnerdal B. *J Pediatr Gastroenterol Nutr* 2: 497; 1983.
6. Dewey K. G., Heinig M. J., Nommsen L. A., et al. *J Pediatr* 119: 538; 1991.
7. Whitehead R. G., Paul A. A., Cole T. J. *Acta Paediatr Scand* 299: 43S; 1982.
8. Kylberg H., Hofvander Y., Sjolin S. *Acta Paediatr Scand* 75: 932; 1986.
9. Persson L. A., Johansson E., Samuelson G. *Human Nutrition — Applied Nutrition* 38: 247; 1984.
10. Heinig M. J., Nommsen L. A., Peerson J. M., et al. *Am J Clin Nutr* 58: 152; 1993.
11. Zlotkin S. H., Anderson G. H. *Pediatr Res* 16: 65; 1982.
12. Pohlandt P. *Acta Paediatr Scand* 63: 801; 1974.
13. Gaull G. E., Rassin D. K., Raiha N. C., et al. *J Pediatr* 90: 348; 1977.
14. Rassin D. K., Gaull G. E., Jarvenpaa A. L., et al. *Pediatrics* 71: 179; 1983.
15. Jarvenpaa A. L., Rassin D. K., Raiha N. C., et al. *Pediatrics* 70: 221; 1982.
16. World Health Organization. Energy and protein requirements. WHO Technical Report Series No. 742, Geneva, WHO. 98, 1985.
17. Fomon S. J., Haschke F., Ziegler E. E., Nelson S. E. *Am J Clin Nutr* 34(5): 1169S; 1982.
18. Wong W. W., Hachey D. L., Insull W., et al. *J Lipid Res* 34: 1403; 1993.
19. Bitman J., Wood L., Hamosh M., et al. *Am J Clin Nutr* 38: 300; 1983.
20. Harzer G., Haug M., Dieterich I., et al. *Am J Clin Nutr* 37: 612; 1983.
21. Hibberd C. M., Brooke O. G., Carter N. G., et al. *Arch Dis Child* 57: 658; 1982.
22. Jensen R. G. *The Lipids of Human Milk.* Boca Raton: CRC Press, 1989.
23. Prentice A., Prentice A. M., Whitehead R. G. *Br J Nutr* 45: 495; 1981.
24. Hachey D. L., Thomas M. R., Emken E. A., et al. *J Lipid Res* 28: 1185; 1987.
25. Hachey D. L., Silber G. H., Wong W. W., Garza C. *Pediatr Res* 25: 63; 1989.
26. Koletzko B., Thiel I., Abiodun P. O. *Z Ernahrungwiss* 30: 289; 1991.
27. Harris W. S., Conner W. E., Lindsey S. *Am J Clin Nutr* 40: 780; 1984.
28. Genzel-Boroviczeny O., Wahle J., Koletzko B. *Eur J Paediatr* 156: 142; 1997.
29. Joint FAO/WHO Codex Alimentarius Commission, 1984; Food and Drug Administration 1985; Commission of European Communities, 1991.
30. Lifshitz F., Moses N. *Am J Dis Child* 143: 537; 1989.
31. Michaelsen K. F., Jorgensen M. H. *Eur J Clin Nutr* 49: 467; 1995.

32. Bhatia J., Bucher C., Bunyapen C. *Pediatr Ann* 27: 525; 1998.
33. Dallman P. R., Siimes M. A., Stekel A. *Am J Clin Nutr* 33: 86; 1980.
34. Yip R. In *Dietary Iron: Birth to Two Years.* (Filer L. J. Jr., Ed): New York: Raven Press, 1989, pg 37.
35. Ferguson B. J., Skikne B. S., Simpson K. M., et al. *J Lab Clin Med* 119: 385; 1992.
36. Ziegler E. E., Fomon S. J., Nelson S. E., et al. *J Pediatr* 116: 11; 1990.
37. Fomon S. J., Ziegler E. E., Nelson S. E., et al. *J Pediatr* 98: 540; 1981.
38. Pizarro F., Yip R., Dallman P. R., et al. *J Pediatr* 118: 687; 1991.
39. Siimes M. A., Vuori E., Kuitunen P. *Acta Paediatr Scand* 68: 29; 1979.
40. Haschke F., Vanura H., Male C., et al. *J Pediatr Gastroenterol Nutr* 16: 151; 1993.
41. Lozoff B., Brittenham G. M., Viteri F. E., et al. *J Pediatr* 100: 351; 1982.
42. Lozoff B., Brittenham G. M., Wolf A. W., et al. *Pediatrics* 79: 981; 1987.
43. Lozoff B., Jiminez W., Wolf A. W. *N Eng J Med* 325: 687; 1991.
44. Walter T. In: *Nutritional Anemias.* (Fomon S. J., Zlotkin S., Eds) Nestle Nutrition Workshop Series, 30. New York: Raven Press; 1990, pg 81.
45. Pollitt E. *Ann Rev Nutr* 13: 521; 1993.
46. Hambraeus L. *Pediatr Clin N Am* 24: 17; 1977.
47. Fomon S. J., Bier D. M., Mathews D. E., et al. *J Pediatr* 113: 515; 1988.
48. Cho F., Bhatia J., Rassin D. K. *Nutrition* 6: 449; 1990.
49. Lindblad B. S., Alfven G., Zetterstrom R. *Acta Paediatr Scand* 67: 659; 1978.
50. Rassin D. K. In: *Protein Requirements in the Term Infant.* (Barness L., Ed) Princeton: Excerpta Medica: 1988, pg 3.
51. Goldman A. S., Cheda S., Keeny S. E., et al. *Sem Perinatol* 18: 495; 1994.
52. Hanson L. A., Ahlstedt S., Andersson B., et al. *Pediatrics* 75: 172; 1985.
53. Neville M. C., Keller R. P., Seacat J., et al. *Am J Clin Nutr* 40: 635; 1984.
54. Neuringer M., Conner W. E., Van Patten C., et al. *J Clin Invest* 73: 272; 1984.
55. Uauy R., Quan R., Gil A. *J Nutr* 124(8): 1436S; 1994.
56. Jyonouchi H. *J Nutr* 124(1): 138S; 1994.
57. Carver J. D. *J Nutr* 124(1): 144S; 1994.
58. Pickering L. K., Granoff D. M., Erickson J. R., et al. *Pediatrics* 101: 242; 1998.
59. Dewey K. G., Heinig M. J., Nommsen-Rivers L. A. *J Pediatr* 126: 696; 1995.
60. Wright A. L., Holberg C. J., Taussig L. M., et al. *Arch Pediatr Adolesc Med* 149: 758; 1995.
61. Kovar M. G., Serdula M. K., Marks J. S., et al. *Pediatrics* 74: 615; 1984.
62. Takala A. K., Eskola J., Palmgren J., et al. *J Pediatr* 115: 694: 1989.
63. Cochi S. L., Fleming D. W., Hightower A. W., et al. *J Pediatr* 108: 887; 1986.
64. Arnon S. S. *Rev Infect Dis* 6, 193S.
65. Pisacane A., Graziano L., Mazzarella G., et al. *J Pediatr* 120: 87; 1992.
66. Lucas A., Cole T. J. Lancet 336: 1519; 1990.
67. Goldfarb J. *Clin Perinatol* 20: 225; 1985.
68. Food and Drug Administration: Rules and regulations. Nutrient requirements for infant formulas (21 CFR part 107), Fed Reg 50:45106, 1985.
69. American Academy of Pediatrics, Committee on Nutrition. *Pediatrics* 101: 148; 1998.
70. American Academy of Pediatrics, Committee on Nutrition. *AAP News* 8: 18; 1992.
71. Martinez G. A., Ryan A. S., Malec D. J. *Am J Dis Child* 139: 1010; 1985.
72. Anderson T. A., Ziegler E. E. In: *Weaning, Why, What and When?* (Ballabriga A., Ray J., Eds) Nestle Nutrition Workshop Series, 10, New York: Raven Press, 1987, pg 153.
73. Ballabriga A., Schmidt E. In: *Weaning, Why, What and When?* (Ballabriga A., Ray J., Eds) Nestle Nutrition Workshop Series, 10, Raven Press, New York, 1987, pg 129.
74. Ahmad A. In: *Weaning, Why, What and When?* (Ballabriga A., Ray J., Eds) Nestle Nutrition Workshop Series, 10, New York: Raven Press, 1987, pg 197.
75. Zumrawi F. Y., Min Y., Marshall T. *Ann Human Biol* 19: 165; 1992.
76. Healy M. J. R., Yang M., Tanner J. M., Zumrawi F. Y. In: *Linear Growth Retardation in Less Developed Countries.* (Waterlow, J. C., Ed) New York: Raven Press, 41, 1988.
77. Nelson S. E., Rogers R. R., Ziegler E. E., et al. *Early Hum Devel* 19: 223; 1989.
78. Garza C., Frongillo E., Dewey K. G. *Acta Paediatr* 404: 4S; 1994.

8

Nutrition for Healthy Children and Adolescents Ages 2 to 18 Years

Suzanne Domel Baxter

Physical Growth and Development

A child's first year of life is marked by rapid growth, with birth weight tripling and birth length increasing by 50%. After the rapid growth of the first year, physical growth slows down considerably during the preschool and school years, until the pubertal growth spurt of adolescence. Birth weight does not quadruple until two years of age, and birth length does not double until four years of age. A one-year-old child has several teeth, and his/her digestive and metabolic systems are functioning at or near adult capacity. By one year of age, most children are walking or beginning to walk; with improved coordination over the next few years, activity increases dramatically. Although increased activity in turn increases energy needs, a child's rate of growth decreases. Growth patterns vary in individual children, but each year children from two years to puberty gain an average of 4 1/2 to 6 1/2 pounds (2 to 3 kg) in weight and 2 1/2 to 3 1/2 inches (6 to 8 cm) in height. As the growth rate declines during the preschool years, a child's appetite decreases and food intake may become unpredictable and erratic. Parents and other caregivers need to know that these changes are normal so that they can avoid struggles with children over food and eating.

After the first year of life, more significant development occurs in fine and gross motor, cognitive, and social-emotional areas than during the first year of life. During the second year of life, children learn to feed themselves independently. By 15 months of age, children can manage a cup, but with some spilling. At 18 to 24 months of age, children learn to tilt cups by manipulating their fingers. Children are able to transfer food from bowls to their mouths with less spilling by 16 to 17 months of age, when well-defined wrist rotation develops. However, two-year-old children often prefer foods that can be picked up with their fingers without having to chase it across their plates.

The normal events of puberty and the simultaneous growth spurt are the primary influences on nutritional requirements during the second decade of life. During puberty, height and weight increase, many organ systems enlarge, and body composition is altered due to increased lean body mass and changes in the quantity and distribution of fat. The

0-8493-2705-9/01/$0.00+$1.50

timing of the growth spurt is influenced by genetic as well as environmental factors. Children who weigh more than average for their height tend to mature early, and vice versa. Although stature tends to increase most rapidly during the spring and summer, weight tends to increase either at a fairly steady rate over the entire year or undergoes a more rapid increase during the autumn. The most rapid linear growth spurt for an average American boy occurs between 12 and 15 years of age. For the average American girl, the growth spurt occurs about two years earlier, between 10 and 13 years of age. The growth spurt during adolescence contributes about 15% to final adult height, and approximately 50% to adult weight. During adolescence, boys tend to gain more weight than girls, and gain it at a faster rate. Furthermore, the skeletal growth of boys continues for a longer time than that of adolescent girls. Adolescent boys deposit more muscle mass, and adolescent girls deposit relatively more total body fat. Menarche, which is closely linked to the growth process, has a lasting impact on nutritional requirements of adolescent girls.

Adolescence is a period of various cognitive challenges. For example, when an adolescent realizes that his or her body is in the process of maturing, he or she may begin to assess changes in his or her own body size and shape, compare them with those of others, and form opinions about any differences. Adolescent girls and boys may be very self-conscious, especially during early and mid-adolescence. According to Piaget's developmental levels, it is usually during adolescence that abstract thinking supersedes concrete thinking. Thus, an adolescent may consider his or her body not just as it is, but also as it *might* be. In addition, an adolescent can contemplate new or different ways of combining or eating food. Furthermore, an adolescent can more easily conceptualize nutrients such as calories and fat, and skillfully manipulate their dietary intake.

Energy and Nutrient Needs

Dietary Reference Intakes and Recommended Dietary Allowances

The Dietary Reference Intakes (DRIs) expand and replace the series of Recommended Dietary Allowances (RDAs) published beginning in 1941 through 1989 by the Food and Nutrition Board.[1] Although previous RDAs focused on preventing classical nutrient deficiencies, the DRIs go beyond this to include current knowledge about the role of nutrients and food components in long-term health. The DRIs are reference values that are quantitative estimates of nutrient intakes to be used for planning and assessing diets for healthy people in America and Canada.[2] The DRIs include RDAs as goals for intake by individuals, but also present the following new types of reference values: Estimated Average Requirement (EAR), Adequate Intake (AI), and Tolerable Upper Intake Level (UL); these are discussed in detail in another section. Briefly, within the DRI framework, the RDA serves as a goal for individuals; it is the average daily dietary intake level that is sufficient to meet the nutrient needs of almost all (97 to 98%) healthy individuals in a lifestage and gender group. The EAR is a nutrient intake value that is estimated to meet the nutrient needs of 50% of the healthy individuals in a lifestage and gender group; it is used to assess adequacy of intakes of population groups, and to develop RDAs. The AI is used instead of an RDA when sufficient scientific evidence is not available to calculate an EAR; the AI is based on observed or experimentally determined approximations of nutrient intake by a lifestage and gender group (or groups) of healthy people. The UL is the highest level of nutrient intake per day that is likely to pose no risks of adverse health effects to almost all individuals in the general population. The risk of

TABLE 8.1

Recommended Levels for Individual Intake[a] for Children and Adolescents

	Children		Boys		Girls	
	1–3 years	4–8 years	9–13 years	14–18 years	9–13 years	14–18 years
Calcium (mg/d)	500*	800*	1300*	1300*	1300*	1300*
Phosphorus (mg/d)	460	500	1250	1250	1250	1250
Magnesium (mg/d)	80	130	240	410	240	360
Vitamin D (μg/d)[b,c]	5*	5*	5*	5*	5*	5*
Fluoride (mg/d)	0.7*	1*	2*	3*	2*	3*
Thiamin (mg/d)	0.5	0.5	0.9	1.2	0.9	1.0
Riboflavin (mg/d)	0.5	0.6	0.9	1.3	0.9	1.0
Niacin (mg/d)[d]	6	8	12	16	12	14
Vitamin B_6 (mg/d)	0.5	0.6	1.0	1.3	1.0	1.2
Folate (μg/d)[e,f]	150	200	300	400	300	400
Vitamin B_{12} (μg/d)	0.9	1.2	1.8	2.4	1.8	2.4
Pantothenic acid (mg/d)	2*	3*	4*	5*	4*	5*
Biotin (μg/d)	8*	12*	20*	25*	20*	25*
Choline (mg/d)[g]	200*	250*	375*	550*	375*	400*
Vitamin C (mg/d)	15	25	45	75	45	65
Vitamin E (mg/d of α-tocopherol)[h]	6	7	11	15	11	15
Selenium (μg/d)	20	30	40	55	40	55
Vitamin A (μg/d)	300	400	600	900	600	700
Vitamin K (μg/d)	30*	55*	60*	75*	60*	75*
Chromium (μg/d)	11*	15*	25*	35*	21*	24*
Copper (μg/d)	340	440	700	890	700	890
Iodine (μg/d)	90	90	120	150	120	150
Iron (mg/d)[i]	7	10	8	11	8	15
Manganese (mg/d)	1.2*	1.5*	1.9*	2.2*	1.6*	1.6*
Molybdenum (μg/d)	17	22	34	43	34	43
Zinc (mg/d)	3	5	8	8	11	9

[a] Recommended Dietary Allowances (RDAs) are presented in bold type and Adequate Intakes (AIs) in ordinary type followed by an asterisk (*). RDAs and AIs may both be used as goals for individual intake. RDAs are set to meet the needs of almost all (97-98%) individuals in a group. The AI for other life-stage and gender groups is believed to cover needs of all individuals in the group, but lack of data or uncertainty in the data prevent being able to specify with confidence the percentage of persons covered by this intake. Adapted from: Food and Nutrition Board, Institute of Medicine, *Dietary Reference Intakes for Calcium, Phosphorus, Magnesium, Vitamin D, and Fluoride*, National Academy Press, Washington, DC, 1997; Food and Nutrition Board, Institute of Medicine, *Dietary Reference Intakes for Thiamin, Riboflavin, Niacin, Vitamin B_6, Folate, Vitamin B_{12}, Pantothenic Acid, Biotin, and Choline*, National Academy Press, Washington, DC, 1998; Food and Nutrition Board, Institute of Medicine, *Dietary Reference Intakes for Vitamin C, Vitamin E, Selenium, and Carotenoids*, National Academy Press, Washington, DC, 2000; Food and Nutrition Board, Institute of Medicine, *Dietary Reference Intakes for Vitamin A, Vitamin K, Arsenic, Boron, Chromium, Copper, Iodine, Iron, Manganese, Molybdenum, Nickel, Silicon, Vanadium, and Zinc*, National Academy Press, Washington, DC, 2001.

[b] As cholecalciferol. 1 μg cholecalciferol = 40 IU vitamin D.

[c] In the absence of adequate exposure to sunlight.

[d] As niacin equivalents (NE). 1 mg niacin = 60 mg tryptophan.

[e] As dietary folate equivalent (DFE). 1 DFE = 1 μg food folate = 0.6 μg folic acid (from fortified food or supplement) consumed with food = 0.5 μg synthetic (supplemental) folic acid taken on an empty stomach.

[f] In view of evidence linking folate intake with neural tube defects in the fetus, it is recommended that all women capable of becoming pregnant consume 400 μg synthetic folic acid from fortified foods and/or supplements in addition to intake of food folate from a varied diet.

[g] Although AIs have been set for choline, there are few data to assess whether a dietary supply of choline is needed at all states of the life cycle, and it may be that the choline requirement can by met by endogenous synthesis at some of these stages.

[h] DRIs for vitamin E are based on α-tocopherol only and do not include amounts obtained from the other seven naturally occurring forms historically called vitamin E. RDAs and AIs apply only to intake of 2*R*-stereoisomeric forms of α-tocopherol from food, fortified food, and multivitamins.

[i] For girls under 14 years who have started to menstruate, one might advise an increased intake to approximately 2.5 mg/d to what would be advised for a girl of the same characteristics before menarche.

TABLE 8.2

Tolerable Upper Intake Levels[a,b] (ULs) for Children and Adolescents

	1–3 years	4–8 years	9–13 years	14–18 years
Calcium (g/d)	2.5	2.5	2.5	2.5
Phosphorus (g/d)	3	3	4	4
Magnesium (mg/d)[c]	65	110	350	350
Vitamin D (μg/d)	50	50	50	50
Fluoride (mg/d)	1.3	2.2	10	10
Niacin (mg/d)[d]	10	15	20	30
Vitamin B6 (mg/d)	30	40	60	80
Synthetic folic acid (μg/d)[d]	300	400	600	800
Choline (g/d)	1.0	1.0	2.0	3.0
Vitamin C (mg/d)	400	650	1200	1800
Vitamin E (mg/d α-tocopherol)[e]	200	300	600	800
Selenium (μg/d)	90	150	280	400
Vitamin A (μg/d performed A)	600	900	1700	2800
Copper (μg/d)	1000	3000	5000	8000
Iodine (μg/d)	200	300	600	900
Iron (mg/d)	40	40	40	45
Manganese (mg/d)	2	3	6	9
Molybdenum (μg/d)	300	600	1100	1700
Zinc (mg/d)	7	12	23	34
Boron (mg/d)	3	6	11	17
Nickel (mg/d soluble nickel salts)	0.2	0.3	0.6	1.0
Vanadium (mg/d)[f]				

[a] UL = the maximum level of daily nutrient intake that is likely to pose no risk of adverse effects. Unless otherwise specified, the UL represents total intake from food, water, and supplements. Currently, ULs are not available for other nutrients. In the absence of ULs, extra caution may be warranted in consuming levels above recommended intakes.

[b] Adapted from: Food and Nutrition Board, Institute of Medicine, *Dietary Reference Intakes for Calcium, Phosphorus, Magnesium, Vitamin D, and Fluoride*, National Academy Press, Washington, DC, 1997; Food and Nutrition Board, Institute of Medicine, *Dietary Reference Intakes for Thiamin, Riboflavin, Niacin, Vitamin* B_6, *Folate, Vitamin* B_{12}, *Pantothenic Acid, Biotin, and Choline*, National Academy Press, Washington, DC, 1998; Food and Nutrition Board, Institute of Medicine, *Dietary Reference Intakes for Vitamin C, Vitamin E, Selenium, and Carotenoids*, National Academy Press, Washington, DC, 2000; Food and Nutrition Board, Institute of Medicine, *Dietary Reference Intakes for Vitamin A, Vitamin K, Arsenic, Boron, Chromium, Copper, Iodine, Iron, Manganese, Molybdenum, Nickel, Silicon, Vanadium, and Zinc*, National Academy Press, Washington, DC, 2001.

[c] The UL for magnesium represents intake from a pharmacological agent only and does not include intake from food and water.

[d] The ULs for niacin and synthetic folic acid apply to forms obtained from supplements, fortified foods, or a combination of the two.

[e] DRIs for vitamin E are based on α-tocopherol only and do not include amounts obtained from the other seven naturally occurring forms historically called vitamin E. The ULs apply to any form of supplementary α-tocopherol.

[f] The UL for adults is 1.8 mg/d of elemental vanadium. It was not possible to establish ULs for children for vanadium, but the source of intake should be from food only.[5]

adverse effects increases as intake increases above the UL.[2] Although the DRIs are based on data, scientific judgment was required in setting all reference values because data were often scanty or drawn from studies with limitations; this is especially true in deriving DRIs for children and adolescents.[2]

In 1997, DRIs were published for calcium, phosphorus, magnesium, vitamin D, and fluoride.[2] In 1998, DRIs were published for thiamin, riboflavin, niacin, vitamin B_6, folate, vitamin B_{12}, pantothenic acid, biotin, and choline.[3] In 2000, DRIs were published for vitamin C, vitamin E, and selenium.[4] No DRIs were proposed for carotenoids, although

TABLE 8.3

1989 Recommended Dietary Allowances (RDAs) for Children and Adolescents for Nutrients without Dietary Reference Intakes[a]

		Weight[b]		Height[b]		Calories	Protein	
Category	Age (years)	(kg)	(lb)	(cm)	(in)	(kcal/day)	(g/day)	(g/kg)
Children	1–3	13	29	90	35	1300	16	1.2
	4–6	20	44	112	44	1800	24	1.1
	7–10	28	62	132	52	2000	28	1.0
Boys	11–14	45	99	157	62	2500	45	1.0
	15–18	66	145	176	69	3000	59	0.9
Girls	11–14	46	101	157	62	2200	46	1.0
	15–18	55	120	163	64	2200	44	0.8

[a] Adapted from Food and Nutrition Board, National Research Council, *Recommended Dietary Allowances*, 10th ed, National Academy Press, Washington, DC, 1989. The RDAs, expressed as average daily intakes over time, are intended to provide for individual variations among most normal persons as they live in the U.S. under usual environmental stresses. Diets should be based on a variety of common foods in order to provide other nutrients for which human requirements have been less well defined. The RDAs are designed for the maintenance of good nutrition of practically all healthy people in the U.S.

[b] The median weights and heights of those under 19 years of age were taken from Hamill, P. V. V., Drizd, T. A., Johnson, R. B., et al., *Am J Clin Nutr*, 32, 607, 1979. The use of these figures does not imply that the height-to-weight ratios are ideal.

existing recommendations for increased consumption of carotenoid-rich fruits and vegetables are supported. However, β-carotene supplements are not advisable.[4] In 2001, DRIs were published for vitamin A, vitamin K, boron, chromium, copper, iodine, iron, manganese, molybdenum, nickel, vadadium, and zinc.[5] No DRIs were set for arsenic or silicon.[5] For boron, nickel, and vanadium, ULs were proposed, but EARs, RDAs, or AIs were not set.[5] The RDAs and AIs for children and adolescents are provided in Table 8.1. The ULs for children and adolescents are provided in Table 8.2. Additional groups of nutrients and food components slated for review over the next several years include energy and macronutrients, electrolytes, and other food components.[2]

Energy

Daily energy needs depend on three major factors: energy expended when at rest, during physical activity, and as a result of thermogenesis. Resting energy expenditure is the largest of the three factors unless the physical activity level is very high; thermogenesis is the smallest. In turn, these factors are affected by individual variables which include age, sex, body size and composition, genetics, energy intake, physiologic state (e.g., growth, pregnancy, lactation), coexisting pathological conditions, and ambient temperature.

Recommended energy allowances for children and adolescents from the 1989 RDAs are stipulated as kilocalories (kcal)/day based on reference weights for children ages 1 to 10 years in three age groups for both genders combined, and for adolescents ages 11 to 18 years in two age groups for boys and girls separately (see Table 8.3). According to Heald and Gong, the best way to calculate individual energy requirements for adolescents may be to use kcal/centimeter (cm) of height; thus, boys 11 to 14 years of age need 15.9 kcal/cm, boys 15 to 18 years of age need 17.0 kcal/cm, girls 11 to 14 years of age need 14.0 kcal/cm, and girls 15 to 18 years of age need 13.5 kcal/cm.[6] In Table 8.4, energy requirements for children and adolescents from Pellett[7] are stipulated in terms of kcal/day (mean

TABLE 8.4

Energy Requirements for Children and Adolescents[a]

Age (years)	Weight[b] (kg)	Height (cm)	Estimated Energy Allowance By Time (kcal/d (range))	By Weight (kcal/kg)	By Height (kcal/cm)
Children					
1–1.9	11	82	1200 (900–1600)	105	14.0
2–3.9	14	96	1400 (1100–1900)	100	14.6
4–5.9	18	109	1700 (1300–2300)	92	15.6
6–7.9	22	121	1800 (1400–2400)	83	14.9
8–9.9	28	132	1900 (1400–2500)	69	14.4
Boys					
10–11.9	36	143	2200 (1700–2900)	61	15.4
12–17.9[c]	57	169	2700 (2000–3600)	47	16.0
Girls					
10–14.9	44	155	2200 (1700–2900)	50	14.2
15–17.9[c]	56	162	2300 (1700–3000)	41	14.2

[a] Adapted from Pellett, P. L., *Am J Clin Nutr*, 51, 711, 1990. Data originate from original median weights and heights (see original document).
[b] Weight is rounded to nearest kilogram for age.
[c] During these years, individual growth rates can vary enormously; thus, allowances should be based on individual weights and the requirements per kg body weight.

and range), kcal/kilogram (kg), and kcal/cm for children ages 1 to 9.9 years in five groups for both genders combined, for adolescent boys ages 10 to 17.9 years in two groups, and for adolescent girls ages 10 to 17.9 years in two groups.

Physical activity patterns are quite variable among children and adolescents, and there is considerable variability in both the timing and magnitude of the growth spurt. Thus, recommended energy allowances for children and adolescents assume a wide range within which energy can be adjusted individually to account for body weight, activity, and rate of growth. An accepted and practical method for assessing the adequacy of a child's or adolescent's energy intake is to monitor growth by tracking height and weight on growth charts developed by the National Center for Health Statistics; these charts are provided in Section 32.

Protein

Protein is essential for growth, development, and maintenance of the body; it also provides energy. Protein yields 4 kcal/gram (g). Food sources of protein include meat, fish, poultry, milk, cheese, yogurt, dried beans, peanut butter, nuts, and grain products. Animal proteins are called "high-quality" or "complete" because they contain all the essential amino acids in the proportions needed by humans. Vegetable proteins, with the exception of soybeans, are called "low-quality" or "incomplete" because they have low levels of one or more essential amino acids. A vegetable protein may be paired with another vegetable protein or with a small amount of animal protein to provide adequate amounts of all the essential amino acids. For example, black-eyed peas can be paired with rice, peanut butter with wheat bread, pasta with cheese, or cereal with milk.

Proteins in the body are continuously being degraded and resynthesized. Because the process is not entirely efficient and some amino acids are lost, a continuous supply of amino acids is needed to replace these losses, even after growth has stopped. The primary factor that influences protein needs is energy intake because when energy intake is insufficient, protein is used for energy. Thus, all protein recommendations are based on the assumption that energy needs are adequately met. In addition, protein recommendations are based on high-quality protein intakes; appropriate corrections must be made for diets which customarily provide low-quality proteins.

Table 8.3 provides the 1989 RDAs for high-quality protein in g/day and g/kg of body weight for children and adolescents. As Table 8.3 indicates, requirements slowly decline relative to weight during the preschool and elementary school-age years. During the adolescent years, protein recommendations do not emphasize the growth spurt because it is small relative to body size. A 14-year-old adolescent who weighs 54 kilograms (kg) (118.8 pounds) needs 54 g of protein each day; assuming that energy needs are met, this protein need is met by eating a hamburger (3-ounce meat patty on a bun) and two slices of cheese pizza.

According to Heald and Gong,[6] the most useful method for determining protein needs for adolescents is to use the 1989 RDAs for protein as they relate to height. For adolescent boys ages 11-14 and 15-18 years, the protein daily recommendation based on height is 0.29 and 0.34 g/cm height, respectively. For adolescent girls ages 11-14 and 15-18 years, the protein daily recommendation based on height is 0.29-0.27 g/cm height, respectively.[6]

Carbohydrates

Children and adolescents should get 55-60% of their daily calories from carbohydrates.[8] Complex carbohydrates (starchy foods such as pasta, breads, cereals, rice, and legumes) should provide the majority of kcal from carbohydrates, and simple carbohydrates (naturally occurring sugars in fruits and vegetables) should provide the rest. Carbohydrate yields 4 kcal/g. A 4- to 6-year-old child who needs 1800 kcal/day would need about 990 to 1080 kcal (or 248 to 270 g) from carbohydrates daily. An 11- to 14-year-old adolescent who needs 2500 kcal/day would need about 1375 to 1500 kcal (or 344 to 375 g) from carbohydrates daily.

Fat and Cholesterol

To promote lower cholesterol levels in all healthy U.S. children ages 2-18 years, the American Academy of Pediatrics recommends that children older than two years should gradually adopt a diet that by the age of five years reflects the following five guidelines.[9]

1. Nutritional adequacy should be achieved by eating a wide variety of foods.
2. Caloric intake should be adequate to support growth and development and to reach or maintain desirable body weight.
3. Total fat intake over several days should be no more than 30% of total calories and no less than 20% of total calories.
4. Saturated fat intake should be less than 10% of total calories.
5. Dietary cholesterol intake should be less than 300 milligrams (mg) per day.[9]

These recommendations are consistent with those of the Dietary Guidelines for Americans, which were designed to provide advice for healthy Americans age two years and over about food choices that promote health and prevent disease.[10] A precise percentage of dietary fat intake that supports normal growth and development while maximally reducing atherosclerosis risk is unknown. Thus, a range of appropriate values averaged over several days for children and adolescents is recommended based on the available scientific information. More information regarding the safety of low-fat diets for children is found in "Low Fat Diets" in this section.

Fat yields 9 kcal/g. Dietary sources of fat include oils, margarine, butter, fried foods, egg yolks, mayonnaise, salad dressings, ice cream, hard cheese, cream cheese, nuts, fatty meats, chips, and doughnuts. Table 8.5 provides the fat, saturated fat, and cholesterol content of various foods.

TABLE 8.5

Total Fat, Saturated Fat, and Cholesterol Content of Various Foods

Food	Amount	Total Fat (g)	Saturated Fat (g)	Cholesterol (mg)	Kcal
Almonds, roasted, salted	1 oz	15.3	1.1	0	172
Bacon	2 slices	6.3	2.2	11	73
Bread, white	1 slice	0.9	0.0	0	64
Butter	1 t	4.1	2.5	11	36
Cheese, American	1 oz	8.9	5.6	27	106
Cheese, cheddar	1 oz	9.4	6.0	30	114
Chicken breast with skin, roasted	1/2 breast	7.6	2.2	83	193
Chicken breast without skin, roasted	1/2 breast	3.1	0.9	73	142
Coconut, dried, sweetened, flaked	1/3 c	8.1	7.2	0	115
Corn oil	1 t	13.6	1.7	0	120
Cottonseed oil	1 t	13.6	3.5	0	120
Egg, whole, boiled	1 large	5.3	1.6	213	77
Egg, white only, boiled	1 large	0.0	0.0	0	17
Egg, yolk only, boiled	1 large	5.1	1.6	213	59
Fish, flounder or sole, cooked	3 oz	1.3	0.3	58	99
Ground beef, regular, broiled	3.5 oz	19.5	7.7	101	292
Ground beef, extra lean, broiled	3.5 oz	15.8	6.2	99	265
Ice cream, vanilla, 10% fat	1/2 c	7.3	4.5	29	132
Ice milk, vanilla	1/2 c	2.8	1.7	9	92
Lard (pork fat)	1 t	12.8	5.0	12	115
Margarine, corn & hydrogenated corn	1 t	3.8	0.7	0	34
Margarine, liquid oil	1 t	3.8	0.7	0	34
Milk, whole	1 cup	8.2	5.1	33	150
Milk, 2%	1 cup	4.7	2.9	18	121
Milk, 1%	1 cup	2.6	1.6	10	102
Milk, skim	1 cup	0.4	0.3	4	86
Olive oil	1 t	13.5	1.8	0	119
Peanut butter	2 t	16.0	3.1	0	188
Peanuts, dry roasted	1 oz	13.9	1.9	0	164
Pecans, raw	1 oz	19.0	2.0	0	190
Pork, lean, roasted	3.5 oz	4.8	1.7	93	166
Safflower oil	1 t	13.6	1.2	0	120
Shrimp, boiled	3 oz	0.9	0.2	166	84
Soybean oil	1 t	13.6	2.0	0	120
Tuna fish, oil pack, drained	3 oz	7.0	1.3	15	169
Tuna fish, water pack, drained	3 oz	0.7	0.2	25	99
Turkey breast with skin, roasted	3.5 oz	3.5	1.0	42	126
Yogurt, frozen, vanilla, soft serve	1/2 c	4.0	2.5	2	114

Adapted from Bowes, A. D. P., *Bowes and Church's Food Values of Portions Commonly Used*, 16 ed, revised by Pennington, J. A. T., J. B. Lippincott Company, Philadelphia, 1994.

TABLE 8.6

Fiber Content of Foods that Most U.S. Children and Adolescents Will Eat

Food source	Serving size	Approximate grams of dietary fiber
Baked Beans	1 c	13
Chili with beans	1 c	7
Refried beans	4 oz	6
Brown rice	1 c	4
Peanuts (dry roasted)	2 oz	4
Strawberries	1 c	4
Whole-wheat bread	2 slices	4
Potato, baked, with skin	1 medium	3.5
Apple	1 medium	3
Banana	1 large	3
Carrot (raw)	1 medium	3
Corn	1/2 c	3
Kiwi	1 large	3
Raisins	1/3 c	3
Whole-grain crackers	1/2 oz	2–3
Cereal	1 c	2–3[a]
Applesauce	1/2 c	2
Broccoli	1/2 c	2
Orange	1 medium	2
Peanut butter	2 Tbsp	2

[a] Dietary fiber content of cereal varies widely. Best fiber choice for children has 3+ g per cup.

[b] Adapted from Williams, C. L., *J Am Diet Assoc*, 95, 1140, 1995.

Fiber

Fiber has important health benefits such as promoting normal laxation which can be a problem for many children. In addition, fiber may help reduce the risk of certain chronic diseases of adulthood such as some cancers, cardiovascular disease, and diabetes. The American Health Foundation recommends that children ages two years and older consume a minimal amount of fiber equal to their age plus 5 g/day, and a maximum amount of age plus 10 g/day, to achieve intakes of a maximum of 35 g/day after the age of 20 years.[11,12] This range is thought to be safe even if intake of some vitamins and minerals is marginal. According to the American Academy of Pediatrics,[13] a reasonable daily fiber intake for children is 0.5 g/kg of body weight to a maximum of 35 g/day. The two recommendations are similar for children up to age 10 years, but the age plus 5 recommendation is lower for older adolescents than the recommendation for 0.5 g/kg of body weight.

Fiber intake should be increased gradually through consumption of a variety of fruits, vegetables, legumes, cereals, and other whole-grain products such as breads and crackers. Fiber supplements for children are not recommended as a means of meeting dietary fiber goals.[11] Increased intakes of dietary fiber should be accompanied by increased intakes of water because dietary fiber increases water retention in the colon, which leads to bulkier and softer stools.[11] For most children and adolescents, dietary fiber goals can be met if the daily diet includes two servings of vegetables, three servings of fruits, two slices of whole wheat bread, and a serving of breakfast cereal containing three or more grams of fiber.[12] Table 8.6 provides a list of foods containing fiber that most U.S. children and adolescents will eat.

High-fiber diets do have the potential for reduced energy density, reduced kcal intake, and poor growth, especially in very young children. Furthermore, high-fiber diets may reduce the bioavailability of minerals such as iron, calcium, and zinc. However, the potential health benefits of a moderate increase in dietary fiber intake in childhood are thought to outweigh the potential risks significantly, especially in highly industrialized countries such as the U.S.[11]

Selected Vitamins and Minerals

Vitamin D

Throughout the world, the major source of vitamin D for humans is the exposure of the skin to sunlight; vitamin D that is synthesized in the skin during the summer and fall months can be stored in the fat for use in the winter, which minimizes requirements for vitamin D. In nature, very few foods contain vitamin D; thus, children and adolescents who live in far northern latitudes (e.g., northern Canada and Alaska) may need vitamin D supplements. Food sources of vitamin D include some fish liver oils, eggs from hens that have been fed vitamin D, the liver and fat from aquatic mammals such as seals and polar bears, and the flesh of fatty fish. Foods fortified with vitamin D include milk products and other foods such as margarine and breakfast cereals; the majority of human intake of vitamin D is from fortified foods. Fortified milk is supposed to contain 10 μg (400 IU) per quart regardless of the fat content of milk; however, several recent surveys have indicated that many milk samples contained less than 8 μg per quart. Although it is well recognized that vitamin D deficiency causes abnormalities in calcium and bone metabolism, it is premature to suggest that cancer risk is increased by vitamin D deficiency. The AIs for vitamin D for children and adolescents (see Table 8.1) were set to cover the needs of almost all children and adolescents regardless of exposure to sunlight. Currently, there is no scientific evidence that demonstrates an increased requirement for vitamin D during puberty even though metabolism of vitamin D increases during puberty to enhance intestinal calcium absorption to provide adequate calcium for the rapidly growing skeleton.[2]

Folate

Folate is important during periods of increased cell replication and growth due to its role in DNA synthesis and the formation of healthy red blood cells; thus, the 1998 RDAs for folate are 1.5 times greater for children age 9 to 13 years than for children age 4 to 8 years (see Table 8.1). There is strong evidence that the risk of having a fetus with a neural tube defect decreases with increased intake of folate during the periconceptional period; thus, it is recommended that all women capable of becoming pregnant take 400 μg of synthetic folic acid daily, from fortified foods and/or supplements, in addition to consuming food folate from a varied diet. Folate fortification became mandatory for enriched grain products in the U.S. effective January 1, 1998. Besides fortified grains and cereals, other food sources of folate include leafy green vegetables, orange juice, liver, cantalope, yeast, and seeds.[3]

Calcium

Over 99% of total body calcium is found in teeth and bones. Approximately 45% of adult skeletal mass is accounted for by skeletal growth during adolescence; thus, achieving and maintaining adequate calcium intake during adolescence is necessary for the development of a maximal peak bone mass which may help reduce the risk of osteoporosis later in adulthood.

TABLE 8.7

Approximate Calcium Content for One Serving of Various Foods

Food	Serving Size	Approximate Calcium Content (mg)
Cheese (Swiss)	1.5 oz	405
Cheese (cheddar or jack)	1.5 oz	310
Milk (whole, 1%, 2%, or buttermilk)	1 c	300
Yogurt	8 oz	300
Cheese (part skim mozzarella)	1.5 oz	280
Tofu, raw, firm	1/2 c	260
Cheese (American)	2 oz	250
Calcium-fortified orange juice	6 oz	200
Canned sardines (with bones)	2 oz	180
Canned salmon (with bones)	3 oz	180
Cooked greens (collards)	1/2 c	180
Pudding	1/2 c	150
Spinach (cooked)	1/2 c	120*
Frozen yogurt (vanilla, soft serve)	1/2 c	100
Ice cream (vanilla, 10% fat)	1/2 c	85
Cooked greens (mustard, kale)	1/2 c	80
Cottage cheese	1/2 c	75
Spinach (raw)	1 c	60*
Orange	1 medium	55
Beans, canned (baked, pinto, or navy)	1/2 c	50
Sweet potatoes (mashed)	1/2 c	40
Broccoli (cooked)	1/2 c	35
Broccoli (raw)	1/2 c	20

* The calcium from spinach is essentially nonbioavailable.

Adapted from Bowes, A. D. P., *Bowes and Church's Food Values of Portions Commonly Used*, 16th ed, revised by Pennington, J. A. T., J. B. Lippincott Company, Philadelphia, 1994.

The calcium AIs for adolescents are higher than for children because from age 9 through 18 years (see Table 8.1), calcium retention increases to a peak and then declines. However, the calcium AIs remain the same for adolescents from age 9 to 18 years because calcium absorption efficiency decreases. Thus, during this developmental period, measures of sexual maturity are better predictors of calcium retention than chronological age.[2]

Major food sources of calcium include milk, yogurt, cheese, and green leafy vegetables. Calcium-fortified orange juice is also an excellent source of calcium, as is tofu. Table 8.7 contains approximate calcium contents for one serving of various common foods. Vitamin D (discussed previously in this section) is needed for the body to absorb calcium.

The calcium content of food is generally of greater importance than bioavailability when evaluating food sources of calcium. The efficiency of calcium absorption is fairly similar from most foods, including milk and milk products and grains, which are major food sources of calcium in North American diets. Calcium may be poorly absorbed from foods such as spinach, beans, sweet potatoes, and rhubarb which are rich in oxalic acid, and from unleavened bread, raw beans, seeds, nuts and grains, and soy isolates which are rich in phytic acid. Calcium absorption is relatively high from soybeans, although they contain large amounts of phytic acid. Compared to calcium absorption from milk, calcium absorption from spinach is about one tenth, and from dried beans is about half.[2]

When developing the AIs for calcium, the Food and Nutrition Board of the Institute of Medicine reviewed concerns regarding factors that affect the calcium requirement.[2] For example, they discussed racial differences in calcium metabolism, that sodium and calcium excretion are linked in the proximal renal tubule and that many commonly consumed processed foods are high in sodium, that protein increases urinary calcium excretion, that caffeine has a modest negative impact on calcium retention, that calcium bioavailability is reduced in vegetarian diets due to the high oxalate and phytate content, and that exercise and calcium both influence bone mass. However, the Board concluded that available evidence did not warrant different calcium intake requirements for individuals according to their race, sodium consumption, protein intake, caffeine intake, level of physical activity, or for individuals who consume a vegetarian diet.[2]

Children and adolescents (and adults) with lactose intolerance develop symptoms of diarrhea and bloating after ingesting large doses of lactose such as the amount present in a quart of milk (~46 g). People who generally are lactose digesters include Northern Europeans, Finns, Hungarians, probably Mongols, the Fulani and Tussi tribes of Africa, and the Punjabi of India; the remainder of the world's population are lactose nondigesters.[14] However, as digesters intermix reproductively with nondigesters, the rate of lactose malabsorption falls.[14] In general, evidence for lactose malabsorption as a clinical problem is not manifest until after five to seven years of age, although this age can vary.[14] Individuals with lactose intolerance can increase their tolerance to dairy products by drinking smaller doses of milk (such as eight ounces), or by ingesting fermented products such as yogurt, hard cheeses, cottage cheese, and acidophilus milk.[14] In addition, lactose-free dairy products are available. Although lactose intolerance may influence intake, lactose-intolerant individuals absorb calcium normally from milk; thus, there is no evidence to suggest that it influences the calcium requirement.[2]

Iron

According to the American Academy of Pediatrics,[15] iron deficiency is the most common nutritional deficiency in the U.S. Children aged one to two years are the most susceptible to iron deficiency due to increased iron needs related to rapid growth during the first two years of life and a relatively low iron content in most infant diets when iron is not added by supplementation or fortification. Children age 3 to 11 years are at less risk for iron deficiency until the rapid growth of puberty. Preadolescent school-age children who consume a strict vegetarian diet are at greater risk for iron deficiency anemia. Adolescent boys are at risk for iron deficiency anemia during their peak growth period when iron stores may not meet the demand of rapid growth; however, the iron deficiency anemia generally corrects itself after the growth spurt. Adolescent girls are at greater risk for iron deficiency anemia due to blood losses during menstruation. A major consequence of iron deficiency is that significant iron deficiency adversely affects child development and behavior. Furthermore, iron deficiency leads to enhanced lead absorption, and childhood lead poisoning is a well-documented cause of neurologic and developmental deficits. These consequences, along with evidence that dietary intake during infancy is a strong determinant of iron status for older infants and younger children, emphasize the importance of prevention. Significant improvements have been made in the iron nutritional status of infants and young children in the U.S. during the past two decades, perhaps because during this same time frame, several changes were made in infant feeding patterns.[15] These changes included increased dietary iron content or iron bioavailability, increased incidence of breastfeeding, increased use of iron-fortified formula, and reduced use of whole milk and low-iron formula during the first year of life.[15]

Dietary iron is classified as "heme" or "non-heme" iron. Heme iron is found in foods from animals such as meat, fish, and poultry. Non-heme iron is provided by plants; good sources include dark-green leafy vegetables, tofu, lentils, white beans, dried fruits, and iron-fortified breads and cereals. On average, healthy people absorb about 5 to 10% of the iron consumed, and people who are iron deficient absorb about 10 to 20%. Heme iron is more easily absorbed than non-heme iron. About 20% of heme iron consumed is absorbed regardless of how it is prepared and served; however, the absorption rate of non-heme iron can be increased by eating foods with non-heme iron with either meat, foods rich in vitamin C, or foods that contain some heme iron at the same meal. Non-heme iron absorption can be hindered by as much as 50% when tannins, phytates, and calcium (which are found in foods such as tea, bran, and milk, respectively) are eaten at the same meal.

The RDAs for iron for children and adolescents are included in Table 8.1. Because the amount of iron available in the American diet is estimated to be about 5 to 7 mg/1000 kcal, it may be difficult for adolescent girls to obtain 15 mg of iron from dietary sources alone if their caloric intake is between 2000 and 2400 kcal/day. Groups of adolescents at special risk of iron deficiency include 1) older adolescent girls due to their increased iron need and their low dietary intake, 2) pregnant adolescents, and 3) girl athletes such as runners who may lose iron through occult gastrointestinal bleeding.

The Committee on the Prevention, Detection, and Management of Iron Deficiency Anemia Among U.S. Children and Women of Childbearing Age was established under the Food and Nutrition Board of the Institute of Medicine; its recommended guidelines were published in 1993.[16] The committee concluded that iron enrichment and fortification of the U.S. food supply should remain at current levels rather than increasing or decreasing the levels. Furthermore, it was recommended that dietary sources of iron be consumed instead of supplemental sources when possible. Iron supplements should be kept out of reach of children because iron is a very common cause of poisoning in children.[16]

Zinc

Zinc is needed for protein synthesis, wound healing, and sexual maturation; thus, zinc is especially important during adolescence due to the rapid rate of growth and sexual maturation.[6] (See Table 8.1 for the RDAs for zinc for children and adolescents.) Adolescents undergoing rapid growth are at risk for inadequate zinc levels, and should be encouraged to include zinc-rich foods in their daily diet. Foods high in zinc include red meats, certain seafood, and whole grains; many breakfast cereals are fortified with zinc. The bioavailability of zinc in foods varies widely. Zinc from whole grain products is less available than zinc from meat, liver, eggs, and seafood (especially oysters). Furthermore, consumption of phytate-rich foods limits absorption and maintenance of zinc balance.[5]

Food Guide Pyramid for Young Children

Figure 8.1 illustrates the Food Guide Pyramid for Young Children released by the United States Department of Agriculture (USDA) in March, 1999.[17] The pyramid targets children two to six years of age; it is an adaptation of the original Food Guide Pyramid[18] released in 1992. The purpose of the new pyramid is to simplify educational messages and focus on young children's food preferences and nutritional needs. The new pyramid was developed by adapting existing food guidance recommendations to meet the specific needs of young children after actual food patterns of young children were analyzed by USDA's Center for Nutrition Policy and Promotion. Table 8.8 provides an overview of changes made in the new pyramid. The new pyramid continues to emphasize eating a variety of foods. However, it de-emphasizes fat restriction, recognizing that some fats are necessary for early growth and development.

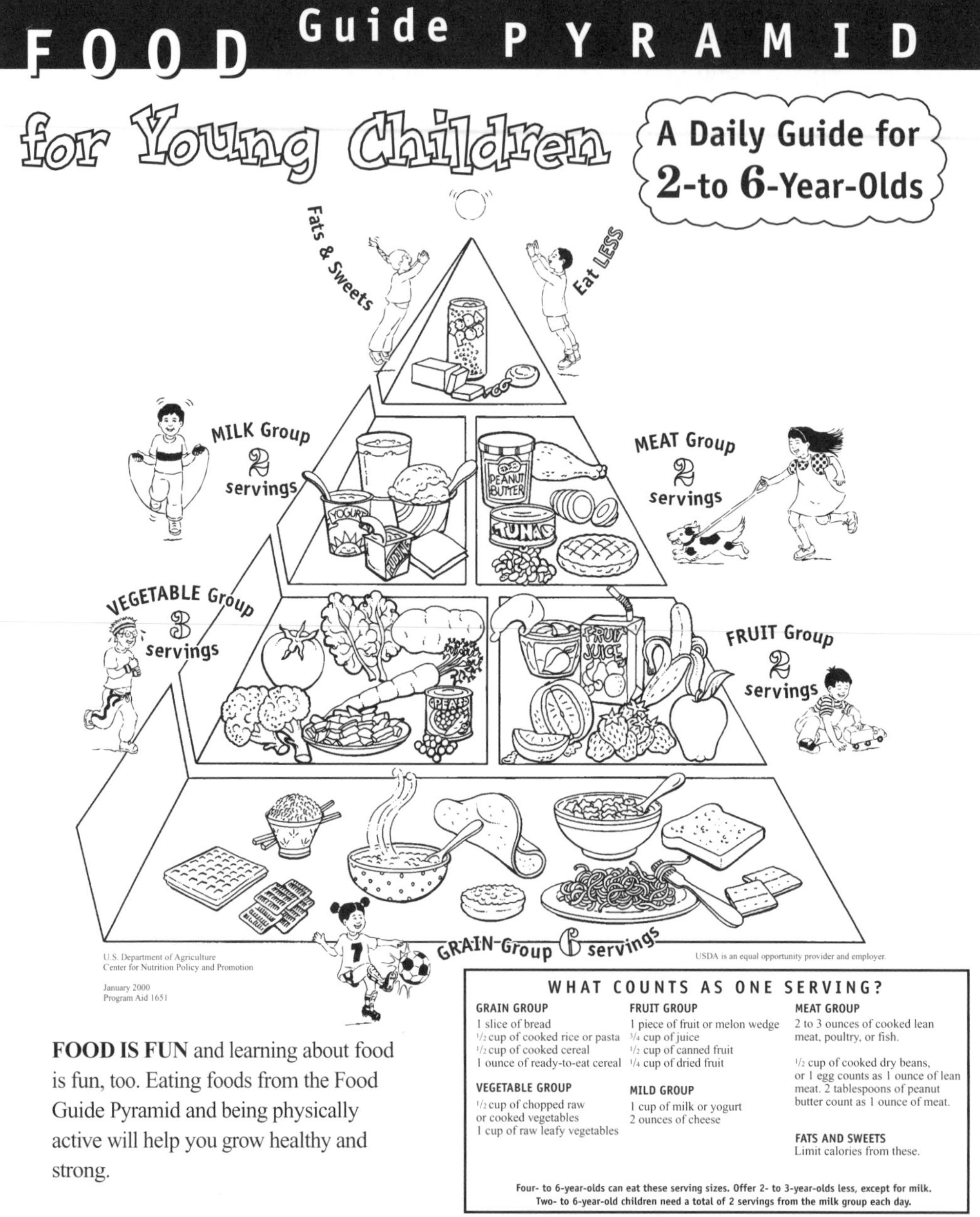
FOOD Guide PYRAMID
for Young Children
A Daily Guide for 2-to 6-Year-Olds
Fats & Sweets
Eat LESS
SODA POP
MILK Group
2 servings
YOGURT
PUDDING
MEAT Group
2 servings
PEANUT BUTTER
TUNA
VEGETABLE Group
3 servings
PEAS
FRUIT Group
2 servings
FRUIT JUICE
GRAIN-Group 6 servings
U.S. Department of Agriculture
Center for Nutrition Policy and Promotion
January 2000
Program Aid 1651
USDA is an equal opportunity provider and employer.
FOOD IS FUN and learning about food is fun, too. Eating foods from the Food Guide Pyramid and being physically active will help you grow healthy and strong.
WHAT COUNTS AS ONE SERVING?
GRAIN GROUP
1 slice of bread
1/2 cup of cooked rice or pasta
1/2 cup of cooked cereal
1 ounce of ready-to-eat cereal
VEGETABLE GROUP
1/2 cup of chopped raw or cooked vegetables
1 cup of raw leafy vegetables
FRUIT GROUP
1 piece of fruit or melon wedge
3/4 cup of juice
1/2 cup of canned fruit
1/4 cup of dried fruit
MILD GROUP
1 cup of milk or yogurt
2 ounces of cheese
MEAT GROUP
2 to 3 ounces of cooked lean meat, poultry, or fish.
1/2 cup of cooked dry beans, or 1 egg counts as 1 ounce of lean meat. 2 tablespoons of peanut butter count as 1 ounce of meat.
FATS AND SWEETS
Limit calories from these.
Four- to 6-year-olds can eat these serving sizes. Offer 2- to 3-year-olds less, except for milk.
Two- to 6-year-old children need a total of 2 servings from the milk group each day.
EAT a variety of FOODS AND ENJOY!

FIGURE 8.1
Food guide pyramid for young children.

TABLE 8.8

Changes Made in the New Food Guide Pyramid for Young Children

- The food groups have shorter names.
- A single number of servings is given for each food group rather than a range of servings.
- Foods are drawn in a realistic style.
- Foods are illustrated in single serving portions when possible.
- Foods included are those commonly eaten by young children such as fruit juice, green beans, breads, cereals, and pasta. (Although the baked potato is not the most commonly served form of potato, it is illustrated to encourage children to consume a lower fat version of potato. Also, dark-green leafy vegetables and whole-grain products are illustrated to encourage children to eat them more often.)
- Abstract symbols for fat and added sugars in the original pyramid have been eliminated.
- The tip of the pyramid has drawings of food items rather than symbols.
- The pyramid is surrounded with illustrations of children engaged in active pursuits, to show the importance of physical activity.

From *Tips for Using the Food Guide Pyramid for Young Children 2 to 6 Years Old*, USDA, Center for Nutrition Policy and Promotion, Washington, DC, 1999, Program Aid 1647.

A booklet entitled *Tips for Using the Food Guide Pyramid for Young Children 2 to 6 Years Old* was developed to go along with the new pyramid.[19] It includes tips to encourage healthful eating, basic information about the new pyramid, "child-size" serving sizes, lists of foods by group to encourage children to eat a variety of foods, suggested kitchen activities for parents to do with children, snack and meal planning ideas, a chart to track foods eaten over several days, and "hands-on" food activities for home or child care centers.

Both the original and the new pyramid show how adults, adolescents, and children can make food choices for a healthful diet as described in the *Dietary Guidelines for Americans*.[10] The five food groups in the pyramid include grains, vegetables, fruits, milk, and meat. Each group provides some, but not all, of nutrients and energy that children need. No one food group is more important than another. The grain group forms the base of the pyramid because the largest number of servings needed each day comes from this group. Grain products provide vitamins, minerals, complex carbohydrates, and dietary fiber. Foods from the fruit and vegetable groups provide vitamins, minerals, and dietary fiber. Foods from the milk group provide calcium. Foods from the meat group (meat, poultry, fish, eggs, dry beans/peas, and peanut butter) provide protein, iron, and zinc. The small tip of the pyramid shows fats and sweets (e.g., salad dressing, cream, butter, margarine, soft drinks, and candy); these foods contain kcal but few vitamins and minerals.

Table 8.9 contains young children's serving sizes by food group, along with the number of servings needed from each food group each day. Two- to three-year-olds need the same variety of foods as four- to six-year-olds but fewer kcal, so offer them smaller amounts (about 2/3 serving). The one exception is that two- to six-year-olds need a total of two servings from the milk group each day. Offer children a variety of foods from the five food groups, and let children decide how much to eat. Table 8.10 contains a sample meal and snack plan according to food group for one day for four- to six-year-old children.

What are Children and Adolescents Eating?

1989–1991 Continuing Survey of Food Intakes by Individuals (CSFII)

The 1989–1991 CSFII sample consisted of individuals residing in households in the 48 contiguous United States; it included two separate samples, basic and low income. All

TABLE 8.9

Young Children's Serving Sizes by Food Group

Grain Group (6 servings each day)
Offer whole or mixed grain products for at least 3 of the 6 grain group servings each day.

Whole grain:	*Enriched:*
1/2 cup cooked brown rice	1/2 cup cooked rice, pasta, or grits
2-3 graham cracker squares	1/2 English muffin or bagel
5-6 whole grain crackers	1 slice white, wheat, French or Italian bread
1/2 cup cooked oatmeal	1/2 hamburger or hot dog bun
1/2 cup cooked bulgur	1 small roll
3 cups popped popcorn*	6 crackers (saltine size)
3 rice or popcorn cakes*	1 4-inch pita bread or 1 4-inch pancake
1 ounce ready-to-eat whole grain cereal	1/2 cup cooked farina or other cereal
1 slice pumpernickel, rye, or whole wheat bread	9 3-ring pretzels*
2 taco shells*	1 7-inch flour tortilla
1 7-inch corn tortilla	1 ounce ready-to-eat, unfrosted cereal
Grain products with more fat and sugars:	
1 small biscuit, muffin, or piece of cornbread	
1/2 medium doughnut	
9 animal crackers	

Vegetable Group (3 servings each day)

1/2 cup of chopped raw or cooked vegetable
1 cup raw leafy greens
1/2 cup tomato or spaghetti sauce
3/4 cup vegetable juice
1 cup vegetable soup
1 medium (ear of corn, potato)
2 cooked broccoli spears
7-8 raw carrot or celery sticks (3" long)*
10 french fries
5 cherry tomatoes*

Fruit Group (2 servings each day)

1 medium orange, apple, banana, or peach
1/2 grapefruit
1/2 cup cut-up fresh, canned, or cooked fruit
3/4 cup fruit juice
1/4 cup dried fruit*
12 grapes or 11 cherries*
7 medium strawberries
1/2 cup blueberries or raspberries
1 large kiwi
1 small pear

Milk Group (2 servings each day)

For this amount of food ...	*Count this many milk group servings*
1 cup milk or 1 cup soy milk (calcium fortified)	1
1/2 cup milk	1/2
1 cup yogurt (8 ounces)	1
1.5 ounces natural cheese	1
2 ounces processed cheese	1
1 string cheese (1 ounce)	2/3
1/2 cup cottage cheese	1/4
1/2 cup ice cream	1/3
1/2 cup frozen yogurt or 1/2 cup pudding	1/2

TABLE 8.9 *(Continued)*

Young Children's Serving Sizes by Food Group

Meat Group (2 servings each day)
Two to three ounces of cooked lean meat, poultry, or fish equal one serving of meat. Amounts from the meat group should total 5 ounces a day for 4- to 6-year-olds and about 3 1/2 ounces a day for 2- to 3-year-olds.

For this amount of food ...	*Count this many ounces*
2 ounces cooked lean meat, poultry, or fish	2 ounces
1 egg (yolk and white)	1 ounce
2 tablespoons peanut butter*	1 ounce
1 1/2 frankfurters (2 ounces)*	1 ounce
2 slices bologna or lunchmeat (2 ounces)	1 ounce
1/4 cup drained canned salmon or tuna	1 ounce
1/2 cup cooked kidney, pinto, or white beans	1 ounce
1/2 cup tofu	1 ounce
1 soy burger patty	1 ounce

* May cause choking in 2- and 3-year-old children.

Adapted from *Tips for Using the Food Guide Pyramid for Young Children 2 to 6 Years Old*, USDA, Center for Nutrition Policy and Promotion, Washington, DC, 1999, Program Aid 1647.

household members were asked to provide intake information. Each individual provided three consecutive days of dietary data which consisted of one 24-hour recall and a two-day food record. A knowledgeable adult (usually the primary meal planner/preparer) reported the food intakes of household members younger than 12 years.[20]

Data from the 1989–1991 CSFII have been analyzed numerous ways to provide insight into what children and adolescents are eating. For example, data were analyzed to determine dietary sources of nutrients among 4008 U.S. children age 2 to 18 years.[21] Results indicated that fortified foods (e.g., ready-to-eat cereals) were influential contributors of many vitamins and minerals. Furthermore, low nutrient-dense foods were major contributors of energy, fats, and carbohydrate, which compromises intakes of more nutrient-dense foods, and may impede compliance with current dietary guidance.

Data from CSFII 1989–1991 were also analyzed to determine fruit and vegetable consumption among 3148 U.S. children age 2 to 18 years.[22] Results indicated that only one in five children met the recommendation of consuming five or more servings of fruits and vegetables per day. Intakes of all fruits and of dark green and/or deep yellow vegetables were very low compared with recommendations. Furthermore, almost one-fourth of all vegetables consumed by children and adolescents were french fries.

Finally, data from the CSFII 1989–1991 were analyzed to determine what percentage of children ages 4-6 (n = 603) and 7-10 (n = 782) met the American Health Foundation's age plus 5 recommendation for fiber,[11,12] and what the leading contributors to total dietary fiber intake were.[23] Results indicated that only 45% of 4- to 6-year-olds and 32% of 7- to 10-year-olds met the age plus 5 rule. Children who met the rule did so by consuming significantly more high- and low-fiber breads and cereals, fruits, vegetables, legumes, nuts, and seeds. Furthermore, children who met the rule had significantly higher energy-adjusted intakes of vitamins A and E, folate, magnesium, and iron compared to children with low fiber intakes who had significantly higher energy-adjusted intakes of fat and cholesterol. Surprisingly, low-fiber breads and cereals provided 21 and 19% of total dietary fiber for 4- to 6-year-olds and 7- to 10-year-olds, respectively, whereas high-fiber breads and cereals provided only 6% of total dietary fiber for both age groups. Conclusions from these results include that substituting high-fiber breads and cereals for low-fiber ones would increase children's fiber intakes and should be relatively easy to accomplish.[23]

TABLE 8.10

Sample Meal and Snack Plan according to Food Group for One Day for Four- to Six-Year-Old Children (Offer two- to three-year-old children the same variety but smaller portions.)

	Grain	Vegetable	Fruit	Milk	Meat
Breakfast					
Orange juice, 3/4 cup			1		
Whole-grain toast, 1 slice	1				
Cheerios, 1 oz	1				
Milk, 1/2 cup				1/2	
Mid-Morning Snack					
Graham crackers, 2 squares	1				
Cold water, 1/2 cup					
Lunch					
Tuna Casserole with:					
Tuna fish, 2 oz (1/2 cup)					2 oz
Macaroni, 1/2 cup	1				
Green peas, 1/2 cup		1			
Processed cheese, 1 oz				1/2	
Banana, 1 medium			1		
Milk, 1/2 cup				1/2	
Mid-Afternoon Snack					
Animal crackers, 9	1				
Peanut butter, 2 Tbsp					1 oz
Cold water, 1/2 cup					
Dinner					
Chicken, 2 oz					2 oz
Baked potato, 1 medium		1			
Broccoli, 1/2 cup		1			
Milk, 1/2 cup				1/2	
Evening Snack					
Whole grain crackers (5)	1				
Cold water, 1/2 cup					
Total Food Group Servings	6	3	2	2	5 oz

Adapted from *Tips for Using the Food Guide Pyramid for Young Children 2 to 6 Years Old*, USDA, Center for Nutrition Policy and Promotion, Washington, DC, 1999, Program Aid 1647.

1994–1996 Continuing Survey of Food Intakes by Individuals (CSFII)

The 1994–1996 CSFII sample consisted of individuals residing in households in the 50 United States, and included an oversampling of the low-income population. Only selected household members were asked to provide intake information. Each individual provided two nonconsecutive days of dietary data obtained by the 24-hour recall method through in-person interviews.[20] Proxy interviews were conducted routinely for subjects under 6 years of age, and children 6 to 11 years of age were asked to describe their own food intake assisted by an adult household member (referred to as the assistant). The preferred proxy or assistant was the person responsible for preparing the subject's meals.[24]

To determine how the dietary intake of children and adolescents compared with nutrition recommendations, the Healthy Eating Index (HEI) was used to examine the diets of 5354 American children ages 2 to 18 from USDA's 1994–1996 CSFII.[25] The HEI is computed on a regular basis by USDA as a summary measure of people's diet quality. It consists of 10 components, each representing different aspects of a healthful diet. Components 1 to 5 measure the degree to which a person's diet conforms to USDA's Food Guide Pyramid serving recommendations for the five major food groups: grains, vegetables, fruits, milk, and meat/meat alternatives. Components 6 and 7 measure total fat and saturated fat consumption, respectively, as percentages of total kcal intake. Components 8 and 9 measure total cholesterol and sodium intake, respectively. Component 10 measures the degree of variety in a person's diet. Each component has a maximum score of ten and a minimum score of zero. High component scores indicate intakes close to recommended ranges or amounts; low component scores indicate less compliance with recommended ranges or amounts. The maximum combined score for the 10 components is 100. An HEI score above 80 implies a good diet, a score between 51 and 80 implies a diet that needs improvement, and a score less than 51 implies a poor diet.[25]

Results indicate that most children have a diet that is poor or needs improvement. As children get older, their overall HEI score declines; thus, the percentage of children with a diet that needs improvement or is poor increases, and the percentage of children with a good diet declines. For children ages 2 to 3, 35% have a good diet, and 5% have a poor diet. For boys 15 to 18 years old, only 6% have a good diet, and 21% have a poor diet. The decline in diet quality begins between the 2-3 and 4-6 age groups, with the percentage of children having a good diet falling from 35 to 16%, and the percentage having a diet that needs improvement rising from 60 to 75%. The decline continues between the 7-10 and 11-14 age groups, with the percentage of children having a good diet falling from 14 to 7%. As indicated by the HEI component scores in Table 8.11, the decline in the quality of children's diets as they get older is linked to declines in their fruit and milk consumption. Fifty-three percent of children ages 2 to 3 meet the recommendation for fruit compared to only 11 to 12% of children ages 15 to 18. Although 44% of children ages 2 to 3 meet the recommendation for milk, only 12 and 28% of girls and boys, respectively, ages 15 to 18, do so. Except for cholesterol and variety to a smaller extent, most children do not meet most recommendations.[25]

Further analyses of data from the 1994–1996 CSFII indicated that the quality of a child's diet is related to the income of his or her family.[26] As indicated in Table 8.12, poor children are less likely than nonpoor children to have a diet rated as good. For children ages 2-5, 19% of those in a poor household had a good diet compared to 28% of those in a nonpoor household.

Data from the 1994–1996 CSFII were also analyzed to determine whether carbonated soft drink consumption was associated with consumption of milk, fruit juice, and the nutrients concentrated in these beverages among children and adolescents age 2-18 years (n = 1810).[27] Results indicated that adolescents (13-18 years) were more likely to consume soft drinks than preschool-age children (2-5 years) and school-age children (6-12 years). Among preschool-age children, school-age children, and adolescents, 49.5, 35.9, and 17.5%, respectively, did *not* consume any soft drinks during the two days of dietary recall; furthermore, the majority of children in each age category were nonconsumers of diet soft

TABLE 8.11

Healthy Eating Index (HEI): Overall and Component Mean Scores for Children, 1994–1996[a,b]

Age (years)	Children 2–3	Children 4–6	Children 7–10	Girls 11–14	Boys 11–14	Girls 15–18	Boys 15–18
Overall HEI Score	73.8	67.8	66.6	63.5	62.2	60.9	60.7
1. Grains	8.3	7.2	7.6	6.7	7.2	6.3	7.5
	(54)	(27)	(31)	(16)	(29)	(17)	(34)
2. Vegetables	5.9	4.9	5.1	5.5	5.4	5.8	6.3
	(31)	(16)	(20)	(24)	(23)	(26)	(35)
3. Fruits	7.0	5.3	4.3	3.9	3.5	3.1	2.8
	(53)	(29)	(18)	(14)	(9)	(12)	(11)
4. Milk	7.2	7.4	7.6	5.2	6.2	4.2	6.1
	(44)	(44)	(49)	(15)	(27)	(12)	(28)
5. Meat	6.3	5.3	5.5	5.7	6.5	5.8	6.9
	(28)	(14)	(17)	(15)	(28)	(21)	(36)
6. Total fat	7.4	7.3	7.2	7.2	6.8	7.1	6.8
	(40)	(38)	(35)	(37)	(33)	(38)	(34)
7. Saturated fat	5.4	5.6	5.7	5.8	5.7	6.6	6.0
	(27)	(28)	(28)	(31)	(32)	(42)	(35)
8. Cholesterol	9.0	8.9	8.7	8.5	7.6	8.4	6.7
	(83)	(83)	(80)	(78)	(69)	(77)	(58)
9. Sodium	8.8	8.1	6.8	7.1	5.2	6.9	3.7
	(64)	(53)	(34)	(39)	(21)	(37)	(15)
10. Variety	8.4	7.9	8.1	7.8	8.1	6.7	7.8
	(64)	(53)	(54)	(51)	(58)	(37)	(51)

[a] Parentheses contain % of children meeting dietary recommendations for each component.

[b] From *Report Card on the Diet Quality of Children*. Nutrition Insights, Insight 9, October, 1998, issued by the Center for Nutrition Policy and Promotion, USDA, http://www.usda.gov/cnpp (accessed July 21, 1999).

TABLE 8.12

Percentage of Children Ages 2 to 18 by Age, Poverty Status, and Diet Quality as Measured by the Healthy Eating Index, Three-Year Average 1994–1996

Characteristic	Good Diet[a]	Needs Improvement[a]	Poor Diet[a]
Ages 2-5			
At or below poverty	19	70	11
Above poverty	28	65	7
Ages 6-12			
At or below poverty	10	78	12
Above poverty	12	78	10
Ages 13-18			
At or below poverty	3[b]	72	25
Above poverty	7	74	19

[a] A Healthy Eating Index (HEI) score above 80 implies a good diet, a score between 51 and 80 implies a diet that needs improvement, and a score less than 51 implies a poor diet.

[b] Sample size relatively small to make reliable comparisons.

Adapted from Federal Interagency Forum on Child and Family Statistics, *America's Children: Key National Indicators of Well-Being, 1999.* Federal Interagency Forum On Child and Family Statistics, Washington, DC, US Government Printing Office. The report is also available on the World Wide Web: http://childstats.gov.

drinks (94.9, 89.0, and 85.9%, respectively). White preschool-age children and adolescents were more likely to consume soft drinks than black preschool-age children and adolescents. Among adolescents, boys were more likely than girls to consume soft drinks. Among preschool-age children and adolescents, those who resided in central city metropolitan statistical areas (within a metropolitan area containing the largest population) were more likely to consume soft drinks than those residing in noncentral city metropolitan statistical areas (within a metropolitan area not containing the largest population). No significant differences in soft drink consumption were found by poverty status or region of the country. In general, soft drink consumption was inversely associated with consumption of milk, fruit juice, and the nutrients concentrated in these beverages. For all age groups, energy intake was higher among those in the highest soft drink consumption category compared with nonconsumers. These results indicate that nutrition education messages for children and/or their parents should encourage limited consumption of soft drinks.[27]

1994–1996 and 1998 Continuing Survey of Food Intakes by Individuals (CSFII)

The Supplemental Children's Survey to the 1994–1996 CSFII (CSFII 1998) was conducted to add intake data from 5559 children age birth through 9 years to the intake data collected from 4253 children of the same age who participated in the CSFII 1994–1996. The CSFII 1998 was designed to be combined with the CSFII 1994–1996; thus, approaches to sample selection, data collection, data file preparation, and weighting were consistent.[28]

Analyses of data from the 1994–1996 and 1998 CSFII provide some of the most recent insight into the dietary intake of children and adolescents nationwide. Tables 8.13 through 8.17 include national probability estimates based on all four years of the CSFII (1994–1996 and 1998) for children ages 9 years and under, and on CSFII 1994–1996 only for individuals age 10 years and over.[28] As indicated in Table 8.13, mean intakes as percentages of the 1989 RDAs meet or exceed the RDAs for most nutrients for both girls and boys of all ages. The most notable exception is for calcium for girls ages 12 to 19 years, for which mean intake as a percentage of the RDA for this group is only 64%, down from 102% for girls ages 6 to 11 years. As indicated in Table 8.14, the percentages of children with diets meeting 100% of the 1989 RDAs is around or below 50% for energy, vitamin E, and zinc for both boys and girls, and for vitamin A and calcium for girls. For all nutrients for all ages of children, the percentages of children with diets meeting 100% of the 1989 RDAs is higher for males than females. Furthermore, in general, the percentages of children with diets meeting 100% of the 1989 RDAs decreases as children get older, especially between the 6-11 and 12-19 year age groups, and more so for girls than boys. As indicated in Table 8.15, the mean percentages of kcal from protein, total fat, saturated fat, and carbohydrate in the diets of children and adolescents closely follows nutrition recommendations. However, as indicated in Table 8.16, although the diets of many children do meet recommendations for cholesterol, most children do not meet recommendations for total fat or saturated fat. Breakfast consumption declines as children get older; ~97% of children ages 2 to 5 years eat breakfast, compared to ~93% of children ages 6 to 11 years and ~76% of children ages 12 to 19 years (data not shown). Although ~80% of children of all ages from 2 to 18 years consume vegetables, the percentages of children consuming fruits and fruit juices declines as children get older, from ~73% for children ages 2 to 5 years to ~59% for children ages 6 to 11 years, to ~45% for children ages 12 to 19 years (data not shown).[28]

TABLE 8.13

Nutrient Intakes: Mean Intakes as Percentages of the 1989 Recommended Dietary Allowances Intakes by Individuals 1994–1996, 1998

Sex and Age (Years)	Sample Size	Food Energy	Protein	Vitamin A (µg RE)	Vitamin E	Vitamin C	Thiamin	Riboflavin	Niacin
	Number	Percentages of 1989 RDA							
Boys & Girls									
1–2	2118	102	307	185	79	257	161	213	142
3–5	4574	103	281	179	88	240	170	193	155
Boys									
6–9	787	103	258	147	98	227	175	190	164
6–11	1031	101	244	139	96	226	172	186	161
12–19	737	99	184	108	93	213	150	155	148
Girls									
6–9	704	91	227	127	89	214	150	162	139
6–11	969	91	214	121	91	208	149	160	138
12–19	732	87	145	100	88	171	131	135	126

Adapted from USDA, Agricultural Research Service, *Food and Nutrient Intakes by Children 1994–96, 1998*, 1999, bhnrc/foodsurvey/home.htm (accessed December 22, 1999).

(RDAs), by Sex and Age, Children 19 Years of Age and Under, One Day, Continuing Survey of Food

Sex and Age (Years)	Vitamin B_6	Folate	Vitamin B_{12}	Calcium	Phosphorus	Magnesium	Iron	Zinc	Selenium
	------ Number ------		Percentages of 1989 RDA						
Boys & Girls									
1–2	130	396	457	107	121	234	108	74	299
3–5	144	424	421	108	136	204	132	92	375
Boys									
6–9	136	319	337	122	159	156	158	109	334
6–11	133	298	326	116	152	146	161	107	318
12–19	117	180	292	95	136	92	169	96	263
Girls									
6–9	115	237	307	106	138	140	136	94	297
6–11	114	248	283	102	134	129	130	93	276
12–19	104	138	190	64	92	77	91	82	178

Online, ARS Food Surveys Research Group, available on the "Products" page at http://www.barc.usda.gov/

TABLE 8.14

Nutrient Intakes: Percentage of Children with Diets Meeting 100% of the 1989 Recommended Dietary Individuals 1994–1996, 1998

Sex and Age (Years)	Sample Size	Food Energy	Protein	Vitamin A (μg RE)	Vitamin E	Vitamin C	Thiamin	Riboflavin	Niacin
	------ Number	------------------- Percentage of Children							
Boys & Girls									
1–2	2023	45.1	98.9	78.5	19.0	81.4	85.7	95.1	71.8
3–5	4386	44.6	99.1	75.5	25.2	79.6	89.6	93.1	82.7
Boys									
6–9	758	46.3	98.7	66.3	35.5	77.4	93.4	93.5	87.2
10–11	991	42.9	97.8	63.2	33.4	78.3	90.2	92.2	86.0
12–19	696	39.4	90.4	35.9	35.4	67.5	76.0	76.8	75.8
Girls									
6–9	665	26.3	98.9	53.5	28.0	77.8	83.4	85.7	77.0
10–11	922	27.9	95.3	50.4	27.7	75.1	80.5	83.8	74.7
12–19	702	25.2	76.2	30.6	24.0	57.7	68.0	64.4	61.9

Adapted from USDA, Agricultural Research Service, *Food and Nutrient Intakes by Children 1994-96, 1998*, 1999, bhnrc/foodsurvey/home.htm (accessed December 22, 1999).

Allowances (RDAs), by Sex and Age, Two-Day Average, Continuing Survey of Food Intake by

Sex and Age (Years)	Vitamin B_6	Folate	Vitamin B_{12}	Calcium	Phosphorus	Magnesium	Iron	Zinc	Selenium
	------ Number ------------------- Percentage of Children -------------------								
Boys & Girls									
1–2	65.5	99.0	99.0	49.9	65.6	97.4	44.5	15.2	97.9
3–5	75.7	99.1	98.0	48.4	75.3	95.2	65.7	30.4	99.7
Boys									
6–9	68.9	96.6	97.9	63.0	89.9	85.6	82.9	49.6	99.4
10–11	67.9	95.5	97.8	57.2	83.3	77.2	81.6	47.0	99.1
12–19	53.8	73.2	92.5	36.2	72.9	33.4	83.2	34.6	97.4
Girls									
6–9	56.1	95.6	96.9	47.3	78.9	80.2	69.5	32.7	99.3
10–11	55.1	90.6	93.9	43.2	73.1	68.3	61.5	31.9	98.3
12–19	42.4	58.3	73.9	13.4	33.6	17.8	27.5	23.9	86.4

Online, ARS Food Surveys Research Group, available on the "Products" page at http://www.barc.usda.gov/

TABLE 8.15

Nutrient Intakes: Mean Percentage of Calories from Protein, Total Fat, Saturated Fat, and Carbohydrate, by Sex and Age, One-Day, Continuing Survey of Food Intakes by Individuals 1994–1996, 1998

Sex and Age (Years)	Sample Size Number	Protein	Total Fat	Saturated Fat	Carbohydrate
		Percentage of kcal			
Boys & Girls					
1–2	2118	14.8	32.4	13.3	54.3
3–5	4574	14.2	32.2	12.1	55.2
Boys					
6–9	787	14.0	32.5	12.0	54.9
6–11	1031	14.0	32.6	12.0	54.8
12–19	737	14.4	33.1	11.7	53.2
Girls					
6–9	704	13.9	32.4	11.9	55.2
6–11	969	13.9	32.6	11.9	54.9
12–19	732	14.0	32.2	11.3	55.0

Adapted from USDA, Agricultural Research Service, *Food and Nutrient Intakes by Children 1994-96, 1998*, 1999, Online, ARS Food Surveys Research Group, available on the "Products" page at http://www.barc.usda.gov/bhnrc/foodsurvey/home.htm (accessed December 22, 1999).

TABLE 8.16

Nutrient Intakes: Percentage of Children with Diets Meeting Recommendations for Total Fat, Saturated Fatty Acids, and Cholesterol, by Sex and Age, Two-Day Average, Continuing Survey of Food Intakes by Individuals 1994–1996, 1998

Sex and Age (Years)	Sample Size	Total Fat Intake at or below 30% of kcal	Saturated Fatty Acid Intake below 10% of kcal	Cholesterol Intake at or below 300 Milligrams
		Percentage of Children		
Boys & Girls				
1–2	2023	34.2	18.2	85.5
3–5	4386	33.0	22.6	84.6
Boys				
6–9	758	30.5	22.5	80.4
10–11	991	31.3	24.9	79.1
12–19	696	30.4	27.6	55.9
Girls				
6–9	665	32.6	23.4	86.2
10–11	922	33.5	24.5	85.5
12–19	702	35.4	33.5	80.9

Adapted from USDA, Agricultural Research Service, *Food and Nutrient Intakes by Children 1994-96, 1998*, 1999, Online, ARS Food Surveys Research Group, available on the "Products" page at http://www.barc.usda.gov/bhnrc/foodsurvey/home.htm (accessed December 22, 1999).

Vitamin-Mineral Supplements

According to the Food and Nutrition Board, the "RDAs can typically be met or closely approximated by diets that are based on the consumption of a variety of foods from diverse food groups that contain adequate energy."[1,29] According to the American Dietetic Association,[30] children can best achieve healthful eating habits by consuming a varied diet in moderation[10] that includes foods from each of the major food groups, as illustrated by the Food Guide Pyramid.[18] Routine supplementation is not necessary for healthy growing children who consume a varied diet, according to the American Academy of Pediatrics.[31] If parents wish to give supplements to their children, a standard pediatric vitamin-mineral product with nutrients in amounts no larger than the RDA may be given. Megadose levels should be discouraged due to potential toxic effects. Parents should be cautioned to keep vitamin-mineral supplements out of the reach of children because the taste, shape, and color of most pediatric preparations make them quite appealing to children.

Although the American Academy of Pediatrics advocates that routine vitamin-mineral supplementation is not necessary for healthy growing children who eat a varied diet, it does identify five groups of children at nutritional risk who may benefit from supplementation.[31] These groups are identified in Table 8.17. Dietary intake over several days should be assessed by a Registered Dietitian to determine if an individual child from one of these groups needs to take a supplement.

TABLE 8.17

Five Groups of Children at Nutritional Risk Who May Benefit from Vitamin-Mineral Supplementation

- Children from deprived families or who suffer parental neglect or abuse
- Children with anorexia or an inadequate appetite or who consume a fad diet
- Children with chronic disease (e.g., cystic fibrosis, inflammatory bowel disease, hepatic disease)
- Children who participate in a dietary program for managing obesity
- Children who consume a vegetarian diet without adequate dairy products

From Committee on Nutrition, American Academy of Pediatrics, Feeding from Age One Year to Adolescence, *Pediatric Nutrition Handbook*, 4th ed., Kleinman, R. E., Ed., American Academy of Pediatrics, Elk Grove Village, IL, 1998, pg 125, with permission.

Development of Preschool Children's Food Preferences and Consumption Patterns

Widespread evidence indicates that the nutrition guidelines are not being followed by most children. For example, most children consume far too few fruits and vegetables,[22,32-34] and the majority of children still exceed daily recommendations for total fat, saturated fat, and cholesterol.[35] Furthermore, the incidence of childhood obesity has increased dramatically during the last three decades.[36,37] To help understand why children eat less of what is recommended by nutrition guidelines and more of what is not recommended, and why the incidence of childhood obesity is increasing, Birch and Fisher[38] recommend that consideration be given to factors that impact children's food preferences and consumption patterns. Extensive evidence suggests that children's food preferences are shaped by early experience with food and eating, and that family environment and practices used by parents and other adults (e.g., school staff) may permanently affect dietary practices of children.[39] Birch and colleagues[40] have repeatedly found that exposure to food, as well as the social environment in which it is eaten, are crucial in the development of preschool children's food preferences and consumption patterns. Research indicates that children's food preferences are major determinants of consumption;[41-45] therefore, not eating certain items (such as vegetables) is related to low preferences. Furthermore, research indicates that preschool children's preferences for dietary fat are related to their levels of body fat.[45]

Learning to Eat

During the first years of life, an enormous amount of learning about food and eating occurs as infants transition from consuming only milk to consuming a variety of foods,[38] and from eating when depleted or hungry to eating due to a variety of social, cultural, environmental, and/or physiological cues.[46] According to Birch and Fisher,[38] this transition from univore to omnivore is shaped by the infant's innate preference for sweet and salty tastes and the rejection of sour and bitter tastes,[47] and by the predisposition of infants and children to be neophobic or to reject new foods.[48] A child's experience with food and flavors is shaped beginning with the parents' decision to breastfeed or formula-feed.[38] Limited research indicates that breastfed infants eat more of new foods than formula-fed infants, which suggests that the varied flavors in breastmilk facilitate the breastfed infant's acceptance of new foods during the weaning period.[49]

Exposure to Food and Preschool Children's Food Preferences and Consumption

Table 8.18 includes three studies by Birch and colleagues[50-52] which indicate that preschool children's neophobia or rejection of new foods can be overcome by exposure. Results from

TABLE 8.18

Research Concerning Exposure to Food and Preschool Children's Food Preferences and Consumption

Reference	Authors and Year	Subjects	Study Design	Results
50	Birch and Marlin, 1982	14 two-year-olds	Each child received 2-20 exposures to 5 novel fruits or cheeses over 25-26 days	Later, children ate more of items with higher exposures when given pairs of items and asked to taste both and pick one to eat more of
51	Birch et al., 1987	43 children in 3 age groups: 26, 38, or 64 months old	Each child received 5, 10, or 15 exposures to 7 new fruits; asked to taste some and look at others	For all age groups, preferences increased significantly only when foods were tasted
52	Sullivan and Birch, 1990	39 children, 4-5 years old	Each child tasted 1 of 3 versions of tofu (sweetened, salty, or plain) 15 times over several weeks	Preferences increased with exposure regardless of added sugar, salt, or plain; 10 exposures needed

these studies indicate that preschool children's food preferences are learned through repeated exposure to foods.

Social Environment of Eating and Preschool Children's Food Preferences and Consumption

Although exposure and availability are necessary for children to learn to accept new foods, the social environment of eating is also important. Children learn about what to eat and why to eat, and receive reinforcements and incentives for eating from their families and the larger environment.[53] Most of this learning occurs during routine mealtime experiences, in the absence of formal teaching.[40] For example, adults who want children to eat healthful foods (e.g., vegetables) may bribe children with rewards for eating healthful foods. However, research indicates that such practices actually lead children to dislike the healthful foods, which is not what adults intend. The five studies[54-58] included in Table 8.19 indicate the importance of the social environment of eating and food contingencies (i.e., "if you eat __, then you can __") on preschool children's food preferences and consumption. Results from another study of influential factors of caregiver behavior at lunch in early child-care programs indicated that although caregivers believed they positively influenced children's eating behaviors, observed behaviors of caregivers at mealtimes were inconsistent with expert recommendations.[59]

Adult Influences on Preschool Children's Ability to Self-Regulate Caloric Intake

Infants are born with the ability to self-regulate their kcal intake by adjusting their formula intake when the kcal level of the formula changes[60] and when solid foods are added.[61] Preschool children are able to adjust the kcal eaten in a snack or meal, based on the kcal eaten in a preload snack.[62,63] Furthermore, preschool children are able to adjust the kcal eaten at various meals and snacks during the day so that the number of kcal consumed in a 24-hour period is relatively constant.[64] Although children have the ability to self-regulate their kcal intake, the two studies[65,66] included in Table 8.20 indicate that this ability may be negatively impacted by child-feeding practices that encourage or restrict children's eating. Using observations of family meal times, Klesges and colleagues[67] found that parental prompts, especially encouragements to eat, were highly correlated to preschool children's relative weight, and increased the probability that a child would eat. Furthermore, a child's refusal to eat usually led to a parental prompt to eat more food, whereas a child's food request was not likely to elicit either a parental prompt to eat or subsequent eating by the child.

According to Birch,[46] child feeding practices that encourage children to eat in response to external cues instead of internal cues regarding hunger and satiety "may form the basis for the development of individual differences in styles of intake control that exist among adults. Some of the problems of energy balance seen in adulthood may result from styles of intake control in which hunger and satiety cues are not particularly central." According to the American Dietetic Association,[30] "perhaps some of the best advice regarding child feeding practices continues to be the division of parental and child responsibility advocated by Satter." Satter advocates that parents (or adults) are responsible for presenting a variety of nutritious and safe foods to children at regular meal- and snack-times, as well as the physical and emotional setting of eating; children are responsible for deciding how much, if any, they will eat.[68,69]

TABLE 8.19

Research Concerning Social Environment of Eating and Preschool Children's Food Preferences and Consumption

Reference	Authors and Year	Subjects	Study Design	Results
54	Birch et al., 1980	64 children, 3-4 years old; 16 per context	Children given sweet or nonsweet foods (with initially neutral preferences) over several weeks in 1 of 4 contexts: 1) as reward for behavior, 2) paired with adult greeting, 3) as nonsocial behavior (put in child's locker), or 4) at snack time	Preferences increased when foods presented as rewards, or paired with adult greeting; effects lasted longer than 6 weeks after contexts ended; suggest positive social contexts can be used to increase preferences for foods not liked but more nutritious
55	Birch et al., 1982	12 children, 3-5 years old	Children told if they drank juice, then they could play	Instrumental ("if") use of juice reduced preferences for it
56	Birch et al., 1984	31 children, 3-5 years old	Children told if they drank milk drink, then they received verbal praise or a movie	Instrumental ("if") use of milk beverage reduced preferences for it
57	Newman and Taylor, 1992	86 children, 4-7 years old	Children told that if they ate one snack, then they could eat another snack (with both of neutral preference initially)	"If" snacks became less preferred and "then" snacks became more preferred
58	Hendy, 1999	64 preschool children	To encourage acceptance of 4 new fruits and vegetables during 3 preschool lunches, teachers used 1 of 5 actions: 1) choice-offering ("Do you want any of this?"), 2) reward (special dessert), 3) insisting children try one bite, 4) modeling by teacher, or 5) simple exposure	Choice-offering and reward were more effective than other actions; Hendy concluded that dessert rewards are not needed because the less expensive and more nutritious action of choice-offering works as well

Feeding Toddlers and Preschool Children

Young children cannot innately choose a well-balanced diet. They depend on adults to offer them a variety of nutritious and developmentally appropriate foods. A child's intake at individual meals may vary considerably, but the total daily caloric intake remains fairly constant.[64] Many parents become anxious about the adequacy of their young child's diet or frustrated with their child's unpredictable eating behavior which may include refusals

TABLE 8.20

Research Concerning Adult Influences on Preschool Children's Ability to Self-Regulate Caloric Intake

Reference	Authors and Year	Subjects	Study Design	Results
65	Birch et al., 1987	22 children, 4 years old	Flavored pudding preload of different kcal followed by ad lib snacks; children encouraged to focus on either internal cues (hunger, satiety) or external cues (time of day, amount left, rewards)	Only children encouraged to focus on internal cues showed sensitivity to kcal density of preload by decreasing kcal eaten in snack after preload that was high in kcal (and vice versa)
66	Johnson and Birch, 1994	77 children, 3-5 years old	Preload snacks of different kcal followed by ad lib foods; children's body fat measured; mothers completed questionnaire regarding their degree of control of what and how much their children ate	Children with greater body fat stores were less able to regulate kcal consumption in response to alterations in preload snacks; more controlling mothers had children who showed less ability to self-regulate ($r = 0.67$).

to eat certain foods, and food jags. Parents may resort to feeding tactics such as bribery, clean your plate rules, struggles, or short-order cooking to encourage their child to eat. A more healthful approach is Satter's division of feeding responsibility (see "Adult Influences on Preschool Children's Ability to Self-Regulate Caloric Intake" in this section). Table 8.21 contains suggestions for concerns parents commonly encounter when feeding young children. Table 8.22 contains healthful eating tips to use with young children.

Snacks

Most young children fare best when fed four to six times a day, due to their smaller stomach capacities and fluctuating appetites. Snacks should be considered minimeals by contributing to the total day's nutrient intake. Snacks generally accepted by many children include fresh fruit, cheese, whole-grain crackers, breads (e.g., bagels, tortilla), milk, raw vegetables, 100% fruit juices, sandwiches, peanut butter on crackers or bread, and yogurt.

Choking

Young children should always be watched while eating meals and snacks because they are at risk for choking on food. Children remain at risk for choking on food until around age four years when they can chew and swallow better. Foods most likely to cause problems include ones that are hard, round, and do not readily dissolve in saliva. Table 8.23 contains a list of foods that may cause choking, along with some tips to decrease young children's risk of choking. Any food can cause choking if the child is not supervised while eating, if the child runs while eating, or if too much food is stuffed in the mouth.

TABLE 8.21

Suggestions for Concerns Parents Commonly Encounter when Feeding Children

If a child refuses to try new foods

- Remember, this is normal! Continue to offer each new food twice per week for a total of 10-12 times.
- Serve a new food with familiar ones.
- Ask the child if s/he would like to try some of the new food, but avoid forcing or bribing the child to eat the new food. Be an effective role model and eat some of the new food yourself.
- Involve the child in shopping for and preparing the new food.

If a child refuses to eat what is served

- Remember, children may have strong likes and dislikes, but this does *not* mean they need to be served different foods than the rest of the family.
- Allow the child to choose from the foods available at a meal what s/he will eat, but avoid forcing or bribing him/her to eat.
- Include at least one food at each meal that you know your child will eat, but do not cater to a child's likes or dislikes. Avoid becoming a short-order cook. The less attention paid to this behavior, the better.

If a child is stuck on a food jag or wants to eat the same food over and over

- Children may want to eat only one or two foods day after day, meal after meal; common food jags occur with peanut butter and jelly sandwiches, pizza, macaroni and cheese, and dry cereal with milk.
- Relax, and realize this is normal and temporary. Refuse to call attention to the behavior.
- Continue to offer regular meal, but do not force or bribe the child to eat it.
- Serve the food jag item as you normally would (maybe once or twice a week).

If a child refuses to eat meat

- Tough meat is often difficult for children to chew. Offer bite-size pieces of tender, moist meat, poultry, or fish.
- Use meat in casseroles, meatloaf, soup, spaghetti sauce, pizza, or burritos.
- Try other high-protein foods such as eggs, beans, and peanut butter.

If a child refuses to drink milk

- Offer cheese, cottage cheese, yogurt, or pudding either alone or in combination dishes (such as macaroni and cheese, pizza, cheese sauce, banana pudding).
- Use milk when cooking hot cereals, scrambled eggs, macaroni and cheese, soup, and other recipes.
- Use calcium-fortified juices.

If a child refuses to eat vegetables and fruits

- Offer more fruits if a child refuses vegetables, and vice versa.
- Avoid over-cooking vegetables; serve vegetables steamed or raw (if appropriate). Include dips or sauces (e.g., applesauce with broccoli or carrots).
- Include vegetables in soups and casseroles.
- Continue to offer a variety of fruits and vegetables.

If a child eats too many sweets

- Avoid using sweets as a bribe or reward.
- Limit the purchase and preparation of sweet foods in the home.
- Incorporate sweets into meals instead of snacks for better dental health.
- Try using fruit as dessert.

Adapted from Lucas, B., Normal Nutrition from Infancy through Adolescence, *Handbook of Pediatric Nutrition*, Queen, P. M., Lang, C. E., Eds., Aspen, Gaithersburg, MD, 1993, pg 145.

TABLE 8.22

Healthful Eating Tips to Use with Young Children

Be Patient

Because young children are often afraid to try new foods...
- Offer a new food more than once; food may be accepted when it becomes familiar to the child.
- Offer new foods in small "try me" portions (one to two tablespoons) and let the child ask for more.
- Show the child how the rest of the family enjoys the new food.

Be a Planner

Most children need three regular meals plus one or two snacks each day.
- For breakfast and lunch, offer foods from three or more of the five pyramid food groups.
- For the main meal, offer foods from four or more of the five pyramid food groups.
- For snacks, offer foods from two or more of the five pyramid food groups. Make sure that snacks are not served too close to mealtime.

Be a Healthful Role Model

Remember, what you *do* can mean more than what you *say.*
Children learn about how and what to eat from routine eating experiences.
- Eat meals with children whenever possible.
- Try new foods and new preparation methods.
- Walk, run, and play with children instead of just watching them.

Be Adventurous

- Take children grocery shopping and let them choose a new vegetable or fruit from two or three choices.
- Have a weekly "family try-a-new-food" night.
- At home, allow children to help you wash and prepare food.

Be Creative

- Encourage children to invent a new snack or sandwich from three or four healthful ingredients you provide.
- Try a new bread or whole grain cracker.
- Talk about food groups in the new snack or sandwich, how they taste — smooth, crunchy, sweet, juicy, chewy, and how colorful the items are.

Adapted from *Tips for Using Food Guide Pyramid for Young Children*, USDA, Center for Nutrition Policy and Promotion, Washington, DC, 1999, Program Aid 1647.

Excessive Fruit Juice Consumption

Fruit juice, especially apple, is a common beverage for young children. Although fruit juice is a healthful, low-fat, nutritious beverage, there are some health concerns regarding excessive fruit juice consumption by young children. For example, drinking fruit juice helps fulfill nutrition recommendations to eat more fruits and vegetables. However, as children increase their intake of fruit juices, they may decrease their intake of milk,[70] which can decrease their intake of calcium unless the juice is calcium-fortified. This is a concern because results from the CSFII 1994–1996, 1998 indicated that only ~50% of children ages one to five years met the 1989 RDAs for calcium.[28] Carbohydrate malabsorption is common following the ingestion of several fruit juices in young children with chronic nonspecific diarrhea as well as in healthy young children.[71] In 1991, a policy statement by the Committee on Nutrition of the American Academy of Pediatrics recommended that parents be cautioned about young children's potential gastrointestinal problems associated with the ingestion of excessive amounts of juices containing sorbitol (e.g., apple, pear, and prune), which is a naturally occurring but nonabsorbable sugar alcohol.[72] Excess fruit juice

TABLE 8.23

Choking in Young Children

Foods that May Cause Choking in Young Children

- frankfurters (hot dogs)
- chunks of meat
- nuts and seeds
- peanut butter (spoonful)
- raisins
- whole grapes
- cherries with pits
- large pieces of fruit
- raw carrots or celery
- popcorn
- chips
- pretzels
- marshmallows
- round or hard candy

Tips to Decrease Young Children's Risk of Choking

- Cut frankfurters lengthwise into thin strips.
- Cook carrots or celery until slightly soft and then cut into sticks.
- Cut grapes or cherries into small pieces.
- Spread a thin layer of peanut butter on a cracker instead of allowing young children to eat peanut butter from a spoon.
- Insist that young children sit down while eating so they can concentrate on chewing and swallowing.
- Always watch young children while they eat meals and snacks.
- Discourage allowing a young child to eat in the car if the only adult present is driving because it may be difficult for the adult to quickly aide a choking child.

Adapted from *Tips for Using the Food Guide Pyramid for Young Children 2 to 6 Years Old*, USDA, Center for Nutrition Policy and Promotion, Washington, DC, 1999, Program Aid 1647.

consumption may present a contributing factor in nonorganic failure to thrive.[73] Drinking 12 or more fluid ounces of fruit juice per day is associated with short stature and with obesity in young children;[74] thus, it is recommended that parents and caretakers limit young children's consumption of fruit juice to less than 12 ounces per day.[70,74]

Low-Fat Diets

Emphasis regarding low-fat, low-cholesterol diets has increased during the past decade, as has the debate over whether low-fat diets are appropriate for children.[75-80] Parental concern about later atherosclerosis or obesity has led to failure to thrive in some infants age 7 to 22 months who were fed very low-fat, calorie-restricted diets.[81] The American Academy of Pediatrics Committee on Nutrition supports recommendations that children older than two years follow a diet with a maximum of 30% of calories from fat and no more than 300 mg of cholesterol per day.[9] (Ages two to five years represent a transition between the higher fat intake during infancy and the population-based recommended fat intake). Nonfat and low-fat milks are not recommended for use during the first two years of life.

The Special Turku coronary Risk factor Intervention Project for Babies (STRIP Baby Trial) evaluated the effects of a low-saturated fat diet on growth during the first three years of life in 1062 healthy infants who were randomized at age seven months into an intervention group (n = 540) or control group (n = 522).[82] The intervention consisted of individualized dietary counseling provided to parents at one- to six-month intervals to reduce risk factors to atherosclerosis. Results indicated that mean fat intake of children in both groups was lower than expected, especially during the first two years of life. The true mean of the height of intervention boys was at most 0.34 cm more or 0.57 cm less, and the weight was at most 0.19 kg more or 0.22 kg less than that of control boys. The respective values for girls were at most 0.77 cm more or 0.16 cm less and at most 0.42 kg more or 0.04 kg less.

Furthermore, there were similar numbers of slim children in both groups. The authors concluded that a supervised, low-saturated fat, low-cholesterol diet had no influence on growth of children in the study between 7 and 36 months of age.[82] Follow-up analyses were conducted on intervention and control children who were followed for more than two years (n = 848) to study the fat and energy intakes of children with different growth patterns. Results indicated that relative fat intakes (as percent of energy intake) were similar in children showing highly different height gain patterns. Furthermore, children with consistently low fat intake grew equally to the children with higher fat intake. The authors concluded that moderate supervised restriction of fat intake to values between 25 and 30% of kcal is compatible with normal growth in children ages 7 to 36 months.[83]

The safety and efficacy of lower fat diets in pubertal children have been indicated by results from the Dietary Intervention Study in Children (DISC). The three-year, six-center randomized controlled trial involved 663 children; at baseline, boys (n = 362) and girls (n = 301) had a mean age of 9.7 and 9.0 years, respectively.[84] An intervention group (n = 334) followed a diet with 28% of kcal from total fat, ~10% of kcal from saturated fat, and 95 mg/day of cholesterol. A comparable usual care group (n=329) consumed ~33% of kcal from total fat, ~12% of kcal from saturated fat, and 113 mg/day of cholesterol. The intervention group had significant but modestly lower levels of LDL-cholesterol and maintained a psychologic well-being; however, there were no differences in height, weight, or serum ferritin levels in the two groups. The authors concluded that a properly designed dietary intervention is effective in achieving modest lowering of LDL cholesterol levels over three years while maintaining adequate growth, iron stores, nutritional adequacy, and psychological well-being during the critical growth period of adolescence. Furthermore, "an important public health inference from the DISC results is that current dietary recommendations for healthy children, which are less restricted in total fat than the DISC diet, can be advocated safely, particularly when children are under health care that follows their growth and development."[84] Follow-up analyses were conducted to assess the relationship between energy intake from fat and anthropometric, biochemical, and dietary measures of nutritional adequacy and safety.[85] Results indicated that lower fat intakes during puberty were nutritionally adequate for growth and maintenance of normal levels of nutritional biochemical measures; furthermore, they were associated with beneficial effects on blood folate and hemoglobin. Lower fat diets were related to lower self-reported intakes of several nutrients (i.e., calcium, zinc, magnesium, phosphorus, vitamin B_{12}, thiamin, niacin, and riboflavin); however, no adverse effects were observed on blood biochemical measures of nutritional status. The authors concluded that "current public health recommendations for moderately lower fat intakes in children during puberty may be followed safely."[85]

Further evidence regarding the safety and efficacy of lower fat diets in upper elementary school children (third through fifth grades) has been provided by the Child and Adolescent Trial for Cardiovascular Health (CATCH), which is described more fully later in this section. Results from CATCH failed to indicate any evidence of deleterious effects of the three-year intervention on growth or development of children who were third-graders at the beginning of the intervention.[86]

Group Feeding

Many young children spend some or most days away from home in child care centers, preschools, Head Start programs, or home child care centers, where they may eat up to two meals and two snacks daily. Federal and state regulations or guidelines exist for food service in child care centers, Head Start programs, and preschool programs in public schools. Some centers participate in USDA-sponsored child nutrition programs. When choosing a child care center or preschool, parents should be encouraged to consider the feeding program, including food variety, quality, safety, cultural aspects, and developmental appropriateness. Peer pressure regarding food and eating among preschoolers is evident in a study by Birch which indicated that the food selections and eating behaviors of preschool children influenced the food preferences and eating behaviors of other preschool children.[87]

Portion Sizes

Portion sizes for young children are small, especially when compared with adult portions. A rule-of-thumb method is to initially offer one tablespoon of each food for every year of age for preschool children; more food may be provided according to appetite.

Limited research indicates the effects of portion size on children's food intake.[88] Sixteen younger (three years) and 16 older (five years) preschool children participated in three lunches during their usual lunchtime at day-care. Each lunch consisted of macaroni and cheese served in either small, medium, or large portion sizes, along with set portion sizes of carrot sticks, applesauce, and milk. Results indicated that older preschoolers consumed more macaroni and cheese when served the large portion compared to the small portion ($p<0.002$). However, portion sizes did not significantly affect food intake among younger preschoolers. These results indicate the important role of portion size in shaping children's dietary intake, and imply that portion size can either promote or prevent the development of overweight among older preschool children. Furthermore, these results indicate the importance of encouraging preschool children to focus on their own internal cues of hunger and satiety instead of "eating everything to clean the plate."[88]

Feeding School-Age Children

During the school-age years (ages 6-12), steady growth is paralleled by increased food intake. Although children tend to eat fewer times a day, after-school snacks are common. Studies indicate that eating breakfast is related positively to children's cognitive function and school performance, especially for undernourished children (for a review, see Reference 89). Specifically, schoolchildren who had fasted both overnight and in the morning, particularly children who were nutritionally at risk, demonstrated slower stimulus discrimination, increased errors, and slower memory recall.[90] According to Grantham-McGregor, "studies to date have provided insufficient evidence to determine whether children's long-term scholastic achievement is improved by eating breakfast daily."[91]

Although eating breakfast is important, research indicates that between 6 and 16% of elementary school children skip breakfast.[92-94] Furthermore, between 1965 and 1991, breakfast consumption declined significantly for each age group of children (1-4 years, 5-7 years, 8-10 years) and adolescents (11-14 years and 15-18 years), especially for older adolescents age 15-18 years; breakfast was consumed by 89.7% of boys and 84.4% of girls in 1965, and by 74.9 and 64.7%, respectively, in 1991.[95] Children who skip breakfast tend to have a lower kcal intake and consume fewer nutrients than children who eat breakfast.[92,93] During the upper elementary years, children may skip breakfast due to time constraints, because school starts early, due to the responsibility of getting themselves ready in the morning, or simply because they do not feel like eating. When breakfast nutrient consumption patterns of third graders were examined using baseline data from CATCH, 94% of the 1872 children from 96 public schools in four states reported eating breakfast on the day of the survey.[92] Of the 94% who ate breakfast, 80% ate at home, 13% ate at school, 3% ate at both home and school, and 4% ate breakfast elsewhere.

National School Lunch and Breakfast Programs

One in ten children gets two of their three major meals in school, and more than half get one of their three major meals in school.[96] The National School Lunch Program (NSLP) is a federally assisted meal program available in almost 99% of all public schools and to about 92% of all students in the country.[97] On a typical day, about 58% of the students to whom it is available participate. Regulations stipulate that a NSLP lunch provide one-third of the RDAs for kcal, protein, iron, calcium, and vitamins A and C. Schools may choose one of four systems for planning their menus; two options are based on a computerized nutritional analysis of the week's menu, and the other two options are based on minimum component quantities of meat or meat alternate, vegetables and fruits, grains and breads, and milk.[97]

The School Breakfast Program (SBP) is available to approximately half of the nation's students in more than 70,000 schools.[98] On a typical day, about 7.2 million children participate. Regulations stipulate that a SBP breakfast provide one-fourth of the RDAs for kcal, protein, iron, calcium, and vitamins A and C.[98]

Any child at a participating school may purchase a NSLP lunch or SBP breakfast. Children from families with incomes at or below 130% of the poverty level are eligible for free breakfasts and lunches. Those between 130 and 185% of the poverty level are eligible for reduced-price breakfasts and lunches. The federal government reimburses the schools for each breakfast and lunch that meets SBP and NSLP requirements, respectively.[97,98]

Impact of School Meals on Children's Dietary Intake

The School Nutrition Dietary Assessment Study (SNDAS) collected information on school meals from a nationally representative sample of schools (n=545) and 24-hour recalls from approximately 3350 students from these schools in spring, 1992.[99] Results from the SNDAS regarding dietary intakes of NSLP participants and nonparticipants[100] indicated that 1) NSLP participants had higher lunch intakes of vitamin A, calcium, and zinc, and lower intakes of vitamin C than nonparticipants who ate lunch; 2) NSLP participants' lunches provided a higher percentage of kcal from fat and saturated fat, and a lower percentage of carbohydrate than nonparticipants' lunches; 3) NSLP participants were more than twice as likely as nonparticipants to consume milk and milk products at lunch; and 4) NSLP participants also consumed more meat, poultry, fish, and meat mixtures than nonparticipants.

Results from the SNDAS regarding dietary intakes of SBP participants and nonparticipants[100] indicated that 1) SBP participants had higher average breakfast intakes of kcal, protein, and calcium, and derived a greater proportion of kcal from fat and saturated fat than nonparticipants; 2) SBP participants were three times more likely than nonparticipants to consume meat, poultry, fish, or meat mixtures at breakfast; and 3) SBP participants were also more likely than nonparticipants to consume milk or milk products at breakfast. The most surprising finding from the SNDAS was that the presence of the SBP in schools did not affect the likelihood that a student ate breakfast before starting school. Research is needed to determine the best ways to encourage elementary school students to consume healthful breakfasts. Universal school breakfast, which allows all students to eat school breakfast for free, has been advocated by some as a means to increase the percentage of children who eat breakfast. However, results from the SNDAS indicated that approximately 42% of children who were eligible for free or reduced price school breakfast did not eat it.[94] Perhaps scheduling the SBP for classes to eat as a part of regular school hours (similar to the NSLP) is needed to increase the percentage of children who eat breakfast.

Results from a study by Baranowski et al.[101] indicate the important contribution that school lunch makes in increasing children's consumption of fruits and vegetables. Differences in children's consumption of fruits and vegetables by meal and day of the week were assessed using seven-day food records completed by 2984 third-graders from 48 elementary schools in the Atlanta, Georgia area. Results indicated that fruits and vegetables were most frequently consumed at weekday lunch, and second most frequently at dinner. Participation in school lunch accounted for a substantial proportion of fruits and vegetables consumed at lunch. Few fruits and vegetables were consumed at breakfast or snack.[101]

Impact of Elementary Schools on Older Children's Food Preferences and Consumption Patterns

The impact of exposure and social environment on preschool children's food preferences and consumption is discussed earlier in this section. Limited research indicates that exposure to food also plays a role in older children's food preferences and consumption. Results from a study by Hearn et al.[102] indicated that availability and accessibility to fruits and vegetables (as assessed by telephone interviews with parents) was positively related to upper elementary school children's preferences and consumption. Furthermore, children ate more fruits and vegetables for lunch at schools that offered more fruits and vegetables for lunch.

Research with upper elementary school children indicates that they prefer vegetables less than fruits.[43,103,104] Results from focus groups with ~600 fourth- and fifth-grade students from Georgia, Alabama, and Minnesota indicate that children predominantly believe that vegetables taste "nasty"[104] and "if it's good for you, then it must taste bad"[103,104] which is related to statements made by adults such as "I don't care if they don't taste good; eat your vegetables because they're good for you."[104] Research concerning the influence of a variety of psychological and social factors on children's fruit and vegetable consumption indicates that preferences are the strongest predictors.[44,105] This implies that interventions that alter children's preferences for fruits and vegetables will be more effective in increasing their consumption than other strategies pursued to date. However, intensive school-based interventions designed to specifically increase children's preferences for fruits and vegetables have had limited success.[32,106,107] Furthermore, although some elementary school programs have helped children to improve their dietary intake,[108] intensive interventions specifically designed to increase children's fruit and vegetable consumption have had only limited success.[32,106,107,109-111] Finally, schools may represent a potentially useful setting for preventing childhood obesity, but comprehensive elementary school programs in the U.S. such as CATCH and Know Your Body have not had major effects on children's body weight.[108,112,113] Perhaps the limited success of elementary school-based interventions to date to increase children's preferences for and consumption of fruits and vegetables, and to help prevent childhood obesity is because the interventions have not attempted to educate school staff and parents about how their behaviors impact children's food preferences and consumption patterns.

Children have acquired knowledge about eating and have developed food preferences by the time they enter school; however, their food preferences and consumption patterns are continually modified because they eat daily.[114] More than 95% of children in the U.S. are enrolled in school, where they may eat one or two meals per school day.[115] Thus, elementary schools play a critical role in shaping children's food acceptance patterns and can therefore help to improve their diet.[116] No other public institution has as much continuous and intensive contact with children during their first two decades of life than public schools.[113] Elementary school staff have a greater potential influence on a child's health than any other group outside of the home.[117] School-based programs offer a systematic and efficient means to improve the health of youth in America by promoting positive lifestyles.[118] Health promotion programs in elementary schools have the potential to help prevent chronic diseases in U.S. adults.[117] Although school-based health programs may promote healthful lifestyles, classroom lessons are not sufficient to produce lasting changes in students' eating behaviors.[53] In fact, curriculum-based nutrition education in schools has had minimal effects on student's eating behavior.[119] Children's food preferences and consumption are influenced by the elementary school environment through familiarity and reinforcement.[120] Students of public elementary schools generally attend for 7 hours a day, 180 days a year. Although students have options for obtaining food in schools, the most prominent federally supported programs are the SBP and the NSLP.

Elementary school breakfast and lunch menus typically follow a cycle that repeats several times during the school year; thus, children are provided with repeated exposures to healthful foods (e.g., fruits and vegetables).[121] However, elementary schools also provide children with repeated exposures to other foods (e.g., candy and pizza) which are used by school staff as rewards.[53,122-124] Unfortunately, the social context in which vegetables are often offered at school (e.g., "If you eat your peas, then you can eat your cookie") probably negatively affects preferences for them, thereby potentially decreasing their consumption.[121] However, the social context in which candy and pizza are offered probably positively affects preferences for those foods, thereby potentially increasing their consumption.[121] These repeated exposures to vegetables and foods such as candy and pizza in negative and positive social contexts, respectively, provide the associative learning that help children develop food consumption patterns that are inconsistent with nutrition guidelines[40] which recommend increased intake of vegetables but moderation in sugar and fat intake.[10,29,125,126] In addition, school staff often encourage children to finish all of their food, regardless of whether or not the children are still hungry,[122] which encourages children to disregard their own feelings of hunger and satiety.

Concern regarding the impact of school staff on children's food preferences and consumption patterns has been voiced by several government and professional groups. According to the Centers for Disease Control and Prevention,[116] students need exposure to healthful foods as well as the support of people around them, and teachers need to be discouraged from using food for disciplining or rewarding students. According to the American Dietetic Association, "... the nutrition goals of the National School Lunch Program and School Breakfast Program should be supported and extended through school district policies that create an overall school environment with learning experiences that enable students to develop lifelong, healthful eating habits."[127] Furthermore, the American Dietetic Association recommends that school meals be served in an environment that encourages their acceptance,[128] or a setting and atmosphere that encourages their consumption,[127] which may be interpreted to mean an environment that avoids the use of food contingencies. A joint statement by the American Dietetic Association, Society for Nutrition Education, and the American School Food Service Association indicates that schools are to be healthful environments where the cafeteria and food-related policy allow students the opportunity to make healthful food choices and provide them with models of healthful food practices.[129]

Considerable research has been conducted concerning the impact of exposure and the social context of eating on preschool children's food preferences, consumption, self-regulation of intake, and adiposity. However, research of this type is needed with older children. According to Hill and Trowbridge,[39] insights gained from research concerning children's food preferences and consumption patterns "can assist in developing interventions to improve child-feeding practices, which may lead to development of healthier eating patterns." Parents and school staff need to expose children to healthful foods, provide opportunities for children to learn to like rather than dislike healthful foods, encourage children to respect their own feelings of hunger and satiety, and reduce the extent to which learning and experience potentiate children's liking for high-sugar and/or high-fat foods.[130] Interventions to increase children's consumption of foods consistent with nutrition guidelines and to prevent childhood obesity must educate adults about their role in the development of children's food preferences and consumption patterns, specifically exposure to food, the social context of eating (e.g., food rewards and contingencies), and adult influences on children's ability to self-regulate caloric intake. Table 8.24 provides five practical applications for adults to use when feeding children.

TABLE 8.24

Five Practical Applications for Adults to Use when Feeding Children

- Offer a variety of healthful foods in a positive environment at regular meal and snack times.
- Instead of requiring children to finish all of their food, encourage them to respect their own feelings of hunger and satiety. Use choice-offering statements such as "If you're still hungry, there's more ___" or "If you're full, then you don't have to eat any more."
- To help children learn to eat a variety of foods, continue to offer new foods even if a new food is initially rejected. Ten to 12 exposures at two per week may be needed before a child learns to accept a new food.
- To encourage children to eat or to try new foods, use choice-offering statements such as "Would you like to try/taste your ___?" Avoid rewarding or bribing children for eating. Also, avoid using food contingencies (e.g., "If you eat your ___, then you can ___.")
- Instead of using food as a reward, use non-food items such as stickers or a token economy (e.g., wherein tokens are exchanged for tangible non-food rewards such as shoe laces, wrist bands, play time).

Childhood Obesity

Overwhelming evidence indicates that the incidence of obesity among children and adolescents has increased dramatically during the last three decades.[36,37] According to Dietz, "obesity is now the most prevalent nutritional disease of children and adolescents in the United States."[131] Critical periods during the childhood years for the development of obesity include the period of adiposity rebound that occurs between five and seven years of age, and adolescence.[131] The causes of childhood obesity are multifactorial, including both genetics and environment. Inactivity appears to play a major role in the increasing rate of childhood obesity, as does television viewing. Results from the Third National Health and Nutrition Examination Survey indicated that children ages 8 to 16 years who watched four or more hours of television each day had greater body fat and greater body mass index than children who watched television less than two hours each day.[132] With the advances in technology, especially regarding computers, more children are spending more hours in sedentary states. Preventing childhood obesity is more desirable than trying to treat obesity during adolescence and adulthood. One critical component of obesity prevention is increased physical activity; another is educating adults regarding the development of children's food preferences and food consumption patterns. The topic of childhood obesity is covered thoroughly in Section 70.

Influences from Peers and Media

Children's food preferences and consumption patterns can be altered either positively or negatively by peers and the media. For example, results from the Third National Health and Nutrition Examination Survey indicated that approximately 26% of U.S. children ages 8 to 16 years watched four or more hours of television each day, and that as hours of television viewing increased, so did body fat and body mass index.[132] Unfortunately, research indicates that food advertisements aired during children's Saturday morning television programming are generally contrary to nutrition recommendations.[133]

Sugar and Aspartame

Although there are widespread beliefs that both sugar (i.e., sucrose) and aspartame produce hyperactivity and other behavioral problems in children, both dietary challenge and dietary replacement studies have demonstrated that sugar has little if any adverse effects on behavior.[134] For example, Wolraich et al.[135] conducted a double-blind controlled trial with 25 normal preschool children and 23 school-age children who were described by their parents as sensitive to sugar. The different diets that children and their families followed for each of three consecutive three-week periods were either high in sucrose, aspartame, or saccharin (placebo). Children's behavior and cognitive performance were evaluated weekly. Results strongly indicated that even when intake exceeded typical dietary levels, neither sucrose nor aspartame had discernible cognitive or behavioral effects in normal preschool children or in school-age children who were believed to be sensitive to sugar. Furthermore, the few differences associated with the ingestion of sucrose were more consistent with a slight calming effect than with hyperactivity.[135] Results from a 1995 meta-analytic synthesis of 16 reports containing 23 controlled double-blind challenge studies found that sugar did not affect the behavior or cognitive performance of children; however, a small effect of sugar or effects on subsets of children could not be ruled out.[136]

According to Kanarek,[134] the strong belief of parents, educators, and medical professionals that sugar has adverse effects on children's behavior may be attributed to several factors. First, adults may misconceive the relationship between sugar and behavior. Children in general have difficulty altering their behavior in response to changing environmental conditions, such as shifting from the unstructured nature of a party or snack time at school to the more rigorous demands of classwork. If the party or snack included foods with a high sugar content, adults may relate the child's sugar intake with behavioral problems as the child tries to adapt from an unstructured activity to one with structure. Second, sugar-containing foods such as candy are often forbidden or given to children in very limited amounts; the prohibited nature of these foods may contribute to the belief which associates them with increased activity. Finally, expectations of both adults and children could promote the idea that sugar leads to hyperactivity. Children hear adults comment that "too much sugar makes children hyper" and children believe them and act accordingly to fulfill the prophecy.[134]

Although experimental evidence fails to indicate that sugar affects children's behavior and cognition, children should not have unlimited access to sugar, because undernutrition may occur if foods with essential nutrients are replaced by kcal from sugar; furthermore, sugar (and starch) can promote tooth decay. On the Food Guide Pyramid,[18] sweets are located at the tip along with fats and oils, indicating that these foods should be used sparingly. According to the Dietary Guidelines for Americans,[10] the diet should be moderate in sugars, especially if kcal needs are low. The position of the American Dietetic

Association regarding the use of nutritive and nonnutritive sweeteners[137] is that "consumers can safely enjoy a range of nutritive and nonnutritive sweeteners when consumed in moderation and within the context of a diet consistent with the Dietary Guidelines for Americans."

Feeding Adolescents

Characteristics of Food Habits of Adolescents

Adolescents often experience newly found independence, busy schedules, searches for self-identification, dissatisfaction with body image, difficulty accepting existing values, and a desire for peer acceptance. Each of these events may help explain changes in food habits of adolescents. Common characteristics of food habits of adolescents include an increased tendency to skip meals (especially breakfast and lunch), eating more meals outside the home, increased snacking (especially on candy), consumption of fast foods, and dieting.[138]

Insight regarding adolescents' perceptions about factors influencing their food choices and eating behaviors was provided from focus groups with 141 seventh- or tenth-graders (40% white, 25% Asian-American, 21% African-American, 7% multiracial, 6% Hispanic, 1% Native American) from two urban schools in St. Paul, Minnesota.[139] Factors identified by the adolescents as being most influential on their food choices included hunger and food cravings, appeal of food (primarily taste), time considerations of themselves and their parents, and convenience of food. Factors identified by the adolescents to be of secondary importance included food availability, parental influences on eating behavior (including the family's culture or religion), perceived benefits of food (e.g., for health, energy, body shape), and situational factors (e.g., place, time). Additional factors discussed included mood, body image concerns, habit, cost, media influences, and vegetarian lifestyle choices. A sense of urgency about personal health in relation to other concerns, and taste preferences for other foods were major barriers to eating more fruits, vegetables, and dairy products and eating fewer high-fat foods. Suggestions provided by the adolescents to help adolescents eat a more healthful diet included making healthful food taste and look better, making healthful food more available and convenient, limiting the availability of unhealthful options, teaching them good eating habits at an early age, and changing social norms to make it "cool" to eat healthfully. These results suggest that if interventions to improve adolescent nutrition are to be effective, they need to have adolescent input and address a broad range of factors, especially environmental factors (e.g., increased availability and promotion of appealing, convenient foods in homes, schools, and restaurants).[139]

The Minnesota Adolescent Health Survey (MAHS) was completed by more than 30,000 adolescents from 1986 through 1987. The MAHS was a comprehensive assessment of adolescent health status, health behaviors, and psychosocial factors; although it included relatively few nutrition-related items, a wealth of knowledge about adolescent nutrition was gained. Neumark-Sztainer et al. summarized the knowledge learned from a decade of subsequent analyses of data collected in the MAHS, as well as implications for working with youth.[140] Major concerns identified included overweight status, unhealthful weight-control practices, and high prevalence rates of inadequate intakes of fruits, vegetables, and dairy products. Risk factors for inadequate food intake patterns or unhealthful weight-control practices included low socioeconomic status, minority status, chronic illness, poor school achievement, low family connectedness, weight dissatisfaction, overweight, homosexual orientation among boys, and use of health-compromising behaviors. The results suggest a need for innovative outreach strategies that include educational and environmental approaches to improve adolescent eating behaviors. A critical issue that needs to be addressed is the validity of adolescents' self-reported behaviors.[140]

Youth Risk Behavior Surveillance — United States, 1997

The Youth Risk Behavior Surveillance System (YRBSS) monitors six categories of priority health-risk behaviors among high school youth in grades 9 through 12.[141] In 1997, as part of the YRBSS, the Centers for Disease Control and Prevention conducted a national school-based Youth Risk Behavior Survey (YRBS) that resulted in 16,262 questionnaires completed by students in 151 schools. Table 8.25 provides an overview of results from the YRBS for dietary behaviors including fruit and vegetable consumption, fat consumption, perceived overweight, attempted weight loss, laxative use or vomiting, diet pill use, dieting, and exercising to either lose weight or keep from gaining it.[141]

TABLE 8.25

Results Regarding Dietary Behaviors from the Youth Risk Behavior Survey, United States, 1997

Dietary Behavior	Percentage of Students*
Ate five or more servings of fruits and vegetables (defined as fruit, fruit juice, green salad, or cooked vegetables) during day prior to survey:	
Overall	29
Boys	32[a]
Girls	26[a]
Ate two or fewer servings of foods typically high in fat content (defined as hamburgers, hot dogs, or sausage; french fries or potato chips; and cookies, doughnuts, pie, or cake) during day prior to survey:	
Overall	62
Girls	71[a]
Boys	56[a]
Hispanics	64[b]
Whites	63[b]
Blacks	55[b]
White girls	73[c]
Black girls	63[c]
Hispanic boys	60[d]
Black boys	47[d]
Girls in grade 12	77[e]
Girls in grade 9	65[e]
Boys in grade 12	59[f]
Boys in grade 10	52[f]
Boys in grade 11	61[g]
Boys in grade 9	50[g]
Boys in grade 10	52[g]
Considered themselves overweight:	
Overall	27
Girls	34[a]
Boys	22[a]
Hispanics	30[b]
Blacks	24[b]
Hispanic boys	27[c]
White boys	22[c]
Black boys	15[c]
Tried to lose weight during the 30 days preceding the survey:	
Overall	40
Girls	60[a]
Boys	23[a]

TABLE 8.25 *(Continued)*

Results Regarding Dietary Behaviors from the Youth Risk Behavior Survey, United States, 1997

Dietary Behavior	Percentage of Students*
Hispanics	46[b]
Blacks	36[b]
White girls	62[c]
Hispanic girls	61[c]
Black girls	51[c]
Hispanic boys	33[d]
White boys	22[d]
Black boys	20[d]
Used laxatives or vomited during the 30 days preceding the survey to lose weight or keep from gaining it:	
Overall	5
Girls	8[a]
Boys	2[a]
Hispanics	7[b]
Whites	4[b]
Hispanic girls	10[c]
Black girls	6[c]
Black boys	4[d]
White boys	2[d]
Used diet pills during the 30 days preceding the survey to lose weight or keep from gaining it:	
Overall	5
Girls	8[a]
Boys	2[a]
Dieted to either lose weight or keep from gaining it during the 30 days preceding the survey:	
Overall	30
Girls	46[a]
Boys	18[a]
Hispanics	33[b]
Whites	30[b]
Blacks	25[b]
White girls	48[c]
Hispanic girls	46[c]
Black girls	34[c]
Hispanic boys	23[d]
White boys	17[d]
Black boys	16[d]
Exercised to either lose weight or keep from gaining it during the 30 days preceding the survey:	
Overall	52
Girls	65[a]
Boys	40[a]
Hispanics	56[b]
Whites	52[b]
Blacks	44[b]
White girls	70[c]
Hispanic girls	65[c]
Black girls	49[c]
Hispanic boys	48[d]
White boys	39[d]
Black boys	38[d]

* Percentages with the same letter within a dietary behavior are significantly different.

Adapted from Kann, L., Kinchen, S. A., Williams, B. I., et al, *Youth Risk Behavior Surveillance - United States, 1997,* In CDC Surveillance Summaries, MMWR 47 (No. SS-3), 1998; available at http://www.cdc.gov/.

Health Behaviour in School-Aged Children: A WHO Cross-National Study International Report, 1997–1998

The Health Behaviour in School-Aged Children Study is a unique cross-national research study conducted in collaboration with the World Health Organization (WHO) Regional Office for Europe.[142] The first survey was carried out in 1983–1984; since 1985, surveys have been conducted at four-year intervals in a growing number of countries. The study looks at 11-, 13-, and 15-year old children's attitudes and experiences concerning a wide range of health related behaviors and lifestyle issues. The 1997–1998 survey included more than 123,227 children from 26 European countries and regions, Canada, and the U.S. The 1997–1998 sample of children from the U.S. included 5168 children; of these, there were 2395 boys and 2774 girls, 1558 11-year-olds, 1803 13-year-olds, and 1808 15-year-olds. Results indicated that for the most part, U.S. children were less likely to have a good diet than were children in other countries. Specifically, U.S. children were less likely to eat fruit and vegetables each day than were children in the majority of other countries. Children in the U.S. were more likely to eat potato chips and french fries every day, as well as sweets or chocolate, than were children in most other countries. Children in the U.S. ranked among the top three or four countries for consuming soft drinks every day. For all countries, boys were more likely to drink more milk and eat more junk foods and fried foods, and girls were more likely to eat fruit and vegetables each day. However, fruit and vegetable consumption decreased with age. Concerns about body size and dieting behavior increased with age for girls in all countries, but decreased for boys. Children in the U.S. were more likely than children in any other country to report that they were dieting or should be on a diet (47, 53, and 62% of 11-, 13-, and 15-year-old U.S. girls, respectively, and 34, 33, and 29% of 11-, 13-, and 15-year-old U.S. boys, respectively). For all countries, children with mothers or fathers with high socioeconomic status had the highest levels of daily consumption of healthy food items, and those with mothers or fathers whose status was low had the highest daily consumption of less nutritious food items. These results emphasize important relationships between age, gender, country, and socioeconomic status on food intake and dieting habits.[142]

Feeding Adolescents at School

Some research regarding feeding adolescents at school has been conducted. For example, one study surveyed 2566 adolescents in grades 6, 7, and 8 (which covers ages 10 to 15 years) to assess their perceptions of school food service and nutrition programs.[143] Results indicated that the top predictors of satisfaction were school menus which include food that students like, quality of the food choices, and prices that are acceptable for what students get. Girls were more satisfied with school-prepared foods than boys, perhaps because girls mature faster than boys during these years, which may be reflected as willingness to try new foods at an earlier age. Sixth-grade students were more satisfied than either seventh- or eighth-grade students. This may be because as adolescents move into the early teenage years, they become more independent from their parents and begin making their own decisions instead of eating school meals because their parents want or expect them to do so.[143]

Another study examined the effects of pricing strategies on sales of fruits and vegetables with adolescents in two high schools (1431 students at one urban school and 1935 students at the other suburban school).[144] Fruit, carrot, and salad purchases were monitored in each school cafeteria during an initial baseline period. Next, prices for these items were reduced by 50%, and sales were monitored. Finally, prices were returned to baseline, and sales were monitored for an additional three weeks. Results indicated that even though promotion was minimal, lower pricing significantly increased sales for fruit and carrots but not salads among high school students. However, the magnitude of the intervention effects differed by school, which suggests that contextual factors (e.g., packaging, display) may modify pricing effects. These results imply that adolescents can be encouraged to select fruits and vegetables when the prices of these items are lowered, and that this may occur without measurable changes in the overall a la carte sales revenue or the number of meal pattern customers, which are both important considerations for school food service revenues.[144]

Caffeine

Caffeine is a stimulant for the central nervous system; it tends to decrease drowsiness and reduce the sense of fatigue, but too much can cause palpitations, stomach upset, insomnia, and anxiety. Its effects vary among individuals, depending on the amount ingested, body size of the individual, and personal tolerance. Some people are able to build up a tolerance to caffeine through regular use; others are more sensitive to it. If someone who has regularly consumed caffeine suddenly stops using it, mild withdrawal symptoms (e.g., headaches, craving for caffeine) may occur. Substantial amounts of caffeine are found in several soft drinks, coffee, tea, and some pain relievers; smaller amounts are found in chocolate and foods with cocoa. Consumption of caffeine increases during adolescence with greater intakes of soft drinks, tea, and coffee. This can be a concern because caffeine has a modest negative impact on calcium retention, yet consumption of milk and other foods high in calcium decreases as children get older.[25,28] Furthermore, the stimulating effect of caffeine may set the stage for needing stimulation; although caffeine is classified as a drug, society is very accepting of this stimulant and has not considered it a nuisance.[145]

Vegetarian Diets

During the adolescent years, when there is increased independence and decision making and greater influence by peers and role models, vegetarian diets may be relatively common. There is considerable variation in the eating patterns of vegetarians. For the lacto-ovo-vegetarian, the eating pattern is based on grains, vegetables, fruits, legumes, seeds, nuts, dairy products, and eggs; meat, fish, and poultry are excluded. For the vegan, or total vegetarian, the eating pattern is similar to the lacto-ovo-vegetarian pattern except for the additional exclusion of eggs, dairy, and other animal products. However, considerable variation may exist in the extent to which animal products are avoided within both of these patterns.[146]

According to the American Dietetic Association, "well-planned vegan and lacto-ovo-vegetarian diets are appropriate for all stages of the life cycle, including pregnancy and lactation."[146] Appropriately planned vegan and lacto-ovo-vegetarian diets satisfy nutrient needs of infants, children, and adolescents and promote normal growth.[147] Dietary deficiencies are more common in populations with very restrictive diets. All vegan children need a reliable source of vitamin B_{12}; in addition, vitamin D supplements or fortified foods should be used if sun exposure is limited. Emphasis should be placed on foods rich in calcium, iron, and zinc. Vegetarian children can be helped to meet energy needs through frequent meals and snacks, as well as the use of some refined foods and foods higher in fat.[146] Section 40 contains additional information regarding vegetarian diets.

Eating Disorders

Anorexia nervosa and bulimia may affect about one million adolescents. Eating disorders are thought to occur for a variety of reasons which include poor self-concept, pressure to be thin, body shape and size, depression, and biological errors in organ function or structure. Up to 10% of these adolescents may die prematurely as a result of eating disorders.[145] Most eating disorder patients develop the problem during adolescence; however, it may be difficult to distinguish an adolescent with "normal" eating habits from one with an eating disorder, due to some of the psychologic changes which occur during adolescence.[6] More information regarding eating disorders may be found in Section 68.

Teen Pregnancy

Nutrient needs rise considerably during pregnancy; for adolescents who are pregnant, nutritional considerations are paramount, especially if they are still growing. For adolescent girls, linear growth typically is not completed until approximately four years after the onset of menarche. Some indication of physiologic maturity and growth potential may be obtained from gynecologic age, which is the difference between chronologic age and age at menarche. A young adolescent girl (i.e., gynecologic age of two years or less) who becomes pregnant may still be growing; thus, her nutrient requirements must meet her own needs for growth and development, as well as the extra demands of fetal growth.[6] Eating habits of adolescents (e.g., skipped meals, increased snacking, consumption of fast foods, and dieting) create a health risk for pregnant adolescents because during pregnancy, nutritional needs for the fetus are met before needs of the mother.[145] Adolescents who are pregnant should be cautioned against skipping meals, especially breakfast, because skipping meals may increase the risk of ketosis.[138] More information regarding teen pregnancy may be found in Section 5.

Health Promotion and Disease Prevention

Healthy People 2010 Nutrition Objectives for Children and Adolescents

Table 8.26 includes Healthy People 2010 nutrition objectives, as well as dental objectives related to nutrition, for children and adolescents.[126] The nutrition objectives address reducing weight, reducing growth retardation, improving eating behavior (e.g., increasing consumption of fruit, vegetables, grain products, and calcium products; decreasing consumption of fat, saturated fat, and sodium), reducing iron deficiency, and improving meals and snacks at school. The dental objectives related to nutrition address dental caries, untreated dental decay, and school-based health centers with oral health components.

"5 A Day for Better Health" Program

The national "5 A Day for Better Health" Program was instituted in 1991 to encourage Americans to eat five or more servings of fruits and vegetables every day. The program is a public-private partnership between the National Cancer Institute (NCI) and the Produce for Better Health Foundation (a nonprofit foundation representing the fruit and vegetable industry); it includes retail, media, community, and research components.[148] At

TABLE 8.26

Healthy People 2010 Nutrition Objectives for Children and Adolescents

19-3. Reduce the proportion of children and adolescents who are overweight or obese (defined as at or above the gender- and age-specific 95th percentile of BMI).

Objective	Reduction in Overweight or Obese Children and Adolescents*	2010 Target	1988–1994 Baseline
19-3a.	Children and adolescents aged 6 to 11 years	5%	11%
19-3b.	Children and adolescents aged 12 to 19 years	5%	10%
19-3c.	Children and adolescents aged 6 to 19 years	5%	11%

* Defined as at or above the gender- and age-specific 95th percentile of BMI based on the revised CDC growth charts for the U.S.

19-4. Reduce growth retardation (defined as height-for-age below the fifth percentile in the age-gender appropriate population using the 1977 NCHS/CDC growth charts) among low-income children under age 5 years.
Target: 5% Baseline: 8%

19-5. Increase the proportion of persons age 2 years and older who consume at least two daily servings of fruit.
Target: 75% Baseline: 28%

19-6. Increase the proportion of persons age 2 years and older who consume at least three daily servings of vegetables, with at least one-third being dark green or orange vegetables.
Target: 50% Baseline: 3%

19-7. Increase the proportion of persons age 2 years and older who consume at least six daily servings of grain products, with at least three being whole grains.
Target: 50% Baseline: 7%

19-8. Increase the proportion of persons age 2 years and older who consume less than 10 percent of calories from saturated fat.
Target: 75% Baseline: 36%

19-9. Increase the proportion of persons age 2 years and older who consume no more than 30 percent of calories from total fat.
Target: 75% Baseline: 33%

19-10. Increase the proportion of persons age 2 years and older who consume 2400 mg or less of sodium daily (from foods, dietary supplements, tap water, and salt use at the table).
Target: 65% Baseline: 21%

19-11. Increase the proportion of persons aged two years and older who meet dietary recommendations for calcium (based on consideration of calcium from foods, dietary supplements, and antacids).
Target: 75% Baseline: 46%

19-12. Reduce iron deficiency among young children and females of childbearing age.

Objective	Reduction in Iron Deficiency*	2010 Target	1988-1994 Baseline
19-12a.	Children age 1 to 2 years	9%	5%
19-12b.	Children age 3 to 4 years	1%	4%
19-12c.	Nonpregnant females age 12 to 49 years	7%	11%

* Iron deficiency is defined as having abnormal results for two or more of the following tests: serum ferritin concentration, erythrocyte protoporphyrin, or transferrin saturation.

19-15. (Developmental) Increase the proportion of children and adolescents aged 6 to 19 years whose intake of meals and snacks at school contributes to good overall dietary quality.

21-1. Reduce the proportion of children and adolescents who have dental caries experience in their primary or permanent teeth.

Objective	Reduction of Dental Caries in Primary and/or Permanent Teeth	2010 Target	1988–1994 Baseline
21-1a.	Young children	11%	18%
21-1b.	Children	42%	52%
21-1c.	Adolescents	51%	61%

TABLE 8.26 *(Continued)*

Healthy People 2010 Nutrition Objectives for Children and Adolescents

21-2. Reduce the proportion of children, adolescents, and adults with untreated dental decay.

Objective	Reduction of Untreated Dental Decay	2010 Target	1988-1994 Baseline
21-2a.	Young children	9%	16%
21-2b.	Children	21%	29%
21-2c.	Adolescents	15%	20%

21-13. (Developmental) Increase the proportion of school-based health centers with an oral health component.

Adapted from US Department of Health and Human Services, *Healthy People 2010*, 2nd ed., US Government Printing Office, Superintendent of Documents, Washington, DC, November, 2000. Available online at http://www.health.gov/healthypeople (accessed July 30, 2001).

the beginning of the program in 1991, a baseline survey with adults indicated that only 23% reported consuming five or more daily servings of fruits and vegetables.[149] The NCI funded nine studies in the spring of 1993 to develop, implement, and evaluate interventions in specific community channels to increase the consumption of fruits and vegetables in specific target populations; four of the nine projects used school-based programs to target children or adolescents.[150] Of these four projects, one targeted fourth-grade students and their parents,[110] two targeted fourth- and fifth-grade students,[106,109] and one targeted high school students.[111] Although all four interventions increased daily consumption of fruits and vegetables, the increases were small for three interventions and ranged from 0.2 servings for "Gimme 5 Fruit, Juice, and Vegetables for Fun and Health" in Georgia,[106] 0.4 servings for "Gimme 5: A Fresh Nutrition Concept for Students" in New Orleans,[111] and 0.6 servings for "5 A Day Power Plus" in Minnesota.[109] Increases were larger, at 1.4 servings for "High Five" in Alabama, possibly because classroom lessons were delivered by trained curriculum coordinators instead of classroom teachers.[110] Perhaps the limited success of school-based interventions to date is because they have not attempted to educate school staff about how their behaviors impact children's food acceptance patterns as discussed earlier.

Child Nutrition and Health Campaign

Launched in October, 1995, the Child Nutrition and Health Campaign is sponsored by the American Dietetic Association/Foundation, Kellogg Company, and National Dairy Council.[151] The campaign focuses on five major objectives:

1. Convene a nationally recognized panel of experts on child nutrition to address the nutritional needs of children, provide leadership to the campaign, and guide the development of messages for the campaign.
2. Educate parents, children, and health care professionals about the links among healthful childhood nutrition, classroom performance, and health during the adult years.
3. Publicize the important roles of high-carbohydrate, low-fat breakfast foods and healthful snacks for children's nutrition.
4. Fund research on the behavioral aspects of achieving healthful nutrition in children and on the development of lifelong healthful eating habits.
5. Launch a multi-year, multifaceted campaign to improve children's nutrition and health and to build strategic coalitions to spread the messages of the campaign.[151]

Five papers which review the scientific literature regarding links between nutrition and cognition have been published.[12,35,89,152,153] An intensive media program was developed to bring three key messages to various audiences through publications, public service announcements, news releases, consumer education activities, professional kits, and a video. The three key messages are: 1) give children a healthy start to their day, 2) get children (and adults) moving for the fun of it, and 3) grownups: be a role model.[151]

USDA School Meals Initiative for Healthy Children and Team Nutrition

The USDA School Meals Initiative (SMI) for Healthy Children underscores the national health responsibility to provide children with school meals consistent with the Dietary Guidelines for Americans and current scientific nutrition recommendations; the vision of the SMI is to "improve the health and education of children through better nutrition."[154] Team Nutrition was established by USDA as a nationwide integrated initiative to help implement the SMI; the goal of Team Nutrition is to "improve the health and education of children by creating innovative public and private partnerships that promote food choices for a healthful diet through the media, schools, families, and the community." Team Nutrition exists to empower schools in all 50 states to serve meals that meet the Dietary Guidelines for Americans, and to teach and motivate children in grades pre-kindergarten through 12 to make healthy eating choices. The four Dietary Guidelines for Americans that Team Nutrition focuses on are 1) eat a variety of foods, 2) eat more fruits, vegetables and grains, 3) eat lower fat foods more often, and 4) be physically active. Helping every child in the nation to have the opportunity to learn how to eat for good health is made possible by extensive, strategic public-private partnerships and approximately 300 Team Nutrition Supporters who represent all of the industries that touch children's lives, including nutrition and health, education, food and agriculture, consumer, media and technology, and government.[154] Table 8.27 lists common values shared by supporters of Team Nutrition.

TABLE 8.27

Common Values Shared by Supporters of Team Nutrition

- Children should be empowered to make food choices that reflect the Dietary Guidelines for Americans.
- Good nutrition and physical activity are essential to children's health and educational success.
- School meals that meet the Dietary Guidelines for Americans should appeal to children and taste good.
- Programs must build upon the best science, education, communication and technical resources available.
- Public/private partnerships are essential to reaching children to promote food choices for a healthful diet.
- Messages to children should be age appropriate and delivered in a language they speak, through media they use, in ways that are entertaining and actively involve them in learning.
- The focus should be on positive messages regarding food choices children can make.
- It is critical to stimulate and support action and education at the national, state, and local levels to successfully change children's eating behaviors.

From http://www.fns.usda.gov/tn/Missions/index.htm (accessed January 29, 2000).

The Child and Adolescent Trial for Cardiovascular Health (CATCH)

CATCH was a four-center, randomized field trial that evaluated the effectiveness of a school-based cardiovascular health promotion program.[155] A total of 5106 ethnically diverse students (who were third-graders at baseline and fifth-graders at the end of the intervention) participated in 56 intervention and 40 control public schools in California, Louisiana, Minnesota, and Texas. Of the 56 intervention schools, 28 schools participated in a third-grade through fifth-grade intervention which included school food service modifications, enhanced physical education, and classroom health curricula; the other 28 schools received these components plus family education. Results at the end of the three-year intervention indicated that the percentage of energy from fat in intervention school lunches fell significantly more (from 38.7 to 31.9%) than in control school lunches (from 38.9 to 36.2%) ($p<0.001$). The intensity of physical activity in physical education classes increased significantly in intervention schools compared with control schools ($p<0.02$). The percentage of energy from fat from 24-hour recalls among intervention school students was significantly reduced (from 32.7 to 30.3%) compared with that among control school students (from 32.6 to 32.2%, $p<0.001$). Intervention students reported significantly more daily vigorous activity than controls (58.6 vs. 46.5 minutes, $p<0.003$). However, no significant differences were detected in blood pressure, body size, and cholesterol measures for students at the intervention schools compared to those at the control schools.[86]

A three-year followup was conducted with 3714 students (73%) of the initial CATCH cohort of 5106 students.[156] End-point comparisons were made between students from intervention and control schools to determine whether changes at the end of intervention in grade five were maintained through grade eight. Results for eighth-graders indicated that self-reported daily energy intake from fat remained lower for intervention than control students (30.6 vs. 31.6%, $p = 0.01$). Intervention students maintained significantly higher daily vigorous physical activity than controls ($p = .001$), although differences narrowed over time. Significant differences in favor of intervention students persisted at grade eight for dietary knowledge and dietary intentions, but not for social support for physical activity. No significant differences were noted for BMI, blood pressure, or serum lipid and cholesterol levels. In summary, followup of the CATCH cohort suggests that behavior changes from the intervention were sufficient to produce effects detectable three years later. However, differences between the intervention and control groups were narrowing in magnitude over time. Additional research is needed to determine how best to maintain the intervention effects long-term.[156]

Food Safety

The Fight Bac!™ campaign is a partnership of industry, government, and consumer groups dedicated to reducing the incidence of foodborne illness.[157] The multifaceted campaign includes television and radio public service announcements in several languages, media mailings, newspaper articles, publications, World Wide Web (www.fightbac.org), community action kits, supermarket action kits, exhibit and convention kits, and educator kits for grades kindergarten through three and four through six. Launched in October, 1997, the eye-catching Fight Bac!™ cartoon character teams up with the following four critical messages to teach consumers about safe food handling: clean, separate, cook, and chill.[157] Table 8.28 provides more details regarding these four messages.

Children, adolescents, and adults of all ages need to understand the important role they play in decreasing the incidence of foodborne illnesses through proper hand washing as well as safe food preparation and storage. According to the Hospitality Institute of Technology and Management,[158] hands should be washed with soap, a fingernail brush with soft bristles, and a large volume of flowing warm water to ensure adequate removal of pathogenic microorganisms (e.g., those from fecal sources) from fingertips and under fingernails. Fingernails should be neatly trimmed to less than 1/16 inch to make them easier to clean. When working with food, hand washing without the fingernail brush is sufficient because the pathogen count is much lower. Table 8.29 describes the double and single methods of hand washing. Although young children may be encouraged to wash

TABLE 8.28

Details Regarding the Four Critical Messages of the Fight Bac!™ Campaign

Clean: Wash Hands and Surfaces Often

- Wash hands with hot soapy water before handling food.
- Wash hands with hot soapy water after using the bathroom, changing diapers, and touching animals.
- Wash dishes, utensils, cutting boards, and counter tops with hot soapy water after preparing each food item and before preparing the next food item.
- Use paper towels to dry hands and clean kitchen surfaces.

Separate: Don't Cross-Contaminate

- Keep raw meat, poultry, and seafood separate from other foods in grocery carts and refrigerators.
- Use a different cutting board for preparing raw meats.
- Wash hands, cutting boards, dishes, and utensils with hot soapy water after they come in contact with raw meat, poultry, or seafood.
- Do not place cooked food on a plate or serving dish that previously held raw meat, poultry, or seafood.

Cook: Cook to Proper Temperatures

- To make sure that meat, poultry, casseroles, etc. are cooked all the way through, use a clean thermometer.
- Cook roasts and steaks to at least 145°F; cook whole poultry to 180°F.
- Cook ground beef to at least 160°F. Do not eat ground beef that is still pink inside.
- Cook eggs until the white and yolk are firm.
- Do not eat foods that contain raw eggs or only partially cooked eggs.
- Cook fish until it is opaque and flakes easily with a fork.
- When microwaving foods, make sure there are not cold spots by stirring and rotating food for even heating.
- Reheat sauces, soups, and gravies to a boil. Heat other leftovers thoroughly to at least 165°F.

Chill: Refrigerate Promptly

- Refrigerate or freeze prepared foods and leftovers within two hours or sooner.
- Defrost food in the refrigerator, under cold running water, or in the microwave, but never at room temperature.
- Marinate foods in the refrigerator.
- Divide large amounts of leftovers into small, shallow containers for quick cooling in the refrigerator.
- Avoid packing the refrigerator because cool air must circulate to keep food safe.

Adapted from *Fight Bac!™ Four Simple Steps to Food Safety*, Partnership for Food Safety Education, www.fightbac.org (accessed January 11, 2000).

their hands long enough for them to sing their "A, B, Cs" slowly, the amount of lathering and the volume of water used to wash off the lathering appear to be more important than the length of time spent washing.[158]

Dental Health

Nutrition is an integral component of oral health.[159] Nutrition and diet may affect the development and progression of diseases of the oral cavity. Likewise, oral infectious diseases and acute, chronic, and terminal systemic diseases with oral manifestations, affect diet and nutritional status. The primary factors to be considered in determining the cariogenic, cariostatic, and anticariogenic properties of the diet include the form of the food (liquid, solid and sticky, long lasting), frequency of consumption of sugar and other fermentable carbohydrates, nutrient composition, sequence of food intake, and combinations of foods.[159]

Because children of all ages eat frequently, snacks should emphasize foods that are low in sucrose, are not sticky, and that stimulate saliva flow which helps limit acid production in the mouth.[160] Protein foods such as nuts and cheese may provide nutritional and dental

TABLE 8.29

Two Methods of Hand Washing

Double Wash Procedure (to be used to remove fecal pathogens and other pathogenic microorganisms from skin surfaces when entering the kitchen, after using the toilet, after cleaning up vomitus or fecal material, or after touching sores or bandages):

First wash using the fingernail brush (~7 seconds required to complete):

- Turn on water so it runs at 2 gallons per minute with a temperature of 110 to 115°F. Place hands, lower arms, and fingernail brush under flowing water and thoroughly wet them.
- Apply 1/2 to 1 teaspoon of hand soap or detergent to fingernail brush.
- Brush and lather hand surfaces with tips of bristles on fingernail brush under flowing water, especially fingertips and around and under fingernails. Build a good lather.
- Continue to use fingernail brush under water until there is no more soapy lather on hands, lower arms, or nail brush. Hazardous microorganisms in the lather are only removed to a safe level when all the soap is rinsed off the hands, arms, and fingertips.
- Place nail brush on holder with bristles up so bristles can dry.

Second wash without the fingernail brush (~13 seconds required to complete):

- Apply 1/2 to 1 teaspoon of hand soap or detergent to hands.
- While adding warm water as necessary, rub hands together to produce a good lather; lathering must extend from fingertips to shirt sleeves.
- After lathering, rinse all of lather from fingertips, hands, and arms in flowing water. The volume of water used for rinsing hands, not the time of the wash, is the critical factor.
- Thoroughly dry hands and arms using disposable paper towels. Discard paper towels in waste container without touching container.

Single Wash Procedure (to be used to remove normal low levels of pathogens before and after eating and drinking; after handling garbage; after handling dirty dishes or utensils; between handling raw and cooked foods; after blowing or wiping nose; after touching skin, hair, or soiled clothes; and as often as necessary to keep hands clean after they become soiled):

- Wet hands and lower arms with warm water.
- Follow directions above for "Second wash without the fingernail brush."

Adapted from Snyder, O. P., Hospitality Institute of Technology and Management, 1998, http://www.hi-tm.com/Documents/Safehands.html (accessed January 11, 2000).

benefits because some protein foods are thought to have a protective effect against caries. When desserts are consumed, it is best if they are eaten with meals. Chewing sugarless gum after snacks containing fermentable carbohydrate may benefit school-age children and adolescents. The efforts of dietary control are complemented by good oral hygiene. A fluoride supplement is recommended into the teen years if the water supply is not fluoridated.[160]

Maxillary anterior caries (baby bottle tooth decay or BBTD) is the major nutrition-related dental disease found in infants and preschool children; it appears to be related to feeding behaviors after longer bottle or breastfeeding.[159] The primary cause of BBTD is prolonged exposure of the teeth to a sweetened liquid such as formula, milk, juice, soda pop, or other sweetened drinks.[160] This often occurs when a child is routinely given a bottle at bedtime or naptime, because the liquid pools around the teeth during sleep, saliva flow decreases, and the child may continue to suck liquid over an extended period of time. Toddlers are also at high risk if they hold their own bottle and have access to it anytime throughout the day. The primary strategy to prevent BBTD is education. Parents and child care providers should be encouraged to avoid putting an infant or young child to sleep with a bottle, and to use a cup to offer juices and liquids other than breast milk or formula.[160] Section 54 provides additional information regarding the prevention of dental caries in children and adolescents.

References

1. Food and Nutrition Board, National Research Council, *Recommended Dietary Allowances*, 10th ed, National Academy Press, Washington, DC, 1989.
2. Food and Nutrition Board, Institute of Medicine, *Dietary Reference Intakes for Calcium, Phosphorus, Magnesium, Vitamin D, and Fluoride*, National Academy Press, Washington, DC, 1997. Available online at www.nap.edu (accessed July 13, 2001).
3. Food and Nutrition Board, Institute of Medicine, *Dietary Reference Intakes for Thiamin, Riboflavin, Niacin, Vitamin B6, Folate, Vitamin B12, Pantothenic Acid, Biotin, and Choline*, National Academy Press, Washington, DC, 1999.
4. Food and Nutrition Board, Institute of Medicine, *Dietary Reference Intakes for Vitamin C, Vitamin E, Selenium, and Carotenoids*, National Academy Press, Washington, DC, 2000. Available online at www.nap.edu (accessed July 13, 2001).
5. Food and Nutrition Board, Institute of Medicine, *Dietary Reference Intakes for Vitamin A, Vitamin K, Arsenic, Boron, Chromium, Copper, Iodine, Iron, Manganese, Molybdenum, Nickel, Silicon, Vanadium, and Zinc*, National Academy Press, Washington, DC, 2001. Available online at www.nap.edu (accessed July 13, 2001).
6. Heald, F. P., Gong, E. J. In: *Modern Nutrition in Health and Disease*, 9th ed, (Shils, M. E., Olson, J. A, Shike, M., Ross, A. C., Eds), Williams & Wilkins, Baltimore, 1999, pg 857.
7. Pellett, P. L., *Am J Clin Nutr*, 51: 711; 1990
8. Nutrition Committee, American Heart Association, *Circulation*, 94: 1795; 1996.
9. Committee on Nutrition, American Academy of Pediatrics, *Pediatrics*, 101: 141; 1998.
10. *Nutrition and Your Health: Dietary Guidelines for Americans*, 5th ed, USDA and US Dept of Health and Human Services, 2000, Home and Garden Bulletin No. 232.
11. Williams, C. L., Bollella, M., Wynder, E. L., *Pediatrics*, 96: 985; 1995.
12. Williams, C. L., *J Am Diet Assoc*, 95: 1140; 1995.
13. Committee on Nutrition, American Academy of Pediatrics, Carbohydrates and Dietary Fiber, *Pediatric Nutrition Handbook*, 4th ed, Kleinman, R. E., Ed, American Academy of Pediatrics, Elk Grove Village, IL, 1998, pg 203.
14. Committee on Nutrition, American Academy of Pediatrics, *Pediatrics*, 86: 643; 1990.
15. Committee on Nutrition, American Academy of Pediatrics, Iron Deficiency, *Pediatric Nutrition Handbook*, 4th ed, Kleinman, R. E., Ed, American Academy of Pediatrics, Elk Grove Village, IL, 1998, pg 233.
16. Food and Nutrition Board, Institute of Medicine, *Iron Deficiency Anemia: Recommended Guidelines for the Prevention, Detection, and Management among U.S. Children and Women of Childbearing Age*, National Academy Press, Washington, DC, 1993.
17. *Food Guide Pyramid for Young Children*, USDA, Center for Nutrition Policy and Promotion, Washington, DC, 1999, Program Aid 1649. Also available at http://www.usda.gov/cnpp.
18. *Food Guide Pyramid: A Guide to Daily Food Choice*, USDA, Human Nutrition Service, Home and Garden Bulletin No. 252, 1992.
19. *Tips for Using the Food Guide Pyramid for Young Children 2 to 6 Years Old*, USDA, Center for Nutrition Policy and Promotion, Washington, DC, 1999, Program Aid 1647. Also available at http://www.usda.gov/cnpp.
20. Borrud, L. G., Introduction and Overview, *Design and Operation: The Continuing Survey of Food Intakes by Individuals and the Diet and Health Knowledge Survey*, 1994-96, Tippett, K. S., Cypel, Y. S., Eds, USDA, Agricultural Research Service, NFS Report No. 96-1, December, 1997, pg 1.
21. Subar, A. F., Krebs-Smith, S. M., Cook, A., et al., *Pediatrics* 102: 913; 1998.
22. Krebs-Smith, S. M., Cook, A., Subar, A. F., et al., *Arch Pediatr Adolesc Med*, 150: 81; 1996.
23. Hampl, J. S., Betts, N. M., Benes, B. A., *J Am Diet Assoc*, 98: 1418; 1998.
24. Guenther, P. M., Cleveland, L. E., Ingwersen, L. A., Questionnaire Development and Data Collection Procedures, *Design and Operation: The Continuing Survey of Food Intakes by Individuals and the Diet and Health Knowledge Survey*, 1994-96, Tippett, K. S., Cypel, Y. S., Eds, USDA, Agricultural Research Service, NFS Report No. 96-1, December, 1997, pg 42.

25. Nutrition Insights, Insight 9, October, 1998, issued by the Center for Nutrition Policy and Promotion, USDA, http://www.usda.gov/cnpp (accessed July 21, 1999).
26. Federal Interagency Forum on Child and Family Statistics, *America's Children: Key National Indicators of Well-Being, 1999*, Federal Interagency Forum On Child and Family Statistics, Washington, DC, US Government Printing Office, p 79. The report is also available on the World Wide Web: http://childstats.gov.
27. Harnack, L., Stang, J., Story, M., *J Am Diet Assoc*, 99: 436; 1999.
28. USDA, Agricultural Research Service, *Food and Nutrient Intakes by Children 1994-96, 1998*, 1999, Online, ARS Food Surveys Research Group, available on the "Products" page at http://www.barc.usda.gov/bhnrc/foodsurvey/home.htm (accessed December 22, 1999).
29. Food and Nutrition Board, National Research Council, *Diet and Health: Implications for Reducing Chronic Disease Risk*, Washington, DC, Government Printing Office, 1989.
30. American Dietetic Association, *J Am Diet Assoc*, 99: 93; 1999.
31. Committee on Nutrition, American Academy of Pediatrics, Feeding from Age 1 Year to Adolescence, *Pediatric Nutrition Handbook*, 4th ed, Kleinman, R. E., Ed, American Academy of Pediatrics, Elk Grove, IL, 1998, pg 125.
32. Domel, S. B., Baranowski, T., Davis, H., et al., *J Nutr Educ*, 25: 345; 1993.
33. Domel, S. B., Baranowski, T., Davis, H., et al., *J Am Coll Nutr*, 13: 33; 1994.
34. Wolfe, W. S., Campbell, C. C., *J Am Diet Assoc*, 93: 1280; 1993.
35. Nicklas, T. A., *J Am Diet Assoc*, 95: 1127; 1995.
36. Freedman, D. S., Srinivasan, S. R., Valdez, R. A., et al., *Pediatrics*, 99: 420; 1997.
37. Troiano, R. P., Flegal, K. M., *Pediatrics*, 101: 497; 1998.
38. Birch, L. L., Fisher, J. O., *Pediatrics*, 101: 539; 1998.
39. Hill, J. O., Trowbridge, F. L., *Pediatrics* 101: 570; 1998.
40. Birch, L. L., Johnson, S. L., Fisher, J. A., *Young Child*, 50: 71; 1995.
41. Birch, L. L., *J Nutr Educ*, 11: 189; 1979.
42. Calfas, K., Sallis, J., Nader, P., *J Dev Behav Ped*, 12: 185; 1991.
43. Domel, S. B., Baranowski, T., Leonard, S. B., et al., *Prev Med*, 22: 866; 1993.
44. Domel, S. B., Thompson, W. O., Davis, H. C., et al., *Health Educ Res: Theory Prac*, 11: 299; 1996.
45. Fisher, J. O., Birch, L. L., *J Am Diet Assoc*, 95: 759; 1995.
46. Birch, L. L., *Bull Psychonomic Soc*, 29: 265; 1991.
47. Cowart, B. J., *Psychol Bull*, 90: 43; 1981.
48. Birch, L. L., *J Am Diet Assoc*, 87: S36; 1987.
49. Sullivan, S. A., Birch, L. L., *Pediatrics*, 93: 271; 1994.
50. Birch, L. L., Marlin, D. W., *Appetite: J Intake Res*, 3: 353; 1982.
51. Birch, L. L., McPhee, L., Shoba, B. C., et al., *Appetite*, 9: 171; 1987.
52. Sullivan, S. A., Birch, L. L., *Dev Psychol*, 26: 546; 1990.
53. Lytle, L., Achterberg, C., *J Nutr Educ*, 27: 250; 1995.
54. Birch, L. L., Zimmerman, S. I., Hind, H., *Child Dev*, 51: 856; 1980.
55. Birch, L. L., Birch, D., Marlin, D. W., et al., *Appetite: J Intake Res*, 3: 125; 1982.
56. Birch, L. L., Marlin, D. W., Rotter, J., *Child Dev*, 55: 431; 1984.
57. Newman, J., Taylor A., *J Exp Child Psychol*, 64: 200; 1992.
58. Hendy, H. M., *Ann Behav Med*, 21: 1; 1999.
59. Nahikian-Nelms, M., *J Am Diet Assoc*, 97: 505; 1997.
60. Fomon, S. J., *Nutrition of Normal Infants*, Mosby-Yearbook, St. Louis, MO, 1993, pg 114.
61. Adair, L. S., *J Am Diet Assoc*, 84: 543; 1984.
62. Birch, L. L., Deysher, M., *Learning and Motivation*, 16: 341; 1985.
63. Birch, L. L., Deysher, M., *Appetite*, 7: 323; 1986.
64. Birch, L. L., Johnson, S. L., Andresen, G., et al., *N Eng J Med* 324: 232; 1991.
65. Birch, L. L., McPhee, L., Shoba, B. C., et al., *Learning and Motivation*, 18: 301; 1987.
66. Johnson, S. L., Birch, L. L., *Pediatrics*, 94: 653; 1994.
67. Klesges, R. C., Coates, T. J., Brown, G., et al., *J Appl Behav Anal*, 16: 371; 1983.
68. Satter, E., *How to Get Your Kids to Eat … But Not Too Much*, Bull Publishing, Palo Alto, CA, 1987.
69. Satter, E. M., *J Am Diet Assoc*, 86: 352; 1986.
70. Dennison, B. A., *J Am Coll Nutr*, 15(5): 4S; 1996.

71. Hyams, J. S., Etienne, N. L., Leichtner, A. M., et al., *Pediatrics*, 82: 64; 1988.
72. Committee on Nutrition, American Academy of Pediatrics, *AAP News*, February, 1991, http://www.aap.org/policy/899.html (accessed December 29, 1999).
73. Smith, M. M., Lifshitz, F., *Pediatrics*, 93: 438; 1994.
74. Dennison, B. A., Rockwell, H. L., Baker, S. L., *Pediatrics*, 99: 15; 1997.
75. Olson, R. E., *J Am Diet Assoc*, 100: 28; 2000.
76. Satter, E., *J Am Diet Assoc*, 100: 32; 2000.
77. Dwyer, J., *J Am Diet Assoc*, 100: 36; 2000.
78. Krebs, N. F., Johnson, S. L., *J Am Diet Assoc*, 100: 37; 2000.
79. Lytle, L. A., *J Am Diet Assoc*, 100: 39; 2000.
80. Van Horn, L., *J Am Diet Assoc*, 100: 41; 2000.
81. Pugliese, M. T., Weyman-Daum, M., Moses, N., et al., *Pediatrics*, 80: 175; 1987.
82. Niinikoski, H., Lapinleimu, H., Viikari, J., et al., *Pediatrics*, 99: 687; 1997.
83. Niinikoski, H., Viikari, J., Rönnemaa, T., et al., *Pediatrics*, 100: 810; 1997.
84. The Writing Group for the DISC Collaborative Research Group, *JAMA*, 273: 1429; 1995.
85. Obarzanek, E., Hunsberger, S. A., Van Horn, L., et al., *Pediatrics*, 100: 51; 1997.
86. Luepker, R. V., Perry, C. L., McKinlay, S. M., et al., *JAMA*, 275: 768; 1996.
87. Birch, L. L., *Child Development*, 51: 489; 1980.
88. Rolls, B. J., Engell, D., Birch, L. L., *J Am Diet Assoc*, 100: 232; 2000.
89. Pollitt, E., *J Am Diet Assoc*, 95: 1134; 1995.
90. Pollitt, E., Cueto, S., Jacoby, E. R., *Am J Clin Nutr*, 67: 779S; 1998.
91. Grantham-McGregor, S. M., Chang, S., Walker, S. P., *Am J Clin Nutr*, 67: 785S; 1998.
92. Dwyer, J. T., Ebzery, M. K., Nicklas, T. A., et al., *Fam Econ Nutr Rev*, 11: 3; 1998.
93. Nicklas, T. A., Bao, W., Webber, L. S., et al., *J Am Diet Assoc*, 93: 886; 1993.
94. Gleason, P., *Am J Clin Nutr*, 61(1): 213S; 1995.
95. Siega-Riz, A. M., Popkin, B. M., Carson, T., *Am J Clin Nutr*, 67: 748S; 1998.
96. Dwyer, J., *Am J Clin Nutr*, 61: 173S; 1995.
97. School Lunch Program — Frequently Asked Questions, http://www.fns.usda.gov/cnd/Lunch/AboutLunch/faqs.htm (accessed May 20, 1999).
98. School Breakfast Program — Frequently Asked Questions, http://www.fns.usda.gov/cnd/Breakfast/AboutBFast/faqs.htm (accessed May 20, 1999).
99. Burghardt, J. A., *Am J Clin Nutr*, 61(1): 182S; 1995.
100. Burghardt, J. A., Devaney, B. L., Gordon, A. R., *Am J Clin Nutr*, 61(1): 252S; 1995.
101. Baranowski, T., Smith, M., Hearn, M. D., et al., *J Am Coll Nutr*, 16: 216; 1997.
102. Hearn, M. D., Baranowski, T., Baranowski, J., et al., *J Health Educ*, 29: 26; 1998.
103. Baranowski, T., Domel, S., Gould, R., et al., *J Nutr Educ*, 25: 114; 1993.
104. Kirby, S., Baranowski, T., Reynolds, K., et al., *J Nutr Educ*, 27: 261; 1995.
105. Resnicow, K., Davis-Hearn, M., Smith, M., et al., *Health Psychol*, 16: 272; 1997.
106. Baranowski, T., Davis, M., Resnicow, K., et al., *Health Educ Behav*, 27: 96; 2000.
107. Resnicow, K., Davis, M., Smith, M., et al., *Am J Public Health* 88: 250; 1998.
108. Luepker, R. V., Perry, C. L., Osganian, V., et al., *J Nutr Biochem*, 9: 525; 1998.
109. Perry, C. L., Bishop, D. B., Taylor, G., et al., *Am J Public Health*, 88: 603; 1998.
110. Reynolds, K. D., Franklin, F. A., Binkley, D., et al., *Prev Med*, 30(4): 309; 2000.
111. Nicklas, T. A., Johnson, C. C., Myers, L., et al., *J School Health*, 68: 248; 1998.
112. Donnelly, J. E., Jacobsen, D. J., Whatley, J. E., et al., *Obesity Res*, 4: 229; 1996.
113. Resnicow, K., *Ann N Y Acad Sci*, 699: 154; 1993.
114. Birch, L. L., *Dev Psychol*, 26: 515; 1990.
115. Kennedy, E., *Prev Med*, 25: 56; 1996.
116. Centers for Disease Control and Prevention. *Guidelines for School Health Programs to Promote Lifelong Healthy Eating*. MMWR. No. RR-9, 1996.
117. Berenson, G., Arbeit, M., Hunter, S., et al., *Ann N Y Acad Sci*, 623: 299; 1991.
118. Kolbe, L. J., *Prev Med*, 22: 544; 1993.
119. Contento, I. R., Manning, A. D., Shannon, B., *J Nutr Educ*, 24: 247; 1992.
120. Contento, I., Balch, G. I., Bronner, Y. L., et al., *J Nutr Educ*, 27: 298; 1995.
121. Baxter, S. D., *J Sch Health*, 68: 111; 1998.

122. Gittelsohn, J., Evans, M., Story, M., et al., *Am J Clin Nutr,* 69(4): 767S; 1999.
123. Lytle, L., *Nutrition Education for School-aged Children: A Review of Research.* USDA, Food and Consumer Service, Office of Analysis and Evaluation, Alexandria, VA, 1994.
124. Molnar, A., *Sponsored Schools and Commercialized Classrooms: Schoolhouse Commercializing Trends in the 1990s,* Center for the Analysis of Commercialism in Education (CACE), University of Wisconsin-Milwaukee, 1998, http://www.uwm.edu/Dept/CACE/.
125. The Surgeon General's Report on Nutrition and Health, US Dept of Health and Human Services, Public Health Service, Washington, DC, DHHS (PHS) publication 88-50210, 1988.
126. US Department of Health and Human Services, *Healthy People 2010,* 2nd ed, US Government Printing Office, Superintendent of Documents, Washington, DC, November, 2000. Available online at http://www.health.gov/healthypeople (accessed July 3, 2000).
127. American Dietetic Association, *J Am Diet Assoc,* 100: 108; 2000.
128. American Dietetic Association, *J Am Diet Assoc,* 96: 913; 1996.
129. American Dietetic Association, Society for Nutrition Education, and American School Food Service Association, *J Am Diet Assoc,* 95: 367; 1995.
130. Birch, L. L., *Nutr Rev,* 50: 249; 1992.
131. Dietz, W. H., *Pediatrics,* 101: 518; 1998.
132. Andersen, R. E., Crespo, C. J., Bartlett, S. J., et al., *JAMA,* 279: 938; 1998.
133. Kotz, K., Story, M., *J Am Diet Assoc,* 94: 1296; 1994.
134. Kanarek, R. B., *Nutr Rev,* 52: 173; 1994.
135. Wolraich, M. L., Lindgren, S. D., Stumbo, P. J., et al., *N Eng J Med,* 330: 301; 1994.
136. Wolraich, M. L., Wilson, D. B., White, J. W., *JAMA,* 274: 1617; 1995.
137. American Dietetic Association, *J Am Diet Assoc,* 98: 580; 1998.
138. Committee on Nutrition, American Academy of Pediatrics, Adolescent Nutrition, *Pediatric Nutrition Handbook,* 4th ed, Kleinman, R. E., Ed, American Academy of Pediatrics, Elk Grove Village, IL, 1998, pg 141.
139. Neumark-Sztainer, D., Story, M., Perry, C., et al., *J Am Diet Assoc,* 99: 929; 1999.
140. Neumark-Sztainer, D., Story, M., Resnick, M.D., et al., *J Am Diet Assoc,* 98: 1449; 1998.
141. Kann, L., Kinchen, S. A., Williams, B. I., et al., *Youth Risk Behavior Surveillance — United States, 1997,* In CDC Surveillance Summaries, MMWR 47 (No. SS-3), 1998; available at http://www.cdc.gov/.
142. World Health Organization, *Health and Health Behaviour among Young People.* WHO Policy Series: Health policy for children and adolescents. Issue 1. International Report, 2000. Available at http://www.nih.gov/news/pr/jan2000/nichd-31.htm and http://www.ruhbc.ed.ac.uk/hbsc/download/hbsc.pdf (accessed February 7, 2000).
143. Meyer, M. K., *J Am Diet Assoc,* 100, 100, 2000.
144. French, S. A., Story, M., Jeffery, R. W., et al., *J Am Diet Assoc,* 97: 1008; 1997.
145. Frank, G., Nutrition for Teens, *Promoting Teen Health: Linking Schools, Health Organizations, and Community,* Henderson, A., Champlin, S., Evashwick, W., Eds, Sage Publications, Thousand Oaks, CA, 1998, pg 28.
146. American Dietetic Association, *J Am Diet Assoc,* 97: 1317; 1997.
147. Sanders, T. A. G., Reddy, S. *Am J Clin Nutr,* 59: 1176S; 1994.
148. Havas, S., Heimendinger, J., Reynolds, K., et al, *J Am Diet Assoc,* 94: 32; 1994.
149. Subar, A. F., Heimendinger, J., Patterson, B. H., et al., *Am J Health Promot,* 9: 352; 1995.
150. Havas, S., Heimendinger, J., Damron, D., et al., *Public Health Reports,* 110: 68; 1995.
151. Stedronsky, F. M., *J Am Diet Assoc,* 98: 758; 1998.
152. Rickard, K. A., Gallahue, D. L., Fruen, G. E., et al., *J Am Diet Assoc,* 95: 1121; 1995.
153. Bronner, Y. L., *J Am Diet Assoc,* 96: 891; 1996.
154. http://www.fns.usda.gov/tn (accessed January 29, 2000).
155. Perry, C. L., Stone, E. J., Parcel, G. S., et al., *J Sch Health,* 60: 406; 1990.
156. Nader, P. R., Stone, E. J., Lytle, L. A., et al., *Arch Pediatr Adolesc Med,* 153: 695; 1999.
157. www.fightbac.org (accessed January 11, 2000).
158. Snyder, O., P., Hospitality Institute of Technology and Management, 1998, http://www.hi-tm.com/Documents/Safehands.html (accessed January 11, 2000).
159. American Dietetic Association, *J Am Diet Assoc,* 96; 184; 1996.
160. Lucas, B., Normal Nutrition from Infancy through Adolescence, *Handbook of Pediatric Nutrition,* Queen, P. M., Lang, C. E., Eds, Gaithersburg, MD, 1993, pg 145.

9

The Health-Promoting Diet throughout Life: Adults

Marsha Read

Introduction

The normal diet for adults is based on the need to provide sufficient nutrients to sustain life and an appropriate balance of nutrient intake to support optimal health. The first *Surgeon General's Report on Nutrition and Health* in 1988[1] brought together a substantial body of research that documented that diet, aside from providing the essential nutrients for daily functioning, was a key factor with respect to chronic diseases such as coronary heart disease, cancer, diabetes, and obesity. The underlying premise of the various dietary guidelines/recommendations that have been developed has been to provide adequate nutrient intake while avoiding dietary patterns that might place an individual at greater risk for chronic disease. The following subsections describe the most commonly used dietary guidelines/recommendations, guidelines for counseling healthy adults, information on current food and nutrient consumption patterns of adults, and current research with respect to health implications of inappropriate macronutrient intake.

Dietary Recommendations and Guidelines

Dietary Guidelines

Dietary guidelines have undergone several revisions from the late 1970s to the recently released *Dietary Guidelines for Americans 2000.*[2] The 1970s Dietary Goals provided recommendations with respect to energy intake, carbohydrate, fat, and sodium intakes. Specific percent of calories from carbohydrate and fat were put forth, 48 and 30% respectively. Cholesterol intake was recommended at 300 mg/day and sodium intake was recommended not to exceed 5 g/day.[3] The first set of the U.S. Dietary Guidelines was published in 1980[4] (Table 9.1).

The first guidelines were followed by several revisions. The most recent iteration of dietary guidelines for Americans adopts a basic "ABC" concept — **A**im for Fitness, **B**uild

0-8493-2705-9/01/$0.00+$1.50

TABLE 9.1

1980 U.S. Dietary Guidelines

Eat a wide variety of foods
Maintain ideal weight
Avoid too much fat, saturated fat, and cholesterol
Eat foods with adequate starch and fiber
Avoid too much sugar
Avoid too much sodium
If you drink alcohol, do so in moderation

TABLE 9.2

2000 U.S. Dietary Guidelines[a]

Aim for Fitness
Aim for a healthy weight
Be physically active each day
Build a Healthy Base
Let the Pyramid guide your food choices
Eat a variety of grains daily, especially whole grains
Eat a variety of fruits and vegetables daily
Keep food safe to eat
Choose Sensibly
Choose a diet low in saturated fat and cholesterol, and moderate in total fat
Choose beverages and foods that limit your intake of sugars
Choose and prepare foods with less salt
If you drink alcoholic beverages, do so in moderation

[a] www.ars.usda.gov/dgac/dgacguideexp.pdf

a Healthy Base, and Choose Sensibly as the key constructs[2] (Table 9.2). These current dietary guidelines continue to emphasize sensible dietary choices, variety, and moderation.

From the first edition of the guidelines to the current, the focus has been on a variety of foods to supply adequate nutrient intake, increased complex carbohydrate consumption, moderate fat intake, and moderate alcohol consumption if you drink. A new concept added to the 2000 guidelines deals with the issue of food safety. This introduces a new concept on diet and health and reflects the current issues with respect to maintaining a safe food supply from production to consumption. The concept "Keep Food Safe" adds discussion on prevention of foodborne illness consistent with the concerns arising from several recent food poisoning outbreaks in the United States.

The Food Guide Pyramid

The Food Guide Pyramid sets forth recommendations for a pattern of daily food choices based on servings from five major food groups — bread, cereal, rice and pasta; fruit; vegetable; milk, yogurt and cheese; and meat, poultry, fish, dry beans, eggs and nuts[5] (Figure 9.1). The visual presentation as a pyramid was meant to convey that from the five food groups emphasis should be placed on those shown in the lower three levels/sections of the pyramid. The Food Guide Pyramid was also meant to be used in concert with the dietary guidelines, i.e., to eat a variety of foods and balance the foods eaten with physical activity, and either maintain or improve weight. Each food group suggests a range of servings. Selecting the lower number of recommended servings is estimated to provide approximately 1600 kcals, with the mid-range providing approximately 2200 kcals, and 2800 kcals at the upper range. Refer to Table 9.3 for examples of menu plans at the lower and upper caloric range based on the Food Guide Pyramid. These estimates are intended

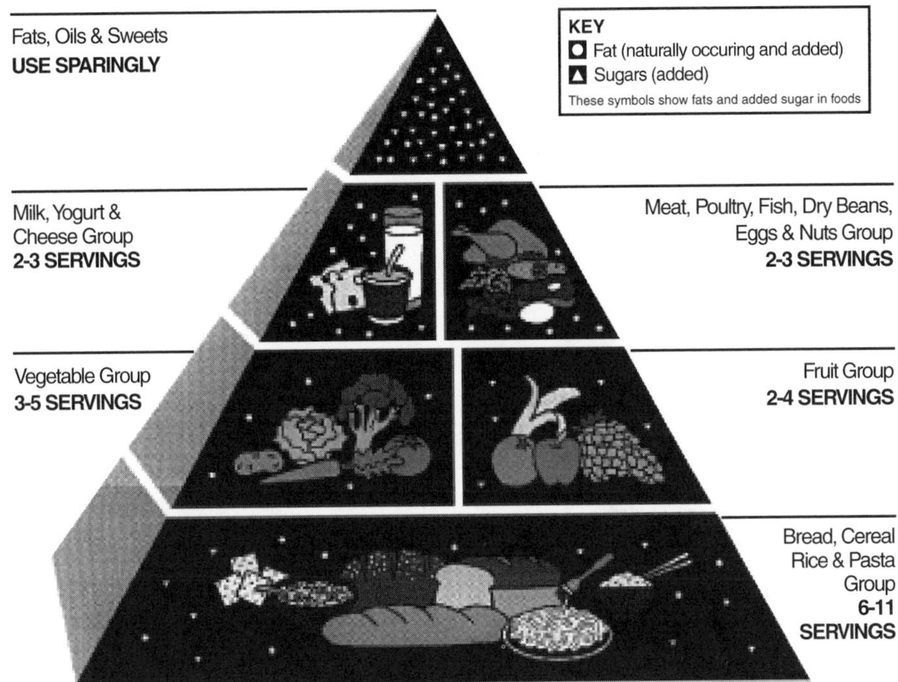

FIGURE 9.1
USDA Food Guide Pyramid.

to help consumers choose an appropriate level of caloric intake while maintaining an appropriate variety of foods to support health. In addition, the visual representation of the food guide as a pyramid was meant to imply that appropriate nutritional choices build upon a *base* of nutrient dense food choices before consuming foods from the less nutrient dense foods of fats, oils, and sweets at the top of the pyramid. Cited advantages and disadvantages of the Food Guide Pyramid according to Kant, Block, Schatzkin, et al.[6] include:

Advantages:

- The pyramid depicts foods, which makes it easier for consumers to relate to rather than nutrients and numbers such as recommended dietary allowances (RDAs).
- The pyramid is relatively simple and easy to read and to remember.
- The pyramid food groups and recommended servings from each food group are likely to represent a variety of foods that can subsequently provide adequate nutrient intake.
- The pyramid food groups allow for personal choice within a food group and thereby supports individual food choices.

Disadvantages:

- Applicability of the food groups within the pyramid to alternate dietary patterns such as vegetarianism and ethnic food patterns may be unclear.
- The Food Guide Pyramid does not address the dietary guideline regarding alcohol intake.

TABLE 9.3

Meal Plans Based on the Food Guide Pyramid

1600 kcalorie Menu (Minimum Servings from Each Food Group)

Breakfast
- 1 cup Raisin Bran cereal
- 4 oz skim milk
- 1/2 grapefruit

Lunch
- Turkey sandwich with mustard
  - 2 pieces of whole wheat bread
  - 3 ounces lean turkey
  - 1 tablespoon mustard
- Carrot sticks (1 medium)
- Apple (1 medium)

Snack
- 1 cup low fat yogurt
- 1/2 sesame bagel

Dinner
- 3 ounces grilled salmon
- Green salad (romaine, iceberg lettuce, tomato, cucumber)
- 1 tablespoon low-fat dressing
- 1/2 cup green beans
- 1 cup wild rice

2800 kcalorie Menu (Upper Serving Recommendations from Each Food Group)

Breakfast
- 1 bowl oatmeal cereal with 1/4 cup raisins
- 4 ounces skim milk
- 2 pieces whole wheat toast
- 2 teaspoons margarine
- 1 tablespoon jam
- 4 ounces orange juice

Lunch
- 1 peanut butter and jelly sandwich
  - 2 pieces whole wheat bread
  - 1 tablespoon jelly
  - 2 tablespoons peanut butter
- Apple (1 medium)
- Celery sticks (1 stalk)

Snacks (a.m. and p.m.)
- 1 ounce low fat cheese
- 4 crackers
- banana
- plain bagel

Dinner
- 3 ounces grilled chicken breast
- 1/2 cup peas
- 1 cup herb rice
- Green salad (romaine, iceberg lettuce, sliced tomatoes, cucumber)
- 1 tablespoon of low-fat dressing
- Melon slices
- Dinner roll

- Interpretation of combination foods as pizza, stews, etc., is not clear within the framework of the pyramid food groups.
- Dietary adequacy may not be obtained if individuals make poor choices within the pyramid food groups.

While there is only one Food Guide Pyramid published by the U.S. Department of Agriculture, variations of the pyramid have arisen. These variations have been constructed to help Americans with alternative dietary preferences build a healthy dietary pattern. These are described in other sections of this handbook (see Section 11 on Guidelines).

Recommended Dietary Allowances (RDA), Estimated Safe and Adequate Daily Dietary Intakes (ESADDIs), Daily Reference Intake (DRI), and Daily Values (DV)

The most common reference standard for nutrient intake has been the recommended dietary allowance (RDA). This standard was first established by the Food and Nutrition Board in 1941, with the most recent edition in 1989.[7] The original intent was to review and revise the RDAs every four to five years, taking into account current research. The constructs used in formulating a specific RDA were: (a) an estimation of how much of each essential nutrient the average healthy person requires to maintain health and how those requirements vary among people; (b) an increase in the average requirement to cover the needs of almost all members of the population, based on a bell curve distribution; (c) an increase in the RDA again to cover cooking losses and inefficient body utilization, as well as provide for cases of greater nutrient need such as in pregnancy and infancy; and (d) use of scientific judgment in establishing the RDA. Three central premises underlie the RDAs:

1. The RDA is an amount intended to be consumed as part of a normal diet
2. The RDA is neither a minimal requirement nor an optimal level of intake, but instead represents a safe and adequate level of intake based on current scientific knowledge
3. The RDA is most appropriately used as a nutrient intake guide applied to subgroups of the population, but can be used to estimate the probable risk of nutrient deficiency for an individual.

For nutrients in which scientific evidence provides support for their essentiality but are insufficient to establish an RDA, there are estimated safe and adequate daily dietary intakes (ESADDIs). Most ESADDIs are shown as a range of intake values that represent the upper and lower limits of safe intake. ESADDIs are established for biotin, copper, manganese, and molybdenum.[7]

The current iteration of recommended intakes includes the dietary reference intake (DRI). DRI encompasses four types of nutrient recommendations for healthy individuals: adequate intake (AI); estimated average intake (EAR); recommended dietary allowance (RDA); and tolerable upper intake levels (UL).[8,9] AI is a nutrient recommendation based on observed or experimentally determined approximation of nutrient intake by a group (or groups) of healthy people when sufficient scientific evidence is not available to calculate an RDA or an EAR. The EAR is the average requirement of a nutrient for healthy individuals in which a functional or clinical assessment has been conducted and measures of adequacy have been made at a specified level of dietary intake. The EAR is an amount of intake of a nutrient at which approximately 50% of subjects would have their needs met and 50% would not. The EAR is intended to be used for assessing nutrient adequacy of populations and not individuals. The new RDA is the amount of a nutrient needed to meet the requirements of nearly all (97 to 98%) of the healthy population of individuals

TABLE 9.4

WHO Dietary Recommendations

Total Energy: sufficient to support normal growth, physical activity, and body weight (body mass index = 20-22)
Total Fat: 15-30% of total energy
Saturated fatty acids: 0-10% total energy
Polyunsaturated fatty acids: 3-7% total energy
Dietary cholesterol: 0-300 milligrams per day
Total Carbohydrate: 55-75% total energy
Complex carbohydrates: 50-75% total energy
Dietary fiber: 27-40 grams/day
Refined sugars: 0-10% total energy
Protein: 10-15% total energy
Salt: upper limit of 6 grams/day (no lower limit set)

for whom it was developed. An RDA for a nutrient should serve as an intake goal for individuals and not as a standard of adequacy for diets of populations. This is different than the previous or old RDA. UL values are established in cases where there is adequate scientific evidence to suggest an upper level of intake that is consistent with adverse or toxic reactions. The UL represents the maximum level of intake for a nutrient that will not cause adverse effects in almost all of the population ingesting that amount.

The daily values (DV) are used as standards in food labeling. DVs provide reference intake standards for nutrients that have an RDA, in which case they are referred to as reference daily intakes (RDIs), and for nutrients for which no RDA exists, in this case referred to as daily reference values (DRVs). DRVs are established for fat, saturated fat, cholesterol, carbohydrate, dietary fiber, sodium, and potassium. As a rule the RDIs are greater than the RDA for specific nutrients and provide a large margin of safety. The term RDI replaces the term U.S. Recommended Daily Allowances (USRDAs) used on earlier food labels.[10]

World Health Organization (WHO) Recommendations

The World Health Organization (WHO) has also published diet recommendations with the goal of reducing risk for chronic disease.[11] WHO recommendations are expressed as a range of average daily intakes from lower to upper limits (Table 9.4).

Food Labels

Food labeling became mandatory in 1993 with the enactment of the Nutrition Labeling and Education Act (NLEA).[10] The legislation required food labeling on most foods with the exceptions of low nutrient-dense foods such as coffee, spices, and ready-to-eat foods prepared on site. Nutrition information remains voluntary on many raw foods. The nutrition facts panel on food labels provides information to help the consumer make more informed choices, including information on calories per serving, calories from fat, saturated fat and cholesterol, and protein among other nutrients (Table 9.5).

American Cancer Society and National Cancer Institute Guidelines

In the 1980s the American Cancer Society issued the following dietary guidelines aimed at reducing cancer risk within the populace:[12]

1. Choose most of the foods you eat from plant sources.
   - Eat five or more servings of fruits and vegetables every day.

TABLE 9.5

Nutrition Facts Panel Information[a]

Serving size (based on amounts commonly used)
Number of servings per container
Kcalories per serving
Kcalories from fat
% Daily value of total fat, saturated fat, cholesterol, sodium, total carbohydrate, dietary fiber, sugars, protein, vitamin A, vitamin C, calcium and iron
Reference values for total fat, saturated fat, cholesterol, sodium, total carbohydrate, and fiber
Kcaloric conversion guide for protein, fat, and carbohydrates

[a] www.healthfinder.gov/searchoptions/topicsaz.htm — search for food labels.

- Eat foods from plant sources, such as breads, cereals, grain products, rice, pasta, or beans several times each day.

2. Limit your intake of high-fat foods, particularly from animal sources.
   - Choose foods low in fat.
   - Limit consumption of meats, especially high-fat meats.
3. Be physically active: achieve and maintain a healthy weight.
   - Be at least moderately active for 30 minutes or more on most days of the week.
   - Stay within your healthy weight range.
4. Limit consumption of alcoholic beverages, if you drink at all.

The National Cancer Institute endorses the following guidelines, which reflect in large part the recommendations of the American Cancer Society:[13]

1. Avoid obesity.
2. Reduce fat intake to 30% of total energy intake as a start. Then consider a reduction closer to 20% of total energy intake if at high risk, such as a family history of cancer.
3. Eat more higher-fiber foods, such as fruits, vegetables, and whole-grain cereals.
4. Include foods rich in vitamins A, E, and C, as well as carotenoids, in the daily diet.
5. If alcohol is consumed, do not drink excessively.
6. Use moderation when consuming salt-cured, smoked, and nitrite-cured foods.

There are also guidelines set forth by the National Cholesterol Education Program and the American Heart Association (refer to the section on cardiovascular disease).

Nutrition Counseling for Adults

Determining Energy Requirements

To plan a diet consistent with dietary guidelines, the nutrition professional should first determine the caloric requirements of a client. The total energy requirements will be the sum of the resting energy requirement, energy needs for physical activity and the energy needed for the thermic effect of foods. To determine the total energy requirement:

Step 1: Estimating Appropriate Body Weight

The Hamwi method is a common tool to estimate appropriate body weight. For females, the estimation is 100 lb for the first 5 feet of height and 5 lb per inch over 5 feet; e.g., a 5′6″ woman would be calculated as: (100 lbs for first five feet) + (5 lbs/inch over 5 ft = 5 × 6 = 30) = 130 lbs. For men the estimation is 106 lbs for the first 5 feet of height and 6 lbs per inch over 5 feet; e.g., a 6′0″ man's desirable weight would be calculated as: (106 lbs for first five feet) + (6 lbs/ inch over 5 feet = 6 × 12 = 72) = 178 lbs. Adjustments are made for a large frame (+10%) or a small frame (–10%).

Step 2: Estimating Energy Needs Based on Body Weight

To estimate energy needs, the first step is to determine resting energy requirements (REE). While several methods exist to calculate energy requirements based on weight, the abbreviated or quick method is probably useful for normal adults. The abbreviated method is as follows:

For adults:	
Women	wt in kg × 23
Men	wt in kg × 24

Step 3: Estimating Energy Required for Physical Activity

Once the REE requirements are determined, an estimate of the energy needs for physical activity must be made. Again there are several alternatives to use to estimate caloric needs for physical activity. The Physical Activity Levels (PALs)[14] method is shown below:

- Seated work with no option of moving around and little or no strenuous leisure activity (PAL factor = 1.4 to 1.5 × REE)
- Seated work with ability or requirement to move around but little or no strenuous leisure activity (PAL factor = 1.6 to 1.7 × REE)
- Standing work (housework, shop clerks) (PAL factor 1.8 to 1.9 × REE)
- Significant amounts of sport or strenuous leisure activity (30 to 60 minutes four to five/week) (PAL factor + 0.3 increment over 1.8 to 1.9 × REE)
- Strenuous work or highly active leisure (PAL factor 2.0 to 2.4)

Step 4: Add REE (Step 2) and Physical Activity (Step 3)

Step 5: Calculate Thermic Effect of Food

To estimate the thermic effect of food multiply the sum of the REE and physical activity by 10% and add that amount to the total.

Determining Protein, Fat, and Carbohydrate Requirements

After the total energy requirements are determined, the contributions from protein, fat, and carbohydrate need to be determined.

1. **Protein:** by converting grams of protein into its caloric equivalent, the percent of protein from total calories can be derived.

2. **Fat:** the recommendation for fat is 30% or less of total energy requirements.
3. **Carbohydrate:** the percent of calories that will come from carbohydrate will be the difference between total energy requirements minus the percent of kcalories from protein and fat.

Estimates of Actual Intakes of Adults for Macronutrients

Nutrition monitoring has been going on since the early 1900s in the United States, when the USDA's Food Supply Series was initiated.[15] Currently the National Nutrition Monitoring and Related Research Program (NNMRRP) is the umbrella for activities that provide regular information about the contribution that diet and nutritional status make to health.[16]

Energy Intake

With respect to total energy intake, for adult men, caloric consumption consistently exceeds that of adult women by approximately 400 kcalories. With one age group exception (ages >70 years), men consumed in excess of 2000 kcalories on average, while women consistently averaged less than 2000 kcalories per day. Fat was contributing slightly above the recommended 30% of kcalories for both men and women. Adult men derive somewhat more kcalories from alcohol compared to women, but women are considerably higher in their carbohydrate intake than men. Men consumed not quite a third of their total energy intake from foods consumed away from home. For women, the contribution of energy from foods eaten away from home is one fourth of their total energy intake. Men were more likely than women to consume a diet that met 100% of the RDA. Table 9.6 provides energy intake data on age cohorts for adult men and women based on the 1994-96 Continuing Survey of Food Intake for Individuals (CSFII). Foods eaten away from home are contributing approximately 30 to 40% of total kcalories consumed by young adults. The percent of kcalories derived from foods eaten away from home decreases with age (Table 9.7).

Total Protein, Carbohydrate, and Fat Intakes

Protein intake is higher for adult men compared to adult women, yet the mean protein intake for both men and women exceeds the 1989 RDA (Table 9.8). With their higher mean protein intake, more men (80.2%) than women (69.2%) met 100% of the 1989 RDA for protein. As with total energy intake, foods consumed away from home contribute at least 25% of the overall protein intake. For men, 29% of the total protein intake was derived from foods eaten away from home. For women, this was 24.6%.

Total carbohydrate intake is higher for men than women, consistent with their higher total energy intake. The mean intake of carbohydrate for adult men was roughly 50 to 60 grams/day higher than the adult female intake (Table 9.8). The mean fiber intake per day for both men and women is below even the lower level of the recommended 24 to 70 grams per day (Table 9.9).

Fat intake for adult men and women, as with protein and carbohydrate intakes, reflects the gender differences in total energy intake pattern, i.e., men consume more than women. The majority of adult men and women exceed the 30% of energy from fat recommendation. Only 29.4% of adult men and 36.8% of adult women maintained a diet within the 30%

TABLE 9.6

Total Energy Intake and Sources of Energy for Adult Men and Women[a]

Age	Males	Females
20–29 yrs	2821	1841
30–39 yrs	2665	1710
40–49 yrs	2435	1682
50–59 yrs	2270	1600
60–69 yrs	2072	1489
70 > yrs	1834	1384
20 < yrs	2455	1646

Sources of Energy Intake (% of Total kcalories)

	Protein		Total Fat		Carbohydrate		Alcohol	
Age	M	F	M	F	M	F	M	F
20–29 yrs	15.2	14.7	32.4	31.8	49.8	63.0	3.4	1.9
30–39 yrs	15.9	15.7	34.0	32.4	48.8	61.8	2.4	1.5
40–49 yrs	16.0	15.6	33.1	33.4	49.2	51.1	2.8	1.4
50–59 yrs	16.3	16.5	33.8	32.4	48.7	51.2	2.5	1.6
60–69 yrs	16.6	16.7	33.5	32.6	49.3	61.2	2.1	1.3
70 > yrs	16.3	16.7	33.0	31.4	50.9	63.3	1.6	1.5
20 < yrs	16.0	15.9	33.3	32.4	49.3	51.9	2.6	1.4

Percent of Individuals Meeting 100% of the 1989 RDA for Energy (2-Day Average)

Age	Males	Females
20–29 yrs	35.4	20.5
30–39 yrs	32.5	17.4
40–49 yrs	26.4	14.0
50–59 yrs	39.0	21.4
60–69 yrs	32.5	15.2
70 > yrs	19.5	12.4
20 > yrs	31.5	17.0

M = males, F = females

[a] http://www.barc.usda.gov/bhnrc/foodsurvey/home.htm

TABLE 9.7

Contribution (% kcal) of Breakfast, Snacks, and Foods Consumed Away from Home to Total Energy Intake (1 day) 1994–1996; M = males; F = females[a]

	Breakfast		Snacks		Foods Away From Home	
Age	M	F	M	F	M	F
20–29 yrs	14.2	16.0	18.2	17.0	40.0	34.3
30–39 yrs	15.5	16.9	15.5	16.9	31.4	26.6
40–49 yrs	16.3	16.9	15.5	17.1	29.4	25.4
50–59 yrs	18.2	19.1	15.4	15.2	26.7	23.0
60–69 yrs	20.9	19.9	15.0	15.1	20.0	17.6
70 > yrs	23.8	23.0	12.2	12.3	14.2	12.5
20 < yrs	17.1	18.2	15.7	15.9	29.4	24.5

[a] http://www.barc.usda.gov/bhnrc/foodsurvey/home.htm

recommendation. Foods eaten away from home contributed 30.9% of the total fat intake for men and 26.2% for women (Table 9.8). Cholesterol intake is considerably less for women than men. Women of all age groups consumed under 300 mg/day, whereas, adult men generally consumed slightly more than 300 mg/day on average (Table 9.10). More

TABLE 9.8

Total Protein, Carbohydrate, and Fat Intakes (gm)[a]

	Protein Intake (gm)		Carbohydrate (gm)		Fat (gm)	
Age	**M**	**F**	**M**	**F**	**M**	**F**
20–29 yrs	104.1	65.9	344.9	241.6	103.3	65.9
30–39 yrs	102.7	65.3	322.3	218.8	102.7	63.2
40–49 yrs	95.3	63.5	294.7	213.8	95.3	63.5
50–59 yrs	90.3	64.1	273.1	201.5	90.3	59.4
60–69 yrs	83.5	60.4	252.5	188.7	83.5	56.2
70 > yrs	72.9	56.6	239.2	183.5	72.9	49.2
20 < yrs	94.9	63.8	298.8	211.7	94.9	50.5

M = males, F = females

[a] http://www.barc.usda.gov/bhnrc/foodsurvey/home.htm

TABLE 9.9

Fiber Intake (gm)[a]

Age	M	F
20–29 yrs	18.3	13.2
30–39 yrs	19.4	13.6
40–49 yrs	18.3	14.0
50–59 yrs	18.5	14.5
60–69 yrs	18.5	14.2
70 > yrs	17.7	14.2
20 < yrs	18.6	13.9

M = males, F = females

[a] http://www.barc.usda.gov/bhnrc/foodsurvey/home.htm

adults consumed a diet consistent with the recommended cholesterol intake (55.1% of men; 79.4% of women) than for total fat, where only 29.4% of adult men and 36.8% of adult women maintained a diet within 30% of the total energy intake. The intake of the types of fat — saturated, polyunsaturated, monounsaturated, and cholesterol is presented in Table 9.10.

Health Implications of Current Macronutrient Intakes

Energy and Obesity Issues

Overweight is associated with several chronic diseases — coronary heart disease, hypertension, noninsulin-dependent diabetes mellitus, and some forms of cancer.[17,18] An estimated 300,000 Americans per year die from obesity-related conditions.[18] Obesity is also an associated risk factor for joint disease, gallstones, and obstructive sleep apnea.[19] In 1995, the economic cost associated with obesity was estimated at $62.3 billion.[20]

From 1976-1980 and 1988-1994, the Centers for Disease Control and Prevention (CDC) reported an increase of 10% in the incidence of overweight in the American population.[21] Data from the CSFII, 1994 (http://www.barc.usda.gov/bhnrc/foodsurvey/home.htm) indicate among adults, both men and women, the incidence of overweight is approximately 30% (Table 9.11). If the incidence of obesity continues to rise at current rates, it is predicted that by 2230, every adult in the U.S. will be overweight.[22]

TABLE 9.10

Intake of Saturated Fatty Acids, Monounsaturated Fatty Acids, Polyunsaturated Fatty Acids, and Cholesterol[a,b]

Age	Saturated Fatty Acids		Monounsaturated Fatty Acids		Polyunsaturated Fatty Acids		Cholesterol	
	M	F	M	F	M	F	M	F
20–29 yrs	35.4	22.3	40.1	25.2	19.6	13.5	348	219
30–39 yrs	35.3	21.3	39.4	24.1	20.1	12.8	362	217
40–49 yrs	30.6	21.0	35.6	24.0	18.3	13.6	331	222
50–59 yrs	28.6	19.1	33.9	22.6	18.1	13.1	332	200
60–69 yrs	25.9	17.9	30.1	20.8	16.5	12.1	307	218
70 > yrs	22.8	15.9	26.4	18.7	13.9	10.6	270	188
20 < yrs	31.3	20.0	36.8	23.0	18.4	12.8	331	213

Percent of Individuals Meeting the Recommendations for Total Fat, Saturated Fat, and Cholesterol

Age	Total Fat		Saturated Fatty Acids		Cholesterol	
	M	F	M	F	M	F
20–29 yrs	29.3	40.1	34.1	42.3	63.1	77.0
30–39 yrs	28.1	35.9	30.7	39.7	62.6	80.9
40–49 yrs	27.4	30.5	31.7	38.5	53.5	76.0
50–59 yrs	28.0	36.5	36.2	46.0	54.2	80.7
60–69 yrs	33.9	38.0	42.1	46.1	58.1	78.7
70 > yrs	34.4	42.2	41.6	47.9	67.1	84.5
20 > yrs	29.4	36.8	34.5	42.7	55.1	79.4

M = males, F = females

[a] Saturated fatty acids, monounsaturated fatty acids, polyunsaturated fatty acids in grams; cholesterol in milligrams.

[b] http://www.barc.usda.gov/bhnrc/foodsurvey/home.htm

TABLE 9.11

Incidence of Overweight (%)[a]

Age	Men	Women
20–29 yrs	21.5	22.1
30–39 yrs	32.3	27.4
40–49 yrs	37.0	36.1
50–59 yrs	39.9	37.8
> 60 yrs	40.7	33.4
< 20 yrs	31.8	31.7

[a] http://www.barc.usda.gov/bhnrc/foodsurvey/home.htm

The prevalence of overweight/obesity among Americans is at odds with the perceptions of the importance of maintaining an appropriate body weight. When Americans were surveyed as part of the 1994-96 USDA Diet and Health Knowledge survey, 68.1% of adult males over 20 years of age reported that "maintaining a healthy weight" was very important. For that same survey, 77% of the adult women over 20 years of age reported maintenance of a healthy body weight as very important. Given the importance Americans place on maintaining healthy body weight and given the high incidence of overweight/obesity, it is little wonder that Americans spend in excess of $33 billion a year on weight loss schemes.[23] Among these are the myriad of weight loss diets that appear on the market every year. In 1992, 33-40% of American women and 20-24% of American men reported being on a diet.[24]

Fad Diets Used for Weight Loss Promotion

While numerous fad diets come and go, several categories tend to remain fairly common. These include high protein/low carbohydrate diet regimens, low fat diets, and very low calorie diets.

High Protein/ Low Carbohydrate

These diets generally restrict the carbohydrate intake to 100 grams or less per day. Restriction of carbohydrate leads to an initial mobilization of glycogen and then to gluconeogenesis and ketosis, all of which promote water loss and some lean tissue loss, which constitute a significant portion of the weight loss. Some of the low carbohydrate diets promote high protein and consequently a higher animal fat intake which is inconsistent with the dietary guidelines for fat intake.[25] Examples of high protein/low carbohydrate diets are Atkins' Diet Revolution, Calories Don't Count, and The Doctor's Quick Weight Loss Diet (Stillman's).

Low Fat Diets

Generally these diets restrict fat intake to 20% or less of total energy intake. Examples of these types of diets include the T-factor Diet, the Pasta Diet, the Pritikin Diet, and Fit or Fat. The average weight loss on these types of diets is 0.1 to 0.2 kg per week. With the limited fat intake, one drawback is the low satiety factor which may prompt noncompliant diet behavior.[26]

Very Low Calorie Diets

These diets arose during the 1970s and were known as protein-sparing-modified fasts or liquid protein diets. These diet plans generally rely on liquid supplements to substitute for food intake and restrict the overall caloric level to less than 800 kcalories per day. These diets may be indicated for moderately to several obese patients (BMI >30). The severe caloric restriction does lead to weight loss, but generally this level of caloric intake cannot be sustained, and weight regain is a potential problem. These diets may also lead to weight loss from lean tissue mass.[23, 27]

The Zone Diet

The Zone Diet is a modified approach to the low carbohydrate-high protein type of diet. The diet promotes a macronutrient intake of 30% protein, 30% fat, and 40% carbohydrate. At this ratio of protein: fat: carbohydrate, the author contends that insulin levels will remain stable, and this, in turn, dampens insulin's potential to promote the conversion of carbohydrates into fat and thereby promote weight gain. The Zone Diet claims go beyond the promise of weight loss via insulin regulation into the realms of disease prevention. The Zone Diet author argues that a high carbohydrate, low fat diet promotes an imbalance in "bad" eicosanoid production that can lead to the development of such diseases as arthritis and coronary heart disease. However, there is no significant body of evidence to support the author's claims.[28, 29]

Putting fad diets aside, an approach to weight management that recognizes overweight obesity as a chronic condition and incorporates the elements of a healthy diet, exercise, and behavior modification, is more likely to be successful over time, and particularly in the maintenance of weight loss.[30]

Protein Intake — Health Issues

The average American diet is very liberal with respect to protein intake. The RDA for protein for women aged 19 to 24 is 46 grams, and for men of the same age the RDA is 58 grams.[7] In contrast, the average protein intake in grams for adults over 20 in the U.S. is 63.8 grams for women and 94.9 grams for men. Some concern has been expressed over the long term health consequences of excessive protein intake. There is some evidence in humans that a lifetime on a high animal protein diet (typical American diet pattern) can aggravate existing renal problems,[31] may increase the risk for cancer of the kidney,[32] and can accelerate adult bone loss.[33, 34] Lastly, higher animal protein intake is associated with higher than desirable levels of total fat and saturated fat intake.

A primary, albeit not exclusive source of protein in the American diet is meat. The U.S. Food Guide Pyramid recommends between 5 and 7 ounces of cooked lean meat or equivalent in meat alternatives per day. To be consistent with the Dietary Guidelines to reduce total fat and saturated fat in the diet, it would be helpful to consume lower-fat types of meat and perhaps a greater amount of some forms of meat alternatives such as soybean products. However, Americans derive the majority of their protein from meat. The 1994-96 CSFII indicated that for adult males over 20 years of age, the average daily intake of meat and meat alternatives was 6.4 ounces, and for women the total was 3.9. With respect to total intake, men were consuming sufficient amounts of meat and meat alternatives when compared to the recommended 5 to 7 ounces. Women, on the other hand, fell below the minimum 5 ounces recommended in the U.S. Food Guide Pyramid. With that in mind, data from the CSFII indicate that regardless of meat servings, protein intake is meeting RDA requirements. Consequently, the source of protein may be an important consideration. The ratio of meat to meat alternatives is skewed heavily in favor of meat (beef, pork, lamb, and veal). For men, of the average 6.4 ounces of lean meat and meat alternatives consumed daily, 2.7 ounces are derived from lean meat and another 1.0 ounce from the higher fat sources of frankfurter and lunch meat. Consequently, 3.7 of the 6.4 ounces, or 58%, was from meat. Only 1.5 ounces and 0.5 ounce, respectively, were contributed by poultry and fish. For women, 1.4 ounces of meat and 0.5 ounces of frankfurter and lunch meat were consumed on a daily average. This accounts for 49% of the total meat or meat alternative consumption. For women, poultry contributed 1.1 ounce and fish 0.4 ounce towards the total meat and meat alternative intake. Some data suggest that an increase in fish and consequently in omega-3-fatty acid intake may be warranted.

Protein Supplements

Protein supplements are quite common among athletes and physically active adults as part of their strength training regimens.[35] Bucci argues that while there is very little research that documents the benefits of protein supplementation, high protein diets are safe.[35] However, the amount recommended for endurance athletes is 70 gm/day, and for strength athletes 112 to 178 gm. The lower range of these recommendations is clearly within the normal intake of American men. This argues against the need for further protein supplementation.

Amino Acid Supplements

Individual amino acid supplements have been promoted on the market periodically. Again, a target audience has often been the athlete or physically active adult, with promises of enhanced performance. There is a dearth of research that can support such claims.[35] In addition, in 1992 a scientific panel convened to address the safety of amino acid supplements concluded that there is little research on which to support making amino acid supplement recommendations, and some amino acid supplementation (serine and proline) can have adverse health effects. Consequently, the panel concluded that no level of amino acid supplementation may be considered safe at this time.[36]

Fat Intake Issues — Amount and Type of Fat

The adult American diet is slightly over the 30% of total energy that is recommended. Data from the 1994-96 CSFII reveals that approximately 25% of the total energy intake is contributed by discretionary fats as cream, butter, margarine, cream cheese, oil, lard, meat drippings, cocoa, and chocolate. Based on the average energy intake of adult males, discretionary fat contributes 614 kcals per day, and for females 412 kcals per day. By cutting back on discretionary fat intake, American adults could conceivably lose 0.8 to 1.0 lb per week. This would be helpful in dealing with the adult obesity rates in the U.S. Simple changes in discretionary fat intake could be helpful. For example:

- Substituting mustard for mayonnaise on sandwiches = 5 gm (45 kcals) fat savings
- Ordering hamburger rather than a cheeseburger = 9 gm fat savings (81 kcals)
- Using salt and pepper instead of sour cream on a baked potato = 3 gm fat savings (27 kcals)

Americans consume more saturated fat than is desirable. In addition, approximately 5% of the total fat intake in the American diet is contributed from trans-fatty acids.[37] Biochemically, trans-fatty acids act similarly to saturated fatty acids, raising LDL levels and decreasing HDL levels.[38] While their effect is not as great as saturated fat, they may contribute to a lipid intake pattern that raises the risk for coronary heart disease.[39] Trans-fatty acids are formed as a result of the hydrogenation process and are found in such food items as margarine, shortening, commercial frying fats, and many high-fat baked and snack foods. Trans-fatty acids also occur naturally in milk and butter as a result of the fatty acids synthesized by rumen flora in the rumen. Concern over trans-fatty acid intake has led some consumers to question whether they should forgo margarine and return to butter. Research suggests that saturated fat, as in butter, still exerts a greater negative effect on a person's lipid profile than do trans-fatty acids. However, use of less hydrogenated forms such as tub rather than stick margarine may be beneficial.

Carbohydrate Intake Issues

Two issues arise with respect to the carbohydrate intake of American adults — low fiber intake and high sugar intake. Low fiber intake is associated with a higher incidence of such chronic diseases as heart disease,[40] cancer,[41] and diabetes.[42] At least partial explanation for the low fiber intake is related to the low fruit and vegetable intake associated with the typical American diet. Data from the 1994-96 CSFII indicated that for adult males the average total servings (based on the Food Guide Pyramid serving recommendations) of vegetables per day was four. For females the average was three servings. For both men and women, one-third of the vegetable servings were accounted for by white potatoes. Average servings of fruit per day for both men and women was 1.5. This is just under the minimum Food Guide Pyramid recommendation for two servings per day. Another contributing factor to the low fiber intake is the lack of whole grain foods in the diet. Adult men consumed on average 8 servings of grain products per day, which is approximately mid-range of the 6 to 11 servings of grain products recommended by the Food Guide Pyramid. Women averaged six servings from grain products. However, for both men and women, only one of these servings was from whole grain products. The health benefits of a higher fiber diet are addressed in other relevant sections of this handbook.

The other carbohydrate intake issue is the consumption of refined sugar, which contributes calories but little other nutritive value to the diet. The 1994-96 CSFII data revealed that approximately 14% of the average energy intake for adult males was from added sugars. For women, the caloric contribution from added sugars was slightly higher at approximately 15%. Foods such as breads, cakes, soft drinks, jam, and ice cream were contributing to the discretionary sugar intake. In 1994 to 1996, soft drink consumption out-paced milk and coffee, and approximately 75% of the soft drink consumption is of the sugar-sweetened variety.[43] During the last decade, consumption of snack foods such as cakes, cookies, pastries, and pies has increased 15%, likely contributing to the high intake of discretionary sugar.[43] These data are in contrast to the importance consumers report they place on a diet moderate in sugar intake. A majority (slightly over 50%) of adults surveyed in the 1994-96 CSFII indicated it was very important to consume a diet moderate in sugar.

Summary

Counseling the normal healthy American adult should focus on dietary intake patterns that promote health and reduce risk for chronic disease, i.e., diet recommendations should follow the U.S. Dietary Guidelines. Therefore, consistent with the 2000 edition of the U.S. Dietary Guidelines, the focus on nutrition counseling should be:

Aim for fitness.

- Aim for a healthy weight:
  1. Calculate the appropriate weight for the individual.
  2. Consider the fat distribution pattern and take a more aggressive posture with individuals whose body fat distribution is more "apple" than "pear" shaped and hence places them at higher health risk.
  3. For individuals whose body weight is inappropriate, initiate counseling to assist in weight reduction. This may include calculation of appropriate caloric intake, recommendations of sources of caloric intake from the macro-nutrients of protein, fat, and carbohydrate, appropriate portion sizes to control caloric intake, and increases in physical activity (second dietary guideline, see below).
- Be physically active each day.

Build a healthy base.

- Let the pyramid guide your food choices. Based on current consumption patterns, the average adult can likely benefit from nutrition counseling that:
  1. Recommends greater restraint with respect to servings of discretionary fats, sweets, and alcohol from the top portion of the pyramid.

2. Recommends somewhat higher intake of fish and meat alternatives such as soy products and a continued reduction of ounces of high fat meats like frankfurters and luncheon meats.

- Eat a variety of grains daily, especially whole grains. Current carbohydrate consumption patterns indicate that the average adult American should be counseled to:
  1. Increase his/her consumption of whole grain products.
  2. Use greater restraint with respect to his/her consumption of less nutrient dense refined sugar.
- Eat a variety of fruits and vegetables daily. Variety as well as an increase in quantity is appropriate when counseling adults. Data indicate that the most common vegetable is the potato. Greater variety of both fruits and vegetables will help contribute a wider range of nutrients and other phytochemicals that might be more appropriate for health promotion.
- Keep food safe to eat. Food safety is as important as nutrient intake with respect to health maintenance. Attention in counseling should be given to insuring the individual's understanding of safe food handling and food preparation techniques.

Choose sensibly.

- Choose a diet low in saturated fat and cholesterol and moderate in total fat. Over-consumption of discretionary fat is common with adult Americans. Counseling that helps identify small dietary changes that can be made to reduce total fat, saturated fat and cholesterol intake is appropriate.
- Choose beverages and foods that limit your intake of sugars. Nutrition counseling for adults should help clients identify sources of sugars in their diet, particularly the sugar contribution that might be coming from soft drinks. Not only are soft drinks widely promoted in the American culture, but popular serving sizes range from 8 to 16 to as high as 32 ounces.
- Choose and prepare foods with less salt. The concerns of a high salt intake are dealt with in other sections of this handbook, which also indicate the need to help adults recognize foods that are contributing to an excessive salt intake.
- If you drink alcoholic beverages, do so in moderation. The average American adult needs to be cognizant of his/her caloric intake. Low nutrient dense alcohol calories may be inconsistent with the caloric intake needed to achieve/maintain a healthy weight. This fact needs to be discussed in a nutrition counseling session.

References

1. United States Department of Health and Human Services, Public Health Service, No. 88-50210, *Surgeon General's Report on Nutrition and Health*. United States Government Printing Office, Washington DC, 1988.
2. *Dietary Guidelines for Americans 2000*, www.ars.usda.gov/dgac
3. US Senate, Select Committee on Nutrition and Human Needs, US Senate, December 1977, 95th Congress — 1st Session.

4. United States Department of Agriculture, United States Department of Health and Human Services, *Nutrition and Your Health. Dietary Guidelines for Americans*. Home and Garden Bulletin No. 232, Washington, DC, 1980.
5. United States Department of Agriculture, *The Food Guide Pyramid.* Home and Garden Bulletin No. 252.a, United States Printing Office, Washington, DC, 1992.
6. Kant, A.K., Block, G., Schatzkin, A., et al., *JADA* 91: 1526; 1991.
7. Food and Nutrition Board, National Research Council, *Recommended Dietary Allowances*, 10th ed., National Academy Press, Washington, DC, 1989.
8. Food and Nutrition Board, Institute of Medicine, *Dietary Reference Intakes for Calcium, Phosphorus, Magnesium, Vitamin D and Fluoride,* National Academy Press, Washington, DC, 1997.
9. Food and Nutrition Board, Institute of Medicine, *Dietary Reference Intakes for Thiamin, Riboflavin, Niacin, Vitamin* B_6*, Folate, Vitamin* B_{12}*, Pantothenic Acid, Biotin, and Choline.* National Academy Press, Washington, DC, 1998.
10. Food and Drug Administration, *Focus on Food Labeling*. Special Issue of FDA Consumer Magazine, May 1993, DHHS Publication No. (FDA) 93-2262, United States Government Printing Office, Washington, DC, 1993.
11. ________________ *Nutrition Reviews*, 49: 291; 1991.
12. ________________ American Cancer Society, *Nutrition and Prevention*, www2.cancer.org/Prevention/index.cfm?prevention=importance.
13. Wardlaw, G. *Contemporary Nutrition: Issues and Insights*. 3rd ed., Brown and Benchmark, Madison, WI, 1997.
14. Shetty, P.S., Henry, C.J.K., Black, A.E., Prentice, A.M.., *Eur J Clin Nutr,* 1006: 11S; 1996.
15. Boyle, M.A., Morris, D.H., *Community Nutrition in Action: An Entrepreneurial Approach,* 2nd ed., Wadsworth Publishing, Belmont, CA, 1999, p. 112.
16. Federation of American Societies for Experimental Biology, Third Report on Nutrition Monitoring in the United States, Vol. 1, United States Government Printing Office, Washington DC, 1995.
17. Centers for Disease Control and Prevention, *National Diabetes Fact Sheet: National Estimate and General Information on Diabetes in the United States,* United States Department of Health and Human Services, Centers for Disease Control and Prevention, Atlanta, GA, Nov. 1, 1977.
18. McGinnis, J.M., Foege, W.H., *JAMA*, 270: 2207; 1993.
19. National Institutes of Health, National Heart, Lung and Blood Institute, Clinical guidelines on the identification, evaluation, and treatment of overweight and obesity in adults — the evidence report, *Ob Res*, 6: 51S, 1998.
20. Colditz G.A., Wolf, A.M., In: *Progress in Obesity Research*, (Anderson, A.H., Bouchard, C., Lau, D., Leiter, L., Mendelson, R., Eds) John Libbey & Co., 7th International Congress on Obesity, 1996.
21. Centers for Disease Control and Prevention, Update: prevalence of overweight among children, adolescents and adults, United States, 1988-94, *Mortality and Morbidity Weekly Report*, 46(9), 199-202, 1997b.
22. Foreyt, J., Goodrick, K., *The Lancet*, 346: 134; 1995.
23. American Dietetics Association, Position of the American Dietetic Association: Weight management. *JADA*, 97: 71; 1997.
24. National Institutes of Health, *Methods for voluntary weight loss and control*, Technology Assessment Conference, Bethesda, MD, 1992.
25. The Low-Carb, High-Protein Craze, *Am Inst Cancer Res Newsl*, Vol. 67, Spring 2000.
26. American Dietetic Association, Position of the American Dietetic Association: Very-low-calorie weight loss diets, *JADA*, 90: 722; 1990.
27. Kendall, A., Levitski, D.A., Strupp, B.J., Lissner, L., *Amer J Clin Nutr,* 53: 1124; 1991.
28. *U.C. Berkeley Wellness Letter,* June, 1998.
29. Liebman, B., *Nutrition Action Health Letter,* July/August, 1996.
30. Rippe, J.M., Crossley, S., Ringer, R., Obesity as a chronic disease: modern medical and lifestyle management, *JADA*, 98: 2: S9; 1998.
31. Ahmed, F.E., *JADA*, 91: 1266; 1991.
32. Chow, W.H., Gridley, G., McLaughlin, J.K., Mandel, J.S., et al., *J Natl Cancer Inst*, 86: 1131; 1994.

33. Hu, J., Zhao, X.H., Parpia, B., *Am J Clin Nutr*, 58: 398; 1993.
34. Hegsted, D.M., *J Nutr*, 116: 2316; 1986.
35. Bucci, L., *Nutrients as Ergogenic Aids for Sports and Exercise*, CRC Press, Boca Raton, 1993.
36. Anderson, S.A., Raiten, D.J., Eds, *Safety of Amino Acids Used as Supplements*, Federation of American Societies for Experimental Biology, Bethesda, MD, 1992.
37. Emken, E.A., *Amer J Clin Nutr*, 62: 659S; 1995.
38. Katan, M.B., Zock, P.L., *Ann Rev Nutr* 15: 473; 1995.
39. Shapiro, S., *Amer J Clin Nutr*, 66: 1011S; 1997.
40. Jenkins, D.J.A., *New Engl J Med*, 329: 21; 1993.
41. Munster, I.P., de Boer, H.M., Jansen, M.C., et al., *Amer J Clin Nutr*, 59: 626; 1994.
42. Salmeron, J., Manson, J.E., Stampfer, M.J., Coldizt, G.A., et al., *JAMA*, 277: 472; 1997.
43. Frazao, E., Ed, *America's Eating Habits*, Economic Research Service Report. Agriculture Information Bulletin No. 750. Washington, DC, 1999.

10

Nutrition in the Later Years

Elaine B. Feldman

Introduction

This section incorporates some nutritional concepts that are described in more detail in the sections on cardiovascular disease, cancer, skeletal disorders, neuropsychiatric disorders (cognitive), and the adult diet. Information will be provided on the varying problems of the successful and healthy free-living older adults and domiciled elderly, the very old (>85 years), and the old old (centenarians).

Background

The elderly are the fastest growing segment of the U.S. population (see below). It is projected that the number of institutionalized elderly will triple in the next few decades, and the number of people over 85 years of age (the very old) as a percent of the total population will quadruple. The nutritional needs and problems of these groups differ from those of their younger cohorts. Specific changes in lifestyle and physiology influence nutritional status. The prevalence of chronic disease increases with age, and the treatment of these diseases with drugs and diet have an additional impact on nutritional status. Dietary recommendations need to be designed for these people in order to obtain their compliance. Surveys have shown that in people over age 75, malnutrition affects 15% of outpatients, 50% of hospitalized patients, and 85% of institutionalized patients.[1]

The Biology of Aging

Aging is characterized by a gradual, cumulative loss in metabolic control. Homeostatic mechanisms that control body function gradually become less efficient. Physiologically

0-8493-2705-9/01/$0.00+$1.50

and biochemically, senescence occurs not in an orderly fashion but at unexpected times and with unanticipated events. Some of these events are predictable, but some are not. For example, the loss of ovarian function is predictable but its timing is not. There is considerable individual variation in the loss of menses among women. Some of the age-related loss in metabolic control can be explained by age-related accumulations of DNA mutations in both the nuclear and mitochondrial genome. Some of these mutations are diet responsive while others are not.

With age there are changes in DNA (base substitutions, deletions, aberrant repair) that result in functional loss in the activity of the gene product(s) the DNA encodes. Changes in the DNA (as well as some of the gene products) are biomarkers of aging.[2] Studies in animals have shown that lifelong food restriction results in a delay in the appearance of DNA aberrations as well as a delay in the changes in the activities of key enzymes. Food–restricted animals live longer than non-restricted animals that are kept under the same conditions, fed the same qualitative diet, and are of the same gender and genetic makeup.[3] The extrapolation of these findings in rats and mice to humans is questionable because of the nature of the experimental conditions used. The animals are genetically similar and they are protected from infectious agents. They are reared under conditions of carefully regulated environments that are temperature, humidity, and light controlled. The food is carefully prepared to contain all the needed nutrients, with the only constraint being the reduction in the energy supply. Humans do not exist under these conditions. They are randomly exposed to environmental insults, their food is seldom consistent from one day to the next, and their genetic backgrounds are highly variable. As social creatures we do not live singly in cages; we experience wars, economic duress, social upheavals, and so forth. Nonetheless, some of the observations in animals have been also made in humans. For example, normal aging in humans is characterized by an accumulation of deletions in mitochondrial DNA in various tissues.[4] This may result from free radical attack on the genome, and may be ameliorated by antioxidants.[5]

Age has a profound effect on membrane saturation and fluidity.[6] An age-related decline in membrane-associated reactions or pathways occurs, independent of changes in the diet or the hormonal milieu. The efficiency of oxidative phosphorylation declines with age (Table 10.1). Mitochondrial damage and loss of function occurs, in part related to increased formation of superoxide and other free radicals.

With age, the efficiency of transmission of hormone and secondary messenger communications decreases (Table 10.2). This is due to numerous structural and functional changes in the endocrine glands, a decline in gene expression, and in the accuracy and efficiency of protein synthesis. The hormones affected regulate the metabolism of carbohydrates, lipid, and protein. The progressive changes in the mitochondria and in gene expression lead to progressive loss in the tight control of intermediary metabolism (Table 10.1). This is coupled with age-related changes in the endocrine and central nervous systems.

Mortality and Aging Statistics

The leading causes of death in the U.S. in 1980 and 1996 are listed in Table 10.3.[7] Over this period the three leading causes of death remain: cardiovascular, neoplastic, and cerebrovascular disease. Chronic obstructive pulmonary disease currently exceeds injuries, followed by diabetes mellitus, human immunodeficiency virus (HIV) infection (not listed in 1980), suicide, and chronic liver diseases. Table 10.4 lists the death rates for 1996.[8] Many

TABLE 10.1

Effects of Age on Intermediary Metabolism and Its Control

Pathway	Control Points	Effects of Age[a]
Glycolysis	Transport of glucose into the cell (mobile glucose transporter)	↓
	Glucokinase	↓
	Phosphofructokinase	↓
	α-Glycerophosphate shuttle	
	Redox state, phosphorylation state	
Pentose phosphate shunt	Glucose-6-phosphate dehydrogenase	↓
	6-phosphogluconate dehydrogenase	↓
Glycogenesis	Stimulated by insulin and glucose	ND
	High-phosphorylation state (ratio of ATP to ADP)	ND
Glycogenolysis	Stimulated by catecholamines	ND
Lipogenesis	Stimulated by insulin	
	Acetyl-CoA carboxylase	
	High-phosphorylation state	
	Malate citrate shuttle	↓
Gluconeogenesis	Stimulated by epinephrine	
	Malate aspartate shuttle	↓
	Redox state	↑
	Phosphoenopyruvate carboxykinase	↓
	Pyruvate kinase	
Cholesterogenesis	HMG CoA reductase	
Ureogenesis	Carbamyl phosphate synthesis	↑,↓
	ATP	ND
Citric acid cycle	All three shuttles	
	Phosphorylation state	↓
Lipolysis	Lipoprotein lipase	↓
Respiration	ADP influx into the mitochondria	↓
	Ca^{2+} flux	
	Shuttle activities	↓
	Substrate transporters	↓
Oxidative phosphorylation	ADP-ATP exchange	↓
	Ca^{2+} ion	
Protein synthesis	Accuracy of gene transcription	↓
	Availability of amino acids	↓
	ATP	↓

[a] ↑ — increased as the animal ages; ↓ — decreased as the animal ages; ND — no data.

From Berdanier, C.D., *Advanced Nutrition: Macronutrients*, 2nd ed., CRC Press, Boca Raton, 2000, pg. 252. With permission.

TABLE 10.2

Hormone Changes with Age

Hormone	Age Effects
Serum thyroxine (T_4)	↓
Serum triiodothyronine (T_1)	↓
Thyroid-binding globulin	No change or ↑
Thyroid-stimulating hormone	↓
Insulin	↑ followed by ↓
ACTH	↓
Epinephrine	↓
Glucagon	↓
Growth hormone	↓
Estrogen	↓
Testosterone	↓
Cortisol (glucocorticoids)	↓
Pancreatic polypeptide	↑

Note: ↑ — increase; ↓ — decrease.

From Berdanier, C.D., *Advanced Nutrition: Macronutrients*, 2nd ed., CRC Press, Boca Raton, 2000, pg. 250. With permission.

TABLE 10.3

Leading Causes of Death and Numbers of Deaths, According to Sex and Race, United States, 1996

Sex, Race, and Rank Order	Cause of Death	Deaths
All Persons		
	All causes	2,314,690
1	Diseases of heart	733,381
2	Malignant neoplasms	539,633
3	Cerebrovascular diseases	159,942
4	Chronic obstructive pulmonary diseases	106,027
5	Unintentional injuries	94,948
6	Pneumonia and influenza	83,727
7	Diabetes mellitus	61,767
8	Human immunodeficiency virus infection	31,130
9	Suicide	30,903
10	Chronic liver disease and cirrhosis	26,047
Male		
	All causes	1,163,569
1	Diseases of heart	360,075
2	Malignant neoplasms	281,898
3	Cerebrovascular diseases	62,475
4	Unintentional injuries	61,589
5	Chronic obstructive pulmonary diseases	54,485
6	Pneumonia and influenza	37,991
7	Diabetes mellitus	27,648
8	Human immunodeficiency virus infection	25,277
9	Suicide	24,998
10	Chronic liver disease and cirrhosis	16,311
Female		
	All causes	1,151,121
1	Diseases of heart	373,286
2	Malignant neoplasms	257,635
3	Cerebrovascular diseases	97,467
4	Chronic obstructive pulmonary diseases	61,642
5	Pneumonia and influenza	45,736
6	Diabetes mellitus	34,121
7	Unintentional injuries	33,359
8	Alzheimer's disease	14,426
9	Nephritis, nephrotic syndrome, and nephrosis	12,662
10	Septicemia	12,177
White		
	All causes	1,992,966
1	Diseases of heart	645,614
2	Malignant neoplasms	489,406
3	Cerebrovascular diseases	138,296
4	Chronic obstructive pulmonary diseases	97,889
5	Unintentional injuries	79,405
6	Pneumonia and influenza	74,194
7	Diabetes mellitus	49,511
8	Suicide	27,856
9	Chronic liver disease and cirrhosis	21,422
10	Alzheimer's disease	20,198

TABLE 10.3 *(Continued)*

Leading Causes of Death and Numbers of Deaths, According to Sex and Race, United States, 1996

Sex, Race, and Rank Order	Cause of Death	Deaths
Black		
	All causes	282,089
1	Diseases of heart	77,841
2	Malignant neoplasms	60,766
3	Cerebrovascular diseases	18,481
4	Human immunodeficiency virus infection	13,997
5	Unintentional injuries	12,656
6	Diabetes mellitus	10,800
7	Homicide and legal intervention	9,983
8	Pneumonia and influenza	7,963
9	Chronic obstructive pulmonary diseases	6,924
10	Certain conditions originating in the perinatal period	4,711

Data based on the National Vital Statistics System, taken from Table 33, *Health*, United States, 1998, page 212.

TABLE 10.4

Leading Causes of Death in the United States, Death Rates and Age-Adjusted Death Rates, 1996

Rank[1]	Cause of Death	% of Total Deaths	Rate/100,000 Population	Age-Adjusted Rate
1	Heart diseases	31.6	276.6	134.6
2	Cancers	23.4	205.2	129.1
3	Stroke	6.9	60.5	26.5
4	Lung diseases	4.5	40.0	21.0
5	Accidents[2]	4.0	35.4	30.1
6	Pneumonia and flu	3.5	31.1	12.6
7	Diabetes mellitus	2.6	23.2	13.6
8	AIDS	1.4	12.3	11.6
9	Suicide	1.3	—	10.8
10	Liver disease	1.1	11.6	7.5
11	Renal diseases	1.1	9.5	4.3
12	Infections	0.9	9.2	4.1

[1] Based on the total number of deaths in 1996 (2,322,421). These 12 causes account for 82.3% of the total.

[2] The preferred term is unintentional death. It includes motor vehicle-related deaths.

Taken from *Morbidity and Mortality Weekly Report,* U.S. Department of Health and Human Services, Vol. 46, Oct. 10, 1997.

of these disorders are nutrition-related in their etiology or treatment, and are discussed in individual sections in this handbook.

These mortality statistics are relatively similar for men and women, with striking differences seen only in the higher prevalence of Alzheimer's disease, renal disease, and septicemia appearing for women, and HIV, suicide, and liver disease replacing these in men.

Life expectancy at birth is expected to exceed 80 years in the first century of this millennium, up from 49 years in 1900. The proportion of people in the U.S. over age 65 increased by 89% between 1960 and 1990, and over age 84 by 232%. The number of centenarians in the U.S. has increased eightfold from 1950 (4447) 1990 (35,808).[9]

Lifestyle and Socioeconomic Changes Affecting the Nutritional Status of the Elderly

Changes with aging include:[10]

- Reduced income with retirement
- Insufficient funds for purchase of food
- Skipping meals
- Illness and increased medical expenses
- Loss of mobility
- Diminished acuity in sensory perceptions (hearing, vision, taste)
- Inability to drive to doctor's appointments or to the grocery store
- Inability to prepare or store food
- Loss of balance
- Diminished self-esteem
- Social isolation

Diseases that are common in the elderly and impact on their nutritional status include:

- Senile dementia of the Alzheimer's type, with cognitive impairment and memory loss
- Arthritis, with limited mobility of joints, and deformities
- Osteopenia, with fractures and deformities
- Parkinson's disease, with rigidity and tremor
- Dental and oral health problems — problems with chewing
- Gastrointestinal disorders — swallowing difficulties
- Neoplasms, with hypercatabolism, anorexia, and cachexia
- Diabetes mellitus, with restrictive diets and medication interactions
- Renal insufficiency, with restrictive diets and dialysis treatment
- Paralysis, limiting mobility
- Depression, leading to anorexia

Some deterioration in mental function may be attributable to malnutrition of protein, energy, and vitamins and/or minerals, either primary or secondary to disease. These aspects are discussed in the sections on the nutrients and the diseases.

A survey of the elderly in South Carolina in 1990[10] showed that 20% skip meals, 33% live alone, 45% use multiple prescription medications. Half of those over 85 years of age are dependent or disabled; 10% over age 65 are cognitively impaired, with 25% so impaired over age 85. Indicators of poor nutritional status were:

- <80% of desirable weight for age
- <10th percentile for triceps skinfold thickness or midarm muscle circumference
- Weight loss >5%/month or 10% loss in 6 months; involuntary weight loss

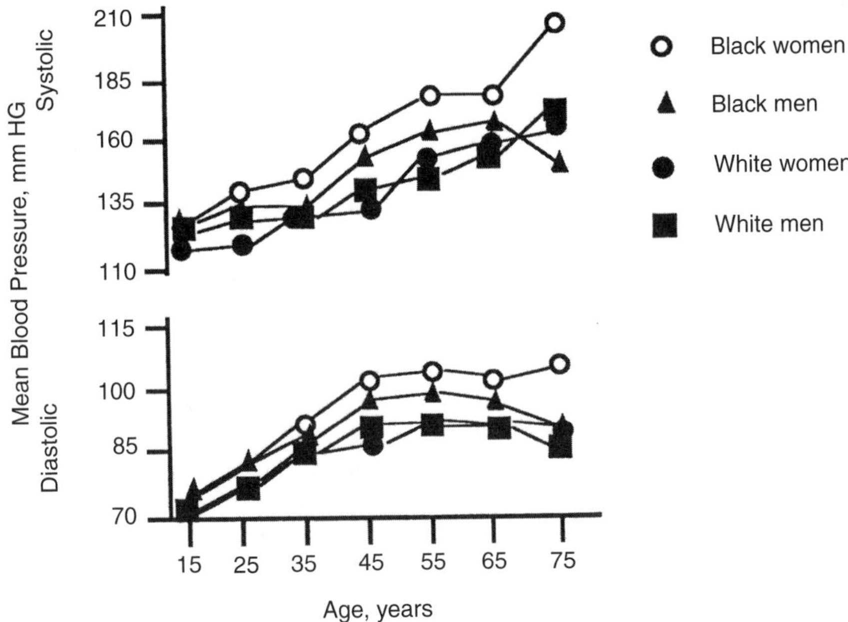

FIGURE 10.1
The change in blood pressure with age. The ordinate represents mean blood pressure, with the upper curves depicting systolic blood pressure and the lower curves diastolic pressure. The circles represent black women, the triangles represent black men, the filled circles represent white women, and the squares represent white men. From Feldman, E.B., *Nutrition in the Middle and Later Years*, Wright-PSG, Littleton, MA, 1983. Data are adapted from Hames, C.G., *Postgrad Med*, 56: 110; 1974, with permission.

- Osteoporosis
- Anemia

Pathophysiology of Aging

The changes with aging and old age that may be nutrition related and/or diet responsive include:

- Blood pressure (Figure 10.1)[11,12] — Both systolic and diastolic blood pressure increase with age, so beyond age 50 half of the population has hypertension. In the Southeast, this is especially prevalent in African-American women.[12] A variety of nutrients affect blood pressure, including energy, sodium, potassium, calcium, magnesium, selenium, lipids, protein, and vitamin C. Consumption of fruits and vegetables (10 servings a day) lowered blood pressure significantly.[13] While the role of sodium has been questioned, recent trials show a beneficial effect of sodium restriction even in the presence of other successful non-pharmacologic interventions.[14]
- Blood lipids — Genetics and lifestyle (diet, exercise) interact to influence the concentration and composition of blood lipids and lipoproteins. To date, there is no convincing evidence that risk factors for cardiovascular disease differ in the elderly, although their impact may differ because of changes in vasculature.

Neither homocysteine levels in relation to age nor the regulation of homocysteine by B vitamins have been adequately studied.[15] Stroke is more common in older adults, and nutrients that affect thrombosis and blood clotting are important in the management of these risk factors. (See section on Cardiovascular Risk.)

- The incidence of cancer and the decline in the immune system with aging may be influenced by many nutrients. Whether advice about diet (plant-based, avoidance of certain foods/nutrients or cooking methods) is equally applicable to the elderly is not known. (See section on Cancer Prevention.)
- Bone density — Bone density declines with aging in women and men, beginning in women around the perimenopausal years, and decades later in men. Bone mineralization is related to the intakes of calcium, vitamin D, and other nutrients, as well as to activity level and alcohol intake. Evaluation with appropriate tests should be part of the geriatric assessment. Women, especially, should be encouraged to achieve a maximum bone density through adequate intake of calcium and physical activity. The greater the bone density at peak, the less serious the effect of estrogen loss that is associated with decreased bone density. Problems with bone and cartilage are being addressed with dietary supplements like glucosamine that are under evaluation. Fish oils and polyunsaturated fatty acids also may be of benefit in various types of arthritis.[16]
- Significant memory loss is not a necessary accompaniment of aging. Nutritional interventions in patients with senile dementia of the Alzheimer type may either ameliorate or slow the progress of the disease, or, more likely, improve the patient's general nutritional status and function.
- The immune system shows impairment, particularly of cellular immunity, and may be improved with B_6, vitamin E, or selenium.[17]

The Geriatric Assessment

Nutrition screening should be part of the geriatric assessment.[18] The clinical nutritional assessment of adults is detailed in the Assessment section. The elderly are a heterogeneous population, so no assumptions should be made about individuals.

Particular attention should be paid to the intake of medications. Polypharmacy is common in the elderly and may lead to drug-nutrient interactions that affect the efficacy and safety of the medication as well as the nutritional status of the patient. Among these are:

- Thiazide diuretics for the management of hypertension. These drugs increase the loss of potassium.
- Antidepressants used for mood management. These drugs may induce dry mouth, altered taste, nausea, vomiting, constipation, and/or reduced appetite.
- Chronic antacids and laxative use (preoccupation with need to have a daily bowel movement) can result in chronic diarrhea and electrolyte imbalance.
- Anti-inflammatory preparations used to relieve muscle or joint pain. These drugs may induce iron-deficiency anemia.
- An annual involuntary weight loss of 4% is a cutpoint that affects 13% of individuals over age 65 whose 2-year mortality is doubled versus weight-stable individuals.[1]

The RDAs for the Elderly

The most recent revisions of the Recommended Dietary Allowances, including the new Dietary Reference Intake values, have added a category for the elderly. Values have been set for males and females for calcium, phosphorus, magnesium, vitamin D, fluoride, thiamin, riboflavin, niacin, vitamin B_6, folate, vitamin B_{12}, pantothenic acid, biotin, and choline. Values for vitamin D have been increased because of concern about deficient intake, decreased metabolism, and the prevalence of bone disease in the elderly (see section on Skeletal Diseases). More recently, values were set for vitamins C and E and selenium for those over 70 years of age (Table of DRIs). The remaining RDAs and the recommendations for intake of essential nutrients dating from 1989 (vitamin A, macronutrients, some trace minerals) are under revision and may set new values for males and females >70 years of age.

A Food Pyramid for those over 70 years of age has been developed by Tufts University nutritionists (Figure 10.2). In contrast to the original Food Pyramid (Section 11), the need for water forms the base of the pyramid for the elderly, while the number of servings in the various food groups has been modified downward, and supplements of calcium, vitamin D, and vitamin B_{12} are recommended.[19]

Body Composition and Aging

Changes in body composition with aging (Figure 10.3) include an increase in the percent of body fat and a decrease in lean body mass.[20] These changes are associated with an age-related decline in metabolic rate and with a quantitatively greater decline in energy expenditure from physical activity[21] (Figure 10.4).

The fat mass in untrained older men (age 69) was significantly higher than in younger subjects (age 31) and correlated negatively with plasma IGF-1 levels. Older trained subjects had a similar fat mass to untrained younger subjects. The lean body mass (skeletal muscle) was lower in older than in younger untrained men, but older trained men did not differ from similarly trained younger men.[22] Investigators have experimented with the use of growth hormone to lessen age-related changes in body composition, with encouraging results.[23] A study in men age 61 to 81 years showed that injections of human growth hormone given over 6 months increased low levels of IGF-1 to the higher levels of the youthful. Lean body mass increased 9%, and fat mass decreased 14%. Data, however, are inadequate to recommend a costly and potentially toxic therapy that is administered by injection.

Nutrient Requirements and Aging

For many nutrients, requirements in the older adult relate more to gender and body size than age. Important changes (increased or decreased need) in a number of nutrients, however, include energy, vitamins B_{12}, D, and calcium.[1]

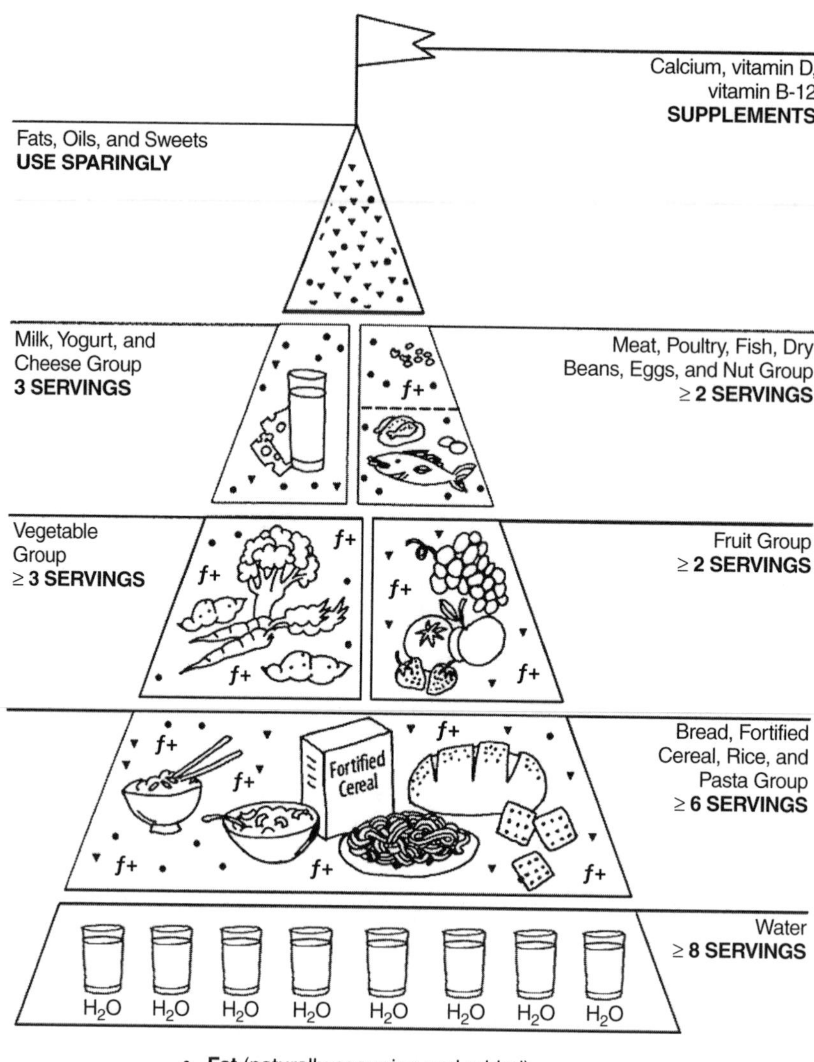

FIGURE 10.2
The Food Pyramid modified for adults 70 years of age and older. From Russell, R.M., Rasmussen, H., and Lichtenstein, A.H. *J. Nutr.* 129: 156; 1999, with permission.

Energy

The decrease with age in the whole body basal metabolic rate (Figure 10.4) is especially pronounced in the cells of the brain, skeletal muscle, and heart that are major contributors to the resting energy expenditure. In combination with the decline in physical activity, overall energy consumption declines on average 10% per decade after age 60. In men between age 28 and 80, energy intake declines by 600 kcal.[21] Women have a lower metabolic rate than men, independent of body size. The resting metabolic rate in women declines

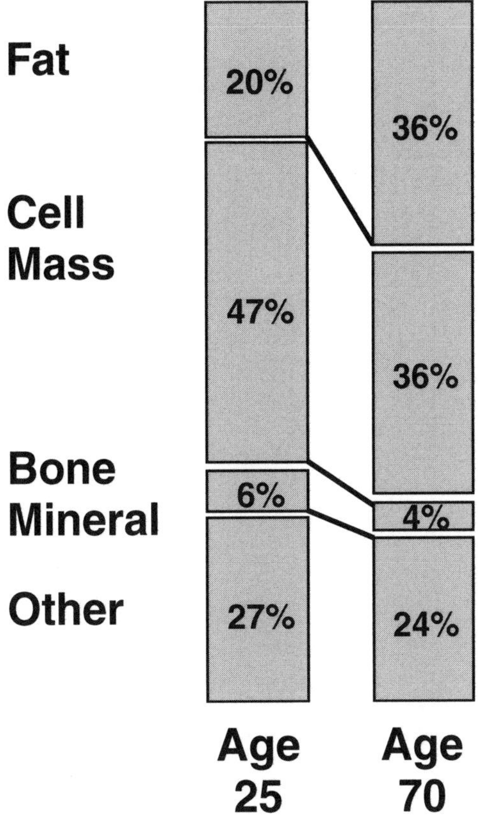

FIGURE 10.3
The age-related change in body composition in men. From Feldman, E.B., *Essentials of Clinical Nutrition*, F.A. Davis, Philadelphia, 1988, with permission.

4% per decade between age 50 and 80, with an increased downward slope after menopause compared to a nonsignificant decline before age 50.[24]

The decline in basal/resting metabolic rate can be lessened somewhat by increased physical activity (Figure 10.5). A combination of strength training and moderate aerobic exercise, e.g., 30 minutes/day or walking 10 to 12 miles per week, can increase the resting metabolic rate by 10%.[25]

Voluntary expenditure can increase significantly with physical activity. An increase in energy expenditure by physical activity in an exercise program will have beneficial effects, improving glucose uptake and metabolism by tissues (Figure 10.6), thereby normalizing glucose tolerance.[26] Studies used the insulin clamp technique and showed no difference in glucose uptake in healthy persons age 21 to 53 years, with significantly lower values in persons over 54 years of age. The relative drop in muscle mass in older subjects may be responsible for this difference.

Fat stores in older men and women can be reduced towards those of younger individuals (Figure 10.7) with an increase in lean body mass.[27] Studies showed that the proportion of body fat was significantly less in 67-year-olds who exercised regularly than in age-matched sedentary controls. The loss of aerobic capacity with aging can be attenuated by 50% with a regular exercise program (Figure 10.8).[27] The maximal aerobic capacity of physically active older subjects was significantly greater than that of persons of comparable age and

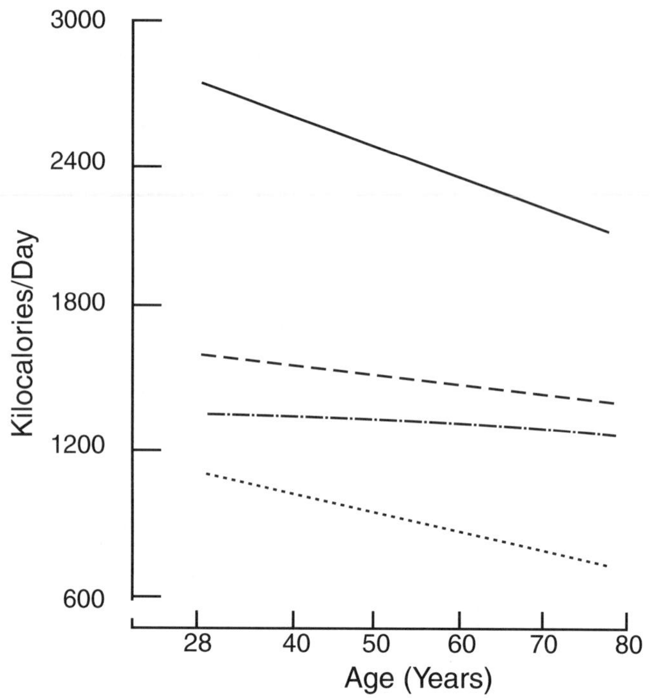

FIGURE 10.4
Energy expenditure and aging. The solid line represents energy expenditure in men, the dashed line indicates basal expenditure in men, the dotted line shows energy expended for activity in men. The resting metabolic rate in women is the dot/dash line. The resting metabolic rate in kcal/minute is the ordinate and age in years is the abscissa. Adapted from Feldman, E.B., In: *Essentials of Clinical Nutrition,* F.A. Davis, Philadelphia, 1988, ch. 9 and Rudman, D., Feller, A.G., Nagrai, H.S., et al. *N Engl J Med,* 323: 11; 1991.

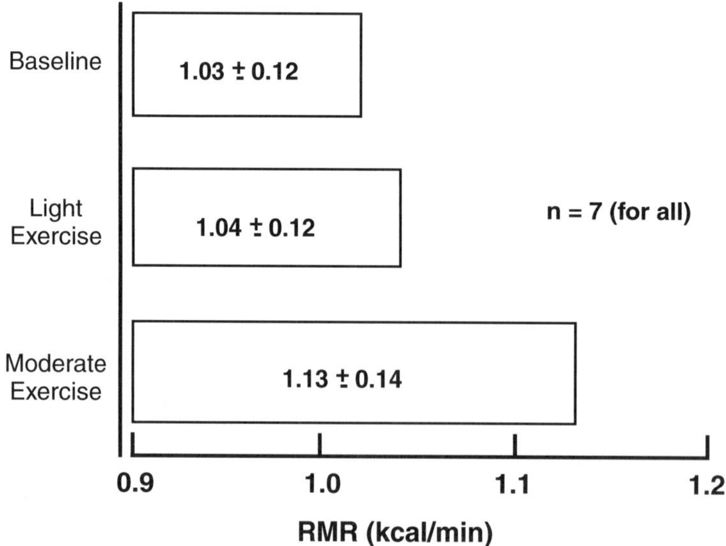

FIGURE 10.5
Exercise and the resting metabolic rate in older persons. The length of the top bar represents the resting metabolic rate in kcalories/minute. The upper bar is the control, the middle bar shows effects of light exercise, and the lowest bar shows the effect of moderate exercise. Adapted from Poehlman, E.T., Gardner, A.W., Goran, M.I., *Betabolism,* 41: 041; 1992.

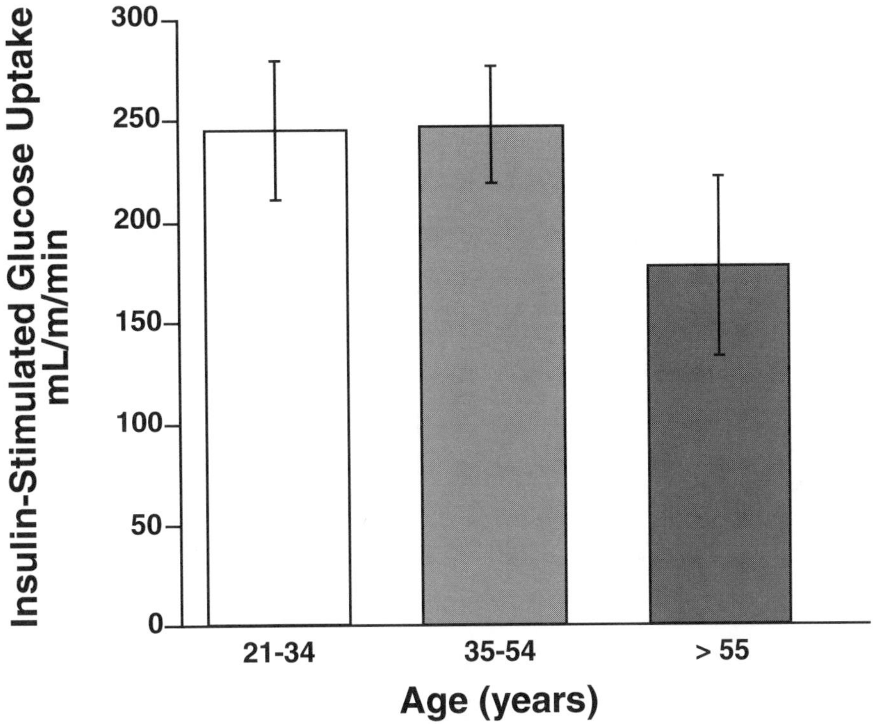

FIGURE 10.6
The effect of age on glucose uptake. The height of the bar represents the mean insulin-stimulated glucose uptake. The error bars represent 2.5 standard deviations from the mean. The lesser glucose uptake in those over age 55 differs significantly from the other two age groups ($p<0.01$). Adapted from Rosenthal, M., Doberne, L., Greenfield, M., et al. *J. Am. Geriatr. Soc.* 30: 562; 1982.

BMI who did not exercise regularly, and was similar to that of young subjects who did not exercise regularly.

An exercise program is important to prevent or limit obesity, diabetes mellitus, and increases in blood pressure, lessen bone loss, and provide a favorable blood lipid profile, increasing HDL-cholesterol and decreasing triglycerides.

To compensate for decreased energy requirements and prevent excessive weight gain, overweight, and obesity, the energy intake of the elderly usually needs to decrease. Older subjects who limit their energy intake, however, must consume more nutrient-dense foods in order to meet protein and micronutrient needs. They should limit their intakes of energy-dense foods such as fats and sweets, and take in adequate amounts of protein-rich foods. A one-a-day multivitamin supplement designed for older adults may be indicated when decreased energy intake is prescribed.

Vitamin B_{12}

Vitamin B_{12} status in the elderly is impaired by achlorhydria and bacterial overgrowth that binds this vitamin, inhibiting absorption. Achlorhydria affects 10 to 30% of the geriatric population, and associated atrophic gastritis further decreases the absorption of vitamin B_{12} from food. The absorption of synthetic B_{12} is not adversely affected. This has led some nutritionists to recommend markedly increasing the level of oral intake for older adults from the RDA of 2.6 to 25 µg/day. This increased amount may be found in some

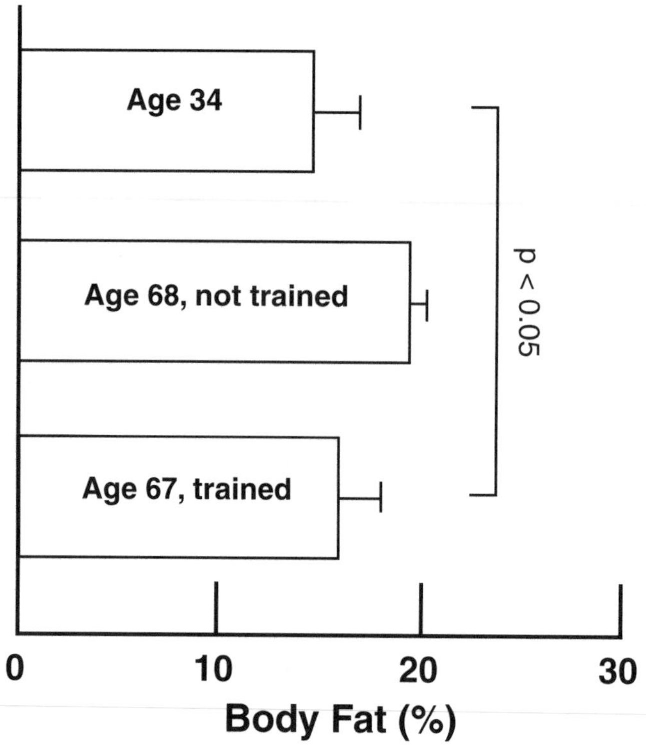

FIGURE 10.7
The effect of aging and physical training on body fat. The length of the top bar indicates values for % body fat in young people, the middle bar represents these values in old people, not physically trained, and the bar at the bottom represents the values in old people who are physically trained. Young people differ significantly from old untrained, and old physically trained differ from old untrained. Adapted from Hollenbeck, C. et al. *J. Am. Geriatr. Soc.* 33: 273; 1985.

vitamin supplements formulated for the older age group. The body's handling of vitamin B_{12} is reviewed in the section on Anemia.

Vitamin D

Vitamin D status in the elderly is impaired by multiple factors that decrease:

- Dietary intake
- Exposure to the sun
- Skin synthesis
- Hepatic and renal hydroxylation
- Receptors in the gastrointestinal tract
- Absorption

Skin synthesis of vitamin D by the elderly is only 30-40% of that of children and young adults.[28] The resulting decreases in vitamin D stores in the body lead to an increase in parathyroid hormone and an increase in bone remodeling and bone loss. These factors are discussed in the section on Skeletal Disorders.

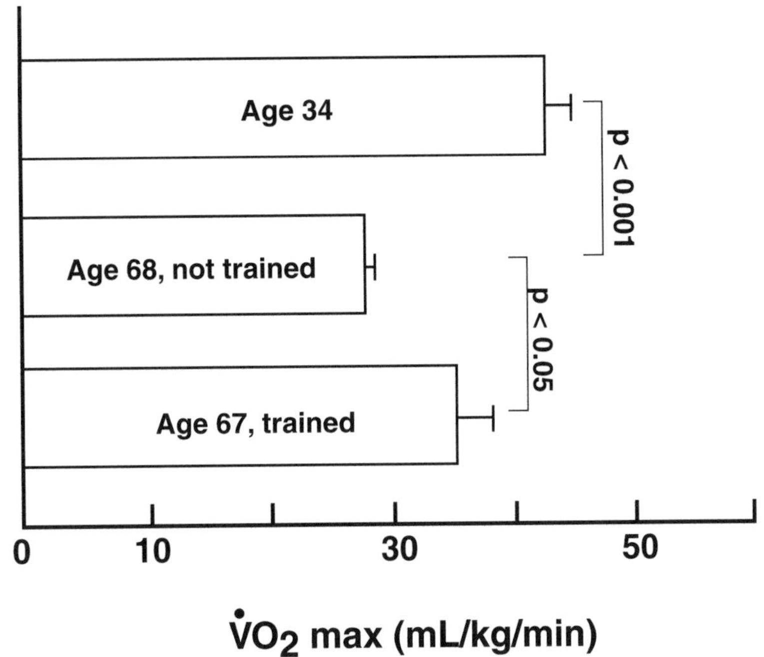

FIGURE 10.8
The effect of aging and physical training on aerobic capacity. The length of the top bar indicates values for maximum oxygen consumption in young people. The middle bar represents these values in old persons not physically trained, and lowest the bar represents the values in old people who are physically trained. Young people differ significantly from old untrained, and old physically trained differ from old untrained. Adapted from Hollenbeck, C. et al. *J. Am. Geriatr. Soc.* 33: 273; 1985.

Multivitamin/Mineral Supplement

A daily multivitamin supplement suitable for the older age group may be indicated to meet general micronutrient needs (vitamins, minerals). This is especially true for small, old people, and whenever energy intake to meet energy expenditure is less than 1300 kcal/day.

Anorexia in the Elderly

Anorexia and weight loss are common in the elderly, especially in patients suffering from medical or mental illness.[29] With normal aging, men and women may decrease their energy intake as they are less active physically and as their resting metabolic rate declines (Figure 10.4). The feeding drive (hunger) may decrease, and satiety may occur more readily. This physiological change with aging, however, may be the precursor of pathological anorexia and weight loss that most commonly is due to depression. Physiological and disease-related anorexia may be mediated by changes in a variety of hormones or cytokines. In order to prevent cachexia, with resultant morbidity and mortality, early recognition by nutritional screening, and aggressive management is needed. Management can include the use of enteral supplements and, if necessary, tube feedings or parenteral nutrition. The underlying medical or psychiatric disorder must also be diagnosed and treated.

Various interventions have been proposed to improve appetite and metabolism in the elderly. Among these is the use of growth hormone supplements. Growth hormone has been shown to have some favorable effects on function, yet it is not without risk and is quite expensive.[23]

Other studies in men comparing subjects with average ages 24 and 70 years showed that aging may be associated with a significant impairment in the ability to control food intake following overeating or undereating. These findings may explain the vulnerability of older persons to unexplained weight loss.[30]

Nutritional Deficiencies in the Elderly

Various recent surveys have shown that 40% of the aged have intakes lower than two-thirds of the RDA for energy and that intakes of calcium, iron, vitamins A, E, and D, water soluble vitamins, and zinc are low.[1] Deficient intakes are especially prevalent in some ethnic groups and older individuals with low income. Osteopenia and iron deficiency anemia are common, and are discussed in the respective sections of this handbook.

Homebound and Institutionalized Elderly

Malnutrition is common in elderly nursing home residents. Of special concern are intakes of calcium, vitamin A, thiamin, riboflavin, and iron. Recommendations to decrease this prevalence include improving the eating environment, searching for early signs of undernutrition, finding treatable causes of poor food intake (depression, dental problems) with appropriate modifications of the diet, and controlling infection.[31] Predictors or mortality within six months were low levels of hemoglobin, cholesterol, and albumin. Socialization improves eating behavior. Spacing meals at five-hour intervals, using multiple smaller meals and snacks, providing a good breakfast, having food at the proper temperature, and attention to adequate light all can improve food intake and meal enjoyment.[32]

Congregate and home delivery feeding programs are crucial for homebound elderly. Water is a major concern in nursing home subjects. Thirst mechanisms are impaired in many elderly, and water needs to be provided and intake insured, especially in hot climates and in hot weather.

Patients should not be over-sedated and should be encouraged to be active, even if bed- or chair-bound. A study of frail, institutionalized 90-year-olds showed that high-resistance weight training lead to significant gains in muscle strength, size, and functional mobility.[33]

The Hospitalized Patient

The severity of nutritional deficits correlates with increased risk of subsequent morbid events in the hospitalized elderly.[34] Risk factors for malnutrition in hospitalized elderly patients should be evaluated promptly on or after admission. These risk factors include a history of inadequate food intake or unexplained, rapid weight loss, body weight or other anthropometric measurements that show depletion, and low serum albumin.

With acute illness, food and water intake may cease. In the presence of hypercatabolism from diseases, especially inflammatory or infectious disease, nutrient needs are increased. Injuries or surgery may have similar effects. The elderly have fewer nutritional reserves, especially if they are already undernourished; attention to feeding is vital. Any deficits may be enhanced by the food deprivation resulting from tests or treatments that withhold meals.

A study in a veterans' hospital of non-terminally ill hospitalized patients indicated that many elderly patients were maintained on inadequate energy intakes that may have contributed to an eightfold increased risk of mortality in this group. These patients with low nutrient intake also exhibited significantly lower serum cholesterol and serum albumin levels on discharge than other patients.[33] The investigators recommend that greater efforts should be made to prevent the development of protein–energy undernutrition during hospitalization. Caregivers should be aware that the food may be unpalatable or unacceptable by some ethnic groups, and this adds to the difficulty of adequate patient nourishment. Illness or medication-related nausea, vomiting, or diarrhea will exacerbate these difficulties.

Enteral supplements or total enteral or parenteral nutrition should be considered when appropriate. An energy-rich, protein-rich beverage (one to two 8-oz servings daily) can improve the outcome of patients with hip fracture and chronic obstructive pulmonary disease, and be associated with diminished falling in frail elderly. Consultation with a dietitian can help immeasurably.

Conclusion

The older population differs from younger adults not only by age but also by health status. The elderly group is not a homogeneous population, and their many different health and social problems impact their nutritional status.[35] Optimal nutrient intake not only meets their needs but prevents some chronic diseases and ameliorates others. Attention must be paid to environmental, psychological, and pathophysiological parameters in evaluating nutritional status and interventions. While there is no panacea for the aged, nor a "fountain of youth," much can be done to recognize their nutritional needs and improve their nutritional health.

References

1. Ausman LA, Russell RM. In: *Modern Nutrition in Health and Disease* (Shils ME, Olson JO, Shike M, Ross AC, Eds), 9th ed., Williams & Wilkens, Baltimore, 1999, ch. 53.
2. Berdanier CD. In: *Encyclopedia of Gerontology* (Birren JE, Ed), Vol 2, Academic Press, New York, 1996, pg 135.
3. Wei EC. In: *Nutrients and Gene Expression: Clinical Aspects* (Berdanier CD, Ed) CRC Press, Boca Raton, 1996, pg 165.
4. Masoro EJ. *Exptl Gerontology* 30: 291; 1995.
5. Carr AC, Frei B. *Am J Clin Nutr* 69: 1086; 1999.

6. Berdanier CD. In: *Fatty Acids in Foods and Their Health Implications* (Chow CK, Ed) 2nd ed, Marcel Dekker, New York, pg 569.
7. Health United States, 1998.
8. *Morbidity and Mortality Weekly Report*, US Department Health and Human Services, Vol. 46, October 10, 1997.
9. Berdanier CD. *Advanced Nutrition: Macronutrients*, 2nd ed., CRC Press, Boca Raton, 2000.
10. White P. *Nutrition Today* 26:142; 1991.
11. Feldman EB. In *Nutrition in the Middle and Later Years* (Wright-PSG, Ed), Littleton, MA, 1983, ch. 6.
12. Hames CG. *Postgrad Med* 56: 110; 1974.
13. Appel LJ, Moore TJ, Obarzanek E, et al. *N Eng J Med* 338: 1117; 1997.
14. Whelton PK, Appel L, Espeland MA, et al. *JAMA* 279: 839; 1998.
15. Selhub J, Jaques PF, Bostom AG, et al. *N Eng J Med* 331: 286; 1995.
16. James MJ, Cleland LG. *Sem Arth Rheum* 27: 85; 1997.
17. Bogden JD, Bendich A, Kemp FW, et al. *Am J Clin Nutr* 60: 137; 1994.
18. Fogt EJ, Bell SJ, Blackburn GL. In: *Geriatric Nutrition, a Comprehensive Review* (Morley JE, Glick Z, Rubenstein LZ, Eds), 2nd ed., Raven Press, New York, 1995, ch. 5.
19. Russell RM, Rasmussen H, Lichtenstein AH. *J Nutr* 129: 156; 1999.
20. Feldman EB. In: *Essentials of Clinical Nutrition*, FA Davis, Philadelphia, 1988, ch. 9.
21. Munro HN. *Br Med Bull* 37: 84; 1981.
22. Horber FF, Kohler SA, Lippuner K, Jaeger P. *Eur J Clin Invest* 26: 279; 1996.
23. Rudman D, Feller AG, Nagrai HS, et al. *N Eng J Med,* 323: 11; 1991.
24. Poehlman ET, Goran MI, Gardner AW, et al. *Am J Physiol* 264: E450; 1993.
25. Poehlman ET, Gardner AW, Goran MI. *Metabolism,* 41: 041, 1992.
26. Rosenthal M, Doberne L, Greenfield M, et al. *J Am Geriatr Soc* 30: 562; 1982.
27. Hollenbeck C, Haskell W, Rosenthal M, Reaven GM, *J Am Geriatr Soc* 33: 273; 1985.
28. Holick MF, Matsuoka LY, Wortsman J. *Lancet* 2: 1104; 1989.
29. Morley JE. *Drugs & Aging* 8: 134; 1996.
30. Roberts S, Fuss P, Heyman MB, et al. *JAMA* 272: 1601; 1994.
31. Rudman D, Feller AG. *J Am Geriatr Soc* 37: 173; 1989.
32. Thomas DR, Verdery RB, Gardner L, et al. *J Parent Ent Nutr* 15: 400; 1991.
33. Fiatarone MA, Marks EC, Ryan ND, et al. *JAMA* 263: 3029; 1990.
34. Sullivan DH, Sun S, Walls R. *JAMA* 281: 2013; 1999.
35. Feldman EB. *Am J Clin Nutr* 58: 1; 1993.

Part V

Human Nutritional Status Assessment

11

Dietary Guidelines, Food Guidance, and Dietary Quality

Eileen Kennedy

The 1969 White House Conference on Food, Nutrition, and Health[1] was instrumental in the development of the first set of U.S. dietary guidelines. Specific recommendations emerged out of this conference advocating that the government examine the links between diet and chronic disease. The 1969 conference was followed in 1977 by the release of the U.S. Senate Dietary Goals;[2] these dietary goals for the first time summarized specific recommendations for diet-related goals for the American public.

The Dietary Guidelines for Americans are the cornerstone of federal nutrition policy in the U.S. Nutrition programs use the Dietary Guidelines as the basis of the nutrition standards; thus programs such as Food Stamps, School Lunch/School Breakfast, and Women, Infants, and Children (WIC) use the dietary guidelines in developing program services. In addition, all nutrition education programs at the federal level must have messages consistent with the Dietary Guidelines. As a result, the impact of the Dietary Guidelines is broad. It is estimated that one of every five Americans participates in at least one federal nutrition program.

History of the Dietary Guidelines for Americans

The Dietary Guidelines attempt to answer the question, "what should Americans eat to stay healthy?" Specifically, the Dietary Guidelines provide advice for healthy Americans age two years and over about food choices that promote health and reduce the risk of disease.

The Dietary Guidelines were first developed in 1980[3] and have been updated every five years since then — 1985, 1990, 1995, and the most recent, Dietary Guidelines 2000.[4-7] The *National Nutrition Monitoring and Related Research Act* of 1990[8] requires the Secretary of Agriculture and the Secretary of Health and Human Services to jointly publish a report every five years entitled "The Dietary Guidelines for Americans." The report must (1) contain nutrition and dietary information and guidelines for the general public, (2) be based on the preponderance of scientific and medical knowledge current at the time of publication, and (3) be prompted by each federal agency in carrying out federal food, nutrition, or health programs. The 1995 Dietary Guidelines were the first to be statutorily mandated by the U.S. Congress.

0-8493-2705-9/01/$0.00+$1.50

Since 1985, the United States Department of Agriculture (USDA) and the Department of Health and Human Services (HHS) have used essentially the same process to prepare the Dietary Guidelines. An external Dietary Guidelines Advisory Committee (DGAC) has been appointed by the two secretaries to review and revise the Dietary Guidelines as necessary. The members of the DGAC are widely recognized nutrition and medical experts. A series of open public meetings are held to review and discuss the guidelines. Upon completion of the DGAC process, a technical report is sent to the two secretaries and reviewed within the two departments. In addition, in 1995 and 2000, consumer research was conducted[9-10] to test consumer reaction to specific design and content elements of the technical report. The consumer research is also used as one element in promoting the Dietary Guidelines.

Dietary Guidelines for Americans

From 1980 to 1995, the Dietary Guidelines have been relatively stable (Table 11.1), maintaining seven guidelines. However, the 1995 guidelines reflected some exciting and important changes. The 1995 guidelines,[6] more than ever before, put an emphasis on total diet; the wording moved away from individual foods in the direction of a total diet based on variety, moderation, and proportionality. The concept of total diet is reflected symbolically through the graphic of the 1995 Dietary Guidelines bulletin that links all seven guidelines together, anchored around "Eat a Variety of Food."

In the 1995 guideline on variety, the bulletin[6] stresses a total diet rather than an individual food approach to healthy eating. The recommendation is to choose foods from each of the five major food groups in the Food Guide Pyramid. Also, an emphasis is placed on

TABLE 11.1

Dietary Guidelines for Americans, 1980 to 2000

1980 7 Guidelines	1985 7 Guidelines	1990 7 Guidelines	1995 7 Guidelines
Eat a variety of foods.	Eat a variety of foods.	Eat a variety of foods.	Eat a variety of foods.
Maintain ideal weight	Maintain desirable weight	Maintain healthy weight	Balance the food you eat with physical activity — maintain or improve your weight
Avoid too much fat, saturated fat, and cholesterol	Avoid too much fat, saturated fat, and cholesterol	Choose a diet low in fat, saturated fat, and cholesterol	
Eat foods with adequate starch and fiber	Eat foods with adequate starch and fiber	Choose a diet with plenty of grain products, vegetables, and fruits	Choose a diet with plenty of grain products, vegetables, and fruits Choose a diet low in fat, saturated fat, and cholesterol
Avoid too much sugar	Avoid too much sugar	Use sugars only in moderation	Choose a diet moderate in sugars
Avoid too much sodium	Avoid too much sodium	Use salt and sodium only in moderation	Choose a diet moderate in salt and sodium
If you drink alcohol, do so in moderation	If you drink alcohol beverages, do so in moderation	If you drink alcoholic beverages, do so in moderation	If you drink alcoholic beverages, do so in moderation

foods from the base of the pyramid (grains) to form the center of the plate, accompanied by food from other food groups.

For the first time, the Dietary Guidelines in 1995 recognized that with careful planning, a vegetarian diet can be consistent with the Dietary Guidelines and the Recommended Dietary Allowances.[11] The guidelines also present a clear message that food sources of nutrients are preferred to supplements. This "food first" strategy is reinforced by a discussion of other healthful substances present in food but not in dietary supplements. However, the 1995 guidelines do provide specific examples of situations where dietary supplements may be needed.

The 1995 guidelines also more forcefully moved in the direction of providing a discussion of the direct link between diet and health. Weight gain with age was discouraged for adults. Weight maintenance is encouraged as a first step to achieving a healthy weight. The benefits of physical activity are emphasized, and for the first time, a statement was included on the benefits of moderate alcohol consumption in reducing the risk of heart disease. On this later point, both HHS and USDA were clear that the alcohol guideline was not intended to recommend that people start drinking.

In the 1995 guidelines there was also direct reference to nutrition education tools that could be used to promote the Dietary Guidelines. The guidelines explain how consumers can use the "three crown jewels" to build a healthy diet — the Dietary Guidelines, the Food Guide Pyramid,[12] and the Nutrition Facts Label.

The Dietary Guidelines 2000, released by President Clinton in May 2000,[7] break with the tradition of seven guidelines and now incorporate ten guidelines. Not only do the Dietary Guidelines 2000 continue to emphasize a total diet approach, they also emphasize a healthy lifestyle approach. This is reflected clearly in three concepts that are used as organizing principals for the 2000 Guidelines aim for fitness, build a healthy base, and choose sensibly.

Three new guidelines have been added to the Dietary Guidelines 2000 (Table 11.2). There is now a separate guideline for physical activity which states, "be physically active every

TABLE 11.2

U.S. Dietary Guidelines 2000 and Countries having Similar Guidelines

U.S. Dietary Guidelines 2000[7]	Countries Having Similar Guidelines[13]
Aim for a healthy weight	Australia, Canada, China, Japan, Korea, Malaysia, The Netherlands, New Zealand, Philippines, Singapore, Thailand, United Kingdom
Let the Pyramid guide your food choices	*Variety*: Australia, Canada, China, France, Germany, Hungary, Indonesia, Korea, Malaysia, New Zealand, Philippines, Singapore, South Africa, Sri Lanka, Thailand, United Kingdom, Japan *Five Steps to Healthy Eating:* India
Eat a variety of grains daily, especially whole grains	Australia, Canada, Denmark, Germany, Hungary (choose potatoes over rice), India, Malaysia, Norway, Singapore, South Africa (starchy foods), Thailand
Choose a diet that is low in saturated fat, and cholesterol, and moderate in total fat	Australia (but low fat diets not suitable for children), Canada, Japan, The Netherlands, New Zealand, Singapore, South Africa
Choose and prepare foods with less salt	Australia, Canada, China, Denmark, Germany, Hungary, India, Japan, Korea, Malaysia, The Netherlands, Singapore, South Africa, Thailand
If you drink alcoholic beverages, do so in moderation	Canada, China, France, Germany, Indonesia (avoid), Hungary (forbidden for pregnant women and children), Korea, The Netherlands, New Zealand, Singapore, South Africa, United Kingdom

day." In addition to help in maintaining a healthy weight, this guideline discusses other health benefits of physical activity. Specific quantitative recommendations are given for amount of physical activity for adults (30 minutes or more) and children (60 minutes or more) per day. For the first time ever, there is a guideline on food safety. Again, this reinforces components of a healthy diet and healthy lifestyle. Finally, there is a separate guideline for fruits and vegetables.

The consumer research conducted as part of the Dietary Guidelines 2000 process[10] influenced the development of the guidelines. One clear message is that consumers preferred simple, action-oriented guidelines. Thus, the guidelines are much more direct and action oriented as evidenced by "aim for a healthy weight" and "keep foods safe to eat."

The guidelines are more consumer friendly, and emphasize practical ways in which the consumers can put the concepts into practice. To that end, a section entitled "Advice for Today" is included at the end of each individual guideline and includes suggestions on key ways to operationalize the guidelines. The consumer research on the 2000 Dietary Guidelines [10] indicated that consumers particularly appreciated sections such as "Advice for Today."

Comparison with Other Dietary Guidelines

A large number of countries — both industrialized and developing — have authoritative sets of dietary guidelines.[13] Despite vastly different geographical and sociocultural contexts, six elements are common to the sets of dietary guidelines (Table 11.2).

A guideline on variety is common; it is often the core element of the different sets of dietary guidelines, and is used to reflect the concepts of dietary diversity. The variety guidelines range from general statements such as, "Eat a variety of foods" to very specific quantifications, such as that as found in the Japanese guideline: "Obtain well-balanced nutrition with a variety of foods; eat 30 foodstuffs a day."

Many of the country-specific dietary guidelines emphasize limiting or moderating total fat and saturated fat intake. Where there is a quantification of limits, this is most commonly a diet containing no more than 30% of total energy from fat and less than 10% of energy from saturated fat.

Countries typically also include a weight guidelines, clearly emphasizing maintaining or achieving a healthy weight; in the French guideline this is more specific, indicating that individuals should weigh themselves monthly.[13] Most of the dietary guidelines worldwide promote a plant-based diet as the building block of healthful eating. To that end, many countries emphasize grains as the basis of good diet. Reduction of salt and/or sodium is emphasized in a number of the sets of dietary guidelines.

Finally, the issue of alcohol consumption is addressed in many sets of dietary guidelines. There is always a level of caution related to the role of alcohol as part of a healthy diet. The most recent 2000 Dietary Guidelines for Americans, for example, indicates that the benefits of alcohol in reducing the risk of heart disease can be achieved in other ways: maintaining a healthy weight, cessation of smoking, increasing physical activity, and reducing the level of fat and saturated fat in the diet. Indeed, countries like Venezuela go even further, and specify that "alcoholic beverages are not part of a healthy diet."[14]

Comparison of U.S. Dietary Guidelines with Disease-Specific Guidelines

A number of professional associations have developed sets of dietary guidelines. Table 11.3 compares the U.S. Dietary Guidelines 2000[7] with guidelines of the American Heart Association (AHA)[15] and American Cancer Society (ACS).[16] Clearly the AHA and ACS have somewhat different objectives in developing their specific sets of guidelines. The AHA guidelines put forward recommendations for a healthful diet which, if followed, reduce the risk of heart disease. Similarly, recommendations from the ACA are for dietary guidelines which reduce the risk of cancer. Given the somewhat differing objectives, there is a remarkable degree of similarly in the three sets of guidelines (Table 11.3). Here again, the USDA/HHS, the AHA, and the ACA each recommend dietary guidelines related to weight, total fat/saturated fat, salt, and alcohol in moderation as the basis of a healthful diet.

Future Directions

Many countries have been successful in developing and promoting food-based Dietary Guidelines. In most cases these guidelines are intended for individuals ages two and older. In the U.S., the Dietary Guidelines from their inception in 1980 have been intended for individuals ages two and older. There is a clear gap in dietary guidelines for children ages two and younger.

A limited number of countries have some parts of their food-based guidelines devoted to children less than two years of age. In most cases the advice for children under two years of age relates to a discussion of breastfeeding. Australia, for example, states: "encourage and support breastfeeding." Similar wording is found in guidelines from the Philippines and Singapore.

Most industrialized countries rely on national pediatric associations to guide the broad policy recommendations for infant feeding and/or feeding practices for the first two years of life. In almost all cases, advice from pediatric associations stresses that human milk is the preferred form of infant feeding.[17]

In devising food-based dietary guidelines for children under two, there would be a clear need to segment this group of children by age groups; birth to 6 months, 6 to 12 months, and 13 to 24 months. The dietary issues addressed across these three age groups would differ.

Dietary Guidance

In the preceeding segment the development of the U.S. Dietary Guidelines was traced. The United States Department of Agriculture (USDA) has a long, rich history of providing science-based nutrition information and education for the general public (Table 11.4). The Organic Act of 1862 not only created USDA but also mandated that the department, "acquire and diffuse among people useful information on subjects connected to agriculture." This led to some of the pioneering work of W.O. Atwater, who in the 1890s began identifying the links between food composition, dietary intake, and health. This seminal

TABLE 11.3

Comparison of Three Sets of Dietary Recommendations

Recommendation	DGA	AHA	ACS
Include a variety of foods in the diet; emphasis on a plant-based diet.	Yes, include food from five major food groups: bread, cereal, rice, and pasta; vegetables, fruits, meat, poultry, fish, dry beans, eggs, and nuts; and milk, yogurt, and cheese. Also provide information on good food sources of nutrients.	Yes, echo DGA recommendations: grains, fruits, and vegetables should supply 55 to 60 percent of total kcalories.	Yes, with emphasis on grains, especially whole grains, fruits, vegetables, and beans as an alternative to meat.
Encourages maintenance of a healthy weight including importance of physical activity.	Yes, defined as Body Mass Index (BMI) of 19 to 25. Recommend gaining no more than 10 pounds after achieving adult height. Recommend moderate activity for 30 minutes/day on most, if not all days.	Yes, healthy weight not specifically defined. Weight gain in adulthood not specifically addressed. Regular physical activity encouraged.	Yes, refers to DGA definition of BMI of 19 to 25. Recommend moderate activity for 30 minutes/day on most, if not all days.
Limit fat intake.	Yes, recommend choosing a diet with no more than 30 percent of calories from total fat and less than 10 percent of kcalories from saturated fat. Refers to Daily Value of 300 mg/day cholesterol on food labels, without making specific recommendation. Briefly discusses use of omega-3 and trans fatty acids.	Yes, recommend choosing a diet with no more than 30 percent of kcalories from total fat, less than 10 percent of kcalories from saturated fat, and less than 300 mg cholesterol/day. Limit intake of omega-5 polyunsaturated fatty acids to no more than 10 percent of total kcalories. Recommend limiting trans fatty acids but do not give quantitative limit.	Yes, do not give quantitative limits. Recommend limiting consumption of meats, especially high-fat meats.
Limit salt and sodium consumption.	Yes, refer to Daily Value on food labels of 2400 mg of sodium/day without making specific recommendation.	Yes, limit salt to 6g/day (equivalent to 2400 mg of sodium).	Not specifically addressed.
Moderate intake of sugars.	Yes, no quantitative limitations given.	Yes, no quantitative limitations given.	Not specifically addressed.
Limit consumption of alcoholic beverages.	Yes, includes caveat to limit to 1 drink/day for women, if you drink at all. Also includes list of those who should not drink at all including children and pregnant women.	Yes, echo DGA recommendations.	Yes, refer to DGA recommendations.

TABLE 11.4
History of USDA Food Guidance

1860s	1862 USDA formed
1870s	
1880s	
1890s	1890 W. O. Atwater — human nutrition research
1900s	1902 Atwater — Variety, Balance, and Moderation
1910s	1914 Cooperative Extension Service
	1916 Caroline Hunt — First food guide
1920s	
1930s	1933 Food Plans at 4 Cost Levels
1940s	1941 National Nutrition Conference for Defense
	1946 School Lunch Program began
1950s	1956 Basic Four Food Guide
1960s	1964 Food Stamp Program began
	1969 White House Conference on Food, Nutrition, and Health
1970s	1970 EFNEP began
	1971 FNIC formed at NAL
	1975 WIC began (WIC pilot projects authorized in 1972)
	1977 Food and Agriculture Act of 1977, NET began; USDA named "lead" agency for nutrition research, extension, and teaching
1980s	1980 Dietary Guidelines for Americans first issued
	1982 JSHNR defines "nutrition education research"
	1986 USDA Comprehensive Plan for HN Research and Education
1990s	1990 National Nutrition Monitoring and Related Research Act
	1990 Nutrition Labeling and Education Act/NEFLE
	1992 Food Guide Pyramid
	1994 Nutrition and Food Safety Education Task Force
	1995 Dietary Guidelines for Americans, 4th edition
2000	May, 2000 National Nutrition Summit

science led to the development of the USDA food guides. Dissemination of the food guides was facilitated by the 1914 Smith-Lever Act which created the Cooperative Extension Service and specified that the Extension Service provide people with, "useful and practical information on subjects relating to agriculture and home economics."

In the 1930s the USDA began developing family food plans at four separate cost levels. The food plans continue to be used with the best known — the Thrifty Food Plan — serving as the nutritional basis of benefits of the Food Stamp Program. Former Secretary of Agriculture Henry Wallace once commented, "the lack of common-sense knowledge of nutrition even among the many well to-do people in the U.S. is appalling."

In 1941 the first set of Recommended Dietary Allowances was released at the National Nutrition Conference for Defense; at this conference USDA scientists noted that consumers spent enough money on food but did not obtain an adequate diet. As a result, the USDA was urged to develop nutrition education and media-type materials to promote good nutrition for the American public. This emphasis on nutrition education continued in the 1950s and 1960s, culminating with the 1969 White House Conference on Food, Nutrition, and Health.[18,19] The 1969 conference reinforced the need for aggressive nutrition promotion activities for all Americans, with a special emphasis on reaching low income populations.

Throughout the 1970s, federal agencies increased funding for nutrition programs and nutrition education activities.[20] New programs were created, including the Special Supplemental Food Program for Women, Infants, and Children (WIC), School Breakfast, and other programs such as Food Stamps and School Lunch were expanded nationwide.

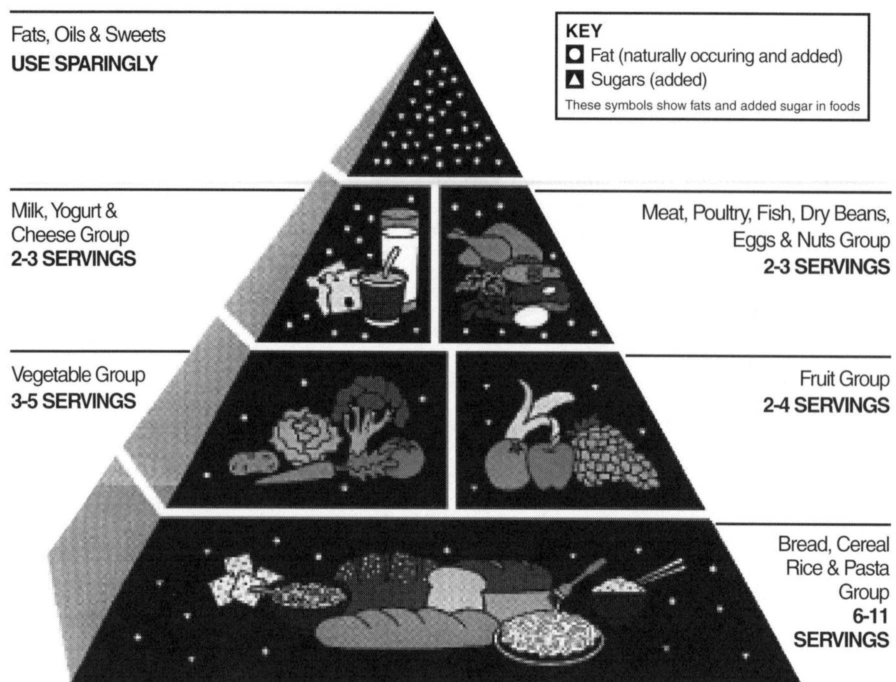

FIGURE 11.1
Food Guide Pyramid: a guide to daily food choices.

The 1977 Food and Agriculture Act named USDA as the lead agency for nutrition research, extension, and teaching. In 1980 USDA and HHS released the first Dietary Guidelines for Americans.[21] Throughout the 1980s and into the 1990s USDA placed a renewed emphasis on developing comprehensive, coordinated efforts to promote nutrition for all Americans.

Food Guide USDA Pyramid

The release of the 1980 Dietary Guidelines for Americans provided the impetus for the development of a new food guide that would allow consumers to put the dietary guidelines into action. Work throughout the 1980s and into the early 1990s culminated in the now well-known 1992 USDA Food Guide Pyramid.[22] The Pyramid has been a popular success, recognized by the majority of Americans. The Pyramid builds on the extensive experience with food guidance systems within USDA. The three essential concepts underlying the Food Guide Pyramid are variety, balance, and moderation. Different visuals were tested with consumers to assess which graphic portrayal most effectively communicated the underlying concepts of balance, variety, and moderation. The graphics were tested first with adults with at least a high school education; consumer testing was expanded later to include children and low-literacy and low-income adults. The Pyramid shape emerged as the most effective graphic, communicating the concepts of variety, balance, and moderation (Figure 11.1).

The USDA Pyramid communicates a wealth of information with little accompanying text. Very complex information is presented in the Pyramid visual. As a result, many consumers are not aware that a more detailed publication on the Food Guide Pyramid exists.[22] This publication discusses the differing energy needs of individuals illustrated at

1600, 2200, and 2800 kcalories. Within the Food Guide Pyramid Bulletin (USDA, 1992) there is an in-depth discussion of "How to Make the Pyramid Work for You." Topics such as what constitutes a serving, different types of fats, and how to use the Pyramid to make low-fat selections are also included in the Pyramid Bulletin.

The Pyramid graphic shown in Figure 11.1 communicates not only balance, variety, and moderation but provides the basis of a healthful diet. The number and amounts of foods recommended in the Pyramid are based on three factors:

- Recommended Dietary Allowances for age and gender groups
- Dietary Guidelines for Americans
- Americans' typical consumption patterns

The advice provided in the Food Guide Pyramid is designed to provide dietary guidance that ensures nutritional adequacy — defined as the RDAs and Dietary Guidelines — within the framework of typical consumption patterns. Thus, while ostensibly an infinite number of food combinations could be used to ensure nutritional adequacy, the five major food groups emphasized in the USDA Pyramid anchor the food selections to current consumption patterns.

A proliferation of pyramids has emerged since the USDA version was published in 1992. However, all of the Pyramids, whether Asian, Mediterranean, or vegetarian, are based on the same building blocks — grains, vegetables, and fruits.[23-25] The similarities in the various pyramids are more dominant than the differences.

In addition, in 1999, USDA released a children's version of the Food Guide Pyramid targeted at children ages two to six years. Here again, the concepts of balance, variety, and moderation underpin the children's graphic (Figure 11.2). The specific icons used in the food groups are based on foods typically consumed by children. Worth noting are the age-specific recommendations for serving sizes at the bottom of the graphic as well as the deliberate inclusion of exercise icons.

The year 2000 Dietary Guidelines for Americans[26] for the first time include the Food Guide Pyramid as part of a specific guideline; "Let the Pyramid Guide Your Food Choices" is the first guideline put forward to build a healthy base. One key reason for including the Pyramid as a direct part of the Dietary Guidelines is the wide-ranging familarity of consumers with the Pyramid and the messages embedded within. The USDA Food Guide Pyramid and the Children's Food Guide Pyramid will continue to be essential parts of the nutrition education and nutrition promotion efforts within the USDA.

Diet Quality Measures

Since the early 1900s, the major areas of concern in public health nutrition have shifted form problems of nutritional deficiency to problems of excesses and imbalances. Problems of relative overconsumption are, on average, more prevalent today than problems of underconsumption. The successive sets of U.S. Dietary Guidelines that have emerged since 1980 have emphasized the links between diet and a range of chronic diseases. An extensive body of scientific literature exists to document the association between diets high in total fat, saturated fat, and low in fiber and complex carbohydrate with coronary heart disease, stroke, diabetes, and certain forms of cancer.

While extensive research has been conducted to link the typical American diet to a range of chronic diseases, less research has been done on methods of measuring diet quality. Until recently, most of the diet quality measures focused on individual nutrients; most

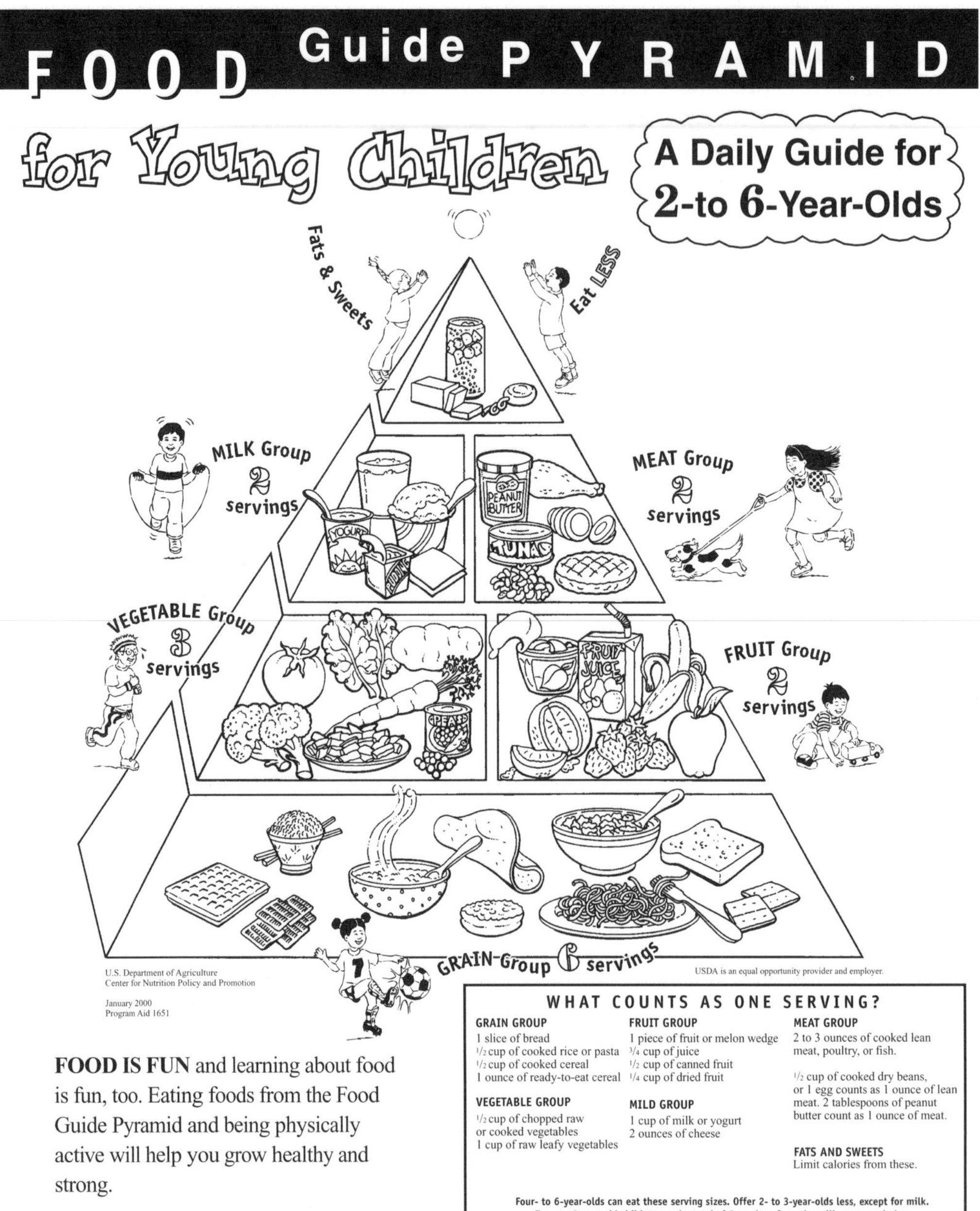

EAT a variety of FOODS AND ENJOY!

FIGURE 11.2
Food Guide Pyramid for Young Children.

TABLE 11.5

Components of the Healthy Eating Index and Scoring System

	Score Ranges[1]	Criteria for Maximum Score of 10	Criteria for Minimum Score of 0
Grain consumption	0–10	6–11 servings[2]	0 servings
Vegetable consumption	0–10	3–5 servings[2]	0 servings
Fruit consumption	0–10	2–4 servings[2]	0 servings
Milk consumption	0–10	2–3 servings[2]	0 servings
Meat consumption	0–10	2–3 servings[2]	0 servings
Total fat intake	0–10	30% or less energy from fat	45% or more energy from fat
Saturated fat intake	0–10	Less than 10% energy from saturated fat	15% or more energy from saturated fat
Cholesterol intake	0–10	300 mg or less	450 mg or more
Sodium intake	0–10	2400 mg or less	4800 mg or more
Food variety	0–10	8 or more different items in a day	3 or fewer different items in a day

1 People with consumption or intakes between the maximum and minimum ranges or amounts were assigned scores proportionately.

2 Number of servings depends on Recommended Energy Allowance.

often these measures were based on measures such as mean percent of the Recommended Dietary Allowances.[27,28]

Despite the U.S. Dietary Guidelines' emphasis on a total diet, indices based on the dietary guidelines have tended to be selective in the components included.[29,30] Few assessment indices have been developed to assess overall diet quality. In an effort to measure how well American diets conform to recommended healthy eating patterns, USDA developed the Healthy Eating Index (HEI) in 1995.

Healthy Eating Index Structure

The Healthy Eating Index (HEI) was designed to measure various aspects of a healthful diet. As shown in Table 11.5; the HEI is a ten-component index; components one through five measure the degree to which a person's diet conforms to the Food Guide Pyramid's serving recommendations for the five major food groups of grains, vegetables, fruits, milk, and meat. The number of recommended servings for each food group varies with the individual's age, gender, physiological status, and energy requirements. The use of food groups rather than nutrients was meant to provide consumers with an easier standard against which to judge their dietary patterns. In addition, there may be as yet unknown components in foods that would not be picked up by measuring simply the nutrients in foods.

Components 6 to 9 measure various aspects of the dietary guidelines, including total fat, saturated fat, cholesterol, and sodium, respectively. Component 10 provides a measure of dietary variety. Despite general agreement that dietary variety is important, it is surprising how few studies have attempted to quantify the concept of variety.[30,31] The HEI counted the total number of different foods that contribute substantially to meeting one or more of the five food group requirements. Foods were counted only if they were eaten in amounts sufficient to contribute at least a half serving in any of the food groups. Identical foods eaten on separate occasions were aggregated before imposing the one-half serving cutoff point. Foods that were similar, such as different forms of potatoes or two different forms of white bread, were counted only once in the variety category.

Each of the ten components has a score ranging from zero to ten; cutoffs for scoring the minimum and maximum scores are shown in Table 11.5. Thus, the HEI can vary from one to 100.

What Are Americans Eating?

The HEI was applied to nationally representative data derived from the Continuing Survey of Food Intake by Individuals (CSFII) for two time periods, 1989 to 1990 and 1994 to 1996. The combined score for 1989 to 1990 was 63.9,[23] contrasted with 63.6, 63.5, and 63.8 for 1994, 1995, and 1996 respectively.[25] Clearly there were not wide variations in the average HEI across this seven-year period.

In addition, the distribution of the average HEI scores did not vary dramatically over the period of 1989 to 1996. Throughout this time period, the majority of individual scores fell in the 51 to 80% range, a category defined as "needs improvement." Only about 11 to 12% of individuals fell in the "good diet" category at any point in time; conversely, approximately 18% of individuals were classified in the "poor diet" category. Scores for the individual HEI components varied with the average score, with the fruit category consistently being the lowest, and the cholesterol score doing best.

The HEI score varied with some economic and demographic factors.[23,25] Females had slightly higher scores than males, and persons in the younger and older groups scored higher than adults in the 19 to 50 age category. Children two to three years had the highest HEI score. Children in this age category scored particularly high on the fruit and dairy component of the HEI when compared with older children, suggesting that changes in dietary habits may play an important role as children age.

Throughout the seven-year period we see a pattern of increasing HEI with increase in income. However the effect of increases in education are more dramatic than the effect of income on increases in HEI. One interpretation is that higher education may enable individuals to translate dietary guidance into improved food patterns.

The scientific rigor of the HEI depends on its ability to accurately measure diet quality. Research has documented that the average HEI in 1989 and 1990 correlated with a range of nutrients and energy intake.[23] For most nutrients, the likelihood of falling below 75% of the RDA for a selected nutrient decreased as the HEI score increased. For example, only 47% of persons with an HEI of 50 or less had vitamin C intake greater than 75% of the RDA, compared to approximately 91% of people scoring 80 or more on the HEI. The data would suggest that as the HEI increases, levels of nutrient intake also increase.

Interestingly, the correlation of the HEI with overall energy intake was modest, suggesting that simply consuming larger quantities of food will not by itself result in a better diet.

Finally, the HEI was compared to individuals' self-rating of their diets.[6] Persons who rated their diets as excellent or good had a significantly higher probability of having an HEI classified as a "good diet." Conversely, individuals who self-rated their diet as fair or poor had an HEI more likely to be classified as "needs improvement."

Policy Implications

The Food Guide Pyramid and the Dietary Guidelines for Americans provide a standard against which to evaluate the total diet. However, neither the Pyramid nor the Dietary Guidelines provide a method for easily assessing total diet. The development of the USDA Healthy Eating Index provided an easy to use, single summary measure of diet quality. The HEI provides a method for monitoring diet quality over time using national survey data. In addition, the HEI has the potential to serve as a tool for individuals to self-evaluate diet quality.

The data from both 1989 to 1990 and 1994 to 1996 indicate that improvements need to be made in the dietary patterns of most Americans. The data obtained from applying the HEI to nationally representative surveys can be one tool to help focus our national nutrition promotion interventions.

Summary

Worldwide major improvements in public health will be accomplished by improvement in dietary patterns. Food-based dietary guidelines have been developed in a broad range of countries. A move toward consensus on food-based dietary guidelines is a practical way to develop core elements of global dietary guidelines that can be effectively promoted by individual countries as well as international health organizations.

References

1. Office of the President, Proceedings of White House Conference on Food, Nutrition and Health. White House, Washington, DC, 1970.
2. US Senate Select Committee on Nutrition and Human Needs. *Dietary Goals for the United States* (2nd ed.), 1977.
3. US Department of Agriculture and US Department of Health and Human Services. *Nutrition and Your Health: Dietary Guidelines for Americans*. Home and Garden Bulletin No. 232, 1980.
4. US Department of Agriculture and US Department of Health and Human Services. *Nutrition and Your Health: Dietary Guidelines for Americans* (2nd ed.). Home and Garden Bulletin No. 232, 1985.
5. US Department of Agriculture and US Department of Health and Human Services. *Nutrition and Your Health: Dietary Guidelines for Americans* (3rd ed.). Home and Garden Bulletin No. 232, 1990.
6. US Department of Agriculture and US Department of Health and Human Services. *Nutrition and Your Health: Dietary Guidelines for Americans* (4th ed.). Home and Garden Bulletin No. 232, 1995.
7. US Department of Agriculture, US Department of Health and Human Services, *Nutrition and Your Health: Dietary Guidelines for Americans* (5th ed.). Home and Garden Bulletin No. 232, 39 pp, May 2000.
8. US Congress, *Public Law 101-445,* 7U.S.C.5341, Library of Congress, Washington DC, 1990.
9. Prospect Associates. Dietary Guidelines Focus Group Report, Final Report, Washington, DC, Nov 1995.
10. Systems Assessment & Research, Inc; Report to USDA of the Initial Focus Groups on *Nutrition and Your Health: Dietary Guidelines for Americans* (4th ed.), Lanham, MD, September 1999.
11. National Research Council, National Academy of Sciences. *Recommended Dietary Allowances* (10th ed.), Washington, DC, National Academy Press, 1989a.
12. US Department of Agriculture, *The Food Guide Pyramid,* Home and Garden Bulletin No. 252, 1992.
13. *Modern Nutrition in Health and Disease* (9th ed.), Williams & Wilkins, Baltimore, MD, 1990.
14. Peng M, Molina V. *Food Dietary Guidelines and Health-Based Promotion in Latin America,* Pan American Health Organization, Washington, DC, April 1999.

15. Krauss RM, Deckelbaum RJ, Ernst N, et al. Dietary guidelines for healthy American adults, a statement for health professionals from the Nutrition Committee, American Heart Association, *Circulation*, 94:1795; 1996.
16. American Cancer Society Advisory Committee on Diet, Nutrition, and Cancer Prevention. Guidelines on diet, nutrition, and cancer prevention: reducing the risk of cancer with healthy food choices and physical activity, *CA Cancer J Clin* 1996; 46: 325-341.
17. American Academy of Pediatrics, *Breastfeeding and the Use of Human Milk*, Pediatrics. 100(6): 1035-1039.
18. *Healthy People: The Surgeon General's Report on Health Promotion and Disease Prevention*, Washington, DC; US Dept of Health, Education, and Welfare, 1979; 177. DHHW (PHS) publication 79-55071.
19. *The Surgeon General's Report on Nutrition and Health*, Washington, DC: US Dept of Health and Human Services; 1988. DHHS (PHS) publication 88-50210.
20. *Healthy People 2000: National Health Promotion and Disease Prevention Objectives*, Washington, DC; US Dept of Health and Human Services; 1991. DHHS (PHS) publication 91-60213.
21. *Nutrition and Your Health: Dietary Guidelines for Americans*, Washington, DC; US Dept of Agriculture/Dept of Health and Human Services; 1980. Home and Garden Bulletin No. 328.
22. *Food Guide Pyramid*, Washington, DC: US Dept of Agriculture, Human Nutrition Information Service; 1992. Home and Garden Bulletin No. 252.
23. Kennedy E, Ohls J, Carlson S, Fleming K. *JADA* 95: 1103; 1995.
24. Kennedy E. Oct, 1998. Building on the pyramid — where do we go from here? *Nutrition Today* 11: 183-185.
25. Kennedy E, Bowman S, Lino M, Gerrior S, Basiotis PP. 1999. Diet Quality of Americans, Chapter 5. In: *America's Eating Habits.* Frazao E, Ed. Economic Research Service, Washington, DC.
26. USDA/HHS. May, 2000. Nutrition and Your Health: Dietary Guidelines for Americans, 5th ed. Home and Garden Bulletin No. 232, Washington, DC.
27. Guthrie HA, Scheer JC. *JADA* 78: 240; 1981.
28. Block GA. *Am J Epidemiol* 115: 402; 1982.
29. Patterson RE, Haines RS, Popkin BM. *JADA* 94: 57; 1994.
30. Kent AK, Schatzkin A, Harris TU, et al. *Am J Clin Nutr* 57: 434; 1993.
31. Krebs-Smith S, Smieiklas-Wright H, Guthrie HA, Krubs-Smith J. *JADA* 87: 807; 1987.

Other References

USDA, Center for Nutrition Policy and Promotion. October, 1996. The State of Nutrition Education in USDA: A Report to the Secretary. USDA: Washington, D.C.

Childrens Food Guide Pyramid, 1999.

12

Dietary Guidelines in Three Regions of the World

Johanna Dwyer, Odilia I. Bermudez, Leh Chii Chwang, Karin Koehn, and Chin-Ling Chen*

Introduction and Overview

Dietary guidelines are "recommendations for achieving appropriate diets, and healthy lifestyles."[1] This section examines the similarities and differences, strengths and weaknesses of dietary guidelines from three regions of the world, concluding with some recommendations for crafting future guidelines.

Effective guidelines have several elements in common. They are designed to address and mitigate the major diet-related nutrition problems of the population. As these problems change over time, the focus of dietary guidance must also shift. Effective guidelines are evidence based, and the strength of supportive evidence is strong. Eating habits, cultural beliefs, and food supplies available are considered. The messages conveyed are tested prior to their finalization to ensure that the guidelines can be communicated effectively. Successful guidelines are integrated with other nutritional guidance of a public health nature. They are recognized as only one of a group of essential components of effective food and nutrition policies. Other factors include access to a variety of safe and affordable foods from available resources. Ideally, successful guidelines are promulgated simultaneously with ways to measure their effectiveness.

In this section we examine guidelines from regions representing different culinary approaches, food customs, and economies. English-speaking North America and Oceania are highly industrialized, affluent countries. Several Asian and Latin American countries that vary in degree of urbanization and standards of living are also examined.

The United States, Canada, Australia, and New Zealand

In English-speaking North America and Oceania, diseases of affluence (i.e., obesity, heart disease, and certain cancers) are common and therefore these issues are given attention.

* This material is based upon work supported by the U.S. Department of Agriculture, under Agreement No. 58-1950-9-001. Any opinions, findings, conclusions, or recommendations expressed in this publication are those of the authors and do not necessarily reflect the views of the U.S. Department of Agriculture. We thank Smita Ghosh for her help in editing the manuscript.

0-8493-2705-9/01/$0.00+$1.50

All of these affluent countries share similar dietary patterns and nutrition-related problems, including a diet excessive in calories, fat, salt, sugars, and alcohol, and too low in fruits, vegetables, and whole grains. Their guidelines have addressed excessive as well as inadequate food consumption, weight, and physical activity since they were first formulated in the late 1970s and early 1980s.

Each of these countries has an ethnically diverse population. In the U.S., according to 1990 census data, 12% of the population was African American and 9% were of Hispanic origin.[2] The Aboriginal and Torres Strait Islander people comprise only about 2% of the Australian population, but they often live under impoverished, overcrowded conditions that put them at nutritional risk,[3] and they have a high prevalence of android pattern obesity, which is associated with many health problems.[4] In New Zealand, 13% of the population belong to the rapidly growing Maori minority, and another 5% are Pacific Islanders.[5] Some of these minority groups have increased risks of chronic degenerative diseases as they move away from traditional customs to modern diets and lifestyles. The information accompanying the Australian and New Zealand dietary guidelines refers to these special problems, although the dietary guidelines are targeted to the general population.

Formulation of Dietary Guidelines for the United States, Canada, Australia, and New Zealand

Table 12.1 shows the approaches used in the development of the dietary guidelines in these countries. All used experts and scientists, and each of the guidelines was endorsed by a relevant government agency. In the U.S., the National Nutrition Monitoring and Related Research Act required that the Dietary Guidelines for Americans be updated every five years and be reviewed by the Departments of Health and Human Services and Agriculture. The law has expired but revisions continue on the same timetable, led by relevant government agencies. Other U.S. federal food guidance for the general public is required to be consistent with these guidelines.

All four countries address their guidelines to both the general population and health professionals or other policy makers. New guidelines usually follow the precedents established in earlier versions (see Table 12.1). Some changes simply involve different wording. For example, the American guideline regarding sugar has evolved from "Avoid too much sugar" in 1980[6] to "Use sugars only in moderation" in 1990[7] and "Choose a diet moderate in sugars" in 1995,[8] to the current "Choose beverages and foods that limit your intake of sugars."[9] Other changes are more innovative. In 1992 Australia added guidelines for two specific nutrients: calcium and iron. The U.S. added a new guideline on food safety in 2000.

Australia and New Zealand have specific guidelines for infants, toddlers, school-age children, adolescents, and the elderly that also address other health recommendations. New Zealand also has dietary guidelines for pregnant or breastfeeding women.

As described in Table 12.1, the U.S., Canada, and Australia all have pictorial representations or graphics for their dietary recommendations. The U.S. has a food guide pyramid graphic that incorporates some of its guidelines.[10] Canada uses a rainbow graphic to depict the components of a healthy diet. Australia has two graphics — a pyramid and a plate.

Similarities and Differences among Dietary Guidelines in the United States, Canada, Australia, and New Zealand

Table 12.2 shows that all of these countries have recommendations for certain nutrients and also for groups of foods, such as fruits/vegetables, grains, dairy, and meats. Food

TABLE 12.1

Development of Dietary Guidelines in the United States, Canada, Australia, and New Zealand

	United States	Canada	Australia	New Zealand
Title of guideline	Dietary Guidelines for Americans	Canada's Guidelines for Healthy Eating	Australian Dietary Guidelines	Food and Nutrition Guidelines
Year	1995, 2000	1991	1992	1991
Endorsing unit	Departments of Agriculture, Health, and Human Services	Department of National Health and Welfare	National Health and Medical Research Council	Nutrition Task Force at the Ministry of Health
Approaches*	1-5, 7	1-5, 7	1-5	1-5
Target audiences**	G, H, P, N	G, H, P, N	G, H, P	G, H, P
Graphic representation	Pyramid	Rainbow	Pyramid	None

* 1 = Experts, scientists views; 2 = Review of former guidelines; 3 = From food groups; 4 = From consumption/nutrition survey; 5 = Definition of nutritional objectives; 6 = Economic data; 7 = Consumer focus groups.

** G = General population; H = Health professionals; P = Policy makers; N = Nutrition education of schoolchildren.

TABLE 12.2

Dietary Guidelines of the United States, Canada, Australia and New Zealand

United States 2000	Canada	Australia	New Zealand
1. Aim for a healthy weight	1. Enjoy a variety of foods	1. Enjoy a wide variety of nutritious foods	1. Eat a variety of foods from each of the four major food groups each day
2. Be physically active each day	2. Emphasize cereals, breads, other grain products, vegetables and fruits	2. Eat plenty of bread and cereals (preferably whole grain), vegetables (including legumes), and fruits	2. Prepare meals with minimal added fat (especially saturated fat), salt, and sugar
3. Let the pyramid guide your food choices	3. Choose lower-fat dairy products, leaner meats, and foods prepared with little or no fat	3. Eat a diet that is low in fat, and in particular, low in saturated fat	3. Choose prepared foods, drinks and snacks that are low in fat (especially saturated fat), salt, and sugar
4. Build a healthy base	4. Achieve and maintain a healthy body weight by enjoying regular physical activity and healthy eating	4. Maintain a healthy body weight by balancing physical activity and food intake	4. Maintain a healthy body weight by regular physical activity and by healthy eating
5. Choose a variety of grains daily, especially whole grains	5. Limit salt, alcohol, and caffeine	5. If you drink alcohol, limit your intake	5. Drink plenty of liquids each day
6. Choose a variety of fruits and vegetables daily		6. Eat only moderate amounts of sugars and foods containing added sugars	6. If drinking alcohol, do so in moderation
7. Keep food safe to eat		7. Choose low salt foods and use salt sparingly	
8. Choose a diet that is low in saturated fat and cholesterol and moderate in total fat		8. Encourage and support breast-feeding	
9. Choose sensibly		9. Eat foods containing calcium; this is particularly important for girls and women	
10. Choose beverages and foods that limit your intake of sugars		10. Eat foods containing iron; this is particularly important for girls and women, vegetarians and athletes	
11. Choose and prepare foods with less salt			
12. If you drink alcoholic beverages, do so in moderation			

based guidelines are easier than nutrient based guidelines for the consumer to implement, since human beings eat foods, not specific nutrients.

In all of these countries, heart disease, hypertension, diabetes with its complications, and cancer are the leading causes of death.[4,9,11-13] Obesity is prevalent and increases the severity of many of these diseases.[13,14]

The core messages in all of these dietary guidelines are similar: eat a variety of foods and include physical activity to achieve/maintain a healthy weight (Table 12.2). All of these countries have recommendations on limiting fat, salt, and alcohol and increasing fruits, vegetables, and whole grains. The U.S., Canada, and New Zealand all suggest limiting alcoholic beverages to less than two drinks per day for men and one for women. Australia has a higher limit — less than four drinks for men and two for women per day.

The background and supporting information accompanying the Dietary Guidelines provides the rationale for quantitative suggestions for intakes of specific nutrients.[4,9,15,16] All of these countries suggest that 50 to 55% of total calories should come from carbohydrates. The U.S., Canada, and Australia recommend less than 30% of total calories from fat and less than 10% from saturated fat. New Zealand is more liberal, suggesting no more than 30 to 35% of kcalories from fat and 12% from saturated fat.

There are some differences in the guidelines. In the most recent U.S. guidelines (2000), food safety is addressed. Australia includes a guideline specifically to encourage and support breastfeeding, and it also has two other nutrient-specific guidelines, "eat foods containing calcium" and "eat foods containing iron."[4] The calcium and iron guidelines are emphasized for both girls and women, and iron is also stressed for vegetarians and athletes.

Most of the guidelines other than alcohol for the U.S. and Canada are for all healthy individuals over age two years. The fat guideline in Canada is not applicable until a child reaches age five.

Other health recommendations included in New Zealand's guidelines are non-smoking related, especially for adolescents, and pregnant and breastfeeding women. The elderly, who may suffer from isolation and therefore poor nutrition, are encouraged to "make mealtime a social time." Australia encourages its elderly to eat at least three meals per day. Elderly people and pregnant women are especially vulnerable to risks associated with foodborne illnesses. Australia's food safety guidelines address food safety in the elderly (care for your food: prepare and store it correctly), and the New Zealand guidelines discuss *Listeria* in the information specifically directed to pregnant women.

Latin America

Dietary guidelines were first formulated in Latin America in the late 1980s.[17] Guidelines from Chile, Guatemala, Mexico, Panama, and Venezuela are provided as examples of dietary guidelines in the region.

Latin America is a region with great inequalities in the distribution of welfare, and also large variations in the nutritional health of its population groups. There has been a shift from dietary deficiency disease to problems of dietary excess in many countries of the region over the past two decades. In Chile, the prevalence of protein–calorie malnutrition in children is declining rapidly. However, the prevalence of chronic degenerative diseases associated with imbalances in food intake and sedentary lifestyles is rising.[18] In contrast, in Guatemala, Mexico, and Panama, poverty-related undernutrition and dietary deficiency diseases are still prevalent, especially among children and women of reproductive age in rural areas. At the same time, the prevalence of diet-related chronic diseases is rising. Venezuela is an oil-exporting country, but it still has large economic inequalities and grapples with poverty-related malnutrition as well as dietary excess.

In most Latin American countries, food consumption patterns are influenced by those of the U.S. Changing cultural and economic influences, rural–urban migration, greater availability of processed foods, and advertising also affect food consumption.[19] Both over- and undernutrition result.[20] The development of poor ghettos in metropolitan areas, short lactation periods, low wages, and low maternal educational levels is associated with undernutrition in young children. The interactions of urbanization, sedentary lifestyles, lack of nutrition education, and excessive consumption of cheap foods low in nutritional value lead to diseases of overconsumption such as obesity, diabetes, and cardiovascular disease.[20]

Formulation of the Dietary Guidelines in Latin America

Most of the Latin American countries are in the implementation stage in formulating dietary guidelines.[21] The dietary guidelines for the Mexican population were issued by the Mexican Institute of Nutrition.[22] Venezuela issued dietary guidelines in the late 1980s that were later revised and updated.[23] The dietary guidelines have been implemented in many ways. For example, they have been incorporated into Venezuelan kindergarten, elementary, and secondary school curricula.[23-25]

Table 12.3 contains details about the dietary guidelines development process. Four of the countries have dietary guidelines for the general population. Some also have guidelines for specific population groups (Chile, Panama, and Venezuela) or target certain groups on specific concerns (Guatemala for food safety among the poor). Governmental or quasi-governmental organizations develop and promulgate the guidelines based on the views and opinions of experts and scientists. Some also use background data on food consumption surveys (Chile, Mexico, Panama) and economic data (Venezuela, Mexico). Most of the countries also refer to food groups in their dietary guidelines.[18,22,23,26,27]

Four of the countries also use graphic representations of food groups and supporting messages (see Table 12.3). Chile, Mexico, and Panama adapted the food guide pyramid used in the U.S. Guatemala summarized its food groups and dietary guidelines in a family pot, or "crockpot" graphic. Venezuela has no graphic but the government has produced an extensive set of educational materials directed at different target groups.[24,25]

Similarities and Differences among Latin American Dietary Guidelines

Table 12.4 summarizes the dietary guidelines for the Latin America. The number of guidelines range from 6 in Panama to 12 in Venezuela; Venezuela also has issued 40 educational messages to facilitate implementation of the guidelines. Mexico has ten dietary guidelines — each one contains several additional messages.

In general, the guidelines are focused on foods, and provide general guidance. Variety is mentioned in all guidelines. Guatemala, Mexico, and Venezuela discuss economic disparities in supporting documents. For example, Guatemala recommends that those with limited resources eat meats, eggs, and dairy products at least once or twice a week, while Venezuela urges prudence in the management of financial resources (see Table 12.4).

TABLE 12.3

Development of Dietary Guidelines in Latin American Countries

	Chile	Guatemala	Mexico	Panama	Venezuela
Title of guideline	Food Guidelines for Chile	Food Guidelines for Guatemala	Food Guidelines — Mexico	Food Guidelines for Panama	Food Guidelines for Venezuela
Year	1997	1998	1993	1995	1991
Endorsing unit	Ministry of Health, the Food Technology and Nutrition Institute, and the Nutrition Center at the University of Chile	Food Guidelines National Committee (inter-institutional)	National Nutrition Institute	Ministry of Health	CAVENDES Foundation, National Institute of Nutrition, several universities
Approaches*	1, 3, 4	1, 3, 6	1, 3, 4, 5, 6	1, 3, 4, 5	1, 2, 5, 6
Target audiences**	G, P, N	G	G	G, P	G, P, N
Graphic representation	Pyramid	Family pot	Pyramid	Pyramid	None
Other guidelines	For school age children and the elderly	Food safety	None	For the first year of age	For the preschooler, school age children, and the elderly

* 1 = Experts, scientists views; 2 = Review of former guidelines; 3 = From food groups; 4 = From consumption/nutrition survey; 5 = Definition of nutritional objectives; 6 = Economic data

** G = General population; H = Health professionals; P = Policy makers; N = Nutrition education of schoolchildren.

TABLE 12.4

Dietary Guidelines of Selected Latin American Countries

Chile	Guatemala	Mexico	Panama	Venezuela
1. Eat different types of foods throughout the day 2. Increase consumption of fruits, vegetables, and green vegetables 3. Prefer vegetable oil and limit animal fats 4. For meat, prefer fish and poultry 5. Increase consumption of low fat milk 6. Reduce salt intake 7. Moderate sugar consumption	1. Include grains, cereals, or potatoes at each meal because they are nutritious, tasty, and have low cost 2. Eat vegetables and greens every day to benefit your body 3. Every day, eat any type of fruit, because they are healthy, easy to digest, and nutritious 4. If you eat tortilla and beans every day, eat one spoonful of beans with each tortilla to make it more nutritious 5. At least twice a week eat one egg or one piece of cheese, or drink one glass of milk, to complement your diet 6. At least once per week, eat a serving of liver (beef) or meat to strengthen your body 7. To stay healthy, eat a variety of foods as indicated in the household pot	1. Avoid monotony by consuming a wide variety of foods; select different foods each day and at each meal, choosing among those available at the market and following the proportions recommended by the food guide pyramid 2. Include at least two servings of fruits and vegetables at every meal 3. Eat variety of grains and grain products, preferably whole grains, at every meal, mixing cereals and legumes 4. Include a moderate serving of animal products at every meal, choosing those with the least fat 5. Limit consumption of fats, including cooking oils and fatty foods, to less than 30% of daily energy intake; limit saturated fats, of animal origin, to less than 10% of total energy; reduce cholesterol intake to less than 300 mg per day	1. Eat a variety of foods 2. Eat sufficient grains, roots, vegetables, and fruits 3. Select a diet low in saturated fat, cholesterol, and oil 4. Eat sugar and sweets in moderation 5. Eat sat and sodium in moderation 6. Maintain a healthy weight	1. Eat a variety of foods every day 2. Eat just enough to maintain a proper weight 3. Eat preferably with your family 4. Practice good hygiene when handling food 5. Manage your money well when selecting and purchasing food 6. Breast milk is the best food for children under 6 months of age 7. Eat only moderate quantities of food of animal origin 8. Use vegetable oils in preparing meals and avoid excess animal fat 9. Get the fiber your body needs from the vegetable products you eat daily 10. Consume salt in moderation 11. Water is essential for life, and drinking water helps to preserve your health 12. Alcoholic beverages are not part of a healthy diet

6. Reduce consumption of salt and sugar, starting by not using salt at the table and reducing sugars in liquids (coffee, tea, or juices)
7. Restrict consumption of products with excess of additives (colorants, flavorings, etc.); avoid alcohol and do not smoke
8. Breastfeed children from birth and start complementary food at the fourth month of age
9. Avoid obesity by monitoring weight according to the suggested weight for stature
10. Increase physical activity, walk briskly or practice any other type of aerobic exercise for about 20-30 minutes, 4 or 5 times a week

Some countries incorporate specific concerns about food consumption (Table 12.4). Guatemala emphasizes the importance of hand washing, and keeping food and water well covered. Venezuela has a guideline emphasizing good hygiene in handling food.

Guidelines directed to over-consumption are included by all the countries. These include specific recommendations to increase physical activity (Mexico), maintain a healthy weight (Mexico, Panama), or to moderate or reduce the use of fats and sugars (Chile, Mexico, Panama, and Venezuela). Chronic disease risks are also addressed. These include recommendations for moderate use of salt (Chile and Venezuela) or sodium (Panama), limiting consumption of fats and sugars (Chile, Mexico, Panama, Venezuela), saturated fats (Mexico, Panama), and cholesterol (Mexico, Panama). Other guidelines are directed to limiting specific foods or nutrients, or to increase other more nutrient-rich foods (fruits, vegetables, whole grains) (See Table 12.4).

The Latin American guidelines focus mostly on foods, not specific nutrients (Table 12.4). However, Panama recommends moderation in the use of sodium along with salt. Guatemala, a country with low literacy rates, also emphasizes nutrients but in simple, short messages; it singles out energy, protein (both animal and vegetable), vitamins A and C, calcium, iron, and zinc, as well as fiber. This emphasis reflects Guatemala's goals of preventing both dietary deficiencies and excesses. Venezuela's guidelines have little emphasis on specific foods (Table 12.4).

All of the Latin American countries include advice on consuming fruits, vegetables, and grains daily. Guatemala specifically mentions beans and tortillas. Other countries (Chile, Mexico, and Venezuela) mention the need for limiting fat. Salt restriction is mentioned in Mexico, Venezuela, and Panama. Both Mexico and Venezuela have a guideline limiting alcohol. Chile and Guatemala include a guideline on use of dairy products; Chile focuses on low-fat milk products; Guatemala urges at least one to two servings of whole fat milk products, since much of the population is poor and does not consume milk. Mexico and Venezuela have specific guidelines stressing the importance of breastfeeding. Panama has special dietary guidelines for infants, recommending exclusive breastfeeding during the first six months of life, and complementary feeding thereafter.[27]

Conclusions about Dietary Guidelines in Latin America

Dietary guidelines for Latin American countries reflect the diversity in socioeconomic situations and nutritional problems in the region, and each country's unique perspectives. They offer the general public, service providers, and policy makers actionable recommendations for improving nutrition and health status. Some of these countries have already identified barriers that limit the use of the dietary guidelines (Chile, Venezuela). Others, such as Mexico, still need to evaluate the applicability of their guidelines to the eating practices of the diverse Mexican population. Dietary guidelines in Guatemala were directed to the poor; problems associated with over-consumption of foods and sedentary lifestyles still need to be addressed.

Asian Countries

Introduction

Asia's diversity is reflected in the many nutritional problems that were evident in the ten countries we reviewed. Until the mid 1950s, poverty-related malnutrition was the major problem. The primary concern was to ensure adequate energy intakes and prevention or control of dietary deficiency diseases.[28,29] Today, nutrition problems in Asia cover the entire spectrum from deficiency disease to excess.

Asian dietary guidelines focus on reducing or preventing both chronic deficiency and chronic degenerative diseases, since both problems are often prevalent.[1,30,31] Presently, India still has high rates of protein–energy malnutrition among some groups. In countries such as Korea, Japan, Taiwan, and Singapore, protein–energy malnutrition has declined dramatically in the past three decades.[29,31,32] Countries such as Thailand and China have low rates of protein–energy malnutrition, but micronutrient deficiencies (iron, iodine, vitamin A, and riboflavin) are still common.[33-36] Indonesia and the Philippines face persistent problems of undernutrition and deficiency disease among the poor coupled with emerging problems of overnutrition and increased chronic degenerative disease, particularly among the affluent.[28,35,37] Filipino guidelines for more affluent populations focus on chronic degenerative diseases and avoiding excess,[38] whereas their guidelines for the relatively less affluent population emphasize achieving sufficiency of nutrient intakes.[37]

Formulation of the Dietary Guidelines in Asia

Table 12.5 shows the various approaches used in developing dietary guidelines in Asia. The guidelines are all intended to provide nutrition education and dietary guidance to the general public in terms that are understandable to most consumers. They are also often used to help officials in the health, agricultural, and education sectors in program planning. All of the countries surveyed rely on government agencies and/or professional societies to develop and endorse their official guidelines.[37] Some countries (the Philippines, Korea, and Japan) formulate guidelines based on findings from national nutrition or food consumption surveys. Others develop their dietary guidelines based on what experts deem appropriate.

Graphics have been adopted by many Asian countries to help the public visualize these dietary guidelines and food guides. These include pyramids (India, Malaysia, Singapore), pagodas (Korea and China), a plum flower (Taiwan), the "Big 6" for the six food groups (Japan), and a six-sided star (Philippines). Another pyramid is also available for the more affluent Filipinos.[38]

Similarities and Differences among Asian Dietary Guidelines

Table 12.6 presents information on representative dietary guidelines from the Asian region. Most of the guidelines are general, and are food- rather than nutrient-based. The exception is Singapore, which has guidelines that are quantitative and nutrient-specific.[39] There are common core food-based messages in all the guidelines; these include: choose a diet composed of a wide variety of foods, eat enough food to meet bodily needs and maintain or improve body weight, select foods that are safe to eat, and enjoy your food.

The guidelines also vary with respect to number and relative emphasis on balance, adequacy, moderation, and restriction. Although all the Asian dietary guidelines recommend eating a variety of foods, they differ on how they suggest achieving a varied pattern (see Table 12.6). Some include recommendations for frequency of consumption. Eating breakfast daily is recommended in the Indonesian guidelines, and having regular meals is recommended in the Korean guidelines.[35,40] Other guidelines recommend specific

TABLE 12.5

Development of Dietary Guidelines in Asian Countries

	India	Indonesia	Philippines	Malaysia	Thailand
Title of guideline	Dietary Guideline for affluent Indians; Dietary Guideline for relatively poor Indians	13 Core Messages for a Balanced Diet	Nutritional Guidelines for Filipinos	Proposed Dietary Guidelines for Malaysia	The Thai Dietary Guidelines for Better Health
Year	1988	1995	1990	1996	1995
Endorsing unit	Indian Council of Medical Research (Expert Committee)	National Development and Planning Coordinating Board	Dept. of Science and Technology (National Guidelines Committee)	Ministry of Health	The Division of Nutrition, Department of Health, Ministry of Public Health
Approaches*	1-6	1	1-5	1, 2 , 3	1
Target audiences**	N	G	G, H	G, H	G
Graphic representation	Pyramid	None	Pyramid, 6-sided star	Pyramid	None

	Korea	Japan	Taiwan	China	Singapore
Title of guideline	National Dietary Guidelines	Guidelines for Health Promotion: Dietary Guidelines	Dietary Guidelines for the Population	Chinese Dietary Guidelines for Chinese Residents	Guidelines for a Healthy Diet
Year	1990	1985	1995	1997	1993
Endorsing unit	Korean Nutrition Society/ Ministry of Health and Welfare	Ministry of Health and Welfare	Department of Health	Chinese Nutrition Society	National Advisory Committee on Food & Nutrition, Ministry of Health
Approaches*	1, 2, 4	1, 2, 3, 5	1	1	1
Target audiences**	G	G, H	G	G	G
Graphic representation	Pagoda	Numeral 6	Plum flower	Pagoda	Pyramid

* 1 = Experts, scientists views; 2 = Review of former guidelines; 3 = From food groups; 4 = From consumption/nutrition survey; 5 = Definition of nutritional objectives; 6 = Economic data.

** G = General population; H = Health professionals; P = Policy makers; N = Nutrition education of school children.

TABLE 12.6

Dietary Guidelines of Selected Asian Countries

India Affluent	India Relatively Poor	Indonesia	Philippines	Malaysia
1. Overall energy should be restricted to levels commensurate with sedentary occupations so that obesity is avoided 2. Give preference to undermilled over highly refined and polished cereals 3. Include green leafy vegetables in the diet 4. Restrict daily edible fat intake to less than 40g, total fat intake to less than 20% of total calories, and intake of ghee (clarified butter) to special occasions only 5. Restrict intake of sugar and sweets 6. Avoid high-salt intake, especially for those prone to hypertension	1. Diet should be the least expensive and conform to traditional and cultural practices as closely as possible 2. Energy derived from cereals should not exceed 75% of the total energy requirement 3. Some pulses should be eaten along with the high-cereal diet, with at least 150 ml of milk and 150 g of vegetables per day 4. Energy from fat and oil should not exceed 10%, and that from refined carbohydrate (sugar or jaggery) should not exceed 5% of total calories	1. Eat a wide variety of foods 2. Consume foods that provide sufficient energy 3. Obtain about half of total energy requirements from complex CHO-rich foods 4. Obtain not more than a quarter of total energy intake from fats or oils 5. Use only iodized salt 6. Consume iron-rich foods 7. Breastfeed your baby exclusively for four months 8. Have breakfast every day 9. Drink adequate quantities of fluids that are free of contaminants 10. Take adequate exercise 11. Avoid drinking alcoholic drinks 12. Consume foods prepared hygienically 13. Read the labels of packaged foods	1. Eat a variety of foods 2. Keep ideal body weight 3. Consume enough protein 4. Keep fat consumption at 20% of energy intake 5. Drink milk every day 6. Reduce salt intake 7. Keep in good dental health 8. Moderate alcohol and caffeine consumption 9. Keep harmony between diet and daily life 10. Enjoy meals	1. Enjoy a variety of foods 2. Maintain healthy body weight by balancing food intake with regular physical activity 3. Eat plenty of rice and other cereal products, fruits, and vegetables 4. Minimize fat in food preparation and choose foods low in fat and cholesterol 5. Choose foods low in salt and sugar 6. Drink plenty of water daily 7. Practice breastfeeding
Thailand	**Korea**	**Japan**	**China**	**Singapore**
1. Eat sufficient and appropriate cereals or whole grain cereal products 2. Eat fish, lean meat, legumes, and their products	1. Eat a variety of foods 2. Keep ideal body weight 3. Consume enough protein 4. Keep fat consumption at 20% of energy intake 5. Drink milk every day	1. Obtain well-balanced nutrition with a variety of foods (30 foods a day); take staple food, main dish, and side dishes together	1. Eat a variety of foods 2. Eat appropriate quantity of foods 3. Moderate oil and fat 4. Eat moderately polished cereals	1. Eat a variety of foods 2. Maintain desirable body weight 3. Restrict total fat intake to 20-30% of total energy intake

TABLE 12.6 *(Continued)*

Dietary Guidelines of Selected Asian Countries

Thailand	Korea	Japan	China	Singapore
3. Be mindful of fat intake of below 30% of total energy intake and make sure that low cholesterol foods are chosen 4. Eat a variety of fruits and vegetables to ensure adequate vitamins and fiber supplies 5. Eat sweets and sugars only in moderation 6. Restrict salt intake 7. Recognize and eat well prepared food which is free of microorganisms and food contaminants 8. Avoid or restrict alcohol consumption	6. Reduce salt intake 7. Keep in good dental health 8. Moderate alcohol and caffeine consumption 9. Keep harmony between diet and daily life 10. Enjoy meals	2. Take energy corresponding to daily activity 3. Consider the amount and quality of fats and oils consumed: avoid too much; eat more vegetable oils than animal fat 4. Avoid too much salt — not more than 10 g a day 5. Happy eating makes for happy family life; sit down and eat together and talk; treasure family taste and home cooking	5. Limit salt intake 6. Eat fewer sweets 7. Limit alcohol balance food distribution through three meals	4. Modify composition of fat in the diet to 1/3 polyunsaturated, 1/3 monounsaturated, and 1/3 saturated 5. Reduce cholesterol intake to less than 300 mg/day 6. Maintain intake of complex carbohydrates at about 50% total energy intake 7. Reduce salt intake to less than 4.5 g a day (1800 mg Na) 8. Reduce intake of salt-cured, preserved, and smoked foods 9. Reduce intake of refined and processed sugar to less than 10% of energy 10. Increase intake of fruit and vegetables and whole-grain cereal products 11. For those who drink alcohol, have no more than 2-3 standard drinks (about 40 g alcohol) per day 12. Encourage breastfeeding in infants until at least 6 months of age

amounts of different kinds of foods. For example, to assure a well-balanced diet, the Japanese guidelines recommend eating thirty or more different kinds of foods daily.[41] Japanese guidelines also suggest balancing main and side dishes around staple foods. Malaysia recommends choosing foods from each of the food groups daily.[42] The Filipino and Chinese guidelines also focus on achieving dietary adequacy, emphasizing food rather than nutrient-based interventions.

Table 12.6 describes the guidelines with respect to nutrients. Virtually all emphasize ensuring adequacy of energy/calorie intake. Korea mentions achieving and maintaining energy balance by balancing intake and expenditure.[35] Most guidelines stress increased intakes of fruits, vegetables, cereal, and dairy food to promote fiber, vitamin, and mineral intakes and geting enough food. Some also indicate the proportion of foods that should be consumed in relation to total energy intake. For example, the Indian guidelines for the low-income population recommend that less than 75% of kcalories should come from cereals.[43] In countries where deficiencies of vitamins and minerals have been identified as public health problems, the guidelines reflect this and emphasize food sources rich in those nutrients. For example, calcium is mentioned specifically in some guidelines; a specific calcium-rich food (milk) is mentioned in the Taiwanese, Chinese, and Korean guidelines, and fish and seaweed in the Japanese guidelines. In Indonesia, people are advised to "consume iron-rich foods, and use only iodized salt."[40] The Filipino guidelines recommend choosing "foods fortified with nutrients."[37] The guidelines for less affluent Indians and Indonesians recommend eating enough food.[40,43]

The guidelines for more affluent countries such as Taiwan, Singapore, Korea, Japan (and also for the more affluent members of the populations in Indonesia and India) emphasize moderation in fat, saturated fat, and/or simple sugars. The major difference between the various guidelines in Asia is in the amounts and the relative balance suggested between dietary constituents. The Asian guidelines on moderation in fat and salt intake vary greatly. Some simply say to avoid excess, or to limit/restrict the use of fat (see guidelines for India, Malaysia, Taiwan, China), while others specify the type of fat to be consumed. For example, the Japanese guidelines recommend use of vegetable oil instead of animal fat, and in the Indian guidelines, ghee (clarified fat, very high in saturated fat) is recommended but only for special occasions for affluent Indians. China, Taiwan, and Singapore are three countries with similar ethnic origins and dietary patterns that share similar dietary guidelines recommending reducing intake of salt and salt-cured foods. Singapore is the most specific, recommending eating less than 5 grams of salt or 2000 mg of sodium per day.[39] General recommendations on limiting salt intake are present in other guidelines throughout the region. The Japanese guidelines recommend eating less than 10 grams of salt per day. Neither Malaysia nor the Philippines mention salt.[39]

The majority of the guidelines stress common nonfood-related healthy behaviors such as not smoking, dental hygiene, stress management, weight control, and physical activity. Asian dietary guidelines also specify the settings (places or environments) or other circumstances surrounding food and eating (Table 12.6). Most countries in this region also acknowledge the impacts of lifestyle changes on health, and emphasize attaining a healthy body weight to prevent diet-related disease. The Indonesian guideline recommends consuming "foods to provide sufficient energy."[40] Some of these differences in emphasis reflect the vastly different levels of affluence within and between countries in Asia. For example, India has two sets of guidelines. One is for the poor and emphasizes nutrient adequacy and avoiding dietary deficiency diseases. The other Indian guideline is for affluent individuals and emphasizes energy balance, restricting energy intakes to levels "commensurate with sedentary occupation, so that obesity is avoided," coupled with moderation and restriction of fat, saturated fat, and sugar to reduce chronic degenerative disease.[43]

Asian guidelines also recognize that eating is more than just "refueling" or nourishment from the physiological standpoint. They recognize that food provides pleasure and has strong links to family, tradition, and culture. Enjoyment of meals is therefore a concern in all countries, but is especially evident in the Japanese and Korean guidelines. In Japan, dietary guidelines that promote family values are included; citizens are advised to "make all activities pertaining to food pleasurable ones." Another Japanese guideline states "enjoy cooking and use mealtimes as occasions for family communication."[44,45] In Korea, eating is viewed as a way of keeping harmony between diet and other aspects of daily life, and this is stated in the guidelines (see Table 12.6).[35]

Conclusions about Dietary Guidelines in Asian Countries

Dietary guidelines for the Asian countries are all directed at the general population. Many countries, including Malaysia, Indonesia, China, and Japan, also have specific guidelines focusing on different ages, sexes, and conditions, such as infants, and pregnant and lactating women.[33,39,44,45] Specific foods are recommended for these population groups. For example, breastfeeding in early infancy is a common recommendation in the dietary guidelines of many Asian countries. Human breast milk is recognized as the best food for infants. Encouragement of breastfeeding and recognition of breast milk's unique properties are included in the guidelines.[41,58] The duration of exclusive breastfeeding ranges from four months (Indonesia) to four to six months (Philippines), and six months in Singapore. Another difference is age of weaning, with introduction of other foods in addition to breast milk. For example, it is recommended at four to six months in the Philippines, but the Malaysian guidelines recommend weaning at no earlier than five to six months, with breastfeeding continuing for up to two years.

Some dietary guidelines are common to all Asian countries. One is to eat clean and safe foods; such recommendations are especially important in areas where the climate is very hot and foods are easily spoiled. The hygienic messages range from "consume food that is hygienically prepared" in Malaysia to "eat clean and safe food to prevent foodborne disease in the family" in the Philippines. Similar guidelines are provided in both the Taiwan and the People's Republic of China's guidelines. "Drink more boiled water" is mentioned in Taiwan, and the guideline for Mainland China is "avoiding unsanitary and spoiled foods."[30,44,46]

Conclusions

Dietary guidelines in the future must continue to take into account local dietary patterns, cultural traditions, and food availability. Guidelines are most effective when they indicate what aspects of diet need to be addressed to promote nutritional health in both the poor and rich. In some countries where disparities in incomes are very large, two sets of guidelines may be necessary.

Dietary guidelines should be flexible so that they can be used by people with different lifestyles as well as by people of different ages, and with different population groups (pregnant, lactating, infants, children, and elderly persons). Different guidelines may be needed for urban and rural populations or for other special groups such as ethnic minorities in some countries.

Messages delivered to the public in dietary guidelines should provide advice on the selection of a nutritionally balanced diet and encourage other suitable lifestyle behaviors to promote health in target groups. It is difficult to include all without making the guidelines so long that their communicability is compromised. Therefore, other ancillary forms of nutrition education are also needed. Graphics allow people to put dietary guidelines and other recommendations about food consumption into action.

Nutrition education using dietary guidelines is only one ingredient for ensuring sufficient knowledge to choose a healthful diet. Motivation and opportunities to change nutrition and health behaviors in favorable directions are also necessary. Knowledge, science, technology, culture, and food sources all change with the times, and so do foodways. Therefore, it is necessary to review guidelines periodically and make appropriate modifications, i.e., every five or ten years.

In conclusion, dietary guidelines can serve multiple purposes. These include providing useful information to the public policy maker; serving as communication tools to nutrition and health professionals, as guides to the food industry in product formulation, and as instructional objectives for those involved in the provision of food, nutrition, and health education. Food is not the only factor that can influence health. Most health problems in modern society are multifactorial in origin. However, people can help themselves by establishing healthy dietary habits and paying attention to other factors (such as physical activity, not smoking, decreasing stress, and improving work environments). Such measures increase the chances for a long and active life. What individuals and families understand, accept, and do in their day-to-day lives matters the most in implementing healthy lifestyles. The Dietary Guidelines help people to ensure their nutritional health.

References

1. Tontisirin K, Kosulwat V. In: Florentino RF, Ed. *Meeting National Needs of Asian Countries in the 21st Century.* Singapore: International Life Sciences Institution Press, 1996: pg 15.
2. United States Census Bureau. Population Estimates, 1999. At: http://www.census.gov, accessed March 15, 2000.
3. Australian Bureau of Statistics. The Health and Welfare of Australian's Aboriginal and Torres Strait people, 1999. At: http://abs.gov.au, accessed March 15, 2000.
4. National Health and Medical Research Council. *Dietary Guidelines for Australians.* Canberra: Australian Government Publishing Service, 1992.
5. Thompson CD. In: C.A. F, Ed. Dietary Guidelines in Asia-Pacific. Philippines, Quezon City: ASEAN-New Zealand IILP Project 5, 1997: pg 69.
6. US Department of Agriculture, US Department of Health, Committee DGA. Report of the Dietary Guidelines Advisory Committee on the Dietary Guidelines for Americans, 1980. Springfield: National Technical Information Service, 1980.
7. US Department of Agriculture, US Department of Health, Committee DGA. Report of the Dietary Guidelines Advisory Committee on the Dietary Guidelines for Americans, 1990. Springfield: National Technical Information Service, 1990.
8. US Department of Agriculture. Report of the Dietary Guidelines Advisory Committee on the Dietary Guidelines for Americans, 1995: Agricultural Research Service, Dietary Guidelines Advisory Committee, 1995.
9. US Department of Agriculture, A Dietary Guidelines Advisory Committee. Report of the dietary guidelines advisory committee on dietary guidelines for American, 2000, to the secretary of Health and Human Services and the Secretary of Agriculture, National Technical Information Service, 2000. Spingfield: Department of Agriculture, US Department of Health, 2000.

10. Food and Nutrition Information Center. Food guide pyramid information. At: http://www. nla.usda.gov/fnic/etext, accessed March 20, 2000.
11. CDC. 1999. Cancer prevention and control. At: http://www.cdc.gov/cancer/nper/register.htm, accessed March 22, 2000.
12. CDC. 1999. Chronic diseases conditions. At: http://www.cdc.gov/nccdphp/major.htm, accessed March 22, 2000.
13. Mokdad AH. *JAMA* 282:1519; 1999.
14. Health Canada on-line. Nature and dimensions of nutrition related problems, 1999. At: http://www.hc-sc.gc.ca, accessed March 15, 2000.
15. Nutrition Taskforce. Food for Health. Wellington: Department of Health (pamphlet), 1991.
16. Department of National Health and Welfare. Canada's Guidelines for Healthy Eating. Ottawa: Department of Health and Welfare, 1990.
17. Bengoa J, Torun B, Behar M, Scrimshaw N. In: *Nutritional Goals and Food Guides in Latin America. Basis for Their Development.* JM Bengoa BT, M Behar, and N Scrimshaw, Eds. Caracas, Venezuela: Arch Latinoam Nutr, 1987: pg 373-426.
18. Chilean Ministry of Health, Institute of Nutrition and Food Technology, Nutrition Center at the University of Chile. Guias de alimentacion para la poblacion Chilena. Santiago, Chile: Ministry of Health, 1997: pg 164.
19. Tagle MA. In: Nutritional goals and food guides in Latin America. Basis for their development. JM Bengoa BT, M Behar, and N Scrimshaw, Eds. Caracas, Venezuela: *Arch Latinoam Nutr* 1987: pg 750-765.
20. Valiente S, Abala C, Avila B, Monckeberg F. In: Nutritional goals and food guides in Latin America. Basis for their development. JM Bengoa BT, M Behar, and N Scrimshaw, Eds. Caracas, Venezuela: *Arch Latinoam Nutr* 1987: pg 445-465.
21. Peña M, Molina V. Food based dietary guidelines and health promotion in Latin America. Washington, DC: Pan American Health Organization and Institute of Nutrition of Central America and Panama, 1999: pg 31.
22. Chavez MMd, Chavez A, Rios E, Madrigal H. Guías de alimentación: Consejos practicos para alcanzar y mantener un buen estado de nutricion y salud. Mexico, DF: Salvador Zubiran National Institute of Nutrition, 1993: pg 58.
23. Instituto Nacional de Nutrición, Fundación Cavendes. Guías de Alimentación para Venezuela. Caracas, Venezuela: Fundación Cavendes, 1991: pg 88.
24. Ministerio de la Familia, Fundación Cavendes. Guías de Alimentación en el Niño Menor de seis Años. Orientacion Normativa. Caracas, Venezuela: Fundación Cavendes, 1997: pg 44.
25. Ministerio de la Familia, Fundación Cavendes. Guías de Alimentación para Venezuela del Niño Menor de seis Años. Manual para hogares y multihogares de cuidado diario. Caracas, Venezuela: Fundación Cavendes, 1996: pg 131.
26. Guatemala NCoDG. Guías alimentarias para Guatemala: Los siete pasos para una alimentacion sana. Guatemala: Dietary Guidelines National Committee, 1998: pg 44.
27. Panamanian Ministry of Health. Guías alimentarias para Panama. Panama City, Panama: Ministry of Health, 1995: pg 40.
28. Florentino RF. In: Dietary Guidelines in Asian Countries: Towards a Food-Based Approach, proceedings of a seminar and workshop on national dietary guidelines. Florentino RF, Ed. *Meeting National Needs of Asian Countries in the 21st Century.* Singapore: International Life Sciences Institution Press, 1996: pg 32.
29. Karyadi D, Karyadi E. In: Dietary Guidelines in Asian Countries: Towards a Food Based Approach, proceedings of a seminar and workshop on national dietary guidelines. Florentino RF, Ed. *Meeting National Needs of Asian Countries in the 21st Century.* Singapore: International Life Sciences Institution Press, 1996: pg 28.
30. Department of Health Taiwan ROC. Daily dietary guidelines for all populations. 1999. At: http://health99.doh.gov.tw/Query/ShowPic.pl?t106.htm, accessed March 23, 2000.
31. WHO. Obesity epidemic puts millions at risk from related diseases. Press release WHO/46. 1997. At: http://www.who.int/dsg/justpub/obesity.htm, accessed March 15, 2000.
32. WHO. Malnutrition — The Global Picture. At: http://www.who.int/nut/ malnutrition_worldwide.htm, accessed March 15, 2000.

33. Chinese Nutrition Society. *Nutrition Today* 1999; 34: 106.
34. Japan Dietetic Association. Recommended Dietary Allowances for Japanese Fifth Revision (1994). Newsletter, Japan Dietetic Association. Tokyo, 1995: 2 pages.
35. Kim SH, Jang YA, Lee HS. In: *Dietary Guidelines in Asia-Pacific.* Florencio CA, Ed. Philippines, Quezon City: ASEAN-New Zealand IILP Project 5, 1997: pg 52.
36. Tanphaichitr V, Leelahagul, P. In: *Dietary Guidelines in Asia-Pacific.* Florencio CA, Ed. Philippines, Quezon City: ASEAN-New Zealand IILP Project 5, 1997: pg 97.
37. Florencio CA. In: *Dietary Guidelines in Asia-Pacific.* C.A. F, Ed. Philippines, Quezon City: ASEAN-New Zealand IILP Project 5, 1997: 77 pages.
38. Orbeta SS. *Nutrition Today* 1998; 33: 210.
39. National Dietary Guidelines. In: Proceedings of a Seminar and Workshop on National Dietary Guidelines: Meeting National Needs of Asian Countries in the 21st Century. Florentino RF, Ed. Singapore: International Life Sciences Institute Press, 1996.
40. Kusharto CM, Hardinsyah, R. In: *Dietary Guidelines in Asia-Pacific.* C.A. F, Ed. Philippines, Quezon City: ASEAN-New Zealand IILP Project 5, 1997: 52 pages.
41. Sakamoto M. In: *Dietary Guidelines in Asia-Pacific.* C.A. F, Ed. Philippines, Quezon City: ASEAN-New Zealand IILP Project 5, 1997: 43 pages.
42. Siong TE, Yusof AM. In: *Dietary Guidelines in Asia-Pacific.* C.A. F, Ed. Philippines, Quezon City: ASEAN-New Zealand IILP Project 5, 1997: 59 pages.
43. Devadas RP. In: *Dietary Guidelines in Asia-Pacific.* C.A. F, Ed. Philippines, Quezon City: ASEAN-New Zealand IILP Project 5, 1997: 28 pages.
44. Ge K. In: *Dietary Guidelines in Asia-Pacific.* C.A. F, Ed. Philippines, Quezon City: ASEAN-New Zealand IILP Project 5, 1997: pg 17.
45. Sakamoto M. In: Dietary Guidelines in Asian Countries: Towards a Food-Based Approach, Proceedings of a Seminar and Workshop on National Dietary Guidelines. In: *Meeting National Needs of Asian Countries in the 21st Century.* Florentino RF, Ed. Singapore: International Life Sciences Institution Press, 1996: pg 43.
46. Department of Health Taiwan ROC. Daily Food Guide. 1999.
At: http://health99.doh.gov.tw/ Query/ShowPic.pl?p048.htm, accessed March 23, 2000.

13

*Healthy People — Goals and Interpretations**

Margaret Tate and Matthew P. Van Tine

Overview

In the 1970s, the United States Department of Health and Human Services began the process of defining specific goals to improve the health of Americans. The first publication, *Healthy People: The Surgeon General's Report on Health Promotion and Disease Prevention,*[1] was released in 1979. This preventive health initiative is now entering its third decade with the January 2000 release of *Healthy People 2010.*[2]

Healthy People: The Surgeon General's Report on Health Promotion and Disease Prevention outlined goals for the nation to reduce premature death and preserve independence for older adults. In 1980, *Promoting Health/Preventing Disease: Objectives for the Nation* was released.[3] This report delineated 15 priority areas and 226 objectives for the country to achieve over the next decade. These objectives were organized under the general heading of prevention services, health protection, and health promotion.

Healthy People 2000: National Health Promotion and Disease Prevention Objectives[4] was released in 1990. This report expanded on the 1980 objectives. Two new focus areas, cancer and HIV, were also added. *Healthy People 2000* consisted of the following three goals:

- Increase the span of healthy life for Americans
- Reduce health disparities among Americans
- Achieve access to preventive services for all Americans

The report was comprised of 22 priority areas organized under the general headings of health promotion, health prevention services, and surveillance and data systems. The report also organized the appropriate objectives in four areas according to age (children, adolescent and young adults, adults and older adults) and special at–risk population groups (low income, minorities, and people with disabilities).

In 1995, *Healthy People 2000 Midcourse Review and 1995 Revisions*[5] was released. This report evaluated the nation's progress on the 2000 objectives and resulted in changes in

* Special thanks to Judy Moreland, Judy Nowak, Sharon Sass, and Geri Tebo for their help in developing this manuscript.

0-8493-2705-9/01/$0.00+$1.50

TABLE 13.1

Healthy People 2010 Focus Areas

1. Access to quality health services
2. Arthritis, osteoporosis, and chronic back conditions
3. Cancer
4. Chronic kidney disease
5. Diabetes
6. Disability and secondary conditions
7. Educational and community-based programs
8. Environmental health
9. Family planning
10. Food safety
11. Health communications
12. Heart diseases and stroke
13. HIV
14. Immunization and infectious disease
15. Injury and violence prevention
16. Maternal, infant, and child health
17. Medical product safety
18. Mental health and mental disorders
19. Nutrition and overweight
20. Occupational safety and health
21. Oral health
22. Physical activity and fitness
23. Public health infrastructure
24. Respiratory diseases
25. Sexually transmitted diseases
26. Substance abuse
27. Tobacco use
28. Vision and hearing

U.S. Department of Health and Human Services, *Healthy People 2010* 2nd ed., Government Printing Office, Superintendent of Documents, Washington, DC, January 2000.

some objectives, as well as incorporation of new objectives. Forty-seven sentinel objectives were selected to track the nation's success in meeting the objectives. At the midpoint review, 33 of the sentinel objectives were moving in the right direction, nine were moving in the wrong direction, and two had not changed. Data was not available on the remaining three objectives.

Healthy People 2010, released in January 2000, provides the nation with its third ten-year blueprint for a healthier population. Over 350 national membership organizations and 270 state and local health agencies contributed to the development of this report.

Healthy People 2010 is organized around the following two goals:

- Increase quality and years of healthy life — defined as "a personal sense of physical and mental health and the ability to react to factors in the physical and social environments."[2]
- Eliminate health disparities — defined as "eliminate disparities among different segments of the population. These include differences that occur by gender, race or ethnicity, education or income, disability, living in rural localities, or sexual orientation."[2]

The two-volume report consists of 467 objectives organized in 28 focus areas. These focus areas are listed in Table 13.1.

TABLE 13.2

Leading Health Indicators

Physical activity
Overweight and obesity
Tobacco use
Substance abue
Responsible sexual behavior
Mental health
Injury and violence
Environmental quality
Immunization
Access to health care

U.S. Department of Health and Human Services, *Healthy People 2010* 2nd ed., Government Printing Office, Superintendent of Documents, Washington, DC, January 2000.

A new addition to *Healthy People 2010* is the identification of leading health indicators (Table 13.2). These represent major public health concerns in the U.S. They are divided into two groups: lifestyle challenges and system enhancement challenges.[6] The lifestyle challenges are physical activity, overweight and obesity, tobacco use, substance abuse, and responsible sexual behavior. The system challenges are mental health, injury and violence, environmental quality, immunizations, and access to health care. Specific objectives will be used to track progress toward improving the leading health indicators.

Nutrition has been one of the focus areas since the beginning of the Healthy People initiative. In *Healthy People 2010,* the goal of the nutrition and overweight focus area is to promote health and reduce chronic disease associated with diet and weight. There are 18 objectives listed in the nutrition section, with 33 other nutrition-related objectives listed in other focus areas.

Table 13.3 delineates the primary nutriton-related objectives from *Healthy People 2000* and *Healthy People 2010.* The table is organized around the *Healthy People 2000* objectives. The first column lists the nutrition objectives from Section 2 as well as key nutrition-related objectives from other *Healthy People 2000* focus areas. The objectives from the nutrition section are bolded. The information in italic print was added at the midcourse review. The second column is the baseline data that was used to evaluate the objectives, and the third column is the source of that data. The fourth column, Outcome, evaluates the success in meeting the *Healthy People 2000* objective. The fifth column lists the corresponding *Healthy People 2010* objectives, if available. It also lists any new objectives. Again, the objectives from the nutrition section (Section 19) are bolded. The last two columns list the baseline data, and data sources for *Healthy People 2010.* The baseline data rates used in *Healthy People 2010* were age-adjusted to the year 2000, whereas the rates used in *Healthy People 2000* were age-adjusted to the 1940 population or are crude rates. If an objective does not have baseline data or a known data source, it is listed as a developmental objective.

Table 13.4 provides the full names for the abbreviations used in the data source columns. The information presented in the chart is taken directly from the references indicated in the footnotes.

Healthy People is truly one of this country's most significant public health initiatives. It is a valuable tool to help Americans promote health and prevent disease, disability, and premature death. To be successful, we must continue to work together to put Healthy People into practice.

TABLE 13.3

Summary of Healthy People 2000 and 2010 Objectives

Healthy People 2000 Objectives	Baseline	Data Source	Outcome	Healthy People 2010 Objectives	Baseline	Data Source
2.1 Reduce coronary heart disease deaths to no more than 100/100,000 people. (4)	Age-adjusted baseline: 135/100,000 in 1987. (4)	NVSS, CDC (4)	In 1996, the death rate from coronary heart disease (CHD) was 105 deaths/100,000 population. (8)	12-1 Reduce coronary heart disease deaths. Target: 166/100,000 people. (2)	208 coronary heart disease deaths/100,000 population (age-adjusted) in 1998. (2)	NVSS, CDC, NCHS (2)
2.2 Reverse the rise in cancer deaths to achieve a rate of no more than 130/100,000 people. (4)	Age-adjusted baseline: 133/100,000 in 1987. (4)	NVSS, CDC (4)	In 1997, the age adjusted cancer death rate was 125 deaths/100,000 population (preliminary data). (8)	3-1 Reduce the overall cancer death rate. Target: 158.7 cancer deaths/100,000 population. (2)	201.4 cancer deaths/100,000 population (age-adjusted) in 1998. (2)	NVSS, CDC, NCHS (2)
2.3 Reduce overweight to a prevalence of no more than 20% among people age 20 and older and no more than 15% among adolescents through 19. (4)	26% for people age 20 through 74 in 1976-80, 24% for men and 27% for women; 15% for adolescents age 12 through 19 in 1976-80. (4)	NHANES, CDC; Hispanic HANES, CDC; IHS; NHIS, CDC (4)	In 1994, the prevalence of overweight was 35% for people 20-74 years and 24% for adolescents 12-19 years. This is a substantial increase over the 1976-80 baseline data. (8)	**19-1 Increase the proportion of adults who are at a healthy weight. Target: 60%. (2)**	42% of adults age 20 years and older were at a healthy weight (defined as a body mass index (BMI) equal to or greater than 18.5 and less than 25) in 1988-94. (2)	NHANES, CDC, NCHS (2)
				19-2 Reduce the proportion of adults who are obese. Target: 15%. (2)	23% of adults age 20 years and older were identified as obese (defined as a BMI of 30 or more) in 1988-94. (2)	NHANES, CDC, NCHS (2)
				19-3 Reduce the proportion of children and adolescents who are overweight or obese. Target: age 6-11 years: 5%; age 12-19 years: 5%; age 6-19 years: 5%. (2)	1988-94 baseline for children age 6-11: 11%; age 12-19: 10%; age 6-19: 11%. (2)	NHANES, CDC, NCHS (2)
2.4 Reduce growth retardation among low-income children age 5 and younger to less than 10%. (4)	Up to 16% among low-income children in 1988, depending on age and race/ethnicity. (4)	Pediatric Nutrition Surveillance System, CDC (4)	The target to reduce growth retardation to less than 10% for all low-income children age 5 years and under has been met, although the target for African-American children under 1 year has not. (7)	**19-4 Reduce growth retardation among low-income children under age 5 years. Target: 5%. (2)**	8% of low-income children under age 5 years were growth retarded in 1997 (defined as height-forage below the 5th percentile in the age-gender appropriate population using the 1977 NCHS/CDC growth charts). (2)	PNSS, CDC, NCCDPHP (2)

2.5 Reduce dietary fat intake to an average of 30% of calories or less and average saturated fat intake to less than 10% of calories among people age 2 and older. (4) In addition, increase to at least 50% the proportion of people age 2 and older who meet the Dietary Guidelines' average daily goal of no more than 30% of calories from fat, and increase to at least 50% the proportion of people age 2 and older who meet the average daily goal of less than 10% of calories from saturated fat. (5)	36% of calories from total fat and 13% from saturated fat for people age 20 through 74 in 1976-80; 36% and 13% for women age 19 through 50 in 1985. (4) Baseline (for the midcourse) addition for people age 2 and older: 21% met the goal for fat and 21% met the goal for saturated fat based on 2-day dietary data from the 1989-91 NHANES; 22% met the goal for fat and 21% met the goal for saturated fat based on the 3-day dietary data from 1989-91 CSFII. (5)	NHANES, CDC; CSFII, USDA (4)	34% of calories from total fat and 12% from saturated fat for people age 20 through 74 from the 1994 NHANES; 34% met the goal for fat and 36% met the goal for saturated fat based on the 3-day dietary data from 1989-91 CSFII. (8)	**19-8 Increase the proportion of persons age 2 years and older who consume less than 10% of calories from saturated fat. Target: 75%. (2)**	36% of persons age 2 years and older consumed less than 10% of calories from saturated fat in 1994-96. (2)	CFSII, USDA (2)
				19-9 Increase the proportion of persons age 2 years and older who consume no more than 30% of calories from fat. Target: 75%. (2)	33% of persons age 2 years and older consumed no more than 30% of daily calories from fat in 1994-96. (2)	CSFII, USDA (2)
2.6 Increase complex carbohydrate and fiber-containing foods in the diets of adults to 5 or more daily servings for vegetables (including legumes) and fruits, and to 6 or more daily servings for grain products. (4) In addition, increase to at least 50% the proportion of people age 2 and older who meet the Dietary Guidelines' average daily goal of 5 or more servings of vegetables/ fruits, and increase to at least 50% the proportion who meet the goal of 6 or more grain products. (5)	2 1/2 servings of vegetables and fruits and 3 servings of grain products for women age 19 through 50 in 1985. (4) Baseline for the midcourse addition): 29% met the goal for fruits and vegetables and 40% met the goal for grain products for people age 2 and older based on 3-day dietary data in 1989-91. (5)	CSFII, USDA (1)	4.7 servings of vegetables and fruits and 6.9 servings of grain products for people age 2 and over; 35% met the goal for fruits and vegetables and 52% met the goal for grain products for people age 2 and older in 1989-91. (8)	**19-5 Increase the proportion of persons age 2 years and older who consume at least 2 daily servings of fruit. Target: 75%. (2)**	28% of persons age 2 years and older consumed at least 2 daily servings of fruit in 1994-96. (2)	CSFII, USDA (2)
				19-6 Increase the proportion of persons age 2 years and older who consume at least 3 daily servings of vegetables, with at least one-third being dark green or deep yellow vegetables. Target: 50%. (2)	3% of persons age 2 years and older consumed at least 3 daily servings of vegetables, with at least one-third of these servings being dark green or deep yellow vegetables in 1994-96. (2)	CSFII, USDA (2)
				19-7 Increase the proportion of persons age 2 years and older who consume at least 6 daily servings of grain products, with at least 3 being whole grains. Target: 50%. (2)	7% of persons age 2 years and older consumed at least 6 daily servings of grain products, with at least 3 being whole grains in 1994-96. (2)	CSFII, USDA (2)

TABLE 13.3 *(Continued)*

Summary of Healthy People 2000 and 2010 Objectives

Healthy People 2000 Objectives	Baseline	Data Source	Outcome	Healthy People 2010 Objectives	Baseline	Data Source
2.7 Increase to at least 50% the proportion of overweight people age 12 and older who have adopted sound dietary practices combined with regular physical activity to attain an appropriate body weight. (4)	30% of overweight women and 25% of overweight men for people age 18 and older in 1985. (4)	NHIS, CDC (4)	In 1995, 15% of the overweight women and 19% of the overweight men age 18 and older have adopted sound dietary practices combined with physical activity to attain an appropriate body weight. (8)	No corresponding objective.		
2.8 Increase calcium intake so at least 50% of youth age 12 through 24 and 50% of pregnant and lactating women consume 3 or more servings daily of foods rich in calcium, and at least 50% of people age 25 and older consume 2 or more servings daily. (4)	7% of women and 14% of men age 19 through 24 and 24% of pregnant and lactating women consumed 3 or more servings, and 15% of women and 23% of men age 25 through 50 consumed 2 or more servings in 1985-86. (4)	CSFII, USDA (4)	15% of people 11-24 years and 13% pregnant and lactating females consumed an average of 3 or more servings daily, and 47% of children 2-10 years and 21% people 25 years and over consumed 2 or more servings in 1996. (8)	**19-11 Increase the proportion of persons age 2 years and older who meet dietary recommendations for calcium. Target: 75%. (2)**	46% of persons age 2 years and older were at or above approximated mean calcium requirements (based on consideration of calcium from foods, dietary supplements, and antacids) in 1988-94. (2)	NHANES, CDC, NCHS (2)
2.9 Decrease salt and sodium intake so at least 65% of home meal preparers prepare foods without adding salt, at least 80% of people avoid using salt at the table, and at least 40% of adults regularly purchase foods modified or lower in sodium. (4)	54% of women age 19 through 50 who served as the main meal preparer did not use salt in food preparation, and 68% of women age 19 through 50 did not use salt at the table in 1985; 20% of all people age 18 and older regularly purchased foods with reduced salt and sodium content in 1988. (4)	CSFII, USDA; Health and Diet Survey, FDA (4)	In 1995, 19% of people 18 years and over regularly purchase foods with reduced salt and sodium content, 58% rarely or never use salt at the table. (8)	**19-10 Increase the proportion of persons age 2 years and older who consume 2,400 mg or less of sodium daily. (2)**	21% of persons age 2 years and older consumed 2400 mg of sodium or less daily (from foods, dietary supplements, tap water, and salt use at the table) in 1988-94. (2)	NHANES, CDC, NCHS (2)

2.10 Reduce iron deficiency to less than 3% among children age 1 through 4 and among women of childbearing age. (4)	9% among children age 1 through 2, 4% for children age 3 through 4, 5% for women age 20 through 44 in 1976-80. (4)	NHANES, CDC; Alaska Native Children, CDC 1988; PNSS, CDC (4)	6% among children age 1-4 years; 9% for children age 1-2 years; 4% for children age 3-4 years; 8% for females age 20-44 years were anemic in 1988-94. (8)	**19-12 Reduce iron deficiency among young children and females of childbearing age. Target for children age 1-2 years: 5%; Children age 3-4 years: 1%; Non-pregnant females age 12-49 years: 7%. (2)**	1988-94 baseline: children age 1-2 years: 9%; Children age 3-4 years: 4%; Non-pregnant females age 12 to 49 years: 11%. (2)	NHANES, CDC, NCHS; NCHS (2)
				19-13 Reduce anemia among low-income pregnant females in their third trimester. Target: 20%. (2)	29% of low-income pregnant females in their third trimester were anemic (defined as hemoglobin <11.0 g/dL) in 1996. (2)	PNSS, CDC, NCCDPHP (2)
				19-14 (Developmental) Reduce iron deficiency among pregnant females. (2)		Potential Data Source: NHANES, CDC, NCHS (2)
2.11 Increase to at least 75% the proportion of mothers who breastfeed their babies in the early postpartum period and to at least 50% the proportion who continue breastfeeding until their babies are 5 to 6 months old. (4)	54% at discharge from birth site and 21% at 5 to 6 months in 1988. (4)	Ross Laboratories Mothers Survey; PNSS, CDC (4)	62% in early postpartum period and 26% at 6 months in 1997. (8)	16-19 Increase the proportion of mothers who breastfeed their babies. Target: in early postpartum period: 75%; at 6 months: 50%; at 1 year: 25%. (2)	1998 baseline: in early postpartum period: 64%; at 6 months: 29%; at 1 year: 16%. (2)	Mothers' Survey, Abbott Laboratories Inc., Ross Products Division (2)
2.12 Increase to at least 75% the proportion of parents and caregivers who use feeding practices that prevent baby bottle tooth decay. (4)	55% for parents and caregivers of children 6-23 months in 1988. (5)	NHIS, CDC (8)	No data beyond baseline. (7)	No corresponding objective.		

TABLE 13.3 *(Continued)*

Summary of Healthy People 2000 and 2010 Objectives

Healthy People 2000 Objectives	Baseline	Data Source	Outcome	Healthy People 2010 Objectives	Baseline	Data Source
2.13 Increase to at least 85% the proportion of people age 18 and older who use food labels to make nutritious food selections. (4)	74% used labels to make food selections in 1988. (4)	Health and Diet Survey, FDA (4)	In 1995, 75% of the people 18 years and over reported using food labels. (8)	No corresponding objective.		
2.14 Achieve useful and informative nutrition labeling for virtually all processed foods and at least 40% of fresh meats, poultry, fish, fruits, vegetables, baked goods, and ready-to-eat carry-away foods. (4)	60% of sales of processed foods regulated by FDA had nutrition labeling in 1988; baseline data on fresh and carry-away foods unavailable. (4)	Food Label and Package Survey, FDA (4)	In 1995, 96% of processed foods had nutrition labeling. In 1996, 73% of fresh produce and 71% of fresh seafood had nutrition labeling. (8)	No corresponding objective.		
2.15 Increase to at least 5000 brand items the availability of processed food products that are reduced in fat and saturated fat. (4)	2500 items reduced in fat in 1986. (4)	Nielsen Company National Scantrack (4)	In 1991, 5618 reduced fat and saturated fat food products were available. (8)	No corresponding objective.		
2.16 Increase to at least 90% the proportion of restaurants and institutional food service operations that offer identifiable low-fat, low-calorie food choices, consistent with the Dietary Guidelines for Americans. (4)	About 70% of fast food and family restaurant chains with 350 or more units had at least one low-fat, low-calorie item on their menu in 1989. (4)	Survey of Chain Operators, National Restaurant Association (4)	In 1990, 75% of large-chain restaurants offering at least one low-fat, low-calorie item. (8)	No corresponding objective.		

2.17 Increase to at least 90% the proportion of school lunch and breakfast services and child care food services with menus that are consistent with the nutrition principles in the Dietary Guidelines for Americans. (4)	1% of schools offered lunches that provided an average of 30% or less of calories from total fat, and less than 1% offered lunches that provided an average of less than 1% of calories from saturated fat. Of the schools participating in the USDA school breakfast program, 44% offered breakfasts that provided an average of 30% or less of calories from total fat, and 4% offered breakfasts that provided an average of less than 10% of calories from saturated fat in 1992. (5)	1992 School Nutrition Dietary Assessment Study; SHPPS, CDC, NCCDPHP (8)	There were no new data beyond the baseline to measure this objective. (7)	**19-15 (Developmental) Increase the proportion of children and adolescents age 6 to 19 years whose intake of meals and snacks at schools contributes proportionally to good overall dietary quality. (2)**	Potential Data Source: CSFII, USDA (2)
2.18 Increase to at least 80% the receipt of home food services by people age 65 and older who have difficulty in preparing their own meals or are otherwise in need of home-delivered meals. (4)	48% in 1991. (8)	NHIS, CDC (8)	50% in 1995. (8)	No corresponding objective.	

TABLE 13.3 *(Continued)*

Summary of Healthy People 2000 and 2010 Objectives

Healthy People 2000 Objectives	Baseline	Data Source	Outcome	Healthy People 2010 Objectives	Baseline	Data Source
2.19 Increase to at least 75% the proportion of the nation's schools that provide nutrition education from preschool through 12th grade, preferably as part of quality school healthy education (4)	60% of states in 1991. (5)	National Survey of School Health Education Activities, CDC, NCCDPHP (8)	The proportion of States that required nutrition education increased from 60% in 1990 to 69% in 1994. (8)	7-2 Increase the proportion of middle, junior high, and senior high schools that provide comprehensive school health education to prevent health problems in the following areas: unintentional injury; violence; suicide; tobacco use and addiction; alcohol or other drug use; unintended pregnancy; HIV/AIDS, and STD infection; unhealthy dietary patterns; inadequate physical activity; and environmental health. Summary objective target: 70%; Unhealthy dietary patterns target: 95%. (2)	Summary objective baseline: 28%; unhealthy dietary patterns baseline: 78% in 1994. (2)	SHPPS, CDC, NCCDPHP (2)
2.20 Increase to at least 50% the proportion of worksites with 50 or more employees that offer nutrition education and/or weight management programs for employees. (4)	17% offered nutrition education activities and 15% offered weight control activities in 1985. (4)	NWHPS, ODPHP (4)	The proportion of worksites with 50 or more employees that offer programs for employees increased from 17% in 1985 to 31% in 1992. (8)	**19-16 Increase the proportion of worksites that offer nutrition or weight management classes or counseling. Target: 85%. (2)**	55% of worksites with 50 or more employees offered nutrition or weight management classes or counseling at the worksite or through their health plans in 1998-1999. (2)	NWHPS, AWHP (2)

2.21 Increase to at least 75% the proportion of primary care providers who provide nutrition assessment and counseling and/or referral to qualified nutritionists or dietitians. (4)	Physicians provided diet counseling for an estimated 40-50% of patients in 1988. (4)	Lewis 1988 (4)	There were no new data beyond the baseline to measure this objective. (7)	**19-17 Increase the proportion of physician office visits made by patients with a diagnosis of cardiovascular disease, diabetes, or hyperlipidemia that include counseling or education related to diet and nutrition. Target: 75%. (2)**	Counseling or education on diet and nutrition was ordered or provided for 42% of physician visits that were related to the diagnosis of cardio-vascular disease, diabetes, or hyper-lipidemia in 1997. (2)	NAMCS, CDC, NCHS (2)
2.22 Reduce stroke deaths to no more than 20/100,000 people. (5)	Age-adjusted baseline: 30.3/100,000 in 1987. (5)	NVSS, CDC (4)	In 1996, the age adjusted death rate from stroke was 26.4/100,000. (8)	12-7 Reduce stroke deaths. Target: 48 deaths/100,000 population. (2)	60 deaths from stroke/100,000 population in 1998. (2)	NVSS, CDC, NCHS (2)
2.23 Reduce colorectal cancer deaths to no more than 13.2/100,000 people. (5)	14.4/100,000 in 1987. (5)	NVSS, CDC (4)	In 1996, the age adjusted death rate was for colorectal cancer 16.3 death/100,000 population. (8)	3-5 Reduce the colorectal cancer death rate. Target: 13.9 deaths/100,000 population. (2)	21.1 colorectal cancer deaths/100,000 pop-ulation in 1998. (2)	NVSS, CDC, NCHS (2)
2.24 Reduce diabetes to an incidence of no more than 2.5/1,000 people and a prevalence of no more than 25/1,000 people. (5)	1986-88, the indence was 2.9/1,000; the prevalance was 28/1,000. (5)	NHIS, CDC; IHS; Hispanic HANES, CDC (4)	In 1994-96, the incidence of diabetes was 3.1/1,000 population and the prevalence was 31/1,000 population. (8)	5-3 Reduce the overall rate of diabetes that is clinically diagnosed. Target: 25 overall cases/1,000 population. (2)	40 overall cases (new and existing) of diabetes/1,000 population (age-adjusted) in 1997. (2)	NHIS, CDC, NCHS (2)
2.25 Reduce the prevalence of blood cholesterol levels of 240 mg/dL or greater to no more than 20% among adults. (5)	27% for people age 20-74 in 1976-80, 29% for women and 25% for men. (5)	NHANES, CDC (4)	The prevalence of high blood cholesterol was 19% among people 20-74 years in 1988-94. (8)	12-14 Reduce the proportion of adults with high total blood cholesterol levels. Target: 17%. (2)	21% of adults age 20 years and older had total blood cholesterol levels of 240 mg/dL or greater in 1988-94. (2)	NHANES, CDC, NCHS (2)
2.26 Increase to at least 50% the proportion of people with high blood pressure whose blood pressure is under control. (5)	11% controlled among people age 18-74 in 1976-80; an estimated 24% for people age 18 and older in 1982-84. (5)	NHANES, CDC; 1982-88 Seven State Survey, NIH (4)	In 1991, the control rate among people 18-74 years with high blood pressure was 29%. (8)	12-10 Increase the proportion of adults with high blood pressure whose blood pressure is under control. Target: 50%. (2)	18% of adults age 18 years and older with high blood pressure had it under control in 1988-94. (2)	NHANES, CDC, NCHS (2)

TABLE 13.3 *(Continued)*

Summary of Healthy People 2000 and 2010 Objectives

Healthy People 2000 Objectives	Baseline	Data Source	Outcome	Healthy People 2010 Objectives	Baseline	Data Source
2.27 Reduce the mean serum cholesterol among adults to no more than 200 mg/dL. (5)	213 mg/dL among people age 20-74 in 1976-80, 211 mg/dL for men and 215 mg/dL for women. (5)	NHANES, CDC (4)	Average total serum cholesterol for people 20-74 years was 203 mg/dL in 1988-94. (8)	12-13 Reduce the mean total blood cholesterol levels among adults. Target: 199 mg/dL. (2)	206 mg/dL was the mean total blood cholesterol level for adults age 20 years and older in 1988-94. (2)	NHANES, CDC, NCHS (2)
				19-18 Increase food security among US households and in so doing reduce hunger. Target: 94%. (2)	88% of all US households were food secure in 1995. (2)	Current Population Survey, US Dept of Commerce, Bureau of the Census; National Food and Nutrition Survey, (beginning in 2001) DHHS and USDA (2)
4.8 Reduce alcohol consumption by people 14 and older to an annual average of no more than 2 gallons of ethanol/person. (4)	2.54 gallons of ethanol in 1987 (4)	NIAAA, ADAMHA (4)	In 1994, 2.21 gallons alcohol/person age 14 years and older were consumed. (8)	26-12 Reduce average annual alcohol consumption. Target: 2 gallon. (2)	2.19 gallons of ethanol/person age 14 years and older were consumed in 1996. (2)	AEDS, NIH, NIAAA (2)
12.1 Reduce infections caused by key foodborne pathogens to incidences of no more than: *Salmonella* species: 16/100,000 *Campylobacter jejuni:* 25/100,000; *Escherichia coli*: 0157:H7: 4/100,000; *Listeria monocytogenes:* 0,5/100,000. (4)	*Salmonella* species:18/100,000; *Campylobacter jejuni:* 50/100,000; *Escherichia coli:* 0157:H7: 8/100,000; *Listeria monocytogenes:* 0.7/ 100,000. (4)	NCID, CDC (4)	In 1996, *Salmonella* species: 15/100,000; *Campylobacter jejuni:* 24/100,000; *Escherichia coli:* 0157:H7: 3/100,000; *Listeria monocytogenes:* 0.5/100,000. (8)	10-1 Reduce infections caused by key foodborne pathogens. Target (cases/100,000): *Campylobacter* species: 12.3; *Escherichia coli* 0157-H7: 1.0; *Listeria monocytogenes:* 0.25; *Salmonella* species: 6.8; *Cyclospora cayetanensis:* developmental; Postdiarrheal hemolytic uremic syndrome: developmental; Congenital *Toxoplasma gondii:* developmental. (2)	In 1997, the case/100,000 population was *Campylobacter* species: 24.6; *Escherichia coli:* 0157-H7:2.1; *Listeria monocytogenes:* 0.5; *Salmonella* species: 13.7. (2)	Foodborne Disease Network (FoodNet), CDC, NCID; FDA, CFSAN; FSIS, OPHS and state agencies. Potential data sources: NNDSS, CDC, NCID (2)

12.2 Reduce outbreaks of infections due to *Salmonella enteritidious* to fewer than 25 outbreaks yearly. (4)	77 Outbreaks in 1989. (4)	NCID, CDC (4)	In 1996, there were 50 outbreaks due to *Salmonella enteritidious.* (8)	10-2 Reduce outbreaks of infections caused by key foodborne bacteria. Target (number of outbreaks/year): *Escherichia coli* 0157-H7:11; *Salmonella* serotype Enteridis: 22. (2)	The number of outbreaks in 1997: *Escherichia coli* 0157-H7-22; *Salmonella* serotype Enteridis-44. (2)	Foodborne Disease Outbreak Surveillance System, CDC, NCID (2)
12.3 Increase to at least 75% the proportion of households in which principal food preparers routinely refrain from leaving perishable food out of the refrigerator for over 2 hours and wash cutting boards and utensils with soap after contact with raw meat and poultry. (4)	For refrigeration of perishable foods, 70%; for washing cutting boards with soap, 66%; and for washing utensils with soap, 55%, in 1988. (4)	Food Safety Survey, FDA; Diet-Health Knowledge Survey, USDA (4)	For refrigeration of perishable foods, 72% (in 1993); for washing cutting boards with soap, 71% (in 1997); washing utensils with soap, no data beyond the baseline. (8)	10-5 Increase the proportion of consumers who follow key food safety practices. Target: 79%. (2)	72% of consumers followed key food safety practices in 1998. (2)	Food Safety Survey, FDA: FSIS, USDA (2)
14.1 Reduce the infant mortality rate to no more than 7/1000 live births. (4)	10.1/1000 live births in 1987. (4)	NVSS, CDC: Linked Birth and Infant Death Data Set, CDC (4)	In 1996, the infant mortality rate was 7.3/1,000 live births. (8)	16-1 Reduce fetal and infant deaths. Target (per 1000 live births plus fetal deaths): 4.1 at 20 or more weeks of gestation; 4.5 during the perinatal period. (2)	In 1997, (per 1000 live births plus fetal deaths) 6.8 for 20 or more weeks of gestation; 7.5 during the perinatal period. (2)	NVSS, CDC, NCHS (2)
14.5 Reduce low birth weight to an incidence of no more than 5% of live births and very low birth weight to no more than 1% of live births. (4)	6.9 and 1.2%, respectively, in 1987. (4)	NVSS, CDC (4)	7.4% and 1.4% respectively, in 1996. (8)	16-10. Reduce low birth weight (LBW) and very low birth weight (VLBW). Target: 5.0% for LBW Target: 0.9% for VLBW. (2)	1998 baseline: 7.6% for LBW 1.4% for VLBW. (2)	NVSS, CDC, NCHS (2)
14.6 Increase to at least 85% the proportion of mothers who achieve the minimum recommended weight gain during their pregnancies. (4)	68% of married females who had a full-term live birth and prenatal care in 1980. (8)	National Natality Survey, CDC, National Maternal and Infant Health Survey, CDC, NCHS (8)	In 1990, 75% of mothers achieved the minimum recommended weight gain during their pregnancies. (8)	16-12. (Developmental) Increase the proportion of mothers who achieve a recommended weight gain during their pregnancies. (2)		Potential data sources: NVSS, CDC, NCHS (2)

TABLE 13.3 *(Continued)*

Summary of Healthy People 2000 and 2010 Objectives

Healthy People 2000 Objectives	Baseline	Data Source	Outcome	Healthy People 2010 Objectives	Baseline	Data Source
15.5 Increase to at least 90% the proportion of people with high blood pressure who are taking action to help control their blood pressure. (4)	79% of aware hypertensives age 18 and older were taking action to control their blood pressure in 1985. (4)	NHIS, CDC (4)	In 1994, 71% of people 18 years and over with high blood pressure were using medication and diet. (8)	12-11 Increase the proportion of adults with high blood pressure who are taking action (for example, losing weight, increasing physical activity, and reducing sodium intake) to help control their blood pressure. Target: 95% (2)	72% of adults age 18 years and older with high blood pressure were taking action to control it in 1998. (2)	NHIS, CDC, NCHS (2)
15.8 Increase to at least 60% the proportion of adults with high blood cholesterol who are aware of their condition and are taking action to reduce their blood cholesterol to recommended levels. (4)	11% of all people age 18 and older, and thus an estimated 30% of people with high blood cholesterol were aware that their blood cholesterol was high in 1988. (4)	Health and Diet Survey, FDA (4) Cholesterol Awareness Survey, NHLBI, NIH. (8)	60% of all people age 18 and older with high blood cholesterol were aware that their blood cholesterol was high in 1995. (8)	No corresponding objective.		
15.15 Increase to at least 75% the proportion of primary care providers who initiate diet and, if necessary, drug therapy at levels of blood cholesterol consistent with current management guidelines for patients with high blood cholesterol. (4)	In 1986, the median cholesterol level when diet therapy was initiated: 240-259 mg/dL; median cholesterol level when drug therapy was initiated: 300-319 mg/dL. (8)	Cholesterol Awareness Survey, NIH, NHLBI (8)	In 1995, the median cholesterol level when diet therapy was initiated: 200-219 mg/dL; median cholesterol level when drug therapy was initiated: 240-259 mg/dL. (8)	No corresponding objective.		

15.16 Increase to at least 50% proportion of worksites with 50 or more employees that offer high blood pressure and/or cholesterol education and control activities to their employees. (4)	16.5% offered high blood pressure activities and 16.8% offered nutrition education activities in 1985. (4)	NWHPS, ODPHP (4)	In 1992, 29% offered high blood pressure activities; 31% offered nutrition education activities; 32% offered blood pressure screening. (8)	No corresponding objective.		
				2-9. Reduce the overall number of cases of osteoporosis Target: 8%. (2)	10% of adults age 50 years and older had osteoporosis as measured by low total femur bone mineral density (BMD) in 1988-94. (2)	NHANES, CDC, NCHS (2)
16.3 Reduce breast cancer deaths to no more than 20.6/100,000 women. (4)	22.9 breast cancer deaths/100,000 females in 1987. (4)	NVSS, CDC (4)	20.2 breast cancer death/100,000 females in 1997. (8)	3-3 Reduce the breast cancer death rate. Target: 22.2 deaths/100,000 females. (2)	27.7 breast cancer deaths/100,000 females in 1998. (2)	NVSS, CDC, NCHS (2)
				4-3 Increase the proportion of treated chronic kidney failure patients who have received counseling on nutrition, treatment choices, and cardiovascular care 12 months before the start of renal replacement therapy. Target: 60%. (2)	45% of newly diagnosed patients with treated chronic kidney failure received counseling on nutrition, treatment choices, and cardiovascular care in 1996. (2)	USRDS, NIH, NIDDK (2)
				5-1 Increase the proportion of persons with diabetes who receive formal diabetes education. Target: 60%. (2)	40% of persons with diabetes received formal diabetes education in 1998. (2)	NHIS, CDC, NCHS (2)
				5-2 Prevent diabetes. Target: 2.5 new cases/1,000 persons/year. (2)	3.1 new cases of diabetes/1000 persons (3-year average) in 1994-96. (2)	NHIS, CDC, NCHS (2)

TABLE 13.3 *(Continued)*

Summary of Healthy People 2000 and 2010 Objectives

Healthy People 2000 Objectives	Baseline	Data Source	Outcome	Healthy People 2010 Objectives	Baseline	Data Source
				7-11 Increase the proportion of local health departments that have established culturally appropriate and linguistically competent community health promotion and disease prevention programs for racial and ethnic minority populations. Target: nutrition and overweight - 50%. (2)	44% for nutrition and overweight in 1996-97. (2)	NHIS, CDC, NCHS (2)
				10-4 (Developmental) Reduce deaths from anaphylaxis caused by food allergies. (2)		Potential data Source: NVSS, CDC, NCHS (2)
				12-9 Reduce the proportion of adults with high blood pressure. Target: 16%. (2)	28% of adults age 20 years and older had high blood pressure in 1988-94. (2)	NHANES, CDC, NCHS (2)
				16-15 Reduce the occurrence of spina bifida and other neural tube defects (NTDs). Target: 3 new cases/ 10,000 live births. (2)	6 new cases of spina bifida or another NTD/ 10,000 live births in 1996. (2)	NBDPN, CDC, NCEH (2)

	16-16 Increase the proportion of pregnancies begun with an optimum folic acid level. Target: 80% for consumption of at least 400 μg of folic acid each day from fortified foods or dietary supplements by non-pregnant women age 15 to 44; 220 ng/ml for median red blood cell (RBC) folate level among non-pregnant women age 15 to 44. (2)	21% for the consumption of folic acid; 161 ng/ml for the median RBC folate level In 1991-94. (2)	NHANES, CDC, NCHS (2)
	16-17 Increase abstinence from alcohol, cigarettes, and illicit drugs among pregnant women. Target: Increase in reported abstinence in past month from substances by pregnant women: 94% for alcohol; 100% for binge drinking; 98% for cigarette smoking; 100% for illicit drugs. (2)	Increase in reported abstinence in past month from substances by pregnant women: 86% for alcohol; 99% for binge drinking; 87% for cigarette smoking; 98% for illicit drugs in 1996-97. (2)	National Household Survey on Drug Abuse; SAMHSA; NVSS, CDC, NCHS (2)
	16-18 (Developmental) Reduce the occurrence of fetal alcohol syndrome. (2)		Potential data sources: FASnet, CDC, NCEH (2)
	18-5 (Developmental) Reduce the relapse rates for persons with eating discorders including anorexia nervosa and bulimia nervosa. (2)		Potential data sources: Prospective studies of patients with anorexia nervosa and bulimia nervosa, NIH, NIMH. (2)

TABLE 13.4
Abbreviations for Data Sources

Abbreviation	Source
ADAMHA	Alcohol, Drug Abuse and Mental Health Administration
AEDS	Alcohol Epidemiologic Data System
ASTDHPPE	Association of State and Territorial Directors of Health Promotion and Public Health Education
AWHP	Association of Worksite Health Promotion
CDC	Centers for Disease Control and Prevention
CFSAN	Center for Food Safety and Applied Nutrition
CSFII	Continuing Survey of Food Intake by Individuals
FASnet	Fetal Alcohol Syndrome Network
FDA	Food and Drug Administration
FSIS	Food Safety and Inspection Survey
IHS	Indian Health Service
NAMCS	National Ambulatory Medical Care Survey
NBDPN	National Birth Defects Prevention Network
NCCDPHP	National Center for Chronic Disease Prevention and Health Promotion
NCEH	National Center for Environmental Health
NCHS	National Center for Health Statistics
NCID	National Center for Infectious Disease
NHANES	National Health and Nutrition Examination Survey
NHIS	National Health Interview Survey
NHLBI	National Heart, Lung and Blood Institute
NIAAA	National Institute of Alcohol Abuse and Alcoholism
NIDDK	National Institute of Diabetes and Digestive and Kidney Disease
NIMH	National Institute of Mental Health
NIH	National Institute of Health
NNDSS	National Notifiable Disease Surveillance System
NVSS	National Vital Statistics System
NWHPS	National Worksite Health Promotion Survey
ODPHP	Office of Disease Prevention and Health Promotion
OPHS	Office of Public Health and Science
SAMHSA	Substance Abuse and Mental Health Services Administration
SHPPS	School Health Policies and Programs Study
USDA	United States Department of Agriculture
USRDS	U.S. Renal Data System

U.S. Department of Health and Human Services, *Healthy People 2010* (conference edition, in two volumes), Washington, DC, January 2000.

References

1. US Department of Health, Education and Welfare (HEW), *Healthy People: the Surgeon General's Report on Health Promotion and Disease Prevention,* Washington, DC, 1979, Superintendent of Documents.
2. US Department of Health and Human Services, *Healthy People 2010,* 2nd ed., Government Printing Office, Superintendant of Documents, Washington, DC: January 2000.
3. US Department of Health and Human Services, Public Health Service: *Promoting Health and Preventing Disease: Objectives for the Nation,* Washington, DC, 1980, U.S. Government Printing Office.
4. US Department of Health and Human Services, *Healthy People 2000: National Health Promotion and Disease Prevention Objectives,* Washington, DC, 1990, U.S. Government Printing Office.
5. US Department of Health and Human Services, *Healthy People 2000: Midcourse Review and 1995 Revisions,* Washington, DC, 1990, U.S. Government Printing Office.
6. *ADA Courier,* Chicago, 2000. The American Dietetic Association, 39: 5; 5.

7. US Department of Health and Human Services, *Healthy People 2010* Objectives: Draft for Public Comment, Washington, DC: September, 1998.
8. National Center for Health Statistics. *Healthy People 2000 Review,* 1998-99, Hyattsville, MD, Public Health Service.

14

Food Labeling: Foods and Dietary Supplements

Constance J. Geiger

Overview

Definition of Food Labeling

Food labeling consists of the information present on all food packages. Nutrition labeling is one component of the food label. Other components include the principal display panel, the information panel, the identity of the food, the list of ingredients, the name and place of business of the manufacturer, packer, or distributor, as well as any claims made.[1]

Progression of the Section

This section reviews the regulatory history of food labeling, the required portions of the nutrition label, labeling of restaurant and fresh foods, definitions of allowed nutrient content claims, and requirements for allowed health claims and structure/function claims. Additional resources for food labeling are provided.

History of Food Labeling

Major Food and Nutrition Labeling Laws and Regulations

Food labeling laws progressed from protecting consumers from economic harm (Pure Food and Drug Act of 1906)[2] to reducing consumers' risk of chronic disease (Nutrition Labeling and Education Act of 1990[3] [NLEA]). The NLEA amended the Food, Drug, and Cosmetic Act of 1938[4] and required that nutrition information be conveyed to consumers so they could readily understand the information and its significance in the context of a total daily diet. The NLEA[3] mandated major revisions in the Food and Drug Administration's (FDA) food labeling regulations, including requiring nutrition labeling on almost all processed foods, a revised list of nutrients to be labeled, standardized serving sizes,

0-8493-2705-9/01/$0.00+$1.50

TABLE 14.1

Major Food and Nutrition Labeling Laws/Selected Regulations

Law	Primary Provisions
Pure Food and Drug Act, 1906[2]	Barred false and misleading statements on food and drug labels.
Federal Food, Drug, and Cosmetic Act, 1938	Replaced the Pure Food and Drug Act of 1906. Created distinct food labeling requirements. Required "common and usual name" of food, ingredient declarations, net quantity information, name and address of manufacturer/distributor. Defined misbranding.[4]
Fair Packaging and Labeling Act, 1966	Provided FDA with authority to regulate provision of label information and package size.[8]
Regulations for enforcement of the Federal Food, Drug, and Cosmetic Act and the Fair Packaging and Labeling Act	Merged existing regulations into one entity. Required nutrition labeling on processed foods that were fortified or carried claims. Provided for labeling of fat and cholesterol. Established standards for dietary supplements. Established regulations for artificially flavored foods and imitation foods per serving. Disallowed nutrient claims unless food contained 10% or more of the US RDA. Incorporated label information: number of servings/container; calories, protein, carbohydrate, and fat content; percentage of adult US RDA for protein and seven vitamins and minerals. Provided for sodium labeling without requirement for the full nutrition label panel.[9-11]
Nutrition Labeling and Education Act, 1990	Provided for mandatory nutrition labeling on almost all food products, expanded required nutrition information in a new format, created standardized serving sizes, provided consistent definitions of nutrient content claims, and defined permissible health claims.[3]
Dietary Supplement Health and Education Act, 1994	Defined dietary supplements, provided for nutrition labeling in a new format, required the name and quantity of every active ingredient, provided for structure/functions claims and good manufacturing practices, encouraged research on dietary supplements, created two new government entities: Commission on Dietary Supplement Labels and the Office of Dietary Supplements.[12]
FDA Modernization Act, 1997	Expanded procedures by which FDA can authorize health claims and nutrient content claims, e.g., provided for a notification process.[13]

nutrient content claims, and for the first time, health claims. In the interest of harmony and uniformity, the U.S. Department of Agriculture's Food Safety and Information Service (FSIS) issued similar regulations for meat and poultry products.[5] Table 14.1 summarizes the major laws and selected regulations dealing with food labeling. (For further details, see Geiger, 1992[6] and Geiger, 1998.[7])

Regulatory Oversight for Labeling

A number of regulatory agencies have jurisdiction over food labeling, including FDA, USDA, Federal Trade Commission (FTC), and Bureau of Alcohol, Tobacco and Firearms (BATF). Table 14.2 shows their responsibilities.

TABLE 14.2

Agencies having Jurisdiction over Food Labeling

Agency	Responsibility
FDA	Mandatory labeling of most packaged foods except products containing certain amounts of meat and poultry, and beverages with certain amounts of alcohol. Voluntary labeling of fresh fruits and vegetables, fresh fish, game, and restaurant foods except those containing certain amounts of meat and poultry
USDA	Mandatory labeling on most processed meat and poultry products, e.g., hot dogs, chicken noodle soup
FTC	Claims made in food advertising
BATF	Voluntary labeling of alcoholic beverages

Required Portions of the Food Label

Required sections of the Nutrition Facts Label (see Figure 14.1) are illustrated here. The nutrition facts information is based on a serving of the product as packaged.

Required Nutrients

The nutrients required to be labeled in the Nutrition Facts Panel are listed in Table 14.3. If a product is fortified with a certain nutrient or a claim is made about a voluntary nutrient, then that nutrient also is required to be labeled. Other nutrients (voluntary nutrients) that may be included on the label are found in Table 14.3.

Serving Size

Standardized serving sizes, known as Reference Amounts Customarily Consumed (RACCs), are established for many categories of foods. RACCs are based on average amounts people usually eat at one time, based on USDA survey data. These uniform serving sizes help consumers compare products. See Table 14.4 for selected RACCs.

Kcalories and Kcalories from Fat

Amount of kcalories and kcalories from fat are required because of public health authorities' concerns with fat in the diet.

Daily Values

The standards for labeling of nutrients are known as Daily Values (DVs). The percent of DV is listed for certain nutrients on the label so that consumers can determine how a serving of a food fits into their total daily diet. The DVs include Daily Reference Values (DRVs) and Reference Daily Intakes (RDIs). DRVs are set for nutrients that previously did not have label standards, such as fat, cholesterol, and saturated fat (see Table 14.5). DRVs are based on a daily intake of 2000 kcalories, which is a reasonable reference number for adults and children over four, and are calculated based on current nutrition recommendations. The

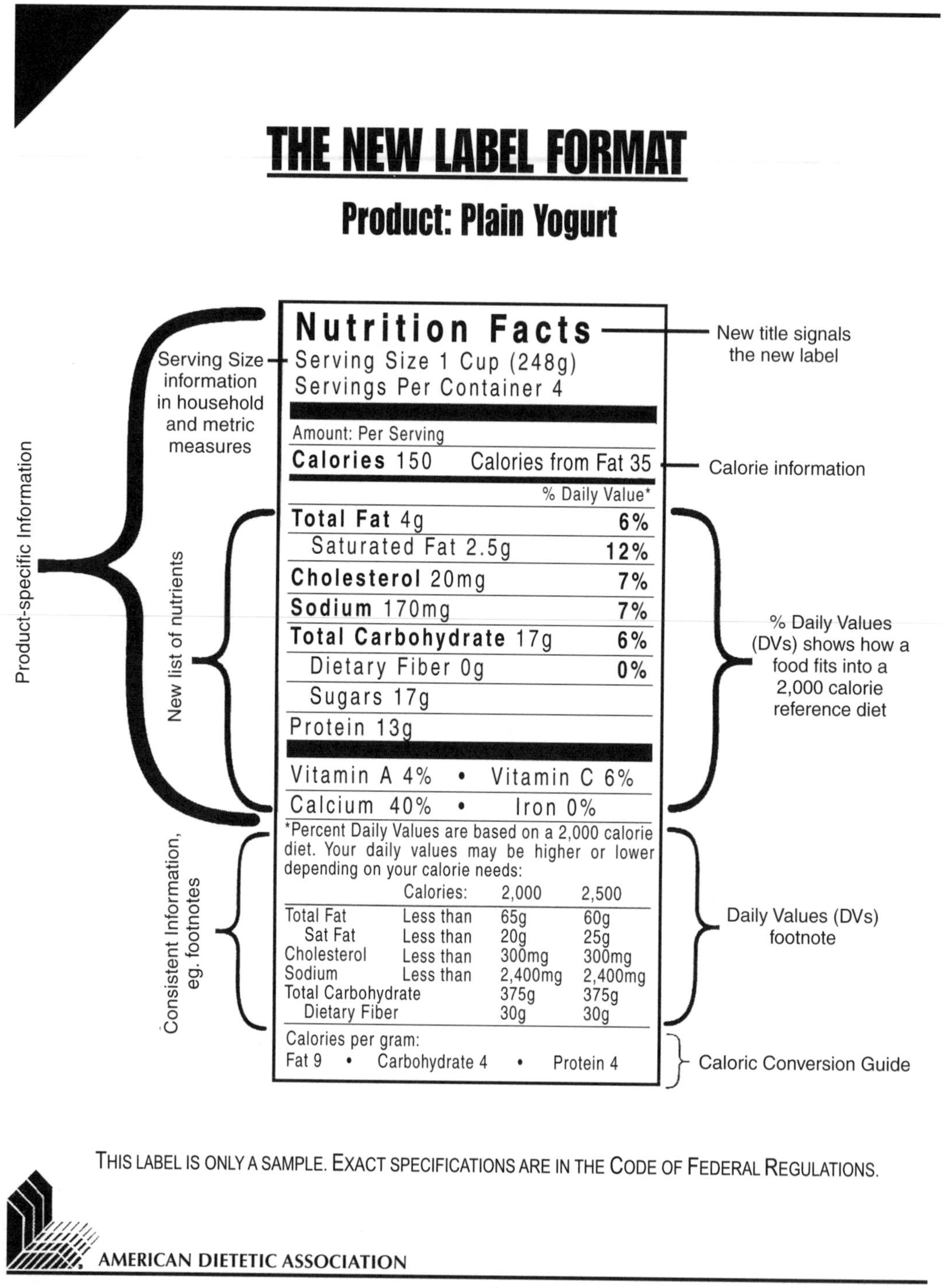

THE NEW LABEL FORMAT

Product: Plain Yogurt

Nutrition Facts — New title signals the new label

Serving Size 1 Cup (248g) — Serving Size information in household and metric measures
Servings Per Container 4

Amount: Per Serving
Calories 150 Calories from Fat 35 — Calorie information

	% Daily Value*
Total Fat 4g	**6%**
Saturated Fat 2.5g	**12%**
Cholesterol 20mg	**7%**
Sodium 170mg	**7%**
Total Carbohydrate 17g	**6%**
Dietary Fiber 0g	**0%**
Sugars 17g	
Protein 13g	

Vitamin A 4% • Vitamin C 6%
Calcium 40% • Iron 0%

*Percent Daily Values are based on a 2,000 calorie diet. Your daily values may be higher or lower depending on your calorie needs:

	Calories:	2,000	2,500
Total Fat	Less than	65g	60g
Sat Fat	Less than	20g	25g
Cholesterol	Less than	300mg	300mg
Sodium	Less than	2,400mg	2,400mg
Total Carbohydrate		375g	375g
Dietary Fiber		30g	30g

Calories per gram:
Fat 9 • Carbohydrate 4 • Protein 4

Product-specific Information
New list of nutrients
% Daily Values (DVs) shows how a food fits into a 2,000 calorie reference diet
Consistent Information, eg. footnotes
Daily Values (DVs) footnote
Caloric Conversion Guide

THIS LABEL IS ONLY A SAMPLE. EXACT SPECIFICATIONS ARE IN THE CODE OF FEDERAL REGULATIONS.

FIGURE 14.1
Nutrition facts panel (© 1994, American Dietetic Association. *Learning the New Food Labels.* Used with permission).

TABLE 14.3

Labeling of Nutrients: Required and Voluntary[1]

Required Nutrients	Voluntary Nutrients
Total kcalories	kcalories from saturated fat
kcalories from fat	kcalories from polyunsaturated fat
Total fat	kcalories from monounsaturated fat
Saturated fat	Potassium
Cholesterol	Soluble fiber
Sodium	Insoluble fiber
Total carbohydrate	Sugar alcohol
Dietary fiber	Other carbohydrates
Sugars	Other essential vitamins and minerals
Protein	
Vitamin A	
Vitamin C	
Calcium	
Iron	

TABLE 14.4

Selected Reference Amounts Customarily Consumed (RACCs)[1,a]

Category	RACC
Bakery products: biscuits, bagels, tortillas, soft pretzels	55 g
Beverages: carbonated and noncarbonated beverages, wine coolers, water; coffee or tea, flavored and sweetened; juice, fruit drinks	240 mL
Breads	50 g
Cereals and other grain products	Varies from 25 g for dry pasta to 140 g for prepared rice
Cheese	30 g
Eggs	50 g
Fats and oils	1 tbsp
Fruits: fresh, canned, or frozen except watermelon	140 g
Meat: entrees without sauce	85 g cooked; 110 g uncooked
Nuts and seeds	30 g
Soups	245 g
Vegetables; fresh, canned, or frozen	85 g fresh or frozen 95 g for vacuum packed 130 g for canned in liquid

[a] See 21 CFR 101.12 for details.

TABLE 14.5

DRVs for Adults: Calculations and Values[1]

Nutrient	Derivation/Calculation	Label Value
Fat	30% of 2000 kcalories from fat = 600 kcalories/9 kcalories/g	65 g
Saturated fat	10% of kcalories from saturated fat = 200 kcalories/9 kcalories/g	20 g
Carbohydrate	60% of kcalories from carbohydrate = 1200 kcalories/ 4 kcalories/g	300 g
Protein	10% of kcalories from protein = 200 kcalories/ 4 kcalories/g	50 g
Fiber	11.5 g per 1000 kcalories	25 g (rounded up)
Cholesterol	NA	<300 mg
Sodium	NA	<2400 mg
Potassium	NA	3500 mg

TABLE 14.6

RDIs for Adults and Children over 4[1]

Nutrient	RDI
Vitamin A	5000 IU
Vitamin C	60 mg
Calcium	1000 mg
Iron	18 mg
Vitamin D	400 IU
Vitamin E	30 IU
Vitamin K	80 μg
Thiamin	1.5 mg
Riboflavin	1.7 mg
Niacin	20 mg
Vitamin B_6	2.0 mg
Folate	400 μg
Vitamin B_{12}	6 μg
Biotin	300 μg
Pantothenic acid	10 mg
Phosphorus	1000 mg
Iodine	150 μg
Magnesium	400 μg
Zinc	15 mg
Selenium	70 μg
Copper	2 mg
Manganese	2 mg
Chromium	120 μg
Molybdenum	75 μg
Chloride	2400 mg

term RDIs replaces the term U.S. Recommended Dietary Allowances (RDAs), but the values are currently the same as the U.S. RDAs, which represent the highest recommended levels of the 1968 RDAs (see Table 14.6). The RDI values will be updated when the National Academy of Sciences completes its latest review of all nutrient recommendations.

A DVs footnote is provided at the bottom of the label to inform consumers of the DVs for both 2000- and 2500-calorie levels. The calorie information at the bottom of the label is voluntary (see Figure 14.1).

Substances without DVs

Substances without DVs, such as sugars and soluble and insoluble fiber, are not required to carry a percent of DV. For dietary supplement labels, substances such as herbs are separated from the nutrients. The amount of the herb must be listed along with a symbol referring to the statement "Daily Value not established."

Labeling of Restaurant Foods and Fresh Foods

Restaurant Foods

Labeling of restaurant foods is voluntary. If a nutrient content claim or health claim is made, then nutrition labeling becomes mandatory. However, the full Nutrition Facts Label does not need to appear. Only the amount of the nutrient that is the subject of the claim needs to be labeled, e.g., "low fat," contains 3 g of fat.

Fresh Fruits, Vegetables, and Seafood

The FDA recommends that food retailers provide nutrition information for raw fruits, vegetables, and fish at point of purchase. Charts, brochures, or signs can be used to depict nutrition information for the 20 most commonly consumed fruits, vegetables, and raw fish. The FDA provides the data for retailers in the *Code of Federal Regulations* (21 CFR 101.45 and Appendix C to Part 101).

Meats and Poultry

The USDA recommends that food retailers provide point-of-purchase information for meat and poultry. As with fresh produce and fish, charts, brochures, or signs can be used to depict the nutrition information.[5]

Nutrient Content Claims Allowed for Foods and Dietary Supplements

Overview

The FDA and USDA have issued regulations for uniform definitions for nutrient content claims. A nutrient content claim characterizes the level of a nutrient in a food, e.g., "high fiber." Two types of nutrient content claims can be made: absolute (free, low, good source, high, lean, extra lean) and comparative (reduced, light, less, more). The regulations establish the allowed terms and the criteria/requirements for their use (see Tables 14.7, 14.8).[1] For additional detail see the *Code of Federal Regulations* (21 CFR 101.13 and 101.54-101.69).

Health Claims Allowed for Foods and Dietary Supplements

Overview

NLEA allowed health claims to be carried on qualified food products. Prior to this time, these claims were considered unauthorized drug claims. A health claim describes the relationship between a food, a nutrient, or other substance in a food, and the risk of a health-related condition or disease.

Health claims can be made through third-party references, such as the American Heart Association, symbols such as a heart, statements, and vignettes or descriptions. Regardless of the manner of presentation, the requirements for the claim must be met in order for a food or supplement to carry the claim on its product packaging or in its advertising. Health claims carry general and specific requirements. General requirements include not exceeding certain amounts of fat (13 g), saturated fat (1 g), cholesterol (40 mg), and sodium (480 mg). The food must be a "good source" of fiber, protein, vitamin A, vitamin C, calcium, or iron. The specific requirements for each health claim are listed in the *Code of Federal*

TABLE 14.7

Allowed Nutrient Content Claims with Definitions[1, a, b]

Claim	Calories	Fat	Saturated Fat	Cholesterol	Sodium	Fiber	Sugar	Protein	Vitamins/Minerals
"Free," "no," "zero," "without"	Less than 5 kcalories	0.5 g or less	0.5 g or less	Less than 2 mg cholesterol and 2 g or less saturated fat and trans fat	Less than 5 mg	NA	Less than 0.5 g	NA	NA
"Very low"	NA	NA	NA	NA	Less than 35 mg	NA	NA	NA	NA
"Low," "contains a small amount," "little"	40 kcalories or less	3 g or less	1 g or less	20 mg or less cholesterol and 2 g or less saturated fat	140 mg or less	NA	NA	NA	NA
"Reduced"	25% lower in kcalories than the comparable food	25% lower in kcalories than the comparable food	25% lower in kcalories than the comparable food	25% lower in kcalories than the comparable food	25% lower in kcalories than the comparable food	NA	25% lower in kcalories than the comparable food	NA	NA
"Light"	1/3 fewer kcalories than the reference foods, only if the reference food contains less than 50% calories from fat	50% less fat than the reference food	NA	NA	50% less sodium than the reference food, food also is low fat and low calorie	NA	NA	NA	NA
"Good source," "provides," "contains"	NA	NA	NA	NA	NA	2.5-4.9 g	NA	5 g or more	10 — 19% of the DV
"High," "excellent source of," "rich in"	NA	NA	NA	NA	NA	5 g or more	NA	10 g or more	20% or more of the DV
"More," "added," "enriched," "fortified"	NA	NA	NA	NA	NA	NA	NA	10% more of the DV (5 g)	10% more of the DV

[a] Definitions vary for meal and main dishes.
[b] Complete definitions are found in 21 CFR 101.13 and 21 CFR 101.54-101.69.

TABLE 14.8

Other Nutrient Content Claims Definitions[a,b]

Claim	Definition
% Fat-free	Must be "low-fat" or "fat-free." Must indicate the amount of fat present in 100 g of food
Lean	Less than 10 g fat, less than 4 g saturated fat, less than 95 mg cholesterol per RACC and per 100 g
Extra lean	Less than 5 g fat, less than 2 g saturated fat, less than 95 mg cholesterol per RACC and per 100 g

[a] Definitions vary for main dish and meal products.
[b] Complete definitions are found in 21 CFR 101.13 and 21 CFR 101.54-101.69.

Regulations (21 CFR 101.14; 101.70-101.81), except for those authorized through FDAMA or by the courts.

Current health claims are authorized in three ways: by FDA as a result of NLEA, which also allowed for petitions for new health claims (12 claims); by notification of FDA through FDAMA (two claims); or through court action as a result of the *Pearson* decision (two claims at time of section submission). FDAMA allowed FDA to authorize a health claim if a scientific body of the U.S. Government that has official responsibility for human nutrition research or public health protection publishes a current authoritative statement. A company or organization must notify FDA at least 120 days prior to the introduction of the food carrying the claim into interstate commerce. FDAMA health claims, unlike the other claims, do not allow an opportunity for public comment. If FDA takes no action within 120 days of the notification, the health claim can be made on the food qualifying for the claim. The *Pearson* decision resulted from a lawsuit filed by Durk Pearson, Sandy Shaw, and the American Preventive Medical Association to allow four previously denied health claims to be made on dietary supplements. The court decision mandated that FDA 1) reconsider whether to authorize the four previously denied health claims, 2) determine if the weight of the scientific evidence in support of the claim is greater than that against it, and 3) if so, then determine if qualifying language would not mislead consumers. FDA is also required to define significant scientific agreement.

FDA authorized seven claims as a result of NLEA. Since that time, FDA has approved an additional three claims submitted as petitions, two claims submitted as notifications through FDAMA, and two claims as a result of the *Pearson* decision.

The health claim model language and requirements are indicated in three tables: those resulting from NLEA and petitions (Table 14.9); those not prohibited by FDA through FDAMA (Table 14.10), and those allowed by court decision that carry extensive qualifying language (Table 14.11). Again, the requirements for the FDAMA and court-mandated (*Pearson* decision) health claims do not appear in the *Code of Federal Regulations*.

Structure Function Claims

Overview

Structure/function claims can be made on dietary supplements (DSHEA 1994).[12] A structure/function claim is characterized as a statement that describes the role of a nutrient or dietary ingredient that affects a function or structure of the body, or such claims can describe how such a substance maintains a structure or function.

TABLE 14.9
Health Claims Authorized through the Regulations Implementing NLEA[1,7]

Health Claim	Model Language	Requirements	Can Be Made On Qualified
Cancer			
Fruits and vegetables and cancer	Low fat diets rich in fruits and vegetables (foods that are low in fat and may contain dietary fiber, vitamin A, and vitamin C) may reduce the risk of some types of cancer, a disease associated with many factors. Broccoli is high in vitamins A and C and is a good source of dietary fiber	Food product must be or must contain a fruit or vegetable; product is "low fat;" product is a "good source" of at least one of the following: vitamin A, vitamin C, or fiber	Foods
Fiber-containing grain products, fruits and vegetables and cancer	Low fat diets rich in fiber-containing grain products, fruits, and vegetables may reduce the risk of some types of cancer, a disease associated with many risk factors	Food product must be or must contain a grain product, fruit, or vegetable; food product is "low fat," and is (prior to fortification) a "good source of dietary fiber"	Foods
Fat and cancer	Development of cancer depends on many factors. A diet low in total fat may reduce the risk for some cancers	Food product is "low fat;" fish and game meats must be "extra lean"	Foods
Coronary Heart Disease			
Fruits, vegetables and grain products that contain fiber, especially soluble fiber, and risk of coronary heart disease	Development of heart disease depends on many factors. Eating a diet low in saturated fat and cholesterol and high in fruits, vegetables, and grain products that contain fiber may lower blood cholesterol levels and reduce risk of heart disease	Food products contains $\geq$ 0.6 g soluble fiber; soluble fiber is listed on Nutrition Facts Panel. Food product must be "low fat," "low saturated fat," and "low cholesterol;" food is, or must contain, a vegetable, fruit, or grain product	Foods
Soluble fiber from certain foods (oats and psyllium) and coronary heart disease	Diets low in saturated fat and cholesterol that include ___ g of soluble fiber per day from (name of food) may reduce the risk of heart disease. One serving of (name of food) supplies ___ g of the ___ g necessary per day to have this effect	Food is "low saturated fat," "low cholesterol," and "low fat;" food contains β-glucan soluble fiber from whole oats; food contains $\geq$0.75 g whole oat soluble fiber; soluble fiber is listed on the Nutrition Facts Panel; or Food is "low saturated fat," "low cholesterol," and "low fat"; food contains $\geq$1.7 g soluble fiber from psyllium husk; soluble fiber is listed on the Nutrition Facts Panel	Foods
Soy protein and coronary heart disease	Diets low in fat and cholesterol that include 25 g of soy protein a day may reduce the risk of heart disease. One serving of (name of food) provides ___ g of soy protein	Food contains $\geq$6.25 g soy protein; food is "low cholesterol," "low saturated fat;" food is "low fat," unless it is derived from or consists of whole soybeans and contains no fat in addition to the fat naturally present in the whole soybeans it contains or from which it is produced	Foods

Saturated fat and cholesterol and coronary heart disease	Development of heart disease depends upon many factors, but its risk may be reduced by diets low in saturated fat and cholesterol and healthy lifestyles	Food must be "low saturated fat," "low fat," and "low cholesterol;" fish and game meats must be "extra lean"	Foods
Plant sterols/stanol esters and coronary heart disease	For plant stanol esters: Diets low in saturated fat and cholesterol that include two servings of foods that provide a daily total of at least 3.4 g of vegetable oil stanol esters in two meals may reduce the risk of heart disease. A serving of [name of food] supplies ___ g of vegetable oil stanol esters For plant sterol esters: Foods containing at least 0.65 g per serving of plant sterol esters, eaten twice a day with meals for a daily total intake of at least 1.3 g, as part of a diet low in saturated fat and cholesterol, may reduce the risk of heart disease. A serving of [name of food] supplies ___ g of vegetable oil sterol esters	Food contains 1.7 g of plant stanol esters/RACC (spreads, salad dressings, snack bars, and dietary supplements in softgel form) or 0.65 g of plant sterol esters/RACC (spreads and salad dressings); food is "low cholesterol" and "low saturated fat;" food must not exceed the fat disqualifying levels (13 g) of health claims unless it is a spread or a salad dressing. Those products (spreads or salad dressings) exceeding 13 g of fat must carry a disclosure statement referring people to the Nutrition Facts Panel for information about fat content; food contains 10% or more of the DV for vitamin A, vitamin C, iron, calcium, protein, or fiber unless the product is a salad dressing[14]	Foods and dietary supplements
Other Health Claims			
Calcium and osteoporosis	Regular exercise and a healthy diet with enough calcium help teen and young adult white and Asian women maintain good bone health and may reduce their high risk of osteoporosis later in life. Adequate calcium intakes are important, but daily intakes above 2000 mg are not likely to provide any additional benefit	Food or dietary supplement must be "high" in calcium	Foods and dietary supplements
Sodium and hypertension	Diets low in sodium may reduce the risk of high blood pressure, a disease caused by many factors	Food must be "low sodium"	Foods
Sugar alcohols and dental caries	Frequent eating of foods high in sugars and starches as between-meal snacks can promote tooth decay. The sugar alcohol used to sweeten this food may reduce dental caries	Food must contain less than 0.5 g sugar; sugar alcohol in the food shall be sorbitol, isomalt, xylitol, lactitol, hydrogenated glucose syrup, hydrogenated starch hydrolysates, or a combination	Foods
Folic acid and neural tube defects	Healthful diets with adequate folate may reduce a woman's risk of having a child with a brain or spinal cord defect	Food or supplements must be a "good source" of folate; claim cannot be made on foods that contain more than 100% of the RDI for vitamin A, such as preformed vitamin A or retinol, or vitamin D	Foods and dietary supplements

TABLE 14.10
Health Claims Allowed to Pass Through FDAMA

Health Claim	Model Language	Requirements	Can Be Made on Qualified
Whole grains and CHD	Diets rich in whole grains and other plant foods and low in total fat, saturated fat, and cholesterol may help reduce the risk of heart disease and certain cancers	Diets rich in whole grain foods and other plant foods and low in total fat, saturated fat, and cholesterol may help reduce the risk of heart disease and certain cancers[15]	Foods
Potassium-containing foods and blood pressure and stroke	Diets containing foods that are good sources of potassium and low in sodium may reduce the risk of high blood pressure and stroke	Foods contain at least 10% DV for potassium/RACC; food is "low sodium," "low cholesterol," "low saturated fat"/RACC; potassium is listed on the Nutrition Facts Panel[16]	Foods

TABLE 14.11
Qualified Health Claims Allowed by the Pearson Decision

Health Claim	Model Language	Requirements	Can Be Made on Qualified
Omega-3 fatty acids and CHD	The scientific evidence about whether omega-3 fatty acids may reduce the risk of coronary heart disease is suggestive, but not conclusive. Studies in the general population have looked at diets containing fish and not omega-3 fatty acids, and it is not known whether diets or omega-3 fatty acids in fish may have a possible effect on a reduced risk of coronary heart disease. It is not known what effect omega-3 fatty acids may or may not have on risk of CHD in the general population	Dietary supplement cannot state the daily dietary intake necessary to achieve a claimed effect because the evidence is not definitive; labeling cannot recommend or suggest intakes of more than 2 g per day, preferable 1 g or less[17]	Dietary supplements
Folic acid, vitamin B_6, vitamin B_{12} and vascular disease	It is known that diets low in saturated fat and cholesterol may reduce the risk of heart disease. The scientific evidence about whether folic acid, vitamin B_6, and vitamin B_{12} may also reduce the risk of heart disease and other vascular disease is suggestive, but not conclusive. Studies in the general population have generally found that these vitamins lower homocysteine, an amino acid found in the blood. It is not known whether elevated levels of homocysteine may cause vascular disease or whether high homocysteine levels are caused by other factors. Studies that will directly evaluate whether reducing homocysteine may also reduce the risk of vascular disease are not yet complete	Dietary supplement cannot state the daily dietary intake necessary to achieve a claimed effect because the evidence is not definitive; products with more than 100% DV (400 µg) of folic acid must identify the safe upper limit of 1000 µg in parentheses[18]	Dietary supplements

Requirements

The general requirements for structure/function claims are: 1) the statement must be truthful and not misleading, 2) the manufacturer of the product carrying the claim must notify the FDA within 30 days of first marketing a dietary supplement, and 3) the dietary supplement must carry the following disclaimer: "This statement has not been evaluated by the FDA. This product is not intended to diagnose, treat, cure or prevent any disease."[12]

Specific requirements for structure/function claims are not found in the *Code of Federal Regulations*. FDA does not approve individual claims.

Resources

Food and Drug Association www.fda.gov

The FDA website provides a wealth of information about FDA regulatory actions and positions, industry guidance, and consumer education materials. The site provides FDA organizational structure and a telephone and email directory so that staff contacts can be made. The "What's New" section lists FDA's latest actions. A separate page is devoted to dietary supplements. Links are provided to other regulatory agencies such as the FTC and the FSIS.

Food Safety and Inspection Service www.fsis.gov

The USDA's FSIS is responsible for overseeing labeling of meat and poultry foods. The agency allows health claims on a case-by-case basis. (USDA requires label approval prior to use on a product.) FSIS's website provides regulatory guidelines and current information.

Code of Federal Regulations (CFR) www.access.gpo/nara/cfr/index.html

The CFR codifies all of the general and permanent rules published in the *Federal Register* by FDA and FSIS, USDA, FTC, and BATF. The CFR is divided into 50 titles, each representing an area of federal regulation, e.g., 21 CFR is Food and Drugs and 9 CFR is USDA. The titles are then divided into chapters that usually bear the name of the responsible agency. Those most pertinent to the food label include 21 CFR 100-169 (FDA, food labeling), 21 CFR 170-199 (FDA, food additives), and 9 CFR 200 to end (FSIS, food labeling). The CFR can be accessed online through the FDA website. The CFR is updated once per year.

Federal Register

The *Federal Register* is one of the most important sources for information on any government agency's activities. Federal government agencies, such as FDA and USDA, publish regulations in the *Federal Register* to implement food and dietary supplement laws in various forms (notice, proposed rule, final rule) on a daily (Monday through Friday) basis. Once a final rule is published it becomes incorporated into the CFR. The *Federal Register* can be accessed through FDA's website. It can be searched by agency, date, date range, or topic.

References

1. Food and Drug Administration, US Department of Health and Human Services. Code of Federal Regulations, Title 21, Parts 100-169. Washington, DC: Superintendent of Documents, US Government Printing Office, 2000.
2. *Federal Food and Drug Act of 1906.* 34 USC § 768.
3. *Nutrition Labeling and Education Act.* P. L. No. 101-535, 104 Stat 2353.
4. *Federal Food, Drug and Cosmetic Act of 1938.* 52 USC § 1040.
5. US Department of Agriculture, Food Safety and Information Service. Code of Federal Regulations, Title 9, Parts 200 to end. Washington, DC: Superintendent of Documents, US Government Printing Office, 2000.
6. Geiger, CJ. Review of nutrition labeling formats. *J Amer Diet Assoc* 91: 808; 1992.
7. Geiger, CJ. Health claims: history, current regulatory status and consumer research. *J Amer Diet Assoc* 98: 1312; 1998.
8. Federal Fair Packaging and Labeling Act 1966. 80 USC § 1966.
9. Food and Drug Administration. Nutrition labeling: proposed criteria for food label information panel. *Federal Register* March 30, 1972; 37(62): 6493-6497.
10. Food and Drug Administration. Nutrition labeling: *Federal Register* January 19, 1973; 38(13): 2124-2164.
11. Food and Drug Administration. Nutrition labeling: *Federal Register* March 14, 1973; 38(49): 6950-6975.
12. *Dietary Supplement Health and Education Act of 1994.* 108 Stat. 4325, 4322.
13. *Food and Drug Administration Modernization Act of 1997.* 21 USC § 301 note.
14. Food and Drug Administration. Food labeling: health claims; plant sterol/stanol esters and coronary heart disease; interim final rule. *Federal Register* September 8, 2000; 65(175): 54686-54739.
15. General Mills. Whole grain foods authoritative statement claim notification. July 1999. Available at http://vm.cfsan.fda.gov/
16. Tropicana Products, Inc. Notification for a health claim based on an authoritative statement for potassium containing foods. Docket No. 00Q-1582. Available at http://vm.cfsan.fda.gov/
17. FDA, Center for Foods Safety and Applied Nutrition. Letter regarding dietary supplement health claim for omega-3 fatty acids and CHD. October 31, 2000. Available at http://vm.cfsan.fda.gov/
18. FDA. Center for Foods Safety and Applied Nutrition. Letter regarding dietary supplement health claim for folic acid, vitamin B_6, vitamin B_{12} and vascular disease. November 28, 2000. Available at http://vm.cfsan.fda.gov/

15

Nutrition Monitoring in the United States

Karil Bialostosky, Ronette R. Briefel, and Jean Pennington

Nutrition monitoring has been defined as "an ongoing description of nutrition conditions in the population, with particular attention to subgroups defined in socioeconomic terms, for purposes of planning, analyzing the effects of policies and programs on nutrition problems, and predicting future trends."[1] The nutrition monitoring program in the United States has evolved over the past century to meet data needs for nutrition policy and nutrition research. This section provides a brief review of the evolution of the nutrition monitoring program, summarizes the program's monitoring and surveillance activities during the past decade, and describes the links between nutrition monitoring, nutrition research, and nutrition policy.

Goal of the Nutrition Monitoring Program

The name of the National Nutrition Monitoring System (NNMS) was changed to the National Nutrition Monitoring and Related Research Program (NNMRRP) with the passage of the National Nutrition Monitoring and Related Research Act of 1990 (P.L. 101-445).[2-5] The goal of the nutrition monitoring program is to have a coordinated, comprehensive system that provides information about the dietary and nutritional status of the U.S. population, conditions that affect the dietary and nutritional status of individuals, and relationships between diet and health.

The program is composed of interconnected federal and state activities that provide information about the relationship between food and health. A general conceptual model representing this relationship is shown in Figure 15.1 and is comprised of five measurement components: nutrition and related health measurements; food and nutrient consumption; knowledge, attitudes, and behavior assessments; food composition and nutrient data bases; and food supply determinations.

0-8493-2705-9/01/$0.00+$1.50

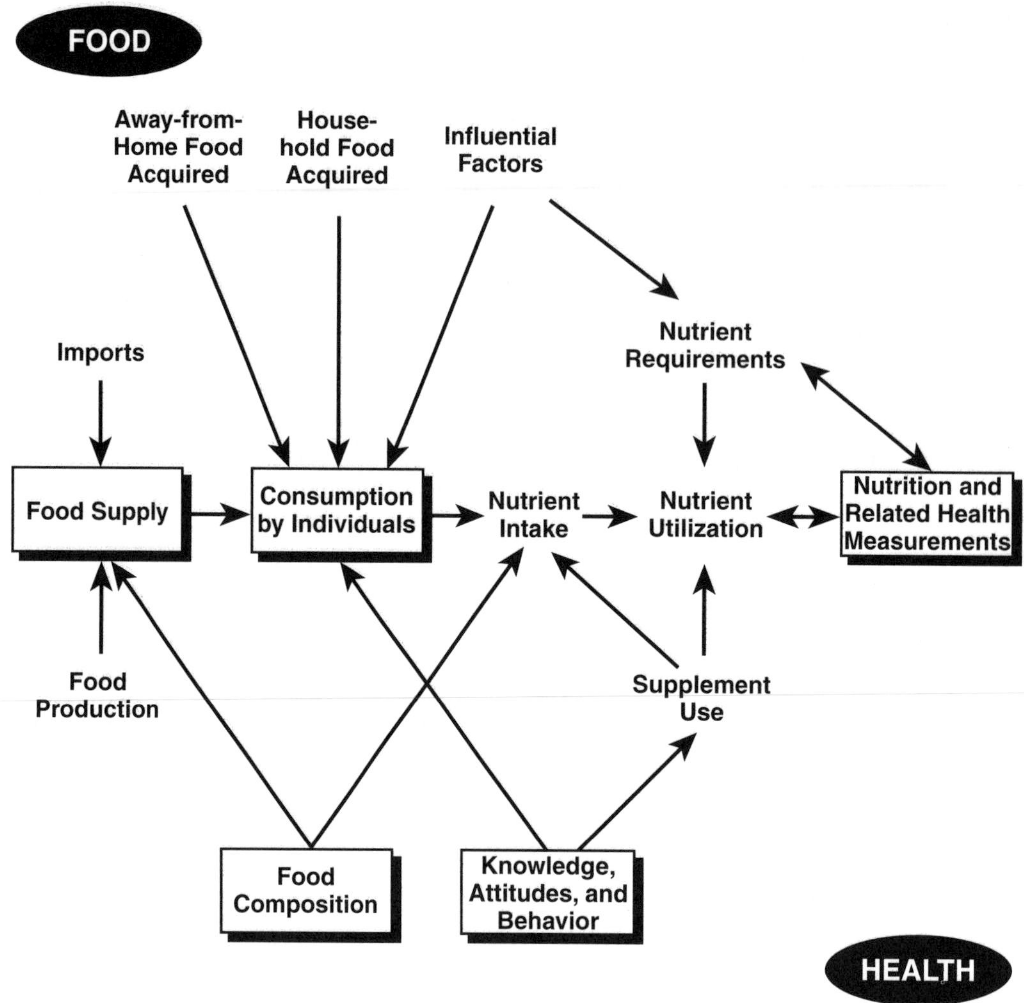

FIGURE 15.1
Food and health relationships. Source: Adapted from U.S. Department of Health and Human Services and U.S. Department of Agriculture. Ten-Year Comprehensive Plan for the National Nutrition Monitoring and Related Research Program. 1993.

Uses of Nutrition Monitoring Data

The nutrition monitoring program provides information for public policy decisions and scientific research (Table 15.1). Monitoring and surveillance data are used to identify high-risk population groups to plan public health intervention programs and target food assistance awareness efforts, establish the national health agenda and evaluate progress towards achieving national health objectives,[6,7] establish guidelines for the prevention, detection, and management of nutritional conditions,[8-14] and evaluate the impact of nutrition initiatives for military feeding systems.[15] Data are also used to monitor food production and marketing programs and their impact on the food supply.[7,16]

TABLE 15.1

Uses of Nutrition Monitoring Data[1]

Public Policy
Monitoring and Surveillance
Identify high-risk groups and geographical areas with nutrition related problems
Assess progress toward achieving the nutrition and health objectives in *Healthy People 2000 and 2010*[6,7]
Recommend guidelines for the prevention, detection, and management of nutrition and health conditions
Evaluate the effectiveness of nutritional initiatives for military feeding systems
Evaluate changes in agricultural policy, food production and marketing, that may affect the nutritional quality and healthfulness of the U.S. food supply
Develop reference standards for nutritional status
Programmatic
Develop nutrition education and dietary guidance (e.g., Dietary Guidelines for Americans and 5 A Day
Plan and evaluate food assistance programs
Plan and assess nutrition intervention programs and public health programs
Regulatory
Develop food labeling policies
Document the need for and monitor food fortification policies
Establish food safety guidelines
Scientific Research
Establish nutrient requirements through the lifecycle (Recommended Dietary Allowances and Dietary Reference Intakes)
Study diet-health relationships and the relationship of knowledge and attitudes to dietary and health behavior
Foster and conduct national and international nutrition monitoring research
Conduct food composition analysis
Study the economic aspects of food consumption and food security

[1] Adapted from the U.S. Department of Health and Human Services and U.S. Department of Agriculture. Ten-Year Comprehensive Plan for the National Nutrition and Related Research Program. 1993.

One example of the use of nutrition monitoring data for the development of population reference standards is the U.S. Growth Charts. Data from the third National Health and Nutrition Examination Survey (NHANES III) were used to develop the revised U.S. Growth Charts which were released in 2000.[17] The revised standards include charts for infants through 19 years of age, as well as a new chart for body mass index (BMI) by age.[17] The charts are included in the Anthro module of the computer software package EpiInfo, providing both z-scores and percentiles for each chart. NHANES trend data on anthropometric measures in children have been used by the U.S. Consumer Product Safety Commission to evaluate the need to revise standards for consumer items such as infant safety seats.[18]

Nutrition monitoring data are also used to estimate food insecurity in the U.S. Food security refers to assured access to nutritionally adequate and safe foods "without resorting to emergency food supplies, scavenging, stealing, and other coping strategies."[19] Efforts spearheaded by the private sector and academia began to pave the way toward a scientific basis for defining and measuring food insecurity and hunger in the mid-1980s.[20-22] Although national surveys such as NHANES and the USDA's food consumption surveys used questions related to a food security construct as early as 1977,[23-27] the Ten-Year Comprehensive Plan for the National Nutrition Monitoring and Related Research Program called for the development of a standard measure of food insecurity.[4] Research and refinement led to an 18-item food security scale that was first included as a supplement to the 1995 Current Population Survey.[23] Using the scale, it is estimated that the prevalence of food security in U.S. households is approximately 88%.[28] A number of nationally representative surveys of the U.S. population have begun to incorporate this standard measure, and a number of state and local surveys are including an abbreviated short form.[29] Policy documents like *Healthy People 2010*[7] and the U.S. Action Plan on Food Security[30] use the food security measure to assess progress, and the scale can also be used as a yardstick by which to evaluate federal food and nutrition assistance programs with respect to welfare reform.

Programmatic uses of nutrition monitoring data include developing and promoting nutrition education activities and programs such as the Dietary Guidelines for Americans[31] and 5 A Day for Better Health,[32] public health programs such as the National Cholesterol Education Program[8] and the National High Blood Pressure Education Program,[9] and federally supported food assistance programs such as the Food Stamp Program and the Special Supplemental Nutrition Program for Women, Infants, and Children (WIC).[33,34]

Regulatory uses of nutrition monitoring data include developing food fortification,[35,36] food safety,[16] and food labeling policies to inform consumers.[37] Nutrition monitoring data have been used by regulatory agencies to examine U.S. food fortification policies[35,36] and to provide dietary exposure estimates for nutrient and non-nutrient food components.[16] For example, dietary intake and serum data collected in NHANES III were used to assess folate status and the relationship between serum determinations, diet, and other nutrition and health variables prior to folate food fortification rulemaking by the Food and Drug Administration (FDA).[36,38]

Scientific research uses of nutrition monitoring data range from revising the standards of human nutrient requirements[39-41] to studying the relationship between diet, nutrition, and health. National data on the population's dietary intakes and serum nutrient levels have been used extensively for the investigation of nutrient requirements throughout the lifecycle and for the development of the Dietary Reference Intakes by the National Academy of Sciences (NAS).[39,40] Continued research to develop nutrition status indicators will be important for future monitoring efforts.

Nutrition monitoring data are essential to identify food and nutrition research priorities of significance to public health.[6,7,13,14,42,43] National nutrition data have been used for scientific reviews such as The Surgeon General's Report on Nutrition and Health[13] and the NAS report on Diet and Health: Implications for Reducing Chronic Disease Risk.[14] Such scientific reviews often form the basis for the development of nutrition policies. Other research is focused on studying the relationships between knowledge and attitudes to dietary and health behavior, the economic aspects of food consumption and food security, and food composition analysis.

The increased prevalence of overweight and obesity in the U.S. is the current focus of public health nutrition efforts. Using standardized international health-based definitions for men and women aged 20 to 74 years, the age-adjusted prevalence of overweight (BMI > = 25) was 59%, and obesity (BMI > = 30.0) was 20% in NHANES III (1988-94), compared to 51 and 12%, respectively, in NHANES II (1976-80).[7,44] This increasing trend has also been observed for adolescents, children, and preschoolers.[45,46] Using the 95th percentile of BMI from NHANES II as the definition of overweight and the 85th to 95th percentile as the definition of risk for overweight, 11% of children and adolescents were overweight and another 14% were at risk for overweight during 1988 to 1994.[45] The prevalence of overweight in children and adolescents increased from about 5% in the 1960s and 1970s.[45]

NHANES III anthropometry data serve as the baseline measures for the *Healthy People 2010* weight objectives.[7] Future NHANES data will be used to track progress in reducing the prevalence of overweight and obesity. The NIH Obesity Initiative is aimed at public health efforts to reduce overweight and foster collaborative research to better understand the etiology and prevention of obesity.[10,47] National and state nutrition monitoring data on dietary intake, physical activity patterns, weight loss efforts, and consumer knowledge, attitudes, and behaviors will be important for public health education and research efforts to reduce the prevalence of overweight and obesity in the U.S.

History of the Nutrition Monitoring Program: Milestones and Publications

Informally, the nutrition monitoring system had its genesis at the end of the 19th century. Early studies on food and nutrition were begun by Dr. W. O. Atwater in the 1890s.[48] These small-scale studies aimed to help the working class achieve good diets at a low cost. The first national survey, the Consumer Purchases Study of 1936-37, provided a comprehensive picture of household food consumption and indicated that one-third of the nation's families had diets that were poor by nutritional standards. In the late 1960s, concerns about the nutritional status of the U.S. population re-emerged as a result of widespread hunger. Not only was Congress concerned about the extent to which people were affected by hunger, but also by the Federal government's inability to document the problem because of a lack of nutrition monitoring coordination. A 1977 act of congress required the U.S. Department of Agriculture (USDA) and the U.S. Department of Health, Education, and Welfare (currently Department of Health and Human Services [HHS]) to develop plans to coordinate the two largest components of the monitoring program, DHHS's National Health and Nutrition Examination Survey and USDA's Nationwide Food Consumption Survey (NFCS).[49] It also mandated the development of a reporting system to translate the findings from these two national surveys and other monitoring activities into periodic reports to Congress on the nutritional status of the American population. A 1986 report, the first progress report on nutrition monitoring, provided an overview of the dietary and nutritional status of the population and recommendations for improvements in the monitoring program.[50] In 1989, the report was updated by an expert panel.[51]

In 1988, the Interagency Committee on Nutrition Monitoring (ICNM) was established to provide a formal mechanism for improving the planning, coordination, and communication among agencies.[52] As a first step, the Directory of Federal Nutrition Monitoring Activities was published in 1989.[53] It was updated and expanded in 1992 to include state surveillance efforts,[54] and in 1998 it became available on the Internet.[55] The most recent version was published on the Internet in 2000.[56] The publication is used extensively as a resource for finding nutrition monitoring data sources, contact persons, and published references.

The *National Nutrition Monitoring and Related Research Act* of 1990 (P.L. 101-445)[3] established several mechanisms to ensure the collaboration and coordination of federal agencies as well as state and local governments involved in nutrition monitoring. Under the act, the Secretaries of DHHS and USDA have joint responsibility for implementation of the coordinated program and the transmission of required reports to Congress via the President. The ICNM was formalized and became the Interagency Board for Nutrition Monitoring and Related Research (IBNMRR), which currently includes 22 agencies that contribute to or use national nutrition monitoring data. The IBNMRR serves as the central coordination point for federal nutrition monitoring activities. The board coordinates the preparation of the annual budget report on nutrition monitoring and biennial reports on progress and policy implications of scientific findings to the President and Congress, and the periodic scientific reports that describe the nutritional and related health status of the population to Congress. In 1993 and 1995, respectively, the Board published Chartbook I: Selected Findings from the National Nutrition Monitoring and Related Research Program[57] and the Third Report on Nutrition Monitoring in the United States.[58]

Three staff working groups (Survey Comparability, Food Composition Data, and Federal-State Relations and Information Dissemination and Exchange [Federal-STRIDE]) were established under the board to improve communication and coordination among member agencies on high-priority issues. After the welfare reform law was enacted in 1996, a fourth group — the Welfare Reform, Nutrition, and Data Needs Working Group — was established to determine whether federal surveys and surveillance systems represented by the IBNMRR could capture the effects of welfare reform on nutrition, hunger, and health status, identify gaps in data collections, encourage use of comparable data collection among surveys, serve as a repository on national nutrition survey efforts related to welfare reform, and foster collaborative research on nutrition and welfare reform. The group has been quite active and now includes federal as well as non-federal members.

The act also established the National Nutrition Monitoring Advisory Council (NNMAC) to provide scientific and technical guidance to the IBNMRR. The council includes nine members (five appointed by the President and four by Congress) with expertise in the areas of public health, nutrition monitoring research, and food production and distribution.

Finally, the 1990 act called for the development of a Ten-Year Comprehensive Plan.[59] The plan includes three primary goals: to provide for a comprehensive National Nutrition Monitoring and Related Research Program (NMRRP) through continuous and coordinated data collection, improve the comparability and quality of data across NNMRRP, and improve the research base for nutrition monitoring. These national goals are complemented by state and local objectives to strengthen data collection capacity, improve the quality of state and local data, and improve methodologies to enhance comparability of NNMRRP data across national, state, and local levels. Table 15.2 includes a summary of the nutrition monitoring program's history.

TABLE 15.2

Milestones and Publications of the National Nutrition Monitoring and Related Research Program

1977	*Food and Agriculture Act* (P.L. 95-113) passed
1978	Proposal for a comprehensive nutritional status monitoring system submitted to Congress
1986	First progress report on Nutrition Monitoring in the United States published
1988	Interagency Committee on Nutrition Monitoring formed
1989	Second progress report on Nutrition Monitoring in the United States and The Directory of Federal Nutrition Monitoring Activities published
1990	*National Nutrition Monitoring and Related Research Act* (P.L. 101-445) passed
1991	Interagency Board for Nutrition Monitoring and Related Research established through incorporation and expansion of the ICNM
	Proposed Ten-Year Comprehensive Plan for the Nutrition Monitoring and Related Research Program published for comment
1992	National Nutrition Monitoring Advisory Council formed
	The Directory of Federal and State Nutrition Monitoring Activities published
1993	Ten-Year Comprehensive Plan for the National Nutrition Monitoring and Related Research Program published
	Chartbook I: Selected Findings from the National Nutrition Monitoring and Related Research Program published
1995	Third progress report on Nutrition Monitoring in the U.S. published
1998	The Directory of Federal and State Nutrition Monitoring and Related Research Activities published
2000	The Directory of Federal and State Nutrition Monitoring and Related Research Activities revised and published

Nutrition Monitoring Measurement Components

The NNMRRP aims to study the relationship between food and health through data collection in five measurement component areas. Since the 1930s, more than 40 surveys and surveillance systems have evolved in response to the information needs of federal agencies and other nutrition monitoring data users. Chronological listings of past nutrition monitoring surveys and activities have been published.[4,5,59-61] Subsumed under each area is a host of studies, surveys, surveillance programs, and related research. Table 15.3 summarizes the major activities since 1990 by measurement area. Brief descriptions of surveys and surveillance systems are summarized below and have been described in detail elsewhere.[4,5,53-58,60,62] The Directory of Federal and State Nutrition Monitoring and Related Research Activities includes additional information. As an Internet publication, each survey synopsis contained in the directory includes a hypertext link for more information on each activity (http://www.cdc.gov/nchs/data/direc-99.pdf).

Nutrition and Related Health Measurements

Nutrition and related health data have a wide variety of policy, research, health and nutrition education, medical care practices, and reference standards applications. The cornerstone of this NNMRRP measurement component, NHANES, provides national data on the nutritional status, dietary intake, and numerous health indices of the U.S. population.[3-5,58,60-64] It also provides national population reference distributions, national prevalences of diseases and risk factors, and trends in nutritional and health status over time. NHANES followup studies allow epidemiologic investigations of the relationships of nutrition and health to risk of death and disability. The current NHANES (1999+) has a continuous annual design, and oversampling of Mexican Americans, blacks, older persons, adolescents, and pregnant females in the first three years.

The National Health Interview Survey provides information about self-reported health conditions annually and about special nutrition and health topics periodically, such as vitamin/mineral supplement usage, youth risk behavior, food program participation, diet and nutrition knowledge, cancer, and disability and food preparation. Other special topical modules relate to tracking of our nation's health and nutrition objectives.

Recently, a number of health care provider record-based surveys were merged and expanded into one integrated survey called the National Health Care Survey. Data on alternative health care settings, such as ambulatory surgical centers, hospital outpatient departments, emergency rooms, hospices, and home health agencies, are being collected through this system. The survey provides information on the availability and utilization of dietary and nutritional services in these types of agencies. For hospital outpatient visits, information is obtained about physician-reported hypertension and obesity, and counseling services for diet, weight reduction, and cholesterol reduction. The survey also provides information on hospitalizations resulting from nutrition-related diseases.

A number of other surveys and surveillance systems, primarily conducted by the Centers for Disease Control and Prevention (CDC), also contribute nutrition-related health information, particularly for low-income pregnant women, infants, and children who participate in publicly funded health, nutrition, and food assistance programs.[62,65,66] These surveillance systems provide data representative of the population in participating states and include physical measures such as height, weight, hemoglobin, and hematocrit.

TABLE 15.3

Federal Nutrition Monitoring Surveys and Surveillance Activities Since 1990

Date (initiated)	Dept.	Survey	Sample Size and Target U.S. Population
Nutrition and Related Health Measurements			
Continuous (1915)	HHS	National Vital Registration System	All births and deaths in the total U.S. population
Annual (1957)	HHS	National Health Interview Survey (NHIS)	Civilian, noninstitutionalized household population (N = 103,477 individuals and N = 39,832 households in 1997)
1985, 1990, 1998	HHS	National Health Interview Survey on Health Promotion and Disease Prevention	Civilian, noninstitutionalized household population in the U.S., ages 18+ y (N = 41,104 households in 1990)
1987, 1992	HHS	National Health Interview Survey on Cancer Epidemiology and Cancer Control	Civilian, noninstitutionalized household population ages 18+ y in the U.S. (N = 12,000 households in 1992)
1991	HHS	1991 National Health Interview Survey on Health Promotion and Disease Prevention	Civilian, noninstitutionalized, household population of the United States, ages 18+ y (N = 43,732 households)
1992–1993	HHS	National Health Interview Survey on Youth Behavior Supplement	Youth ages 12-21 y (N = 10,645 households)
1994	HHS	National Health Interview Survey on Disability	Civilian, noninstitutionalized household population (N = 107,469 households)
1993, 1995	HHS	National Health Interview Survey Year 2000 Objectives Supplement	Civilian, noninstitutionalized household population in U.S., ages 18+ y (N = 17,317 households in 1995)
1990, 1995 (1973)	HHS	National Survey of Family Growth	Women, 15-44 y (N = 10,847 households in 1995)
Continuous (1973)	HHS	Pregnancy Nutrition Surveillance System (PNSS)	Low-income, high-risk pregnant women participating in programs in 18 states, the Navajo Nation, and the Intertribal Council of AZ (N = 599,000 records in 1995)
Continuous (1973)	HHS	Pediatric Nutrition Surveillance System (PedNSS)	Low-income, high-risk children, birth-17 y in participating programs in 43 states and DC, Puerto Rico, and 6 Indian reservations (N = 8,800,000 records in 1995)
1988–1990	HHS	National Maternal and Infant Health Survey	Women, hospitals, and prenatal care providers associated with live births (N = 9953), still births (N = 3309), and infant deaths (N = 5332)
1988–1994	HHS	Third National Health and Nutrition Examination Survey (NHANES III). Followup study is under consideration	U.S. noninstitutionalized, civilian population, 2+ mo; Oversampling of blacks and Mexican-Americans, children 0-5 y, and individuals 60+ y (N = 33,994 individuals interviewed; N = 31,311 individuals examined)
1989–1993	HHS	National Health and Nutrition Examination III Supplemental Nutrition Survey of Older Americans	NHANES III (1988-91) examinees 50+ years (N = 2602 completed NHANES III dietary recall (DR) and 1st SNS interview; N = 2519 completed NHANES III DR and 2nd SNS interview; N = 2261 completed NHANES III DR and 2 SNS interviews)

1990–1991	HHS	Survey of Heights and Weights of American Indian School Children	American Indian school children, ages 5-18 y (N = 9464 children in 1990-91 school year)
1991–1992	HHS	Navajo Health and Nutrition Survey	Persons ages 12+ y residing on or near the Navajo reservation in AZ, NM, and CO (N = 985 examined)
1991–1992	HHS	Longitudinal Followup to the National Maternal and Infant Health Survey	Participants of the 1988 NMIHS (N = 9400 mothers of 3 yr olds; N = 1000 women who had infant deaths; N = 1000 women who had late fetal deaths in 1988
1992	HHS	NHANES I Epidemiologic Followup Study	Individuals examined in NHANES I, 25-74 y at baseline, 1971-74 (N = 9281, 1992 cohort)
Continuous (1992)	HHS	NHANES II Mortality Followup Survey	Individuals examined in NHANES II, 30-74 y at baseline, 1976-80 (N = 9252)
Continuous (1992)	HHS	Hispanic HANES (HHANES) Mortality Followup Survey (in progress)	Individuals interviewed in HHANES, 20-74 y at baseline, 1982-84 (N = NA)
Annual (1992)	HHS	National Health Care Survey (integrates: National Home and Hospice Care Survey (1992-94; 1996), National Nursing Home Survey (since 1973-74) and Followup (1995, 1997), National Hospital Discharge Survey (since 1965), National Ambulatory Medical Care Survey (since 1973), National Hospital Ambulatory Medical Care Survey (1992), and National Survey of Ambulatory Surgery (1994-96)	Record-based health care provider surveys including: visits to hospital emergency and outpatients departments of non-Federal, short-stay, general and specialty hospitals and ambulatory surgical centers; office visits to non-Federal, office-based physicians; and home health agencies and nursing homes (N = 11,396 for 1996 NHHCS; N = 9556 for 1995 NNHS; N = 282,525 for 1995 NHDS; N = 32,978 for 1996 NAMCS; N = 52,194 for 1996 NHAMCS; N = 125,751 for 1996 NSAS)
Continuous (1992)	HHS	NHANES III Mortality Followup Survey	Individuals interviewed and examined in NHANES III, 20+ y at baseline, 1988-94 (N = NA)
1996–1999	HHS	Demonstration Sites for PedNSS and PNSS	Low-income, high risk women, infants, and children that participate in government food assistance programs and participate in PedNSS and PNSS (N = minimum of 1000 children in WIC for PedNSS; N = minimum of 300 women in WIC for PNSS)
1999+	HHS	National Health and Nutrition Examination Survey	Civilian, noninstitutionalized individuals. Oversampling of blacks, Mexican-Americans, adolescents, older persons, and pregnant women in the first 3 years. (N = NA)
Food and Nutrient Consumption			
Continuous (1917)	DOD	Nutritional Evaluation of Military Feeding Systems and Military Populations	Enlisted personnel of the Army, Navy, Marine Corps, and Air Force (N = 20-240 depending on study focus)
Annual supplement (1995)	BLS; CB; USDA	Current Population Survey, Supplement on Food Security	Civilian, noninstitutionalized U.S. population (N = approx. 59,500 for CPS)

TABLE 15.3 *(Continued)*

Federal Nutrition Monitoring Surveys and Surveillance Activities Since 1990

Date (initiated)	Dept.	Survey	Sample Size and Target U.S. Population
Continuous (1980)	DOL	Consumer Expenditure Survey	Civilian, noninstitutionalized, population and a portion of the institutionalized population (N = 5000 in quarterly interview survey of consumer unites; N = 6000 diary surveys of consumer unites kept for 2 consecutive 1-week periods)
Continuous (1983)	DOC	Survey of Income and Program Participation (SIPP)	Civilian, noninstitutionalized population of the U.S. (N = 11,600-36,800 households in a continuous series of panels)
1994, 1996 (1984)	USDA	Study of WIC Participants and Program Characteristics	WIC participants using mail surveys of State and local WIC agencies, record abstractions at local WIC service sites and, in 1988, interviews with participants (N = 7,000,000+ individuals in 1996)
1988–1994	HHS	NHANES III and Supplemental Nutrition Survey of Older Americans	See NHANES III listing above. Individuals ages 50+ y examined in NHANES III with telephones (See listing above for N)
1989–1991, annual 1994–1996, annual (1985-1986)	USDA	Continuing Survey of Food Intakes by Individuals (CSFII) (Intake of Pyramid Servings and Servings database 1994-1996)	Females 19-50 y and their children 1-5 y and males 19-50 y residing in households in 48 conterminous States in 1985-86, individuals of all ages residing in households in 48 conterminous States in 1989-91, and nationwide in 1994-96; oversampling of individuals in low-income households; individuals 2+ y from CSFII 1994-96 (N = 15,303 in 1994-96)
1989-91	HHS	Strong Heart Dietary Survey	American Indian adults ages 45-74 y in SD, OK, and AZ (N = 888)
1991–1992	DOC	Development of a National Seafood Consumption Survey Model	Individuals residing in eligible households and recreational/subsistence fishermen (N = —)
1992	USDA	School Nutrition Dietary Assessment Study	School-age children in grades 1-12 in 48 conterminous States and D.C. (N = 380 school districts; N = 607 schools; N = 4489 students)
1992	USDA	Adult Day Care Program Study	Adult day care centers and adults participating in the Child and Adult Care Food Program (N = 282 CACFP Centers; N = 282 non-CACFP Centers; N = 942 participating adults)
1994–1995	USDA	WIC Infant Feeding Practices Study	Nationally representative sample of WIC mothers and infants living in the 48 contiguous States, the District of Columbia and the 33 WIC agencies on Indian reservations (N = 971)
1995	USDA	Early Childhood and Child Care Study	Child care sponsors, providers, and children participating in the CACFP (N = 566 sponsors; N = 1962 providers; N = 1951 households; N = 2174 child-day observations)
1997–1998	USDA	Supplemental Children's Survey	Noninstitutionalized children 0-9 y in households in the U.S.; oversampling of low-income households (N = approx 5000)
1998	USDA	School Nutrition Dietary Assessment Study II	School-age children in grades 1-12 in 48 conterminous States and D.C. (N = approx 1152 schools)
1999+	HHS	National Health and Nutrition Examination Survey	Civilian, noninstitutionalized individuals. Oversampling of blacks, Mexican-Americans, adolescents, older persons, and pregnant women in the first 3 years (N = approx 3200)

Knowledge, Attitudes, and Behavior Assessments			
Continuous (1984)	HHS	Behavioral Risk Factor Surveillance System	Individuals 18+ y residing in households with telephones in participating States (N = approx 2039 per state in all 50 states for 1995)
1990, 1994 (1982)	HHS	Health and Diet Survey	Civilian, noninstitutionalized individuals in households w/telephones, 18+ y (N = 5005 in 1995)
1989–1991 1994–1996	USDA	Diet and Health Knowledge Survey	Main meal-planner/preparers in households participating in 1989-91 and 1994-96 CSFII (N = 5765 for 1994-96)
Annual (1990)	HHS	Youth Risk Behavior Survey (YRBS)	Youths attending school in grades 9-12 and 12-21 y of age in households in 50 States, D.C., Puerto Rico, and Virgin Islands (N = approx 12,000 for the National surveys and N = approx 2000 for the State and local surveys)
1990	HHS	Cholesterol Awareness Survey — Physicians' Survey	Physicians practicing in the conterminous U.S. (N = 1,604)
1990–1991	HHS	Nationwide Survey of Nurses' and Dietitians' Knowledge, Attitudes, and Behavior Regarding Cardiovascular Risk Factors	Registered nurses and registered dietitians currently active in their professions (N = 7200 registered nurses; N = 1621 occupational health nurses oversample; N = 1782 registered dietitians)
1990–1991	HHS	Nutrition Label Format Studies	Primary food shoppers, ages 18+ y (N = 2676)
1991	HHS	Weight Loss Practices Survey	Individuals currently trying to lose weight, ages 18+ y, in households with telephones (N = 1232 current dieters; N = 205 African American oversample; N = 218 nondieting controls)
1991	HHS	5 A Day for Better Health Baseline Survey	Individuals ages 18+ y with telephones (N = approx. 2059)
1992–1993; 1998	HHS	Consumer Food Handling Practices and Awareness of Microbiological Hazards Screener	Individuals in households w/telephones, 18+ y (N = 1620)
1993–1994	HHS	Infant Feeding Practices Survey	New mothers and healthy, full-term infants 0-1 y (N = 1200)
1994–1995	USDA	WIC Infant Feeding Practices Survey	Prenatal and postnatal women and their infants participating in the WIC program (N = 971)
Food Composition and Nutrient Databases			
Continuous (1892)	USDA	National Nutrient Data Bank Food Composition Laboratory	(N = —)
Annual (1961)	HHS	Total Diet Study	Representative diets of specific age-sex groups (N = —)
1991–1993, 1993–1994, 1995–1996 (1977)	HHS	Food Label and Package Survey	(N = 1250 food brands)

TABLE 15.3 *(Continued)*

Federal Nutrition Monitoring Surveys and Surveillance Activities Since 1990

Date (initiated)	Dept.	Survey	Sample Size and Target U.S. Population
Continuous (1977)	USDA	Survey Nutrient Data Base for CSFII 1989-91, 1994-96; NHANES III 1988-94	(N = —)
1988–1994	HHS	Technical Support Information for the NHANES III, 1988-94 Dietary Interview Data Files	(N = —)
1994–1996	USDA	CSFII 1994-96 Technical Support Files Food Coding Database Recipe Database Survey Nutrient Database and Related Files	(N = —)
Food Supply Determinations			
Annual (1909)	DOC	Fisheries of the United States	(N = —)
Annual (1909)		U.S. Food and Nutrition Supply Series:	(N = —)
	USDA	Estimates of Food Available	
	USDA	Estimates of Nutrients	
Continuous (1985)	USDA	A.C. Nielsen SCANTRACK	(N = 3000 supermarkets since 1988)

Abbreviations: ARS, Agricultural Research Service; ASPE, Assistant Secretary for Planning and Evaluation; BLS, Bureau of Labor Statistics; CACFP, Child and Adult Care Food Program; CB, Census Bureau; CDC, Centers for Disease Control and Prevention; DOC, Department of Commerce; DOD, Department of Defense; DOL, Department of Labor; FDA, Food and Drug Administration; ERS, Economic Research Service; FNS, Food and Nutrition Service; HHS, Department of Health and Human Services; HNIS, Human Nutrition Information Service*; HRSA, Health Resources Services Administration; IHS, Indian Health Service; NCCDPHP, National Center for Chronic Disease Prevention and Health Promotion; NCHS, National Center for Health Statistics; NCI, National Cancer Institute; NHLBI, National Heart, Lung, and Blood Institute; NIH, National Institutes of Health; NA — not applicable; NMFS, National Marine Fisheries Service; NOAA, National Oceanic and Atmospheric Administration; SSA, Social Security Administration; ASARUM, U.S. Army Research Institute of Environmental Medicine; USDA, U.S. Department of Agriculture.

* HNIS was integrated into ARS in 1994.

— = Not applicable

NA = Not available

The Pediatric Nutrition Surveillance System (PedNSS), sponsored since 1973, is used to monitor simple key indicators of nutritional status among low-income, high-risk infants and children who participate in publicly funded health, nutrition, and food assistance programs.[66] Data can be analyzed at individual, clinic, county, state, and national levels. The Pregnancy Nutrition Surveillance System (PNSS), sponsored since 1978, tracks nutrition-related problems and behavioral risk factors associated with low birth weight among high-risk prenatal women.[66] The PNSS is used to identify preventable nutrition-related problems and behavioral risk factors to target interventions.

Food and Nutrient Consumption

Food consumption measurements include estimates of individuals' intakes of foods and beverages (nonalcoholic and alcoholic) and nutritional supplements. Both CSFII and NHANES provide national estimates of food and nutrient intakes in the general U.S. population and subgroups. These surveys and the FDA Total Diet Study provide the potential to assess pesticide levels in diets.

Periodic assessments of food and nutrient consumption of specific population subgroups not adequately covered in national surveys have been conducted for military populations, Native Americans, children, and low income populations. A 1996 Supplemental Children's Survey was conducted specifically to assess pesticide exposures in the diets of infants and young children. Since 1995, a yearly supplement to the Current Population Survey (CPS), conducted by the U.S. Census Bureau, has been devoted to measuring the extent of food insecurity and hunger among people living in U.S. households.[23,28,67]

Evaluations of USDA nutrition and food assistance programs are routinely conducted. The Adult Day Care Program Study and the Early Childhood and Child Care Study each determined the characteristics and dietary intakes of their participants and the features of day care centers participating in the Child and Adult Care Food Program. A number of studies have been conducted to evaluate the nutrition and health effects of participating in WIC, provide current participant and program characteristics of the WIC program, and describe the infant feeding practices of WIC participants. The School Nutrition Dietary Assessment Study assessed the nutrient content of USDA and non-USDA meals offered in U.S. schools and the contribution of the National School Lunch Program to overall nutrient intake.[68] A follow-up study was conducted to compare changes over time.

Knowledge, Attitudes, and Behavior Assessments

National surveys that measure knowledge, attitudes, and behavior about diet and nutrition and how these relate to health were added to the nutrition monitoring program in 1982. In general, the focus of the Health and Diet Surveys is on people's awareness of relationships between diet and risk for chronic disease, and on health-related knowledge and attitudes. The survey has studied consumer use of food labels, the effectiveness of the National Cholesterol Education Program, and weight loss practices.[69,70] The focus of the Diet and Health Knowledge Survey initiated by USDA in 1989 is on the relationship of individuals' knowledge and attitudes about dietary guidance and food safety to their food choices and nutrient intakes.

Surveys addressing specific topics such as infant feeding practices, weight loss practices and progress toward achieving related national health objectives, and cholesterol awareness of health professionals have been periodically conducted to meet specific data needs. The National Cancer Institute (NCI) conducted the 5 A Day Baseline Survey in collaboration with food industry to assess knowledge, behavior, and attitudes about fruits and vegetables.[71] NCI also conducted the Cancer Prevention Awareness Survey and the National Knowledge, Attitudes, and Behavior Survey to measure progress on knowledge, attitudes, and behaviors regarding lifestyle and cancer prevention and risk factors. The FDA conducted a study to assess consumer food handling practices and awareness of microbiological hazards, and also conducted a number of studies to evaluate the Nutrition Facts Label features and usability by consumers.[72]

The focus of the Behavioral Risk Factor Surveillance System (BRFSS) is on personal behavior and its relationship to nutritional and health status. BRFSS has been used by state health departments to plan, initiate, and guide health promotion and disease prevention programs, and to monitor their progress over time.[73] The Youth Risk Behavior Survey monitors priority health risk behaviors among adolescents through national, state, and local surveys.[74]

Food Composition and Nutrient Databases

FDA's Total Diet Study provides annual food composition analysis of core foods of the U.S. food supply, and the Food Label and Package Survey, sponsored by a number of agencies, is conducted to monitor labeling practices of U.S. food manufacturers.[75,76] The survey also includes a surveillance program to identify levels of accuracy of selected nutrient declarations compared to values obtained from nutrient analyses of products.

Since 1892, USDA has maintained the National Nutrient Data Bank (NNDB) for the purpose of deriving representative nutrient values for more than 6000 foods and up to 80 components consumed in the U.S.[77] Data are obtained from the food industry, from USDA-initiated analytical contracts, and from the scientific literature. Values from NNDB are released electronically as the USDA Nutrient Data Base for Standard Reference (SR). The SR is updated periodically to reflect changes in the food supply as well as changes in analytical methodology. The SR nutrient data are used as the core of most nutrient databases developed in the U.S. for special purposes, such as those used in the commercially available dietary analysis programs.[77-79] USDA produces the Survey Nutrient Data Base (SNDB), which contains data for 28 food components and energy for each food item for analysis of NHANES and CSFII.[80] The database is periodically updated. The National Food and Nutrient Analysis Program was initiated in 1997 to produce accurate and current food composition data characterizing the U.S. national food supply. This goal is being achieved through stratified random sample collection and chemical assay of commonly eaten foods accounting for the majority of Americans' nutrient intake. The new data will be incorporated into the NNDB.

Many individuals are consuming nutrients from dietary supplements. To enable the estimation of total nutrient intakes and the impact of dietary supplements on nutrition and health, the National Center for Health Statistics (NCHS) has developed and is maintaining a database on dietary supplements for use with national surveys.[81]

Food Supply Determinations

Since the beginning of this century, U.S. food supply estimates have reflected levels of foods and nutrients available for consumption. These data, updated and published annually by USDA as the U.S. Food and Nutrient Supply Series, are used to assess the potential of the U.S. food supply to meet the nutritional needs of the population and changes in the food supply over time. They are also used to evaluate the effects of technological alterations and marketing changes on the food supply over time, to study the relationships between food and nutrient availability and nutrient-disease associations, and to facilitate management of federal marketing, food assistance, nutrition education, food enrichment and fortification policy. The Fisheries of the United States Survey has been conducted by the National Marine Fisheries Service since 1909 to provide annual estimates of fish and shellfish availability and consumption in the U.S. food system.

Evolution of the Nutrition Monitoring Program

The history of nutrition monitoring in the U.S. is discussed earlier in this section, and notes significant legislative and other events. The current nutrition monitoring program is firmly grounded in USDA and HHS nutrition-related studies and surveys that address pertinent health issues and needs. The future evolution of the program will be based on these and other identified health issues and needs of the population that relate to diet, physical activity, lifestyle, and health. The focus of the program may shift as past health problems are resolved through nutrition education and public policy changes (e.g., food fortification) and as new diet-related health concerns emerge. The studies and surveys within the current monitoring program can be adapted to meet changing needs, and new studies can be added as resources permit. The present and future needs for nutrition monitoring will be defined and clarified based on nutrition-related studies conducted by government, academic, medical, clinical, and private institutions.

Improvements to the nutrition monitoring program will result from research that develops new methodologies and improves existing ones to assess nutrition and health status. New and improved methods may allow more accurate and efficient assessment of food and nutrient intake, assessment of physiological measures of nutrient status, and techniques to relate food and nutrient intake to health status. These improvements will result in more accurate data, and they may result in data that are not comparable to previous data collected with other methods. These newer data may also shift the focus of the nutrition monitoring program.

Changes in Health Needs

Speculation about the future evolution of the nutrition monitoring program requires consideration of the factors that may change the health concerns of the population. Some of the factors are changes in the food supply, in the demographics of the U.S. population, and in individual dietary and other lifestyle behaviors. Innovation to the food supply may alter the nutrient content of existing foods or may result in new food products. In either case, the nutrient intake of the population or of specific population groups may change as these altered or new foods are consumed. Changes in the food supply may result from genetic engineering of plants or animals, changes in agricultural practices, and new manufacturing processes or technologies. Within the past several decades there has been increased access to food from fast-food chains and other restaurants, increased availability of prepared foods from grocery stores that require only microwave heating prior to consumption, and increased consumption of ethnic dishes. Such changes are likely to continue.

Alterations in the demographics of the U.S. population may affect the mean food and nutrient intakes from national surveys, because the surveys reflect the food preferences, patterns, and practices of the population. The number of Hispanics and blacks in the U.S. population is increasing at a rate faster than the white, non-Hispanic population. The population is also becoming older as the baby boomers and their children age. Changes in income levels and income disparities in the population may result in changes in diet and health outcomes reported from surveys. Income disparities among racial and ethnic groups and among age and gender categories will continue to be important in identifying population groups that are more vulnerable to diet and health-related problems.

Modifications in individual dietary and other lifestyle behavior may lead to changes in health. Consumers are encouraged to follow the Dietary Guidelines for Americans and the Food Guide Pyramid, to read Nutrition Facts Labels, and to be more physically active. These nutrition education efforts may help consumers improve their diets and health outcomes. Consumers may become increasingly knowledgeable of the health effects of overweight and obesity and make attempts to alter their eating patterns and physical activity to lose weight. People are also influenced by the nutrition information they receive from other sources (TV, radio, books, magazines, advertisements). They may begin to take (or alter their intake of) dietary supplements, increase intake of functional foods, or become interested in organic produce, herbal products, or botanicals. Such behavior changes could affect health. Hopefully, consumers will adopt behaviors that will improve their health; however, it is possible that poor dietary advice may have the opposite effect. It is also possible that continued sedentary lifestyles and wide access to food will maintain the current problems of overweight and obesity in the U.S. and the health problems related to them.

Preparing for the Future

In December 1999 the National Academy of Sciences (NAS) organized a public symposium entitled "Nutrition Monitoring in the U.S.: Preparing for the Next Millennium." This session convened nutrition scientists from industry, academia, government, and the public sector along with policy makers to discuss current efforts to streamline and integrate the monitoring program and to identify and highlight future diet, nutrition, and health data needs. Conference participants discussed ways to optimize the utility and relevance of the nutrition monitoring program for organizations whose activities depend on the availability and reliability of the data obtained from the program. The National Nutrition Summit, held in May, 2000 in Washington, D.C., focused on several nutrition monitoring themes including obesity, physical activity, and food security.

Additional activities in progress to prepare the nutrition monitoring program for the future include integration of USDA and NHCS nutrition surveys, improving the comparability and quality of survey methods, and providing state and local nutrition-related data, including data for population subgroups.

Survey Integration

Continuous collection of diet- and nutrition-related data in cross-sectional and longitudinal surveys and surveillance systems is needed to assess the health of the U.S. population and plan nutrition services and educational programs. Efforts are under way to integrate and merge the NHANES and the CSFII by 2002. The survey will include a nationally representative annual sample of black, white, and Mexican-American persons for all income and low income households, and a common dietary data collection and processing system. Federal agencies are currently conducting sample design and dietary survey methodology research, evaluating the extent of seasonal and geographic coverage with the combined annual survey, and designing and implementing the integrated sample to better meet nutrition monitoring data needs and develop a "core" (identical) set of demographic, socioeconomic, nutrition, and health-related program questions that are essential to estimate and report dietary intakes for the integrated sample. The two departments are also working to operationalize improvements in sample design, dietary methodologies, and questionnaires. The framework for the survey's design will need to provide flexibility and opportunities for modifications over time.

Comparability and Quality of Methods

An integral part of the coordination of nutrition monitoring activities is the use of standardized or comparable methodologies for the collection, quality control, analysis, and reporting of data. Progress has been made in developing indicators for height and weight to assess growth and overweight, household food security, and folic acid status. Standardized indicators are needed for population descriptors, food security, diet, nutritional, and related health status, and knowledge, attitudes, and behavior assessments. As these indicators are developed, they will be incorporated into existing and planned surveillance systems.

Reliable, valid, and cost-effective measures of nutritional status need to be developed and improved, along with appropriate interpretive criteria. Research is needed on appropriate methods (such as questionnaires, interviewing procedures, physical measures, and biological indicators) for subgroups at increased nutritional risk, practical and efficient measures of diet, biochemical, and clinical parameters, and applied statistical methodologies for the collection and interpretation of nutrition monitoring data. Research to develop and standardize questionnaires for valid and reliable estimators of knowledge, attitudes, and behavior will aid in the development of public health strategies at federal, state, and local levels to improve dietary status, promote health, and prevent nutrition-related disease.

State and Local Data

Nutrition monitoring data are needed at the state and local levels, especially as they relate to welfare reform and other policy changes. Continued improvements to the CDC state surveillance systems, the use of comparable methodologies, and supplemental data collection for defined populating groups will be central to meeting state and local data needs in the future. Improvements will be dependent upon the availability of resources to provide technical assistance and data collection capacity to states.

Data for Population Subgroups

Many surveys of the nutrition monitoring program collect data on population subgroups such as low-income people and minorities. However, data are still limited for select subgroups, such as the homeless, Native Americans, and Asian and Pacific Islanders. NCHS is exploring an initiative known as community HANES to study specific population subgroups for whom national estimates cannot be easily, practically, or cost-effectively made.

The Link between Nutrition Monitoring, Research, and Policy

Research, monitoring, and policy are intertwined by a complex set of interrelationships. As shown in Figure 15.2, nutrition monitoring is vital to policymaking and research.[15,60,82] Monitoring provides information and a database for public policy decision making and

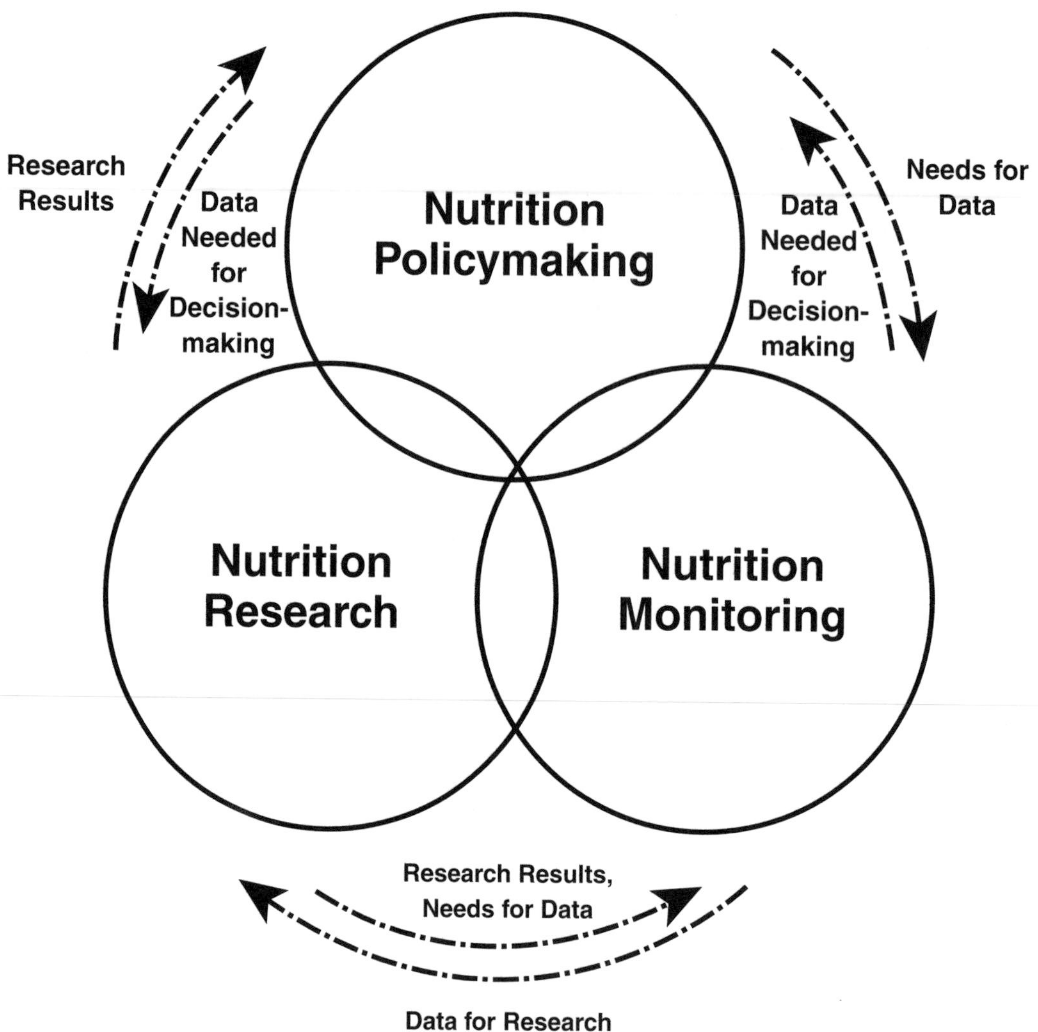

FIGURE 15.2
Overlapping of nutrition monitoring, policy making, and research. Source: Adapted from U.S. Department of Health and Human Services and U.S. Department of Agriculture. Ten-Year Comprehensive Plan for the National Nutrition and Related Research Program. 1993.

establishing research priorities.[42,63,83-85] Nutrition research provides data for policymaking and for identifying nutrition monitoring data needs.[42,63]

The Third Report on Nutrition Monitoring in the United States identified a number of food components of particular public health concern in the U.S. population: food energy, total fat, saturated fatty acids, cholesterol, alcohol, iron, calcium, and sodium. The report also included a range of health issues of particular concern for low-income, high-risk populations including anemia, low birth weight, overweight, high serum total cholesterol, hypertension, osteoporosis, low intakes of a number of nutrients (including folate, calcium, iron, and others), and food insufficiency.[58] Based on these findings, the report also provided recommendations for future nutrition monitoring and nutrition methods research.

To illustrate the link between nutrition monitoring, nutrition research, and nutrition policy, this section explores a current public health issue identified in the Third Report on Nutrition Monitoring in the United States: the relationship of calcium intake and osteoporosis. All dietary components have unique considerations with respect to determining dietary adequacy and measuring physiological status. The example of calcium and osteoporosis illustrates some of the challenges of measuring both dietary and physiological status, drawing conclusions about the relationship between dietary intake and health, and providing guidance to the public to improve health based on the available data and scientific research.

Dietary Assessment of Calcium Status

Assessment of dietary calcium intake has been routinely included in national food consumption surveys such as NHANES and CSFII. The Adequate Intakes (AIs) for calcium established by IOM are 500 mg/day for ages 1 to 3 years, 800 mg/day for ages 4 to 8 years, 1300 mg/day for ages 9 to 18 years, 1000 mg/day for ages 19 to 50 years, and 1200 mg/day for ages 51 years and over.[58]

Mean total (diet, dietary supplements, antacids) intakes of calcium fall short of AIs, especially for teenage girls, women, and older males (Table 15.4). During 1988 to 1994 mean calcium intakes for females decreased from a peak at 2 to 8 years of age (789 mg/day) to about 776 mg/day for women 50 years of age and older. Calcium intakes for males peaked at 9 to 19 years of age (1016 mg/day) and declined to about 851 mg/day for ages 50 years and over.[86] In issuing its recommendations, the Institute of Medicine indicated that there is a great disparity between recommended calcium values and current dietary

TABLE 15.4

Percent of the U.S. Population Meeting the Adequate Intake (AI) for Calcium, 1988–1994

	Dietary Intake (Food)			Total Intake (Food + Supplements + Antacids)		
Age and Sex	Mean (mg)	Median (mg)	% Meeting AI	Mean (mg)	Median (mg)	% Meeting AI
Males						
2–8 y	868	853	88	875	856	89
9–19 y	1003	989	51	1016	994	52
20–49 y	920	872	60	982	906	64
50+ y	778	717	30	851	762	35
2+ y	895	862	55	945	889	58
Females						
2–8 y	780	767	79	789	773	79
9–19 y	728	721	17	746	729	19
20–49 y	657	624	31	759	672	40
50+ y	610	564	13	776	663	27
2+ y	667	637	29	765	696	36
Total						
2–8 y	826	820	84	833	824	84
9–19 y	865	857	34	881	865	35
20–49 y	786	728	45	868	785	52
50+ y	685	633	21	809	708	30
2+ y	777	738	41	852	785	47

Source: NHANES III.

patterns.[39] Many individuals are not consuming sufficient intakes to meet their requirements and reduce the likelihood that they will develop osteoporosis.

Dairy products provide three-fourths of the dietary calcium intake in U.S. diets, and the dietary intake of calcium parallels what is known about intake of dairy products, i.e., that milk consumption begins to decline for females in their teenage years and remain low throughout life (except perhaps during pregnancy and lactation, when women are advised to drink milk). Milk consumption is also generally low among older men and women. Monitoring data from the 1987-88 NFCS showed that 50% of dietary calcium came from milk and milk products, 20% from milk and cheese as ingredients in mixed dishes, and 30% from all other food groups.[87] Additional USDA data indicate that between 1909 and 1990 dairy products comprised approximately 75% of calcium intake, indicating that the major contributing source has not changed a great deal.[58]

Because information on the use of dietary supplements and antacids was collected in NHANES III, it is possible to estimate the total intake of calcium from all sources. About 17% of the population reported the use of supplemental calcium in the diet in 1988 to 1994.[86] Table 15.4 indicates that these additional non-food sources of calcium in the diet have little overall impact on the percentage of the population meeting the AI for calcium. Overall, children ages 2 to 8 years are most likely to meet the recommended adequate intakes of calcium, with food sources providing the majority of calcium intake. In fact, just approximately 52% of calcium for children ages 2 to 18 years is derived from milk. For children 2 to 5 years, milk contributes almost 60% of calcium, for those 6 to 11 years milk contributes about 54% of calcium, and it contributes 46% of calcium to the diets of 12- to 18-year-olds.[88] Other calcium sources for children ages 2 to 18 include cheese (14%), yeast bread (7%), ice cream/sherbet/frozen yogurt (3%), and cakes/cookies/quickbreads/donuts (2.3%).

Physiological Assessment of Calcium Status

About 99% of body calcium is in the skeleton, and its primary function is structural, i.e., to build and maintain bones and teeth. The remaining body calcium is in blood, extracellular fluid, muscle, and other tissues, where it plays roles in vascular contraction and vasodilation, muscle contraction, nerve transmission, and glandular secretion. Blood levels of calcium remain relatively constant even in people with osteoporosis (decreased bone mass). The calcium is removed from the bone to maintain blood levels. Calcium metabolism and bone metabolism are highly integrated and correlated. Osteoporosis takes many years to develop and is usually not diagnosed until later years, such as when a fracture occurs.

Unfortunately, there have not been large-scale survey methods that are both reliable and cost-efficient for determining physiological calcium status until recently. In NHANES III, bone density was measured for the first time in a nationally representative sample of Americans. Among females 50 years of age and older, osteopenia (less than optimal bone density) at the total femur occurred in 42% of non-Hispanic whites, 37% of Mexican-Americans, and 28% of non-Hispanic blacks. Prevalence estimates for osteoporosis at the total femur in these three groups were 17, 12, and 8%, respectively.[89] Research is focused on developing and interpreting biochemical markers related to bone resorption, bone turnover, and osteoporosis risk.[90-92]

Relating Dietary and Physiological Data

Significant bone accretion occurs during adolescence and early adulthood. The low dietary calcium intakes by many adolescents and adults, particularly females, suggest that they are not getting the calcium they need to maintain optimal bone health and prevent age-related bone loss. Low peak bone density coupled with inadequate calcium intake in subsequent years may increase the risk of bone fracture in later years. Osteopenia and osteoporosis are both associated with inadequate bone mineral, especially calcium. Fractures resulting from osteoporosis are a major cause of morbidity in post menopausal caucasian females in the U.S. Osteoporosis develops over several decades of life and may not be apparent until a fracture occurs. Although loss of bone mineral is related to dietary intake of calcium, there are also other important considerations with regard to this condition.

The link between dietary calcium intake and bone status (osteoporosis) is not always direct. Dietary intake of calcium may not be a good predictor of physiological calcium status in some population groups or individuals because of the following confounding factors:

Calcium intake:

- Calcium intake collected in national surveys captures only recent (1 to 2 days) dietary intake, whereas osteoporosis takes several decades to develop. NHANES III and NHANES 1999+ did include questions about the historical consumption of milk, although long-term intake is difficult for many people to report accurately.[93,94] In addition, dietary intake surveys tend to underestimate total food and energy intake, so that calcium intake from surveys may be underestimated as well.[95]
- The use of calcium supplements will increase calcium intake and may affect bone health.

Intake of other nutrients:

- If energy intake has not been adequate (as with malnutrition or severe dieting), there may not be sufficient protein or sufficient amounts of other nutrients to help build or maintain bone. Bone is a complex tissue with a steady turnover rate that requires many nutrients. Even if calcium is adequate, the bone may not form properly if other important nutrients are lacking.
- Excess protein intake, especially from animal sources, may lead to increased excretion of calcium in the urine. IOM (1997) points out that while dietary protein intake increases urinary calcium excretion, inadequate protein intakes (34 g/day) are associated with poor general health and poor recovery from osteoporotic hip fractures.
- Dietary phylloquinone (vitamin K-1) or phylloquinone status may be associated with age-related bone loss.[96-98]
- The effects of caffeine on the skeleton are modest at calcium intakes of 800 mg/day or higher.[39]
- The Institute of Medicine[39] reviewed the relationship between salt intake and bone health, and concluded that indirect evidence indicates that dietary salt has a negative effect on the skeleton, although the effect of a change in sodium intake on bone loss and fracture rates has not been reported. IOM (1997) concluded that available evidence does not warrant different calcium intake requirements for individuals according to their salt consumption.

Role of genetics:

- Blacks and Asians experience more lactose intolerance than whites and tend to eat fewer dairy products than whites. Although blacks and Asians tend to have lower calcium intakes than whites, they do not necessarily show an increase in the prevalence of osteoporosis. In the U.S., older persons of northern European origin have the lowest bone densities and highest fracture risks. About 75% of older blacks have bone densities above the fracture threshold. Thus, it appears that race or genetic background plays a role in the development of osteoporosis.

Physiological status:

- Decreased estrogen production at menopause is associated with accelerated bone loss, particularly from the lumbar spine, for about five years.[99] Estrogen replacement therapy at menopause is one approach to help prevent bone loss and osteoporosis in women for whom no contraindications are present.
- Decreased calcium absorption with age is well recognized and may be due in part to low vitamin D intake. Vitamin D deficiency may play a role in hip fractures of those over 70 years. Older people often have decreased vitamin D intake because most dietary vitamin D comes from vitamin D-fortified milk, a food not preferred by older persons. In addition, older persons have decreased conversion of vitamin D to its active form in the skin. This may be due do decreased vitamin D metabolism, decreased sun exposure (sunlight is required for the conversion), and/or use of sunscreen (which blocks sunlight) to prevent skin cancer.
- Pregnancy and lactation, especially repeated pregnancies and periods of lactation, may create an increased body requirement for calcium, which, if not met, may lead to decreased bone calcium in the mother.
- Some medications interfere with calcium absorption and function.
- Some endocrine disorders may affect calcium balance and status.
- Weight-bearing exercise is very important to maintain bone health. Negative calcium balance may result from immobilization, illness, or lack of exercise.[100,101]

Public Nutrition Policy Regarding Calcium

In addition to the national dietary data, which suggest that calcium intakes are below recommended levels for girls, women, and older adults, and the physiological data regarding the incidence of osteopenia and osteoporosis in the U.S. population, there are also epidemiological data linking age-related osteopenia to lifetime calcium intake. These data support the suspected relationship between dietary calcium intake and bone health. The Third Report on Nutrition Monitoring in the U.S.[58] states,

> Many Americans are not getting the calcium they need to maintain optimal bone health and prevent age-related bone loss. Achieving peak bone mass and maintaining bone mass appear to be related to adequate calcium intake in adolescence and early adulthood. Because of the high rates of bone accretion during adolescence, continued monitoring of calcium intake is important.

The report classifies calcium as a "current public health issue" along with food energy, total fat, saturated fatty acids, cholesterol, alcohol, iron, and sodium and recommends the "development of interpretive criteria to link monitoring data to functional outcomes or health outcomes."

Nutrition monitoring data on calcium intake and calcium-containing foods were used to make scientific recommendations at the 1994 NIH Consensus Conference on Optimal

Calcium Intake.[12] The U.S. policy on calcium is to continue to emphasize the consumption of dairy products through the Dietary Guidelines for Americans[31] and the Food Guide Pyramid, and to suggest alternatives (fish with bones, green leafy vegetables, legumes, calcium-fortified orange juice, calcium supplements) for those who do not consume dairy products (e.g., those who are vegans, lactose intolerant, allergic to milk, those who do not like dairy products, and those whose cultural diets do not include dairy products). The Food Guide Pyramid recommendations are for two servings of dairy products per day for adults 24 years of age and older, and 3 servings per day for children, teenagers, younger adults, and pregnant and lactating women.

Conclusion

The primary goal of the 1990 Ten-Year Comprehensive Plan, "to establish a comprehensive nutrition monitoring and related research program by collecting quality data that are continuous, coordinated, timely, and reliable; using comparable methods for data collection and reporting of results; conducting relevant research; and efficiently and effectively disseminating and exchanging information with data users" is still pertinent a decade later.[39] Nutrition monitoring data are needed to inform both research and policy agendas. It is through this intertwined relationship between monitoring, research, and policy that we can continue to effect change. Given the competing demands for limited national resources and resulting budget limitations, however, the goals for the nutrition monitoring program will continue to be evaluated against other competing national needs. Continued support is necessary to maintain and expand the nutrition monitoring program in the U.S.

References

1. Mason JB, Habicht JP, Tabatabai H, Valverde V. *Nutritional Surveillance.* Geneva: WHO, 1984.
2. Ostenso GL. *JADA* 84:1181; 1984.
3. U.S. Congress. P. L. 101-445. National Nutrition Monitoring and Related Research Act of 1990. Washington, DC: 101st Congress, October 22, 1990.
4. U.S. Department of Health and Human Services and U.S. Department of Agriculture. Ten-year comprehensive plan for the national nutrition monitoring and related research program. Federal Register, 58:32752-32806, June 11, 1993.
5. Kuczmarski MF, Kuczmarski RJ. In: *Modern Nutrition in Health and Disease,* 8th ed. Shils ME, Olson JA, Shike M, Eds. Philadelphia: Lea & Febiger, 1994:1506-1516.
6. U.S. Department of Health and Human Service. *Healthy People 2000: National Health Promotion and Disease Prevention Objectives.* DHHS Publication No. (PHS) 91-50212. Washington, DC: U.S. Government Printing Office, 1991.
7. U.S. Department of Health and Human Services. *Healthy People 2010.* Conference Edition in Two Volumes. U.S. Department of Health and Human Services. Washington, DC: U.S. Department of Health and Human Services, January, 2000.
8. National Cholesterol Education Program. Second Report of the Expert Panel on Detection, Evaluation, and Treatment of High Blood Cholesterol in Adults (Adult Treatment Panel II). NIH Publication No. 93-3095. Bethesda, MD: National Heart, Lung, and Blood Institute, 1993.
9. National Heart, Lung, and Blood Institute. Sixth report of the Joint National Committee on Detection, Evaluation, and Treatment of High Blood Pressure. DHHS Publ. No. 98-4080. Washington, DC: U.S. Department of Health and Human Services, November, 1997.

10. National Institutes of Health. *Obesity Res* 1998;6(2):51S-209S.
11. Centers for Disease Control and Prevention. *Morbidity and Mortality Weekly Report* 1998; 47(RR-3):1-29.
12. National Institutes of Health. NIH Consensus Statement: Optimal calcium intake. Bethesda, MD: National Institutes of Health, June 6-8, 1994;12(4).
13. U.S. Department of Health and Human Services. The Surgeon General's Report on Nutrition and Health. PHS Publication No. 88-50210. Washington, DC: U.S. Department of Health and Human Services, 1988.
14. National Research Council. Diet and Health. *Implications for Reducing Chronic Disease Risk.* Washington, DC: National Academy Press, 1989.
15. Committee on Military Nutrition Research, Food and Nutrition Board, Institute of Medicine. Military Nutrition Initiatives. Washington, DC: Institute of Medicine. IOM Report-91-05, February 25, 1991.
16. Life Sciences Research Office. Estimation of Exposure to Substances in the Food Supply. Anderson SA, ed. Prepared for the Food and Drug Administration. Bethesda, MD: Life Sciences Research Office, 1988.
17. Kuczmarski RJ. *Am Acad Pediatr News* 9:14; 1998.
18. Change in the Physical Dimensions of Children in the U.S.: Results from the National Health and Nutrition Examination Survey from the National Center for Health Statistics. Report to the U.S. Consumer Product Safety Commission. Hyattsville, MD. January 1998.
19. Life Sciences Research Office, Federation of American Societies for Experimental Biology. *J Nutr* 1990; 120S: 1559-1600.
20. Wehler CA. Community Childhood Hunger Identification Project: New Haven Risk Factor Study. Hartford, CT: Connecticut Association for Human Services; 1986.
21. Radimer KL, Olson CM, Campbell CC. *J Nutr* 120:1544; 1990.
22. Guyer B, Wehler C, Anderka M, Friede A, et al. *Mass J Community Health* Fall/Winter 1985-1986: 3-9.
23. Hamilton WL, Cook JT, Thompson WW, et al. *Household Food Security in the United States in 1995: Summary Report of the Food Security Measurement Project*. Alexandria, VA: U.S. Department of Agriculture, Food and Consumer Service; September 1997.
24. Briefel RR, Woteki CE. *J Nutr Educ* 1992; 24: 24S-28S.
25. Alaimo K, Briefel RR, Frongillo EA Jr, Olson CM. *Am J Public Health* 1998; 88: 419-426.
26. Basiotis PP. In: Haldeman VA, ed. *American Council on Consumer Interests 38th Annual Conference: The Proceedings*. Columbia, MO: 1992.
27. Rose D, Oliveira V. *Am J Public Health.* 1997; 87: 1956-1961.
28. Carlson SJ, Andrews MS, Bickel GW. *J Nutr* 1999.
29. Blumberg SJ, Bialostosky K, Hamilton WL, Briefel RR. *Am J Public Health* 1999 Aug; 89(8): 1231-4.
30. U.S. Department of Agriculture. U.S. Action Plan on Food Security: Solutions to Hunger. Washington, DC. March 1999.
31. U.S. Department of Agriculture and Department of Health and Human Services. Nutrition and Your Health: Dietary Guidelines for Americans, 5th ed. USDA Home and Garden Bulletin No. 232. Washington, DC: U.S. Government Printing Office, 2000.
32. Subar AS, Heimindinger J, Krebs-Smith SM, et al. 5 A Day for Better Health: A baseline study of American's fruit and vegetable consumption. Rockville, MD: National Cancer Institute, 1992.
33. Devaney B, Fraker TM. *J Policy Anal Management* 1986; 5(4): 725-41.
34. Centers for Disease Control and Prevention. Nutritional status of children participating in the Special Supplemental Nutrition Program for Women, Infants, and Children — United States, 1988-91. Morbidity and Mortality Weekly Report, Jan 26, 1995; 45(3): 65-69.
35. Crane NT, Wilson DB, Cook DA, Lewis CJ, et al. *Am J Public Health* 1995; 85: 660-666.
36. Lewis CJ, Crane NT, Wilson DB, Yetley EA. *Am J Clinical Nutr* 1999; 70: 198-207.
37. U.S. Department of Health and Human Services, Food and Drug Administration. Notice of final rule: food labeling: health claims and label statements; dietary fiber and cardiovascular disease; dietary fiber and cancer. *Federal Register* 2552-2605; 2537-2552, January 5, 1993.
38. Wright JW, Bialostosky K, Gunter EW, Carroll MD, et al. *Vital Health Stat* 1998; 11(243).

39. Institute of Medicine, Food and Nutrition Board. Dietary Reference Intakes for Calcium, Phosphorus, Magnesium, Vitamin D, and Fluoride. A Report of the Standing Committee on the Scientific Evaluation of Dietary Reference Intakes. Washington, DC: National Academy Press, 1997.
40. Institute of Medicine, Food and Nutrition Board. Dietary Reference Intakes for Thiamin, Riboflavin, Niacin, Vitamin B_6, Folate, Vitamin B_{12}, Pantothenic Acid, Biotin, and Choline: A Report of the Standing Committee on the Scientific Evaluation of Dietary Reference Intakes and its Panel on Folate, Other B Vitamins, and Choline and Subcommittee on Upper Reference Levels of Nutrients. Washington, DC: National Academy Press, 1998.
41. National Research Council. Recommended Dietary Allowances, 10th ed. Washington, D.C.: National Academy Press, 1989.
42. Sims LS. Research aspects of public policy in nutrition generating research questions to determine the impact of nutritional, agricultural, and health care policy and regulations on the health and nutritional status of the public. The Research Agenda for Dietetics Conference Proceedings. Chicago, IL: American Dietetic Association, 1993: 25-38.
43. Office of Science and Technology Policy, Executive Office of the President. Meeting the Challenge. A research agenda for America's Health, Safety, and Food. Washington, DC: Government Printing Office, February, 1996.
44. Pamuk E, Makuc D, Heck K, Reuben C, Lochner K. Socioeconomic status and health chartbook. Health, United States, 1998. Hyattsville, MD: National Center for Health Statistics, 1998.
45. Troiano RP, Flegal KM, Kuczmarski RJ, Campbell SM, Johnson CL. *Arch Pediatr Adolesc Med* 1995 Oct; 149(10): 1085-91
46. Ogden CL, Troiano RP, Briefel RR, Kuczmarski RJ, et al. *Pediatrics* 1997 Apr; 99(4): E1.
47. National Institute of Diabetes and Digestive and Kidney Diseases (NIDDK), National Institutes of Health, Weight-control Information Network (WIN), http://www.niddk.nih.gov/health/nutrit/win.htm.
48. Peterkin BB. *J Nutr* 1994 Sep; 124: 1836S-1842S.
49. *Food and Agriculture Act of 1977* (PL 95-113). Sec. 1428. Cong Rec 123, September 29, 1977.
50. U.S. Department of Health and Human Services, U.S. Department of Agriculture. Nutrition monitoring in the United States: A progress report from the Joint Nutrition Monitoring Evaluation Committee. DHHS Publication No. (PHS) 86-1255. Washington, DC: U.S. Government Printing Office, 1986.
51. Life Sciences Research Office. Nutrition monitoring in the United States: An update report on nutrition monitoring. DHHS Publication No. (PHS) 89-1255. Washington, DC: U.S. Government Printing Office, 1989.
52. U.S. Department of Health and Human Services, Interagency Committee on Nutrition Monitoring. Announcement of committee formation. 53 FR 26505 no. 134. Washington, DC: U.S. Government Printing Office, 1988.
53. Interagency Committee on Nutrition Monitoring. Nutrition monitoring in the United States: The directory of federal nutrition monitoring activities. DHHS Publication No. (PHS) 89-1255-1. Washington, DC: Public Health Service, 1989.
54. Interagency Board for Nutrition Monitoring and Related Research. Wright J, ed. Nutrition monitoring in the United States: The directory of federal and state nutrition monitoring activities. DHHS Publication No. (PHS) 92-1255-1. Hyattsville, MD: Public Health Service, 1992.
55. Interagency Board on Nutrition Monitoring and Related Research. The directory of federal and state nutrition monitoring and related research activities. Bialostosky K, ed. Washington, DC: Public Health Service, 1998.
56. Interagency Board on Nutrition Monitoring and Related Research. The directory of federal and state nutrition monitoring and related research activities. Bialostosky K, ed. Washington, DC: Public Health Service, 2000. http://www.cdc.gov/nchs/data/direc-99/pdf.
57. Interagency Board for Nutrition Monitoring and Related Research. Nutrition Monitoring in the United States. Chartbook I: Selected Findings from the National Nutrition Monitoring and Related Research Program. Ervin B, Reed D, eds. DHHS Publication No. (PHS) 93-1255-2. Hyattsville, MD: Public Health Service, 1993.

58. Life Sciences Research Office, Federation of American Societies for Experimental Biology. Third report on nutrition monitoring in the United States: Vol. 1 and 2. Prepared for the Interagency Board for Nutrition Monitoring and Related Research. Washington, DC: U.S. Government Printing Office, 1995.
59. U.S. Department of Health and Human Services and Department of Agriculture. Proposed Ten-Year Comprehensive Plan for the National Nutrition Monitoring and Related Research Program. Federal Register, October 29, 1991; 91-25967: SS716-55767.
60. Briefel R. Nutrition monitoring in the U.S. In: *Present Knowledge in Nutrition,* 7th edition. EE Ziegler and LLJ Filer, Jr., eds. ILSI Press, Washington, DC. 1996. ch 52.
61. Kuczmarski MF, Moshfegh AJ, Briefel RR. *J Am Diet Assoc* 1994; 94: 753-60.
62. Woteki CE, Wong FL. Interpretation and utilization of data from the National Nutrition Monitoring System. In *Research. Successful Approaches.* Monsen ER, ed. American Dietetic Association, Mexico. 1992.
63. Woteki CE. Conference Proceedings. *J Am Dietetic Assoc* pp 39-48; 1993.
64. U.S. Department of Health and Human Services. National Center for Health Statistics. Third National Health and Nutrition Examination Survey, 1988-94, Reference manuals and reports (CD-ROM). Hyattsville, MD: Centers for Disease Control and Prevention, 1996. Available from the National Technical Information Service (NTIS), Springfield, VA. Acrobat .PDF format; includes access software: Adobe Systems Inc. Acrobat Reader 2.1.
65. Randall B, Bartlett S, Kennedy S. Study of WIC Participant and Program Characteristics, 1996. Alexandria, VA: U.S. Department of Agriculture, Food and Nutrition Service. August, 1998.
66. Centers for Disease Control and Prevention. From Data to Action. CDC's Public Health Surveillance for Women, Infants and Children. Wilcox LS, Marks JS, eds. Public Health Service. Washington, DC. 1994.
67. Hamilton WL, Cook JT, Thompson WW, Buron LF, et al. Measures of food security, food insecurity, and hunger in the United States in 1995: Technical report of the food security measurement study. Alexandria, VA: U.S. Department of Agriculture, Food and Consumer Service, July, 1997.
68. Burghardt JA, Devaney BL, Gordon AR. *Am J Clin Nutr* 1995; 61: 252S-257S.
69. Heaton AW, Levy AS. *J Nutr Educ* 1995; 27: 182-90.
70. Levy AS, Heaton AW. *Ann Intern Med* 1993; 119: 661-6.
71. Heimendinger J, Van Duyn MA, Chapelsky D, Foerster S, et al. *J Public Health Manag Pract* 1996; 2(2): 27-35.
72. Schucker RE, Levy AS, Tenney JE, Mathews O. *J Nutr Educ* 1992; 24(2): 75-81.
73. Serdula MK, Williamson DF, Anda RF, Levy A, et al. *Am J Public Health* 1994; 84: 1821-4.
74. Youth Risk Behavior Surveillance — United States, 1997. MMWR 47 (SS-3). August 14, 1998.
75. O'Brien T. Office of Food Labeling, Center for Food Safety and Applied Nutrition, Food and Drug Administration. Status of Nutrition Labeling of Processed Foods: 1995 Food Label and Package Survey (FLAPS). Washington, DC: Food and Drug Administration. 1996.
76. Brecher S. Office of Food Labeling, Center for Food Safety and Applied Nutrition, Food and Drug Administration. Status of Serving Size in the Nutrition Labeling of Processed Foods: Food Label and Package Survey (FLAPS). Washington, DC: Food and Drug Administration. 1997.
77. Schakel SF, Buzzard IM, Gebhardt SE. *J Food Comp Anal* 10: 102-114. 1997
78. Haytowitz DB, Pehrsson PR, Smith J, Gebhardt SE, et al. *J Food Comp Anal* 1996; 9(4): 331-364.
79. Holden JM, Davis CS. Strategies for sampling: The assurance of representative values. In: Quality and Accessibility of Food-Related Data. Greenfield, H, AOAC International 105-117. 1995.
80. Perloff BP, Rizek RR, Haytowitz DH et al. *J Nutr* 120: 1530-4. 1990.
81. Ervin RB, Wright JD, Kennedy-Stephenson J. *Vital Health Stat 11.* 1999 Jun; (244): i-iii, 1-14.
82. International Conference on Nutrition, Food and Agriculture Organization of the United Nations/World Health Organization Joint Secretariat for the Conference. The International Conference on Nutrition: World Declaration and Plan of Action for Nutrition, Rome; 1992.
83. Calloway CW. *J Am Dietetic Assoc* 1984: 1179-1180.
84. Brown Jr. GE (1984) *J Am Dietetic Assoc* 84: 1185-1188.

85. National Center for Health Statistics. Unpublished data from the third National Health and Nutrition Examination Survey. April 2000.
86. Forbes AL, Stephenson MG. *J Am Dietetic Assoc* 1984; 84: 1189-1193.
87. Fleming KH, Heimbach JT. *J Nutr* 1994; 124: 1426S-1430S.
88. Subar AF, Krebs-Smith SM, Cook A, Kahle LL. 1989-1991. *Pediatrics* 1998 Oct; 102(4 Pt 1): 913-23.
89. Looker AC, Orwoll ES, Johnston CC Jr, Lindsay RL, et al. *J Bone Miner Res* 1997 Nov; 12(11): 1761-8.
90. Garnero P, Hausherr E, Chapuy M-C, Marcelli C, et al. *J Bone Miner Res* 1996; 11: 1531-1538.
91. Rico H, Relea P, Crespo R, Revilla M, et al. *J Bone Joint Surg* 1995; 77-B: 148-151.
92. Hannon R, Blumsohn A, Naylor K, Eastell R. *J Bone Mineral Res* 1998; 13(7): 1124-1133.
93. Murphy S, Khaw KT, May H, Compston JE. *BMJ* 1994 Apr 9; 308(6934): 939-41.
94. Soroko S, Holbrook TL, Edelstein S, Barrett-Connor E. *Am J Public Health* 1994 Aug; 84(8): 1319-22.
95. Bingham SA. *Nutr Abst Rev* 1987; 57: 705-42.
96. Feskanich D, Weber P, Willett WC, Rockett H, Booth SL, Colditz GA. *Am J Clin Nutr* 69: 74-79, 1999.
97. Liu G, Peacock M. *Calcified Tissue Int* 62: 286-289, 1998.
98. Szulc P, Arlot M, Chapuy MC, Duboeuf F, et al. *J Bone Miner Res* 9: 1591-1595, 1994.
99. Gallagher JC, Goldgar D, Moy A. *J Bone Miner Res* 2: 491-496, 1987.
100. Frost HM. *Bone Miner* 2: 73-85, 1987.
101. Specker BL. *J Bone Miner Res* 11: 1539-1544, 1996.

16

Clinical Nutrition Studies: Unique Applications

Marlene M. Most, Valerie Fishell, Amy Binkoski, Stacie Coval, Denise Shaffer Taylor, Guixiang Zhao, and Penny Kris-Etherton

Nutrition research is the hallmark of establishing nutrient requirements and giving dietary guidance to promote health and wellbeing throughout life. Over the years it has been an active area of investigation, leading to the discovery of many important findings that have provided the basis for dietary guidelines and recommendations. Until recently, resources describing the design, implementation, and management of clinical nutrition studies were limited. Because of the growing interest and activities in clinical nutrition research, a number of important resources are now available that describe key aspects of conducting clinical nutrition studies. These resources (i.e., books and journal articles) are listed in Table 16.1. They provide detailed information about all aspects of conducting nutrition research with human participants. Collectively, they are a wealth of information for all researchers interested in and actively involved with human nutrition research. Indeed, these resources are a true "goldmine" to the field for standard studies, including those that employ either a single- or multicenter model. However, there are many studies that are uniquely different, presenting what may seem to be insurmountable challenges with respect to the experimental design, diet design, participant population studied, and feeding model utilized. For the most part, these have not been discussed in detail in the publications listed in Table 16.1.

Thus, the purpose of this section is to describe unique challenges in human nutrition research applications and provide guidance about how they can be effectively managed to maintain tight experimental control. First, we have included a variety of forms that were developed for different nutrition studies we have conducted that are not available in other resources. These forms deal with important aspects of conducting a well-controlled feeding study. They can be adapted to other human nutrition studies that vary in design from more typical protocols. Second, we provide descriptions of studies that illustrate challenges in the design and conduct of clinical nutrition studies, with notes on how these were handled.

Forms and Documentation for Assuring Dietary Protocol Compliance

Essential to all controlled feeding studies is recruiting participants who not only meet the eligibility criteria that have been defined, but are also willing to adhere to all aspects of

0-8493-2705-9/01/$0.00+$1.50

TABLE 16.1

Resources for Information on the Conduct of Clinical Nutrition Studies

Dennis, BH, Ershow, AG, Obarzanek, E, Clevidence, BA. *Well-Controlled Diet Studies in Humans.* The American Dietetic Association, Chicago, IL, 1999.
Dennis, BH, Kris-Etherton, PM. Designing and Managing a Small Clinical Trial. In: *Research, Successful Approaches,* pp. 151-170. Edited by E. Monsen. The American Dietetic Association, Chicago, IL, 1992.
Dennis, BH, Stewart, P, Hua-Wang, C, Champagne, C, Windhauser, M, Ershow, A, Karmally, W, Phillips, K, Stewart, K, Van Heel, N, Farhat-Wood, A, Kris-Etherton, PM. Diet design for a multicenter controlled feeding trial: The DELTA Program. *JADA* 1998; 98: 766-776.
Obarzanek, E, Moore, TJ. The Dietary Approaches to Stop Hypertension (DASH) Trial. *JADA* 1999; 8: S1-S104.

the experimental protocol. Hence, they serve as partners in research with the investigative team. Also important are the day-to-day operations that depend largely on the proper preparation, delivery, and consumption of the diets and adherence to study protocol by the participants. For many studies the diets are the treatments, and therefore must be strictly delivered as set forth by the protocol. Forms to assist with participant selection and documentation of diet adherence activities are needed to assure quality.

Recruiting Participants

The major goal of recruitment is to enroll the required number of participants necessary for the study within the projected timeline and within the budget constraints. The recruitment of potential study participants can be accomplished in many ways, and will be guided by inclusion/exclusion criteria set forth in the study protocol. Reaching the target study population is key. For example, post-menopausal women would more likely see an advertisement in a community weekly than, obviously, in a high school newspaper. Therefore, recruitment tactics focus on the groups that need to be recruited, and are planned accordingly. The Institutional Review Board (IRB) must clear all recruiting materials before use to assure that the information is not misleading and the study is accurately represented. Detailed information about recruiting is available elsewhere (see Table 16.1), but is briefly discussed below.

Advertisements in the local media are effective recruitment tools. Newspaper advertisements can be general in nature or contain specific information about the study (see example, Figure 16.1). An advantage of a newspaper advertisement is that it reaches a large audience, while a disadvantage is that it can be expensive. The ability to target a specific audience may be somewhat limited unless the newspaper audience is narrow, such as for business reports or campus newspapers. Radio and television advertisements also can be expensive and are limited in the amount of information that can be disseminated about the study. However, it may be possible to obtain free radio and television advertising by submitting the material as a public service announcement. Local morning or early evening magazine-format programs often welcome an interview with the study investigator, who can describe the study and ask for volunteers.

Other recruiting tools include speaking about the study to different local community organizations, such as the Lions clubs or church groups. Although time consuming, it targets a specific audience. Health fairs provide a community service as well as a recruitment opportunity. For example, free blood pressure screenings will help identify potential participants for a study examining blood pressure-lowering diets. Distributing and posting flyers on bulletin boards in supermarkets, drug stores, or doctors' offices is an excellent avenue for communicating the need for study participants. Mass mailings of a brochure, postcard, or letter describing the study can be sent to a target population. This tends to

Is Eating Cocoa and Chocolate Good for You??

We are currently recruiting participants for a nutrition study aimed at determining whether cocoa and chocolate contain antioxidants that may be good for you.

The study dates are June 1–June 29 and July 12–Aug 10. You must complete both 4 week periods.

(There is a break from June 29 to July 12th)

You may qualify if you meet all of these criteria:

- You must be healthy and between the ages of 20–67 (male or pre-menopausal female);
- You must not be a smoker and cannot consume alcohol, coffee, or tea during the study;
- You must be willing to eat only foods (including cocoa and chocolate) provided for the study and come to the study center on University Park campus for breakfast and dinner 5 days/week — food for lunches and the weekend will be packed for takeout;
- You must not have diabetes mellitus or uncontrolled (> 140/95) high blood pressure or other serious health conditions;
- You must not be pregnant, nursing, or planning to get pregnant.

All food will be provided during the study along with monetary compensation. If you are interested in participating in this study, please call (814) 863-3168, give your name, mention that you are interested in the Cocoa Study, and give us a number where you can be reached.

FIGURE 16.1
Sample subject recruitment advertisement.

be an effective tool but is labor-intensive and costly for the materials, mailing list, and postage. Email also can be used for recruitment but, like mass mailings, it sometimes requires the purchase of the mailing list.

Regardless of the recruitment method used, careful records are required to track the recruitment progress, and more importantly, to document that the eligibility criteria are being met.

Screening Potential Participants

Once a person expresses interest and contacts the recruiter, the screening process begins. The initial contact should be used to exclude those who do not meet the most easily identifiable criteria (see Telephone interview form, Figure 16.2). Obviously, a smoker who calls to ask about a study that is recruiting only non-smokers would be excluded quickly during the telephone screening process. Another example would be the screening of a post-menopausal woman who is taking hormone replacement therapy (HRT) when the study protocol excludes women on HRT. These initial exclusions early in the recruiting process prevent bringing people in for the more expensive clinic visits, and thus prevent

Folate Study
TELEPHONE INTERVIEW FORM
Pennsylvania State University

Subject ID: ____________
Today's Date: __/__/__
Reviewer's Initials: ______

Before asking any questions, please read the following paragraph to obtain verbal consent to conduct the telephone interview:
"We received your message that you are interested in participating in the Folate Study. I would like to ask you a series of questions about your willingness to participate in the study, your past medical history, and your current lifestyle behaviors. If you agree to answer these questions, and it is then determined that you meet the criteria for this study, we will schedule you for a screening visit. Are you willing to answer a series of questions, which will take about 15 minutes?"
1. ☐ Yes (continue with interview)
2. ☐ **No** (thank them for their time and interest)

Full Name w/middle initial ______________________________ DOB ____________
Local address ____
Home # ____________ Work # ______________

1.	Are you a female between the ages of 19–35 years inclusive?	☐ Yes	☐ **No**
2.	Do you plan to remain in the area for the duration of the study?	☐ Yes	☐ **No**
3.	Are there any personal reasons (e.g., family problems, vacations, child care difficulties, etc.) that would keep you from participating in the study?	☐ **Yes**	☐ No
4.	Are there any professional reasons (e.g., job-related travel, irregular work schedule, conferences, etc.) that would keep you from participating in the study?	☐ **Yes**	☐ No
5.	There is a variety of foods in the Folate Study. Are there any foods you refuse to eat, are allergic to, or for whatever reason have to avoid?	☐ **Yes**	☐ No

Go to Food List

Listed are foods included on the diet for this study. I will go through the list — tell me if there is any food you cannot or would not eat.

FOODS	Ok?	FOODS	Ok?
Turkey breast		Penne pasta	
Zucchini (fresh)		Celery	
Green olives		Mayo dressing	
Potatoes		Radishes	
Dill pickles		Onion	
Tuna		Sweet relish	
Mayonnaise		Canned pears	
Canned peaches		Applesauce	
Grapes (fresh)		Watermelon (fresh)	
Canned pineapple		Blueberries	
Jello		Potato chips (regular/barbecue)	
Banana muffin		Cinnamon-apple muffin	
Blueberry muffin		Pineapple-orange muffin	
Beef		Mashed potatoes w/ gravy	
Chicken breast		Seasoned rice (thyme, oregano, parsley flakes)	

FIGURE 16.2
Telephone interview form.

Spaghetti		Meatballs & marinara sauce	
Ground turkey		Taco seasoning	
Cornbread muffin		Skim milk	
Crackers		Pretzels	

6. Do you currently smoke?	☐ **Yes**	☐ No
a. If No, have you ever smoked before?	☐ **Yes**	☐ No
1. If Yes, how long since your last cigarette? ________		
7. Are you willing to discontinue your consumption of alcohol for the entire 8 weeks of the study?	☐ **Yes**	☐ No
8. Do you have access to the following appliances at home/apartment/dorm:		
Refrigerator	☐ Yes	☐ **No**
Freezer	☐ Yes	☐ **No**
Microwave or oven or toaster oven	☐ Yes	☐ **No**
Explain that they will take Sat/Sun meals home on Friday and will need a place to store/cook their food		
9. It is important to maintain your current body weight for the duration of the study. Are you willing to maintain your current body weight?	☐ Yes	☐ **No**

Medical and Lifestyle Information

Do you have any of the following medical conditions:

1. Heart disease	☐ **Yes**	☐ No
2. Diabetes	☐ **Yes**	☐ No
3. High blood pressure (hypertension) treated with medication	☐ **Yes**	☐ No
4. Renal or kidney failure	☐ **Yes**	☐ No
5. Gastrointestinal condition such as Crohn's disease, irritable bowel syndrome, ulcer, or history of bowel surgery	☐ **Yes**	☐ No
6. History of blood clotting disorder	☐ **Yes**	☐ No
7. Liver disease such as cirrhosis	☐ **Yes**	☐ No
8. Condition that requires the use of steroid medication	☐ **Yes**	☐ No
9. Gout requiring treatment	☐ **Yes**	☐ No
10. Recent history of depression or mental condition requiring medication within the last 6 months	☐ **Yes**	☐ No
11. Anemia	☐ **Yes**	☐ No
12. Sickle cell anemia	☐ **Yes**	☐ No
13. Lung disease such as chronic bronchitis or emphysema	☐ **Yes**	☐ No
14. Cancer, active within the last 10 years	☐ **Yes**	☐ No
15. Thyroid disease or thyroid problem requiring treatment such as iodine or surgery, or taking medication for your thyroid	☐ **Yes**	☐ No
16. Do you have any other medical condition not previously mentioned?		
If Yes, specify: ________	☐ Yes	☐ **No**
a. **If Yes, is the subject eligible?**	☐ **Yes**	☐ No
17. Do you take any type of doctor-prescribed medication?	☐ **Yes**	☐ No
If Yes, specify medication and reason: ________		
a. If Yes, is the subject eligible?	☐ Yes	☐ **No**
b. If she takes birth control, explain she has to be willing to forego its use for the duration of the study (8 weeks) and has to have a 2-week wash-out period before starting. This means she has to finish her entire packet of pills and from that last day she starts the 2-week wash-out period.	☐ Yes	☐ **No**

FIGURE 16.2
Continued.

18. Do you take any type of self-prescribed medication, vitamin, mineral, or other supplement (including garlic or ginseng?)	☐ **Yes**	☐ No
If Yes, specify medication/supplement: ________		
a. If Yes, are you willing to discontinue? ________	☐ Yes	☐ **No**
19. Are you on a special diet prescribed by a doctor or self-prescribed?	☐ **Yes**	☐ No
If Yes, specify: ________		
________	☐ Yes	☐ No
a. If Yes, is the subject eligible? ________		
20. Do you exercise more than 8 hours a week or play sports regularly?	☐ **Yes**	☐ No
If Yes, please describe: ________		
21. Are you willing to have a pregnancy test 3x during the 8-week study?	☐ Yes	☐ **No**
22. In order to assess folate, red blood cells, and homocysteine, blood will be taken at the beginning of the study and once every week after that. There will be a total of 9 blood draws, with no more than 2 tubes of blood taken each time. Are you willing to do this?	☐ Yes	☐ **No**

Note: This form has to be reviewed by the Study Coordinator		
If any of the bolded boxes are marked, the subject is ineligible.		
Is the subject eligible?	☐ Yes	☐ **No**
a. If Yes, go to Women's History Form and then schedule clinic visit.		
b. If No, thank subject for his/her time and terminate the interview.		

FIGURE 16.2
Continued.

wasting resources in terms of staff time and money. For those who pass the initial telephone interview, further screening is required. They will come to the study site for clinical laboratory tests or other measurements to assure that they are relatively healthy and meet all the study eligibility criteria.

To assist with identifying whether someone would be able to adequately follow the dietary protocol, general dietary information may be gathered in questionnaire form during the study screening visits. The questions identify participants who cannot or will not eat any foods due to religious reasons, allergies, or severe physical discomfort. A complete list of study foods or a copy of the study menus in layman's terms may be reviewed with potential participants. This information is especially important when particular foods in the menu cannot be substituted.

Other useful screening information includes whether a person can safely store and prepare foods to be consumed away from the clinical site, and environmental, family, or work situations that may make adherence to the protocol difficult (see General dietary questionnaire, Figure 16.3). For persons whose adherence may appear to be questionable, a meeting with the study dietitian may help to determine if reasonable provisions can be made within the protocol requirements, or they may be deemed ineligible. For example, participants who have lactose intolerance may be allowed to use lactose digestive aids and be eligible. Someone who does not have adequate facilities in their home to store and prepare study foods would be ineligible to participate in the study.

The following questions are related to your overall eating environment. Your answers will help the staff determine ways they can make your participation in the study more enjoyable.

	Yes	No
1. Do you foresee any problems transporting, storing, refrigerating, and warming your study foods when you are away from our center?		
2. Do you participate in activities where food is served, such as sporting events, religious gatherings, business meetings, etc.?		
3. Will any holidays, birthdays, family reunions, vacations, etc., occur during the period you are on the study?		
4. If you are responsible for preparing meals in your household, will this make it difficult for you to meet study requirements?		
5. Will anyone in your household be affected or inconvenienced by your participation in this study? If yes, who are they and how will they be affected?		
6. Will your employment (e.g., job transfer) or work hours (e.g., moving to a night shift) change during the study?		
7. Do you, or anyone in your household, work in the food service industry (cafeteria, bakery, restaurant, etc.)? If yes, do you eat any meals or snacks at work either as a requirement of your job or as a matter of convenience?		
8. If you have any concerns about the study, please write them in the space provided below (use the back of this page if you need additional space).		

Reviewed by (staff ID): ________

FIGURE 16.3
General dietary questionnaire.

Orientation Session

When taking part in a feeding study, it is important that each participant carefully follow the dietary protocol. An orientation form that lists these guidelines may be developed and reviewed immediately prior to the actual study start date during an orientation session. Helpful information for the form would be instructions to finish all foods and beverages provided, squeeze condiment packets until empty, use a rubber spatula or bread to clean the plate, and eat fruit and vegetable peels as appropriate. Reminders to complete the daily forms, check for accuracy of the meals, and not make substitutions may be listed. A guideline stating what to do if participants find that they are too full or hungry is useful. Heating directions for takeout foods could also be included. A list of contact persons with telephone numbers is imperative for when questions or problems arise. Participants appreciate a copy of the beverage and seasoning guidelines that specify the types and amounts that may be consumed. If there are restrictions on mints or gum, these should be listed. Participants must be instructed in the safe handling of foods provided to be consumed off site. For example, a simple handout may be given that reminds participants to use a cooler to transport foods for longer than one hour, to refrigerate all perishable foods as soon as possible, and to not eat suspected spoiled foods, but to notify the staff immediately to avoid a missed meal.

Assuring Participant Diet Adherence

Participant adherence to the diet protocol is collected, usually on a daily basis (see Daily checklist, Figure 16.4) by the participant, and is subject to review by study staff. For this

Fat Challenge 2 **Pennington Biomedical Research Center**

Name ______________________ Date ______________

Please answer all questions below and place an "X" in appropriate column. Please fill in the additional information requested when necessary. Please return this form each day to the Pennington Metabolic Kitchen.

1. ______ Yes ______ No Were there any study foods you did not eat/drink on this day? Reasons include missing, spilled, or inedible food, illness or other.

Food/Drink	**Amount**	**Reason**

2. ______ Yes ______ No Did you eat or drink any foods that were not provided by the Metabolic Kitchen today? If yes, please give the food/drink (be very specific), the amount, and reason consumed.

Food/Drink	**Amount**	**Reason**

3. ______ Yes ______ No Did you consume any decaffeinated sugar-free beverages on this day? Record all beverages, including those provided by the Metabolic Kitchen.

Food/Drink	**Amount**
	oz.

4. **Did you eat any of the "unit foods" today?** **Y ____N ____**
How may "unit foods" did you eat? 0 1 2 3 4 5 Other ____

5. ______ Yes ______ No Is there anything you would like us to know in relation to your participation in this study?

FIGURE 16.4
Daily checklist.

reason, the participants must be encouraged to record honestly and must not feel that their participation is threatened in any way. The data, which document diet adherence and deviations, may be used to calculate daily energy and nutrient intakes and to compute a compliance score. The form, called a daily diary, daily log, or food and beverage intake form, may gather information for the following broad categories:

- The type and amount of study foods not eaten
- The type and amount of non-study foods eaten
- The type and amount of discretionary or "allowed" food items consumed
- The type and amount of beverages consumed, including coffee, tea, soft drinks, and alcoholic beverages
- The number of unit foods or calorie adjusters eaten
- Dietary supplements or over-the-counter medications taken
- Feedback regarding concerns or questions related to participation in the study

The forms should provide the participant's identification number and date for which diet information is obtained. It may also contain the kcalorie level for the participant, coded

ILSI
Weekly Monitoring Form
Pennsylvania State University

Subject ID: ________
Today's Date: __/__/__
Reviewer's Initials: ________

Week 1 2 3 4 5 6 7 8 9 10 11 12 13 14

Blood Draw Date

Date of blood draw 1: ___/___/___ **Date of blood draw 2:** ___/___/___

1. In the past week has your exercise level changed? ☐ **Yes** ☐ No
   a. If Yes, was it ☐ More Active ☐ Less Active ☐ No Exercise

2. Have you taken any vitamin, mineral, or other supplements in the past week? ☐ **Yes** ☐ No
   a. If Yes, specify: description ________ amount ________

3. Have you been ill in the past week? ☐ **Yes** ☐ No
   a. If Yes, describe illness: ________________

4. If you were ill in the past week, did your eating change as a result? ☐ **Yes** ☐ No
   a. If Yes, describe: ________________

If any of the bolded boxes are checked, please notify Study Coordinator

FIGURE 16.5
Weekly monitoring form.

treatment diet, a field for entering the participant's weight, and for females, menstruation information. The information gathered then may be coded by the study staff, either on the same form or another form, for data entry.

Another form for staff documentation of diet deviations may be used. This would provide a record of deviations observed during on-site meals or those called in to staff during times of off-site meals, such as weekends. If any study food or beverage is left on the meal tray and was unnoticed during the meal tray check, information regarding the food (i.e., type and amount) is recorded. Similarly, if a participant calls a staff member to report a deviation for an off-site meal (i.e., missing, lost, or spoiled food), the appropriate information is recorded. If discrepancies between the kitchen staff observations and information reported by the participant are found, the study dietitian should adjudicate those. In addition, the study protocol may require the participant to return uneaten portions of study-provided foods. The type and amount of food returned would be recorded on this form. Additional information may be collected regarding what was done with the food not consumed. For example, was the food given back to the participant to eat, replaced at the next meal and eaten, not replaced or not eaten? The data then may be coded for compliance measures and energy or nutrient calculations.

Usually on a weekly basis, the participant will complete another form that asks about general health-related items that might influence food intake or study outcomes (see Weekly monitoring form, Figure 16.5). For example, changes in exercise, any illnesses, and any medications or supplements taken may be reported. Queries for possible symptoms,

Diet D Menu 1						
Date: ___/___/___ Mm dd yy Day: M T W T F S S	Staff Initials	1500	2000	2500	3000	3500
Breakfast						
Orange juice		124.0	124.0	124.0	124.0	248.0
Puffed rice cereal		23.0	23.0	23.0	46.0	46.0
White bread		22.7	45.4	90.4	90.4	90.4
Butter		8.0	9.0	15.0	20.0	20.0
Sweets; jellies		0.0	10.0	10.0	10.0	10.0
Jellies, dietetic		14.2	0.0	0.0	0.0	0.0
Milk, whole		245.0	245.0	245.0	490.0	490.0
Lunch						
Sandwich package:						
*Turkey breast meat		35.0	50.0	56.7	56.7	75.0
*Mayonnaise, regular		4.3	5.0	6.0	9.0	9.0
*Iceberg lettuce		0.0	0.0	0.0	10.0	10.0
*White bread		45.4	45.4	45.4	45.4	90.8
Iceberg lettuce		24.0	24.0	24.0	40.0	40.0
Olive oil		0.0	2.0	2.0	10.0	8.0
Peaches, juice pack		127.6	127.6	127.6	127.6	127.6
Ginger Cookie		14.0	22.0	22.0	22.0	22.0

FIGURE 16.6
Food production form. Foods are indicated in grams for each energy level diet.

such as poor appetite, stuffy nose, fatigue, diarrhea, constipation, nausea, or headache could also be included as appropriate.

Food Production and Meal Assembly

Used in conjunction with standardized recipes, a food production form is followed for the preparation and portioning of all menu items (see Food production form, Figure 16.6). There will be a separate form for each diet and menu. It is usually helpful to color-code the forms according to diet treatment. An established menu sequence will determine which menu is to be served on each day of the study. For each menu, the portion sizes for the various kcalorie levels are listed. The number of participants receiving each kcalorie level for the corresponding diet is listed in the box above each kcalorie designation so that the kitchen staff knows how many servings are required. The food is prepared and portioned according to the list, and then the staff member responsible initials the item in the space provided. At times, it might be necessary to substitute a food item. Documentation of the deviation on the food production form or a separate form, to include the type of food and when it was used may be informative later when detailed diet information is required.

A tray assembly check sheet is valuable for assuring that all participants receive each menu item (see Tray assembly check sheet, Figure 16.7). Separate sheets may be needed for each kcalorie level, menu, and diet, and could be color-coded similar to the food production forms. As the tray is assembled, the item is checked off in the corresponding box for each participant and initialed by the staff to verify that all food items are provided. If the food production forms are used to assemble the foods, a tray assembly check sheet may be used as a quality assurance check. Similar procedures are followed for packed meals, checking off each item as it is placed in the takeout container.

Diet D Menu 1 1500 Kcal								
Date: ____/____/____ Mm dd yy Day: M T W T F S S	Name or I.D. #							
Breakfast								
Orange juice								
Puffed rice cereal (1 PC)*								
White bread (1 slice)								
Butter								
Dietetic jelly (1/2 oz.)								
Whole milk (1 PC)								
Staff Initials								
Lunch								
Turkey sandwich package								
Salad								
Salad dressing								
Peaches (1 PC)								
Ginger cookie (1 small)								
Staff Initials								
Snack								
Trail mix								
Staff Initials								

FIGURE 16.7
Tray assembly check sheet. * PC = portion control.

Another practical form for packed meals and/or snacks is a checklist of the menu items that participants use to verify that all items have been packed in their takeout containers (see Packed meal form, Figure 16.8). The form is attached to or placed inside the container, and the participant is instructed to contact a kitchen staff member if any item on the form is missing from the container. Menu cards also could be used in place of the form. These,

Diet D Menu 1

Name ____________________ **I.D.** ____________________ **Telephone Contact (__)___-___**
Day M T W T F Sa Su **Date** ___ ___ ___ **Packed by** ________________ **Meal B L D S**
(Circle One) **mm dd yy**

Breakfast	Lunch	Dinner
Packed	**Packed**	**Packed**
☐ Orange juice	☐ Turkey sandwich package	☐ Sirloin tips with gravy
☐ Puffed rice cereal (1 box)	☐ Salad	☐ Corn
☐ White bread (1 slice)	☐ Salad dressing	☐ Salad
☐ Butter	☐ Peaches (1 can)	☐ Salad dressing
☐ Dietetic jelly	☐ Ginger cookie (1 small)	☐ Roll
☐ Milk (1 carton)	☐	☐ Butter
☐	☐	☐ Applesauce

Unit Foods		Snack
# of Units	**Packed**	**Packed**
________	☐	☐ Trail mix
________	☐	☐

FIGURE 16.8
Packed meal form.

when placed on the on-site meal trays, also provide a means for the participant to double-check the accuracy of the menu items.

Training Dietary/Kitchen Staff

It is imperative that all staff members who will be involved in the preparation and delivery of research diets understand the strict procedures necessitated by the protocol. For example, they must know the acceptable ranges for gram weights when portioning various food items, how to read the food production forms, and cooking procedures. Those who will be interacting with the participants must know the dietary guidelines, such as allowed beverages and seasonings. The development of a training manual is useful so that staff can periodically review the standard procedures and have a reference available to answer any questions that may arise during the course of a study. Actual observation and/or a written test may be utilized to assess staff competencies. In addition, routine quality control checks are essential, and kitchen staffs who do not consistently meet the rigorous standards set for delivering the experimental diets must be relieved of this responsibility.

Quality Assurance of Diets

During the regular production of the menus, duplicate meals should be prepared and collected for monitoring quality assurance and for chemical analysis of target nutrients. The food should be prepared and weighed following the standard procedures. Ideally, food preparation staff should not know that these will be used for quality checks, but this may be difficult to disguise. One way to overcome possible bias is for the staff to prepare a meal for analysis identical to one prepared for a participant, and the two may be switched prior to serving. For portion weight checks, as each food for one menu is placed into a container, the weight of that food item is recorded and compared to what should be present. Any discrepancies should be noted. The person who made a mistake when weighing the food or assembling the meal can be identified by looking for his/her initials on the production sheets. Retraining of that individual may be necessary to alleviate any further errors. Once the entire menu is in the container it can be blended, and aliquots taken or frozen for later analysis. When the analysis is completed, the actual nutrient values may be compared to the expected nutrient values (from the database), especially for those being controlled.

A spot-checking procedure may be employed to monitor the accuracy of meals distributed to participants. Randomly selected meals and/or food items are checked for completeness and accuracy. If a problem is found, it is described, a plan of action for correction of the problem is detailed, and documentation of the action plan or followup is provided. Again, the person making the mistake should be retrained.

Miscellaneous Forms

The use of a food service sanitary inspection checklist for personnel, food handling, equipment, storage practices, dishwashing, and department areas is standard. Inspection of refrigerator and freezer temperatures also should be conducted on a regular basis. In a research kitchen, regular accuracy checks of the electronic balances should be documented. Use of a form that lists acceptable ranges is a practical way to indicate whether to recalibrate a balance. If foods are donated to the study, their expected delivery, date received, and accuracy may be tracked on a form that also includes a description of the food items, company, address, contact person, and telephone number.

Exit Interview

At the end of the study, an exit interview may be planned for each individual or for a group of participants. Information offered could include laboratory data gathered during the study, health risk assessments, and appropriate educational materials. In addition, anonymous input from completing participants about their experiences and views is helpful for planning future studies. For example, questions asking about favorite foods, disliked foods, and about the menus in general that were served during the study can provide information for improving future menus. Factors that made it easy or difficult to follow the study protocol may be assessed. Additional questions include how study staff treated participants and whether the subjects would recommend participating in a study to their friends. This information can be invaluable for improving future studies by increasing menu acceptability and making study participation a more enjoyable experience.

Unique Study Challenges and Strategies for Addressing Them

Clinical nutrition studies may present challenges at every stage; for example, with menu development, recruitment of participants, and finally, preparation and delivery of the experimental diets. Obstacles must be overcome for a successful outcome. For illustration, studies will be described that have dealt with unique and challenging situations with the population studied, experimental design employed, and experimental diet(s) fed to study participants. The conduct of multiple center clinical nutrition trials present their own challenges, which are discussed elsewhere (see Table 16.1).

Recruitment and Retention

A study was designed to evaluate the effects of diets high in polyunsaturated fatty acids/n-3 fatty acids (PUFA/n-3FA, accounting for 12% of energy), derived from walnuts and walnut oil with different levels of n-6/n-3 FA ratios (9:1 vs. 4:1), on multiple risk factors for cardiovascular disease (CVD). In this crossover study, we recruited 30 males and females, ages 45 to 65, so that the results could be somewhat generalized to a middle-aged population. Various study endpoints, including serum cytokines and the release of TNFα and IL-6 by polymorphonuclear cells, are affected by the menstrual cycle, so this dictated that premenopausal or postmenopausal females on hormone replacement therapy (HRT) be excluded to minimize confounding. All participants were to be healthy, overweight or mildly obese, having moderate hypercholesterolemia, and taking no medications. These eligibility criteria made recruitment efforts challenging. First, many people within this age group were taking nutrient supplements, cholesterol-lowering drugs, or medications for hypertension, diabetes, or rheumatoid arthritis, so were not eligible for the study. Second, many have families and it is difficult for one or both parents to come to the clinical site for breakfast and dinner each weekday for three six-week dietary periods. Third, postmenopausal women without HRT account for only a small proportion of this population.

Various recruitment strategies were used such as advertising by posters, in newspapers and on television, and sending advertising fliers to churches, senior or retired communities, and to individuals between the ages of 45 to 65. We even agreed to feed a couple in order to recruit one of them who qualified to be a study participant while the other did not. To overcome similar problems with recruiting persons in this age group, other clinical centers provide guest meal passes so that family members or friends may regularly join the study participants for meals.

Two studies that needed young females presented unique recruiting and retention situations. Participants with low iron status were required to observe the overloading effect of an iron supplement. Females, who generally have a lower iron status than males due to menstruation, were targeted. Therefore, participants were females, ages 19 to 47, with regular menstrual periods, in good general health and from all ethnic groups. Difficulties in recruiting occurred for several reasons in a college town. During the summer months the overall student population at the university diminishes greatly, presenting a problem by reducing the potential participant pool. Also, the prospect of strictly adhering to a controlled diet during the relaxing summer months provided another hurdle. The two-week break between diet periods was planned around the July 4 holiday and a summer arts festival to avoid further recruiting obstacles.

For this study and one that required females 18 to 22 years of age, weight concerns proved to be a barrier for recruiting. Many young women were trying to lose weight and did not want to maintain their current weight as required by the study protocols. In addition, women in this age group tend to be "fat phobic" and careful about their fat consumption. They were hesitant to consume diets that may have contained more fat than their usual diets. Therefore, it was important that the fats and oils were discreetly added to the study diets. This was accomplished by choosing meals such as turkey with dressing and mashed potatoes or stuffed flounder, which would readily accept the oils and fats without drawing attention.

Both recruitment and retention of participants were challenged in a study that compared whole-food diets with formula diets. For recruitment, potential participants sampled the formula diets. It was emphasized that the formula was all they would consume during two of the four diet periods. Once enrolled, participant retention became the paramount issue. One way of maintaining their participation in the study was to conduct a raffle during each diet period. Raffle items included tickets to a football game, a movie, and a Broadway show that came to campus. Another way was to prepare a portion of the daily formula as "ice cream." The "flavor of the day" was posted, and chocolate and strawberry flavors were always available. For the participants, this alleviated the boredom from having to always drink their meals. Many enjoyed telling their friends that they were on an "ice cream diet."

Providing specialized, prepackaged meals or foods to participants for daily consumption may make recruiting easier (i.e., more participants are willing to eat prepackaged foods at home, rather than having all meals served through a metabolic kitchen), yet challenges still abound as in other clinical nutrition studies. As one site of a year long, multicenter study testing the effect of a prepackaged meal plan on multiple CVD risk factors, 70 men and women with hyperlipidemia, hypertension, and/or Type 2 diabetes mellitus were recruited. Finding participants who met the entry criteria proved to be difficult in a small college town. Thus, the study was conducted simultaneously in a more urban location 90 miles away, where the university's medical school is located. Once all of the participants were recruited, problems arose with the weekly home delivery of the prepackaged, frozen meals. The food could not be left without a signature, which proved to be an obstacle. Participants sometimes received meals different than those they ordered, and they became bored with their limited food selection during the year-long study.

Food Products and Menu Planning

Cocoa powder is a rich source of antioxidants in the form of flavonoids. The Cocoa Study was conducted to evaluate the effects of a diet high in cocoa powder (22 g/day) and dark chocolate (16 g/day) on LDL oxidative susceptibility and total antioxidant capacity of plasma. The study employed a two-period, crossover design. Using a randomized diet treatment assignment, participants were fed the cocoa powder/dark chocolate diet (CP/DC) and an Average American Diet (AAD, control) for four weeks each. The cocoa powder and dark chocolate were incorporated into only one experimental diet, making it impossible to employ a blinded experimental diet design. Planning a study of chocolate would appear to be easy, but the cocoa powder and menu development actually presented some challenges.

First, it was necessary to control for components present in the cocoa powder and dark chocolate to "isolate" the flavonoids for testing their contribution to a possible antioxidant benefit. To do this, the cocoa butter present in the dark chocolate was included in a similar amount in the AAD. Other components included caffeine, theobromine, and fiber, since cocoa powder and dark chocolate contain these in addition to the flavonoids. The caffeine was supplemented in the AAD with diet cola, and 431 mg/day of pure theobromine in a gel capsule was provided. The fiber was equilibrated with bran cereal. In addition, the diets were designed to be low in non-CP/DC flavonoids. Thus, foods that were limited or excluded included tea, coffee, wine, onions, apples, beans, soybeans, orange juice, and grape juice.

Second, there was a fair amount of cocoa powder in the experimental diet, so the participants were sometimes required to add cocoa powder (about 15 g) to their milk (or any other menu item). They also could add a non-caloric sweetener to the "chocolate milk" if they chose to do so. The resulting beverage was notably different from commercially available chocolate milk and that prepared from chocolate syrups. Nonetheless, it was a menu item that the participants found acceptable, albeit different from what they were accustomed to drinking, and they were willing to consume it throughout the study.

Third, the cocoa powder and dark chocolate were incorporated into the diets in different ways to avoid monotony. The daily allotment of cocoa powder was also baked into cookies, muffins, and brownies that would be served at meals. This assured that the cocoa powder and dark chocolate would be consumed throughout the day.

A soy study evaluated the effects of 31 g/day of an isoflavone-rich soy powder (equivalent to 25 g soy protein) on plasma lipids and lipoproteins and vascular reactivity in hypercholesterolemic but otherwise healthy male and female participants. All participants were first fed a Step-I (run-in) diet followed by either a Step-I diet plus soy protein or a Step-I diet with milk protein. Isoflavones are cleared rapidly from the plasma after ingestion, so soy-containing menu items were incorporated throughout the day in an attempt to achieve maximal effects. The barrier to overcome was incorporation of the soy or milk protein into baked products at an acceptable level without sacrificing the quality and acceptability of the product. Acknowledging the importance of this, we worked with a faculty member with expertise in food product design who prepared several great-tasting soy products for the study. With considerable product development effort it was possible to employ a blinded study design.

Similar barriers to flavor were overcome in a study that examined the effects of defatted rice bran on blood lipids and lipoproteins in moderately hypercholesterolemic men and women. Participants were randomly assigned to a reference diet with typical levels of dietary fiber (approximately 15 g/day) or one that contained defatted rice bran to increase dietary fiber to the recommended intake level (30 g/day). Foods were developed with the intention of incorporating the highest amount of defatted rice bran possible. The defatted rice bran had a nutty flavor, a somewhat grainy texture, and imparted a brown color to all the products to which it was added. After much experimentation, we found that one gram beyond a certain amount would yield an unacceptable food product. Because of the color, food products that are expected to be brown, such as spice muffins and ginger cookies, were ideal for the addition of the defatted rice bran.

Folate fortification of foods in the U.S. created some obstacles in menu development for a study that examined the effects of a low-folate diet with milk (8 oz milk, 3 times/day) or with no milk (8 oz apple juice, 3 times/day) on folate absorption and blood homocysteine levels. For a low-folate diet, it was necessary to purchase foods from countries that did not fortify their food products. Pasta imported from Italy became a staple in these menus and was used for lunch salads and dinner items. Foods which are manufactured for individuals with celiac sprue are naturally low in folate because they are made with rice flour and corn starch rather than wheat flour. Some of these items included crackers, pretzels, and a delicious chocolate truffle brownie. The sources of these low-folate foods were obtained by searching shops that specialize in imported foods. Furthermore, information available on the Worldwide Web was immensely helpful to make these menus appealing. One limitation with the menus was that there was only a four-day rotation because of the lack of foods that are naturally low in folate. A short menu rotation may contribute to monotony and boredom, so encouraging adherence may require extra effort.

The Worldwide Web also proved to be useful in finding food items for other studies, such as one that manipulated the glycemic load of a low-fat, high-carbohydrate diet. The number of food items with a known glycemic index is relatively low, and therefore limited the food choices for the menus. Some of the foods are not routinely eaten in the U.S. For example, chana dal, a dried baby garbanzo bean, is a staple in Indian food and has a glycemic index of 8 compared to glucose at 100. Locating a source of the chana dal was made easy by searching various websites. It was used as the carbohydrate source for several meals for the low glycemic index menus.

Participant Adherence and Protocol Acceptability

High monounsaturated fatty acid (MUFA) diets have been studied extensively in the context of evaluating their effects on plasma lipids and lipoproteins. Previous studies have used mainly olive oil as the MUFA source, while other MUFA-rich food sources have not been evaluated. The peanut study was conducted to evaluate the effects of experimental diets high in peanuts and peanut products (e.g., peanut butter and peanut oil) that are rich MUFA sources, on lipid and lipoprotein risk factors for CVD. The greatest challenge with this study was its duration. Although there were five test diets, six 24-day diet periods were scheduled. This schedule necessitated that participants commit to the study for a period of approximately six months.

In a long-term study such as this, it is imperative that special efforts be made to sustain the commitment of the participants. The participants selected one diet period off to allow time for vacations, family activities, or celebrations. Despite participants' initial enthusiasm, some found it difficult to complete the study. Nonetheless, providing some scheduling flexibility did help with adherence. Incentives for the participants, such as t-shirts, coffee mugs, and movie tickets were also advantageous in maintaining long-term adherence. Interestingly, as the study progressed, it was increasingly challenging for the staff to maintain their enthusiasm as well. Theme parties without food (i.e., Halloween night, Thanksgiving celebration) helped participants and staff members maintain a positive attitude throughout the study.

Similarly, some flexibility was given in a nine-month study designed to test the hypothesis that replacement of a fat substitute for dietary fat would significantly decrease body fat relative to a 33% fat diet or a 25% reduced-fat diet. Testing days were scheduled at three-month intervals. Participants were given a three-day break from eating the study meals for the Easter, July 4, and Labor Day holidays. In addition, they were allowed to take a total of seven "vacation" days within the six weeks immediately following the testing days. As for the previously described study, incentives were provided throughout the time period for encouragement.

A study designed to achieve weight maintenance after a weight loss phase presented interesting situations with participant adherence to and acceptability of the protocol. Participants who were moderately overweight were placed on one of two energy-restricted diets to achieve a weight loss of two pounds per week. Following a six-week weight loss period, they were fed the same diets, but with enough energy to maintain their weight. Despite using a metabolic cart to calculate energy needs, about 20% of the participants continued to lose weight during the weight maintenance phase. Because of this, periods longer than four weeks were necessary to establish a stable body weight.

In general, people enjoy participating in controlled weight loss studies, and consequently, adherence is ideal. For this study, the weight loss aspect generally was motivation enough for the participants, although weekly incentives were provided. The hardest part of the study was getting the participants to eat all of their food during the weight maintenance phase of the study. Most wanted to continue to lose weight and had to be encouraged to adhere to the study protocol.

Several people enrolled in the weight loss study had unrecognized eating disorders, making it difficult for them to comply with the protocol, where kcalories were restricted for a portion of the study and then increased for the remainder of the study. This problem pointed out the need for a screening questionnaire that would help identify people with eating disorders so that they would not be enrolled in the study.

In the following series of studies, each of which incorporated a particular food product, it is important that participants like the food, or at least tolerate it and be willing to eat large amounts or more "realistic" quantities daily. While efforts are made to incorporate the food product into a number of tasty products, it would be difficult for participants to adhere to the experiment diet if they dislike the particular food product or the foods that serve as a major delivery vehicle (i.e., milk for cocoa powder).

Studies were conducted using chocolate as a vehicle to assess the effects of stearic acid on plasma lipids, lipoproteins, and platelet function. Our approach was to first evaluate a large dose of the major fat in chocolate (i.e., cocoa butter) and subsequently assess a large dose of milk chocolate (i.e., 10 oz/day), as well as the fat mixture found in chocolate (cocoa butter and dairy butter — 4:1). Our rationale for using large doses was first to determine if there was any effect of chocolate on the study endpoints of interest. Then, more realistic intakes that reflect usual consumption practices would be examined. Initially we needed to assess whether a large dose of chocolate would cause any significant adverse side effects, such as gastrointestinal distress, headaches, or skin problems. Thus, a small pilot study evaluated six participants who were fed large amounts of chocolate (10 oz/day) for approximately one month. Having seen no adverse symptoms, two studies were conducted to evaluate the effects of cocoa butter and milk chocolate on plasma lipids, lipoproteins, and platelet function.

A subsequent study evaluated the incorporation of more realistic amounts of milk chocolate (1 candy bar/day) to a Step-I diet. Moreover, we wanted to mimic real-world chocolate consumption practices. Since a peak time for consumption of chocolate is in the mid-afternoon, participants were required to eat their candy bar at that time. They were required to return the wrapper to the study staff at the dinner meal for adherence assessment and for communicating an important message that participants needed to consume the chocolate bar as well as follow all aspects of the experimental protocol.

Conclusions

Well-controlled clinical nutrition studies have been invaluable in generating results that have advanced our understanding of diet–disease relationships and have provided information that has formed the basis for making nutrient recommendations. A number of recent publications have comprehensively described the process of how to conduct well-controlled feeding studies in humans that employ quality control standards at each step (Table 1). Inherent to conducting these studies is the associated myriad of challenges, not discussed in depth in the literature, that need to be resolved in order to conduct successful studies. This section has presented an overview of these, which relate globally to subject recruitment and compliance/adherence, and maintenance of subject and staff enthusiasm during the feeding study. In addition, we have provided a "forms library" that provides specific forms or a description for virtually every aspect involved in carrying out these studies. Specific examples from the many clinical studies that we have conducted are presented herein, and the approaches we implemented to resolve these problems are described. This information will help readers to overcome the challenges that can arise during the conduct of a well-controlled feeding study. Avoiding inherent pitfalls in feeding studies will facilitate conducting high quality clinical nutrition research efficiently and effectively, and therefore help advance the field.

17

Nutrition Monitoring and Research Studies: Observational Studies

Suzanne E. Perumean-Chaney and Gary Cutter

Purpose

The purpose of this section is to provide an overview and examples of observational studies; specifically, cohort observational studies that incorporate nutritional assessment. After a brief review of the various types of observational studies and their corresponding purposes, a detailed description of the characteristics, advantages, and disadvantages of a cohort study is provided. Next, in order to demonstrate the use of the cohort design in the area of nutrition, a description of six cohort studies that utilized nutritional assessments is provided. Finally, selected nutrition-related publications from the six cohort examples are referenced, along with the corresponding measured nutritional variables.

Observational Studies

Epidemiology is classically known as the study of the distribution of disease in populations; however, this definition expands and often overlaps with other areas of research. We are concerned with two types of research here: clinical studies and observational studies. The primary difference between these two types of research is the randomization of subjects into groups. Clinical studies allow for the randomization of subjects into various treatment or control groups, whereas observational studies examine the subjects according to their natural selection into groups.

Observational studies include natural history studies, case-control studies, prevalence (cross-sectional or population) studies, and cohort (incidence) studies. The research question of interest would generally dictate which of the various observational studies would be used (see Table 17.1). For example, the diagnosis or prevalence of a disease would be facilitated by using the prevalence study design. Cohort studies provide the opportunity to observe populations prospectively, thereby enabling observation of incidence rates as well as prevalence rates. Risk factors and prognosis of a disease can be identified through several different types of observational studies.

0-8493-2705-9/01/$0.00+$1.50

TABLE 17.1

The Question and Appropriate Design

Question	Observational Studies
Diagnosis	Prevalence
Prevalence	Prevalence
Incidence	Cohort
Risk factors	Cohort, case/control, prevalence
Prognosis	Cohort, natural history

TABLE 17.2

Characteristics of a Cohort or Incidence Study

Characteristic
Selection of a study cohort WITHOUT disease
Follow study cohort over time (prospective)
Measurement of incidence and/or absolute risk (new cases developed in a time period)
Comparison of incidence in those with and without the risk factor (relative risk and attributable risk)

Cohort Studies

As noted in Table 17.1, the purpose of cohort studies is to identify the risk factors associated with a disease of interest and obtain the incidence of disease[1] and/or its prognosis. Overall, cohort studies allow the development of a disease to be described, and are therefore typically a favorite among the various types of observational studies.[2]

The defining characteristics of a cohort study are shown in Table 17.2. The first characteristic is identification of a study cohort who currently does not have the disease of interest. Any group of individuals who have either been exposed to the same occurrence, live in a defined geographic area, or have the same risk factors may be identified as a cohort.[1-3] When similar risk factors identify a cohort, a second similar cohort without the identified risk factors and the disease of interest must be obtained for comparison purposes.[2]

The second characteristic is that the study cohort(s) is followed over time. Because the study cohort(s) are disease free, the cohort(s) are followed over time to see which individuals in the cohort(s) actually develop the disease of interest.[1-4] The new cases of the particular disease which developed within a specified time period are then measured to obtain the incidence and absolute risk of the particular disease. Finally, a comparison between the incidence in those individuals who had the risk factors and those individuals who did not produce a relative risk and attributable risk of these risk factors on the development of the disease of interest.

Advantages and Disadvantages of the Cohort Studies

There are several advantages and disadvantages of using cohort studies over other types of observational studies (see Table 17.3). With respect to the advantages, cohort studies make it easier to distinguish cause from association. Because the risk factors are measured

TABLE 17.3

Advantages and Disadvantages of a Cohort Study

Advantages	Disadvantages
Easier to distinguish cause from association	Results are delayed for low incidence or long incubation
Incidence can be obtained	Large number may be needed
Multiple outcomes can be studied	Expensive in resources
Standard questions and measurements can be used	Losses may bias results
May lead to identification of variables which can be experimentally examined	Methods, criteria, and exposure status may change over time

TABLE 17.4

Factors Associated with Causality

Magnitude of the association's strength
Ability to show the association's consistency through replication
Association's identification of one risk factor to one outcome
Risk factor must precede outcome
Outcome is sensitive to different levels of risk factor
Association's logical adherence to current theory
Association's consistency with other information about the outcome
Association's correspondence to other causal associations

prior to the development of the disease of interest, temporal order is established. Temporal order is just one of eight factors associated with causality (see Table 17.4)[4] and strengthens a causal conclusion instead of simply an association between risk factors and outcome often found in other study designs.[1,4] On the other hand, the comparison of cohorts based on risk factors makes the assumption that both cohorts are similar except for the suspected risk factor. However, such an assumption rarely is completely supported and, hence restricts causal implications.[1]

Another important advantage of cohort studies is the ability to obtain the incidence of a disease which in turn can provide estimates of new incidences that preventive programs can use to identify programmatic needs and support budgetary plans.[4] Further, multiple outcomes can be studied, and standard questions and measurements can be used to compare results found in this study to previously completed studies. For example, the Framingham study[5] has provided important information on blood pressure, cholesterol, diet, eye disease, and a number of other risk factors and outcome measures. Other studies, such as the Coronary Artery Risk Development in Young Adults (CARDIA)[6] have emulated Framingham. In this study, variables were selected for inclusion in the baseline examination because of their known or suspected relationships to cardiovascular disease. The availability of multiple endpoints in the same populations further enables one to study the temporal development of the components and their interrelationships. Finally, cohort studies may permit the identification of additional variables related to specific outcome measures which can then be further examined experimentally.[3]

One of the most obvious disadvantages of the cohort studies is that length has to be adequate for development of the disease or a surrogate of the disease of interest.[1,4] For example, blood pressure and cardiovascular disease: cardiovascular disease is the ultimate outcome of interest, but the surrogate, blood pressure, is sufficiently linked to the outcome to make it a viable outcome in its own right. For these diseases or surrogates with low incidence or long incubation periods, the results are delayed. With low disease incidence rates, the sample size for each study cohort may need to be extremely large in order to make the necessary comparisons.[1,4] With both a lengthy process and large sample size, another disadvantage is the expense associated with conducting the study.[4] The length of the study may also influence the ability to recapture all of the subjects at the end of the study. This ability to recapture the study participants depends on their geographic mobility, interest in continuing the study, and death.[4] The inability to capture all study participants may bias the results[1,2] by so-called informative censoring. In addition, the length of the study dictates other potential concerns. Methods, criteria, and exposure status may change over time. For example, environmental, cultural, or technological changes may influence the risk factors identified and the measurement of the variables under study.[2,4]

Summary of Observational Studies

Observational studies are an important part of epidemiological research, in that diseases are studied in their natural environments. Of the various types of observational studies, cohort studies provide the most valuable approach for identifying temporal relationships between risk factors and outcomes. The primary characteristic of cohort studies is that they enable the cohort (or a subgroup of them) to be identified disease-free at the beginning of the study, facilitating study of the incidence of disease. The development of the disease of interest can then be measured and compared across cohorts. Like all observational studies, cohort studies have advantages and disadvantages. The primary advantage is the cohort study's ability to distinguish cause from association, while the primary disadvantage is the cost in time, money, large sample size, and loss of subjects which can lead to substantive biases in the inferences.

The remainder of this section focuses on six selected examples of cohort studies that utilized some form of nutritional assessment (see Table 17.5). Although there are many cohort studies available and additional cohort studies that include nutritional assessments, the following examples were selected to provide a wide range of nationally recognized studies, unique uses of the cohort design, and, most importantly, different methods of collecting nutritional data. The selected examples include the following:

1. Coronary Artery Risk Development in Young Adults (CARDIA)
2. Framingham Study: Heart and Vascular Disease Program
3. Framingham Offspring and Their Spouse Study
4. The RENO (Relationship of Energy and Nutrition to Obesity) Diet-Heart Study
5. The Nurses' Health Study
6. The Health Professionals Follow-Up Study

Examples of Cohort Studies Utilizing Nutrition Assessment

Coronary Artery Risk Development in Young Adults (CARDIA)

The purpose of the CARDIA study was to identify risk factors that either contributed to or protected young adults from coronary heart disease.[6] The sample consisted of 5116 black and white men and women from four cities, who were 18 to 30 years of age.[6,10] Measurements were taken at baseline (1985 through 1986), at two years (1987 through 1988), and biannually thereafter.[7,9,10] Baseline measurements included a sociodemographic

TABLE 17.5

Examples of Cohort Studies Utilizing Nutrition Assessments

Cohort Study	Years Conducted	Sample Studied	Outcome	Nutrition Intake Measurement
Coronary Artery Risk Development in Young Adults (CARDIA)	Baseline: 1985-1986 Year 2: 1987-1988	5116 sampled men and women blacks and whites 18-30 years old	Coronary heart disease risk factors	Baseline: Diet History Questionnaire (interview-administered) Year 2: NCI (Block) Food Frequency Questionnaire
Framingham Study: Heart and Vascular Disease Program	1949-1989	5209 sampled men and women primarily whites 30-62 years old	Cardiovascular risk factors	Semi-Quantitative Food Frequency Questionnaire (Willet)
Framingham Offspring and Their Spouse Study	1971-1988	5135 sampled men and women primarily whites 12-60 years old	Cardiovascular risk factors	24-hr dietary recall
The RENO (Relationship of Energy and Nutrition to Obesity) Diet-Heart Study	1985-1993	508 sampled men and women primarily whites 20-69 years old normal/overweight	Cardiovascular risk factors	1. 24-hr dietary recall 2. 7-Day food record 3. NCI (Block) Food Frequency Questionnaire
The Nurses' Study	1976-1996	121,700 sampled female registered nurses primarily whites 30-55 years old	Cancer risk factors	Semi-Quantitative Food Frequency Questionnaire (Willet)
The Health Professionals Follow-Up Study	1986-1994	51,529 sampled male health professionals primarily whites 40-75 years old	Heart disease and cancer risk factors	Semi-Quantitative Food Frequency Questionnaire (Willet)

questionnaire, medical (family history, current medical history, use of medications), anthropometrics (weight, height, skinfolds, and various circumferences), lab work (lipids, apolipoprotein, insulin, cotinine), blood pressure, lifestyle (treadmill test, questions on tobacco and marijuana use, nutrition intake), and psychosocial questionnaires (type A/B personality, life satisfaction, hostility, social support, and job demand or latitude).[6]

Nutrition intake was assessed with an interview-administered Diet History Questionnaire at baseline and the NCI (Block) Food Frequency Questionnaire at year two.[9,10] Reliability and validity of the Diet History Questionnaire were assessed. Reliability was measured through the correlation between a one-month test-retest method of the Diet History Questionnaire.[7,8]

The nutrient intakes and mean caloric intakes of the Diet History Questionnaire were compared to the same variables derived from 24-hour recalls,[7,8] NCI (Block) Food Frequency Questionnaire,[9] NHANES II,[7] and RDA's Body Mass Index[7] as an assessment of concurrent validity. For both reliability and validity, the Diet History Questionnaire appears to be more applicable for whites than for blacks. The relationship between diet and disease will await the results for this cohort to enter the risk period and show disease development.

Framingham Study: Heart and Vascular Disease Program

The purpose of the Framingham Study was to provide a population-based prospective examination of the development of cardiovascular disease and its risk factors.[11,12] The sample consisted of 5209 primarily white men and women between the ages of 30 to 62 years, who lived in Framingham, Massachusetts.[5,11] Measurements were taken biennially from 1949 through 1989. Measurements included blood labs, medical history, and a physical examination.[5] Additional assessments of stress, nutrition intake, and physical activity were added to the study at a later time. The latest nutrition intake was assessed through the Willet Semi-Quantitative Food Frequency Questionnaire.[11]

Framingham Offspring and Their Spouse Study

The purpose of the Framingham Offspring and Their Spouse Study was to examine the impact of genetic and familial influences on the development of cardiovascular disease and its risk factors.[12-14] The sample consisted of 5135 primarily white men and women who were 12 to 60 years of age.[12,13] Subjects were either the offspring or the offsprings' spouses of the Framingham Study participants.[12-14] Measurements were also taken biennially from 1971 through 1988.[12,14] Measurements included those similar to the original study.[12] For this study, however, nutrition intake was assessed with 24-hour recalls, one-fourth of which were collected during the weekend, and the remaining three-fourths of the subjects were collected during a weekday.[13,14]

The RENO (Relationship of Energy and Nutrition to Obesity) Diet-Heart Study

The purpose of the RENO Diet-Heart Study was to examine prospectively over a five year period the behavioral patterns with respect to weight between normal-weight and mildly to severely obese individuals.[15] The sample consisted of 508 healthy primarily white men and women between the ages of 20 to 69. Subjects were stratified by gender, weight (overweight and normal weight), and five age decades. Measurements were taken over an eight year period (1985 through 1993). Measurements included history questionnaires (weight, activity, health, and demographics), anthropometrics, energy expenditure, laboratory analyses, blood pressure, pulse, weight and dieting measures, activity data (Caltrac Monitors and activity diary), nutrition intake and attitudes, cancer questionnaire, and psychosocial questionnaires (general wellbeing, depression, cohesion, locus of control, hostility inventory, social support, perceived stress).[16]

Nutrition intake was assessed through several measures. The first nutrition assessment was the 24-hour dietary recalls measured at years one and five.[17] The NCI (Block) Food Frequency Questionnaire[18] was used to measure nutrition intake at years two, three, and five. Finally, a seven-day food record that collected information about the day, time, location, and the amount and type of food eaten was measured at years one, three, and five.[19,20]

The Nurses' Health Study

Initially, the purpose of the Nurses' Health Study was to examine the relationship between oral contraceptives and breast cancer.[21,22] The study was then expanded to examine other female-related cancers, lung cancer, and life-style factors such as diet and exercise.[21,22] The sample consisted of 121,700 registered female nurses who were 30 to 55 years of age.[21,22]

Selected from 11 states, nurses were chosen because they were expected to be more accurate in reporting the incidence of diseases and lifestyle factors, and in addition were expected to have higher participation and retention rates.[21-23]

Measurements were requested biennially from 1976 to 1996. Unique to this study, the study researchers did not have personal contact with the nurse participants; instead, all contact was maintained through the mail. That is, study participants were required to mail in their bodily samples, anthropometric information, and the various questionnaires.[21-25] Only when a participant was nonresponsive to mailing in measurements were telephone interviews conducted. Measurements included basic demographics, medical history including the use of medications, blood and toenail samples, anthropometrics, lifestyle factors such as diet, exercise, and cigarette smoking, and quality of life and social support questionnaires.[21,22] In order to confirm the presence of a specified outcome (e.g., cancer, myocardial infarction, diabetes, or fractures), medical chart reviews were conducted when participants indicated an outcome's existence.[21,23,25] Nutrition intake was measured with Willett's semi-quantitative food frequency questionnaire, which assessed the consumption frequency of specified portions of food within the last year.[21,23-25] In 1980, the food frequency questionnaire identified only 61 common foods,[21] while the 1984, 1986, 1990, and 1994 measures were expanded to include 120 common foods, and both vitamin and mineral supplementations.[23]

The Health Professionals Follow-Up Study

The purpose of the Health Professionals Follow-Up Study was to examine the relationship between diet and two chronic diseases: heart disease and cancer.[26] The sample consisted of 51,529 primarily white male health professionals 40 to 75 years of age.[25-27] The health professions included dentists, optometrists, osteopaths, pharmacists, podiatrics, and veterinarians.

Measurements were taken biennially from 1986 through 1994.[25-27] Similar to the Nurses' Health Study, the measures were all self-administered, mailed, and the outcome identifications were verified through medical chart reviews.[25,27-29] The measurements included demographics, medical history, anthropometrics (height, weight, body mass index), chronic disease risk factors (heart disease and cancer in particular), and lifestyle factors such as diet, physical activity, cigarette smoking, and alcohol use.[26-30]

Nutrition intake was assessed with Willett's 131-item semi-quantitative food frequency questionnaire used as the expanded version in the Nurse's Health Study.[25,28] As in the Nurse's Health Study, the food frequency questionnaire assessed the consumption frequency of specified portions of food within the last year.[25,28,30] Nutrition intake was assessed in 1986 and 1990.[27]

Selected nutrition-related publications from the aforementioned studies and their respective measured nutrient variables are shown in Table 17.6.

Summary

This section has focused on the benefits of the cohort study and has provided examples of several studies that have used this form of design. There are certainly other forms that can be utilized to assess the impact of diet on disease or health. The value of

TABLE 17.6

Selected Nutrition-Related Publications from the Six Cohort Examples

Reference	Nutrient Variables
Slattery, M.L., Dyer, A., Jacobs, D.R., Jr., Hilner, J.E., Cann, B.J., Bild, D.E., Liu, K., McDonald, A., Van Horn, L., Hardin, M. (1994). A comparison of two methods to ascertain dietary intake: The CARDIA Study. *J Clin Epidemiol*, 47, 701-711.	Total kcals, macronutrients, and selected micronutrients by gender and race.
Liu, K., Slattery, M., Jacobs, D. Jr., Cutter, G., McDonald, A., Van Horn, L., Hilner, J.E., Caan, B., Bragg, C., Dyer, A., Havlik, R. (1994). A study of the reliability and comparative validity of the CARDIA dietary history. *Ethnicity & Disease*, 4, 15-27.	Total kcals, macronutrients, and selected micronutrients by gender and race.
Bild, D.E., Sholinsky, P., Smith, D.E., Lewis, C.E., Hardin, J.M., Burke, G.L. (1996). Correlates and predictors of weight loss in young adults: The CARDIA Study. *Int J Obesity*, 20, 47-55.	Baseline caloric and fat intake, change in caloric and fat intake at year 2 by gender and race.
Tucker, K.L., Selhub, J., Wilson, P.W.F., Rosenberg, I.H. (1996). Dietary intake pattern relates to plasma folate and homocysteine concentrations in the Framingham Heart Study. *Hum Clin Nutr*, 126, 3025-3031.	Folate intake, ranking of dietary contributors to folate intake by gender and age (67-95 years old). Folate intake through supplements and breakfast cereals, orange juice, green leafy vegetables.
Posner, B.M., Cupples, L.A., Franz, M.M., Gagnon, D.R. (1993). Diet and heart disease risk factors in adult American men and women: The Framingham Offspring-Spouse nutrition studies. *Int J Epidemiol*, 22, 1014-1025.	Total kcals, macronutrients, and selected micronutrients by gender. Ranking of dietary contributors to total fat, saturated fat, cholesterol, calories, carbohydrate, protein, oleic acid, and linoleic acid.
Posner, B.M., Cupples, L.A., Gagnon, D., Wilson, P.W.F., Chetwynd, K., Felix, D. (1993). Healthy People 2000: the rationale and potential efficacy of preventive nutrition in heart disease: The Framingham Offspring-Spouse study. *Arch Intern Med*, 153, 1513-1556.	Total kcals, macronutrients, and selected micronutrients by gender.
Dodds, M.P., Silverstein, L.J. (1997). The 24-Hour Dietary Recall, in S. St. Jeor (Ed.). *Obesity Assessment: Tools, Methods, Interpretations*, New York: Chapman and Hall. RENO Diet-Heart Study	Total kcals, macronutrients, and selected micronutrients by gender and weight status. Total kcals, macronutrients, and selected micronutrients by BMI and age.
Scott, B.J., Reeves, R.B. (1997). Seven Day Food Records. In S. St. Jeor (Ed.). *Obesity Assessment: Tools, Methods, Interpretations*, New York: Chapman and Hall. RENO Diet-Heart Study	Total kcals, macronutrients, and selected micronutrients by gender and weight status.
Benedict, J.A., Block, G. (1997). Food Frequency Questionnaires, in S. St. Jeor (Ed.). *Obesity Assessment: Tools, Methods, Interpretations*, New York: Chapman andHall. RENO Diet Heart Study	Total kcals, macronutrients, and selected micronutrients by gender and weight status. Total kcal, macronutrients, and selected micronutrients by BMI and age.
Silverstein, L.J., Scott, B.J., St. Jeor, S.T. (1997). Eating Patterns, in S. St. Jeor (Ed.). *Obesity Assessment: Tools, Methods, Interpretations*, New York: Chapman and Hall. RENO Diet Heart Study	Number of foods per day, caloric density, number of meals per day and number of eating incidents per day by age group. Number of foods per day, caloric density, eating incidents per day, calories per eating incident, percent fat and total calories by gender and weight status. Breakfast eating variables by gender and weight status.

TABLE 17.6 *(Continued)*

Selected Nutrition-Related Publications from the Six Cohort Examples

Reference	Nutrient Variables
Colditz, G.A. (1995). The Nurses' Health Study: A cohort of U.S. women followed since 1976. *JAMWA*, 50, 40-63.	Selected macronutrients and selected micronutrients by breast cancer, CHD/stroke, colon cancer, fracture, diabetes, and other diseases. Fruits and vegetables by CHD/stroke, red meat by colon cancer, and caffeine by fractures.
Hu, F.B., Stampfer, M.J., Manson, J.E., Ascherio, A., Colditz, G.A., Speizer, F.E., Hennekens, C.H., Willett, W.C. (1999). Dietary saturated fats and their food sources in relation to the risk of coronary heart disease in women. *Am J Clin Nutr*, 70, 1001-1008. The Nurses' Health Study	Saturated fat consumption over ten years. Saturated fat top 5 contributors. Saturated fat consumption by coronary heart disease risk factors. Red meat, white meat, high-fat and low-fat dairy consumption by coronary heart disease.
Liu, S., Willett, W.C., Stampfer, M.J., Hu, F.B., Franz, M., Sampson, L., Hennekens, C.H., Manson, J.E. (2000). A prospective study of dietary glycemic load, carbohydrate intake, and risk of coronary heart disease in U.S. women. *Am J Clin Nutr*, 71, 1455-1461. The Nurses' Health Study	Selected macronutrients, selected micronutrients, and selected food sources by glycemic load. Energy-adjusted dietary glycemic load by CHD. Energy-adjusted total carbohydrate, type of carbohydrate and glycemic index by CHD.
Michels, K.B., Giovannucci, E., Joshipura, K.J., Rosner, B.A., Stampfer, M.J., Fuchs, C.S., Colditz, G.A., Speizer, F.E., Willett, W.C. (2000). Prospective study of fruit and vegetable consumption and incidence of colon and rectal cancers. *J Nat Cancer Inst*, 92, 1740-1752. The Nurses' Health Study and The Health Professionals' Follow-Up Study	Frequency of fruit and vegetable intake by colorectal cancer age-standardized risk factors. Selected categories of fruit and vegetables by relative risk of colon cancer and rectal cancer. Selected categories of fruits and vegetables stratified by vitamin supplement useage by relative risk of colon cancer.
Van Dam, R.M., Huang, Z., Giovannucci, E., Rimm, E.B., Hunter, D.J., Colditz, G.A., Stampfer, M.J., Willett, W.C. (2000). Diet and basal cell carcinoma of the skin in a prospective cohort of men. *Am J Clin Nutr*, 71, 135-141. The Health Professionals' Follow-Up Study	Demographics related to nutrient intake, energy-adjusted dietary fat intake by relative risk of basal cell carcinoma of the skin, energy-adjusted intake of select micronutrients and relative risk of basal cell carcinoma of the skin.
Platz, E.A., Willett, W.C., Colditz, G.A., Rimm, E.B. (2000). Proportion of colon cancer risk that might be preventable in a cohort of middle-aged U.S. men. *Cancer Causes and Control*, 11, 579-588. The Health Professionals' Follow-Up Study	Mean alcohol intake, mean red meat intake, mean folic acid intake by colon cancer risk factors.
Giovannucci, E., Rimm, E.B., Colditz, G.A., Stampfer, M.J., Ascherio, A., Chute, C.C., Willett, W.C. (1993). A prospective study of dietary fat and risk of prostate cancer. *J Nat Cancer Inst*, 85, 1571-1579. The Health Professionals' Follow-Up Study	Fat intake by cancer-free members and by relative risk of prostate cancer. Levels of fat from various animal sources by relative risk of advanced prostate cancer.
Giovannucci, E., Rimm, E.B., Wolk, A., Ascherio, A., Stampfer, M.J., Colditz, G.A., Willett, W.C. (1998). Calcium and fructose intake in relation to risk of prostate cancer. *Cancer Res*, 58, 442-447. The Health Professionals' Follow-Up Study	Low and high intake of total calcium, total fructose, fruit fructose and non-fruit fructose by age-standardized selected characteristics. Total calcium intake and total fructose intake by total, advanced and metastatic prostate cancer.

prospective observational studies relative to cross-sectional studies, where incidence cannot be estimated, only prevalence, must be weighted against the real difficulty in obtaining funding for them. Many such studies today are either sponsored by the government through direct funding via a contract, or as add-ons to multicenter clinical trials. It is difficult to convince funding sources that observational studies, especially in disease areas where a good deal of information already exists, are worth the investment. Thus, sometimes adding components to existing studies such as a clinical trial can be done to gather prospective information. However, in this type of observation add-on, care must be taken to consider generalizability due to the eligibility criteria in the primary study.

References

1. Monsen ER, Cheney CL. *J Am Diet Assoc* 88: 1047; 1988.
2. Friedman GD. *Primer of Epidemiology,* McGraw-Hill, New York, 1987.
3. Zolman JF. *Biostatistics: Experimental Design and Statistical Inference,* Oxford University Press, New York, 1993.
4. Slome et al. *Basic Epidemiological Methods and Biostatistics: A Workbook,* Wadsworth Health Sciences Division, Monterey, 1982.
5. Dawber TR. *The Framingham Study: The Epidemiology of Atherosclerotic Disease,* Harvard University Press, Cambridge, 1980.
6. Friedman, GD, et al. *J Clin Epidemiol* 41: 1105; 1988.
7. McDonald A, et al. *J Am Diet Assoc* 91: 1104; 1991.
8. Liu K, et al. *Ethnicity Disease* 4: 15; 1994.
9. Slattery ML, et al. *J Clin Epidemiol* 47: 701; 1994.
10. Bild DE, et al. *Int J Obesity* 20: 47; 1996.
11. Tucker KL, et al. *Hum Clin Nutr* 126: 3025; 1996.
12. Kannel WB, et al. *Am J Epidemiol* 110: 281; 1979.
13. Posner BM, et al. *Int J Epidemiol* 22: 1014; 1993.
14. Posner BM, et al. *Arch Intern Med* 153: 1993.
15. St. Jeor ST, Dyer AR. In *Obesity Assessment: Tools, Methods, Interpretations,* St Jeor ST, Ed, Chapman and Hall, New York, 1997, ch. 1.
16. St. Jeor ST, Ed, *Obesity Assessment: Tools, Methods, Interpretations,* Chapman and Hall, New York, 1997.
17. Dodds MP, Silverstein LJ. In *Obesity Assessment: Tools, Methods, Interpretations,* St Jeor ST, Ed, Chapman and Hall, New York, 1997, ch. 17.
18. Benedict JA, Block G. In *Obesity Assessment: Tools, Methods, Interpretations,* St Jeor ST, Ed, Chapman and Hall, New York, 1997, ch. 19.
19. Scott BJ, Reeves RB. In *Obesity Assessment: Tools, Methods, Interpretations,* St Jeor ST, Ed, Chapman and Hall, New York, 1997, ch. 18.
20. Silverstein LJ, Scott BJ, St Jeor ST. In *Obesity Assessment: Tools, Methods, Interpretations,* St Jeor ST, Ed, Chapman and Hall, New York, 1997, ch. 22.
21. Colditz GA. *JAMWA* 50: 40; 1995.
22. Colditz GA, Coakley E. *Int. J. Sports Med* 18: S162; 1997.
23. Hu FB, et al. *Am J Clin Nutr* 70: 1001; 1999.
24. Liu S, et al. *Am J Clin Nutr* 71: 1455; 2000.
25. Michels KB, et al. *J Natl Cancer Inst* 92: 1740; 2000.
26. Rimm EB, et al. *The Lancet* 338: 464; 1991.
27. Van Dam RM, et al. *Am J Clin Nutr* 71: 135; 2000.
28. Giovannucci E, et al. *J Natl Cancer Inst* 85: 1571; 1993.
29. Platz EA, et al. *Cancer Causes Control* 11: 579; 2000.
30. Giovannucci E, et al. *Cancer Res* 58: 442; 1998.

18

Nutrition Monitoring and Research Studies: Nutrition Screening Initiative

Ronni Chernoff

The Nutrition Screening Initiative

Screening for Malnutrition

Malnutrition is not a condition that occurs rapidly; it is a chronic condition that develops slowly over time. It is widely accepted that malnutrition from any etiology is not a positive factor in health status, and may have a negative impact on other health conditions. There have been many reports of the health consequences of malnutrition, particularly in hospitalized individuals where poor nutritional status has been associated with increased lengths of hospital stay, co-morbidities, complications, readmissions, and mortality.[1-6] This is particularly profound because it has been estimated that 85% of noninstitutionalized older adults have one or more chronic conditions, many of which are related to nutritional status.[7] If it is possible to identify indicators of risk for the development of malnutrition, and these factors are reversible conditions, then interventions that will alleviate risk can be instituted before malnutrition becomes overt and worsens chronic conditions.

Nutritional screening is of value if 1) it reliably identifies the existence of risk factors for malnutrition; 2) it recognizes the existence of poor nutritional status; 3) it contributes to the avoidance of malnutrition; 4) it will minimize suffering; and 5) the condition of malnutrition can be reversed.[6,8] Reuben et al.[8] describe criteria necessary to define the potential effectiveness of interventions; these criteria are whether or not identification of malnutrition can be achieved more accurately with screening than without it, and whether or not individuals who have malnutrition detected early have a better outcome than those who have malnutrition detected later in the course of their illness.

Rush[9] defines the role of nutrition screening in older adults in different terms. He describes another criteria set for screening including specificity, sensitivity, inexpensive screening devices, and interventions where health benefit is not sacrificed by not treating those who are at moderate or low risk. He indicates that screening is appropriate where there is a relatively small but important proportion of the population that is affected, where those who are affected can be identified by an easily applied tool, and where there is an effective intervention.

0-8493-2705-9/01/$0.00+$1.50

Developing a Tool

Keeping these criteria in mind, and looking for a way to make both professional and volunteer care providers more attentive to the malnutrition risks encountered by older adults, the Nutrition Screening Initiative (NSI) was established in 1990 as a public awareness tool for use by community and health care workers who have regular contact with older adults. The tools were developed as a joint venture of the American Dietetic Association, the American Academy of Family Physicians, and the National Council on the Aging. The premise of the Nutrition Screening Initiative is that if factors associated with malnutrition risk are identified early, interventions can be instituted that may delay or avoid the progression of the risk factors towards overt malnutrition.[10]

The NSI was developed as a nested set of tools that identify risk factors for poor nutritional status and then diagnose malnutrition. There are three tiers: a checklist, level II, and level III screens.[11] The items on the tools were developed by reviewing the literature and developing consensus by a technical advisory committee of experts. The checklist was tested using a follow-up sample from a previous study of nutritional status in older people.[12]

The Checklist

The checklist was created as a public awareness screening tool for use by health care and social services personnel and other providers who work in community-based programs in which older adults participate. It was conceived and designed to bring awareness to nutritional issues that may impact on the health status of elderly clients. The checklist is widely available for reproduction and information collection, and permission to use it in non-profit settings is not required.[11]

The checklist was titled "Determine Your Nutritional Health" based on a mnemonic that contains the risk factors for malnutrition listed on the reverse side of the checklist. (Figures 18.1a and b). The checklist is a one-page questionnaire that can be used in community, long term care, or acute health settings by volunteers, health aides, or health professionals. The objective of awareness of potential nutritional problems in older people was easily achieved; those who have been critical have built their criticisms on the basis of assumptions that have gone farther than the original intent of the tool or the NSI campaign.[13]

The items on the checklist were developed using reference literature, expert opinion, existing databases, and pilot testing.[12] Using biochemical or laboratory parameters to define nutritional status may be misleading because the most commonly used measures, such as serum proteins, are affected by so many different factors independent of diet or nutritional status.[9]

Implementation Strategies

Screening can be conducted in many settings, and by health professionals as well as health care workers or lay volunteers. Involving interested participants (nurses, aides, admission clerks, etc.) will increase the likelihood that data collection (weights, heights, completion of screening instruments) will be more complete.

Modifications that allow the screening tools to be used in different settings and for unique purposes make this approach and this instrument user friendly, applicable, and relevant. A tool that is flexible, valid, and reliable and allows different applications in diverse settings is very valuable. The easier and less time consuming it is to collect data that give insights into an individual's nutrition and health status, the more valuable the

Determine Your Nutritional Health

The warning signs of poor nutritional health are often overlooked. Use this checklist to find out if you or someone you know is at risk.

Read the statements below. Circle the number in the yes column for those that apply to you or someone you know. For each yes answer, score the number in the box. Total your nutritional score.

	YES
I have an illness or condition that made me change the kind and/or amount of food I eat.	2
I eat fewer than 2 meals per day.	3
I eat few fruits or vegetables, or milk products.	2
I have 3 or more drinks of beer, liquor, or wine almost every day.	2
I have tooth or mouth problems that make it hard for me to eat.	2
I don't always have enough money to buy the food I need.	4
I eat alone most of the time.	1
I take 3 or more different prescribed or over-the-counter drugs a day.	1
Without wanting to, I have lost or gained 10 pounds in the last 6 months.	2
I am not always physically able to shop, cook, and/or feed myself.	2
TOTAL	

Total Your Nutritional Score. If it's -

0-2 Good! Recheck your nutritional score in 6 months.

3-5 You are at moderate nutritional risk. See what can be done to improve your eating habits and lifestyle. Your office on aging, senior nutrition program, senior citizens counter, or health department can help. Recheck your nutritional score in 3 months.

6 or more You are at high nutritional risk. Bring this checklist the next time you see your doctor, dietitian, or other qualified health or social service professional. Talk with them about any problem you may have. Ask for help to improve your nutrition health.

These materials developed and distributed by the Nutrition Screening Initiative, a project of:

AMERICAN ACADEMY OF FAMILY PHYSICIANS

THE AMERICAN DIETETIC ASSOCIATION

NATIONAL COUNCIL ON THE AGING

Remember that warning signs suggest risk, but do not represent diagnosis of any condition. Turn this page to learn more about the warning signs of poor nutritional health.

FIGURE 18.1
Determine your nutritional health.

The Nutrition Checklist is based on the Warning Signs described below. Use the word DETERMINE to remind you of the Warning Signs.

DISEASE

Any disease, illness, or chronic condition which causes you to change the way you eat, or makes it hard for you to eat, puts your nutritional health at risk. Four out of five adults have chronic diseases that are affected by diet. Confusion or memory loss that keep getting worse is estimated to affect one out of five or more older adults. This can make it hard to remember what, when, or if you've eaten. Feeling sad or depressed which happens to about one in eight older adults, can cause big changes in appetite, digestion, energy level, weight, and well-being.

EATING POORLY

Eating too little and eating too much both lead to poor health. Eating the same foods day after day or not eating fruit, vegetables, and milk products daily will also cause poor nutritional health. One in five adults skips meals daily. Only 13% of adults eat the minimum amount of fruit and vegetables needed. One in four older adults drinks too much alcohol. Many health problems become worse if you drink more than one or two alcoholic beverages per day.

TOOTH LOSS/MOUTH PAIN

A healthy mouth, teeth, and gums are needed to eat. Missing, loose, or rotten teeth, or dentures which don't fit well or cause mouth sores make it hard to eat.

ECONOMIC HARDSHIP

As many as 40% of older Americans have incomes of less that $6000 per year. Having less - or choosing to spend less - than $25 to 30 per week for food makes it very hard to get the foods you need to stay healthy.

REDUCED SOCIAL CONTACT

One-third of all older people live alone. Being with people daily has a positive effect on morale, well-being, and eating.

MULTIPLE MEDICINES

Many older Americans must take medicines for health problems. Almost half of older Americans take multiple medicines daily. Growing old may change the way we respond to drugs. The more medicines you take, the greater the chance for side effects such as increased or decreased appetite, change in taste, constipation, weakness, drowsiness, diarrhea, nausea, and others. Vitamins or minerals when taken in large doses act like drugs and can cause harm. Alert your doctor to everything you take.

INVOLUNTARY WEIGHT LOSS/GAIN

Losing or gaining a lot of weight when you are not trying to is an important warning sign that must not be ignored. Being overweight or underweight also increases your chance of poor health.

NEEDS ASSISTANCE IN SELF CARE

Although most older people are able to eat, one of every five has trouble with walking, shopping, and buying and cooking food, especially as they get older.

ELDER YEARS ABOVE AGE 80

Most older people lead full and productive lives, but as age increases, risk of frailty and health problems increase. Checking your nutritional health regularly makes good sense.

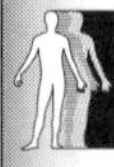

The Nutrition Screening Initiative, 1010 Wisconsin Avenue, NW, Suite 800, Washington, D.C. 20007
The Nutrition Screening Initiative is funded in part by a grant from Ross Laboratories, a division of Abbott Laboratories.

FIGURE 18.1
Determine your nutritional health. (*Continued.*)

information. One example is the slight modifications made to the Nutrition Screening Initiative Checklist for use in a dental office[14,15] (Figure 18.2). Dental professionals are in a unique position to monitor their patients' nutritional status since many of the consequences of poor nutrition manifest themselves in the oral cavity (bleeding or swollen gums; pain in mouth, teeth, gums; angular cheilosis; alterations in the surface of the tongue). Additionally, oral health problems may contribute to the development of inadequate nutritional status due to lesions, loose or missing teeth, poorly fitting dentures, dry mouth, tooth decay or disease, and difficulty in chewing or swallowing.

The warning signs of poor nutritional health are often overlooked. A checklist can help determine if someone is a nutritional risk:

Read the statements below. Circle the number in the **yes** column for those that apply to you. For each **yes** answer, score the number in the box. Total your nutritional score.

	YES
An illness or condition makes me change the kind and/or amount of food I eat.	2
I avoid eating a food group, i.e., meat, dairy, vegetables, and/or fruit.	2
I have two or more drinks of beer, liquor, or wine almost every day	2
I have tooth pain or mouth sores that make it hard to eat or make me avoid certain foods.	2
I snack or drink sweetened beverages two or more times per day between meals.	2
I had three or more new cavities at a recent dental check-up	2
I don't always have enough money to buy the food I need.	4
I eat alone most of the time.	1
I have a dry mouth, which makes me drink or use gum, hard candy, cough drops, or mints to moisten my mouth two or more times per day.	1
I take three or more different prescription or over-the-counter drugs daily.	1
Without wanting to, I have lost or gained 10 pounds in the last six months.	2
I am not always physically able to shop, cook, and/or feed myself.	2
TOTAL	

Total your nutritional Score. If it is:

0–2	**Good!** Recheck your nutritional score in 6 months.
3–5	**You are at moderate nutritional risk.** Try to improve your eating habits and lifestyle.
6 or more	**You are at high nutritional risk.** Talk with your doctor, dental hygienist, or dietitian about any problems you may have. Ask for help to improve your nutritional health.

FIGURE 18.2
Determine your nutritional health checklist, modified for use in a dental office.

The checklist can also be modified for use in specialized community or clinical settings. One example is use in a rural community setting as reported by Jensen et al.[16] They found that the checklist items indicating poor appetite, eating problems, low income, eating alone, and depression were associated with functional limitation.

Implementation Partners

Nurses are essential partners and participants in nutrition screening. They are the best individuals to gather anthropometric data and health history information. They are well-positioned to evaluate individuals' functional status by assessing ability to engage in activities of daily living (self care) and instrumental activities of daily living (managing independence). Clinical nurse specialists (CNS) are uniquely positioned to conduct health and nutrition screenings in clinic settings, particularly to identify risk factors that are modifiable before nutritional status begins a slippery slope downward. The advantage of implementing health promotion programs before or concurrently with the emergence of risk-associated conditions should be apparent.[17]

Other health practitioners (dentists, social workers, physical therapists, speech pathologists, etc.) may also use the screening tool for clients who may have risk factors for the development of malnutrition. Community workers who run senior centers, senior meal programs, home health agencies, etc. can also use the checklist to help identify clients who may require more attention to their dietary intake, social circumstance, and chronic disease management.

Subjective Global Assessment (SGA)

Another tool devised by a group of clinicians in Canada uses a brief set of history and physical assessment items to make an evaluation of nutritional status.[18] The Subjective Global Assessment (SGA) includes an analysis of weight changes, dietary change, gastrointestinal symptoms, functional capacity, medical status, and physical assessment (Figure 18.3). This tool relies on a subjective rating by using clinical judgment on weight loss, dietary intake, loss of subcutaneous tissue, functional capacity, fluid retention, and appar-

(Select appropriate category with a checkmark, or enter numerical value where indicated by "#.")

A. History
1. Weight change
   Overall loss in past 6 months: amount = # ________ kg; % loss = # ________
   Change in past 2 weeks: ________ increase
   ________ no change
   ________ decrease
2. Dietary intake change (relative to normal)
   ________ No change
   ________ Change Duration = # ________ weeks
   Type: ________ suboptimal solid diet ________ full liquid diet
   ________ hypocaloric liquids ________ anorexia
3. Gastrointestinal symptoms (that persisted for >2 weeks)
   ________ none ________ nausea ________ vomiting ________ diarrhea ________ anorexia
4. Functional capacity
   ________ No dysfunction (e.g., full capacity)
   ________ Dysfunction Duration = # ________ weeks
   Type: ________ working suboptimally
   ________ ambulatory
   ________ bedridden
5. Disease and its relation to nutritional requirements ________________
   Primary diagnosis (specify) ________
   Metabolic demand (stress): ________ no stress ________ low stress
   ________ moderate stress ________ high stress

B. Physical (for each trait specify: 0 = normal, 1+ = mild, 2+ = moderate, 3+ = severe)
   # ________ loss of subcutaneous fat (triceps, chest)
   # ________ muscle wasting (quadriceps, deltoids)
   # ________ ankle edema
   # ________ sacral edema
   # ________ ascites

C. SGA rating (select one)
   ________ A = Well nourished
   ________ B = Moderately (or suspected of being) malnourished
   ________ C = Severely malnourished

FIGURE 18.3
Features of Subjective Global Assessment (SGA).

ent muscle wasting.[8,18] This tool has been successfully adopted and used by physicians and nurses in clinical settings. It has been tested in the clinical setting with different assessors, with a high degree of interrater reliability (0.91).[19,20] Most of validity reports of the SGA were conducted on hospitalized subjects with mean ages of 50 years or older, which may contribute to some questions about its general applicability. However, the addition of laboratory values to the SGA did not improve its validity.[19]

Although the SGA is a short tool that can be used successfully by health practitioners, there are limitations to its use as a screening tool. It requires a trained clinician to administer, since there is some clinical judgment involved that would not be expected in someone who is not a health professional. It requires that the individual being assessed is undressed and able to be turned, which does not lend itself to community-based assessment programs. Also, its validation has been demonstrated on middle-aged, rather than elderly, subjects.[8]

Mini Nutritional Assessment (MNA)

The Mini Nutritional Assessment (MNA) is a tool developed to easily evaluate the nutritional status of frail elderly individuals.[21] This instrument was developed to meet a perceived need to go beyond the DETERMINE checklist developed by the NSI, which was designed to raise the awareness of potential malnutrition risks, and the SGA, which was designed for use with hospitalized individuals. The MNA, therefore, was created to complement the screening tools already described.

The objectives for the MNA were to meet the following criteria:

- Be a reliable instrument
- Define thresholds
- Be used with minimal training
- Be free of rater bias
- Be minimally intrusive to patients
- Be inexpensive

The tool was designed to collect 18 items that combine objective and subjective data. These data include simple anthropometric measures (height, weight, arm and calf circumferences, and weight loss), general geriatric assessment items, a brief general dietary assessment, and self-assessment of health and nutrition perception (Figure 18.4).

This tool has been validated in several studies by comparing the scores to the judgments of trained nutrition clinicians and to a comprehensive nutritional assessment that collected in-depth data about the nutritional status of the subjects.[22] These studies found that the threshold for well-nourished on this instrument with a 30-point scale was 22 to 24 points; the threshold for malnutrition was 16 to 18 points on this scale.

The MNA meets its objectives of being a practical, non-invasive tool that contributes to the rapid evaluation of an elderly subject's nutritional status, contributing early intervention to correct nutritional deficits. This tool is easily used in a variety of settings including hospitals, nursing homes, physician offices, or clinics.

MINI NUTRITIONAL ASSESSMENT
MNA™

ID# ____________

Last Name: ____________ First Name: ____________ M.I. ____ Sex: ____ Date: ____________

Age: ____ Weight,kg: ____________ Height, cm: ____________ Knee Height, cm: ____________

Complete the form by writing the numbers in the boxes. Add the numbers in the boxes and compare the total assessment to the Malnutrition Indicator Score.

ANTHROPOMETRIC ASSESSMENT

	Points
1. Body Mass Index (BMI) (weight in kg) / (height in m)^2 a. BMI < 19 = 0 points b. BMI 19 to < 21 = 1 points c. BMI 21 to < 23 = 2 points d. BMI ≥ 23 = 3 points	☐
2. Mid-arm circumference (MAC) in cm a. MAC < 21 = 0.0 points b. MAC 21 ≤ 22 = 0.5 points c. MAC > 22 = 1.0 points	☐.☐
3. Calf circumference (CC) in cm a.CC < 31 = 0 points b. CC ≥ 31 = 1 point	☐
4. Weight loss during last 3 months a. weight loss greater than 3kg (6.6 lbs) = 0 points b. does not know = 1 point c. weight loss between 1and 3 kg (2.2 and 6.6 lbs) = 2 points d. no weight loss = 3 points	☐

GENERAL ASSESSMENT

5. Lives independently (not in a nursing home or hospital) a. no = 0 points b. yes = 1 point	☐
6. Takes more than 3 prescription drugs per day a. yes = 0 points b. no = 1 point	☐
7. Has suffered psychological stress or acute disease in the past 3 months a. yes = 0 points b. no = 2 points	☐
8. Mobility a. bed or chair bound = 0 points b. able to get out of bed/chair but does not go out = 1 point c. goes out = 2 points	☐
9. Neuropsychological problems a. severe dementia or depression = 0 points b. mild dementia = 1 point c. no psychological problems = 2 points	☐
10. Pressure sores or skin ulcers a. yes = 0 points b. no = 1 point	☐

DIETARY ASSESSMENT

	Points
11. How many full meals does the patient eat daily? a. 1 meal = 0 points b. 2 meals = 1 point c. 3 meals = 2 points	☐
12. Selected consumption markers for protein intake • At least one serving of dairy products (milk, cheese, yogurt) per day? yes ☐ no ☐ • Two or more servings of legumes or eggs per week? yes ☐ no ☐ • Meat, fish, or poultry every day? yes ☐ no ☐ a. if 0 or 1 yes = 0.0 points b. if 2 yes = 0.5 points c. if 3 yes = 1.0 points	☐.☐
13. Consumes two or more servings of fruits or vegetables per day? a. no = 0 points b. yes = 1 point	☐
14. Has food intake declined over the past three months due to loss of appetite, digestive problems, chewing or swallowing difficulties? a. severe loss of appetite = 0 points b. moderate loss of appetite = 1 point c. no loss of appetite = 2 points	☐
15. How much fluid (water, juice, coffee, tea, milk,...) is consumed per day? (1 cup = 8 oz.) a. less than 3 cups = 0.0 points b. 3 to 5 cups = 0.5 points c. more than 5 cups = 1.0 points	☐.☐
16. Mode of feeding a. Unable to eat without assistance = 0 points b. self-fed with some difficulty = 1 point c. self-fed without any problem = 2 points	☐

SELF ASSESSMENT

17. Do they view themselves as having nutritional problems? a. major malnutrition = 0 points b. does not know or moderate malnutrition = 1 point c. no nutritional problem = 2 points	☐
18. In comparison with other people of the same age. how do they consider their health status? a. not as good = 0.0 points b. does not know = 0.5 points c. as good = 1.0 points d. better = 2.0 points	☐.☐

ASSESSMENT TOTAL (max.30 points): ☐☐.☐

MALNUTRITION INDICATOR SCORE

≥ 24 points	well-nourished	☐
17 to 23.5 points	at risk of malnutrition	☐
< 17 points	malnourished	☐

FIGURE 18.4
The Mini Nutritional Assessment form.

Nutritional Assessment in Older Adults

The descriptions of the screening tools used to define nutritional status among elderly people highlight the fact that one of the more difficult determinations in elderly people is the accurate assessment of their nutritional status. This evaluation is more challenging in older adults because of the physiologic changes that occur with normal aging. Many of the commonly used assessment standards are not reliable in this population for a variety of reasons.[23]

Anthropometric Measures

Anthropometric measures, including height, weight, and skinfold measures, are usually important components of a nutritional assessment. These parameters are the ones most affected by the aging process.[24] The most apparent age-related change occurs in height. Height decreases as people get older due to changes in skeletal integrity, most noticeably affecting the spinal column. Loss of height may be due to thinning of the vertebrae, compression of the vertebral discs, development of kyphosis, and the effects of osteomalacia and osteoporosis.[25] Loss of height occurs in both males and females, although it may happen more rapidly to elderly women with osteoporosis. Therefore, stature changes and body appearance may be altered and, as older people lose their ability to stand erect, the organs in the thoracic cavity will become displaced and breathing and gastrointestinal problems may ensue.[26,27]

Height is difficult to measure in individuals who are unable to stand erect, cannot stand unaided, cannot stand at all due to neuromuscular disorders, paralysis, or loss of lower limbs, or are bedbound due to other medical problems. One estimate of stature in these individuals is to measure their recumbent height or the bone lengths of extremities.[23,28] This estimate of stature may not be very reliable, but it provides some estimate of height to help determine whether body weight is appropriate for height.

Weight is another important anthropometric measure that is altered with advancing age. Weight changes occur at different rates among elderly people. Use of most standard height and weight tables is not valid in older people since most reference tables do not include elderly people in their subject pool, and most are not age-adjusted.

Body mass index (BMI) is a commonly-used measure to evaluate relative weight for height using a mathematical ratio of weight (in kilograms) divided by height (in square meters).

$$\text{Wt (Kg)/Ht (M)}^2$$

This formula yields a whole number that should be greater than 21 and less than approximately 35.[10] Nomograms and tables are available that minimize the need for calculation. There is some controversy among experts regarding the range of acceptable BMI measures in elderly people.[4,29]

Skinfold measurements (triceps, biceps, subscapular, suprailiac, thigh) are often included in a thorough nutritional assessment. However, loss of muscle mass, shifts in body fat compartments, changes in skin compressibility and elasticity, and lack of age-adjusted references serve to decrease the reliability of skinfold measures in the assessment of nutritional status in elderly people.[30]

Biochemical Measures

Biochemical assessment parameters are also affected by advancing age.[23] Laboratory measures may reflect an age-related decline in renal function, fluid imbalances or hydration status, or the effects of long-term chronic illnesses. Among the commonly used biochemical markers of nutritional status, serum transferrin is one that is markedly affected by advancing age. Since tissue iron stores increase with age, circulating serum transferrin levels are reduced. A lower than normal serum transferrin should be evaluated in relation to other biochemical measures and serum iron levels, if obtainable.[31]

The most reliable predictor of nutritional status in elderly people is serum albumin. A serum albumin below 4.0 g/dl (depending on local laboratory normal ranges) is not usual in an older person unless the subject is overhydrated, has cancer, renal or hepatic disease, or is taking medications that may interfere with hepatic function. Recent evidence suggests that serum albumin is a prognostic indicator of potential infectious complications and other nosocomial problems in hospitalized, frail, or dependent elderly individuals.[32] A depressed serum albumin seems to be a primary prognostic indicator of rehospitalization, extended lengths of stay, and other complications associated with protein energy malnutrition in elderly people.[33,34] Unless there are medical reasons, most biochemical measures should remain within normal limits.

Serum cholesterol has been considered in the risk for coronary heart disease, but a depressed serum cholesterol is also associated with poor health status in older people.[35] It may be predictive of impending mortality[36] and should be evaluated carefully within the context of other health measures.

Immunologic Assessment

Tests for immunocompetence are often included as part of a nutritional assessment because malnutrition results in compromised host-defense mechanisms. However, the incidence of anergy is reported to increase with advanced age, and the response to skin test antigens appears to peak after longer intervals in older people.[37] The value of these tests is limited in elderly people.

Socioeconomic Status

Social history, economic status, drug history, oral health condition, family and living situations, and alcohol use should be evaluated along with the physical and physiologic measures usually assessed.[23] It is also useful to assess elderly individuals using instruments that evaluate how well they perform activities of daily living. Available tools assess the capability of an individual in managing the activities necessary for independence; these tools add another valuable dimension to the assessment of elderly people.[38,39] (See Tables 18.1 and 18.2.)

Summary

Nutrition monitoring, screening, and assessment in the older adult population pose challenges to health care professionals due to the heterogeneity of this group. It has been said that the older we become, the more unique we are. The difficulty in using the tools

TABLE 18.1

Activities of Daily Living

Toileting

Cares for self; no incontinence
Needs to be reminded or needs help with cleanliness; accidents rare
Soiling or wetting at least once a week
No control of bladder or bowels

Feeding

Eats without assistance
Eats with minor assistance or with help with cleanliness
Feeds with assistance or is messy
Requires extensive assistance with feeding
Relies on being fed

Dressing

Independent in dressing and selecting clothing
Dresses and undresses with minor assistance
Requires moderate assistance with dressing and undressing
Needs major assistance with dressing but is helpful
Completely unable to dress and undress oneself

Grooming

Always neatly dressed and well groomed
Grooming adequate; may need minor assistance
Requires assistance in grooming
Needs grooming care but is able to maintain groomed state
Resists grooming

Ambulation

Totally independent
Ambulates in limited geographical area
Ambulates with assistance (cane, wheelchair, walker, railing)
Sits unsupported in chair or wheelchair but needs help with motion
Bedridden

Bathing

Bathes independently
Bathes self with help getting into bath or shower
Washes hands and face but needs help with bathing
Can be bathed with cooperation
Does not bathe and is combative with those trying to help

Adapted from M.P. Lawton, The functional assessment of elderly people, *Journal of the American Geriatrics Society* 19: 4465, 1971.

TABLE 18.2

Instrumental Activities of Daily Living

Instrumental Activities of Daily Living
Ability to use telephone
Shopping
Food preparation
Housekeeping
Laundry
Mode of transportation
Responsibility for own medications
Ability to handle finances

Adapted from M.P. Lawton, The functional assessment of elderly people, *Journal of the American Geriatrics Society* 19: 4465, 1971.

discussed here is that people age at different rates and in different ways related to their health status, their lifestyle, and their genetic inheritance. Although a variety of reasonable approaches to nutrition assessment and monitoring in the older population exist, it is wise for the clinician to understand that the definitive tool or definition of malnutrition in older people has yet to be reported and that there are vast opportunities for research in this area.

References

1. Bienia R, Ratcliff S, Barbour GL, et al. *J Am Geriatr Soc* 30: 433; 1982.
2. Herrmann FR, Safran C, Levkoff SE, et al. *Arch Int Med* 152: 125; 1992.
3. Harris T, Cook EF, Garrison R, et al. *JAMA* 259: 1520; 1988.
4. Galanos AN, Pieper CF, Cornoni-Hunt JC, et al. J *Am Geriatr Soc* 42: 368; 1994.
5. Epstein AM, Read JL, Hoefer M. *Am J Pub Health* 77: 993; 1987.
6. MacLellan DL, Van Til LD. *Can J Pub Health* 89: 342; 1998.
7. Millen B, Levine EL. In: *Geriatric Nutrition: A Health Professional's Handbook,* (Chernoff R, Ed). Gaithersburg, MD: Aspen Publishers, 1999.
8. Reuben DB, Greendale GA, Harrison GG. *J Am Geriatr Soc* 43: 415; 1995.
9. Rush D. *Ann Rev Nutrition* 17: 101; 1997.
10. Lipschitz DA, Ham RJ, White JV. *Am Fam Phys* 45: 601; 1992.
11. Wellman, NS. *Nutrition Today* (II), 44S; 1994.
12. Posner BM, Jette AM, Smith KW, Miller DR. *Am J Pub Health* 83: 972; 1993.
13. Rush D. *Am J Pub Health* 83: 944; 1993.
14. Boyd LD, Dwyer JT. *J Dental Hyg* 72: 31; 1998.
15. Saunders MJ. *Special Care in Dentistry* 15: 26; 1995.
16. Jensen GL, Kita K, Fish J, et al. *Am J Clin Nutr* 66: 819; 1997.
17. Curl PE, Warren JJ. *Clin Nurse Spec* 11: 153; 1997.
18. Detsky AS, McLaughlin JR, Baker JP, et al. *J Parent Enteral Nutr* 11: 8; 1987.
19. Detsky AS, Baker JP, Mendelson RA, et al. *J Parent Enteral Nutr* 8: 153; 1984.
20. Baker JP, Detsky AS, Wesson D, et al. *N Engl J Med* 306: 969; 1982.
21. Guigoz Y, Vellas B, Garry PJ. *Nutr Rev* 54: S59; 1996.
22. Guigoz Y, Vellas B, Garry PJ. *Facts Res Gerontol* 4: 15; 1994.
23. Mitchell CO, Chernoff R. In*: Geriatric Nutrition: The Health Professional's Handbook,* 2nd ed. (Chernoff R, Ed). Gaithersburg MD, Aspen Publishers, 1999.
24. Mitchell CO, Lipschitz DA. *Am J Clin Nutr* 35: 398; 1982.
25. Chumlea WC, Garry PJ, Hunt WC, et al. *Hum Biol* 60: 918; 1988.
26. Silverberg SJ, Lindsay R. *Med Clin N Am* 71: 41; 1987.
27. Heaney RP. In: *Nutrition in Women's Health* (Krummel DA, Kris-Etherton PM, Eds) Gaithersburg MD, Aspen Publishers, 1996.

28. Martin AD, Carter JEL, Hendy KC, et al. In: *Anthropometric Standardization Reference Manual* (Lohman TG, Roche AF, Martorell R, Eds) Champaign IL, Human Kinetics Publishers, 1988.
29. Nutrition Interventions Manual for Professionals Caring for Older Adults. Washington DC, Nutrition Screening Initiative, 1992.
30. Chumlea WC, Guo SS, Glasser RM, et al. *Nutrition, Health and Aging* 1: 7; 1997.
31. Fleming DJ, Jacques PF, Dallal GE, et al. *Am J Clin Nutr* 67: 722; 1998.
32. Finucane P, Rudra T, Hsu R, et al. *Gerontology* 34: 304; 1988.
33. Ferguson RP, O'Connor P, Crabtree B, et al. *J Am Geriatr Soc* 41: 545; 1993.
34. Sullivan DH, Walls RC, Lipschitz DA, *Am J Clin Nutr* 53: 599; 1991.
35. Wilson PWF, Anderson KM, Harris T, et al. *J Gerontol Med Sci* 49: M252; 1994.
36. Rudman D, Mattson DE, Nagraj HS, et al. *J Parent Enteral Nutr* 12: 155; 1988.
37. Cohn JR, Buckley CE, Hohl CA, et al. *J Am Geriatr Soc* 31: 261; 1983.
38. Katz S. *J Am Geriatr Soc* 31: 721; 1983.
39. Spector WD. In: *Quality of Life Assessments in Clinical Trials* (Spilker B, Ed) New York, Raven Press, 1990.

19

Dietary Intake Assessment: Methods for Adults

Helen Smiciklas-Wright, Diane C. Mitchell, and Jenny H. Ledikwe

Introduction

There has been longstanding interest in assessing diets of individuals.[1,2] Early in the 20th century, nutritionists studied food and nutrient intakes in order to provide guidance in food selection,[3,4] to interpret clinical and laboratory findings,[5] and to establish dietary requirements.[6,7] Interest in dietary assessment was stimulated in the latter part of the century with the increasing evidence for the role of diet in promoting health and reducing chronic disease risk.[8-11]

Early investigators were concerned with many of the issues that continue to be important for dietary assessment:

1. Selecting appropriate methods for collecting dietary data[5,12-15]
2. Assessing the day-to-day variability of intakes by individuals[12,16,17]
3. Establishing procedures for data analysis[18-20]
4. Estimating food/food group and nutrient intake[5,21]

The following statement appears in the National Research Council's report on diet and chronic disease: "One of the most difficult tasks in nutrition research is documenting the actual or habitual food and nutrient intake of individuals or groups."[8] We should not be surprised that obtaining information about what individuals consume and analyzing for dietary components is a challenging undertaking. Food intake can be a complex behavior.[22] In any day, an individual may consume many different foods, at several eating occasions, both at home and away from home. Willingness and ability to report what is consumed can be influenced by social and environmental events and cognitive abilities.[23-25] Furthermore, food composition databases must continuously be updated to reflect an expanding food marketplace and an increasing number of dietary components associated with health.[26]

This section is organized to review the methods most commonly used to assess intakes by individuals. Attention is given to methodologic validity as well as to the current emphasis on food pattern analysis, dietary supplements, and functional foods.

0-8493-2705-9/01/$0.00+$1.50

Methods of Dietary Assessment

The common methods for assessing intakes by individuals are food records, recalls, and food frequencies/diet histories. There have been several reviews of dietary assessment methods, their appropriate uses, modes of administration, and sources of error.[1,27-31] Methods are generally characterized either by the reference period in which respondents are asked to provide information (i.e., retrospective and prospective methods)[31] or by the time frame for which data are collected (i.e., quantitative daily and food frequency methods).[27,28,30]

There is no single optimal dietary assessment method. The objectives of an assessment should be used as a guide in selecting the most appropriate method. Some 30 years ago, Christakis advised that the assessment method selected should be no more detailed, no more cumbersome, and no more expensive than necessary.[32] This advice is still sound.[31] Assessment protocols, regardless of method, may need to provide highly quantitative and detailed data on food consumption. This would be the case for research studies such as clinical trials.[33] More qualitative data is likely to be appropriate when food intake information is used for dietary guidance and counseling.[34]

Food Record

Food records, also known as food diaries, provide a prospective account of foods and beverages consumed in a defined period of time. Generally, records are kept for brief time periods (one to seven days),[28] but they have been kept for up to a month[35] and even a year.[36] To be representative of usual intake, multiple days of records are needed.[27,37]

Food records may be used to meet a variety of objectives. Records are useful for detecting imbalances in food intake and making dietary change recommendations.[38] They are used as self-management tools in weight loss interventions and may be valuable in predicting successful weight loss.[39] Food records have been used extensively to calibrate other dietary assessment methods.[40-45] Records are also useful for documenting compliance of an individual's food intake with a feeding protocol in studies where adherence to a specific diet regimen is important.[46] Intervention studies may use food records to document effectiveness.[47-49]

Food portions may be either weighed or estimated depending on the subjects and the purpose(s) of the assessment.[50] While weighing foods will increase the accuracy of the portion size recorded, it can also increase respondent burden. Sophisticated scales that do not disclose food weights are available, decreasing respondent recording burden[51] but increasing cost. A variety of portion size aids, listed in Table 19.1, are available when portion sizes are to be estimated.

While records are usually kept by respondents, they may also be kept by observers. When food intake is recorded by observation, trained personnel visually estimate dietary intake.[52,53] Observation is particularly useful when circumstances preclude self-reporting of food intake. Thus, observation has been used in assessing intake of nursing home residents. The Omnibus Budget Reconciliation Act[54] requires that all Medicare and Medicaid certified nursing facilities implement a standardized comprehensive assessment, including a measure of nutrient intake, for all residents. Observers visually estimate the portion of served items consumed (i.e., from all to none) by a resident.[55]

When using food records, consideration should be given to the record forms to be used as well as instructions and training for subjects, particularly regarding portion size. Instructions should include guidance on completing the record form as well as directives encouraging subjects to record foods at the time of consumption and not to alter normal eating patterns. Table 19.2 provides sample instructions for the administration of a food record.

TABLE 19.1

Tools for Portion Size Estimation

Type	Examples
Household measures	Measuring cups and spoons[161]
	Rulers[161]
Food models	Food replicas[165]
	Graduated food models[166]
	Thickness sticks[161]
Pictures	2-Dimensional portion shape drawings[124,161]
	Portion photos of popular foods[167]
	Portion drawings of popular foods[161]
Food labels	Nutrition facts label
	Food package weights

TABLE 19.2

Sample Instructions for the Administration of a Food Record

To help us do the best analysis of your food intake, please follow these instructions.

Maintain Your Usual Eating Pattern. Try not to modify your food intake because you are keeping a record.
Record Everything You Eat or Drink. Be sure to include all snacks and drinks. Also include any vitamin or mineral supplements and the dosage for each day.
Write Foods Down As Soon As You Eat Them. Three daily record pages are provided for each day; however, you may not need to use all three. Try to write clearly.

Details are Important!

Completing the food record form

Date. Please record the date at the top of each form.
Name. Please write your name in the space at the top of the form.
Time of Day. Record the time of the day you ate each meal, including AM or PM.
Meal/Where Prepared? Record the name of the meal eaten (i.e., breakfast, lunch, dinner, supper, or snack) and where the meal was prepared (i.e., at home, at a restaurant).
Food Item. Write the name of each food item eaten.
Description/Preparation. Include information on how each food was prepared.
Amount. Record the amount of each food either by using the poster provided or common household measures.

After records have been completed, they should be reviewed to ensure completion. If reviewed with the subject, probing questions may be used to clear up ambiguities and ensure the completeness of the record. This is termed interviewer-assisted food records. When data from food records are compiled and analyzed, records will need to be coded using a standard method.

As subject burden can be high for food records, participant willingness and abilities are considerations when using this method. Literacy is required for completion of records; therefore, the method may not be appropriate for all individuals. The act of keeping food records can affect dietary intake,[56,57] which may be critical for estimates of usual intake. Cost is an additional consideration, as reviewing records for completeness, data entry, and data analysis can be expensive.[31]

Recall

Dietary recall provides a retrospective record of intake over a defined time period. While dietary recall may be for any length of time, this method is almost always administered to cover a 24-hour time period and is generally termed the 24-hour recall.[30] Data can be collected either for the previous day or for the 24 hours preceding the interview. To estimate the usual intake of individuals, multiple recalls are needed, preferably on random, nonconsecutive days.[36,58] Typically, an individual is asked to recall all foods eaten during the reference time period, describe the foods, and estimate the quantities consumed.

The 24-hour recall has become a favored way of collecting dietary data,[33,47,59] as recalls can be administered easily and quickly with low respondent burden. Depending on the objectives of the recall, the amount and depth of information collected will vary. This method is becoming the gold standard, particularly as methodological improvements[60-62] and technological capabilities[63,64] increase validity. With the emergence of technological aids in dietary assessment, it is becoming more common for interviewers to collect intake data using interactive software, entering intake data directly into a computer as it is collected.

Recalls may be obtained either in person or by telephone-administered interview. Because recalls by telephone interview have been shown to be practical, valid, and cost-effective,[63-68] they are becoming an increasingly popular mode of data collection, especially for research purposes.

Prior to conducting recalls, training of interviewers is important. This is particularly relevant when more quantitative data are required, increasing the need to use multiple pass and probing techniques. Figure 19.1 provides a sample probing sequence to elicit detailed information regarding one specific food (i.e., macaroni and cheese). The complexity of this probing sequence exemplifies the potentially complex nature of probing questions and the need for good interviewer training. More qualitative food intake data can be achieved with more limited questions.

The 24-hour recall has been criticized because of accuracy related to portion size estimation and subject memory. Portion size estimation aids are available to facilitate quantity estimation (Table 19.1). While 24-hour recalls are not designed to affect the "encoding" of food information, they can incorporate strategies to facilitate memory retrieval. Those strategies include standardized data collection protocols, structured probes to ensure standardized collection, and interactive interview systems.[29,47] The multiple pass technique, which will be discussed later in this section, has also been designed to facilitate memory retrieval.

Food Frequency Questionnaire

Food frequency questionnaires (FFQs) are designed to obtain information about usual food consumption patterns. They provide estimates on intake over a specified time period, ranging from as little as a week[69] to as much as one year.[70] FFQs consist of a list of foods and frequency-of-use response categories. Questionnaires may also include portion size response categories. Food lists may be extensive in order to provide estimates of total intake or they may be focused on foods, groups of foods, or nutrients. Several nutrient specific FFQs have been developed which allow for the examination of selected nutrients such as fat,[71] vitamin A,[72] and vitamin B_6.[73] While not necessarily appropriate for identifying precise nutrient intake, these instruments can provide a rapid, cost-effective way to estimate an individual's usual intake.[74]

Questionnaires may be abbreviated when used to screen for nutritional risk. Screening instruments are typically brief, self-administered, and can be scored quickly, providing an efficient way to monitor eating patterns of individuals. Examples of screening tools include the instruments developed as part of the Nutrition Screening Initiative, which were designed to identify older adults who may need nutrition services and to provide diag-

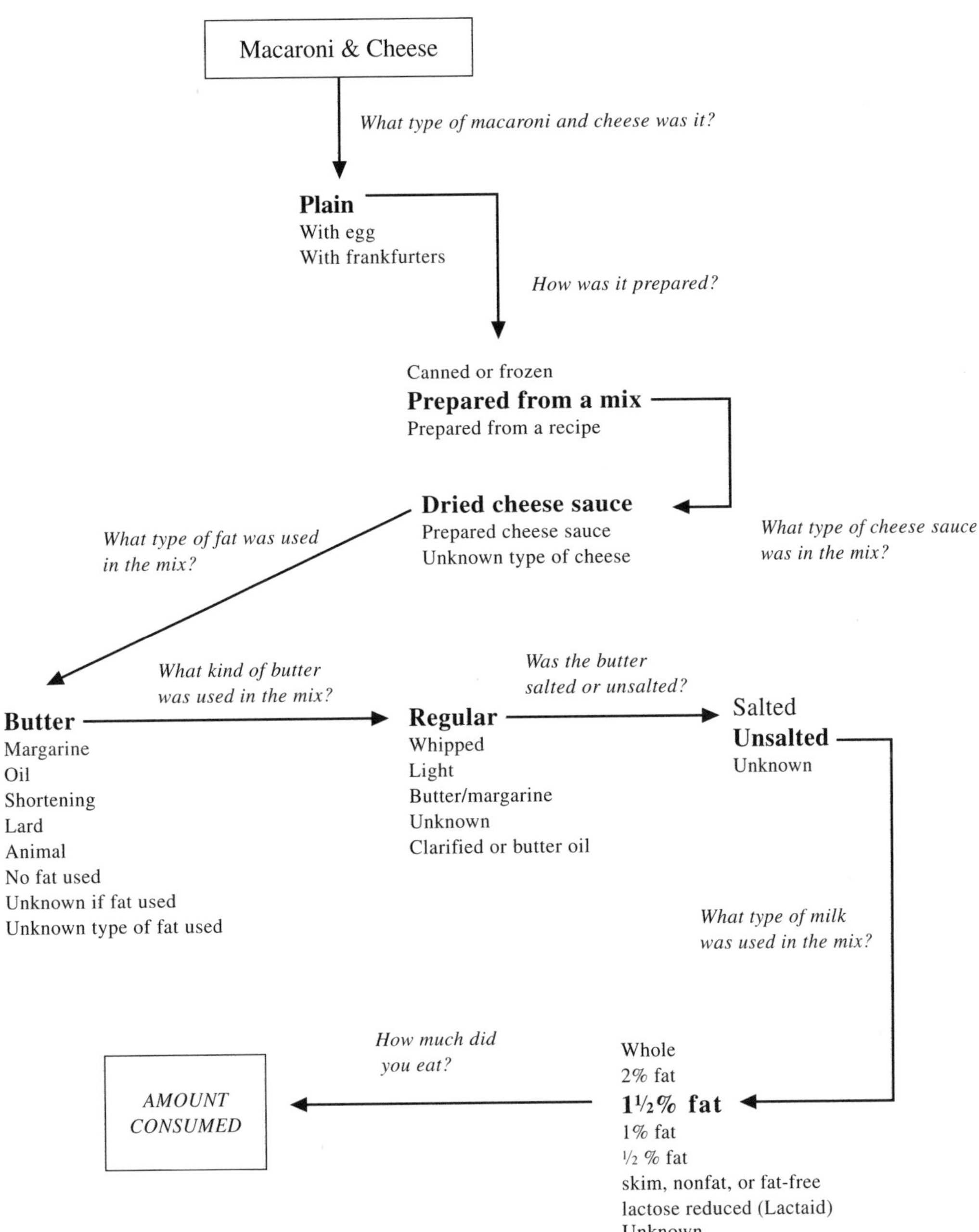

FIGURE 19.1
A sample probing scheme. This scheme could be used with recalls to elicit more information from a respondent who consumed macaroni and cheese. Bold print indicates respondent's reply. Probing questions, which are specific for each response, are italicized. (Adapted from Nutrition Data System for Research [NDS-R] software, developed by the Nutrition Coordinating Center [NCC], University of Minnesota, Minneapolis, MN.)

nostic information on nutrition status.[75,76] Very abbreviated instruments may not be valid representations of true intake.[77]

Creating a food frequency questionnaire is an intensive process,[78] thus, there is heavy reliance on instruments that have already been developed. Validity is a critical issue and is generally determined by calibration with other assessment methods.[73,79-84] When using an FFQ, it is important to ensure that the questionnaire is valid for use in the population of interest, as the performance of an instrument may vary between subgroups. Questionnaires have been validated in specific populations such as adolescents,[85] pregnant women,[42] and low-income black women.[86]

Several cognitive issues could compromise the validity of an FFQ. Subjects may have difficulty recalling foods consumed over a lengthy time period. Additionally, participants may need to perform arithmetic computations to average usual consumption of foods to fit into the response categories for consumption frequency. The cognitive demands of the FFQ may be reduced by a new variation in questionnaire administration, termed the picture sort approach, in which participants sort food cards into categories.[87,88]

While FFQs generally provide qualitative data, if portion size estimation is included on the questionnaire, semi-quantitative information can be deduced from these instruments. In some cases, inclusion of portion size may yield only small differences in data as compared to FFQs analyzed using only medium portions.[89]

Diet History

Food frequency questionnaires are sometimes referred to as diet histories. The classic diet history method was designed to estimate an individual's usual intake over a relatively long period of time. Originally developed by Burke,[90] the method consists of several components, including a 24-hour recall and questions about usual eating patterns, a cross-check questionnaire with a list of foods and questions about likes, dislikes, and usages, and a three-day food record. This method is not used commonly today. Administration requires a highly trained dietitian and can be time consuming.

Summary

Several methods have been listed which can be used to assess the usual dietary intake of adults. Well-designed quality control procedures are particularly important in research studies to ensure consistency of data across time and subjects.[33] Additionally, the advantages and disadvantages of data collection modes (i.e., self- or interviewer-completed) should be considered (See Table 19.3). The success of any assessment method is based upon a partnership between the individual respondent and the assessment staff. Care should be taken to ensure the appropriateness of the method and the level of detail collected. Respecting participants' abilities and ensuring that their dignity is not compromised is salient in establishing a successful partnership.

Issues Affecting Validity

In his address at the First International Conference on Dietary Assessment Methods, Beaton stated, "In the past decade there has been a great deal published about the errors

TABLE 19.3

Self-Completed and Interviewer-Completed Data Collection

Collection Mode	Advantages	Disadvantages
Self	Interviewer training not needed Sense of privacy Data collection time may be reduced	Response rate may be low Respondent burden may be high Tasks may be misinterpreted Respondent training needed for more complete data Data preparation and entry time may be high
Interviewer by phone	Good Response rate Opportunities for probing Low respondent burden Relatively quick Interviewer anonymity	Contact times may be inconvenient Hearing problems for some subjects Availability of portion aids Data collection may be more expensive for toll calls Potential for interviewer bias
Interviewer in person	Good response rate Opportunities for probing Low respondent burden Respondent interviewer rapport	Contact times may be inconvenient Potential for interviewer bias

in dietary data…this is understandable, but unfortunate because it can easily leave the impression that dietary data are worthless."[91] He reminded his audience that, while dietary intake data cannot and never will be estimated without error, a serious limitation is not the errors themselves, but failure to understand the nature of the errors and the consequent impact on data analysis and interpretation. Several recent reviews have delineated potential sources of error for different assessment methods.[28,31,51] Consideration of strategies to minimize error is pertinent in yielding accurate intake data, regardless of assessment method (see Table 19.4).

Recent attention to the accuracy of dietary intake data has focused on the underreporting of energy by 10 to almost 40%.[59,92-97] These findings are based on an extensive literature comparing intakes to energy needs estimated using doubly-labeled water,[98] weight maintenance data,[59] and applying age- and sex-specific equations to estimate energy requirements.[99] Underreporting has been found to be more common among women[99-101] and older persons[99,100,102] as well as overweight,[99-101] post-obese,[92] and weight-conscious individuals.[99,100] Literacy[103] and depression[104] have been associated with underreporting. Selective underreporting has also been associated with certain food types such as fats[95,99,105] and sweets.[105]

While underreporting of energy is common in groups of individuals,[59,94,95,99,100,106-108] both underreporting and overreporting can occur.[44,59,100] Individuals who possess characteristics

TABLE 19.4

Benefits Derived from Minimizing Assessment Error

Clinical Setting	Research Setting
Improve ability to detect inadequate, imbalanced, or excessive dietary intake	Improve accuracy of nutrient intake estimations
Provide a better basis for nutrition counseling and interventions	Decrease attenuation between intake data and biomarkers
Improve ability to monitor dietary changes	Provide a better basis for nutrition education program
	Provide a better basis for elucidation of diet-disease relationships

associated with underreporting may actually report intake accurately or overreport intake. However, the magnitude of underreporting may be even greater for individuals as error due to overestimation can reduce underestimation bias in groups.[102]

Due to the complex nature of intake data and the variability of under and over reporting, it is unlikely that a single correction factor will be derived that could be applied to self-reported energy intake.[109] The purpose of this section is to review components of assessment that may be modified to reduce sources of error.

Memory

Food recall is a cognitively demanding task. Understanding of dietary recall accuracy is derived from advances in cognitive psychology.[23] Classic work in this area described memory processes: encoding or learning information, transmission to long-term memory, and retrieval.[110-112] Early studies described strategies for encoding information as well as strategies for retrieving memories, such as free recall, recognition, and cued recall.

The memory model of cognitive psychology is applicable to dietary recall.[25] To accurately report intake, people must be able to remember what foods were consumed, how the foods were prepared, and the quantities of foods eaten. This requires the acquisition of specific food memories and the ability to retrieve these memories. Individuals who pay little attention to foods consumed, people who have difficulty storing information in memory, and those who lack the cognitive ability to retrieve food memories may not be able to accurately recall dietary intake.

Several techniques have been developed to reduce memory-related error in dietary data. For the 24-hour recall, techniques such as probing (See Figure 19.1),[113] encoding strategies,[25] memory retrieval cues,[25] and a multiple pass system[59,62] have been employed to improve memory. Campbell and Dodd's[113] classic paper showed that probing elicited additional information with significant impact on total caloric intake. Ervin and Smiciklas-Wright found that older adults were able to remember more foods when a deeper processing strategy was used during encoding and a recognition task was used for memory retrieval.[25] Record-assisted recalls may be used to help reduce memory-related error in food records.[114,115]

Recent work suggests that 24-hour recalls which incorporate a multiple pass technique into a standardized interview protocol with structured probes can reduce the commonly observed underestimation of intake for groups of individuals.[62] A multiple pass technique provides respondents several opportunities (i.e., passes) to recall foods eaten using both free recall and cued (probed recall) strategies.[59,62,116,117] As generally administered, the strategy involves three recall passes: an introductory opening sequence in which a respondent is asked to recall all items eaten, an interactive, structural probe sequence to elicit food descriptions and amounts, and a final review of the recall. The multiple pass technique is theoretically sound,[117] and when incorporated into a well-structured interactive interview process may decrease underreporting for groups of individuals.[59,62] While these studies are encouraging for the presentation of group data, there is room for improvement in assessing individuals' intakes.[59] Little data exists, however, on alternative modes of administering a multiple pass strategy and the "gains" at each pass.

A multiple pass technique can be facilitated by the use of interactive software.[118] This allows for a greater level of detail and facilitates data collection, but the technology is generally expensive and is not used commonly in clinical settings. However, written tools, such as probing guides, may be used to mimic this process when quantitative analysis is critical.

Portion Sizes

It is well documented that individuals have difficulty estimating amounts of foods and beverages.[61,119-121] There is a tendency toward overestimation of smaller portion sizes and underestimation of larger portion sizes which can lead to the "flat slope syndrome."[121,122] Portion size estimation aids (Table 19.1) have been shown to reduce portion size estimation error.[123] Estimation aids vary in sophistication and cost. Choice of tools is dictated partially by feasibility. In a clinical setting, aids such as food replicas, real foods, and food picture books may be appropriate. For interviews conducted by phone, tools that are compact for mailing, such as a chart with two-dimensional portions,[124] would be more appropriate.

A number of investigators have investigated whether training subjects to "judge" portion sizes improves quantity estimates.[61,125-130] These studies suggest that training effects may be retained for some days after training and may have significant impact on some, but not all foods. For example, amorphous foods (e.g., salads) are more resistant to training effects.

Variability of Intake

Day-to-day variation of food intake has been well documented in the literature.[36,131,132] Accordingly, assessment of an individual's total dietary intake, particularly by quantitative daily methods, at any one time may not yield an accurate measure of usual intake.[36] Basiotis et al. found that over 100 days of dietary data may be needed to accurately estimate an individual's typical intake for certain nutrients, such as vitamin A.[133] To lessen the effect of day-to-day dietary variation when using 24-hour recalls, assessment should be done on multiple, random, nonconsecutive days[36,58,134] that include both weekend and weekdays. For food records and 24-hour recalls, increasing the number of assessment days will decrease error related to variation in food intake; however, this must be balanced with subject tolerability and assessment objectives.

Consumption Frequency

Accurate estimation of how often foods are consumed is particularly important for retrospective assessment methods. For food frequency questionnaires, frequency of consumption estimates may contribute more error than portion size estimates.[135] The cognitive demands required to mathematically calculate consumption frequency contribute to the error involved with this measure. It has been suggested that the precision of food frequency questionnaires can be increased by not using predefined consumption frequency categories, such as three to four times per week, instead allowing participants to simply enter a number to reflect intake.[135] Ability to accurately recall the frequency of consumption of foods deteriorates as the amount of time between intake and assessment increases, yet longer reference time periods yield more accurate results than questionnaires with shorter reference periods.[136]

Response Bias

All assessment methods are subject to response bias. Social desirability may lead some individuals to selectively omit foods that may be regarded as unacceptable (e.g., alcohol, high fat foods),[23] while others may report eating a healthier diet than that which was actually consumed.[137,138] Self-reported assessment data may also be biased by participation in a dietary intervention.[139]

For both interviewer-assisted and self-completed assessment, questions should be reviewed for face validity to help ensure that participant comprehension of the questions is appropriate. When using interviewers to collect data, training to avoid leading questions and verbal and nonverbal cues that may appear to be judgmental can decrease response bias. Quality control procedures can ensure that interviewer questioning is consistent and nonbiasing.[140,141] Conducting interviews by telephone may reduce bias compared to face-to-face interviews.[63]

In regard to particular assessment methods, food frequency questionnaires may be subject to response bias, as current diet may influence recall of dietary intake in the past,[142] especially for individuals with diet-related illnesses.[143] Response bias can also be induced by methods with a high participant burden. For example, the burden of keeping food records may lead subjects to submit incomplete records, introducing a response bias.[144] Techniques that reduce respondent burden, such as interviewer-assisted food records, can reduce this effect and may improve the quality of data collected.

Data Entry

Data entry is the link between the information provided by a respondent and analysis of the data. Data entry often requires decisions by coders to adjust information provided to meet the demands of a specific data analysis program.[145] If the respondent provides incomplete data or the database does not include all diet items, coders must decide on reasonable substitutions for portion size or food items. Thus, the quality of the data provided by respondents, the quality of the database, and the default assumptions by coders can all contribute to variability in the final food and nutrient data descriptions.[145]

Decisions about amounts of foods eaten may be guided by U.S. Department of Agriculture (USDA) publications on portions commonly consumed in the United States. The USDA has published several reports on foods commonly eaten and the quantities consumed at an eating occasion.[146,147] These reports provide data on amounts eaten by participants in nationwide food consumption surveys.

Food Composition Tables

Food composition databases provide values for the nutritional content of foods. Errors in these databases will introduce systematic biases during data analysis. Further research to improve the validity of the nutrient values within food composition databases will further increase the accuracy of any dietary assessment methodology. This topic will be covered in more detail in Section 23.

Summary

Dietary assessment is a dynamic field, with novel approaches being developed, such as computer-assisted self-interviews.[148] Various techniques to improve validity have been developed (See Table 19.5), but much work still needs to be done to decrease both systematic and random errors. Refinement of current methods and the development of new techniques will improve confidence in the accuracy of dietary data.

TABLE 19.5

Considerations to Reduce Error when Collecting Assessment Data

Potential Error Sources	24-Hour Recalls	Food Records	Food Frequency Questionnaire
Memory	Multiple pass technique Probing questions Encoding strategies	Interviewer assisted records Encouraging adherence to appropriate instructions	Memory retrieval techniques
Portion size	Portion size estimation aids Subject training Interviewer training	Portion size estimation aids Weighing scale Subject training	Portion size estimation aids Subject training
Day-to-day variability	Multiple recall days Nonconsecutive days of data Include weekdays & weekends Collect data in different seasons	Multiple days of records Include weekdays & weekends Collect data in different seasons	N/A
Response bias	Interviewer training Clearly worded, open-ended questions Objective interviewer responses Recalls on unannounced, random days	Objective instructions Reduce respondent burden Limit days of data collection	Objective responses for interviewer mode
Data entry	Documentation of decisions Interactive software with detailed probes and automatic coding	Strict coding and data entry rules Interviewer assisted records Detailed probing guides and instructions	Strict coding and data entry rules Computer scannable forms for automatic coding

Current Issues in Assessment and Analysis

Dietary Quality Scores and Food Pattern Analysis

Historically, dietary quality scores have been a method of interpreting nutrient intakes of an individual by comparison with a dietary standard such as the Recommended Dietary Allowances[149] or, more recently, the Daily Reference Intakes.[150] The nutrient adequacy ratio (NAR), the amount of a particular nutrient in the diet divided by the dietary standard, has been commonly used for a number of years.[30,151] A mean adequacy ratio (MAR) can also be calculated and represents the mean of the NAR for several nutrients of interest.[30] Another way to examine the quality of an individual's diet is to calculate the number of servings from each food group and compare this with food grouping standards such as the USDA Food Guide Pyramid.[152] However, depending on the food group scheme used, serving sizes and placement of foods into groups may vary considerably. Approaches to food group analyses also differ.[153] For individuals, a behavioral approach, in which food group changes are based on nutrition education strategies, is more appropriate. This approach usually defines specific nutritional education programs for health promotion, such as the National Cancer Institute's 5 A Day Program.

With the introduction of the USDA Food Guide Pyramid,[152] other dietary quality scores have been developed which take into account not just nutrients or food group servings alone, but an aggregation of these two assessments into one score. The Healthy Eating

Index score, created by the USDA, takes into account servings from the major food groups of the Food Guide Pyramid as well as a dietary variety and health risk-related nutrient intakes.[154] This more comprehensive approach, as well as others that have been developed,[155] is becoming an increasingly popular approach to interpretation of the dietary intakes of groups or individuals. According to a recent article, identifying food patterns in groups and in individuals might be a better determinant of risk for disease as well as mortality.[156] This is based on the premise that diets are not comprised of single nutrients or foods but combinations of nutrients and nonnutrient components. The interactions of all these dietary components make it difficult to determine the effects of single dietary components. Additionally, dietary behaviors are complex and many different patterns of intake may be occurring simultaneously, such as decreasing fat intake while increasing fruits and vegetables.

Any method of assessing an individual's dietary intake is dependent on the methods of interpretation. More comprehensive methods of interpretation may facilitate the identification of more specific patterns of intake and their relationship to disease.

Dietary Supplements

Increased nutrient intakes from supplements have been related to certain disease risk such as cardiovascular disease (vitamin E), neural tube defects (folate), osteoporosis (calcium), and cancer (antioxidants such as vitamin C and beta-carotene). Approximately 40 to 50% of the general population over the age of two years in the U.S. takes a dietary supplement (see Table 19.6).[157,158] These numbers continue to rise especially for more non-traditional or complementary therapies such as herbal or botanical supplements. Supplement use is higher in non-Hispanic white females, and increases with age in some segments of the population.[157,159] The supplement intake of special populations such as individuals with cancer diagnosis are much higher, up to 80% in some studies.[159,160] Knowledge of dietary supplements as well as an understanding of assessment methods is critical to the overall assessment of nutrient and other dietary components.

Supplement intake data can be assessed in a variety of ways and is usually collected by questionnaire, including food frequency questionnaires, or as part of intake data such

TABLE 19.6

Categories of Supplements

Category	Examples
Vitamins (single or multiple formulations)	Vitamin C, E, D, B_6
Minerals (single or multiple formulations)	Iron, calcium, chromium, zinc
Vitamin(s) with mineral(s)	Calcium with vitamin D; vitamin E with selenium
Herbs and other botanicals	St. John's Wort, ginkgo biloba, ginseng, saw palmetto
Flavonoids	Quercetin, rutin, hesperidin, diadzin
Carotenoids	Lycopene, zeaxanthin, lutein, dried carrot extract, other vegetable extracts
Fatty acids/fish oils, other oils	Linoleic acid, omega 3 fatty acids, DHA EPA
Amino acids/nucleic acids/proteins including co-enzymes, enzymes & hormones	L-glutamine, coenzyme Q-10, bromelain, tryptophan
Microbial prepartions/probiotics	*Lactobacillus acidophilus, B. bifidus, L. bulgaris*
Glandular and other organ preparations	Dessicated glands such thyroid and adrenal
Miscellaneous	Shark cartilage, pycogenol, chrondoitin sulfate

as by 24-hour dietary recall or by food records. When collected by the latter methods it is important to recognize that the intake of supplements for the day of data collection may not reflect the pattern of intake over an extended period of time. Detailed questionnaires, which are better for capturing long-term intake and frequency of intake, are used frequently in research studies, clinical practice, and nutrition monitoring and surveys.[161,162]

Quantifying supplement intake is a difficult and tedious process. When collecting supplement information, it is important to identify what level of detail is needed to describe or quantify dietary intakes with dietary supplements. Strategies may include having those individuals bring in their supplement labels, or photocopy the labels. Other strategies include having the participants respond to questionnaires that provide lists of single vitamins and minerals as well as common brand names for multiple formulations. For herbal and botanical ingredients and other components not typically found in common formulations, it might be necessary to identify the active components and, above all else, to obtain brand name and label information.

Functional Foods

According to the Institute of Medicine of the National Academy of Sciences (1994) the definition of functional foods is "any food or food ingredient that may provide a health benefit beyond the traditional nutrients it contains."[163] Currently, there is a major research emphasis to identify physiologically active components, or phytochemicals, and their potential for decreasing disease risk. Functional foods can consist of foods or food ingredients, including fruits and vegetables to more specialized products such as those containing soy or phytostanols (i.e., margarines with claims of reducing blood cholesterol levels).

Since many of the phytochemicals in foods are still under investigation, it is premature to emphasize quantification of single functional food components in dietary assessment. However, improvements in individual assessment methods will make it possible to quantify and link these components in functional foods with their potential health benefits. Examples of where individual assessment plays a significant role in providing this linkage can be found in the literature examining fruit and vegetable intakes. There are now databases that can accurately quantify the carotenoid content of foods.[118,164] As cooking methods, storage, and exposure to air and water are known to affect the carotenoid content of fruits and vegetables, the development of these databases has been a challenge. In the case of assessing carotenoids, for example, it is important to distinguish between pink and white grapefruit (i.e., pink grapefruit has 3740 mg lycopene, whereas white grapefruit has 0 mg). This one simple observation in assessing an individual's intake can have a significant impact on determining the relationship between dietary carotenoids and blood carotenoids and the potential role they may have in cancer risk in groups of individuals.

In assessing diets for research purposes it is important to consider the level of detail required for other components in foods as well. The assessment issues outlined in this section are the same for assessing functional foods. As more components are identified and quantification is possible, databases need to be developed that make analysis of functional foods and their components possible. The knowledge gained in the study of functional foods will drive the type and level of detail in methodology and database development.

References

1. Bingham S. *Nutr Abstr Rev (Series A)* 57: 705; 1987.
2. Medlin C, Skinner JD. *JADA* 88: 1250; 1988.
3. Mudge GG. *J Home Ec* 15: 181; 1923.
4. Mudge GG. *JADA* 1: 166; 1926.
5. Turner D. *JADA* 16: 875; 1940.
6. Widdowson EM. *J Hygiene* 36: 269; 1936.
7. Widdowson, EM. *J Hygiene* 36: 293; 1936.
8. National Research Council, *Diet and Health: Implications for Reducing Chronic Disease Risk,* National Academy Press 46; 1989.
9. Public Health Service, *Healthy people: Surgeon General's Report on Health Promotion and Disease Prevention,* US Department of Health and Human Services, Washington DC; 1979.
10. Public Health Service, *Promoting Health/Preventing Disease: Objectives for the Nation,* US Department of Health and Human Services, Washington DC; 1980.
11. US Department of Health and Human Services, *Healthy People 2010 (Conference Edition),* US Department of Health and Human Services, Washington DC; 2000.
12. Leverton RM, Marsh AG. *J Home Ec* 31: 111; 1939.
13. Huenemann RL, Turner D. *JADA* 18: 562; 1942.
14. Young C, et al. *JADA* 28: 124; 1952.
15. Young C, et al. *JADA* 28: 218; 1952.
16. Wait B, Roberts LJ. *JADA* 8: 323; 1932.
17. Yudkin J. *Brit J Nutr* 5: 177; 1951.
18. Hunt CL. *J Home Ec* 5: 212; 1918.
19. Burke BS, Stuart HC. *J Pediatr* 12: 493; 1938.
20. Donelson EG, Leichsenring JM. *JADA* 18: 429; 1942.
21. Tigerstedt R. *Skand Arch Physiol* 24: 97; 1910.
22. Blundell JE. *Am J Clin Nutr* 71: 3; 2000.
23. Dwyer JT, Krall EA, Coleman KA. *JADA* 87: 1509; 1987.
24. Smith AF. *Eur J Clin Nutr* 47: S6; 1993.
25. Ervin RB, Smiciklas-Wright H. *JADA* 98: 989; 1998.
26. Roberfroid MB. *J Nutr* 129: 1398S; 1999.
27. Life Sciences Research Office, *Guidelines for Use of Dietary Intake Data,* Federation of American Societies for Experimental Biology, Bethesda, MD; 1996.
28. Gibson RS. *Principles of Nutritional Assessment,* Oxford University Press, New York; 1990.
29. Thompson FE, Byers T. Dietary assessment resource manual, *J Nutr* 124: 2245S; 1994.
30. Smiciklas-Wright H, Guthrie HA. *Nutrition Assessment: A Comprehensive Guide for Planning Intervention,* 2nd ed, Simko MD, Cowell C, Gilbride, JA Eds, Aspen Publishers, Gaithersburg, MD: 165; 1995.
31. Dwyer J. *Modern Nutrition in Health and Disease,* 9th ed, Shils ME, Olson JA, Shike M, Ross AC, Eds, Williams & Wilkins, Philadelphia: 937; 1999.
32. Christakis G. *Am J Public Health* 63: 1S; 1973.
33. Copeland T, et al. *JADA* in press.
34. Olendzki B, et al. *JADA* 99: 1433; 1999.
35. St. Jeor ST, Guthrie HA, Jones MB. *JADA* 83: 155; 1983.
36. Tarasuk V, Beaton GH. *Am J Clin Nutr* 54: 464; 1991.
37. Craig MR, et al. *JADA* 100: 421; 2000.
38. Tian HG, et al. *Eur J Clin Nutr* 49: 26; 1995.
39. Streit KJ, et al. *JADA* 91: 213; 1991.
40. Achterberg C, et al. *J Can Diet Assoc* 52: 226; 1991.
41. Block G, Hartman AM, Naughton D. *Epidemiology* 1: 58; 1990.
42. Brown JE, et al. *JADA* 96: 262; 1996.
43. Cummings SR, et al. *Am J Epidemiol* 126: 796; 1987.

44. Domel SB, et al. *J Am Coll Nutr* 13: 33; 1994.
45. Kristal AR, et al. *Am J Epidemiol* 146: 856; 1997.
46. Jackson B, et al. *JADA* 86: 1531; 1986.
47. Buzzard IM, et al. *JADA* 96: 574; 1996.
48. Gorbach SL, et al. *JADA* 90: 802; 1990.
49. Kuehl KS, et al. *Prev Med* 22: 154; 1993.
50. Moulin CC, et al. *Am J Clin Nutr* 67: 853; 1998.
51. Bingham SA, *Ann Nutr Metab* 35: 117; 1991.
52. Gittelsohn J, et al. *JADA* 94: 1273; 1994.
53. Dubois S. *JADA* 90: 382; 1990.
54. Omnibus Budget Reconciliation Act of 1990, P. L. 101-508; 1990.
55. Morris JN, et al. *The Gerontologist* 30: 293; 1990.
56. Rebro SM, et al. *JADA* 98: 1163; 1998.
57. Pekkarinen M. *World Rev Nutr Diet* 12: 145; 1970.
58. Larkin FA, Metzner HL, Guire KE. *JADA* 91: 1538; 1991.
59. Jonnalagadda SS, et al. *JADA* 100: 303; 2000.
60. Lyons GK, et al. *JADA* 96: 1276; 1996.
61. Howat PM, et al. *JADA* 94: 169; 1994.
62. Johnson RK, Driscoll P, Goran, MI. *JADA* 96: 1140; 1996.
63. Fox TA, Heimendinger, J, Block G. *JADA* 92: 729; 1992.
64. Derr JA, et al. *Am J Epidemiol* 136: 1386; 1992.
65. Casey PH, et al. *JADA,* 99: 1406; 1999.
66. Krantzler NJ, et al. *Am J Clin Nutr* 36: 1234; 1982.
67. Pao EM, Sykes KE, Cypel VS. *USDA Methodological Research for Large Scale Dietary Intake Surveys, 1975-88,* Home Economics Research Report no. 49, US Department of Agriculture, Human Nutrition Information Service, US Government Printing Office, Washington, DC: 181; 1989.
68. Morgan KJ, et al. *JADA* 87: 888; 1987.
69. Cullen KW, et al. *J Am Coll Nutr* 18: 442; 1999.
70. Hartman AM, et al. *Nutr Cancer* 25: 305; 1996.
71. Retzlaff BM, et al. *Am J Public Health* 87: 181; 1997.
72. Sloan NL, et al. *Am J Public Health* 87: 186; 1997.
73. Brants HA, et al. *Eur J Clin Nutr* 51: S12; 1997.
74. Briefel RR, et al. *JADA* 92: 959; 1992.
75. White JV, Dwyer JT, Posner BM, et al. *JADA* 92: 163; 1992.
76. The Nutrition Screening Initiative, *Incorporating Nutrition Screening and Interventions into Medical Practice,* The Nutrition Screening Initiative, Washington, DC; 1994.
77. Posner BM, et al. *Am J Public Health* 83: 972; 1993.
78. Subar AF, et al. *FASEB J* 14: A559; 2000.
79. Block G, et al. *J Clin Epidemiol* 43: 1327; 1990.
80. Longnecker MP, et al. *Epidemiology* 4: 356; 1993.
81. Musgrave KO, et al. *JADA* 89: 1484; 1989.
82. Willett WC, et al. *JADA* 87: 43; 1987.
83. Potischman N, et al. *Nutr Cancer* 34: 70; 1999.
84. Lund SM, Brown J, Harnack L. *Eur J Clin Nutr* 52: 53S; 1998.
85. Rockett HR, Wolf AM, Colditz GA. *JADA* 95: 336; 1995.
86. Coates RJ, et al. *Am J Epidemiol* 134: 658; 1991.
87. Kumanyika SK, et al. *Am J Clin Nutr* 65: 1123S; 1997.
88. Kumanyika S, et al. *JADA* 96: 137; 1996.
89. Laus MJ, et al. *J Nutr Elder* 18: 1; 1999.
90. Burke BS. *JADA* 23: 1041; 1947.
91. Beaton GH. *Am J Clin Nutr* 59: 253S; 1994.
92. Black AE, et al. *Eur J Clin Nutr* 51: 405; 1997.
93. Bandini LG, et al. *Am J Clin Nutr* 65: 1138S; 1997.
94. Champagne CM, et al. *JADA* 98: 426; 1998.
95. Goris AH, Westerterp-Plantenga MS, Westerterp KR. *Am J Clin Nutr* 71: 130; 2000.

96. Martin LJ, et al. *Am J Clin Nutr* 63: 483; 1996.
97. Kroke A, et al. *Am J Clin Nutr* 70: 439; 1999.
98. Schoeller DA, Fjeld CR. *Annu Rev Nutr* 11: 355; 1991.
99. Briefel RR, et al. *Am J Clin Nutr* 65: 1203S; 1997.
100. Johansson L, et al. *Am J Clin Nutr* 68: 266; 1998.
101. Stallone DD, et al. *Eur J Clin Nutr* 51: 815; 1997.
102. Black AE, et al. *Eur J Clin Nutr* 45: 583; 1991.
103. Johnson RK, Soultanakis RP, Matthews DE. *J Am Diet Assoc* 98: 1136; 1998.
104. Smiciklas-Wright H, et al. *FASEB J* 13: A263; 1999.
105. Bingham S. *Am J Clin Nutr* 59: 227S; 1994.
106. Champagne CM, et al. *JADA* 96: 707; 1996.
107. Kortzinger I, et al. *Ann Nutr Metab* 41: 37; 1997.
108. Mertz W, et al. *Am J Clin Nutr* 54: 291; 1991.
109. Schoeller DA. *Metabolism* 44: 18; 1995.
110. Wessells MG. *Cognitive Psychology,* Harper & Row, New York; 1982.
111. Craik FIM. *Philos Trans R Soc Lond B Biol Sci* 302: 341; 1993.
112. Schaie KW, Willis SL. *Adult Development and Aging,* 2nd ed, Schaie KW, Willis SL, Eds, Little, Brown and Company, Boston; 324; 1986.
113. Campbell VA, Dodds ML. *JADA* 51: 29; 1967.
114. Eldridge AL, et al. *JADA* 98: 777; 1998.
115. Lytle LA, et al. *JADA* 93: 1431; 1993.
116. De Maio TJ, Ciochetto T, Davis W. *American Statistical Association: Survey Methods:* 1021; 1993.
117. Wright JD, Ervin RB, Briefel RR, Eds. *Consensus Workshop on Dietary Assessment: Nutrition Monitoring and Tracking the Year 2000 Objectives,* Department of Health and Human Services, National Center for Health Statistics, Hyattsville, MD, 1993.
118. Nutrition Coordinating Center, *Nutrient Data System for Research (NDS-R) software,* University of Minnesota, Minneapolis, MN.
119. Blake AJ, Guthrie HA, Smiciklas-Wright H. *JADA* 89: 962; 1989.
120. Smiciklas-Wright H, et al. *Progress Report 390,* Northeastern Cooperative Regional Research Publication, Pennsylvania State University, Agriculture Experiment Station: 1; 1988.
121. Young LRN. *Nutr Rev* 53: 149; 1995.
122. Faggiano F, et al. *Epidemiology* 3: 379; 1992.
123. Cypel YS, Guenther PM, Petot GJ. *JADA* 97: 289; 1997.
124. Nutrition Consulting Enterprises, *Food Portion Visual,* Nutrition Consulting Enterprises, Framingham, MA, 1981.
125. Rapp SR, et al. *JADA* 86: 249; 1986.
126. Bolland JE, Yuhas JA, Bolland TW. *JADA* 88: 817; 1988.
127. Yuhas JA, Bolland JE, Bolland TW. *JADA* 89: 1473; 1989.
128. Bolland JE, Ward JY, Bolland TW. *JADA* 90: 1402; 1990.
129. Weber JL, et al. *JADA* 97: 176; 1997.
130. Slawson DL, Eck LH. *JADA* 97: 295; 1997.
131. Guthrie HA, Crocetti AF. *JADA* 85: 325; 1985.
132. McAvay G, Rodin J. *Appetite* 11: 97; 1988.
133. Basiotis PP, et al. *J Nutr* 117: 1638; 1987.
134. Hartman AM, et al. *Am J Epidemiol* 132: 999; 1990.
135. Flegal KM, et al. *Am J Epidemiol* 128: 749; 1988.
136. Smith A. *Cognitive Processes in Long-Term Dietary Recall, DHHS Publication No. 92-1079,* Series 6, No. 44, Department of Health and Human Services, National Center for Health Statistics, Hyattsville, MD; 1991.
137. Hebert JR, et al. *Int J Epidemiol* 24: 389; 1995.
138. Hebert JR, et al. *Am J Epidemiol* 146: 1046; 1997.
139. Kristal AR, et al. *J Am Diet Assoc* 98: 40; 1998.
140. Edwards S, et al. *Am J Epidemiol* 140: 1020; 1994.
141. Smiciklas-Wright H, et al. *JADA* 81: 28S; 1991.
142. Dwyer JT, Coleman KA. *Am J Clin Nutr* 65: 1153S; 1997.

143. Malila N, et al. *Nutr Cancer* 32: 146; 1998.
144. Gersovitz M, Madden JP, Smiciklas-Wright H. *JADA* 73: 48; 1978.
145. Lacey JM, et al. *Coder Variability in Computerized Dietary Analysis*, Research Bulletin Number 729, Massachusetts Agricultural Experiment Station, Massachusetts; 1990.
146. Pao EM, et al. *Foods Commonly Eaten by Individuals: Amounts Per Day and Per Eating Occasion*, Home Economics Research Report Number 44, Consumer Nutrition Center, Human Information Service, Hyattsville, MD; 1982.
147. Krebs-Smith SM, et al. *Foods Commonly Eaten in the United States: Quantities Consumed Per Eating Occasion and in a Day, 1989-91*, NFS Report No. 91-3, US Department of Agriculture, Agriculture Research Service, Washington, DC; 1997.
148. Kohlmeier L, et al. *Am J Clin Nutr* 65: 1275S; 1997.
149. Food and Nutrition Board, *Recommended Dietary Allowances*, 10th ed, National Academy Press, Washington, DC; 1989.
150. Food and Nutrition Board, *Dietary Reference Intakes for Thiamin, Riboflavin, Niacin, Vitamin B_6, Folate, Vitamin B_{12}, Pantothenic Acid, Biotin, and Choline*, National Academy Press, Washington, DC; 1998.
151. Guthrie HA, Scheer JC. *JADA* 78: 240; 1981.
152. US Department of Agriculture, *The Food Guide Pyramid: A Guide to Daily Food Choices*, US Department of Agriculture, Nutrition Information Service; 1992.
153. Cullen KW, et al. *JADA* 99: 849; 1999.
154. Bowman SA, et al. *The Healthy Eating Index: 1994-96, CNPP-5*, US Department of Agriculture, Center for Nutrition Policy and Promotion; 1998.
155. Haines PS, Siega-Riz AM, Popkin BM. *JADA* 99: 697; 1999.
156. Kant AK, et al. *JAMA* 283: 2109, 2000.
157. Ervin RB, Wright JD, Kennedy-Stephenson J. *Use of Dietary Supplements in the United States, 1988-94*, Series 11, No. 244, Department of Health and Human Services, National Center for Health Statistics, Hyattsville, MD; 1999.
158. Slesinski MJ, Subar AF, Kahle LL. *J Nutr* 126: 3001; 1996.
159. Newman V, et al. *JADA* 98: 285; 1998.
160. Winters BL, et al. *FASEB J* 13: A253; 1999.
161. Tippett KS, Cypel YS, Eds. *Design and Operation: the Continuing Survey of Food Intakes by Individuals and the Diet and Health Knowledge Survey, 1994-96*, Nationwide Food Survey Report No. 91-1, US Department of Agriculture, Agricultural Research Service; 1998.
162. Rock CL, et al. *Nutr Cancer* 29: 133; 1997.
163. Milner JA. *J Nutr* 129: 1395S; 1999.
164. US Department of Agriculture, *USDA-NCC Carotenoid Database for U.S. foods, 1998-1999.*
165. NASCO, *Nasco nutrition teaching aids, 1999-2000 catalog* Fort Atkinson, WI: 437; 1999.
166. National Center for Health Statistics, *Dietary Intake Source Data: United States, 1976-80. (DHHS publication no. PHS 83-1681)*, Series 11, no. 231, US Department of Health and Human Services, Washington, DC; 1983.
167. Hess MA, Ed. *Portion Photos of Popular Foods*, American Dietetic Association: 128; 1997.

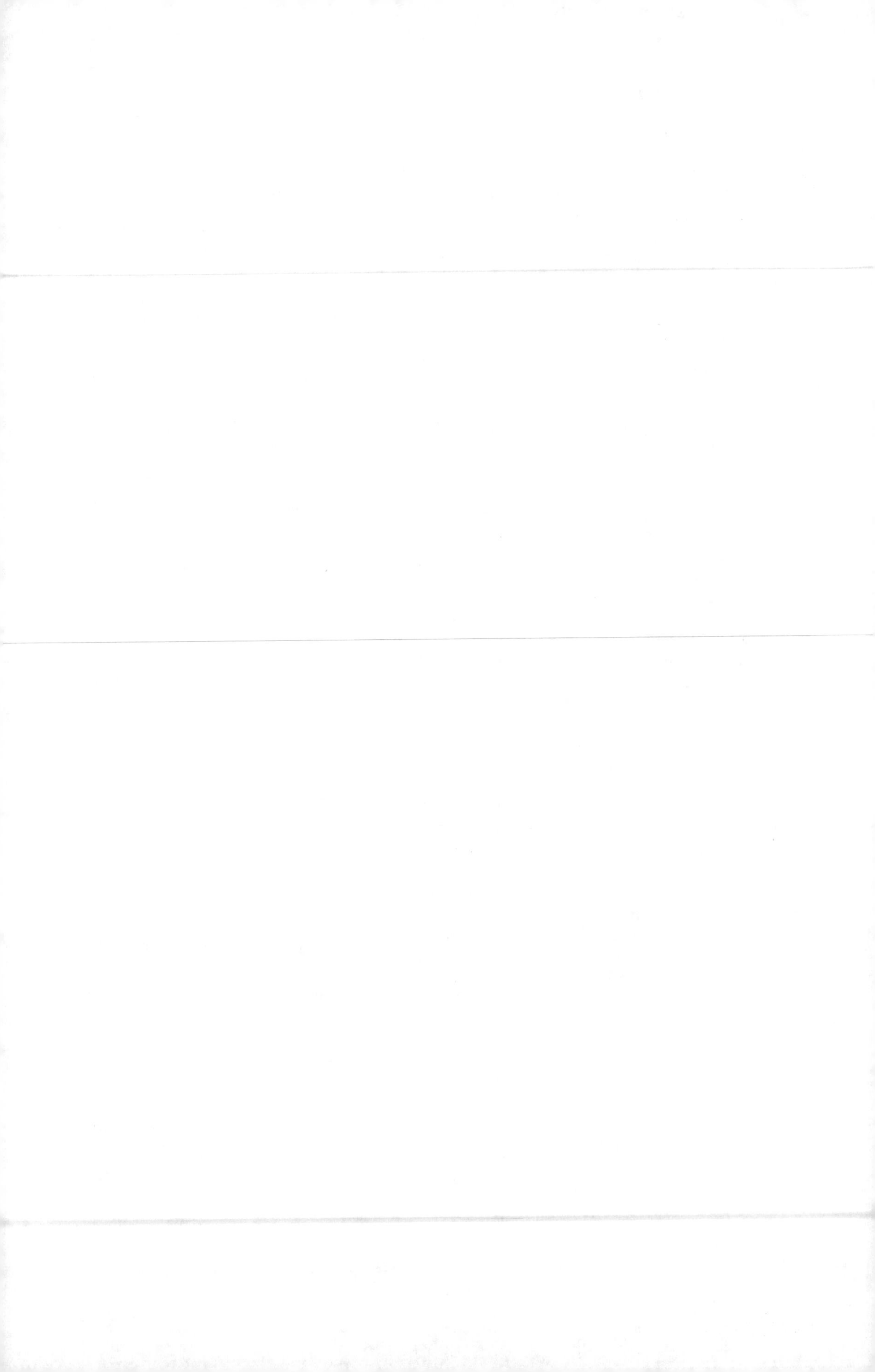

20

Validity and Reliability of Dietary Assessment in School-Age Children

R. Sue McPherson, Deanna M. Hoelscher, Maria Alexander, Kelley S. Scanlon, and Mary K. Serdula

Introduction

This review of 50 studies examines the validity and/or reliability of dietary assessment methods used for school-age children during the last three decades, and discusses the challenges of measuring children's dietary behaviors. This section is an update from previously published work of the referenced authors.[67] Recommendations on the use of available assessment methods are discussed and gaps in our knowledge of dietary assessment in children are outlined, along with suggestions for future research.

Review Methodology

The studies included in this review cover a variety of dietary assessment methods including the 24-hour recall, food record, food frequency questionnaire, diet history, and observation. A total of 41 validity and 9 reliability studies used at least one of these methodologies and met the three review criteria: 1) publication in a peer-reviewed English journal article between January 1970 and August 2000; 2) inclusion of school children age 5 to 18 years living in an industrialized country; and 3) reporting of specific reliability and/or validity tests from a minimum sample of 30 children in either the main study sample or a subsample (denoted by age, gender, or ethnic), after the publishing author's exclusions for analyses. Studies were identified by Medline searches using key words and supplemented by cross-referencing from author reference lists. Studies that did not specifically use the words validity, reliability, reproducibility, or repeatability in the results or discussion may not have been identified. The degree of reliability or validity of the instrument reported was not considered an inclusion factor. Multiple validity or reliability studies that were included in a single article were considered separately and are repeated in the descriptions of results.

0-8493-2705-9/01/$0.00+$1.50

TABLE 20.1

Definitions and Explanation of Tables

General

Study entries are listed in ascending order by age.
Multiple validity or reliability studies included in a single journal article are presented as separate entries in the appropriate table.

Definitions

Adults required — Adults provided all of the intake information or were required to supplement and assist the child's report.
Quantitative — Quantity of food consumed was estimated using weights, measures, or food models. Responses were open-ended.
Semi-quantitative — Quantity of food consumed was estimated using a standard portion size, serving, or a predetermined amount, and respondent was asked about the number of portions consumed.
Non-quantitative — Quantity of food consumed was not assessed.
Self-administered — Child completed the dietary assessment without assistance.
Group-administered — Child completed the dietary assessment with help from a proctor, teacher, or caregiver in a group setting.
Interviewer-administered — A trained interviewer elicited the dietary assessment information from the child in a one-on-one setting.

Results Section

Omission of any of the following components indicates it was not provided in the article or was from a sample of less than 30 children. Statistical significance of measures is noted with clarifications as to whether significance testing was shown in the article or only reported via a statement from the publishing authors. The results are ordered as follows:

Correlations for energy, protein, and total fat between methodologies or administrations.
Range of correlations between methodologies or administrations for the nutrients assessed.
For validity studies: the absolute values and percent difference in energy intake between the validation standard and the instrument ([instrument-validation standard]/validation standard × 100).
For reliability studies: the absolute values and percent difference in energy intake between the first and follow-up assessment ([follow-up instrument-first instrument]/follow-up instrument × 100).
Comparison of mean intake of nutrients assessed.
Comparison of foods or food groups consumed.
Comparison of portion size.
Results by age, gender, or ethnicity.

Dietary Assessment Methodologies

The following topics define each dietary method and refer its tables of results of validity and reliability studies, thereby providing a summary of the current state of each field. The format of entries in Tables 20.2 through 20.6, which contain the validity and reliability studies for the various methods, is explained in Table 20.1.

24-Hour Recall (Table 20.2)

The 24-hour recall consists of a structured interview in which a trained nutritionist or other professional asks the child and/or adult caregiver to list everything the child ate or

TABLE 20.2

Recall Validity Studies Among School-Age Children

Reference	Sample	Age/Grade	Instrument	Validation Standard	Design	Results
Basch et al. 1990[16]	18 M[b] 28 F[b] Latino	4-7 y Adults required[c]	Evening meal recall; quantitative	Observation	Compared mothers' recall of what child ate at evening meal on the previous day against observation of the meal. Excerpted evening meal from 24-hour recall.	Energy-adjusted Pearson correlations between recalled evening meal and observed evening meal were 0.71 for energy, 0.50 for protein, and 0.52 for total fat. Range of correlations for 18 nutrients assessed was –0.10 for phosphorus to 0.82 for iron. Recalled energy intake was 9% higher than observed intake (507 vs. 465 kcal/meal). Seven nutrients were significantly overestimated by recalled intake of the meal (significance testing not shown). Range of mothers reporting fewer items consumed as compared to the number of items observed consumed was between 4 and 30%. 15.5% of reported portion sizes were smaller and 33.5% of portions were greater than those observed (significance testing not shown).
Eck et al. 1989[11]	33 M&F	4-9.5 y Adults required	Lunch recall; quantitative	Observation	Compared mother's, father's, or both parents plus child's (consensus) recall of lunch against observation of lunch on the previous day. Excerpted lunch meal from 24-hour recall.	Pearson correlations between consensus recall of lunch and observed lunch were 0.87 for energy, 0.91 for protein as % of kcal and 0.85 for total fat as % of kcal. Range of correlations for 9 nutrients assessed was 0.75 for carbohydrate as % of kcal to 0.91 for protein as % of kcal. Pearson correlations between observed intake and fathers' recall were 0.83 for energy, 0.79 for protein as % of kcal and 0.72 for total fat as % of kcal. Pearson correlations between observed intake and mother's recalled intake were 0.64 for energy, 0.56 for protein as % of kcal and 0.65 for total fat as % of kcal. Recalled energy intake from the consensus, fathers' and mothers' recalls was 2% (558 kcal/meal), 5% (545 kcal/meal) and 4% (550 kcal/meal) lower than observed intake (572 kcal/meal), respectively. Only mothers' recall of energy from dairy foods/beverages and snacks/desserts were significantly different from observed intake. There were no significant differences in mean nutrient intake between any pairs compared. Qualitative comparison of number of items recalled revealed that only fathers' recalls of non-dairy beverages and snacks/desserts differed significantly from observed intake. Consensus approach appeared to reduce the tendency to overreport low intakes and underreport high intakes (flattened slope phenomenon).

TABLE 20.2 *(Continued)*

Recall Validity Studies Among School-Age Children

Reference	Sample	Age/Grade	Instrument	Validation Standard	Design	Results
Lindquist et al. 2000[65]	17 M[b] 13 F[b] 17 White 13 Black	6.5-11.6 y Adults required	Three 24-hour recalls, one phone, two interview	TEE[f] by doubly-labeled water	Compared average of 3 child's parent-assisted recalls against 14-d TEE.	Pearson correlation between average recalled intake and TEE was 0.32 for energy. Recalled energy intake was 0.5% higher than TEE from doubly-labeled water (7.90 vs 7.86 mJ/day). Inaccuracy in energy reporting was not predicted by age, gender, ethnicity, social class, or adiposity.
Reynolds et al. 1990[17]	18 M&F 25 M&F 31 M&F	7-8 y 9-10 y 11-12 y	Daytime recall; non-quantitative	Observation	Compared average of 3 child's recalls of daytime meals against observation of daytime meals. Exchange units of foods that were developed from the recalls for analyses.	Recalled energy intake was 34% lower for 7-8 year olds (1818 vs. 2751 kcal/daytime meals), 21% lower for 9-10 year olds (2291 vs. 2887 kcal/ daytime meals) and 17% lower for 11 year olds (2643 vs. 3185 kcal/daytime meals) than observed intake. Children significantly underestimated their energy, carbohydrate and fat consumption as compared to observers, with younger children having larger differences. Exact agreement for the 9 exchange groups ranged from 94% for lean fat meat to 17% for the fat group. Girls were significantly more accurate in reporting medium fat meat exchange units than boys, 62% versus 50% respectively (significance testing not shown).
Lytle et al. 1993[7]	49 M&F	3rd Grade	24-hour recall assisted by food record; quantitative	Observation	Compared food record-assisted recalls completed by children against observation of school lunch and breakfast by trained personnel and of other meals at home by parents.	Pearson correlations between recalled and observed intakes were 0.59 for energy, 0.62 for protein as % of kcal and 0.64 for total fat as % of kcal. Range of correlations for the 8 nutrients assessed was 0.41 for polyunsaturated fat as % of kcal to 0.79 for saturated fat as % of kcal. Recalled energy intake was 10% higher than observed intake (1823 vs. 1650 kcal/day). There was an overall 77.9% agreement in the types of food items recalled and observed. Food portions were recalled within 10% of observed portions 35% of the time; overestimation occurred 42% and underestimation occurred 23% of the time.

Van Horn et al. 1990[8]	18 M 14 F	8-10 y	24-Hour recall by phone; quantitative	1-Day food record	Compared child's recall of intake against parent's observation recorded as a food record.	Pearson correlations between recalled intake and record of intake were 0.76 for energy, 0.74 for protein as % of kcal and 0.73 for total fat as % of kcal. Range of correlations for the 10 nutrients assessed was 0.64 for saturated fat as % of kcal to 0.93 for iron. Recalled energy intake was 2% lower than recorded intake (1799 vs. 1836 kcal/day). There were no significant differences between child and parent reports of nutrient intake (significance testing not shown).
Todd & Kretsch 1986[a10]	30 M&F Chinese 31 M&F Hispanic	8-11 y	Breakfast and lunch recall; quantitative	Observation	Compared child's recall of intake of school breakfast and lunch against observation of school meals with plate waste subtracted. Excerpted breakfast and lunch meals from 24-hour recall.	Pearson correlations between recalled lunch and observed lunch for Chinese were 0.49 for energy, 0.62 for protein and 0.25 for total fat, and for Hispanics were 0.53 for energy, 0.51 for protein and 0.46 for total fat. Range of correlations for the 15 nutrients assessed for Chinese was –0.10 for sodium to 0.63 for thiamin, and for Hispanics was 0.34 for niacin to 0.81 for vitamin C. Chinese children's recalled energy intake was 10% lower than observed intake (686 vs. 765 kcal/2 meals). Chinese children recalled consistently less food than consumed, which was significantly lower for 4 of the 15 nutrients. Hispanic children's recalled energy intake was 6% higher than observed intake (665 vs. 630 kcal/2 meals). Hispanic children recalled intake versus consumed intake was inconsistent and was significantly higher for 2 nutrients and lower for 1 of the 15 nutrients assessed. For Chinese, food item omissions ranged from 4% for milk to 35% for vegetables. For Hispanics, food item omissions ranged from 0% for juice and milk to 35% for vegetables.
Samuelson 1970[13]	56 M&F 43 M&F	8 y 13 y	Lunch recall; quantitative	Chemical analysis of food	Compared child's recall of lunch against weighed chemical analyses of a double portion of lunch, with plate waste subtracted. Excerpted lunch meal from 24-hour recall.	Spearman correlations between recall of lunch and chemical analyses of lunch for 8- and 13-year olds for energy were 0.68 and 0.71, respectively. Correlations for protein of 8- and 13-year olds were 0.55 and 0.45, respectively. Correlations for total fat of 8- and 13-year olds were 0.61 and 0.69, respectively. Range of correlations for the 4 nutrients assessed for 8-year-olds was 0.55 for protein to 0.68 for energy. Range of correlations for 13-year-olds was 0.45 for protein to 0.71 for energy. Among 8-year-olds, recalled energy intake was 18% higher than chemical analyses (472 vs. 399 kcal/meal). Among 13-year-olds, recalled energy intake was 1% higher than chemical analyses (494 vs. 491 kcal/meal). Median portion size estimated by child compared to weighing was not significantly different for 8-year-olds and was 14% lower among 13-year-olds (significance testing not shown).

TABLE 20.2 *(Continued)*

Recall Validity Studies Among School-Age Children

Reference	Sample	Age/Grade	Instrument	Validation Standard	Design	Results
Lytle et al. 1998[14]	238 M 248 F 253 White 146 Asian 73 Black 14 Other	4th Grade	Lunch recall; quantitative	Observation	Compared child's recall of school lunch against observation of lunch. Excerpted lunch meal from 24-hour recall.	Pearson correlations between recall and observed intake for energy was 0.44. Range of correlations for the 5 nutrients assessed was 0.39 for beta-carotene to 0.61 for vitamin C. Recalled energy intake was 14% higher than observed intake (600 vs. 526 kcal/meal). There were significant differences between recalled and observed nutrient intake for all nutrients except beta-carotene (borderline significant). The highest correlation was for servings of fruit, 0.65, and lowest for servings of vegetables, 0.42. No ethnic specific analyses provided.
Baxter et al. 1997[a15]	120 M 117 F 58 White 179 Black	4th Grade	Lunch recall; quantitative	Observation	Compared child's recall of food items from school lunch either the same day or the following day against observation of that lunch.	Average matched food rates from recall of lunch and observation of lunch were 84% and 68% for same day and next day intervals, respectively. Rates for omitted and added (phantom) foods were significantly lower for the same day (16% vs. 5%) than next day recalls (32% vs. 13%). Children were least likely to omit beverages and main dishes and most likely to omit condiments and miscellaneous foods. There were no significant gender, ethnic, or time interval differences in the accuracy of recalling the amount of food consumed (significance testing not shown).
Mullenbach et al. 1992[9]	22 M 18 F	6-9th Grade Adults required	24-Hour recall by phone; quantitative	3-day food record	Compared adolescents' parent-assisted recall against adolescents' parent-assisted 3-day food records completed 2-4 weeks prior to recalls.	Pearson correlations between recall and food records were 0.42 for energy, 0.42 for protein, and 0.33 for total fat. Range of correlations for the 19 nutrients assessed was 0.09 for cholesterol to 0.57 for riboflavin. Recalled energy intake was 12% lower than recorded energy intake (1835 vs. 2097 kcal/day). There were no significant differences between recalled and recorded average nutrient intake, although the 24-hour recall estimates were all lower than those from the food record.

[a] Results of all subgroups not reported due to samples below the N=30 criterion
[b] Males (M), females (F)
[c] Adult assistance required for instrument administration
[d] N/A — not applicable
[e] FFQ — food frequency questionnaire
[f] TEE — total energy expenditure

drank during a specified time period, typically the previous day.[5] The 24-hour recall is an estimate of actual intake that incorporates a detailed description of the food, including brand names, ingredients of mixed dishes, food preparation methods, and portion sizes consumed. Because of the detail provided, complete nutrient intake can be calculated for the designated day. When conducted with a random sample population, a single 24-hour recall is appropriate for estimating group means, but is not a tool to predict individual-level health outcomes such as serum cholesterol levels. Because of intra-individual variation in intake, multiple recalls are needed to accurately estimate usual nutrient intake. Nelson and colleagues have addressed how to calculate the number of days of recording required to estimate intakes of individual nutrients for children age 2 to 17 years.[6] Collection of 24-hour recall data can occur via paper records or with a computer-assisted program. Prompts for quantification of portion size such as two- or three-dimensional food models are typically employed.

Food Record (Table 20.3)

Food records are written accounts of actual intake of the food and beverages consumed during a specified time period, usually three, five, or seven days.[5] A single food record is a measure of actual intake and, like the 24-hour recall, is appropriate for estimating group means but is not a tool to predict individual-level health outcomes. The work of Nelson and colleagues can be used to calculate the number of days of records necessary to determine nutrient intake with precision.[6] Respondents record detailed information about their dietary intake, such as brand names, ingredients of mixed dishes, food preparation methods, and estimates of amounts consumed. By collecting the information at the time of consumption, error due to memory loss is reduced, and thus food records often serve as a validation standard. Prompts for quantification of food portions, such as two- or three-dimensional food models are frequently used to aid respondents. Audiotaping food records has been explored as an alternative to handwritten records.[8]

Food Frequency Questionnaires (Tables 20.4 and 20.5)

Food frequency questionnaires (FFQs) which measure usual food intake are often used for epidemiological studies, since they are relatively easy to administer, less expensive than other assessment methods, and easily adapted for population studies. These measures of usual intake can be used to rank respondents by intake levels and are useful for predicting health outcomes at both group and individual levels. Respondents are asked to report frequency of consumption and sometimes portion size for a defined list of foods; the questionnaire can be self-administered or conducted with individual or group assistance. Respondents report their usual intake over a defined period of time in the past year, month, or week, although frequency of intake on the previous day has also been assessed. FFQs can be classified as quantitative, semi-quantitative, or non-quantitative. Data from non-quantitative FFQs are generally used to assess frequency of consumption of food; however, these frequencies may also be associated with standard portions to estimate nutrient amounts. The burden of work for the researcher is on the front end, developing the food list for inclusion on the FFQ. The appropriateness of the food list for the FFQ often needs to be population specific to accurately assess usual intake.

Diet History (Table 20.6)

Diet histories assess the past diet of an individual in the form of usual meal patterns, food intake, and food preparation practices through an extensive interview or questionnaire.[5]

TABLE 20.3

Food Record Validity Studies Among School-Age Children

Reference	Sample	Age/Grade	Instrument	Validation Standard	Design	Results
Lindquist et al. 2000[65]	17 M[b] 13 F[b] 17 White 13 Black	6.5-11.6 y Adults required[c]	3-Day audio-taped food record	TEE[f] by doubly-labeled water	Compared average of 3 child's parent-assisted reports of intake from audiotaped food records against 14-d TEE.	Mean recorded energy intake from 3-day audiotaped records was 14% lower than TEE from doubly-labeled water (6.73 vs. 7.86 mJ/day). Age was significantly related to reporting accuracy with underestimation of energy intake from audiotaped food records increasing with age.
Knuiman et al. 1987[21]	30 M	8-9 y Adults required	3-Day lunch food record; quantitative	Observation	Compared child's parent-assisted record of lunch intake against observation of lunch with weighed duplicate portions. Excerpted lunch meal from 7-day non-consecutive food records collected over 15 days.	Correlations between mean values from recorded and observed lunch intake were 0.71 for energy, 0.66 for protein, and 0.63 for total fat. Range of correlations for 14 nutrients (i.e., both absolute and density values) assessed was 0.62 for saturated fatty acids as % of kcal to 0.92 for polyunsaturated fat as % of kcal. Recorded energy intake was 25% higher than observed intake (456 vs. 365 kcal/meal). Ten nutrients were significantly overestimated by recorded intake of lunch as compared to observation.
Knuiman et al. 1987[21]	68 M	8-9 y Adults required	7-Day dinner food record; quantitative	Chemical analysis of food	Compared mothers' record of dinner intake against chemical analyses of duplicate portions of dinner. Excerpted dinner from 7-day non-consecutive food records collected over 15 days.	Correlations between mean values from recorded dinner intake and chemical analyses of dinner were 0.52 for energy, 0.56 for protein, and 0.58 for total fat. Range of correlations for the 14 nutrients (i.e., both absolute and density values) assessed was 0.45 for polyunsaturated fat as % of kcal to 0.85 for cholesterol. Recorded energy intake was 31% higher than chemical analysis of food (647 vs. 495 kcal/meal). Nine nutrients were significantly overestimated by mother's record of dinner as compared to chemical analysis of dinner.

Van Horn et al. 1990[8]	33 M&F	8-10 y	1-Day food record audio-taped; quantitative	Observation	Compared child's report of intake from taped food record against parent's observation recorded as a food record.	Pearson correlations between child's and parent's records were 0.68 for energy, 0.82 for protein as % of kcal, and 0.82 for total fat as % of kcal. Range of correlations for the 10 nutrients assessed was 0.68 for energy to 0.96 for iron. Child's recorded energy intake was 2% lower than parents' recorded energy intake (1882 vs. 1913 kcal/day). There were no significant differences between child and parent reports of nutrient intake (significance testing not shown).
Bandini et al. 1997[19]	109 F[b] White, Black, Hispanic, other	8-12 y Adults required	7-Day food record; quantitative	TEE by doubly labeled water	Compared child's adult-assisted food record against 14-day TEE.	Mean recorded energy intake was 13% lower than TEE from doubly labeled water (7.00 vs. 8.03 mJ/day). Age was significantly related to reporting accuracy with underestimation of energy intake from food records increasing with age. There were no significant differences by ethnicity.
Champagne et al. 1998 [a20]	60 M[b] 58 F 56 Black 62 White	9-12 y Adults required	8-Day food record; quantitative	TEE by doubly-labeled water	Compared child's parent assisted record of intake against TEE.	Mean recorded energy intake was 24% lower than TEE from doubly labeled water for boys (1953 vs. 2555 kcal/day) and 27% lower for girls (1633 vs. 2232 kcal/day). Mean recorded energy intake was 28% lower than TEE from doubly labeled water for blacks (1678 vs. 2346 kcal/day) and 22% lower for whites (1909 vs. 2441 kcal/day).
Green et al. 1998[18]	14 F 19 F 29 F 43 F	16 y 17 y 18 y 19 y	3-Day food record; quantitative	Serum folate, red blood cell (RBC) folate, and serum vitamin B_{12}.	Compared adolescent's report of folate and vitamin B_{12} intake on weighed record against serum micronutrient levels collected 1 week before food records.	Pearson correlations between recorded folate intake and serum folate were 0.65, between recorded folate intake and RBC folate were 0.50, and between recorded vitamin B_{12} intake and serum B_{12} were 0.32.

[a] Results of all subgroups not reported due to samples below the N=30 criterion
[b] Males (M), females (F)
[c] Adult assistance required for instrument administration
[d] N/A — not applicable
[e] FFQ — food frequency questionnaire
[f] TEE — total energy expenditure

TABLE 20.4

Food Frequency Questionnaire (FFQ) Validity Studies Among School-Age Children

Reference	Sample	Age/Grade	Instrument	Response Categories (Range)	Validation Standard	Design	Results
Blom et al. 1989[a22]	13 M[b] 17 F	2-16 y Adults required[c]	36 Items; (sucrose, protein, fat, fiber, nitrite, vitamin C) self-administered; referent period not specified; non-quantitative	Unknown (<1/ week to ≥4 times/day)	7-Day food record	Compared child's parent-assisted report of intake of foods with high content of sucrose, protein, fat, fiber, nitrite, and vitamin C against child's parent- and other adult-assisted report of intake on 7-day consecutive food record completed 6-8 weeks before the FFQ.	Spearman correlations between FFQ and food records for frequency of food groups with high content of protein and fat were 0.69 and 0.69, respectively. Range of correlations for 6 food groups assessed was 0.52 for sucrose to 0.76 for vitamin C. Compared to the food record, 2 food groups were significantly overestimated and 3 significantly underestimated by the FFQ. Of 34 food items, 5 were significantly overestimated and 8 significantly underestimated by the FFQ.
Taylor et al. 1998[23]	26 M 41 F	3-6 y Adults required	35-Items; (calcium) self-administered; past year; semi-quantitative	Open-ended (never to number of times/month)	4-Day diet record	Compared parent's report of child's intake of calcium against parent's report of child's 4-day diet record.	The FFQ significantly overestimated mean calcium intake by 18% compared to the food record (942 mg vs. 798 mg/day).
Kaskoun et al. 1994[a]30	22 M 23 F white & Native American	4-6 y Adults required	<111-Items; self-administered; past year; semi-quantitative; adult portions	9 (<1/month to ≥6 times/day)	TEE by doubly-labeled water	Compared parent's report of child's energy intake against 14-day TEE completed after or at the same time as the FFQ.	The FFQ significantly overestimated total energy intake by 59% compared to TEE (9.12 vs. 5.74 mJ/day).
Persson et al. 1984[31]	477 M[b]&F[b]	4 & 8 y Adults required	27 Items; interviewer administered; referent period not specified; non-quantitative	8 (None to ≥4 times/day)	7-Day food record	Compared parent's report of child's frequency of intake of foods against parent's report of child's intake on 7-day food records. Foods from the records were translated into food categories of the FFQ.	Of the 27 food items, the frequencies of intake of 15 were significantly overestimated, and 9 were significantly underestimated by the FFQ compared to the food record.

Hammond et al. 1993[24]	150 M&F	5-11 y Adults required	35 Items (fat, energy, fiber); self-administered; past month; non-quantitative	10 (None to 7 days/week)	14-Day food checklists	Compared child's parent-assisted report of frequency of intake of foods against child's parent-assisted report of intake on 14-day food checklists. Food checklists consisted of 2 sets of 7-day consecutive food records 1 and 2 months after the FFQ, respectively, and contained the same food categories as the FFQ.	For the 35 foods, the median difference in days/week consumption between the FFQs and food checklists was: equal to 0 for 17 foods, >0 for 5 foods, and <0 for 13 foods (significance testing not shown). Differences ranged from –1 (cakes, chips) to 1 (green vegetables). Percentage of responders classified by FFQ to within ± 1 day per week of frequencies reported on checklists ranged from 46.8% for low-fiber cereal to 99.3% for lamb, fish, and liver.
Byers et al. 1993[25]	43 M 54 F white & black	6-10 y Adults required	35 Items (15 fruits, 20 vegetables); self-administered; past 3 months; semi-quantitative; adult portions	9 (None or <1 time/month to ≥6 times/day)	Serum carotenoids vitamins A, C, and E	Compared parent's report of child's fruit and vegetable intake against child's serum micronutrient levels.	Spearman correlations between serum and dietary nutrients were 0.16 for carotene, 0.39 for vitamin C, 0.14 for vitamin A, and 0.32 for vitamin E. Correlations between serum levels of carotene, vitamin C, vitamin A, and vitamin E and frequencies of intake of total fruits and vegetables were 0.24, 0.29, 0.14, and 0.17, respectively. There were no differences by gender or ethnicity (significance testing not shown).
Bellu et al. 1996[32]	165 M[b] 158 F[b]	8-10 y Adults required	116 Items; self-administered; past 6 months; semi-quantitative; "average" portions	Unknown	24-Hour recall	Compared parent's report of child's nutrient intake against mother's report of child's intake on 24-hour recall.	Mean energy estimates from the FFQ were 27% higher than the 24-hour recall for girls (2156 vs. 1703 kcal/day) and 25% higher for boys (2281 vs. 1821 kcal/day). Among girls, of the 10 nutrients, the FFQ significantly overestimated 1 nutrient and significantly underestimated 2 nutrients. Among boys, 3 nutrients were significantly overestimated and 1 was significantly underestimated by the FFQ.

TABLE 20.4 *(Continued)*

Food Frequency Questionnaire (FFQ) Validity Studies Among School-Age Children

Reference	Sample	Age/Grade	Instrument	Response Categories (Range)	Validation Standard	Design	Results
Arnold et al. 1995[33]	77 F	7-12 y Adults required	160 Items; self-administered; past year (inferred); semi-quantitative; adult portions	Open-ended (none to number of months/year)	14-Day food record	Compared child's parent-assisted report of nutrient intake from 2 administrations against child's parent-assisted report of intake on 14-day food records. Records, consisting of 2 sets of 7-day consecutive food records were completed 1 month after the first FFQ and 6 months later.	Pearson correlations (log-transformed, energy-adjusted) between the first FFQ and the first food record and the second FFQ and second food record were 0.13 to 0.22 for energy, 0.20 to 0.30 for protein, and 0.28 to 0.46 for fat, respectively. Range of correlations for 16 nutrients assessed was 0.06 for starch to 0.61 for vitamin B_2. For the first FFQ, energy intake was 24% higher than the first food record (2319 vs. 1861 kcal/day). For the second FFQ, energy intake was 16% higher than the second food record (2205 vs. 1902 kcal/day). Both administrations of the FFQ overestimated intake for all 16 nutrients compared to the corresponding food records (significance testing not shown).
Baranowski, Smith et al. 1997[26]	1530-1570 M[b]&F[b] black & white	3rd Grade	7 Items (3 fruit, 4 vegetables); group-administered; past month; semi-quantitative; "serving" portions	10 (None to ≥5 times/day)	7-Day food record	Compared child's report of servings of fruits and vegetables against child's report of intake on 7-day food records. Foods from the records were abstracted into the FFQ categories by a dietitian.	Pearson correlations between FFQ and food records for fruits and vegetables, fruits and juices, and vegetables were 0.20, 0.24, and 0.15, respectively. Total servings of fruits and vegetables/week as measured by the FFQ was 50.9; by food record was 15.9. The FFQ significantly overestimated intake of food items in all 7 food categories, both aggregate and individual items (significance testing not shown).

Bellu et al. 1995[34]	39 M 49 F	9-12 y Adults required	116 Items; self-administered; past 6 months; semi-quantitative; "average" portions	Unknown	14-Day food record	Compared parent's report of child's nutrient intake against parent's report of child's intake on 14-day weighed food records. Records consisted of 2 sets of 7-day consecutive food records at the beginning of the study and 6 months later, respectively, before and after the FFQ.	Pearson correlations between FFQ and food records were 0.46 for energy, 0.34 for protein, and 0.39 for fat. Range of correlations for 18 nutrients assessed was 0.07 for vitamin A to 0.52 for carbohydrates. FFQ energy intake was 40% higher than the diet record (2620 vs. 1865 kcal/day). The FFQ significantly overestimated 6 nutrients and significantly underestimated 5 nutrients compared to the food records.
Rockett et al. 1997[35]	122 M[b] 139 F[b] 96% White	9-18 y	131 Items Youth/Adolescent Questionnaire; self-administered; past year; semi-quantitative; child portions	Dependent on type of food	24-Hour recall	Compared child's report of nutrient intake (mean of 2 administrations 1 year apart) against child's report of intake on three 24-hour recalls. Recalls were collected via telephone by research dietitians in the year between FFQ administrations.	Pearson correlations (unadjusted log-transformed values) between FFQs and recalls were 0.35 for energy, 0.30 for protein, and 0.41 for fat. Range of correlations for 28 nutrients assessed was 0.09 for copper to 0.46 for vitamin C. Deattenuated correlations (adjusted for energy and within-person variation) were 0.43 for protein and 0.57 for total fat. Range of deattenuated correlations for 29 nutrients assessed was 0.24 for sodium to 0.75 for vitamin C. FFQ energy intake was 1% higher than the recalls (2196 vs. 2169 kcal/day). Of 31 nutrients assessed, 16 were overestimated by the FFQ and 8 were underestimated (significance testing not shown). Correlations did not show a consistent pattern by gender or age (significance testing not shown).

TABLE 20.4 *(Continued)*

Food Frequency Questionnaire (FFQ) Validity Studies Among School-Age Children

Reference	Sample	Age/Grade	Instrument	Response Categories (Range)	Validation Standard	Design	Results
Domel et al. 1994[27]	160-165 M&F black & white	4-5th Grade	45 Items (15 fruit, 30 vegetables); group-administered; past month; semi-quantitative; "serving" portions	7 (None or <1/ month to several per day)	22-Day food record	Compared child's report of frequency of fruit and vegetable intake (mean of 2 administrations) against child's report of intake on 22 consecutive days of food records. Records were collected between FFQ administrations; foods from the records were abstracted by a dietitian into servings of fruit and vegetables.	Spearman correlations between month 1 FFQ and food records and month 2 FFQ and food records were 0.12 and 0.17 for total fruit, –0.04 and 0.02 for total vegetables, and –0.05 and 0.01 for total fruit and vegetable. Range of correlations for 8 fruit/vegetable groupings assessed was –0.05 for total fruit and vegetables to 0.32 for fruit and vegetable juice. Mean daily servings of total fruit and vegetables were 409% higher for the month 1 FFQ compared to the corresponding food records (11.7 vs. 2.3), and 135% higher for the month 2 FFQ compared to the food records (5.4 vs. 2.3). Both administrations of the monthly FFQ significantly overestimated mean daily servings for all 8 fruit/vegetable groupings compared to the corresponding food records.
Domel et al. 1994[27]	154-156 M[b]&F[b] black & white	4-5th Grade	45 Items (15 fruit, 30 vegetables); group-administered; past week; semi-quantitative; "serving" portions	5 (None or <1/ week to several per day)	2-Week food record	Compared child's report of frequency of fruit and vegetable intake (mean of 2 administrations) against child's report of intake on 7-day food records. Records were collected between FFQ administrations; foods from the records were abstracted by a dietitian into servings of fruit and vegetables.	Spearman correlations between week 1 FFQ and food records and week 2 FFQ and food records were 0.18 and 0.18 for total fruit, –0.01 and 0.11 for total vegetable, and 0.00 and 0.05 for total fruit and vegetable. Range of correlations for 8 fruit/vegetable groupings assessed was –0.01 for total vegetable to 0.25 for total legumes and fruit. Mean daily servings of total fruits and vegetables were 295% higher for week 1 FFQs compared to the corresponding food record (8.3 vs. 2.1) and 306% higher for week 2 FFQ (7.3 vs. 1.8). Both administrations of the weekly FFQ significantly overestimated mean daily servings for all 8 fruit and vegetable groupings compared to the corresponding food records.

Koehler et al. 2000[66]	66 M 54 F American Indian, non-hispanic-white, Hispanic	5-8th Grade	33 Items Yesterday's Food Choices-YFC; self-administered; past day; non-quanitative	Yes, not sure, and no	24-Hour recall	Compared child's reported intake of particular foods against child's 24-hour recall, both completed on same day.	Spearman correlations between scores on the FFQ and 24-hour recall were 0.71 for low fat foods, 0.35 for high fiber foods, 0.29 for fruits and vegetables, and 0.40 for high fat foods.
Jenner et al. 1989[36]	61 M 57 F	~11-12 y	175 Items; group-administered; past week; non-quantitative	6 (None to every day)	14-Day food record	Compared child's report of nutrient intake against child's report of intake on 14-day diet records. Seven sets of 2 consecutive day records were collected in the 3 months following administration of the FFQ. Nutrient estimates from FFQ completed by parents were also compared to the 14-day diet records.	Pearson correlations (log-transformed) between the children's FFQs and diet records were 0.25 for energy, 0.18 for protein, and 0.19 for total fat. Range of correlations for 13 nutrients assessed was 0.11 for monounsaturated fat to 0.42 for complex carbohydrates. Correlations between the parents' FFQs and diet records were 0.38 for energy, 0.26 for protein and 0.30 for total fat. Range of correlations was 0.26 for protein to 0.47 for complex carbohydrates. Children's FFQ energy intakes were 36% higher than diet records (10.9 vs. 8.0 mJ/day). Parents' FFQ estimates of children's energy intake were 21% higher than the children's diet records (9.7 vs. 8.0 mJ/day). All 13 nutrients were overestimated by both the child and the parent FFQ (significance testing not shown).
Kinlay et al. 1991[28]	57 M[b] 48 F[b]	13-17 y Adults required	12 Items (fat, saturated fat); self-administered; past week; semi-quantitative	Dependent on type of food	FFQ[e]	Compared child's parent-assisted report of fat intake against child's parent assisted report of fat intake on FFQ.	Spearman correlations between the brief FFQ and the FFQ were 0.40 for total fat as % of kcal and 0.54 for saturated fat as % of kcal.
Field et al. 1998[29]	102 M&F 50% M 50% F 35% White 24% Black 15% Hispanic	9-12th Grade	27 Items (12 fruit, 15 vegetables) Youth/Adolescent Questionnaire; self-administered; past year; semi-quantitative	Unknown (<1/month to ≥2 times/day)	Three 24-hour recalls	Compared child's report of fruit and vegetable intake against child's report of intake on 3 nonconsecutive 24-hour recalls completed 2 weeks apart. FFQ was administered 2-4 weeks after the third recall.	Spearman correlations between the brief FFQ and mean of three 24-hour recalls were 0.33 for fruit only, 0.29 for fruit juice, 0.33 for fruit and juice, 0.32 for vegetables, and 0.41 for fruit (including juice) and vegetables.

TABLE 20.4 *(Continued)*

Food Frequency Questionnaire (FFQ) Validity Studies Among School-Age Children

Reference	Sample	Age/Grade	Instrument	Response Categories (Range)	Validation Standard	Design	Results
Field et al. 1998[29]	102 M&F 50% M 50% F 35% White 24% Black 15% Hispanic	9-12th Grade	4 Items (2 fruit, 2 vegetable) Youth Risk Behavior Surveillance System Questionnaire (YRBSS); self-administered; past day; semi-quantitative	Unknown (none to ≥3 times/day)	Three 24-hour recalls	Compared child's report of fruit and vegetable intake against child's reported mean intake of fruits and vegetables calculated with an algorithm using 3 nonconsecutive 24-hour recalls completed 2 weeks apart. YRBSS was administered 2-4 weeks after the third recall.	Spearman correlations between YRBSS items and mean of 24-hour recalls were 0.17 for fruit only, 0.07 for fruit juice, 0.21 for fruit and juice, 0.24 for vegetables, and 0.28 for fruit (including juice) and vegetables.
Field et al. 1998[29]	102 M&F 50% M 50% F 35% White 24% Black 15% Hispanic	9-12th Grade	6 Items (2 fruit, 4 vegetable) Behavioral Risk Factor Surveillance System Questionnaire (BRFSS); self-administered; past day; semi-quantitative	Unknown (none to ≥3 times/day)	Three 24-hour recalls	Compared child's report of fruit and vegetable intake against child's reported mean intake of fruits and vegetables calculated with an algorithm using 2 nonconsecutive 24-hour recalls completed 4 weeks apart. BFRSS was administered halfway between the two recalls.	Spearman correlations between past day BRFSS and mean of 24-hour recalls were 0.33 for fruit only, 0.30 for fruit juice, 0.34 for fruit and juice, 0.14 for vegetables, and 0.30 for fruit (including juice) and vegetables.

Field et al. 1998[29]	100 M&F 50% M 50% F 35% White 24% Black 15% Hispanic	9-12th Grade	6 Items (2 fruit, 4 vegetable) BRFSS; self-administered; past year; semi-quantitative	Unknown (none to ≥5 times/day)	Three 24-hour recalls	Compared child's report of fruit and vegetable intake against child's reported mean intake of fruits and vegetables calculated with an algorithm using 3 nonconsecutive 24-hour recalls completed 4 weeks apart. BFRSS was administered preceding the third recall.	Spearman correlations between past year BRFSS and mean of 24-hour recalls were 0.36 for fruit only, 0.36 for fruit juice, 0.35 for fruit and juice, 0.33 for vegetables, and 0.43 for fruit (including juice) and vegetables.
Green et al. 1998[18]	14 F 19 F 29 F 43 F	16 y 17 y 18 y 19 y	116 Items; self-administered; past year; semi-quantitative	Unknown	Serum folate, red blood cell (RBC) folate, and serum vitamin B_{12}	Compared child's report of folate and vitamin B_{12} intake against serum micronutrient levels.	Pearson correlations were 0.48 between folate intake from the FFQ and serum folate, 0.42 between folate intake from the FFQ and RBC folate, and 0.25 between vitamin B_{12} intake from the FFQ and serum B_{12}.
Andersen et al. 1995[37]	13 M 36 F	11th Grade Adults required	190 Items; group-administered; past year; semi-quantitative	Dependent on type of food	7-Day food record	Compared child's parent assisted report of nutrient intake against child's report of intake on 7-day weighed food records completed 2-3 months after FFQ administration. Records consisted of 4 consecutive days, a 1-week interval, and 3 consecutive days.	Spearman correlations between FFQ and food records were 0.51 for energy, 0.48 for protein, 0.57 for total fat. Range of correlations for 18 nutrients assessed was 0.14 for vitamin D to 0.66 for monounsaturated fat. FFQ energy intake was 24% higher than diet records (10.7 vs. 8.6 mJ/day). The FFQ significantly overestimated 16 of the 18 nutrients. The FFQ significantly overestimated intake of 8 of 13 food items as compared to diet records.

[a] Results of all subgroups not reported due to samples below the N=30 criterion
[b] Males (M), females (F)
[c] Adult assistance required for instrument administration
[d] N/A — not applicable
[e] FFQ — food frequency questionnaire
[f] TEE — total energy expenditure

TABLE 20.5

Food Frequency Questionnaire (FFQ)[e] Reliability Studies Among School-Age Children

Reference	Sample	Age/ Grade	Instrument	Response Categories (Range)	Design	Results
Basch et al. 1994[39]	166 M&F[b] Latino	4-7 y Adults required[c]	~116 Items; interviewer-administered; past 6 months; semi-quantitative; child portions	9 (None or <1/ month to ≥6/ day)	Compared both 3-month and 1-year test-retest reproducibility of nutrient estimates from FFQs completed by the parent.	Pearson correlations (log-transformed) between the 2 FFQs at 3 months were 0.53 for energy, 0.49 for protein, and 0.56 for total fat. Range of correlations for 12 nutrients assessed at 3 months was -0.06 for sucrose to 0.61 for crude fiber. At 1 year, correlations were 0.46 for energy, 0.40 for protein, and 0.47 for total fat. Range of correlations for 12 nutrients assessed at 1 year was 0.06 for sucrose to 0.57 for polyunsaturated fat.
Arnold et al. 1995[33]	77 F	7-12 y Adults required	160 Items; self-administered; past year; semi-quantitative; adult portions	5 (Open-ended, none to number of months/ year)	Compared 6-month test-retest reproducibility of nutrient estimates from FFQs completed by the parent and child.	Pearson correlations (log-transformed, energy adjusted) between the 2 FFQs were 0.60 for energy, 0.51 for protein, and 0.14 for total fat. Range of correlations for 16 nutrients assessed was 0.14 for total fat to 0.71 for fiber. Mean energy intake was 5% higher in the first FFQ compared to the second (2319 vs. 2205 kcal/day). Mean intake of 15 nutrients was higher in the first FFQ compared to the second; 1 nutrient was lower (significance testing not shown).
Domel et al. 1994[27]	146 M&F black & white	4-5th Grade	45 Items (15 fruit, 30 vegetable); group-administered; past week; semi-quantitative; "serving" portions	5 (None or <1/ week to several per day)	Compared 1-week test-retest reproducibility of fruit and vegetable intake from FFQs completed by the child. Order of fruit (15 items) and vegetables (30 items) was reversed between first and second administrations.	Spearman correlations between the 2 FFQs were 0.50 for total fruit, 0.48 for total vegetable, and 0.54 for total fruit and vegetable intake. Range of correlations for 8 fruit and vegetable groupings assessed was 0.39 for fruit and vegetable juice to 0.54 for total fruit and vegetables. Mean daily servings of total fruits and vegetables was 12% higher for Week 1 FFQ compared to Week 2 FFQ (8.3 vs. 7.3). Mean daily servings of 6 fruit and vegetable groupings of 8 assessed were higher for Week 1 FFQ compared to Week 2 FFQ (significance testing not shown).
Domel et al. 1994[27]	156 M&F black & white	4–5th Grade	45 Items (15 fruit, 30 vegetable); group-administered; past month; semi-quantitative; "serving" portions	7 (None or <1/ month to several per day)	Compared 1-month (3.5-week) test-retest reproducibility of fruit and vegetable intake from FFQs completed by the child. Order of fruit (15 items) and vegetables (30 items) was reversed between first and second administrations.	Spearman correlations between the 2 FFQs were 0.43 for total fruit, 0.37 for total vegetable and 0.47 for total fruit and vegetable intake. Range of correlations for 8 fruit and vegetable groupings assessed was 0.28 for fruit and vegetable juice to 0.47 for both legumes and total fruit and vegetable intake. Mean daily servings of total fruits and vegetables was 54% higher for Month 1 FFQ compared to Month 2 FFQ (11.7 vs. 5.4). Mean daily servings of 8 fruit and vegetable groupings were higher for Month 1 FFQ compared to Month 2 FFQ (significance testing not shown).

Rockett et al. 1995[38]	75 M 101 F 3 N/A[d] multi-ethnic	9-18 y	151 Items Youth/Adolescent Questionnaire; self-administered; past year; semi-quantitative; adult portions	9 (None or <1/month to ≥6/day)	Compared 1-year test-retest reproducibility of nutrient estimates from FFQs completed by the child.	Pearson correlations (log-transformed, energy-adjusted) between the 2 FFQs were 0.49 for energy, 0.26 for protein, and 0.41 for total fat. Range of correlations for 7 nutrients assessed was 0.26 for protein and iron to 0.58 for calcium. Mean energy intake was 10% higher in the first FFQ compared to the second (2477 vs. 2222 kcal/day). Mean intake of 6 nutrients assessed was significantly higher in the first FFQ compared to the second. Range of correlations for 8 food groups assessed was 0.39 for meats to 0.57 for soda. Pearson correlations (log-transformed) for servings/day were 0.49 for fruits, 0.48 for vegetables, and 0.48 for fruits and vegetables. Of 8 food groups, mean serving frequencies of 5 were significantly higher in the first FFQ compared to the second. Reproducibility of nutrient intake was significantly higher for girls than boys (mean correlation for all nutrients was 0.44 and 0.34, respectively). There were no significant differences by age or ethnicity.
Frank et al. 1992[40]	189 M&F black & white	12-17 y	64 Items; group-administered; past week; semi-quantitative; adult portions	6 (None to >3 times/day)	Compared 2-week test-retest reproducibility of food intake from FFQs completed by the child.	Two-thirds of the children reported similar responses for the frequency of consumption of low-fat milk, diet carbonated soft drinks and shellfish. Twelve food groups had percent agreement of 50% or better (significance testing not shown).
Andersen et al. 1995[37]	53 M 50 F	11th Grade Adults required	190 items; group-administered; past year; semi-quantitative	Dependent on type of food	Compared 6-week test-retest reproducibility of nutrient estimates from FFQs completed by the child and parent.	Spearman correlations (energy-adjusted) between the 2 FFQs were 0.87 for energy, 0.86 for protein, and 0.86 for total fat. Range of correlations for 18 nutrients assessed was 0.72 for vitamin C to 0.91 for alcohol. Median energy intake was 11% higher in the first FFQ compared to the second (12.3 vs. 10.9 mJ/day). Median intake of 15 nutrients was significantly higher in the first FFQ compared to the second FFQ. Differences in median correlations for nutrient intake were not significant between girls and boys (0.78 vs. 0.74, respectively).

[a] Results of all subgroups not reported due to samples below the N=30 criterion
[b] Males (M), females (F)
[c] Adult assistance required for instrument administration
[d] N/A — not applicable
[e] FFQ — food frequency questionnaire

The diet history provides a measure of usual intake appropriate for ranking individuals and predicting health outcomes. In contrast to other methods of dietary assessment, a diet history is usually more qualitative than quantitative, allowing detailed information about food preparation, eating habits, and food consumption to be collected by a highly trained interviewer. This method requires children and/or parents to recall dietary intake from the past, understand spatial relationships, be able to apply math skills, and have the stamina to complete the typically one- to two-hour interview. Because of the respondent burden, diet histories are not often used to assess children's diets.

Observation (Table 20.6)

Observation is useful for assessing preliterate children (third grade or younger), either in a lunchroom setting with school meals or in controlled school or group activities. Intensively trained observers unobtrusively watch the children, sometimes many at a time, to ascertain foods, brand names and portion sizes consumed. A single observation provides a measure of actual intake that is appropriate for estimating group means and cannot be used to predict health outcomes. Multiple observations can provide a measure of usual intake. The recordings are interpreted after the collection process and coded to a nutrient database to calculate nutrient intake for each child. Observations are often used as the validation standard for studies among school-age children.

Discussion

Ideally, a comprehensive review of validity and reliability studies such as this one would direct researchers to the best assessment technique for a particular setting. Unfortunately, as this report indicates, dietary assessment techniques for children are difficult to evaluate and generalize because the validation standards against which the instruments have been compared are frequently beset with shortcomings. These validation standards may have inconsistent validity, or use a referent period that differs from that used for the instrument. Heterogeneity of the studies also makes it difficult to draw conclusions; the differences in study administrations and study populations make comparisons uncertain both within a type of assessment method and between methods. Noting these challenges to interpretation, the correlations between the validation standard and the dietary assessment tool were almost always higher for recalls or records than for FFQs.

This review may serve best to facilitate comparison of dietary methods to determine the most effective data collection instruments to use with particular quantitative or qualitative research questions.[43-44] The reader may, for example, scan each table for instruments with higher or lower nutrient correlations with a particular validity standard, instruments that children can complete without adult assistance, those with no portion size estimation, and instruments specific to assessing intake of food groups — all by age or grade. Applications of the dietary assessment methods are summarized in Table 20.7 which provides advantages and disadvantages for using the dietary assessment methodologies, applicable study designs, and brief highlights of their validity from this review. Using this series of tables, the reader can select a dietary assessment tool that is appropriate for specific research questions.

It is evident that many of the validation standards used in the reviewed articles are imperfect, especially for children. Food records or recalls were the most common choices

TABLE 20.6

Diet History and Observation Reliability Studies Among School-Age Children

Reference	Sample	Age/ Grade	Instrument	Design	Results
Rasanen, 1979[41]	47 M&F[b] 50 M&F 37 M&F	5 y 9 y 13 y Adults required[c]	Diet history; past year; interviewer administered; quantitative	Compared 7-month test-retest reproducibility of nutrient intake from a diet history completed by child and parent.	Pearson correlations between the first and second interviews were 0.59 for energy, 0.60 for protein, and 0.57 for total fat. Range of correlations for 11 nutrients assessed was 0.41 for ascorbic acid to 0.60 for protein. Mean daily energy intake was 27% higher in the first diet history interview as compared to the second interview (3256 vs. 2573 kcal/day).
Simons-Morton et al. 1992[42]	45 M&F	3-5th Grade Adults required	Observation; lunch only; quantitative	Compared 2 simultaneously collected adult observers' estimates of nutrient intake and food items from observation of lunch.	Intraclass correlations between paired observers ranged from 0.81-0.90 for energy and from 0.74-0.88 for fat. Of the 6 nutrients assessed, intraclass correlations were lowest for total fat (0.74-0.88) and highest for vitamin A (0.96-0.98). Inter-observer percent differences in mean energy intake ranged from 0.1%-6.8%. Overall agreement on food items between observers was 84%; percent agreement was highest for chips and condiments, and lowest for desserts. Differences in portion size estimates accounted for most of the energy and nutrient differences between observers.

[a] Results of subgroups not reported due to samples below the N=30 criterion
[b] males (M), females (F)
[c] adult assistance required for instrument administration
[d] N/A — Not applicable
[e] FFQ — Food frequency questionnaire

TABLE 20.7

Summary of Reviewed Dietary Assessment Methods for School-Age Children

Method and Number of Studies Reviewed	Ages Evaluated	Energy & Macro-Nutrient Validity[a]	Energy Intake Compared with Standard[b]	Type of Diet Measure	Study Design Applications	Advantages	Disadvantages
FOOD RECALL Validity — 12 Reliability — 0	4-14 y Adult assistance needed for <9 y	Energy 0.23-0.87 Protein 0.05-0.82 Total fat 0.25-0.46	–34 to 18%	One recall measures group intake Multiple recalls measure individual or group intake	• Cross-sectional • Intervention • Monitoring • Clinical • Epidemiologic	• Short administration time • Defined recall time • Intake can be quantified • Procedure does not alter habitual dietary patterns • Low respondent burden • Can be telephone administered • Procedure can be automated	• Recall depends on memory • Portion size difficult to estimate • Trained interviewer required • Expensive to collect and code
FOOD RECORD Validity — 7 Reliability — 0	8-19 y Adult assistance needed for <9 y	Energy 0.52-0.71 Protein 0.56-0.66 Total fat 0.58-0.63	–28 to 31%	One record measures group intake Multiple records measure individual or group intake	• Cross-sectional • Intervention • Monitoring • Clinical • Epidemiologic	• Record does not rely on memory • Defined record time • Intake can be quantified • Training can be group administered • Procedure can be automated	• Recorder must be literate • High respondent burden • Food eaten away from home less accurately recalled • Procedure alters habitual dietary patterns • Validity may decrease as recording days increase • Expensive to collect and code
FOOD FREQUENCY Validity — 22 Reliability — 7	2-19 y Adult assistance needed for <9 y	Energy 0.13-0.51 Protein 0.18-0.34 Total fat 0.19-0.39	1 to 59%	One FFQ measures usual intake	• Cross-sectional • Intervention • Monitoring • Epidemiologic	• Trained interviewers not needed • Interviewer or self-administered • Relatively inexpensive to collect • Procedure does not alter habitual dietary habits • Low respondent burden • Total diet or selected foods or nutrients can be assessed • Can be used to rank according to nutrient intake • Procedure can be automated	• Recall depends on memory • Period of recall imprecise • Quantification of intake imprecise because of poor recall or use of standard portion sizes • Specific food descriptions not obtained

DIET HISTORY Validity — 0 Reliability — 1	5-13 y Adult assistance needed for all ages	N/A	N/A	One history measures usual intake	• Monitoring • Clinical • Epidemiologic	• Literacy not required • Procedure does not alter habitual dietary habits • Can obtain highly detailed descriptions of foods and preparation methods	• Recall depends on memory • Highly trained interviewers required • Period of recall imprecise • Very high respondent burden • Requires long interview time • Quantification of intake imprecise because of poor recall or use of standard portion sizes • Expensive to administer
OBSERVATION Validity — 0 Reliability — 1	8-10 y	N/A	N/A	One observation measures group intake Multiple observations measure individual or group intake	• Intervention • Monitoring • Epidemiologic	• Literacy not required • Procedure does not alter habitual dietary habits • Procedure does not rely on memory • Defined observation time • Intake can be quantified • Multiple days give measure of individual or group intake	• Highly trained observers required • Requires long observation period • Expensive to administer

[a] Pearson correlation
[b] Calculation of percentage = ([instrument-validation standard]/validation standard)

for validation standards here, and information on the validity of these methods in children is mixed. Recalls both over- and underestimated energy, and food records underestimated energy intake. Most recall validity studies used observation of the child as the standard, but the majority of the studies only considered individual meals or daytime intakes to determine validity of the 24-hour recall. Accurate completion of food records is greatly dependent on the ability of the child to read and write. Because young children have not been shown to accurately complete food records independently, caution is suggested when interpreting studies that use records as the validation standard. The validity of food records or recalls for measuring long term or usual food intake improves with more days of recording,[5] indicating that multiple records may be needed. Multiple food records/recalls can introduce compliance issues for children because of the high respondent burden. Since a high degree of cooperation is required from children for food records and recalls, it is essential for both methods that children be motivated to participate, and in particular be cognitively able to complete the records.

In evaluating validation studies, the effect of correlated errors between the method evaluated and the validation standard should be considered. All dietary assessment methods have inherent errors; for validation studies, it is important that these errors be as independent as possible.[45] For example, if errors between the methods are similar (e.g., both methods rely on dietary information from a respondent such as FFQ and recalls), correlations between the two methods will be artificially inflated. In contrast, errors inherent in physiologic measures (e.g., doubly labeled water measurements or serum micronutrients) or observational data do not rely on information provided by respondents, and would be a more independent comparison to a respondent-based measure.[46] Comparisons of physiologic endpoints, such as blood nutrient levels, to dietary assessment methods have not been widely used with school-age children and offer other problems, since food intake may not be directly correlated with physiologic endpoints.

Selecting a validation standard can be a difficult task, because there is often no dietary assessment tool available with the same referent period as the assessment tool. Thus, a compromise may be needed in the study design. For example, an FFQ measures usual food consumption over a period of six months to a year, while a food record generally is used to measure food consumption on a day-to-day basis. In order to validate an FFQ, it would be necessary to complete several sets of food records over the referent period for the FFQ. Clearly, validation studies that use a week of continuous consecutive food records may not capture seasonal variation in diet. Similarly, a food recall, which is generally used to measure one complete day of consumption, should be validated by a method that assesses an entire day, not just a portion of the day.

The problem of referent periods also influences the experimental design for reliability studies. Because there is much day-to-day variation in diet, re-administration should be close enough in time to reflect the same referent period. Since some methods reflect diet over a short span of time (e.g., 1-day records and 24-hour recalls), theoretically the reliability testing should be completed on the same day as the assessment tool, which may allow memory effects from the first assessment to bias the re-administration. Studies that examine reliability should alternate administrations in order to eliminate bias as much as possible. Because FFQs usually include a longer referent period, it is easier to develop reproducibility studies for this method.

In all the studies reviewed, adult dietary assessment methods were adapted for administration to a pediatric population. Specific adaptations included incorporating parental or adult assistance, adjusting portion size information, using shorter referent times, and administering the instrument in the school setting. Children younger than nine years of age need adult assistance to provide accurate dietary information because they usually have limited reading skills and adults control most of the food offered, as well as the timing and frequency of eating occasions.[47-48] This review found that almost all of the validity and reliability studies among children less then nine years of age, with the exception of a few of the recall and FFQ studies, included adult participation. This participation varied from completion of the form entirely to obtaining only supplemental information from parents or surrogates, such as childcare providers, or secondary sources such as school food service observations.

Children generally have difficulty in estimating portion sizes.[30,49,50] A recent review of portion size aids was unable to make guidelines for portion size estimation for children or adults.[51] Both two- and three-dimensional models have been used to enhance children's portion size estimation.[7-9,11,16,21,39,41-42,52-54] Pictures of food and portions have been incorporated in assessments to enhance children's understanding; however, the addition of pictures did not increase accuracy among third-graders.[55] Among the newer tools for dietary assessment are reference books with life-size photographs of portion sizes, which have been credited as being both easy and accurate.[56-59] Training to improve portion size estimation among children has been attempted with significant improvements in estimation; however, even with training, some errors were reported as high as 100%.[60]

Semi-quantitative FFQs have not generally used portion sizes adjusted for children's level of intake. This may have enhanced the lack of agreement between the FFQ and validation standard, if the validation standard allowed for collection of specific portions consumed by the child. These FFQs may have systematically overestimated intake due to portion size miscalculations.

Because the school provides a natural means of regularly accessing school-age children, several researchers continue to explore ways of using this setting to collect dietary intake data. Methods such as using a group workbook to collect 24-hour recall information[61] have been developed to expand the number of eating occasions that can be evaluated, while trying to minimize the respondent burden for multiple records or recalls.

Recommendations

Despite the extensive dietary intake data available to nutritionists, epidemiologists, and pediatricians, this review identifies methodological concerns associated with the assessment tools currently used to determine dietary intake of school-age children. Generally, comparisons across studies were limited by differences in instruments, research design, validation standards, and populations. The paucity of data in many areas also made it difficult to draw generalized conclusions.

In the last three decades the most extensive body of validation work among children has occurred with FFQs, with only a limited number of validation studies and even fewer reliability studies of the other methods among school-age children. In the future, evaluations of dietary assessment techniques for children need to be conducted that give particular attention to experimental design, careful use of validation standards, and inclusion of different age, gender, and ethnic subgroups. As with adults, there is no perfect method of assessing dietary intake in children. Special consideration must be given to the age and cognitive ability of the child as well as methodological issues associated with nutrient analyses, food coding, and portion sizes. Both age and cognitive ability relate to the child's understanding of the method used and the thought processes that contribute to self-reporting of food choices.

What needs to be done? Ideally, studies need to examine the validity and reliability of each dietary assessment method by age, gender, and ethnic subgroup to understand the best application of each tool. Selection of the measure of truth for validation studies will be challenging, since there is not always a good choice when the referent periods differ so markedly between instruments, and the potential effect of correlated errors is considered. Physiologically based measures, such as doubly labeled water or serum micronutrient concentrations, represent a type of standard with considerable appeal and merit further study, since these measures are not affected by respondent error. In addition, studies that compare multiple validation standards for a particular assessment method would allow comparisons of the validation standards best suited for particular situations. Future studies need to address the timing of the referent period that best suits the assessment instrument in the design phase.

New approaches and modifications to existing approaches for dietary assessment among school-age children are needed. The dietary habits of children, especially young children who are preliterate, are inherently difficult to study. Unfortunately, assessment techniques that work reasonably well among adult men and women may not be useful for children, especially those less than nine years of age, who may need assistance from a proxy or special prompting techniques to estimate portion size. Creative measures must be developed to better estimate children's portion sizes and enhance researchers' ability to capture details of their dietary intake. Systematic evaluations of children's ability to estimate portion size utilizing various approaches by age are needed.

Researchers are urged to investigate how variables such as age, gender, ethnicity, socioeconomic status, and obesity affect the validity of dietary assessment methods. This review found little research on the effects of age, gender, or ethnicity. Given the multiplicity of minority groups in the U.S., there is a need for research to determine whether group-specific dietary assessment tools are necessary. Other areas, such as the effect of body size on reporting of dietary intake, require further study. For example, a recent study suggested that children with central fat distribution had higher rates of underreporting energy intake than lean or obese children, or those with peripheral fat distribution.[20] Another study reported that energy intake was significantly lower in obese children than non-obese children when compared to doubly labeled water as a percentage of energy expenditure.[62] Underreporting of dietary intake by obese adolescents is consistent with recent findings that obese adults tend to underreport their dietary intake.[62] With the increasing prevalence of obesity among children and adolescents, it is essential to determine whether body size differences significantly affect completion of dietary assessment instruments.[64]

In summary, much remains to be learned about the dietary intake of American youth. This review serves as a guide to the state of dietary assessment among school-age children. Recalls and records generally agreed more with the validation standards than did FFQs. Administration protocols differed greatly, the recalls and records often represented only meals or portions of the day, and the FFQ food lists varied from a few items to the total diet. This review can also serve as a foundation for initiating new studies and as a resource for developing research questions from the gaps identified in the current methodologies. The key to advancing the field is to build on our current base of methods, refine techniques that are useful, and develop new approaches to overcome obstacles that have been identified in study designs and data collection procedures. In the new millenium we must be able to accurately assess the dietary intake of our school-age children so that we can monitor dietary intake trends, make accurate research and policy decisions, and develop and effectively evaluate nutrition interventions.

Acknowledgment

The authors would like to thank Heidi Nowak for assisting with manuscript preparation.

References

1. McPherson RS, Montgomery DH, Nichaman MZ. *J Nutr Ed* 27: 225; 1995.
2. Kennedy E, Goldberg J. *Nutr Rev* 53: 111; 1995.
3. US Department of Health and Human Services. Healthy people 2000: national health promotion and disease prevention objectives. DHHS Publication No. (PHS) 91-50212, US Gov. Printing Office, Washington, DC, 1990.
4. Ferro-Luzzi A, Martino L. In *Implementing Dietary Guidelines for Healthy Eating*, (Wheelock V, Ed), Blackie A&P, London, 1997, pg 3.
5. Thompson FE, Byers T. *J Nutr*, 124: 2245S, 1994.
6. Nelson M, et al. *Am J Clin Nutr* 50: 155; 1989.
7. Lytle LA, et al. *JADA* 93:1431; 1993.
8. Van Horn LV, et al. *JADA* 90: 412; 1990.
9. Mullenbach V, et al. *JADA* 92: 743; 1992.
10. Todd KS, Kretsch MJ. *Nutr Res* 6: 1031; 1989.
11. Eck LH, Klesges RC, Hanson CL. *JADA* 89: 784; 1989.
12. Emmons L, Hayes M. *JADA* 62: 409; 1973.
13. Samuelson G. *Nutr Metabol* 12: 321; 1970.
14. Lytle LA, et al. *JADA*, 98: 570; 1998.
15. Baxter SD, et al. *JADA* 97: 1293; 1997.
16. Basch CE, et al. *Am J Pub Health* 81: 1314; 1990.
17. Reynolds LA, Johnson SB, Silverstein J. *J Ped Psych* 15: 493; 1990.
18. Green TJ, Allen OB, O'Connor DL. *J Nutr* 128, 1665, 1998.
19. Bandini LG, et al. *Am J Clin Nutr* 65: 1138S; 1997.
20. Champagne CM, et al. *JADA* 98: 426; 1998.
21. Knuiman JT, et al. *JADA* 87: 303; 1987.
22. Blom L, et al. *Acta Pediatr Scand* 78: 858; 1989.
23. Taylor RW, Goulding A. *Eur J Clin Nutr* 52: 404; 1998.
24. Hammond J, et al. *Eur J Clin Nutr* 47: 242; 1993.
25. Byers T, et al. *Epidemiology* 4: 350; 1993.
26. Baranowski T, et al. *JADA* 97: 66; 1997.
27. Domel SB, et al. *J Am Col Nutr* 13: 33; 1994.
28. Kinlay S, Heller RF, Halliday JA. *Prev Med* 20: 378; 1991.
29. Field AE, et al. *Am J Pub Health* 88: 1216; 1998.
30. Kaskoun MC, Johnson RK, Goran MI. *Am J Clin Nutr* 60: 43; 1994.
31. Persson LA, Carlgren G. *Int J Epidemiol* 13: 506; 1984.
32. Bellu R, et al. *Nutr Res* 16: 197; 1996.
33. Arnold JE, et al. *Ann Epidemiol* 5: 369; 1995.
34. Bellu R, et al. *Nutr Res* 15: 1121; 1995.
35. Rockett HRH, et al. *Prev Med* 26: 808; 1997.
36. Jenner DA, et al. *Eur J Clin Nutr* 43: 663; 1989.
37. Andersen LF, et al. *Eur J Clin Nutr* 49: 543; 1995.
38. Rockett HRH, Wolf AM, Colditz GA. *JADA* 95: 336; 1995.
39. Basch CE, Shea S, Zybert P. *Am J Pub Health* 84: 861; 1994.
40. Frank GC, et al. *JADA* 92: 313; 1992.
41. Rasanen L. *Am J Clin Nutr* 32: 2560; 1979.
42. Simons-Morton BG, et al. *JADA* 92: 219; 1992.
43. Cullen KW, et al. *JADA* 99: 849; 1999.
44. Eldridge AL, et al. *JADA* 98: 777; 1998.

45. Willett W. *Nutritional Epidemiology,* 2nd ed, Oxford University Press, New York, 1998.
46. Bingham SA. *Am J Clin Nutr* 59: 227S; 1994.
47. Frank GC. *Am J Clin Nutr* 59: 207S; 1994.
48. Baranowski T. In *Handbook of Health Behavior Research I: Personal and Social Determinants,* (Grochman DS, Ed), Plenum Press, New York, 1997, pg 179.
49. Buzzard IM, Siever YA. *Am J Clin Nutr* 59: 275S; 1994.
50. Contento I, et al. *J Nutr Educ* 27: 284; 1995.
51. Cypel YS, Guenther PM, Petot GJ. *JADA* 97: 289; 1997.
52. Crawford PB, et al. *JADA* 94: 626; 1994.
53. Frank GC, et al. *JADA* 71: 26; 1977.
54. McPherson RS, et al. *Pediatrics* 86: 520; 1990.
55. Baranowski T, et al. *JADA* 86: 1381; 1986.
56. Nelson M, Atkinson M, Darbyshire S. *Br J Nutr* 72: 649; 1994.
57. Nelson M, Atkinson M, Darbyshire S. *Br J Nutr* 76: 31; 1996.
58. Faggiano F, et al. *Epidemiology* 3: 379; 1992.
59. Hess MA, Ed. *Portion Photos of Popular Foods.* The American Dietetic Association & Center for Nutrition Education, University of Wisconsin-Stout, 1997.
60. Weber JL, et al. *Am J Clin Nutr* 69: 782S; 1999.
61. Farris RP, et al. *JADA* 85: 1315; 1985.
62. Bandini LG, et al. *Am J Clin Nutr* 52: 421; 1990.
63. Schoeller DA. *Metabolism* 44: 18S; 1995.
64. Goran MI. *Pediatrics* 101: 505S; 1998.
65. Lindquist CH, et al. *Obesity Res* 8: 2; 2000.
66. Koehler KM, et al. *JADA* 100: 205, 2000.
67. McPherson RS, et al. *Prev Medicine* 31: 11S; 2000.

21

Methods and Tools for Dietary Intake Assessment in Individuals vs. Groups

Ruth E. Patterson

Introduction

Dietary intake is an important, modifiable determinant of health and longevity. Comprehensive reviews of the literature have consistently concluded that clear, causal links exist between food intake and major causes of morbidity and mortality, such as coronary heart disease, cancer, diabetes, and obesity.[1-3] In addition, undernutrition continues to be a substantial health problem in many countries.[4]

Given the importance of diet in human health, assessment of dietary intake plays a pivotal role in efforts to improve the health of individuals and populations throughout the world. Dietary intake data are used for three major purposes:

1. At the individual level, assessment of dietary intake is necessary for determining a person's dietary adequacy or risk, assessing adherence to recommended dietary patterns, and tailoring education and counseling efforts.
2. Dietary intake assessment is an integral part of research studies investigating how diet determines the health of individuals and populations. Etiologic studies assess dietary intake as an exposure for association with disease outcomes. Behavioral research assesses dietary intake (or change in intake) as an outcome in studies designed to develop and test strategies that encourage adoption of healthful eating patterns.
3. Finally, at the population level, assessment of dietary intake is necessary to identify national health priorities and develop public health dietary recommendations. These data are used to determine the success of public health interventions in improving dietary patterns and for identification of population subgroups at risk or in need of special assistance. Nutrition monitoring also serves a key role in food assistance programs, fortification initiatives, food safety evaluations, and food labeling programs.

0-8493-2705-9/01/$0.00+$1.50

It is clear that dietary assessment is a cornerstone of efforts to improve the health of individuals and groups. However, there are significant concerns about the accuracy and usefulness of self-reported dietary data. The challenges associated with assessing dietary intake are well known and have to do with day-to-day variation in intake, respondent reporting errors and biases, limitations of the assessment instruments, and error in food composition tables.[5] Several different assessment methods and tools have been developed to address these difficulties, and each method has different strengths and weaknesses with regard to the type and quality of data produced. In addition, there are significant differences among these assessment methods in practical matters of respondent burden and cost. Therefore it is necessary to carefully consider the specific objectives of the dietary assessment as a precursor to choosing the best or most appropriate method. Perhaps the first and most important question is whether the data will be used for assessing intake in individuals or groups.

Here we describe the three major types of dietary assessment methods: 1) food records and 24-hour dietary recalls, 2) food frequency questionnaires, and 3) brief assessment instruments. We summarize the scientific and practical advantages and disadvantages of each of these methods. Then we consider the use of these three dietary assessment methods for assessing diet in individuals versus groups; when they are used for determination of an individual's dietary adequacy for purposes of counseling, research studies of dietary intake and disease risk, and nutrition monitoring of populations.

Description of the Three Major Dietary Assessment Methods

Food Records and Dietary Recalls (Records/Recalls)

For many years, food records were considered the "gold standard" of dietary assessment methods. Food records require individuals to record everything consumed over a specified period of time, usually one to seven days. Respondents are typically asked to carry the record with them and to record foods as eaten. Some protocols require participants to weigh and/or measure foods before eating, while less stringent protocols use models and other aids to instruct respondents on estimating serving sizes. The food consumption information is entered into a specialized software program for calculation of nutrient intakes. This data entry step is a time-consuming task and requires trained data technicians or nutritionists.

A dietary recall is a 20 to 30 minute interview in which the respondent is asked to recall all foods and beverages consumed over the past 24 hours. These interviews can be conducted in person or by telephone. In some settings, the information is captured on paper forms and subsequently entered into the software program for nutrient analysis. However, ideally the interview will be conducted simultaneously with direct data entry into the software program. The record/recall analysis program provides specific prompts about foods, preparation methods, and portion sizes; therefore this protocol results in greatly increased standardization of the information received.

Advantages and Disadvantages of Records/Recalls

Both records and recalls provide the same type of data: detailed information on all foods and beverages consumed on specified days. In theory, a food record provides a "perfect" snapshot of intake. In practice, there are significant limitations associated with this method for assessing food intake. The principal problems are the large respondent burden of recording food intake and the impact on usual food consumption caused by record keeping. Respondents may alter their normal food choices merely to simplify record keeping or because they are sensitized to food choices. The latter reason appears more likely among women,[6] restrained eaters,[7] obese respondents,[8] or participants in a dietary intervention.[9] Other sources of error by respondents include mistakes or omissions in describing foods and assessing portion sizes.

Unannounced, interviewer-administered 24-hour dietary recalls are often recommended because respondents cannot change what they ate retrospectively.[10] One major disadvantage of dietary recalls is that they rely on the respondent's memory and ability to estimate portion sizes. In addition, it cannot be verified that social desirability does not influence self-report of the previous day's intake. A noteworthy benefit of recalls is that they are appropriate for low literacy populations.

Both records and recalls are expensive and time-consuming. However, the major scientific issue with records/recalls concerns the issue of day-to-day variability in intake, which means that several days of records/recalls are required to characterize usual intake. Using data on variability in intake from food records completed by 194 participants in the Nurses Health Study, [11] the number of days needed to estimate the mean intakes for individuals within 10% of "true" means would be 57 days for fat, 117 days for vitamin C, and 67 days for calcium. For estimating food consumption for individuals, variability can be even greater. For example, the number of days needed to estimate the following foods within 10% of "true" means would be 55 days for white fish and 217 days for carrots. Unfortunately, research has shown that reported energy intake, nutrient intake, and recorded numbers of foods decreases with as few as four days of recording dietary intake.[12] These changes may reflect reduced accuracy and completeness of recording intake or actual changes in dietary intake to reduce the burden of recording intake. In either case, there are considerable limitations on the usefulness of this methodology for characterizing usual intake in individuals.

Food Frequency Questionnaires (FFQs)

FFQs were developed for conducting research on dietary intake and chronic diseases such as heart disease and cancer. Because these diseases develop over 10 or more years, the biologically relevant exposure is long-term diet consumed many years prior to disease diagnosis. Therefore, instruments that only capture data on short-term or current intake (i.e., food records or recalls) are generally of limited usefulness in nutritional epidemiology research.

FFQs are designed to capture standardized, quantitative data on current or past, long-term diet. Although these questionnaires vary, they usually include three sections: 1) adjustment questions, 2) the food list, and 3) summary questions. Adjustment questions assess the nutrient content of specific food items. For example, participants are asked what type of milk they usually drink and are given several options (e.g., whole, skim, soy), which saves space and reduces participant burden compared to asking for the frequency of consumption and usual portion sizes of many different types of milk. Adjustment questions also permit more refined analyses of fat intake by asking about food preparation practices (e.g., removing skin from chicken) and types of added fats (e.g., use of butter versus margarine on vegetables).

The main section of an FFQ consists of a food or food group list, with questions on usual frequency of intake and portion size. To allow for machine scanning of these forms, frequency responses are typically categorized from "never or less than once per month" to "2+ per day" for foods and "6+ per day" for beverages. Portion sizes are often assessed by asking respondents to mark "small," "medium," or "large" in comparison to a given medium portion size. However, some questionnaires only ask about the frequency of intake of a "usual" portion size (e.g., 3 ounces of meat).

The food list in an FFQ is chosen to capture data on major sources of energy and nutrients in the population of interest, between-person variability in food intake, and specific scientific hypotheses. The choice of a food list is part data-driven and part scientific judgment. One data-based approach uses record/recall data to determine the major nutrient sources in the diet (i.e., the contribution of specific foods to the total population intake of nutrients). Information on food sources of nutrients in the American population have been published[13,14] but are often unavailable for specific population groups (e.g., Hispanics). However, a food is only informative if intake varies from person to person such that it discriminates between respondents. Therefore, another data-based approach to choosing the food list is to start with a extensive list of foods that is completed by a representative sample of the larger population. Stepwise regression analysis is performed where the dependent variable is the nutrient and the independent variable is frequency of consumption of foods.[15] In this process the computer algorithm ranks foods by the degree to which they explain the most between-person variance in nutrient intake, which is reflected in change in cumulative R^2. In addition to these two data-driven methods, items are often added to a questionnaire because of specific hypotheses (e.g., does consumption of soy foods reduce breast cancer risk).

A particularly challenging issue in FFQ food lists has to do with assessing intake of mixed dishes. For example, many FFQs ask about frequency of pizza consumption. However, from a nutrient perspective there is no accurate way to define "pizza." Depending on whether it is meat or vegetarian, thick or thin crust, tomato or pesto sauce, and so forth, pizza may be either low-fat and high-carbohydrate or extremely high-fat and high-protein. However, it is unreasonable to ask individuals to disaggregate their pizza into servings of breads, vegetables, meats, cheese, and added fats. Therefore FFQs typically strike an uneasy compromise between asking about some mixed dishes (e.g., pizza, hamburgers, tacos) while also asking the respondent to provide information on foods contained in their mixed dishes: "cheese, including cheese added to foods and in cooking." Unfortunately, asking about both "lasagna" and "cheese in cooking" presents the peril of double counting. There are little or no data to guide an investigator in making these judgments.

Finally, to save space and reduce respondent burden, similar foods are often grouped into a single line item (e.g., white bread, bagels, and pita bread). When grouping foods, important considerations include whether they are nutritionally similar enough to be grouped and whether the group will make cognitive sense to the respondent. For example, a food group composed of rice, macaroni, and cooked breakfast cereal may be nutritionally sensible. However, this question could be difficult to answer because it requires summing food consumption across different meal occasions.

Finally, FFQ summary questions that ask about usual intake of fruits and vegetables are often included in the questionnaire because the long lists of these foods needed to capture micronutrient intake can lead to overreporting of intake.[16]

Assessing the Reliability and Validity of Food Frequency Questionnaires

Because records and recalls are open-ended, they can (in theory) be applied in a standardized manner across populations with markedly different eating patterns. However, as noted above, FFQs are closed-ended forms with limited food lists. Because the food list varies from questionnaire to questionnaire, every FFQ will have different measurement characteristics. In addition, a questionnaire with appropriate foods and portion sizes for one population group (e.g., older caucasian men) may be wholly inappropriate for another subgroup (e.g., teenage African-American females). Finally, given changes in the food supply over time, such as the introduction of specially manufactured low-fat foods, questionnaires can become obsolete. Therefore the measurement characteristics (i.e., reliability and validity) of an FFQ need to be assessed for each new questionnaire and each new population group assessed.

Reliability generally refers to reproducibility, or whether an instrument will measure an exposure (e.g., nutrient intake) in the same way twice on the same respondents. Validity, which is a higher standard, refers to the accuracy of an instrument. Generally a validity study compares a practical, epidemiologic instrument (e.g., an FFQ) with a more accurate but more burdensome method (e.g., dietary recalls).

Reliability and validity of an FFQ are typically investigated using measures of bias and precision. Bias is the degree to which the FFQ accurately assesses mean intakes in a group. Lack of bias is especially important when the goal is to measure absolute intakes for comparison to dietary recommendations or some other objective criteria. For example, when the aim is to estimate how close Americans are to meeting the dietary recommendation to eat five servings of fruits and vegetables per day, it is critical to know whether the assessment instrument used under- or overestimates fruit and/or vegetable intake. Precision concerns whether an FFQ accurately ranks individuals from low to high nutrient intakes, which is typically the information needed to assess associations of dietary intake with risk of disease. It is important to remember than an instrument can be reliable without being accurate. That is, it can yield the same nutrient estimates two times and be wrong (e.g., biased upward) both times. Alternatively, an instrument can be reliable and consistently yield an accurate group mean (e.g., unbiased), but have poor precision such that it does not accurately rank individuals in the group from low to high in nutrient intake.

A reliability study compares intake estimates from two administrations of the FFQ in the same group of respondents. If an instrument is reliable, the mean intake estimates should not vary substantially between the two administrations. In addition, correlation coefficients between nutrient intakes estimated from two administrations of the FFQ in the same group of respondents should be high, and are generally in the range of 0.6 to 0.7. Reliability is easy to measure and gives an upper bound as to the accuracy of an instrument. While a high reliability coefficient does not imply a high validity coefficient, a low reliability coefficient clearly means poor validity. That is, if an instrument cannot measure a stable phenomenon (such as usual nutrient intake) the same way twice, it clearly cannot be accurate.

In a validity study, bias is assessed by comparing the mean estimates from an FFQ to those from multiple days of records/recalls in the same respondents. This comparison allows us to determine whether nutrient intake estimates from an FFQ appear to be under- or overreported in comparison to the criterion measure. Precision is measured as the correlation coefficients between nutrient intake estimates from the FFQ in comparison to a criterion measure, and typically range from 0.4 to 0.6. However, lower correlation coefficients (<0.4) are not unusual for nutrients that are poorly estimated with an FFQ, such as energy.[17] In addition, inclusion of dietary supplement use will often improve correlation coefficients (>0.8) because supplement use may be more accurately assessed and/or because supplement doses can be extraordinarily high compared to dietary intake, and thereby markedly increase the variability in intake for a nutrient. Some studies also assess precision by ranking nutrient intake estimates, dividing them into categories (e.g., quartiles) and comparing these to similar categories calculated from another instrument. However classifying a continuous exposure into a small number of categories does not reduce the effects of measurement error, and therefore this analysis does not provide additional information above correlation coefficients.[18]

The theory behind these (so-called) validity studies is that the major sources of error associated with FFQs are independent of those associated with records and recalls, which avoids spuriously high estimates of validity resulting from correlated errors. The errors associated with FFQs are the limitations imposed by a fixed list of foods and the respondents' ability to report usual frequency of food consumption (and usual portion sizes) over a broad time frame. In contrast, diet records are open-ended, do not depend on memory, and permit measurement of portion sizes. Errors in food records result from coding errors and changes in eating habits while keeping the records. Error in recalls results from estimation of portion sizes, participant memory, and coding errors.

Nonetheless, it is apparent that there are correlated errors between FFQs and records or recalls. Social desirability could influence how participants record or recall food intake across all types of dietary assessment instruments.[6,9] Participant error in estimating portion sizes could bias recall and FFQ estimates of intake in similar ways. There are also correlated errors in nutrient databases. Finally, research using doubly-labeled water to determine energy requirements have demonstrated significant underreporting of energy intakes from food records that may vary by participant characteristics.[8] It is important to be aware of the limitations of records and recalls as criterion measures of dietary intake, and cautiously interpret results based on these measures.

A final note is that an FFQ cannot, in and of itself, be validated. Only individual nutrient intake estimates can be validated by comparison of a nutrient estimate from the FFQ to a more accurate measure.

Advantages and Disadvantages of Food Frequency Questionnaires

The major advantage of FFQs is that they attempt to assess usual, long-term diet; either current or in the past. In addition, they have relatively low respondent burden and are simple and inexpensive to analyze because they can be self-administered and are machine scannable. A disadvantage of these questionnaires is that respondents must estimate usual frequency of consumption of approximately 100 foods and the associated usual portion sizes. These types of questions (i.e., this cognitive task) can be exceedingly difficult for many respondents, as evidenced by the prevalence of energy estimates from FFQs well outside the realm of what is plausible.[19] For example, it is not unusual for respondents to report usual energy intakes that are less than 500 kcals per day or greater than 5000 kcals per day. In addition, the format of the questionnaire is not user-friendly. Because FFQs are machine scannable, respondents must indicate their responses by filling in circles in a food-by-frequency matrix similar to that used in standardized testing. Some population groups may be unfamiliar or uncomfortable with such data collection methods. As might be hypothesized, validity studies of FFQs suggest that these forms may be less valid in less educated respondents.[20]

Another major disadvantage of these questionnaires is related to the close-ended nature of the form. The limited food list will not be appropriate for all individuals in a population and as noted above, different forms have different measurement characteristics in different populations. Therefore data from different FFQs are not directly comparable, nor are data from the same FFQ used in different populations, or data from the same FFQ used at different points in time (because of changes in the food supply). Finally, dependent upon the food list chosen by the investigator, the validity of nutrient intake estimates will vary from nutrient to nutrient.

Brief Dietary Assessment Instruments

Comprehensive dietary assessments (records/recalls and FFQs) are not always necessary or practical, which has led to the development of a diverse collection of brief assessment instruments. These include three general types: 1) ecologic-level measures such as food disappearance data or household food inventories, 2) short instruments that target a limited number of foods and/or nutrients, and 3) questionnaires that assess dietary behavior.

Ecologic-Level Measures

One well-known ecologic assessment of dietary intake is per capita food consumption estimated using national data on the total food supply. Publications from the Food and Agricultural Organization provide data on a country's total food supply from which non-consumption uses (such as exports and livestock feed) are subtracted, after which the total remaining food available can be divided by the population to obtain the per capita estimate of intake. These population intakes have been correlated with disease incidence across countries in provocative hypothesis-generating studies.[21-24]

Other ecologic measures, such as supermarket sale receipts,[25] have been developed and evaluated. Household food inventories are another example. In one study, the presence (in the house) of 15 high-fat foods was found to correlate with household members' dietary fat intake at 0.42 ($p<0.001$).[26] Individuals with ≤ 4 high-fat foods in their house had a mean of 32% energy from fat compared to 37% for those with ≥ 8 high-fat foods. Poor household food availability has also been shown to be significantly associated with greater individual-level measures of food insecurity.[27]

Targeted Instruments

Dietary assessment instruments that measure a limited number of foods and/or nutrients are most useful when the target food/nutrient is not distributed throughout the food supply. For example, dietary fat is widely distributed in dairy foods, meats, added fats, desserts, prepared foods, etc. Therefore, short instruments that attempt to estimate fat intake tend to be biased and imprecise.[28,29] Alternatively, intake of the isoflavones genestein and daidzain, which are largely limited to soy foods, can be captured with a relatively short instrument (15 foods).[30]

Behavioral Instruments

The development of diet behavioral instruments was motivated by problems with assessing dietary intervention effectiveness, particularly low-fat interventions. Traditional comprehensive instruments, such as records and FFQs, yield fairly imprecise estimates of fat intake that may not be sensitive to an intervention focused on changing participants' dietary behavior. One of the best known instruments of this type is the fat-related diet habits questionnaire.[31] This instrument was based on an anthropologic model that described low-fat dietary change as four types:

1. Avoiding high-fat foods (exclusion)
2. Altering available foods to make them lower in fat (modification)
3. Using new, specially formulated or processed, lower-fat foods instead of their higher-fat forms (substitution)
4. Using preparation techniques or food ingredients that replace the common higher-fat alternative (replacement)

Although originally developed for intervention assessment, the diet-habits questionnaire has since been used as a short assessment instrument in other research settings.[32,33]

Advantages and Disadvantage of Brief Assessment Instruments

The principal advantage of ecologic measures is that they are simple, inexpensive, nonintrusive, and objective measures of nutritional status. However these environmental indicators do not provide precise measures of individual intake.

Targeted questionnaires also tend to yield rather imprecise food and/or nutrient estimates. For example, short questionnaires for assessing fruit and vegetable intake have been extensively used in surveillance and intervention research. The typical approach uses two summary questions to capture consumption of most fruits and vegetables: "How often did you eat a serving of fruit (not including juices)?" and "How often did you eat a serving of vegetables (not including salad and potatoes)?," to which are added usual consumption of juice, salad, and potatoes.[34] Comparison of this brief measure with food records, food frequency estimates, and serum carotenoids indicates that this method yields particularly biased (underestimated) and imprecise measures of vegetable intake, likely because vegetables in mixed foods such as casseroles or sandwiches may be forgotten and unreported.[16]

The major advantage of the behavioral questionnaires is that they are short and simple (i.e., low respondent burden) and can be easily data-entered and scored. The disadvantage is that the diet "score" derived from these measures can be difficult to interpret because it is not comparable to nutrient or food intake measures. In addition, because these questionnaires have typically been "validated" in relation to records or recalls, which have many sources of error and bias, the degree to which they accurately reflect dietary intake is unknown.

Use of Dietary Assessment Methods in Individuals vs. Groups

Determination of an Individual's Dietary Adequacy for Purposes of Counseling

Records/Recalls

Records and recalls are used in clinical and counseling settings to assess dietary intake and are often used in a qualitative fashion. That is, respondents are asked to describe a usual day's intake and the nutritionist simply "eyeballs" the eating pattern for estimating dietary adequacy or risk, adherence to a prescribed diet, and/or areas for improving eating habits. The individualized nature of the interview can allow for probing and personalization of the feedback.

Whether these methods are used in a quantitative or qualitative manner, records and recalls can provide useful and understandable information to a respondent. The respondent can observe that the dietary recommendations are based directly on the food intake information provided and can use the advice to alter future food choices, food preparation techniques, or portion sizes. Therefore, on an individual level, records and recalls can serve an important teaching function. In addition, there is considerable literature indicating that the act of keeping records (i.e., self-monitoring) is a significant predictor of success in achieving weight loss or making other dietary changes.[29]

Food Frequency Questionnaires

FFQs tend to produce imprecise dietary intake estimates because of respondent error and inappropriate food lists. In addition, the data input (usual frequency of intake and portion sizes) and nutrient calculation algorithms are a black box to the respondent. Therefore the respondent cannot easily use this information to make more healthful food choices. For these reasons, FFQs are not generally useful for assessing an individual's nutrient intake for purposes of counseling.

However, data on *food consumption* from FFQs has been used for individual feedback. For example, Kristal et al. developed computer programs for tailored feedback to participants in a self-help dietary intervention that used FFQ data to provide food-specific recommendations to reach nutritional goals (e.g., "if you use low-fat mayonnaise instead of regular mayonnaise you will cut your fat by 28 g per week").[35] Because the feedback provided to the participants is food based and taken directly from their responses (e.g., type of mayonnaise used and frequency consumed), this approach avoids the black box problems associated with using FFQs to estimate nutrient intake.

Brief Assessment Instruments

These instruments are diverse, and therefore it is difficult to generalize regarding their use. Ecologic measures are intended to be environmental indicators and therefore are generally not appropriate for individuals. However, it is clear that some simple targeted instruments can be very useful for individual counseling. For example, a rather short set of questions can likely assess usual fruit and vegetable consumption sufficiently for purposes of advising a respondent whether his/her intake appears to be adequate or inadequate.

Research Studies of Dietary Intake and Disease Risk

Records/Recalls

Records and recalls have limited usefulness in research studies of diet and disease risk for both scientific and practical reasons. Scientifically, records/recalls only assess current, short-term diet, and in most etiologic studies usual long-term (and often past) diet is the exposure of biologic significance. Practically, records and recalls are infeasible because of costs and respondent burden. However, records and recalls are often used in subsamples of the parent study for the following purposes:

1. FFQ reliability and validity substudies
2. Evaluating dietary interventions where the goal is to compare mean intakes in the intervention versus the control group
3. As a check of the main study assessment instrument (such as an FFQ)

Food Frequency Questionnaires

As noted above, the major advantage of an FFQ is that it attempts to assess the exposure of interest in most applications: usual dietary intake in an individual. The main use of these instruments is to rank study participants from low to high intake of many foods and nutrients for comparison (on the individual level) with disease risk. However, these questionnaires produce food and nutrient estimates containing considerable random error resulting from inadvertently marking the wrong frequency column, skipping questions, and failures in judgment. These errors introduce noise into nutrient estimates such that our ability to find the "signal," such as an association of dietary fat and breast cancer, is masked or attenuated (i.e., biased toward no association).

However, a more important concern in research studies is systematic error. Systematic error refers to under- or overreporting of intake across the population, and person-specific sources of bias. For example, studies indicate that obese women are more likely to underestimate dietary intake than normal-weight women.[8] Systematic error may result in either null or spurious associations. Prentice used data from FFQs collected in a low-fat dietary intervention trial to simulate the effects of random and systematic error on an association of dietary fat and breast cancer, where the true relative risk (RR) was assumed to be 4.0.[36] Assuming only random error exists in the estimate of fat intake, the projected (i.e., observed) RR for fat and breast cancer would be 1.4. Assuming both random error and systematic error exists, the projected RR would be 1.1, similar to that reported in a recent meta-analysis on dietary fat and breast cancer.[37] Data on systematic error from biomarker studies, combined with these types of statistical simulations, clearly suggest that measures of self-reported dietary intake may not be adequate to detect many associations of diet with disease, even when a strong relationship exists. It is important to note that records/recalls are not exempt from these biases.

Finally, FFQs cannot provide detailed information on specific foods (e.g., brand names) or eating patterns (e.g., meals per day or consumption of breakfast) that may be important in some research studies.

Brief Assessment Instruments

Most brief instruments were developed for very specific research applications. The biggest concern when using a brief instrument is that it is often impossible to anticipate all the questions regarding diet that may become important by the end of a study. Therefore, the choice of a brief instrument limits future questions that can be addressed. Nonetheless, data collection for research purposes is a compromise between what is ideal and what is practical, and a comprehensive dietary assessment may not always be possible.

Nutrition Monitoring of Populations

Records/Recalls

Records and recalls have proven very useful for nutrition monitoring. A single day's intake can provide estimates of the average intake of large groups that are comparable to those obtained with more burdensome techniques.[38] Because these methods are open-ended, they are especially useful for assessing mean intake across population groups with markedly different eating patterns.

However, a single day's intake cannot be used to study distributions of dietary intake because on any one day, an individual's diet can be unusually high (e.g., a celebratory meal) or low (e.g., a sick day). These days are not representative of an individual's intake even though they may be perfectly recorded. This day-to-day variation in intake is random and does not bias the mean intake for a group, although this variability does result in an increased distribution of observed intake (i.e., a wide standard deviation). However, if multiple measures (per person) are collected on a subsample of the population, it is possible to obtain an estimate of the within- vs. between-person variance and calculate the "true" standard deviation around the mean for the population. This procedure allows the investigator to determine the percent of individuals above (or below) a specified cut-point.[15]

Although the use of records/recalls in nutrition monitoring appears straightforward, there is actual considerable subtlety about the data needed to address public health dietary objectives. For example, assume that a public health objective is to reduce total fat intake to less than or equal to 30% energy from fat. A critical clarification of this objective is whether:

1. The population mean intake should be 30% energy from fat, in which case approximately half of the group will have intakes exceeding that level, or

2. The entire population should have intakes less than or equal to 30% energy from fat, in which case the group mean will be several percentage points below 30%.

If the public health objective is the first goal listed, then nutrition monitoring can be appropriately performed with a single 24-hour record/recall for determination of mean intake in the population. Alternatively, if the public health objective is the second, then multiple records/recalls (per person) will need to be collected for assessment of intake distribution in the population to determine the proportion of individuals consuming more than 30% energy from fat.

Food Frequency Questionnaires

FFQs have proven most useful in nutritional epidemiologic studies when the objective is to rank individuals from low to high intake for a food or nutrient. However, as described above, FFQs are close-ended forms with limited food lists, and the accuracy of FFQs will vary considerably across groups with different eating patterns. Therefore when the goal is to assess mean intakes in population subgroups with markedly different dietary patterns, or to track changes in intake over long periods of time, the FFQ is not the instrument of choice.

Brief Assessment Instruments

The accuracy of several of these instruments is particularly sensitive to differences in dietary patterns across population groups. For example, the validity of a fat-related behavioral questionnaire depends entirely on knowledge of those dietary behaviors that influence fat intake. In populations with different dietary patterns, the instrument would be useless for assessment of fat intake. Overall, it is useful to remember that brief dietary assessment instruments are developed for very specific objectives and caution needs to be taken when applying them to other populations or using them for other purposes.

Summary

Much of what has been presented here is summarized in Tables 21.1 through 21.3. Specifically, Table 21.1 summarizes the major scientific and practical advantages and disadvantages of the major dietary assessment methods. Table 21.2 provides an overview of the issues regarding use of data from dietary intake assessment methods. Table 21.3 gives a summary of consideration regarding use of dietary intake assessment in individuals versus groups.

The use of sophisticated computerized technologies and internet accessibility has the potential to address many of the practical and logistic limitations of the major dietary intake assessment methods. For example, a computer screen could provide life-size pictures of foods to help respondents more accurately estimate serving sizes. A user-friendly computer-administered dietary recall could eliminate the costs associated with this method of collecting data. A touch-screen FFQ program, with algorithms for limiting questions to foods eaten with some minimal frequency, could eliminate the unfriendly format of the questionnaire and tailor the food list. Nonetheless, these practical advances will not eliminate the scientific problems inherent in dietary self-report. In particular, the issues of systematic and person-specific biases in self-report can likely only by addressed by use of objective biomarkers for identification, quantification, and correction of random and systematic error.[39]

It is clear from this brief overview that choosing the appropriate dietary assessment method is a complex decision based on the specific objective, with an eye toward the competing demands of accuracy and practicality. There is no right or wrong approach, only the best possible measure given the specific objectives of the assessment. In spite of all the challenges and limitations of dietary assessment methods, these data will continue to serve an essential role in efforts to improve the health and longevity of individuals and groups.

TABLE 21.1

Summary of the Major Advantages and Disadvantages of Dietary Assessment Methods

Characteristics	Single Record/Recall	Multiple Record/Recalls per Person	Food Frequency Questionnaire (FFQ)	Brief Assessment Instruments
Brief Description	Detailed recording of everything consumed in one day	Multiple days (per person) of recording of everything consumed	Measure of usual intake determined from frequencies of consumption of about 100 foods (or food groups)	Diverse group of short tools developed to target limited number of foods, nutrients, and/or dietary behavior
Scientific Features				
Advantages	Open-ended format appropriate for all types of eating patterns Provides detailed information on foods consumed Provides data that are comparable across populations and time Recalls can't affect (past) food choices	(Same as single records/recalls) 3-4 days of records/recalls have been used to characterize usual intake in individuals	Captures data on usual, long-term intake Can be used retrospectively	Ideal for studies where comprehensive assessment is not needed Some are non-intrusive and therefore relatively objective Behavioral assessments may be more sensitive to dietary interventions than nutrient estimates
Disadvantages*	Can only capture information on current intake, and one day's intake does not characterize usual intake Records can change eating behavior Recalls depend on respondent memory	(Same as single records/recalls) Because of day to day variability in intake, even 3-4 days of intake only roughly approximates usual intake	Accurate reporting of usual intake of foods is very difficult for some respondents Limited food list will not be appropriate for all respondents Different questionnaires are needed for different populations and therefore do not produce comparable nutrient estimates	Typically provide fairly imprecise estimates of nutrient intakes Because of targeted nature of these instruments, future scientific questions on other foods or nutrients cannot be addressed
Practical Features				
Advantages	Recalls do not require literate respondents Because recalls are interviewer administered, data can be collected in a standardized way	(Same as single records/recalls)	Fairly low respondent burden Once developed, scannable FFQs are inexpensive and easy to analyze	Low respondent burden Usually simple and inexpensive to code and analyze
Disadvantages	Expensive to collect, code, and analyze	(Same as single records/recalls) Multiple records or recalls are extremely burdensome for participants	FFQ development costs are extremely high	

* All types of dietary self-report are subjective and are subject to under-reporting and person-specific biases associated with sex, obesity, social desirability, etc.

TABLE 21.2

Summary of the Issues Regarding Use of Data from Dietary Intake Assessment Methods

Data	Single Record/Recall	Multiple Record/Recalls per Person	Food Frequency Questionnaire (FFQ)	Brief Assessment Instruments
Appropriate use of data	To estimate absolute mean values for intakes of foods and nutrients Group means and standard deviations for comparison to other groups	As an approximation of usual intake in an individual if used with caution and recognition that there will be considerable attenuation of associations with other variables	Ranking individuals from low to high intakes for foods or nutrients	Ranking individuals from low to high intakes for the specific food or nutrient being targeted
Inappropriate use of data*	Ranking respondents from low to high intakes For determination of the percent of population above (or below) some cut-point		Estimation of absolute nutrient intakes for comparison to other questionnaires or populations Just because an FFQ has been "validated" does not mean that it assesses all nutrients with good, or equal, accuracy	Estimation of absolute intakes for nutrients
Data not available	These methods cannot be used to assess dietary intake in the past	(Same as single record/recall)	Eating pattern information (e.g., meals per day). Detailed information on foods consumed, such as brand names	(Same as FFQ)

* Because of considerable random and systematic error, no forms of dietary self-report data should be regarded as "truth."

TABLE 21.3

Summary of Considerations Regarding Use of Dietary Intake Assessment in Individuals vs. Groups

	Single Record/Recall	Multiple Record/Recalls per Person	Food Frequency Questionnaire (FFQ)	Brief Assessment Instruments
Individual Assessment				
Appropriate Use	Qualitative use in clinical setting Teaching tool regarding food composition For self-monitoring	(Same as single record/recall) 3-4 days can be used as an approximation of usual intake	To provide feedback regarding respondent consumption of a food vs. recommended intake	Targeted instrument may be appropriate for individual counseling for the food or nutrient being assessed
Inappropriate Use	As estimate of usual intake		Nutrient intake estimates too imprecise for individual counseling	Reliable estimate of absolute intakes
Research Studies				
Appropriate Use	For comparing mean intakes in control vs. intervention group As a check of FFQ mean intake estimates for a group	(Same as single record/recall) Validity substudies for comparison of nutrient intake estimates to FFQ	For ranking individuals from low to high intakes for determination of associations with disease risk	Where costs or logistic realities prohibit use of a comprehensive assessment instrument
Inappropriate Use	When characterization of usual, long-term diet is the exposure of interest	(Same as single record/recall) In study population where respondent burden will result in poor quality data	For estimation of absolute intakes When comparable data needed across markedly different populations	In cases where there is the potential for important, new research questions to emerge
Nutrition Monitoring of Populations				
Appropriate Use	Nutrition monitoring of group means, including trends analyses Descriptive data on population eating patterns For international comparisons of food and nutrient intake	(Same as single record/recall) 3-4 days can approximate usual intake in individuals		
Inappropriate Use	To determine percentage of population meeting a dietary recommendation or at risk		For estimation of absolute intakes For time trends analyses because changing food supply cam make questionnaires obsolete	To estimate absolute intakes

References

1. National Research Council and Committee on Diet and Health, *Diet and Health: Implications for Reducing Chronic Disease*, National Academy Press, Washington, DC, 1989.
2. US Dept of Health and Human Services, Public Health Service, DHHS (PHS) publication 88-50210, *The Surgeon General's Report on Nutrition and Health*, Washington, DC, 1988.
3. World Cancer Research Fund and the American Institute for Cancer Research, *Food, Nutrition, and the Prevention of Cancer: A Global Perspective.* Potter J. Ed, American Institute for Cancer Research, Washington DC, 1997.
4. Torun B, Chew F. In *Modern Nutrition in Health and Disease, 8th ed* (Shils ME, Olson JA, Shike M, Eds.), Lea & Febiger, Philadelphia, PA, 1994, pg 950.
5. Patterson RE. In *Nutrition in the Prevention and Treatment of Disease*, Coulston M, Rock CL, Monson E, Eds, Academic Press (in press).
6. Hebert JR, Clemow L, Pbert L, et al. *Int J Epidemiol* 24: 389; 1995.
7. Jansen A. *Br J Clin Psychol* 35: 381; 1996.
8. Black AE, Prentice AM, Goldberg GR, et al. *JADA* 93: 572; 1993.
9. Kristal AR, Andrilla CAH, Koepsell TD, et al. *JADA* 98: 40; 1998.
10. Buzzard IM, Faucett CL, Jeffery RW, et al. *JADA* 96: 574; 1996.
11. Willet W. *Nutritional Epidemiology*, Oxford University Press, New York, 1990.
12. Rebro S, Patterson RE, Kristal AR, Chaney C. *JADA* 98: 1163; 1998.
13. Block G, Dresser CM, Hartman AM, Carrol MD. *Am J Epidemiol* 122: 13; 1985.
14. Block G, Dresser CM, Hartman AM, Carrol MD. *Am J Epidemiol* 122: 27; 1985.
15. Willet W. *Nutritional Epidemiology.* 2nd ed., Oxford University Press, New York, 1998.
16. Kristal AR, Vizenor NC, Patterson RE, et al. *Cancer Epidemiol Biomarkers Prev* 9: 939; 2000.
17. Patterson RE, Kristal AR, Carter RA, et al. *Ann Epidemiol* 9: 178; 1999.
18. Armstrong BK, White E, Saracci R. In: *Monographs in Epidemiology and Biostatistics*, Oxford University Press, Oxford, 1994.
19. Black AE. *Eur J Clin Nutr* 54: 395; 2000.
20. Kristal AR, Feng Z, Coates RJ, et al. *Am J Epidemiol* 146: 856; 1997.
21. Armstrong B, Doll R. *Int J Cancer* 15: 617; 1975.
22. Gray GE, Pike MC, Henderson BE. *Br J Cancer* 39: 1; 1979.
23. Prentice RL, Sheppard L. *Cancer Causes Control* 1: 81; 1990.
24. Roberts DC. *Prostaglandins Leukotrienes Essential Fatty Acids* 44: 97; 1991.
25. Kerr GR, Amante P, Decker M, Callen PW. *Am J Clin Nutr* 37: 622; 1983.
26. Patterson RE, Kristal AR, Shannon J, et al. *Am J Pub Health* 87: 272; 1997.
27. Kendall A, Olson CM, Frongillo EA. *J Nutr* 125: 2793; 1995.
28. Neuhouser ML, Kristal AR, McLerran D, et al. *Cancer Epidemiol Biomarkers Prev* 8: 649; 1999.
29. Tinker LF, Patterson RE, Kristal AR, et al. *JADA* (in press).
30. Kirkley P, Patterson RE, Lampe J. *JADA* 99: 558; 1999.
31. Kristal AR, Shattuck AL, Henry HJ. *JADA* 90: 214; 1990.
32. Patterson RE, Kristal AR, White E. *Am J Pub Health* 86: 1394; 1996.
33. Neuhouser ML, Kristal AR, Patterson RE. *JADA* 98: 45; 1998.
34. Thompson FE, Subar AF, Kipnis V, et al. *Eur J Clin Nutr* 52: S45; 1998.
35. Kristal AR, Curry SJ, Shattuck AL, et al. *Prev Med* 31: 380; 2000.
36. Prentice RL. *J Natl Cancer Inst* 88: 1738; 1996.
37. Hunter DJ, Speigelman D, Adami HO, et al. *N Engl J Med* 334: 356; 1996.
38. Beaton GH, Milner J, Corey P. *Am J Clin Nutr* 32: 2546; 1979.
39. Prentice RL, Sugar E, Wang CY, et al. *Pub Health Nutr* (in press).

22

The Use of Food Frequency Questionnaires in Minority Populations

Rebecca S. Reeves

Food frequency questionnaires (FFQs) are selected by investigators to assess the usual food or nutrient intakes of groups or individuals because they are relatively easy to administer, less expensive than other dietary assessment methods, and can be adapted to all racial and ethnic populations in the United States.[1] Investigators can also modify these dietary instruments for telephone interviews or self-administered mailed surveys. FFQs are commonly used in epidemiological studies on diet and disease, but are also chosen by investigators as the dietary assessment instrument in clinical intervention studies. The use of these questionnaires in minority populations in the U.S. is increasing for several reasons: the country is becoming more racially and ethnically diverse,[2] government agencies have placed emphasis on including minority population in health-related research,[3] and variations in disease incidence and dietary practices within and across ethnic minorities offer important opportunities for examining the role of diet in relation to risk for chronic disease.[4]

This section reviews 12 published studies evaluating the validity and/or reliability of FFQs used in measuring dietary intakes in adult minority populations in the U.S. over the last 20 years. Also included are selected samples of FFQs and information on obtaining copies. Recommendations on the use of these FFQs are discussed.

A search of the National Library of Medicine's (Bethesda, MD) MEDLINE system was conducted using various terms such as *validity, reliability, reproducibility, diet, food frequency questionnaire, minority, Hispanic, black, Asian, Pacific-islander* and *native America* to identify articles published between 1980 and 2000. These searches were supplemented by cross-referencing from author reference lists. Articles were selected that described the evaluation of any FFQ that assessed the usual daily diet and provided data on the validity and/or reliability of the instrument in a specific U.S. ethnic minority population or a diverse population representing at least 40% minority persons. The degree of reliability or validity of the instrument reported was not considered an inclusion factor. Validity and reliability studies that were reported in the same article were considered separately and are referenced in different tables. The measures of performance chosen were reliability, comparison of means (when available), and validity, because these are usually reported to describe the results of the evaluation of the FFQ. Correlation coefficients were selected as indicators of reliability and validity because they are commonly used and are more easily summarized. Factors that can influence correlation coefficients are the number of days between the times the questionnaire is administered (reliability coefficients) and the number of

0-8493-2705-9/01/$0.00+$1.50

days of food records or 24-hour recalls used for the referent period (validity coefficients). Unadjusted correlation coefficients if available are reported in the tables because of the considerable variation in the kinds of adjustment procedures that were used in these studies and the lack of standardization across studies for methods used.

Terms used to describe FFQs in the tables:

- *Quantitative* — Quantity of food consumed was estimated using weights, measures, or food models. Responses were open-ended.
- *Semi-quantitative* — Quantity of food consumed was estimated using a standard portion size, serving, or a predetermined amount and the respondent was asked about the number of portions consumed.
- *Nonquantitative* — Quantity of food was not assessed.
- *Self-administered* — An adult completed the dietary assessment without assistance.
- *Interviewer-administered* — A trained interviewer collected the dietary information from the adult in a one-on-one setting.
- *Diverse studies* — Publications that include various combinations of racial or ethnic groups
- *Minority studies* — Publications that include only one racial or ethnic group

The twelve studies reviewed for this section were divided into two groups based on ethnic participation. Within the group labeled Minority studies, two consisted of only black subjects,[5,6] one of Asian,[7] and one of Hispanic subjects.[8] In the group labeled Diverse, two studies included black and white subjects,[9,10] three studies black, Hispanic, and white subjects,[11,12,13] one study Hispanic and white,[14] one study Asian and white,[15] and one recruited Asian, black, Hispanic, and white subjects.[16]

The review of the validation studies on FFQs was not conclusive. The median correlations (Table 22.1) between questionnaire–based estimates of nutrient intakes and estimates derived from referent methods were not consistent for ethnic groups, but trends were suggested. The median correlations for black males and females across validation studies were in the range of 0.23 to 0.46; for Hispanic females, 0.32 to 0.49 except for one study conducted in Starr County, Texas which reported a median correlation of 0.75; for white males and females, 0.53, and for Asian males and females, 0.53. If you consider a measure of ≥0.05 as satisfactory or good, 0.30 to 0.49 as fair, and <0.30 as poor,[15] then these median correlations suggest that black and Hispanic groups do not perform extremely well on FFQs.

The validation correlations for total energy, total fat, and vitamin A were inconsistent and in some cases very low across studies. In Table 22.2 the correlation coefficients for total fat ranged from 0.23 to 0.65, with the higher correlations usually found in the Asian or white populations. A similar trend was found for energy among the various groups. The correlation coefficients for Hispanic and black populations were commonly in the range of 0.24 to 0.43, but in the white and Asian groups the coefficients ranged from 0.41 to 0.61. Values for vitamin A were more inconsistent, ranging from 0.15 to 0.67 across all groups. The number of days of food records and recalls that are compared against FFQs can explain some of these low correlations, especially for vitamin A. Many days are required to provide a precise estimate of vitamin A intake, and in these studies the greatest number of daily recalls or records collected over one year was 28. Even in this study, certain subgroup correlations for vitamin A were still 0.23 and 0.29.

The study[5] that reported serum nutrient concentrations of carotenoids, vitamin E, lycopene, and lutein as a referent reported correlations that were much lower for smokers

TABLE 22.1

Median and Reported Range of Correlation Coefficients

Study	Median and Reported Range Validity Coefficients	Reliability Coefficients
Diverse Groups		
Baumgartner et al.[14]	0.50 (0.21–0.57) HF+WF (adjusted value)	0.62 (0.40–0.71) Unadjusted
Hankin et al.[15]	0.63 (0.58–0.67) Chinese females	
	0.46 (0.38–0.64) White females	
	0.56 (0.49–0.60) Filipino females	
	0.38 (0.29–0.41) Hawaiian females	
	0.60 (0.23–0.68) Japanese females	
	0.58 (0.38–0.68) Chinese males	
	0.45 (0.34–0.64) White males	
	0.57 (0.21–0.84) Filipino males	
	0.36 (0.26–0.62) Hawaiian males	
	0.55 (0.46–0.77) Japanese males	
Kristal et al.[11]	Baseline	
	0.31 (0.26–0.46) Black females	0.51(0.37–0.60) Black females
	0.35 (0.25–0.48) Hispanic females	0.51(0.19–0.75) Hispanic females
	Six months (control group)	
	0.40 (0.29–0.49) Black females	
	0.37 (–0.01–0.48) Hispanic females	
Larkin et al.[9]	0.43 (0.26–0.62) White males	
	0.23 (0.09–0.41) Black males	
	0.44 (0.27–0.57) White females	
	0.32 (0.24–0.43) Black females	
Liu et al.[10]	0.64 (0.50–0.86) White males	0.70 (0.60–0.91) White M+F
	0.53 (0.13–0.68) White females	0.58 (0.45–0.85) Black M+F
	0.42 (0.23–0.67) Black males	
	0.27 (0.04–0.53) Black females	
Mayer-Davis et al.[12]	0.58 (0.30–0.77) White females, urban	0.71 (0.43–0.82) White females
	0.38 (0.22–0.62) Black females, urban	0.62 (0.26–0.69) Black females
	0.57 (0.24–0.68) White females, rural	0.64 (0.25–0.88) White females, rural
	0.32 (0.21–0.44) Hispanic females, rural	0.58 (0.33–0.66) Hispanic females, rural
Stram et al.[16]	Average correlation for amount	
	0.30 (0.16–0.41) Black M+F	
	0.48 (0.27–0.62) Hispanic M+F	
	0.57 (0.48–0.64) White M+F	
Suitor et al.[13]	0.32 (0.12–0.52) All females combined	0.88 (0.80–0.94) All females
Minority Groups		
Coates et al.[5]	0.34 (–0.02–0.45) Nonsmokers	
	0.08 (–0.02–0.20) Smokers	
Forsythe et al.[6]		0.88 (0.69–0.98) Black females
Lee et al.[7]	0.46 (0.21–0.66) Chinese females	
McPherson et al.[8]	0.75 (0.53–0.77) Hispanic M+F	0.85 (0.84–0.90) Hispanic M+F

(≤0.02) than for nonsmokers (<0.40). The investigators summarize that their FFQ is reasonably valid for use in a Southern, urban, low-income black population, except for the analysis of lutein and lycopene.

In most of the studies reviewed, the FFQ overestimated the mean of the referent recall or records, and in some cases by nontrivial amounts. One explanation for this difference was, again, the number of days of recalls or records collected for comparison to the FFQ. Depending on which nutrient is of interest in the study and the time period the participant

TABLE 22.2

Food Frequency Questionnaire (FFQ) Validity Studies among Diverse Adult Populations in the U.S.

Reference	Sample	Instrument	Response Categories	Validation Standard	Design	Results
Baumgartner et al.[14]	43 HF (Hispanic) 89 NHF	140 Items; interviewer-administered; open-ended; referent period was previous 4 weeks	Included per month, week or day	4-Day food records	Compared subject's report of past month's food intake against 4 randomly selected nonconsecutive day food records; third FFQ taken 6 months after 1st FFQ to recall original month, then compared against subject's 4 day FR	Pearson correlation coefficients (log transformed and energy adjusted); nutrients which differed significantly by ethnicity between FFQ2 + FFQ3 and food records: Protein(g) HF 0.40 NHF 0.35 Vitamin A (RE) HF 0.67 NHF 0.38 Vitamin C (mg) HF 0.34 NHF 0.64 Calcium (mg) HF 0.49 NHF 0.58
Hankin et al.[15]	Japanese 29M + 29F Chinese 29M + 26 F Filipino 22 M + 25 F Hawaiian 19 M + 28 F Caucasian 29 M + 26 F	Hawaiian Cancer Research Center 47 items, semi-quantitative; administered; covers past twelve months; color photographs showing S, M, L portion sizes were used by subjects to estimate intake on FFQ and FR	8 (Never or hardly ever to 2 or more times/day)	Four 1-week food records at approximately 3-month intervals	Compared subject's report of nutrient intake (FFQ) against average of 4, 1 week FR collected at 3 month intervals during a 1-year period. FFQ collected at end of 12 month period	Intraclass correlations (log transformed) between the subjects' reports on FFQs and average 7 day FR Total fat: JapM 0.55, WM 0.34, ChinM 0.39, FilM 0.60 HawM 0.26 JapF 0.68, WF 0.58, ChinF 0.67, FilF 0.55, HawF 0.40. Vitamin A: JapM 0.74, WM 0.38, ChinM 0.65, FilM 0.53, HawM 0.35, JapF 0.23, WF 0.40, ChinF 0.64, FilF 0.53, HawF 0.29 Intraclass correlation for total fat for all males was 0.48 and for all females 0.60. FFQ overestimated means of FR by large amounts but results on the agreement of the FFQ with FR were generally satisfactory

Kristal et al [11]	555 White F, 271 black F, 159 Hispanic F recruited at three clinical centers. Because Hispanics recruited at Miami clinic only, their data were compared with WF from same clinic; data for WF and BF at two other centers were collapsed and compared	100 Items, self-administered, semi-quantitative; covering last three months; portion sizes were S, M, L. FFQ collected at screening, baseline and six months. Printed in both English and Spanish	9 (Never or <once/mo to 2 or more times/day for foods and 6+/day for beverages)	4-Day food records collected at baseline and 6 months	Compared subjects; recall of baseline FFQs with the baseline food records and at six months, the 6-month FFQ with the 6-month food records	FFQ overestimated % of energy from fat compared with FR. Pearson correlations (log transformed) between FFQ and 4 day FR: Baseline: Fat (% energy, adjusted) BF — 0.26 WF — 0.49 HF — 0.35 WF — 0.35 Saturated fat (% energy adjusted) BF — 0.32 WF — 0.50 HF — 0.37 WF — 0.56 Beta-carotene (unadjusted) BF — 0.42 WF — 0.32 HF — 0.26 WF — 0.30 Correlations at baseline were significantly larger among whites than blacks and tended to be larger for whites than Hispanics. Six Months — Control group Fat (% energy) BF — 0.49 WF — 0.52 HF — 0.48 WF — 0.61 Saturated fat (% energy) BF — 0.47 WF — 0.53 HF — 0.48 WF — 0.68 Beta-carotene (unadjusted) BF — 0.34 WF — 0.23 HF — 0.27 WF — 0.57 Educational level associated with poor validity of FFQ and/or FR measures.

TABLE 22.2 *(Continued)*

Food Frequency Questionnaire (FFQ) Validity Studies among Diverse Adult Populations in the U.S.

Reference	Sample	Instrument	Response Categories	Validation Standard	Design	Results
Larkin et al. [9]	43 BM 48 BF 64 WM 73 WF (40% subjects black)	In Michigan FFQ-113 food items based on data from NFCS 77-78; semiquantitative; collected food intake over past 12 months	9 (Not in past year to more than once a day)	One 24-hr recall + 3-day food record collected 4 times/yr about 3 months apart. FR's administered and reviewed in subject's home. FFQ administered in subject's home about 3 months after 4th set of records had been completed	Compared by sex and ethnic group (BM, BF, WM, WF) report of food intake (4 sets of food record) against the FFQ	Pearson correlation (nonadjusted) values between FFQ and 16 days of FR: Energy: BM — 0.23 BF — 0.26 WM — 0.41 WF — 0.43 Protein (gm): BM — 0.30 BF — 0.40 WM — 0.41 WF — 0.36 Total fat (gm): BM — 0.23 BF — 0.35 WM — 0.44 WF — 0.39 Vitamin A(IU): BM — 0.15 BF — 0.28 WM — 0.26 WF — 0.27 FFQ showed larger mean nutrient intakes compared to FR. Black M+F had lower coefficients between FFQ and FR than white M+F

Liu et al. [10]	33 BM 32 BF 30 WM 33 WF	About 300 items in 20 categories; Interviewer-administered quantitative FF based on the Western Electric dietary history; referent period is past month.	Open-ended	Seven 24-hr food recalls collected by phone	Compared subject's recall of last 30 days against seven 24-hr food recalls	Mean nutrient values for WM are similar between 2 methods; for WF values from FFQ are generally higher than recalls (VitA significantly different); for BM + BF values from history are much higher than recalls (VitA+ Kcal significantly different); Pearson correlations (log transformed) Total Calories: WM — 0.64 WF — 0.47 BM — 0.43 BF — 0.21 Total Fat: (g) WM — 0.65 WF — 0.37 BM — 0.36 BF — 0.23 Vitamin A: (IU) WM — 0.67 WF — 0.62 BM — 0.62 BF — 0.32

TABLE 22.2 *(Continued)*

Food Frequency Questionnaire (FFQ) Validity Studies among Diverse Adult Populations in the U.S.

Reference	Sample	Instrument	Response Categories	Validation Standard	Design	Results
Mayer-Davis et al.[12]	32 WF (urban) 63 BF (urban) 30 WF (rural) 61 HF (rural)	114-Item, interviewer-administered FFQ; modified from NCI-HHHQ to include regional and ethnic food choices; past year	9 (Never or <1/month to 2 or more times/day)	Eight 24-hr recalls over course of 1 year (randomly selected days, about every 6 weeks)	Compared subject's report of frequency of intake from FFQ2 to average of eight 24-hr recalls;	Pearson correlations (log-transformed) between FFQ2 and food recalls were: Energy: WF (urban) — 0.61 BF (urban) — 0.37 WF (rural) — 0.56 HF (rural) — 0.27 Total fat: (g) WF (urban) — 0.66 BF (urban) — 0.59 WF (rural) — 0.58 HF (rural) — 0.40 Vitamin A: (IU) WF (urban) — 0.38 BF (urban) — 0.28 WF (rural) — 0.24 HF (rural) — 0.28 Correlations by educational status: Total fat: (g) <12 grade — 0.05 12 grade — 0.59 Total CHO: (g) <12 grade — 0.19 12 grade — 0.53 Saturated fat: (g) <12 grade — 0.07 12 grade — 0.63 Vitamin A: (IU) <12 grade — 0.31 12 grade — 0.21

Stram et al.[16]	African-Am 151BM, 186 BF Japanese 224 JM, 222 JF Hispanics 136 HM, 123 HF Caucasians 264 WM, 264 WF	Based on Hawaiian Cancer Research Center FFQ; quantitative by placing serving size photos beside the amount category; 8 frequency categories for food and 9 for beverages	Unknown; highest response for food is >2 times/day; for beverages, 4 times/day	Three random 24-hr recalls conducted by phone	An initial FFQ was mailed to random sample of prospective subjects; 3-24 hr recalls were collected by phone after the initial contact; a second FFQ was sent 4-6 weeks after the recalls were completed; the subjects' responses on the 2nd FFQ were compared against the 24-hr recall values	Corrected correlations for the regression of mean 24-hr recalls on the 2nd FFQ by ethnic sex/group for following nutrients: Total kcals: BM — 0.16 BF — 0.17 JM — 0.34 JF — 0.19 HM — 0.33 HF — 0.40 WM — 0.48 WF — 0.28 Total Protein: (g) BM — 0.17 BF — 0.22 JM — 0.31 JF — 0.25 HM — 0.27 HF — 0.35 WM — 0.51 WF — 0.38 Total Fat: (g) BM — 0.29 BF — 0.24 JM — 0.41 JF — 0.32 HM — 0.33 HF — 0.57 WM — 0.57 WF — 0.39 Vitamin A: (IU) BM — 0.30 BF — 0.22 JM — 0.45 JF — 0.49 HM — 0.62 HF — 0.52 WM — 0.59 WF — 0.58
Suitor et al.[13]	Initially who provided 3 diet recalls: WF — 54 BF — 20 HF — 18 Subjects who provided FFQ2 and FR = 62 but no ethnic breakdown	Willett (Harvard Un.) 111 items, self-administered (edited foods, portion size information deleted); developed as a prenatal FFQ	Unknown (recall of past 2 weeks)	Three 24-hr recalls conducted by phone	Compared female's report of food intake between food recalls and FFQ2 which were mailed	Pearson correlation (unadjusted, log transformed values) between FFQ2's and recalls Energy — 0.41 Protein — 0.33 Vitamin A — 0.12 Calcium — 0.52

TABLE 22.2 *(Continued)*

Food Frequency Questionnaire (FFQ) Validity Studies among Diverse Adult Populations in the U.S.

Reference	Sample	Instrument	Response Categories	Validation Standard	Design	Results
Coates et al.[5]	91 BF	HHHQ-original 98 item FFQ revised to include 19 ethnic/regional foods resulting in 117 item FFQ; past year	4 (Times/day, week, month or year)	Serum carotenoids, alpha-tocopherol, lycopene, crytoxanthin, lutein/xeaxanthin	Compared female's FFQ responses to 15-ml nonfasting venous blood sample	Pearson correlations (log transformed, unadjusted) between FFQ and serum for nonsmokers: Alpha-tocopherol (food only) — 0.19 Provitamin A carotenoids — 0.37 Beta-carotene — 0.34 Cryptoxanthin — 0.37 Lycopene — (-0.02) Lutein — 0.12 Person correlations (log transformed, unadjusted) for smokers were: Alpha-tocopherol — (–0.12) Provitamin A carotenoids — 0.07 Beta-carotene — 0.11 Cryptoxanthin — 0.18 Lycopene — (–0.02) Lutein — 0.11 Results suggest that FFQ was reasonably valid for black females. Analysis of lycopene and lutein may not reflect validity of the assessment of these nutrients

Forsythe et al.[6]	80 BF ethnic mix of African blacks, Asian Indians, Caribbean whites, Guyanese Amerindians, and Caribbean Chinese	FFQ-82 items compiled from Caribbean food tables, Willett FFQ, Stower prenatal food guide, and regional recipes	Unknown (weekly intake patterns)	Three 24-hr recalls	Compared female's report of intake against 3, 24-hr recalls, one recall at prenatal visit and two others by phone during next 7 days. 2nd FFQ administered 3 weeks later	Paired t-tests examined differences between the food recall means and the means of the FFQ at time 1. Most of the 14 nutrients were significantly different using the two instruments, with the exception of saturated fat, vitamin A and caffeine. The percentage of energy from protein, CHO, and fat showed no significant differences on either method of assessment. Mean difference scores were computed between food recalls and time 2 FFQ responses in the subsample. Significant differences were found for energy , CHO and vitamin C and the percentage of energy from CHO. The 24-hr recalls did not fully support the responses provided on the FFQ's.
Lee et al.[7]	74 Chin W	84 Items; interviewer administered; past year; portion size asked for foods eaten >1/week; 3-dimensional actual size food models used; type of fat used in cooking asked	5 (Day, week, month, year or not at all)	One 24-hr recall (typical day during past month)	Compared female's report of frequency of intake against the 1-24 recall;	Pearson correlations between the FFQ and the food recall: Total kcal — 0.05 Total fat — 0.21 Protein — 0.56 Vitamin A — 0.46. Nutrient intakes by FFQ that were significantly higher than 24-hr recall were total kcal, total fat, vitamin A, saturated fat, cholesterol and beta carotene. Use of only 1-24 hr recall could explain the modest correlations.
McPherson et al.[8]	33 HM+F	38 Mutually exclusive food types; interviewer administered; referent period last 4 weeks	Unknown	Three random nonconsecutive food records	Compared subject's report of past month's food intake against 3-24 hr food records	Pearson correlation coefficients (unadjusted) between FFQ and records Energy — 0.77 Total fat — 0.76 Cholesterol — 0.61 None of the differences between nutrients on FFQ1 and FR were significant.

is asked to recall on the FFQ, more than four to seven days may be required to capture the actual intake of the individual.

The reliability coefficients across all diverse and minority studies were much higher than the validity coefficients (Table 22.3). The median correlations for black males and females across studies were in the range of 0.51 to 0.88; for Hispanic females, 0.51 to 0.58 except for one study conducted in Starr County, Texas which reported a median correlation of 0.85; for white males and females, 0.64 to 0.71. These coefficients would suggest that within minority and diverse populations, the FFQ can usually describe with some consistency the food or nutrient intakes of individuals when administered at two points in time.

In most of the studies reviewed, the investigators made suggestions and recommendations for improving the performance of the FFQ in minority populations. It was repeatedly mentioned that a "gold standard" referent method was not available, so collecting valid dietary intake data remains challenging. The need to identify a complete food list on the FFQ that captures all of the foods in the usual diet of the study population was highly recommended. Depending on the study, the food list should include foods that will contribute substantially to the nutrients under investigation. This importance of a food list capturing the usual intake of study participants was demonstrated in the study conducted in Starr County, Texas. Because of the limited number of overall foods that the participants consumed, the food list of the FFQ was able to reflect the major sources of food and nutrient intake of these individuals. Because of this unique situation, the nutrient values from the FFQ were more likely to agree with the values from the food records.

Several suggestions were made regarding administration of the dietary assessment forms in minority populations. It is recommended that any staff person who is responsible for interviewing a subject for any dietary assessment measure, whether the conversation takes place in person, or over the phone should be of the same ethnic background as the subject.

Educational attainment of participants appeared to be a major determinant of the validity of the dietary assessment measures in several studies. Agreement between the food frequency and the criterion measure of 24-hour dietary recalls was substantially compromised among individuals with less than a high school education. This was particularly true within a Hispanic group of one study. In another study, it was found that increasing validity with increased education suggested that poor education is a barrier to accurate completion of the FFQ, the food record, or both. In this same study, low educational levels did not affect reliability measures. These findings would suggest that special efforts are needed when using dietary assessment tools with participants of low educational status or culturally diverse dietary habits. Small group instruction and practice in using the dietary tools could improve the dietary information collected. Instructing participants by videotape on completing dietary forms is another method to help improve the accuracy of information.

This section includes examples of the food frequency questionnaires that have been used or adapted for studies of minority populations. This is not intended to be a complete list of all the questionnaires that were used in the 12 studies reviewed, nor is inclusion in this set of examples an implied endorsement of one instrument. The FFQs included are those that are widely available. The FFQs in this set were originally selected by an investigator for modification to his/her population, or the FFQ is the actual instrument used to assess dietary intake. Readers who are interested in using or adapting these dietary assessment tools should contact the resource people listed with each tool.

In selecting a food frequency questionnaire, the reader should consider several points:

1. What is the primary purpose of the project or study you are planning to conduct and how does the food intake data relate to the outcome?

TABLE 22.3

Food Frequency Questionnaire (FFQ) Reliability Studies among Adult Minority Populations in the U.S.

References	Sample	Instrument	Response Categories (range)	Design	Results
Baumgartner et al.[14]	43 HF (Hispanic) 89 WF	140-items; interviewer administered; semi-quantitative; referent period was previous 4 weeks	Included per month, week or day	Compared 6-month test-retest reproducibility of nutrient estimates from FFQ2 and FFQ3. Reproducibility coefficients were not reported by ethnic group except for 2 nutrients	Pearson coefficients (log transformed, adjusted) by ethnic group between the 2 FFQ's for 2 nutrients: Saturated fat: HF — 0.57 WF — 0.77 Retinol: HF — 0.50 WF — 0.80
Forsythe et al.[5]	80 BF ethnic mix of African blacks, Asian Indians, Caribbean whites, Guyanese Amerindians, and Caribbean Chinese	FFQ- 82 items compiled from Caribbean food tables, Willett FFQ, Stower prenatal food guide, and regional recipes	Unknown (weekly intake patterns)	Compared 3 wk test-retest reproducibility of nutrient estimates from FFQs and food recalls	Paired t-tests examined differences between the food recall means and the means of the FFQ at time 1. Most of the 14 nutrients were significantly different using the two instruments, with the exception of saturated fat, Vitamin A and caffeine. The percentage of energy from protein, CHO, and fat showed no significant differences on either method of assessment. Mean difference scores were computed between food recalls and time 2 FFQ responses in the subsample. Significant differences were found for energy, CHO and Vitamin C and the percentage of energy from CHO Pearson correlations between the 2 FFQs were: Energy — 0.91 Protein — 0.97 Total fat — 0.89 Vitamin A — 0.73
Kristal et al.[11]	555 WF 271BF 159 H F recruited at three clinical centers. Because Hispanics recruited at Miami clinic only, their data was compared with WF from same clinic; data for WF and BF at two other centers were collapsed and compared	100 items, self-administered, semi-quantitative; last three months; portion sizes were S, M, L. FFQ collected at screening, baseline and six months	9 (never or <once/month to 2 or more times/day)	Compared 6-month test-retest reproducibility of selected nutrient estimates from baseline and 6 month FFQ's in the control group only Analyses were also stratified on level of education	Pearson coefficients (log transformed) between the 2 FFQ's were: Fat (% energy): BF — 0.37 WF — 0.51 HF — 0.45 WF — 0.34 Vitamin C (unadjusted): BF — 0.60 WF — 0.67 HF — 0.75 WF — 0.44 Beta-carotene (unadjusted): BF — 0.54 WF — 0.61 HF — 0.62 WF — 0.46 Little evidence that reliability was affected by poor education

TABLE 22.3 *(Continued)*

Food Frequency Questionnaire (FFQ) Reliability Studies among Adult Minority Populations in the U.S.

References	Sample	Instrument	Response Categories (range)	Design	Results
Liu et al.[10]	33 black M 32 black F 30 white M 33 white F	About 300 items in 20 categories; interviewer-administered; quantitative history based on the Western Electric dietary history; referent period is past month	Open-ended	Compared subject's history of last 30 days against baseline history	Sex-adjusted partial correlation coefficients (log transformed, not calorie adjusted) between the first and last histories Energy: W M+F — 0.76 B M+F — 0.50 Total fat: (g) W M+F — 0.73 B M+F — 0.56 Protein: (g) W M+F — 0.70 B M+F — 0.57 Vitamin A: (IU) W M+F — 0.77 B M+F — 0.74
McPherson et al.[8]	20 H M+F	38 mutually exclusive food types; interviewer administered; referent period last 4 weeks	Unknown	Compared 1 month test-retest reproducibility of nutrient estimates between FFQ2 and 3 and FFQ 2 and 4	Absolute nutrient intake from FFQ2 was greater than those of FFQ3 and FFQ4. Pearson coefficients (unadjusted) between FFQ2 and FFQ3: Energy: 0.90 Total fat: 0.85 Cholesterol: 0.85 Coefficients (unadjusted) between FFQ2 and FFQ4 were Energy: 0.84 Total fat: 0.70 Cholesterol: 0.79

Mayer-Davis et al.[12]	32 WF (Urban) 63 BF (Urban) 30 WF (Rural) 61 HF (Rural)	114-item, 1st FFQ interviewer-administered and 2nd was conducted over phone; modified from NCI-HHHQ to include regional and ethnic food choices; past year	9 (never or <1/month to 2 or more times/day)	Compared 2-4 year test-retest reproducibility of baseline FFQ1 with FFQ2	Pearson coefficients (log transformed, unadjusted) between 2 FFQ's were: Energy: WF (urban) — 0.81 BF (urban) — 0.64 HF (rural) — 0.83 WF (rural) — 0.61 Total fat: (g) WF (urban) — 0.81 BF (urban) — 0.69 HF (rural) — 0.87 WF (rural) — 0.63 Vitamin A: (IU) WF (urban) — 0.67 BF (urban) — 0.26 HF (rural) — 0.63 WF (rural) — 0.53 Reproducibility of FFQ's was similar across all subgroups evaluated including educational attainment
Suitor et al.[13]	Initially who provided 3 diet recalls: WF 54 BF 20 HF 18 Subjects who provided FFQ1 and FFQ2 = 43 but no ethnic breakdown	Willett (Harvard Un.) 111 items, self-administered (edited foods, portion size information deleted); developed as a prenatal FFQ	Unknown (recall of past 2 weeks)	Compared female's report of food intake between baseline FFQ1 which was completed in the clinic and FFQ2 which was mailed. Those returning FFQ2 were unrepresentative of the original sample	Pearson correlation (unadjusted, log transformed values) between FFQ1 and FFQ2: Energy — 0.92 Protein — 0.87 Vitamin A — 0.89 Calcium — 0.80

2. What length of time are you interested in assessing food intake? 12 months, 3 months?
3. How current is the food list? Does it reflect the current food supply?
4. Does the food list contain foods that contribute significantly to the nutrients you are interested in assessing?
5. Does the food list reflect the traditional or cultural foods eaten by your population?
6. Is the nutrient software analysis program updated on a regular basis to reflect the changing composition of our food supply?
7. Can you individualize the food list of the FFQ to your specific population? How much latitude do you have to modify the existing questionnaire? Can the existing software be modified to reflect the changes you wish to make?
8. Request a list of the validity and reliability studies that investigators have conducted using the FFQ you are considering. Were these studies conducted with populations similar to the groups of persons you wish to recruit into your study?

Diet History Questionnaire

Investigators at the National Cancer Institute have developed a new self-administered, scannable food frequency questionnaire, the Diet History Questionnaire (DHQ). The instrument was designed with particular attention to cognitive ease, and has been updated with respect to the food list and nutrient database using national dietary data (USDA's 1994-96 Continuing Survey of Food II). This instrument is available on the internet and can be downloaded from the site http://www-dccps.ims.nci.nih.gov/arp. The data analysis program that accompanies this questionnaire will become available for downloading from this site in 2001. Validity studies are in progress, but not within minority populations.

At this internet site, information is provided regarding the original Health Habits and History Questionnaire (HHHQ) developed by Gladys Block and updated in 1987 and 1992. Recommendations are provided for the continued use of this questionnaire and the software analysis program that accompanies it. Both the questionnaire and the software can be downloaded from the site.

Harvard University Food Frequency Questionnaire (Willett Questionnaire)

Several food frequency questionnaires are available from the Harvard School of Public Health including this current version designed for use in African American populations. This is a scannable, self-administered FFQ referred to as the "green version." Validity studies of this FFQ among black male prostate cancer survivors will be completed very soon. This questionnaire contains a section on the assessment of vitamin and mineral intake followed by approximately 174 food items. The assessment period of the FFQ is the past 12 months, and respondents are asked to average seasonal use of foods over the entire year. This tool is designed to enhance an individual's ability to respond more appropriately to the food items. For example, the response categories are individualized for each item ranging from never to six or more times per day, and probing questions are asked regarding specific characteristics of foods consumed. (Resource: Laura Sampson, M.S., R.D. Harvard School of Public Health — Nutrition, Bldg. #2, Room 335, 665 Huntington Ave., Boston, MA 02115.)

Fred Hutchinson Cancer Research Center Food Frequency Questionnaire (Kristal Questionnaire)

This questionnaire links answers from an extensive list of food questions to specific food frequency items to derive more precise nutrient estimates for those items. The FFQ is machine-readable and is accompanied by a software system to process the questionnaire. The format has nine frequency categories and small, medium, and large portion sizes. The food list is composed of 122 foods and is preceded by 19 behavioral questions related to preparation techniques and types of food selected. Answers to these questions are used directly in the program to choose more appropriate nutrient composition values for certain foods in the food list. This questionnaire is available in Spanish. (Resource: Alan R. Kristal, Dr. P.H., Cancer Prevention Research Unit, Fred Hutchinson Cancer Research Center, 1124 Columbia St. MP 702, Seattle, WA 98104.)

Cancer Research Center of Hawaii's Dietary Questionnaire (The Hawaii Cancer Research Survey)

The Cancer Research Center of Hawaii, part of the University of Hawaii, has developed a variety of quantitative FFQs for use with the multiethnic population of Hawaii. A questionnaire was recently developed to assess the diets of the five main ethnic groups in the Hawaii-Los Angeles Multiethnic Cohort Study: Hispanics, African-Americans, Japanese, Hawaiians, and Caucasians. Unlike previous questionnaires, the cohort questionnaire was designed to be self administered. Three-day measured food items were collected from all ethnic groups in advance and were used to identify food items for inclusion in the questionnaire. To ensure more accurate specifications of amounts usually consumed, photographs showing three portion sizes were printed on the questionnaire. A customized, an in part ethnic-specific, food composition table was developed for the cohort questionnaire. A calibration study comparing questionnaire responses to the three 24-hour recalls for the same subjects showed highly satisfactory correlations, particularly after the energy adjustment. For more information about the The Cancer Research Center of Hawaii questionnaires, please contact Suzanne P. Murphy, Ph.D., R.D., Cancer Research Center of Hawaii, University of Hawaii, 1236 Lauhala St., Suite 407, Honolulu, HI 96813. Phone: 808-586-2987. Fax: 909-586-2982. Email: Suzanne@crch.hawaii.edu.

New Mexico Women's Health Study, Epidemiology and Cancer Control Program, University of New Mexico Health Sciences Center

This FFQ was developed for an adjunct trial to the New Mexico Women's Health Study, a population-based case-control study of breast cancer in non-Hispanic and Hispanic women. The 140-item FFQ was a modified version of a questionnaire developed by the Human Nutrition Center, University of Texas School of Public Health — Houston for a Texas Hispanic population. The FFQ was revised to include important food sources of energy, macronutrients, and vitamins that were identified following an analysis of food intake recalls. Emphasis was placed on specific rather than grouped food items because recall is considered better for specific items. Usual portion size, based on two-dimensional food models, included data on number of servings, type of food model, and thickness of food. Common serving descriptions were included for each food item and were based either on food models or defined portion size. This FFQ was translated into Spanish. For further information contact R. Sue McPherson, Ph.D., Director, Human Nutrition Center, Associate Profession of Epidemiology and Nutrition, University of Texas — Houston School of Public Health, 1200 Herman Pressler, Houston, TX 77030. Phone: 713-500-9317.

Insulin Resistance Atherosclerosis Study FFQ, School of Public Health, University of South Carolina

The Insulin Resistance Atherosclerosis Study (IRAS) provided the opportunity to evaluate the comparative validity and reproducibility of a FFQ within and across subgroups of non-Hispanic white, Hispanic, and African-American individuals. The 114-item questionnaire was modified from the National Cancer Institute — Health Habits and History Questionnaire originally created by Gladys Block, Ph.D. This interviewer-administered FFQ was modified to include regional and ethnic food choices that were commonly consumed by the participants of the study. The FFQ contains nine categories of possible responses ranging from "never or less than once per month" to "two or more times per day." Portion sizes are determined simply as "small, medium, or large compared to other men/women about your age." At the end of the FFQ, an open-ended question is asked to describe foods that are usually eaten "at least once per week" that were not listed on the FFQ. Also, nine additional questions probe for information regarding common food preparation methods, specific fats used in cooking, and frequency of consumption of fruits and vegetables. For further information about the IRAS FFQ, contact Mara Z. Vitolins, Dr. P.H., R.D., Research Assistant Professor, Wake Forest University School of Medicine, Department of Public Health Sciences, Medical Center Blvd., Winston-Salem, N.C. 27157-1063. Phone: 336-716-2886. Fax: 336-713-4157. Email: mvitolin@wfubmc.edu.

References

1. Coates RJ, Monteilh CP. *Am J Clin Nutr* 65: 1108S; 1997.
2. Spencer G. *Projections of the Hispanic Population: 1983-2089*. US Department of Commerce, Bureau of Census, (Series P-25), Washington, DC, 1989.
3. National Institutes of Health, NIH guidelines on the inclusion of women and minorities as subjects in clinical research, *Fed Reg* 59: 14508; 1994.
4. Hankin JH, Wilkens LR. *Am J Clin Nutr* 59: 198S; 1994.
5. Coates RJ, Eley JW, Block G, et al. *Am J Epidemiol* 15: 658; 1991.
6. Forsythe HE, Gage B. *Am J Clin Nutr* 59: 203S; 1994.
7. Lee MM, Lee F, Ladenla SW, Miike R. *Ann Epidemiol* 4: 188; 1994.
8. McPherson RS, Kohl HW, Garcia G, et al. *Ann Epidemiol* 5: 378; 1995.

9. Larkin FA, Metzner HL, Thompson FE, et al. *JADA* 89: 215; 1989.
10. Liu K, Slattery M, Jacobs D, et al. *Ethnicity Dis* 4: 15; 1994.
11. Kristal AR, Feng Z, Coates RJ, et al. *Am J Epidemiol* 146: 856; 1997.
12. Mayer-Davis JE, Vitolins MZ, Carmichael SL, et al. *Ann Epidemiol* 9: 314; 1999.
13. Suitor C, Gardner J, Willett WC. *JADA* 89: 1786; 1989.
14. Baumgartner KB, Gilliland FD, Nicholson CS. *Ethnicity Dis* 8: 81; 1998.
15. Hankin JH, Wilkens LR, Kolonel LN, Yoshizawa CN. *Am J Epidemiol* 15: 616; 1991.
16. Stram DO, Hankin JH, Wilkens LR. *Am J Epidemiol* 15: 358; 2000.

23

Computerized Nutrient Analysis Systems

Judith M. Ashley and Sue Grossbauer

Introduction

Since the early 1980s, nutrient analysis software programs have taken advantage of microcomputer technology to offer an effective and time-efficient method for calculating dietary intake for a variety of users.[1,2] For health professionals, the computerized dietary analyses can be used as a persuasive tool to provide feedback for clients about current food choices as well as healthful alternatives. For nutrition educators, the hands-on applications of dietary analysis programs are an integral part of student education. For researchers and government agencies, the computerized dietary results are an essential component for documenting and analyzing the usual food intake of individuals and groups or target populations. Computerized nutrient analysis software is also important for recipe development by chefs and caterers, as well as for label information provided by food manufacturers.

Nutrient analysis systems convert individual food choices entered from a food record or food frequency to nutrients.[3,4] Computerized data processing includes creating a data file with a food code and an amount consumed for each food item reported. The computer software then links the nutrient composition of each food, stores that information, and sums across all foods for each nutrient. Dietary analysis software is provided by a large number of companies and organizations today. These companies continually update the quality and scope of their services to stay competitive in the marketplace. However, their computer programs vary considerably in cost, ease of use, features, and capabilities. For the prospective user, the choice of software requires careful consideration of needs and available resources of staff, and financial support for computer hardware and peripherals. Characteristics and general operating features of a number of widely used commercial nutrient software programs with extensive database development are included in Table 23.1.

Primary Characteristics and Operating Features of Software Programs

Primary features of software nutrient analysis programs include 1) nutrient components of interest (e.g., macronutrients, fatty acids, amino acids, sugars, antioxidants), 2) national

0-8493-2705-9/01/$0.00+$1.50

TABLE 23.1

Comparison of Features in Five Selected Programs Available Nationwide

Company	Product Name(s)	Targeted End Users*	Total Number of Unique Foods/Items in Database	Diet Comparisons**	Support***	Operating Requirements	Cost of Product	Current Number of Users or Installations	Other Important Features
Computrition, Inc. Chatsworth, CA 818-701-5544 www.computrition.com	Nutritional Software Library	C, H, M	4200, small database 20,000+, large database	N, M	CE, U	WindowsNT, 98, and 2000	$495 small database $995 large database (single user system only)	N/A	Integrated with foodservice and nutrition management software systems
ESHA Research, Inc. Salem, OR 800-659-3742 www.esha.com	The Food Processor®: Nutrition analysis & fitness software	C, H, M, R	25,000+, includes the Canadian Nutrient File	N, FC, FG, M	C, CE, U	WindowsNT, 98, and 2000	$599 Educational prices available (cost to add stations)	3200	Menu analysis, recipe analysis Exercise planning
First DataBank San Bruno, CA 800-633-3453 (East); 800-428-4495 (West) www.firstdatabank.com	Nutritionist Pro Nutritionist Pro Food Labeling	H, M, R	18,000	N, FC, FG, M Food groups using diabetic exchanges	C, CE, U	WindowsNT, 98, and 2000	$595	Thousands	Professionally designed reports Ability to create menu templates to make data entry faster Ability to generate food labels
Nutrition Coordinating Center (NCC) University of Minnesota 612-626-9450 www.ncc.umn.edu	Nutrition Data System for Research (NDS-R) Academic NDS-R (for teaching purposes) Grad-Pack NDS-R (for graduate students)	R	18,000	N, FC, M System generates 12 standard reports	C, CE, U	WindowsNT, 98, and 2000	$8500 initial, $2500 additional years $690 Academic $495 Grad-Pack	Over 700 installations	Prompts for complete food descriptions, recipe ingredients, and food preparation methods Interview facilitated by multiple-pass system
University of Texas School of Public Health 713-500-9775 www.sph.uth.tmc.edu:8052/hnc/software/soft.htm	Food Intake Analysis System 3.99	R	7320	Comparison standards input by the individual user	C, U	DOS	$3500	60	Commercial version of USDA's Survey Net, used in the Continuing Survey of Food Intakes (CSFI)

* C = Consumers, H = Health Professionals, M = Medical Centers or Hospitals, R = Research
** N = Nutrients using DRI/RDA, FC = Other Food components, FG = Food Guide Pyramid food groups, M = Meals
*** C = Company Support Included in Cost, CE = Company Support Extra Cost, U = Updates available

TABLE 23.2

Examples of Dietary Components Available from Computerized Nutrient Analysis

Energy Sources	**Fiber**	**Fatty Acids**
Energy (kilocalories)	Total dietary fiber	SFA 4:0 to 22:0
Total protein	Soluble fiber	MUFA 14:1 to 22:1
Total fat	Insoluble fiber	PUFA 18:2 to 22:6
Total carbohydrate	Pectins	Trans FA 16:1 to 18:2
Alcohol		
Animal protein	**Vitamins**	**Amino Acids**
Vegetable protein	Vitamin A RE	Tryptophan
% Calories protein	Beta-carotene RE	Threonine
% Calories fat	Retinol	Isoleucine
% Calories carbohydrate	Alpha-tocopherol RE	Leucine
% Calories alcohol	Beta-tocopherol RE	Lysine
	Gamma-tocopherol RE	Methionine
Fat and Cholesterol	Delta-tocopherol RE	Cystine
Cholesterol	Vitamin C	Phenylalanine
Total sat fatty acids (SFA)	Vitamin D	Tyrosine
Total mono fatty acids (MUFA)	Vitamin K	Valine
Total poly fatty acids (PUFA)	Thiamin	Arginine
Total trans fatty acids (TFA)	Riboflavin	Histidine
% Cal SFA	Niacin	Alanine
% Cal MUFA	Folate	Aspartic acid
% Cal PUFA	Vitamin B_6	Glutamic acid
	Vitamin B_{12}	Glycine
Carbohydrates	Pantothenic acid	Proline
Starch	Biotin	Serine
Fructose		
Galactose	**Minerals**	**Other**
Glucose	Calcium	Aspartame
Lactose	Chromium	Saccharin
Maltose	Copper	Ash
Sucrose	Magnesium	Caffeine
	Manganese	Oxalic acid
	Phosphorous	Phytic acid
	Potassium	Sucrose polyester
	Selenium	3-methylhistidine
	Sodium	Water
	Zinc	

standards or guidelines used for evaluation (e.g., DRI/RDAs, U.S. Dietary Guidelines, National Cholesterol Education Program), and 3) comparison by food groups, diabetic exchanges, selected food items, or meal patterns. Many programs begin with client profile information such as gender, age, height, weight, pregnancy or lactation status for women, and tracking information (name, address, phone number, case number). With some program packages, dietary standards can be tailored to fit a specific client's needs, such as calculating energy needs or targeted weight goals. The final presentation of the data may take the form of two- and three-dimensional pie and bar charts, Food Pyramid or DRI comparisons, nutrient summaries, or ranking foods in descending or ascending order based on any nutrient. Data may be collected and averaged for individuals or groups for a specified period, from days to weeks. Nutrients commonly included in software systems results are listed in Table 23.2.

Additional features that may be relevant to users include the software program's ability to provide food–drug interaction data; to incorporate nutrition support regimens; to incorporate a recipe database; to add and/or modify foods, nutrients, and recipes; to scale and/or cost recipes; to provide a shopping list; to plan meals and/or provide sample menus;

and to compare a meal with one-third RDA values (for menu planning). The software may have data export capability (for export into statistical analysis software packages or word processing programs so that text can be edited, or logos or other graphics added), support for scannable questionnaires (useful for health surveys, food frequency checklists, or entering calorie count data from inpatient menus), support for multi-user application, and interface capability with foodservice management software.

Basic Questions to Ask When Considering Different Software Systems

Depending on the projected use of a nutrient analysis system, many or all of the following basic questions may apply when evaluating individual programs:

- *What are the operating system and hardware requirements?* Would this involve an investment in new equipment and peripherals?
- *Who is the target audience of the output?* Are consumers, health professionals, Medical Centers or Hospitals and/or Research included?
- *What are the total number and types of foods contained in the database?* How many foods are included? Are baby foods, convenience foods, fast foods, regional specialties, ethnic specialties, and nutritional supplements included?
- *What specific nutrients or food components are in the database?* Are only a dozen or more than 100 nutrients or other components calculated? Can the database be altered?
- *How complete is the database?* What is the extent of missing values? When data for specific nutrients are missing, are they estimated or left as zero (reducing the usefulness of nutrient reports)? Are missing nutrient values identified on reports, so that they are not misleading?
- *How is the quality of database maintained?* As new nutrient data become available, how often does the software vendor respond?
- *What is the ease of inputting for foods and amounts?* Are there numeric code, food name, and search feature options for entering a food? Is online help provided to distinguish food listings and store frequently used food or meal categories for ready access? Does flexible entry of portions allow choices by weight, volume, and/or dimensions?
- *Is there an accommodation to support food frequency data?* Is this available in a scannable form?
- *Which nutrient standards are used, and are they up to date?* Are the latest DRIs used? Are standards omitted for subpopulations (children, pregnant or lactating women)?
- *What is the variety and quality of on-screen feedback for viewing reports?* Can on-screen reports be used for client counseling? Is the software interactive, allowing a user to experiment with dietary choices while offering instantaneous feedback about the bottom-line impact on nutrient intake?
- *What is the variety and quality of printed reports?* Does the program provide easy-to-understand graphics (e.g., bar graphs, pie charts) in comparing intake with designated standards? Are graphical comparisons available with several stan-

dards, such as the Food Pyramid or NCEP, included? Is the report's final message well formatted and descriptive?

- *Can the reports be customized?* Can reports be reformatted or can specific information and comments be added?
- *Is the report capable of using different measures for comparison?* Does the report include food groups, diabetic food exchanges, glycemic index values?
- *Can multiple-day intakes be summarized?* Can the report include several days or weeks for comprehensive analysis?
- *What are the formulas used for calculating ideal body weight and energy requirements?* Are current and reasonable standards used?
- *Can exercise data be incorporated into caloric requirements?* Does the report include exercise recommendations?
- *Can key sources of each nutrient be identified in the food records?* Can lists of food sources of key nutrients be generated?
- *What is the quality of software documentation, on-line help, and tutorials?* Are they easy to understand and specific to user needs?
- *What is the quality of product support and ongoing maintenance?* Is there sufficient technical support provided to answer user needs?
- *What are the system utilities?* Are there utilities for backing up valuable data and reports?
- *Finally, what does the complete system, with updates and service, cost?* Are there additional costs to add stations or for multiple users?

Importance of Nutrient Databases

Dietary intake data collected using both food records and food frequency questionnaires or checklists rely heavily on food databases. Multiple factors affect the accuracy of the database, including the source of nutrient information, the number of foods and nutrients in the database, the method of handling missing values, and the frequency of updating the database. Several published reports have compared nutrient calculations among a limited number of database systems.[5-12] When the database calculations have been compared to a standard[13-15] or tested against chemical analyses from a single source,[16-18] most found nutrients to be within 15% of reference values. For example, a recent comparison from 4 different databases and their deviations from chemically analyzed values of 36 menus showed that the database values for the nutrients examined had relatively good accuracy: 7 nutrients deviated by values <10%, 5 by 10 to 15%, and only one by 15 to 20%.[19] There are several potential reasons for these variations, including:

1. Nutrient variability in the food supply
2. Frequent changes in the nutrient content of processed foods
3. Nutrient information from food labels is permitted to vary from actual nutrient content by a large margin
4. Estimated or imputed values for missing nutrient information by database developers is a source of error in nutrient estimates

5. Food substitutions or misidentification of foods entered
6. Constraints of chemically determined nutrient values used for comparison (e.g., sample collection, assayed values)

It is important to note that no standardized benchmarks have been established for comparing nutrient calculation output.

Most nutrient analysis systems in the U.S. contain the USDA National Nutrient Database (NNDB) complemented by nutrition information from other scientific sources and food companies.[20] The NNDB was developed and implemented in 1985, and includes the most recent USDA Nutrient Database for Standard Reference and the Primary Nutrient Data Set for USDA Nationwide Food Surveys. The USDA's National Nutrient Databank System (NDBS) is the repository of several types of food information, including food names, food descriptors, food formulations and recipes, the composition of foods, food yields, nutrient retentions, factors for deriving energy, protein, and fatty acid values of foods, and weights for various measures of foods. It currently contains data for over 6200 foods and up to 82 nutrients. The NDBS contains systematic and common food names, source information, and information about analytical methods. The development of representative food composition values involves the acquisition, documentation, evaluation, and aggregation of food composition data compiled from a wide variety of sources. The USDA does not have dedicated intramural analytical laboratories to support the NDBS, and limited data are provided by ongoing research programs. Thus, to meet user needs it is dependent on other sources including the scientific literature, food industry, academia, other government agencies, and contracts sponsored by the Nutrient Data Laboratory. The latest 1999 USDA Nutrient Database, Release #13, includes added food composition data for several hundred new items and added data on selenium and vitamin D compared to the 1998 Release.[21] An online database search program is available on the USDA Nutrient Data Laboratory home page: www.nal.usda.gov/fnic/foodcomp.

Limitations of Nutrient Analysis Software Reports

Nutrient analysis software has its own unique limitations.[4] The calculations of nutrient intake are not exact because there are too many variables in the analysis, including the database and the program's calculation methods. However, these software-related variables are minor in comparison to the larger human challenges to accuracy. Clients and subjects tend to give inaccurate reports of actual food intake using both food records and food frequencies. Data entry is also highly dependent on interpreting and selecting the right match from the food database.

Individuals may also misinterpret the results. Computer-generated printouts tend to convey an authoritative tone, often leading to the perception that the reports are more precise than they really are. Individuals unfamiliar with DRI/RDA comparisons may easily misinterpret them as minimal nutrient needs, assuming that they should be at 100% to avoid deficiencies. Even professionals may have difficulty drawing specific conclusions from the new DRI/RDA comparisons for individuals.

To use nutrient analysis reports effectively, a health professional should provide individual counseling, including:

1. Specific comments and/or supplementary resources for interpreting printouts

2. Explanations of the limitations of the analysis
3. Suggestions for ways to improve dietary intake (e.g., list food sources for specified vitamins or minerals)
4. Specific comments about the appropriateness of different nutrition supplements
5. Other resources for further guidance, as appropriate.

Conclusion

Nutrient or dietary analysis software designed to aid in calculations offers an important adjunct for improving dietary intake and health for individuals and population. However, health professionals and consumers alike need to be aware of both the benefits and limitations of the various systems and reports available.

References

1. Hoover LW. *Clin Nutr* 6: 198; 1987.
2. Feskanich D, Buzzard IM, Welch BT, et al. *JADA* 88: 1263; 1988.
3. Byers T, Thompson FE. *J Nutr* 124: 2245S; 1994.
4. Grossbauer S. In *Communicating as Professionals* (2nd ed), Chernoff R, Ed, The American Dietetic Association: Chicago, IL. 1994, pg 56.
5. Adelman MO, Dwyer JT, Woods M, et al. *JADA* 83: 421; 1983.
6. Hoover LW. *JADA* 83: 501; 1983.
7. Frank GC, Farris RP, Hyg MS, Berenson GS. *JADA* 84, 818; 1984.
8. Taylor ML, Kozlowski BW, Baer MT. *JADA* 85: 1136; 1985.
9. Shanklin D, Endres JM, Sawicki M. *JADA* 85: 308; 1985.
10. Eck LH, Klesges RC, Hanson CL, et al. *JADA* 88: 602; 1988.
11. Stumbo PJ. *JADA* 92: 57; 1992.
12. LaComb RP, Taylor ML, Noble JM. *JADA* 92: 1391; 1992.
13. Nieman DC, Nieman CN. *JADA* 87: 930; 1987.
14. Nieman DC, Butterworth DE, Nieman CN, et al. *JADA* 92: 48; 1992.
15. Lee RD, Nieman DC, Rainwater M. *JADA* 95: 858; 1995.
16. Pennington JAT, Wilson DB. *JADA* 90: 375; 1990.
17. Obarzanek E, Reed DB, Bigelow C, et al. *Int J Food Sci Nutr* 44: 155; 1993.
18. McKeown NM, Rasmujssen HM, Charnley JM, et al. *JADA* 100: 1201; 2000.
19. McCullough ML, Karanja NM, Lin PH, et al. *JADA* 99: S45; 1999.
20. Schakel SF, Sievert YA, Buzzard IM. *JADA* 88: 1268; 1988.
21. US Dept of Agriculture. Agricultural Research Service. 1999. USDA Nutrient Database for Standard Reference, Release 13. Nutrient Data Laboratory home page, http://www.nal.usda.gov/fnic/foodcomp.

24

Nutrient Data Analysis Techniques and Strategies

Alan R. Dyer, Kiang Liu, and Christopher T. Sempos

Overview

Analyses of nutrient data pose special challenges to investigators. In such analyses, investigators need to consider:

1. Possible over- or under-reporting of intakes, leading to "impossible" or extreme values in the data set
2. How to adjust for total energy intake
3. How to model nutrients, e.g., as continuous or categorical variable
4. How to avoid multicollinearity, particularly when nutrients are expressed in absolute amounts, e.g., grams/day
5. How to analyze dietary supplement data
6. How to account for large day-to-day variability in intakes, which can lead to misclassification of individuals with respect to usual intake

The objectives of this section are to examine various approaches to addressing the above issues; to briefly describe the common types of observational and experimental studies that collect nutritional data; and to describe the most common methods of analysis used in the types of studies described.

Quality Control

Whether investigators use a validated food frequency questionnaire or single or multiple 24-hour recalls to collect dietary data, the importance of quality control in such data collection cannot be overemphasized. The phrase GIGO (garbage in, garbage out) serves as a stark reminder of the importance of ensuring that dietary data are of the highest

0-8493-2705-9/01/$0.00+$1.50

quality when they are submitted for analysis. No amount of analytic sophistication can make up for poor quality data.

To improve the quality of collected data, investigators should:

- Develop a Manual of Operations for nutrient data collection
- Train and certify dietary interviewers in collection of data and use of the manual
- Tape interviews with the consent of the participant
- Immediately review a printout of the data collected, including nutrient totals if the system being used permits
- Develop range limits for important nutrients that result in careful review of the questionnaire or 24-hour recall with the participant, if limits are exceeded
- Make inquiries to cooks for clarifying information when needed
- Query the participant for a 24-hour recall on whether the amount consumed was typical, and if atypical, the reason the amount consumed was unusually low or high, e.g., lower than usual due to illness
- Use food composition data to estimate nutrient composition for foods not found in a data base when using 24-hour recalls
- Randomly select tape recordings for repeat completion of questionnaires or re-entry of data, with assessment of discrepancies and correction of incorrect data
- Develop criteria for re-certifying interviewers based on the randomly selected recordings

Interviewers may also be requested to indicate whether they believe the participant has provided reliable data. Persons deemed by the interviewer as not providing reliable data should be excluded from the analyses.

Prior to conducting analyses, investigators might wish to set limits on total caloric intake above or below which persons would be excluded. For example, in the Coronary Artery Risk Development in (young) Adults Study (CARDIA),[1] men who reported intake of >8000 kcals or <800 kcals and women who reported intake of >6000 kcals or <600 kcals on food frequency questionnaires were excluded from analyses, because values outside these limits were not considered consistent with a normal lifestyle.[2] The INTERMAP study of macronutrients and blood pressure also established exclusionary cutoffs for caloric intake obtained from 24-hour recalls.[3,4] Food frequency questionnaires generally have larger standard deviations in total energy intake than 24-hour recalls, and thus are more likely to have individuals with "impossible" or extreme values.[5] Hence, investigators using food frequency questionnaires need to be particularly attentive to establishing exclusionary cutoffs for total energy intake, such as those used in CARDIA. Investigators using 24-hour recalls should consider whether or not to exclude persons reporting that their 24-hour intake was unusual.

Identifying Outliers or Extreme Values

Prior to conducting any analyses, investigators should examine the distribution of each variable of interest for outliers or extreme values. The procedure Proc Univariate in SAS is particularly useful in this regard.[6] In addition to providing the standard descriptive statistics, e.g., mean, median, standard deviation, range, etc., this procedure also identifies the five largest and five smallest values for each variable, and the 1st, 5th, 95th, and 99th percentiles. The user can also request a box plot of the data, which can be very helpful in identifying extreme values. The box plot helps indicate how discrepant the largest and smallest values are from the rest of the data.

The fact that a statistical software package identifies values as large or extreme relative to other values in the distribution should not be taken as prima facie evidence that such values are invalid or that an error was made in data collection or data entry. Values so identified should be examined for such problems. However, if the values are biologically plausible and no error appears to have been made, they should not be arbitrarily excluded from the analysis. Neter, Wasserman, and Kutner[7] suggest that a safe rule is "to discard an outlier only if there is direct evidence that it represents an error in recording, a miscalculation, a malfunctioning piece of equipment, or a similar type of circumstance." When outliers are retained in a data set, the investigator needs to take special steps to assess any influence they may have on the results of the analysis. This can include analyses with and without the outlying value or values, use of nonparametric statistical methods, e.g., the Spearman rank correlation instead of the usual Pearson correlation coefficient, transformations of the data which bring the outlying value closer to the other values, e.g., the log or square root transformation, specific tests for influential observations,[7] or use of robust regression methods.[8]

Adjustment for Total Energy Intake

Adjustment for total energy intake is of particular relevance for epidemiologic studies in which investigators use some form of regression model to examine the associations of specific nutrients with an outcome variable, e.g., blood pressure or cholesterol in multiple linear regression, case-control status in logistic regression, or coronary heart disease incidence in Cox proportional hazards regression. Thorough discussions on adjustment for total energy intake can be found in Willett, Howe, and Kushi,[9] or in Willett.[10] Only the major issues addressed by these authors are described here. The rationale for adjusting for total energy intake is that most nutrients are correlated with total energy intake. This is because they contribute directly to total energy intake, e.g., total fat or carbohydrate, or because persons who consume more kcalories also eat more, on average, of all nutrients, e.g., dietary cholesterol or sodium. For example, in participants of the Multiple Risk Factor Intervention Trial (MRFIT),[11] the baseline correlations of 10 energy contributing nutrients with total energy intake ranged from 0.29 for alcohol intake to 0.87 for total fat intake. Among 24 non-energy contributing nutrients, the correlations ranged from 0.05 for retinol to 0.78 for phosphorus, with a median of 0.52. No nutrient had a negative correlation with total energy intake. Thus, if total energy intake is positively associated with a dependent variable, almost all specific nutrients will also be positively associated with that variable. Hence, in regression analyses involving specific nutrients, there is a need to adjust associations with specific nutrients for the potential confounding effects of total energy intake.

The most common methods of adjustment for total energy intake are typically referred to as the nutrient density method, the standard multivariate method, the residual method, and the multivariate nutrient density method.[9,10,12] The nutrient density method has been the traditional method of adjusting for total energy intake. In this approach, nutrient intake is divided by total energy intake, with energy-contributing nutrients expressed as percent of kcalories, and non-energy contributing nutrients expressed as intake per 1000 kcal. The strengths of this approach include ease of calculation, familiarity by nutritionists, and use in national guidelines.[9] For example, the Committee on Diet and Health of the National Research Council recommends that total fat intake be less than 30% of total energy intake and that saturated fat intake be less than 10%.[13] The primary problem with the nutrient density method is that it does not completely eliminate potential confounding with total energy intake, since nutrients expressed as nutrient density often remain correlated with total energy intake. For example, in the MRFIT, the correlations of percent kcalories from protein, fat, and carbohydrate intake with total energy intake at baseline were –0.23, 0.18, and –0.11, respectively.[11] However, with these three nutrients expressed as g/day, the corresponding correlations were 0.73, 0.87, and 0.77 in these men.

In the standard multivariate method, total energy intake is included in the multivariate regression model along with the nutrient or nutrients of interest. In this model, the regression coefficient for the nutrient of interest represents the effect of changing the nutrient by one unit while maintaining a constant total energy intake. For energy-containing nutrients this can only be accomplished by making changes in other energy-contributing nutrients equal to the amount of energy contained in one unit of the nutrient of interest. Similarly, the regression coefficient for total energy intake does not represent the effect of changing total energy intake by 1 kcal, but the effect of changing energy intake from all other energy contributing nutrients by 1 kcal. For example, if the nutrient in the model is total protein intake, then total energy intake represents fat and carbohydrate intake. In using this approach, estimates of the effect of changing intake of the nutrient by a specific amount should use variation in the nutrient with total energy intake held constant, i.e., the nutrient residual (see below) as the basis for the estimates of effect. Failure to do so can result in estimates of effect based on unrealistic differences in intake of the nutrient.

In the residual method, the investigator regresses each nutrient of interest on total energy intake, and then computes a nutrient residual for each individual by subtracting from the individual's actual intake of that nutrient, the amount predicted based on his/her total energy intake. Because the mean of these residuals is equal to zero, it may be desirable to add a constant to each residual, e.g., the mean intake for the nutrient. The resulting value does not, however, represent the individual's actual intake, and in fact has no "biological" or public policy meaning. The residual method is simply one means by which investigators can adjust for total energy intake. Nutrient residuals are independent of total energy intake. Models that use nutrient residuals can also include total energy intake. The regression coefficient for a nutrient expressed as a nutrient residual is identical to the regression coefficient for the nutrient in the standard multivariate model. However, the regression coefficient for total energy intake will not be identical to that in the standard multivariate model. In the residual model, the association of total energy intake with the dependent variable is not adjusted for intake of the specific nutrient, which could result in an inaccurate estimate of the association of total energy intake with the dependent variable.

In the multivariate nutrient density model, total energy intake is included in the model along with nutrient density. This approach addresses the problem of potential confounding by total energy intake in such analyses. In this model, the regression coefficient for the nutrient estimates the effect of a 1% difference in energy from the nutrient with total caloric intake held constant. As noted by Willett et al.,[9] a major strength of the multivariate nutrient density approach is that it separates diet into two components: composition and total amount.

Modeling Nutrient Intake

Investigators typically model nutrient intake as a continuous variable or a series of dummy variables corresponding to quantiles of the nutrient, e.g., quartiles or quintiles. The advantages of categorizing nutrient intake include reduction of the potential effects of outlying or extreme values, and elimination of the need to assume a linear relation between the nutrient of interest and the dependent variable. Categorization is also more informative to readers since it allows estimation of relative risks in logistic regression and Cox proportional hazards regression for persons in each exposure category relative to a referent category, and in multiple linear regression the mean difference in the dependent variable for persons in each exposure category relative to the referent category. The main weakness in categorizing a continuous variable is that when the relationship is linear, the categorization results in a loss of power. However, regardless of how nutrient intake is modeled in the definitive analysis, categorization is still an extremely useful tool and should be part of any analysis plan. This is because categorization allows the investigator to examine the shape of the relation between the nutrient and the dependent variable, and thus whether the relation is sufficiently linear to support inclusion of the nutrient as a continuous variable in the regression model.

When nutrient intake is categorized, one defines k-1 dummy variables for each individual for the k categories of the variable. For example, if nutrient intake is divided into quartiles, three dummy variables are defined. In defining the dummy variables, it is necessary to define a referent category. This is the category against which the risks or means for the other exposure categories are compared. If nutrient intake is divided into quartiles and the first quartile is to be the referent category, the three dummy variables corresponding to quartiles 2 to 4 are defined as follows:

$$X_1 = \begin{cases} 1 \text{ if intake in second quartile} \\ 0 \text{ otherwise} \end{cases}$$

$$X_2 = \begin{cases} 1 \text{ if intake in third quartile} \\ 0 \text{ otherwise} \end{cases}$$

$$X_3 = \begin{cases} 1 \text{ if intake in fourth quartile} \\ 0 \text{ otherwise} \end{cases}$$

These definitions produce the following values on each of the variables for individuals in the first through fourth quartiles:

Quartile of intake	X_1	X_2	X_3
1	0	0	0
2	1	0	0
3	0	1	0
4	0	0	1

In defining categories for a nutrient, investigators should adjust for total energy intake by defining the categories based on nutrient residuals or nutrient densities, rather than absolute intake.[12] While the standard multivariate method and the nutrient residual method provide identical regression coefficients for the nutrient of interest when the nutrient is entered as a continuous variable, this is not the case when nutrient intake is categorized.[12] In this case, the standard multivariate method should be avoided. It is also desirable to model total energy intake as a continuous variable in such analyses rather than as a second categorical variable, particularly if nutrient density is the variable being categorized.[10,12]

Multicollinearity

Multicollinearity in a regression model can occur when highly intercorrelated variables are entered simultaneously into the model, or when a linear combination of several variables essentially equals a constant. For example, multicollinearity would occur with nutrient data if the model included percent of kcalories from total fat, protein, and carbohydrate, since the sum of these three variables is often 100 or quite close to 100. Hence, investigators should not attempt to enter more than two of these variables simultaneously into a regression model. Similarly, multicollinearity would also occur if these same three variables were entered into a model as g/day along with total energy intake. In this case, only three of these four variables should be entered simultaneously. In general, investigators need to ensure that they do not include in the same model variables representing total intake for a nutrient and all individual components of that intake, e.g., total fat plus saturated fats, polyunsaturated fats, and monounsaturated fats. However, even if investigators are careful to ensure that the types of multicollinearity described above do not occur, multicollinearity can still be a problem when multiple intercorrelated variables are included in a model, e.g., nutrients that come from the same sources. In this situation it may be impossible to determine the separate and independent associations of the multiple variables with the dependent variable. For example, in a study on the associations of potassium, calcium, protein, and milk intakes with blood pressure, the investigators found that while potassium had a relatively stronger association with blood pressure than the other three dietary factors, the high correlations of potassium intake with intakes of the other three made it impossible to determine the independent association of potassium intake with blood pressure.[14]

The use of nutrient residuals and nutrient densities help to reduce the likelihood of multicollinearity, since energy-adjusted nutrients generally have lower intercorrelations than nutrients expressed as absolute amounts.[10] Methods for assessing and detecting multicollinearity, as well as remedial measures, can be found in Neter, Wasserman, and Kutner.[7]

Some investigators may believe that procedures that select variables for inclusion in regression models based on whether or not the variable is significantly related to the dependent variable are appropriate approaches for preventing multicollinearity. Such procedures include forward selection or backward elimination of variables, and stepwise regression. In forward selection of variables, variables are entered into the model one at a time, beginning with the variable that has the strongest association with the dependent variable, followed sequentially by those having the strongest residual associations with the dependent variable, i.e., after taking into account the association of the entering variable with the variables previously entered and their associations with the dependent variable. Variables are entered into the model until no remaining variable would have a statistically significant association with the dependent variable, if it were to enter the model next. In backward elimination of variables, all available variables are entered into the model, and those with the weakest association are sequentially removed until only variables significantly related to the dependent variable remain. Stepwise regression combines forward selection and backward elimination of variables by removing those that are no longer significant when a new variable is entered into the model, so that the final model only contains variables significantly related to the dependent variable.

These variable selection procedures should be avoided for a number of reasons. First, the final model selected will not necessarily be optimal, e.g., maximize R^2. Second, the hypothesis tests used to determine which variables remain in the model are correlated.[8] Third, if a large number of variables is involved, initial entry of all variables may not be possible if one or more is a linear combination of the other variables. Fourth, stepwise procedures may not select possible confounders that should be included whether or not the confounder has a significant association with the dependent variable, e.g., age and sex, or total energy intake in the multivariate nutrient density approach. Fifth, the results of these procedures are often not unique, i.e., they yield final models that do not include the same variables. For example, in a logistic analysis involving the associations of total energy intake and intakes of protein, fat, and carbohydrate with CHD incidence, McGee, Reed, and Yano[15] found that only carbohydrate intake had a significant association with CHD incidence if forward selection of variables was used. When backward elimination was used instead, the final model included fat intake and total energy intake as the only variables significantly and independently related to CHD incidence.

Dietary Supplements

The use of dietary supplements poses a number of complexities for analyses involving nutrient intake, which are not easily resolved. The first question that must be addressed is whether supplement-based intake should be included or excluded. The approach recommended here is to analyze the data with and without inclusion of the supplement-based intake, since this is likely to provide the most complete information on the association of the nutrient with outcome. It may also be beneficial to treat the intake from supplements and food-based intake as separate nutrients. Such an approach is likely to be particularly appropriate if it is difficult to determine the separate and independent effects of food-based intake of the nutrient, or the separate and independent effects of the supplement due to its high correlation with supplemental intake of other nutrients, or where food-based intake and supplement-based intake have very different correlations with other nutrients. If such an analysis is done, food-based intake should be energy adjusted using nutrient residuals or nutrient densities, with supplement-based intake not energy adjusted, except through inclusion of total energy intake in the model. Hence, the analysis for food-based intake would be based on the residual or nutrient density model, whereas the analysis for supplement-based intake would follow the standard multivariate model. If intake is categorized, the categorization of food-based intake should use the nutrient residuals or nutrient densities, whereas the categories for supplement-based intake would be based on absolute amounts. The reason for not suggesting that supplement-based intake be adjusted for total energy intake through calculation of nutrient residuals or nutrient densities is a likely low correlation between total energy intake and supplement-based intake, particularly if the nutrient does not contribute to energy intake.

If analyses are to be conducted in which food- and supplement-based intakes are combined, the investigator needs to decide whether to simply add the two intakes together or to add supplement-based intake to the energy-adjusted intake from foods.[9] It is unclear how, or if, results between these two approaches will differ. If the intake from supplements represents a large proportion of the total intake and thus the correlation between total intake of the nutrient and total energy intake is low, the easiest and probably best approach is to simply combine the supplement-based intake with the food-based intake, and then use the standard multivariate model, whether or not nutrient intake is categorized. If the supplement-based intake does not represent a large proportion of the total intake, it may be worthwhile to examine the associations using both approaches, since it is unclear how the results might differ, of if they will differ in any practical way.

Within-Person Variability in Intake

The goal of examining associations of nutrients with an outcome is to estimate the association of usual intake with that outcome. However, information on nutrient intake collected from a single 24-hour recall is subject to substantial within-person variability due to day-to-day variability in intake in most individuals. Hence, nutrient intake in a single 24-hour recall often does not reflect the individual's average or usual intake. This day-to-day variability in nutrient intake is often referred to as "measurement error." Measurement error typically results in underestimation of associations of nutrients with outcomes. For example, for MRFIT men[11] it was estimated that with one 24-hour recall, the association between a dependent variable and percent of kcalories from total fat would be underestimated by 77.7% in simple linear regression.

Error can generally be divided into two types: random and systematic. If error is random, the average of a large number of repeated measurements approaches the true value, or for nutrient intake, the individual's usual intake. To reduce measurement error, studies will often collect multiple 24-hour recalls. Liu et al[16] describe methods for estimating the number of 24-hour recalls required to achieve a suitable degree of accuracy. In MRFIT men[11] it was estimated that the association between a dependent variable and percent of kcalories from total fat would be underestimated by 46.7% with four 24-hour recalls, compared to the 77.7% underestimation with one 24-hour recall.

If error is systematic, for example due to systematic over- or underreporting of intake, the average of a large number of repeated measurements will not reflect the individual's usual intake. Food frequency questionnaires may also have systematic error if specific foods eaten by an individual are not included in the questionnaire.

Methods are available for correcting or adjusting regression coefficients for measurement error. However, the assumptions that underlie such corrections can be quite strong and may not be strictly applicable to nutrient data. In particular, it is typically assumed that error is random and independent of the true value or usual intake, and that error and usual intake are normally distributed. However, for nutrient data it is likely that error is correlated with usual intake. For example, an individual with a usual intake of 3000 kcal is likely to vary more about his/her usual intake than an individual with a usual intake of 1000 kcal. Correcting for measurement error should be done with care and caution, and with attention to the assumptions underlying such corrections. A thorough discussion on correcting for measurement error in linear regression models is given by Fuller.[17] Willett[10] and Clayton and Gill[18] also discuss measurement error in the context of nutrient data. Spiegelman, McDermott, and Rosner[19] describe the regression calibration method for adjusting point and interval estimates for measurement error in linear regression, logistic regression, and Cox proportional hazards regression. The regression calibration method is appropriate when a gold standard is available in a validation study and a linear measurement error with a constant variance applies, or when replicate measurements are available in a reliability study and linear random within-person error can be assumed. These authors also describe SAS macros that can be used to adjust regression coefficients in these models when the assumptions underlying use of the regression calibration method appear appropriate.

Types of Epidemiologic Studies

A discussion of types of epidemiologic studies with particular reference to nutrition can be found in Sempos, Liu, and Ernst,[20] while a more general review of the topic is given in Hennekens and Buring.[21] There are generally two types of epidemiologic studies: observational and experimental. The main difference between an experimental and an observational study is the control that the investigator exercises over participants, procedures, and exposures. In an experiment, the investigator controls who enters the study, what drugs or procedures are given to participants, and how the study is carried out. In a nutritional intervention study, the investigator would manipulate or attempt to manipulate some or all participants' dietary intake. An observational study does not involve an intervention or manipulation. In such a study, the investigator does not control who enters the study or the factors or drugs to which participants are exposed. Observational studies of individuals include cross-sectional, case-control, and prospective studies, while studies of groups are referred to as ecologic studies. In nutritional epidemiologic studies, nutrient intake is measured but not manipulated, the frequency and pattern of outcomes observed, and associations between nutrients and outcomes estimated using statistical methods.

In a cross-sectional study the question asked is, "What is the correlation or association between nutrient intake and the outcome?" Individuals are included in the study without regard to their status on the outcome or nutrient intake. In these studies, nutrient intake and the outcome are both measured at the same point in time. For example, INTERMAP is a cross-sectional study of the associations of macronutrients with blood pressure.[3,4] In this study, each participant had blood pressure measured twice on each of four occasions and completed a 24-hour recall on each day that blood pressure was measured.

Case-control studies, also referred to as retrospective and case-referent studies, are designed to answer the question, "Do persons with disease (cases) have different nutrient intake than persons who have not been diagnosed with the disease (controls)?" For example, do persons with heart disease consume more dietary cholesterol and saturated fatty acids than persons without heart disease? In case-control studies, recently diagnosed persons with the disease and a set of persons without the disease are interviewed concerning their dietary habits. The goal is to determine usual nutrient intake before the onset of disease.

Prospective studies are also referred to as cohort, incidence, follow-up, and longitudinal studies. The question asked in prospective studies when a nutrient is thought to be related to increased risk of disease is, "Do persons with higher intake develop or die from the disease more frequently or sooner than persons with lower intake?" Alternatively, if a nutrient is thought to be related to decreased risk of disease, the question asked is, "Do persons with lower intake develop or die from the disease more frequently or sooner than persons with higher intake?" For example, are persons who consume more than 50 g/day of alcohol more likely to have a stroke than persons who consume less alcohol? Persons found to be disease free at the time of the cross-sectional survey are followed over time to determine who develops the disease and when the disease occurs.

Ecologic studies compare aggregate data representing entire populations. A common example of this type of study is one in which disease-specific mortality rates for different countries are correlated with nutrient measurements based on food disappearance data.[22] The INTERSALT study included ecologic analyses on associations of urinary electrolytes and other factors with blood pressure, as well as cross-sectional analyses on electrolyte-blood pressure associations within individuals.[23,24]

Experimental studies involving nutritional interventions include feeding or metabolic ward studies and randomized clinical trials. Feeding studies involve feeding groups of individuals precisely measured diets with one or more components varied, with an effect on a biologic variable then measured. The Keys equation for predicting change in total cholesterol from changes in intakes of saturated and polyunsaturated fatty acids and dietary cholesterol was determined from a metabolic ward study.[25] A common design for feeding studies is the crossover design, in which each participant serves as his/her own control. The randomized clinical trial is a prospective study in which individuals are randomly assigned to intervention and control groups. After randomization, both groups are followed over time to assess the efficacy and safety of the intervention. For example, the trial on the Primary Prevention of Hypertension was a randomized, controlled clinical trial on the effects of weight loss, reduction in sodium intake, decreased alcohol intake, and increased exercise on the five-year incidence of hypertension in men and women with high normal blood pressure.[26]

Methods for Comparing Groups in Cross-Sectional Studies

Table 24.1 lists methods of analysis that can be used to compare nutrient intake between two groups, e.g., men and women, or among three or more groups, e.g., African-Americans, Hispanics, and whites. For nutrient intake considered as a continuous variable, the goal of the analysis is to determine whether mean or median intake differs significantly between or among groups. For such analyses, the table indicates the usual method of

TABLE 24.1

Methods for Comparing Nutrient Intake among Groups in Cross-Sectional Studies

Description	Number of Groups (k)	
	k = 2	k > 2
Nutrient Intake Continuous		
Usual method	Two-sample t-test	Analysis of variance
Nonparametric alternative	Wilcoxon rank-sum test	Kruskal-Wallis test
Adjustment for other variables	Analysis of covariance or multiple linear regression	
Nutrient Intake Categorical (c categories)		
Usual method	Chi-square test for 2 x c contingency table	Chi-square test for k x c contingency table

analysis, the nonparametric alternative, and methods that can be used to adjust for potential confounders of differences between groups, e.g., age or total energy intake. Nonparametric tests make fewer assumptions about the shape of the distributions of variables than parametric tests such as the two-sample t-test or analysis of variance. In the Wilcoxon rank-sum test and the Kruskal-Wallis test, the actual observations are replaced by their ranks in the combined sample of all observations. If nutrient intake is divided into categories, the goal of the analysis is usually to determine whether the distributions of intake are homogeneous across groups. The methods listed in Table 24.1 can also be used to compare nutrient intake at baseline in an experimental study; for example, to determine whether in a randomized clinical trial randomization has provided comparable groups with respect to intake of specific nutrients. A useful text on these methods and those described below is that of Rosner.[27]

Methods for Comparing Cases and Controls in Case-Control Studies

Table 24.2 lists methods of analysis that can be used to compare nutrient intake between cases and controls in unmatched and matched case-control studies. Matching is often done in case-control studies to make cases and controls comparable on variables that could confound associations of the variable of interest with disease. For unmatched case-control studies, the methods listed are identical to those for comparing nutrient intake between two groups in cross-sectional studies. For matched case-control studies, the methods of analysis need to take into account the matching. Hence, for a simple comparison of means between cases and controls, the investigator should use a paired t-test rather than a two-sample t-test, or the Wilcoxon signed-rank test rather than the Wilcoxon rank sum test. When multiple regression is used to adjust the mean difference between cases and controls for other variables in matched case-control studies, the investigator needs to ensure that the dependent and independent variables in the model are defined correctly. In such studies, the dependent variable is the difference in nutrient intake for each case-control

TABLE 24.2

Methods for Comparing Nutrient Intake between Cases and Controls in Case-Control Studies

Description	Unmatched	Matched
Nutrient Intake Continuous		
Usual method	Two-sample t-test	Paired t-test
Nonparametric alternative	Wilcoxon rank-sum test	Wilcoxon signed-rank test
Adjustment for other variables	Analysis of covariance or multiple linear regression	Multiple linear regression*
Nutrient Intake Categorical (c categories)		
Usual method	Chi-square test for 2 x c contingency table	McNemar's test for c = 2

* In this model, differences in each variable for the case-control pair are used, with the difference in the nutrient of interest serving as the dependent variable. The test of significance for the adjusted mean difference is the test of the hypothesis that the intercept of the model is equal to zero.

TABLE 24.3
Methods for Assessing Associations in Epidemiologic Studies

Dependent Variable	Nutrient Intake	Unadjusted	Adjusted for Other Variables
Cross-Sectional or Ecologic Study			
Continous	Continous	Pearson correlation Spearman correlation Linear regression	Partial correlation Linear regression
Continous	Categorical	Linear regression	Linear regression
Dichotomous	Continuous, categorical	Logistic regression	Logistic regression
Unmatched Case-Control Study			
Case-control status	Continuous, categorical	Logistic regression	Logistic regression
Matched Case-Control Study			
None	Continuous, categorical	Conditional logistic regression	Conditional logistic regression
Prospective Study			
Time to event	Categorical	Log rank test Cox regression	Cox regression
Time to event	Continuous	Cox regression	Cox regression

pair, while the independent variables are the within-pair differences for the potential confounding variables. The test of significance for the adjusted mean difference is the test of the hypothesis that the intercept in the model is equal to zero.

Methods for Assessing Associations in Epidemiologic Studies

Table 24.3 lists methods for assessing associations of nutrient intake with outcome variables in cross-sectional or ecologic studies, matched and unmatched case-control studies, and prospective studies. For each type of study, the table indicates methods that can be used when nutrient intake is modeled as a continuous variable or as a categorical variable. The table also lists the dependent variable for each type of analysis. For example, in Cox proportional hazards regression, the dependent variable is the time to some event, e.g., death from coronary heart disease. In unmatched case-control studies, the dependent variable is typically case-control status. Since cross-sectional and ecologic studies can have both continuous and dichotomous dependent variables, methods are listed for both types of dependent variable. No dependent variable is listed for conditional logistic regression, since there is no outcome variable that varies from individual to individual in this model. In conditional logistic regression, the independent variables are the case-control difference in each variable, and the model does not include a constant term. A useful text on logistic and Cox regression methods is that of Kahn and Sempos.[28]

The Spearman correlation is listed for use in cross-sectional and ecologic studies, since it is the nonparametric alternative to the Pearson product-moment correlation coefficient. The Pearson-product moment correlation coefficient should not be used if either nutrient intake or the second variable has a very skewed distribution, since the assumption underlying its use is that each variable has a normal distribution for each value of the other variable.

In analyses involving linear regression, interest focuses on the difference in the mean of the dependent variable for a one-unit or greater difference in the independent variable. Hence, the focus is on the regression coefficient. In logistic and Cox regression, interest focuses on estimates of relative risk. In logistic regression, the relative risk is given by the odds ratio, and in Cox regression the hazard ratio. In both models, relative risk estimates are obtained by exponentiation of the regression coefficient or the regression coefficient times some convenient multiplier. For example, if total energy intake is the dietary variable of interest, exponentiation of the regression coefficient gives the relative risk of the outcome for two persons who differ in total energy intake by 1 kcal. Since this is not a particularly meaningful difference for calculating relative risk, an investigator might multiply the regression coefficient by 500 to obtain the relative risk of the outcome for two persons who differ in total energy intake by 500 kcal. When nutrient intake is categorized and dummy variables are included in the regression model, exponentiation of the regression coefficient for a dummy variable gives the risk of the outcome for those in the category corresponding to the dummy variable relative to the referent category, e.g., quartile 4 relative to quartile 1.

In analyses based on Cox regression, true associations between diet and disease may not be found if there are substantial changes in nutrient intake between the baseline assessment of diet and the development of disease, or if there are substantial changes in the rank ordering of study participants with respect to intake over the course of followup.

Analyses of Intervention Studies with Change in Nutrient Intake as Outcome

In nutritional intervention studies, investigators often wish to examine the effects of the intervention on intakes of specific nutrients following completion of the intervention. Investigators can use three approaches to determine whether intake of specific nutrients changed in an intervention group relative to a control group or among three or more groups:

1. Compare intake among groups at followup, ignoring pre-intervention intake using the methods for cross-sectional studies in Table 24.1.
2. Compare the change in intake from pre-intervention to followup among groups using the methods for cross-sectional studies.
3. Compare intake among groups at followup, adjusting for pre-intervention intake with multiple linear regression or analysis of covariance.

Investigators typically use the second approach for intervention studies, even though it tends to be less powerful than analysis of covariance. Assumptions in regard to the analysis of covariance may or may not be met in an intervention study. The first approach may, however, be preferable to the second, if there are no differences in intake among the groups compared at the pre-intervention assessment, and the correlation between the pre-intervention and followup assessments for the nutrient of interest is less than 0.5. Correlations smaller than 0.5 are not uncommon for many nutrients assessed on two occasions.[11]

Hence, for nutrient intake the best approach may be to ignore pre-intervention intake. Prior to conducting analyses in nutritional intervention studies, investigators should examine the correlations of the nutrients from pre-intervention to followup and be prepared to ignore pre-intervention intake in the analyses.

References

1. Slattery ML, et al. *J Am Coll Nutr* 14: 635; 1995.
2. Goldberg GR, et al. *Eur J Clin Nutr* 45: 569; 1991.
3. INTERMAP Cooperative Research Group *Canad J Cardiol* 13: 235B; 1997.
4. INTERMAP Research Group. *Canad J Cardiol* 13: 80B; 1997.
5. Liu K. *Am J Clin Nutr* 59: 262S; 1994.
6. SAS Procedures Guide, Release 6.03 Edition. Cary, NC: SAS Institute, 1988.
7. Neter J, Wasserman W, Kutner MH. *Applied Linear Regression Models.* Homewood, IL: Richard D. Irwin, Inc., 1983.
8. Ryan TP. *Modern Regression Methods.* New York, NY: John Wiley & Sons, 1997.
9. Willett WC, Howe GR, Kushi LH. *Am J Clin Nutr* 65: 1220S; 1997.
10. Willett W. *Nutritional Epidemiology.* New York, NY: Oxford University Press, 1990.
11. Grandits GA, Bartsch GE, Stamler J. In: *Dietary and Nutritional Methods and Findings: The Multiple Risk Factor Intervention Trial (MRFIT)* (Stamler J, et al. Eds.) *Am J Clin Nutr* 65: 211S; 1997.
12. Brown CC, et al. *Am J Epidemiol* 129: 323; 1994.
13. National Research Council. *Diet and Health: Implications for Reducing Chronic Disease Risk.* Washington, DC: National Academy Press, 1989.
14. Reed D, McGee D, Yano K, Hankin J. *Hypertension* 7: 405; 1985.
15. McGee D, Reed D, Yano K. *J Chron Dis* 37: 713; 1984.
16. Liu K, et al. *J Chron Dis* 31: 399; 1978.
17. Fuller WA. *Measurement Error Models.* New York, NY: John Wiley & Sons, 1987.
18. Clayton D, Gill C. In: *Design Concepts in Nutritional Epidemiology.* Margetts BM, Nelson M, Eds, Oxford, UK: Oxford University Press, 1991, pp. 79-96.
19. Spiegelman D, McDermott A, Rosner B. *Am J Clin Nutr* 65: 1179S; 1997.
20. Sempos CT, Liu K, Ernst N. *Am J Clin Nutr* 69: 1S; 1999.
21. Hennekens CH, Buring JE. *Epidemiology in Medicine* (Mayrent SL, Ed) Boston, MA: Little, Brown, 1987.
22. Stamler J, Shekelle R. *Arch Pathol Lab Med* 112: 1032; 1988.
23. The INTERSALT Cooperative Research Group. *J Hypertens* 4: 781; 1986.
24. The INTERSALT Cooperative Research Group. *Br Med J* 297: 319; 1988.
25. Keys A, Anderson JT, Grande F. *Metabolism* 65; 776; 1965.
26. Stamler R, et al. *JAMA* 262: 1801; 1989.
27. Rosner B. *Fundamentals of Biostatistics,* 5th ed. Belmont, CA: Duxbury Press, 1999.
28. Kahn HA, Sempos C. *Statistical Methods in Epidemiology.* New York, NY: Oxford University Press, 1989.

25

Medical Nutritional Evaluation

Elaine B. Feldman

Introduction

Family physicians, pediatricians, and internists are the usual providers of primary medical care for adults, with gynecologists increasingly performing that task for women. The assessment of nutritional status should be carried out in their offices and in hospital settings.[1] The most common reasons for office visits that may require nutritional intervention are problems related to hypertension, diabetes mellitus, degenerative joint disease, heart disease, asthma, abdominal pain, and pregnancy care, as well as part of a general medical examination.[2]

Nutrition science should be applied to many aspects of primary care delivery.[1,3,4] The history, physical examination, and laboratory tests are used to assess nutritional status. As a result, patients may be categorized as normal, malnourished, or at risk of malnutrition. Dietary history, anthropometric measurements, and specific physiologic and biochemical laboratory tests should be appropriately elaborated in patients with malnutrition or at nutritional risk. These usually require referrals. In order to communicate effectively with their patients, physicians should know the components of a healthy diet in terms of foods as well as nutrients and the patterns of consuming food in meals. Details of food composition, however, are more likely in the knowledge base of dietitians and nutritionists.

The physician should obtain specific information about the patient's body weight and its change over time, the patient's recent meal intake (e.g., foods eaten the previous day), appetite, food preferences, level of physical activity, special diets, and intake of supplements. Height and weight are vital signs that should be measured accurately under standardized conditions (not self-reported) in all patients, and body weight should be measured at followup visits. The complete blood count (CBC) and serum albumin provide clues to nutritional anemias and protein status. The patient who is starved, or with gastrointestinal diseases, malabsorption, hepatic and pancreatic disease, renal failure, trauma, sepsis, cancer, or requiring critical care should be given special attention in assessing nutritional status and developing nutritional therapy.[5] A registered dietitian is an invaluable resource in assessing dietary intake by dietary recalls, prospective food records, or food frequency questionnaires.

0-8493-2705-9/01/$0.00+$1.50

The use of dietary supplements of vitamins and minerals is common in our population to meet nutritional needs, optimize nutritional health, and prevent disease. Over-the-counter remedies are available and are marketed with little restriction. Since patients often do not report supplement use to the physician, toxicity or possible drug–nutrient interactions can be overlooked with serious adverse consequences. Unsubstantiated health claims may lead to problems because of toxicity, adverse interactions with other medications or foods, and avoidance of orthodox effective remedies.

The health professional should be aware of good food sources for vitamins and minerals (Section 1, 5-10), appropriate serving sizes, and the facts of nutrient fortification and enrichment of foods, especially as they evolve into newer modalities for nourishment. Encouraging patients to read food labels will result in improving their nutrition knowledge and health (see Section 14). Proper food/nutrient intake lessens the risk of cardiovascular and cerebrovascular diseases (atherosclerosis, hypertension) and cancer.

In the practice of primary care, a miscellany of special circumstances, when suspected, may warrant nutritional interventions. While serious nutritional deficiencies have disappeared in affluent countries, physicians should be aware of their occurrence in patients with alcoholism. That diagnosis should be recognized and the substance abuse treated. Special nutritional needs of women should be addressed. These include replacing iron loss from menstruation to prevent or treat anemia, ameliorating accelerated menopause-related calcium loss from bone, and the special needs of pregnant and lactating women including meeting the periconceptual need for folic acid to prevent neural tube defects, and recognizing the greater susceptibility of women to obesity and alcoholism because of their size, body composition, and metabolic/hormonal differences compared to men. Dementia is increasing as the population ages. More than one-half of cognitive deficiencies in the elderly are attributable to vascular disease and increasingly result from thromboembolism. Risk of vascular disease is increased by a diet high in saturated fats, low in antioxidants, vitamin B_{12}, and choline — especially important in the patient in the middle years. Vegetarians not ingesting any animal products may be at nutritional risk, and vitamin supplementation may be recommended. Patients who cannot or will not eat should be evaluated for possible enteral or parenteral nutrition support and referred to a dietitian or nutrition support team. Caregivers must be wary of dietary fads, most prevalent with regard to weight reduction. Finally, all physicians should be educated in the principles of a health-promoting diet.[6]

Patient Evaluation

The medical history will provide 80 to 90% of the information leading to a diagnosis.[5,7,8] The evaluation of nutritional status will emphasize certain elements of the medical history and social background that will differ depending on the patient's gender, age, and the presenting problem. The usual level of physical activity and the degree of stress should be noted. It is imperative to distinguish whether any impairment of nutritonal status is caused by a patient's disease or is directly related to abnormal intake of nutrients or an unbalanced diet. Malnutrition resulting from disease can be managed effectively only if the underlying disease is controlled or cured. For example, is there physiological or anatomic loss of gastrointestinal function, or is the degree of weight change out of proportion to food intake indicating hyper- or hypometabolism? Does the patient have diabetes mellitus? Is there excessive blood loss from menstruation?

Medical History

The elements of a medical history include the present illness, past medical and surgical history, family history, a medication list, and review of systems.

Pertinent questions to ask are:

- What is the patient's usual weight?
- Has there been any recent change in weight?
- If so, how much and over what period of time?
- What are the maximum and minimum weights?
- What was the weight one year ago, five years ago?

A rapid and profound weight loss is probably the single most important clue to malnutrition. This leads the history taker into an evaluation of normal or abnormal food and nutrient intake. Are there

- Change in smell or taste
- Depression, alcoholism
- Dental problems, poor dentition, sore tongue or swallowing difficulties, affecting appetite or enjoyment of eating
- Poverty, low socioeconomic status, limited access to food
- Special diet prescriptions
- Food idiosyncrasies, (e.g., pica), food fads, excessive use of dietary supplements
- Mechanical problems in eating due to muscle weakness, joint deformities, tremors
- Altered memory or dementia interfering with food and water intake
- Digestion and absorption problems
  - Medications such as antacids, laxatives, oral contraceptives, anticonvulsants
  - Parasites
  - Surgical resection of the gastrointestinal tract
  - Malabsorption syndromes
- Utilization
  - Anticonvulsants, oral contraceptives, antimetabolites, isoniazid
  - Inborn errors of metabolism
- Losses
  - Blood loss
  - Diarrhea (change in bowel habits)
  - Vomiting
  - Draining wounds, fistulas, ostomies
  - Burns
  - Proteinuria, dialysis
- Destruction
  - Fever, sepsis

  - Hypermetabolism
  - Multiple trauma, burns
  - Constipation, obstipation
- Special requirements
  - Chronic disease
  - Recent major surgery
  - Alcohol abuse
  - Hormone replacement therapy
  - Chemotherapy
  - Immunosuppressive therapy
  - Behavior
  - Excessive use of caffeine
  - Alcohol abuse
  - Fad diets
  - Excessive use of dietary supplements
- Miscellaneous
  - Neurologic symptoms, e.g., numbness, dizziness, weakness
  - Skin rash, dryness, flaking, hair loss

Socioeconomic History

The psychosocial evaluation should generate information concening the patient's income and living conditions. This is especially important in the elderly.

- Does the patient live alone?
- Does he or she have access to shopping?
- Are the facilities for storing and cooking food adequate?
- Does the patient have a history of smoking?
- Are financial resources adequate?
- Are there assistance programs available?

Family History

Many nutritional disorders are familial or inherited. Thus, history of cancer, cardiovascular disease, metabolic diseases, gastrointestinal or liver disease, obesity, etc., should alert the examiner in the patient evaluation.

Diet History and Evaluation

An extensive assessment is best done by the professionally trained dietitian, and is required in patients who have nutritional problems or appear at risk of malnutrition. Nevertheless, the physician should acquire basic knowledge of the patient's food intake, meal pattern, and dietary habits. including use of dietary supplements in order to assess general nutritional adequacy and identify potential problems that may need to be addressed.

The physician has the opportunity to practice preventive nutrition by evaluating the patient's energy balance (intake, activity) and the consumption of dietary components predisposing to vascular disease, cancer, or other chronic diseases.

In the inpatient setting it is important to note the diet prescribed and whether the time constraints of diagnostic tests or interventional therapies preclude the patient's eating the meals that were ordered.

General Physical Examination

Height and weight should be considered vital signs and should be measured and recorded with careful attention to accuracy and precision. Height should be measured annually, and weight at most office visits and at regular intervals in the hospitalized patient. The Body Mass Index (BMI) is a useful parameter for monitoring body size. Table 3.20, Section 3, provides BMIs for a wide variety of body sizes. A body weight that is decreased profoundly alerts the physician to increasing morbidity or mortality. A weight loss to <80% of ideal increases chances of infection, while weight loss to 60% of ideal predicts dying, and few individuals survive a loss of 50% of body weight.[9]

Observation, inspection, and measurement are the primary tools of the examination. The physical signs of malnutrition are listed and categorized according to anatomic site and organ system in Table 25.1.

Finding abnormalities provides leads rather than a diagnosis, and alerts the examiner to further measurements and laboratory tests. Easily recognized abnormalities indicate advanced disease.

Laboratory Tests

Some routine laboratory tests can assist in the nutritional assessment and diagnosis. These include CBC, blood chemistries (glucose, electrolytes, minerals, liver and kidney function tests), and tests of blood coagulation (Table 25.2).

Hemoglobin levels will show the presence of anemia that may be vitamin-specific or mineral related, and can indicate chronic disease. The red blood cell size and hemoglobin content and concentration can provide clues to liver disease, alcoholism, and specific nutritional deficiencies. While serum albumin is not a sensitive indicator of protein status, it does provide a clue. Low levels may indicate a limiting amount of substrate for hepatic protein synthesis. On the other hand, non-nutritional factors may be responsible for hypoalbuminemia such as expanded extracellular fluid, accelerated protein breakdown, and impaired liver and kidney function. Albumin levels also may be unreliable indicators

TABLE 25.1
Physical Signs of Malnutrition

System	Sign	Deficiency/Abnormality
Hair	Luster, texture (dull, dry)	Protein
	Depigmentation (flag sign)	
	Color (reddening)	
	Easily plucked	
	Areas of hair loss (alopecia)	
Face	Rash, seborrhea	Riboflavin
	Pallor	Iron, folate, B_{12}
Eyes	Luster of cornea decreased, Bitot spots,	Vitamin A, riboflavin
	xerosis, keratomalacia, night blindness	Iron, B_{12}, folate
	Conjunctival injection	Hypercholesterolemia
	Conjunctival pallor	Wilson's disease, copper excess
	Corneal arcus, eyelid xanthelasma	Wernicke's syndrome, thiamin
	Kayser-Fleischer ring	
	Nystagmus	
Lips	Cheilosis (swelling), angular stomatitis (fissures)	Riboflavin
Tongue	Glossitic (smooth, red)	B_{12}, folate, riboflavin
	Pallor, atrophy	Iron
	Decreased taste	Zinc
Gums	Bleeding, hypertrophy	Vitamin C
Neck	Goiter (enlarged thyroid)	Iodine
Skin	Rash, edema	Protein
	Pigmentation or depigmentation	Niacin
	Flakiness, peeling, dry	Protein, zinc
	Bleeding	Vitamin K
	Perifollicular hemorrhage	Vitamin C
	Hyperkeratoses	Vitamin A
Nails	Spooning	Iron
	Brittle	Protein
Muscles	Atrophy	Protein
	Weakness	Protein, iron, B_{12}, folate
Bones, joints	Fractures, deformities, tenderness	Vitamin D
	Deformities	Vitamin C
Heart	Enlargement	Selenium
	Failure	Thiamin
	Arrhythmias	Calcium, magnesium, potassium
Abdomen	Ascites	Protein
	Hepatomegaly	Alcohol abuse
Neurologic	Mental status/dementia	Thiamin, B_{12}, folate, niacin
	Cranial nerves	Thiamin
	Gait, ataxia	Thiamin, B_{12}, pyridoxine
	Sensory	Thiamin
	Diminished reflexes	Iodine
	Tetany	Calcium, magnesium
	Paralysis	Potassium

TABLE 25.2

Laboratory Tests Useful in Clinical Nutritional Assessment[a]

Laboratory Test	Body Compartment/ Organ System Function
Hemoglobin, hematocrit, red and white blood cell counts and indices, differential (calculate total lymphocyte count)	Protein, visceral Anemia
Urea, creatinine, glucose, sodium, potassium, chloride, carbon dioxide	Renal function Diabetes mellitus Acid-base balance
Cholesterol, triglycerides, lipoproteins	Lipid disorders
Total protein, albumin, uric acid	Liver, kidney function
Calcium, phosphate, magnesium, bilirubin, alkaline phosphatase	Minerals, skeleton
Aminotransferases, iron, ferritin	Liver function Anemia
Transferrin, transthyretin, retinol-binding protein	Iron Protein, visceral
Prothrombin time, partial thromboplastin time	Vitamin K, blood clotting

[a] Adapted from Feldman, E.B. In *Laboratory Medicine; the Selection and Interpretation of Clinical Laboratory Studies.* Noe, D.A., Rock, R.C., Eds. Williams & Wilkins. Baltimore, 1993, ch. 10.

of protein status in the postoperative or acutely injured patient. Some enzyme tests are indicators of nutritional cofactor status, e.g., alkaline phosphatase and zinc, or aminotransferase for Vitamin B_6.

Nutrition Diagnosis and Prescription

The initial nutritional assessment will use information from the history, physical examination, and laboratory tests that may be supplemented by consultation with a dietitian, a clinical nutrition specialist, or other medical specialists or subspecialists. The patient's route of feeding, energy intake, and proportion and amount of macronutrients will be prescribed. The needs to replete or restrict and to supplement will be decided.

A single, ideal prognostic indicator of nutritional risk remains elusive. Rather, multiple parameters must be determined and interpreted in the light of the patient's medical status. One example of a global assessment[7] utilizes elements from the history (weight change, dietary intake change, persistent gastrointestinal symptoms, functional capacity, diseases) and the physical examination (subcutaneous fat, muscle bulk and tone, edema, ascites) to categorize patients as in good nutritional status, with moderate or suspected malnutrition, or with severe malnutrition.

Educating Physicians in Nutrition

Nutrition plays an important role in the etiology, prevention, or treatment of many chronic diseases. Thus, an appropriate knowledge of nutrition principles should be part of the education and training of physicians, especially those in primary care.[4,10] Family medicine specialists have developed guidelines for incorporating nutrition into their medical education and residency training programs.[11-13] The current guidelines are presented in Table 25.3 and can be accessed on the Web site of the American Academy of Family Physicians, www.afp.org.

TABLE 25.3

Recommended Nutrition Guidelines for Family Practice[a]

Develop Attitudes that Recognize

Nutrition is a major part of wellness, disease prevention and treatment of disease
Poor nutrition can cause disease
Family, ethnic and religious attitudes affect nutrition behavior
Socioeconomic factors are important in nutritional excess and deficiency
Different nutritional considerations at different times are required in the life cycle
Nutritionists and dietitians are important in the area of the patient's nutritional status, education and disease prevention

Develop Knowledge Of

Basic nutritional requirements/recommended allowances and intakes
Nutritional content of food and the food pyramid
Nutritional information from public and private sources
The role of qualified nutritional professionals as consultants
The changing nutritional requirements of infancy, childhood, adolescence, pregnancy, lactation, menopause, aging
Nutritional requirements of disease processes and exercise
Clinical effects of dietary fat, carbohydrate, proteins, and fiber
Basic concepts of vegetarianism
The role of nutrition in the treatment and prevention of disease: hypertension, heart, dental, gastrointestinal, liver and renal diseases, diabetes, alcoholism, anemia, cancer
Signs and symptoms of nutrient deficiencies
Breast feeding and formula feeding
Use of vitamin and mineral supplements
Weight reduction and dieting
Food and drug interactions
Allergies and food intolerance
Eating disorders
Refeeding syndromes
Nutrition quackery

Develop Skills In

Assessing nutritional status during the history and physical examinations
Assessing nutritional status and needs of hospitalized patients
Ordering laboratory and metabolic studies to detect nutritional deficiencies and assess adequacy of the nutrition provided
Counseling patients and family about specific nutritional needs related to their life cycle stage and disease process, the role of diet in preventing disease, safe weight reduction and dieting, including health benefits
Educating patients about food marketing and nutritional quackery
Prescribing and managing oral supplementation, tube feeding, peripheral nutrition, and total parenteral nutrition
Preventing and managing refeeding syndromes
Recognizing and appropriately referring patients with disordered eating habits

[a] Adapted from *Physician's Curriculum in Clinical Nutrition.* STFM, Kansas City, 1995.

References

1. Feldman EB. In *Laboratory Medicine; the Selection and Interpretation of Clinical Laboratory Studies.* Noe DA, Rock RC, Eds, Williams & Wilkins, Baltimore, 1993, ch 10.
2. Kolasa KM. *Eur J Clin Nutr* 53: S89; 1999.
3. Feldman EB. *Southern Med J* 88: 204; 1995.
4. Feldman EB. *Nutrition* 16: 649; 2000.

5. Feldman EB. In *Essentials of Clinical Nutrition.* FA Davis, Philadelphia, 1988, ch 3.
6. Nutrition Screening Initiative. *Incorporating Nutrition Screening and Interventions into Medical Practice. A Monograph for Physicians.* 1010 Wisconsin Ave, NW Suite 800, Washington DC 20007. The Nutrition Screening Initiative, 1994.
7. Newton JM, Halsted CH. In *Modern Nutrition in Health and Disease,* Shils ME, Olson JA, Shike M, Ross, AC, Eds, 9th ed, Williams & Wilkins, Baltimore, 1999, ch 55.
8. Owen GM. In *Nutrition Assessment, a Comprehensive Guide for Planning Intervention,* Simko MD, Cowell C, Gilbride JA, Eds, 2nd ed, Aspen Publishers, Inc., Gaithersburg, MD, 1995, chap 6.
9. Feldman EB. In *Essentials of Clinical Nutrition.* FA Davis, Philadelphia, 1988, ch 13.
10. Feldman EB. *Am J Clin Nutr* 54: 618; 1991.
11. Society for Teachers of Family Medicine Working Group on Nutrition Education, *Physician's Curriculum in Clinical Nutrition.* STFM, Kansas City, 1995.
12. American Academy of Family Physicians (AAFP) *Recommended Core Educational Guidelines on Nutrition for Family Practice Residents.* American Academy Family Physicians, Kansas City, 1989, revised 1995.
13. Society for Teachers of Family Medicine. *Physicians Guide to Outpatient Nutrition,* in press.

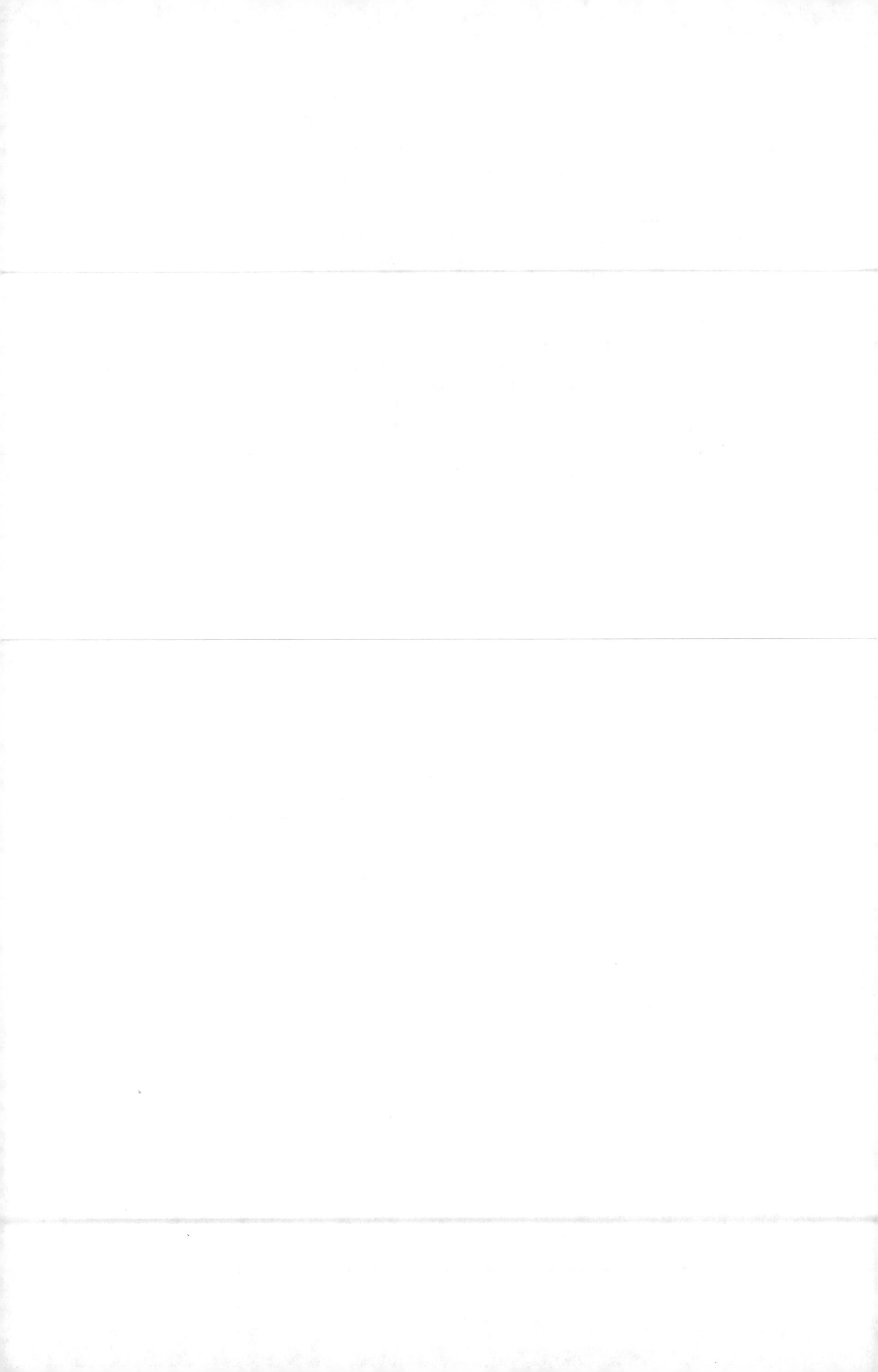

26

Assessment of Lipids and Lipoproteins

Elaine B. Feldman

Introduction

The circulating lipids include free cholesterol, cholesterol esterified with long-chain fatty acids, triacylglycerols (triglycerides, TG), phospholipids, and unesterified or free fatty acids. Lipids are transported in the blood plasma in the form of lipoproteins. The lipoproteins include:

- Chylomicrons
- Very low-density lipoproteins (VLDL)
- Intermediate-density lipoproteins (IDL, beta-VLDL)
- Low-density lipoproteins (LDL)
- High-density lipoproteins (HDL)

The chemical and physical properties of the lipoproteins[1] are shown in Table 26.1. This section summarizes biological factors influencing lipid and lipoprotein levels, describes methodology for assays in common clinical use in laboratories or health care facilities, and provides data on the range of normal values.

Cholesterol

Cholesterol is synthesized by all animal cells (endogenous) and by no plants. It also is derived from animal products in the diet (exogenous). Food sources are listed in Table 51.6 in Section 51. Circulating cholesterol levels vary with age, increasing in men from puberty to the fifth decade of life, and in women until the seventh decade[2] (Table 26.2). Levels in women are lower than in men from age 30 to 50. Mean cholesterol levels vary

0-8493-2705-9/01/$0.00+$1.50

TABLE 26.1

Plasma Lipoproteins in Humans[a]

Class	Particle Diameter (nm)	Flotation Density	Electrophoretic Mobility	Major Apoproteins	Chemical Composition, %				
					Surface			Core	
					Proteins	Phospholipids	Cholesterol	Cholesterol Esters	Tryglycerides
Chylomicrons	80–500	<0.95	α2	B, E, A-1 A-IV, C	2	7	2	3	86
VLDL	30–80	0.95–1.006	pre-β	B, E, C	8	18	7	12	55
IDL	25–35	1.006–1.019	slow pre-β	B, E	19	19	9	29	23
LDL	18–28	1.019–1.063	β	B	22	22	8	42	6
HDL_2	9–12	1.063–1.125	α1	A-I, A-II	40	33	5	17	5
HDL_3	5–9	1.125–1.210	α1	A-I, A-II	55	25	4	13	3

Note: VLDL, Very low-density lipoprotein; IDL, intermediate-density lipoprotein; LDL, low-density lipoprotein; HDL, high-density lipoprotein.

[a] Modified from Feldman, E.B. *Essentials of Clinical Nutrition*, F.A. Davis, Philadelphia, 1988, p. 433.

TABLE 26.2

Average Levels of Circulating Lipids[a,b]

	Total C		LDL C		HDL C		TG	
Age, yr	**mmol/L**	**mg/dl**	**mmol/L**	**mg/dl**	**mmol/L**	**mg/dl**	**mmol/L**	**mg/dl**
White Men								
15–19	3.95	152	2.42	93	1.20	46	0.77	68
20–24	4.13	159	2.63	101	1.17	45	0.88	78
25–29	4.58	176	3.02	116	1.14	44	0.99	88
30–34	4.94	190	3.22	124	1.17	45	1.15	102
35–39	5.04	194	3.41	131	1.12	43	1.23	109
40–44	5.30	204	3.51	135	1.12	43	1.39	123
45–49	5.46	210	3.67	141	1.17	45	1.34	119
50–54	5.49	211	3.72	143	1.14	44	1.45	128
55–59	5.56	214	3.77	145	1.20	46	1.32	117
60–64	5.59	215	3.72	143	1.27	49	1.25	111
65–69	5.54	213	3.80	146	1.27	49	1.22	108
70+	5.56	214	3.69	142	1.25	48	1.30	115
White Women								
15–19	4.08	157	2.42	93	1.33	51	0.72	64
20–24	4.29	165	2.65	102	1.33	51	0.90	80
25–29	4.6	178	2.81	108	1.43	55	0.86	76
30–34	4.63	178	2.83	109	1.43	55	0.82	73
35–39	4.84	186	3.02	116	1.38	53	0.94	83
40–44	5.02	193	3.17	122	1.46	56	0.77	68
45–49	5.30	204	3.30	127	1.51	58	1.06	94
50–54	5.56	214	3.48	134	1.61	62	1.16	103
55–59	5.95	229	3.77	145	1.56	60	1.25	111
60–64	5.88	226	3.87	149	1.59	61	1.18	105
65–69	6.06	233	3.93	151	1.61	62	1.33	118
70+	5.88	226	3.82	147	1.56	60	1.24	110

[a] See Table 26.1 for abbreviations of lipoproteins; C, cholesterol; TG, triglycerides.
[b] Adapted from Lipid Research Clinics Program, *JAMA* 251, 351, 1984.

between 4.2 and 6 mmol/L, depending on age and gender. Population levels have been declining over recent decades. About two-thirds of the plasma cholesterol is transported as LDL and levels of LDL cholesterol parallel those of total cholesterol (Table 26.2). HDL transports about one-quarter of the plasma cholesterol, with levels averaging about 1.17 mmol in men, and are 0.23 to 0.44 mmol higher in women (Table 26.2). Table 26.3 provides data on the upper limits of normal for LDL- and HDL-cholaterol. Table 26.4 provides data on mean values for lipids and lipoproteins in men and women from NHANES III data.[3]

Cholesterol assays and the reference method[4-7] are provided in Table 26.5. Clinical laboratories are automated for the lipid analyses. Specific methods are provided as kits by the manufacturer of the analytical instrument in use. Desktop methodologies also are available for outpatient facilities (physicians' offices, clinics) but are not as accurate or precise as the commercial or hospital laboratory procedures. The latter are regulated and supervised by accrediting organizations such as the College of American Pathologists, and laboratories are regulated by the government (CLIA).

TABLE 26.3

Levels of Circulating Lipids Warranting Attention[a,b]

	LDLC		HDLC		TG	
	75th percentile		25th percentile		90th percentile	
Age, yr	mmol/L	mg/dl	mmol/L	mg/dl	mmol/L	mg/dl
White Men						
15–19	2.83	109	1.01	39	1.41	125
20–24	3.07	118	0.99	38	1.64	146
25–29	3.59	138	0.96	37	1.92	171
30–34	3.74	144	0.99	38	2.41	214
35–39	4.00	154	0.94	36	2.81	250
40–44	4.08	157	0.94	36	2.84	252
45–49	4.24	163	0.99	38	2.84	252
50–54	4.21	162	0.94	36	2.74	244
55–59	4.37	168	0.99	38	2.36	210
60–64	4.29	165	1.07	41	2.17	193
70+	4.26	164	1.04	40	2.27	202
White Women						
15–19	2.89	111	1.12	43	1.26	112
20–24	2.07	118	1.14	44	1.52	135
25–29	3.28	126	1.22	47	1.54	137
30–34	3.33	128	1.20	46	1.58	140
35–39	3.61	139	1.14	44	1.91	170
40–44	3.80	146	1.25	58	1.81	161
45–49	3.90	150	1.22	47	2.02	180
50–54	4.16	160	1.30	50	2.14	190
55–59	4.37	168	1.30	50	2.6	229
60–64	4.37	168	1.33	51	2.36	210
65–69	4.78	184	1.27	49	2.49	221
70+	4.42	170	1.25	48	2.13	189

[a] See Table 26.1 for abbreviations.
[b] Adapted from Lipid Research Clinics Program, *JAMA* 251, 351, 1984.

Triacylglycerols (TG)

Circulating TG levels average about 1.13 mmol/L in young adults after overnight fasting. Levels increase from 50 to 75% with age, and are lower in women compared to men. (Tables 26.2 and 26.3). Median TG values range from 0.90 to 1.47 mmol/L. TG levels are labile, varying by up to 50% daily depending on the recent diet. In the fasting state, TG are transported in the VLDL, whereas chylomicrons transport newly absorbed fat. Upper limits of normal for TG are given in Table 26.3.

Triacylglycerol assays and reference method[9-11] are listed in Table 26.5.

Lipoproteins

Lipoprotein assays[12-15] are given in Table 26.5.

TABLE 26.4

Lipid Levels U.S. NHANES III Population[a,b]

Lipid Level (mg/dL)	Mean ± SD (mg/dL)
Mean total cholesterol	225 ± 45
Men	218 ± 42
Women	237 ± 47
Mean LDL-C	142 ± 37
Men	139 ± 35
Women	147 ± 40
Mean HDL-C	50 ± 16
Men	47 ± 14
Women	56 ± 17
Median TG	140 ± 120
Men	137 ± 129
Women	144 ± 108
Mean total-C/HDL-C	4.9 ± 2.1
Men	5.1 ± 1.7
Women	4.7 ± 2.6
Mean LDL-C/HDL-C	3.1 ± 1.5
Men	3.2 ± 1.2
Women	2.9 ± 1.9
Apolipoprotein A1	147 ± 27
Men	139 ± 23
Women	158 ± 29
Apolipoprotein B	116 ± 26
Men	115 ± 24
Women	119 ± 27

[a] See Table 26.1 for abbrevations.

[b] DHHS NCHS. *Third National Health and Nutrition Examinations Survey*, 1988-94, NHANES III, Hyattsville, MD, 1996.

Chylomicrons

These particles originate in the small intestine when fat is absorbed, and are absent in plasma from fasting subjects. They are visibly present in blood when TG levels exceed 7.90 mmol/L, and the refrigerated plasma may appear turbid (Figure 52.8, Section 52). At higher TG levels the standing plasma will show a creamy top layer. Chylomicrons are transported into the lymphatic system, delivered into the blood, and removed by the action of the enzyme lipoprotein lipase (LPL) to produce remnant particles that are taken up by specifc receptors in the liver. (Figure 26.1). The composition of chylomicrons is listed in Table 26.1.

VLDL

These particles are produced in the liver and result from *in vivo* synthesis from carbohydrate precursors or from free fatty acids mobilized from adipose tissue and delivered to the liver. VLDL composition is given in Table 26.1. The standing plasma begins to appear diffusely turbid when TG levels exceed 2.25 mmol/L (Figure 52.8, Section 52). Lipoprotein lipase action produces VLDL remnants, or IDL, that are rapidly removed from the blood by receptors in the liver (Figure 26.1). An assay for VLDL remnants that has been developed for research studies[12] is under consideration by laboratory manufacturers for clinical applications.

TABLE 26.5

Tests for Plasma Lipids, Lipoproteins, and Lipolytic Enzymes

Assay	Principle of Method	Reference Method	Clinical/Usual Method	Performance Criteria
Total cholesterol	Chemical	Abell-Kendall[5]		CV ≤3%
	Spectrophotometric			Bias <3%
	Modified Liebermann-Burchard[4a,b]			
	Automated enzymatic		Allain[6]	
	Colorimetric		Rautela[7]	
Triacylglycerol (TG)	Glycerol assay	Van Handel-Zilversmit[8]		CV <5%
	Spectrophotometric			Bias <5%
	Automated enzymatic			
	Spectrophotometric		Sampson[9]	
			Hagen[10]	
VLDL			Rautela[11]	
VLDL remnant	Ultracentrifugation		Nakajima[12]	
LDL-calculate	TC-{HDL-C + TG/5}		Friedewald[13]	CV <4%
LDL ultracentrifuge	C in d<1.006 – HDL-C	Beta-quant	Havel-Eder-Bragdon[14]	Bias <4%
LDL direct	Precipitation of chylomicrons, VLDL IDL, HDL by antibodies to apo-E and apo A-I		McNamara[15]	
Lp(a)	ELISA		Marcovina[17]	
HDL	Heparin-Mn or dextran-Mg precipitation of VLDL, LDL; analyze C in supernatant		Burstein[19]	CV <4%
			Warnick[20]	Bias <5%
Apo A-I	Immunoassay	Not available	Albers[24]	CV 6%
Apo B	Immunoassay	Not available	Warnick[25]	
Phospholipids	Lipid phosphorus (lipid extract)		Bartlett[26]	
Free fatty acids	Titration of extracted plasma		Dole-Meinertz[27]	
Fatty acid composition	Gas-liquid chromatography of fatty acid methyl esters		Nelson[28]	
Lipoprotein lipase (LPL)	Hydrolysis of radioactive lipid emulsion by post-heparin plasma		Olivecrona[30]	3-5% accuracy
				Plasma pool
Hepatic lipase (HL)	Antiserum to HL		Huttunen[31]	Values lower in women
	NaCl inhibition of LPL			
Lecithin-cholesterol acyl transferase (LCAT)	Double antibody radioimmunoassay		Albers[32]	

Note: CV = coefficient of variation.

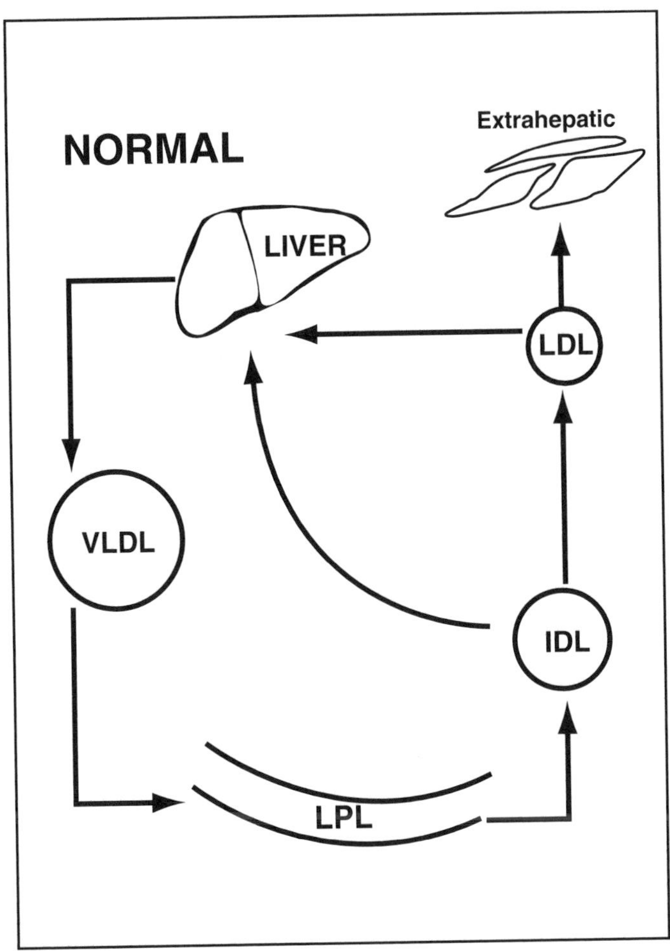

FIGURE 26.1
Production of lipoproteins, delivery into blood, and removal by tissues. See Table 26.1 for abbreviations. LPL = lipoprotein lipase.

IDL

This TG-rich particle is relatively enriched in the proportion of cholesterol esters compared to its precursor VLDL (Table 26.1). The atherogenic beta-VLDL is a related cholesterol-rich particle with interactions with the LDL and remnant receptors (Figure 26.1). This particle is evanescent in the plasma of healthy normolipidemic subjects.

LDL

This particle is the main transporter of cholesterol in the blood and is considered the most atherogenic lipoprotein. The LDL cholesterol level reflects changes in lipoprotein composition. LDL delivers cholesterol to cells and is taken up by specific cell surface receptors (Figure 26.2). LDL assays are listed in Table 26.5. LDL cholesterol may be calculated as:

$$\text{LDL} = [\text{Total cholesterol}] - [\text{HDL-cholesterol}] - [\text{TG}/5]$$ [13]

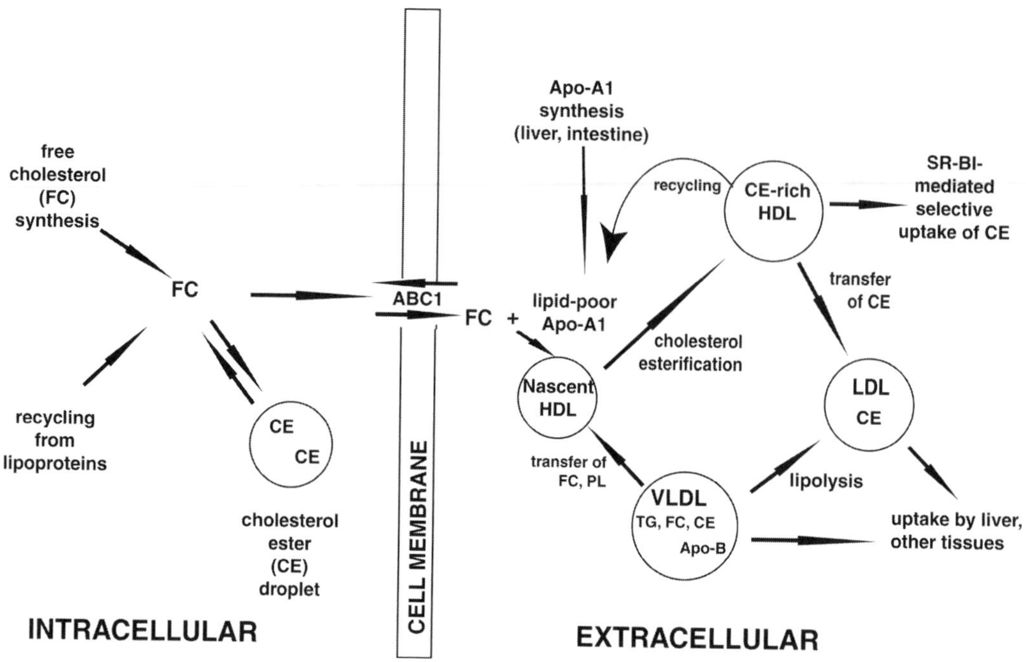

FIGURE 26.2
The generation of HDL and the interrelations of the lipoproteins, their production, and removal. ABC 1 = ATP-binding-cassette transporter. SRB 1 = Scavenger receptor binder. Adapted from Young S. G., and Fielding C. J., *Nature Genetics*, 22, 316, 1999.

Alternatively, LDL can be measured by ultracentrifugation (beta-quantification, or beta-quant)[14] or directly, using an immunologic procedure[15] (Table 26.5).

LDL particle size is variable, ranging from large and buoyant to small and dense (Table 26.6). The small dense particle, oxidative changes in LDL, and the presence of a variant of LDL, Lp(a), raise the atherogenicity of LDL. Lp(a) levels range from undetectable to 1000 mg/L. The risk of atherosclerosis increases as values exceed 300 mg/L. The Lp (a) assay[17] is listed in Table 26.5.

HDL

The HDL particle is generated by the transfer of surface lipids from TG-rich lipoproteins during lipolysis[18] (Figure 26.2). The HDL2 and HDL3 particles differ in size and composition, and particles vary in their content of the specific apolipoproteins, apo A-I and A-II (Tables 26.1 and 26.6). HDL is protective against atherosclerosis, enhancing removal mechanisms by reverse cholesterol transport. Methods of assay[19, 20] are described in Table 26.5.

Standardization of Assays

Blood samples for assays of serum or plasma lipids and lipoproteins should be obtained under standardized conditions of a stable diet, avoiding alcohol, and in the morning after an overnight fast. Serum and plasma values differ as do values of cholesterol when the

TABLE 26.6

Lipoprotein Subclasses[a]

Particle	Diameter	nm	Association with Risk of CVD
VLDL 1	Large	80	Higher
2	Medium	70	Intermediate
3	Small	60	Lower
IDL 1	Large	40	Higher
2	Small		
LDL I	Large	30	Lower
II a			
II b			
III a	Medium		Intermediate
III b			
IV a	Small		Higher
IV b		20	
HDL 2 b	Large	10	Negative risk
2 a		9	
3 a	Small	8	Positive risk
3 b		7	
3 c		6	

[a] See Table 26.1 for abbreviations.

subject is supine, sitting, or standing. A recent meal has minor effects on cholesterol and predominantly cholesterol-containing lipoproteins (LDL, HDL), but has a major influence on levels of TG and TG-containing lipoproteins (VLDL). Optimally, determinations should be carried out on plasma samples obtained by using EDTA as anticoagulant and prepared and stored carefully. The biological variation of cholesterol, within the normal range, approximates 16%.[21] Laboratory accuracy and precision should be standardized with reference materials or reference laboratories.[22] Because of variability, more than one sample of plasma or serum lipids should be drawn, with an interval of several weeks of unchanged lifestyle, and analyzed in order to evaluate lipid status or therapy.[23]

A simple clue to lipid/lipoprotein values is provided by the standing plasma test (Figure 52.8, Section 52). Plasma is refrigerated overnight and examined for turbidity. Hypercholesterolemia does not cause the plasma to become cloudy, whereas elevated TG, either as VLDL, remnants, or chylomicrons will produce diffuse turbidity with or without a creamy supernatant layer (see Section 52).

Apoproteins

The apolipoproteins or apoproteins determine the metabolic fate of the lipoprotein particles and the solubility of lipoprotein lipids in plasma. They include:

- Apo A-I
- Apo A-II
- Apo A-IV
- Apo B-100
- Apo B-48

- Apo C-I
- Apo C-II
- Apo C-III
- Apo-D
- Apo E-2
- Apo E-3 {E-phenotype: E2/2, 2/3, 2/4, 3/3, 3/4, 4/4}
- Apo E-4
- Apo-F
- Apo-G
- Apo-H
- Apo-J
- Apo (a)

Their distribution among the lipoproteins is shown in Table 26.1.

The assay methods available in some clinical laboratories[24,25] are provided in Table 26.5. The mean values in plasma are provided in Table 26.7. The apoprotein level indicates the number of lipoprotein particles in plasma (i.e., concentration). The apoprotein composition and levels are determined in some genetic and lipid laboratories using electrophoretic and immunologic methods.

Other Lipid Assays

- Phospholipids are determined by measuring lipid phosphorus after lipid extraction.[26]
- Free fatty acids in plasma can be analyzed, usually in relation to metabolic abnormalities, such as diabetes mellitus, and related to values of glucose and insulin. The assay is listed in Table 26.5.[27]
- The fatty acid composition of plasma lipids, and separated and isolated free fatty acids, cholesterol esters, phospholipids, or TG can be quantified.[28] This may be useful in the diagnosis of essential fatty acid deficiency and some inborn errors of metabolism.
- Fecal fat can be measured as free fatty acids or TG fatty acids in order to test for malabsorption syndromes.[29]

Regulators of Lipid Metabolism

Enzymes, receptors, and transporters involved in the regulation of lipid and lipoprotein metabolism are listed in Section 52, Table 52.1. Their values are determined primarily in lipid research laboratories rather than as part of the usual clinical lipid profile for patient

TABLE 26.7

Average Levels of Apoproteins in Plasma (mg/L)[a,b]

Apoprotein	Mean ± SD
A-I	1,200 ± 200 (men)
	1,350 ± 250 (women)
A-II	330 ± 50 (men)
	360 ± 60 (women)
B	1,000 ± 200
C-I	70 ± 20
C-II	40 ± 20
C-III	130 ± 50
D	60 ± 10
E	50 ± 20

[a] SD = standard deviations.
[b] From Albers, in *Eleventh International Congress of Clinical Chemistry.* Keuser, E., Giabal, F., Muller, M. M., et al., Eds., Walter de Greyter, Berlin, 1982, with permission.

assessment. Methods for the determination of post-heparin lipolytic activity, lipoprotein lipase,[30] hepatic lipase,[31] and lecithin:cholesterol acyltransferase[32] are listed in Table 26.5.

References

1. Feldman EB. *Essentials of Clinical Nutrition* FA Davis, Philadelphia, 1988.
2. Lipid Research Clinics Program, *JAMA* 251, 351, 1984.
3. NHANES III, *JAMA* 269, 3000, 1993.
4a. Liebermann C. *Ber Deut Chem Ges* 18, 1803, 1885.
4b. Burchard H. *Chem Zentraalbl* 610, 25, 1890.
5. Abell LL, Levy BB, Brodie BB, Kendall FE. *J Biol Chem* 195, 357, 1952.
6. Allain CC, Pool NS, Chan CSG, et al. *Clin Chem* 20, 470, 1974.
7. Rautela SS, Liedtke RJ. *Clin Chem* 24, 108, 1978.
8. Van Handel E, Zilversmit DB. *J Lab Clin Med* 50P, 152, 1957.
9. Sampson EG, Demers LM, Kreig AF. *Clin Chem* 21, 1983, 1975.
10. Hagen JR, Hagen PB. *Can J Biochem Physiol* 40, 1129, 1962.
11. Rautela SS. *Clin Chem* 20, 857, 1974.
12. Nakajima K, Sato T, Tamura A, et al. *Clin Chim Acta* 223, 53, 1993.
13. Friedewald WT, Levy RI, Fredrickson DS. *Clin Chem* 18, 499, 1972.
14. Havel RJ, Eder HA, Bragdon JH. *J Clin Invest* 34, 1345, 1955.
15. McNamara JR, Cole TG, Contols JH, et al. *Clin Chem* 46, 232, 1995.
16. Krauss RM, Burke DJ. *J Lipid Res* 12, 97, 1983.
17. Marcovina SM, Albers JJ, Gabel B, et al. *Clin Chem* 41, 246, 1995.
18. Young SG, Fielding CJ. *Nature Genetics* 22, 316, 1999.
19. Burstein M, Scholnick HR, Mortin R. *J Lipid Research* 11, 283, 1970.

20. Warnick GR. *Clin Chem* 28, 1379, 1982.
21. Cooper GR, Myers GL, Smith SJ, Schlant RC. *JAMA* 267, 1652, 1992.
22. *Handbook of Lipoprotein Testing,* Ed. Rifai N, Warnick GR, Dominiczak MH. AACC Press, Washington, DC, 1997.
23. Smith SJ, Cooper GR, Myers GL, Sampson EJ. *Clin Chem* 39, 1012, 1993.
24. Albers JJ. The determination of apoproteins and their diagnostic value in clinical chemistry. 11th International Congress of Clinical Chemistry, Kaiser E, Gabal F, Muller MM, et al, Eds., Walter de Gruyter, Berlin, 1982.
25. Warnick GR, Cheung MC, Albers JJ. *Clin Chem* 25, 596, 1979.
26. Bartlett GR. *J Biol Chem* 223, 466, 1959.
27. Dole VP, Meinertz H. *J Biol Chem* 231, 2959, 1960.
28. *Blood Lipids and Lipoproteins Quantitation, Composition and Metabolism,* Nelson GH, Ed., Wiley Interscience, NY, 1972.
29. Van de Kamer JH, Huinink HTB, Weijers HA. *J Biol Chem* 177, 347, 1949.
30. Bengtsson-Oivecrona O, Olivecrona T. Assay of lipoprotein lipase. In *Lipoprotein Analysis. A Practical Approach,* Skinner RE, Converse CA, Eds., Oxford University Press, Oxford, 1992, p 169.
31. Huttunen Y, Enholm C, Kinnunen PKJ, Nikkila EA. *Clin Chim Acta* 63, 335, 1975.
32. Albers JJ, Chen C-H, Lacco AG. *Methods in Enzymology* 129, 763, 1986.

27

Genetics of Energy and Nutrient Intake

Treva Rice, Louis Pérusse, and Claude Bouchard

Introduction

The study of the role of genetic variation on energy intake and nutrient intake is broad and has considerable public health implications. Genetic differences influence behavioral and biological affectors of food intake. They are also thought to impact on several nutritionally influenced risk factors (e.g., dyslipoproteinemia) and morbid conditions (e.g., diabetes). These issues have been the topic of much research in the past few decades, as evidenced by the multiple review articles cited in this section. In the behavioral domain, the questions are relatively simple. Do genes determine eating behaviors such as how much one eats, preferences for certain types of foods, and frequency or pattern of eating? The current research suggests that there is resemblance among family members for these behaviors, although it is unclear if they are determined by genes, shared environments, or both.[1] In the physiological domain the questions center on the physical and hormonal mechanisms leading to such things as taste preferences, hunger, and satiety. For instance, taste receptors are clearly genetically determined, although the gene(s) may not be all identified yet,[2] and a growing number of genes encoding hormones and proteins that regulate hunger and satiety have been identified recently.[3]

The genetics of energy and nutrition intake invoke complex issues from the fields of genetic and molecular epidemiology, involving both genetic and environmental interactions. Gene-gene (GxG) interactions occur when the effect of one gene is modified by or depends on the effects of another. For example, leptin is a hormone involved in the signaling between adipose tissue and the hypothalamus. The gene (LEP) that synthesizes leptin has been identified and mapped to chromosome 7. However, multiple factors influence the circulating levels of leptin, and some of these (such as insulin levels) have their own genetic determinants. Thus, the measurable levels of circulating leptin can be influenced by interactions with other genes.

Another complex issue from genetic and molecular epidemiology involves gene-environment interactions (GxE). In this situation, energy and nutrient intake are considered environmental factors which impact on other traits that may have a profound interest from a public health perspective. For example, the exposure of individuals with certain

0-8493-2705-9/01/$0.00+$1.50

genetic mutations to high-fat/cholesterol environments may predispose them to develop disease, while other individuals with alternative gene forms promoting genetic protection remain free of disease in the same high-risk environment. Such gene-diet interaction questions have been addressed in the fields of genetic and molecular epidemiology and constitute the major focus of this review.

This section does not claim to extensively review every topic relating to the genetics of energy and nutrient intake. Rather, an attempt is made to give an overview of the breadth of the problem, some interesting findings, and suggestions for further study. A short review of genetic and molecular epidemiology methods is followed by overviews of the familial factors underlying the behavioral aspects of macronutrient intake, and gene-diet interaction effects on risk factors for coronary disease.

Genetic and Molecular Epidemiology

Before investigating the complex issues of GxE interactions, it must first be established that the trait of interest is heritable, or that it runs in families. Familial resemblance for a trait arises when members within families are more similar than are unrelated pairs of individuals and may be estimated in terms of correlations (or covariances) among family members. Methods for estimating familial resemblance range from relatively simple to very complex.[4,5] However, the cause of the familial resemblance may be due to shared genes, shared environments, or both. In the case where the gene is not known, or not measured, familial resemblance is indexed by comparing the degree of phenotypic (trait) sharing among family members of varying degrees of relatedness. For example, sibling, parent-offspring and dizygotic (DZ) twins share 50% of their genes in common, monozygotic (MZ) twins share 100% of their genes in common, and spouse pairs share few or no genes in common if there is random mating for the trait under study. Depending on cohabitation effects, all of these relative pairs may share some degree of family environments.

Maximal heritability quantifies the strength of the familial resemblance. It represents the percentage of variance in a trait that is due to all additive familial effects, and can include both genetic and familial environmental sources. Depending on the complexity of the study design, this may be partitioned into separate estimates of genetic versus cultural (familial environmental) heritabilities. Each of the genetic and familial environmental sources may be partitioned further. For example, complex traits (phenotypes) may be due to one or more genes with moderate to major effects (oligogenic), many genes each having small effects (polygenic), and/or familial environments that are specific to certain relative pairs such as sibling, twin, or spouse.

In addition to these main effects of genes and familial environments, there may be interactions among these factors such as gene-gene (epistasis) and GxE. These effects are generally non-additive and thus may not be identified in heritability studies described above. Of major interest in this review are GxEs that arise when the phenotypic expression of a trait corresponding to a particular genotype depends, in part, on exposure to particular environmental factors. For example, GxE may occur if the fat mass response to dietary intervention depends on (or is modified by) an individual's genotype. In the hypothetical case of Figure 27.1, an absence of GxE is depicted in panel (a), where the body fat response to increasing fat intake is consistent across genotypes, with a simple mean shift by genotype. In contrast, GxE is present in panel (b), where some genotypes show very different patterns of fat mass accumulation with increasing levels of energy intake.

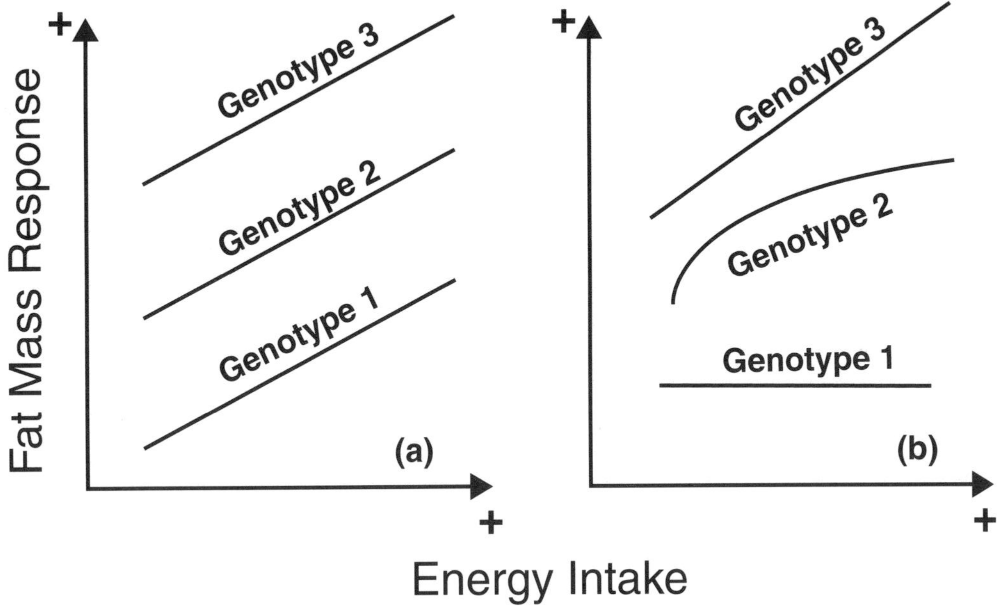

FIGURE 27.1
Hypothetical example of three genotypes plotted by energy intake (X-axis) and fat mass (Y-axis) values. In panel (a), there is no gene-diet interaction since the lines depicting the responses by genotype are parallel. In panel (b), gene by diet interaction is demonstrated, since there is a differential response in fat mass due to energy intake as a function of the genotype. That is, the genotypes respond differently.

Two major approaches are used to study GxE, unmeasured genotype (genetic epidemiology) and measured genotype (molecular epidemiology), as recently reviewed by Pérusse and Bouchard.[6] The twin methodology is a very useful unmeasured genotype approach for testing GxE. One important assumption underlying the twin method is that MZ and DZ twins have equal environmental covariances. Variances can be tested for significant differences across twin types using classical analysis of variance approaches. If the variances are different prior to but not after adjustment for pertinent environmental covariates, then there is indirect evidence of GxE interaction. Alternatively, the twins can be stratified according to degree of environmental sharing, and heritability estimates may be compared across the strata.

The above twin method is cross-sectional and therefore an indirect assessment of the GxE effects. Another unmeasured genotype approach that more directly indexes GxE is the twin intervention study, where MZ pairs (who share 100% of their genes in common) are challenged under standardized treatments (environments). A comparison of the within- and between-pair variances of the response to treatment provides an indication of whether genetic factors underlie the response. That is, a greater variability between- than within-pairs suggests a greater correlated response to environmental challenge for the same genotype.

The second major approach for detecting GxE involves measured genotypes,[6] with the preponderance of evidence for measured gene-nutrition interactions arising from intervention studies. This method is usually applied to association analysis of candidate genes. However, it can be applied to association or linkage analysis of candidate genes or genome scan data.[7] Linkage studies seek identification of loci that cosegregate with the trait (e.g., dietary response) within families, while association studies seek identification of particular variants that are associated with the response at the population level. In other words, linkage analysis is often useful in localizing gene effects but requires family data, while association analysis can provide information about the functional variants that ultimately give rise to the observed phenotypic variability and may be applied to family or individual data. These complementary methods provide the means to probe the genome and describe the complex genetic etiologies underlying the responses to interventions. In association analysis of candidate genes, the phenotypic responses to intervention are compared among groups stratified by genotypes. If individuals with a particular allele form tend to respond to the intervention differently than do individuals with alternative allele forms, then there is evidence of GxEs. GxG interactions are simply incorporated in association analysis by including the main effects of multiple candidate genes, as well as the interaction terms between them.

Although association analysis may be applied to either individual or family data, the dependencies among related individuals should be considered, since failure to adjust for nonindependence can inflate the association evidence. Methods for dealing with this problem range from complex, such as bootstrapping[8] where the model is repeatedly fit to subsets of the data, to relatively simple, such as sandwich estimators.[9,10] The sandwich method asymptotically yields the same parameter estimates as ordinary least squares or regression methods, but the standard errors (and consequently hypothesis tests) are adjusted for the dependencies.

Familial Factors Underlying Macronutrient Intake

In the last few decades, the familial factors underlying macro- and micronutrient intake have been characterized. These studies differed in many respects, making direct comparisons difficult. For example, study designs (twin vs. family), statistical methods of analysis and how macronutrient intake was measured (diaries ranging from 3 to 9 days, 24-hour recall) and reported (absolute vs. percent of kcalories, and adjusted vs. unadjusted for covariates) varied.[1,11] The major conclusion drawn from a review of these studies is that there is familial resemblance, although the source of the resemblance is unclear. For example, deCastro,[12] using a twin design, reported that additive genetic effects accounted for 40 to 65% of the variance for each macronutrient examined, and that there was no contribution from familial environmental sources. On the other hand, two family studies [13,14] suggested that most of the resemblance (30 to 50% of the variance) was due to familial environmental factors. An early study, involving the largest sample sizes reported to date,[15] reflects the most probable answer to the question of genetic vs. environmental determination of food intake: people who live together come to resemble each other whether they are genetically related or not. This conclusion is based on the fact that correlations between genetically unrelated pairs of individuals who live together are as large as those for genetically related cohabitating individuals. Similar conclusions were drawn from both twin[12,16] and family studies.[13,14,17,18]

The magnitude of the familial effect for macronutrient intake generally centers between 30 to 50% in family studies, with higher estimates derived from many twin studies. However, as shown in Table 27.1, there is a considerable range in estimates across studies. Moreover, resemblance tends to be higher for nutrients expressed in percent of total caloric intake as compared to absolute amounts, both across studies and within studies that indexed both types of measures.[13,19] This suggests that the familial effect may be specific to food selection or preference (nutrient concentrations) rather than for amount of foods consumed. Results from twin studies [20,21] and from animal models showing differences in

TABLE 27.1

Range of Heritability Estimates (%) for Macronutrients*

Macronutrient	Genetic	Cultural	Combined
Total kcalories	0–78	23–45	24–51
Absolute values			
Protein	0–70	26–41	8
Total fat	0–56	26–50	9–24
Saturated fat	50–60		10–27
Monounsaturated fats			33–41
Polyunsaturated fats	10–40		3
Saturated/unsaturated ratio			3–12
Total carbohydrates	0–68	20–26	31–36
Simple carbohydrates	12–60		8–20
Complex carbohydrates	22–62		55–56
Sodium			10–71
Dietary Na/K			20–68
Urinary Na/K			18–53
Percent of total kcalories			
Protein	10–70	25–61	61
Total fat	18–48	8–51	27–54
Saturated fat			10–70
Monounsaturated fats			50
Polyunsaturated fats			47
Total carbohydrates	15–67	12–47	52
Dietary cholesterol			66
Sodium			51
Potassium			24
Calcium			52

* Estimates extracted from References 12-14, 16-19, 102.

macronutrient selection among various mouse strains[22] also suggest that food preferences are partly explained by genetic factors. From this review it appears likely that there are substantial familial effects underlying nutrient intake, but whether this effect is due to genetic, familial environmental, or both factors is unclear.

Gene-Diet Interactions

While an appropriate diet is recommended for reducing the risks of many common diseases, it is well known that there is a great deal of variability in people's responses to dietary change. For example, atherogenic diets may carry little risk for some people, but for others dietary changes generally have a good outcome. While the causes for this heterogeneity across people are not completely understood, there is convincing evidence that genes play a role. Phenylketonuria (PKU), an inborn error of metabolism causing an accumulation of phenylalanine in the blood leading to mental retardation, is a classic example. Restriction of dietary phenylananine in individuals who are homozygous for the mutation reduces the phenylalanine accumulation and mental retardation.

The following summary of gene-diet interactions is organized around two general topics: 1) adiposity and 2) lipids and lipoproteins. A summary of some of the genes that may interact with dietary intake to influence these phenotypic domains is given in Table 27.2. Most of the molecular work investigating specific genes has centered on the latter domain.

TABLE 27.2

Summary of Measured Gene-Diet Interactions

Gene*	Cytogenic Location*	Intervention**	Response Phenotype	Study
MTHFR	1p36.32	Cross-sectional, folate	Homocysteine	Jing Ma et al., 1996[92]
TNFR2	1p36.23	High fat	Wt, insulin, leptin in mice	Schreyer et al., 1998[39]
		Cross-section, diet-treated diabetic vs nondiabetic	BMI, leptin	Fernandez-Real et al., 2000[40]
Dob1	1p35-1p31	High fat	Mice bred for diet response	West et al., 1994a, 1994b[29,30]
LEPR	1p22.3	Overfeeding	Fasting insulin, leptin, HDL-c	Ukkola et al., 2000b[46]
HSD3B1	1p12	Aging (longitudinal)	Skinfold sum	Vohl et al., 1994[103]
APOB	2p22.3	Crossover, high vs low saturated fat and cholesterol	CH, LDL-c	Friedlander et al., 2000[59]
		Crossover, saturated vs monounsaturated fat	ApoAI, LDL-c, ApoB, HDL-c	Dreon et al., 1994; 1995[88,89]
		Crossover, high saturated vs NCEP vs high monounsaturated	TG	Lopez-Miranda et al., 2000[83]
IRS1	2q36.3	Optifast wt loss program: diet, exercise, and support group	Wt loss	Benecke et al., 2000[38]
Dob2	3p21	High fat	Mice bred for diet response	West et al., 1994a, 1994b[29,30]
PPARG	3p25.2	Aging (longitudinal) obese vs lean	BMI change	Ek et al., 1999[49]
FABP2	4q26	Crossover, insoluble vs soluble fiber	Total cholesterol, LDL-c, ApoB	Hegele et al., 1997[45]
UCP1	4q28.2	Low kcalorie	Wt and BMI loss	Fumeron et al., 1996[104]
		Low kcalorie + exercise	Wt loss	Kogure et al., 1998[44]
GRL	5q31.3	Overfeeding	Wt, AVF, SBP, CH	Ukkola et al., 2000a[36]
ADRB2	5q32	Overfeeding	Wt, leptin, SF8, OGTT insulin area, abdominal total fat	Ukkola et al., 2000c[37]
		Crossover, saturated vs monounsaturated fats	TG	López-Miranda et al., 2000[83]
LEP	7q31.33	Low kcalorie	Leptin	Mammes et al., 1998[45]
		Low kcalorie	Wt loss	Oksanen et al., 1997[105]
LPL	8p21.3	Low kcalorie	TG, VLDL-tg, ApoB	Jemaa et al., 1997[74]
		Crossover, high saturated vs low saturated and high polyunsaturated	CH	Humphries et al., 1996[75]
		Crossover, high vs low saturated fat and cholesterol	TG, HDL-c	Friedlander et al., 2000[59]

ADRB3	8p11.22	Aging morbid obese vs normal wt	Wt gain	Nagase et al., 1997[53]
			Wt gain	Clément et al., 1995[54]
		Optifast wt loss program: diet, exercise, and support group	Wt loss	Benecke et al., 2000[38]
Dob3	8q23-q24	High fat	Mice bred for diet response	West et al., 1994a, 1994b[29,30]
Dob1	9p13	High fat	Mice bred for diet response	West et al., 1994a, 1994b[29,30]
UCP3	11q14.1	Cross-sectional, morbidly obese vs nonobese	BMI, max BMI, Wt, diabetes	Otabe et al., 1999[43]
APOCIII	11q23.2	Crossover, saturated vs monounsaturated fats	CH, LDL-c, Apo B	López-Miranda et al., 1997[82]
APOAI	11q23.2	Crossover, saturated vs monounsaturated fats	LDL-c	López-Miranda et al., 1994[78]
APOAIV	11q23.2	Reduced fat	HDL-c, TG	Dreon et al., 1994; 1995[88,89]
		High cholesterol	LDL-c	McCombs et al., 1994[79]
		Crossover, NCEP vs average	LDL-c, HDL-c, TG	Mata et al., 1994[80]
		Crossover, saturated vs monounsaturated fats	CH, LDL-c, Apo B	Jansen et al., 1997[81]
CETP	16q21	Cross-sectional, alcohol	HDL-c	Fumeron et al., 1995[96]
LDLR	19p13.2	Fiber	ApoB, total cholesterol, LDL-c	Hegele et al., 1993[84]
APOE	19q13.32	Reduced fat	LDL particle size	Dreon et al., 1994; 1995[88,89]
		Crossover, low vs high cholesterol	HDL-c, CETP	Martin et al., 1993[86]
		Crossover, low vs high fat	HDL-c subclasses and LDL particle size	Williams et al., 1995[87]

* MTHFR = 5,10-methylenetetrahydrofolate reductase (NADPH); TNFR2 = tumor necrosis factor alpha, receptor 2; Dob1 = Dietary obese; HSD3B1 = hydroxy-delta-5-steroid dehydrogenase, 3 beta- and steroid delta-isomerase 1; APOB = apolipoprotein B; IRS1 = insulin receptor substrate 1; Dob2 = Dietary obese; PPARG = peroxisome proliferative activated receptor, gamma; FABP2 = fatty acid binding protein 2; UCP1 = uncoupling protein 1; GRL = glucocorticoid receptor locus; ADRB2 = beta 2 adrenergic receptor; LEP = leptin; LPL = lipoprotein lipase; ADRB3 = beta 3 adrenergic receptor; Dob3 = Dietary obese; Dob1 = Dietary obese; UCP3 = uncoupling protein 3; APOCIII = apolipoprotein C-III; APOAI = apolipoprotein A-I; APOAIV = apolipoprotein A-IV; CETP = cholesteryl ester transfer protein, plasma; LDLR = low-density lipoprotein receptor; APOE = apolipoprotein E.

** Cross-sectional = different subjects across groups; Crossover = same subjects with repeated measured across groups; NCEP = National Cholesterol Education Program diet (total fat < 30%, saturated fat < 10%, cholesterol intake < 300 mg/d)

Regarding the twin intervention method, one series of studies dominates the literature. This was an overfeeding experiment involving MZ twin pairs. In the long-term experiment, 12 pairs of male MZ twins were submitted to a 1000 kcal surplus diet 6 days a week for a period of 100 days.[23] The nutrient content of the diet was 50% carbohydrate, 35% lipid, and 15% protein. During the course of the protocol the excess energy intake was 84,000 kcal. In the short-term experiment, 6 pairs of male MZ twins were given the same protocol for a period of 22 consecutive days[24] In both the long-term and short-term experiments, a variety of physical and metabolic measurements spanning the phenotypic domains listed above were measured before and after the dietary interventions. Genetic epidemiology results from both the long-term and short-term studies have been reported in several publications and provide evidence for GxE interaction. More recently, association studies of the responses to overfeeding for a few candidate genes have been reported.

Adiposity

It is not surprising that overfeeding has an adverse effect on adiposity. In general, an increase in caloric intake leads to an increase in adiposity, and this effect appears to be more pronounced in some individuals, depending on genotypes. Evidence for these conclusions arises from several sources using different study designs.[6,25-27]

More direct evidence of GxE on adiposity was obtained in both the short-term[24] and long-term[23] MZ intervention experiments. In the long-term intervention experiment, there was a mean increase in body mass of 8.1 kg, with a threefold difference between the lowest and highest gainers, ranging from 4 to 12 kg.[23] The variability in response for weight was at least three times greater (F-ratio of 3.4) between unrelated individuals than within twin pairs, suggesting a significant genotype–overfeeding interaction. Similar magnitudes of results were found for body mass index (BMI), percent body fat, fat mass measured with underwater weighing, and subcutaneous fat measured by summing across six skinfolds. Moreover, the variance was six times greater between than within pairs for abdominal visceral fat (measured with computed tomography scan) after adjusting for total fat mass. These findings indicate that some individuals tend to store fat predominantly in selected fat depots in response to caloric surplus primarily as a result of genetic factors. In another MZ twin intervention study,[28] the opposite dietary treatment was conducted. Fourteen pairs of female MZ twins were strictly supervised for 28 days on a very low calorie diet. The diet provided for 1.6 MJ/day and included 37 g protein, 50 g carbohydrates, and 3.8 g fat. Significant diet-induced reductions were seen for several measures of body composition, including weight, BMI, percent fat, fat mass, abdominal fat, and several skinfold measures. Moreover, the variance was 11 to 17 times higher among unrelated individuals than between twin pairs, suggesting a significant GxE interaction effect. Together, these twin studies suggest that the changes in body composition due to dietary intervention (both overfeeding and underfeeding) are due in part to the genotype.

Some of the evidence for gene-diet interactions on adiposity comes from the measured genotype approach. Given the obvious connection between food intake and obesity, there is nevertheless a paucity of measured gene-by-diet interaction studies of obesity. West et al. provided early evidence of gene-diet interaction on obesity in mice.[29,30] Nine strains of mice were selectively bred for their responses to a high-fat diet; there was a sixfold difference in adiposity gain between strains that were sensitive (AKR/J) and resistant (SWR/J) to weight gain. Three dietary obese loci (Dob1, Dob2, and Dob3) were found to underlie these differences, and they have been mapped to syntenic human chromosomes on 1p35-p31 and 9p13 for Dob1, 3p21 for Dob2, and 8q23-q24 for Dob3. No studies were found reporting linkage or association of these genes to dietary responses in humans. However, linkage of nearby anonymous markers (D1S476, D1S200, D1S193,

D1S197 on chromosome 1 and D8S592 and D8S556 on chromosome 8) with several adiposity measures (BMI, sum of skinfolds, fat mass, percent fat, and leptin) has been reported.[31,32]

The lipoprotein lipase (LPL) gene has been implicated in gene-diet interactions in several reports. LPL plays a role in the regulation of plasma lipoprotein composition and concentrations, and in partitioning triglycerides between the adipose tissue for storage and the skeletal muscle for oxidation, and is thus an obvious candidate. Overexpression of LPL in skeletal muscle of transgenic mice was shown to protect against diet-induced obesity.[33] While no studies were found linking the changes in adiposity following dietary intervention with LPL in humans, it has been related to lipid responses (reviewed below). Moreover, the Hind III polymorphism was shown to modulate the relation between visceral fat and plasma triglycerides,[34] providing evidence of pleiotropy (i.e., a single gene impacting on multiple traits).

The glucocorticoid receptor locus (GRL) is also involved in the regulation of LPL activity and lipolysis, and glucocorticoids are insulin antagonists.[35] The Bcl I variant of the GRL locus was associated with the overfeeding response in weight and abdominal visceral fat in the MZ twin overfeeding study.[36] Individuals homozygous for the 2.3 kb allele had a greater increase in response to overfeeding. A similar result was noted for plasma total, LDL cholesterol, and systolic blood pressure responses in the same report, suggesting pleiotropy and that the GRL locus has an impact on the overall atherogenic profile response to overfeeding.

Another genetic factor related to lipolysis is the adrenergic system. Adrenergic receptors (ADR) can stimulate (B1, B2, B3) or inhibit (A2) lipolysis by modulating triglyceride breakdown in the adipocytes. Data from the MZ overfeeding study was used to investigate the effects of ADRA2, ADRB2, and ADRB3 polymorphisms on adiposity and fat distribution responses to overfeeding.[37] Results indicate a significant GxE effect for ADRB2 on weight, plasma leptin, sum of skinfolds, and insulin area under the OGTT (oral glucose tolerance test) curve. Greater weight gain in response to overfeeding occurred in Glu27Glu/Gln27Gln than Gln27Gln carriers of the ADRB2 gene. As with the LPL and GRL loci, ADRB2 impacted the response to overfeeding for multiple traits (i.e., pleiotropy). There were too few subjects with the rare alleles for the ADRA2 and ADRB3 loci in this study for a comprehensive investigation. However, in another study the response in obese women to a weight loss program was investigated for rare mutations at both the ADRB3 (Trp64Arg) and IRS1 (Gly972Arg) loci.[38] Carriers of both rare mutations lost less weight and had a higher frequency of type 2 diabetes than noncarriers. Thus, there is evidence of both pleiotropy (i.e., these loci affect both body composition and insulin levels) and oligogenic effects (i.e., multiple genes affect body composition) between these two genes.

Pleiotropy was also observed for the tumor necrosis factor alpha receptor, which may play a key role in the metabolic syndrome involving both diabetes and obesity. TNFA is expressed in adipose and muscle tissues and blocks the action of insulin. In a study of mice lacking one of the TNF receptors (TNFR2), weight, insulin, and leptin level responses to diet were all modulated by the TNFR genotype.[39] Although this marker has not been reported in gene-diet studies of humans, the presence of the A2 allele was seen to predispose subjects to obesity, higher leptin levels, and insulin resistance.[40] It is interesting to note that the TNFR2 locus is closely linked to the Dob1 (dietary obese) locus on chromosome 1p (Table 27.2).

The above findings for TNFR2, ADRB2, and ADRB3 suggest that each impacts on both adiposity and insulin responses to diet. Insulin is a lipogenic hormone regulating transcription of lipogenic genes, and can act directly or in conjunction with glucose metabolites. In animals, insulin inhibits food intake via receptors in the hypothalamus. The insulin response to diet was examined in the long-term MZ twin overfeeding experiment, in which an OGTT was administered.[41] The between-pair variance in response to overfeeding was 2.5 to 5 times higher than the within-pair variance for measures of fasting insulin and glucose and insulin sensitivity from the OGTT, suggesting gene-diet interactions. Thus, some individuals are more prone than others to modify their insulin and glucose levels and perhaps insulin sensitivity in response to overfeeding.

The number of studies looking for the genes underlying adiposity is currently in a rapid growth stage. For example, 48 different candidate genes have been associated with obesity-related phenotypes in the past few years, as recently reviewed by Pérusse et al.[42] Of these, at least seven candidates (HSD3B1, IRS1, PPARG, UCP1, LEP, ADRB3, and UCP3) were associated with changes in adiposity over time, although only four these (LEP, UCP1, UCP3, and IRS1) were investigated for responses to dietary intervention. All of these markers are good candidates for GxE interactions. The uncoupling proteins have a role in releasing stored energy as heat. UCP3, which is abundant in skeletal muscle tissue, was recently associated with weight change in the morbidly obese during diet therapy.[43] The G polymorphism of the UCP1 gene was also associated with weight loss after a treatment program that included a low-calorie diet and exercise in obese Japanese women.[44] Leptin is a hormone secreted primarily by adipose tissue and is generally considered to act as a satiety signal in a feedback loop with the brain. Several mutations in the LEP gene were associated with plasma leptin responses to dietary intervention in one study.[45] Those authors concluded that LEP may be a gene regulating the variability of responses to nutritional environments rather than for obesity per se. In the long-term MZ twin overfeeding experiment, the Gln223Arg variant of the leptin receptor (LEPR) was associated with several metabolic variables,[46] including plasma leptin, insulin, and HDL-c, but not body composition measures. The insulin receptor substrate 1 (IRS1) gene has a role in controlling cellular growth and metabolism, and was associated with longitudinal changes in BMI.[47] As previously outlined, rare mutations at both the IRS1 and ADRB3 loci led to less weight loss and higher type 2 diabetes in response to a weight loss program in obese women.[38]

The remaining markers listed above are also good candidates in gene-diet interaction effects on obesity, although few reports regarding gene-diet interactions were found. For example, the peroxisome proliferator-activated receptors (PPARs) are expressed in adipose tissue, and the gamma subtype (PPARG) has been implicated in adipose cell function, including lipid composition of the membrane and sensitivity to insulin.[48] PPARG was linked to longitudinal changes in BMI.[49] The adrenergic system (discussed above) has a role in regulating energy balance through thermogenesis and lipid mobilization in adipose tissue. The beta 3 adrenergic receptor (ADRB3) is thought to play a minor role in catecholamine-induced lipolysis. However, reports of linkage or association of ADRB3 to obesity and weight changes in humans have been inconsistent.[50-54]

Lipids, Lipoproteins, and Apolipoproteins

The lipid, lipoprotein, and apolipoprotein response to dietary intervention is the most extensively studied area of those reviewed in this section. A great deal of evidence[55-59] suggests that plasma lipid level responses are under genetic control. Individual differences in the plasma lipid profile response to dietary fats and cholesterols are found in several species, including mouse,[60] rat,[61] and monkey.[62,63] Some individuals are quite sensitive to changes (high-responders) and others are relatively insensitive (low-responders), as confirmed in a meta-analysis of 27 studies.[64] For example, early evidence of environmental (including dietary) effects on total cholesterol (CH), high density lipoprotein-cholesterol (HDL-c), HDL-c subfraction 2 (HDL2-c), and low density lipoprotein-cholesterol (LDL-c) using the twin design was reported by O'Connell et al.[65] Heritability estimates, although remaining significant, were decreased after adjusting for environmental factors, and by stratifying the sample based on nutritional variables. In another study of children with elevated LDL-c levels, the effect of a nutrition-education program was investigated.[66] Greater reductions in plasma total and LDL-c were observed in children with less family history of coronary heart disease.

Evidence for gene-diet interactions on HDL-c subfractions (HDL1-c, HDL2-c, and HDL3-c) were also reported in a baboon population.[67] The baboons were measured under a basal diet and again after being fed a high cholesterol and saturated fat challenge diet. The results suggested that there were both pleiotropic effects (i.e., the same gene(s) influencing multiple traits) and GxE interactions. The authors concluded that although a similar set of genes influenced the variation in each of the three subfractions under both diet conditions, the expression of the genes influencing HDL1-c and HDL2-c were altered by the high-fat diet (i.e., a GxE interaction).

Additional evidence of GxE effects come from the short-term MZ twin overfeeding intervention study. Plasma responses in CH, triglycerides (TG), LDL-c, HDL-c, and the HDL-c/CH ratio were investigated.[68] Although overfeeding induced significant changes only in CH and LDL-c, there were large interindividual differences in the responses of all of these variables. GxE interactions were detected for TG, HDL-c, and HDL-c/CH. It was noted that TG changes were negatively correlated with HDL changes, and that the correlated responses may be related to the susceptibility to develop hypertriglyceridemia, which is known to be under genetic control and related to changes in insulin concentrations.

Much of the evidence for GxE interactions on lipids, lipoproteins, and apolipoproteins involve the measured gene approach.[59,69-71] Genetic variations in several apolipoprotein genes (A-I, A-IV, B, CIII, E), the LDL receptor (LDLR) and LDL subclasses (patterns A and B) have been implicated in the dietary response of lipids.

The LPL gene discussed above, involved in partitioning exogeneous triglycerides between storage and oxidation, has been associated with plasma lipid levels and CHD risk.[72,73] In humans, several mutations have been implicated in the gene-diet interaction. For example, the Hind III polymorphism was associated with variability in plasma cholesterol, LDL-c, LDL-triglyceride, and Apo B responses to diet.[70,74,75] The N291S mutation showed a significant effect on TG and HDL-c responses to diet.[59] Other evidence from a MZ twin study (non-intervention) suggests GxE involvement of the Ser447Ter mutation.[76] Intrapair variances were different across twin types for CH, TG, and HDL-c levels, although the environmental source using this method is not specified. The authors suggested that this LPL variant acts as a restrictive variability gene, so that individuals without the mutation are more susceptible to fluctuations in plasma cholesterol and HDL-c.

Several of the apolipoprotein genes have been implicated in gene-diet interactions.[71,77] The APO A-I, A-IV, and C-III complex of genes is involved in lipid metabolism. A mutation in the A-I gene promoter region ($G \rightarrow A$) was associated with the plasma LDL-c response to a high monounsaturated fat diet.[78] Apo A-IV is an intestinal glycoprotein with two allele forms (A-IV-1 and A-IV-2); its synthesis is stimulated by dietary lipids and it may act centrally to inhibit food intake. Although conflicting reports are found, individuals homozygous for the A-IV-1 allele generally have lower HDL-c and higher TG.[71] In a crossover intervention study, subjects consumed a low-cholesterol diet for two weeks, then three weeks of a high-cholesterol diet.[79] In the high-cholesterol diet condition, plasma LDL-c increased more in the A-IV-1 group than the A-IV-2 group, with no change in HDL-c or TG levels for either genotype. Similar results were found in men (but not women) in another report combining data from three intervention studies.[80] In another study,[81] an $A \rightarrow T$ mutation in position 347 affected the total CH, LDL-c, and Apo B responses to a high fat diet. Lipid changes due to dietary intervention were found to be similar for the Apo C-III gene. For example, the SstI polymorphism interacted with diet to produce genotype-dependent responses in total CH, LDL-c, and Apo B levels.[82] Thus, for this cluster of apolipoprotein genes located on chromosome 11q within 1 cM of each other, there is consistent evidence of a gene-diet interaction effect on LDL-c, although the results for HDL-c and TG are not as clear.

The APOB gene is involved in the synthesis and secretion of chylomicrons and very low density lipoprotein (VLDL), and is a ligand for the interaction of LDL-c with the LDL receptor. Several variants have been associated with lipid responses to dietary intervention. While there are inconsistencies in the literature, genetic variations at both the Mspl and XbaI RFLPs have been reported to influence the plasma Apo A-I, LDL-c, Apo B, and HDL-c[71] and TG[83] responses to dietary fat and cholesterol. Moreover, an insertion/deletion polymorphism of the APOB gene was related to the lipoprotein response to increases in dietary fiber.[84]

Several studies investigated the role of APOE polymorphisms in the response of plasma LDL-c levels to dietary interventions.[85] Apo E is a protein associated with several lipoproteins, mediates the lipoprotein interaction with specific cell surface receptors, and has an important role in CH and TG metabolism. APOE has three common isoforms (E2, E3, and E4), with E3 the most common. APOE represents the most widely studied candidate, and although there are conflicting results in the literature,[55,71,85] most conclude that carriers of the E4 variant respond well to dietary intervention. Several possible explanations were suggested for the differences across studies; for example, expression of the response in absolute versus fractional levels. Since individuals with the E4 phenotype usually have higher initial plasma LDL-c levels, there is likely to be a larger absolute change, while the fractional change may be consistent across APOE phenotypes. Additional factors leading to inconsistencies across studies include low sample sizes leading to reduced power for testing hypotheses, and the sex ratio of subjects, since dietary responsiveness differs between sexes. Other factors include whether the intervention protocol reduced dietary fat, cholesterol, or fiber.[86,87] For example, a meta analysis of 16 studies showed that a greater lipid response in carriers of the E4 allele was only found when the dietary modification reduced total fat intake, irrespective of dietary cholesterol.[70] In another study, the increase in dietary fiber was associated with greater reductions in LDL-c in carriers of the E2 allele. Other studies also suggest a difference in the APOE gene association with plasma LDL-c response, depending on LDL particle size.[88,89] That is, the diet-induced change in LDL-c levels may not be due to reduced particle number but rather to a shift from larger cholesterol-rich LDL particles to smaller, denser LDL particles.

The LDL particles vary in size, density and lipid content. Subjects with small, dense LDL particles (subclass pattern B) exhibit higher levels of TG and Apo B and lower levels of HDL-c compared to subjects with a predominance of larger LDL particles (pattern A). Population studies have shown that about 30 to 35% of adult men exhibit the more atherogenic pattern B which is associated with a threefold higher risk of myocardial infarction. This lipoprotein phenotype is under strong genetic determination, with heritability levels of about 50% and evidence of a major gene effect.[90] The plasma lipoprotein response to changes in dietary fat in relation to the LDL subclass pattern was investigated in a dietary crossover experiment.[88,89] In this study, 105 men were randomly assigned to either a high fat (46%) or low fat (24%) diet for six weeks and then switched to the alternate diet for an additional six weeks. Subjects were categorized as pattern A (n=87) or pattern B (n=18), and the lipoprotein responses were analyzed as the changes from the high- to low-fat diets. After this dietary intervention, pattern B subjects exhibited a threefold greater reduction in LDL-c compared to pattern A subjects, while only men with pattern B exhibited a reduction in Apo B levels. These group differences were independent of BMI, Apo E phenotype, and plasma lipid levels. The decrease of LDL-c observed in pattern A subjects was due primarily to a shift in LDL particle mass from larger to smaller cholesterol-depleted LDL, without a change in LDL particle number. This shift in LDL distribution with the low fat diet induced expression of pattern B phenotype in 36 of the 87 pattern A subjects who did not express it on a high fat diet. Thus, in response to a low fat diet 41% of the pattern A subjects exhibited the more atherogenic pattern B lipoprotein profile. The results of this study provide a good example of genotype-diet interaction and show that dietary recommendations may not be equally good for every individual in the population.

LDLR mediate cholesterol uptake and are located on cells of many tissues. LDLR polymorphisms within the exon have been related to reductions in plasma concentrations of ApoB, total, and LDL cholesterol response to dietary fiber,[84] but not to the response of LDL-c concentrations to dietary fatty acids.[91]

MTHFR is an enzyme involved in folate production and in remethylation of homocysteine. Elevated levels of homocysteine are due to enzymatic deficiencies or to low intake of vitamins B_6, B_{12}, and folic acid, and are risk factors for coronary heart disease. Gene-diet interactions on homocysteine levels have been reported.[92] A MTHFR polymorphism was associated with increased homocysteine levels, but only in men with low folate intake. Thus, low folate intake may increase the risk of hyperhomocysteinemia in subjects with the MTHFR mutation. The MTHFR locus is closely linked to both the TNFR2 and Dob1 loci involved with adiposity responses to dietary intervention.

The FABP2 gene produces the intestinal fatty acid binding protein. It plays a role in absorption and intracellular transport of saturated and unsaturated long chain fatty acids.[93,94] The FABP2 T54 allele has been associated with insulin resistance and an atherogenic metabolic profile. In a crossover study of the effects of dietary soluble and insoluble fiber, the T54 allele was associated with a significant decrease in total and LDL cholesterol and Apo B during a period when the diet was high in soluble fiber.[95]

Finally, the cholesteryl ester transfer protein (CETP) gene mediates the transfer of cholesteryl ester from HDL-c to triglyceride-rich lipoproteins. It also has a role in reverse cholesterol transport and in the catabolism of HDL-c. CETP isoforms were associated HDL-c levels and risk for myocardial infarction, but only in subjects who drank 25 g/day of alcohol.[96] Thus, there is evidence of a gene-alcohol interaction effect on HDL-c levels.

Gene-Gene (GxG) Interactions

Interactions between genes also have a role in determining the susceptibility to diseases. Gene-gene interactions occur when the impact of a gene is mediated by genetic variation at another gene locus. For example, it has been suggested that variation in total CH and LDL-c is influenced by interactions between the linked LDLR and APOE genes.[97] The cholesterol-raising and lowering effects of the E4 and E2 alleles, respectively, were seen only in individuals with a particular LDLR genotype. These two genes are located about 40 cM apart on chromosome 19p13.2-p13.32. Another example of GxG was reported by Helbecque et al.[98] A significant interaction between the VLDL receptor genotype (VLDLR) and the Apo E phenotype was found for plasma TG levels. Interactions among GRL, LPL, and ADRA2[99] were also reported. GRL and ADRA2 interactions were detected for LDL-c levels, while GRL and LPL interactions were found for HDL-c levels. Interestingly, none of the main effects were significant. This is a classical example of GxG interaction, where there is no association in the presence of either locus separately, but jointly they have an effect. Although the exact mechanism is not clear, the interaction may influence rates of lipolysis and release of free fatty acids (FFA) from adipose tissue.

Other examples of GxG interactions are found in the body composition domain. For example, indirect evidence for two pleiotropic loci affecting fat mass and BMI was reported by Borecki et al.[100] using segregation analysis. One locus apparently affected extreme overweight, while the other influenced variation only in the "normal" range. Evidence for multiple loci affecting body composition has also been explored using the measured gene approach. Since each of the LPL, GRL, and ADRA2 loci had similar effects on several correlated body composition traits, the hypothesis of GxG interaction was investigated.[101] Previous studies had reported that the ADRA2 Dra I variant and the GRL Bcl I variant were each associated with abdominal fat. When the three candidates (GRL, ADRA2, and LPL) were considered simultaneously, significant interactions on overall and abdominal adiposity were observed that accounted for a small but significant percentage of the variance.

Only one study was found investigating GxG interactions for responses to dietary intervention, involving the APO A-I and A-IV loci.[81] Male subjects were fed three consecutive diets, each lasting for four weeks, which differed in amounts of saturated and monounsaturated fats. The G → A mutation in APOAI and the 347Thr/Ser mutation in APOAIV were examined. Each locus showed a gene-diet interaction effect on responses in total cholesterol, LDL-c, and Apo B levels. However, the GxG effect on the response was not significant, resulting in a simple additive effect of the two loci on the lipid responses.

Conclusions

This section is not intended to be an exhaustive summary of the genetics of nutrition. Rather, we have attempted to show the broad scope of behavioral and physiological factors underlying the genetics of nutrition. The general findings may be summarized as follows. First, there are familial factors underlying food intake and preferences. However, whether this effect is due to genes, familial environments, or some combination of both is not clear. Second, it is obvious that nutrition plays an important role in the development of certain diseases leading to morbidity and mortality such as obesity, dyslipidemia, and diabetes, and that genes underlie this effect to some extent. Third, there are multiple complex etiologies that lead to increased risk for these diseases.

A great deal of work remains to be done on several fronts. First, very little was found regarding gene-diet interactions for many of the peptides and hormones[3] that have been implicated in food intake. Some of these include cholecsytokinin (CCK), glucagon-like peptide 1, agouti-related peptide, CART, corticotropin releasing factor (CRF), pro-opiomelanocortin (POMC), opioids, neuropeptide Y (NPY), and others. These inhibit food intake, while others stimulate appetite and thus may contribute significantly to the responses to energy intake. More extensive candidate genotyping of existing intervention data would be helpful in this regard. Second, it is highly unlikely that the genes identified to date are the only ones affecting the traits discussed here, even in the lipid domain, for which much is already known. While candidate gene studies are useful in confirming the effects of these known genes, linkage analysis of genome scan data are needed in order to locate novel chromosomal regions that may lead to identification of new genes. In this regard, large-scale diet intervention studies of family data are needed. While this may be impractical in human populations, genome scans from intervention studies of closely related species such as the baboons are feasible. Third, in addition to gene-diet interactions, models that incorporate the possibility of other complex etiologies such as pleiotropy and oligogenic and epistatic actions are needed. Since candidate genes for lipids (e.g., LPL) may also influence other traits such as diabetes and obesity, we should not limit our candidate gene investigations to one type of trait. This field is ripe for an explosion of studies that probe the genome and describe the complex genetic etiologies underlying responses to nutrition. It is obvious that nutrition plays a large role in several traits of public health interest such as those involved in the metabolic syndrome and discussed here. An understanding of the factors involved in this syndrome should take nutritional factors into account.

References

1. Pérusse L, Bouchard C. In: *The Genetics of Obesity* (Bouchard C, Ed) Boca Raton: CRC Press, 1994, p 125.
2. Prutkin J, Fisher EM, Etter L, et al. *Physiol Behav* 69:161; 2000.
3. Smith GP. *Neuropeptides* 33: 323; 1999.
4. Rice TK, Borecki IB. In: *Genetic Dissection of Complex Traits* (Rao DC, Province MA, Eds) San Diego: Academic Press, 2001, p 35.
5. Rao DC, Rice T. In: *Encyclopedia of Biostatistics,* Vol 4. (Armitage P, Colton T, Eds) Sussex, UK: Wiley, 1998, p 3285.
6. Pérusse L, Bouchard C. *Nutr Rev* 57: 31S; 1999.
7. Borecki IB, Suarez BK. In: *Genetic Dissection of Complex Traits* (Rao DC, Province MA, Eds) San Diego: Academic Press, 2001, p 45.
8. Effron B. Philadelphia, PA: *SIAM*. 1982
9. Huber PJ. Proceedings of the 5th Berkeley Symposium on Mathematical Statistics and Probability. Berkeley, CA: University of California Press, Vol I: 221; 1967.
10. White M. *Econometrica* 48: 817; 1980.
11. Woods SC, Schwartz MW, Baskin DG, Seeley RJ. *Ann Rev Psychol* 51: 255; 2000.
12. DeCastro JM. *Physiol Behav* 54: 677; 1993.
13. Pérusse L, Tremblay A, Leblanc C, et al. *Am J Clin Nutr* 47: 629; 1988.
14. Vauthier J-M, Lluch A, Lecomte E, et al. *Int J Epidemiol* 25: 1030; 1996.
15. Garn SM, Cole PE, Bailey SM. *Hum Biol* 51: 565; 1979.
16. Fabsitz RR, Garrison RJ, Feinleib M, Hjortland M. *Behav Genet* 8: 15; 1978.
17. Patterson TL, Rupp JW, Sallis JF, et al. *Am J Prev Med* 4: 75; 1988.
18. Oliveria SA, Ellison RC, Moore LL, et al. *Am J Clin Nutr* 56: 593; 1992.
19. Wade J, Milner J, Krondl M. *Am J Clin Nutr* 34: 143; 1981.
20. Reed DR, Bachmanov AA, Beauchamp GK, et al. *Behav Genet* 27: 373; 1997.
21. Faith MS, Rha SS, Neale MC, Allison DB. *Behav Genet* 29: 145; 1999.
22. Smith BK, Andrews PK, West DB. *Am J Physiol* 278: R797; 2000.
23. Bouchard C, Tremblay A, Després J-P, et al. *N Engl J Med* 322: 1477; 1990.
24. Bouchard C, Tremblay A, Després J-P, et al. *Prog Food Nutr Sci* 12: 45; 1988.
25. Leibel RL, Bahary N, Friedman JM. *World Rev Nutr Diet* 63: 90; 1990.
26. Weinsier RL, Hunter GR, Heini AF, et al. *Am J Med* 105: 145; 1998.
27. Pérusse L, Bouchard C. *Ann Med* 31S: 19; 1999.
28. Hainer V, Stunkard AJ, Kunesova M, et al. *Int J Obes* 24: 1051; 2000.
29. West DB, Waguespack J, York B, et al. *Mamm Genome* 5: 546; 1994.
30. West DB, Goudey-Lefevre J, York B, Truett GE. *J Clin Invest* 94; 1410; 1994.
31. Chagnon YC, Pérusse L, Lamothe M, et al. *Obes Res* 5: 115; 1997.
32. Chagnon YC, Rice T, Pérusse L, et al. *J Appl Physiol* 90: 1777; 2001.
33. Jensen DR, Schlaepfer IR, Morin CL, et al. *Am J Physiol* 273; R683, 1997.
34. Vohl M-C, Lamarche B, Moorjani S, et al. *Arterioscler Thromb Vasc Biol* 15: 714; 1995.
35. Cigolini M, Smith U. *Metabolism* 28: 502; 1979.
36. Ukkola O, Rosmond R, Tremblay A, Bouchard C. *Atherosclerosis* 157: 221; 2001.

37. Ukkola O, Tremblay A, Bouchard C. *Int J Obes* (in press).
38. Benecke H, Topak H, von zur Mühlen A, Schuppert F. *Exp Clin Endocrinol Diab* 108: 86; 2000.
39. Schreyer SA, Chua SC Jr, LeBoeuf RC. *J Clin Invest* 102: 402; 1998.
40. Fernandez-Real J-M, Vendrell J, Ricart W. *Diabetes Care* 23: 831; 2000.
41. Oppert J-M, Nadeau A, Tremblay A, et al. *Metabolism* 44: 96; 1995.
42. Pérusse L, Chagnon YC, Weisnagel SJ, et al. *Obes Res* 9: 135; 2001.
43. Otabe S, Clement K, Dubios S, et al. *Diabetes* 48: 206; 1999.
44. Kogure A, Yoshida T, Sakane N, et al. *Diabetologia* 41: 1399; 1998.
45. Mammes O, Betoulle D, Aubert R, et al. *Diabetes* 47: 487; 1998.
46. Ukkola O, Tremblay A, Després J-P. *J Intern Med* 248: 435; 2000.
47. Lei H-H, Coresh J, Shuldiner, et al. *Diabetes* 48: 1868; 1999.
48. Zeghari N, Vidal H, Younsi M, et al. *Am J Physiol* 279: E736; 2000.
49. Ek J, Urhammer SA, Sørensen TIA, et al. *Diabetologia* 42: 892; 1999.
50. Hegele RA, Harris SB, Hanley AJG, et al. *Diab Care* 21: 851; 1998.
51. Gagnon J, Mauriege P, Roy S, et al. *J Clin Invest* 98: 2086; 1996.
52. Mitchell BD, Cole SA, Comuzzie AG, et al. *Diabetes* 48: 1863; 1999.
53. Nagase T, Aoki A, Yamamoto M, et al. *J Clin Endocrinol Metab* 82: 1284; 1997.
54. Clement K, Vaisse C, Manning B St. J, et al. *N Engl J Med* 333: 352; 1995.
55. Humphries SE, Peacock RE, Talmud PJ. *Clin Endocrinol Metab* 9: 797; 1995.
56. Simopoulos AP. *Biomed Env Sci* 9: 124; 1996.
57. Ordovas JM. *Proc Nutr Soc* 58: 171; 1999.
58. Ellsworth DL, Sholinsky P, Jaquish C. *Am J Prev Med* 16: 122; 1999.
59. Friedlander Y, Leitersdorf E, Vecsler R, et al. *Atherosclerosis* 152: 239; 2000.
60. Kuan SI, Dupont J. *J Nutr* 119: 349; 1989.
61. Van Zutphen LFM, Den Bieman MGCW. *J Nutr* 111; 1833; 1981.
62. Eggen DA. *J Lipid Res* 17: 663; 1976.
63. Rudel LL. *J Am Coll Nutr* 16: 306S; 1997.
64. Hopkins PN. *Am J Clin Nutr* 55: 1060; 1992.
65. O'Connell DL, Heller RF, Roberts DCK, et al. *Genet Epidemiol* 5: 323; 1988.
66. Dixon LB, Shannon BM, Tershakovec AM, et al. *Am J Clin Nutr* 66: 1207; 1997.
67. Mahaney MC, Blangero J, Rainwater DL, et al. *Arterioscler Thromb Vasc Biol* 19: 1134; 1999.
68. Després J-P, Poehlman ET, Tremblay A, et al. *Metabolism* 36: 363; 1987.
69. Abbey M. *Cur Opin Lipidol* 3: 12; 1992.
70. Ordovas JM, López-Miranda J, Mata P, et al. *Atherosclerosis* 118: 11S; 1995.
71. Dreon DM, Krauss RM. *J Am Coll Nutr* 16: 313S; 1997.
72. Jemaa R, Tuzet S, Portos C, et al. *Int J Obes* 19: 270; 1995.
73. Abbey M, Belling B, Clifton P, Nestel P. *Nutr Met Cardiovasc Dis* 1: 10; 1991.
74. Jemaa R, Tuzet S, Betoulle D, et al. *Int J Obes* 21: 280; 1997.
75. Humphries SE, Talmud PJ, Cox C, et al. *Quart J Med* 89: 671; 1996.
76. Thorn JA, Needham EWA, Mattu RK, et al. *J Lipid Res* 39: 437; 1998.
77. Ordovas JM, Schaefer EJ. *Br J Nutr* 83: 127S; 2000.
78. López-Miranda J, Ordovas JM, Espino A, et al. *Lancet* 343: 1246; 1994.
79. McCombs RJ, Marcadis DE, Ellis J, Weinberg RB. *N Engl J Med* 331: 706; 1994.
80. Mata P, Ordovas JM, López-Miranda J, et al. *Arterioscler Thromb* 14: 884; 1994.
81. Jansen S, López-Miranda J, Salas J, et al. *Arterioscler Thromb Vasc Biol* 17: 1532; 1997.
82. López-Miranda J, Jansen S, Ordovas JM, et al. *Am J Clin Nutr* 66: 97; 1997.
83. López-Miranda J, Marín C, Castro P, et al. *Eur J Clin Invest* 30: 678; 2000.
84. Hegele RA, Zahariadis G, Jenkins AL, et al. *Clin Sci* 85: 269; 1993.
85. Kesäniemi YA. *Cur Opin Lipid* 7: 124; 1996.
86. Martin LJ, Connelly PW, Nancoo D, et al. *J Lipid Res* 34: 437; 1993.
87. Williams PT, Dreon DM, Krauss RM. *Am J Clin Nutr* 61: 1234; 1995.
88. Dreon DM, Fernstrom HA, Miller B, Krauss RM. *FASEB J* 8: 121; 1994.
89. Dreon DM, Fernstrom HA, Miller B, Krauss RM. *Arterioscler Thromb Vasc Biol* 15: 105; 1995.
90. Rotter JI, Bu X, Cantor RM, et al. *Am J Hum Genet* 58: 585; 1996.
91. Friedlander Y, Berry EM, Eisenberg S, et al. *Clin Genet* 47: 1; 1995.

92. Jing Ma, Stampfer MJ, Hennekens CH, et al. *Circulation* 94: 2410; 1996.
93. Baier LJ, Sacchettini JC, Knowler WC, et al. *J Clin Invest* 95: 1281; 1995.
94. Hegele RA. *Clin Biochem* 31: 609; 1998.
95. Hegele RA, Wolever TMS, Story JA, et al. *Eur J Clin Invest* 27: 857; 1997.
96. Fumeron F, Betoulle D, Luc G, et al. *J Clin Invest* 96: 1664; 1995.
97. Pedersen JC, Berg K. *Clin Genet* 35: 331; 1989.
98. Helbecque N, Dallongeville J, Codron V. *Arterioscler Thromb Vasc Biol* 17: 2759; 1997.
99. Ukkola O, Pérusse L, Weisnagel SJ, et al. *Metabolism* 50: 246; 2001.
100. Borecki IB, Blangero J, Rice T, et al. *Am J Hum Genet* 63: 831; 1998.
101. Ukkola O, Pérusse L, Chagnon YC, et al. *Int J Obes* (in press) 2001.
102. Heller RF, O'Connell DL, Roberts DCK. *Genet Epidemiol* 5: 311; 1988.
103. Vohl M-C, Dionne FT, Pérusse L, et al. *Obes Res* 2: 444; 1994.
104. Fumeron F, Durack-Bown I, Betoulle D, et al. *Int J Obes* 20: 1051; 1996.
105. Oksanen L, Ohman M, Heiman M, et al. *Hum Genet* 99: 559; 1997.

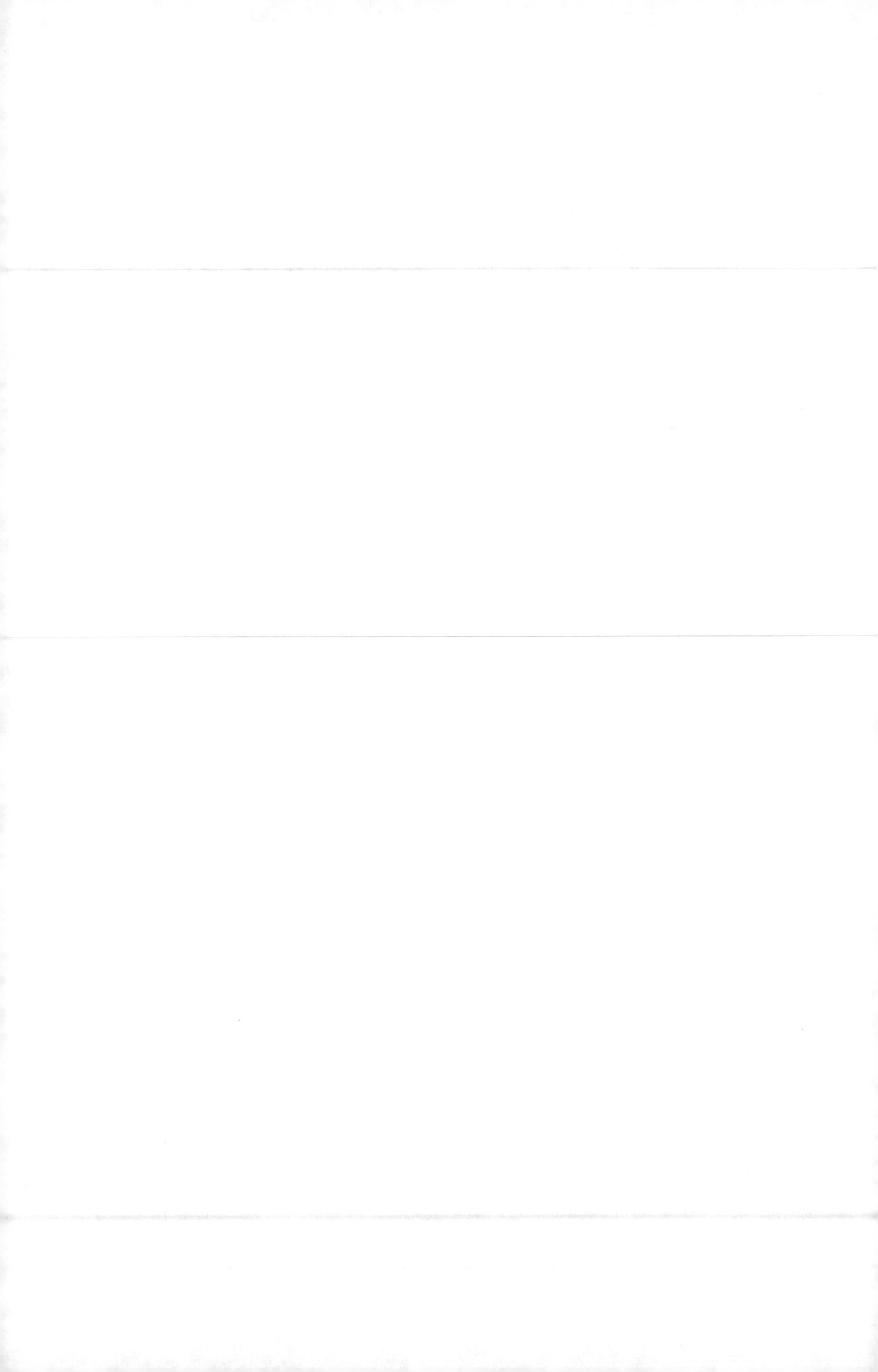

28

Documentation to Improve Medical Assessment Access and Reimbursement

Jessica A. Krenkel

Introduction

Nutrition and nutrition-related medical diagnoses are the basis for medical assessment and the administration of patient nutrition care. Standards of nutrition care are directed to quality treatment but reimbursement issues drive treatment access, and reimbursement is being closely tied to outcomes and costs versus benefits. The recent emphasis on evidence-based medicine and outcomes has stimulated the collection of data to reinforce the cost benefit for professional nutrition services, usually provided by a registered dietitian. Registered dietitians are currently the single identifiable group with the standardized education, clinical training, continuing education, and national credentialing requirements necessary to be directly reimbursed as a provider of nutrition therapy. Professional services may include counseling for preventing disease (primary prevention), for detecting asymptomatic disease or risk factors at early, treatable stages (secondary prevention), for disease treatment (tertiary prevention), and to promote normal growth and development.[1] The approach taken by the National Institute of Medicine (IOM) in making recommendations for future Medicare coverage included two nutrition service categories or levels: nutrition therapy and basic education or advice.[2] Nutrition therapy was identified by the IOM to include the assessment of nutritional status, evaluation of nutritional needs, intervention that ranges from counseling on diet prescriptions to the provision of enteral and parenteral nutrition, and follow-up care as appropriate. Since nutrition therapy is an intensive approach to the management of chronic diseases and requires significantly more training in food and nutrition science than is commonly provided in the curriculum of other health professions, the registered dietitian is the most common reimbursable provider, while basic nutrition could be provided by many health professionals.

The American Dietetic Association (ADA) uses the designation medical nutrition therapy (MNT) for assessment and interventions to treat illness and injury based on clinical research and experience. MNT involves the assessment and analysis of medical and diet history, blood chemistry lab values, and anthropometric measurements. Components of MNT include: 1) Diet modification and counseling and 2) specialized nutrition therapies

0-8493-2705-9/01/$0.00+$1.50

TABLE 28.1

Nutrition Diagnoses

260	Failure to thrive, kwashiorkor
261	Marasmus
263.8	Hypoalbuminemia with malnutrition
262-263.9	Mixed protein-kcalorie malnutrition and
263.0, 263.1	Malnutrition of mild to moderate degree
269.9	Nutritional deficiencies, unspecified
278	Obesity
281.9	Anemia, nutritional
646.1	Obesity/Pregnancy
646.8	Weight Loss/Pregnancy
733.1	Failure to thrive, child
783.1	Abnormal weight gain
783.2	Abnormal weight loss
733.0	Anorexia
307.1	Anorexia nervosa
783.6	Bulimia
307.50	Eating disorder, NOS

such as medical foods through food intake, enteral nutrition delivered via tube, or parental nutrition delivered via intravenous infusion.[3]

Nutrition Diagnosis

Medical diagnoses are officially coded by the International Classification of Diseases, Ninth Revision, Clinical Modification, ICD-9-CM, codes.[4] The codes identify the reasons services, equipment, or supplies are ordered. Diseases and injuries are arranged into 17 groups with 3 to 5 numeric descriptors. These include only a few codes specific to a nutrition diagnosis (Table 28.1) but many that are nutrition-related (Table 28.2) and therefore may require medical nutrition therapy as part of the treatment. A clinical modification of ICD-10-CM has been developed as a replacement for ICD-9-CM but has not been implemented yet.

There are 24 disease management protocols for the most common nutrition-related diagnoses provided by the ADA publication, Medical Nutrition Therapy across the Continuum of Care.[5] When coding the diagnosis for reimbursement, the code of choice should agree with the M.D.-identified diagnosis. For example, the ICD-9-CM codes for diabetes are very specific for complications and control (250.01 — diabetes mellitus without mention of complication, type 1; 250.02 — diabetes mellitus without mention of complication, type 2, uncontrolled). Familiar nutrition diagnoses are the codes related to malnutrition: failure to thrive, kwashiorkor (260), marasmus (261), hypoalbuminemia with malnutrition (263.8), mixed protein-calorie malnutrition (262-263.9), and malnutrition of mild to moderate degree (263, 263.1). There are suggestions for further clarification of malnutrition and weight loss diagnoses by describing body compartments: wasting (involuntary weight loss), cachexia (involuntary loss of body cell mass or fat-free mass when this compartment is reduced by little or no weight loss), and sarcopenia (involuntary loss of muscle mass). An increased degree of specificity for malnutrition may have value to increase the perception of nutrition as medical treatment for the future and to focus treatment on identified patient needs. Submitting codes to the American Medical

TABLE 28.2

Nutrition-Related ICD-9 Diagnosis Code Examples

042	AIDS/HIV
693.1	Allergies — food related
626	Amenorrhea
429.2	ASCVD
239.6	Breast cancer
579.0	Celiac sprue
574	Cholelithiasis
558.9	Colitis/Ileitis
558.10	Colon cancer
428	Congestive heart failure
564	Constipation
555.9	Crohn's disease
250	Diabetes mellitus
250.91	Diabetes mellitus, I, complications
250.01	Diabetes mellitus, I, uncomplicated
250.90	Diabetes mellitus, II, complications
250.0	Diabetes mellitus, II, uncomplicated
648.8	Diabetes, gestational
251.0	Diabetic ketoacidosis
558.9	Diarrhea
271	Disorders of lipid metabolism
562.10	Diverticulitis
536.8	Dyspepsia
535.5	Gastritis
553.3	Hiatal hernia
272.03	Hypercholesterolemia
643.0	Hyperemesis gravidarum
272.1	Hyperglycemia
272.3	Hyperlipidemia
275.42	Hypercalcemia
276.7	Hyperkalemia
276.0	Hypernatremia
252.0	Hyperparathyroidism
275.41	Hypocalcemia
250.80	Hypoglycemia, diabetic, unspecified
251.2	Hypoglycemia, nondiabetic, unspecified
276.8	Hypokalemia
276.1	Hyponatremia
272.4	Hyperlipidemia
401-405	Hypertension
564.1	Irritable bowel
271.3	Lactose intolerance
579.9	Malabsorption syndrome
581.9	Nephrotic syndrome
733	Osteoporosis
239	Stomach cancer

Association and participating in the development of diagnosis codes related to nutrition are new roles for nutrition professionals. Whether the diagnosis codes or the more specific descriptors would improve reimbursement and outcomes is unknown. Ways to diagnose nutrition problems or diseases are only one part of a multidimensional concept needed for clinical nutrition practice today.

Care Standards

Clinical practice tools including practice guidelines, protocols, clinical pathways, care maps, and algorithms integrate clinical expertise and scientific evidence to reduce fragmentation of care, and to guide nutrition practice and nutrition-related diagnoses. The development of these tools begins with the most costly and frequent medical conditions. Professional organizations, insurance companies, government agencies, accrediting organizations, and corporation policies and procedures may establish standards of practice. Standards of practice are gaining importance for justifying treatment approaches for patients and for providing legal justification for time, billing, and counseling content.

Professional organizations that provide standards of practice include the American Dietetic Association, American Society for Parenteral and Enteral Nutrition, American Public Health Association, American Diabetic Association, and other professional associations and practice groups. Government agencies provide standards for various practice settings, which are published in the *Federal Register.* Additionally, interpretive guidelines and survey procedures provide additional sources for practice expectations. The Health Care Financing Administration (HCFA), with responsibility for Medicare, influences healthcare facility standards as well as the reimbursement system for private and public health plans. Additionally, the Agency for Health Care Policy and Research (AHCPR) was created by the U.S. Congress to enhance the quality, appropriateness, and effectiveness of clinical practice guidelines.[6] Accrediting organizations such as the Joint Commission on Accreditation of Healthcare Organizations (JCAHO), dictate expectations for quality nutrition care for many types of facilities. Corporations have relied on many published standards of practice to establish contracts, competencies, and policies and procedures for nutrition practitioners. Employer or professional liability may be determined by adherence to practice standards. Lawsuits related to practice guidelines in the medical profession have not permitted a lower standard for different rural communities, geographical areas, or resource availability, and this would be predicted to be the case for nutrition practice standards as well. Whether established practice guidelines will foster increased lawsuits against practitioners who fail to follow recommendations is unknown.[7]

Medical Assessment Access

Access to quality health care is important in order to eliminate health disparities and increase the quality and years of healthy life for all Americans.[1] Recent major changes in the U.S. health care system include welfare reform, an emphasis on market forces, the use of case management, and altered payment and delivery systems. Adequate access to nutrition care may increase use of these services and improve health outcomes. Conse-

TABLE 28.3

Major Classifications and Models of Managed Care Systems

Classification/Model	Characteristics
Health maintenance organization (HMO)	A managed care organization that provides or arranges for specific health care services for plan members for a fixed, prepaid premium or dollar amount.
Staff model	The HMO owns and operates all facilities needed for the care of plan members and directly hires providers to work in HMO facilities. Closed panel with tight control over practice and benefits.
Group model	The HMO contracts with physician groups to care for plan members instead of directly employing these physicians. These physician groups are managed independently from the HMO and are paid at negotiated, capitated rates.
Network model	The HMO contracts with several single- or multispecialty physician groups.
Independent practice association (IPA)	The HMO contracts directly with individual, independent physicians, who are paid on a capitated basis. These physicians work in their own offices and serve both HMO and non-HMO patients.
Mixed-model	A combination of the above four distinct HMO models and fee-for-service plans to accommodate the different preferences of providers and health plan members.
Preferred provider organization (PPO)	The HMO contracts with individual providers or networks of providers to provide health care, such as nutrition services or dental care, for plan members at discounted fee-for-service rates. Plan members are not matched with gatekeepers and can go to specialists without referrals.
Point-of-service (POS) plan	Plan members are coupled with primary care providers but can seek care directly from other providers for higher copayments.

quently, measures of nutrition access across a continuum of care are an important way to evaluate quality of care.

A significant measure of the trend of decreased access is the proportion of people who have health insurance. In 1997, 85% of persons under 65 years of age had health insurance. Health insurance may be either private or public health plans.[8] Private insurance includes fee-for-service (FFS) plans, single-service hospital plans, or coverage by managed care organizations. Managed care is divided into three major classifications (See Table 28.3): health maintenance organizations (HMOs), preferred provider organizations (PPOs), and point-of-service (POS) plans.[9,10] Public insurance includes Medicaid or other public assistance, Aid for Families with Dependent Children (AFDC), Supplemental Security Income (SSI), Indian Health Service, Medicare, or military health plan coverage.

Medicare Part A (hospital insurance) covers inpatient hospital, home care, and hospice services, skilled nursing facility care, and end-stage renal disease services. Medicare is managed by the Health Care Financing Administration (HCFA) which contracts with 46 fiscal intermediaries who are private insurance companies to process claims. Under Medicare Part A there are no payments specifically for dietitian services, as facility reimbursement is related to complexity of care for different diagnoses and conditions. For hospitals, the HCFA classification scheme is called Diagnosis Related Groups (DRGs), while for skilled nursing facilities the classifications are called Resource Utilization Group (RUGs). The DRGs and RUGs provide the basis for a Prospective Payment System (PPS) or "bundled" approach for hospitals since 1983, skilled nursing facilities since 1998, and home health agencies as of October 2000.[11]

Medicare Part B (medical insurance) provides coverage for outpatient physician and hospital services, laboratory services, durable medical equipment, and other medical services. Part B professional services are administered by 33 carriers. Part B equipment and supplies are administered by four regional durable medical equipment carriers (DMERCs).[11] While there is not a benefit for nutrition counseling under Part B, this is the focus of current legislative efforts by the ADA.

Medicare Part C (Medicare + Choice) offers alternate health plan options in addition to the traditional fee-for-service plan. Medicaid is a federal–state matching entitlement program for certain individuals and families with low income and resources. State participation in the Medicaid program is optional as long as the state has a similar program for this population. Each state has varying coverage of nutrition services for Medicaid recipients.[11]

Although lack of health insurance is clearly a major factor impeding access to care, having health insurance does not guarantee that health care will be accessible or affordable. Managed care has become the dominant form of healthcare delivery in the U.S. replacing the traditional FFS or indemnity system.[12] Managed care shifts financial risk from employers, insurance companies, and self-paying patients to healthcare systems and providers. Providers are paid set or predetermined fees under capitation and bundled fee systems regardless of services ultimately rendered. Managed care attempts to control costs by preventing duplication of services, restricting choices of providers, and increasing efficiency. Access to service is provided by precertification, utilization review, and credentialing. Gatekeepers to the system vary, but the case manager has a key role in complex medical cases. Educating case managers to showcase the benefits of medical nutrition therapy, improved patient care, and cost containment is essential for improved nutrition service access. Nutrition professionals potentially impact preventive services, screening programs, health risk assessments, and case management if they become more knowledgeable about how the systems operate.

Reimbursement for some care settings over others causes an uneven distribution of access to service. Access sites should include the entire continuum of care: acute care, ambulatory care, home care, skilled nursing, and long-term care. While nutrition counseling is generally more effective outside the hospital setting, coverage for nutrition therapy in ambulatory settings is at best inconsistent, but most often nonexistent.[2] This lack of access is a significant barrier to improved patient outcomes associated with nutrition care.

Outcomes

Analysis of the effectiveness of the practice guidelines for medical nutrition therapy is a focus of outcomes research. The outcomes determine reimbursement for clinical practice in our health care system as evidence-based medicine is becoming a controlling factor in determining the distribution of healthcare dollars.[13] The outcome is the result of a process of healthcare that weighs options as to cost and effects. The two major categories of outcomes are health and cost. Outcomes data provide health care payers information on the effectiveness of care to help them "1) reduce health care costs, 2) prioritize care and make reimbursement decisions, 3) establish guidelines, and 4) make purchasing decisions."[14] Decisions such as which tests to run first, or whether to try enteral or parenteral feeding, require knowledge of the evidence which supports nutrition decisions. Acceptance of clinical nutrition by the plan practitioners may be enhanced by the realization that cost-effective medical practice is optimized by wider application of nutrition principles to health maintenance and patient care.[15]

Health outcomes include clinical outcomes such as lab results and length of stay, functional outcomes such as quality of life, and general outcomes such as patient satisfaction and interventions.[14] Clinical research, as well as continuous quality improvement (CQI) or other in-house quality measurements, utilize health outcomes to determine results.[16] These need to be coupled with the cost outcomes of cost-effectiveness, cost-benefit, and charges. Cost-effectiveness is a ratio measure of the number of dollars spent for the

TABLE 28.4

Types of Outcomes

Clinical Outcomes

Primary

Anatomic or Anthropometric — weight, height, % body fat, etc.
Physiologic —
Biochemical labs, such as albumin, hemoglobin, cytokines
Healing, such as pressure ulcers, wounds, burns
Metabolic rate
Study or Disease Specific
Such as stool analysis in cystic fibrosis, or residuals in enteral feeding studies

Secondary

Morbidity
Mortality
Length of stay
Rates of infection
Re-admissions
Drug utilization
Number of doctor visits
Home health care nursing visits

General Outcomes

Patient satisfaction and expectations
Learning outcomes — enrollment, knowledge, behavioral change, improvements
Interventions — type, frequency or usage, acceptance by patient, timeliness
Acceptance of recommendations — M.D., interdisciplinary team, patient
Meal, food, nutrient intake

Functional Outcomes

Quality of life
Activities of daily living
Mental/emotional health
Family interaction
Self-assessed health care status
Pain

Economic Outcomes

Costs — cost-benefit, cost-effectiveness
Revenue
Reimbursement

improvement in an outcome (e.g., dollars spent for a therapy/HbA1c improvement), whereas cost-benefit is a ratio of the dollars spent on a therapy or program service to the number of dollars saved by implementing the program. In Congress, a cost-benefit (COB score) estimates the cost of legislation over a five-year period.[17] Medicare reimbursement is being considered for diseases where there are estimates for economically significant benefits to beneficiaries and reduced Medicare program health care expenditures. A lack of systems to track quality and cost of nutrition care has resulted in increased involvement of the ADA in collecting outcome data.[24] National outcome data for a larger range of medical conditions and preventive care will allow providers and administrators to identify nutrition services and populations that are in need of improved delivery and funding.

Quantification of patient satisfaction and quality of life is difficult, but these outcomes are of importance to the National Committee on Quality Assurance (NCQA) that accredits health maintenance organizations. The NCQA publishes a Health Plan Employer Data Information Set (HEDIS). The 3.0 version had 8 domains with 71 total performance measures to help employers and consumers compare managed care organizations.[18] Patient satisfaction is domain 3, and increased satisfaction has been associated with positive clinical outcomes.[19]

Reimbursement

The value of the dietitian is determined by income generation and by contribution to the goals of the organization in the private and public sectors of society. A lack of reimbursement is a specific barrier to more consistent delivery of diet counseling and to employment of nutrition professionals.

Reimbursement issues have become a barrier for clinical nutrition in hospitals, clinics, and educational and other settings that have begun to operate their clinics with more of a business approach. Reimbursement has been poor to variable, with a wide range of experience expressed nationwide. The Health Care Financing Team at ADA has encouraged registered dietitians to develop skill understanding medical nutrition therapy coding and the coverage issues that surround reimbursement.[20] Recent efforts by ADA offer potential for increased reimbursement. The ADA has had three MNT current procedural terminology (CPT) codes accepted by the American Medical Association and published in the 2001 CPT Code.[21] Under HCFA's coding system, CPT codes are considered Level I HCPCS codes (acronym for HCFA's Common Procedure Coding System). These represent levels of service for individual new (97802) and established (97803) patients and group (97804) that may be used in the private sector (e.g., with third party payers); however, they have not been assigned relative value units (RVU). The RVUs will determine possible payment for MNT levels of service by Medicare and HCFA. The RVU represent a fair and reasonable fee structure based on geographical location, work required/resources consumed to perform service, other operating expenses, and other related factors. The AMA Health Care Professional Advisory Committee (HCPAC) has not accepted ADA's recommended work values which were based on practitioner data collected in March 2000, due to their unfamiliarity with the content and complexity of nutrition services. ADA has notified the AMA and HCFA that the Association will extend development of codes by seeking additional codes and reformatting the present codes to separate the tasks of assessment and intervention. Similar problems have occurred with the codes and RVUs being used for diabetes counseling, as the time needs and complexity are unfamiliar to the AMA. The acceptance of AMA codes and RVU for nutrition provider services is crucial in obtaining reimbursement from Medicare. Medicare decisions set precedents often followed by insurance companies, and add to the credibility of nutrition professionals as providers. The CPT codes and RVUs specific for recognized nutrition providers would be expected to become the basis of reimbursement for Medicare and insurance companies.[22]

Recent bills before congressional committees, the Medical Nutrition Therapy Act of 1999 (H.R. 1187/S.660) and the Medicare Wellness Act of 2000 (S.2225/H.R. 3887), which include some preventive services for Medicare beneficiaries, demonstrate a climate of change for Medicare reimbursement. The Medical Nutrition Therapy Act provides coverage for medical nutrition therapy under Medicare Part B furnished by registered dietitians and qualified nutrition professionals. A compromise is being considered that would be a five-year demonstration project for Medicare coverage of diabetes and renal disease.[23] The major reforms, including prescription drugs, will delay consideration of the controversial Medicare Wellness Act until at least 2001. These bills have gained momentum due to the study of the National Academy of Sciences Institute of Medicine, The Role of Nutrition in Maintaining Health in the Nations Elderly: Evaluating Coverage of Nutrition Services for the Medicare Population, which recommends that medical nutrition therapy — with physician referral — be a covered benefit under the Medicare program.[2]

Presently, numerous CPT codes are used for clinical nutrition services.[10,24,25] Codes and reimbursement vary from state to state, among the various payors, and in different care settings, but commonly used codes include physician codes for new patients (99201 series), established patient or follow-up (99211 series), and consultation codes (99241 series). There is considerable controversy about the use of these codes by non-physician providers with and without "incident to" a physician billing. "Incident to" a physician billing requires supervision by the physician and billing under his tax ID, and is primarily used in states without dietitian licensure. Legal opinion has questioned the use of this billing practice by non-physicians for Medicare patients except at the lowest level of service and payment.[26] Health insurance companies with provider agreements continue to accept "incident to" billing. Hospital-based outpatient clinics bill under the hospital tax ID instead of the physician or the licensed dietitian certified provider ID.

Other codes such as the new MNT codes (97802, 97803, and 97804), or preventive medicine codes (99381, 99391, and 99401 series) are available but may often have low reimbursement, as the RVU are minimal to none. Group counseling for preventive counseling (99411 and 99412) is seldom reimbursed, and also has RVU minimal to none. There has been some progress with the use of G-codes (G0108, G0109) for diabetes counseling, but numerous criteria must be met to bill when using these codes, including the need for services to be provided "incident to" a physician's services and under the physician's supervision. The G codes are provisional codes for a new benefit.[10] The HCPCS Level II manual includes a series of temporary national non-Medicare S codes and descriptors: S9465 — Diabetic management program, dietitian visit, S9470 — Nutritional counseling, dietitian visit.[27]

Articles and previously published information about which codes to use may not meet legal challenge and claims of fraud, as there has not been an easily understandable definition of how dietitians should use the codes. "Practice" does not mean that Medicare will accept the coding if investigated. This has recently been emphasized with Medicare's vigorous monitoring for fraud and abuse,[28] although thus far dietitians have not faced prosecution. Requests for clarification from Medicare are often verbal, and there has been resistance to putting interpretations in writing that are not in the published standards. These numerous inconsistencies and the increasing legal environment emphasize the need to have professional organizations such as the ADA involved in coding issues and supporting bills to clarify services.

Contracts with insurance companies and health maintenance organizations may closely follow Medicare guidelines or may be negotiated for acceptable codes and reimbursement/billing rates. Working with the clinic personnel responsible for these contracts has been beneficial compared to spending time calling each company to get approval for individual patients or to become a provider. The provider forms for dietitians are usually the same as for physicians, but many of the questions are not applicable, and dietitians are not credentialed the same as physicians, especially in states without licensure. Nutrition provider or credentialing information for contracts and provider agreements varies between health insurance companies, and within the same company there may be different benefits, interpretations, and provider agreements by region. A negative complication to payment for nutrition services is the idea of health insurance companies approving professionals for "access." The nutrition professionals on the list are recommended but the health insurance company does not provide payment, and the insured have to self-pay.

The billing level does not reflect the reimbursement level. It is important to have a set fee for any code that is being used, no matter what the reimbursement level. If rates are set at the expected level of payment the reimbursement will most likely be disappointing, as most schedules are discounted by payors. Published fees cannot be varied for different payors, but the fee schedule can be discounted at a set amount for ability to pay or cash payment. A good practice is to keep track of all patients seen, diagnosis, referring physician, and charges or amount billed for future use. Certainly the collectibles are only part of services billed, and nutrition services should be documented to justify diagnosis codes used on reimbursement claims and provide support for medical necessity.[10,11]

Key staff in insurance, billing, or information systems can help track billing and code results and develop procedures to maximize reimbursement. Private practice nutrition professionals may want to contract out insurance and billing tasks until they become more familiar with these systems. Claim forms and processing are integral to reimbursement. Physician offices and some individual certified hospital providers submit claims using

HCFA-1500 and electronic filing. Hospital clinics typically use the HCFA 1450 (UB-92) form for hospital-employed providers, and most hospital outpatient programs use HCFA 1450 form.

Data on the payor mix is important for assessing contracts, marketing, and reimbursement potential. Cost data analysis helps evaluate if your claims are 80 or 30 cents on the dollar. A streamlined approach to analysis in a large center with many payors would be to start with Medicare and the other top four payors.[29] Reimbursement may not always cover costs, but this is important information for decision making and to lobby for changes in rates. Knowing ahead of time that the dietitian costs are not being covered, such as in capitated contracts, allows time to present evidence to clinic or facility administrators that consults are saving physician time or preventing hospitalization and therefore reducing overall costs.

Conclusion

Medical assessment of nutrition contributes to the diagnosis and interventions that improve the quality of health care for patients. Access to nutrition care by the patient and reimbursement of the nutrition professional are inexorably tied to quality outcomes with cost effectiveness. Nutrition professionals need to actively communicate that medical assessment and nutrition care are essential components of quality health care with a low cost versus substantial benefit worthy of healthcare dollars.

Terminology

Capitated Fee — A fixed sum of money per enrollee, paid in advance, for a specified period of time.

Continuum of care — The array of health services and care settings that address health promotion, disease prevention, and the diagnosis, treatment, management, and rehabilitation of disease, injury and disability. Included are primary care and specialized clinical services provided in community and primary care settings, hospitals, trauma centers, and rehabilitation and long-term care facilities.

Managed care — According to the Institute of Medicine, "a set of techniques used by or on behalf of purchasers of health care benefits to manage health care costs by influencing decisionmaking through case-by-case assessments of the appropriateness of care prior to its provision."

Primary care — According to the Institute of Medicine, "The provision of integrated, accessible health care services by clinicians who are accountable for addressing a large majority of personal health care needs, developing a sustained partnership with patients, and practicing in the context of family and community."

Primary prevention — Measures such as health care services, medical tests, counseling, and health education designed to prevent the onset of a targeted condition. Routine immunization of healthy individuals is an example of primary prevention.

Secondary prevention — Measures such as health care services designed to identify and treat individuals who have a disease or risk factors for a disease but who are not yet experiencing symptoms of disease. Pap tests and high blood pressure screening are examples of secondary prevention.

Tertiary prevention — Preventive health care measures or services that are part of the treatment and management of persons with clinical illnesses. Examples of tertiary prevention include cholesterol reduction for patients with coronary heart disease and insulin therapy to prevent complications of diabetes.

Providers — Those providing health care — both individuals (physicians and other health care providers) and the entities that employ them (hospitals, outpatient clinics, physician practices, durable medical equipment suppliers).

Payors — Those assuming the financial risk of health claim losses and/or administering reimbursement for health care claims.

References

1. US Department of Health and Human Services, Office of Public Health and Science, *Healthy People 2010,* National Institute of Medicine, Washington, DC, 2000.
2. National Academy of Science's Institute of Medicine Committee on Nutrition Services for Medicare Beneficiaries, The Role of Nutrition in Maintaining Health in the Nation's Elderly: Evaluating Coverage of Nutrition Services for the Medicare Population, National Academy Press, Washington, DC, 2000.
3. What is medical nutrition therapy? www.eatright.com/gov/mnt/html, November 30, 2000.
4. US Department of Health and Human Services. International Classification of Diseases, 9th Revision, Clinical Modification, 6th ed, DHHS Publication No (PHS), 96-1260, US Department of Health and Human Services, Public Health Service, Health Care Financing Administration, Washington, DC, 1997.
5. The American Dietetic Association, *Medical Nutrition Therapy Across the Continuum of Care,* 2nd ed, The American Dietetic Association and Morrison Healthcare, Chicago, 1998.
6. Rodriguez DJ. *Support Line,* 21(5), 8, 1999.
7. CDC, National Center for Health Statistics. National Health Interview Survey. Hyattsville, MD: National Center for Health Statistics, unpublished data, 1999.
8. Donaldson MS, Yordy KD, Kohr KN (Eds.) Institute of Medicine. *Primary Care: America's Health in a New Era,* National Academy Press, Washington, DC, 1996.
9. Ransom SB, Pinsky WW. Clinical Resource and Quality Management, American College of Physician Executives, Tampa, FL, 1999.
10. American Association of Diabetes Educators, *Reimbursement Primer,* American Association of Diabetes Educators and Roche Diagnostics Corporation, Alexandria, VA, 2000.
11. The Medicare program and nutrition services, www.eatright.com/gov/mntcoverrage.html, December 12, 2000.
12. Kohn L, Corrigan J, Donaldson M. To Err is Human: Building a Safer Health System, Committee on Quality Healthcare in America, Institute of Medicine, Washington, DC, 1999.
13. US Preventive Services Task Force. Guide to Clinical Preventive Services, 2nd ed, US Department of Health and Human Services, Washington, DC, 1995.
14. Voss AC. *The Consultant Dietitian,* 23: 1; 1999.
15. Halsted CH. *Am J Clin Nutr* 67: 192; 1998.
16. Byham-Gray LD. *Today's Dietitian* April, 31, 2000.
17. Andrews M, Karras, C. *STAT Line* VII(3): 1; 2000.
18. Committee on Performance Measurement. Health Plan Employer Data and Information Set. HEDIS 3.0. Washington, DC: National Committee on Quality Assurance; 1997.

19. Clearly PD, McNeil BJ. *Inquiry* 25: 25; 1988.
20. Larson E. *JADA* 100: 881; 2000.
21. American Medical Association. *CPT 2001: Current Procedural Terminology,* Professional Edition, American Medical Association, Chicago, 2000.
22. American Dietetic Association, *Courier,* 39(4): 1; 2000.
23. Congressional Negotiations Underway on MNT in Balanced Budget Act Revisions — Action Alert, Pulse@eatright.org, October 4, 2000.
24. Hodorowicz MA. *Money Matters in Managed Care: How to Increase Reimbursement Success in a Hospital-Based Outpatient Medical Nutrition Therapy Clinic,* Lifestyle Nutrition Education and Counseling; Palos Heights, IL, 1999.
25. Stollman L. *Nutrition Entrepreneur's Guide to Reimbursement Success: A Publication of the Nutrition Entrepreneurs Dietetic Practice Group,* 2nd ed, The American Dietetic Association, Chicago, 1999.
26. How to code for diabetes education services in physician offices without ADA recognition, Diabetes Education Reimbursement and Policy Report, II(2), October, 2000. Reimbursement@aadenet.org/gov_frame.html.
27. American Medical Association, *HCPCS 2000: Medicare's National Level II Codes,* 12th ed, American Medical Association, Dover, DE, 1999.
28. Smith D. *Medicare Nursing Home Enteral Reimbursement Manual: Fraud and Abuse,* 5th ed, Ross Products Division, Columbus, OH, 2000.
29. Maleski PA. Diabetes care center: how to go from a cost center to a profit center, *Diabetes Education Reimbursement and Policy Report,* II(1), September, 2000.

29

Body Composition Assessment

Carolyn D. Berdanier

Mammals, including man, consist of water, protein, fat, and mineral matter. The assessment of this composition can be direct or indirect. Few studies exist on the direct assessment of body composition of man. Analyses of bodies donated for medical research have been published.[1,2] A total of eight such analyses are available. They were done using gravimetric analysis methods, with discrete tissue samples held to be representative of the whole body. Gravimetric methods are those that directly measure the water content of the sample as the difference in sample weight before and after drying. Fat content is difference in tissue weight before and after solvent extraction of the sample. Mineral content (ash content) is the weight of the sample after combustion in a muffle furnace. Protein content is the amount of nitrogen in the sample multiplied by 6.25 under the assumption that most samples are 16% protein. The results of these studies are shown in Table 29.1.

Direct body composition methods are unwieldy for large animals. There is considerable sampling error because of difficulty in preparing a homogeneous body mixture for sampling. In some instances dissection data (Table 29.2) have been accumulated.[3] Direct analysis is possible for small species, i.e., rodents, but even with these species there are difficulties attributed to the preparation of a whole body homogenate and sampling errors associated with nonhomogeniety.

The indirect methods for assessing body composition are more practical. These are listed in Table 29.3. These methods do not require the death of the donor, and can be used at intervals to determine whether a given treatment has an effect on certain body components. For example, bone mass and density (the mineral component of the body) can be assessed using an instrument called a dual energy x-ray absorptiometry (DXA). This machine passes an x-ray through the body and compares the strength of the excitement of the electrons with a known excitement base. The difference in signal strength is attributed to the density of the bone through which the x-ray passes. Changes (losses) in bone mass/density can occur with age, especially in females. Interventions that interfere with this age-related loss are desirable and can be documented using DXA. For example, Deng

TABLE 29.1

Proximate Body Composition of Adult Humans

% Water	50–70
% Fat	4–27
% Protein	14–23
% Mineral	4.6–6

0-8493-2705-9/01/$0.00+$1.50

TABLE 29.2

Size and Body Composition of Adult Men and Women

	Men	Women
Age	57 ± 22	76 ± 15
Height (cm)	170 ± 9	158 ± 6
Weight (kg)	64 ± 14	57 ± 11
Skin (kg)	3.9 ± 1.1	3.2 ± 0.6
Adipose (kg)	13.0 ± 7.3	20.8 ± 10.0
Muscle (kg)	25.3 ± 6.7	16.4 ± 3.8
Bone (kg)	10.2 ± 1.5	7.6 ± 1.3
Residual (kg)	11.6 ± 3.5	9.3 ± 5.5
Body mass index (kg/m^2)	21.9 ± 3.7	23.2 ± 4.6

Source: Clarys JP, Martin AD, Martell-Jones MJ, et al. *Am J Hum Biol* 11: 167; 1999 (with permission).

TABLE 29.3

Indirect Methods for Determining Body Composition

Total body water: dilution of heavy water
Muscle mass: dilution of labeled creatine
Lean body mass: body content of K^{40} (requires use of whole body counter)
% Body fat: specific gravity (weight of body in air versus under water)

% Body fat, calculated: $\frac{2.118 - 1.354 - 078}{\text{density}} \times$ (% total body water/body weight)

% fat = (5.548 – 5.044)/specific gravity
% fat = 100 – total body water/0.732

et al.[4] have reported that the effectiveness of hormone replacement therapy is associated with vitamin D and estrogen receptor genotypes. They documented this association with periodic DXA determinations of bone mass.

Body fat content can be calculated using either DXA or computer-assisted tomography.[5] Investigators have used this technology and compared it with the measurement of skinfold thickness, and have found a good correlation. Skinfold thicknesses are measured using calipers at designated places in the body. The most frequent are the skinfold under the upper arm, the fold over the iliac crest, and the abdominal fold. Using equations (Table 29.4), body fat stores can be estimated.

The body minus its fat store is defined as the lean body mass. This is an arbitrary designation that assumes that the fat store is not metabolically active, but it is not a correct assumption from a metabolic point of view. The adipose tissue is a very active tissue,

TABLE 29.4

General Formulas for Calculating Body Fatness from Skinfold Measurements

Males:

% Body Fat = $29.288 \times 10^{-2}(X) - 5 \times 10^{-4}(X)^2 + 15.845 \times 10^{-2}$ (Age)

Females:

% Body Fat = $29.699 \text{ X } 10^{-2}(X) - 43 \times 10^{-5}(X)^2 + 29.63 \times 10^{-3}(\text{Age}) + 1.4072$

X = sum of abdomen, suprailiac, triceps, and thigh skinfolds; age is in years.

Source: Jackson, A. S. and Pollack, M. L. 1985. *Phys Sports Med* 13: 76-90 (with permission).

having a role in the control of energy balance and a role in the food intake regulatory system. However, from the body composition point of view, these roles are ignored. Lean body mass (LBM) can be estimated if one assumes that the fat-free body has a water content of 72%. The total body water can be measured using heavy water (deuterium) as a diluent. This water distributes itself throughout the total body and through the application of the formula $C_1V_1 = C_2V_2$ the total body water can be calculated. C_1 is the concentration of the deuterium in the infusate; V_1 is the volume of the infusate. C_2 is the concentration of deuterium in the volume of blood withdrawn after a fixed interval (usually 30 minutes). One then solves for V_2, which is the volume of the total body water. The LBM is then calculated:

$$\text{LBM} = \text{total body water}/0.72$$

The details of body composition measurement have been published, and the reader is referred to these sources for further information.[6-8]

References

1. Forbes RM, Cooper AR, Nitchell HH. *J Biol Chem* 203: 359; 1953.
2. Forbes RM, Mitchell HH, Cooper AR. *J Biol Chem* 223: 969; 1956.
3. Clarys JP, Martin AD, Marfell-Jones MJ, et al. *Am J Hum Biol* 11: 167; 1999.
4. Deng H-W, Li J, Li J-l, et al. *Hum Genet* 103: 576; 1998.
5. Malina RM, Koziell S, Bielicki T. *Am J Hum Biol* 11: 189; 1999.
6. Jebb SA, Elia M. *Int J Obesity* 17: 611; 1993.
7. Withers RT, Laforgia J, Heymsfield SB. *Am J Hum Biol* 11: 175; 1999.
8. Lee RD, Nieman DC. *Nutritional Assessment* WCB Brown & Benchmark, Madison WI, 1993; pg 121.

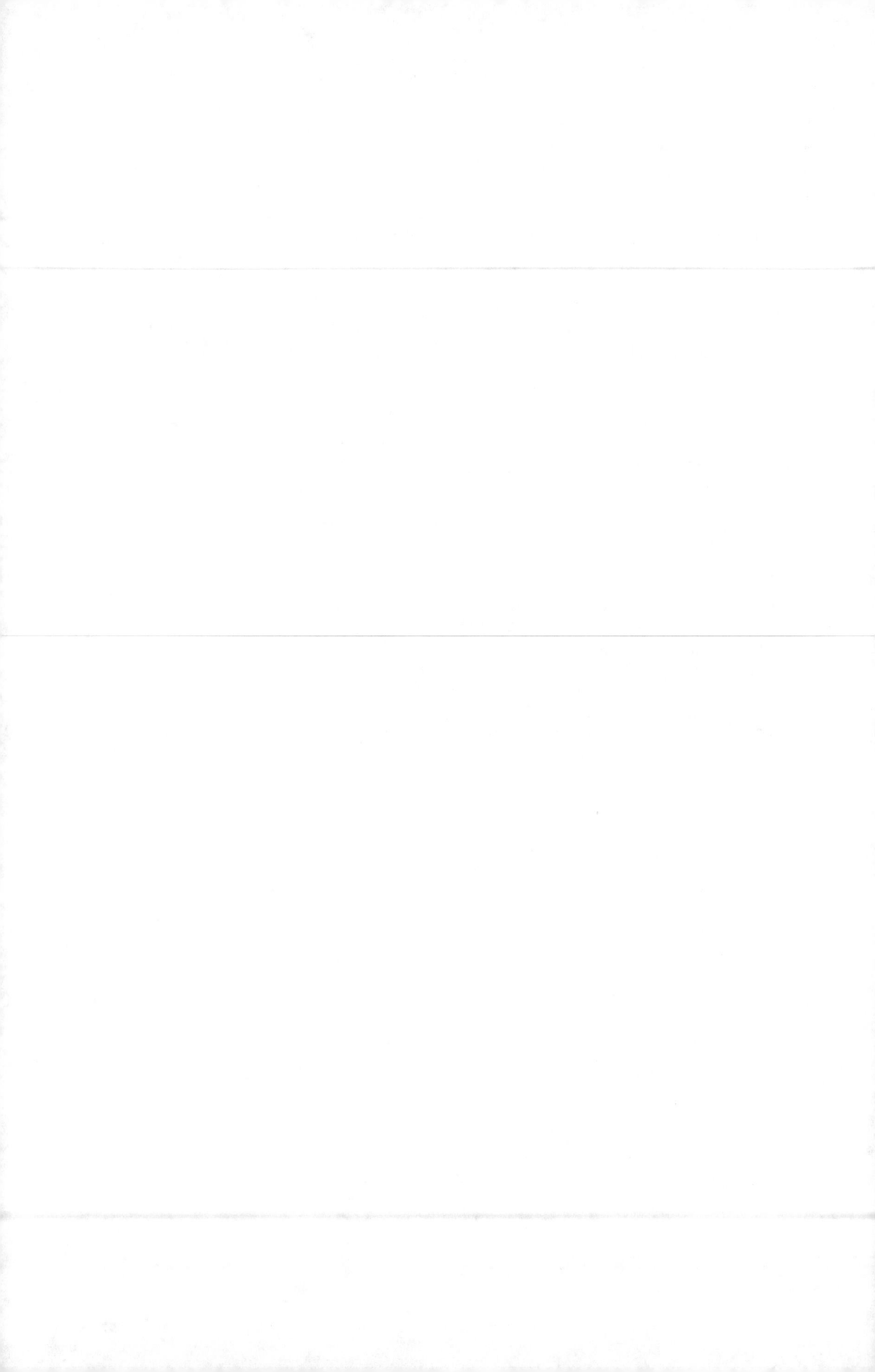

30

The How and Why of Body Composition Assessment

Marta D. Van Loan

Introduction

When it comes to body composition assessment and availability of methods, exercise specialists, health practitioners, and clinicians must consider the demographic characteristics of their clients. Age, ethnicity, sex, degree of adiposity, and physical activity are a few important factors in the selection of appropriate methods and instruments for obtaining the most accurate results. Many methods rely on prediction equations developed from validation groups with specific characteristics. When these instruments and equations are used on individuals or groups with characteristics different from those of the validation group, the accuracy of the results may be questioned. It is also important when selecting a body composition method to assess the relative worth of the method in terms of the criterion or reference method used to evaluate the technique of choice. Acceptable reference or criteria methods include hydrodensitometry (underwater weighing), hydrometry (isotope dilution), or dual energy x-ray absorptiometry (DXA). These reference methods, however, are not without errors and assumptions, and cannot be considered "gold standards" for *in vivo* body composition assessment.

Reference methods typically focus on the body as a two-compartment system consisting of the fat-free mass (FFM) and fat mass (FM), and can be of limited use for individuals whose fat-free mass density and hydration levels differ from the assumed values for this model. Methods that have been validated against the reference two-compartment model will systemically underestimate body fatness for American Indian women, black men and women, and Hispanic women, because the average density of the FFM in these groups exceeds the assumed value of 1.1 g/cc. This can be avoided, however, if one uses methods that have been validated against a multi-compartment model which makes corrections for differences in the hydration level and bone mineral content of the FFM.

Not all body composition assessment is done for the purpose of determining FFM or FM. Other reasons may include but are not limited to determination of 1) osteoporosis risk for older women, 2) fluid balance in individuals with renal disease or other disorders, or 3) monitoring changes in FFM during medical treatment such as AIDS-associated wasting. In this section a variety of body composition methods will be reviewed and evaluated regarding their uses, applications, and limitations.

0-8493-2705-9/01/$0.00+$1.50

Ultrasound

Principles

Ultrasound for the assessment of subcutaneous adipose tissue thickness (SAT) was introduced by Booth et al. in 1966.[1] The ultrasound method, as its name implies, uses high frequency sound waves produced by piezoelectrical crystals in a transducer or probe. The sound waves are "injected" into the skin by placing the transducer over the area of interest. As the waves pass through the skin they are reflected back or "bounce back" to the transducer probe when the waves hit different tissue interfaces. When the reflected sound waves hit the transducer they create a pressure stress on the transducer which is converted to an electrical signal. A-mode ultrasound instruments (no longer in use) measure the delay from when the sound was "injected" into the skin until it "bounced" back to the transducer probe. SAT thickness was then calculated based on the assumption that the speed of ultrasound transmission through different tissue layers was a constant 1500 m/sec. Measurements with the A-mode ultrasound had limited precision and were compromised by the occurrence of numerous echos from connective tissue layers within the SAT. This was especially problematic over the abdomen, the region of most interest.

B-mode and Subcutaneous Adipose Tissue Thickness (SAT)

B-mode ultrasound was an advancement which constructed cross-sectional images of the tissue thickness from the reflected sound waves. These instruments provide images in which measurement of the SAT thickness, muscle thickness, and abdominal depth can be estimated using calipers to measure the thickness of the different tissue layers. Additionally, in the case of pregnancy, images are provided which obstetricians use to assess fetal development. For SAT measurements a frequency of 5 MHZ is used with an 85 mm transducer and a wavelength between 0.3 and 1.5 mm. The cross-sectional images can be saved or "frozen" to allow close examination and assessment of tissue thickness using electronic calipers that digitally mark the boundaries of the tissue of interest. A monitor is often used so that images can be enlarged for better viewing and improved accuracy when placing electronic markers on the tissue edges. In addition, the ultrasound operator can adjust the black and gray scale levels to allow for brighter images and ease of measurement, especially for abdominal scans of obese individuals and estimation of SAT.

Precision of B-mode ultrasound and calipers is about equal, but ultrasound has a slight advantage in that a printed hard copy of the image exists which allows for reexamination if needed. When assessment of body composition of obese individuals is of interest, skinfold calipers do not always have the necessary range of measurement; often the subcutaneous layer of adipose tissue is larger than the width that calipers are capable of opening. This problem does not exist with ultrasound measurements; however, ultrasound does have two drawbacks: 1) it is moderately expensive, and 2) it lacks portability for use in field studies.

Ultrasound measurement for SAT in the limbs and trunk has been reported as excellent, with technical errors of less than 0.2 mm and coefficients of reliability as high as 91 to 98% for most sites.[2,3] When making B-mode ultrasound measurement of SAT, ultrasound gel is applied to the skin surface, to the transducer, and to a bag of gel placed on the skin to separate the transducer from the skin. The transducer is held at a 90° angle to the skin surface and with just enough pressure to ensure good contact between the transducer, the bag of gel, and the skin. Blurred images can be the result of the transducer not aligned at right angles to the skin surface. To make SAT measurements, the right and left sides of the transducer are matched with the corresponding sides of the subject, but measurements of the limb and paraspinal sites are made with the transducer parallel to the limbs and trunk. Similarly, ultrasound measurements over the suprailiac are made with the transducer in a direction toward the pubis symphysis. Variations in the alignment of the transducer are necessary to match the direction of the skinfold measurements.

The use of B-mode ultrasound for the measurement of SAT is similar to that of skinfold measurements for the estimation of body fat.[4] Studies using B-mode ultrasound report mixed results. Equations to estimate body density from ultrasound measurements of SAT were reported by Abe et al.[5] with an error of 0.0006 g/cc for men and women, as well as an equation to predict FFM from the muscle thickness measurement of the ultrasound image. The equations for predicting FFM had errors of 4.4 kg for men and 2.5 kg for women.

Ultrasound for Assessment of Bone Mineral Density

In recent years, ultrasound equipment has been designed for assessment of bone mineral density of the heel. These instruments measure the velocity or transmission of the speed of sound (SOS) through the os calcis bone in the heel. The attenuation of the signal at specific frequencies is related to the density of the bone. One advantage of ultrasound of the heel, unlike the forearm or hand, is that it is a weight-bearing bone and consists of a significant amount of trabecular bone. Additionally, ultrasound of the trabecular bone of the os calcis has little interference from overlying soft tissue. Ultrasound measurements of the heel provide three basic measurement units: 1) SOS, 2) stiffness, and 3) broadband ultrasound attenuation (BUA). When done correctly, ultrasound measurements of the heel are predictive of failure loads of both the proximal femur and vertebra.[6] Instruments vary somewhat among manufacturers; some instruments require the use of a gel as a conductive medium while others use a small amount of water (100 cc). Additionally, some instruments require the use of a "shim" under the foot so that all feet, regardless of size, are positioned in the same location relative to the source of the ultrasound wave. Instruments also vary in that some have a fixed transducer with a water bath while others have contact ultrasound devices with moving transducers. The precision error of the fixed transducer ultrasound appears to be about half that of the moving transducer;[7] therefore, contact ultrasounds may be appropriate for determining individuals at risk for osteoporosis, but they lack enough precision to monitor bone loss or the response to intervention or therapy.

Bioelectrical Impedance Analysis (BIA), Multiple Frequency Impedance (MF-BIA), and Bioimpedance Spectroscopy (BIS)

BIA Theory and Assumptions

The use of BIA for the assessment of body composition has become very popular during the past decade because it is noninvasive, reliable, and easy to use. This technique relies on differences in electrical properties of the FFM and the FM. Impedance (Z) is the resistance of a conductor to the flow of an alternating current and is composed of two components, resistance (R) and reactance (Xc). Resistance is the opposite of conduction, and reactance is the storage of an electrical charge by a condenser for a brief moment. So, impedance is defined as the square root of the sum of the squares of resistance and reactance:

$$Z = \sqrt{R^2 + Xc^2} \quad (30.1)$$

In biological systems, cell membranes function as condensers, and briefly retain some of the electrical charge. This practice is of little or no consequence for single frequency BIA but is of some importance for MF-BIA use and will be addressed further in the MF-BIA section.

In the BIA literature, Z and R are used interchangeably because the reactance component in biological systems is relatively small. The impedance of the lean body is a function of the specific resistivity of the lean tissue, the cross-sectional area of the tissue, and the length of the conductor. This relationship is expressed in the following equation:

$$Z = \rho\ L/A \quad (30.2)$$

where Z is impedance in ohms (Ω), ρ is volume resistivity in ohms* centimeters (Ω × cm), L is conductor length in centimeters squared (cm^2), and A is cross-sectional area. Multiplying both sides of the equation by L/L gives:

$$Z = \rho L^2/AL \quad (30.3)$$

where AL is equal to volume (V). Substituting gives:

$$Z = \rho L^2/V \quad (30.4)$$

In biological systems, electrical conduction is related to water and electrolyte distribution in the conductor. Since FFM contains virtually all the water and electrolytes in the body, conductivity is much greater in the FFM than the FM. Nyboer[8] demonstrated that electrically determined biological volumes were inversely related to Z, R, and Xc. Xc is a small component compared to R, and since R is a better predictor of Z than Xc, the expression for the determination of V has become:

$$V = \rho L^2/R \quad (30.5)$$

A simple compartment model would consist of cells in extracellular fluid. The electrolytes within the intra- and extracellular fluid are highly conductive, while the cell membranes act as an insulating layer of proteins and lipids. This model is present in Figure 30.1 as parallel conductive paths where R_E and R_I represent the resistance of the intra- and extracellular compartments, and C_M is the capacitance of the cell membrane.

Because the human body consists of multiple body parts with differing shapes, sizes, and geometry as well as differing electrical characteristics, the principles of BIA do not completely apply. However, the empirical relationship in Eq. 30.5 has been validated and is used extensively for body composition assessment.

Multiple Frequency BIA (MF-BIA) Theory and Assumptions

The theory behind MF-BIA is not different from that of BIA in terms of the body water and electrolyte content being means by which electrical current is conducted through the body. The one difference with MF-BIA is that at least two different frequencies are used. The theory is that low frequency current can not pass through the cell membrane due to its capacitance. Therefore, low frequency currents are conducted only through the extracellular fluid (ECF) compartment of the body. Conversely, high frequency current (≥50

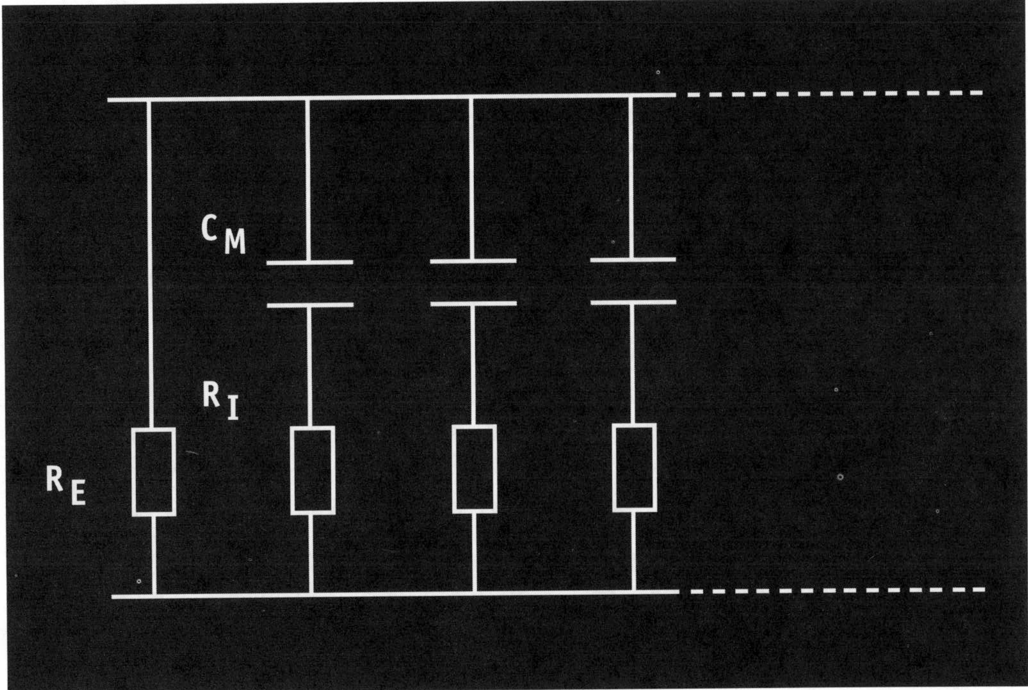

FIGURE 30.1
A circuit equivalent model for conduction of an electrical current through the body, where R_E represents the resistance of the extracellular fluid, R_I is the resistance of the intracellular fluid, and C_M is the capacitance of the cell membrane.

kHz) is capable of passing through the cell membrane, and thus is conducted through the total body water compartment of the body. So, MF-BIA has the potential for distinguishing ECF from total body water (TBW) and, by difference, estimating intracellular fluid, as shown in Figure 30.2.

This approach, however, still depends on the development of prediction equations using standard laboratory methods such as isotope dilution for TBW and tracer dilution for ECF. Again, these prediction equations will vary based on the sample studied, the physical characteristics of the sample subjects, and whether the individuals represent a "normal" healthy population or a specific clinical population. There are numerous clinical conditions for which accurate estimation of fluid compartments can provide valuable information.

Bio-impedance Spectroscopy (BIS) Theory and Assumptions

The basic principle of BIS is similar to MF-BIA in that low frequency current is conducted primarily through the ECF space, while high frequency current is conducted through TBW. The difference of these two fluid compartments allows for the estimation of intracellular fluid, which can be considered the same as body cell mass (BCM). The basic difference between MF-BIA and BIS is that BIS typically operates at 20 to 50 different frequencies ranging from about 5 kHz to 1 mHz. For each of these frequencies, measurements of resistance, reactance, impedance, and phase are recorded. The values derived from these measurements when plotted form a curve called an impedance locus, as seen in Figure 30.3.

The mathematical model to describe this plot is called the Cole-Cole Model.[9] This model produces a semicircular relationship between resistance and reactance with a depressed

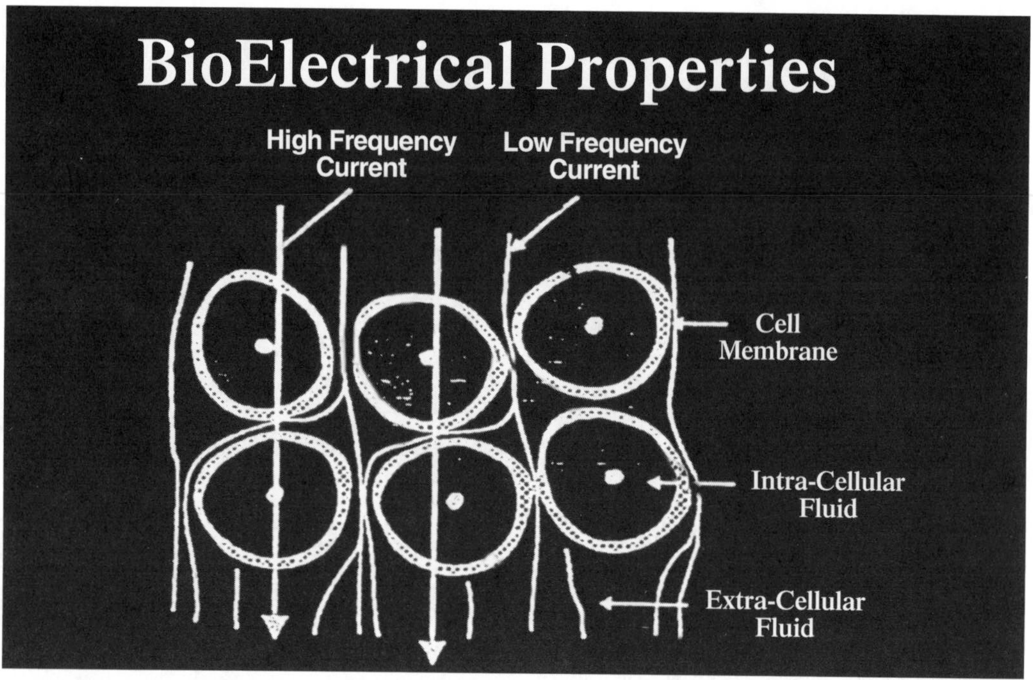

FIGURE 30.2
Conduction of low and high frequency currents through the extracellular fluid and the total body water compartments, respectively.

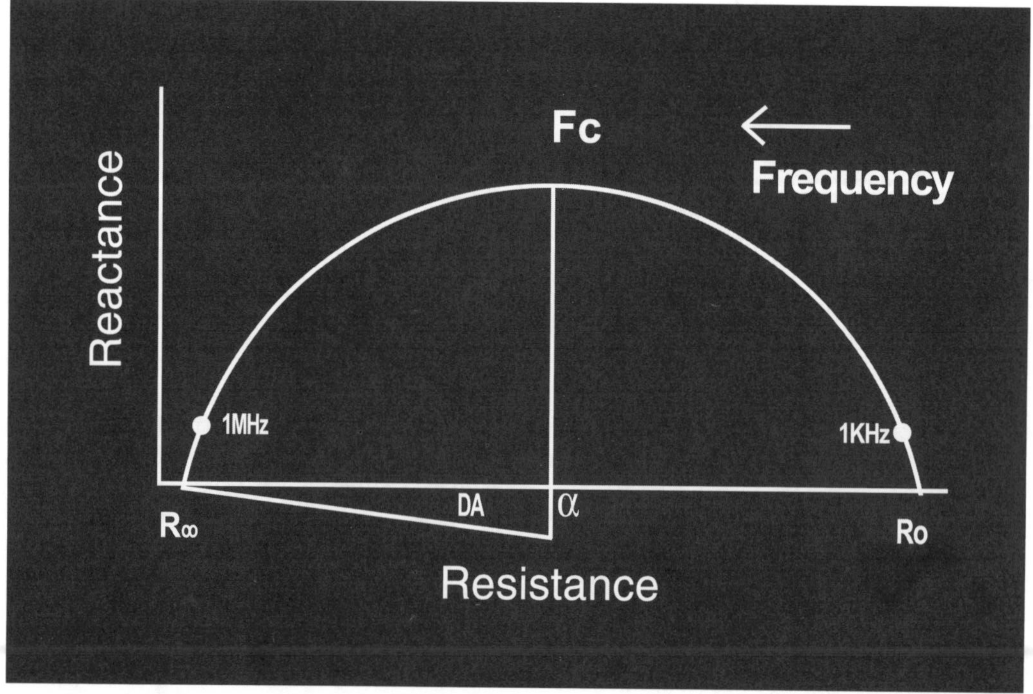

FIGURE 30.3
Cole-Cole Model of an impedance locus plot with resistance vs. reactance at increasing frequencies.

center. In the BIS technique, this modeling is essentially the only way of independently analyzing the components of a heterogeneous material, such as the human body.

The prediction of fluid volumes must be adjusted for the mixture effect of having materials of differing conductive capacity within the fluid being measured. This is done using mixture theory,[10,11] which adjusts for the nonlinear relationship between R and water volume in a mixed medium system. The mixture effects are greatest at low frequency because the conductive volume, presumably ECF, is a smaller proportion of the total volume. Hanai[10] developed an equation to describe the effect on the conductivity of a conducting material having nonconductivity entities in suspension, and hypothesized that the theory could be applied to tissues with non-conductivity materials ranging from 10 to 90%. This theory requires that at low frequencies, the ECF be considered the conductive medium, with all other materials as nonconductive. At high frequencies, the combined fluid compartments of extra- and intracellular fluids are the conductive medium and all other materials nonconductive.[11] This approach has been used successfully by a number of investigators to monitor changes in ECF, TBW, and FFM under a variety of conditions.[12-15]

BIA Measurement Procedures

All single frequency BIA instruments are essentially the same, consisting of an alternating electrical current source, cables and electrodes for introducing the current into the body, and a device for measuring the impedance and reactance. Although two electrodes have been used for making BIA measurements, this practice is not common because the two-electrode configuration requires the use of needle electrodes inserted into the subcutaneous layer of the skin to overcome the skin impedance. The most commonly used approach includes a four- (tetrapolar) electrode arrangement with electrodes placed on the dorsal surfaces of the hand, wrist, ankle, and foot. This configuration allows for the introduction of the current into the body through the more distal electrodes (hand and foot), while the measurement of the impedance to the current is taken from the proximal electrodes (wrist and ankle). A variety of four-electrode single frequency instruments is available, and most operate at a fixed frequency of 50 kHz, but amplitudes may differ between manufacturers. The two most commonly used devices are the RJL model 101 or 103, and the Valhalla Scientific 1990B, which operate at currents of 800 and 500 μA, respectively.[16] Additional BIA devices include hand-held BIA models[17] as well as models that look like bathroom scales, on which one stands while barefoot. Although all these instruments measure resistance and reactance, the values among the devices are not always in agreement;[16] therefore, one must be careful when picking a prediction equation for body composition assessment to use equations developed for a specific instrument.

Measurement devices for MF-BIA are not all alike. Some instruments use three frequencies set at 5, 50, and 100 kHz while others use two frequencies set at either 5 and 50 kHz or 5 and 100 kHz. Again, use of any prediction equations from MF-BIA devices should be matched with the instrument used when the prediction equation was developed.

Few commercially available BIS instruments use Cole-Cole model as the method for measuring fluid compartment. The two most often cited instruments are the 4000B or Hydra-4000 by Xitron Technologies, Inc. (San Diego, CA) and the SEAC (Brisbane, Australia). Both of these instruments have been reported to give acceptable results.

BIA Precision and Accuracy

Reliability (getting the same answer when repeat measurements are made on an individual at a given time) of most instruments is very good, but can be influenced by skin preparation prior to electrode placement, electrode placement, and test conditions. Variation from day to day in weight-stable individuals is good, and has been reported to vary by 3 to 10 ohms or 1 to 2%.[16,18] Precision when measuring electronic resistors of known resistance is excellent, and is reported to be less than 0.5%. Other factors that can effect the accuracy of measurement include time of measurement relative to food consumption, strenuous exercise, alcohol consumption, or other conditions resulting in dehydration. Recommended guidelines for impedance testing have been standardized, and are outlined in a report from the National Institutes of Health (NIH).[19] Standardized measurement procedures for single-frequency BIA also apply to MF-BIA and BIS.

BIA Application

Bioelectrical Impedance Analysis (BIA)

Research studies on the validation of BIA for the assessment of FFM and FM are extensive, and are beyond the limits of this section. However, a brief overview of research with BIA for the general population, ethnic groups, and children is in order. One of the early studies which demonstrated the application of a tetrapolar arrangement of electrodes for the assessment of body composition was that of Lukaski. [20] Lukaski found that the impedance index, height squared divided by resistance, (HT^2/R) was the single best predictor of body weight, FFM, TBW, and total body potassium (TBK). Numerous other research studies have documented a strong relationship between the impedance index (HT^2/R) or R and FFM, or components thereof. The single largest set of published BIA data for body composition assessment was reported by Segal et al. [21] and consisted of 1567 adults (1069 men, 498 women) ages 17 to 62 years. In this study hydrodensitometry was used as the criterion method for determination of FFM and FM. Data from four laboratories were pooled and prediction equations developed for the estimation of lean body mass (LBM) based on body fatness; over or under 20% fat for men and over or under 30% for women. Initial fatness level was determined by the sum of four skinfold measurements. Prediction errors ranged from 1.97 kg LBM for women to 2.47 and 3.03 kg LBM for normal weight and obese men, respectively. Because the sample size was so large, the Segal study has proven to be robust and has been successfully cross-validated by other researchers.[22,23]

The use of BIA for the prediction of TBW and FFM of children has also been studied by numerous investigators. Typical of these results are the findings of Davies and Preece[24] and Houtkooper et al.[25] The research conducted by Davies and Preece[24] included 26 children and adolescents in whom TBW measurements were made as an indicator of FFM. Results included the development of a prediction equation for TBW. TBW was highly correlated ($r = 0.97$) with the impedance index (HT^2/R), and had a prediction error of 1.67 liters. Research by Houtkooper and colleagues[25] included an original sample of 94 children, with cross-validation samples of 68, 25, and 38 from three other research laboratories. The final prediction equation for children age 10 to 19 years included 225 boys and girls, and used the impedance index and weight to predict FFM with an $R^2 = 0.95$ and a standard error of estimate of 2.1 kg.

Prediction equations for use of BIA with different ethnic groups includes white, black, and Asian adults,[26] Hispanic women,[23] and West Indians,[27] to name a few. The Hispanic women who were studied were 20 to 39 years of age and had an average body fat of 27% and a FFM of 43.5 kg. The investigators compared six different BIA prediction equations in the literature and found that the Segal equations[21] and equations published by Lohman et al.[28] and Gray et al.[29] gave results comparable to those obtained from hydrodensitometry. The study by Wang et al.[26] included 778 healthy adult men and women ranging from 18 to 94 years and from three ethnic groups: whites 371, blacks 182, and Asians 225. Again, strong correlations were obtained between the HT^2/R and measurements of TBW, FFM, and TBK. The research conducted on the West Indian volunteers included men, women, and children ranging in age from 8 to 20 years. The BIA equation used was included in the standard software package that accompanies the instrument (RJL, Model 103). The investigators found that the body fat estimates provided by the BIA were similar to those obtained from hydrodensitometry, and the errors were lower than previously reported. They concluded that the equations provided in the RJL instrument were appropriate for a West Indian population residing in the West Indies.

MF-BIA Application

A variety of studies have been conducted to examine the use of MF-BIA for estimation of body fluid compartments and body composition. An early report by Segal et al.[30] used a trifrequency instrument (TVI-10, Daniger Medical Technology, Columbus, OH) with frequencies of 5, 50, and 100 kHz. Segal and co-workers found a strong relationship between ECF and HT^2/R at 5 kHz, and between TBW and HT^2/R at 100 kHz. The prediction equations developed from this study had an error of estimate of 1.94 and 2.64 L for ECF and TBW, respectively. Similarly, Van Loan and Mayclin[31] also studied multiple frequencies in an attempt to predict ECF. Using the Xitron-4000 impedance analyzer (Xitron Technologies Inc., San Diego, CA) they measured R, Xc, Z, and phase angle at 25 frequencies ranging from 1 kHz to 1.35 mHz. They found that the same frequency that was the best predictor of TBW was also the best predictor of ECF. In this particular study the impedance index at a frequency of 224 ohms was the best predictor of both ECF and TBW. In both of these investigations healthy research volunteers were used. In healthy individuals, where fluid balance is maintained by normal physiological mechanisms, TBW and ECF are intricately linked. Therefore, if ECF either increases or decreases, then TBW will also increase or decrease. In other words, a frequency that is found to accurately predict ECF will also predict TBW, as in the case of the Van Loan and Mayclin study. In a study with MF-BIA for predicting water compartments in patients with non-ascitic liver cirrhosis, Borghi et al.[32] used equations developed by Segal et al.[30] and Deurenberg et al.[33] These equations used low frequency impedance for the prediction of ECF and a high frequency current for estimation of TBW. Although the Segal and Deurenberg equations used different low frequency currents for the prediction of ECF (5 and 1 kHz, respectively), results from the two equations were similar to each other and to standard laboratory dilution methods. Likewise, the Segal and Deurenberg equations measured the impedance index at a frequency of 100 kHz for the prediction of TBW and achieved results similar to those obtained from laboratory dilution techniques. Although the MF-BIA technique appears to give results equivalent to those obtained from standard laboratory techniques for the prediction of ECF and TBW, there is a shortcoming. Because multiple regression prediction equations are used to make estimations for groups, estimates for ECF and TBW compartments on an individual basis have an error associated with them. Multiple regression analysis results in smaller individuals being regressed upward toward the group average while larger individuals are regressed downward toward the group average. Thus, at the low end of the spectrum the result is an over-prediction of the value, be it ECF, TBW or FFM, while at the upper end an under-prediction occurs. So, to get the best results possible the user must be aware of the various prediction equations in the scientific literature and select the equation that best represents the sample being studied.

BIS Application

More and more studies are available in the scientific literature in which BIS was the technique by which fluid compartments or FFM were estimated. Four such studies will be briefly reviewed. Van Loan et al.[13] were the first to successfully report the use of BIS in humans for the assessment of ECF, TBW, ICF, and FFM. Using the Cole-Cole modeling technique and the Hanai mixture theory, results reported by Van Loan and co-workers were not different from those obtained by standard laboratory methods. Group averages for ECF and FFM were identical (14.6 and 45.5 L, respectively), while group averages for TBW and ICF differed by only 0.1 L or 100 ml. Never before had such close agreement between a noninvasive bioimpedance method and standard laboratory methods been reported. A similar experiment was conducted by Cornish et al.[34] in healthy adults using the BIS technique and an SEAC analyzer (Brisbane, Australia). The results of Cornish and colleagues demonstrated that the estimation was only slightly better than results obtained by single-frequency BIA and anthropometric measurements. The variability associated with the SEAC's estimation of TBW and ECF was 5.2 and 10%, respectively. The difference between findings reported by Van Loan et al.[13] and those of Cornish may be due to different BIS instruments, instrument sensitivity, variability in the standard techniques for assessing TBW and ECF, test conditions, etc.; it's difficult to say. However, the data suggest that better accuracy was obtained using the Xitron Technologies, Inc. BIS device. Van Loan et al.[14] also used the BIS technique to monitor fluid changes in a group of women prior to conception, during pregnancy, and postpartum. At 34 to 36 weeks of conception, when fluid volume is at a maximum, BIS results for ECF and TBW were within about 1 L of values obtained by standard lab methods; they were about 5% different for ECF and 1% different for TBW. More recently, Van Loan and co-workers[15] reported on the nitrogen accretion of lean tissue in AIDS-wasted patients using BIS. Based on classic nitrogen balance techniques, cumulative nitrogen retention over a 12-week period was 5 kg. At 6 weeks, nitrogen retention was 2.5 kg; BIS results indicated an accretion of 2.8 kg; by 12 weeks cumulative accretion by nitrogen balance methods was 5.0 kg, and by BIS was 5.3 kg. These data, in conjunction with other studies, demonstrate that the BIS technique, using Cole-Cole modeling and Hanai mixture theory, can accurately assess changes in TBW, ECF, and lean tissue accretion.

Dual Energy X-Ray Absorptiometry (DXA)

Basic Principles and History

Absorptiometry requires a photon or energy source and a detector or counting device. Early researchers used radionuclide sources such as ^{125}I or ^{153}Gd, but now x-rays are used to generate the photon energy. Each nuclide source has a characteristic photon energy spectrum and a half-life of decay. As photons travel through the target tissue, interactions take place that reduce the beam intensity. This reduction in beam intensity is referred to as attenuation. Attenuation occurs as photons are either absorbed or scattered when passing through tissue. It occurs by two main interactions *in vivo*: Compton scattering and photoelectric effects. Attenuation of photons passing through a homogenous substance is a function of photon intensity, mass attenuation coefficient (μ_m), and mass per unit area (M). With the DXA method, M represents total mass of the system's volume element. For heterogeneous absorbers, like human tissue, transmitted photon intensity is related to the substance's fractional mass. Basically, attenuation decreases as photon energy increases and is greater for substances with larger μ_ms. When photons of two different energies pass through an absorber, attenuation at the lower energy level can be expressed as a ratio (R) to attenuation observed at the higher energy level.[35] All elements have a characteristic μ_m

at specific energy levels. For example, hydrogen, with an atomic number of 1, has a μ_m of 0.3458 at 40 keV (kilelectron Volts) and a μ_m of 0.3175 at 70 keV, giving a R value of 1.0891. Elements with higher atomic numbers have larger R values. Thus elements found in soft tissue, like Na, K, Cl, have higher atomic numbers and larger R values. There are, however, other elements *in vivo* with even higher numbers, such as Ca, found primarily in bone. Thus, it is the R value which allows for the distinction between soft tissue, lower attenuation coefficients, and bone with higher attenuation coefficients. So, the R value of an unknown element can be used to identify the element because of the known and specific R values for each element. DXA measurements assume that the body is composed of two basic compartments, bone and soft tissue. Again, based on attenuation coefficients, soft tissue can be further divided into two compartments, fat or lean. Therefore, it is the R value that is used to determine the amount of bone and soft tissue and also the amount of fat and lean within the soft tissue.

Early devices for the assessment of bone mineral content (BMC) and density (BMD) used radioisotopes and were either single photon (SPA) or dual photon absorptiometers (DPA). SPA used iodine-125 (^{125}I) as the photon source (Figure 30.4). This instrument allowed for the measurement of BMD, BMC, and bone width in the distal end of the radius and ulna. Cameron and Sorenson[36] and Mazess and co-workers[37] conducted research which provided the foundation for validation, standardization, and comparative data for this early technique.

The second phase of method development for BMD and BMC measurements was the development of DPA using gadolinium –153 (^{153}Gd) as the photon source. The use of DPA advanced the technology from a single energy emission to an isotope with gamma emis-

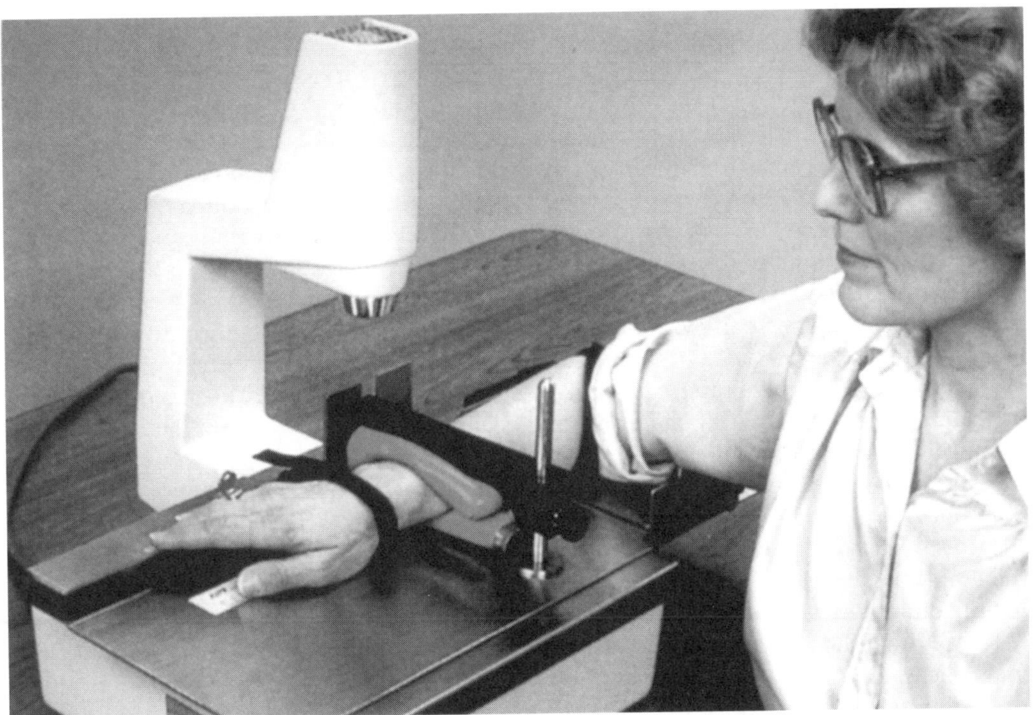

FIGURE 30.4
Single photon absorptiometer using radionuclide source from ^{125}I. Measurement of bone mineral content, bone width, and bone density is being made of the 1/3 distal radius and ulna of the forearm. Material around the forearm is "tissue equivalent" material to equalize the size among different individual forearms.

sions at two energy levels, 44 and 100 keV.[38,39] This method now included a measurement surface large enough for an individual to recline and have measurements taken of the total body, lumbar spine, and femur. In addition to the measurements of BMD and BMC, this technique now allowed for the assessment of total body composition.[40,41] As with all techniques, this method is not without its limitations. First, the constant decay of the radioisotope over time resulted in a lack of precision in the BMD measurement for the same individual and a constant correction of the attenuation coefficient for soft tissue because of the decaying radionuclide. Another method was needed that was not dependent upon a radioisotope as the energy source for the measurement technique.

Dual energy x-ray absorptiometry (DXA) was the third wave in the development of this technique for the assessment of bone parameters as well as body composition parameters. DXA consists of an x-ray tube, as the replacement for previously used radioisotopes, and a filter to split the x-ray beam into two distinct low and high energy levels. The use of two energy levels allows for greater precision in the measurement and estimation of soft tissue composition, and therefore, greater precision in the measurement of BMC and BMD. This technical advance resulted in the use of DXA for both bone metabolism studies and body composition studies. Thus, use of DXA allows for the estimation of numerous parameters for bone: total body bone mineral content and density (TBBMC or TBBMD) plus specific sites such as lumbar spine (Figure 30.5) and proximal femur BMC and BMD. Numerous estimates for body composition can also be made, including total body soft tissue mass (STM), which consists of lean tissue mass (LTM) and fat mass (FM) (STM = LTM + FM). Additionally, soft tissue masses can be examined over different regions of the body.

Measurement of Bone Mineral Mass and Soft Tissue Mass

Estimation of bone mineral mass (g) or bone mineral content (g/cm) can be obtained as well as bone area (cm). BMD is estimated from these basic units. Since the DXA is only a two-dimensional scan, actual density can not be determined; rather, bone mineral content of a given area is measured and adjusted for the width of the bone area, giving g/cm^2. This approach, however, has been validated against neutron activation analysis for the determination of total body calcium, and has provided the foundation for acceptance of the DXA estimate of bone mineral content.[38] In addition, some animal research has been done in which chemical analysis of pig carcasses served as the reference by which DXA was validated. Svendsen et al.[42] found good agreement between Lunar DPX (3.2 software) and fat content with pigs ranging from 35 to 95 kg in body weight. The standard error of estimate between the DXA estimate and chemical analysis was 2.9%. A similar comparison, chemical versus instrument, with a Hologic QDR-1000/W and pediatric software (version 6.01) used on small piglets was not as promising;[43] the estimates of lean mass were within 6%, bone mineral content was underestimated by 30%, and fat was overestimated by 100%. In larger piglets (average weight 6 kg) there was good agreement for lean tissue and bone mineral, but fat was still overestimated by 36%. Since this early work, however, DXA manufacturers have continued to upgrade instrumentation and software.

The DXA methodology for the measurement of BMC and BMD has its limitations. Jebb and colleagues[44,45] reported that estimates of BMD were affected by tissue depth or thickness, with an increasing error when measuring BMD in tissue greater than 20 cm in depth.

Results reported by Van Loan and co-workers examined how DXA estimates of BMD and BMC change when body weight changes.[46] They observed that when body weight declined as a result of a weight loss intervention, the DXA measurement of bone area (BA) changed, presumably because bone edge detection was now easier with less soft

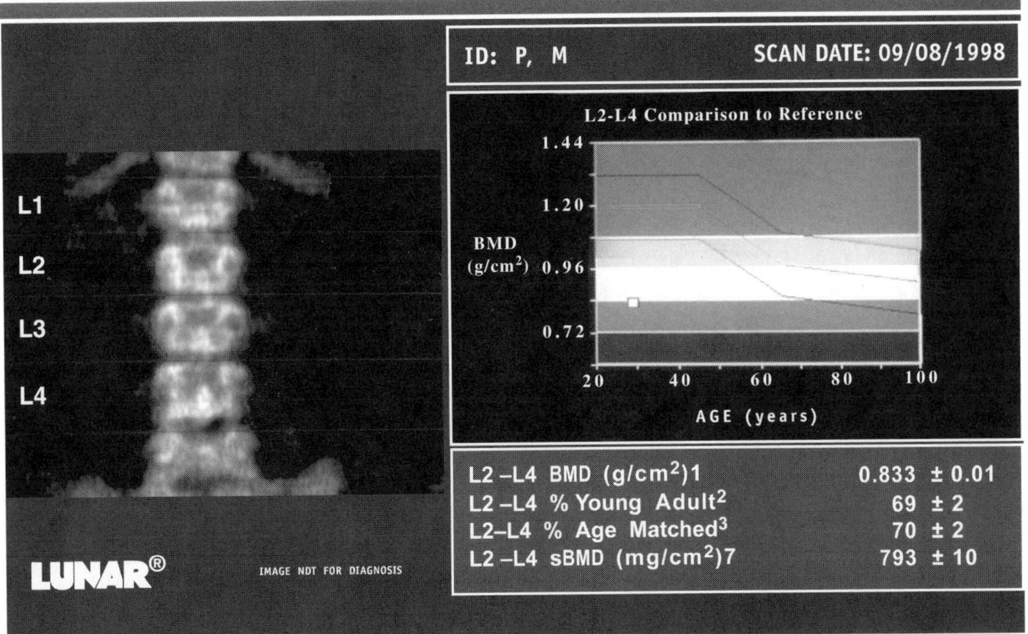

FIGURE 30.5
Image of the spine from a dual energy x-ray absorptiometer (DXA).

tissue attenuation. The net result was a change in the calculation of BMD without a corresponding change in the BMC. In weight-stable individuals, measurement of soft tissue composition has been reported to be similar to reference techniques. One such report was that of Van Loan and Mayclin,[47] who compared DXA estimates of body fat and lean masses to those determined using a four-compartment model for body composition assessment. DXA body composition assessment was in agreement with the results obtained using this model. These results have been confirmed by others.[48] In addition, DXA has reportedly been useful in the determination of intraabdominal adipose tissue (IAAT). Treuth and colleagues [49] derived a prediction equation for estimating IAAT using DXA scans analyzing the upper trunk, lower trunk, and pelvis regions. Anthropometric variables such as waist circumference and sagittal diameter were also made. These variables were used in a multiple regression equation to predict the IAAT mass based on images from computed tomography. This equation can be used in women of varying ages and body composition.

Equipment

Commercially available DXA instruments have been manufactured primarily by three companies in the U.S.: Lunar Corp., Madison, WI; Hologic, Waltham, MA; and Norland, Fort Atkinson, WI. The basis of the measurements for all three instruments is the mass attenuation ratio (R) discussed above. However, all three instruments do not provide the same result. Tothill[50] reported significant differences among the instruments in the estimate of percent body fat. When anthropometric models were tested, no differences were observed between manufacturers; however, there was significant differences in percent body fat between pairs of instruments when research volunteers were tested, varying 2.6 to 6.3%. Differences in regional body composition indicated trunk percent fat was underestimated by Hologic compared to Lunar and Norland, and standard deviations of 4% suggested inadequate agreement between instruments. Tothill and co-workers concluded that differences in body fat estimates among the instruments were great enough to preclude interchanging of instruments on individual subjects and within clinical investigations. Research reported by Van Loan et al.[51] not only found differences in the body composition assessment between Lunar and Hologic instruments but also found significant differences in the BMC and BMD values for the two devices. Some of these differences may be due to physical variations among the instruments. The Hologic model QDR 1000 uses photon energies at 45 and 100 keV, the Lunar model DPX uses 38 and 70 keV, and the Norland XR model has energy levels set at 44 and 100 keV. Differences may also be due to variations in scan areas, pixel area, and calibration procedures. In the ensuing years, DXA technology has moved from the collimated pencil beam approach of the above three instruments to a fan beam mode, with the x-ray fan sweeping the measurement area. This fan beam approach is touted as providing better resolution and precision, shorter scan times, and less radiation exposure compared to the pencil beam mode. Research by Faulkner et al.[52] included cross-validation of Hologic instruments using pencil beam modes QDR-1000W, QDR-2000, and fan beam modes. They determined that results from the three instruments were comparable and had low standard errors of estimate. However, research in this area is limited and requires further investigation to determine how pencil beam and fan beam results compared with a given company and between the different companies.

Accuracy of DXA

A variety of DXA issues have been discussed here regarding the accuracy of DXA in measuring different body compartments. The basic tenet has been that DXA does provide an accurate measure of BMC compared to neutron activation. Several studies have shown that DXA estimates of soft tissue lean and fat compartments are equivalent to results obtained from reference methods when used in weight-stable individuals; however, concerns do arise when using the DXA technique for determining BMD in larger individuals, especially when these individuals engage in a weight loss intervention. DXA has been shown to be a valuable tool in the estimation of IAAT. Despite these positive outcomes, all DXA instruments are not "created equal." Several studies have demonstrated that differences exist in soft tissue and bone parameters between manufacturers and between software versions within a given manufacturer. Therefore, one must use caution when using this technique to monitor individuals longitudinally. In summary, DXA can be used as a component in multiple-compartment body composition assessment by using just the BMC values. It can also be used separately as a stand-alone technique for the estimation of bone mineral, lean tissue, and fat mass. A significant amount of research has been done to suggest that pencil beam DXA may be viewed as a reference method; however, the newer fan beam mode of operation has not yet been thoroughly examined. More research is needed to validate the results using this new approach and determine what, if any, differences exist between the fan beam mode and the pencil beam mode of operation.

Computed Tomography

Basic Principles

Computed tomography (CT) is another x-ray device used commonly in medical diagnosis. However, in the 1980s several studies indicated that the technique could be used for the determination of body composition because images of adipose tissue, muscle, and bone could be obtained with this technique.[53] In this technique, like the DXA, attenuation of an x-ray signal is the process by which different tissues are distinguished. Many people are familiar with the "large tunnel" of a CT scanner. Within the structure of the tunnel is an x-ray tube and detectors. The detectors and x-ray tube are placed opposite one another so that the detectors can rapidly measure the x-ray attenuation as the x-ray photons pass through the individual. For a CT scan, the patient lies on a moveable table which positions the patient in the tube at the appropriate position for the needed image. For example, a brain CT scan would require specific positioning of the head within the CT tunnel. Once properly positioned, the x-ray tube rotates around the table while the detectors collect the necessary attenuation data. A computer then generates an image based on the specific attenuation coefficient characteristics of the different tissues, thus allowing for the separate imaging of bone, adipose tissue, and lean tissue. The differences in the attenuation coefficients allow CT to be used for body composition assessment.[54,55] The CT attenuation score, referred to as Hounsfield units (HU) depends on the level of absorption of the emitted x-ray, and may range from –1000 HU for air to +1000 HU for bone. Research by Sjöström[56] demonstrated that the attenuation score for adipose tissue (AT) was between –190 and –30 HU.

Accuracy

CT scans are expensive, and this cost has no doubt limited the number and extent of validation studies. One study, however, conducted by Rössner et al.[54] compared direct adipose tissue thicknesses from cadavers to CT images from 21 cross-sectional abdominal images and found a significant relationship between the two methods for total adipose tissue ($r = 0.94$) and intraabdominal adipose tissue ($r = 0.83$). Work by Ross and colleagues on rats demonstrated a relationship between CT images and chemical analysis of lipids ($r = 0.98$).[57] Validation and accuracy check with this technique are very limited due primarily to the need for cadaver analysis of humans or chemical analysis of animals.

Body Composition and Visceral Adipose Tissue (VAT) by CT

Whole body composition using CT was investigated by Tokunaga et al.[58] using multiple scans. First, the area within the scan was measured, and then the area between adjacent scans was measured. Total volume was then calculated. Second, adipose tissue within the scan area was measured, providing a determination of total adipose tissue within the region. More extensive work by Sjöström and Kvist[59] using 22 scans from head to foot found that CT estimates of adipose tissue volume were highly correlated to body fat estimates from tritium dilution, hydrodensitometer, and whole body potassium counting. These two studies support the use of CT scans for assessment of total body fat as well as lean tissue that does not rely upon assumptions regarding the constancy of body compartments. This method, however, does involve a significant amount of radiation exposure, requires highly trained technical staff, instrumentation is expensive, and it is not readily available for body composition studies. Consequently, researchers have tried to limit the number of scans needed for accurate estimates of abdominal adipose tissue. Després and co-workers[60] demonstrated that the adipose tissue mass in a cross-sectional scan at the level of lumbar L4-L5 vertebrae was correlated to the total adipose tissue mass in both men and women. As a result of this work and the work of others, it has been determined that a single abdominal scan does provide an acceptable estimate of total abdominal adipose tissue mass.

A major focus of researchers using CT technology for the estimation of adipose tissue is the association between body fat and chronic disease. More specifically, determination of at risk individuals for diabetes mellitus, cardiovascular diseases, and elevated plasma lipid profiles, to name a few, can be improved using CT scans. Investigations[61,62] have shown that obesity with increased levels of VAT was associated with a higher glycemic response even with hyperinsulinemia, suggesting insulin resistance. VAT was also correlated with glucose tolerance and plasma insulin levels in both men and women. These relationships were independent of total body fat. Furthermore, obese subjects will smaller amounts of VAT showed only marginally higher plasma insulin levels compared to control subjects. It appears that the assessment of total body fat alone can be a misleading indicator of individuals at risk, and that the more important concern is the amount of adipose tissue that is sequestered intraabdominally.

Magnetic Resonance Imaging (MRI)

Basic Principles, Acquisition, and Quantification

MRI involves an interaction between the magnet field, generated by the MRI instrument, and the nucleus of the hydrogen atom. Hydrogen is the most abundant element in biological systems, and the proton in the hydrogen nucleus acts like a tiny magnet with a nonzero magnet moment. Typically, an individual is positioned on a moving table and placed inside the magnetic field. The magnetic field of the MRI instruments is about 10,000 times stronger than the magnetic field of the Earth, and is used to align the hydrogen protons in a known direction, at which time a pulsed radio frequency (RF) is applied to the body part within the magnetic field. The hydrogen protons absorb the energy of the RF and change alignment or directional orientation, like a spinning gyroscope falling out of position. Once the RF is turned off, the protons release the absorbed energy and gradually return to their normal position or orientation. The released energy also gives off an RF signal which is detected. The RF signal from the released energy that is used to develop the MR images using computer software.

Proton density and the rate at which the absorbed energy is released, referred to as relaxation time, differs among the different body tissues. The dark and light contrasts in an MR image are due to the different time parameters associated with the energy release: 1) the time to repeat (TR), and 2) the time to echo (TE) the RF pulse. Variation in the RF pulse sequence results in manipulation of the TR and TE times. One such variation in the pulse sequence is called spin-echo, and adjusts the TR parameter for maximum contrast between adipose tissue and muscle tissue. It is the spin-echo sequence that is routinely used to assess adipose tissue. All of this takes time, which can be a limitation of this technique for body composition assessment. The average time needed for abdominal MRI is about eight minutes, and then the image may include motion artifacts from breathing and even cardiac contractions (see Figure 30.6). Consequently, new MRI techniques have included the development of TR and TE so that images can be obtained in a matter of seconds while an individual holds his breath. These faster techniques are known as FLASH (Fast and Low Angle Shot) or GRASS (Gradient Recalled Acquisition at Steady State). The accuracy of these faster techniques has not been thoroughly investigated, but they do allow for a shorter time period for data acquisition and thus less movement artifact in the image.

Quantification of the tissue masses from the MR image requires a variety of steps. The image is divided into squares comprising several hundred rows and columns. Each square

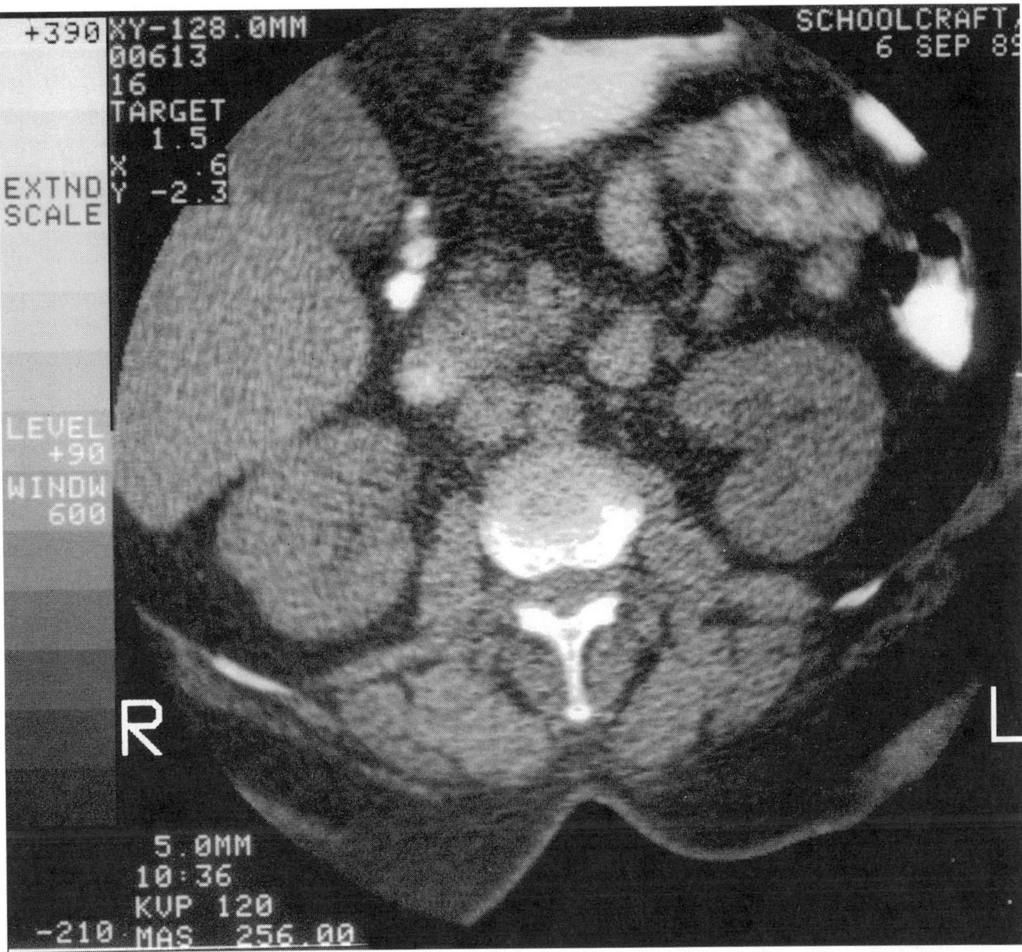

FIGURE 30.6
Magnetic resonance image of the abdominal cavity of an individual. Lighter images around the perimeter represent skin and subcutaneous adipose tissue. Lighter images within the body cavity are visceral adipose tissue depots. The adipose tissue mass can be quantified by digital analysis of the individual image pixels.

is referred to as a pixel. Pixel values in an MRI are dependent upon 1) the excitation pulse used, 2) the proton density, and 3) tissue relaxation times, which may vary among individuals. Additionally, signal intensity may vary within the same tissue in a single acquisition. This is referred to as "ghosting," and can result in tissue being excluded from the analysis. This phenomenon has been improved in recent years. However, changes in signal intensity do require that software programs allow for visual verification and, when necessary, adjustments to include all appropriate tissue. Therefore, adipose tissue quantification cannot be done by simply setting an adipose tissue threshold and using software to count pixels either above or below the designated threshold without manual verification and correction.

Accuracy

Foster and co-workers[63] first reported that MRI could measure adipose tissue and adjacent muscle tissue. This work was confirmed by carcass and cadaver analysis in which direct measurements were made of the tissues. Work by Abate et al.[64] demonstrated that MRI measurement of adipose tissue in humans was similar to direct measurement of visceral and subcutaneous adipose tissue on cadavers. Similar supporting documentation for the accuracy of MRI has been done by comparing MRI to CT scan results.[55] In general, the relationship between CT and MRI for the assessment of adipose tissue is good, with correlations ranging from 0.79 for SAT to 0.98 for VAT, and 0.99 for total adipose tissue.

MRI for Body Composition

Unlike CT scans, MR images do not involve a radiation dose, thus making them more appealing to research volunteers as a method for body composition assessment. MR images, however, like CT scan, are expensive and generally require multiple scans in order to obtain adipose tissue distribution information. The number of researchers who have used MRI is limited. Two different research teams used multiple MRI images over the entire body. Fowler and colleagues[65] acquired 28 images from head to foot, while Ross and co-workers[66] obtained 40+ images from head to foot to determine adipose tissue and lean tissue distribution in both males and females. Fowler demonstrated that as few as four MR images could be used, while Ross showed that one image at the level of L4-L5 lumbar vertebrae could be used to predict total adipose tissue volume. MRI has also been shown to discriminate between visceral and subcutaneous adipose tissue. Measurement of VAT has been shown to be strongly correlated with complications associated with obesity. Although MRI has promise as a "reference" method for adipose tissue composition, more research is needed relative to its accuracy for tissues other than VAT and SAT. Like CT, the need for highly qualified technical personnel to obtain the images, and the cost of instrumentation make this technique beyond the reach of most researchers and clinicians for body composition assessment.

Summary

The techniques discussed in this section are high tech methods, and may not be suitable for all situations. So, how does one decide which method to use, especially when costs and technical expertise vary widely among the methods? Appropriate questions might include the following:

Do I need the information for research or clinical diagnosis?

If for research, do I need greater accuracy and precision to see changes in small groups of people or are large group trends sufficient?

Will individuals come to the test facility or is the work done in a "field" setting?

For either research or clinical intervention, what body composition parameter(s) do I need to know?

- Fat Mass
- FFM
- Bone Mass (BMC or BMD)
- Fluid Volumes
- Adipose tissue distribution

What level of technical expertise is needed to get accurate results?

- Does the procedure require highly trained staff and/or licensed staff?
- Can I get my staff adequately trained with minimal difficulty?
- Can I get my staff licensed with minimal expense?

How much will it cost?

- Do I have to contract with a medical facility to do the measurement?
- Can I purchase the instrument and collect the data myself?

More often than not, time and money will be overriding factors in consideration of a body composition methodology. Thankfully, all the methods discussed in this section do provide reliable and accurate results when used appropriately.

References

1. Booth RA, Goddard BA, Paton A. *Br J Nutr* 20: 719; 1966.
2. Bellisari A. *J Diag Med Sonography* 19: 15; 1993.
3. Bellisari A, Roche AF, Siervogel RM. *Internat J Obesity* 17: 475; 1993.
4. Roche AF. In *Human Body Composition* (Roche AF, Heymsfield SB, Lohman TG, Eds) Human Kinetics Publishers, Champaign, IL, 1996, p 167.
5. Abe T, Kondo M, Kawakami Y, Fukunagg T. *Am J Human Biol* 6: 1661; 1994.
6. Lochmuller E-M, Zeller J-B, Kaiser D, et al. *Osteoporosis Internat* 8: 591; 1998.
7. Adams JE, Harrison EJ, Alsop CW, Selby PL. *Osteoporosis Internat* 8: 55S; 1998.
8. Nyboer J, Bagno S, Nims LF. The electrical impedance plethysmograph, an electrical volume recorder. National Research Council, Committee on Aviation, Report No. 149. Washington, DC, 1943.
9. Cole KS. *Membranes, Ion, and Impulses: A Chapter on Classical Biophysics.* University of California Press, Berkeley, CA, 1972.
10. Hanai T. In: *Emulsion Science* (Sherman PH, Ed), Academic Press, London, 1968, p 354.
11. MacDonald JR. *Impedance Spectroscopy: Emphasizing Solid Materials and Systems.* John Wiley & Sons, New York, 1987.
12. De Lorenzo A, Andreoli A, Matthie J, Withers P. *J Applied Physiol* 82: 1542; 1997.
13. Van Loan MD, Withers P, Matthie J, Mayclin PL. In: *Human Body Composition:* In Vivo *Methods, Models, and Assessment.* (Ellis KJ, Eastman JD, Eds) Plenum Publishers, New York, 1993, p 67.
14. Van Loan MD, Koop LE, King JC, et al. *J Applied Physiol* 78: 1037; 1995.
15. Van Loan MD, Strawford A, Jacob M, Hellerstein M. *AIDS* 13: 241; 1999.
16. Graves JE, Polock ML, Colvin AB, et al. *Am J Human Biol* 1: 803; 1989.
17. Loy SF, Likes EA, Andrews PM, et al. *ACSM's Health & Fitness Journal* 2: 16; 1998.
18. Van Loan MD, Mayclin PL. *Human Biol* 59: 299; 1987.
19. *Bioelectrical Impedance Analysis in Body Composition Measurement.* National Institutes of Health Technology Assessment Conference Statement. December 12-14, 1994.
20. Lukaski HC, Johnson PE, Bolonchuk WW, Lykken GI. *Am J Clin Nutr* 41: 810; 1985.
21. Segal KR, Van Loan MD, Fitzgerald PI, Hodgdon JA. *Am J Clin Nutr* 47: 7; 1988.
22. Stolarczyk LM, Heyward VH, Van Loan MD, et al. *Am J Clin Nutr* 66: 8; 1997.
23. Stolarczyk LM, Heyward VH, Goodman JA, et al. *Med Sci Sports Exerc* 27: 1450; 1995.
24. Davies PSW, Preece MA. *Ann Hum Biol* 15: 237; 1988.
25. Houtkooper LB, Going SB, Lohman TG, et al. *J Applied Physiol* 72: 366; 1992.
26. Wang J, Thornton JC, Burastero S, et al. *Am J Hum Biol* 7: 33; 1995.
27. Young RE, Sinha DP. *Am J Clin Nutr* 55: 1045; 1992.
28. Lohman TG. *Advances in Body Composition Assessment.* Human Kinetics Publishers, Champaign, IL, 1992, p 53.

29. Gray DS, Bray GA, Gemayel N, Kaplan K. *Am J Clin Nutr* 50: 225; 1989.
30. Segal KR, Burastero S, Chun A, et al. *Am J Clin Nutr* 54: 26; 1991.
31. Van Loan MD, Mayclin PL. *Eur J Clin Nutr* 46: 117; 1992.
32. Borghi A, Bedogni G, Rocchi E, et al. *Br J Nutr* 76: 325; 1996.
33. Deurenberg P, Schouten FJM, Andreoli A, De Lorenzo A. In: *Human Body Composition.* In Vivo *Methods, Models and Assessment* (Ellis KJ, Eastman JD, Eds) Plenum Press, New York, 1993, p 129.
34. Cornish BH, Ward LC, Thomas BJ, Elia M. *Eur J Clin Nutr* 50: 159; 1996.
35. Pietrobelli A, Formica C, Wang Z, Heymsfield SB. *Am J Physiol* 271: E941; 1996.
36. Cameron JR, Sorenson JA. *Science* 142: 230; 1963.
37. Mazess RB, Cameron JR, Miller H. *Internat J Applied Rad Isotopes* 23: 471; 1972.
38. Mazess RB, Peppler WW, Chestnut CH, et al. *Calcified Tissue Internat* 33: 361; 1981.
39. Mazess RB, Peppler WW, Gibbons M. *Am J Clin Nutr* 40: 834; 1984.
40. Gotfredsen A, Jensen J, Borg J, Christiansen C. *Metabolism* 35: 88; 1986.
41. Heymsfield SB, Wang J, Heshka S, et al. *Am J Clin Nutr* 49: 1283; 1989.
42. Svendsen OL, Haarbo J, Hassager C, Christiansen C. *Am J Clin Nutr* 57: 605; 1993.
43. Brunton JA, Bayley HS, Atkinson SA. *Am J Clin Nutr* 58: 839; 1993.
44. Jebb SA, Goldberg GR, Jennings G, Elia M. In: *Human Body Composition.* In Vivo *Methods, Models and Assessment.* (Ellis KJ, Eastman JD, Eds) Plenum Press, New York, 1993, p 129.
45. Jebb SA, Goldberg GR, Jennings G, Elia M. *Clin Sci* 88: 319; 1995.
46. Van Loan MD, Johnson HL, Barbieri TF. *Am J Clin Nutr* 67: 734; 1998.
47. Van Loan MD, Mayclin PL. *Eur J Clin Nutr* 46: 125; 1992.
48. Tothill P, Han TS, Avenell A, et al. *Eur J Clin Nutr* 50: 747; 1996.
49. Treuth MS, Hunter GR, Kekes-Szabo T. *Am J Clin Nutr* 62: 527; 1995.
50. Tothill P, Avenell A, Love J, Reid D. *Eur J Clin Nutr* 48: 781; 1994.
51. Van Loan MD, Thompson J, Butterfield G, et al. *Med Sci Sports Exerc* 26: 40S; 1994.
52. Faulkner G, Gleur CC, Engelke K, Genant HK. *J Bone Min Res* 7: 518S; 1992.
53. Borkan GA, Hults DE, Gerzof SF, et al. *Ann Hum Biol* 10: 537; 1983.
54. Rössner S, Bo WG, Hiltbrandt E, et al. *Internat J Obesity* 14: 839; 1990.
55. Seidell JC, Bakker CJ, van der Kooy K. *Am J Clin Nutr* 51: 953; 1990.
56. Sjöström L, Kvist H, Cederblad A, Tylén U. *Am J Physiol* 250: 736E; 1986.
57. Ross R, Léger L, Guardo R, et al. *J Applied Physiol* 70: 787; 1991.
58. Tokunaga K, Matsuzawa Y, Ishikawa K, Tarui S. *Internat J Obesity* 7: 437; 1983.
59. Sjöström L, Kvist H. *Acta Medicia Scan* 723: 169; 1988.
60. Deprés J-P, Prud'homme D, Pouliot MC, et al. *Am J Clin Nutr* 54: 474; 1991.
61. Deprés J-P, Nadeau A, Tremblay A, et al. *Diabetes* 38: 304; 1989.
62. Pouliot MC, Deprés J-P, Lemieux S, et al. *Am J Cardiol* 73: 460; 1994.
63. Foster MA, Hutchinson JMS, Mallard JR, Fuller M. *Magnetic Res Imaging* 2: 187; 1984.
64. Abate N, Burns D, Peshock RM, et al. *J Lipid Res* 35: 1490; 1994.
65. Fowler MA, Fuller MF, Glasbey CA, et al. *Am J Clin Nutr* 54: 18; 1991.
66. Ross R, Léger L, Morris D, et al. *J Applied Physiol* 72: 787; 1992.

31

Frame Size, Circumferences, and Skinfolds

Barbara J. Scott

Introduction

Numerous studies conducted over the past 70 years provide a large body of knowledge and evidence that simple methods of quantifying body size and proportions can be used in many settings to predict body composition and regional fat distribution. This section discusses the strengths, weaknesses, and potential best applications of three field anthropometric methods: frame size, skin folds, and circumferences. These methods have been widely studied and are commonly used because they yield valid and reliable results when applied correctly and because they are noninvasive, inexpensive, portable, and relatively simple to perform.

Applications to Practice

Important applications for the measurement and analysis of body composition and body dimensions using the above methods include:

- Evaluating how individuals or groups are faring in general or in response to changing economic or political situations (new leadership, prolonged drought or famine, war, decreased expenditures for health services, increase in number of individuals or families living in poverty, increased cost of food) (surveillance)
- Monitoring individual response to specific therapeutic interventions (surgery, medication, chemotherapy)
- Making comparisons of actual with "ideal" (weight for height, waist-to-hip ratio, level of body fatness)
- Formulating exercise or dietary programs/regimens
- Providing prognostic indicators in certain disease states linked to body composition (diabetes, certain types of cancer, osteoporosis, cystic fibrosis, HIV/AIDS)
- Providing periodic feedback regarding achievement of goals resulting from lifestyle modifications (diet, exercise, smoking cessation)

0-8493-2705-9/01/$0.00+$1.50

- Assessing level of potential risk for chronic disease (cardiovascular, cancer, diabetes, osteoporosis) and monitoring relative risk over time

The method chosen depends most often on practical considerations of availability of equipment, staff (number and expertise of personnel), time, and facilities. The degree of accuracy or precision needed based on the sample size and purpose for which the information is being collected must also be considered. For example, less precision may be accepted if the purpose is risk assessment or monitoring changes with initiation of an exercise program than if the information is needed for establishing health policy or making clinical decisions about treatment or disease prognosis.

Application to Different Populations

Many variables have been found to affect the validity of measurements of body composition, including age, gender, ethnicity, measurement site selection, weight status, and health status.[1] Therefore, it is imperative that the methods selected are those best suited to the persons or population being studied. Depending on the setting and application, it may be necessary to use different methods, different anatomical sites, or to apply different equations to the same methods.

Reference Methods: AKA "Gold Standards"

Many different methods have been employed over the past seven decades to measure the composition of the human body,[2] and new technologic developments and findings from validation studies both inform and complicate decisions about which method(s) to select for a given purpose. A primary consideration in the selection of a method is whether it can provide valid information for the specific application and population being studied. Many different tests have been employed to compare body composition from experimental methods with those from the "gold standard" including: analysis of variance (examining differences), correlation coefficients (examining similarities), standard error, coefficient of variation (examining the size of the standard deviation relative to the mean), level of bias (difference between "gold standard" and experimental measure), regression analyses to examine unique and additive contributions of different measures in improving the predictive power of body composition equations, and intra- and interobserver variance.

There is no absolutely perfect method to measure and find the true value for body composition in living humans. Thus, indirect methods, most commonly hydrodensitrometry (underwater weighing) and dual-energy x-ray absorptiometry (DXA), have been used as the "gold standards" against which the majority of measures of frame size, circumferences, and skinfolds have been evaluated.[3] The validation studies using underwater weighing were based on a two-compartment model that divides body composition into fat and fat-free components and assumes constant densities for these tissues that are not universally applicable. The more recent availability of DXA technology has provided a three-compartment method free of assumptions about tissue densities but dependent on assumptions of software used with the equipment. Differing results from comparisons of these two methods (ranging from close agreement to significantly higher or lower values) probably reflect differences in the subjects studied (ethnicity, age, level of activity, gender, etc). Therefore, even though it is not clear which method yields a "true" value, it appears that more investigators are leaning toward using DXA as the new standard

TABLE 31.1

Data Quality and Anthropometric Measurement Error[7,8]

Goal of Quality Measurement	Terminology, Definitions, and Causes or Contributing Factors
Repeated measures give the same value	Reliability: Differences between measures on a single subject (within subject variability) are not caused by errors in measurement (site or technique) or physiologic variation.
	Imprecision: Different results are obtained for a single subject when measurements are done either by one person (intra-observer differences) or two or more persons (interobserver differences) and reflect measurement errors.
	Undependability: Different results are due to physiologic factors (such as differences over the course of a day in weight [due to weight of food eaten or fullness of the bladder] or height [due to compression of the spine]).
	Unreliability: The sum of errors due to imprecision and undependability.
Measurement represents a "true" value	Inaccuracy: A systematic bias is present due to instrument errors or errors of measurement technique.
	Validity: Measurement is as close to the true value as it is possible to determine.

because it is more acceptable and easier for the subjects, and because it does not rely on assumptions about bone mineral content. More recent studies suggest the simultaneous use of multiple methods is best suited to measuring or accurately examining different body compartments to establish and/or validate field methods on diverse populations.[4]

Measurement Error

Once the field method has been selected as appropriate to the purpose or study at hand, adherence to guidelines for achieving acceptable levels of measurement error[5,6] are needed to evaluate the quality of data collected. (See Table 31.1).

Guidelines for training and certification of measurers direct a repeated-measures protocol where the trainee and trainer measure the same subjects until the difference between them is very small. However, the definition of "small difference" is constrained to some extent by the technique itself (how precise can it be), equipment (how exactly can it be calibrated, how fine is the scale), and by the magnitude of the potential size of the measurement itself (measured in many centimeters, such as height versus in few millimeters, such as some skinfolds).

Some targets for difference to be achieved to certify competency have been proposed (Table 31.2).[9] Given the limits of what accuracy level is possible, investigators must also be aware of the proportion of the total measurement represented by the acceptable difference.[10]

TABLE 31.2

Recommendations for Evaluating Measurement Differences between Trainer and Trainee

	Difference between Trainer and Trainee			
Measurement	Good	Fair	Poor	Gross Error
Height (length) (cm)	0–0.5	0.6–0.9	1.0–1.9	2.0 or >
Weight (kg)	0–0.1	0.2	0.3–0.4	0.5 or >
Arm circumference (cm)	0–0.5	0.6–0.9	1.0–1.9	2.0 or >
Skinfolds (any) (mm)	0–0.9	1.0–1.9	2.0–4.9	5.0 or >

Methods

Even though literally hundreds of anthropometric studies have been done comparing methods and developing predictive equations,[11] there is neither clear evidence nor scientific consensus as to which methods, sites, or equations should be used. Thus, the best practice is to select a method with a preponderance of supporting evidence for the specific setting, population, and application, use good equipment, train staff well, understand the limitations, and be able to interpret the results within these limitations. Specific instructions for taking measurements or locating anatomical sites will not be covered in this section as detailed anthropometric manuals are available.[12,13]

Once a method and/or site of measurement has been selected as appropriate to the purpose for which the information is needed, the next steps include the logistics of selecting, calibrating, and using equipment, and training and certifying staff in the measurement procedures.

Frame Size

It seems intuitive that fat weight is unhealthy, and that persons with larger frames can weigh more and still be healthy. While there is general agreement that frame is a valid consideration in the assessment of weight for height, identifying an exact method for classifying frame size has been problematic.[14] The literature includes a variety of different concepts of frame size: body type and body proportions (length of trunk relative to total height), bone and skeletal size and thickness, and muscularity. There are two general schools of thought, one that frame is primarily a skeletal concept, and the other that it encompasses the fat-free mass (everything that is not fat including bone and muscle). Most researchers agree that a valid measure of frame must be independent of body fatness, while others believe that it must also be somewhat independent of height to be of value in the assessment of weight. However, studies have shown varying degrees of correlation of different measures of skeletal size and dimension with height (the linear dimension of the skeleton) and correlation of measures of both bone and muscle with body weight and fatness. Therefore, additional criterion for validity of frame size measures have been proposed:

1. The correlation of the measure with fat free mass (FFM) should be greater than the correlation of height alone with FFM
2. The measure should have little or no association with body fat beyond that accounted for by the association of FFM with fat[15]

Other studies have proposed more generalized methods or observations for classifying frame according to body type or morphology. The categories of leptomorph, metromorph, and pyenomorph[16] follow the idea that the human body is like a cylinder, and its mass is determined by height, breadth, and depth.

The main purpose for assessing frame size is to evaluate weight and recommend an optimal weight that would be associated with the best present state of health and longest life expectancy. One of the first proposed common uses of frame size was with weight tables published by the Metropolitan Life Insurance Company in 1954, based on mortality rates of insured adults in the U.S. and Canada.[17] These early tables suggested "ideal"

TABLE 31.3

Approximation of Frame Size by 1983 Metropolitan Height and Weight Tables

Women		Men	
Height (inches) in 1″ heels	**Elbow Breadth (inches)**	**Height (inches) in 1″ heels**	**Elbow Breadth (inches)**
58–59″ (4′10″–4′11″)	2 1/4–2 1/2″	62–63″ (5′2″–5′3″)	2 1/2–2 7/8″
60–63″ (5′0″–5′3″)	2 1/4–2 1/2″	64–67″ (5′4″–5′7″)	2 5/8–2 7/8″
64–67″ (5′4″–5′7″)	2 3/8–2 5/8″	68–71″ (5′8″–5′11″)	2 3/4–3″
68–71″ (5′8″–5′11″)	2 3/8–2 5/8″	72–75″ (6′–6′3″)	2 3/4–3 1/8″
72″ (6′0″)	2 1/2–2 3/4″	76″ (6′4″)	2 7/8–3 1/4″

TABLE 31.4

Frame Size by Elbow Breadth by Gender and Age

Age (years)	Males			Females		
	Small Frame	**Medium Frame**	**Large Frame**	**Small Frame**	**Medium Frame**	**Large Frame**
18–24	≤ 6.6	> 6.6 and <7.7	≥7.7	≤5.6	> 5.6 and <6.5	≥6.5
25–34	≤ 6.7	> 6.7 and <7.9	≥7.9	≤5.7	> 5.7 and <6.8	≥6.8
35–44	≤ 6.7	> 6.7 and <8.0	≥8.0	≤5.7	> 5.7 and <7.1	≥7.1
45–54	≤ 6.7	>6.7 and <8.1	≥8.1	≤5.7	> 5.7 and <7.2	≥7.2
55–64	≤ 6.7	> 6.7 and <8.1	≥8.1	≤5.8	> 5.8 and <7.2	≥7.2
65–74	≤ 6.7	> 6.7 and <8.1	≥8.1	≤5.8	> 5.8 and <7.2	≥7.2

Source: Frisancho, A.R., *Am. J. Clin. Nutr.*, 40: 808; 1984.

weights by gender and by ranges of height and frame size (small, medium, and large), but provided no method or instructions for assessing frame.[18] The tables were updated in 1983 and provided instructions for measuring elbow breadth and applying cutoffs for classifying frame size using data from the U.S. National Health and Nutrition Examination Survey (HANES, 1971-75) that were to result in approximately 50% of persons falling in medium frame and 25% in small and large frame categories, respectively (see Table 31.3).[19] When these cutoffs were subsequently tested on a large Canadian sample (n = 12,348 males and 6957 females), they were found to classify only a small percent of the sample as having large frames, thereby increasing the probability of misclassification into incorrect frame size categories and consequent unrealistic weight recommendations.[20]

Practical evaluation of measures of frame size is complicated by several factors including a lack of national reference standards for any measure except elbow breadth (see Table 31.4). Because frame size can not be directly measured by any single parameter, there is no "gold standard" by which to judge proposed surrogate measures, nor is there consensus on how to assign cut points for small, medium, or large frame or a standard upon which to base expectations of how frame size is (should be) distributed in a normal population. Different conceptualizations include:

- Distribution by percentiles:
  - Terciles (equal numbers in each of three frame categories)
  - Distribution by quartiles where the lowest and highest quartiles constitute the small and large frame categories, respectively, with the middle two quartiles combined to indicate medium frame
  - Distribution by varying "border values" defined at the 15th, 20th , or 25th and 75th, 80th , or 85th percentiles for small and large frame

- Defining cut-points by standard deviations with medium frame falling within plus or minus one standard deviation of the mean and those with small and large frames falling below or above these values.

Many different skeletal measurements, including segmental lengths, breadths, circumferences, and radiographs have been examined for assessing frame size. (See Table 31.5) These include:

- Wrist and arm circumference
- Elbow, knee, shoulder, chest, hip, wrist and ankle breadths
- Combination measurements:
  - Ratio of wrist circumference to height,
  - Frame index ([elbow breadth (mm)/height (cm)] × 100)
  - Regression of the sum of bitochanteric and biacromial breadths (large calipers) on height; and
  - Ratio of sitting to standing height.

Circumferences

Circumference measurements have been widely examined because they are relatively easy to perform, inexpensive, noninvasive, and require only a tape measure and minimal training of personnel. Primary applications include:

- Monitoring brain growth in children
- Monitoring effectiveness of treatments (including physical exercise) to measure reduction or increase in selected body areas
- As a marker of protein-energy malnutrition
- Estimation of the relative proportion of body weight from fat versus lean both as an independent measure and as a measure of frame size
- Describing body shape or the relative distribution of body weight using ratios such as waist to hip or head to chest (children)

Techniques for taking circumference measures are relatively simple. However, significant errors can result from improper positioning or placement of the tape and from differences in tension applied. In general, the tape is placed perpendicular to the long axis of the body, but exceptions include the head and neck, where the measurement is made at the widest and narrowest points, respectively. In almost all cases except the head, the tension on the tape is just enough to place it snug against the skin without causing an indentation. However, if the purpose of the circumference is to estimate frame size (or skeletal size), it is not entirely clear whether the tape should be pulled more tightly to get as close to the bone as possible. Equipment includes a flexible, nonstretchable, relatively narrow (0.7 cm) tape measure that has metric measures on one side and English on the other. Special anthropometric tapes are available, such as those already interlocked to slip over the arm or head, with arrows to make reading the measurement or finding the midpoint of the back of the arm easier. Detailed instructions for technique for measurement

TABLE 31.5

Selected Validation Studies of Determinants of Frame Size (FS)

Frame Size Measure	Subjects[a]	Methods and Criterion[b,d]	Results
Bony chest breadth[21]	n = 2201, ♂, Scotland.	a. Bony chest breadth measured by x-ray b. Criterion tested: 1, 3, and sig ↑ in wt with ↑ in FS	a. Correlation of bony chest breadth to wt > correlation of ht to wt b. Wt ↑ about 3.7 kg per each cm ↑ in bony chest breadth c. Wt ↑ about 12 kg per FS (S → M → L) d. Wt: bony chest breadth ratio correlated with FFM
Ratio of height (cm) to wrist circumference (cm)[23]	100 ♂ and ♀ adult patients at a university medical center, USA	a. Wrist measured distal to styloid process at wrist crease on right arm b. Frame size (S, M, L) assigned using this ratio by gender	a. Method for assigning frame size not stated. It appears that some sort or "normal" distribution was applied, but no other criteria of validity were tested. b. FS assigned by Ht:wrist ratio: ♂ S > 10.4; M 9.6-10.4; L < 9.6; ♂ S > 11.0; M 10.1-11.0; L < 10.1
Elbow and bitrochanteric breadths[24]	n = 16,494 ; age range: 18 to 74; ♂ and ♀; black and white; USA NHANES 1971-1974.	a. Criterion tested: 1, 3, and 4 b. Body fat determined by sum of triceps and subscapular skinfolds	a. Correlation coefficients of weight, elbow, bitrochanteric breadth to log-transformed sum of skinfold values done by gender by 3 age groups by race demonstrate lowest correlation with elbow breadth. b. Categories of SML FS established for elbow breadths with cut points at the 15th and 85th percentiles (values given by gender, race, and age group) demonstrate significant gender differences and some racial differences. c. Greater differences were observed for mean weights of subjects when they were categorized by FS (S, M, L) versus height (short, medium, tall) demonstrating that FS is more effective in weight discrimination
Elbow breadth[21]	n = 21,752; "adults" age range: 25-54; "elderly" age 55-74; ♂ and ♀; multiracial; USA NHANES I and II.	Based on this large data set, percentiles of weight, skinfolds (triceps, and subscapular), and bone-free upper arm muscle were developed by height, gender, and FS (using elbow breadth) for two age groups	a. Values of elbow breadth for S, M, L FS are given for males and females by age. (See Table 31.4) b. These standards can be used to identify persons who are at risk of being undernourished or overfat.
Height (H) and sum of biacromial (A) and bitochanteric (T) (HAT method) Body fatness estimated by hydrostatic weighing[25]	mean age = 22; n = 113 ♂, 182 ♀; H; university students; Ht and Wt representative of US population for this age group; Caucasian, USA.	a. Criterion: 3,5 b. Bivariate model developed based on height (H) and sum of biacromial (A) and bitochanteric (T) breadths c. Boundaries for FS (S, L) set by gender using mean ht ± 1 sd	a. Criterion satisfied. b. For ♂ differences in wt between FS primarily due to differences in FFM c. For ♀ there was small but sig. increase in FM per FS but no increase in FFM per FS d. FS equations: ♂ ht (8.239) + (A + T); ♀ ht (10.357) + (A + T) e. HAT FS boundaries: ♂ S <1459.3; M 1459.4-1591.9; L > 1592.0; ♀ S <1661.9; M 1662.0-1850.7; L >1850.8

TABLE 31.5 *(Continued)*

Selected Validation Studies of Determinants of Frame Size (FS)

Frame Size Measure	Subjects[a]	Methods and Criterion[b,d]	Results
Wrist, biacromial, elbow, hip, knee, and ankle breadths Body fatness estimated by hydrostatic weighing[15]	n = 225 ♂ and 215 ♀; age range =18-59; Canada, Quebec City, French descent. Tended to be leaner than either Canadian or US reference populations.	a. Criterion: 5-6 b. Differences in lean weight between FS categories (assigned by terciles) > differences in % body fat	a. All bone breadth measures were shown to be associated with FFM. b. Biacromial, elbow, hip, and knee did not meet criterion 6. c. Both criterion satisfied for wrist and ankle breadths. (Data not shown for FS cut points.)
Actual FS (AFS)[c] Body composition determined by JP, Br[26]	n = 17; $\overline{x}$ age = 20.9 ± 1.4; H; ♂; Caucasian; UK	a. Criterion: 1-5 and correlation with proposed measure AFS	a. Lack of agreement in assigning FS between methods 2-5. b. Criterion satisfied: ankle breadth and elbow breadth 1-5; AFS and hand length 1-3 and 5; HAT 1-3; chest breadth 1-4; wrist breadth 2,3; height:wrist 3. c. Additional correlations: ht → wt r = 0.68 (s); ht → FFM r = 0.70 (s); FFM → FM r = 0.20 (ns)
Frame index[5,27]	n = 21,648 ♂; 21,391 ♀ (sample size planned for 96% statistical confidence); age range = 18-70; Germany	Developed: a. Percentile curves for weight, height, BMI by gender and age b. Three categories of frame index using 20th and 80th percentiles as border values c. Median values for BMI and % BF by gender and age for each FS	a. Graph of median curves for frame-specific BMI by age (18-64) demonstrate important differences with age and gender and consistently higher BMI with for larger frame. b. Graph of median curves for frame-specific % BD by age (18-64) also demonstrate age and gender differences and consistently higher body fat with larger FS. c. Values used for cut points for frame index (at the 20th and 80th percentiles by gender and age) are not given for this sample. However, those published by Frisancho (derived from US NHANES data) could be used for other studies.
Biacromial, bi-iliocristal, wrist, and knee diameters and sitting height Body composition: DW[28]	n = 2512 ♂ age range = 45-59 South Wales	a. Criterion of effectiveness, improvement in correlation of BMI with body fatness when BMI is adjusted for FS	a. All 4 breadth frame measures were positively associated with BF (range of r = 0.16 [wrist] – 0.45) and height (range of r = 0.32 – 0.43). (Correlation of sitting height with BF or total ht not reported.) b. Adjusting BMI for FS did not improve the association of BMI with BF. c. Correlations of the BMI adjusted for FS by wrist and sitting height (both r = 0.74) were essentially the same as for BMI alone (r = 0.76). d. Correlations of the BMI adjusted for FS by biacromial, bi-iliocristal and knee diameters (range of r = 0.60 – 0.66) were lower than for BMI alone (r = 0.76), indicating a possible inflating effect of subcutaneous fat on these diameter measures.

Elbow breadth and height:wrist ratio Body composition: BIA-Lu[29]	n = 42 ♀; 38 ♂ age range = 18-55; USA	a. Criterion tested: 3, measures result in normal distribution of FS, and produce the same FS in an individual	a. Criterion 3 met for ♂ but not ♀. b. Both measures resulted in a FS distribution highly skewed to small frame (53-73% of subjects) with 0-3% in large frame. c. These two FS measures produced the same FS in 69% of the subjects.
Arm and wrist circumferences; ankle, elbow and wrist breadths; subscapular skinfolds; frame index 2; ht and wt; visual assessment.[30]	n = 300 (71 ♂ and 229 ♀); mean age = 72.6 ± 5.1; H; Caucasian; Midwest, USA	a. Criterion tested: 3 and agreement across methods in classifying FS	a. Distribution of FS designation varied by determinant but was not influenced by age. b. Visual assessment and elbow breadth[19] classified about 75% of subjects as medium frame. Elbow breadth[21] and Frame Index 2[5] resulted in more even distribution of FS. c. Association with "fatness" (subscapular skinfold) was noted for women with elbow breadth and for men with height:wrist. d. Ankle and wrist breadth had lowest correlations with subscapular skinfold, but lack of population-based standards limits their application.
Wrist and knee width used as FS measures; ht and wt; sitting ht Slenderness index (ht/wrist + knee width) % BF measured by UWW and BIA.[31]	n = 120, matched for age, gender, and BMI. China (Singapore and Beijing Chinese) and Netherlands (Caucasian)	a. Measured % BF compared by matched BMI between ethnic groups b. % BF calculated from BMI compared to measured c. Skeletal mass calculated from ht, wrist, and knee width	a. % BF differences observed between groups for the same BMI, with % BF ↑ with ↑ FS. b. % BF calculated vs. measured not different for Beijing Chinese and Dutch. c. % BF calculated underpredicted true value by 4% in Singapore Chinese. d. Differences in FS are at least partially responsible for differences in relationship of BMI → % BF among different ethnic groups.

[a] Footnotes: Subjects (all information provided in the original reference is given): n = number of subjects; age in years; health status: H = healthy; gender: ♂ = male; ♀ = female.

[b] Criterion applied: 1 = highly correlated with weight; 2 = highly correlated with fat free mass (FFM); 3 = minimally correlated with body fatness; 4 = minimally correlated with height; 5 = correlation with FFM is greater than the correlation of height alone with FFM; 6 = little or no association with body fat beyond that accounted for by the association of FFM with fat.

[c] In this study, the authors propose a reference measure "actual FS" comprised on the sum of a battery of 22 different skeletal measures (11 breadths, 9 lengths, and 2 depths) as described in text of Logman et al.[12]

[d] Methods for determing body composition: UWW = underwater weighing; BIA = bioelectrical impendance analysis; JP = regression equations of Jackson and Pollack;[32,33] Br = formula of Brozek et al.;[34] DW = regression equation of Durnin and Wormersley;[35] BIA-Lu = bioelectrical impedance analysis using the equations of Lukaski et al.[36]

[e] Abbreviations: FS = frame size; S, M, L= small, medium, large; ht = height; wt = weight; FFM = fat free mass; FM = fat mass; % BF = percent body fat; r = correlation coefficient; sig = statistically significant; ns = not statistically significant; sd = standard deviation.

of the head, neck, chest, waist, abdomen, hips or buttocks, thigh, calf, ankle, forearm, and wrist are described by Callaway et al., who recommend intra- and intermeasurer limits of agreement of 0.2 cm for relatively small sites (calf, ankle, wrist, head, arm, forearm) and 1.0 for the large sites (waist, abdomen, buttocks, chest).[37]

One of the most commonly measured and clinically practical anthropometric methods is the arm muscle area. This method was originally developed for use in the field for the evaluation of undernourished children.[38] Arm circumference and tricep skinfold measurement can be used to compare an individual to a reference population[39] and estimate the relative proportion of fat and muscle[40] or to estimate the severity of undernutrition in seriously ill hospitalized patients.[41] The use of arm circumference has importance when either undernutrition or overnutrition are of concern, and it can be easily used in the field, hospital, or community setting. Similarly, head circumference is a common measurement for infants in the first two to three years of life and can be plotted on standard growth charts to be compared with population norms.

Because of some of the difficulties of applying traditional height-weight tables to individuals who are either very lean or very fat and because of the practicality of doing circumference measurements, various researchers have evaluated the validity of using circumferences to estimate body composition and physical fitness (see Table 31.6). Using underwater weighing as the "gold standard," tables have been developed to estimate percent body fat within 2.5 to 4% for women and men using the following circumferences:

Young Women (ages 17–26)	Older Women (ages 27–50)	Young Men (ages 17–26)	Older Men (ages 27–50)
Abdomen	Abdomen	Right upper arm	Buttocks
Right thigh	Right thigh	Abdomen	Abdomen
Right forearm	Right calf	Right forearm	Right forearm

Source: Katch, F.I. and McArdle, W.D. in *Nutrition, Weight Control, and Exercise,* Lea & Febiger, Philadelphia, 1988.

The U.S. Navy requires personnel to pass certain physical fitness screening tests including having an appropriate weight for height. In this setting it is quite important to use a method that provides more specific information than traditional height-weight indices in differentiating individuals who have excess lean weight from those individuals with excess fat. Because of the large numbers of potential recruits and enlisted personnel being measured, practicality is also very important. Equations using circumference measures have been used to estimate percent body fat and body density since the early 1980s.

Skinfold Measurements

The skinfold (sometimes referred to as fatfold) technique is performed by pinching the skin and underlying fat at a given location between the thumb and forefinger, pulling the fold slightly away from the body, placing calipers on the fold, and measuring its thickness. Some skinfold sites are relatively easy to locate and measure, while others are not. Many individual factors can affect the accuracy of skinfold measurements:

- Degree of leaneness or fatness
- Muscle tone (including presence of muscle wasting)
- Changes with growth
- Younger or older age (as they affect accuracy of assumptions about tissue composition, muscle tone, skinfold compressibility, and elasticity)

TABLE 31.6

Selected Validation Studies of Circumference Measures

Circumference Site(s)	Subjects[a]	Methods	Results
Waist, hip[43]	n = 18 ♂ and 22 ♀, BMI ≥30; Scotland.	IAF measured by MRI, and central abdominal fat measured by DXA.	In obese ♀, DXA, waist and hip were equally well correlated with IAF (r = 0.74, 0.75, 0.70, respectively) In obese ♂, only DXA was moderately correlated with IAF (r = 0.46)
Neck, abdomen, thigh[44]	n = 5710 ♂ and 477 , Navy personnel, USA	% BF estimated from standardized Navy equations for men {% Body Fat = (0.740 × abdomen) – (1.249 × neck) + 0.528[a] 2. Body Density = –[.19077 × Log10 (abdomen – neck)] + [.15456 × Log10 (height)] + 1.0324; Percent body fat = [(4.95/body density) – 4.5] × 100[a]} and women {% Body Fat = (1.051 × Biceps) – (1.522 × forearm) – (0.879 × neck) + (0.326 × abdomen) + (0.597 × thigh) + 0.707[a]} % BF estimates correlated with 3 measures of physical fitness	Estimates of percent body fat derived from these circumference measurements and equations correlated better with performance on the Navy's physical fitness tests than did commonly used weight-height indices
Waist, hip[48]	n = 32,978; age range = 25-64; participants in 19 ♂ and 18 ♀ populations participating in a WHO MONICA project.	Identification of obesity compared by cut points for waist circumference at 2 levels (1. ♂ ≥ 94 cm; ♀ ≥ 80 cm; 2. ♂ ≥ 102 cm; ♀ ≥ 88 cm) vs cut points for BMI (≥ 25 kg/m^2) and WHR (♂ ≥ 0.95; ♀ ≥ 0.80).	Sensitivity was lowest in populations with fewer overweight individuals and highest in populations with more overweight. Use of waist cut points vs BMI or WHR cut points would correctly identify most people without obesity but miss some with obesity. Optimal screening cutoff points for waist circumference may be population specific.
Waist, hip umbilical[49]	n = 91, ♀; age range 20-54; BMI: 18-34 kg/m2	% BF by DXA compared with %BF from predictive equations.	Comparability and precision of % BF estimates from predictive equations can be improved by adjusting for umbilical circumference and BMI.
Waist, hip[50]	n = 385 (140 ♂ and 245 ♀); mean age = 80 (range = 65-96); USA.	% BF by DXA and BIA. BF distribution by skinfolds.	% BF < % vs &, upper body obesity > % vs & even in older age; Strong age adjusted correlations among obesity measures (BMI, %BF [DXA & BIA], skinfolds) were observed for both % and &; Weak associations among measures of upper body obesity differed by gender .

[a] Subjects (all information provided in the original reference is given): n = number of subjects; $\overline{x}$ age = mean age (years); gender: ♂ = male; ♀ = female.
[b] Methods for determining intra-abdominal fat: MRI = magnetic resonance imaging.
[c] Methods for determining body composition: UWW = underwater weighing; DXA = dual energy x-ray absorptiometry; DD = deuterium dilution; TBK = total body potassium; BIA = bioelectrical impedance analysis; SKF = JP = regression equation of Jackson and Pollack;[32,33] Br = formula of Brozek et al.;[34] DW = regression equation of Durnin and Wormersley;[35] BIA-Lu = bioelectrical impedance analysis using the equations of Lukaski, et al.[36]
[d] Abbreviations: IAF = intraabdominal fat; WHR = waist to hip ratio; ht = height; wt = weight; BMI = body mass index; ffm = fat free mass; fm = fat mass; % BF = percent body fat; r = correlation coefficient; sig = statistically significant; ns = not statistically significant; sd = standard deviation.

- Subject cooperation (small children may be frightened or uncooperative)
- Ethnicity
- Health status (bedridden vs. ambulatory)
- Hydration status

Use of this method relies on two main assumptions: 1) skinfolds provide good measures of subcutaneous fat; and 2) there is a good relationship between subcutaneous fat and total body fat. The ability to predict total body fat varies by site, with some sites highly correlated with total fat and others relatively independent of total fat. Studies show that the relationship between subcutaneous and total body fat (ranging from 20 to 70%) is affected by age, gender, degree of fatness, and race.[51-53] Thus, it is important to review the literature carefully and select sites and predictive equations that have been validated for the population being measured and provide sufficient precision for the desired application.

Guidelines for skinfold measurement technique, location of measurement sites, and information on reliability of measurement at the various sites have been published.[54] Considerable supervised practice is required before an individual can take accurate skinfold measurements. Training by an experienced person should be conducted, and measures practiced until consistency is achieved between the expert and trainee and by the trainee on within-subject repeated measures. Experts agree on the importance of using standardized techniques in both locating the site and using calipers to take the measurement, yet some argue that in light of the many biologic variables affecting body composition, technical errors in skinfold measurement are of comparatively little importance.[55] Nonetheless, given a standard level of training and care in measurement, high levels of reliability can be achieved (see Table 31.7).

Many different models of skinfold calipers are available, but only those designed to maintain a constant tension (10 g/mm) between the jaws should be used. However, even with the higher quality calipers, there is a difference in the pressure exerted by the jaws and therefore in the degree of compression of the skinfold.[56] Differences in compression have also been attributed to differences in caliper jaw surface area such that calipers with smaller surface area and lighter spring tension (such as the Lange) give larger values than

TABLE 31.7

Reliability of Selected Skinfold Measurement Sites

Site	Intermeasurer Error	Intrameasurer Error
Subscapular	SEM: 0.88 to 1.53 mm	SEM: 0.88 to 1.16 mm
Midaxillary	SEM: ± 0.36; 1.47 mm (children); ± 0.64 mm (adults)	SEM: Children: ± 0.95 mm Adults: ± 1.0,1.22, 2.08 mm
Pectoral (chest)	R: .9, .93, .97; SEM: 2.1 mm	R: .91 to .97 mm; SEM: ± 1-2 mm
Abdominal		R: .979; SEM: 0.89 mm
Suprailiac	SEM: 1.53 mm (children); 1.7 mm (adults)	R: .97; SEM: 0.3-1.0 mm
Thigh	R: > .9, .97, .975; SEM: ± 2.1, ± 2.4, 3-4 mm	R: .91, .98, .985; SEM: 0.5-0.7 mm, 1-2 mm
Medial calf		R: .94, .98, .99; SEM: 1.0-1.5 mm
Tricep	SEM: 0.8-1.89 mm	SEM: 0.4-0.8 mm
Bicep	SEM: ± 1.9 mm	SEM: 0.2-0.6, ± 1.9 mm

[a] Information in this table has been summarized from Harrison GG, Buskirk ER, Carter JEL, et al. Skinfold Thickness and Measurement Technique. In: Lohman TG, Roche AF, Martorell R. *Anthropometric Standardization Reference Manual.* (1988) Champaign, IL: Human Kinetics. pp 55-80. This chapter includes the specific citations for the reliability studies.

[b] Abbreviations used: SEM: Standard error of measurement; R: reliability coefficient.

[c] Multiple error estimates represent differing results from different studies.

calipers with larger surface area and tighter spring tension (Holtain and Harpenden).[57] Because of these differences attributable to the calipers themselves, it is important to calibrate often,[58] and to consistently use the same equipment in order to compare data within or across subjects.

Importance of Frame Size, Skinfolds, and Circumferences to Disease Risk

A variety of approaches have been employed to better understand the validity of using these field measurements for the assessment of risk for the most prevalent and serious diseases: heart disease, diabetes, cancer, and osteoporosis. Major interest has been in evaluating these measures for their ability to measure, estimate, or predict:

- Total fat or percent body fat
- Fat or weight patterning or distribution
- Skeletal size or density
- Biochemical markers such as lipids and insulin sensitivity/resistance
- Health outcomes such as elevated blood pressure, morbidity or mortality (cancer, diabetes, coronary artery disease, myocardial infarction)

The preponderance of studies relating anthropometric measures to disease have been in the area of cardiovascular disease (CVD) in an attempt to identify potentially modifiable body factors and to understand potential markers for and predictors of disease. An extensive summary of studies done in men illustrates the methodological and statistical difficulties that are encountered when assessing the relationship between CVD and various body measurements.[59] In general, studies have not shown a consistent relationship between obesity and CVD using a variety of measures (weight for height, relative weight, total body fat, etc.). The strength of association between central fat distribution and CVD is stronger than that of body fat alone, yet a large percent (30 to 50%) of the variation remains unexplained. Potential sources of difficulty in conducting these studies include inability to identify adequate surrogates for obesity, confounding effects of cigarette smoking or subclinical disease, short followup periods, and inadequate methodology for identifying subgroups of obese persons who are at risk. For example, several studies suggest that persons who have undesirable patterns of body fat distribution that develop early in life may be at increased risk.[60,61] While one study of three distinct populations found a consistent direct association between abdominal obesity as measured by waist circumference and waist:hip ratio and dyslipidemia,[62] others have found the sagittal abdominal diameter to be a better predictor of risk than BMI, waist circumference, or waist-to-hip ratio.[63,64]

Several studies evaluating the ability of simple anthropometric measures to identify those at risk for low bone mass and fractures have found a strong association between weight and bone mineral density (BMD), while others have not. (See Table 31.8). Possible factors affecting the relationship between body weight and/or size and bone mineral density include simple mechanical loading (a larger and heavier body will need a stronger skeletal support), the influence of endogenous sex steroids, and possibly muscularity (either directly by its contribution to total body weight or indirectly by its association with increased activity). For these reasons, anthropometric measures related to gender-related weight distribution (central versus lower body), FS, and measures of muscularity/adiposity have been investigated for their value in estimating BMD.

TABLE 31.8

Selected Studies Examining the Relationships between Anthropometric Measures and Bone Mass or Bone Mineral Density

Anthropometric Measures	Subjects	Methods	Results
a. Frame: biacromial, biiliac, bicofemoral, bicohumeral, and wrist breadths; b. Skinfold: triceps, biceps, forearm, subscapula, suprailium, calf, abdomen, thigh; c. Circumferences: calf, waist, upper arm, abdomen d. Height and weight[65]	n = 342; mean age = 44.1 (range = 25-79); ♀; USA	Correlation of anthropometric measures to: a. Measured (photon absorptiometry) bone mineral density (g/cm^2) at the radius, femoral neck, Ward's triangle, trochanter, lumbar spine b. Constructed summary bone density score (radius, spine, femoral neck) Muscle mass (termed "muscularity") estimated from circumferences and skinfolds[a] Multiple regression models constructed to test the usefulness of measures in predicting bone mass.	a. For all skeletal sites one frame measure (biacromial width [BW]), one skinfold (subscapular[SSF]) and one circumference (calf[CC]) provided the strongest correlations. b. The greater trochanter was more strongly correlated with all anthropometric measures than any other skeletal site. c. After inclusion of age, BW, SSF, and muscularity in multiple regression model, BW was a significant predictor for all sites except the radius, and SSF and muscularity were significant for all sites. d. Neither height nor weight contributed significantly to the model after BW, SSF, and CC or muscularity were included. e. Despite the strength of the associations, none of the models accounted for more than 40-45% of the variability in bone mass at any site and therefore are not adequate to predict bone mass for individuals. f. No measures of distribution of body fat were significantly associated with bone mass. g. Cross-sectional data not adequate to address questions of rates of bone loss.
a. Elbow breadth b. Height, weight and BMI c. Waist:Hip ratio[67]	n = 6705; ♀ mean age = 71.2 ± 5, Non-black, USA	Bone mineral density (BMD) measured by single-photon (proximal and distal radius and calcaneus) and dual-energy x-ray absorptiometry (lumbar spine and proximal femur) Adiposity measured by bioelectrical impedance	a. Weight was the major determinant of BMD at all sites, explaining 6-20% of the variability. (Weight explained more of the variability at direct weight bearing sites — proximal femur and os calcis.) Effect of weight on BMD did not seem to vary with age. (Age had independent significant effect on BMD decline.) b. Although the measures of BMI, elbow breadth, height, and waist:hip ratio resulted in statistically significant ($P<0.001$) improvements in fit of the model, they added very little explanatory power over weight alone. c. A modest proportion of the weight effect was explained by adiposity (36-63% at weight bearing sites and 8-12% at forearm sites). d. These data suggest that both mechanical loading and metabolic mechanisms affect BMD.
Waist:Hip ratio, wt, BMI, arm muscle and fat area	n = 1873 ♀ (97% post-menopausal), Italy	Bone mineral content (BMC) and density (BMD) evaluated by DXA as normal (N), osteopenic (OPN) or osteoporotic (OPR)	Body wt., BMI, arm muscle and fat sig > in N than either OPN or OPR groups. WHR not different between groups. Wt and age sig predictors of BMC and BMD but high levels of variation in BMC for the same level of wt (under, normal, over) negate its usefulness as a predictive indicator.

Conclusion

Even though there is an extensive body of literature examining the validity of using measures of frame size, circumferences, or skinfolds to predict disease risk or disease outcomes, conclusive findings and consensus on which measures are best remain elusive. Nonetheless, the ability of researchers to build on the lessons learned from these early studies and apply emerging new technologies give reason for optimism about reaching the goal of using simple, inexpensive techniques to improve individual and public health.

References

1. Wang J, Thornton JC, Kolesnik S, Pierson RN. *Ann NY Acad Sci* 904: 317; 2000.
2. Sutcliffe JF. *Phys Med Biol* 41: 791; 1996.
3. Wagner DR, Heywood VH. *Res Q Exec Sport* 70: 135; 1999.
4. Heywood VH. *Sports Med* 22: 146; 1996.
5. Frisancho AR. *Anthropometric Standards for The Assessment of Growth and Nutritional Status* University of Michigan Press, Ann Arbor, 1990.
6. Ulijaszek SJ, Mascie-Taylor CGN (Eds). *Anthropometry: The Individual and The Population* Cambridge University Press, Cambridge 1994.
7. Ulijaszek SJ, Kerr, DA. *Br J Nutr* 82: 165; 1999.
8. Nordhamm K, Sodergren E, Olsson E, et al. *Int J Obes* 24: 652; 2000.
9. Zerfas AJ. *Manual for Anthropometry* University of California Press, Los Angeles, 1985.
10. Ulijaszek SJ, Lourie JA. *Coll Antropol* 21: 429; 1997.
11. Fuller NJ, Sawyer MB, Elia M. *Int J Obesity* 18: 503; 1994.
12. Lohman TG, Roche AF, Martorell R. *Anthropometric Standardization Reference Manual* University of Illinois Press, Champaign, 1988.
13. Heyward VH, Stolarczyk LM. *Applied Body Composition Assessment* University of Illinois Press, Champaign, 1996.
14. Van Itallie TB. *Am J Public Health* 75: 1054; 1985.
15. Himes JH, Bouchard C. *Am J Public Health* 75: 1076; 1985.
16. Kretschmer E, *Korperbautypus und Charakter* Springer, Berlin 1921.
17. Metropolitan Life Insurance Co. *Statistical Bulletin* 40: 1; 1959.
18. Weigley ES, *JADA* 84: 417; 1984.
19. Metropolitan Life Insurance Co. *Statistical Bulletin* 64: 2; 1983.
20. Faulkner RA, Dailey DA. *Can J Public Health* 80: 369; 1989.
21. Frisancho AR. *Am J Clin Nutr* 40: 808; 1984.
22. Garn SM, Pesick SD, Hawthorne VM. *Am J Clin Nutr* 37: 315; 1983.
23. Grant JP. *Handbook of Total Parenteral Nutrition* WB Saunders, Philadelphia, 1980.
24. Frisancho AR, Flegel PN. *Am J Clin Nutr* 11: 418; 1983.
25. Katch VL, Freedson PS. *Am J Clin Nutr* 36: 669; 1982.
26. Peters DM, Eston R. *J Sports Sci* 11: 9; 1993.
27. Greil H, Trippo U. *Coll Anthropol* 2: 345; 1998.
28. Fehily AM, Butland BK, Yarnell JWG. *Eur J Clin Nutr* 44: 107; 1990.
29. Nowak RK, Olmstead SL. *JADA* 87: 339; 1987.
30. Mitchell MC. *JADA* 93: 53; 1993.
31. Deurenberg P, Deurenberg YM, Wang J, et al. *J Obes Relat Metab Disord* 23: 537; 1999.
32. Jackson AS, Pollock ML. *Br J Nutr* 40: 497; 1978.
33. Jackson AS, Pollock ML, Ward A. *Med Sci Sports Exerc* 12: 175; 1980.
34. Brozek J, Grande F, Anderson JT, et al. *Ann NY Acad Sci* 110: 113; 1963.
35. Durnin JVGA, Womersley J. *Brit J Nutr* 32: 77; 1974.

36. Lukaski HC, Johnson PE, Bolonchuk WW, Lykken GI. *Am J Clin Nutr* 41: 1985; 1984.
37. Callaway CW, Chumlea WC, Bouchard C, et al. *Anthropometric Standardization Reference Manual* University of Illinois Press, Champaign, 1988.
38. Jelliffe EFP, Jelliffe DB. *J Trop Pediatr* 15: 179; 1969.
39. Frisancho AR. *Am J Clin Nutr* 34: 2540; 1981.
40. Gurney JM, Delliffe DB. *Am J Clin Nutr* 26: 912; 1973.
41. Heymsfield SB, McManus C, Smith J, et al. *Am J Clin Nutr* 36: 680; 1982.
42. Katch FI, McArdle WD. *Nutrition, Weight Control and Exercise* Lea & Febiger, Philadelphia, 1988.
43. Kamel EG, McNeill G, Van Wijk MC. *Obes Res* 8: 36; 2000.
44. Conway TL, Cronan TA, Peterson KA. *Aviat Space Environ Med* 60: 433; 1989.
45. Wright HF, Dotson CO, Davis PO. *US Navy Med* 72: 23; 1981.
46. Hodgdon JA, Beckett MB. *Technical Report No. 84-29* Naval Health Research Center, San Diego, 1984.
47. Wright HF, Dotson CO, Davis PO. *US Navy Med* 71: 15; 1980.
48. Molarius A, Seidell JC, Sans S, et al. *J Clin Epidemiol* 52: 1213; 1999.
49. Rutishauser IHE, Pasco JA, Wheeler CE. *Eur J Clin Nutr* 49: 248; 1995.
50. Goodman-Gruen D, Barrett-Connor E. *Am J Epidemiol* 143: 898; 1996.
51. Vickery SR, Cureton KJ, Collins MA. *Hum Biol* 60: 135; 1988.
52. Behnke AR. *Obesity* FA Davis, Philadelphia, 1969.
53. Lohman TG. *Hum Biol* 53: 181; 1981.
54. Harrison GG, Buskirk ER, Carter JEL, et al. *Anthropometric Standardization Reference Manual* University of Illinois Press, Champaign, 1988.
55. Durnin JVGA, DeBruin H, Feunekes GIJ. *Br J Nutr* 77: 3; 1997.
56. Schmidt PK, Carter JEL. *Hum Biol* 62: 369; 1990.
57. Gruber JJ, Pollack ML, et al. *Res Q* 61: 184; 1990.
58. Gore CJ, Woolford SM, Carlyon RG. *J Sports Sci* 13: 355; 1995.
59. Williams SRP, Jones E, Bell W, et al. *Eur Heart J* 18: 376; 1997.
60. Freedman DS. *Am J Med Sci* 310: S72; 1995.
61. Van Lenthe FJ, Kemper HCG, Van Mechelen W, Twist JWR. *Int J Epidemiol* 25: 1162; 1996.
62. Paccaud F, Schluter-Fasmeyer V, Wietlisbach V, Bovet P. *J Clin Epidemiol* 53: 393; 2000.
63. Ohrval M, Berglund L, Vessby B. *Int J Obesity* 24: 497; 2000.
64. Gustat J, Elkasabany A, Srinivasan S, Berenson GS. *Am J Epidemiol* 151: 885; 2000.
65. Slemenda CW, Hui SL, Williams CJ, et al. *Bone Miner* 11: 101; 1990.
66. Ross WD, Crawford SM, Kerr DS, et al. *Am J Phys Anthropol* 77: 169; 1988.
67. Glauber HS, Vollmer WM, Nevitt MC, et al. *J Clin Endocrinol Metab* 80: 1118; 1995.
68. Bedogni G, Simonini G, Viaggi S, et al. *Ann Hum Biol* 26: 561; 1999.

32

Height, Weight, and Body Mass Index (BMI) in Childhood

Christine L. Williams and Mary Horlick

Introduction

In childhood, height (stature) and weight are the two most frequently used measures of growth and nutritional status. In addition, indices of weight-for-height, especially BMI, are used as a proxy for body fatness or obesity. Since growth is the most sensitive indicator of overall health in childhood, it is essential that accurate measurements be made on a regular basis during routine health supervision of children and adolescents to identify and address significant deviations in a timely manner.

Pediatric health professionals take two basic anthropometric measurements on each child: *recumbent length* (for children *under* two years of age) or *standing height* (for children *over* two years of age) and *weight*. From these two measurements, *body mass index (BMI)* can be derived from a reference chart or calculated by formula. This section will focus on these three measures: height (or length), weight, and BMI. For each measurement the following aspects will be discussed: definition, normal patterns of change, measurement techniques, and interpretation of values using reference growth charts. Since most practicing pediatricians in the U.S., as well as other health professionals who care for children, record their measurements in inches and pounds, these units will be used in the discussion.

Height

Description

Height, or stature, is a linear measure from the base on which the child is standing, to the firm top of the child's head. Height is measured in children over two years of age. It is measured with the child standing with erect posture, and without shoes. From birth to two years of age, the infant or toddler's stature is measured as recumbent length. This is the total length of the child from the bottom of the feet (positioned at a 90-degree angle) to the top of the head. Recumbent length is slightly greater than standing height measured in the same individual.

0-8493-2705-9/01/$0.00+$1.50

Normal Patterns of Linear Growth in Childhood

Normal changes in height (or length): during the first year of life, babies increase in recumbent length about 10 inches on average, from about 20 inches long at birth to 30 inches by their first birthday. During the second year of life their length increases by 4 to 5 inches, or about 1/4 inch per month. After age 2 years, height is measured in the standing position. Growth continues at a slower but steady rate of about 2 1/2 inches per year until about the age of 11 in girls and 13 in boys, when the growth spurt associated with puberty and adolescence usually begins. Puberty is characterized by a greater rate of growth, culminating in a peak height velocity (inches grown per year) comparable to the rate of growth during the second year of life. The peak height velocity for girls is about 2 1/2 to 4 1/2 inches/year, and for boys is about 3 to 5 inches/year. For both boys and girls, however, puberty and the pubertal "growth spurt" may occur several years earlier or later than average and still be within a normal range. Normal growth stops when the growing ends of the bones fuse, which usually occurs between 14 and 16 years of age for girls, and between 16 and 18 years of age for boys.

Normal Growth Rates During Childhood and Adolescence

Age	Growth Rate (per year)	
	Inches (in)	Centimeters (cm)
0–1 year	7–10	18–25
1–2 years	4–5	10–13
2 years to puberty	2–2 1/2	5–6
Girls: pubertal growth spurt	2 1/2–4 1/2	6–11
Boys: pubertal growth spurt	3–5	7–13

Measuring Length

The stature of subjects less than two years of age is measured as recumbent length. This is done most accurately with a measuring "box" or "board" that has an inflexible headpiece against which the top of the head is positioned, and a moveable footboard against which the feet are placed at a 90-degree angle. If possible, the child should be relaxed, the legs should be fully extended, and the head should be positioned so that a line connecting the outer margin of the eyes with the ears is at a 90-degree angle with the bottom of the measuring box. Recumbent length is measured from the top of the head to the bottom of the feet. It should be measured to the nearest quarter inch and recorded in the child's chart. Measurement of recumbent length on an examining table without a "box" should also be from the top of the head to the bottom of the feet, which are positioned at a 90-degree angle. It is recommended that the same examiner measure the child at each visit to minimize inter-examiner variability.

Because recumbent length is slightly greater than standing height, it is recommended that measurements of both length and height be obtained for two visits between two and three years of age. With these simultaneous recumbent length and standing height values, measurement discrepancy can be distinguished from actual change in growth rate.

Measuring Height

The height of subjects older than two years of age is measured, without shoes, with a stadiometer. A stadiometer consists of a measuring tape affixed to a vertical surface, such as a wall or a rigid free-standing measuring device, and a movable block, attached to the vertical surface at a right angle, that can be brought down to the crown of the head. In the absence of a stadiometer, height can be measured on a platform scale, but this is less accurate than the stadiometer. In either case, the subject should stand with heels together and back as straight as possible; the heels, buttocks, shoulders, and head should touch the wall or the vertical surface of the measuring device. The weight of the subject is distributed evenly on both feet and the head is positioned in the horizontal plane. The arms hang freely by the sides with the palms facing the thighs. The subject should be asked to inhale deeply and maintain a fully erect position. The examiner positions the movable block until it touches the head; applying sufficient pressure to compress the hair. The height marker is read while pressing firmly on the headpiece. The number on the height bar immediately behind the indicator line of the height marker is read. The examiner's eyes should look directly at the indicator line at about the same height in order to avoid parallax in reading the measurement. The height is measured to the nearest quarter inch, and then recorded on the child's chart. It is recommended that a second reading be taken to check accuracy.

Height has diurnal variation. Children are tallest in the morning, and shrink as much as a centimeter during the course of a day as the fibrous intervertebral cartilaginous disks are compressed. Diurnal variation in height is completely due to changes in the height of the vertebral column, and full height is regained when the child lies down flat for about 30 minutes.

Interpretation of Height Measurements

Depending on the statural genes that a child inherits from their parents, children tend to gravitate toward a specific percentile or channel of the standard height (or length) charts during the first two to three years of life. Thereafter, most children track close to that percentile or channel, maintaining a stable position relative to their peers.

Children who track consistently along the lowest height percentiles may have *familial short stature* in which the parents are short and the child has simply inherited the same statural genes. Other short children may have *constitutionally delayed growth* characterized by a slower rate of growth in the first two or three years of life, followed by normal growth velocity that tracks along a height percentile or channel lower than expected for the family. These children often have later onset of puberty and its accompanying growth spurt, as well as a parent who followed a similar pattern of growth as a child. Final adult height is generally appropriate for parental height expectations.

Children whose linear growth decelerates and shifts gradually downward to a lower percentile deserve medical evaluation. Poor linear growth may reflect inadequate nutrition, an underlying disease affecting a major organ system, or a genetic abnormality. Children whose linear growth accelerates and shifts upward to a higher percentile also deserve medical evaluation. Increased rate of linear growth may reflect overnutrition, early or precocious onset of puberty, or another endocrine or genetic abnormality.

Reference Charts for Height (and Length)

Growth charts are simple grids which are used to plot out a child's height according to age and sex. Pediatric health professionals should measure and plot height on a growth chart at every visit, at least every six months before school age, and annually thereafter. Growth charts are derived from the heights of large numbers of healthy children of all ages, separating the wide range of normal heights into percentiles by statistical techniques. The spaces between the percentile lines are called channels. Age in years is plotted along the horizontal axis at the bottom of the chart and height in inches (or centimeters) is plotted along the vertical axis on the left of the chart. The 50th percentile, representing the average height for a given age, is drawn as a heavy line. Growth charts are commonly drawn for values between the 5th and 95th or 3rd and 97th percentiles of the population distribution values.

The Center for Disease Control (CDC) has published Growth Charts for boys and girls, for birth to 36 months of age and for ages 2 to 20 years. These include charts for plotting linear growth including Length-for-Age (age 2 years of age and under), Height-for-Age (age 2 years and older), Weight-for-Length, and Weight-for-Height. These charts may be downloaded from the CDC internet website: http://www.cdc.gov/growthcharts.

Weight

Description

Body *weight* is a measure of body mass, which is a composite of each contributing tissue (e.g., fat, muscle, bone, etc). Although weight should ideally be measured without clothing, this is often impractical. Most commonly, weight is measured with the child in underwear only, or in light indoor clothing, without shoes.

Normal Patterns of Weight Gain in Childhood

Newborn infants commonly double their birth weight by six months of age, and triple it by their first birthday. Boys on average increase from 8 pounds at birth to 23 pounds at 1 year; while girls on average increase from slightly less than 8 pounds at birth to about 21 pounds at age 1 year. From 1 to 2 years of age, toddlers who are tracking along the 50th pecentile for weight gain about 5 to 6 pounds, or about 1/2 pound per month, and during the third year of life weight gain averages about 4 pounds. Children tracking along higher percentile zones will gain more, and those tracking on the lower percentiles gain proportionately less.

Measurement Techniques

Weight should be measured in the clinical setting using a standard balance beam scale with moveable weight or with an instrument of equivalent accuracy. It is recommended that the scale be calibrated at least monthly using standard weights. It is preferable to weigh the child without clothing, or in light indoor clothing, but at least the child's shoes and heavy outer clothing should be removed. With older children, heavy belts should be removed and their pockets should be emptied. The beam of the platform scale must be graduated so that it can be read from both sides. The subject stands still over the center of the platform with body weight evenly distributed between both feet. Weight is recorded to the nearest quarter pound.

Weight, like height, has diurnal variation. In contrast to height, however, weight is lowest in the morning after emptying the bladder, and increases gradually through the day, depending on diet and physical activity.

Interpretation of Weight Measurements

Body weight and patterns of weight gain and adiposity in childhood are the result of gene-environment interactions. A child's genotype reflects the genes inherited from his or her parents. The phenotype expressed, however, with respect to body weight and fatness, is also heavily influenced by environmental factors such as diet and physical activity. Most children will gravitate toward a specific percentile curve of the standard weight charts during the first few years of life. However, with the increasing prevalence of childhood obesity in the U.S., it is not uncommon for children's weights to gradually cross upward across percentiles, rather than maintain a consistent percentile position relative to their peers. It is recommended that body weight, height, and calculated BMI values all be monitored carefully during routine health supervision, so that children and adolescents who begin to deviate from normal growth patterns may receive further evaluation and treatment.

Children's weight percentiles may be similar to their height percentiles, or may be somewhat above or below, and still be "normal" or healthy if the BMI is below the 85th percentile for age.

Healthy children who consistently track along the lower weight percentiles throughout childhood are considered normal if their weight is proportionate to their height (close to the same percentile) and consistent with parental heights and weights.

Children whose weight gain decelerates and shifts gradually downward to a lower percentile, or who actually lose weight (with the exception of overweight children on medically supervised diets), should be medically evaluated to determine the cause. Poor weight gain or unexplained weight loss may reflect inadequate nutrition, an eating disorder, an underlying disease affecting a major organ system, or depression or other psychological problems.

Overweight children who are placed on a medically supervised diet to slow down the rate of weight gain or to lose weight should be carefully monitored so adequate intake of essential nutrients is assured through a balanced calorie-controlled diet, and caloric intake is adequate to maintain linear growth throughout treatment.

Reference Charts for Weight

Weight charts are available to plot out a child's weight according to age and gender, similar to height charts. Weight charts are also constructed from the weights of large numbers of healthy children of all ages, separating the wide ranges of weights into percentiles by statistical techniques. As for the height charts, the spaces between percentile lines are called channels. Age in years is plotted along the horizontal axis at the bottom of the chart and weight in pounds (or kilograms) is plotted along the vertical axis on the left of the chart. The 50th percentile, representing the average weight for a given age, is drawn as a heavy line. Weight charts most commonly provide percentile channels between the 5th and 95th percentile, but are also available now for a distribution between the 3rd and 97th percentiles.

The CDC has published Growth Charts for boys and girls for birth to 36 months of age and for ages 2 to 20 years. These include charts for plotting weight, weight-for-age, and weight-for-height. These charts may be downloaded from the CDC website: http://www.cdc.gov/growthcharts.

Body Mass Index (BMI)

Body Mass Index

Body Mass Index, or BMI (wt/ht^2) provides a guideline based on weight and height to determine underweight or overweight status. BMI is not an exact measure of fatness because levels of fatness vary among children at a given BMI. This is true because BMI reflects (1) frame size, (2) leg length, and (3) amount of lean and fat tissue. Although BMI correlates less well with the percent of body weight that is fat than other more direct measures of fat such as triceps skinfold thickness or other body composition techniques, the readily available weight and height data make BMI a more useful tool for assessment of overweight or underweight.

BMI in children and adolescents compares well to laboratory measurements of body fat. Children and adolescents with a BMI-for-age above the 95th percentile are classified as overweight. BMI values above the 95th percentile, applied as a definition of overweight in children and adolescents

1. Reflects adiposity
2. Is consistent across age groups
3. Is predictive of morbidity

The percentage of children and adolescents who are overweight in the U.S. has more than doubled in the past 30 years, and the sharpest increase has occurred in the last 20 years, since the late 1970s. For 6 to 17 year old youth, about 12.5% (or 5.3 million) are overweight (BMI >95th percentile reference value).

The rationale for proposing a pediatric BMI classification is based on studies indicating that BMI is related to health risks. Overweight children are likely to become overweight adults, with risk increasing with severity and duration of the problem. Sixty percent of youth with a BMI-for-age above the 95th percentile have at least one risk factor for cardiovascular disease, while twenty percent have two or more risk factors. High blood pressure, abnormal blood lipid levels (elevated total cholesterol, LDL-cholesterol, and/or triglycerides; low HDL-cholesterol), insulin resistance, and Type II diabetes mellitus are some of the risk factors observed in overweight children and adolescents. Overweight children are also at increased risk for a wide range of other medical and psychological problems.

Normal Patterns of BMI during Childhood and Adolescence

For U.S. children, BMI increases rapidly during the first year of life and then declines to its lowest value on average between four and six years of age. After reaching this nadir, BMI again begins a slow increase throughout the rest of childhood and adolescence. The upward shift of the BMI curve, after reaching the lowest point, has been termed "adiposity rebound." Studies suggest that children who begin their adiposity rebound at younger ages are at greater risk for being overweight as older adolescents and young adults.

Measurement of BMI

BMI, also known as the weight-height index or Quetelet index, is calculated as the quotient of weight divided by height squared:

The *English formula* (in inches and pounds) is as follows:

Weight in pounds ÷ Height in inches ÷ Height in inches × 703 = BMI

The *Metric formula* (in meters and kilograms) is as follows:

Weight in kilograms ÷ Height in meters ÷ Height in meters = BMI

Interpretation of BMI Values

Interpretation of BMI depends on the sex and age of the child, since boys and girls differ in their body fatness as they mature. Therefore BMI is plotted on age and sex-specific charts. Established cutoff points are used to identify children and adolescents who are underweight or overweight. BMI values which should raise clinical concern are the following:

Underweight	BMI-for-Age <5th percentile
"At-Risk" of Overweight	BMI-for-Age 85th–95th percentile
Overweight	BMI-for-Age ≥95th percentile

Reference Charts for Body Mass Index (BMI)

The CDC has published BMI-for-age charts; one chart for boys ages 2 to 20 years, and another chart for girls 2 to 20 years of age. These charts may be downloaded from the CDC internet website: http://www.cdc.gov/nccdphp/dnpa/bmi/bmi-for-age.htm. At the same site, a CDC "Table for Calculated Body Mass Index Values for Selected Heights and Weights for Ages 2 to 20 Years" may also be downloaded. Clinicians can avoid having to calculate BMI values by using this extensive set of tables covering heights from 29 to 78 inches and weights from 18 to 250 pounds.

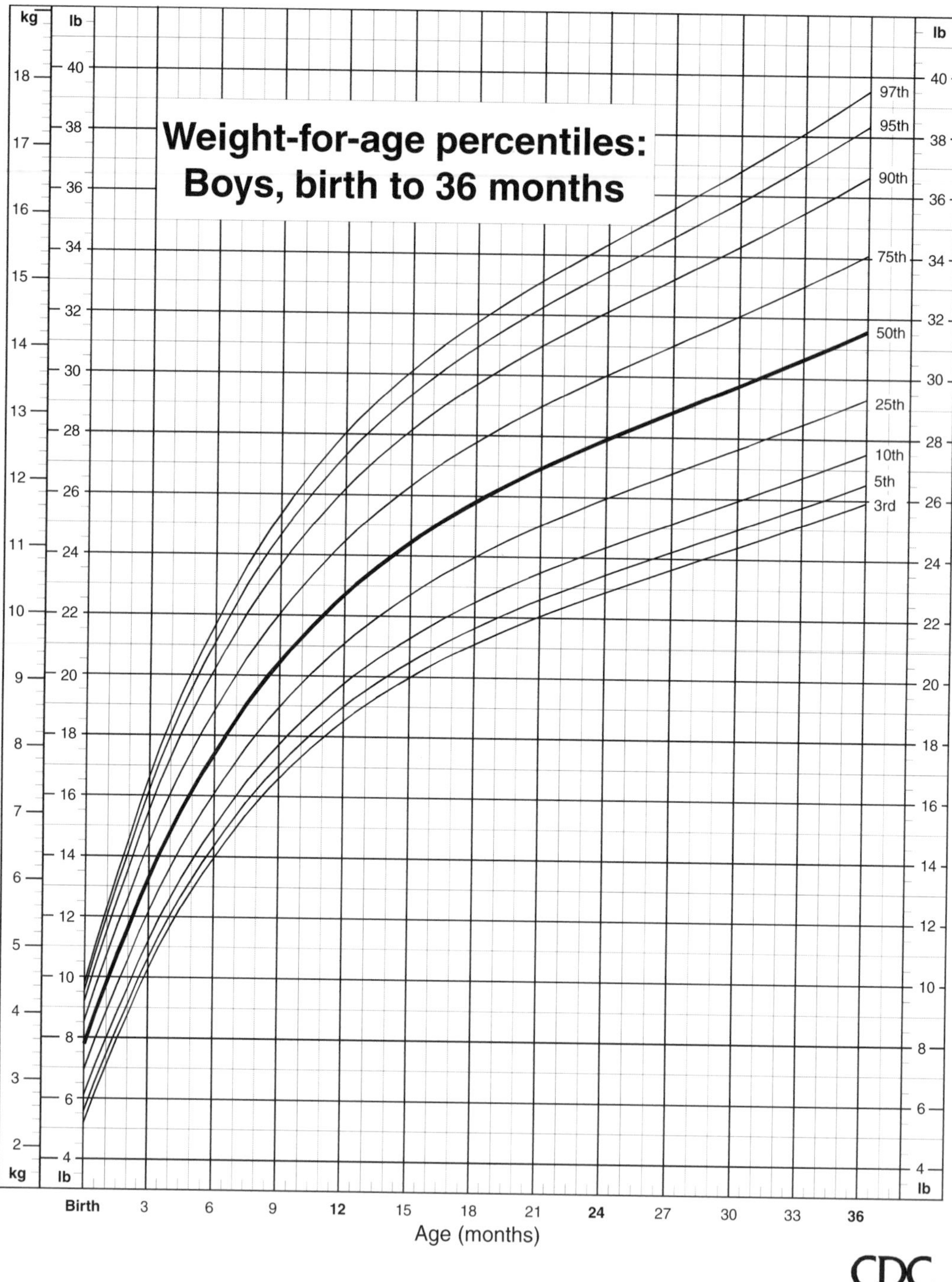

FIGURE 32.1
Weight-for-age percentiles, boys, birth to 36 months, CDC growth charts: United States. Source: Developed by the National Center for Health Statistics in collaboration with the National Center for Chronic Disease Prevention and Health Promotion (2000).

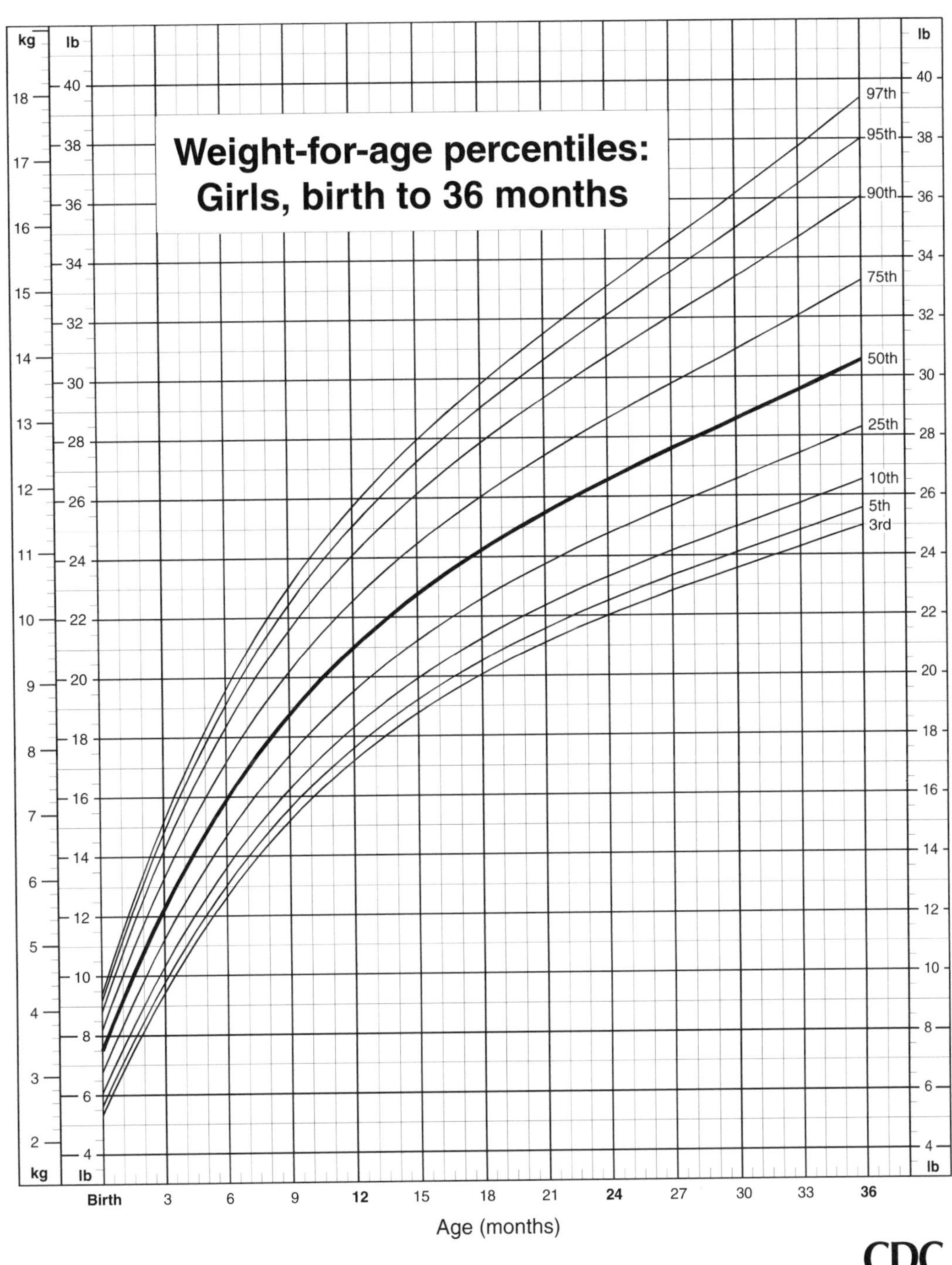

FIGURE 32.2
Weight-for-age percentiles, girls, birth to 36 months, CDC growth charts: United States. Source: Developed by the National Center for Health Statistics in collaboration with the National Center for Chronic Disease Prevention and Health Promotion (2000).

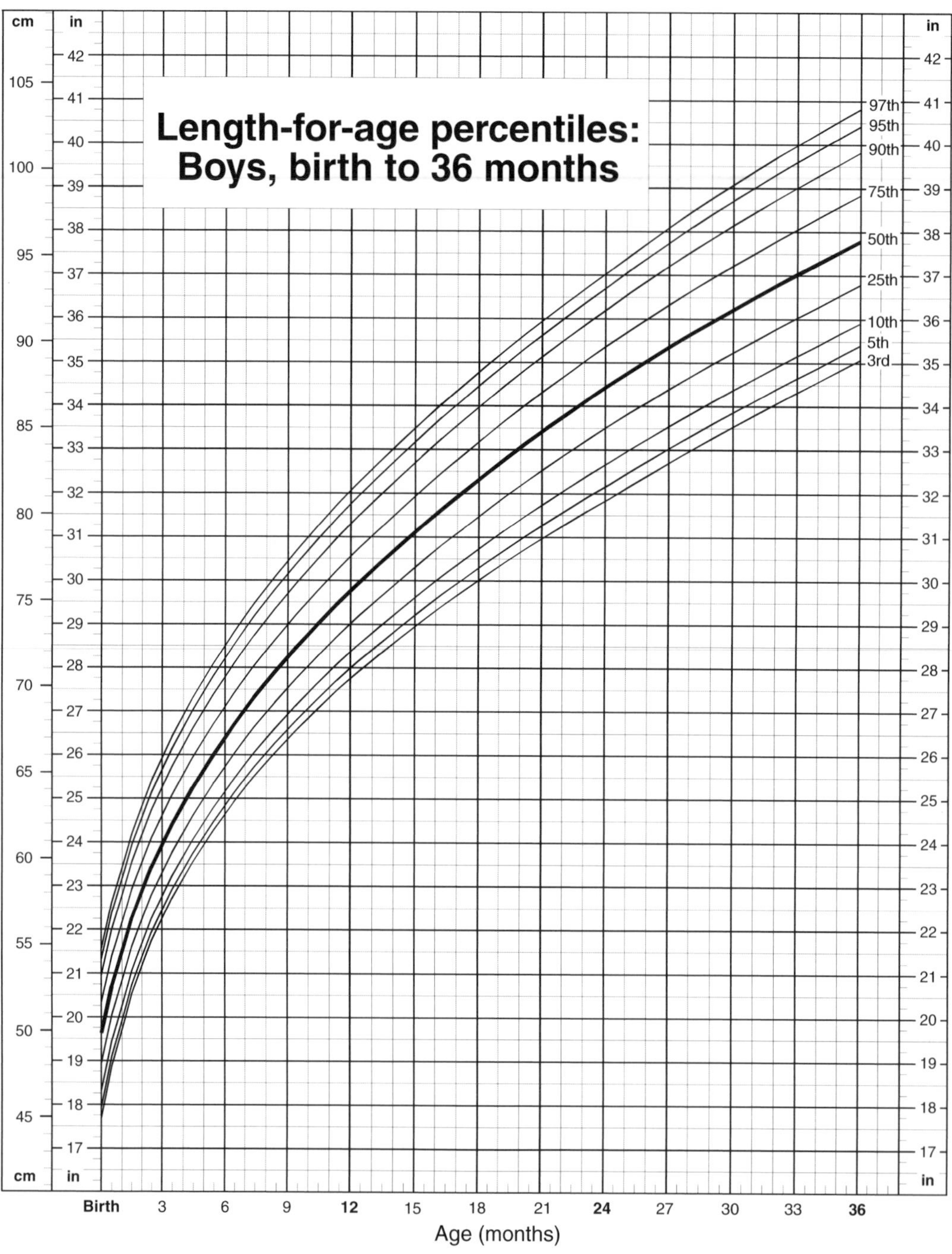

FIGURE 32.3
Length-for-age percentiles, boys, birth to 36 months, CDC growth charts: United States. Source: Developed by the National Center for Health Statistics in collaboration with the National Center for Chronic Disease Prevention and Health Promotion (2000).

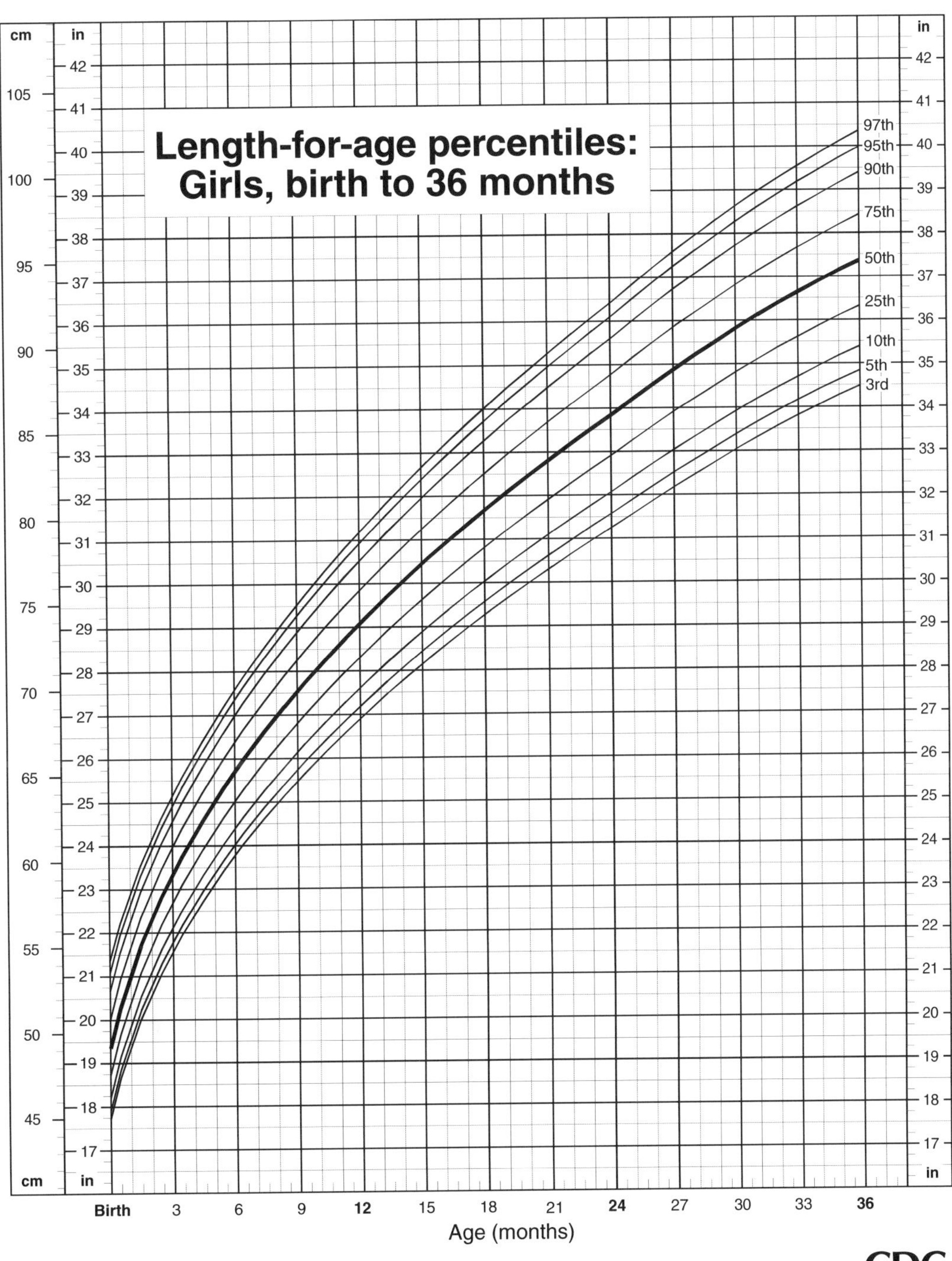

FIGURE 32.4
Length-for-age percentiles, girls, birth to 36 months, CDC growth charts: United States. Source: Developed by the National Center for Health Statistics in collaboration with the National Center for Chronic Disease Prevention and Health Promotion (2000).

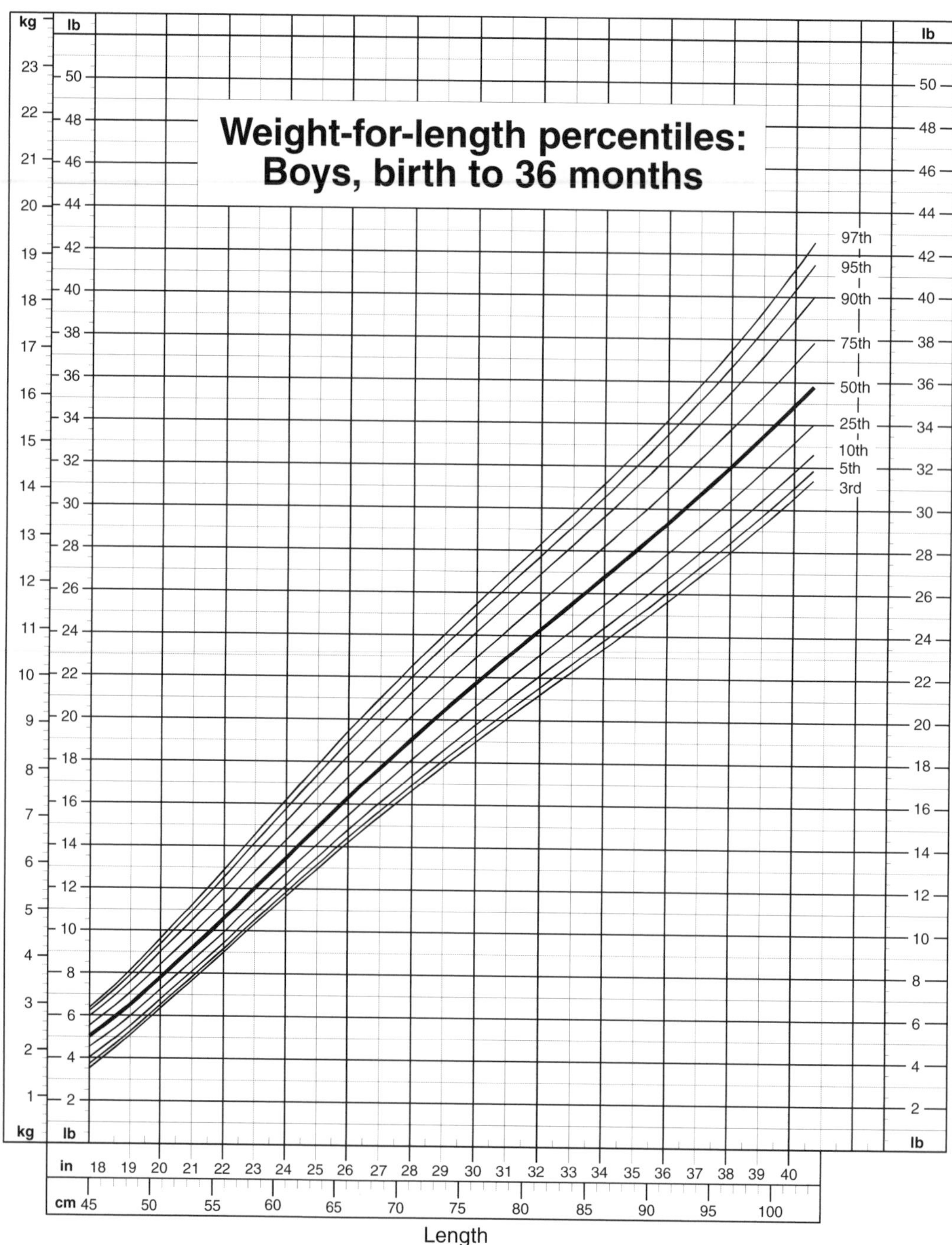

FIGURE 32.5
Weight-for-length percentiles, boys, birth to 36 months, CDC growth charts: United States. Source: Developed by the National Center for Health Statistics in collaboration with the National Center for Chronic Disease Prevention and Health Promotion (2000).

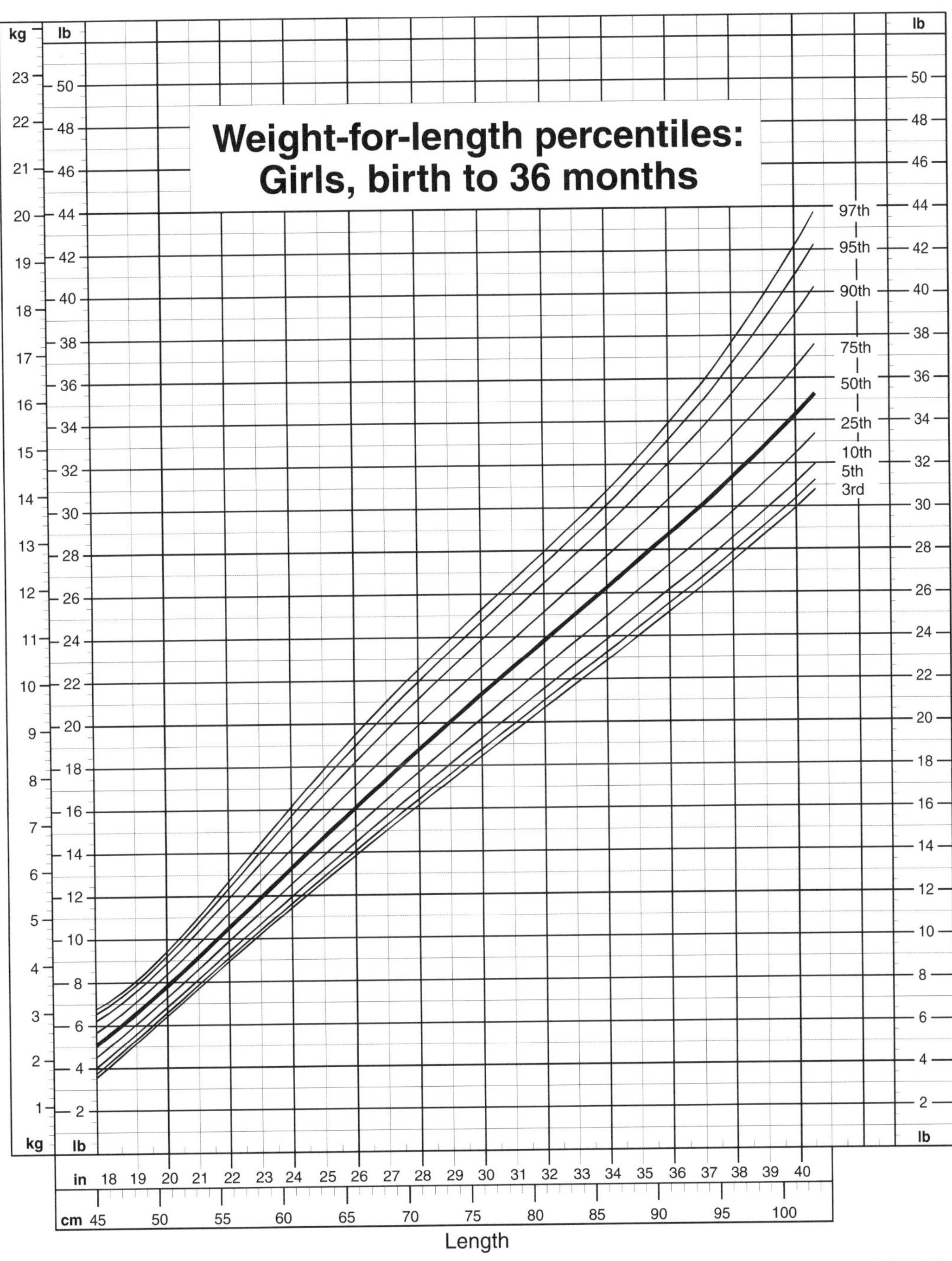

FIGURE 32.6
Weight-for-length percentiles, girls, birth to 36 months, CDC growth charts: United States. Source: Developed by the National Center for Health Statistics in collaboration with the National Center for Chronic Disease Prevention and Health Promotion (2000).

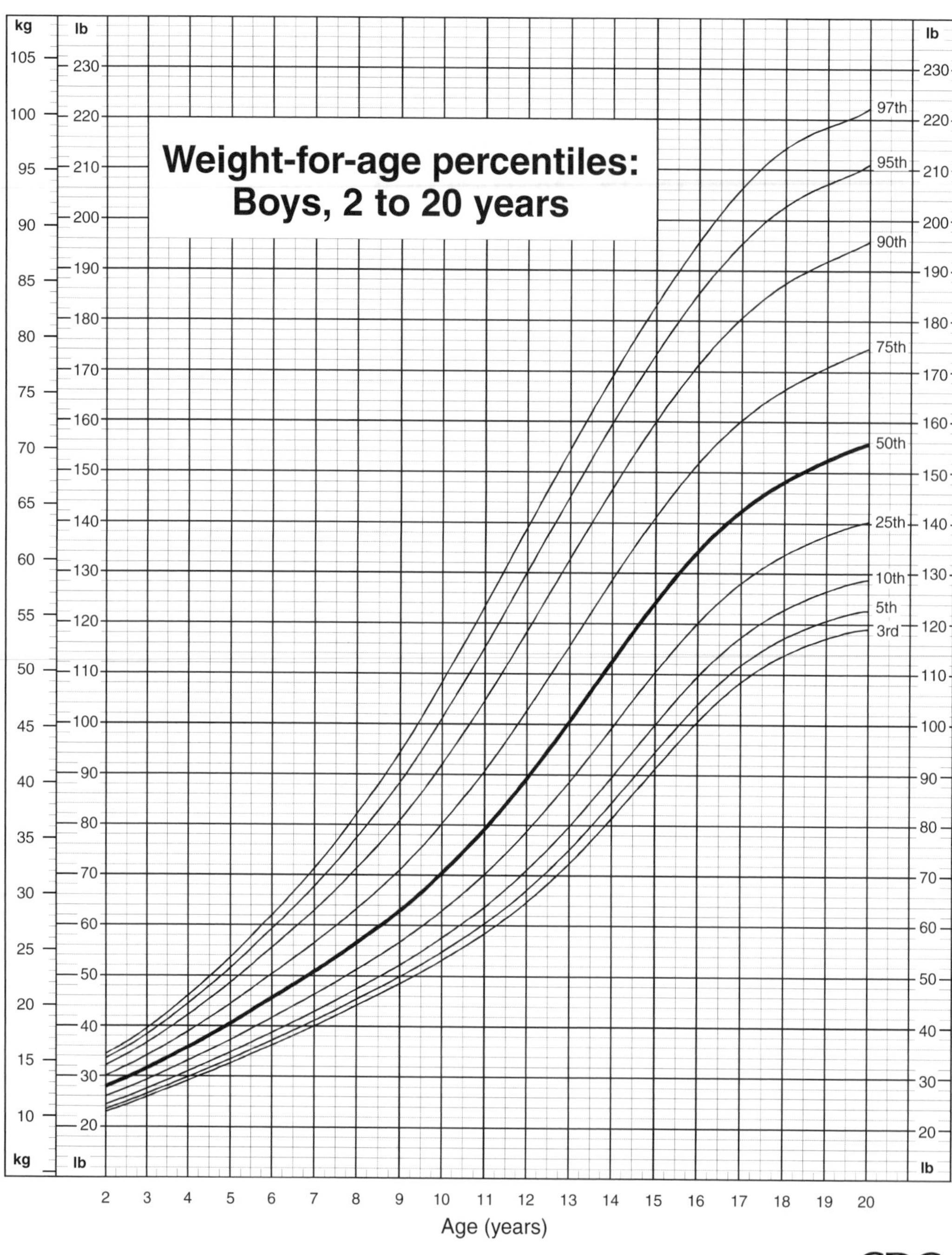

FIGURE 32.7

Weight-for-age percentiles, boys, 2 - to 20 years, CDC growth charts: United States. Source: Developed by the National Center for Health Statistics in collaboration with the National Center for Chronic Disease Prevention and Health Promotion (2000).

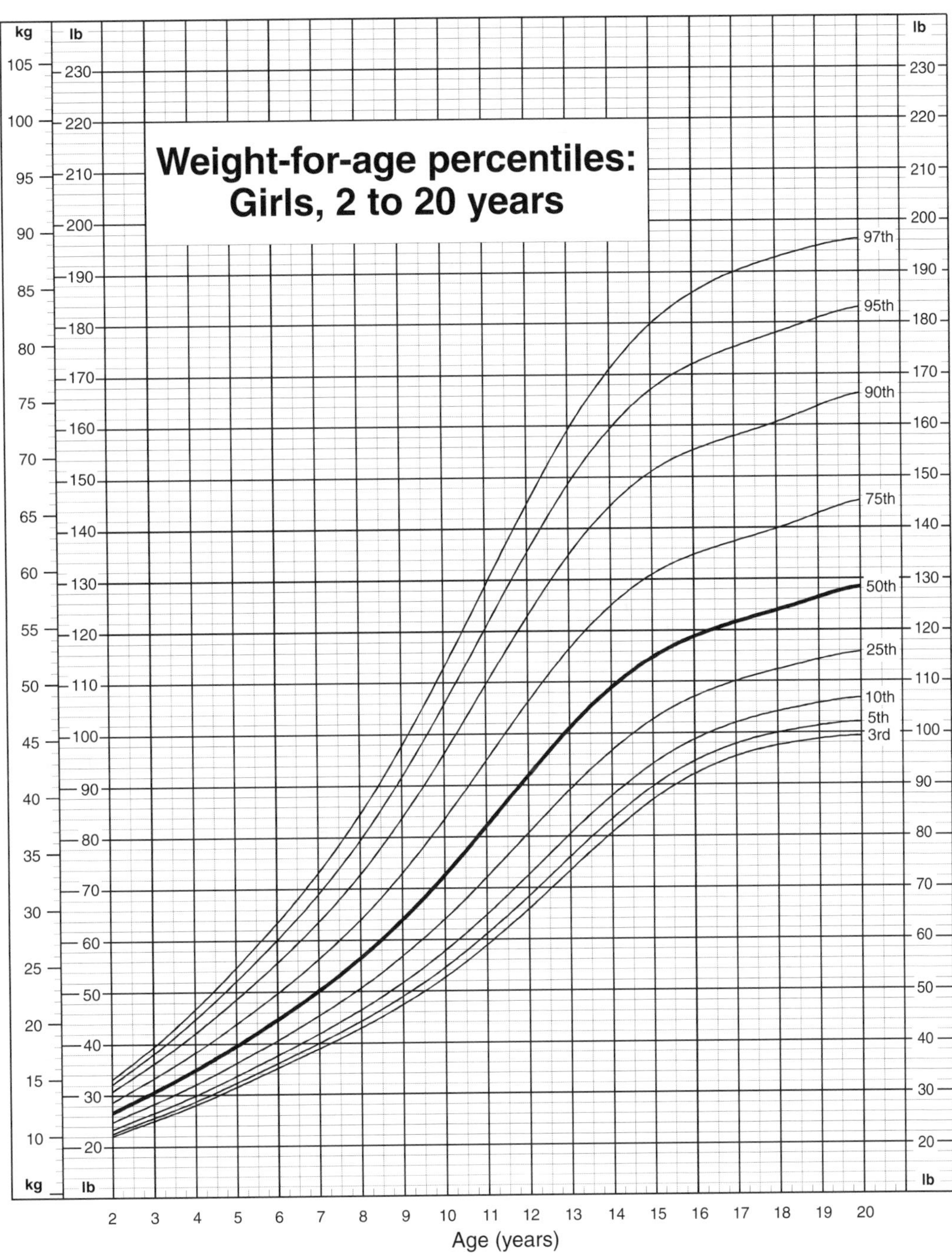

FIGURE 32.8
Weight-for-age percentiles, girls, 2 to 20 years, CDC growth charts: United States. Source: Developed by the National Center for Health Statistics in collaboration with the National Center for Chronic Disease Prevention and Health Promotion (2000).

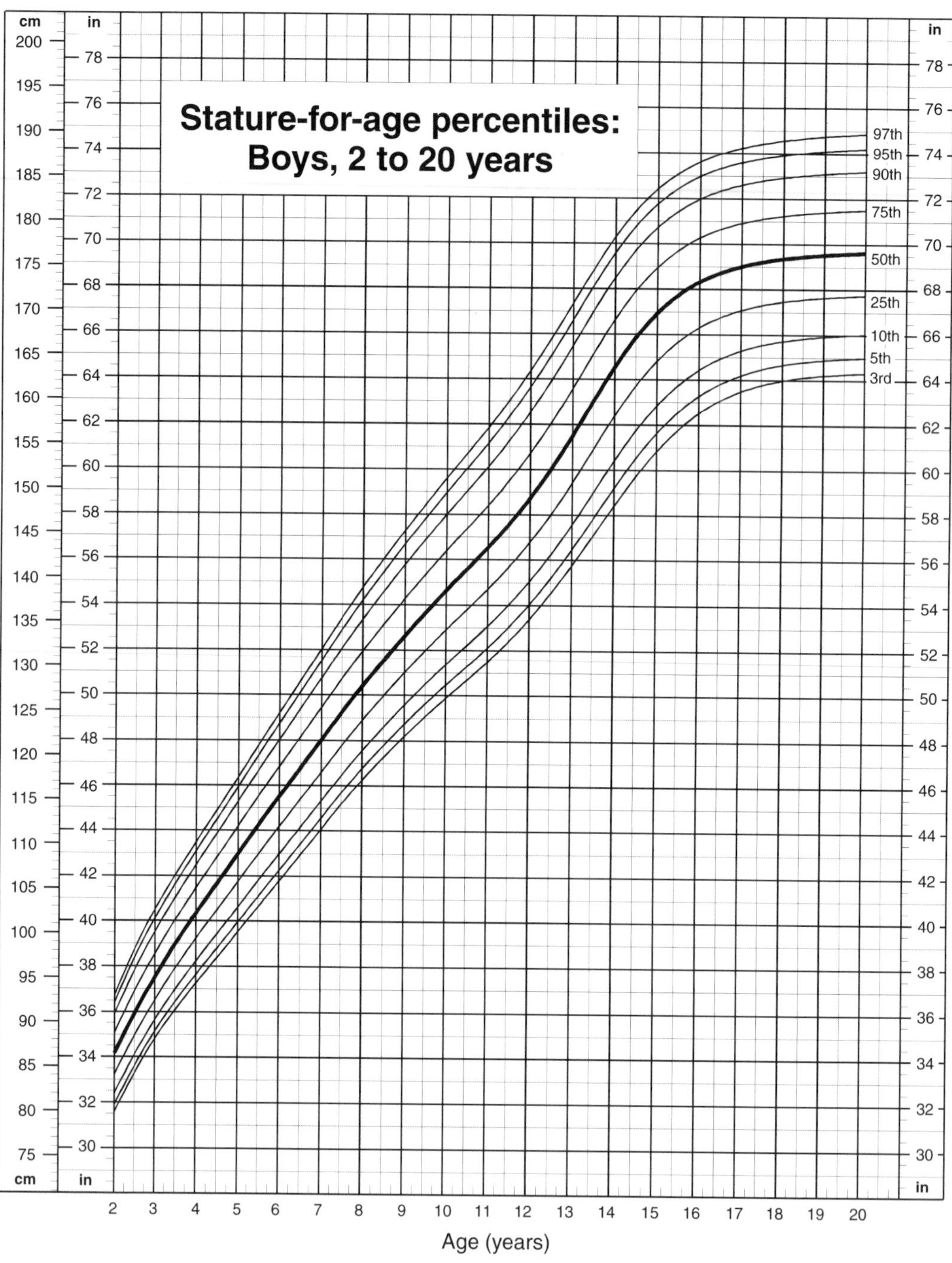

FIGURE 32.9
Stature-for-age percentiles, boys, 2 to 20 years, CDC growth charts: United States. Source: Developed by the National Center for Health Statistics in collaboration with the National Center for Chronic Disease Prevention and Health Promotion (2000).

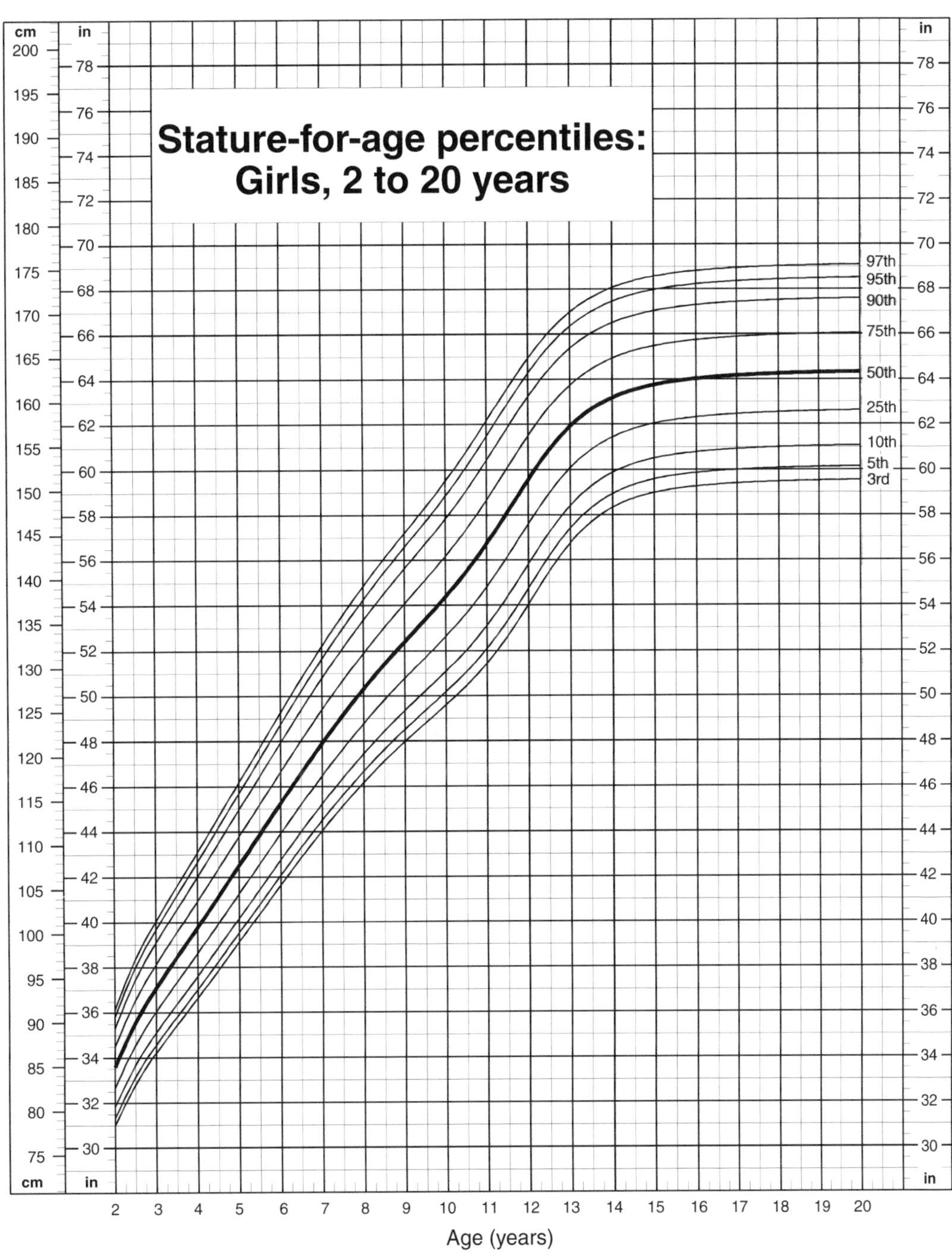

FIGURE 32.10
Stature-for-age percentiles, girls, 2 to 20 years, CDC growth charts: United States. Source: Developed by the National Center for Health Statistics in collaboration with the National Center for Chronic Disease Prevention and Health Promotion (2000).

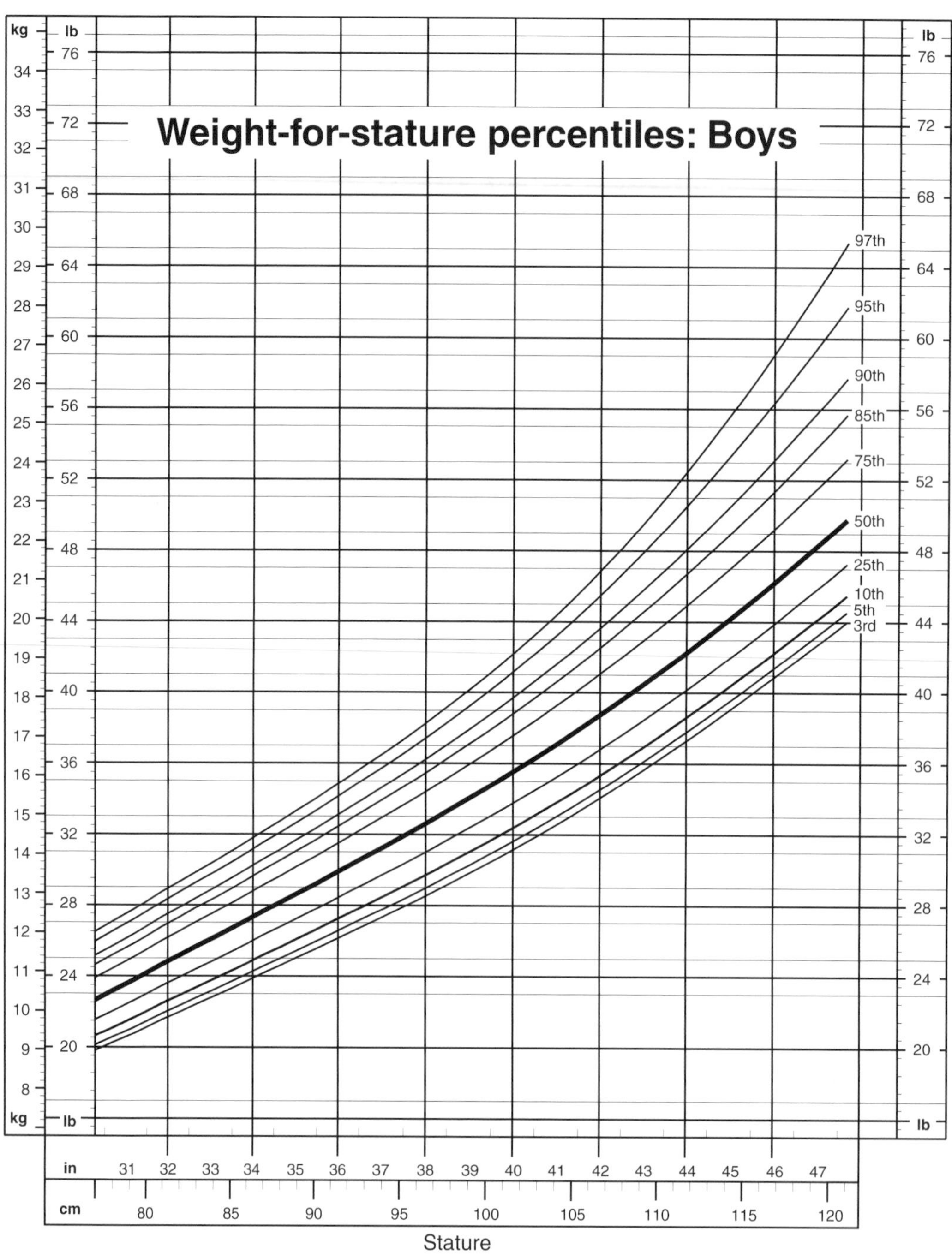

FIGURE 32.11
Weight-for-stature percentiles, boys, CDC growth charts: United States. Source: Developed by the National Center for Health Statistics in collaboration with the National Center for Chronic Disease Prevention and Health Promotion (2000).

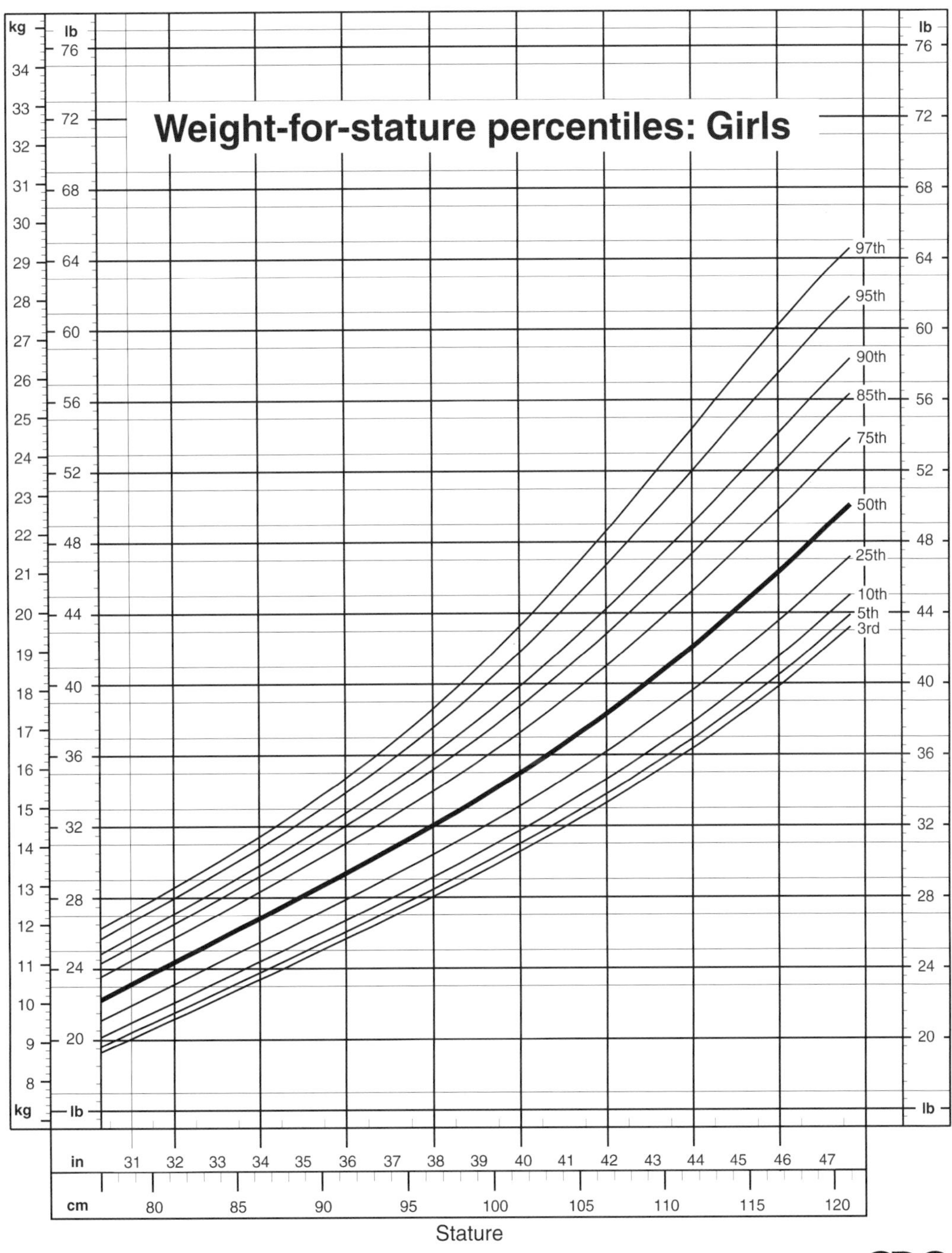

FIGURE 32.12
Weight-for-stature percentiles, girls, CDC growth charts: United States. Source: Developed by the National Center for Health Statistics in collaboration with the National Center for Chronic Disease Prevention and Health Promotion (2000).

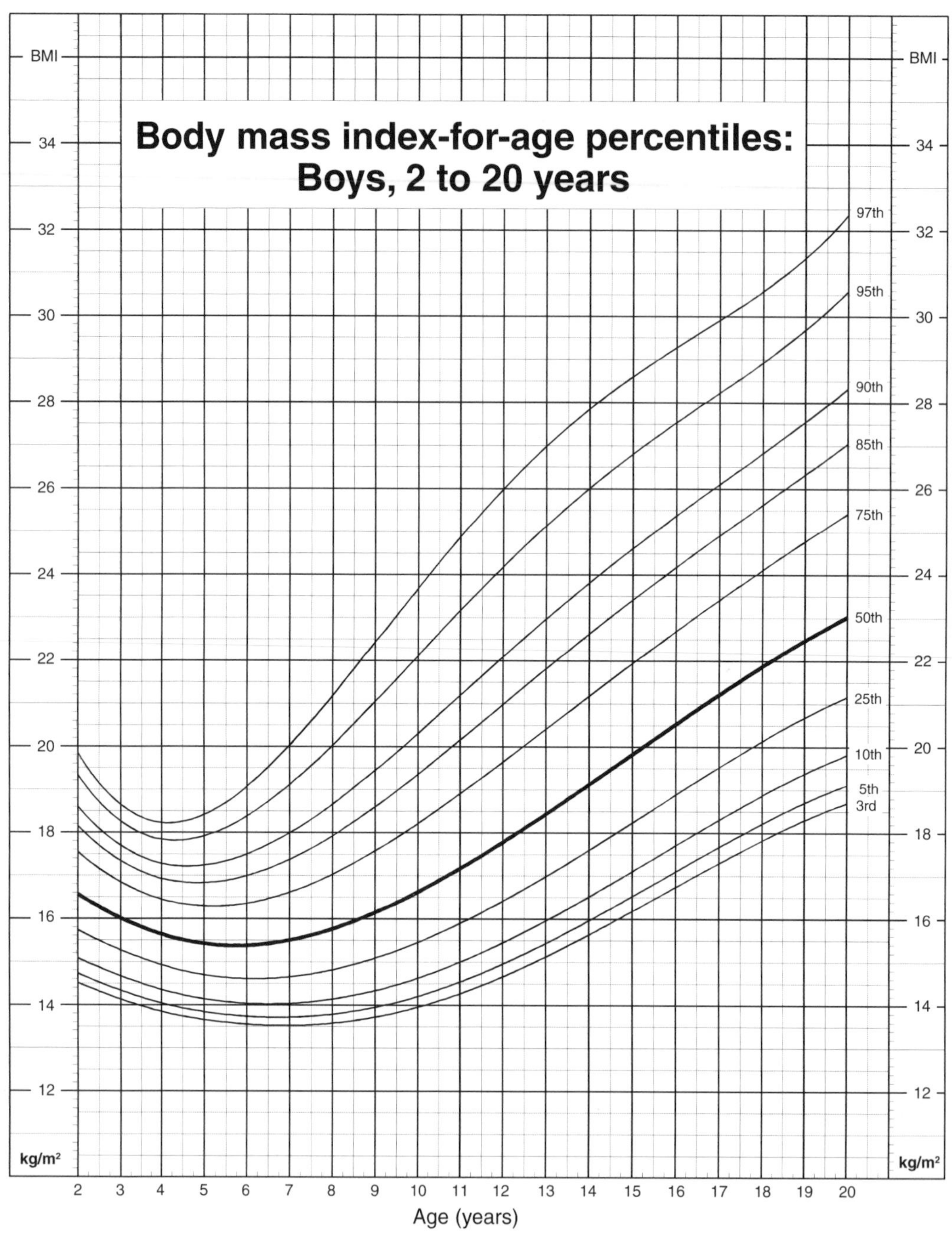

FIGURE 32.13
Body mass index-for-age percentiles, boys, 2 to 20 years, CDC growth charts: United States. Source: Developed by the National Center for Health Statistics in collaboration with the National Center for Chronic Disease Prevention and Health Promotion (2000).

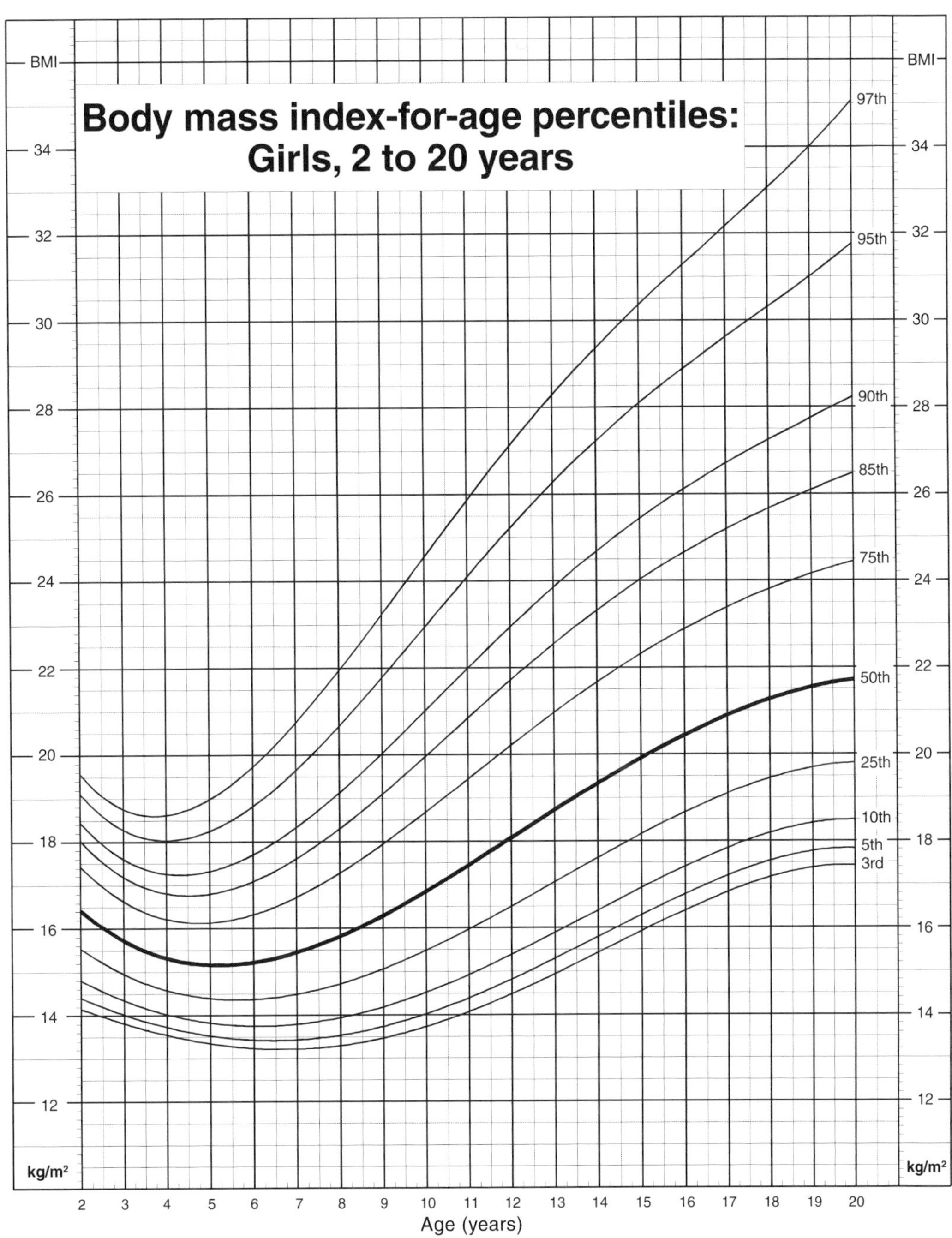

FIGURE 32.14
Body mass index-for-age percentiles, girls, 2 to 20 years, CDC growth charts: United States. Source: Developed by the National Center for Health Statistics in collaboration with the National Center for Chronic Disease Prevention and Health Promotion (2000).

Sources of Further Information

Kuczmarski RJ, Ogden CL, Grummer-Strawn LM, et al. CDC growth charts: United States. Advance data from vital statistics; no. 314. National Center for Health Statistics. 2000.

Whitaker RC, Pepe MS, Wright JA, Seidel KD, Dietz WH. Early adiposity rebound and the risk of adult obesity. *Pediatrics* 998;101(5). http://www.pediatrics.org/cgi/content,/full/101-3/e5.

Himes JH, Deitz WH. Guidelines for overweight in adolescent preventive services: recommendations from an expert committee. *Am J Clin Nutr* 1994; 59: 307-316.

Pietrobelli A, Faith M, Allison DB, Gallagher D, Chiumello G, Heymsfeld SB. Body Mass Index as a measure of adiposity among children and adolescents: a validation study. *J Ped* 1998; 132: 204-210.

Lazarus R, et al. BMI in screening for adiposity in children and adolescents: systematic evaluation using receiver operating *curves. Am J Clin Nutr* 1996; 63: 500-506.

Freedman DS, et al. The relation of overweight to cardiovascular risk factors among children and adolescents: the Bogalusa Heart Study. *Pediatrics* 1999; 103: 1175-1182.

Guo SS, et al. The predictive value of childhood BMI values for overweight at age 35 years. *Am J Clin Nutr* 1994: 59: 810-819.

Dietz WH, Bellizzi MC. Introduction: the use of BMI to assess obesity in children. *Am J Clin Nutr* 1999; 70: 123-5S.

Guo SS, Chumlea WC. Tracking of BMI in children in relation to overweight in adulthood. *Am J Clin Nutr* 1999; 70: 145-148S.

Barlow SE, Dietz, WH. Obesity evaluation and treatment: expert committee rcommendations. *J Ped* 1998; 102(3): 29E.

Gutin B, Basch C, Shea S, et al. Blood pressure, fitness, and fatness in 5- and 6-year-old children. *JAMA* 1990; 264: 1123-1127.

Shear CL, Freedman DS, Burke GL, et al. Body fat patterning and blood pressure in children and young adults — the Bogalusa Heart Study. *Hypertension* 1987; 9: 236-244.

Rames LK, Clark WR, Connor WE, et al. Normal blood pressures and the evaluation of sustained blood pressure elevation in childhood: the Muscatine study. *Pediatrics* 1978; 61: 245-251.

Deschamps L, Desleuz JF, Machinot S, et al. Effects of diet and weight loss on plasma glucose, Insulin, and free fatty acids in obese children. *Ped Res* 1978; 12: 757-760.

Parra A, Schultz RS, Graystone JE, et al. Correlative studies in obese children and adolescents concerning body composition and plasma insulin and growth hormone levels. *Ped Res* 1971; 5: 606-613.

Tracy W, De NC, Harper JR. Obesity and respiratory infection in infants and young children. *BMJ* 1971; 1: 16-18.

Gam SM. Continuities and changes in fatness from infancy through adulthood. *Curr Prob Ped* 1985; 15: 1-47.

Kelsey JL, Acheson RM, Keggi KJ. The body build of patients with slipped capital femoral epiphysis. *Am J Dis Child* 1972; 124: 276-281.

Dietz WH. Health consequences of obesity in youth: childhood predictors of adult disease. *Pediatrics* 1998; 101: 518-525.

Morrison JA, Payne G, Barton BA, Khoury PR, Crawford P. Mother-daughter correlations of obesity and cardiovascular disease risk factors in black and white households: the NHLBI Growth and Health Study. *AJPH* 1994; 84: 1761-1767.

Guo SS, Khoury PR, Sprecker B. Prediction of fat-free mass in black and white preadolescent girls from anthropometry and impedance. *Am J Hum Biol* 1993; 5: 735-745.

33

Anthropometric Assessment: Height, Weight, Body Mass Index (Adults)

George A. Bray

Historical Perspective

Quetelet

Lambert-Adolf-Jacques Quetelet is credited with the concept of the body mass index (BMI).[1] The proposal was made in a monograph in 1835 on the development of the human body. As Freudenthal says, "With Quetelet's work in 1835 a new era in statistics began … The work gave a description of the average man as both a static and dynamic phenomenon."[2] It was Quetelet who introduced the concept of quantitation in measurement of the human being, thus providing a framework for progess in epidemiology and statistics. Quetelet, with his mathematical background, took statistical methods into new arenas. He was a pioneer in the application of statistics to human biology, anthropology, and criminology.

Quetelet was interested in the underlying factors that determined the distribution of such events as births, marriages, deaths, and the prevalence of various types of crime. In his work he noted the seasonal distribution of births, deaths, and marriages. He also noted a seasonal distribution of crime, and that crimes against property appeared more frequently in cold months while crimes against the person were more common in the summer. Commenting on the constancy of crimes from year to year, he said, "Thus we pass from one year to another with the sad perspective of seeing the same crimes reproduced in the same order and calling down the same punishments in the same proportions. Sad condition of humanity …".[1] Fortunately, the human being has been able to change this apparent constancy by education, laws, and better government. Much of the work in the volume *Sur l'Homme* deals with means and distributions of the measurements he made. It was not until a later publication in 1845 in the *Bulletin de la Commission de Statistique (de Belgique)* that he dealt with the concept of the binomial distribution in detail. In his work, Quetelet devoted a significant amount of space to the issues of height and weight. The concept of the "average man" originated with Quetelet, and is one of his seminal contributions. To quote from Chapter 2 of his work, Quetelet says:

> If man increased equally in all his dimensions, his weight at different ages would be as the cube of his height. Now, this is not what we really observe. The increase in weight

0-8493-2705-9/01/$0.00+$1.50

> is slower, except during the first year after birth; then the proportion which we have just pointed out is pretty regularly observed. But after this period, and until near the age of puberty, the weight increases nearly as the square of the height. The development of the weight again becomes very rapid at the time of puberty, and almost stops at the 25th year. In general, we do not err much when we assume that, during development, the square of weight at different ages are as the fifth powers of the height; which naturally leads to this conclusion, in supposing the specific gravity constant, that the transverse growth of man is less than the vertical.
>
> However, if we compare two individuals who are fully developed and well-formed with each other, to ascertain the relations existing between the weight and stature, we shall find that the weight of developed persons, of different heights, is nearly as the square of the stature. Whence it naturally follows, that a transverse section, giving both the breadth and thickness, is just proportioned to the height of the individual. We furthermore conclude that, proportion still being attended, width predominates in individuals of small stature.[1]

These two paragraphs succinctly summarize the concept of the body mass according to Quetelet, and the rationale on which he developed his concept.

Life Insurance

Nearly 70 years after Quetelet, the life insurance industry in the United States began to weigh in on the importance of excess weight as a risk for early death.[3] It was also noted that a central distribution of weight was important. The 1922 *Statistical Bulletin of the Metropolitan Life Insurance Company*[4] says:

> It is generally recognized that weight of the human body in relation to its height plays a part in determining the health and longevity of the individual. It is only recently, however, that the long experience of the insurance companies has made possible the crystallization of this impression into a series of definite propositions. We know now, for example, that overweight is a serious impairment among insured lives, the gravity increasing with the excess in weight over the average for the height and age. But, even this statement has its exceptions because, at younger ages, a limited amount of overweight is apparently an advantage. Such persons have uniformly lower death rates from tuberculosis. It is after the age of 35 that overweight, even in relatively small amounts, begins to be dangerous. The seriousness increases with advancing age and with the amount of overweight.

From this point forward until the last decade of the 20th century, there were "weight tables" of appropriate, desirable, or ideal weight proposed by the life insurance industry. The Framingham Study, which was the first American effort at a long-term population-based evaluation of health risks, used the Metropolitan Life Insurance Table of 1959 as the basis for comparing the weights of people living in Framingham with some standard. The term came to be called the Metropolitan Relative Weight, which was the weight for height of an individual to the expected weight for height from the Metropolitan Life Insurance Table median frame grouping.

Various Indices

Several indices relating height to weight were proposed in the middle of the 20th century. The BMI, or what might be appropriately called the Quetelet Index (QI), was compared against several other indices by Keys et al.[5] They evaluated three indices of weight and height: the Wt/Ht, the $Wt/[Ht]^2$ (QI), and the $Ht/[Wt]^{1/3}$ (Ponderal Index) against skinfold estimates of fat. Of these three, the QI had a slightly better correlation with fatness than Wt/Ht. The Ponderal Index was clearly the worst.

Gradual Adoption of the BMI

Benn reopened this question again in 1971.[6] He showed that a simple index of weight/$(Ht)^p$ could be derived for each population, in which p was a power where weight had the lowest relation to height for that population. For most populations this number is between 1 and 2. The ratio that Quetelet proposed in 1835 had a power of 2 $[wt/(Ht)^2]$. Lee, Kolonel, and Hinds,[7] in an effort to apply a weight/height index to a variety of populations in Hawaii, found different indices useful for ranking the different populations. However, these authors did not measure fatness, and since all of these weight-to-height indices are strongly related to weight,[8] their data are not helpful in resolving the value of the QI versus the Benn Index as estimates of fat. Keys et al.[5] examined the relationship of weight-to-height indices in 12 populations. The best correlations with body fat as estimated from skinfolds were found with $[wt/(Ht)^2]$. He found that the QI had correlations ranging between .611 and .850 when related to skinfold thickness. In a detailed evaluation of four large study populations, Garn and Pesick [8] showed a strong correlation between any index and weight which approximated $r = 0.90$. In this study, the population-specific indices, as proposed by Benn $[wt/(Ht)^2]$, ranged between 1.18 and 1.83. These population-specific indices provided no advantage over the $Wt/(Ht)^2$ when related to skinfolds.

Garrow and Webster[9] have examined the QI as a measure of fatness in a group of obese subjects. Fat was measured by three separate techniques including densitometry, measurement of total body water, and measurement of total body potassium using γ-emission from naturally occurring ^{40}K. As Garrow and Webster point out, there is considerable variation in estimating fat between the methods that they selected for this study.[9] The accuracy for measuring fat was greater for men than for women by all methods used by Garrow and Webster. The standard deviations for estimating fat by the QI, however, were only slightly larger than those for density, body water, and body potassium. The relationship of $FAT/(Ht)^2$ plotted against $[wt/(Ht)^2]$ yielded very similar slopes for men (0.715) and women (0.713). This indicates that men and women of similar height differ in weight by tissue which is approximately 75% fat and 25% non-fat. In their data analysis there was an important difference in the fatness between men and women, such that a woman with 0 (zero) body fat would have a QI of 13.7 kg/m^2, whereas a man with 0 body fat would have a QI of 16.9 kg/m^2. Garrow and Webster thus conclude that "Quetelet's Index has been underrated as a measure of obesity in adults. It … provides a measure of fatness not much less accurate than specialized laboratory methods." As they point out, this index can be applied over the entire weight range, while such measurements as skinfold thickness are severely limited in obese individuals and nearly useless in very obese individuals.

An additional feature of the QI is the similarity of the mortality and morbidity curves plotted against QI for men and women. Whether related to excessive deaths or to morbidity from various disease entities, the minimum QI (BMI) is similar for both sexes at comparable ages. Yet at all ages, the quantity of body fat in women is higher than men for any given height/weight combination. This implies that the extra fat in women (the zero fat BMI values noted above) is not associated with increased risk of excess morbidity or mortality. A similar conclusion, ushering in the era of studies in body fat distribution,[1] suggests that for comparable increases in risk indices such as blood pressure, women have approximately 20 kg more adipose tissue stores of fat than men.[2]

In summary, the relationship between height and weight [wt/(Ht)^2] proposed by Quetelet in 1835 has stood the test of time. In tribute to his contribution and its validation from a number of sources, it would be appropriate to refer to it as the Quetelet Index, or QI, and replace the frequently used body mass index, or BMI, with this new nomenclature.

Measurement of Weight

Recommended Technique

During infancy, a leveled pan scale with a beam and movable weights is used to measure weight. The pan must be at least 100 cm long so that it can support a 2-year-old infant at the 95th percentile for recumbent length. A quilt is left on the scale at all times, and the scale calibrated to zero and across the range of expected weights when only a quilt is on it, using test objects of known weights. Calibration is performed monthly and whenever the scales are moved. Similar procedures are used to calibrate the scales used for older individuals. When the scales are not in use, the beam should be locked in place or the weights shifted from zero to reduce wear.

The infant, with or without a diaper, is placed on the scales so that the weight is distributed equally on each side of the center of the pan. Weight is recorded to the nearest 10 g with the infant lying quietly, which may require patience. When an infant is restless, it is possible to weigh the mother when holding the infant and then weigh the mother without the infant, but this procedure is unreliable, partly because the mother's weight will be recorded to the nearest 100 g. It is better to postpone the measurement and try later. The measurement is repeated three times, and the average recorded after excluding any clearly erroneous value. If a diaper is worn, the weight of the diaper is subtracted from the observed weight, because most reference data for infants are based on nude weights.

In a clinic, the measured weight is recorded in tabular form in addition to being plotted. This plotting is done while the subject is present. Irregularities may be noted in the serial data for a subject or there may be major discrepancies between the percentile levels for highly correlated variables. When this occurs, the measurer checks the accuracy of the plotting and remeasures the subject if the plotting is correct.

A subject able to stand without support is weighed using a leveled platform scale with a beam and moveable weights or an electronic balance. The beam on the scale must be graduated so that it can be read from both sides and the scale positioned so that the measurer can stand behind the beam, facing the subject, and can move the beam weights without reaching around the subject. The movable tare is arranged so that a screwdriver is needed to shift it. The subject stands still over the center of the platform with the body weight evenly distributed between both feet. Light indoor clothing can be worn, excluding shoes, long trousers, and sweater. It is better to standardize the clothing, for example, a disposable paper gown. The weight of this clothing is not subtracted from the observed weight when the recommended reference data are used. Weight is recorded to the nearest 100 g.*

Handicapped subjects, other than infants, who cannot stand unsupported can be weighed using a beam chair scale or bed scale. If an adult weighs more than the upper limit on the beam, a weight can be suspended from the left-hand end of the beam, after

* For electronic scales, the subject stands in the center of the platform in appropriate clothing and the weight is recorded when stable.

which the measurer must determine how much weight must be placed on the platform for the scale to record zero when there is no weight on the platform. This weight is added to the measured value when a scale modified in this fashion is used. In studies to assess short-term changes, weights must be recorded at times standardized in relation to ingestion, micturition, and defecation, but for single weight this is not necessary.

Purpose

Weight is the most commonly recorded anthropometric variable, and generally is measured with sufficient accuracy. Accuracy can be improved, however, by attention to details of the measurement technique. Strictly, this measurement is of mass rather than weight, but the latter term is too well established to be replaced easily. Weight is a composite measure of total body size. It is important in screening for unusual growth, obesity, and undernutrition.

Literature

There is general agreement that weight should be measured using a beam scale with movable weights or a calibrated electronic balance. A pan scale is needed for measurements made during infancy. The use of a spring scale is not recommended, despite its greater mobility, except in field conditions where there may be no practical alternative. Automatic scales that print the weight directly onto a permanent record are available but expensive. The scale should be placed with the platform level and in a position where the measurer can see the back of the beam without leaning around the subject. Scales with wheels to facilitate movement from one location to another are not recommended because they need calibration every time they are moved.

Weight is best measured with the subject nude, which is practical during infancy.[10] At older ages, nude measurements may not be possible.[10] If not, standardized light clothing, for example, a disposable paper gown, should be worn in preference to "light indoor clothing."[10]

There are diurnal variations in weight of about 1 kg in children and 2 kg in adults. Therefore, recording the time of day at which measurements are made is necessary.[10] Usually it is not practical to measure at a fixed time, but a narrow range may be achievable.

Reliability

Intermeasurer differences (M) from the Fels Longitudinal Study are as follows:[10]

M = 1.2 g (SD = 3.2 g) at 5 to 10 years
M = 1.5 g (SD = 3.6 g) at 10 to 15 years
M = 1.7 g (SD = 3.8 g) at 15 to 20 years
M = 1.5 g (SD = 3.6 g) for adults

In the Health Examination Survey by the National Center for Health Statistics, the intermeasurer and intrameasurer technical errors were about 1.2 kg, when pairs of measurements were made 2 weeks apart.[10] About 10% of the observed error would have been due to growth.

Measurement of Stature (Standing Height)

Recommended Technique

Measurement of stature requires a vertical board with an attached metric rule and a horizontal headboard that can be brought into contact with the most superior point on the head. The combination of these elements is called a stadiometer. Fixed and portable models are available, and plans for fabrication of a stadiometer by an investigator are available from the Field Services Branch, Division of Nutrition, Centers for Disease Control, Atlanta, Georgia 30333.

The subject is barefoot or wears thin socks and little clothing so that the positioning of the body can be seen. The subject stands on a flat surface that is at a right angle to the vertical board of the stadiometer. The weight of the subject is distributed evenly on both feet, and the head is positioned in the Frankford Horizontal Plane. The arms hang freely by the sides of the trunk, with the palms facing the thighs. The subject places the heels together, with both heels touching the base of the vertical board. The medial borders of the feet are at an angle of about 60°. If the subject has knock knees, the feet are separated so that the medial borders of the knees are in contact but not overlapping. The scapulae and buttocks are in contact with the vertical board. The heels, buttocks, scapulae, and the posterior aspect of the cranium of some subjects cannot be placed in one vertical plane while maintaining a reasonable natural stance. These subjects are positioned so that only the buttocks and the heels or the cranium are in contact with the vertical board.

The subject is asked to inhale deeply and maintain a fully erect position without altering the load on the heels. The movable headboard is brought onto the most superior point on the head with sufficient pressure to compress the hair. The measurement is recorded to the nearest 0.1 cm, and the time at which the measurement was made is noted.

Recumbent length is measured in place of stature until the age of two years. Between two and three years, recumbent length or stature can be measured, and the choice made between these variables must be noted because they differ systematically. Two measurers are needed to measure stature in children aged two to three years. One measurer places a hand on the child's feet to prevent lifting of the heels and keep the heels against the vertical board, and he or she makes sure that the knees are extended with the other hand. The second measurer lowers the headboard and observes its level.

When there is lower limb anisomelia (inequality of length), the shorter side is built up with graduated wooden boards until the pelvis is level, as judged from the iliac crests. The amount of the buildup is recorded because it can alter the interpretation of weight-stature relationships.

Purpose

Stature is a major indicator of general body size and bone length. It is important in screening for disease or malnutrition and in the interpretation of weight. Variations from the normal range can have social consequences, in addition to their association with disease.

When stature cannot be measured, recumbent length can be substituted and, depending on the purpose of the study, adjustments for the systematic differences between these highly correlated measurements may be desirable.[10] Arm span may be used in place of stature when stature cannot be measured and it is not practical to measure recumbent length. The measurement of arm span is described in the section on segment lengths. Also, stature can be estimated from knee height, as described in the section on recumbent anthropometry.

Literature

Stature can be measured using a fixed or movable anthropometer. An anthropometer consists of a vertical graduated rod and a movable rod that is brought onto the head. An anthropometer can be attached to a wall or used in a free-standing mode, utilizing a base plate to keep the vertical rod properly aligned. Measurements of stature with a movable anthropometer tend to be less than those with a stadiometer.[10] It is not recommended that stature be measured against a wall, but if this must be done, a wall should be chosen that does not have a baseboard, and the subject should not stand on a carpet. An apparatus that allows stature to be measured while the subject stands on a platform scale is not recommended.

Some workers do not ask subjects to stretch to the appropriate extent. This is likely to lead to less reproducible positioning and less reliability than the recommended procedure. Some workers ask the subjects to assume a position of military attention; this is inappropriate for young children and for the elderly. In one alternative technique, a measurer exerts upward force under the mastoid processes to keep the head at the maximum level to which it was raised when the subject inhaled deeply. A second measurer lowers the headboard and observes its level, while a third person records the value. The need for three measurers reduces the practicality of this technique, but when it is applied the diurnal variation in stature is reduced.[10]

Some workers place the head in a "normal" position, with the eyes looking straight ahead; this is less precise than positioning in the Frankfort Horizontal Plane. Others tilt the head backwards and forwards and record stature when the head is positioned so that the maximum value is obtained. It is difficult to apply the latter procedure while the subject maintains a full inspiration.

It is general practice to place the subject's heels together, but the angle between the medial borders has varied from study to study. If these borders are parallel, or nearly so, many young children and some obese adults are unable to stand erect.

Reliability

Intermeasurer differences (M) for large samples in the Fels Longitudinal Study are as follows:[10]

M = 2.4 mm (SD = 2.1 mm) at 5 to 10 years
M = 2.0 mm (SD = 1.9 mm) at 10 to 15 years
M = 2.3 mm (SD = 2.4 mm) at 15 to 20 years
M = 1.4 mm (SD = 1.5 mm) at 20 to 55 years
M = 2.1 mm (SD = 2.1 mm) at 54 to 85 years

Comments

BMI and Gender

Women are fatter than men at any BMI. On average, this number is 11-12% higher for the same BMI and age group. Yet this extra fatness in women is not associated with extra risk to health. Thus, because the component units of the BMI, height, and weight can be measured with great reliability compared to total body fat, measuring body fat is not recommended. Rather, BMI is preferred because it is gender neutral. Table 33.1 shows BMI.

BMI and Ethnic Groups

A recent study compared percent body fat at different ages in men and women of three ethnic groups (Table 33.2). Ethnic differences are obvious, and imply that using the BMI to evaluate risk requires an adjustment related to ethnic differences. This is one of many adjustments to BMI in arriving at the risk from obesity for individuals.[11]

BMI Curves and Children

BMI curves have been developed for children by the Centers for Disease Control and Prevention (www.CDC.gov). The principle behind this table for children was to take the height for BMI 25 and 30 for 18-year-olds and then take corresponding height deviations at various ages. The BMI of 30 for children is close to the 95th percentile of height for weight. The BMI of 25 in children is close to the 85th percentile of weight for height in children.

Misclassification

Since BMI measures height and weight, it is an imperfect tool for evaluating fat. Correlations of fat with BMI vary from <0.1 to >0.8 depending on initial percent of fat, level of physical training, and age. Older people tend to lose height, and this elevates the BMI inappropriately. Body builders, Sumo wrestlers, and professional athletes will have high BMI values for low body fat. However, the purpose and value of the BMI is not to assess athletes, but to provide a starting point in risk assessment of overweight in sedentary people.

BMI and Central Fat

Body fat and visceral fat are related, but BMI as an index of body fatness cannot assess central fat. A measure of waist circumference can be a valuable addition in the assessment of risk. To have a clear picture of the steps in this process, it would be helpful to examine the natural history of the change in BMI. Figure 33.1 shows the increasing percentage of the population with a BMI >25 (top line) or >30 (lower line). Both lines rise until age 50 to 60 years. This means that an increasing percentage of the population is moving from the pre-overweight category with a BMI <25 to overweight or obese. Thus, the natural history of overweight is a gradual transition of the potentially or pre-overweight into overweight or clinical overweight categories. In addition, there appears to be about 25% of the population who will never become overweight. This is shown in Figure 33.1.

Risk Evaluation — Know Your BMI

The BMI is a useful tool in assessing the risk from overweight. In epidemiological studies, the risk of many diseases increases as BMI increases. This is shown in Figure 33.2, along with the cut points used for determining overweight and clinical overweight.

The curvilinear relationship shown is for overall mortality. The steepness of the curve varies for different diseases. For diabetes mellitus there is a very steep relationship. For

TABLE 33.1
Body Mass Index (BMI) Values

	Good Weights							Overweight					Obese									
	BMI																					
Height	19	20	21	22	23	24	25	26	27	28	29	30	31	32	33	34	35	36	37	38	39	40
4′10″	91	96	100	105	110	115	119	124	129	134	138	143	148	153	158	162	167	172	177	181	186	191
4′11″	94	99	104	109	114	119	124	128	133	138	143	148	153	158	163	168	173	178	183	188	193	198
5′	97	102	107	112	118	123	128	133	138	143	148	153	158	163	168	174	179	184	189	194	199	204
5′1″	100	106	111	116	122	127	132	137	143	148	153	158	164	169	174	180	185	190	195	201	206	211
5′2″	104	109	115	120	126	131	136	142	147	153	158	164	169	175	180	186	191	196	202	207	213	218
5′3″	107	113	118	124	130	135	141	146	152	158	163	169	175	180	186	191	197	203	208	214	220	225
5′4″	110	116	122	128	134	140	145	151	157	163	169	174	180	186	192	197	204	209	215	221	227	232
5′5″	114	120	126	132	138	144	150	156	162	169	174	180	186	192	198	204	210	216	222	228	234	240
5′6″	118	124	130	136	142	148	155	161	167	173	179	186	192	198	204	210	216	223	229	235	241	247
5′7″	121	127	134	140	146	153	159	166	172	178	185	191	198	204	211	217	223	230	236	242	249	255
5′8″	125	131	138	144	151	158	164	171	177	184	190	197	203	210	216	223	230	236	243	249	256	262
5′9″	128	135	142	149	155	162	169	176	182	189	196	203	209	216	223	230	236	243	250	257	263	270
5′10″	132	139	146	153	160	167	174	181	188	195	202	209	216	222	229	236	243	250	257	264	271	278
5′11″	136	143	150	157	165	172	179	186	193	200	208	215	222	229	236	243	250	257	265	272	279	286
6′	140	147	154	162	169	117	184	191	199	206	213	221	228	235	242	250	258	265	272	279	287	294
6′1″	144	151	159	166	174	182	189	197	204	212	219	227	235	242	250	257	265	272	280	288	295	302
6′2″	148	155	163	171	179	186	194	202	210	218	225	233	241	249	256	264	272	280	287	295	303	311
6′3″	152	160	168	176	184	192	200	208	216	224	232	240	248	256	264	272	279	287	295	303	311	319
6′4″	156	164	172	180	189	197	205	213	221	230	238	246	254	263	271	279	287	295	304	312	320	328

TABLE 33.2

Percent Body Fat for Men and Women of Different Ethnic Groups and Three Age Ranges According to Body Mass Index*

	Females (% fat)			Males (% fat)		
BMI (kg/m²)	African American	Asian	Caucasian	African American	Asian	Caucasian
Age 20–39						
18.5	20	25	21	8	13	8
25	32	35	33	20	23	21
30	38	40	39	26	28	26
Age 40–59						
18.5	21	25	23	9	13	11
25	34	36	35	22	24	23
30	39	41	41	27	29	29
Age 60–79						
18.5	23	26	25	11	14	13
25	35	36	38	23	24	25
39	41	41	43	29	29	31

* Adapted from Gallagher, D et al. *Am J Clin Nutr* 2000 Sep; 72(3): 694-701.

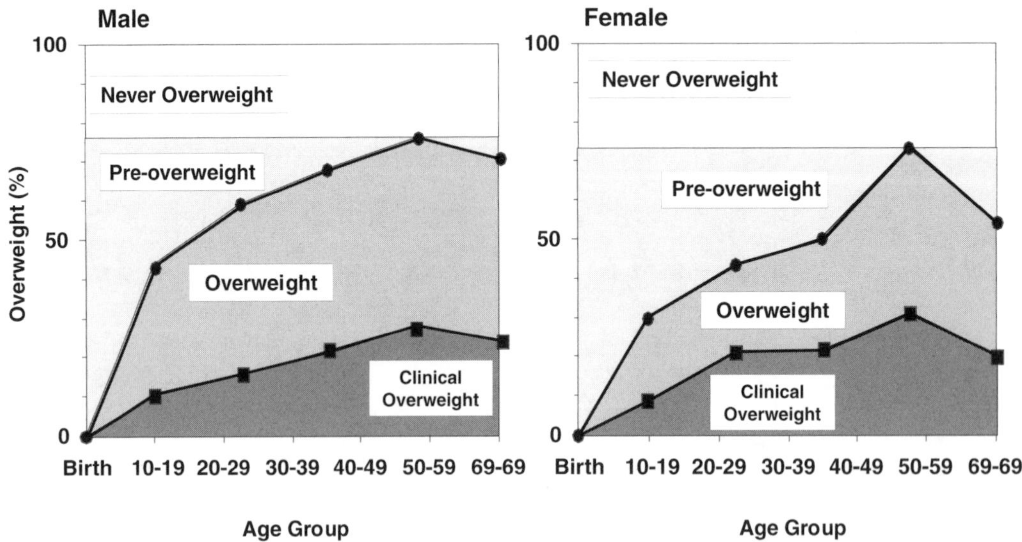

FIGURE 33.1
The natural history of overweight is a gradual transition of the potentially, pre-overweight into overweight, or clinical overweight categories. In addition, there appears to be about 25% of the population who will never become overweight.

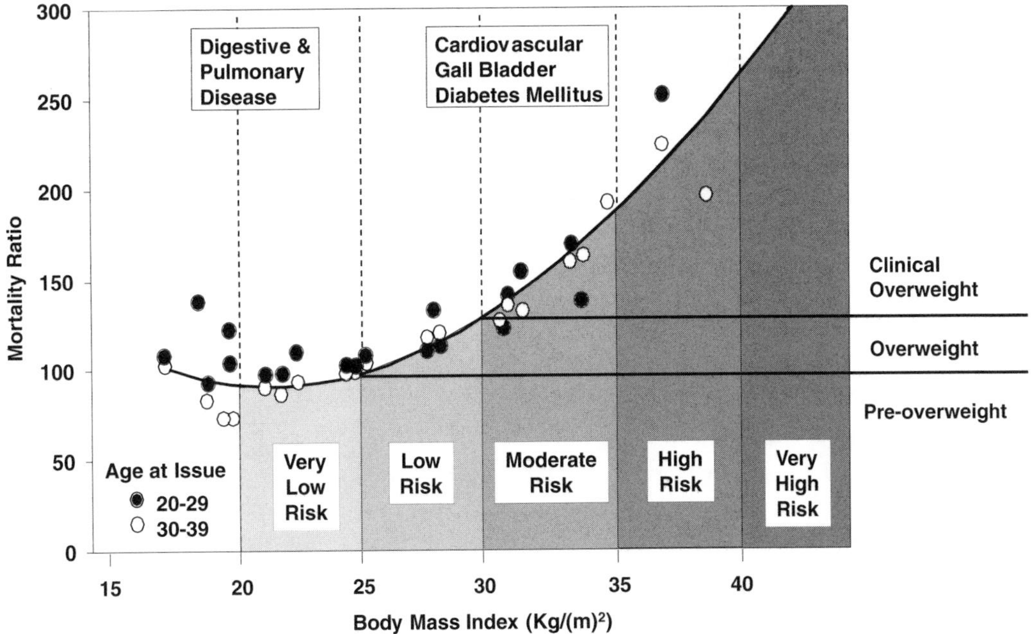

FIGURE 33.2
In epidemiological studies, the risk of many diseases increases as BMI increases. The curvilinear relationship shown here is for overall mortality. The steepness of the curve varies for different diseases.

this disease, individuals with a BMI of 23 to 24 are already at higher risk than those with a BMI of 20.

The curvilinear relationship of BMI has a similar shape to that of diastolic blood pressure and risk of death, or cholesterol concentrations and the risk of death. This is shown for all three in Figure 33.3. The dashed vertical lines in this figure represent the arbitrary cut points that separate low from moderate and high risk.

Starting with an accurately determined BMI, a clinician can sort through an algorithm such as that developed by the National Heart, Lung, and Blood Institute (Figure 33.4). Using this algorithm points the clinician and patient along the path of effectively evaluating the patient's BMI. "Know Your BMI" could serve as an effective public health campaign. If the public began to learn their BMI, it would be incumbent upon health professionals to be able to guide their patients in its use.

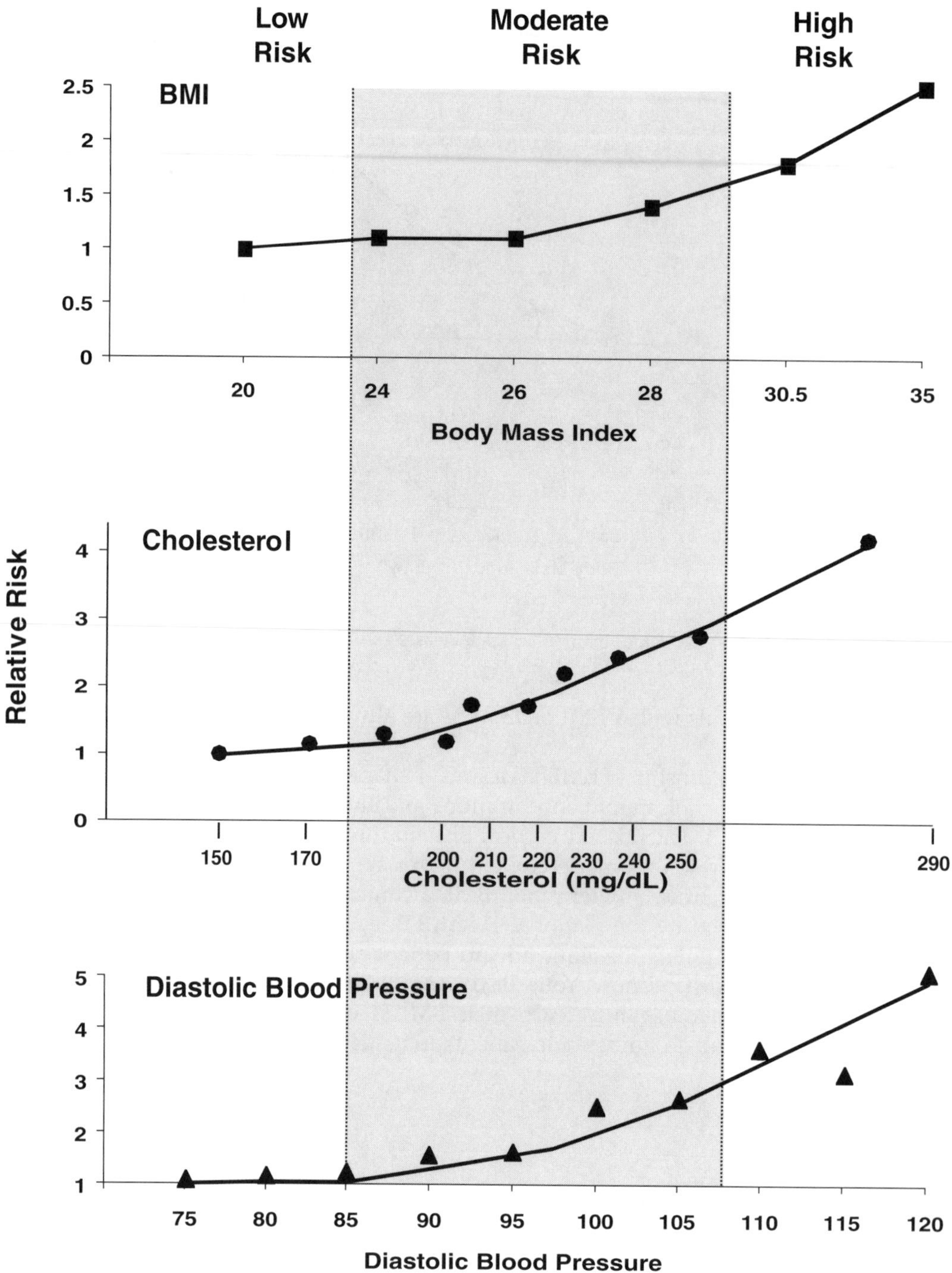

FIGURE 33.3
The curvilinear relationship of BMI has a similar shape to that of diastolic blood pressure and risk of death or cholesterol concentrations and the risk of death. The dashed vertical lines represent the arbitrary cut points that separate low from moderate and high risk.

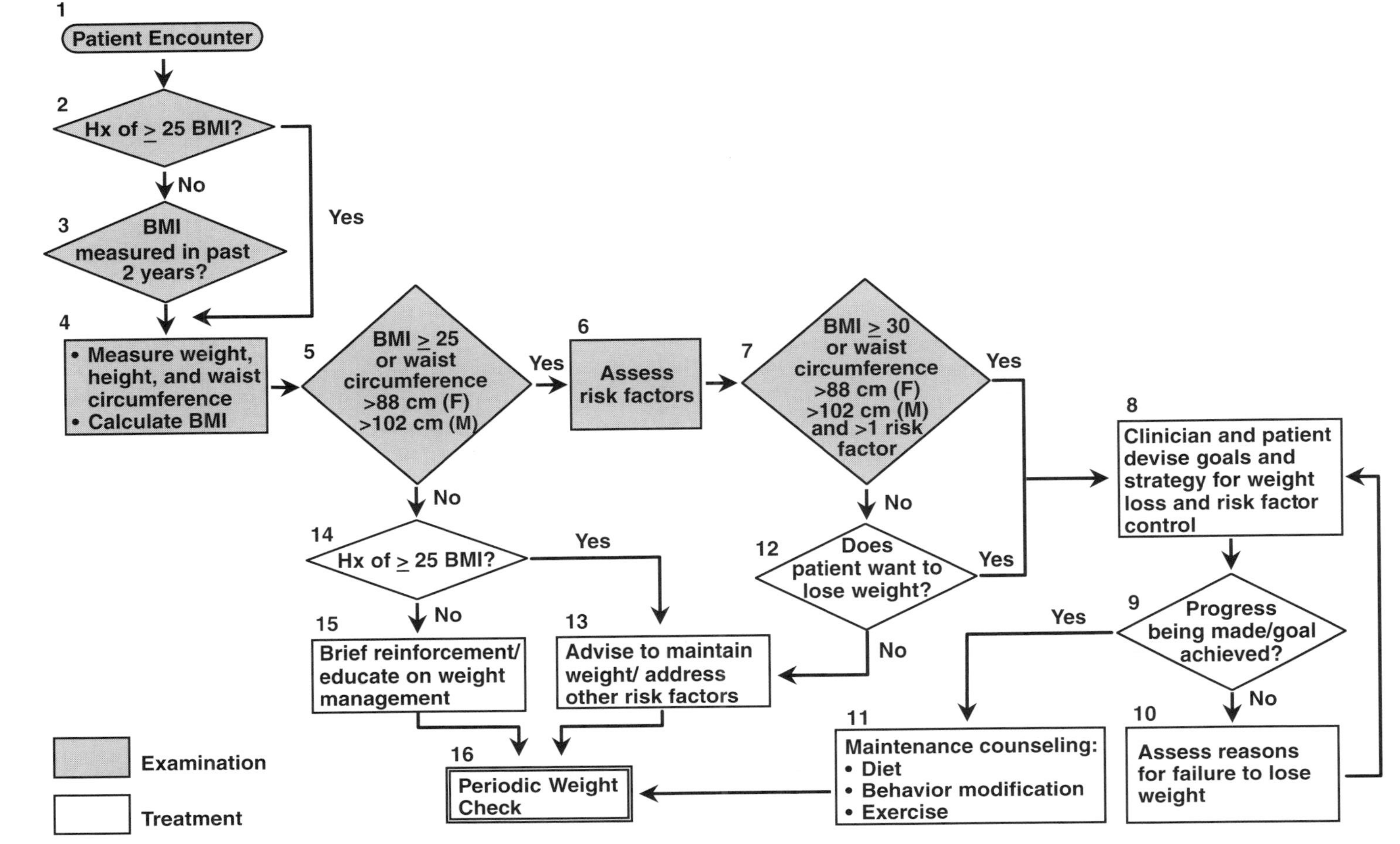

FIGURE 33.4
This algorithm developed by the National Heart, Lung, and Blood Institute can point the clinician and patient along the path of effectively evaluating the patient's BMI.

References

1. Quetelet, A. Sur l'homme et le developpement de ses facultes, ou essai de physique sociale; Paris: Bachelier, 1835.
2. Freudenthal H. In: *Dictionary of Scientific Biography* (Gillespie CC, Ed). New York: Charles and Sons; 1975; pg 236.
3. Bray GA. *Obes Res* 3: 97; 1885.
4. Metropolitan Life Insurance Company. *Stat Bull Met Life Ins* 1922; 3: 3-4.
5. Keys A, Fidanza F, Karvonen MJ, et al. *J Chronic Dis* 25: 329; 1972.
6. Benn RT. *Brit J Prev Soc Med* 25: 42; 1971.
7. Lee J, Kolonel N, Hines MW. *Int J Obes* 6: 233; 1982.
8. Garn SM, Pesick SD. *Am J Clin Nutr* 36: 573; 1982.
9. Garrow JS, Webster JD. *Int J Obes* 9: 147; 1985.
10. Gordon CC, Chumlea WC, Roche AF. In: *Anthropometric Standardization Reference Manual.* Champaign, IL: Human Kinetics Books, 1988, pg 3.
11. Gallagher D, Heymsfield SB, Heo M, Jebb SA, Murgatroyd PR, Sakamoto Y. *Am J Clin Nutr* 2000 Sep;72(3):694-701.

34

Glossary of Terms Used in Energy Assessment

Carolyn D. Berdanier

All living things require energy to sustain life. If a plant, that energy comes from the sun. If an animal, the energy must be provided by the food that is consumed. Warm-blooded animals are kept warm by their metabolisms. All the reactions that comprise intermediary metabolism release heat as a byproduct. Some reactions are exogonic; that is, they release more heat than they consume. Others are endogonic; they consume more energy than they release. None of the reactions in a living system are 100% efficient. The reaction produces a product(s) plus heat. This is the heat that sustains the body temperature and yet also escapes from the body via radiation or evaporation (insensible water loss and sweating) from the body surface. If a body is neither gaining nor losing weight, the energy released as heat is equal to that needed by the body to sustain its metabolism. Thus, the heat that is produced is equal to the total food energy (corrected for digestive loss and internal energy conversion to mechanical, chemical, and electrical energy) that must be provided on a daily basis to sustain the body. Altogether, the living system is a heat-generating system. That heat can be measured directly using a calorimeter or indirectly by measuring the oxygen consumed and the carbon dioxide produced. Using equations that relate heat production to the gas exchange (CO_2 and O_2), the energy used by the body can be calculated.

The measurement of energy need and energy production has been the subject of nutritional investigation since the time of Lavoisier. A number of terms have evolved that refer to discrete portions of the energy equation. These are listed in Table 34.1 along with other terms relevant to energy balance in man and other species.

The standardization of energy terms has been published by the National Academy of Sciences.[1] Nutrition scientists (as well as other scientists interested in energy metabolism) are encouraged to use these terms.

0-8493-2705-9/01/$0.00+$1.50

TABLE 34.1

Terms of Reference in Energy Metabolism

Anabolism: the totality of reactions that account for the synthesis of the body's macromolecules; heat is a byproduct of these reactions.

Android obesity: a form of obesity where fat distribution is mainly in the shoulders and abdomen; sometimes referred to as the "apple" shape.

Anthropometry: Measurements of body features, i.e., weight, height, etc.

Apparent digested energy (DE): energy of the consumed food (IE) less the energy of the feces (FE); DE = IE – FE.

Archimedes principle: an object's volume when submerged in water equals the volume of the water it displaces. If the mass and volume are known, the density can be calculated. This principle is used to determine body fatness.

Balance: When energy intake (EI) equals energy expenditure (EE), energy balance is zero. When energy intake exceeds expenditure, balance is positive and weight is gained. When intake is less than expenditure, balance is negative and weight is lost. (EI = EE; balance = 0)

Basal metabolic rate (BMR): the energy required to sustain life; measured in a resting animal in a thermoneutral environment (neither sweating nor shivering), at sexual repose, and in the postabsorptive (but not starving) state. Expressed as heat units/hour/unit body surface or per unit body weight ($Kg^{0.75}$). A less stringent measurement of this basal energy requirement is the resting metabolic rate (RMR). RMR is measured under clinical conditions to provide an approximation of the BMR and provide a basis for diet recommendations.

Body cell mass: the metabolically active, energy-requiring mass of the body.

Body density: mass (weight) per unit volume.

Calorie: a unit of heat energy; a calorie is defined as the amount of heat required to raise the temperature of one gram of water one degree Celsius; this is the physicist's unit. The nutritionist's unit is the calorie or kilocalorie (abbreviated, kcal), and refers to the heat needed to raise the temperature of one kilogram of water rather than one gram of water. The term kilojoule is the preferred term for expressing the energy need for living systems because it accounts for not only heat energy but also other forms of energy (mechanical, electrical, etc.) that living systems use. The kcal can be converted to the kilojoule by multiplying kcal × 4.184.

Calorimetry: the measurement of heat production by the body. This measurement can be either direct (using a whole body calorimeter) or indirect (using measurements of oxygen consumed and carbon dioxide produced).

Catabolism: the totality of those reactions that reduce macromolecules to usable metabolites, CO_2, and water. Heat is a byproduct of these reactions.

Digestive energy (DE): the energy of food after the energy losses of digestion are subtracted. Similar to apparent ingestive energy (see above).

Gaseous products of digestion (GE): the energy of combustible gases produced in the digestive tract incident to fermentation of food by microorganisms. In ruminants, that can account for a substantial energy lost from the system. In nonruminents this loss is relatively minor.

Gynoid obesity: excess body fat deposited mainly on the hips and thighs; sometimes referred to as the "pear" form of obesity.

Heat of activity (HjE): the heat produced through muscular activity; an active person can have a very large percent of their energy need accounted for by HjE. A sedentary person can have the reverse. The energy need for different activities has been determined, and some of these are listed in Table 34.2. Sometimes TEA (total energy from activity) is used for this term.

Heat of digestion and absorption (HdE): the heat produced as a result of the action of the digestive enzymes, and the heat produced when the products of digestion are absorbed. Expressed in heat units (see DE above). Sometimes DIT (diet-induced thermogenesis) is used.

Heat of fermentation (HfE): the heat produced in the digestive tract as a result of microbial action. Expressed in heat units (see GE above).

Heat of product formation (HrE): the heat produced in association with metabolic processes of product formation from absorbed metabolites. In its simplest form, HrE is the heat produced by a biosynthetic pathway. Expressed as heat units.

Heat of thermal regulation (HcE): the additional heat needed to maintain body temperature when the environmental temperature falls below or rises above the zone of thermic neutrality. Expressed in heat units. Sometimes CIT (cold-induced thermogenesis) or BAT (brown fat thermogenesis) is used. It is thought that the heat generated upon cold exposure emanates primarily from the brown fat depots. There is some argument about this role of the brown fat.

Heat of waste formation and excretion (HwE): the additional heat production associated with the synthesis and excretion of waste products. For example, the synthesis and excretion of urea is energetically expensive in mammals and results in a measurable increase in total heat production. Expressed in heat units.

TABLE 34.1 *(Continued)*

Terms of Reference in Energy Metabolism

Heat increment (HiE): the increase in heat production following the consumption of food. Includes the heat lost through digestion and absorption and the heat of fermentation. Expressed as heat units. The heat increment is usually considered non-useful energy loss, but under special circumstance (cold environments) it helps to maintain the body temperature.

IBW: ideal body weight.

Indirect calorimetry: the calculation of energy production through the measurement of oxygen consumed. It is predicated on the relationship of the heat lost when substrates are oxidized to CO_2 and water. With this oxidation via the mitochondrial respiratory chain, some energy is trapped in the high-energy bond of ATP. The rest of the energy is released as heat. Because there is a relationship between oxygen used and the energy trapped plus energy released as heat, measuring the oxygen consumed is an indirect measure of heat production. Thus, at zero energy balance, heat production (oxygen consumed) can predict the energy need of the body at rest or when actively involved in a variety of tasks. There are several systems available for this measurement. The closed system uses a reservoir of gases, and the oxygen consumed is measured. The open system measures the carbon dioxide exhaled without measuring oxygen consumed.

Metabolizable energy (ME): the energy in food minus the energy lost through digestion and absorption, the energy of undigested residues (FE), and the energy lost through fermentation. ME = IE – (FE + UE + GE).

N-corrected metabolizable energy (MnE): ME adjusted for total nitrogen retained or lost from body tissue. MnE = ME – (k × TN). For birds or monogastric mammals, gaseous energy is usually not considered. The correction for mammals is generally k = 7.45 kcal/g/nitrogen retained in body tissue (TN). The factor 8.22 kcal/g TN is used for birds, representing the energy equivalent of uric acid/g nitrogen.

NPU: net protein use.

NDp cal %: net protein kcalories percent; the percent of the total energy value of the diet provided by protein.

Nutrient density: the nutrient composition of food expressed in terms of nutrient quantity/100 kcal.

Nutritional assessment: measurement of indicators of dietary status and nutrition-related health status of individuals or populations.

Obesity: excess fat stores; overweight individuals have more than 15 but less than 20% of their body mass as fat; obese individuals have more than 20% of their body mass as fat. Body fatness may not always be reflected by the body weight of the individual.

Postprandial: after a meal.

Quantitative computed tomography: an imaging technique consisting of an array of x-ray sources and radiation detectors aligned opposite each other. As x-ray beams pass through a body they are weakened or attenuated by the tissues of that body. The signals are then compared with a computer that uses the information to construct a model of the body and estimate its fatness as well as its composition. This instrument is a very sophisticated (and expensive) way to determine body fatness.

Respiratory quotient (RQ): ratio of CO_2 produced to O_2 consumed.

Skinfold thickness: a double fold of skin and underlying tissue that can be used to estimate body fatness.

Thermic effect of food: heat production upon food consumption; sometimes referred to as diet-induced thermogenesis (DIT).

Thermogenesis: heat production; when stimulated by exposure to cold it is referred to as cold-induced thermogenesis and represents the extra energy the body generates to maintain body temperature. In rodents this extra heat is thought to be produced by the brown fat cells. In man there is evidence that both supports and denies this response of specialized fat cells to cold exposure.

Total heat production (HE): the energy lost from the body as a result of its metabolism. It can be measured directly or estimated from the gas exchange. The commonly accepted equation for the indirect computation of heat production from the respiratory exchange is HE (kcal) = 3.866 (liters O_2) + 1.200 (liters CO_2) – 1.431 (g urinary nitrogen) – 0.518 (liters CH_4).

True digestive energy (TDE): the intake of energy minus the fecal energy of food origin (FiE = FE – FeE – FmE) minus heat of fermentation and digestive gaseous losses (TDE = IE – FE + FeE + FmE – HfE – GE).

True metabolizable energy (TME): the intake of food energy corrected for fecal loss and urine energy loss (TME = TDE – UE + UeE).

Urinary energy (UE): the gross energy of the urine. Represents the energy of nonutilized absorbed compounds from food (UiE), endproducts of metabolic processes (UmE), and endproducts of endogenous origin, i.e., creatinine, urea, uric acid, etc.(UeE).

TABLE 34.2

Methods and Equations Used for Calculating Basal Energy Need

Method	Equation
1. Heat production, direct calorimetry	kcal (kJ)/m^2 (surface area)
2. Oxygen consumption; indirect	O_2 cons./$W^{0.75}$
3. Heat production; indirect	Insensible Water Loss (IWL) = Insensible Weight Loss (IW) + (CO_2 exhaled – O_2 inhaled) $\text{Heat production} = \text{IWL} \times 0.58 \times \left(\frac{100}{25}\right)$
4. Energy used; indirect	$\text{Basal energy} = \frac{\text{Creatinine N (mg / day)}}{0.00482\ (\text{W})}$
5. Estimate (energy need not measured) (Harris Benedict equation)	BMR = 66.4730 + 13.751W + 5.0033L – 6.750A (men)
6. Estimate (energy need not measured)	BMR = 655.9055 + 9.563W + 1.8496L – 4.6756A (women) $\text{BMR} = 71.2\text{W}^{0.75}\left[1 + 0.004(30 - \text{A}) + 0.010\left(\frac{\text{L}}{\text{W}^{0.33}} - 43.4\right)\right]$ (men) $\text{BMR} = 65.8\text{W}^{0.75}\left[1 + 0.004(30 - \text{A}) + 0.018\left(\frac{\text{L}}{\text{W}^{0.33} - 42.1}\right)\right]$ (women)

Abbreviations are as follows: W = weight in kg; L = height in cm; A = age in years.

See Heshka, S., Feld, K., Yang, M et al. *JADA* 93: 1031, 1993 for a comparison of various prediction equations.

Reference

1. Subcommittee on Biological Energy, National Research Council, *Nutritional Energetics of Domestic Animals* Nat. Acad. Press, Washington, DC, 1981.

35

Metabolic Assessment of the Overweight Patient

Shawn C. Franckowiak, Kim M. Forde, and Ross E. Andersen

Introduction

Clinicians often see overweight patients seeking weight loss, and those seeking weight loss implore advice from nutrition specialists and dietitians on the quantity of calories they should consume each day. To produce weight loss, a negative energy balance needs to exist whereby the patient consumes less energy than he or she expends in a day. The total energy need of a person is expressed as:

Total daily energy needs (TDEE) = BMR + TEF + TEA + energy needed for growth, reproduction, lactation or healing from injury.

BMR: Basal Metabolic Rate
TEF: Thermic Effect of Feeding
TEA: Thermic Effect of Activity

The total amount of energy a person expends daily during the waking hours is termed Total Daily Energy Expenditure (TDEE) and is composed of three different components: the Resting Metabolic Rate (RMR), the Thermic Effect of Feeding (TEF), and the Thermic Effect of Activity (TEA) (see Figure 35.1). RMR is the energy expenditure needed to sustain the basic biochemical reactions of the body in a resting state. A resting state is when a person is fasting (not starving), awake in a thermoneutral environment (not sweating or shivering), and lies still without any skeletal muscle movement. The TEF is the energy expenditure attributed to the digestion and absorption of food. The energy needed for the digestion and absorption of foods is greater than that needed for resting, and therefore is designated as TEF. It is the difference in energy use between the fed and fasting states. The TEA is the energy expenditure associated with skeletal muscle movement. TEA is the most influenced component of TDEE because a person can choose to do variable amounts of physical activity that ultimately involve skeletal muscle movement. The RMR accounts for approximately 60 to 75% of TDEE, the TEF constitutes approximately 10%, and the TEA comprises 15 to 30% of energy expenditure.

0-8493-2705-9/01/$0.00+$1.50

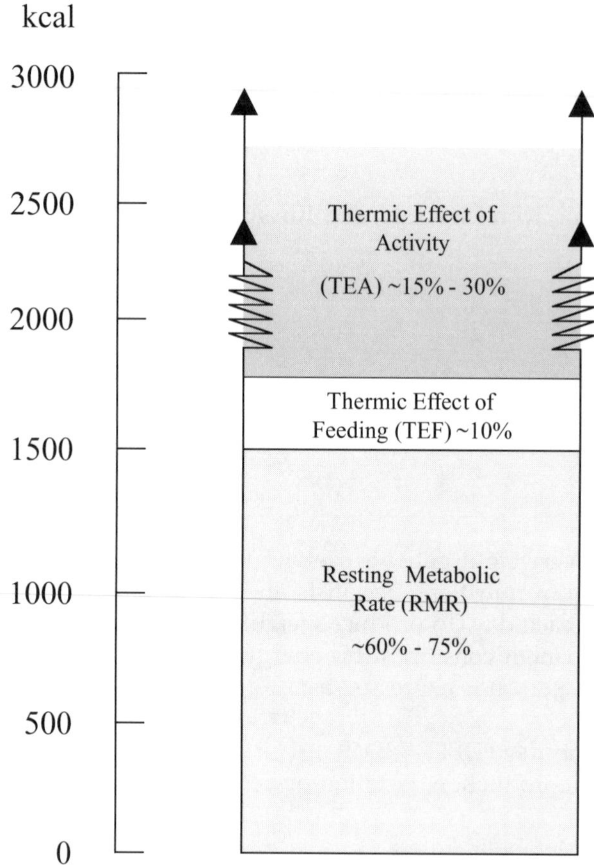

FIGURE 35.1
The three major components of the total daily energy expenditure (TDEE). RMR: Resting Metabolic Rate, TEF: Thermic Effect of Feeding, TEA: Thermic Effect of Activity. Adapted from Poehlman, E.T. *Med Sci Sports Exerc*, 21; 516, 1989.

Definitions of Energy Units and Components of Metabolism

Before introducing the definition of resting metabolic rate, it is important to define the energy unit. This is the "kilocalorie" or "kilojoule." The kilocalorie is the amount of heat content or energy required to raise the temperature of 1 kg of water 1 degree Celsius at 15 degrees Celsius; it is used in measurements of the heat production of chemical reactions including those of biological systems.[1] At any given time, there are continuous biochemical reactions consisting of the breakdown of adenosine triphosphate (ATP) to a smaller molecular of adenosine diphosphate (ADP) + ENERGY to serve the functional element of cells.[2] This reaction produces the energy that is measurable in kilocalories. The word kilocalorie may be used to define the amount of energy in the food a person consumes; it can also quantify the amount of energy a person expends.

RMR is presented as a measure of energy expressed as the amount of kcalories expended in a day, represented as kcal/d. However, the kilocalorie can also be expressed as the kilojoule to achieve uniformity of SI unit measuring system.[1] One kilocalorie equals 4.184 kilojoules. Although the joule may be a uniform standard unit that scientists use, the layperson will be better served when measurement of energy intake and expenditure is presented as kilocalories in order to make the term relevant to food labels and packaging used in everyday life. Those seeking to lose weight pursue a negative energy balance whereby they expend more kilocalories than consumed. A negative energy balance can be achieved by increasing TDEE or decreasing the amount of kcalories consumed during the weight loss period. Calorie is a word that many people associate with food labels to define the energy richness of a food item; it is often seen on exercise machinery stating the quantity of calories expended for a person of a given body weight for each minute of exercise. When investigating energy balance, it is important to understand the concept that a kcalorie is a measure of energy, and energy that is expended is measurable using different techniques. This section will be devoted to defining RMR and several components that make up TDEE, and it shall provide an overview of the methodology, implementation, and interpretation of the RMR.

TDEE

TDEE in free-living populations can be measured using doubly-labeled water ($^2H_2{}^{18}O$). Measurement of TDEE by doubly-labeled water involves using stable isotopes of hydrogen and oxygen. A specimen of urine is collected from the subject at baseline; the administered dosage of doubly-labeled water is determined by body weight. Although this is the gold standard for the measurement of TDEE , doubly-labeled water is very costly and is almost exclusively used by scientists involved in measuring TDEE and various components of the metabolism for clinical research studies.

Usually, clinicians do not have the option of estimating TDEE by doubly-labeled water. Therefore, TDEE is typically estimated by measuring the RMR and estimating the energy expenditure of physical activity. Physical activity patterns may be assessed using accelerometers or by administering a valid questionnaire.

RMR

RMR is one of the three components that comprise total daily energy expenditure.[3] RMR can be defined as the energy required to sustain bodily functions and maintain body temperature at rest, and is quantitatively the largest component of energy expenditure in humans. Typically it can account for 60 and 75% of the total daily expenditure.[4] RMR is often used to estimate the daily energy needs of individuals for population-based studies. It is a useful tool in the clinical management of obesity.[4] Researchers have defined RMR as being different from that of BMR; BMR is the energy expenditure of a person at rest (not asleep) in a fasting state, at sexual repose in a thermoneutral environment (neither shivering nor sweating). The RMR is defined as the energy expenditure measured on an outpatient basis.[5] For clinical purposes, the RMR can be assumed to be similar to the BMR.[5] It is less expensive and intrusive for the participant.

The RMR is the component of metabolism that is difficult to influence. Clinicians working with overweight patients will be quick to point out that their overweight clients often believe that they have a low or sluggish RMR, and consequently feel that this is the reason for their inability to lose or maintain weight. Often, RMR values are not as low as the patient believes. RMR measurements are frequently within the normal range for the patient's age, gender, height, and weight.

TEF

TEF is occasionally called diet-induced thermogenesis, and accounts for 10% of the TDEE of a person. TEF represents the energy expenditure associated with the ingestion, digestion, and absorption of food. There is an increase in the metabolic rate when a person has eaten food. This is why the assessment of RMR typically requires individuals to be fasted for a minimum of 12 hours prior to the assessment of that component of the metabolism. TEF can be measured by taking the measurements of a valid RMR assessment and comparing these to values attained using the same testing procedures after the ingestion of a meal of known energy value and composition. The difference between the RMR and the energy used for digestion and absorption is the TEF (TEF + RMR = energy expended after a meal is consumed).

TEA

The TEA is the only component of the TDEE that we can directly influence. TEA is the amount of energy expended as a direct result of voluntary skeletal muscle movement. TDEE differs between active and sedentary persons. Sedentary persons expend less energy than active persons, and thus their TEA as a percent of their total energy expenditure is less than that of active persons.

Techniques for Measuring RMR

RMR can be measured using two different methods: direct calorimetry and indirect calorimetry. Direct calorimetry is the measurement of overall heat liberated by a body mass. Heat production is proportional to the body surface area available (kilocalories/m^2) for the release of heat by radiation or transvection.

Indirect calorimetry involves measuring oxygen consumption (O_2) and carbon dioxide production (CO_2) to determine RMR by using a calculated equation of Weir.[6] To produce measurement values for indirect calorimetry in kilocalories per day, the measurement of one liter of oxygen consumed generates 3.9 kilocalories, and one liter of carbon dioxide produced generates 1.1 kilocalorie.[7] The original Weir equation involves measurement of gases that are consumed and produced at rest plus the collection of total 24-hour urine nitrogen during the same day of measurement. However, a second abbreviated Weir equation has been developed that is less than 2% measurement error when compared to the longer equation.[6] This equation is below.

Abbreviated Weir Formula:

$$RMR = [3.9(V_{O_2}) + 1.1\ (V_{CO_2})]1.44$$

variables: V_{O_2} = oxygen consumption in mL/min

V_{CO_2} = carbon dioxide production in mL/min

Note: this equation is to determine resting energy expenditure, so for determining RMR the patient must be in a 12-hour fasted state.

Direct Calorimetry

The measurement of energy need of an adult who is neither gaining nor losing weight can be made using a whole body calorimeter. This instrument measures the heat released by the body as a result of its metabolism.[7-9] It is a composite value in that it is not only the result of baseline metabolic reactions that produce heat, but also the heat that results from the ingestion, digestion, and absorption of foods, plus that which results from muscular activity. Subjects must remain in the whole body calorimeter for hours at a time so that sufficient data can be accumulated. This technique is extremely expensive and has limited clinical potential.[7]

Indirect Calorimetry

For most, a viable alternative is the indirect calorimeter or metabolic cart. Indirect calorimetry measures the gas exchange of an individual.[8,10] The gases detected by the metabolic cart are compared to the environmental conditions of the surrounding room's gases at standard temperature, pressure, and humidity (STPD). STPD is a symbol indicating that a gas volume has been expressed as if it were at standard temperature (0° Celsius), standard pressure (760 mm Hg absolute), and 0% humidity; under these conditions, a mole of gas occupies 22.4 liters. The testing environment should be controlled for temperature, barometric pressure, and humidity. Depending on the instrumentation, the measurement conditions are entered prior to beginning the assessment, and correction factors are applied to standardize the results. The room temperatures should also be kept between 68 and 74° Fahrenheit. Furthermore, the room should be dimly lit, and spare blankets should be offered to individuals who may experience coldness when sitting for prolonged periods of time.

The measurement of gas exchange allows for the calculation of the respiratory quotient (RQ). ($RQ = CO_2/O_2$). The RQ reflects cellular metabolism and is a reflection of heat production (direct calorimetry). The RQ indicates the fuel mixture being oxidized.[8] Different fuels such as fats, carbohydrates, and proteins require different amounts of oxygen for oxidation to CO_2 and water. Thus, the RQ varies depending on the ratio of fat to carbohydrate in the fuel mixture.[11] In starvation, the major fuel is fat, and the RQ is 0.70. Usually a mixture of fuels (carbohydrate and fat) is oxidized. The various substrates and their RQ values are shown in Table 35.1.

TABLE 35.1

Respiratory Quotient and Energy Content of Various Substrates

Fuel (Substrate)	Energy Content ($Kcal \cdot g^{-1}$)	Respiratory Quotient (RQ)
Carbohydrate	4.1	1.00
Fat	9.3	0.70
Protein	4.3	0.80

Adapted from American College of Sports Medicine. *Guidelines for Exercise Testing and Prescription.* Malvern, PA: Lea & Febiger, page 14, 1991.

Instrumentation Available

There are two indirect calorimetry systems: open-circuit and closed-circuit systems. Both techniques require devices to measure the concentration of O_2, CO_2, gas volume or flow

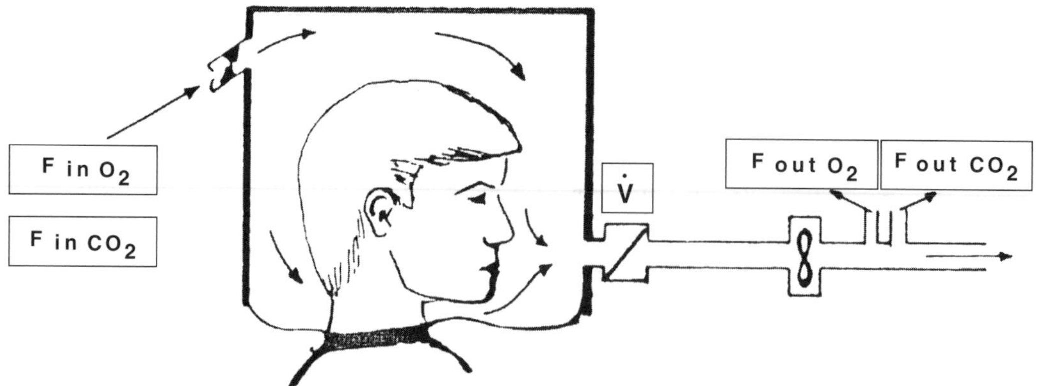

FIGURE 35.2
Open Circuit technique of Indirect Calorimetry using a canopy hood. From Ferrenini E. *Metabolism*, 37; 296, 1988. With permission.
Labels: $FinO_2$: Forced Inspiratory Oxygen; $FinCO_2$: Forced Inspiratory Carbon Dioxide; : Gas Flow; $FoutO_2$: Forced Expiratory Oxygen; $FoutCO_2$: Forced Expiratory Carbon Dioxide.

rate, temperature, and time. In the closed-circuit system, the patient breathes from a reservoir (a mixture of gases resembling ambient air), and the decrease in oxygen over time is used to calculate $\dot{V}_{O_2}$. Closed-circuit systems are usually simpler in design and less costly than open systems. Open-circuit systems are more versatile and can be more easily used in the clinical setting.[7] The patient breathes from a reservoir of air of known composition in the closed-circuit system; the depletion of oxygen, $\dot{V}C_{O_2}$ and $\dot{V}_{O_2}$ are calculated.[7] In the open-circuit technique (see Figure 35.2), the patient breathes room air and expires into a gas sampling system which eventually vents the expired air back into the room. Open-circuit systems are more commonly used to measure RMR in the clinical setting, since they are more versatile and can be used in a variety of clinical conditions. The techniques described in this section will therefore focus on the open-circuit indirect calorimetry system.

Types of Collection Systems

Many types of accessories allow for the collection of consumed and expired gases of the person being tested, including face masks, mouth pieces, chambers, and ventilated hoods.

Face Masks

Similar to the face masks used by firefighters and military personnel, face masks provide a sealed environment around the nose and mouth in order to collect all gases. The face mask has an elastic head harness which encompasses the back of the head. These work well for collection of gases; however, they may be more awkward for some patients than other collection systems, and it is important to have several sizes of masks on hand to optimize fit. Although not as comfortable as some of the other collection devices, the face mask is very easily used with portable gas analyzers and is useful for field settings or where exercise-induced energy expenditure is measured.[12]

Mouthpieces

These are similar to the snorkel that is used to allow breathing underwater. The mouthpieces used for RMR measurement are usually identical to mouthpieces used for maximal V_{O_2} testing. In order for the mouthpiece to work correctly, the subject being tested needs to maintain a tight seal around the mouthpiece and have a nose clip sealing off the nasal passageway. A certain amount of discomfort may be experienced from a static contraction of the jaw muscles to keep a tight seal around the mouthpiece. Therefore, this collection system is not often used to assess RMR.

Ventilated (Canopy) Hood

The ventilated hood is the most widely used collection system. It is advantageous for a number of reasons — it allows for easy spontaneous breathing in apparently healthy individuals, there is no error associated with facial features such as beard or facial hair of the test subject, it has been found to be accurate in long term measurement of RMR, and it is a relatively noninvasive gas collection system. The hood drapes over the entire head of the subject in a semirecumbent position.

Comparison of Collection Devices

There are advantages and disadvantages for each collection device. In the clinical setting, the ventilated hood may offer a more relaxed and unobtrusive measurement environment. However, for patients that may be claustrophobic, the lights of the laboratory may need to be dimmed to reduce feelings of being confined. The face masks work well for collection of gases; however, structural differences in the size of the face may make it necessary to use different sized masks for the variety of structural differences found in patients. Furthermore, face masks are expensive, and for valid measurements a variety of masks is necessary. Finally, although mouthpieces may seem to have no limitations, they are difficult for patients when the measurements last for long periods of time. Moreover, a nose clip must be placed on the nose during measurement to prevent any escape of nonmeasured gas, and this can be extremely invasive for the patient as well.

Clinical Applications and Usefulness of RMR

Understanding the energy requirement of an individual can be useful in prescribing a personal dietary intake. The interpretation of the values attained by RMR measurements should be done by an experienced clinician. Typically, university hospitals and established university weight loss centers will have access to metabolic carts to perform RMR assessments. An accurate measure of RMR will allow the clinician to tailor the energy intake of the individual (and increase overall energy expenditure via the thermic effect of activity) in order to produce a negative energy balance.

This information may also be important in the estimation of TDEE. The values of RMR may be multiplied by an activity factor to produce best estimates of TDEE, as outlined in Table 35.2. It may be helpful get detailed recent exercise histories from patients to help assess the appropriate level of general activity. Bear in mind that most people overestimate their activity levels.

TABLE 35.2

Factors for Estimating Total Daily Energy Needs of Activities for Men and Women (Age 19 to 50)

Level of General Activity	Activity Factor (Multiplied by REE†)	Energy Expenditure (Kcal/kg/day)
Very light		
Men	1.3	31
Women	1.3	30
Light		
Men	1.6	38
Women	1.5	35
Moderate		
Men	1.7	41
Women	1.6	37
Heavy		
Men	2.1	50
Women	1.9	44
Exceptional		
Men	2.4	58
Women	2.2	51

From Food and Nutrition Board, National Research Council, NAS: Recommended Dietary Allowances, 10th ed. Washington, DC. National Academy Press, 1989, p. 29 (with permission). See Heshka S., Feld K., Yang M.U. et al. Resting energy expenditure in the obese: A cross-validation and comparison of prediction equations. *J. Am. Diet. Assoc.* 93, 1031-1036, 1993 for a comparison of various prediction equations.

† REE = resting energy expenditure.

Helping Patients Gain Weight

RMR values attained from indirect calorimetry can also be used for certain anabolic circumstances. Often, hospital clinicians will measure RMR in patients suffering from severe burns or frail, elderly patients as a result of the onset of disease. For these instances, the values attained at bedside are important in tailoring meal plans to facilitate weight gain in life-threatening medical situations.

Those individuals seeking to gain weight for performance purposes can also benefit from accurate measures of RMR. Individuals who seek to increase overall lean body mass (or fat-free mass) may wish to understand how much energy is required above maintenance to produce a safe rate of weight gain. The values attained from RMR in conjunction with counseling on an appropriate activity and exercise program may be helpful to individuals training for body-building or sports performance-related events. Two case studies depicting the usefulness of values attained from assessment or prediction of RMR are described below.

Case Studies

Person Seeking Weight Loss

A 40-year-old woman with a height of 5′6″ and weight of 185 pounds (BMI of 30 kg/m^2) seeks to lose 20 pounds. This person seeks treatment from a dietician in a hospital that has no metabolic cart. Therefore, an equation to predict resting metabolic rate will be used. Using a prediction equation that has a table with value of kcals based on age and gender multiplied by body surface area,[13] the RMR is predicted to be 1498 kcal/d. Furthermore, the woman participates in 30 minutes of vigorous aerobic exercise 4 days per week. Therefore, to determine her predicted TDEE, we multiply her RMR by an activity factor that is equal to a moderately active person. This activity factor is 1.5. Multiplying 1498 by 1.5 yields a TDEE of 2247 kcal/d. To predict a safe rate of weight loss of 1.5 pounds per week, the energy intake needs to be restricted by 750 kcals per day, equaling a consumption of approximately 1447 kcal/d (if 3500 kcal equals one pound of weight loss).

Person Seeking Weight Gain

A 20-year-old man who is weight training and agility training over a 15-week period seeks to gain 15 pounds for the start of fall football season. He is 6′5,″ weighs 270 pounds, and has 18% body fat. Fortunately, he lives near a university hospital that has dieticians who specialize in sports nutrition and have access to a metabolic cart. When assessed for RMR, the man has a baseline RMR of 2653 kcal/d. The man's training habits, which involve two hours of strength and agility training each day, warrant that his RMR be multiplied by an activity factor of 1.7. His determined TDEE is therefore 4510 kcal/d. However, he seeks to gain weight and not remain weight stable. Therefore, in order to predict an average of 1 pound of weight gain per week, the man needs to ingest 500 kcal/d more than his predicted TDEE. This value is equal to 5010 kcal/d.

Predicting RMR

Often, technology for direct measurement of RMR is not readily available to healthcare professionals who provide treatment plans based on RMR values. As an alternative, clinicians frequently use prediction equations to estimate RMR. These prediction equations have mostly been developed using regression equations to fit functions according to gender, age, height, weight, and other available clinical variables.[14] A majority of these equations were developed using normal-weight persons who were relatively sedentary. Unfortunately, this poses a problem when predicting RMR in the obese population, considering that RMR is directly related to the fat-free mass (FFM) of the individual,[15-18] and the obese person has a larger distribution of adipose tissue and a decreased proportion of FFM when compared to their normal-weight counterparts.[19] Equations are available for the prediction of RMR for the normal weight and overweight populations (Table 35.3).

Harris-Benedict Equation

For normal-weight individuals (determined by BMI or body composition analysis), the prediction equation of Harris and Benedict[20] offers an appropriate equation:

$$\text{Men: kcal/d} = 66.4730 + 13.751W + 5.0033L - 6.750A$$
$$\text{Women: kcal/d} = 655.0955 + 9.563W + 1.8496L - 4.6756A$$

where W = weight (kg); L = height (cm); A = age (years)

These equations were developed in 1919 and are currently widely used by clinicians. However, given the increased prevalence of overweight in industrialized countries like the U.S.,[21] it may be necessary for the clinician to use prediction equations that have been validated using overweight persons.

TABLE 35.3

Equations for Estimating Resting Metabolic Rate (RMR) kcal/24 hours[a]

Reference	Equations	Reference
Bernstein et al.	W: 7.48(kg) – 0.42(cm) – 3.0(yr) + 844 M: 11.0(kg) + 10.2(cm) – 5.8(yr) – 1,032	81
Cunningham	501.6 + 21.6(LBM); where for W: LBM = [69.8 – 0.26(kg) – 0.12(yr)] × kg/73.2 for M: LBM = [79.5 – 0.24(kg) – 0.15(yr)] × kg/73.2	82
Harris and Benedict	W: 655 + 9.5(kg) + 1.9(cm) – 4.7(yr) M: 66 + 13.8(kg) + 5.0(cm) – 6.8(yr)	20
Fleisch[a]	W/M: kcal's/m² of BSA from Fleisch table × $[[0.007184 \times (kg)]^{0.425} \times (cm)^{0.725}]] \times 24$	22
James	W: 18 – 30yr: 487 + 14.8(kg) 30 – 60yr: 845 + 8.17(kg) >60yr: 658 + 9.01(kg) M: 18 – 30yr: 692 + 15.1(kg) 30 – 60yr: 873 + 11.6(kg) >60yr: 588 + 11.7(kg)	83
Mifflin et al.	W: 9.99(kg) + 6.25(cm) – 4.92(yr) – 161 M: 9.99(kg) + 6.25(cm) – 4.92(yr) + 5	23
Owen et al.	W: 795 + 7.18(kg) M: 879 + 10.2(kg)	84
Pavlou et al.	M: –169.1 + 1.02(pRMR)	85
Robertson and Reid[a]	W/M: kcals/m² of BSA from Robertson and Reid table × $[[0.007184 \times (kg)]^{0.425} \times (cm)^{0.725}]] \times 24$	13

Key. W = Women, M = Men, pRMR = predicted RMR from the Harris and Benedict equation,[a]this equation uses tabled values for kcals/m². From Heshka S., Feld K., Yang M.U. et al. Resting energy expenditure in the obese: A cross-validation and comparison of prediction equations. Copyright The American Dietetic Association. Reprinted with permission from *J. Am. Diet. Assoc.* 93, 1031-1036, 1993.

Robertson-Reid and Fleisch Equations

Three prediction equations may potentially offer reasonable predictions of RMR for the overweight patient. The prediction equations of Robertson and Reid[13] and the equation of Fleisch[22] have been recommended for obese populations.[14] The Robertson and Reid and Fleisch equations will be presented in this section as viable prediction equations for the obese patient. The Robertson and Reid equation was derived from the actual measurement of RMR of 987 men and 1323 women age 3 to 80. The equation requires that the clinician find a value for heat output (in table form) based on the patient's age and gender. Subsequently, this value is multiplied by the body surface area of the person (in m²) to determine kcal/hr; this number is then multiplied by 24 to yield daily RMR. The basis of this prediction equation is that there is constant heat output that corresponds to surface area within people who are the same gender and age:

RMR in kcal/d = heat output in kcal × body surface area in m² × 24 hours
heat output = value derived for men and women from a table developed by Robertson and Reid[13]
body surface area (BSA) = $(([0.007184 \times (\text{wt in kgs})]^{0.425} \times (\text{ht in cms})^{0.725}))$
time = 24

The equation of Fleisch uses the same concept as the Robertson and Reid equation. However, the values of heat output differ, and Fleisch provides a separate table to calculate the predicted RMR.[22]

Mifflin et al. Equation

A third prediction equation for the obese population comes from Mifflin et al.[23] This equation was derived using linear regression analysis on a subset of patients (247 females, 251 males) who had their RMRs measured using indirect calorimetry. In an unpublished research study at the Johns Hopkins School of Medicine, the equation has provided predicted RMR values in obese patients at a university weight loss center that are not different than those produced by actual measurement. The equation is as follows:

$$\text{Men (kcal/d)} = 9.99(\text{kg}) + 6.25(\text{cm}) - 4.92(\text{years of age}) + 5$$
$$\text{Women (kcal/d)} = 9.99(\text{kg}) + 6.25(\text{cm}) - 4.92(\text{years of age}) - 161$$

Pretesting Procedures for Measurement of RMR

The testing procedures for determining RMR necessitate that a strict protocol be followed to ensure that the measurement is accurate. Individuals should be provided with pretesting requirements for the RMR estimate. The subject should be questioned about his/her adherence to pretest procedures prior to the test. If one or more of these procedures are not followed, the individual should be rescheduled at a later date to reduce measurement error.

Weight Stable

If the subject has experienced recent weight loss, measurement of RMR may not be valid. Measurement should be avoided if the person being tested is on a weight loss program or has lost or gained more than one pound in the past week. To reduce error associated with physiological responses to weight loss, a period of weight stabilization of two weeks is necessary prior to an RMR assessment.

Well Rested

RMR measurement should be administered as close to the time a person awakes as possible. Additionally, the individual being tested should get a restful night's sleep prior to coming to the clinic or hospital for the RMR assessment. If an individual has had an uneasy night's rest prior to RMR assessment, confounding environmental influences may unduly increase the metabolic expenditure of the individual. Measurement should occur before 10:00 am; measurements taken in the late morning may be suspect to increased metabolic activity.

Fasted

Measurements should be taken first thing in the morning after a 12-hour overnight fast.[24] A light meal the night before measurement should be encouraged; RMR is the energy expended at rest in a fasted state, and therefore any lasting effects of food or drink would contribute additional energy expenditure from diet-induced thermogenesis. Early morning coffee or tea should be avoided, and only water should be ingested prior to measurement. Clinicians can determine whether the patient is fasting by examining the RQ values during testing.

Measurement in Relation to Last Exercise Bout

Testing should be performed at least 24 hours after rest from exercise to eliminate any residual effects from the most recent training session.[25] Hence, the person being testing should be instructed to abstain from programmed exercise for at least one day prior to measurement of RMR.

Location and Acclimation to the Testing Environment

Studies have shown that there are no differences in measurements of RMR performed with or without an inpatient overnight stay.[5] Therefore, to avoid excessive costs associated with inpatient stays, an outpatient procedure is usually recommended. Upon arrival to the lab where the RMR assessment will occur, the subject should be instructed to rest in a sedentary supine or semirecumbent position for at least 30 minutes prior to the assessment. During this time, the subject should remain still. The subject should be asked if they need to void, since it is necessary that they are comfortable during the entire test. Some laboratories will further acclimatize the individual by placing the collection system (canopy hood) over him/her to ensure that he/she is comfortable with the measurement setting.

Analysis

The metabolic cart will often express resting metabolic rate as the mean of multiple minute measurements. However, the cart will also provide continuous measurements of V_{O_2} and V_{CO_2}. Many researchers suggest that the calculation of RMR be the average of five of these continuous minute measurements of steady state.[18,26] Steady state is 5 minutes of measurement of V_{O_2} and V_{CO_2} that possess an intravariability of 5% or less.[26]

Table 35.4 is a simple checklist to ensure that the assessment of RMR is valid.

Factors Affecting RMR

A variety of factors have been shown to influence RMR, including genetics, age, gender, total body weight, fat-free weight, aerobic fitness level, total energy flux through the body, body and/or environmental temperature, hormonal factors, drugs, and stress.[27] Of these factors, the strongest correlation exists between an individual's FFM and RMR,[27] and collectively, fat-free mass, age, sex, and physical activity account for 80 to 90% of the variance in resting metabolic rate.[28]

Exercise

Since exercise training has been associated with increases in fat-free mass, this is one factor which can be manipulated to potentiate resting metabolism. Cross-sectional studies have

TABLE 35.4
Checklist for RMR Testing

Pre-Testing Subject Requirements
✓12 hour fast. Water is allowed ad libitum.
✓Refrain from strenuous physical activity/exercise for 48 hours prior to testing.
✓Well Rested. Make sure subject has at least 8 hours of sleep.
✓Minimize activity the morning of test. Light grooming allowed. Shower the night prior.
✓Keep food diaries for 48 hours prior to testing. Dinner meal should be <1000 kcals night prior.
Laboratory Requirements
✓Room should be isolated to reduce any external noise.
✓Room should be dimly lit, but not dark.
✓Temperature should be controlled and ideally at 22° to 24° Celsius. Blankets should be used if subject is cold.
✓The bed or comfortable chair should be semi-recumbent and not flat; having a slight incline of approximately 10 degrees.
Testing Procedures
✓Monitor subject during testing. Direct subject to avoid any: talking, fidgeting, and sleeping.
✓Acclimate patient to test. Possibly perform practice test prior to actual procedure.
✓Rest subject in semi-recumbent position for at least 30 minutes prior to testing.
✓If able to, use HR monitor to track HR the day before, morning of and during test.

Authors would like to thank Dr. Jack Wilmore for the helpful suggestions for the RMR checklist.

demonstrated that aerobically trained individuals have higher resting metabolic rates for their metabolic size than their untrained counterparts.[29-32]

Age

Age is another variable that has been found to have a significant impact on an individual's resting metabolism. In fact, the decline in resting metabolic rate is one of the most consistent physiological changes that occurs with age.[33] Recent studies have suggested a curvilinear reduction in RMR with advancing age that is accelerated beyond middle-age and post-menopausal years.[33] Several studies attribute the age-related decline in RMR primarily to the loss of fat-free mass that often accompanies aging; however, there remains uncertainty whether other physiological factors may also contribute to the reduction of RMR.[33]

Gender

Gender differences in resting metabolism have also been reported, with males having a higher RMR than females by approximately 50 kcal/day.[28] This difference is independent of the gender difference in fat-free mass, and is consistent across the life span.[28] Menopausal status has also been pinpointed as an influence on RMR in women. Studies have found lower RMR in postmenopausal women relative to premenopausal women, which was again primarily attributable to reductions in lean mass and a decline in aerobic fitness.[33-35]

Environment

Environmental factors also influence RMR, with the resting metabolism of people in tropical climates typically 5 to 20% higher than that of their counterparts living in more temperate areas.[36] Cold climates also have a significant impact on resting metabolic rate that is dependent on an individual's body fat content and the amount and type of clothing worn.[36] During extreme cold stress at rest, metabolic rate can double or triple with shivering as the body attempts to maintain a stable core temperature.[36]

Cigarette Smoking

Some studies have documented the influence of such substances as cigarettes, caffeine, alcohol, and certain medications on resting metabolism. Many lay persons believe that cigarette smoking may be helpful in maintaining body weight,[37] and many smokers are unwilling to quit because of their fear of weight gain. Over time, studies have demonstrated that the increase in metabolic rate resulting from cigarette smoking is transient.[37] One study found no effect in habitual smokers when assessment of metabolic rate did not begin until 25 to 30 minutes after smoking. Thus, it is thought that the acute metabolic effects of cigarettes are not significant beyond 30 minutes after smoking. Yet, given the typical ~30 minutes between cigarettes for most smokers, RMR may remain slightly elevated throughout the day as a result of these "acute" effects.[37]

Caffeine

Caffeine has been identified as a substance that elevates metabolic rate, and caffeine ingestion has also been shown to increase work performance and promote lipid oxidation during prolonged exercise.[38-40] In a study investigating the influence of caffeine on the resting metabolic rate of exercise-trained and inactive subjects it was found that metabolic rate was increased in response to a stimulus of approximately two cups of coffee (300 mg).[38] This study also compared regular and non-regular caffeine consumers to investigate the effects of consumption levels on metabolic response. This investigation confirmed previous findings that with regular consumption, the physiological and stimulatory effects of caffeine were not diminished.[38]

Alcohol

Alcohol is another substance that has been found to influence resting metabolic rate. Alcohol is decidedly the most commonly consumed psychoactive drug in the U.S., and because of its energy density, it is widely believed to be a causal factor in the development and maintenance of obesity.[41] However, in a study utilizing data gathered in two national cross-sectional surveys — the Second National Health and Nutrition Examination Survey (NHANES II; n = 10929) — and the Behavioral Risk Factor Surveys (BRFS; n = 18388), it was found that alcohol consumption had a slight negative effect on the body weights of men, and a profound negative effect on the body weights of women.[41,42] This negative effect was not a result of lowered dietary intake among drinkers. In fact, in controlled isoenergetic dietary studies, subjects tended to lose weight on alcohol-containing regimens.[43,44] This has lead to the hypothesis that alcohol intake may increase resting energy expenditure.[41] Early studies found inconsistent evidence regarding the effects of alcohol on resting energy expenditure.[41,45] However, recent studies have found evidence in support of the hypothesis that alcohol may increase resting energy expenditure,[41,46] although further investigations are needed to explain the mechanism by which alcohol suppresses body weight.[41]

Medications

Medications are also known to impact resting metabolism. Beta-blocking medications, for example, are prescribed to several million Americans with cardiovascular disease to treat conditions such as hypertension and angina.[47] Unfortunately, despite their widespread use in medical practice, beta-blocking medications have many side effects. One such side effect is the influence on resting energy expenditure. Research indicates that resting energy expenditure and perhaps the energy needs of individuals treated with beta-blockers are reduced.[47] The magnitude of this reduction in resting metabolic rate has been found to vary between 8 and 17%.[47] One study reported a reduction in resting metabolism of approximately 17% or 4 kcal/kg/day in a group of healthy subjects taking 80 mg of propranolol twice daily for 5 days.[47] This could result in significant weight gain in a patient receiving beta-blockers long-term if no changes were made to both dietary and exercise habits.[47]

RMR and Weight Loss

America currently has a preoccupation with weight loss and as a result, for many years scientists have been interested in identifying interventions that might potentiate RMR to facilitate weight loss in overweight and obese patient populations.[27] Factors causing a decrease in resting metabolic rate would make weight maintenance or weight loss difficult, or possibly result in weight gain. Conversely, anything that increases resting metabolic rate would potentially facilitate weight loss and maintenance of the weight lost.[48]

Energy Restriction and RMR

Over the past decade, there has been a dramatic increase in the prevalence of overweight and obesity in adults as well as children and adolescents. Using data from the National Health and Nutrition Examination Survey (NHANES III) it has been reported that more that 33.4% of U.S. adults are overweight,[21,49] representing an increase of 8% over the past 10 years;[50,51] paradoxically, dieting has become a way of life for many Americans. In a study utilizing data from the 1996 state-based Behavioral Risk Factor Surveillance System, it was reported that 28.8 and 43.6% of men and women, respectively, trying to lose weight at any given time.[52] Researchers have been exploring the consequences of dieting — particularly those related to changes in the resting metabolic rate.[26] Several investigators have found that a restrictive diet depresses resting metabolic rate, which may contribute to the regaining of weight often observed after treatment. One such study found that the RMR of obese individuals decreased during a protein-sparing modified fast, and remained depressed for two months after treatment despite increased energy consumption to a level that allowed body weight stabilization.[53] Similar findings were reported by Heshka et al.[19] in participants of a conservative weight-loss program. It was found that resting metabolic rate declined to a greater degree than would be expected from loss of lean mass alone.[19] Other investigators have found no adverse effects on RMR, and have concluded that any decline in resting metabolism is fully explained by an anticipated reduction in fat-free mass accompanying weight loss.[26] A study examining the short-term and long-term effects of very low-calorie diets (VLCDs) observed a 17.3% decrease from baseline of resting energy expenditure after patients consumed 500 kcal/d for just 2 weeks.[54] This reduction in resting metabolism was associated with a weight reduction of only 5.8%. There was, however, an observed rebound in RMR accompanying the patients' return to a 1000 to 1200 kcal/d balanced diet, and the 11% end-of-treatment decline in RMR was paralleled by a 12% reduction in body weight.[54]

It appears that RMR declines rapidly in response to energy restriction. Reductions as great as 30% have been reported in some individuals.[27] Very low-energy diets, in particular, have been found to be associated with substantial short-term reductions in RMR.[26] This decline, however, appears to be attributable primarily to the caloric restriction, and is largely reversed when dieting is stopped.[26] With weight stability, reductions in RMR have been found to be modest, and are highly related to the changes in fat-free mass.[26] It is thought that physical activity, energy deficit, macronutrient distribution, and rate of weight loss may be key factors in the retention of fat free mass, and by extension, RMR.

Exercise and RMR

Many effects of exercise are thought to be beneficial to weight loss and weight maintenance. A single bout of exercise produces an increase in energy expenditure, the magnitude of which is dependent on the intensity, duration, and type of exercise.[15] Weight-bearing activities such as walking, jogging, and cross-country skiing lead to energy expenditure that is directly related to body weight, and may be of particular benefit to obese individuals.[15] Muscle-strengthening exercises may produce an added advantage by maintaining or increasing muscle mass. Some investigators have proposed a carryover effect of exercise on metabolic rate; however, if any long-term effect exists, it is thought to only occur after very vigorous and sustained physical activity.[15]

Both resistance and endurance training have therefore been proposed as interventions that might potentiate RMR to facilitate weight loss in overweight and obese patient populations. Findings from several cross-sectional studies have indicated that athletes demonstrate a higher RMR than sedentary individuals, and training studies indicate that sedentary individuals who are not restricting energy can increase their RMR by beginning a regular exercise program.[4] Despite these findings, the research literature regarding the effects of resistance and endurance training, separately or in combination, on elevating the RMR is mixed, and whether exercise training enhances RMR remains a controversial question.[25]

Resistance Training and RMR

Resistance training is thought to have the potential to increase RMR by increasing fat-free mass.[25] This belief is founded on the significant relation between fat-free mass and RMR. Heavy resistance training promotes skeletal-muscle development, which could have a favorable impact on a person's RMR by increasing the total amount of metabolically active tissue.[27] However, the extent to which resistance training is able to increase RMR has not been well documented, and studies evaluating the impact of high-intensity resistance exercise on body composition and other physiological adaptations during weight loss have reported inconsistent findings. In one longitudinal study comparing the effects of strength training and aerobic exercise on body composition, body weight, and RMR in healthy, non-dieting young men, the resistance training was associated with increased strength and FFM, but body weight and RMR did not change significantly.[27] These findings were corroborated by a similar study with untrained female subjects in which a statistically significant increase in RMR was not observed despite favorable alterations in body composition.[18] Further studies of longer duration are needed to determine whether a significant increase in RMR would be observed with a longer resistance training program.[18]

Endurance Training and RMR

Physical activity, especially in the form of endurance exercise, significantly affects energy intake and expenditure, and is therefore a key regulatory component in the energy balance equation.

After exercise, oxygen consumption decreases rapidly but may remain above resting levels for several hours or even days after the bout of activity.[4] The repair of damaged muscle tissue and the resynthesis of substrates such as CP, ATP, and glycogen partially account for the excessive post-exercise oxygen uptake (EPOC) in the exercised muscles, and may be the cause of the elevated muscle oxygen uptake in recovery. Bullough[55] reported that RMR was greater in trained than untrained subjects only when trained subjects were in a state of recovery from vigorous exercise. Their data indicate that RMR is influenced by exercise, energy intake, and their interaction, and suggest that higher RMR in trained versus untrained individuals results from acute effects of high-intensity exercise rather than from a chronic adaptation to exercise training.

Phelain et al.[56] have examined the effects of low- and high-intensity aerobic exercise of similar energy output on post-exercise energy expenditure and substrate oxidation in fit eumenorrheic women. They used continuous indirect calorimetry performed during cycle ergometry exercise and for three hours after low-intensity exercise (500 kcal at 50% VO_2 max) or high-intensity exercise (500 kcal at 75% VO_2 max). Mean EPOC for the three-hour post-exercise period for high-intensity exercise (9.0 ± 1.7 L, 41 kcals) was significantly greater than that for the lower intensity activity (4.8 ± 1.6 L, 22 kcals). Oxygen consumption (VO_2) following the higher intensity exercise remained elevated at the end of the three-hour post-exercise period, but was not with the low intensity group. Quinn et al.[57] reported that exercise duration increases EPOC significantly, and that a 60-min bout of aerobic exercise yields approximately twice the EPOC than either 20 or 40 min in trained younger women. However, Almuzaini et al.[58] examined the effects of splitting a 30-min exercise bout of cycling into two equal sessions versus a single uninterrupted session. They compared the effects of these two exercise trials on EPOC and resting metabolic rate (RMR) and concluded that dividing a 30-min exercise session into two parts for these individuals significantly increases magnitude of EPOC but does not affect RMR.

Short and Sedlock[59] also found that fit individuals have faster regulation of post-exercise metabolism when exercising at either the same relative or absolute work rate than their untrained counterparts. Gillette and colleagues[60] also compared strenuous resistive exercise to steady-state endurance exercise of similar estimated energy cost. They found that the resistance training resulted in a greater excess post-exercise V_{O_2} compared to the aerobic exercise.

Energy Restriction Combined with Exercise Training: The Effects on RMR

Dietary restriction without exercise does not appear to be an optimal strategy to promote weight loss and weight maintenance.[61] Additionally, in clinical practice, exercise when used alone has not been viewed as an optimal means of weight reduction.[61] This may be attributed in part to the difficulty many patients have in maintaining an appropriate program of physical activity.

Ballor and Poehlman[62] performed a meta-analysis to examine how exercise training and gender influence the composition of diet-induced weight loss. They found that diet-plus-exercise training (DPE) groups did not differ from dietary-restriction-only (DO) groups with respect to either the amount of body weight lost (mean = –10 ± 1.4 kg) or fat mass lost (mean = –8 ± 1.1 kg). Exercise training, however, attenuated the amount of body weight lost as fat-free mass compared to DO for the same sex. The percentage of weight

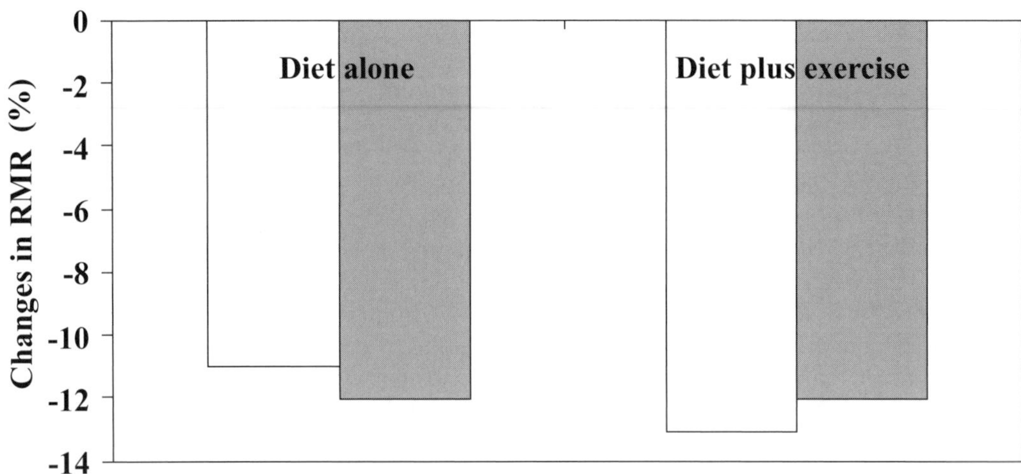

FIGURE 35.3
Changes in resting metabolic rate following interventions of diet plus exercise training or dietary restriction alone. Data adapted from Ballor, D.L. and Poehlman, E.T. *Eur J Appl Physiol*, 71; 535-42, 1995.

lost as fat-free mass for DPE subjects was approximately half (P <0.05) of that for DO subjects of the same sex. The DO males lost 28 ± 4% of weight as fat-free mass, while DPE males lost 13 ± 6%. The DO females lost 24 ± 2% of their weight from lean mass compared to the DPE females, who only lost 11 ± 3% of their weight from the FFM. These data provide evidence that exercise training reduces the amount of fat-free mass lost during diet-induced weight loss. In addition, gender differences do not seem to exist with respect to body composition changes of weight reduction.

The decline of RMR in response to energy restriction has been well documented, and is suspected to decrease the rate of weight loss during periods of energy restriction.[63] Exercise is frequently advocated in the treatment of obesity as a means of increasing energy expenditure and potentially counteracting the negative effects of dietary restriction.[16] Several studies based on the addition of a component of exercise to dietary restriction have been published.[15,16,49,61,64] Some studies have continued to report similar decreases in RMR, whereas others have shown an attenuation of the decrement, or an increase in RMR when an element of exercise was added. Ballor and Poehlman conducted a meta-analysis to examine the independent and interactive effects of dietary restriction, endurance exercise training, and gender on RMR.[65] Collectively, weight loss was greater (P <0.05) for men (18 kg) than for women (12 kg). They found no exercise training or gender effects on RMR during weight loss. Collectively, dietary restriction resulted in a –0.59 kJ min^{-1} (approximately –12%) decrease in RMR (P <0.05). When normalized to body weight, RMR was reduced by less than 2% (P <0.05). These data suggest that exercise training does not differentially affect RMR during diet-induced weight loss. In addition, decreases in resting metabolism appear to be proportional to the loss of the metabolically active tissue (Figure 35.3).

Energy Restriction Combined with Resistance Training: The Effects on RMR

In theory, strength training should attenuate the decline of RMR if it preserves fat free mass by preventing atrophy of skeletal muscle. Skeletal muscle contributes more than

50% of the fat free mass of the body.[64] It is for this reason that resistance training was initially added to weight-loss programs: to reduce or prevent the loss of muscle during energy restriction, which, in theory, should attenuate the drop in RMR typically seen with weight loss.

Few studies have been conducted that combined diet with heavy resistance exercise, and studies evaluating the impact of high-intensity resistance exercise on body composition and other physiological adaptations during weight loss have reported inconsistent findings.[61] Conflicting results regarding the impact dietary restriction combined with resistance training has on lean body mass have been reported. An additional problem in evaluating the impact of resistance training is the fact that many investigators fail to examine all the physiological variables of interest simultaneously. Two studies incorporating strength training during energy restriction found contradictory results. One study reported an increase in fat free mass (RMR was not measured),[64,66] whereas the second found no effect of strength training on fat free mass or RMR, indicating that there are no advantages of a resistance training program to maintenance of lean body mass and attenuating reductions in resting metabolic rate.[64,67] The lack of an effect on fat free mass in this study may have been attributable to the relatively low energy intake of 522 kcal/d overriding the potential benefits of strength training.[64]

In the case of VLCDs, a limited number of studies have combined resistance training with a VLCD.[68] Most studies have found that incorporating resistance training into the very low energy diet regimen does not attenuate the loss of fat free mass or decrease in RMR.[68] It has, however, been reported that significant muscle hypertrophy is possible in an individual undergoing severe energy restriction.[68,69] Hypertrophy was observed only in the exercised muscles, and the resistance training was unable to prevent the loss of overall fat free mass any better than diet alone.[68,69] In a study comparing the benefits of aerobic and resistance training when combined with an 800 kilocalorie liquid diet, it was found that the addition of an intensive, high-volume resistance training program resulted in preservation of fat free mass and RMR during weight loss.[68]

The results of studies examining both moderate and severe dietary energy restriction have lead to the following hypothesis: there may be a minimum level of dietary intake necessary for significant muscle hypertrophy to occur with resistance training.[68] Researchers have reported that a dietary intake of at least 1000 to 1500 kcal/day is required to attain the positive benefits that exercise training can have on RMR and fat free mass.[68,70,71] Further studies are therefore necessary to determine whether a diet adequate in protein, fiber, and vitamins and minerals, but low in total energy, can help mediate the expected chronic adaptations to heavy resistance training.[61]

Caloric Restriction Combined with Endurance Training: The Effects on RMR

Aerobic exercise not only increases energy expenditure, but may also minimize the reductions in resting energy expenditure (REE) that accompany dieting by potentially increasing sympathetic nervous system activity.[66,70,72] It has also been found to attenuate the loss of fat-free mass.[66,73] In turn, this should prevent reduction in REE. Several studies have been undertaken to examine the effects of incorporating endurance training into weight loss regimens, with the hypothesis that its addition would attenuate losses of FFM and, by extension, reductions in RMR.[72] Studies have documented favorable effects of aerobic activity on REE in participants who consumed diets providing 1200 to 1500 kcal/day.[72,74-76] In a study designed to examine the effects of diet and exercise training on resting metabolic rate, participants were placed on a program combining moderate energy restriction and supervised aerobic exercise.[74] It was found that REE, when adjusted for body weight, increased 10% in this group of obese women.[74] In another study examining the effects of exercise on weight, body composition, REE, appetite, and mood in obese women, it was found that participants who consumed diets providing 1200 to 1500 kcal/day and engaged in aerobic activity experienced favorable changes in REE.[72] In addition, the study confirmed the findings of previous investigators regarding the effect of aerobic training in participants consuming VLCDs.[77,78] When participants were prescribed a 925 kcal/day diet, there was no effect of aerobic training on REE. However, when participants terminated their marked dietary energy restriction, a positive effect was observed.[72] In contrast, there have been studies that have found no attenuation of the reduction in RMR in patients consuming a balanced deficit diet consisting of 1200 to 1500 kcal/day. In a study examining the physiologic changes after weight reduction with vigorous exercise and moderate intensity physical activity, there were no differences between groups in decreases in RMR.[79] In this study, vigorous aerobic activity did not attenuate reductions in RMR in patients consuming a self-selected diet.[79] There have also been studies which have failed to find any positive effect on RMR of aerobic training in participants consuming VLCDs. In fact, one study found that participants who exercised vigorously while consuming 720 kcal/day had significantly greater reductions in REE than did nonexercising dieters.[77] Similar findings were reported by Heymsfield et al.[78] This reduction in REE appears to be a consequence of compounding the marked caloric deficit introduced by the VLCD with that introduced by exercise.[72] It has therefore been suggested that the most favorable findings for weight loss are obtained when exercise was combined with diets of 1000 to 1500 kcal/day rather than with VLCDs providing 400 to 800 kcal/day.[72]

Summary

The research literature regarding the effects of dieting resistance and endurance training, separately or in combination, on RMR is mixed. (Table 35.5 shows a collection of studies.) Despite the numerous reported benefits of exercise training, many studies have failed to show significant benefits of exercise on changes in weight and body composition or RMR. Consequently, the significance of many of the effects of exercise remains questionable.[16]

The precise cause of the discrepancy among longitudinal studies investigating the effects of exercise training on RMR is unknown. There are, however, several factors which have been suggested as playing a role in the inconsistent findings. The timing of the RMR measurement in regard to the last bout of exercise training, as well as differences in training mode, exercise intensity, duration, frequency, and total training load have been highlighted as potential factors which may account for some of the discrepancies among studies.[27] Thus, more rigorous, well-controlled longitudinal studies are needed to elucidate the impact of exercise training, both resistance and endurance as well as combined strength and endurance, on RMR.

Despite the equivocal findings regarding the impact of exercise training on resting metabolic rate of dieting individuals, exercise appears to be the single most important behavior for long-term weight control in obese individuals.[80] In addition to the well-known benefits of both resistance and endurance training, it has been found, almost universally, that persons who maintain their weight loss report that they exercise regularly, whereas weight regainers do not. Exercise should therefore remain a cornerstone in the treatment of overweight and obesity.

TABLE 35.5

Collection of Some of the Studies Investigating Changes in Physiological Variables Associated with Treatment

Study	Intervention	# of Participants	Weight Change (kg)	Fat Change (kg)	FFM Change (kg)	RMR Change (kcal/day)
Belko et al., 1987[86]	diet only	5	–7.78	–5.1	–2.68	–109.9
	diet + aerobic	6	–5.70	–4.7	–0.96	–10.0
Broeder et al., 1992[87]	control	19	0.3	0.1	0.2	–17.2
	strength only	13	0.00	–2.1	2.10	58.5
	aerobic only	15	–1.10	–1.4	0.30	30.9
van Dale et al., 1987[88]	diet only	6	–12.2	–9.4	–2.80	–533.66
	diet + aerobic	6	–13.2	–10.9	–2.30	–371.53
van Dale et al., 1989[89]	diet only (no yo-yo)	7	–15.20	–11.9	–3.30	–389.0
	diet + aerobic (no yo-yo)	7	–18.90	–15.2	–3.70	–374.0
	diet + aerobic (no yo-yo)	6	–19.40	–15.4	–4.00	–302.0
Frey-Hewitt et al., 1990[90]	control	41	0.38	–0.27	0.64	27.1
	diet only	36	–6.68	–5.52	–1.16	–149.0
	aerobic only	44	–4.10	–4.12	0.01	–22.8
Hill et al., 1987[91]	diet only	3	–7.90	–4.48	–3.44	–211.2
	diet + aerobic	5	–8.30	–6.13	–2.13	–252.0
Keim et al., 1990[92]	diet + aerobic	5	–13.08	–7.30	–4.70	–139.0
	aerobic only	5	–5.61	–3.90	–1.30	18.0
Lennon et al., 1985[74]	diet only	22	–6.90	–6.01	–0.89	
	diet + aerobic (self-selected)	23	–6.70	–6.40	–0.30	
	diet + aerobic (prescribed)	20	–9.70	–8.60	–1.10	
Wadden et al., 1990[26]	diet (BDD) + aerobic	9	–18.20	–16.3	–0.70	–203.3
	diet (VLCD) + aerobic	6	–21.60	–15.6	–1.90	–166.5
Geliebter et al., 1997[64]	diet only	22	–9.50	–6.80	–2.70	–88.2
	diet + strength	20	–7.80	–6.70	–1.10	–127.2
	diet + aerobic	23	–9.60	–7.20	–2.30	–148.9
Pavlou et al., 1989[15]	diet + aerobic	15	–8.30	–6.91	–1.30	1.0
	diet only	16	–6.40	–5.47	–0.80	–176.0
Mathieson et al., 1986[93]	diet + aerobic (high carb VLCD)	5	–6.70	na	na	–333.0
	diet + aerobic (low carb VLCD)	7	–8.00	na	na	–207.0
Svendson et al., 1993[94]	control	20	0.50	0.50	0.60	63.0
	diet only	50	–9.50	–7.80	–1.20	–86.25
	diet + aerobic	48	–10.30	–9.60	0.00	–45.95
Wilmore et al., 1998[25]	aerobic only	77	0.00	–0.60	0.70	16.72
Kraemer et al., 1997[61]	control	6				132.0
	diet only	8	–6.2			–75.0
	diet + aerobic	9	–6.8			–30.0
	diet + aerobic + strength	8	–7.0			–143.0
Wadden et al., 1997[72]	diet only	29	–14.40	–11.6	–2.80	–106.0
	diet + aerobic	31	–17.20	–10.6	–3.20	–46.0
	diet + strength	31	–13.70	–14.0	–3.10	–20.0
	diet + aerobic + strength	29	–15.20	–13.4	–1.80	–7.0
Racette et al., 1995[16]	diet only	13	–8.30	–6.1	–2.2	–129.0
	diet + aerobic	10	–10.50	–8.8	–1.7	–129.0
Sum et al., 1994[95]	aerobic + strength	42	–16.10	1.70	–17.8	109.3
Donnelly et al., 1991[96]	diet only	26	–20.4	–4.70	–16.1	–138.3
	diet + aerobic	16	–21.4	–4.80	–16.6	–158.6
	diet + strength	18	–20.9	–4.70	–16.1	–186.9
	diet + aerobic + strength	9	–22.9	–4.10	–18.0	–217.0

TABLE 35.5 *(Continued)*

Collection of Some of the Studies Investigating Changes in Physiological Variables Associated with Treatment

Study	Intervention	# of Participants	Weight Change (kg)	Fat Change (kg)	FFM Change (kg)	RMR Change (kcal/day)
Kraemer et al., 1999[61]	control		–0.35	–0.80	-4.84	–93
	diet only	8	–9.64	–6.68		–80
	diet + aerobic	11	–8.99	–7.00		–122
	diet + aerobic + strength	10	–9.90	–9.57		–136
Henson et al., 1987[97]	diet + aerobic	7	–9.50	–8.59	–1.1	–247.0
Heymsfield et al., 1989[78]	diet only	5	–7.0	–4.4	–2.60	–115.2
	diet + aerobic	6	–7.5	–5.3	–2.20	–278.4
Bryner et al., 1999[68]	diet + aerobic	10	–18.1	–12.8	–4.1	–210.7
	diet + strength	10	–14.4	–14.5	–0.8	63.3
Doucet et al., 1999[98] (men)	diet only (phase 1)	10	–11.9	–10.7	–1.2	–304
	diet + aerobic (phase 2)	9	–2.0	–3.3	1.3	134
Doucet et al., 1999[98] (women)	diet only (phase 1)	7	–7.6	–5.8	–1.8	–148
	diet + aerobic (phase 2)	7	–1.2	–2.2	1.0	–199
Franckowiak et al., 1999[79]	diet + aerobic	18	–7.03	–5.99	–1.03	–185.4
	diet + lifestyle	21	–5.42	–4.71	–0.72	–170.5

Acknowledgment

The authors would like to acknowledge the support from NIH Grant M400-215-2111 RO1 (Dr. Andersen).

References

1. *Stedman's Medical Dictionary.* Baltimore, MD: Williams & Wilkins; 1995, pg 262.
2. Moffett DF, Moffett SB, Schauf CL. *Human Physiology: Foundations and Frontiers.* St. Louis, MO: Mosby-Yearbook, 1993, ch 4.
3. Poehlman ET. *Med Sci Sports Exerc* 21: 515; 1989.
4. Andersen, RE. In: *Lifestyle and Weight Management Consultant Manual.* Cotton RT, Ed. San Diego, CA: American Council on Exercise; 1996, pg 95.
5. Bullough RC, Melby CL. *Ann Nutr Metab* 37: 24; 1993.
6. Weir JBdV. *J Physiol* 109: 1; 1949.
7. Matarese LE. *J Am Diet Assoc* 97: 154S; 1997.
8. Webb P. In: *Obesity* (Björntorp P, Brodoff BN, Eds). Philadelphia, PA: J.B. Lippincott; 1992, pg 91.
9. Jéquier E. In: *Substrate and Energy Metabolism,* Garrow JS, Halliday D, Eds. London: Libbey; 1985, pg 82.
10. Ferrannini E. *Metabolism* 37: 287; 1988.
11. American College of Sports Medicine. *Guidelines for Exercise Testing and Prescription.* Malvern, PA: Lea and Febiger; 1991, pg 14.
12. National Institutes of Health. Consensus conference on physical activity and cardiovascular health. 276, 241-246. 1996.
13. Robertson JD, Reid DD. *Lancet* 1: 940; 1952.

14. Heshka S, Feld K, Yang MU, et al. *JADA* 93: 1031; 1993.
15. Pavlou KN, Whatley JE, Jannace PW, et al. *Am J Clin Nutr* 49: 1110; 1989.
16. Racette SB, Schoeller DA, Kushner RF, et al. *Am J Clin Nutr* 61: 486; 1995.
17. Seefeldt VD, Harrison, GG. In: *Anthropometric Standardization Reference Manual,* Lohman TG, Roche AF, Martorell R, Eds. Champaign, IL, Human Kinetics Books, 1988: pg 111.
18. Cullinen K, Caldwell M. *JADA* 98: 414; 1998.
19. Heshka S, Yang M-U, Wang J, et al. *Am J Clin Nutr* 52: 981; 1990.
20. Harris JA, Benedict FG. *Biometric Studies of Basal Metabolism in Man.* Washington, DC: Carnegie Institute of Washington; 1919.
21. Kuczmarski RJ, Flegal KM, Campbell SM, et al. *JAMA* 272: 205; 1994.
22. Fleisch A. *Helv Med Acta* 1: 23; 1951.
23. Mifflin MD, St.Jeor ST, Hill LA, et al. *Am J Clin Nutr* 51: 241; 1990.
24. Berke EM, Gardner AW, Goran MI, et al. *Am J Clin Nutr* 55: 626; 1992.
25. Wilmore JH, Stanforth PR, Hudspeth LA, et al. *Am J Clin Nutr* 68: 66; 1998.
26. Wadden TA, Foster GD, Letizia KA, et al. *JAMA* 264: 707; 1990.
27. Broeder CE, Burrhus KA, Svanevick LS, et al. *Am J Clin Nutr* 55: 795; 1992.
28. Goran MI. *Med Clin N Am* 2: 347; 1984.
29. Poehlman ET, Gardner AW, Ades PA, et al. *Metabolism* 41: 1351; 1992.
30. Poehlman ET, McAuliffe TL, Van Houten DR, et al. *Am J Physiol* 259: E66; 1990.
31. Poehlman ET, Melby CL, Badylak SF. *Am J Clin Nutr* 47: 793; 1988.
32. Poehlman ET, Melby CL, Badylak SF, et al. *Metabolism* 38: 85; 1989.
33. Poehlman ET, Arciero PJ, Goran MI. *Exerc Sport Sci Rev* 22: 251; 1994.
34. Arciero PJ, Goran MI, Poehlman ET. *J Appl Physiol* 75: 2514; 1993.
35. Poehlman ET, Goran MI, Gardner AW, et al. *Am J Physiol* 264: 450E; 1993.
36. McArdle WD, Katch FI, Katch VL. *Exercise Physiology: Energy, Nutrition, and Human Performance.* Philadelphia: Lea & Febiger; 1991, ch 9.
37. Perkins KA. *J Appl Physiol* 72: 401; 1992.
38. Poehlman ET, Despres JP, Bessette H, et al. *Med Sci Sports Exerc* 17: 689; 1985.
39. Costill DL, Dalsky GP, Fink WJ. *Med Sci Sports* 10: 155; 1978.
40. Ivy JL, Costill DL, Fink WJ, et al. *Med Sci Sports Exerc* 11: 6; 1979.
41. Klesges RC, Mealer CZ, Klesges LM. *Am J Clin Nutr* 59: 805; 1994.
42. Williamson DF, Forman MR, Binkin NJ, et al. *Am J Publ Health* 77: 1324; 1987.
43. McDonald JT, Margen S. *Am J Clin Nutr* 29: 1093; 1976.
44. Pirola RC, Lieber CS. *Pharmacology* 7: 185; 1972.
45. Lieber CS. *Nutr Rev* 46: 241; 1988.
46. Suter PM, Schutz Y, Jequier E. *N Engl J Med* 326: 983; 1992.
47. Lamont LS. *J Cardiopulm Rehabil* 15: 183; 1995.
48. Connolly J, Romano T, Patruno M. *Fam Pract* 16: 196; 1999.
49. Andersen RE, Wadden TA, Bartlett SJ, et al. *JAMA* 281: 335;1 999.
50. Coulston AM. *JADA* 98: 6S; 1998.
51. Mokdad AH, Serdula MK, Dietz WH, et al. *JAMA* 282: 1519; 1999.
52. Serdula MK, Mokdad AH, Williamson DF, et al. *JAMA* 282: 1353; 1999.
53. Elliot DL, Goldberg L, Kuehl KS, et al. *Am J Clin Nutr* 49: 93; 1989.
54. Foster GD, Wadden TA, Feurer ID, et al. *Am J Clin Nutr* 51: 167; 1990.
55. Bullough RC, Gillette CA, Harris MA, et al. *Am J Clin Nutr* 61: 473; 1995.
56. Phelain JF, Reinke E, Harris MA, et al. *J Am Coll Nutr* 16: 140; 1997.
57. Quinn TJ, Vroman NB, Kertzer R. *Med Sci Sports Exerc* 26: 908; 1994.
58. Almuzaini KS, Potteiger JA, Green SB. *Can J Appl Physiol* 23: 433; 1998.
59. Short KR, Sedlock DA. *J Appl Physiol* 83: 153; 1997.
60. Gillette CA, Bullough RC, Melby CL. *Int J Sport Nutr* 4: 347; 1994.
61. Kraemer WJ, Volek JS, Clark KL, et al. *Med Sci Sports Exerc* 31: 1320; 1999.
62. Ballor DL, Poehlman ET. *Int J Obes Relat Metab Disord* 18: 35; 1994.
63. Henson LC, Poole DC, Donahoe CP, et al. *Am J Clin Nutr* 46: 893; 1987.
64. Geliebter A, Maher MM, Gerace L, et al. *Am J Clin Nutr* 66: 557; 1997.
65. Ballor DL, Poehlman ET. *Eur J Appl Physiol* 71: 535; 1995.

66. Ballor DL, Katch VL, Becque MD, et al. *Am J Clin Nutr* 47: 19; 1988.
67. Donnelly JE, Pronk NP, Jacobsen DJ, et al. *Am J Clin Nutr* 54: 56; 1991.
68. Bryner RW, Ullrich IH, Sauers J, et al. *J Am Coll Nutr* 18: 115; 1999.
69. Donnelly JE, Sharp T, Houmard J, et al. *Am J Clin Nutr* 58: 561; 1993.
70. Poehlman ET, Melby CL, Goran MI. *Sports Med* 11: 78; 1991.
71. Sweeney ME, Hill JO, Heller PA, et al. *Am J Clin Nutr* 57: 127; 1993.
72. Wadden TA, Vogt RA, Andersen RE, et al. *J Consult Clin Psychol* 65: 269; 1997.
73. King AC, Haskell WL, Taylor CB, et al. *JAMA* 266: 1535; 1991.
74. Lennon D, Nagle F, Stratman F, et al. *Int J Obes Relat Metab Disord* 9: 39; 1985.
75. Tremblay A, Fontaine E, Poehlman ET, et al. *Int J Obes Relat Metab Disord* 10: 511; 1986.
76. Nieman DC, Haig JL, de Guia ED, et al. *J Sports Med* 28: 79; 1988.
77. Phinney SD, LaGrange BM, O'Connell M, et al. *Metabolism* 37: 758; 1988.
78. Heymsfield SB, Casper K, Hearn J, et al. *Metabolism* 38: 215; 1989.
79. Franckowiak SC, Andersen RE, Bartlett SJ, et al. *Med Sci Sports Exerc* 31: 345S; 1999.
80. Kayman S, Bruvold W, Stern JS. *Am J Clin Nutr* 52: 800; 1990.
81. Bernstein RS, Thornton JC, Yang M-U, et al. *Am J Clin Nutr* 37: 595; 1983.
82. Cunningham JJ. *Am J Clin Nutr* 33: 2372; 1980.
83. James WPT. *Postgrad Med J* 60: 50; 1984.
84. Owen OE, Kavle E, Owen RS, et al. *Am J Clin Nutr* 44: 1; 1986.
85. Pavlou KN, Hoeffer MA, Blackburn GL. *Ann Surg* 203: 136; 1986.
86. Belko AZ, Van Loan M, Barbieri TF, et al. *Int J Obes Relat Metab Disord* 11: 93; 1987.
87. Broeder CE, Burrhus KA, Svanevick LS, et al. *Am J Clin Nutr* 55: 802; 1992.
88. van Dale D, Saris WHM, Schoffelen PFM, et al. *Int J Obes Relat Metab Disord* 11: 367; 1987.
89. van Dale D, Saris WHM. *Am J Clin Nutr* 49: 409; 1989.
90. Frey-Hewitt B, Vranizan KM, Dreon DM, et al. *Int J Obes Relat Metab Disord* 14: 327; 1990.
91. Hill JO, Sparling PB, Shields TW, et al. *Am J Clin Nutr* 46: 622; 1987.
92. Keim NL, Barbieri TF, Belko AZ. *Int J Obes Relat Metab Disord* 14: 335; 1990.
93. Mathieson RA, Walberg JL, Gwazdauskas FC, et al. *Metabolism* 35: 394; 1986.
94. Svendsen OL, Hassager C, Christiansen C. *Am J Med* 95: 131; 1993.
95. Sum CF, Wang KW, Choo DCA, et al. *Metabolism* 43: 1148; 1994.
96. Donnelly JE, Pronk NP, Jacobsen DJ, et al. *Am J Clin Nutr* 54: 56; 1991.
97. Henson LC, Poole DC, Donahoe CP, et al. *Med Sci Sports Exerc* 46: 893; 1987.
98. Doucet E, Imbeault P, Almeras N, et al. *Obes Res* 7: 323; 1999.

36

Energy Assessment: Physical Activity

M. Joao Almeida and Steven N. Blair

Introduction

Measuring physical activity is one of the most difficult tasks in physical activity research due to its complexity and the fact that it is based on individual behavior characterized by daily variability in practices and routines. A recent conference at the Cooper Institute focused on the Measurement of Physical Activity.[1] A major conclusion was that for field studies there is no single measure able to accurately assess physical activity in all groups of the population, in all settings, and for all aspects of physical activity. Although some methods are highly accurate and valid, it may not be feasible to use them in field settings, as the cost may be prohibitive. Another problem is the lack of a field criterion measure capable of testing the concurrent validity of current or newly developed methods for assessing physical activity. Choosing a method to assess physical activity is difficult and requires finding the balance between objectives of the study or project and the accuracy, validity, and feasibility of available instruments.

Concepts and Definitions

Physical activity is defined as bodily movement resulting in energy expenditure.[2] Total daily energy expenditure (TEE) has three components: resting metabolic rate (RMR), thermic effect of food (TEF), and energy expenditure by physical activity. Although RMR and TEF account for 60 to 80% of TEE, within-subject variability is very small. Physical activity energy expenditure is the component that can vary greatly from day to day for every individual; therefore, only activity-related energy expenditure will be considered in this section. Physical activity includes all types of bodily movement, from complex sports performance or hard labor in occupational tasks to simply fidgeting. However, physical activity is commonly characterized by its dimensions such as type, frequency,

0-8493-2705-9/01/$0.00+$1.50

intensity, and duration. Some authors also consider the importance of the circumstances and purpose of activity[3] or its efficiency.[4]

Although physical activity results in energy expenditure, the latter can remain constant, whereas the activity may vary immensely; this may result in different physiological effects and health outcomes for various activities. Energy expenditure varies with body size, so individuals of different body sizes might be expending different amounts of calories while performing the same activity. Activity-related energy expenditure is determined by frequency, intensity, and duration and may be expressed in total kilocalories (or kilojoules) or kilocalories per kilogram of body mass.

- Type is a qualitative parameter of physical activity and can be categorized as:
  - In adults: occupational physical activity, leisure-time physical activity, or house and yard work
  - In children: formal vs. informal activities, or school vs. outside school activities.
- Intensity of activity can be defined as a qualitative (light, moderate, or vigorous) or quantitative (specific rate of energy expenditure [METs, Watts, or oxygen uptake]) variable of activity. Although it can be used as an outcome measure, intensity is more often used as an independent variable.
- The frequency of physical activity behaviors is usually expressed as bouts or sessions per day or per week.
- Duration of activity is generally described in minutes, hours, or percentage of time spent engaging in an activity.

Why it is Important to Assess Physical Activity

Epidemiological studies carried out over the past few decades strongly support a causal association between low levels of physical activity and increased risk of several chronic diseases such as cardiovascular disease, type 2 diabetes mellitus, obesity, and some forms of cancer.[5] These relationships have largely been established using self-reported physical activity, although aerobic fitness is used in some studies.[6,7] Reviews of studies examining the association between physical activity and breast cancer[8] and studies of physical activity determining the characteristics and effects of interventions[9] show that inconsistent findings could be related to the lack of precision of some physical activity measures. These authors emphasized the need to utilize standardized methods, and Melanson and Freedson[10] also emphasized the need for valid, reliable, non-reactive, and precise methods. Such instruments will facilitate determination of the specific type and amount of habitual physical activity necessary to gain protective effects against degenerative diseases. Further evaluation of existing methods and the development of new or alternative methods of activity assessment are required if we are to improve our understanding of critical activity-disease relationships.

It also is important to assess physical activity for surveillance purposes. We need to determine whether individuals of all ages are meeting public health physical activity recommendations and whether or not patterns are changing over time. Assessing physical activity will provide valuable information to public health professionals, teachers, researchers, policymakers, and others responsible for physical activity interventions.

Movement Pattern (Day, Week, Season, Year)

It may be important to know how the patterns of activity vary at different times. The majority of health benefits are acquired as chronic adaptations to exercise, which requires habitual patterns of physical activity to be measured. Adults generally have relatively regular daily patterns which may only change for different seasons or during holidays. They may not need to be assessed over longer periods as may be necessary for children. Climate may influence greatly the type and frequency of activities undertaken. Significant differences have been found between weekdays and weekends in type and amount of activity.

Underlying Mechanism of Effect

There are several health-related dimensions of physical activity such as caloric expenditure, aerobic intensity, weight bearing, flexibility, and strength.[17] A similar caloric expenditure in different activities may have a different effect on health outcome (i.e., weight training and swimming). Selecting an activity measure that will accurately assess the different health-related dimensions is required to find the true associations between physical activity and health outcomes. This is analogous to selecting different dietary measures for studies of cardiovascular disease, where saturated fat in the diet may be of prime importance, and for cancer, where fruit and vegetable intake may be of great interest.

Nature of the Study Population (Age, Gender, Culture)

The nature of the population to be examined is relevant for the choice of method. Methods developed for adults may not be appropriate for children. One reason for this is that children appear to have more variation than adults in patterns of activity. Children also often do not perform activities over extended periods. They may play at one activity for a few minutes, then abruptly switch to another activity for a few minutes before going on to something else. This intermittent and frequently changing pattern of activity requires that children's physical activity be assessed by using different intervals of assessment and outcome measures.[18] Physical activity has been assessed in children and adolescents by various methods including self-report by questionnaire or interview and report by proxies such as parents or teachers. Children have lesser ability than adolescents or adults to recall their activities accurately, which renders self-report questionnaires in children of limited value. Objective methods such as heart rate monitors, motion sensors, DLW, and indirect calorimetry have been used frequently in small-scale studies. A comprehensive approach to measurement issues in assessing children's physical activity was presented recently by Welk et al.[18] Points to be considered when selecting a physical activity measurement for children and adolescents are that seven days of monitoring are required to obtain stable estimates of overall activity patterns,[19] both weekend and weekdays need to be included in the assessement,[20] and motion sensors need to be worn for the entire day or at least for multiple times over the course of the day.[19]

Age and gender also need to be considered when selecting a physical activity assessment method for adults, and socioeconomic factors also may often be important. For example, activity patterns between female and male executives may be similar, whereas women who are homemakers with child care responsibilities may have very different activity patterns than men of the same social class. There has been little work on specific activity assessment methods for specific racial or ethnic groups, although such work is beginning to appear.[21] It is important to consider the various types of activity that are likely to be present in a population when planning what assessment method to use. If the study group is a general population sample, it will probably be necessary to include a wide range of activities, including occupational, household, caretaking, leisure time, walking or cycling for transportation to work or on errands, and sports. If the project is to be conducted in a group of business executives, it is probably reasonable to evaluate leisure time physical activity in detail, since these are activities that provide most of the energy expenditure beyond RMR and TEF in this group. For these executives, it is reasonable to give only limited attention to occupational and household activities.

Physical activity varies with age, with general population data showing a gradual decline and the highest prevalence of sedentary behavior observed in elderly persons, especially women.[5] However, there may be substantial differences in activity patterns in retired individuals. For some, most of the activity might be housework and yard work, for others it might be walking, and perhaps for those living in retirement centers the major activities might be recreational activities such as golf or dancing. It is not possible to select a single activity assessment method for use with older individuals, but it is important to consider the type of older population that will be included in the project.

In summary, the nature of the population to be monitored is important to consider when selecting a physical activity assessment method. In general, younger persons are more active than older individuals, men are more active than women, and members of minority groups tend to be less active than non-Hispanic whites. Nonetheless, it is not possible to simply select a method based on age, gender, or racial/ethnic group status. Many other factors such as educational level, health status, geography, climate, and occupational group must be considered. Ideally, it would be useful to collect some pilot data, perhaps by open-ended questionnaires, to obtain information on types of activity most often reported by the target population.

Sample/Population Size

The characteristics or the size of a sample must be taken into account before selecting the activity measure. A national survey or a large population study is not likely to use labor-intensive or high-cost techniques. A validation study or clinical trial with a relatively small sample means that the cost, time, logistical complexity, and other resources per person can be increased allowing the use of more sophisticated, time-consuming, and accurate techniques.

Period of Measurement

For instruments that measure activity over periods of time, an important question is the length of the monitoring period. This may differ for adults as compared with children and adolescents. According to Janz et al.,[22] four or more days of activity monitoring are needed to achieve satisfactory reliability, although Gretebeck and Montoye[23] suggested that at least five or six days of monitoring are needed to minimize intra-individual variance. More recently, Trost et al.[19] concluded that a seven-day monitoring period was required for accelerometers to assess usual activity in children and adolescents and account for apparent differences between weekday and weekend activity behaviors in the same way as within daily differences.

In addition to considering the length of the monitoring period, it also is necessary to consider whether multiple periods need to be monitored over the course of a year. It is obvious that seasonal or climatic effects could have an influence on physical activity, but this has not been studied adequately. Most epidemiological studies on physical activity and health have obtained activity measurements at one time point. However, some of these approaches have asked about activity over periods of various lengths — past week, past month, past three months, past year, or usual activity. It is not clear whether any single approach is better than any other, so at this time investigators should simply select the recall period that seems logical for their specific population.

Cost and Feasibility

Although objective measures are probably more accurate than self-reports for assessing physical activity, the high cost of these methods does not allow for them to be used in some studies. For example, the use of methods such as DLW is virtually impossible in epidemiological studies because of cost, participant burden, and the limited availability of the isotopes. Motion sensors (reviewed in more detail later) are objective and show promise, and the cost of such instruments has been decreasing. However, they still may be too expensive for use in some large studies, and technical support may be required, which further increases the cost. Many of the objective methods also impart a greater participant burden than questionnaire approaches. Use of DLW or motion sensors requires multiple visits to the study laboratory and requires participant cooperation and involvement over longer periods.

Summary

It is not possible to give a few simple guidelines for selecting a physical activity assessment method, and we have presented several factors that need to be considered when making a decision. The purpose of the study, type of physical activity that is of interest, nature of the study group, size and complexity of the study, and the available resources are all essential elements to be evaluated in order to select the most appropriate method for measuring physical activity. It is important to spend sufficient time in planning and selecting an assessment method to avoid later problems.

Methods Available

Extensive research has been carried out on methods for assessing physical activity, which has resulted in a great number of methods being developed and made available. We review several categories of activity assessment methods here. Techniques available for assessing physical activity can be grouped into two broad categories:

- Objective measures — calorimetry, direct observation, physiological markers, and motion sensors
- Subjective measures — self-report (self-administered questionnaire, interviews, diaries, or proxy reports)

Objective measures assess activity directly. They have been used in many studies to assess levels of physical activity in all age groups, and also have been used extensively to validate self-report measures. Continuing development and refinement of the different devices are beginning to overcome their high cost and complexity, facilitate their use in wider samples, and provide easier data entry, manipulation, and analyses. Subjective methods have been most frequently used in population surveillance and large population studies. These methods typically result in assigning individuals to one of a few broad categories of habitual activity — perhaps sedentary, low active, moderately active, or highly active.

Several recent reviews are available on the different techniques for assessing physical activity and energy expenditure in both field and laboratory settings.[1,3,10-15,24] Some of the available methods will be discussed here, with particular emphasis on methods that have been tested for validity and reliability.

Subjective Assessments

Subjective physical activity assessments rely principally on self-report of activity patterns by the study participant. This information may be obtained by structured interview, self-completed questionnaires, or diaries. Self-report methods have been widely used in studies on physical and health outcomes and for population surveillance of physical activity.

Self-report techniques such as physical activity diaries, recall surveys, quantitative history surveys, and proxy report (e.g., provided by parents, spouses, or teachers) are widely used to assess typical levels of physical activity. They rely on the subject (or proxy) to recall activities performed over a period of time that can vary from one day to one year (more often one week to one month) on the assumption that this period represents the individual's typical activity for most of the time. The complexity of the self-report measures may also vary immensely, in which the subject may be asked a few simple questions to very detailed information regarding type, frequency, time, duration, intensity, and perceived exertion. As result, levels of activity are expressed in different scoring systems, which makes it difficult to interpret and compare among studies.

Self-report methods are useful for adolescents and adults, but are not particularly appropriate for children. Self-report methods are unreliable in young children as they do not have the cognitive ability needed to recall and record type, duration, and intensity of physical activity, particularly over extended periods of time.[25] Furthermore, children seem to expend energy in diverse contexts and styles, such as those involved in spontaneous play. This diversity ranges between brief but frequent bouts of vigorous activity to activities of a longer duration such as walking or biking to school, and this diversity makes accurate recall difficult. According to Sallis et al.,[26] reliability and validity improve with increasing age, and validity is improved when the recall interval (i.e., time from the physical activity to the moment of report) is as short as possible. They conclude that recall instruments should only be used with children 10 years old or older.

Advantages of self-report methods are that they are:

- Useful to assign individuals to broad activity categories, which is appropriate in epidemiological studies and population surveys
- Relatively inexpensive
- Time efficient and have a low participant burden
- Applicable to mail-back or telephone surveys

Disadvantages of self-report methods are that:

- Accuracy is affected by the individual's recall errors and incorrect perceptions of activities

- Validity is limited by the ability of the subject (or proxy) to recall and report activity behaviors accurately[12]
- Intensity of activity is difficult to obtain

Interviews

Structured physical activity interviews may facilitate the recall of type, amount, frequency, duration, and intensity of activity episodes. However, even with this structure and guidance by the interviewer, it is still difficult for participants to recall and report all details of physical activity participation. A major problem is accurately classifying activity intensity and accurately reporting actual minutes spent in an activity. For example, a person may report swimming for an hour, when in fact they were at the beach for an hour and only swam for 10 minutes. When reporting minutes spent in an activity, it is difficult to know the minimum length of the bout that should be counted. It is reasonably easy to identify activity bouts of 10 to 15 minutes, but should repeated bouts of five minutes or two minutes be counted and summed over the course of the day? One of the most widely used structured interviews is the seven-day physical activity recall, which has been used in both community surveys and clinical trials.[27,28] A major disadvantage with the interview method for large studies is the increased cost incurred by the interviewers' time.

Self-Completed Questionnaires

Questionnaires are the most common instruments used in large-scale studies because of their low cost and ease of administration in large groups of subjects. One problem with the self-completed questionnaire approach is that study participants often overestimate the amount of their physical activity. However, even with their limitations, a large body of evidence from studies on physical activity and health outcomes has been based on self-completed activity questionnaires. There is good consensus from these studies, with the clear finding that sedentary individuals are more likely than their more active peers to develop chronic disease or die prematurely during followup. Thus, the relatively crude classifications of activity status by the questionnaires appear to be valid for predicting health outcomes. The various recent reviews of physical activity assessment methods include a detailed listing of questionnaires.[3,24] We encourage investigators to review these various instruments and select the one that logically appears to be best suited to the specific purposes and needs of the planned study. Most of the published questionnaires have acceptable reliability and validity for assigning individuals into broad activity categories.

One of the problems faced by public health officials is surveillance of physical activity in the population. Issues that can be addressed with a good surveillance system include trends in population physical activity over time and comparisons of activity in different regions. Many times it also would be desirable to make cross-national comparisons. Unfortunately, physical activity surveys in different countries have been performed with different methods and measurement strategies. In order to help standardize definitions and physical activity assessments across countries, the World Health Organization and the U.S. Centers for Disease Control and Prevention have convened an international group of experts to develop an International Physical Activity Questionnaire (IPAQ). Short and long versions of the questionnaire have been developed, reviewed, and revised, and are currently being tested for reliability and validity. Preliminary results of these studies are now available and are encouraging. The short and long versions of IPAQ can be administered by interview, self-completed questionnaire (in person or by mail-back survey), or by a telephone interview. Although the IPAQ may be revised in light of the ongoing studies, the final version should be available by 2001. Contact information for the Chair of the International Working Group and the U.S. coordinator is:

- Michael Booth
  mikeb@pub.health.su.oa.zu
- Michael Pratt
  mxp4@cdc.gov

Diaries

Some investigators have used physical activity diaries to classify study participants.[29] According to Bratteby et al.,[30] the activity diary method provides a reasonable estimate of total energy expenditure and physical activity levels in population groups. However, Sallis concluded that diary measures have strong validity but that the burden on subjects is high and compliance varies with the population being studied.[31] Diaries are not considered feasible in young children. Physical activity diaries are likely to be most useful when used in small studies or clinical trials. Participants in these studies are likely to be more motivated than participants in large population studies to accept the high participant burden involved in keeping a diary. Diaries are more likely to be successful when used for relatively short periods of a few days.

Objective Assessments

Several methods of physical activity assessment using objective approaches are available. These methods tend to require a higher participant burden than the subjective approaches, and the cost for objective methods is higher, often much higher. Nonetheless, these objective methods are extremely useful, especially for small and highly controlled clinical trials.

Calorimetry

Calorimetry involves measurement of calories expended. This can be done by directly measuring heat production by the body, but such methods are costly and are most applicable to a few studies where highly accurate measures of energy expenditure are required.[3] Indirect calorimetry is a method that determines energy expenditure from VO_2 consumption and VCO_2 production, and is frequently used in the laboratory to measure exercise metabolism. Calorimetry is usually used to validate other physical activity assessment methods in laboratory settings. Recent advances in instrumentation for portable metabolic analyzers have made these devices more suitable for field settings to evaluate the metabolic rate, and thus the energy cost of various free-living activities. These methods are still intrusive, have a high participant burden, require technically trained laboratory staff, and are relatively expensive. These approaches can be quite useful to validate other physical activity assessments in field settings, but have limited applicability in most clinical settings where activity assessment is desired.

Doubly-Labeled Water

DLW is considered the gold standard for validating other field methods of assessing total energy expenditure. The measurement of average daily metabolic rate, combined with a measurement of resting metabolic rate and an estimate of TEF, permits the calculation of energy expenditure for physical activity under normal daily living conditions.[32] This technique consists of administering an oral dose of $^2H_2{}^{18}O$, after which carbon dioxide production over time is calculated from the difference in the elimination rates of ^{2}H and ^{18}O, because the ^{2}H label is eliminated from the body only as water, while the ^{18}O label is eliminated as water and carbon dioxide. Goran et al.[33] indicate that studies examining the validity of the DLW method show the technique to be accurate within 5 to 10% when compared with data from subjects living in metabolic chambers. Although the DLW technique is considered the gold standard for validating field methods to assess energy expenditure, it is notable that it has never been validated in field settings because of the lack of a suitable reference criterion.[3]

The advantages of the DLW method are:

- It is unobtrusive and is unlikely to influence daily behaviors
- It allows for determination of energy expenditure in free-living conditions
- It provides an accurate quantification of the energy expenditure of physical activity over several days

Disadvantages of the DLW method are that:

- It requires specialized equipment and personnel, which makes it expensive
- The isotopes are very expensive and there is limited availability[34]
- It is necessary to ingest an isotope which may not be accepted by some individuals
- It provides no information about the type, frequency, duration, or intensity of specific bouts of activity

Therefore, although the method provides an integrated measure of energy expenditure over time, it does not provide information about how energy expenditure was accomplished. For example, total energy expenditure can be increased by small elevations in activity intensity over many hours or by participating in vigorous intensity activity over a few minutes, and these two patterns might have very different effects on health or functional outcomes.

Overall, the DLW method has the potential to be used as the criterion measure to validate more practical field methods.[3] It has already been used to validate some field methods such as activity diaries,[30] heart rate monitoring,[35] and accelerometers.[32,36]

Direct Observation

Direct observation consists of an observer coding the activities (type and intensity) performed by an individual during short periods of time. The observation usually takes place during specific periods such as playtime at school or physical education classes. It may be done in real time or by viewing videotapes. Direct observation has been used mainly to assess physical activity in children. It does not interfere directly with the activities, assesses multiple dimensions of physical activity, and can include information concerning contextual variables such as physical and social environments. Although the physical activity data collected are objective and reliable, times and places available to observe participants are limited. Thus, observation studies are done more often on preschool[37,38] than on school-age children.[39] Another disadvantage of direct observation studies is the fact that they require intensive training and monitoring of observers to maintain quality control. Direct observation is time-consuming and costly, which may explain its infrequent use. The method is used primarily with small samples, and also as a criterion measure to validate other instruments.

Heart Rate Monitoring

Heart rate monitoring is an objective method based on the well-established relationship between heart rate and metabolic demand; that is, as physical work increases, heart rate increases to provide increased circulation to the working muscles and the heart. There is a linear association between heart rate and energy expenditure over much of the heart rate range. Heart rate monitors are available that provide minute-by-minute recordings of heart rate over the course of the day, or even several days. This allows for plotting heart rate over time, and records physical activity at different intensities in short periods of time (e.g., minute by minute) and continuously over several days.

Heart rate is a common index of activity intensity that has been used in several studies in both adults and children.[22,25,40-43] However, the use of heart rate as an unbiased indicator of physical activity intensity has been questioned.[42,44] Heart rate monitoring provides useful information about physical activity amount and intensity within individuals, but is less useful for comparisons between individuals. This is because heart rate for a standard task, say walking at 3 mph on the level, is strongly influenced by a person's cardiorespiratory fitness. The fit individual might have a heart rate of 90 beats/minute during this walk, and the unfit person might have a heart rate of 120 beats/minute. The method can be used to compare an individual's activity from day to day, but not to compare multiple individuals unless the heart rate energy expenditure relationship is calibrated for each person by laboratory testing.

Riddoch and Boreham[15] reviewed 13 studies that used heart rate to assess activity levels in children, and they concluded that at higher exercise intensities, when heart rates tend to be high, heart rate monitoring could provide valid estimates of energy expenditure. However, at lower exercise intensities when fear, excitement, and other emotional states can significantly affect heart rates, the method was less accurate. Thus, if measurement of light and moderate intensity activities is intended, heart rate monitoring presents significant limitations.

In summary, heart rate monitoring is useful to determine whether an individual is changing his activity patterns from day to day, such as might be expected in a physical activity intervention study. Heart rate monitoring can be used to compare individuals if the individual heart rate energy expenditure curves are established, and it is especially useful for detecting moderately vigorous to vigorous activities. The heart rate monitoring approach is time consuming, requires close cooperation from study participants, requires equipment and technical expertise, and is not especially feasible for large population studies. The method is objective and can provide important information about the intensity of physical activity, and if summed over the course of the day provides an indication of overall amount of activity.

Activity Monitors

In the last few years, activity monitors have been increasingly investigated and used in cross-sectional and intervention studies and to validate other physical activity assessment instruments. Activity monitors can be simple, such as pedometers or step counters, or more complex, such as accelerometers.

Pedometers

Pedometers record the number of steps taken, which is provided as total volume during a period of time, such as one or several days' activity. Earlier pedometers operated on a pendulum principle, and there were major problems with reliability and validity of these instruments. Some more recent pedometers are electronic devices, which are substantially more accurate than the older pendulum models.

Advantages of the electronic pedometers are that they are:

- Inexpensive, with reliable instruments costing $20 or less
- Small and light in weight, no more than an ounce or two
- Unobtrusive
- Simple to operate

Disadvantages are that they:

- Do not provide chronological information regarding the distribution of steps over the recording period
- Do not provide data on physical activity intensity
- Do not provide data on pattern of activity over the course of the day
- Are not resistant to tampering

Overall, we find these devices useful for self-monitoring of physical activity in behavioral intervention programs and think that they provide objective data that allows for assignment to broad activity categories. Ordering information for a frequently used pedometer that has undergone extensive reliability and feasibility testing is given here.

Yamax DigiWalker
New LifeStyles, 5900 Larson Avenue, Kansas City, MO 64133 USA
Phone: U.S. 888-748-5377, outside U.S. 816-353-1852; Fax 816-353-9808
E-mail teresa@digiwalker.com; Website www.digiwalkerinfo.com

Accelerometers

Accelerometers are motion sensors that detect movement of the body. There has been extensive research and development of these instruments over the past several years, and several devices are currently available. Major advantages of accelerometers are:

- Their ability to record and store activity data on a minute-by-minute basis for extended periods of time under free-living conditions
- The objective measure of total body movement or limb movement respectively depending on whether they are placed on the torso or on the limbs
- The chronological recording of acceleration allows for evaluation of frequency, intensity, and duration of body movement; time spent in sedentary activities can also be determined
- The estimates of total energy expenditure

However, these devices also present limitations such as:

- They cannot be worn during any water activities since they are not developed to be exposed to water
- They are unable to discriminate the energy cost of activities such as carrying loads or walking upstairs, and do not distinguish between uphill and downhill walking or hiking[45]

- The cost of the equipment and the time needed to download and manipulate the data for some of these devices are too great for use in large-scale studies
- They have not been validated for the assessment of upper body activities such as throwing, catching, and lifting

When all things are considered, we think accelerometers offer great potential for physical activity assessment, especially for smaller studies such as clinical trials or clinical interventions. Because of the potential of these instruments and the large amount of recent and ongoing research on accelerometer measurement of physical activity, we will provide a more extensive review of this approach than we have for other methods presented in this section.

Accelerometers are available for measurement of movement in a single plane (usually the vertical plane) or in all three planes. The unidimensional Caltrac is the accelerometer that has been used most widely in physical activity research.[10] A second unidimensional accelerometer has been developed by Computer Science and Applications (CSA, Shalimar, FL). Janz et al.[22] found correlations of r = 0.50 to 0.74 between the CSA accelerometer and heart rate telemetry, with higher correlations found for more vigorous activities.

Presently, there are two tridimensional accelerometers, the Tracmor and the TriTrac-R3D (Hemokinetics, Inc., Madison, WI); however, only the latter is commercially available. Bouten et al.[46] report that tridimensional accelerometers predicted activity-related energy expenditure better than unidimensional accelerometers when young adults performed different types of activity (sedentary activities, walking). Tridimensional accelerometers should more accurately record activities that include extensive horizontal motion, bending, and twisting. However, some investigators find little difference between unidimensional and tridimensional accelerometers.

In a study of college students, Matthews and Freedson[47] compared results from the Tritrac accelerometer with self-reports of activity on a three-day log (r = 0.82) and a seven-day recall (r = 0.77). They concluded that although the Tritrac accelerometer underestimated daily energy expenditure, it provided more accurate results than the Caltrac accelerometer. The Tritrac accelerometer correctly classified 84% of the students into two groups: low active and high active. The ability of the Tritrac accelerometer to measure activity in one-minute intervals makes it possible to analyze data from specific time segments and allows determining total time spent at different activity intensities as well as sustained periods of moderate or vigorous activity.

There have been few investigations using the TriTrac-R3D with children and adolescents. Results of accelerometer studies may be different in adults than in children, because children are more likely than adults to expend vertical energy through jumping and climbing and have more frequent but short bouts of moderate to vigorous activity.[48] Welk and Corbin were among the first to report the use of the Tritrac accelerometer in children.[49] In a sample of 35 children (9 to 11 years old), they evaluated the TriTrac-R3D against heart rate monitoring and the unidimensional Caltrac accelerometer. The TriTrac-R3D was moderately correlated (r = 0.58) with the heart rate monitor and highly correlated (r = 0.88) with the Caltrac. The correlation of accelerometer data with heart rate was highest during free play and lowest when activity was more limited or structured.

Ordering information for accelerometers is included here.

- TriTrac-R3D
  StayHealthy, Inc, 222 East Huntington Drive, Suite 213, Monrovia, CA 91016
  Phone 626-256-6152
  Email pbylsma@stayhealthy.com; Website www.stayhealthy.com

- CSA
  Computer Science and Applications, Inc., 2 Clifford Drive, Shalimar, FL 32579
  Phone 850-651-4991; Fax 850-651-2816
  Email csainc@fwb.gulf.net; Website www.csa-ucc.com

Summary

Motion sensors and heart rate monitors overcome problems associated with inaccurate subject recall of activity and are less costly than direct observation. Objective measurements provided by heart rate monitors and accelerometers can be used across all age groups as long as their output is provided in raw scores. This is because estimates of energy expenditure provided by some devices have substantial errors due to the fact that the population from which the equations were derived is specific and may not represent the population to be studied. Investigators may need to develop their own energy expenditure equations based on their own study group. It is important to remember that these instruments can be prone to technical problems, are expensive, and they provide no information concerning specific activities or the context in which activities are performed.[12] Although they provide an objective measure of physical activity, accurate assessment relies on each participant complying to wear the device throughout the monitoring period.

Conclusions

We have reviewed several categories of physical activity assessment methods and discussed the strengths and weaknesses of each approach. Table 36.1 includes a listing of several physical activity assessment methods and indications of how each meets various factors that need to be considered when selecting the most appropriate method. The table combines information presented in preceding sections and should be a useful summary tool to help investigators and clinicians make decisions regarding physical activity assessment.

All physical activity assessment methods and instruments have strengths, limitations, advantages, and disadvantages. Our major recommendation is that the choice of a method to assess physical activity depends primarily on the purpose of the study and the dimensions to be assessed in order to answer the relevant questions. Other critical factors to be taken into account include the population to be evaluated, the size of the study group, and cost and feasibility issues.

Acknowledgments

We thank Melba Morrow for editorial assistance and Stephanie Parker for administrative assistance. The work reported here was supported in part by grants from the National Institutes of Health (AG06945 and HL58608).

TABLE 36.1
Methods for Assessing Physical Activity

Instrument	Format of Assessment	Units of Measurement	Period of Measurement	Field Measure	Characteristics of Activity Assessed						Context in which Activity Occurs				Population				Cost	Sample Size
					Type	Frequency	Intensity	Duration	Total Volume of Activity	Sedentary	Leisure	Work	Household	Transport	Children	Adolescents	Adults	Older adults		
Objective Measures																				
DLW[1-3]	Ingestion of a known concentration of isotopes	EE (kj or kcal)	7 to 14 days	✓					✓						✓	✓	✓	✓	H	S
Whole-room indirect calorimeter	Re-create free-living conditions in a confined space	EE through measurement of heat production and/or respiratory gas exchange	A few days			✓	✓	✓	✓						✓	✓	✓	✓	H	S
Indirect calorimetry	Standardized protocols of exercise in a controlled environment	VO2 uptake EE	Minute or less intervals	✓			✓	✓	✓		✓	✓	✓	✓	✓	✓	✓	✓	H	S
HR monitor[4]	Wearing the monitor for all the measurement period	Beats/min	Intervals of 1 minute or less for up to several days	✓		✓	✓	✓	✓						✓	✓	✓	✓	M	M
Pedometer Yamax Digiwalker[5]	Wearing the device for all the measurement period	Steps		✓					✓							✓	✓	✓	L	L
Caltrac[6,7]	Wearing the monitor for all the measurement period	Movement counts/kcal		✓					✓						✓	✓	✓	✓	M	L
CSA[8-10]	Wearing the monitor for all the measurement period	Counts		✓					✓						✓	✓	✓	✓	M	L

Method	Procedure	Outcome	Period	1	2	3	4	5	6	7	8	9	10	11	12	13	14	15	Cost	Sample size
TriTrac-R3D[11,12]	Wearing the monitor for all the measurement period	Movement Counts/ kcal		✓					✓						✓	✓	✓	✓	M	
Tracmor[13]	Wearing the monitor for all the measurement period	Counts		✓					✓								✓	✓	M	
Direct Observation[14]	Observer rates the activity and intensity	Minutes of activity		✓	✓	✓	✓	✓	✓						✓	✓			H	S
Subjective Measures																				
7-Day Physical Activity Recall (PAR)[15]	Interview	Kcal/kg or kcal/day	7 days	✓		✓	✓	✓	✓		✓	✓				✓	✓		L	L
PAQ-C[16]				✓											✓	✓			L	
Leisure Time Exercise Quest. (LTEQ)[17]				✓											✓	✓				
PDPAR[18,19]		After school		✓											✓	✓				
Self-administered PA checklist (SAPAC)[20]				✓											✓	✓				
Child/Adol Activity Log (CAAL)[21]				✓											✓	✓				
4 x 1 day recalls	Interview		1 day repeated four times	✓		✓	✓	✓			✓				✓	✓			M	S
Diary[22]		Can be minutes, kcal, or other measures, depending on how diary structured		✓	✓	✓	✓	✓	✓	✓	✓	✓	✓	✓		✓	✓	✓	M	M

Cost: L = Low; M = Medium; H = High

Sample size: S = Small (this is typically a few dozen participants); L = Large (can be up to a few 100 participants)

1. Schoeller DA. *J Nutr* 118:1278; 1988. 2. Schoeller DA. *J Nutr* 129:1765; 1999. 3. Seale JL, Conway JM, Canary JJ. *J Appl Physiol* 74:402; 1993. 4. Murayama N, Ohtsuka R. *Am J Hum Biol* 11:647; 1999. 5. Eston RG, Rowlands AV, Ingledew DK. *J Appl Physiol* 84:362; 1998. 6. Bray MS, Wong WW, Morrow JR, Jr., et al. *Med Sci Sports Exerc* 26:1524; 1994. 7. Nichols JF, Patterson P, Early T. *Can J Sport Sci* 17:299; 1992. 8. Janz KF. *Med Sports Exerc* 26:369; 1994. 9. Melanson ELJ, Freedson PS. *Med Sci Sports Exerc* 27:934; 1995. 10. Trost SG, Ward DS, Moorehead SM, et al. *Med Sci Sports Exerc* 30:629; 1998. 11. Welk GJ, Corbin CB. *Res Q Exerc Sport* 66:202; 1995. 12. Nichols JF, Morgan CG, Sarkin JA, et al. *Med Sci Sports Exerc* 31:908; 1999. 13. Bouten CV, Westerterp KR, Verduin M, Janssen JD. *Med Sci Sports Exerc* 26:1516; 1994. 14. Rowe PJ, Schuldheisz JM, vanderMars H. *Pediatr Exerc Sci* 9:136; 1997. 15. Sallis JF, Buono MJ, Roby JJ, et al. *Med Sci Sports Exerc* 25:99; 1993. 16. Crocker PR, Bailey DA, Faulkner RA, et al. *Med Sci Sports Exerc* 29:1344; 1997. 17. Raudsepp L, Pall P. *Biol Sport* 14:199; 1997. 18. Trost SG, Ward DS, McGraw B, Pate RR. *Pediatr Exerc Sci* 11:341; 1999. 19. Weston AT, Petosa R, Pate RR. *Med Sci Sports Exerc* 29: 138; 1997. 20. Sallis JF, Strikmiller PK, Harsha DW, et al. *Med Sci Sports Exerc* 28:840; 1996. 21. Garcia AW, George TR, Coviak C, et al. *Internat J Behav Med* 4:323; 1997. 22. Bratteby LE, Sandhagen B, Fan H, Samuelson G. *Eur J Clin Nutr* 51:585; 1997.

References

1. _________ *Res Q Exerc Sport* 71(2), 1S. 2000.
2. Caspersen CJ, Powell KE, Christenson GM. *Pub Health Rep* 100:126; 1985.
3. Montoye HJ. *Measuring physical activity and energy expenditure*, Human Kinetics, Champaign, IL: 1996.
4. Goran MI, Sun M. *Am J Clin Nutr* 68: 944S; 1998.
5. _________ US Department of Health and Human Services. *Physical Activity and Health: A Report of the Surgeon General*, Atlanta, GA: US Department of Health and Human Services, Centers for Disease Control and Prevention, National Center for Chronic Disease Prevention and Health Promotion; 1996.
6. Blair SN, Kohl HW, III, Paffenbarger RS, Jr, et al. *JAMA* 262: 2395; 1989.
7. Blair SN, Kohl HW, III, Barlow CE, et al. *JAMA* 273: 1093; 1995.
8. Ainsworth BE, Sternfeld B, Slattery ML, et al. *Cancer* 83:611; 1998.
9. Stone EJ, McKenzie TL, Welk GJ, Booth ML. *Am J Prev Med* 15:298; 1998.
10. Melanson EL, Jr., Freedson PS. *Crit Rev Food Sci Nutr* 36: 385; 1996.
11. Baranowski T, Bouchard C, Bar-Or O, et al. *Med Sci Sports Exerc* 24: 237S; 1992.
12. Heath GW, Pate RR, Pratt M, *Pub Health Rep* 108(1): 42; 1993.
13. Wareham NJ, Rennie KL. *Int J Obes Relat Metab Disord* 22: 30S; 1998.
14. Rowlands AV, Eston RG, Ingledew DK. *Sports Med* 24: 258; 1997.
15. Riddoch CJ, Boreham CA. *Sports Med* 1995; 19: 86; 1995.
16. Freedson PS. *Pediatr Exerc Sci* 1: 8; 1989.
17. Paffenbarger RS, Jr, Lee I-M, Kampert JB. *World Rev Nutr Diet* 82: 210; 1997.
18. Welk GJ, Corbin CB, Dale D. Measurement issues in the assessment of physical activity in children. *Res Q Exerc Sport* 71: 59S; 2000.
19. Trost SG, Pate RR, Freedson PS, Sallis JF, Taylor WC. *Med Sci Sports Exerc* 32: 426; 2000.
20. Sallis JF. *J Sch Health* 61: 215; 1991.
21. Masse LC, Fulton JE, Watson KL, et al. *Res Q Exerc Sport* 70: 212; 1999.
22. Janz KF, Witt J, Mahoney LT. *Med Sci Sports Exerc* 27: 1326; 1995.
23. Gretebeck RF, Montoye HJ. *Med Sci Sports Exerc* 24: 1167; 1992.
24. FitzGerald SJ, Kriska AM, Pereira MA, de Courten, MP. *Med Sci Sports Exerc* 29: 910; 1997.
25. Sallis JF, Buono MJ, Roby JJ, et al. *Med Sci Sports Exerc* 22: 698; 1990.
26. Sallis JF, McKenzie TL, Alcaraz, JE. *Am J Dis Child* 147: 890; 1993.
27. Blair SN, Haskell WL, Ho P, et al. *Am J Epidemiol* 122: 794; 1985.
28. Sallis JF, Haskell WL, Wood PD, et al. *Am J Epidemiol* 121: 91; 1985.
29. Bouchard C, Tremblay A, Leblanc C, et al. *Am J Clin Nutr* 37: 461; 1983.
30. Bratteby LE, Sanhagen B, Fan H, Samuelson GA. *Eur J Clin Nutr* 51: 585; 1997.
31. Sallis JF, Buono MJ, Roby JJ, et al. *Med Sci Sports Exerc* 25: 99; 1993.
32. Westerterp KR, Bouten CV. *Z Ernahrungswiss* 36: 263; 1997.
33. Goran MI, Poehlman ET, Danforth EJ, Nair KS. *Int J Obes Relat Metab Disord* 18: 622; 1994.
34. Stager JM, Lindeman A, Edwards J. *Sports Med* 19: 166; 1995.
35. Racette SB, Schoeller DA, Kushner RF. *Med Sci Sports Exerc* 27: 126; 1995.
36. Bouten CV, Verboeket-van d V, Westerterp KR, et al. *J Appl Physiol* 81: 1019; 1996.
37. Danner F, Noland M, McFadden M, et al. *Pediatr Exerc Sci* 3: 11; 1991.
38. DuRant RH, Baranowski T, Davis H, et al. *Med Sci Sports Exerc* 24: 265; 1992.
39. Bailey RC, Olson J, Pepper SL, et al. *Med Sci Sports Exerc* 27: 1033; 1995.
40. McKenzie TL, Sallis JF, Nader PR, et al. *J Appl Behav Anal* 24: 141; 1991.
41. Welk GJ, Corbin CB. *Res Q Exerc Sport* 66: 202; 1995.
42. Maffeis C. Pinelli L, Zaffanello M, et al. *Int J Obes Relat Metab Disord* 19: 671; 1995.
43. Sallis JF, Strikmiller PK, Harsha DW, et al. *Med Sci Sports Exerc* 28: 840; 1996.
44. Freedson PS. *J Sch Health* 61: 220; 1991.
45. DeVoe D, Gotshall RW. *J Hum Movement Studies* 34: 271; 1998.
46. Bouten CV, Westerterp KR, Verduin M, Janssen JD. *Med Sci Sports Exerc* 26: 1516; 1994.

47. Matthews CE, Freedson PS. *Med Sci Sports Exerc* 27: 1071; 1995.
48. Corbin SB. *J Am Coll Dent* 61: 17; 1994.
49. Welk GJ, Corbin CB. *Res Q Exerc Sport* 66: 202; 1995.

37

Thermogenesis

Bryan C. Bergman and James O. Hill

Introduction

This section deals with thermogenesis, which we define as energy expenditure (EE) above resting metabolic rate (RMR) not associated with physical activity. Other sections in this volume deal with both RMR and physical activity individually, and therefore these subjects will not be addressed. As defined for discussion in this section, thermogenesis can be produced from diet, drugs, and cold exposure. This section will discuss factors that may enhance thermogenesis, followed by a discussion of potential implications of thermogenesis in determining total energy expenditure (TEE), and how modulations in thermogenesis may influence the obesity epidemic now facing the United States and other countries.

Thermic Effect of Food

The thermic effect of food (TEF) is the acute increase in metabolic rate above resting metabolic rate after meal ingestion which can last for up to six hours (Figure 37.1). The TEF has also been called dietary-induced thermogenesis (DIT), but this term is less specific and could refer to the chronic effect of overfeeding on thermogenesis, which will be discussed in a later section. Thermic effect of food accounts for approximately 7 to 10% of daily EE under mixed meal conditions,[2,3] and thus could be an important determinant of daily EE. Factors which influence TEF are controversial, largely because of methodological differences between studies and questions about the applicability of laboratory studies to real-life situations.[4] Investigators often do not monitor TEF for sufficient time to quantitate the full effect of a meal on EE, which may explain much of the disagreement between studies.[1] IT is influenced by many variables, including meal size and frequency, meal composition, age, gender, obesity, and previous exercise.

0-8493-2705-9/01/$0.00+$1.50

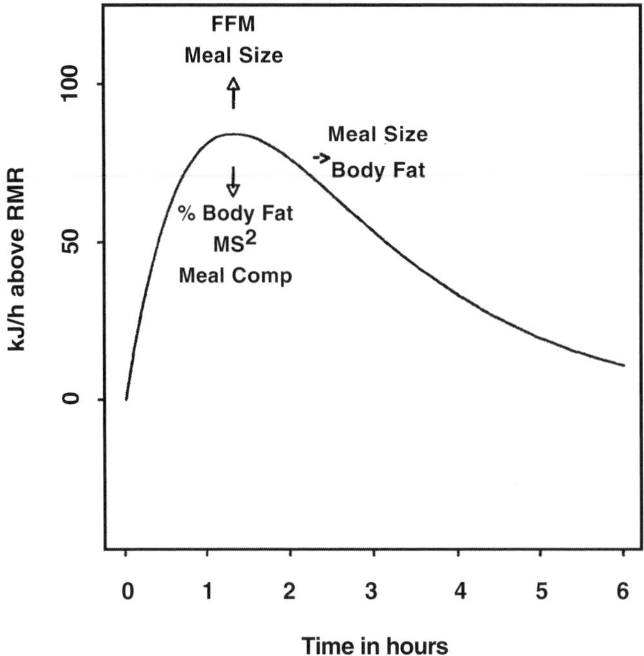

FIGURE 37.1
An illustration of how the TEF (thermic effect of food) curve shifts depending on subject and meal characteristics. Meal size and fat-free mass (FFM) tend to increase the peak; subject's body fat and meal size squared (MS^2) tend to lower the peak; meal size and subject's body fat tend to move the time of the peak further out. There is some evidence that increased fat in the meal may decrease the peak. Illustrated curve equation: $175.9 \times T \times e^{-T/1.3}$, where T is time and e is the base of the natural logarithm. RMR, resting metabolic rate. Reprinted with permission from: Reed, G. W. and Hill, J. O. Measuring the thermic effect of food. *Am J Clin Nutr* 63: 164-9, 1996.

Meal Size and Frequency

It should not be surprising that meal size is positively correlated with magnitude of TEF, due to increased energy requirements necessary to digest, transport, and store the greater energy load (Figure 37.1).[1] Increasing meal size enhances TEF in young women,[5] adult non-obese women,[6] and lean and obese men.[7,8] The greater the number of kcalories consumed during a meal, the more dramatic the increase in TEF.

The effect of meal frequency on TEF is unclear. Enhanced TEF has been reported when a meal is consumed in one bolus compared the same meal consumed at 30-minute intervals over a 3-hour period,[9] and is unchanged when a meal is consumed as one meal compared to two smaller meals.[10] The potential absolute change in TEF comparing an isocaloric load consumed as one meal or several meals is small, and is not likely to significantly affect daily EE. Thus, any role of meal pattern in overall energy balance is not likely due to differences in TEF.

Meal Composition

Macronutrient composition of the meal influences the magnitude of TEF. Meals containing a high percentage of protein invoke a greater TEF compared to isoenergetic meals with a high percentage of carbohydrate,[11-14] which are more thermogenic than a meal containing a greater percentage of fat,[13,15-17] although there is data to the contrary.[6] Additionally, higher fiber content in isoenergenic- and macronutrient-matched meals may result in enhanced TEF compared with low fiber meals.[18]

An important question to consider is whether alterations in TEF can modulate daily EE. If a high-protein diet increases TEF compared to a high-carbohydrate or high-fat diet, it is possible that high protein diets may increase daily EE, which may explain some of the anecdotal success of high-protein diets for weight loss. However, Westerterp et al.[17] found that changes in TEF from alterations in macronutrient content did not significantly affect daily EE determined by whole room calorimetry. Moreover, others have also reported isoenergetic high-carbohydrate and low-carbohydrate diets did not change TEE measure by whole room calorimetry.[19,20] Therefore, because TEF is such a small percentage of TEE, alterations in TEF induced by changes in macronutrient composition do not appear to increase daily EE, and thus will not enhance weight loss or weight maintenance.

Age, Gender, and Obesity

Effects of age on TEF are unclear, as few studies have examined this directly. From TEF data on 471 subjects, Tataranni et al.[21] reported no overall relationship between the magnitude of TEF and age in men and women, and in women alone, and only a slight negative relationship between age and TEF in men alone. Moreover, other studies have found decreased TEF in older, compared to younger men,[22] but no relationship between age and TEF in women.[23] While there may be a small decrease in TEF in men but not women with increasing age, the absolute change in EE is small, and therefore not likely to impact weight stability in older individuals. More studies are needed to elucidate mechanisms of why TEF decreases with age in men, but not women.

Gender does not seem to change the magnitude of thermogenesis in response to a meal.[21,24] Potential alterations in TEF with menstrual cycle phase are unclear, as investigators have reported increased TEF during luteal phase,[25] decreased TEF during luteal phase,[26] and no change in TEF with menstrual cycle phase.[27] Additional studies are needed to more clearly elucidate whether menstrual cycle phase, or alterations in sex steroid hormones via utilization of birth control pills, have an effect on TEF.

The role of reduced TEF in the etiology of obesity remains controversial. Some report that obesity is associated with decreased TEF compared to age-matched control subjects,[28-33] but others report data to the contrary.[8,12] Potential factors influencing confounding results for effects of obesity on TEF have been reviewed by de Jonge and Bray,[34] who suggested that obesity does decrease TEF. Additionally, obese type II diabetic men[29] have lower TEF compared to age-matched obese men, and insulin-resistant lean men exhibit decreased TEF compare to insulin-sensitive lean men.[35] However, when obese subjects lose weight, TEF is either partially normalized[36] or not different from age-matched lean subjects.[37,38] These data suggest that alterations in TEF are a result of the obese state and not a predisposing factor promoting accumulation of adiposity.

Effects of Exercise on TEF

Acute exercise prior to meal ingestion has been reported to increase TEF in normal-weight men and women,[5,39] or not change TEF in lean men.[35] The magnitude of enhanced TEF post exercise is quantitatively small, with enhanced EE of 4.5 kcal/hr for 4 hours reported by Nichols et al.[39] and 5 and 6 kcal/hr for 2 hours reported by Young[5] with a 630 and 1260 kcal meal, respectively. Mechanisms for elevations in TEF following exercise are unclear, as further research is necessary to elucidate mechanisms responsible for enhanced TEF. Due to the small absolute increase in TEF post exercise, meal consumption after exercise is not likely to increase whole-body EE or help promote weight loss or maintenance.

In obese subjects, enhanced post-exercise TEF occurs following an acute one-hour bout of cycle ergometry.[32,35] After exercise, TEF was elevated 3.3 and 7.6 kcal/hr for 3 hours in insulin-sensitive and non-insulin-sensitive obese men, respectively. While TEF was elevated after exercise in obese men, values were lower than lean men with similar insulin sensitivity.[35] Thus, dampened TEF is a consequence of obesity both at rest and immediately following exercise.

The literature is also unclear with respect to effects of chronic endurance exercise training on TEF. Investigators have reported endurance exercise training to both decrease,[40] and increase TEF[41] by 30% (4.5 kcal/hr for 2 hrs) in men and rats.[42] Additionally, enhanced TEF has been reported in obese and diabetic men following 12 weeks of cycle ergometer training.[29] While TEF was not normalized compared to age-matched lean subjects, these data suggest that chronic endurance exercise training may increase TEF. Thus, while most data suggest that chronic endurance exercise training increases TEF, the absolute change relative to daily EE is small.

Thermogenesis with Chronic Overfeeding

The previous discussion of TEF has not dealt with potential alterations in RMR with chronic dietary alterations such as overfeeding. The literature is unclear as to the effect of overfeeding on RMR. Some investigators have reported enhanced RMR during overfeeding in humans,[43-46] while an equal number have not shown an effect.[47-51] This confusion is not due to diet composition, as there does not appear to be a relationship between macronutrient composition of overfeeding and alterations in RMR.

While the response of RMR to overfeeding is unclear, the effect on TEF is less ambiguous. Overfeeding increases TEF due to the greater total amount of food consumed, as TEF is determined by energy content of the diet.[8] However, it is less clear if TEF to a given energy load is increased during overfeeding. Overfeeding has been reported to enhance TEF during an isoenergetic meal before and after overfeeding in some,[47,51] but not all studies.[49]

The notion of "luxoconsumption" originally proposed by Neumann,[52] and revisited by Miller et al.,[53] where excess ingested energy is "wasted" to minimize weight gain, has not been proven. Several investigators have determined all aspects of energy balance during overfeeding and accounted for the vast majority of ingested energy. They measured enhanced TEF due to a greater total volume of food consumed, facultative energy requirements of excess energy storage, and increased cost of activity due to greater total body weight.[44,49,50] However, 85 to 90% of excess energy consumed is stored and not oxidized.[50] Thus, overfeeding may enhance TEF to an isoenergetic challenge, and potentially increase RMR. However, there is no evidence for "luxoconsumption" in overeating humans, where excess ingested energy is dissipated as heat and not stored.

Cold-Induced Thermogenesis

During cold exposure, the first method of maintaining body heat is shunting of blood from the periphery to the body core to reduce heat loss. As body temperature drops slightly, shivering is initiated to generate heat through contraction of pilo-erectile muscles in the skin, followed by involuntary contraction of skeletal muscle. Chronic cold exposure may lead to cold acclimatization and the development of non-shivering thermogenesis (NST), where other body tissue begins to produce heat which replaces shivering thermogenesis. While NST is well documented in rodents, its role in human thermoregulation during chronic cold exposure is less clear.

Cold exposure in rats results in increased rates of heat production due, in part, to increased sympathetic nervous system activity.[54] Enhanced norepinephrine release[55] and concentration[56] persist for the duration of cold exposure, and serve to increase brown adipose tissue (BAT) thermogenesis for maintenance of body temperature. BAT is a mitonchondrially dense specialized tissue for heat generation found in rodents and animals which hibernate. Heat is generated from uncoupling of oxygen consumption to the phosphorylation of ADP to ATP such that oxygen is consumed, but ATP is not produced. The metabolic energy is released as heat instead of captured in high-energy phosphate bonds.

Norepinephrine is thought to be a vital component to the development of cold tolerance, as daily injections of norepinephrine improve cold tolerance in animals which had never before been exposed to cold.[57] Acute exposure of rats to cold results in loss of body weight, and initiation of energetically inefficient shivering thermogenesis for warmth.[58] However, continued exposure results in normalization of weight as animals eat more when shivering abates due to enhanced activity of BAT for heat production.[58,59]

Humans, however, respond much differently than rats when exposed to cold. There has been little evidence to suggest that humans have the capacity for BAT thermogenesis. Humans have a small amount of BAT, and compared to rodents this tissue is less active. Thus, compared to rodents, humans exhibit different adaptive mechanisms to tolerate cold exposure. Following cold acclimatization, humans tolerate lower core body temperature during cold exposure without enhanced thermogenesis seen in the rat model.[59] As a result, humans acclimatized to cold shiver less during a cold challenge, and adaptive heat production is reduced. One study has shown that it is possible to induce NST through chronic cold exposure in humans;[60] however, others have not replicated this result, as shivering thermogenesis was maintained after cold acclimatization with no evidence for NST.[48] Cold acclimatization is largely an academic question, as it generally does not occur in humans except under extreme circumstances. Normally, human behavior can be changed to get out of the cold or alter the microenvironment to prevent a drop in body temperature.[61]

Over-the-Counter Weight Loss Stimulants

There are numerous products on the market and natural substances in foods and beverages which may increase whole-body EE. While many products claim to have thermogenic properties, the extent to which these drugs enhance EE is often tenous. An added difficulty when assessing thermogenic properties of substances, especially those marketed as an over-the-counter stimulants, is the large variety of different concentrations available to the consumer, both between different products and between batches of one individual product. Additionally, supplements exhibit great variability in drug bioavailability, especially when the stimulant in question is consumed with other foods and/or drugs. Here we will attempt to cover the main thermogenic substances on the market, as well as potential summation or synergy when using these drugs in combination.

Caffeine

Caffeine is a stimulant of EE in both rats and humans. Caffeine ingestion alone has been reported to increase EE by 3 to 7% for up to three hours.[62-64] Dulloo et al.[63] reported that a single 100 mg caffeine dose increased resting metabolic rate by 3 to 4% over 150 minutes in both lean and post-obese humans. Thus, caffeine ingestion may have utility in enhancing daily EE for weight loss. However, some investigators have not observed increased EE with caffeine ingestion alone,[65] likely due to small dose administration, as caffeine's effects on thermogenesis are dose dependent.[66] The mechanism of action of caffeine's stimulatory effect on EE may be a result of the energy cost of enhanced lipolysis from phosphodiesterase inhibition and/or antagonism of adenosine action.[67] In addition to thermogenic properties of caffeine ingested alone, caffeine also increases TEF when consumed with a meal in both young and old men and women.[68] Additionally, caffeine ingestion with a meal partially normalizes the attenuated TEF observed in post-obese subjects.[63]

Not all population groups exhibit similar increases in thermogenesis following caffeine consumption. Thermogenic effects of caffeine appear to be similar in men and women,[68] and in habitual and non-habitual consumers of caffeine.[69] However, older men and women tend to exhibit less of an increase in thermogenesis when compared to young controls.[70] Caffeine-stimulated thermogenesis may also be attenuated in endurance-trained subjects compared to sedentary control subjects.[69] Differences in the magnitude of caffeine-induced thermogenesis in obese compared to lean individuals is unclear. Some investigators reported less of an effect of caffeine to increase thermogenesis in obese compared to lean women,[71] while others reported no difference in the thermogenic response to caffeine in lean and obese women.[72,73]

Following repeated administration of caffeine, Dulloo et al.[63] reported that the net increase in daily EE in post-obese subjects was roughly half that observed in lean controls. This study found that 100 mg of caffeine ingested at 2-hour intervals for 12 hours promoted an 11 and 8% increase in EE in lean and post-obese subjects, respectively, during that 12-hour period, with no effect of caffeine on subsequent 12-hour EE (Figure 37.2).[63] Caffeine administration repeated for 12 hours resulted in an increase in daily EE of 150 kcal/day in lean, and 79 kcal/day in post-obese subjects. Thus, this study suggested that caffeine consumption throughout the day may have utility in promoting weight loss or weight maintenance. However, the effects of caffeine supplementation on weight loss in obese subjects during an energy-restricted diet were evaluated in a 24-week double-blind trial by Astrup et al.[74] These authors reported no significant difference in weight loss during 200 mg caffeine supplementation administered three times per day compared to placebo in obese subjects (Figure 37.3). Subjects supplemented with caffeine reported side effects which included dizziness, headache, and insomnia which abated after eight weeks, with no effects on systolic or diastolic blood pressure or heart rate. Thus, these data suggest that caffeine alone in combination with energy restriction offers no benefit for added weight loss compared to placebo control. Considering the small effect of caffeine to stimulate thermogenesis, it is not surprising that caffeine ingestion alone does enhance weight loss via enhanced thermogenesis. However, based on data from Dulloo et al.,[63] caffeine supplementation may be needed more times per day than performed by Astrup

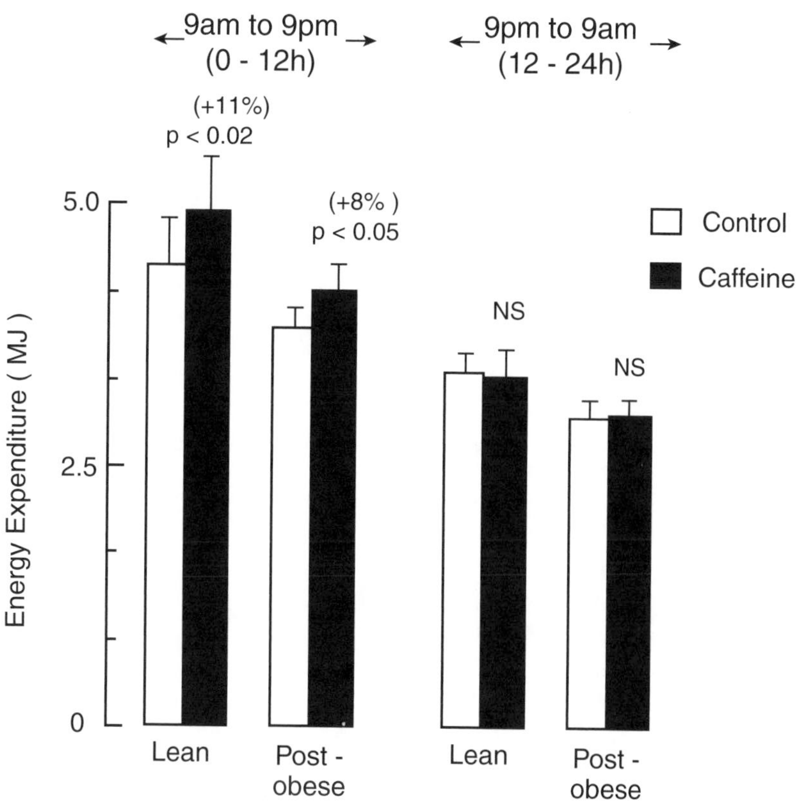

FIGURE 37.2
Energy expenditure compartmented into the first 12-h d period (0 to 12 h) and the subsequent 12-h night period (12 to 24 h) in lean (n = 5) and postobese (n = 6) subjects during a control study (open bars) and during administration of caffeine. Vertical bars represent the SEM values. The probability level for significant differences is for paired data. MG values can be converted to kcal by multiplying them by 239. Reprinted with permission from: Dulloo, A. G., Geissler, C. A., Horton, T., Collins, A., and Miller, D. S. Normal caffeine consumption: influence on thermogenesis and daily energy expenditure in lean and postobese human volunteers. *Am J Clin Nutr* 49: 44-50, 1989.

et al.[74] to significantly increase daily EE. If true, repeated caffeine supplementation for 12 hours during the day may be useful in promoting enhanced EE for weight loss. While not discussed in this section, caffeine ingestion may be beneficial for assisting weight loss via appetite suppression, regardless of effects on thermogenesis.

Ephedrine

Ephedrine is a sympathomimetic agent which increases energy expenditure by enhancing norepinephrine release from sympathetic nerve endings with stimulation of all three beta receptor subtypes.[75] Ephedrine administration alone via intravenous injection has been reported to increase resting energy expenditure by 16% in dogs[76a] and 17% in obese premenopausal women.[76] Moreover, chronic oral ephedrine administration in female subjects induced a sustained 10% increase in resting metabolic rate compared to pretreatment values.[77] Similarly, chronic administration of ephedrine alone to mice increased EE by 9% and induced an 18% decrease in body weight.[78] Chronic ephedrine supplementation may increase the magnitude of enhanced EE compared to acute ephedrine administration.[79]

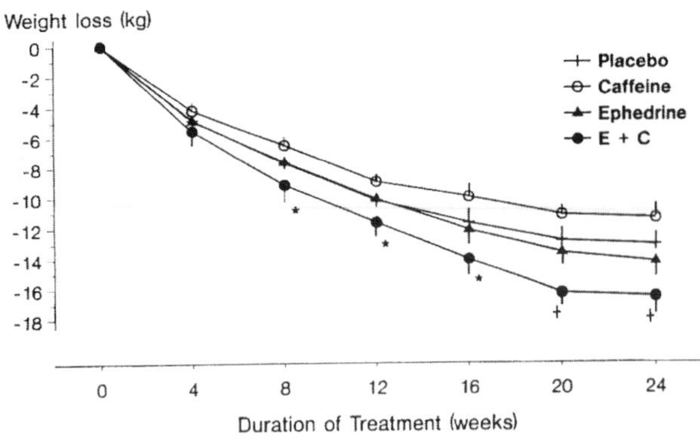

FIGURE 37.3
Changes in body weight of diet plus placebo, caffeine (C), ephedrine (E) or E + C. Means ± SEM are presented. E + C versus placebo: *P<0.04 †P<0.01. Reprinted with permission from: Astrup, A., Breum, L., Toubro, S., Hein, P., and Quaade, F. The effect and safety of an ephedrine/caffeine compound compared to ephedrine, caffeine, and placebo in obese subjects on an energy restricted diet. A double blind trial. *Int J Obes Relat Metab Disord* 16: 269-77, 1992.

These data suggest that chronic ephedrine administration may be a useful adjunct to promote weight loss in obese individuals.

Despite evidence suggesting ephedrine alone can increase RMR, experimental evidence is lacking for ephedrine supplementation alone in enhancing weight loss when combined with energy restriction. Astrup et al.[74] reported that ephedrine supplementation of 20 mg three times per day during energy restriction for 24 weeks did not enhance weight loss compared to placebo (Figure 37.3). Subjects reported significantly more side effects compared to caffeine-only supplementation, which also did not enhance weight loss, with symptoms including insomnia, tremor, and dry mouth most prevalent for the first four weeks of treatment. Additionally, Pasquali et al.[80] reported no enhancement of weight loss with two doses of ephedrine compared to placebo during a three-month intervention.

While evidence suggests ephedrine administration alone does not enhance weight loss compared to placebo, several studies have investigated ephedrine combined with other potentially thermogenic agents on RMR and weight loss. A combination of ephedrine and caffeine administration is more effective in enhancing thermogenesis compared to either caffeine or ephedrine alone,[81] with above additive synergism observed at a dose of 20 mg ephedrine and 200 mg caffeine.[82,83] Additionally, data suggest that addition of ephedrine and caffeine to an energy-restricted diet enhances weight loss in obese women compared to caffeine or ephedrine administered separately during isocaloric energy restriction,[74] or compared to energy restriction alone.[84] Astrup et al.[71] reported supplementation with ephedrine plus caffeine during a 6-month energy-restricted diet enhanced weight loss by 3.4 kg compared with placebo, caffeine alone, or ephedrine alone (Figure 37.3). Similarly, Dulloo and Miller[81] reported that daily administration of 22 mg ephedrine, 30 mg caffeine, and 50 mg theophylline to post-obese subjects decreased energy intake by 16% and increased EE 8%. These data are corroborated by animal studies reporting decreased body weight during eight weeks of daily ephedrine and caffeine supplementation due to decreased energy intake and increased EE in monkeys.[85] These data suggest that ephedrine plus caffeine supplementation decreases appetite and enhances TEE, which may be beneficial for weight loss practices in the obese.

Ephedrine supplementation has also been combined with aspirin, which doubled ephedrine's thermogenic action in mice[78] and enhanced ephedrine stimulation of TEF in obese, but not lean women.[86] Aspirin acts only to enhance the thermogenic effects of ephedrine, as chronic aspirin administration alone had no effect on energy balance in mice.[78] However, addition of aspirin to an ephedrine and caffeine mixture does not further potentiate TEF induced by ephedrine and caffeine alone in lean and obese women.[86] The drug combination of ephedrine, caffeine, and aspirin taken before meals for two months has been reported to induce weight loss without controlled energy restriction in a double-blind experiment in obese humans.[87]

These data suggest that administration of caffeine and ephedrine in combination, with or without aspirin, may increase daily EE and enhance weight loss during energy restriction. The increase in metabolic rate is small and may promote weight loss from appetite suppression when these drugs are used in combination.[84,85]

Nicotine

Anecdotal evidence suggests that smoking either increases metabolic rate, decreases appetite, or both, as weight gain frequently occurs with smoking cessation. Many investigations support the former, as resting EE in men has been found to increase 5% for one hour after smoking 2 cigarettes in 20 minutes (.8 mg nicotine yield),[88] 3.3% over a 3-hour period after smoking 4 cigarettes (3.2 mg nicotine yield),[62] 6.5% over 2 hours following nicotine nasal spray administration,[89] and 6% increase in RMR in male habitual smokers after smoking 2 cigarettes in 20 minutes.[90] While an increase in RMR may be advantageous for weight loss or weight maintenance, the absolute increase in EE from nicotine administration is not convincing. Collins et al.[62] reported the most dramatic increase in RMR (6%) for 3 hours after smoking 2 cigarettes in 20 minutes. However, the absolute increase in EE was only an additional 12.5 kcals over the 3-hour period, which is unlikely to promote substantial weight loss, even if smoking was maintained throughout the day. DIT is not enhanced following nicotine administration via nasal inhalation at 15 micrograms/kg body weight.[89] Additionally, habitual smoking does not appear to influence nicotine-induced thermogenesis in men.[90] Thus, data are lacking to suggest nicotine administration, either from cigarette smoking or nasal spray inhalation, may have weight loss effects via enhancement of EE.

Nicotine may be more potent in appetite suppression than in enhancement of EE. Miyata et al. [91] reported that systemic nicotine infusion decreased body weight in rats via reductions in energy intake, with the most dramatic effects on reduction in meal number. Gender differences were not observed for the alterations in meal size and number and body weight reduction during nicotine administration in rats.[92] Increased concentrations of serotonin and dopamine were found in the lateral hypothalamus following nicotine administration, which suggested that nicotine may exert anorectic effects in part by alterations in these brain neurotransmitters. Appetite supressive effects of nicotine are not as clear in humans. Perkins et al.[93] administered nicotine via nasal spray inhalation at three doses and then monitored subsequent meal size following an overnight fast. Suprisingly, the authors reported meal caloric intake was increased following nicotine administration in both men and women compared to placebo controls. However, the same authors reported that nicotine reduced appetite in men during a subsequent meal test when nicotine was administered following consumption of a morning meal.[94] More studies are needed to determine if nicotine is an anorectic agent in humans.

Only one study investigated gender differences in thermogenic effects of nicotine, where nicotine was administered via nasal spray inhalation.[89] Nicotine was administered once every 30 minutes for 2 hours at 20 micrograms nicotine/kg for each dose. Nicotine increased resting EE in men, but not women. Since nicotine intake is associated with lower body weights in both men and women, the authors speculated that nicotine exerts anorectic effects in women via more dramatic appetite suppression compared to men.

Obviously, cigarette smoking should not be used to promote weight loss, due to well documented health risks caused by smoking. However, since smoking cessation should be a health goal for the population, understanding the expected alterations in appetite and/or RMR following nicotine withdrawl will be vital to attenuate weight gain often reported with smoking cessation. The literature suggests that clinicians and health professionals may expect a slight decrease in RMR, potentially as dramatic as 6% in chronic smokers, upon cessation of smoking.[62] Assuming that smoking only occurs during waking hours, 8 hours sleep/night, a caloric equivalent for oxygen of 4.85 kcal/L O_2, and RMR of 3.5 ml/kg/min; a 6% decrease in RMR in a 70 kg individual would be predicted to decrease EE by only 70 kcal/day. While the accumulation of 70 kcal/day positive energy balance may promote slight weight gain, this simple calculation suggests that enhanced appetite following smoking cessation may be more powerful for promoting weight gain, and thus behavioral therapy may be indicated to help control energy intake.

Prescription Drugs for Weight Loss

Several prescription medications are currently available to physicians to enhance weight loss. Two of these medications, sibutramine and fenfluramine, are systemic agents which are putatively thought to only affect appetite. Orlistat, a pancreatic lipase inhibitor, is not systemic and thus is unlikely to have thermogenic action. The potential thermogenic role of both sibutramine and fenfluramine for enhancing weight loss is discussed here.

Sibutramine

Sibutramine is a serotonin and norepinephrine reuptake inhibitor[95] which enhances weight loss compared to placebo both with[96,97] and without[95] behavior modification. However, thermogenic effects of sibutramine are less clear. Studies in rats suggest that sibutramine increases resting EE via beta adrenergic stimulation of BAT.[98] However, human data suggests that sibutramine increases resting metabolic rate,[99] or does not change RMR or TEF.[96,97] Several investigators have reported that sibutramine attenuates the decline in RMR that occurs during weight loss.[100,101] Thus, effects of sibutramine on thermogenesis in humans are unclear; however, evidence indicates that sibutramine does decrease appetite and/or increase satiety, which promotes weight loss.[99,100]

Fenfluramine

Fenfluramine is a serotonin-releasing agent and reuptake inhibitor[102] which enhances weight loss compared to placebo in both rats[103] and humans.[104-106] Effects of fenfluramine on thermogenesis are not clear, and there appear to be species differences which further cloud data interpretation. Investigations on rats suggested fenfluramine promotes a transient decrease in energy intake, with maintenance of weight loss via enhanced TEF, as there were no changes in resting energy expenditure.[103,107] Others, however, reported that fenfluramine decreased energy intake throughout the treatment period[108] in rats. In humans, fenfluramine appears to act as an appetite suppressant, with decreased energy intake compared to placebo reported for treatment groups.[105] Most investigators report unchanged RMR and TEF following fenfluramine treatment in humans.[105,109-111] However, enhanced TEF has been reported in humans following acute administration of fenfluramine in men.[112] Thus, fenfluramine appears to have little, if any, thermogenic action, with enhancement of weight loss in humans predominately via appetite suppression.

Uncoupling Proteins and Thermogenesis

Uncoupling proteins (UCP) are proteins located in the inner mitochondrial membrane. These proteins dissipate the proton gradient by allowing proton leaking across the inner mitochondrial membrane. This results in a disassociation of respiration from ATP production, with the result of an increase in heat production.[113] Thus, oxygen is consumed and heat is produced but there is no ATP synthesis. UCP are an exiting area of research, as they may be potential weight loss drug targets to promote a less efficient metabolism and subsequent increase in TEE.

The first uncoupling protein, now termed UCP1, was isolated from BAT in 1978 by Heaton and colleagues,[114] subsequently purified by Lin et al.[115] in 1980, and molecularly cloned in 1985.[116] UCP1 is only found in BAT, and the inhibition by purine nucleoside di- and tri-phosphates and stimulation by free fatty acids was initially described in isolated BAT mitochondria.[117] Humans exhibit minimal BAT, therefore alterations in BAT thermogenesis cannot explain changes in whole-body energy expenditure or the propagation of the current obesity epidemic.

Since the discovery of UCP1, proteins with similar homology have been identified. UCP2 is expressed in most tissues, and exhibits 55% homology with UCP1 based on initial cloning in 1997.[118,119] There was considerable excitement over the discovery of UCP3 in skeletal muscle, BAT, and heart in 1997, as it was thought to be a potential regulator of thermogenesis which could partly explain susceptibility to, or development of obesity. However, excitement abated after publications reported UCP2 and 3 mRNA responded unintuitively following various perturbations, suggesting that UCP2 and 3 are not regulators of thermogenesis *in vivo*. Fasting increased UCP2 and 3 mRNA expression in rats[120-122] and in lean and obese humans[123] during a time when whole-body EE was decreased,[124] suggesting that UCP2 and 3 were not involved in altering thermogenesis in response to dietary intervention. However, food restriction downregulated UCP3, but not UCP2 mRNA expression in skeletal muscle.[120,121,125,126] Data showing upregulation of UCP3 mRNA in response to conditions associated with enhanced lipid oxidation,[120-123] in addition to results which have shown upregulation of UCP3 mRNA in rats during intralipid and heparin infusion,[127] suggest a role of UCP3 in fat metabolism and not thermogenesis. It is important to consider that mRNA expression does not necessarily represent alterations in protein content due to post-transcriptional regulation of the mRNA transcript. Thus, measures of protein content and activity are necessary to fully elucidate the potential role of UCP2 and 3 in thermogenesis. However, initial research suggests that they do not behave similarly to UCP1 in BAT and thus may not determine susceptibility to obesity.

UCP Up-Regulation and Knockout Experiments

Knockout mice for UCP1 cannot maintain body temperature during cold exposure, confirming the role of BAT in determining NST.[127] Interestingly, UCP1 knockout mice are not obese, which suggests that UCP1 is not a determinant of obesity.[128] Recent reports indicate that UCP3 knockout mice are also not obese, and they do not show alterations in fatty acid oxidation, exercise tolerance, or cold-induced thermogenesis.[129,130] These knockout mice do exhibit more tightly coupled mitochondria (state 3/state 4 ratio) as well as reduced production of reactive oxygen species. Thus, these data suggest that neither UCP1 nor 3 solely determine metabolic rate or body weight regulation.

Thermogenesis and Obesity

There is no strong evidence that alterations in thermogenesis contribute to obesity. Thermogenesis, excluding resting metabolic rate and physical activity, only contributes roughly 10% to total daily EE. Thermic effect of food is the majority of this 10% of TEE, which has been reported to be slightly decreased in obese compared to lean subjects in some,[28,29-33,131] but not all studies.[8,12] More importantly, it is not known whether alterations in TEF promoted the obese state, or whether the obese state promotes alterations in TEF. Insight into this question arises from investigations on subjects before and after weight reduction. When subjects are studied after weight loss, TEF is either not different from age-matched lean subjects[38] or partially normalized,[36] suggesting that decreased TEF is a result of weight gain, and not a causative factor in the development of obesity. Therefore, it is unlikely that alterations in thermogenesis can explain the increased prevalence of obesity today.

Thermogenesis, NEAT, and Alterations in Daily Energy Expenditure

Thermogenesis induced by drugs, food consumption, or cold exposure is of questionable importance in determining TEE due to their transient nature and the relatively small effect on increasing whole body oxygen consumption. However, fidgeting behavior has recently been described and may contribute significantly to enhance whole-body EE.[132] Levine et al.[132] quantitated EE during 8 weeks of overfeeding 1000 kcal/day in 16 non-obese men. They coined the term Nonexercise Activity Thermogenesis (NEAT) to account for EE not associated with physical activity or TEF. The authors reported that changes in NEAT predicted resistance to fat gain during overfeeding, while no relationship was observed between fat gain and changes in TEF or RMR (Figure 37.4). This NEAT exhibited marked intra-individual variability and may partially explain why some individuals are more susceptible to obesity than others.

Currently, we don't have a conclusive idea of what determines the magnitude of NEAT, or why there is up to tenfold variability in NEAT from person to person.[132] However, NEAT is an interesting avenue for future research which may suggest possible lifestyle interventions or drug targets which could potentiate NEAT and promote greater whole-body EE. One should not discount the importance of energy expended by NEAT activities. Levine et al.[133] recently reported on the energetics of gum chewing, a component of NEAT. The authors reported that gum chewing increased energy expenditure by 11 kcal/hour, a 20% increase over RMR. If gum chewing occurred during the waking hours throughout

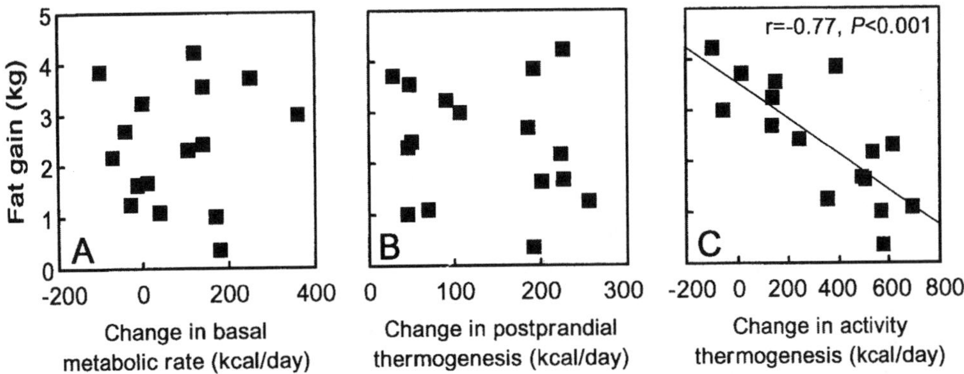

FIGURE 37.4
The relation of the change in (A) basal metabolic rate, (B) postprandial thermogenesis, and (C) activity thermogenesis with fat gain after overfeeding (27-33). Exercise levels and the thermic efficiency of exercise were unchanged with overfeeding, so that changes in activity thermogenesis represent changes in NEAT. Reprinted with permission from: Levine, J. A., Eberhardt, N. L., and Jensen, M. D. Role of nonexercise activity thermogenesis in resistance to fat gain in humans [see comments]. *Science* 283: 212-4, 1999.

the day with no other lifestyle changes, the authors predicted weight loss of up to 5 kg body weight in one year. Thus, NEAT activities increase EE only slightly, but may have important implications for long-term energy balance.

Thermic effect of food has the largest influence in dictating changes in whole-body EE excluding physical activity and NEAT. However, diet composition is the most influential moderator of TEF, more so than age, gender, or weight.[11-17] Thus, differences between individuals in TEF are mostly due to alterations in macronutrient composition of the diet (see "Meal Composition" under TEF) and have very small effects on changing whole body EE. It is therefore unlikely that alterations in TEF are responsible for changes in daily EE in most people. Rather, the amount of planned physical activity far exceeds any small increment in thermogenesis induced by drugs, cold, or diet in determining daily EE.

Conclusions

Thermogenesis, as defined in this section, is an increase in whole body EE above RMR which is not due to physical activity. Meal consumption increases EE, called TEF, which accounts for up to 10% of daily EE and therefore is the most important element in determining thermogenesis. Over-the-counter stimulants such as caffeine, ephedrine, and nicotine are also important in enhancing thermogenesis and reducing appetite, and may be beneficial in enhancing weight loss during energy restriction. Cold exposure also can induce thermogenesis to maintain body temperature. But in humans, this process is largely unimportant except under extraordinary circumstances, as behavior can be changed to alter our microenvironment to prevent prolonged cold exposure necessary to induce shivering and non-shivering thermogenesis observed in rodents. Alterations in thermogenesis are also unlikely to play a major role in the development of obesity and the growing problem of obesity around the world, since thermogenesis is a relatively minor determinant of whole-body EE.

References

1. Reed GW, Hill JO. *Am J Clin Nutr* 63: 164; 1996.
2. Horton ES. *Am J Clin Nutr* 38: 972; 1983.
3. Schutz Y, Bessard T, Jequier E. *Am J Clin Nutr* 40: 542; 1984.
4. Weststrate JA. *Am J Clin Nutr* 58: 592; 1993.
5. Young JC. *Eur J Appl Physiol* 70: 437; 1995.
6. Kinabo JL, Durnin JV. *Br J Nutr* 64: 37-44, 1990.
7. Belko AZ, Barbieri TF, Wong, EC. *Am J Clin Nutr* 43: 863; 1986.
8. D'Alessio DA, Kavle EC, Mozzoli MA, et al. *J Clin Invest* 81: 1781; 1988.
9. Tai MM, Castillo P, Pi-Sunyer FX. *Am J Clin Nutr* 54: 783; 1991.
10. Kinabo JL, Durnin, JV. *Eur J Clin Nutr* 44: 389; 1990.
11. Karst H, Steiniger J, Noack R, Steglich HD. *Ann Nutr Metab* 28: 245; 1984.
12. Nair KS, Halliday D, Garrow JS. *Clin Sci* 65: 307; 1983.
13. Tappy L. *Reprod Nutr Dev* 36: 391; 1996.
14. Zed C, James WP. *Int J Obes* 10: 391; 1986
15. Labayen I, Forga L, Martinez JA. *Eur J Nutr* 38: 158; 1999.
16. Schwartz RS, Ravussin E, Massari M. et al. *Metabolism* 34: 285; 1985.
17. Westerterp KR, Wilson SA, Rolland V. *Int J Obes Relat Metab Disord* 23: 287; 1999.
18. Raben A, Christensen NJ, Madsen J, et al. *Am J Clin Nutr* 59: 1386; 1994.
19. Abbott WG, Howard BV, Ruotolo G, Ravussin E. *Am J Physiol* 258: E347; 1990.
20. Hill JO, Peters JC, Reed GW, et al. *Am J Clin Nutr* 54: 10; 1991.
21. Tataranni PA, Larson DE, Snitker S, Ravussin E. *Am J Clin Nutr* 61: 1013; 1995.
22. Schwartz RS, Jaeger LF, Veith RC. *Metabolism* 39: 733; 1990.
23. Armellini F, Zamboni M, Mino A, et al. *Metabolism* 49: 6; 2000.
24. Murgatroyd PR, Van De Ven ML, Goldberg GR, Prentice AM. *Br J Nutr* 75: 33; 1996
25. Piers LS, Diggavi SN, Rijskamp J, et al. *Am J Clin Nutr* 61: 296; 1995.
26. Tai MM, Castillo TP, Pi-Sunyer FX. *Am J Clin Nutr* 66: 1110; 1997.
27. Melanson KJ, Saltzman E, Russell R, Roberts SB. *J Nutr* 126: 2531; 1996.
28. Nelson KM, Weinsier RL, James LD, et al. *Am J Clin Nutr* 55: 924; 1992.
29. Segal KR, Blando L, Ginsberg-Fellner F, Edano A. *Metabolism* 41: 868; 1992.
30. Segal KR, Chun A, Coronel P, et al. *Metabolism* 41: 754; 1992.
31. Segal KR, Edano A, Tomas MB. *Metabolism* 39: 985; 1990.
32. Segal KR, Gutin B, Albu J, Pi-Sunyer FX. *Am J Physiol* 252: E110; 1987.
33. Swaminathan R, King RF, Holmfield J, et al. *Am J Clin Nutr* 42: 177; 1985.
34. de Jonge L, Bray GA. *Obes Res* 5: 622; 1997.
35. Segal KR, Albu J, Chun A, et al. *J Clin Invest* 89: 824; 1992.
36. Schwartz RS, Halter JB, Bierman, EL. *Metabolism* 32: 114; 1983.
37. Bukkens SG, McNeill G, Smith JS, Morrison DC. *Int J Obes* 15: 147; 1991.
38. Weinsier RL, Nelson KM, Hensrud DD. *J Clin Invest* 95: 980; 1995.
39. Nichols J, Ross S, Patterson P. *Ann Nutr Metab* 32: 215; 1988.
40. Poehlman ET, Melby CL, Badylak SF. *Am J Clin Nutr* 47: 793; 1988.
41. Witt KA, Snook JT, O'Dorisio TM, et al. *Int J Sport Nutr* 3: 272; 1993.
42. McDonald RB, Wickler S, Horwitz B, Stern JS. *Med Sci Sports Exerc* 20: 44; 1988.
43. King RF, McMahon MJ, Almond DJ. *Clin Sci* 71: 31; 1986.
44. Klein S, Goran M. *Metabolism* 42: 1201; 1993.
45. Poehlman ET, Tremblay A, Despres JP, et al. *Am J Clin Nutr* 43: 723; 1986.
46. Welle SL, Nair KS, Campbell RG. *Am J Physiol* 256: R653; 1989.
47. Hill JO, Peters JC, Yang D, et al. *Metabolism* 38: 641; 1989.
48. Poehlman ET, Tremblay A, Fontaine E, et al. *Metabolism* 35: 30; 1986.
49. Ravussin E, Schutz Y, Acheson KJ, et al. *Am J Physiol* 249: E470; 1985.
50. Roberts SB, Young VR, Fuss P, et al. *Am J Physiol* 259: R461; 1990.
51. Weststrate JA, Hautvast JG. *Metabolism* 39: 1232; 1990.

52. Neumann RO. *Arch Hyg* 45: 1; 1902.
53. Miller DS, Mumford P, Stock MJ. *Am J Clin Nutr* 20: 1223; 1967.
54. Hsieh A, Carlson L, Gray C. *Am J Physiol* 190: 247; 1957.
55. Leduc J. *Acta Physiol. Scand.* 183: 1S; 1961.
56. Bergh U, Hartley H, Landsberg L, Ekblom B. *Acta Physiol Scand* 106: 383; 1979.
57. LeBlanc J, Pouliot M. *Am J Physiol* 207: 853; 1964.
58. Foster DO, Frydman ML. *Experientia Suppl* 32: 147S; 1978.
59. LeBlanc J. *Int J Sports Med* 13: 169S; 1992.
60. Davis T, Johnson S. *J App Physiol* 16: 231; 1961.
61. Bittel J. *Int J Sports Med* 13: 172S; 1992.
62. Collins LC, Cornelius MF, Vogel RL, et al. *Int J Obes Relat Metab Disord* 18: 551; 1994.
63. Dulloo AG, Geissler CA, Horton T, et al. *Am J Clin Nutr* 49: 44; 1989.
64. Koot P, Deurenberg P. *Ann Nutr Metab* 39: 135; 1995.
65. Dulloo AG, Duret C, Rohrer D, et al. *Am J Clin Nutr* 70: 1040; 1999.
66. Astrup A, Toubro S, Cannon S, et al. *Am J Clin Nutr* 51: 759; 1990.
67. Dulloo AG, Seydoux J, Girardier, L. *Int J Obes* 15: 317; 1991.
68. Fukagawa NK, Veirs H, Langeloh G. *Metabolism* 44: 630; 1995.
69. Poehlman ET, Despres JP, Bessette H, et al. *Med Sci Sports Exerc* 17: 689; 1985.
70. Arciero PJ, Bougopoulos CL, Nindl BC, Benowitz NL. *Metabolism* 49: 101; 2000.
71. Bracco D, Ferrarra JM, Arnaud MJ, et al. *Am J Physiol* 269: E671; 1995.
72. Jung RT, Shetty PS, James WP, et al. *Clin Sci* 60: 527; 1981.
73. Yoshida T, Sakane N, Umekawa T, Kondo M. *Int J Obes Relat Metab Disord* 18: 345; 1994.
74. Astrup A, Breum L, Toubro S, et al. *Int J Obes Relat Metab Disord* 16: 269; 1992.
75. Liu YL, Toubro S, Astrup A, Stock MJ. *Int J Obes Relat Metab Disord* 19: 678; 1995.
76. Jaedig S, Henningsen NC. *Int J Obes* 15: 429; 1991.
77. Astrup A, Madsen J, Holst JJ, Christensen NJ. *Metabolism* 35: 260; 1986.
78. Dulloo AG, Miller DS. *Am J Clin Nutr* 45: 564; 1987.
79. Astrup A, Lundsgaard C, Madsen J, Christensen NJ. *Am J Clin Nutr* 42: 83; 1985.
80. Pasquali R, Baraldi G, Cesari MP, et al. *Int J Obes* 9: 93; 1985.
81. Dulloo AG, Miller DS. *Int J Obes* 10: 467; 1986.
82. Astrup A, Toubro S. *Int J Obes Relat Metab Disord* 17: 41S; 1993.
83. Astrup A, Toubro S, Cannon S, et al. *Metabolism* 40: 323; 1991.
84. Astrup A, Breum L, Toubro S. *Obes Res* 3: 537S; 1995.
85. Ramsey JJ, Colman RJ, Swick AG, Kemnitz JW. *Am J Clin Nutr* 68: 42; 1998.
86. Horton TJ, Geissler CA. *Int J Obes* 15: 359; 1991.
87. Daly PA, Krieger DR, Dulloo AG, et al. *Int J Obes Relat Metab Disord* 17: 73S; 1993.
88. Walker JF, Collins LC, Vogel RL, Stamford BA. *Int J Obes Relat Metab Disord* 17: 205; 1993.
89. Perkins KA, Sexton JE, DiMarco A. *Physiol Behav* 60: 305; 1996.
90. Perkins KA, Epstein LH, Stiller RL, et al. *Am J Clin Nutr* 52: 228; 1990.
91. Miyata G, Meguid MM, Fetissov SO, et al. *Surgery* 126: 255; 1999.
92. Blaha V, Yang ZJ, Meguid M, et al. *Acta Medica* 41: 167; 1998.
93. Perkins KA, Epstein LH, Sexton JE, et al. *Psychopharmacology* 106: 53; 1992.
94. Perkins KA, Epstein LH, Stiller RL, et al. *Psychopharmacology* 103: 103; 1991.
95. Stock MJ. *Int J Obes Relat Metab Disord* 21: 25S; 1997.
96. Bray GA, Blackburn GL, Ferguson JM, et al. *Obes Res* 7: 189; 1999.
97. Seagle HM, Bessesen DH, Hill JO. *Obes Res* 6: 115; 1998.
98. Connoley IP, Liu YL, Frost I. *Br J Pharmacol* 126: 1487; 1999.
99. Hansen DL, Toubro S, Stock MJ, et al. *Am J Clin Nutr* 68: 1180; 1998.
100. Hansen DL, Toubro S, Stock MJ, et al. *Int J Obes Relat Metab Disord* 23: 1016; 1999.
101. Walsh KM, Leen E, Lean ME. *Int J Obes Relat Metab Disord* 23: 1009; 1999.
102. McTavish D, Heel RC. *Drugs* 43: 713; 1992.
103. Stallone DD, Levitsky DA. *Int J Obes Relat Metab Disord* 18: 679; 1994.
104. Andersen T, Astrup A, Quaade F. *Int J Obes Relat Metab Disord* 16: 35; 1992.
105. Lafreniere F, Lambert J, Rasio E, Serri O. *Int J Obes Relat Metab Disord* 17: 25; 1993.

106. O'Connor HT, Richman RM, Steinbeck S, Caterson ID. *Int J Obes Relat Metab Disord* 19: 181; 1995.
107. Levitsky DA, Stallone D. *Clin Neuropharmacol* 11: 90S; 1988.
108. Vickers SP, Benwell KR, Porter RH, et al. *Br J Pharmacol* 130: 1305; 2000.
109. Durnin JV, Womersley J. *Br J Pharmacol* 49: 115; 1973.
110. Garrow JS, Belton EA, Daniels A. *Lancet* 2: 559; 1972.
111. Recasens MA, Barenys M, Sola R, et al. *Int J Obes Relat Metab Disord* 19: 162; 1995.
112. Troiano RP, Levitsky DA, Kalkwarf HJ. *Int J Obes* 14: 647; 1990.
113. Ricquier D, Bouillaud F. *Biochem J* 345(2): 161; 2000.
114. Heaton GM, Wagenvoord RJ, Kemp Jr, A, Nicholls DG. *Eur J Biochem* 82: 515; 1978.
115. Lin CS, Hackenberg H, Klingenberg EM. *FEBS Lett* 113: 304; 1980.
116. Jacobsson A, Stadler U, Glotzer MA, Kozak LP. *J Biol Chem* 260: 16250; 1985.
117. Nicholls DG. *Biochim Biophys Acta* 549: 1; 1979.
118. Fleury C, Neverova M, Collins S, et al. *Nat Genet* 15: 269; 1997.
119 Gimeno RE, Dembski M, Weng X, et al. *Diabetes* 46: 900; 1997.
120. Boss O, Samec S, Kuhne F, et al. *J Biol Chem* 273: 5; 1998.
121. Brun S, Carmona MC, Mampel T, et al. *FEBS Lett* 453: 205; 1999.
122. Samec S, Seydoux J, Dulloo AG. *FASEB J* 12: 715; 1998.
123. Millet L, Vidal H, Andreelli F, et al. *J Clin Invest* 100: 2665; 1997.
124. Ma SW, Foster DO. *Can J Physiol Pharmacol* 64: 1252; 1986.
125. Esterbauer H, Oberkofler H, Dallinger G, et al. *Diabetologia* 42: 302; 1999.
126. Vidal-Puig A, Rosenbaum M, Considine RC, et al. *Obes Res* 7: 133; 1999.
127. Weigle DS, Selfridge LE, Schwartz MW, et al. *Diabetes* 47: 298; 1998.
128. Enerback S, Jacobsson A, Simpson EM, et al. *Nature* 387: 90; 1997.
129. Weststrate JA, Hautvast JG. *Metabolism* 39: 1232; 1990.
130. Witt KA, Snook JT, O'Dorisio TM, et al. *Int J Sport Nutr* 3: 272; 1993.
131. Segal KR, Gutin B, Nyman AM, Pi-Sunyer FX. *J Clin Invest* 76: 1107; 1985.
132. Levine JA, Eberhardt NL, Jensen MD. *Science* 283: 212; 1999.
133. Levine J, Baukol P, Pavlidis I. *N Engl J Med* 341(27): 2100, 1999.

38

Environmental Challenges and Assessment*

Gary D. Foster and Suzanne Phelan

Introduction

Several environmental changes, including advances in technology, research, and education, as well as economic improvements have brought about the near disappearance of many nutritional disorders such as pellagra, beriberi, scurvy, and rickets.[1] However, while these nutritional problems have declined, other nutritional disorders have increased. For example, the prevalence of overweight and obesity has increased from 43 to 54% of the U.S. population since 1980 (Figure 38.1).[2] Similar increases have occurred in Europe and other industrialized countries.[3]

In this section, the major environmental factors that have contributed to the rise in obesity are examined. In addition, methods of assessing environmental influences at the population and clinical levels are reviewed.

Etiology of Obesity

Obesity is the result of an energy imbalance in which intake exceeds expenditure. Both biological and behavioral factors play a role in the development of obesity.[4] Research over the past 15 years has underscored the importance of genetic factors.[5,6] However, it is unlikely that changes in the gene pool could account for the significant increase in obesity that has occurred since 1980 in both adults and children (Figures 38.1 and 38.2).[2,3,7-9] People of the same genetic makeup who move to industrialized cultures from less industrialized cultures have a corresponding increase in body weight, suggesting the importance of environmental factors in the development of obesity.[10]

Indeed, the environment of industrialized countries has been viewed as so severely promoting obesity that it has been labeled "toxic."[11,12] In order to combat this toxic environment, extreme measures have been proposed, including a tax on high-fat, low-nutrition foods.[13-15] Clearly, the environment of industrialized nations is obesity-promoting.[4,16,17] In

* Preparation of this article was supported, in part, by NIH Grant DK-5614.

0-8493-2705-9/01/$0.00+$1.50

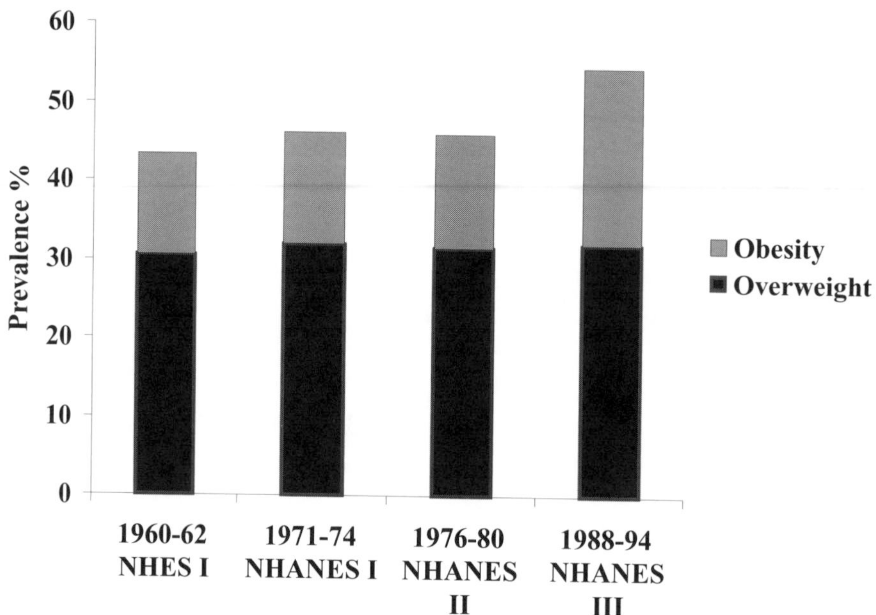

FIGURE 38.1
Prevalence of overweight (BMI ≥ 25–29.9 kg/m^2) and obesity (BMI ≥ 30 kg/m^2) in the U.S. from 1960 to 1994. NHES = National Health Examination Survey; NHANES = National Health and Nutrition Examination Survey. Flegal, K.M., et al., *Int. J. Obes. Relat. Metab. Disord.*, 22: 39; 1998, with permission.

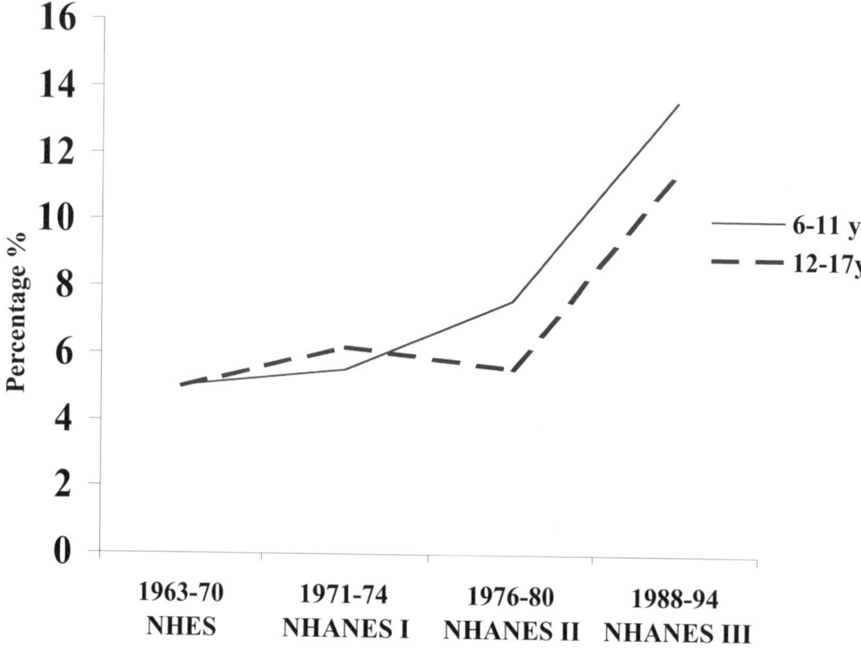

FIGURE 38.2
Prevalence of overweight and obesity (BMI ≥ 95th percentile) in children and adolescents in the U.S., 1963–1994. *Third Report on Nutrition Monitoring in the United States*, U.S. Government Printing Office, Washington, D.C., 1995, 1–51; Troiano, R.P. et al., *Arch. Pediatr. Adolesc. Med.*, 149: 1085; 1995.

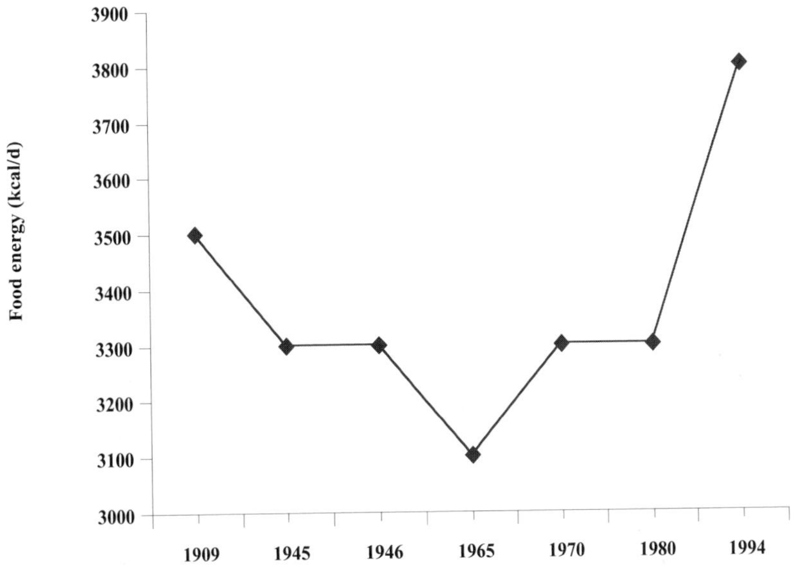

FIGURE 38.3
Food energy per capita per day in the U.S. USDA Center for Nutrition Policy and Promotion, Washington, D.C., 1996, 1–10.

order to better understand the environmental influences on obesity, both energy intake and expenditure must be examined.

Environmental Factors

Energy intake

Despite the increasing prevalence of obesity, U.S. data on food intake suggest only a slight increase or modest decline in energy intake over the past two to three decades.[18,19] Similarly, daily energy intake in England appears to have decreased.[20] However, the interpretation of these data is compromised given the consistent inaccuracy of self-reported food intake.[21-23]

Several other key indicators suggest that energy consumption may have increased. Data from the U.S. Department of Agriculture (USDA) indicate that the food supply has increased substantially over the past century and most significantly over the past few decades (Figure 38.3). Specifically, the amount of food available for consumption per capita per day has increased from 3300 kcalories in 1980 to 3800 kcalories in 1994.[24] Although these data do not measure energy consumption, other indicators, including increases in portion sizes and the widespread availability of high-fat, energy-dense foods, further suggest that increases in energy intake likely account, in part, for the rising prevalence of obesity.[25]

Larger Portions and Decreased Costs

Although little empirical data exist examining secular trends in portion sizes, the "supersizing" of America is ubiquitous. Whereas once only 8 oz servings of soft drinks were

TABLE 38.1

Typical vs. Recommended Serving Sizes

	Typical	USDA
Medium baked potato	7 oz	4 oz
Medium bagel	4 oz	2 oz
Medium muffin	6 oz	2 oz

USDA = United States Department of Agriculture

Young, L.R. and Nestle, M., *JADA*, 98: 458; 1998, with permission.

available, today 16, 32, and 64 oz drinks can be purchased at convenience stores and restaurants nationwide.[11] A McDonald's "medium" serving of French fries was re-classified to "small" in order to make room for a new supersized serving of French fries. In addition, recommended serving sizes are often much smaller than people's perceptions. For example, research participants selected a "medium" bagel that was twice the size of the recommended USDA serving, and chose a "medium" muffin that was three times the recommended serving size (Table 38.1).[26]

Consumption of larger portions is further enhanced by attractive size/quantity discounts. "Value meals" offering larger burgers, fries, and soft drinks for only a small increase in cost have continued to gain in popularity. Similarly, a 22 oz soft drink at a movie theatre costs $2.50 while a drink twice the size (i.e., 44 oz) costs only 50 cents more. In addition, marketing data suggest that supersizing and multiple unit pricing (i.e., "2 for $1.00" instead of "50 cents each") translate into greater food consumption.[11] In one study,[27] subjects poured themselves 20% more bottled water when it came in a two-liter container than when it came in a one-liter container. Interestingly, when the containers were labeled "tap water," participants poured the same amount from each container, suggesting that consumption is influenced by perceived cost/value. Other research has shown that reducing the price of health foods increases sales of these items.[28,29]

High-Fat, Energy-Dense Foods

Of all the nutrients, fat is the most energy dense, providing 9 kcalories per gram compared to 7 for alcohol and 4 for protein and carbohydrate. Since fat is the most energetically dense macronutrient, its consumption is likely to increase the risk of subsequent weight gain.[30-33]

Surprisingly, secular data on food consumption show that the percentage of kcalories from fat has actually declined steadily over the past 30 years in the U.S.[34] and Britain.[20] However, other indicators suggest that consumption of high-fat foods is on the rise. For example, the amount of fats and oils in the food supply has nearly doubled in the U.S. since 1909 (Figure 38.4).[24] In addition, the increased availability of high-fat, energy-dense food is observable in the proliferation of food courts, service station minimarts, fast food restaurants, and drive-through windows. Increasingly, fast food restaurants are found in schools and hospital cafeterias. McDonald's stated goal is to have no American more than four minutes from one of their restaurants. Furthermore, an estimated three new McDonald's restaurants are opened each day.[12]

Food retailers spend billions of dollars each year advertising high-fat, energy-dense foods that bring in the most profit.[17] Correspondingly, consumer purchases of high-fat foods are on the rise. The proportion of money spent at fast-food and other restaurants has risen from 26.9% in 1974 to 38.2% in 1994.[35] A recent study suggests that eating food away from home, controlling for multiple other factors, is associated with higher weights.[36] In addition, home purchases of high-fat, energy-dense foods have risen. Specifically, the

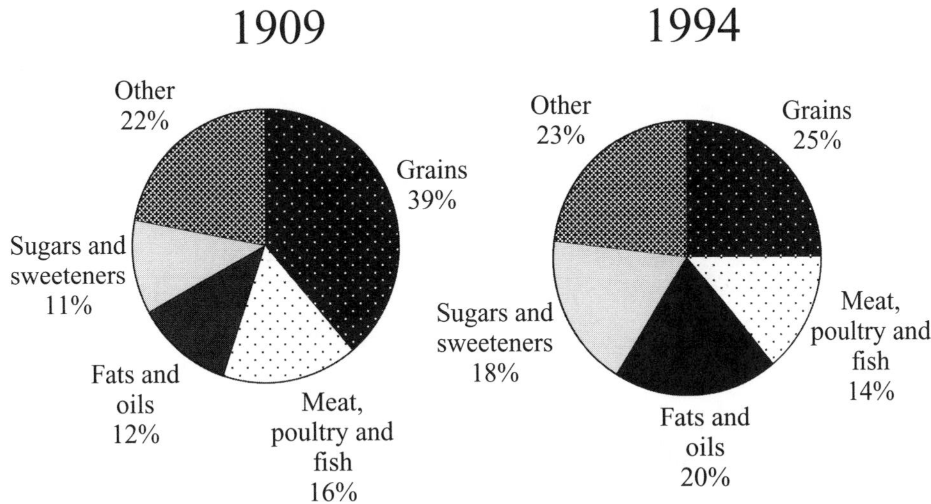

FIGURE 38.4
Sources of food energy in the U.S. food supply. USDA Center for Nutrition Policy and Promotion, Washington, D.C., 1996, 1–10.

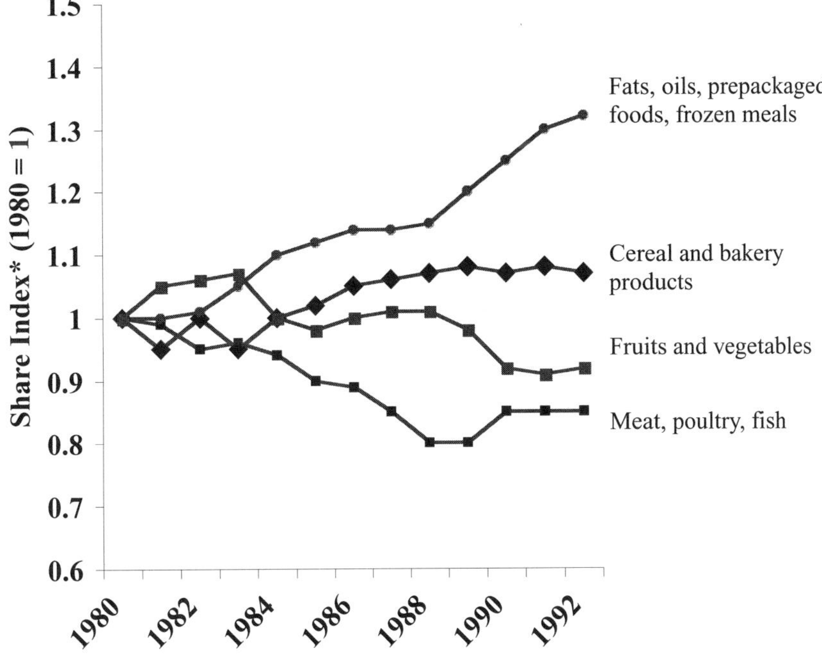

FIGURE 38.5
Relative changes in amount of home foods purchased, 1980 to 1992. U.S. Bureau of Labor Statistics, *Monthly Labor Review,* December: 3–32. * reflects food purchasing habits adjusted for price changes.

proportion of home food purchases of fats, oils, prepackaged foods, and frozen meals has increased more than any other category of food since the 1980s, even after controlling for changes in food prices.[37] The second largest increase was in cereal and bakery products, including cookies, cakes, and doughnuts (Figure 38.5). Interestingly, the percentage of Americans consuming low-fat products has also increased from 19% in 1978 to 76% in

1991.[38] The added sugars in low-fat foods and the belief that larger portions are more acceptable may offset any caloric benefit of consuming low-fat products.[39]

Summary

The available research, based principally on self-report, does not reveal significant increases in dietary intake over the past few decades. However, several indicators suggest that the environment has promoted increased energy intake. Two principal factors appear to be responsible: 1) increasing portion sizes; and, 2) accessibility to high-fat, energy-dense foods at affordable prices.

Energy Expenditure

Although about one-fourth of U.S. adults do not engage in any physical activity during their leisure time, there is little evidence that physical activity levels have changed significantly over the past decade (Figure 38.6).[40] Nonetheless, it is generally accepted that with the modernization of society, energy expenditure has decreased and is at least partly responsible for the increasing prevalence of obesity.[20,41,42] The decrease in energy expenditure is most likely due to changes in activities of daily living.[41] While data in the U.S. are lacking, evidence from Finland and Britain support that decreases in energy spent on activities of daily living and work have indeed occurred.[43]

Table 38.2 lists some of the ways time (and energy) is saved each day. While little data have documented trends in the use of such energy-saving devices, consumer purchases suggest a proliferation. Automobiles are clearly the preferred mode of travel over walking in both the U.S. (Figure 38.7)[44] and the United Kingdom.[45] Purchases of cable television and videocassette rentals have increased dramatically (Figure 38.8).[46] While longitudinal

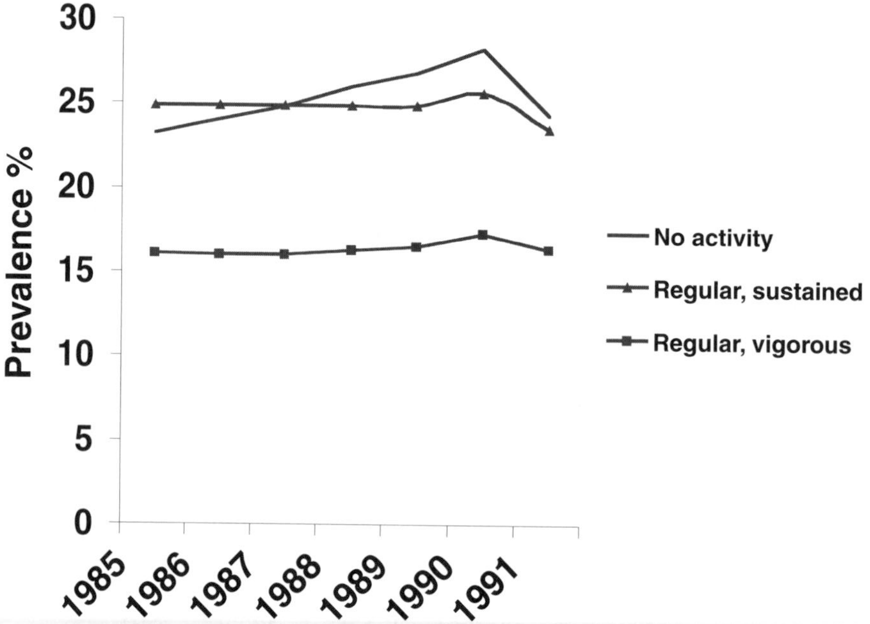

FIGURE 38.6
Trends in leisure-time physical activity of adults age 18+ years. U.S. Department of Health and Human Services, Washington, D.C., 1996, 88-50210, Government Printing Office.

TABLE 38.2

Energy Savers

Personal computers
Telecommuting
Cellular phones
E-mail/Internet
Shopping by phone
Food delivery services
Phone extensions
Dishwashers
Escalators/Elevators
Cable movies
Drive-thru windows
Computer games
Intercoms
Moving sidewalks
Remote controls
Garage door openers

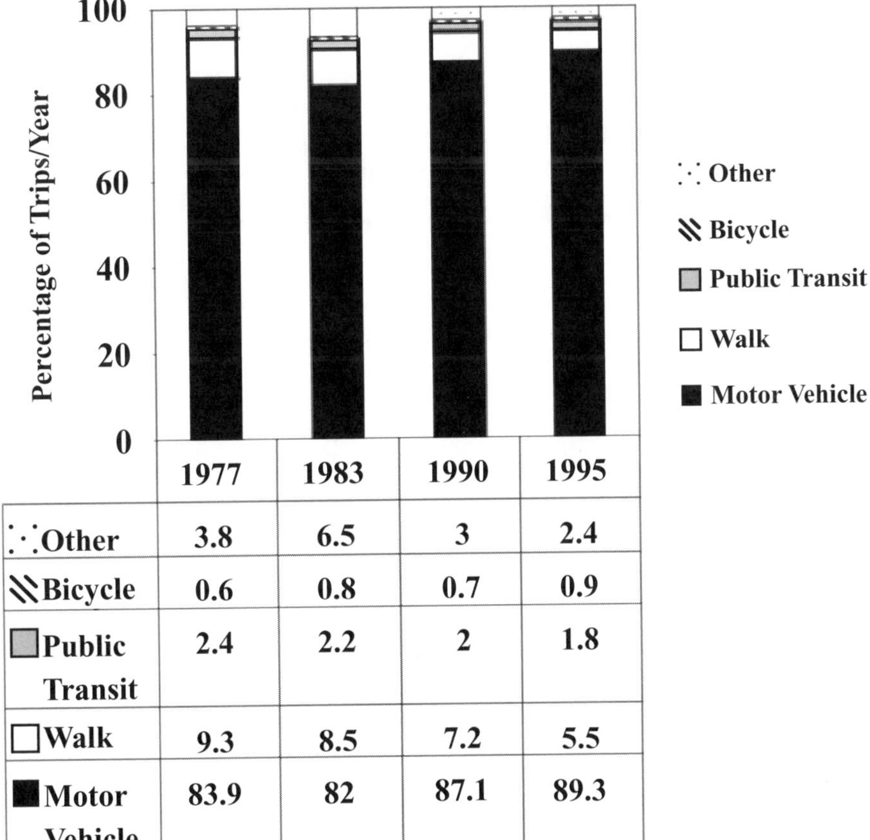

	1977	1983	1990	1995
Other	3.8	6.5	3	2.4
Bicycle	0.6	0.8	0.7	0.9
Public Transit	2.4	2.2	2	1.8
Walk	9.3	8.5	7.2	5.5
Motor Vehicle	83.9	82	87.1	89.3

FIGURE 38.7
Mode of travel in the U.S. from 1977 to 1995. Pickrell, D., and Schimek, P., *Nationwide Personal Transportation Survey,* Dept. of Transportation, Washington, D.C., 1998.

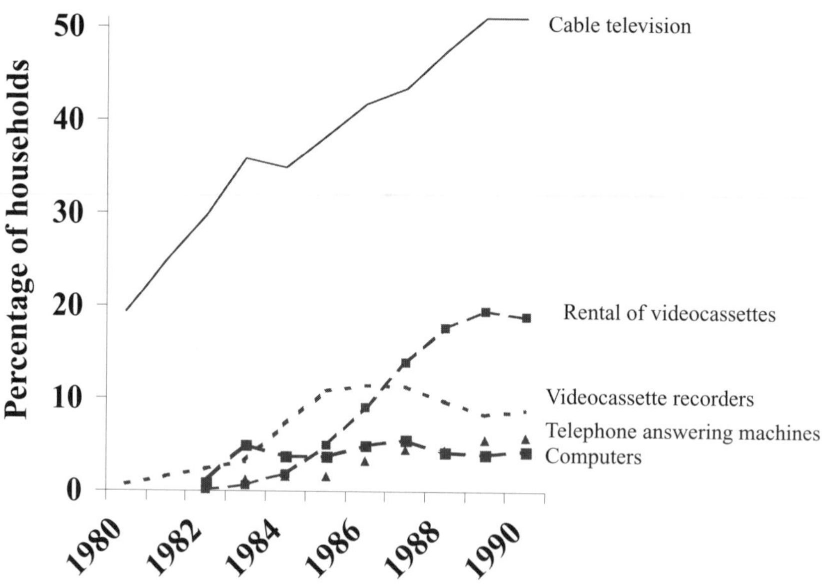

FIGURE 38.8
Percentage of households reporting expenditures, 1980 to 1990. U.S. Bureau of Labor Statistics, *Monthly Labor Review*, May 18–26, 1992.

data on television viewing in the U.S. are lacking, television viewing in England has increased from 13 hours per week in the 1960s to 26 hours per week today.[20] In the U.S., television viewing is strongly related to the increasing prevalence of obesity among children[47-49] and to the level of obesity in adults.[50,51] Research is needed from other countries and for other sedentary activities such as video watching and computer work.

Cultural and Social Factors

The increasing prevalence of overweight is also associated with cultural and social factors. The prevalence of obesity in the U.S. is greatest among non-Hispanic blacks and Mexican-American women (Figure 38.9).[8] This may reflect cultural values and beliefs that limit the motivation for weight control and effectiveness of weight control programs or specific behaviors such as lower levels of physical activity.[52,53] Recent research also suggests that metabolic factors play a role, including decreased energy expenditure among obese African-American women relative to Caucasian women.[54]

Obesity is also more common among low-income populations.[55] Low-income populations often experience differential access to health care services[56,57] due to cost barriers, unavailability of health insurance, and discrimination in health care.[58,59] Economic status may also impact families' nutritional patterns, level of concern about nutrition, and knowledge of foods to purchase and consume.[1,60,61]

Assessment of Environmental Challenges

A detailed review of measures of food intake and physical activity can be found in Sections 3 and 7 of this book and other comprehensive texts (e.g., St. Jeor, 1997[62]). Therefore, only a brief review of assessment tools will be provided here.

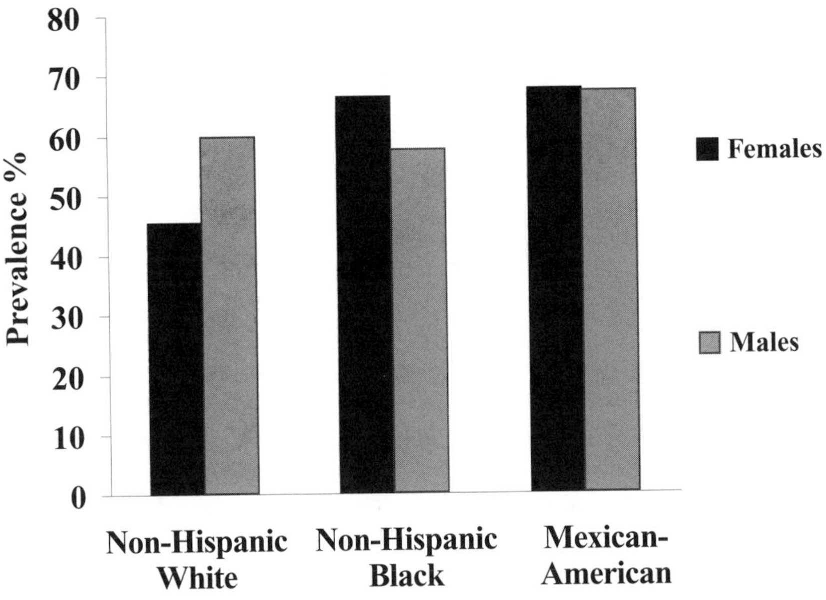

FIGURE 38.9
Prevalence of overweight (BMI ≥ 25 kg/m²) in the U.S. by race-ethnic group for men and women age 20–74 years, 1998–1994. Flegal, K.M., et al., *Int. J. Obes. Relat. Metab. Disord.*, 22: 39; 1998, with permission.

Epidemiologic Assessment

Physical Activity

Although physical activity tends to be over-reported,[23,40] questionnaires are frequently used in epidemiologic studies to classify levels of physical activity.[63,64] Although several physical activity measures exist (e.g., diaries, retrospective histories), recall surveys appear to be the least likely to influence behavior and generally require the least amount of effort by respondents.[40,63] Among the most frequently used measures are the Physical Activity Recall (PAR)[65] and the Paffenbarger.[66] The PAR is available in interviewer- and self-administered versions[65] and categorizes activities by their intensity; the Paffenbarger is a one-page questionnaire that evaluates habitual daily and weekly activity. Measures of sedentary-promoting behaviors, such as television viewing and computer use, are only beginning to be utilized and validated. However, sedentary behavior can be simply assessed by the number of reported minutes per day spent in sedentary behaviors (e.g., watching television, using the computer, video games, and driving).

Food Intake

As noted earlier, food intake tends to be underreported, particularly in obese individuals.[22] Nonetheless, several methods of assessment exist to measure nutrient intake. The 24-hour recall has been used in many large-scale studies (e.g., the National Health and Nutrition Examination Surveys) to assess nutrient intake. The 24-hour recall is typically administered by trained interviewers. It takes about 20 minutes to complete, requires no record keeping on the part of respondents, and, unlike other measures (e.g., food diaries), does not cause subjects to alter their intake.[67] Alternatively, if assessment of subjects' average, long-term intake is needed (rather than a more precise measurement of short-term consumption), food frequency questionnaires (FFQ) are an appropriate alternative. FFQ (e.g., the Block[68]) assess the frequency and quantity of habitual consumption of food items listed on a questionnaire in reference to the past week or month. These are easy to administer and do not require trained interviewers.

Clinical Assessment

Physical Activity

The questionnaires reviewed above (i.e., PAR[65] and the Paffenbarger[66]) may also be useful in assessing physical activity in the clinical setting. Alternatively, a few simple questions may provide a practical and efficient means of assessing physical activity. These include: "How many minutes do you spend each week in planned physical activity?"; "Approximately how many city blocks do you walk each day?"; and "How many flights of stairs do you climb each day?" Television viewing, computer and video game use, and driving time may also be evaluated in the clinical setting by weekly number of minutes for each activity. Finally, pedometers, which provide a count of the total number of steps taken each day, can be very useful in monitoring changes in physical activity.

Food Intake

The most commonly used means to assess energy and nutrient intake in the clinical setting is the food record. Food records are patients' daily notations of the type, quantity, and calories of food and liquid consumed. Patients are instructed to record all meals, drinks, and snacks immediately after eating. Patients may also record the number of fat grams consumed, place of consumption, and minutes of television viewing per day. It should also be noted that food records are commonly used as an intervention tool.[69] If a less reactive and more immediate assessment of intake is required, FFQ or 24-hour recalls may be used. Restaurant eating can be assessed at the time of the clinic assessment with the question, "How many times per week, on average, do you eat at restaurants?".

Assessment Model

The ultimate challenge of environmental assessment is to integrate the multiple factors that influence obesity. As Figure 38.10 illustrates, food intake and physical activity may result from a combination of influences (e.g., large portion sizes, use of labor-saving devices) that interact with cultural and social factors to promote obesity. In this model, excess food intake may be due to larger portion sizes at restaurants, but other factors must also be considered. For example, cultural taste preferences and economic status may also influence restaurant selection. Although distinguishing among the several overlapping environmental influences can be difficult, an awareness of such interrelationships is critical for designing public health and clinical interventions aimed at decreasing the prevalence of obesity.

Summary and Conclusion

In summary, obesity is due to an imbalance of energy intake and expenditure. Both biological and behavioral factors are implicated. Several environmental changes have

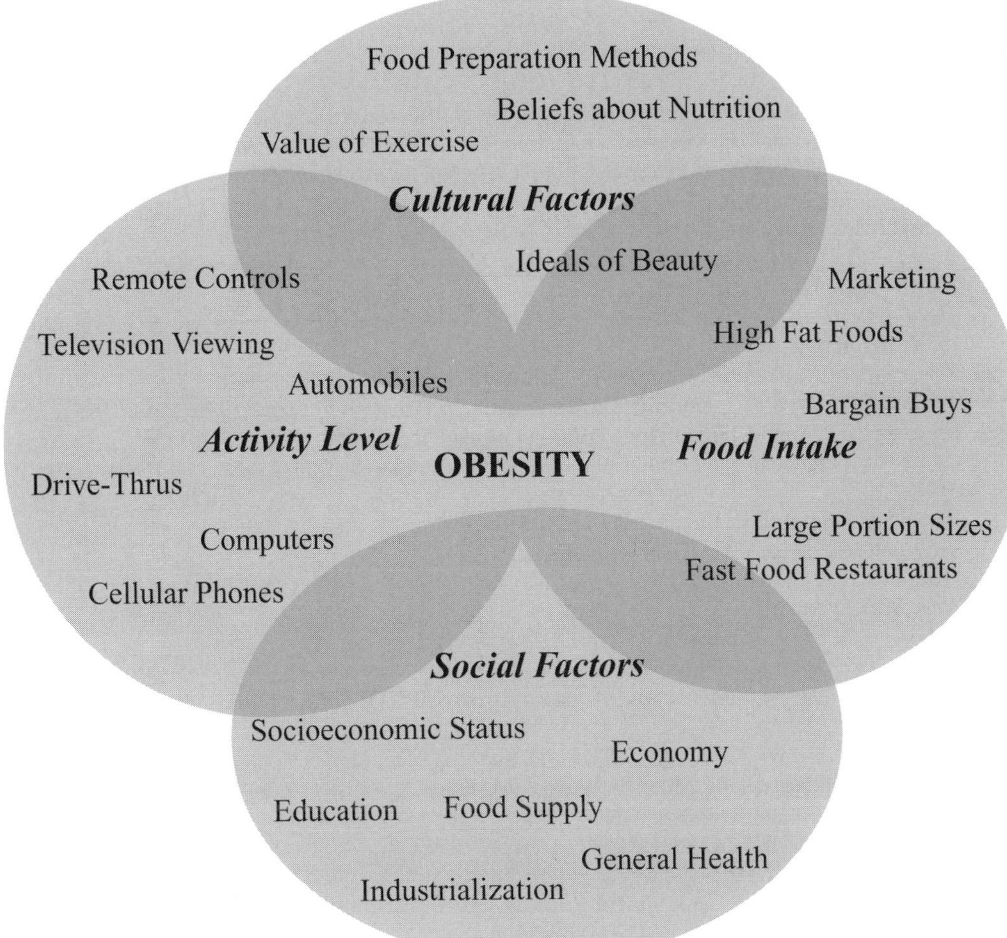

FIGURE 38.10
Environmental influences on obesity.

occurred over the past few decades that appear to contribute to the increase in obesity in industrialized nations. In particular, portion sizes are larger, and high-fat, energy-dense foods are heavily marketed and readily available at a low cost. In addition, the amount of energy expended in activities of daily living appears to have declined.

The problem of obesity may be instructive to understanding other nutrition-related disorders affected by environmental factors, including high cholesterol, hypertension, and osteoporosis. As in the case of obesity, it is likely that a combination of cultural, societal, and other environmental forces leads to the development of nutritional problems in the world today. Clearly, promoting healthy nutrition will require targeting multiple environmental components and encouraging a partnership among various sectors of society, including the government, food industry, and the media.[3]

References

1. *Food, Nutrition, and Diet Therapy,* W.B. Saunders, Philadelphia, 1984.
2. Flegal KM, Carroll MD, Kuczmarski RJ, Johnson CL. *Int J Obes Relat Metab Disord,* 22: 39; 1998.
3. WHO. *Obesity: Preventing and Managing the Global Epidemic,* Geneva, 1998.
4. Brownell KD, Wadden TA. *J Consult Clin Psychol* 60: 505; 1992.
5. Stunkard AJ, Sorenson T, Hanis, C et al. *N Engl J Med,* 314: 193; 1986.
6. Bray GA. In *Contemporary Diagnosis and Management of Obesity,* Bray G.A, Ed, Handbooks in Health Care, Newtown, 1998, pg 35.
7. *Third Report on Nutrition Monitoring in the United States,* US Government Printing Office, Washington, DC, 1995, 1-51.
8. Kuczmarski RJ, Flegal K, Campbell S, Johnson C. *JAMA* 242: 205; 1994.
9. Troiano RP, Flegal KM, Kuczmarski RJ, et al. *Arch Pediatr Adolesc Med* 149: 1085; 1995.
10. Bhatnagar D, Anand IS, Durrington PN, et al. *Lancet* 345: 405; 1995.
11. Center for Science in the Public Interest, The pressure to eat, *Nutrition Action Health Letter,* 25: 3; 1998.
12. Battle KE, Brownell KD. *Addict Behav* 21: 755; 1996.
13. Brownell KD. New York Times, A29, Dec. 15, 1994.
14. Horgan KB, Brownell KD. In *Treating Addictive Behaviors,* Miller and Heather, Eds, Plenum, New York, 1998; pg 105.
15. Ahmad S. *U.S. News and World Report,* 62-63, 1997.
16. Brownell KD,Wadden TA. In: *The Handbook of Eating Disorders: The Physiology, Psychology, and Treatment of Obesity, Bulimia, and Anorexia,* Brownell KD, Foreyt JP, Eds, Basic Books, New York, 1986.
17. Wadden TA, Brownell KD. In *Behavioral Health: A Handbook of Health Education and Disease Prevention,* Matarazzo JB, Miller N, Weiss SM, Herd A, Weiss S, Eds, Wiley, New York, 1984; pg 608.
18. Ernst N, Obarzanek E, Clark MB. *JADA* 97: S47; 1997.
19. Federation of American Societies for Experimental Biology, *Third Report in Nutrition Monitoring in the Unites States,* US Government Printing Office, Washington, DC, 1995, pg 148.
20. Prentice AM, Jebb SA. *Br Med J* 311: 437; 1995.
21. Schoeller DA, Fjeld CR. *Ann Rev Nutr* 11: 355; 1991.
22. Schoeller DA. *Metabolism* 44: 18; 1995.
23. Lichtman SW, Pisarka K, Berman ER, et al. *N Engl J Med,* 327: 1893; 1992.
24. US Department of Agriculture's Center for Nutrition Policy and Promotion, *Nutrient Content of the U.S. Food Supply, 1909-94: A Summary,* Washington, DC, 1996, 1-10.
25. Wadden TA, Brownell KD, Foster GD. *J Consult Clin Psychol* (in press).
26. Young LR, Nestle M. *JADA* 98: 458; 1998.
27. Wansink B. *J Marketing,* 60: 1; 1996.
28. French SA, Jeffery RW, Story M, et al. *Am J Publ Health* 87: 849; 1997.
29. Jeffery RW, French SA, Raether C, Baxter JE. *Prev Med,* 23: 788; 1994.
30. Golay A, Bobbioni E. *Int J Obes Relat Metab Disord* 21: S2; 1997.
31. Lissner L, Levitsky DA, Bengtsson C. *Am J Clin Nutr* 46: 886; 1987.
32. Stubbs RJ, Harbron CG, Murgatroyd PR. *Am J Clin Nutr* 62: 316; 1995.
33. Thomas CD, Peters JC, Reed GW. *Am J Clin Nutr* 55: 934; 1992.
34. Kennedy ET, Bowman SA, Powell R. *J Am Coll Nutr* 18: 207; 1999.
35. Kinsey JD. *J Nutr* 124: 1878S; 1994.
36. Binkley JK, Eales J, Jekanowski M. *Int J Obes Relat Metab Disord* 24: 1032; 2000.
37. Bureau of Labor Statistics, The changing food-at-home budget: 1980 and 1992 compared, *Monthly Labor Review,* December: 3-32, 1998.
38. Heini AF, Weinsier RL. *Am J Med* 102: 259; 1997.
39. Rolls BJ, Miller DL. *J Am Coll Nutr* 16: 535; 1997.

40. US Dept of Health and Human Services, *The Surgeon General's Report on Nutrition and Health.* 88-50210. 1996. Washington, DC, Government Printing Office.
41. Hill JO, Wyatt HR, Melanson EL. *Med Clin North Am* 84: 333; 2000.
42. Weinsier RL, Hunter GR, Heini AF, et al. *Am J Med* 105: 145; 1998.
43. Fogelholm M, Mannisto S, Vartiainen E. *Int J Obes Relat Metab Disord* 20: 1097; 1996.
44. Pickrell D, Schimek P. *Trends in Personal Motor Vehicle Ownership and Use: Evidence From the Nationwide Personal Transportation Survey,* US Department of Transportation, Washington, DC, 1998.
45. DiGuiseppi C, Roberts I, Li L. *Br Med J* 314: 710; 1997.
46. Bureau of Labor Statistics, Consumer spending on durables and services in the 1980s, *Monthly Labor Review,* May: 18-26, 1992.
47. Dietz WH, Gortmaker SL. *Pediatrics* 75: 807; 1985.
48. Gortmaker SL, Must A, Sobol AM, et al. *Arch Pediatr Adolesc Med* 150: 356; 1996.
49. Andersen RE, Crespo CJ, Bartless SJ, et al. *JAMA* 279: 938; 1998.
50. Tucker LA, Friedman GM. *Am J Pub Health* 79: 516; 1989.
51. Tucker LA, Bagwell M. *Am J Pub Health* 81: 908; 1991.
52. Kumanyika S, Morssink C, Agurs T. *Ethnicity and Disease* 2: 166; 1992.
53. Kumanyika S, Wilson JF, Guilford-Davenport M. *JADA* 93: 416; 1993.
54. Foster GD, Wadden TA, Swain RM, et al. *Am J Clin Nutr* 69: 13-17, 1999.
55. Sobal J, Stunkard AJ. *Psychol Bull* 105: 260; 1989.
56. Ginzberg E. *JAMA* 262: 238; 1991.
57. Finucane TE, Carrese JA. *J Gen Intern Med* 5: 120; 1990.
58. Wenneker MB, Epstein AM. *JAMA* 261: 253; 1987.
59. Carlisle DM, Leake BD, Shapiro MF. *Am J Pub Health* 85: 352; 1995.
60. *Ten-State Nutrition Survey, 1968-1970,* US Department of Health, Education, and Welfare, Center for Disease Control, Washington, DC, 1972.
61. Hulshof KF, Lowik MR, Kik FJ, et al. *Eur J Clin Nutr* 45: 441; 1991.
62. St. Jeor ST. *Obesity Assessment: Tools, Methods, Interpretations,* Chapman & Hall, New York, 1997.
63. LaPorte RE, Montoye HJ, Caspersen CJ. *Pub Health Rep* 100: 131; 1985.
64. Caspersen CJ. *Exerc Sport Sci Rev* 17: 423; 1989.
65. Blair SN. In: *Behavioral Health: A Handbook of Health Enhancement and Disease Prevention,* Matarazzo JD, Weiss SM, Herd JA, Miller NE, Eds, John Wiley & Sons, New York, 1984, pg 424.
66. Foreyt JP, Poston WSC. *Obes Res* 6: 18S; 1998.
67. Wolper C, Heshka S, Heymsfield SB. In: *Handbook of Assessment Methods for Eating Behaviors and Weight-Related Problems. Measures, Theory, and Research,* Allison DB, Ed, Sage,Thousand Oaks, 1995, pg 215.
68. Block G, Woods M, Potosky A, Clifford C. *J Clin Epidemiol* 43: 1327; 1990.
69. Wadden TA, Foster GD. *Med Clin North Am* 84: 441; 2000.

39

Psychological Tests

Victor R. Pendleton and John P. Foreyt

Psychological factors play a significant role in many nutritional abnormalities. These factors include mood (depression, anger, anxiety), emotional eating, distorted body image, low self-esteem, poor self-efficacy, dietary restraint, stress, susceptibility to external cues to eat, locus of control, and stage of change (see Table 39.1). They contribute to a number of nutritional abnormalities including obesity, anorexia nervosa, bulimia nervosa, and binge eating disorder. In this section we discuss instruments that assess psychological factors relevant to nutritional goals and concerns.

Obesity

Obesity is epidemic in our modern society.[1] In the U.S. from 1960 to 1994 the prevalence of obesity has increased from 10 to 20% in men, and from 15 to 25% in women.[2] The abundance of good tasting, energy-dense food is a significant factor fueling this increasing prevalence of obesity. Aromas, advertisements, and social gatherings are some of the environmental cues that trigger eating behavior. An individual's susceptibility to external cues to eat, perceptions of ability to control behavior, and feelings of self-efficacy and self-esteem are factors that interact with the environment to determine behavioral responses.

Despite awareness of the problem of obesity in the U.S., and the chronic and debilitating conditions related to it, many people do not attempt to change behaviors that contribute to the problem.[1] Of those who do attempt change, the majority fail to maintain their weight loss goals. Researchers have speculated as to why this is the case. One theory is that, in general, interventions do not match the way people change. This theory, known as the *Stages of Change* or the *Transtheoretical Model*,[3] posits that people move through various levels of readiness to change, from not interested (precontemplation), to thinking about it (contemplation), to planning to do it one day (preparation), to making concrete efforts to change (action), to maintaining successful change (maintenance). The criticism is that traditional interventions are overwhelmingly action-oriented and offer no help to individuals in the precontemplation and contemplation stages who might benefit from more

0-8493-2705-9/01/$0.00+$1.50

TABLE 39.1

Psychological Factors Contributing to Nutritional Abnormalities

Depression, anger, anxiety
Emotional eating
Distorted body image
Low self-esteem
Poor self-efficacy
Dietary restraint
Stress
Susceptibility to external cues to eat, locus of control
Stage of change

TABLE 39.2

Psychological Instruments and What They Measure

	Mood	Body Image	Self-Esteem	Self-Efficacy	Eating Disorders	Restricted Eating	Locus of Control	Stage of Change
RLCQ	X							
SCL90-R	X							
BECK	X							
FRS		X						
EDI2		X			X			
RSE			X					
ESES				X			X	
BES				X	X			
EDE					X			
EI						X		
DEBQ						X	X	
DBS							X	
SOCA								X
URICA								X

RLCQ — Recent Life Change Questionnaire; SCL90-R — System Checklist 90 — Revised; BECK — Beck Depression Inventory; FRS — Figure Rating Scale; EDI2 — Eating Disorders Inventory 2; RSE — Rosenberg Self-Esteem Scale; ESES — Eating Self-Efficacy Scale; BES — Binge Eating Scale; EDE — Eating Disorders Examination; EI — Eating Inventory; DEBQ — Dutch Eating Behavior Questionnaire; DBS — Diet Beliefs Scale; SOCA — Stages of Change Algorithm; URICA — University of Rhode Island Change Assessment Scale

consciousness-raising efforts. Some researchers suggest that this is a contributing factor to the high relapse rate in traditional weight loss programs.

The ability to measure psychological states and traits may facilitate the planning of treatment for disordered eating. We have identified instruments that measure these characteristics (Table 39.2) and describe each of them in this section. Each description explains what the instrument measures, how it measures it, why it is important, administration and scoring procedures, norms, psychometrics, and availability. Many of the instruments do not provide norms for obese populations; however, in light of the evidence indicating no significant differences in levels of psychopathology between obese and non-obese individuals, the lack of obesity-specific norms may not be a major problem.[4]

Eating Disorders

Anorexia nervosa (AN), bulimia nervosa (BN), and binge eating disorder (BED) are eating disorders described in the Diagnostic and Statistical Manual, 4th edition, (DSM-IV) published by the American Psychiatric Association (1994). Anorexia nervosa is marked by a failure to maintain a minimal healthy body weight and a fear of gaining weight. Bulimia nervosa is characterized by the uncontrollable eating of unusually large amounts of food (binge eating) followed by compensatory behavior such as vomiting. Binge eating disorder was proposed as an eating disorder for inclusion in the DSM-IV. Although it was not accepted as a formal disorder, the DSM-IV included research criteria to encourage further investigation of the condition.[5] BED is characterized by recurrent episodes of eating unusually large amounts of food within discrete periods of time, which are associated with feelings of being out of control. Three of the following features must also be present to meet the DSM-IV criteria for BED: rapid eating; eating until uncomfortably full; eating when not physically hungry; and feelings of embarrassment, disgust, depression, and/or guilt. Additionally, the behavior must occur at least two days per week for a period of six months.[5]

These eating disorders are often comorbid with other psychological abnormalities. For example, the cardinal features of anorexia nervosa include fear of being out of control and distorted body image.[6] Comorbid major depression or dysthymia has been reported in 50 to 75% of anorexia nervosa patients.[7] According to Maxmen and Ward,[6] 75% of bulimics develop major depression. Increased rates of anxiety were reported in 43% of bulimics.[7] Restrained eating and emotional eating due to stress are believed to be related to binge eating disorder.[8] Large and unplanned changes in body weight are symptoms of depression.[5] Instruments assessing these eating disorders are also described in this section.

Mood

Recent Life Changes Questionnaire (RLCQ)

Overeating has been identified as a compensatory behavior used by some individuals to cope with stress.[9-11] Life events can be a major source of stress. Some individuals experiencing high amounts of stress in their lives find it particularly difficult to control their eating behavior. Rahe[12] reported that overweight women experienced more recent stress than normal controls. The Recent Life Changes Questionnaire (RLCQ)[13,14] estimates the amount of stress experienced by determining the number of significant events that have recently occurred in the person's life.

The RLCQ is a popular 74-item questionnaire that quantifies the occurrence of specific events in the areas of health, work, home/family, personal/social, and finance. It has been used to assess the relation between stress and general illness susceptibility.[13,14] For each event identified, the RLCQ asks the respondent to give a value on a 100-point scale representing an appraisal of the degree of stressfulness associated with the event. The values are added together for a subjective life change unit (SLCU) total. Normative values (i.e., weights or LCUs) are also available for these 74 items.[15]

Descriptions of the psychometric properties of the RLCQ are limited. Two studies address test-retest reliability. Using SLCU values (weights), Rahe[16] reported an alpha correlation of 0.90 for the RLCQ when given one week apart and 0.56 when given eight months apart. Pearson and Long[17] found the alpha reliability of the RLCQ using SLCU values to be 0.84 ($p<.001$) over a one-month interval. The RLCQ can be found in Rahe.[14]

Symptom Checklist 90-R (SCL90-R)

The Symptom Checklist 90-R (SCL90-R)[18] is a 90-item self-report instrument designed to assess current pathology along 9 dimensions: somatization, obsessive-compulsive, interpersonal sensitivity, depression, anxiety, hostility, phobic anxiety, paranoid ideation, and psychosis. The scales of particular interest to clinicians are anxiety, hostility, and depression because they measure characteristics that may be related to abnormal eating behaviors.[6] The items describe physical and psychological conditions, and subjects are asked to assess the degree to which the conditions have affected them over the past seven days. Responses are selected from a five-point Likert scale that ranges from "not at all" (0) to "extremely" (4). The subscale scores are determined by averaging the scores of the items comprising each subscale.

The SCL-90-R has extensive normative data for psychiatric and non-psychiatric populations, white and non-white subjects, men, women, and adolescents.[18] The subscales have good internal consistency with alpha coefficients ranging from .77 to .90.[19] Investigations yielded Pearson Product Moment Coefficients in the range from .78 to .90, which indicate good test-retest reliability.[19]

A weakness of the SCL90-R is a lack of evidence supporting the discriminant validity of the subscales. The test appears to have the ability to measure general distress; however, its ability to discriminate between types of distress is not supported. The SCL-90-R is available from National Computer Systems, Inc. in Minneapolis, Mn. Their email address is assessment@ncs.com.

Beck Depression Inventory (BDI)

The comorbidity of depression and eating disorders is well documented.[20,21] Depressive symptoms are more severe among obese subjects who also binge eat than among non-bingers.[22] Its assessment in people receiving treatment for these conditions is important because the depression may have a negative impact on program adherence.[23] Intervention outcome for depressed patients receiving treatment for eating-related disorders may be improved by treating the depression first.[24,25]

BDI[26] is a 21-item instrument commonly used to measure depression. The items explore changes in mood, activity level, self-concept, and feelings of self-worth. The BDI has been used with a broad array of subjects ranging from young adolescents through adults. It is easy to understand and takes only about 10 minutes to complete.

Each item offers a choice of four self-descriptive statements that range in severity from 0 to 3. The instrument is scored by summing the values of the individual items. The range of possible scores is from 0 to 63. Cutoff scores for interpretation of the instrument are: 0 to 9 normal; 10 to 18 mild to moderate depression; 19 to 29 moderate to severe depression; and 30 to 63 severe depression.[27] Individuals scoring above 16 should receive further screening.

The reliability of the BDI is good. The test-retest reliabilty has been consistently reported in the range of .60 to .84[27] in nonpsychiatric populations. Internal consistency is in the .73 to .92 range.[27] The BDI is available from The Psychological Corporation, San Antonio, Texas. Their email address is customer_service@harcourtbrace.com.

Body Image

Figure Rating Scale (FRS)

The FRS[28] is a popular instrument used to assess an individual's level of dissatisfaction with physical appearance. Dissatisfaction with aspects of physical appearance is very common among people suffering with weight and eating problems. Indeed, it is part of the DSM-IV criteria for diagnosing anorexia and bulimia.[5]

The instrument consists of a set of nine figures of increasingly larger size. Administration is done in two parts. First, respondents are asked to select the figure that most closely resembles their current size. They are then asked to select the figure that most closely resembles their ideal size. The difference (discrepancy score) between selections represents their level of body dissatisfaction.

Despite its popularity, little reliability and validity data exist for this instrument. Measurement of internal consistency is not applicable with this type of scale. Two-week test-retest reliability was .82 for ideal size and .92 for current size in a sample of 34 men, and .71 for ideal size and .89 for current size in a sample of 58 women.[29] In a sample of 146 women, correlations between discrepancy scores and other measures of self-image were moderate to strong.[29] These results suggest that the FRS has adequate validity and good test-retest reliability. The scale appears in Stunkard, Sorenson, and Schlusinger.[28]

Eating Disorders Inventory — 2 (EDI2)

The EDI2[30] is a popular 91-item self-report instrument used to assess eating attitudes and behaviors along three subscales: drive for thinness, bulimia, and body dissatisfaction. Measurement of these factors is important because of their relation to serious nutrition-related conditions such as anorexia and bulimia.

The drive for thinness and the bulimia subscales assess attitudes and behaviors toward weight and eating, respectively. The body dissatisfaction scale is most related to body image. It assesses attitudes and behaviors toward the shapes of nine different body parts. Subjects indicate the degree to which they relate to statements by choosing from six possible choices ranging from "never" to "always." The three most pathological responses are scored 3, 2, and 1 in order of descending severity. The three least pathological responses are not scored. Scores are computed by summing all responses for each subscale.

Normative data are available for male and female college-age eating-disordered and non-eating-disordered subjects[31] as well as for adolescents. The body dissatisfaction subscale has been found reliable with children as young as eight years old.

In reports on internal consistency, alpha coefficients range from .69 to .93 for the three scales.[31] One-year test-retest reliability in a sample of non-disordered subjects ranged from .41 to .75.[32] Test-retest reliability after a three-week span was above .8 on all scales in a similar sample.[33] The EDI2 is available from Psychological Assessment Resources, Odessa, FL. Their email address is custserv@parinc.com.

Self-Esteem

Rosenberg Self-Esteem Scale (RSE)

The RSE[34] is a ten-item Likert scale that measures global self-esteem. This construct refers to a person's general feelings of self-worth. Low self-esteem is related to various eating disorders[35,36] and may confound efforts to correct dysfunctional eating behavior. Identifying and treating low self-esteem may improve outcome in the treatment of some eating disorders.[37]

The items are statements of self-perception. Respondents are presented with a choice of four responses ranging from "strongly agree" to "strongly disagree." The scale is scored by assigning a zero to low self-esteem responses and a one to high self-esteem responses. Individual item scores are summed to arrive at the scale score. A score of 10 indicates high self-esteem across all items.

The RSE is a mature instrument with norms available from many samples. However, several scoring approaches have been used, which sometimes makes comparisons tricky. For example, the aforementioned scoring method is suggested in the RSE available from the University of Maryland.[38] Descriptive statistics for a Guttman-scale version of the RSE are reported by Wylie.[39] In the Guttman-scale version, higher scores represent lower self-esteem and lower scores represent higher self-esteem. Conversely, Poston et al.[40] suggest that a scoring method resulting in scores ranging from 10 to 40 is the most widely used method. In this method, lower scores represent lower self-esteem and higher scores represent higher self-esteem.

The RSE has good internal consistency. Rosenberg[34] reported an alpha coefficient of .77 for a sample of 5024 high school juniors and seniors. In a survey of seven studies, Wylie reported alpha coefficients in the range from .72 to .87.[39] Two-week test-retest reliability for a sample of 28 college students was .85. With a sample of 990 Canadian high school students, test-retest correlation after a seventh-month interval was .63.[39]

The RSE is available free of charge for educational and research purposes. It can be downloaded directly from the University of Maryland website.[38] The University of Maryland website address (URL) for the scale is http://www.bsos.umd.edu/socy/rosenberg.htm.

Self-Efficacy

Eating Self-Efficacy Scale (ESES)

The ESES[41] is a self-report instrument designed to measure perceived ability to control eating behavior in 25 challenging situations. Perceived ability to control eating is evaluated along two subscales: control in socially acceptable situations and control when experiencing negative affect. For many people, today's environment is filled with opportunities and encouragement to consume large quantities of food, and this is especially challenging for those who eat in response to stress. Understanding a person's behavioral response in the presence of gastronomical opportunities and stress is important in the design of programs to normalize eating.

The ESES is a 25-item Likert scale that presents answers in a 7-point format. Ten of the items make up the social acceptability subscale and the other 15 make up the negative affect subscale. Subscale scores are computed by summing the scores of the associated items.

The instrument appears to have good internal consistency across subscales. Alpha coefficients for a sample of 484 female undergraduates were .85 for the negative affect subscale and .85 for the social acceptability subscale.[41] Seven-week test-retest reliability computed using a sample of 85 female undergraduates was .70.[41] The ESES appears in Glynn and Ruderman.[41]

Binge Eating Scale (BES)

The BES[42] is a 16-item scale designed to assess binge eating in obese subjects. It has also been used with non-obese populations. Eight items of the BES measure binge eating behavior and the other eight measure associated feelings and thoughts. Each item consists of a cluster of self-statements. Respondents are asked to select the statement that most closely resembles their feelings. Responses are given different weights. The scale score is computed by summing weighted scores of the 16 items. The BES does not assess all of the information necessary to make a clinical diagnosis, but does measure behavioral features and cognitions associated with binge eating. The scale score has been interpreted as an indication of severity of binge eating.[43] The range of potential scores is 0 to 46. The higher the score, the more severe the binge eating. A score above 27 suggests severe binge eating.

The original work by Gormally et al.[42] suggests that the BES has adequate internal consistency. The scale discriminates well between people with bulimia nervosa (non-purging) and normal controls.[43] The BES has good test-retest reliability.[44] The BES, along with norms and instructions for scoring, appears in Gormally et al.[42]

Eating Disorders

Eating Disorders Examination (EDE)

The EDE[45] is a 62-item semistructured interview that measures the presence of disorders along four subscales: shape concern, weight concern, eating concern, and dietary restraint. Shape concern is related to general feelings of dissatisfaction and preoccupation with issues related to body image. Weight concern relates to the desire to lose weight and the importance given to it. The eating concern subscale measures fear and guilt about eating as well as any preoccupation with food. The dietary restraint scale attempts to quantify the degree to which the subject is guided by strict rules concerning type and quantity of food.

In addition to subscale items, the examination also has diagnostic items used in making a clinical diagnosis of eating disorders. The EDE was originally developed with individuals suffering from bulimia and anorexia nervosa. Hence, the examination is useful in determining specific areas of concern as well as in making formal clinical diagnosis of eating disorders. It is a mature instrument that underwent many revisions before publication.

The items used in calculating the four subscales are scored using a severity indicator expressed by a seven-point Likert scale value that ranges from zero to seven. These items are organized within a set of 23 higher-order categories such as pattern of eating, restraint, and fear of losing control. The 4 subscales are comprised of these 23 higher order items, with the restraint scale consisting of 5 items, the eating concern scale 5, the weight concern scale 5, and the shape concern scale 8. Subscale values are computed by summing the severity indicators of the related items and then dividing by the number of valid items. A global score, defined as the sum of the individual subscale scores divided by the number of valid subscales, may also be computed. The diagnostic items are scored in terms of frequency; e.g., frequency of binge days over the preceding two months.

The EDE has become the preferred method for the assessment of binge eating. It measures eating behavior using a 28-day recall method, although some questions extend out to the previous 3 and 6 months. Even when administered by trained interviewers, requiring subjects to recall what they ate more than 14 days prior is problematic.

The EDE is designed to be administered and scored by trained interviewers familiar with eating disorders. Administration may take one hour or more when properly administered. The authors of the instrument recommend that the interviewer first seek to develop a rapport with the subject. The belief is that good rapport and a feeling of trust facilitates disclosure and contributes in a positive way to the validity of the process.

The EDE appears to have satisfactory internal consistency. With a sample of 100 eating disordered patients and 42 controls, Cooper et al.[46] reported alpha coefficients ranging from .68 to .82 for the four subscales. Another study measuring internal consistency in a sample of 116 eating-disordered people reported alpha coefficients ranging from .68 to .78.[47] In studies of inter-rater reliability, very good correlations were reported across all items.[48,49] The EDE appears in Fairburn and Cooper.[45]

Restrained Eating

Eating Inventory (EI)

The EI,[50] also known as the Three-Factor Eating Questionnaire (TFEQ-R), is a 51-item self-report instrument that was developed as a measure of behavioral restraint in eating. Measuring restraint is important in the nutritional context of obesity because severe caloric restriction may lead to binge eating and increased metabolic efficiency, promoting weight gain.[51,52] Restriction also has nutritional sequelae such as vitamin deficiency and related morbidity.

The instrument is divided into two parts. The first part consists of 36 true/false questions. The second part has 14 questions presented in a four-level Likert format with choices ranging from *rarely* to *always,* plus an additional question that is a six-point rating of perceived self-restraint. Questions ask about cues to eat, ability to control eating, and willingness to diet. Respondents are asked to indicate how often each statement applies to their personal behavior patterns.

The questionnaire has three subscales:

1. Cognitive control of eating
2. Disinhibition
3. Susceptibility to hunger

The first subscale is related to one's awareness of, and ability to cognitively control or restrain, eating behavior. The second subscale refers to one's tendency to periodically lose control of eating, and the third relates to one's ability to resist cues to eat.

Scoring is described in the Eating Inventory Manual.[53] The control sub-scale has 21 questions, the disinhibition subscale has 16, and the hunger subscale has 14. Each question has a value of zero or one. Individual subscale scores are calculated by summing the scores of the related questions. Scores above 13, 11, and 10 are considered to be in the clinical range for the control, disinhibition, and hunger subscales, respectively.

The EI appears to have good construct validity. Food diaries and doubly-labeled water techniques have been used to assess the construct validity of the subscales. These studies have shown that high scores on the restraint scale are correlated in the hypothesized direction with low levels of caloric intake.[54,55]

The test has good internal consistency (>.80)[50] and test-retest reliability of .91 over 2 weeks.[56] The inventory appears in Stunkard and Messick (1985).[50] The inventory and related scoring materials are available from The Psychological Corporation, San Antonio, Texas. Their email address is customer_service@harcourtbrace.com.

Dutch Eating Behavior Questionnaire (DEBQ)

The DEBQ[57] is a 33-item self-report instrument that measures eating behavior along three subscales: restrained eating, emotional eating, and eating in response to external cues. The diagnostic capabilities of this instrument are useful for identifying overeating triggers when designing effective behavioral interventions, as well as for the identification of individuals with restrained eating patterns.

The instrument consists of questions related to eating behavior. Each item is presented in a five-point Likert response format with possible answers being: *never, seldom, sometimes, often,* and *very often*. Some of the items have an additional *not relevant* category. Subscale scores are computed by summing the scores of the related items and dividing by the number of items. Items scored as not relevant are omitted from the subscale score.

The restraint scale has received most of the research attention. Some norms are available for the restraint scale.[58] In general, they indicate that women have higher restraint scores than men, and that obese people have higher restraint scores than non-obese. Internal consistency of the scales was reported in the range from .80 to .95.[58] Two-week test-retest reliability of the restraint scale was .92.[56] The DEBQ is published in Van Strien et al.[57] and in Wardle.[59]

Locus of Control

Dieting Beliefs Scale (DBS)

The DBS[60] is a 16-item scale that measures weight-specific locus of control. Weight locus of control is a method for categorizing beliefs about factors influencing weight. Individuals with an internal locus of control have the expectancy that they can control, to some extent, their own weight. An external locus of control implies a more fatalistic orientation marked by beliefs that weight is determined by factors outside of personal control, e.g., genetics, environment, and/or social context.

The utility of this instrument is in the planning of treatment for obese and overweight people. Theoretically, individuals who believe they have control over factors determining their weight would be expected to have greater success in weight management programs. Identifying individuals with an external locus of control might be valuable in the process of treatment planning because it would cue the counselor to be particularly mindful to avoid interventions that might inadvertently reinforce pre-existing negative expectations. For example, very modest and frequently measured short term goals may be set for people with external loci of control in an effort to encourage them toward more positive expectations.

The 16 items are statements expressing either internal or external locus of control viewpoints: eight are internal and eight are external. The items are presented in a six-point Likert format ranging from *not at all descriptive of my beliefs* (1) to *very descriptive of my beliefs* (6). Eight of the items are reverse scored. The instrument is scored in the internal direction so that high scores indicate more of an internal locus of control.

The DBS has three subscales: internal control, uncontrolled factors, and environmental factors. The internal control subscale is related to the belief that individuals can control their weights through internal means such as willpower and effort. The uncontrolled factors subscale is associated with belief in the importance of factors such as genetics and fate. The environmental factors subscale is related to beliefs in the importance of context and social setting. The subscales are scored by summing the scores of the individual items that make up the scale.

This scale demonstrates moderate internal consistency (Chronbach's alpha = .69) and good stability in a sample of undergraduate students.[60] The DBS is published in Stotland and Zuroff.[60]

Stage of Change

Stages of Change Algorithm (SOCA)

The SOCA[61] is a self-report instrument that assesses weight loss activities and intentions. The instrument is based on the transtheoretical model,[62] which conceptualizes change as a five-stage process. The stages are precontemplation, contemplation, planning, action, and maintenance. The purpose of the model is to maximize successful behavior change. The model posits that optimal intervention strategies vary according to a person's position in the change process. The purpose of the SOCA is to facilitate treatment planning by identifying the individual's position in the process. Persons in the precontemplation stage may not be at all concerned with their condition. These individuals might benefit from efforts to raise their awareness and to personalize their risk factors. People in the contemplation stage may be concerned but not yet decided on taking action. Such people might benefit from information regarding possible treatment alternatives. The preparation stage is characterized by people who have decided to do something about their condition but who have not yet begun. Encouragement to take action and to make a commitment to their health may help people in this stage to move to the action stage. Individuals who are ready to take action, or who have recently begun taking action, may benefit most from behavioral interventions such as goal setting and self-monitoring. Moral support and recognition might be best for people in the maintenance stage. The SOCA uses only four of the stages: precontemplation, contemplation, action, and maintenance. The model is of particular interest in the context of nutrition because of the refractory nature of dysfunctional eating behavior.

The SOCA consists of four yes/no items. The scoring is simple and the determination of the person's stage of change is quickly determined.[61] Data describing the reliability of the SOCA for weight loss are not available. The SOCA was found to be reliable when applied to similar problems. For example, in their investigation of the processes of change in smoking-related behavior, Prochaska et al. observed alpha coefficients ranging from .69 to .92, with the majority being above .80.[63] The SOCA is published in Rossi et al.[61]

University of Rhode Island Change Assessment Scale (URICA)

The URICA[64,65] is a 32-item Likert scale designed to measure a person's position in the four-stage change process: precontemplation, contemplation, action, and maintenance. It is similar in concept to the SOCA. It is different in that it has 28 more items, and each stage of change is implemented as a scale. The URICA produces a score for each scale. When viewed together, the scale scores can be interpreted as a profile. This approach is richer than the SOCA because it provides a framework that allows attitudes and behaviors characteristic of different stages of change to coexist in a single individual. Thus, the URICA may be able to detect gradual shifts from one stage to another. The URICA is general in format and not specific to any particular problem area. It has been widely used across an array of problem areas, including a sample of 184 people in a weight control program.

Items are presented in a five-point format. Scale scores are computed by summing the responses to the scale items. Good internal consistency is indicated by numerous studies reporting alpha coefficients ranging from .69 to .89 across all scales.[64-66] The general version of the URICA is published in McConnaughy et al.[64] A version designed for use in a weight control context is available in Rossi et al.[61]

References

1. Mokdad AH, Serdula MK, Dietz WH, et al. *JAMA* 282: 1519; 1999.
2. AACE/ACE Obesity Task Force. AACE/ACE *Position Statement on the Prevention, Diagnosis and Treatment of Obesity,* Am Assoc Endocrinol Am Coll Endocrinol, 1998.
3. Prochaska JO, Norcross JC, DiClemente CC. *Changing for Good: The Revolutionary Program that Explains the Six Stages of Change and Teaches You How to Free Yourself From Bad Habits.* W. Morrow, New York; 1994.
4. Perri MG, Nezu AM, Viegener BJ. *Improving the Long-Term Management of Obesity: Theory, Research, and Clinical Guidelines.* John Wiley & Sons, New York; 1992.
5. Am Psychiatric Assoc *Diagnostic and Statistical Manual of Mental Disorders* (4th ed). Washington, DC, 1994.
6. Maxmen JS, Ward NG. *Essential Psychopathology and Its Treatment.* Norton, New York 1995.
7. Halmi KA, Eckert E, Marchi P, et al. *Arch Gen Psychiatry* 48: 712; 1991.
8. Polivy J, Herman CP. In: *Binge Eating: Nature, Assessment and Treatment.* Fairburn CG, Wilson GT, Eds, Guilford, New York 1993; pg 173.
9. Heatherton TF, Baumeister RF. *Psych Bull* 110: 86; 1991.
10. Pendleton VR, et al. *Eat Disord* (in press).
11. Striegel-Moore R. *Addict Behav* 20: 713; 1995.
12. Rahe RH. In: *Obesity Assessment: Tools, Methods, Interpretations.* St. Jeor ST, Ed, Chapman & Hall, New York, 1997; pg 400.
13. Rahe RH. *Internat J Psychiat Med* 6: 133; 1975.
14. Rahe RH. In: *Comprehensive Textbook of Psychiatry,* Kaplan HI, Sadock BJ, Eds, Williams & Wilkins, Baltimore 1995; pg 1545.
15. Miller GD, Harrington ME. In: *Obesity Assessment: Tools, Methods, Interpretations.* St. Jeor, ST Ed) Chapman & Hall, New York 1997; pg 457.
16. Rahe RH. *Psychosomatic Med* 40: 95; 1978.
17. Pearson JE, Long TJ. *Eval Counsel Devel* 18: 72; 1985.
18. Derogatis LR. *Symptom Checklist-90-R Administration, Scoring and Procedures Manual* National Computer Systems, Minneapolis, 1994.
19. Derogatis LR, Cleary PA. *J Clin Psychol* 33: 891; 1977.
20. Garner DM, Olmstead MP, Davis R, et al. *Internat J Eat Disord* 9: 1; 1990.
21. Strober M, Katz JL. *Internat J Eat Disord* 6: 171; 1987.
22. Marcus MD. In: *Binge Eating: Nature, Assessment, and Treatment.* Fairburn CG, Wilson GT, Eds, Guilford Press, New York; 1993; pg 77.
23. Webber EM. *J Psychol* 128: 339; 1994.
24. Clark MM, Niaura R, King TK, Pera V. *Addict Behav* 21: 509; 1996.
25. Tanco S, Linden W, Earle T. *Internat J Eat Disord* 23: 325; 1998.
26. Beck AT, Ward C, Mendelson M, et al. *Arch Gen Psychiat* 4: 53; 1961.
27. Beck AT, Steer RA, Garbin MG. *Clin Psychol Rev* 8: 77; 1988.
28. Stunkard A, Sorenson T, Schlusinger F. In: *The Genetics of Neurological and Psychiatric Disorders.* Kety S, Rowland LP, Sidman RL, Matthysse SW, Eds, Raven, New York, 1983; pg 115.

29. Thompson JK, Atalbe MN. *Internat J Eat Disord* 10: 615; 1991.
30. Garner DM, Olmnsted MP, Polivy J. *Internat J Eat Disord* 2: 15; 1983.
31. Garner DM. *Eating Disorder Inventory-2 Manual* Psychological Assessment Resources Inc, Odessa, FL; 1991.
32. Crowther JH, Lilly RS, Crawford PA, et al. Am Psychol Assoc Nat Convention, Boston; 1990.
33. Wear RW, Pratz O, *Internat J Eat Disord* 6: 767; 1987.
34. Rosenberg M. *Society and the Adolescent Self Image* Princeton University Press, Princeton NJ; 1965.
35. Herman CP, Polivy J. In: *The Psychobiology of Bulimia*. Pirke K, Vandereycken W, Ploog D, Eds, Springer-Verlag, Munich; 1988.
36. Polivy J, Heatherton TF, Herman CP. *J Abnormal Psychol* 97: 354; 1988.
37. Fairburn CG, Marcus MD, Wilson GT. In: *Binge Eating: Nature, Assessment, and Treatment.* Fairburn CG, Wilson GT, Eds, Guilford, New York 1993; pg 361.
38. Rosenberg M. *The Rosenburg Self-Esteem Scale* University of Maryland, College Park, 1965.
39. Wylie RC *Measures of Self-Concept* University of Nebraska Press, Lincoln, 1989.
40. Poston WSC, Goodrick GK, Foreyt JP. In: *Obesity Assessment: Tools, Methods, Interpretations.* St. Jeor ST, Ed, Chapman & Hall, New York, 1997; 425.
41. Glynn SM, Ruderman AJ. *Cognitive Therapy Res* 10: 403; 1986.
42. Gormally J, Black S, Daston S, Rardin D. *Addictive Behav* 7: 47; 1982.
43. Marcus MD, Wing RR, Hopkins JJ. *Consult Clin Psychol* 3: 433; 1988.
44. Wilson GT. In *Binge Eating: Nature, Assessment, and Treatment.* Fairburn CG, Wilson GT, Eds, Guilford, New York, 1993; pg 227.
45. Fairburn CG, Cooper Z. In: *Binge Eating: Nature, Assessment, and Treatment.* Fairburn CG, Wilson GT, Eds, Guilford, New York, 1993; pg 317.
46. Cooper Z, Cooper PJ, Fairburn CG. *Br J Psychiat* 154: 807; 1989.
47. Beumont PJ, Kopec-Schrader EM, Touyz SW. *Aus N Zea J Psychiat* 27: 506; 1993.
48. Cooper Z, Fairburn CG. *Internat J Eat Disord* 6: 1; 1987.
49. Wilson GT, Smith D. *Internat J Eat Disord* 8: 173; 1989.
50. Stunkard AJ, Messick S. *J Psychosomat Res* 29: 71; 1985.
51. Klesges RC, Isbell TR, Klesges LM. *J Abnormal Psychol* 101: 668; 1992.
52. Polivy JH, Herman CP. *Am Psychol* 40: 193; 1985.
53. Stunkard AJ, Messick S. *Eating Inventory Manual* Harcourt Brace Jovanovich San Antonio 1988.
54. Tuschi RL, Platte P, Laessie RG, et al. *Am J Clin Nutr* 52: 81; 1990.
55. Laessie RG, Tuschi RJ, Kotthaus BC, Pirke KM. *J Abnormal Psychol* 98: 504; 1990.
56. Allison DB, Kalinsky LB, Gorman BS. *Psychol Assess* 4: 391; 1992.
57. Van Strien T, Frijters JE, Bergers GP, Defares PB. *Internat J Eat Disord* 5: 295; 1986.
58. Gorman BS, Allison DB. In: *Handbook of Assessment Methods for Eating Disorders and Weight Related Problems*. Allison DB, Ed, Sage, London 1995; pg 149.
59. Wardle J. *J Personal Assess* 31: 161; 1987.
60. Stotland S Zuroff, DC. *J Personal Assess* 54: 191; 1990.
61. Rossi JS, Rossi SR, Velicer WF, Prochaska JO. In: *Handbook of Assessment Methods for Eating Behaviors and Weight Related Problems.* Allison DB, Ed, Sage, London 1995; pg 387.
62. Prochaska JO, DeClemente CC, Norcross JC. *Am Psychol* 47: 1102; 1992.
63. Prochaska JO, Velicer WF, DiClemente CC, Fava J. *J Clin Consult Psychol* 56: 520; 1988.
64. McConnaughy EA, DiClemente CC, Prochaska JO, Velicer WF. *Psychotherapy* 26: 494; 1989.
65. McConnaughy EA, Prochaska JO, Velicer WF. *Psychotherapy* 20: 368; 1983.
66. DiClemente CC, Hughes SO. *J Substance Abuse* 2: 217; 1990.

Part VI

Modified Diets

40

Vegetarian Diets in Health Promotion and Disease Prevention

Claudia S. Plaisted and Kelly M. Adams

Overview/Introduction

Vegetarianism is rapidly growing in popularity. Technically defined, vegetarians are individuals who do not eat any meat, poultry, or seafood.[1,2] Estimates on the number of vegetarians in the United States vary greatly according to the definition of vegetarianism provided in the survey. True vegetarians make up about 1% of the population, representing approximately two million people, according to a 1997 poll.[3] A higher percentage of teenagers than adults follow a vegetarian diet — almost 2%.[3]

Vegetarian dietary patterns can represent an exceptionally healthy way of eating. They are typically rich in vitamins, minerals, phytochemicals, and fiber while often also low in fat, saturated fat, and cholesterol.[1,4] However, each individual diet will need to be assessed for its nutritional adequacy. This section provides some guidance in characterizing vegetarian dietary patterns, health benefits, and concerns as well as identifying sources of various nutrients that may be marginal in many vegetarian diets.

Characteristics of Vegetarian Eating Styles

When working with someone who follows a vegetarian diet, it is important to ask him a variety of questions about his usual dietary patterns. Many people consider themselves to be vegetarian if they eat non-flesh foods several days a week. Others claim to be vegetarians when they consume fish or poultry. Table 40.1 lists the types of vegetarian diets and describes what foods fall into each category.

In popular culture, many diets incorporate principles of vegetarianism and may represent more restrictive ways of eating, as described in Table 40.2. For the purposes of this section, "vegetarian" will refer to an individual following a lacto and/or ovo or vegan dietary pattern.

0-8493-2705-9/01/$0.00+$1.50

TABLE 40.1
Types of Vegetarian Diets

Vegan	Consumes nuts, fruits, grains, legumes, and vegetables. Does not consume animal-based food products, including eggs, dairy products, red meats, poultry, or seafood. Some vegetarians may avoid foods with animal processing (honey, sugar, vinegar, wine, beer).
Lacto-Vegetarian	Consumes milk and other dairy products, nuts, fruits, grains, legumes, and vegetables. Does not consume eggs, red meats, poultry, or seafood.
Ovo-Vegetarian	Consumes eggs, nuts, fruits, grains, legumes, and vegetables. Does not consume milk or dairy, red meats, poultry, or seafood.
Lacto-Ovo Vegetarian	Consumes milk and other dairy products, eggs, nuts, fruits, grains, legumes, and vegetables. Does not consume red meats, poultry, or seafood.
Pollo-Vegetarian[a]	Not technically considered a vegetarian type of diet, although often referred to as "vegetarian" in popular culture. Consumes milk and other dairy products, eggs, nuts, fruits, grains, legumes, vegetables, and poultry.
Peche-Vegetarian also called pesco- and pecto-vegetarian[a]	Not technically considered a vegetarian type of diet, although often referred to as "vegetarian" in popular culture. Consumes milk and other dairy products, eggs, nuts, fruits, grains, legumes, vegetables, and seafood.
Omnivore	Consumes from a wide variety of foods, including meats, grains, fruits, vegetables, legumes and dairy products. Individuals who consume red meats (beef, pork, lamb, etc.), poultry, seafood, or any still or once living non-plant-based matter are not vegetarians.

[a] This is not technically a vegetarian diet, although it is often referred to as such.

TABLE 40.2
Types of Popular Diets Incorporating Various Principles of Vegetarianism[a]

Fad diets	Popular weight loss diets often incorporate various principles of vegetarianism, although not generally in nutritious, balanced ways. The cabbage soup diet is an example, which is based on consuming only a vegetable soup based on cabbage as a weight-loss technique.
Fruitarian	Consumes botanical fruits (including nuts and seeds); avoids meats, poultry, seafood, dairy, eggs, and vegetables. May avoid legumes.
Macrobiotic	Largely based on grains and in-season foods, including vegetables (except those of the nightshade family), sea vegetables, soups, and beans. Nuts and seeds are not consumed on a daily basis; fruits are included with the exception of tropical fruits. Seafood is sometimes included as well. Asian foods contribute significantly to food choices. This is an example of a diet following a food-combining philosophy.
Natural hygiene or raw foods diet	Generally raw vegetables, fruits, whole grains or sprouted grains (in some cases may be cooked), sprouted or non-sprouted legumes, nuts, and seeds. Some individuals may consume raw dairy products. There is great variation in this diet plan: many followers do consume cooked foods, and some consume meat as well. This is an example of a diet following a food-combining philosophy, but has many variations among followers.

[a] Many variations exist on each of these types of diets. This is not intended as a comprehensive listing.

Individuals following restrictive diets are more susceptible to dietary deficiencies and imbalances.[1,2] Table 40.3 describes the nutrients that may be of concern in many vegetarian diets.

Health Benefits and Risks of Vegetarianism

Most health risks associated with a vegetarian diet are found with strict vegetarianism (veganism) only, not with the more liberal forms of intake found in lacto-vegetarians, ovo-

TABLE 40.3

Nutrients Potentially at Risk in Vegetarian Diets; Dietary Reference Intakes (DRIs), Functions and Sources[2,27-29]

Vitamin/ Mineral	DRI: adult value 19–50 yr old, non-pregnant	Function	Good Sources in Vegetarian Diet
Vitamins			
Vitamin B_{12}	M: 2.4 μg F: 2.4 μg	Works with folic acid to make red blood cells; important in maintaining healthy nerve fibers; helps the body use fat and protein.	Dairy products, eggs, fortified cereals, fortified soy products/ meat substitutes, fortified nutritional yeast.
Vitamin D	Adequate Intake (AI): M: 5 μg F: 5 μg	Promotes absorption of calcium and phosphorus and helps deposit them in bones and teeth.	Fortified milk; made in body when skin is exposed to sunlight.
Riboflavin (B_2)	M: 1.3 mg F: 1.1 mg	Helps the body release energy from protein, fat, and carbohydrates.	Fortified dairy products, fortified breads and cereals, tomatoes, lima beans, raisins, avocado, beans, and legumes.
Minerals			
Calcium	AI: M: 1000 mg F: 1000 mg	Used to build bones and teeth and keep them strong; important in muscle contraction and blood clotting.	Dairy products, broccoli, mustard and turnip greens.
Iron[a]	M: 8 mg F: 18 mg	Carries oxygen in the body, both as a part of hemoglobin (in the blood), and myoglobin (in the muscles).	Whole-grain and enriched cereals, some dried fruits, soybeans.
Zinc	M: 11 mg F: 8 mg	Assists in wound healing, blood formation, and general growth and maintenance of all tissues; component of many enzymes.	Plant and animal proteins.
Manganese[b]	AI: M: 2.3 mg F: 1.8 mg	Found in most of body's organs and tissues, particularly in bones, liver, and kidneys. Serves as a cofactor in many metabolic processes. Deficiency not seen in human populations.	Whole grains, cereal products, tea, some fruits and vegetables.
Iodine	150 μg/d	Constituent of thyroid hormones (regulation of metabolic rate, body temperature, growth, reproduction, making body cells, muscle function, nerve growth).	Fortified in salt, found widely in processed foods and grains where soil concentration is adequate.
Copper[c]	900 μg	Necessary for the formation of hemoglobin; keeps bones, blood vessels, and nerves healthy.	Nuts, legumes, whole grains.
Selenium	55 μg	Antioxidant functions, role in eicosanoid metabolism, regulation of arachadonic acid and lipid peroxidation, some hormone conversions.	Eggs, whole grains, legumes, brazil nuts.
Macronutrients and Other Dietary Components			
Protein	RDA: Male: 63 g Female: 50 g or 0.8 gm/kg	Building of nearly all body tissues, particularly muscle tissue, energy.	Dairy products, legumes, meat analog products often made from soy; whole grains and vegetables are poorer sources.

TABLE 40.3 *(Continued)*

Nutrients Potentially at Risk in Vegetarian Diets; Dietary Reference Intakes (DRIs), Functions and Sources[2,27-29]

Vitamin/ Mineral	DRI: adult value 19–50 yr old, non-pregnant	Function	Good Sources in Vegetarian Diet
Omega-3 fatty acids	Optimal intake estimated at 1-2 g/d; fatty acids should make up at least 3% of day's energy intake.	One is called linolenic acid. Energy source, cell wall structure, may play a role in disease prevention. Fats also play a role in the absorption and transport of fat-soluble vitamins. Linolenic acid cannot be made by the body. Omega-3 series fatty acids can be found in grains, seeds, nuts, and soybeans, and the body can manufacture eicosapentaenoic acid (EPA) and docosahexaenoic acid (DHA) from these precursors.	Fats and oils (bean, nut, and grain oils), nuts and seeds (butternuts, walnuts, soybean kernels), soybeans, flax seeds, and flax seed oil.

[a] There is some evidence that vegetarian diets tend to be quite high in iron and that iron deficiency anemia is no more common among vegetarians than in meat eaters.[1]

[b] Manganese is not necessarily at risk for deficiency in vegetarians. Some research has indicated that vegetarians have a higher intake of this nutrient; however, bioavailability may be a concern.[14,17]

[c] Copper is not necessarily at risk for deficiency in vegetarians. Some research has indicated that vegetarians have a higher intake of this nutrient; however, bioavailability may be a concern.[14,17]

vegetarians, or lacto-ovo vegetarians.[1,5,6] Table 40.4 lists the health risks of vegetarianism, most of which are related to the potential for nutrient deficiencies found with this type of diet. These health risks are not unique to vegetarians, however, as they can be quite common in people following an imbalanced omnivorous diet.

Many vegetarians follow a dietary pattern that reduces their risks for common chronic diseases, as noted in Tables 40.5 and 40.6.[4] New vegetarians, in particular, however, may rely heavily on dairy products which may actually increase risk for cardiovascular disease. Other practical concerns for new vegetarians are found in Table 40.7.

Table 40.8 compares the typical dietary intake of vegans and lacto-ovo vegetarians with omnivores; the health risks/outcomes associated with specific kinds of vegetarian diets are mentioned in Table 40.9. The nutrients of special concern will vary depending on the

TABLE 40.4

Health Risks of Vegetarianism[1,5,7,13,22-26,30,31]

Dietary Factor	Risk
Calcium	Low calcium intake in vegan or macrobiotic diet can lead to low bone mineral density.
Iodine	A strict vegan consuming no iodized salt or processed food products can develop goiter.
Vitamin B_{12}	In strict vegans or in the offspring of vegan mothers only, deficiency can lead to anemia, or in far more severe cases, neuropathy.
Energy	Impaired growth can result in infants and children with inadequate energy intake or those weaned to "homemade" formulas.
Docosahexaenoic acid (DHA)	Greatest concern for fetus and young infants. DHA is needed for neural and retinal development.
Dairy products	Limited evidence exists linking high consumption of dairy products to diabetes (type 1) primarily in infants and children, and to ovarian cancer in adults with galactose-1-phosphate uridyltransferase defects.

TABLE 40.5

Health Benefits of Vegetarianism[1,2,4,10-13,19,32-34]

Lower Risk Of

Cancer (particularly colon and lung)
Obesity
Heart disease
Type 2 diabetes
Hypertension
Constipation and hemorrhoids
Kidney stones
Gallstones

Potential Lower Risk For (Limited Evidence Suggesting)

Arthritis
Gout
Dementia
Tooth decay
Duodenal ulcers

TABLE 40.6

Protective Factors in the Typical Lacto-Ovo Vegetarian Diet[1,4,10,18,20]

Higher fiber
Lower fat, saturated fat, and cholesterol
Higher folate intake
Higher intake of antioxidants
Higher intake of phytochemicals
Lower intake of total and animal protein

TABLE 40.7

Practical Concerns about Vegetarianism

New vegetarians or those who are vegetarian for philosophical (as opposed to health) reasons may rely heavily on the use of dairy products and eggs.

Whole milk cheeses, 2% and higher fat content milk, eggs and whole milk yogurts are rich in fat, saturated fat, and in some cases cholesterol. These can contribute to higher risks for cardiovascular disease in particular, and should be evaluated.

Some adolescents with eating disorders may use vegetarianism as a rationalization for avoiding foods or entire food groups.

TABLE 40.8

Nutrient Differences between Omnivore, Lacto-Ovo and Vegan Dietary Patterns[1,2,33]

Dietary Component	Vegan	Lacto-ovo	Omnivore
Total fat	~30% fat	30-36% fat	34-38% fat
Saturated fat	Generally low saturated fat intake	Generally moderate saturated fat intake	Generally higher saturated fat intake
P/S ratio	High P/S	Mod P/S	Poor P/S
Cholesterol	0 mg	150-300 mg	400 mg
Fiber (g/d range)	Generally 50-100% higher than omnivores and higher than lacto-ovo vegetarians. (range: 16.1-55.3 g/d)	Generally 50-100% higher than omnivores (range: 5.2-74.4 g/d)	Generally low (range: 3.5-33.8 g/d)

TABLE 40.8 *(Continued)*

Nutrient Differences between Omnivore, Lacto-Ovo and Vegan Dietary Patterns[1,2,33]

Dietary Component	Vegan	Lacto-ovo	Omnivore
Carbohydrate (% total kcalories)	50-65%	50-55%	<50%
Protein	10-12% of calories (none from animal sources)	12-14% of calories (~1/2 from animal sources)	14-18% of calories (~2/3 from animal sources)
Cholesterol levels (mmol/L)	4.29	4.88	5.31
Folate (mcg/d ranges)	170-385	214-455	252-471
Blood pressure	112.5/65.3	111.8/68.8	120.8/76.4

TABLE 40.9

Health Risks of Individuals Following Various Types of Vegetarian Diets[1,2,33]

Type of Vegetarian Diet	Health Risk Profile	Nutrients at Greatest Risk
Vegan	Low risk of obesity, heart disease, cancer, hypertension, and diabetes. Vegans may have a lower health risk than lacto-ovo vegetarians due to the typical lower fat and higher fiber content than either lacto-ovo or non-vegetarians.	Vitamin B_{12} Vitamin D Calcium Zinc Energy Potentially Iron
Lacto-vegetarian	Generally low risk of obesity, heart disease, cancer, hypertension, and diabetes. Unskilled or new vegetarian may rely heavily on whole-milk based products, thus consuming high fat, saturated fat, and cholesterol intakes which could increase the risk of cardiovascular-related diseases.	Zinc Potentially Iron
Ovo-vegetarian	Generally low risk of obesity, heart disease, cancer, hypertension, and diabetes. Unskilled or new vegetarian may rely heavily on eggs and egg-based products, thus consuming high fat, saturated fat, and cholesterol intakes which could increase the risk of cardiovascular-related diseases.	Zinc Potentially Iron
Lacto-ovo vegetarian	Generally low risk of obesity, heart disease, cancer, hypertension, and diabetes. Unskilled or new vegetarian may rely heavily on whole-milk or egg-based products, thus consuming high fat, saturated fat, and cholesterol intakes which could increase the risk of cardiovascular-related diseases.	Zinc Potentially Iron

type of vegetarian diet followed. As discussed in Table 40.10, some nutrients are more critical during specific developmental phases; deficiency of a particular nutrient at a particular stage of the life cycle can have dramatic consequences.[5,7-9]

Energy and Macronutrients in the Vegetarian Diet

A common misconception about a vegetarian diet concerns protein. Many new vegetarians are frequently confronted with the question: "So how do you get your protein?" Individuals following a lacto-ovo vegetarian diet rarely have to worry about protein. Even vegans eating a reasonably balanced diet with adequate kcalories can easily meet their protein needs.[1,4] In reality, it is much more likely that the individual is suffering from a dietary

TABLE 40.10

Critical Periods of Importance for Selected Nutrients[2,25,27]

Nutrient	Critical Periods during Lifecycle
Vitamin B_{12}	Throughout, particularly critical during pregnancy, infancy, and childhood
Riboflavin (B_2)	Pregnancy, periods of growth
Vitamin D	Childhood and pre-puberty, pregnancy, elderly
Calcium	Childhood and pre-puberty, elderly
Iron	Infancy, childhood, adolescence, pregnancy, adulthood (women particularly)
Zinc	Puberty, pregnancy, elderly
Iodine	Adolescence, pregnancy, lactation
Protein	Infancy, childhood, adolescence, pregnancy
Omega-3 fatty acids (especially DHA)	Pregnancy, infancy
Energy	Periods of growth, especially toddlers/preschoolers, due to small stomach capacity

TABLE 40.11

Definitions Related to Protein Complementation[2]

Complete protein	Contains all essential amino acids in ample amounts; amino acid pattern is very similar to humans
Incomplete protein	May be low in one or more amino acids; amino acid pattern is very different from humans
Limiting amino acid	The essential amino acid(s) that are in the smallest supply in the food
Essential amino acid	Cannot be synthesized by the human body. Include: Arginine, Histidine, Isoleucine, Leucine, Lysine, Methionine, Phenylalanine, Threonine, Tryptophan, Valine

TABLE 40.12

Limiting Essential Amino Acids and Vegan Sources[1,2]

Food	Limiting Amino Acids	Vegan Sources of the Limiting Amino Acids
Legumes	Methionine, Cysteine	Grains, nuts, seeds, soybeans
Cereals/grains	Lysine, Threonine	Legumes
Nuts and seeds	Lysine	Legumes
Peanuts	Methionine, Lysine, Threonine	Legumes, grains, nuts, seeds, soybeans
Vegetables	Methionine	Grains, nuts, and seeds, soybeans
Corn	Tryptophan, Lysine, Threonine	Legumes, sesame and sunflower seeds, soybeans

deficiency of a micronutrient, such as calcium or zinc, than a protein deficiency. Energy and protein can be of concern in some adult vegetarian diets, particularly if the individual follows severe dietary restrictions, and in children.[8]

Tables 40.11 through 40.13 provide information about essential and non-essential amino acids and protein complementation. In the 1970s, carefully complementing proteins at each meal was thought to be the only way for vegetarians to avoid protein deficiency. We now know that it is not necessary to combine proteins at each meal,[1,4] yet it is important to understand the terminology related to the body's protein needs and the principles of complementation.

Table 40.14 compares average protein intakes in the U.S., while Tables 40.15 and 40.16 provide information about protein and nutrient- and energy-dense food sources. As an arbitrary guideline, foods with 2 g or less of protein were not included. Information about nutrient- and energy-dense foods can be useful for young children who may fill up quickly on a bulky vegetarian diet without meeting their kcalorie and nutrient needs.[9]

TABLE 40.13

Guidelines for Protein Complementation[1,2]

Type of Vegetarian Diet	Guidelines for Complementation[a]
Lacto-ovo	Dairy and eggs provide complete protein, as do other animal products.
Vegan	A vegan diet that contains a variety of grains, legumes, vegetables, seeds, and nuts over the course of a day in amounts to meet a person's calorie needs will provide adequate amino acids in appropriate amounts. Soybeans match human needs for essential amino acids as precisely as animal foods, and are thus a complete protein.
Any	It is not necessary to combine proteins in each meal. Young children, however, may need to have the complementary proteins consumed within a few hours of each other.

[a] All proteins except gelatin provide all of the amino acids. Some protein sources have relatively low levels of some amino acids, so a large amount of that food would need to be consumed if it were the only source of those "limiting" amino acids.[1]

TABLE 40.14

Protein Intakes in the United States[1]

Type of Diet	Percent of Calories from Protein	Sufficient to Meet RDA?
Typical U.S. diet	14–18%	Yes
Lacto-ovo vegetarians	12–14%	Yes, provided adequate calories are consumed
Vegans	10–12%	Yes, provided adequate calories are consumed

TABLE 40.15

Protein: Vegetarian Sources and Amounts[27,35,36]

Adult RDA: Males 63 g/day Females 50 g/day[a]

Food	Portion Size	Protein (g)	Kcal
Cereals/Grains			
Quinoa	0.5 cup	11.1	318
Millet, cooked	1 cup	8.4	286
Wheat germ, toasted	0.25 cup	8.4	111
Bagel, plain	1 bagel	7.5	195
Couscous, cooked	1 cup	6.8	200
Macaroni, enriched, cooked	1 cup	6.7	197
Pita, whole wheat	1 pita	6.3	170
Grape-Nuts, Post	0.5 cup	6.0	200
Oatmeal Crisp, almond, General Mills	1 cup	6.0	220
Oatmeal, old fashioned, Quaker	0.5 cup dry	5.5	148
Oat bran, raw	0.33 cup	5.4	76
Brown rice, medium grain, cooked	1 cup	4.5	218
English muffin, plain	1 muffin	4.4	134
Barley, pearled, cooked	1 cup	3.5	193
Whole wheat bread	1 slice	2.7	69
Corn grits, instant, white, enriched	1 oz. packet dry	2.4	96
Vegetables			
Peas, green, canned	0.5 cup	3.8	59
Corn, yellow, boiled	0.5 cup	2.7	89
Broccoli, boiled	0.5 cup	2.3	22

TABLE 40.15 *(Continued)*

Protein: Vegetarian Sources and Amounts[27,35,36]

Adult RDA: Males 63 g/day Females 50 g/day[a]

Food	Portion Size	Protein (g)	Kcal
Fruits			
Prunes, dried	10 prunes	2.2	201
Dairy/Soymilk			
Cottage cheese, 1% fat	1 cup	28.0	164
Yogurt, lowfat (1.5% milk fat), plain, Breyers	1 cup	11.0	130
Simple Pleasures, chocolate	0.5 cup	8.9	134
Gruyere cheese	1 oz.	8.5	117
Milk, low fat (1%)	1 cup	8.0	102
Cheddar cheese	1 oz.	7.1	114
Soymilk	1 cup	6.6	79
American processed cheese	1 oz.	6.3	106
Pudding, all flavors, from instant mix Jell-O brand	0.5 cup	4.0	155
Frozen yogurt, soft serve	0.5 cup	2.9	115
Ice cream, vanilla, regular (10% fat)	0.5 cup	2.3	133
Beans/Legumes			
Soybean nuts, roasted	0.5 cup	30.3	405
Lentils, boiled	1 cup	17.9	230
Lima beans, boiled	1 cup	14.7	216
Kidney beans, canned	1 cup	13.3	207
Garbanzo beans, canned	1 cup	11.9	286
Soy Products/Meat Substitutes			
Tofu, raw, firm	0.5 cup	19.9	183
Tempeh	0.5 cup	15.7	165
Pepperoni from meat substitute	16 slices	14.0	70
Better 'n Burger, Morningstar Farms	1 patty	11.3	75
Soybeans, green, boiled	0.5 cup	11.1	127
Ground meatless, frozen, Morningstar Farms	0.5 cup	10.3	60
Meatless deli turkey	3 slices	9.0	40
Nuts/Seeds			
Peanut butter, chunk style/crunchy	2 T	7.7	188
Sunflower seeds, dried	1 oz.	6.2	160
Almonds, blanched	1 oz.	6.0	174
Sesame butter (tahini)	2 T	5.0	174
Cashews, dry roasted	1 oz.	4.3	163
Eggs			
Egg substitute, frozen	0.25 cup	6.8	96
Egg, chicken, whole, fresh/frozen	1 large	6.2	75
Egg, chicken, yolk fresh	1 large	2.8	61
Mixed Foods			
Frozen French bread pizza, vegetarian	6 oz. pizza	17.0	270
Shells & cheese, from mix	1 cup	16.0	360
Burritos w/ beans	2 burritos	14.1	447
Biscuit w/ egg	1 item	11.1	316
Potato, baked, w/ sour cream & chives	1 potato	6.7	393

[a] Taking into account the lower digestibility and amino acid profile, a reasonable RDA for vegans is approximately 10% more protein than omnivores.[1]

TABLE 40.16

Vegetarian Sources of Energy-Dense, Nutrient-Dense Foods[35,36]

Food	Portion Size	Kcal
Cereals/Grains		
Granola, low-fat	1 cup	422
Quinoa	0.5 cup	318
Millet, cooked	1 cup	286
Pancakes, Bisquick, blueberry	3 each	220
Oatmeal Crisp	1 cup	210
Grape-Nuts, Post	0.5 cup	200
Macaroni, enriched, cooked	1 cup	197
Bagel, plain	1 bagel	195
Raisin bran, dry	1 cup	175
Corn muffin (2.5 x 2.25 inch)	1 muffin	174
Pita, whole wheat	1 pita (6.5 in diameter)	170
Banana nut muffin, from mix	1 muffin	160
Oat bran muffin	1 muffin	154
Vegetables		
Tater Tots, frozen, heated	4 oz.	204
Potatoes, mashed from granules	1 cup	166
Fruits		
Avocado, California, raw	0.5 medium	153
Raisins, golden, seedless	0.66 cup	302
Mixed fruit, dried, diced, Delmonte	0.66 cup	220
Dairy/Soymilk		
Milkshake, thick vanilla	1 cup	256
Yogurt, flavored, lowfat, 1% milkfat, Breyers	1 cup	251
Ricotta cheese, part-skim	0.5 cup	171
Cottage cheese (1% fat)	1 cup	164
Pudding, all flavors, from instant mix Jell-O	0.5 cup	155
Milk, whole	1 cup	150
Yogurt, lowfat (1.5 % milk fat), plain, Breyers	1 cup	130
Cheddar cheese	1 oz.	114
Milk, low fat (1%)	1 cup	102
Soymilk	1 cup	79
Beans/Legumes		
Soybean, dried, boiled, mature	1 cup	298
Garbanzo beans, canned	1 cup	286
Lentils, boiled	1 cup	230
Soy Products/Meat Substitutes		
Soybean nuts (roasted)	0.5 cup	405
Tempeh	1 cup	330
Soyburger w/ cheese	1 each	316
Chicken nuggets, meatless	5 pieces	245
Frankfurter, meatless	1 each	102
Nuts/Seeds		
Peanut butter, chunky style	2 T	188
Almonds, blanched	1 oz.	174

TABLE 40.16 *(Continued)*

Vegetarian Sources of Energy-Dense, Nutrient-Dense Foods[35,36]

Food	Portion Size	Kcal
Sesame butter (tahini)	2 T	174
Sunflower seeds, dried	1 oz.	160
Mixed Foods		
Egg salad	1 cup	586
Burritos, w/ beans	2 burritos	447
Potato, baked, w/ sour cream and chives	1 potato	393
Shells & cheese, from mix	1 cup	360
Peanut butter and jam sandwich on wheat	1 each	344
Cheese enchilada	1 item	320
Biscuit w/ egg	1 item	316
Lasagna, no meat, recipe	1 piece	298
Chili, meatless, canned	0.66 cup	190
Trail mix, regular	0.25 cup	150
Vegetable soup	1 cup	145
Pizza, cheese	1/8 of 12-inch	140
Pasta with marinara sauce	1 cup	180-450

Micronutrients in the Vegetarian Diet

Although vegetarian dietary patterns can be extremely healthful,[1,10,11-13] certain micronutrients can be challenging to obtain in sufficient quantities, depending on the specific dietary restrictions the individual follows. Tables 40.17 through 40.28 provide information about sources of micronutrients that can be of concern for some vegetarian individuals.[1,4-7,11,13-17] As a guideline, foods with less than 5 to 10% of the recommended amount of that particular nutrient per serving were not included in the tables.

Bioavailability of minerals can influence the amount available for absorption. Tables 40.24 and 40.28 list factors that may enhance or inhibit the absorption of iron and zinc.

Non-Nutritive and Other Important Factors in the Vegetarian Diet

Typical vegetarian diets are rich in many beneficial non-nutritive factors such as dietary fiber and phytochemicals.[18-20] Tables 40.29 and 40.30 provide information about sources of these beneficial but non-nutritive factors.

Omega-3 fatty acids are a type of polyunsaturated fatty acid thought to reduce the risk of cardiovascular disease through their effects on triglyceride levels and platelet aggregation.[2,21] One type of omega-3 fatty acid, alpha-linolenic acid, is an essential fatty acid and must be consumed in the diet to prevent deficiency. Two other types of omega-3 fatty acids are eicosapentaenoic acid (EPA) and docosahexaenoic acid (DHA). Omega-3 fatty acids may be of concern to vegetarians because although alpha-linolenic acid is found in many plant foods, EPA and DHA are not.[1] For healthy adults this is not usually a concern, because the body has the ability to manufacture EPA and DHA from alpha-linolenic acid,

TABLE 40.17

Riboflavin:[a] Vegetarian Sources and Amounts[28,35,36]

Adult RDA: Males 1.3 mg/day Females 1.1 mg/day

Food	Portion Size	Riboflavin (mg)	Kcal
Cereals[bc]/Grains			
Raisin bran	1 cup (2.1 oz.)	0.678	175
Bran flakes	0.66 cup (1 oz.)	0.43	91.5
Corn flakes, Kellogg's	1 cup (1 oz.)	0.375	90
Bagel, plain	1 bagel (3.5 inch)	0.22	195
Sesame breadsticks	2 sticks	0.22	120
Pita, white	1 pita (6.5 inch diameter)	0.20	165
Lasagna noodles	2 oz. dry	0.20	210
Cornbread, homemade from low-fat milk	1 slice	0.19	173
Corn muffin (2.5 x 2.25 inch)	1 muffin	0.19	174
English muffin, wheat	1 muffin	0.17	127
English muffin, plain	1 muffin	0.16	134
Muffin, blueberry, homemade (2.75 x 2 inch)	1 muffin	0.16	163.5
Macaroni, enriched, cooked	1 cup	0.14	197
Wild rice, cooked	1 cup	0.14	166
Rye bread	1 slice	0.11	83
Vegetables			
Mushrooms, boiled	0.5 cup	0.23	21
Tomato puree, canned	1 cup	0.14	100
Sweet potatoes, baked, with skin	1 medium	0.14	117
Tomato, red, sun-dried	0.5 cup	0.13	69.5
Garden cress, boiled	0.5 cup	0.11	16
Fruits			
Raisins, golden seedless	0.66 cup	0.19	302
Banana	1 medium	0.11	105
Raspberries, raw	1 cup	0.11	60
Avocado, Calif. raw	0.5 medium	0.105	153
Dairy/Soymilk			
Yogurt, plain, lowfat	1 cup	0.493	209
Milk, whole	1 cup	0.395	150
Cottage cheese, 1% fat	1 cup	0.37	164
Milk, nonfat	1 cup	0.34	86
Feta cheese	1 oz.	0.24	75
Ricotta cheese, part-skim	0.5 cup	0.23	171
Soymilk	1 cup	0.17	79
Cheddar cheese, reduced fat	1 oz.	0.14	80
Cheddar cheese	1 oz.	0.11	114
Goat cheese, soft	1 oz.	0.11	76
Beans/Legumes			
Soybeans, boiled	1 cup	0.49	298
Kidney beans, canned	1 cup	0.18	207
Great northern beans, canned	1 cup	0.16	299
Pinto beans, boiled	1 cup	0.16	234
Lentils, boiled	1 cup	0.14	230

TABLE 40.17 *(Continued)*

Riboflavin:[a] Vegetarian Sources and Amounts[28,35,36]

Adult RDA: Males 1.3 mg/day Females 1.1 mg/day

Food	Portion Size	Riboflavin (mg)	Kcal
Soy Products/Meat Substitutes			
Chicken nuggets, meatless	5 pieces	0.30	245
Vegetarian burger, grilled, Morningstar Farms	1 patty	0.24	140
Breakfast links, Morningstar Farms	2 links	0.22	63
Tofu, raw, firm	0.5 cup	0.13	183
Nuts/Seeds			
Almonds, dry roasted	1 oz.	0.17	166
Eggs			
Egg, chicken, boiled	1 large	0.298	89.9
Egg substitute, frozen	0.25 cup	0.188	52.8
Mixed Foods			
Bean burrito	2 each	0.61	447
Cheese enchilada	1 each	0.42	319
Egg omelet w/ onion, pepper, tomato, mushroom	1 each	0.344	125
Vegetarian chili, fat-free w/black beans, Health Valley	5 oz.	0.255	70
Beverages			
Coffee substitute w/ milk	0.75 cup	0.298	120
Miscellaneous			
Brewers yeast	1 T	0.342	22.6

[a] Also called vitamin B_2.
[b] Most fortified breakfast cereals contain 0.43-0.51 mg per serving.
[c] Many "100% Natural" breakfast cereals are not enriched and contain 0.03-0.12 mg per serving.

although vegetarians still have lower levels of blood DHA.[1,22] The fetus and young infant have a dramatically reduced ability to perform this conversion.[23] Because DHA is needed for brain and retinal development, some pregnant or breastfeeding vegetarian women may need to reduce their intake of linoleic acid (an omega-6 fatty acid) relative to their intake of alpha-linolenic acid to increase DHA levels, or they may choose to try DHA-enriched eggs or DHA supplements derived from microalgae, although the safety of this has not been established.[22-26] Table 40.31 lists vegetarian dietary sources of the omega-3 fatty acid alpha-linolenic acid.

The Effects of Cooking, Storage, and Processing on the Critical Nutrients

Cooking, storage, and processing methods can influence the amount of a nutrient present in a food. Table 40.32 presents the effects of cooking, storage, and processing on the nutrients that may be of concern in a vegetarian diet.

TABLE 40.18

Vitamin B_{12}: Vegetarian Sources and Amounts[28,35,36]

Adult RDA: 2.4 µg/day

Food	Portion Size	Vitamin B12 (µg)	Kcal
Cereals[a]/Grains			
Total, wheat	1 cup	7.00	116
Waffle, whole grain	2 each	3.11	154
Bran flakes	1 cup	2.49	152
Granola, lowfat	0.33 cup	1.50	120
Kix	1.5 cup	1.50	110
Corn flakes, dry	1 cup	1.27	92.9
Waffle, frozen, toasted	1 each	0.882	92.4
Dairy/Soymilk[b]			
Soymilk, Edensoy Extra	1 cup	3.0	130
Cottage cheese, 1% fat	1 cup	1.43	164
Milk, skim	1 cup	0.93	86
Yogurt, flavored, lowfat 1% milkfat, Breyers	1 cup	0.90	251
Milk, whole	1 cup	0.87	150
Yogurt, whole, plain	1 cup	0.84	139
Yogurt, nonfat, flavored w/ aspartame, Light 'n Lively Free 70 Cal	1 cup	0.60	70
Buttermilk, cultured	1 cup	0.54	99
Feta cheese	1 oz.	0.479	74.8
Swiss cheese	1 oz.	0.476	107
Ricotta cheese, part-skim	0.5 cup	0.36	171
Havarti cheese	1 oz.	0.357	105
American processed cheese food	1 oz.	0.235	68.9
Cheddar cheese	1 oz.	0.23	114
Soy Products/Meat Substitutes[c]			
Breakfast links	2 each	3.41	63
Soyburger w/cheese	1 each	1.72	316
Soyburger	1 each	1.70	142
Tempeh	1 cup	1.66	330
Breakfast patties	1 each	1.49	68
Chicken, meatless, breaded, fried patty	1 piece	0.95	177
Eggs			
Egg, chicken, boiled	1 large	0.56	78
Mixed Foods			
Spinach soufflé	1 cup	1.37	219
Cheese pizza	1 piece (1/8 of a 15-inch pie)	0.53	223
Miscellaneous			
Fortified nutritional yeast (Red Star T6635)	1 T	4.0	40

[a] Some commercial cereals are not fortified with vitamin B_{12}; check labels carefully.
[b] Subject to fortification; unfortified soymilk contains no vitamin B_{12}.
[c] Subject to fortification; check labels of individual products carefully.

TABLE 40.19

Vitamin D: Vegetarian Sources and Amounts[28,35-37]

Adult Adequate Intake: 5 µg cholecalciferol (200 IU per day)

Food	Portion Size	Vitamin D (IU)[a]	Kcal
Cereals/Grains			
Raisin Bran	1 cup (2.1 oz.)	56	175
Corn Pops	1 cup	50	110
Lucky Charms	1 cup	44.8	125
Corn flakes	1 cup (1 oz.)	44	90
Granola, lowfat	0.33 cup	39.9	120
Wheat bran muffin from recipe w/ 2% milk	1 muffin (57 g)	25.1	161
Waffles, plain, recipe	1 each (75 g)	23.5	218
Vegetables			
Mushrooms, boiled	0.5 cup	59.3	21.1
Dairy/Soymilk			
Soymilk, Soy Moo, fat free, Health Valley	1 cup	100	110
Milk, nonfat	1 cup	98	85.5
Milk, whole	1 cup	97.6	150
Pudding, vanilla, instant, w/ whole milk	0.5 cup	49.0	162
Eggs			
Egg, chicken, boiled	1 large	26	78
Egg yolk, cooked	1 each	24.6	59.2
Mixed Foods			
Soup, tomato bisque, with milk	1 cup	49.2	198
Egg salad	0.5 cup	38.5	293
Egg omelet w/ mushroom	1 each (69 g)	36.4	91.2
Fats/Oils/Dressings			
Margarine, hard, hydrogenated soybean[b]	1 tsp.	19.9	29.8
Desserts			
Egg custard pie, frozen, baked	1 piece (105 g)	40.1	221
Chocolate-filled crepe	1 each (78 g)	28.1	119
Coffee cake, from mix	1 piece (72 g)	22.2	229

[a] 1 IU vitamin D = 0.025 µg cholecalciferol.

[b] Subject to fortification; check labels.

TABLE 40.20

Calcium: Vegetarian Sources and Amounts[28,30,35,36]

Adult AI: Males 1000 mg/day Females 1000 mg/day

Food	Portion size	Calcium (mg)	Kcal
Cereals/Grains			
Calcium fortified cereal bars	1 bar (37 g)	200	140
Vegetables			
Collards, frozen, boiled	0.5 cup	179	31
Kale, frozen, boiled	1 cup	179	39
Turnip greens, canned	0.5 cup	138	16
Squash, acorn, baked	1 cup	90.2	115
Okra, boiled	0.5 cup	88	34
Squash, butternut, baked	1 cup	84	82
Broccoli, cooked	1 cup	72	44
Peas, green, cooked, from frozen	0.5 cup	19.2	62.4
Fruits			
Calcium-fortified orange juice	8 oz	300	120
Dairy/Soymilk			
Soy milk, fortified	8 oz (1 cup)	400	110
Malted milk, chocolate (Ovaltine)	8 oz	384	225
Evaporated milk, skim	4 oz	372	100
Evaporated milk, whole	4 oz	329	169
Goat's milk	8 oz (1 cup)	327	168
Yogurt, tofu yogurt, frozen	8 oz	309	254
Cow's milk, skim	8 oz (1 cup)	302	86
Cow's milk, 1/2%	8 oz (1 cup)	300	90
Cow's milk, 1%	8 oz (1 cup)	300	102
Yogurt, fat-free	8 oz	300	100
Yogurt, lowfat	8 oz	300	200
Yogurt, regular	8 oz	300	250
Cow's milk, 2%	8 oz (1 cup)	297	121
Cow's milk, whole	8 oz	290	150
Swiss cheese	1 oz	272	107
Cheddar cheese	1 oz	204	114
American cheese	1 oz	174	106
Mozzarella cheese, part skim	1 oz	183	72
Feta cheese	1 oz	140	75
Soy milk, non-fortified	8 oz (1 cup)	79.3	150
Cottage cheese, 1% fat	0.5 cup	69	82
Beans/Legumes			
Great northern beans	0.5 cup	60	105
Soy Products/Meat Substitutes			
Tofu, raw, firm	0.5 cup	258	183
Tempeh	1 cup	154	330
Nuts/Seeds			
Almonds, dried	1 oz (about 24 nuts)	75	167
Desserts			
Custard, 2% milk	1 cup	394	298
Sherbet, orange	1 cup	264	104
Soft serve ice cream, French vanilla	1 cup	226	370
Frozen yogurt, soft serve	1 cup	212	230
Ice cream, vanilla, regular, 10% fat	1 cup	168	226
Miscellaneous			
Blackstrap molasses	1 Tbsp	172	47

TABLE 40.21

Copper:[a] Vegetarian Sources and Amounts[b] [27,35,36]

Adult RDA: 900 μg/day

Food	Portion Size	Copper (mg)	Kcal
Cereals/Grains			
100% Bran	1 c	1.04	178
Granola, lowfat, Kellogg's	0.5 c	0.655	211
Vegetables			
Potatoes, baked, stuffed w/cheese	1 ea (254 g)	0.671	373
Vegetable juice cocktail, V-8	1 c	0.484	46.0
Potatoes, Baked, w/skin	1 ea (122 g)	0.372	133
Fruits			
Avocado, California	1 ea	0.460	306
Prunes, dehydrated, cooked	0.5 c	0.286	158
Dairy/Soy Milk			
Soy milk	1 c	0.288	79.2
Beans/Legumes			
Beans, adzuki, canned, sweetened	0.5 c	0.384	344
Garbanzo beans, boiled	0.5 c	0.289	135
Soy Products/Meat Substitutes			
Tempeh	1c	1.11	330
Scallops, meatless, breaded, fried	0.5 c	0.819	257
Luncheon slice, meatless	1 piece (67 g)	0.608	188
Soyburger w/cheese	1 ea	0.559	316
Tofu, raw, firm, calcium sulfate	0.5 c	0.476	183
Nuts & Seeds			
Cashew, dry roasted	0.25 c	0.76	197
Sunflower seeds, toasted	0.25 c	0.61	208

[a] Severe copper deficiency is rare in humans with no dietary deficiency documented. Generally this is only seen with extended supplemental feeding/total nutrition through manufactured nutrition such as total parenteral nutrition, or impaired utilization.[36]

[b] High zinc intake (from supplements) can cause copper deficiency.[2]

TABLE 40.22

Iodine: Vegetarian Sources and Amounts[27,35,36]

Adult RDA 150 μg males and females

Food	Portion Size	Iodine (μg)	Kcal
Cereals/Grains			
Rice, white, enriched, cooked, long grain	0.5 c (82.5 g)	52	81
Bread, cornbread, homemade	1 piece (65 g)	44.2	176
Fruit-flavored, sweetened	1.1 oz (32 g)	41	120
Roll, white	2 rolls (38 g)	31	100
Muffin, blueberry/plain	1 ea (50g)	28.5	150
Tortilla, flour, 7-8″ diam	1 ea (35 g)	26.3	114
Corn flakes	1 oz (28 g)	26	102
Bread, white	1 slice (28.4 g)	25.8	76.4
Pancakes, from mix, 4″	1ea (38 g)	21	74
Crisped rice	1 oz (28 g)	18.5	111
Noodles, egg, enriched, boiled	1 c (160 g)	17.6	213
Bread, whole wheat	1 slice (28 g)	17.6	69
Bread, rye, American	1 slice (32 g)	15.7	83
Vegetables			
Potato, boiled w/peel	1 ea (202g)	62.6	220
Fruit cocktail, heavy syrup, canned	0.5 c (128 g)	42.24	93
Potato, scalloped, homemade	0.5 c (122 g)	37.8	105
Navy beans, boiled	0.5 c (91 g)	35.5	129
Lima beans, baby, frozen, boiled	0.5 c (90 g)	27.9	95
Orange breakfast drink (from dry)	1 cup	27.3	114
Prunes, heavy syrup	5 ea (86 gm)	25.8	90
Cowpeas/blackeye peas	0.5 c (85 g)	22.1	112
Dairy/Soymilk			
Yogurt, lowfat, plain	1 cup	87.2	155
Buttermilk, skim, cultured	1 cup	60.0	99.0
2% fat milk	1 cup	56.6	137
Cottage cheese 1% fat	1 cup	56.5	164
Nonfat milk	1 cup	56.4	85.5
Whole milk, 3.3%	1 cup	56.1	150
Fruit yogurt, lowfat	1 cup	45.3	250
Eggs			
Fried in margarine	1 ea (46 g)	29	91.5
Scrambled, w/milk, in margarine	1 large, (61 g)	25.6	101
Soft-boiled	1 ea (50 g)	24	78
Mixed Foods			
Grilled cheese on wheat	1 ea (118 g)	28.9	392
Macaroni & cheese, box mix	0.5 c	17.3	199
Condiments/Seasonings			
Salt, Morton lite salt mixture	1 tsp	119	0

TABLE 40.23
Iron: Nonheme Sources in the Vegetarian Diet[27,35,36,38]

Adult RDA: Male 8 mg/Female: 18 mg

Food	Portion Size	Total Iron (mg)	Available Iron (mg) (where info available)	Kcals
Cereals/Grains				
Raisin Bran, dry	0.75 cup	Range: 18.54 to 3.7	0.19	200
Quinoa	1 cup	13.4	—	576
Corn flakes, dry	0.75 cup	6.5	0.32	90
Oatmeal, instant, fortified	0.5 cup	4.2	0.21	145
Special K	0.75 cup	3.4	—	75
Bran muffin	1 med	2.4	0.12	
Oatmeal, instant, regular	1 cup	1.59	—	145
Shredded Wheat, dry	1 oz	1.2	0.06	102
Bagel, enriched	1/2, 3.5" diameter	1.2	0.06	154
Vegetables				
Potato, baked, skin	1 med	2.8	0.14	220
Asparagus, pieces, canned	0.5 cup	2.21	—	23
Peas, cooked	0.5 cup	1.3	0.06	59
Spinach, boiled	0.5 cup	3.21	—	21
Fruits				
Prune juice	8 oz	3.02	—	182
Figs, dried	5 ea (93.5 g)	2.1	—	239
Raisins	2/3 c (100 g)	2.08	—	300
Prunes, dried	5 ea (42 g)	1.04	—	100
Beans/Legumes				
Split pea & carrot soup	7.5 oz	4.5	—	90
Lentil & carrot soup	7.5 oz	4.5	—	90
Black bean and carrot soup	7.5 oz	4.5	—	70
Kidney beans, boiled	0.5 cup	2.6	0.13	112
Navy beans, canned	0.5 cup	2.44	—	148
Chickpeas, boiled	0.5 cup	2.4	0.12	134
Soybeans, green, boiled	0.5 cup	2.25	—	127
Pinto beans, boiled	0.5 cup	2.23	—	117
Lima beans, cooked	0.5 cup	2.09	—	104
Pinto beans, canned	0.5 cup	1.94	—	93.6
Kidney beans, canned	0.5 cup	1.6	0.08	103
Chickpeas, canned	0.5 cup	1.6	0.08	143
Soy Products/Meat Substitutes				
Tofu, raw, regular,	~4 oz	6.65	0.32	94
Chili, made with meat substitute	0.67 cup	5.59	—	186
Garden burger	3.4 oz	2.89	—	186
Scallops, meatless, breaded, fried	.5 cup	1.77	—	257
Soyburger	1 each	1.49	—	142
Breakfast patties	1 each	1.42	—	97.3

TABLE 40.23 *(Continued)*

Iron: Nonheme Sources in the Vegetarian Diet[27,35,36,38]

Adult RDA: Male 8 mg/Female: 18 mg

Food	Portion Size	Total Iron (mg)	Available Iron (mg) (where info available)	Kcals
			—	
Nuts/Seeds				
Pumpkin seed kernel, roasted	.25 cup	8.45	—	296
Sunflower seeds, kernels, dry	.25 cup	2.44	—	205
Cashew, dry roasted	.25 cup	2.1	—	197
Coconut milk, canned	.25 cup	1.9	—	111
Almonds, dried, whole	.25 cup	1.3	—	209
Mixed nuts, dry roasted w/peanuts	.25 cup	1.27	—	204
Miscellaneous				
Molasses, blackstrap	1 Tbsp	3.5	—	47

TABLE 40.24

Iron: Absorption Enhancers and Inhibitors[1,2,38]

Class of Inhibitors	Examples	Found in	Effect on Iron Absorption
Polyphenols	Tannic acid, gallic acid, and catechin	Coffee, tea, red wines, certain spices, fruits, and vegetables	Coffee-35-40% Tea-60% Red wine-50%
Phytates	Substances that form insoluble complexes with nonheme iron	Whole grains, bran, soy products	
EDTA (ethylenediamine-tetraacetic acid)	Food additive used as sodium EDTA, calcium EDTA (prevents color changes and oxidation in foods)	Used broadly	Possibly up to 50% in some cases
Calcium	Calcium chloride (naturally occurring sources of calcium in self selected diets did not show an inhibitory effect; however there is a potential effect of other forms of calcium)	Additive to bread products, potential effect of other forms of calcium	Possibly up to 30-50% in some cases found with calcium chloride fortification
Fiber	Insoluble fibers, Phytate content may be responsible	Whole grains	Possibly 30-50%

Class of Enhancers[a]	Examples	Found in	Effect on Iron Absorption
Organic acids	Malic, ascorbic, citric, and bile acids	Found widely in foods	Enhances absorption
Amino acids	Some amino acids such as cysteine	Protein foods, also found widely in vegetables and grains	Enhances absorption

[a] The presence of these acids with a meal will significantly improve iron absorption and in some cases potentially overcome the inhibitory effects of other components in foods.

TABLE 40.25

Manganese:[a] Vegetarian Sources and Amounts[27,35,36]

Adult AI: Male 2.3 mg/Female 1.8 mg

Food	Portion Size	Manganese (mg)	Kcal
Cereals/Grains			
100% Bran	1 c	5.96	178
Most cereal	1 c	3.63	175
Grape Nuts	1 c	2.65	389
Bran Chex	1 c	2.53	156
All-Bran	0.33 c	2.39	70.7
Raisin Bran	1 c	2.16	175
Noodles, cooked, spinach	1 c	2.1	182
Noodles, cooked, macaroni, whole wheat	1 c	1.93	174
Rice flour, brown	0.25 c	1.59	144
Noodles, cooked, lasagna, whole wheat	2 ea	1.52	136
Wheat Chex	1 c	1.34	169
Vegetables			
Lima beans, boiled	0.5 c	1.07	105
Fruits			
Pineapple, chunks	1 c	2.56	76.0
Blackberries	1 c	1.86	74.9
Soy Products/Meat Substitutes			
Tofu, raw, firm, w/Nigari	0.5 c	1.49	181
Tempeh	0.5 c	1.19	165

[a] Manganese is not necessarily at risk for deficiency in vegetarians. Some research has indicated that vegetarians have a higher intake of this nutrient; however, bioavailability may be a concern.[14,17]

TABLE 40.26

Selenium:[a] Vegetarian Sources and Amounts[27,35,36,39]

Adult RDA: 55 μg/day

Food	Portion Size	Selenium (μg)	Kcal
Cereals/Grains			
Special K, Kellogg's	1 cup	54.9	100
Bagel, plain, toasted	1 each	22.7	195
Granola, lowfat	1 cup	22.5	422
Pita pocket, 100% whole wheat, toasted	1 each	20.2	120
Barley, whole, cooked	0.5 cup	18.2	135
Pita pocket, white	1 each	18	165
Egg noodles, cooked	0.5 cup	17.4	107
Spaghetti/macaroni, enriched, cooked	0.5 cup	14.9	98.5
Puffed wheat	1 cup	14.8	44.4
Whole wheat bread	1 slice	12.8	86.1
Oatmeal, instant, prepared	0.5 cup	12.68	159
Buns, hamburger-style	1 each	12.5	129
English muffin, plain	1 each	11.5	134
Cheerios	1.25 cup	10.6	111
Matzo, whole wheat	1 each	9.89	99.5

TABLE 40.26 *(Continued)*

Selenium:[a] Vegetarian Sources and Amounts[27,35,36,39]

Adult RDA: 55 μg/day

Food	Portion Size	Selenium (μg)	Kcal
Brown rice, long grain	0.5 cup	9.6	108.5
Vegetables			
Brussels sprouts, boiled	1 cup	21.1	60.8
Cucumbers, slices with peel	0.5 cup	6.19	6.76
Mushrooms, raw	5 pieces	14.3	32.4
Fruits			
Grapes, Thompson seedless	0.5 cup	7.7	57
Applesauce, canned	0.5 cup	6.5	52.5
Dairy/Soymilk			
Cottage cheese, 1%	1 cup	13.6	164
Yogurt, fruit, lowfat (12 g protein/8 oz.)	1 cup	8.09	155
Milk, nonfat	1 cup	5.15	85.5
Frozen yogurt, chocolate, nonfat	1 cup	5.02	208
Beans/Legumes			
Black beans, dry, boiled	1 cup	13.7	227
Lima beans, cooked	1 cup	8.19	229
Great northern beans, cooked	1 cup	7.26	209
Chickpeas, boiled	1 cup	6.10	269
Soy Products/Meat Substitutes			
Tofu	0.5	1.79	94.2
Nuts/Seeds			
Brazil nuts, dried	0.25 cup	1036	230
Sunflower seeds, kernels, dry	0.25 cup	21.4	205
Cashew, dry roasted, unsalted	0.25 cup	8	197
Eggs			
Egg, hard cooked	1 each	10.7	77.5
Egg yolk, cooked	1 each	7.50	59.2
Egg white, cooked	1 each	5.88	16.6
Mixed Foods			
Lasagna, no meat, recipe	1 piece (218 g)	29.9	298
Avocado & cheese sandwich on wheat bread	1 each	25.2	456
Peanut butter and jam sandwich on wheat	1 each	24.3	344
Pizza, cheese	1/8 of 15-inch (120 g)	20.0	268
Bean burrito	1 each	14.1	223.5
Cucumber & vinegar salad	1 cup	11.1	47.8
Desserts			
Coffee cake, from mix	1 piece (72 g)	11.0	229
Carrot cake, w/ cream cheese icing, recipe	1 piece (112 g)	9.91	488

[a] Selenium content of foods can vary widely, according to the selenium content of the soil.[39]

TABLE 40.27

Zinc: Vegetarian Sources and Amounts[27,35,36,40]

Adult RDA: Males 11 mg/Females 8 mg

Food	Portion size	Zinc (mg)[a,b]	Kcal
Cereals/Grains			
Just Right	1 cup	22.8	152
Product 19, Kellogg's	1 cup	15	100
Complete bran	1 cup	8.07	195
100% Bran	1 cup	5.74	178
Raisin bran, dry	1 cup	5.71	175
Bran flakes	1 cup	5.15	127
Cap'n Crunch	1 cup	4.00	156
Granola, lowfat	0.33 cup	3.74	120
Quinoa	1 cup	3.4	576
Muffin, wheat bran, from recipe with 2% milk	1 each (57 g)	1.57	161
Noodle, spaghetti, spinach, cooked	1 cup	1.53	182
Bagel, oat bran	1 each	1.42	173
Pancakes, Aunt Jemima, blueberry	3 each (106 g)	1	246
Vegetables			
Palm hearts, cooked	1 cup	5.45	150
Dairy/Soymilk			
Soymilk	1 cup	2.90	150
Frozen, nonfat, chocolate yogurt	1 cup	2.18	208
Ricotta cheese, part-skim	0.5 cup	1.66	170
Edam/ball cheese	1 oz.	1.07	101
Buttermilk, cultured	1 cup	1.03	99
Beans/Legumes			
Adzuki, cooked	1 cup	4.07	294
Lentils, cooked	1 cup	2.52	230
Blackeye peas, boiled from dry	1 cup	2.22	198
Soybean, dried, boiled	1 cup	2.0	298
Kidney beans, red, cooked	1 cup	1.89	225
Chickpeas, canned	0.5 cup	1.28	143
Soy Products/Meat Substitutes			
Natto	1 cup	5.32	371
Miso	0.5 cup	4.60	284
Tempeh	1 cup	3.02	330
Tofu, raw, firm	0.5 cup	1.98	183
Chili with meat substitute	0.66 cup	1.67	186
Meatless scallops, breaded, fried	0.5 cup	1.24	257
Luncheon slice, meatless	1 piece	1.07	188
Nuts/Seeds			
Pumpkin seeds, kernel, dry roasted	0.25 cup	2.58	187
Cashew, dry roasted,	0.25 cup	1.9	197
Almonds, dry roasted	0.25 cup	1.7	203
Sunflower seeds, kernels, dry roasted	0.25 cup	1.7	186
Sesame butter/tahini from unroasted kernels	1 T	1.58	91.1
Peanuts, dry roasted	0.25 cup	1.2	214
Peanut butter, natural	2 T	1.06	187

TABLE 40.27 *(Continued)*

Zinc: Vegetarian Sources and Amounts[27,35,36,40]

Adult RDA: Males 11 mg/Females 8 mg			
Food	**Portion size**	**Zinc (mg)[a,b]**	**Kcal**
Eggs			
Egg substitute	0.5 cup	1.6	74
Mixed Foods			
Cheese enchilada	1 each	2.51	319
Avocado & cheese sandwich on wheat bread	1 each	1.83	456
Pizza, cheese	1/8 of 15-inch	1.56	268
Desserts			
Nutrigrain bar, fruit filled	1 each	1.5	150
Pecan pie, 1/8 of a 9″ pie	1 piece (122 g)	1.26	503
Trail mix, regular	0.25 cup	1.21	173
Doughnut, eggless, carob-coated, raised	1 piece (78 g)	1.14	285

[a] Zinc content of foods is influenced by genetic breeding and fertilizer and soil conditions.
[b] Bioavailability is greater from animal than plant sources.[40]

TABLE 40.28

Zinc: Absorption Enhancers and Inhibitors[1,2,40]

Possible Absorption Enhancers[a]	Sources	Possible Absorption Inhibitors[b]	Sources
Yeast (acts by reducing phytates)	Fermented bread dough	Phytates	Whole grains (rye, barley, oatmeal, wheat), soy products
Animal protein	Animal products	Oxalate	Spinach, Swiss chard, leek, kale, collard greens, okra, rhubarb, raspberries, coffee, chocolate, tea, peanuts, pecans
Histidine	Amino acid widely distributed in foods containing protein	Fiber	Whole grains, fruits, vegetables, legumes
Albumin	Widely distributed in foods containing protein, egg white	Non-heme iron	Legumes, fortified cereals, leafy greens
		Copper	Legumes, whole grains, nuts, seeds, vegetables
		Calcium supplements	Over-the-counter supplements, multivitamins, some antacids
		High iron intakes relative to zinc intake	

[a] Yeast is the only non-controversial zinc absorption enhancer.
[b] Phytates are the only non-controversial zinc absorption inhibitor.

TABLE 40.29

Fiber: Types, Functions, and Sources[1,2,36]

Type of Fiber	Fiber Type	Food Sources	Function
Cellulose	Insoluble	Whole wheat flour, bran, cabbage, peas, green beans, broccoli, cucumbers, peppers, apples, carrots	Increases stool bulk and water absorption, decreases transit time through the GI system
Hemicellulose	Insoluble	Bran cereals, whole grains, brussels sprouts, greens, beet root	
Lignin	Insoluble	Breakfast cereals, bran, older vegetables, strawberries, eggplant, pears, green beans, radishes	
Gums	Soluble	Oatmeal, oat products, dried beans, oat bran, barley	Binds to bile acids and certain lipids to help lower blood cholesterol levels, metabolized to short chain fatty acids in gut which may play a role in signaling hepatic slowed cholesterol production
Pectin	Soluble	Squash, apples, citrus fruits, cauliflower, cabbage, dried peas and beans, carrots, strawberries	

TABLE 40.30

Common Phytochemicals[a] in Foods[18]

Chemical Names	Sources	Proposed Mechanism of Action
Sulforaphane	Isothiocyanates found in broccoli, cauliflower, cress, cabbages, radishes	Activates phase II enzymes in liver (removes carcinogens from cells)
Flavonoids	Citrus fruits and berries	Blocks the cancer-promotion process
Monoterpenes (polyphenols)	Perillyl alcohol in cherries Limonene in citrus Ellagic acid in strawberries & blueberries	May inhibit the growth of early cancers
Genistein	Soybeans, tofu	Prevents the formation of capillaries required to nourish tumors
Indoles	Cruciferous vegetables (broccoli, cauliflower, cress, cabbages, radishes)	Increase immunity, facilitate excretion of toxins
Saponins	Kidney beans, chickpeas, soybeans, lentils	May prevent cancer cells from multiplying
Lycopene	Tomatoes	May fight lung cancer

[a] More than 10,000 phytochemicals are thought to exist. This table represents only a partial listing.

General Vitamin and Mineral Deficiency and Toxicity Symptoms

It is important for practitioners to be aware of the symptoms of nutrient deficiencies in any patient. As a group, vegetarians tend to be more health-conscious and knowledgeable about nutrition than the general public.[1] Some vegetarians choose megadoses of vitamins or minerals to combat real or perceived threats to their health. Therefore, toxicity may be more of a risk than a nutrient deficiency. Table 40.33 presents deficiency and toxicity symptoms of the nutrients potentially deficient in a vegetarian diet.

TABLE 40.31

Omega-3 Fatty Acids: Vegetarian Sources and Amounts[2,29,41]

Reasonable intake: 0.5%-1% of total calorie intake
(represents 1.1-2.2 g on a 2000 kcal diet)

Food	Portion Size	Alpha-linolenic Acid (18:3) (mg)	Kcal
Cereals/Grains			
Oats, germ	0.25 cup	0.4	119
Wheat germ	0.25 cup	0.2	104
Barley, bran	0.25 cup	0.1	115
Vegetables			
Soybeans, green, raw	0.5 cup	4.1	188
Kale, raw, chopped	1 cup	0.13	21
Broccoli, raw, chopped	1 cup	0.1	24
Cauliflower, raw	1 cup	0.1	26
Fruits			
Avocados, California, raw	1 medium	0.173	306
Dairy/Soymilk			
Cheese, Roquefort	1 oz.	0.2	105
Beans/Legumes			
Soybeans, dry	0.5 cup	1.5	387
Beans, pinto, boiled	1 cup	0.2	234
Nuts/Seeds			
Butternuts (dried)	1 oz.	2.4	174
Walnuts, dried, English/Persian	1 oz.	1.9	182
Fats/Oils/Dressings			
Linseed oil	1 T	7.5	124
Flax seed	1 T	2.2	124
Canola oil (rapeseed oil)	1 T	1.6	124
Walnut oil	1 T	1.5	124
Salad dressing, comm., mayonnaise, soybean	2 T	1.38	116
Soybean oil	1 T	1.0	124
Wheat germ oil	1 T	1.0	124
Salad dressing, comm., Italian, regular	2 T	1.0	140

TABLE 40.32

Effects of Cooking, Storage, and Processing on the Critical Nutrients[2]

Nutrient	Cooking	Storage	Processing
Riboflavin	Stable to heat	Destroyed by light and irradiation	—
Vitamin B_{12}	Some losses (30%)	Stable	Small losses (10%)
Copper	Increased content using water from copper pipes	Canning with copper adds content to the food	—
Iron	Cooking in iron vessels increases iron content of foods	—	—
Omega 3 fatty acids (a polyunsaturated fatty acid)	Stable in baking; unstable if smoking point is reached	May go rancid with prolonged storage	—

TABLE 40.33

General Vitamin and Mineral Deficiency and Toxicity Symptoms[2,14,27,37]

Vitamin/Mineral[a]	Deficiency Symptoms[b]	Toxicity Symptoms[c]
Vitamins		
Vitamin D	Children — rickets Adults — osteomalacia	Excessive bone and soft tissue calcification (lung, kidney, kidney stones, tympanic membrane) Hypercalcemia with symptoms of headache, weakness, nausea and vomiting, constipation, polyuria, polydipsia In infants: retarded growth, gastrointestinal upsets, and mental retardation
Vitamin B_{12}	Pernicious (megaloblastic) anemia Smooth red tongue Fatigue Skin hypersensitivity (numbness, tingling and burning of the feet, stiffness and generalized weakness of the legs) Degeneration of peripheral nerves progressing to paralysis Other (glossitis, hypospermia)	Physiological stores substantial (~2000 μg). Stores and enterohepatic recycling may prevent deficiency symptoms for several years (~5) in the absence of intake None known up to 100 μg/d. No known benefit to high doses
Riboflavin (vitamin B_2)	Anemia (normocytic, normochromic) Neuropathy Purple/magenta tongue General B-vitamin deficiency symptoms (soreness and burning of lips, mouth, and tongue) Cheilosis, glossitis, angular stomatitis, seborrheic dermatitis of nasolabial fold, vestibule of the nose, and sometimes the ears and eyelids, scrotum, and vulva	None known
Minerals		
Calcium	Bone deformities including osteoporosis, tetany, hypertension	Hypercalcemia of soft tissues and bone (children and adults) Poor iron and zinc absorption (of particular concern during pregnancy)
Iron	Hypochromic, microcytic anemia Seen across populations, particularly in women, children, and those from low socioeconomic status Fatigue Spoon-shaped nails	Seen at 100 mg intake Constipation Liver toxicity Infections Hemochromatosis Potential increased risk for heart disease and myocardial infarction
Zinc	Growth retardation resulting in short stature, mild anemia, low plasma zinc levels, and delayed sexual maturation Possible in diets very rich in fiber and phytate, which chelates the zinc in the intestine, thus preventing absorption Poor taste acuity, poor wound healing, night blindness, baldness, and skin lesions have also been reported	Toxicity is rare (300 mg/d) Continuous supplementation with high dose zinc can interfere with copper absorption Supplementation of 50 mg/c may decrease HDL Zinc sulfate at 2 g/d can result in nausea, vomiting, diarrhea, dizziness Iron and copper losses in urine with doses as low as 25 mg/day and if large doses (10-15× the RDA) are taken for even short periods of time

TABLE 40.33 *(Continued)*

General Vitamin and Mineral Deficiency and Toxicity Symptoms[2,14,27,37]

Vitamin/Mineral[a]	Deficiency Symptoms[b]	Toxicity Symptoms[c]
Copper	Severe copper deficiency: rare in humans Adults: neutropenia and microcytic anemia Children: neutropenia and leukopenia Decrease in serum copper and ceruloplasmin levels followed by failure of iron absorption leading to microcytic, hemochromic anemia Neutropenia, leukopenia, and bone demineralization are later symptoms Deficiencies have not been reported in otherwise healthy humans consuming a varied diet.	Rare — seen in genetic diseases such as Wilson's disease (genetic deficiency in liver synthesis of ceruloplasmin)

[a] Absorption of some nutrients is affected by concentration of others; intestinal absorption of some nutrients is competitive.

[b] Deficiency can result from inadequate provision in the diet or via inadequate absorption.

[c] Toxicity is typically from overuse of nutritional supplements, although in some cases can be the cause of improper food fortification procedures (such as milk vitamin D fortification problems that arose in 1992).

Sample Meal Plans

Tables 40.34 through 40.37 present sample meal plans for adults and children following a lacto-ovo or vegan diet. These menus provide the Recommended Dietary Allowances (RDA) for energy and protein while presenting an appropriate macronutrient breakdown.

TABLE 40.34

Sample Meal Plan for Lacto-Ovo Vegetarian Adult[35,36]

Kcals: 2218; Carbohydrate: 374 g (67.35%); Protein: 100 g (18.%); Fat: 55 g (22.29%)

Breakfast	*Lunch*	*Dinner*
Raisin Bran (1 cup, 2.15 oz)	Whole wheat bread, 2 slices	Bean burrito
Milk, 1% fat, .75 cup (for cereal)	Griller veg. burger patty, 1 each	Black beans, 1 cup
Milk, 1% fat, 1 cup (beverage)	Mustard	Corn tortilla, 2 each, 6"
Orange juice, 1 cup	Tomato, sliced, 1/2 tomato	Rice, brown, 1 cup
Banana, 1 med	Jack cheese, 1 oz	Salsa, 2 Tbsp
	Apple, 1 med	Sour cream, 1 Tbsp
		Cheddar cheese, 1 oz
		Green salad, 2 cups
		Vinegar & oil dressing (1 tsp olive oil)
		Broccoli, 1 cup
		Milk, 1% fat, 1 cup
Snack		
Cereal bar, raspberry		
Dried apricots, 10 halves		

TABLE 40.35

Sample Meal Plan for Vegan Adult[35,36]

Kcals: 2217; Carbohydrate: 350g (63%); Protein: 90g (16%); Fat: 62g (25%)		
Breakfast	*Lunch*	*Dinner*
Raisin Bran (1 cup, 2.15 oz) Soy milk, 1% fat, 1 cup (for cereal) Soy milk, 1% fat, 1 cup (beverage) Orange juice, 1 cup, Ca fortified Banana, 1 med	Whole wheat bread, 2 slices Griller veg. burger patty (Morningstar Farms), 1 each, cooked Mustard Tomato, sliced, 1/2 tomato Almonds, slivered, blanched, 1 oz Apple, 1 med	Bean Burrito Black beans, 1 cup Corn tortilla, 2 each, 6″ Rice, brown, 1 cup Salsa, 2 Tbsp Walnuts, ground, .5 oz Green salad, 2 cups Vinegar & oil dressing (1 tsp olive oil) Broccoli, 1 cup Soy milk, 1 cup
Snack		
Cereal Bar, raspberry Dried Apricots, 10 halves		

TABLE 40.36

Sample Meal Plan for Vegan Child Age 4 to 6[35,36]

Kcals: 1864; Carbohydrate: 283 g (60.8%); Protein: 68 g (14.5%); Fat: 62 g (30%)		
Breakfast	*Lunch*	*Dinner*
1 packet instant oatmeal 8 oz soymilk fortified with calcium and vitamin B_{12} 1 banana	0.5 cup hummus spread made from chickpeas and sesame butter 2 slices whole wheat bread 6 oz. 100% orange pineapple banana juice carrot sticks 2 molasses cookies	veggie hot dog on bun 0.5 cup mashed potatoes 0.5 cup cooked "creamed" spinach 0.5 cup applesauce 8 oz soymilk
Snack	*Snack*	
4 oz fortified soymilk 4 graham crackers	1.5 oz (approx. 0.25 cup) trail mix 4 oz fortified soymilk	

TABLE 40.37

Sample Meal Plan for Lacto-Ovo Vegetarian Child Age 4 to 6[35,36]

Kcals: 1794; Carbohydrate: 255 g (57%); Protein: 63 g (14%); Fat: 63 g (31.5%)		
Breakfast	*Lunch*	*Dinner*
1 cup Honey Nut Cheerios with 4 oz milk on cereal 4 oz 1% milk to drink orange slices	0.5 cup homemade macaroni and cheese celery sticks and 2 Tbsp peanut butter 2 fruit cookies	burrito with salsa and sour cream, made with vegetarian chili 0.5 cup rice 4 oz 1% milk 0.5 cup green salad with broccoli 0.5 cup applesauce
Snack	*Snack*	
1.5 oz cheese 5 Ritz crackers 4 oz 1% milk	fruit smoothie made with juice, frozen yogurt, and fruit	

Summary

In summary, the term "vegetarianism" may mean different things to different people. Before making or accepting generalizations about vegetarianism, it is important to define the term. A person following a vegetarian lifestyle can have significantly lower risks of many chronic diseases, such as heart disease or cancer, than an omnivore does. However, some nutrients are more difficult to easily obtain from a vegetarian diet and may be a concern for deficiency, especially in children or during other critical life-cycle periods.

References

1. Messina M, Messina V. *The Dietitian's Guide to Vegetarian Diets: Issues and Applications,* Aspen Publishers, Gaithersburg, 1996.
2. Mahan LK, Escott-Stump S. *Krause's Food, Nutrition, and Diet Therapy,* 9th ed, WB Saunders, Philadelphia, 1996.
3. Miller GD, Jarvis JK, McBean LD. *Handbook of Dairy Foods and Nutrition,* 2nd ed, CRC Press, Boca Raton, 2000 pg 252.
4. Messina VK, Burke KI. *J Am Diet Assoc* 97: 1317; 1997.
5. Parsons TJ, Van Dusseldorp M, van der Vliet M, et al. *J Bone Mineral Res* 12: 1486; 1997.
6. Draper A, Lewis J, Malhotra N, Wheeler E. *Br J Nutr* 69: 3; 1993.
7. Remer T, Neubert A, Manz F. *Br J Nutr* 81: 45; 1999.
8. Sanders TA. *Pediatr Clin N Am* 42: 955; 1995.
9. Sanders TA, Reddy S. *Am J Clin Nutr* 59: 1176S; 1994.
10. Alexander H, Lockwood LP, Harris MA, Melby DL. *J Am Coll Nutr* 18: 127; 1999.
11. Craig WJ *Am J Clin Nutr* 59: 1233S; 1994.
12. Burr ML, Butland BK. *Am J Clin Nutr* 48: 840; 1988.
13. Harman SK, Parnell WR. *NZ Med J* 111: 91; 1998.
14. Gibson RS. *Am J Clin Nutr* 59: 1223S; 1994.
15. Nieman DC, Underwood BC, Sherman KM, et al. *J Am Diet Assoc* 89: 1763; 1989.
16. Donovan UM, Gibson RS. *J Adol Health* 18: 292; 1996.
17. Kadrabova J, Madaric A, Kovacikova Z, Ginter E. *Biol Trace Element Res* 50: 13; 1995.
18. Craig WJ. *J Am Diet Assoc* 97: 199S; 1997.
19. Tham DM, Gardner CD, Haskell WL. *J Clin Endocrinol Metab* 83: 2223; 1998.
20. Bingham SA, Atkinson C, Liggins J, et al. *Br J Nutr* 79: 393; 1998.
21. Uauy-Dagach R, Valenzuela A. *Nutr Rev* 54: 102S; 1996.
22. Sanders TAB. *Am J Clin Nutr* 70: 555S; 1999.
23. Gordon N. *Brain Devel* 19: 165; 1997.
24. Gibson RA, Neumann MA, Makrides M. *Lipids* 31: 177S; 1996.
25. Kretchmer N, Beard JL, Carlson S. *Am J Clin Nutr* 63: 997S; 1996.
26. Conquer JA, Holub BJ. *Vegetarian Nutrition: An Internation Journal,* 1-2: 42; 1997.
27. National Research Council, *Recommended Dietary Allowances,* 10th ed, National Academy Press, Washington, DC, 1989.
28. Yates AA, Schlicker SA, Suitor CW. *J Am diet Assoc* 98: 699; 1998.
29. Health and Welfare Canada. *Nutriton Recommendations: The Report of the Scientific Review Committee,* Authority of the Minister of Health and Welfare, Ottawa, 1990.
30. Drezner MK, Hoben KP. *Eating Well, Living Well with Osteoporosis.* Viking Press, New York, 1996.
31. Thaler SM, Teitelbaum I, Berl T. *Am J Kidney Dis* 31: 1028; 1998.
32. Toohey ML, Harris MA, DeWitt W, et al. *J Am Coll Nutr* 17: 407; 1998.
33. Thorogood M, Carter R, Benfield L, et al. *Br Med J* 295: 351; 1987.

34. Key TJA, Thorogood M, Appleby PN, Burr ML. *Br Med J* 313: 775; 1996.
35. Pennington JAT. *Bowes & Church's Food Values of portions Commonly Used,* 17 ed, Lippincott-Raven, Philadelphia, 1998.
36. Hands ES. *Food Finder: Food Sources of Vitamins and Minerals,* ESHA Research, Salem, 1995.
37. Holick MF, Shao Q, Liu WW, Chen TC. *N Engl J Med* 326: 1178; 1992.
38. Morris DH. *Iron in Human Nutrition,* 2nd ed, National Cattlemen's Beef Association, 1998.
39. Holben DH, Smith AM. *J Am Diet Assoc* 99: 836; 1999.
40. McBean LD. *Zinc in Human Nutrition,* National Cattlemen's Beef Association, 1997.
41. United States Department of Agriculture, Agricultural Research Service, Nutrient Data Laboratory, *USDA Nutrient Database for Standard Reference, Release 13,* www.nal.usda.gov/fnic/foodcomp/.

41

Allergic Disorders

Scott H. Sicherer

Definition of Food Allergy

Because individuals ingest food throughout the day, potentially any malady could be falsely associated with eating. In fact, surveys of adults have shown that 18 to 22% believe that they have a food allergy,[1-3] and 28% of parents suspect a food allergy in their infants and young children.[4] However, true food allergy affects 6 to 8% of children[4] and approximately 2% of adults.[3-5] The discrepancy between suspected and true allergy is due, in part, to the manner in which food allergy is defined. Technically, a food allergy is an adverse *immune response* toward protein in food.[6] This is in contrast to a larger number of non-immune mediated adverse reactions to food. These non-immune-mediated reactions include those caused by toxins in foods that would affect anyone ingesting the tainted food, and those caused by a particular condition of the affected individual (*food intolerance*). Examples of food intolerance/reactions to toxins are listed in Table 41.1.

Pathophysiology of Food Allergic Reactions

A vast number of potentially immunoreactive food proteins pass through the gut, but the normal response to these foreign proteins is tolerance. That is, the immune system recognizes these proteins (antigens), but does not process these proteins in a manner that results in adverse reactions. In fact, approximately 2% of ingested food enters the blood stream in an immunologically intact form,[7] but causes no symptoms in the normal individual. It remains unclear why some individuals develop food allergies, but a genetic predisposition toward allergic responses plays a role.[8] For those individuals predisposed to food allergies, food allergens can elicit specific responses in several ways.

The most common immunologic basis for food allergic responses involves the generation of proteins, IgE antibodies, that mediate immediate food hypersensitivity reactions.[9,10] When a protein enters the intestine, immune cells termed antigen presenting cells (APC) process the protein (usually a glycoprotein) and present a small portion of

0-8493-2705-9/01/$0.00+$1.50

TABLE 41.1

Examples of Food Intolerance/Toxic Reactions (Non-Immunologic, Adverse Reactions to Food)[21,140,141]

Disorder/Sensitivity	Pathophysiology/Symptoms
Lactase deficiency (lactose intolerance)	Bloating, diarrhea from inability to digest the lactose in cow's milk; may be dose-related
Tyramine sensitivity	Tyramine in hard cheeses, wine may trigger migraine headache
Scombroid fish poisoning	Oral pruritus, flushing, vomiting, hives from histamine released from spoiled dark meat fish (tuna, Mahi-Mahi)
Caffeine	Pharmacologic effects of jitteriness, heart palpitations
Myristicin	Hallucinogen in nutmeg
Gallbladder disease	Pain following ingestion of fatty foods

the protein to T-cells that specifically recognize the protein fragment (Figure 41.1). Cellular interactions between the APC and T-cell may direct the T-cell toward allergic responses (termed Th-2 responses). The sensitized T-cells replicate and then interact with B-cells in the context of further exposure to the food antigen, leading these B-cells to produce IgE antibodies that specifically bind a portion of the food protein (epitope). These IgE antibodies bind to specific receptors found on mast cells in body tissues and basophils in the bloodstream. The mast cells and basophils have preformed mediators (e.g., histamine) that, when released from the cell, cause tissue swelling (edema from capillary leakage of fluid) and pruritus. When the mast cell or basophil armed with the food-specific IgE antibody comes in contact with the particular allergenic protein, the IgE antibodies attach to the protein and crosslink, resulting in release of the mediators and the onset of the food-allergic reaction.

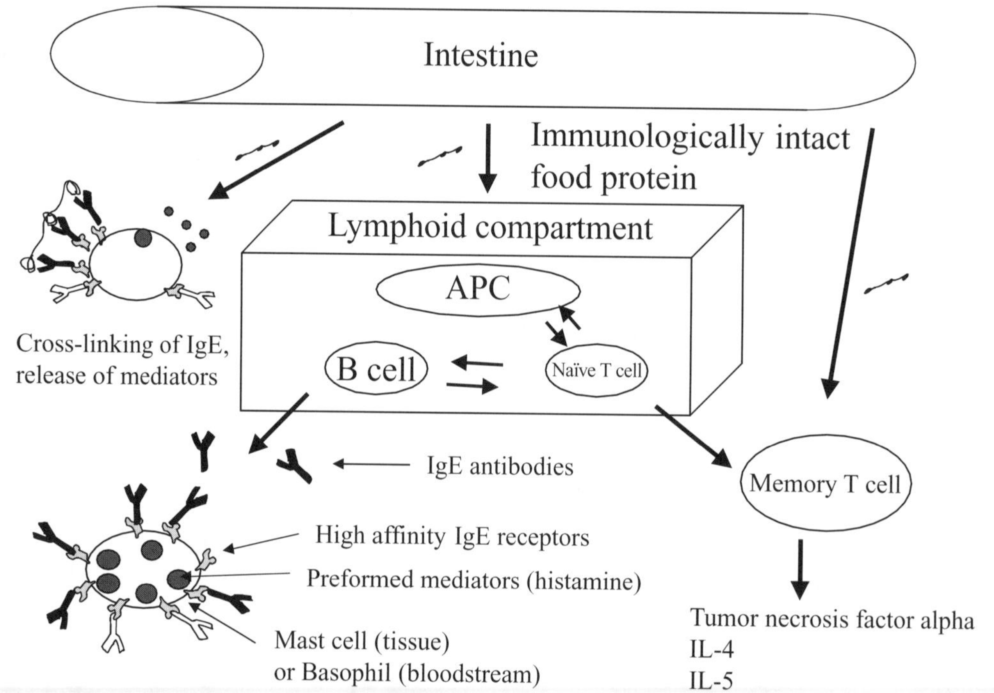

FIGURE 41.1
APC-antigen presenting cells, IL-interleukin. See text for details.

TABLE 41.2

Foods Responsible for the Majority (85 to 90%) of Significant Allergic Reactions[3,5,12,13]

Infants/Young Children	Older Children/Adults
Egg	Peanut
Cow's milk	Tree nuts
Soy bean	Shellfish
Peanut	Fish
Wheat	
Fish	
Tree nuts (walnut, Brazil, hazel, almond, cashew, etc.)	
Shellfish	

A second way in which the immune system may react adversely toward a food protein does not involve the generation of IgE antibody (non-IgE-mediated). In this case the T-cell may, through direct interaction with specific receptors on the cells, elaborate mediators (cytokines) with direct effects. An example is the release of tumor necrosis factor alpha that causes gut edema in certain forms of cow's milk allergy.[11] Further research is under way to better delineate the mechanisms of non-IgE-mediated food allergy.

Food Allergens

Many studies have indicated that a rather short list of foods accounts for the majority (85 to 90%) of food-allergic reactions: chicken egg, cow's milk, wheat, soybean, peanut, tree nuts, fish, and shellfish.[3,12-15] However, virtually any food protein could elicit an allergic response. Many of the allergenic food proteins have been characterized and are generally heat-stable, water-soluble glycoproteins from 10 to 70 kd in size.[16,17] For many of these proteins, the particular allergenic epitopes that bind IgE or T-cell receptors have been mapped.

Epidemiology

Population-based studies utilizing oral food challenges to confirm reactivity have determined that food allergy affects 6 to 8% of young children[4] and almost 2% of adults.[3] The foods causing significant allergic reactions in different age groups are listed in Table 41.2. Most children outgrow their sensitivity to milk, egg, soy, and wheat, but allergy to peanut, tree nuts (e.g., walnut, cashew, Brazil nut, etc.), fish, and shellfish account for the majority of significant food allergies in adults, and are foods for which tolerance rarely develops.[12,18] Peanut and tree nut allergy alone affects 1.3% of the general population of the U.S.[19] Allergic reactions to food dyes and additives are comparatively rare, affecting up to 0.23% of the population.[20] Food allergy is a cause of a number of particular illnesses, as shown in Table 41.3.

TABLE 41.3

Epidemiologic Role of Food Allergy in Various Disorders

Disorder	Prevalence of Food Allergy as a Cause of the Disorder
Anaphylaxis[95,96,142]	34-52%
Asthmatic children[91]	6%
Asthmatic adults[92]	<1%
Atopic dermatitis (moderate-severe) in children[30]	37%
Atopic dermatitis in adults[34]	Rare
Acute urticaria[143]	20%
Chronic urticaria[144]	1.4%
Infantile refractory reflux[145]	42%
Childhood refractory constipation[73]	68%

Food Allergic Disorders

Food allergic disorders affect the skin and the gastrointestinal and respiratory tracts.[21] The pathophysiologic basis of the disorders may be IgE-mediated, non-IgE-mediated, or combined. In general, disorders with acute onset occurring within minutes to an hour after food ingestion are mediated by IgE antibody, while those that are more chronic and occur hours after ingestion are not IgE-mediated. Particular food allergic disorders are discussed below.

Disorders Affecting the Skin

Acute Urticaria

Urticaria, or hives, are characterized by pruritic, transient, erythematous raised lesions with central clearing and a surrounding area of erythema. The rash should leave no residual lesions after resolution. Hives may sometimes be accompanied by localized swellng (angioedema). Although there are many causes of acute urticaria, food allergy accounts for up to 20% of episodes.[22] The immediate onset of hives is mediated by specific IgE to food protein. Lesions usually occur within an hour of ingestion or skin contact with the causal food.[23]

Chronic Urticaria

This disorder of longstanding hives lasting over six weeks is rarely associated with food allergy. Only 1.4% of chronic/persistent urticaria is caused by food allergy, so a search for a causative food in the initial evaluation of this illness is often futile.[24]

Contact Urticaria

In some cases, topical exposure to a food (e.g., on the skin of the face) can cause a local reaction either through irritation or through specific immune mechanisms.[25]

Atopic Dermatitis (AD)

This rash usually begins in early infancy. It is characterized by a typical distribution on the extensor surfaces and faces of infants, or creases in older children and adults, with extreme pruritis and a chronic and relapsing course.[26] Atopic dermatitis is frequently associated with allergic disorders (asthma, allergic rhinitis) and with a family history of allergy.[27] Evidence suggests that, particularly in children, IgE-mediated food allergy plays a pathogenic role,[27] although non-IgE-mediated food allergy has also been implicated.[28] Clinical studies utilizing double-blind, placebo-controlled food challenges (DBPCFCs) have shown a prevalence rate of food allergy in 33 to 37% of children with moderate to severe AD.[29,30] Studies of dietary elimination have repeatedly shown improvement in AD symptoms.[12,31,32] The more severe the rash, the more likely that food allergy is associated;[33] however, AD is rarely associated with food allergy in adults.[34,35]

Dermatitis Herpetiformis (DH)

DH is a chronic papulovesicular skin disorder with lesions distributed over the extensor surfaces of the elbows, knees, and buttocks.[36] Immunohistologic examination of the lesions reveals the deposition of granular IgA antibody at the dermoepidermal junction.[37] The disorder is associated with a specific non-IgE-mediated immune response to gluten (a protein found in grains such as wheat, barley, and rye). Although related to celiac disease, there may be no associated gastrointestinal complaints; however, up to 72% may show villus atrophy on intestinal biopsy.[37] The rash abates with elimination of gluten from the diet.

Disorders Affecting the Gastrointestinal Tract

Immediate Gastrointestinal Hypersensitivity

In this syndrome, ingestion of the causal protein results in immediate (minutes to up to one to two hours) gastrointestinal symptoms that may include nausea, vomiting, abdominal pain, and diarrhea. Considered here as a distinct syndrome, it is more commonly associated with reactions in other organ systems, such as during systemic anaphylaxis in patients with other atopic diseases. For example, children with atopic dermatitis undergoing oral food challenges with foods to which they have specific IgE antibody will sometimes manifest only gastrointestinal symptoms.[13,38]

Oral Allergy Syndrome

Symptoms include pruritus and angioedema of the lips, tongue, and palate, and are of rapid onset, typically while eating certain fresh fruits and vegetables.[39] The reaction occurs primarily in adults with pollen allergy (hay fever) sensitized to crossreacting proteins in particular fruits and vegetables as shown in Table 41.4. Up to 71% of adults with pollen allergy experience these symptoms.[40] The proteins are labile, and cooked forms of the fruits and vegetables generally do not induce symptoms.

Dietary Protein-Induced Proctitis/Proctocolitis of Infancy

Food allergy is the most common cause of rectal bleeding due to colitis in infants.[41] Infants with this disorder are typically healthy, but have streaks of blood mixed with mucus in their stool. The most common causal food is cow's milk or soy, and even breastfed infants can develop this reaction from small amounts of protein passed through breast milk in mothers ingesting the causal protein.[42] Although peripheral eosinophilia and positive radioallergosorbent tests (RASTs; serum tests to determine specific IgE antibody) to milk have been reported, they are not consistent findings.[41,43-45] In cow's milk- or soy formula-fed infants, substitution with a protein hydrolysate formula generally leads to cessation

TABLE 41.4

Cross-Reactions Due to Proteins Shared by Pollens and Foods Leading to Symptoms of the Oral Allergy Syndrome[39,146,147,150]

Birch Pollen	Ragweed Pollen	Grass Pollen
Apple	Melons	Peach
Carrot		Potato
Cherry		Tomato
Apricot		Cherry
Plum		
Celery		

of obvious bleeding within 72 hours. The majority of infants who develop this condition while ingesting protein hydrolysate formulas will experience resolution of bleeding with substitution of an amino acid-based formula.[46]

Dietary (Food) Protein-Induced Enteropathy

This disorder affects primarily infants and young children and is characterized by failure to thrive, diarrhea, emesis, and hypoproteinemia usually related to an immunologic reaction to cow's milk protein.[47-50] The syndrome may also occur following infectious gastroenteritis in infants.[48,51] Patchy villous atrophy with cellular infiltrate on biopsy is characteristic. Diagnosis is based upon the combined findings from endoscopy/biopsy, allergen elimination, and challenge. While this syndrome resembles celiac disease, resolution generally occurs in one to two years.[48]

Dietary (Food) Protein-Induced Enterocolitis Syndrome (FPIES)

FPIES as defined by Powell[52,53] describes a symptom complex of profuse vomiting and diarrhea diagnosed in infancy during chronic ingestion of the causal food protein — usually cow's milk or soy. Since both the small and large bowel are involved, the term enterocolitis is used. When the causal protein is reintroduced acutely after a period of avoidance with resolution of symptoms, symptoms characteristically develop after a delay of two hours, with profuse vomiting and later diarrhea.[53,54] There is also an accompanying increase in the peripheral polymorphonuclear leukocyte count and, in some cases, severe acidosis and dehydration.[54,55] Confirmation of the allergy included a negative search for other causes, improvement when not ingesting the causal protein, and a positive oral challenge resulting in the characteristic symptoms/signs. Approximately 50% of the infants react to both cow's milk and soy. Sensitivity to milk is lost in 60% and to soy in 25% of the patients after two years from the time of presentation.[54,56] Treatment with a hydrolyzed cow's milk formula is advised, although some patients may react to the residual peptides in these formulas, requiring an amino acid-based formula.[57]

Allergic Eosinophilic Gastroenteritis (AEG)/Allergic Eosinophilic Esophagitis (AEE)

These disorders are characterized by infiltration of the esophagus (AEE), gastric, and/or intestinal walls (AEG) with eosinophils, peripheral eosinophilia (in 50 to 75%) and absence of vasculitis.[58] Patients with AEG present with postprandial nausea, abdominal pain, vomiting, diarrhea, protein-losing enteropathy, and weight loss, and depending upon the obstruction ascites can also develop.[59,60] Those with AEE may present with symptoms of severe reflux disease.[61] The diagnosis rests upon biopsy showing eosinophilic infiltration, although there may be patchy disease and infiltration may be missed.[62] Formal trials of food elimination in adults have had mixed success, but large groups have not been evaluated for depth of infiltration and abdominal bloating,[60,63,64] and those studied clearly represent a heterogeneous group. In children with AEE, significant success from dietary elimination has been achieved.[61] AEE was associated with positive tests for food-specific IgE antibody in some of the children, but most with this disorder do not have IgE-mediated food allergy.

Celiac Disease

Celiac disease is a dietary protein enteropathy characterized by an extensive loss of absorptive villi and hyperplasia of the crypts leading to malabsorption, chronic diarrhea, steatorrhea, abdominal distention, flatulence, and weight loss or failure to thrive. As the disease represents an immune response to a food protein, it may be considered a food allergic disorder.[65] Patients with celiac disease are sensitive to gliadin, the alcohol-soluble portion of gluten found in wheat, oat, rye, and barley. Endoscopy typically reveals total villous atrophy and extensive cellular infiltrate. The prevalence of Celiac disease has been reported between 1:3700 and 1:300.[66] Chronic ingestion of gluten-containing grains in Celiac patients is associated with increased risk of malignancy, especially T-cell lymphoma.[67]

Other Disorders Possibly Associated with Food Allergy

Gastroesophageal Reflux (GER)

GER has been associated with cow's milk allergy (CMA) in infants. Forget and Arenda[68] demonstrated that infants who appear to have GER but do not respond to medical therapy may have CMA. Cavataio, Iacono, and colleagues[69-71] have investigated these issues in several prospective controlled trials. They have demonstrated that up to 42% of infants under one year of age with GER also have CMA.

Constipation

Constipation has also been associated with cow's milk allergy in young children.[72,73] Investigators have demonstrated the presence of eosinophilic proctitis in children with chronic constipation, resolution of constipation after withdrawal of cow's milk from the diet (and substitution with soy-based formula), and recurrence upon reintroduction of cow's milk.

Occult Blood Loss from the Gastrointestinal Tract/Iron Deficiency Anemia

Ingestion of whole cow's milk by infants less than six months of age may lead to occult blood loss from the gastrointestinal tract and iron deficiency anemia.[74] The use of infant formulas generally results in resolution of symptoms.

Infantile Colic

There is limited evidence that infantile colic is associated with food (cow's milk) allergy in a subset of patients (sometimes on an IgE-mediated basis), but more studies are needed to define the relationship.[75-77]

Inflammatory Bowel Disease

A role for food allergy in inflammatory bowel disease has been suggested because elemental diets have been shown to induce remission in Crohn's disease. [78,79] However, meta-analyses of elemental diets for Crohn's disease have demonstrated that they are inferior to steroids at inducing and maintaining remission, despite their popularity in some countries.[80-82]

TABLE 41.5

Gastrointestinal Diseases Associated with Food Allergy

Disorder	Age Onset	Duration	Symptoms/Features	Foods
Food protein-induced enterocolitis syndrome [53,54]	1 day-9 months	Usually 1-3 years	Vomiting, diarrhea, failure to thrive, villus injury, dehydration, acidosis	Cow's milk, soybean, (rare grains, poultry)
Enteropathy [15,48]	2-18 months	Usually 1-3 years	Failure to thrive, edema, diarrhea, villus injury, malabsorption	Cow's milk, soy
Celiac disease[152]	Any	Lifelong	Villus injury, malabsorption	Gluten
Proctocolitis [42]	Infants	1 year	Bloody stools	Cow's milk, soybean
Allergic eosinophilic gastroenteritis/ esophagitis[59,61]	Any	Long-lived	Vomiting, abdominal pain, diarrhea, eosinophilic infiltration of gut	Multiple foods

Irritable Bowel Syndrome

The relationship of irritable bowel syndrome to food allergy has not been systematically studied.[83-85] A summary of the gastrointestinal diseases associated with food allergy is given in Table 41.5.

Disorders Affecting the Respiratory Tract

Allergic Rhinitis

Symptoms of congestion, rhinorrhea, and nasal pruritus are usually associated with hypersensitivity to airborne allergens, not foods. Rarely, isolated nasal symptoms may occur as a result of an IgE-mediated allergy to ingested food proteins.[86] The prevalence of this illness, even among patients referred to allergy clinics, appears to be under 1%. On the other hand, 25 to 80% of patients with documented IgE-mediated food allergy experience nasal symptoms during oral food challenges that result in systemic symptoms.[86] In contrast to immune-mediated rhinitis, *gustatory rhinitis* refers to rhinorrhea caused by spicy foods. This reaction is mediated by neurologic mechanisms.[87]

Asthma

Lower airway symptoms of wheezing, cough, and dyspnea induced by lower airway inflammation and bronchoconstriction can be related to food allergy. Reactions may occur based upon IgE-mediated reactions from ingestion of the causative food or from inhalation of vapors released during cooking or in occupational settings.[88-90] The prevalence of food-related asthma in the general population is unknown, but studies utilizing DBPCFCs report a prevalence of 5.7% among children with asthma,[91] 11% among children with atopic dermatitis,[88] and 24% among children with a history of food-induced wheezing.[89] The prevalence of food-induced wheezing among adults with asthma is under 2%.[92]

Heiner's Syndrome

This is a rare, non-IgE-mediated adverse pulmonary response to food, affecting infants. The disorder is characterized by an immune reaction to cow's milk proteins with precip-

TABLE 41.6

Symptoms Occurring in Anaphylaxis[14,15,94,96]

Organ System	Symptoms
Respiratory	Throat tightness, wheezing, repetitive coughing, nasal congestion rhinitis, hypoxia/cyanosis
Gastrointestinal	Obstructive tongue edema, nausea, vomiting, diarrhea, abdominal pain, oral pruritus, lip edema
Skin	Pruritus, urticaria, angioedema, morbiliform rash
Cardiovascular	Hypotension, syncope, dysrhythmia
Other	Sense of "impending doom," uterine contractions

itating antibodies (IgG) to cow's milk protein resulting in pulmonary infiltrates, pulmonary hemosiderosis, anemia, failure to thrive, and recurrent pneumonias.[93] Elimination of cow's milk protein is curative.

Multisystem Disorders

Anaphylaxis

Clinically, anaphylaxis refers to a dramatic, severe multi-organ systemic allergic reaction associated with IgE-mediated hypersensitivity that may be life-threatening. Anaphylaxis has been defined technically as an immediate, systemic reaction caused by rapid, IgE-mediated immune release of potent mediators from mast cells and basophils.[94] Food is the most common cause of out-of-hospital anaphylaxis.[95-97] Symptoms may affect the skin, respiratory tract, and gastrointestinal tract (Table 41.6). Symptoms can be severe, progressive, and potentially fatal. Fatal food-induced anaphylaxis appears to be more common among teenage patients with underlying asthma.[14,15] In addition, patients who experienced fatal or near fatal anaphylaxis were unaware that they had ingested the incriminated food, had almost immediate symptoms, had a delay in receiving adrenaline, and in about half of the cases there was a period of quiescence prior to a respiratory decompensation.[14] The foods most often responsible for food-induced anaphylaxis are peanut, tree nuts, and shellfish.[14,15,98,99]

Food-Associated, Exercise-Induced Anaphylaxis

This uncommon disorder refers to patients who are able to ingest a particular food or exercise without a reaction. However, when exercise follows the ingestion of a particular food, anaphylaxis results.[100-102] In some cases, exercise after any meal results in a reaction. Treatment depends upon elimination of the causal food for 12 hours prior to exercise.

Disorders not Clearly Related to Food Allergy

Patients may relate a variety of ailments to food allergy (headaches, seizures, behavioral disorders, fatigue, arthritis, etc.), but many of these are either false associations or adverse reactions that are not immunologic in nature. Food allergy may play a role in a minority of patients with migraine headaches,[103] although the pharmacologic activity of certain chemicals that are found in some foods (i.e., tyramine in cheeses) is more often responsible. The role of food allergy in childhood behavioral disorders is also controversial. Although a small subset of patients with behavioral disorders may be affected by food dyes, there is no convincing evidence that food allergy plays a direct role in these disorders,[104,105] and children are not allergic to "sugar." On the other hand, for individuals with these ailments who also have bona fide allergies, treatment to relieve symptoms of asthma, atopic dermatitis, and hay fever should be pursued in parallel to treatment directed at the unrelated disorder.

Diagnostic Approach to Food Allergic Disorders

The diagnosis of food allergy often rests simply upon a history of an acute onset of typical symptoms, such as hives and wheezing, following the isolated ingestion of a suspected food, with confirmatory laboratory studies indicating the presence of specific IgE antibody to the suspected food. However, the diagnosis is more complicated when multiple foods are implicated or when chronic diseases such as asthma[106] or atopic dermatitis[107] are evaluated. The diagnosis of food allergy and identification of the particular foods responsible is also problematic when reactions are not mediated by IgE antibody, as is the case with a number of gastrointestinal food allergies.[54] In these latter circumstances, well-devised elimination diets followed by physician-supervised oral food challenges are critical in the identification and proper treatment of these disorders.

General Approach to Diagnosis

The history and physical examination must review general medical concerns to exclude nonimmunologic adverse reactions to foods or to consider other allergic causes for symptoms (e.g., cat allergy causing asthma). In relation to foods, a careful history should focus upon the symptoms attributed to food ingestion (type, acute versus chronic), the food(s) involved, consistency of reactions, quantity of food required to elicit symptoms, timing between ingestion and onset of symptoms, the most recent reaction/patterns of reactivity, and any ancillary associated activity that may play a role (i.e., exercise, alcohol ingestion). The information gathered is used to determine the best mode of diagnosis, or may lead to dismissal of the problem based upon the history alone.

For acute reactions after isolated ingestion of a particular food, such as acute urticaria or anaphylaxis, the history may clearly implicate a particular food, and a positive test for specific IgE antibody would be confirmatory. If the ingestion was of mixed foods and the causal food was uncertain (e.g., fruit salad), the history may help to eliminate some of the foods (those frequently ingested without symptoms), and specific tests for IgE may help to further narrow the possibilities. In chronic disorders such as atopic dermatitis or asthma, it is more difficult to pinpoint causal food(s).[107] The approach to diagnosis in these chronic disorders usually requires elimination diets and oral food challenges to confirm suspected associations. This is particularly the case for the non-IgE-mediated reactions or those attributed to food dyes/preservatives in which ancillary laboratory testing is not helpful.

Tests for Specific IGE Antibody

In the evaluation of IgE-mediated food allergy, specific tests can help to identify or exclude responsible foods. One method to determine the presence of specific IgE antibody is prick-puncture skin testing. While the patient is not taking antihistamines, a device such as a bifurcated needle or lancet is used to puncture the skin through a glycerinated extract of a food and appropriate positive (histamine) and negative (saline-glycerine) controls. A local wheal and flare response indicates the presence of food-specific IgE antibody (a wheal >3 mm is considered positive). Prick skin tests are most valuable when they are negative, since the negative predictive value of the tests is very high (over 95%).[108,109] Unfortunately, the positive predictive value is on the order of only 50%.[108,109] Thus, a positive skin test in isolation cannot be considered proof of clinically relevant hypersensitivity. Intradermal allergy skin tests with food extracts give an unacceptably high false-positive rate, have been associated with systemic reactions including fatal anaphylactic reactions, and should not be used.[109] An additional issue is that the protein in commercial extracts of some fruits and vegetables are prone to degradation, so fresh extracts of these foods are more reliable[110] and the "prick-prick" manner of testing may be indicated, where the probe is used to first pierce the food being tested (to obtain liquid) and then the skin of the patient.

RASTs

In vitro tests for specific IgE (RASTs) are also helpful in the evaluation of IgE-mediated food allergy.[111] Unlike skin tests, RASTs can be used while the patient is taking antihistamines and does not depend on having an area of rash-free skin for testing. Like skin tests, a negative result is very reliable in ruling out an IgE-mediated reaction to a particular food, but a positive result has low specificity. Recent studies have been evaluating improved RASTs that may have added predictive value for clinical reactivity.[111-113]

In addition to the high false positive rate of tests for food-specific IgE antibodies, several other issues complicate interpretation. It is not uncommon for patients to have positive skin tests and RASTs to several members of a botanical family or animal species. This usually represents immunologic cross-reactivity but may not represent clinical reactivity. For example, most peanut-allergic patients will have positive skin tests to at least a few of the other members of the legume family, but only 5% will have clinical reactions to more than one legume.[114] Further testing with oral challenges, if the history does not resolve the issue, would be required. More importantly, the foods selected for testing should be carefully selected to include only those suspected to be at issue in order to avoid false positive tests that inappropriately lead to questions about foods that have been previously tolerated. Lastly, one should be wary of tests such as measurement of IgG_4 antibody, provocation-neutralization, cytotoxicity, applied kinesiology, among other unproved methods.[115]

Food Elimination Diets

As an adjunct to testing, the first step in proving a cause-and-effect relationship with a particular illness and food allergy (whether IgE-mediated or not) is to show resolution of symptoms with elimination of the suspected food(s). In many cases, one or several foods are eliminated, which may be the obvious course of action when an isolated food ingestion (i.e., peanut) causes a sudden acute reaction and there is a positive test for IgE to the food. This would also represent a therapeutic intervention. However, eliminating one or a few suspected foods from the diet when the diagnosis is not so clear (asthma, atopic dermatitis, chronic urticaria) can be a crucial step in determining whether food is causal in the disease process. If symptoms persist, the eliminated food(s) is (are) excluded as a cause of symptoms. Alternatively, and as is more likely the case for evaluating chronic disorders without acute reactions, eliminating a large number of foods suspected to cause a chronic problem (usually including those that are common causes of food-allergic reactions as described above) and giving a list of "allowed foods" may be the preferred approach. The primary disadvantage of this approach is that if symptoms persist, the cause could still be attributed to foods left in the diet. Thus, a third type of elimination diet is an elemental diet in which calories are obtained from a hydrolyzed formula, or preferably from an amino acid-based formula. A variation is to include a few foods likely to be tolerated (but, again this adds the possibility that persistent symptoms are caused by these foods). This diet is extremely difficult to maintain in patients beyond infancy. In extreme cases, nasogastric feeding of the amino acid-based formula can be achieved, although some patients can tolerate the taste of these formulas with the use of flavoring agents provided by the manufacturers. This diet may be required when the diets mentioned above fail to resolve symptoms, but suspicion for food-related illness remains high. It is also required in disorders associated with multiple food allergies such as allergic eosinophilic gastroenteritis. With AEG, prolonged dietary elimination for three to six weeks is sometimes needed to determine whether resolution of symptoms will occur.[61]

Food Challenges

An oral food challenge is performed by feeding the patient the suspected food under physician observation. There are several settings in which physician-supervised oral food challenges are required for diagnosis of food-allergic disease (Table 41.7). Because food challenges may elicit severe reactions, they are usually conducted under physician supervision, with emergency medications to treat anaphylaxis immediately available.[116] Challenges can be performed "openly" with the patient ingesting the food in its native form, "single-blind" with the food masked and the patient unaware if they are receiving the test food, or as DBPCFCs where neither patient nor physician knows which challenges contain the food being tested. While open and single-blind challenges are open to patient or observer bias, the DBPCFC is considered the gold standard for diagnosis, since bias is removed.[116]

In all of these challenges, the food is given in gradually increasing amounts that may be individualized both in dose and timing, depending on the patient's history. For most IgE-mediated reactions, experts suggest giving 8 to 10 grams of the dry food or 100 ml of wet food (double amount for meat/fish) at 10 to 15 minute intervals over about 90 minutes followed by a larger, meal-size portion of food a few hours later.[116] Starting doses may be a minute amount applied to the inner lip followed by 1% of the total challenge, followed by gradually increasing amounts (4, 10, 20%, etc.). However, challenges may be individ-

TABLE 41.7

Indications for Performing Physician-Supervised Oral Food Challenges

To confirm a food allergy when history is unclear and tests not confirmatory
To exclude a food allergy
To monitor for development of tolerance

ualized to parallel the clinical history (i.e., feeding over consecutive days for chronic disorders with delayed symptoms). Similarly, higher risk challenges may start at extremely low doses with very gradual increases over longer time intervals.

Symptoms are recorded and frequent assessments are made during the challenge for symptoms affecting the skin, gastrointestinal tract, and/or respiratory tract. Challenges are terminated when a reaction becomes apparent, and emergency medications are given as needed. Generally, antihistamines are given at the earliest sign of a reaction, with epinephrine and other treatments given if there is progression of symptoms or any potentially life-threatening symptoms.

The practical issues in preparing food challenges include palatability and masking foods in appropriate vehicles, with placebos for DBPCFCs. In many cases, dry forms of the food (flour, powdered egg whites, etc.) can be hidden in puddings or liquids. Bulkier foods may be hidden in pancakes or ground beef. Flavoring agents such as mint can be added for further masking. Hiding the food in opaque capsules is a convenient method to administer blinded challenges for patients who are able to ingest these capsules.

Non-IgE-mediated reactions (e.g., AEG, enterocolitis, etc.) are more difficult to diagnose since there are no specific laboratory tests to identify particular foods that may be responsible for these illnesses. In many cases, a biopsy may be needed (e.g., AEG) to establish an initial diagnosis. Elimination diets with gradual reintroduction of foods and supervised oral food challenges are often needed to identify whether diet plays a role in the disorder, and to identify the causal food(s). Specific challenge protocols have been advised for food-induced enterocolitis syndrome.[53] Oral challenges can be used to evaluate reactions to food additives (coloring and flavoring agents and preservatives) or virtually any complaint associated with foods. When used to evaluate behavioral disorders or other complaints not convincingly associated with food allergy, DBPCFCs are advised to avoid bias.

Treatment of Food Allergy

The mainstay of treatment for food allergy is dietary elimination of the offending food. The elimination of particular dietary food proteins is not a simple task. Table 41.8 lists a variety of possible pitfalls in dietary management of food allergy. A primary issue in avoidance is the ambiguity of food labeling practices. In a cow's milk-free diet, for example, patients must be instructed to not only avoid all cow's milk products, but also to read ingredient labels for key words which may indicate the presence of cow's milk protein. Terms such as casein, whey, lactalbumin, caramel color, "natural flavoring," and nougat may, for example, signify the presence of cow's milk protein. In many cases, the allergic individual must query companies for further product information, although product labeling is improving. Patients and parents must also be made aware that the food protein, as opposed to sugar or fat, is the ingredient being eliminated. For example, lactose-free cow's milk contains cow's milk protein, and many egg substitutes contain chicken egg proteins. Conversely, peanut and soy oil do not generally contain the food protein, unless the processing method is one in which the protein is not completely eliminated (as with cold pressed or "extruded" oil). Lay organizations such as The Food Allergy Network (800-929-4040; www.foodallergy.org) assist families and physicians in the difficult task of eliminating the allergenic foods. When multiple foods are eliminated from the diet, it is prudent to enlist the aid of a dietitian in formulating a nutritionally balanced diet.

TABLE 41.8
Pitfalls in Dietary Allergen Avoidance

Pitfall	Examples
Unfamiliar terms on food labels	Various terms indicating particular food proteins such as casein (milk), whey (milk), ovalbumin (egg)
Ambiguous terms on food labels	"Natural flavoring" may indicate cow's milk
Religious labels	"Pareve" may indicate non-dairy but does not guarantee absence of milk protein
Cross-contamination	In processing lines (e.g., milk protein found in juice boxes) or in the home setting (shared utensils)
Ingredient switching	Large size of a product may have different ingredients than a small size, despite similar packaging design
Hidden ingredients	Egg white to make a pretzel shiny, peanut butter to seal the end of egg rolls, peanut butter to thicken sauces

In addition to elimination of the offending food, an emergency plan must be in place to treat reactions caused by accidental ingestion. Injectable epinephrine and oral antihistamine should be readily available and administered without delay to treat patients at risk for severe reactions.[15,94,117] Caregivers must be familiarized with indications for the use and method of administration of these medications.

Natural History

Most children outgrow their allergies to milk, egg, wheat, and soy by age three years.[18] However, patients allergic to peanuts, tree nuts, fish, and shellfish are much less likely to lose their clinical reactivity,[14,96,118,121] and these sensitivities may persist into adulthood. Approximately one-third of children with AD and food allergy "lost" (or "outgrew") their clinical reactivity over one to three years with strict adherence to dietary elimination, believed to have aided in a more timely recovery.[12] Elevated concentrations of food-specific IgE may indicate a lower likelihood of developing tolerance in the subsequent few years.[113,122] However, tests for food-specific IgE antibody (prick skin tests, RAST) remain positive for years after the food allergy has resolved and cannot be followed as the sole indicator of tolerance.[12] Thus, it is recommended that patients with chronic disease such as atopic dermatitis be rechallenged intermittently (e.g., egg: every two to three years; milk, soy, wheat: every one to two years; peanuts, nuts, fish, and shellfish: if tolerance is suspected; other foods every one to two years) to determine whether their food allergy persists, so that restriction diets may be discontinued as soon as possible.

Prevention of Food Allergy

Dietary modification with the goal of allergy prevention has been attempted during pregnancy, lactation, and early feeding of infants who are at risk for atopic disease based upon strong family histories of allergy. In several series, infants from atopic families whose mothers excluded highly allergenic foods from their diets during lactation had significantly less AD and food allergy compared to infants whose mothers' diets were unrestricted.[123,126] However, the differences may not may not extend beyond early childhood.[126,127]

The delayed introduction of solid foods has also been associated with reduction in allergic disease. In a study of 1265 unselected neonates, the effect of solid food introduction was evaluated over a ten-year period.[128,129] A significant linear relationship was found between the number of solid foods introduced into the diet by four months of age and subsequent AD, with a threefold increase in recurrent eczema at ten years of age in infants receiving four or more solid foods compared to infants receiving no solid foods prior to four months of age. A prospective, nonrandomized study comparing breastfed infants who first received solid foods at three or six months of age revealed reduced AD and food allergy at one year of age in the group avoiding solids for the six-month period,[130] but no significant difference in these parameters at five years.[131] Since these series did not randomize patients, the studies must be considered suggestive until further randomized trials confirm the findings.

Future Therapies

Currently, strict avoidance of causal foods and treatment of accidental ingestion is the only available therapy for food allergy. Immunotherapy ("allergy shots") has not proven practical for treatment[132] except in the case of the oral allergy syndrome, in which immunotherapy with the pollens responsible for the cross-reactivity may provide relief.[133] Toward a goal of more definitive therapies for food allergic disorders, a multitude of experimental therapies is under investigation.

Humanized anti-IgE antibodies for injection into patients have been developed that are able to bind and remove free-floating IgE antibodies from the bloodstream and may reduce or abolish allergic responses. Anti-IgE may, therefore, provide treatment for many IgE-mediated allergic disorders (not just food allergy). More allergen-specific novel therapies include vaccination with proteins altered such that the epitopes that bind IgE are removed while areas of the protein are left intact so that T-cells can still mount a response leading, potentially, to tolerance.[134-137] Another approach to induce tolerance to specific food allergens is vaccination with DNA sequences that code for the production of food allergens,[138,139] and the use of immune modulators (cytokines, specific DNA sequences) that can direct the immune system away from allergic responses and toward tolerance of the proteins. It is hoped that these novel approaches will provide relief from chronic disease and prevent anaphylaxis for food allergic individuals.

References

1. Altman DR, Chiaramonte LT. *J Allergy Clin Immunol* 97: 1247; 1996.
2. Sloan AE, Powers ME. *J Allergy Clin Immunol* 78: 127; 1986.
3. Young E, Stoneham MD, Petruckevitch A, et al. *Lancet* 343: 1127; 1994.
4. Bock SA. *Pediatrics* 79: 83; 1987.
5. Sicherer SH, Furlong TJ, DeSimone J, Sampson HA. *J Allergy Clin Immunol* 103: 186; 1999.
6. Bruijnzeel-Koomen C, Ortolani C, Aas K, et al. *Allergy* 50: 623; 1995.
7. Husby S, Jensenius J, Svehag S. *Scand J Immunol* 22: 83; 1985.
8. Zeiger R, Heller S, Mellon M, et al. *Pediatr Allergy Immunol* 3: 110; 1992.

9. Geha RS. *J Allergy Clin Immunol* 90: 143; 1992.
10. Vercelli D, Geha R. *J Allergy Clin Immunol* 88: 285; 1991.
11. Heyman M, Darmon N, Dupont C. et al. *Gastroenterology* 106: 1514; 1994.
12. Sampson HA, Scanlon SM. *J Pediatr* 115: 23; 1989.
13. Burks AW, James JM, Hiegel A, et al. *J Pediatr* 132: 132; 1998.
14. Yunginger JW, Sweeney KG, Sturner WQ, et al. *JAMA* 260: 1450; 1988.
15. Sampson HA, Mendelson LM, Rosen JP. *N Engl J Med* 327: 380; 1992.
16. Spuergin P, Mueller H, Walter M, et al. *Allergy* 51: 306; 1996.
17. Burks AW, Shin D, Cockrell G, et al. *Eur J Biochem* 245: 334; 1997.
18. Bock SA. *J Allergy Clin Immunol* 69: 173; 1982.
19. Sicherer SH, Munoz-Furlong A, Burks AW, Sampson HA. *J Allergy Clin Immunol* 103: 559; 1999.
20. Young E, Patel S, Stoneham MD, et al. *J R Coll Physicians Lond* 21: 241; 1987.
21. Sicherer SH. *Am Fam Physician* 59: 415; 1999.
22. Sehgal VN, Rege VL. *Ann Allergy* 31: 279; 1973.
23. Sicherer SH, Burks AW, Sampson HA. *Pediatrics* 102: 46; 1998.
24. Champion RH. *Br J Dermatol* 119: 427; 1988.
25. Hanifin JM. *J Dermatol* 24: 495; 1997.
26. Hanifin JM, Rajka G. *Acta Dermatol Venereol* 92: 44S; 1980.
27. Sampson HA. *Ann Allergy* 69: 469; 1992.
28. Isolauri E, Turjanmaa K. *J Allergy Clin Immunol* 97: 9; 1996.
29. Burks AW, Mallory SB, Williams LW, Shirrell MA. *J Pediatr* 113: 447; 1988.
30. Eigenmann PA, Sicherer SH, Borkowski TA, et al. *Pediatrics* 101: 48; 1998.
31. Lever R, MacDonald C, Waugh P, Aitchison T. *Pediatr Allergy Immunol* 9: 13; 1998.
32. Atherton DJ, Soothill JF, Sewell M, et al. *Lancet* 1: 401; 1978.
33. Guillet G, Guillet MH. *Arch Dermatol* 128: 187; 1992.
34. deMaat-Bleeker F, Bruijnzeel-Koomen C. *Monogr Allergy Basel Karger* 32: 157; 1996.
35. Munkvad M, Danielsen L, Hoj L, et al. *Acta Dermatol Venereol* 64: 524; 1984.
36. Fry L, Seah PP. *Br J Dermatol* 90: 137; 1974.
37. Egan CA, O'Loughlin S, Gormally S, Powell FC. *Ir J Med Sci* 166: 241;1997.
38. Sampson HA, McCaskill CC. *J Pediatr* 107: 669; 1985.
39. Ortolani C, Ispano M, Pastorello E, et al. *Ann Allergy* 61: 41; 1988.
40. Bircher AJ, Van MG, Haller E, et al. *Clin Exp Allergy* 24: 367; 1994.
41. Jenkins HR, Pincott JR, Soothill JF, et al. *Arch Dis Child* 59: 326; 1984.
42. Lake AM, Whitington PF, Hamilton SR. *J Pediatr* 101: 906; 1982.
43. Goldman H, Proujansky R. *Am J Surg Pathol* 10: 75; 1986.
44. Anveden HL, Finkel Y, Sandstedt B, Karpe B. *Eur J Pediatr* 155: 464; 1996.
45. Pittschieler K. *J Pediatr Gastroenterol Nutr* 10: 548; 1990.
46. Vanderhoof JA, Murray ND, Kaufman SS, et al. *J Pediatr* 131: 741; 1997.
47. Iyngkaran N, Yadav M, Boey C, Lam K. *J Pediatr Gastroenterol Nutr* 8: 667; 1988.
48. Walker-Smith JA. *J Pediatr* 121: 111S; 1992.
49. Iyngkaran N, Robinson MJ, Prathap K, et al. *Arch Dis Child* 53: 20; 1978.
50. Yssing M, Jensen H, Jarnum S. *Acta Paediatr Scand* 56: 173; 1967.
51. Kleinman RE. *J Pediatr* 118: S111; 1991.
52. Powell GK. *J Pediatr* 93: 553; 1978.
53. Powell G. *Comp Therapy* 12: 28; 1986.
54. Sicherer SH, Eigenmann PA, Sampson HA. *J Pediatr* 133: 214; 1998.
55. Murray K, Christie D. *J Pediatr* 122: 90; 1993.
56. Burks AW, Casteel HB, Fiedorek SC, et al. *Pediatr Allergy Immunol* 5: 40; 1994.
57. de Boijjieu D, Matarazzo P, Dupont C. *J Pediatr* 131: 744; 1997.
58. Katz A, Goldman H, Grand R. *Gastroenterology* 73: 705; 1977.
59. Talley NJ, Shorter RG, Phillips SF, Zinsmeister AR. *Gut* 31: 54; 1990.
60. Caldwell JH, Mekhjian HS, Hurtubise PE, Beman FM. *Gastroenterology* 74: 825; 1978.
61. Kelly KJ, Lazenby AJ, Rowe PC, et al. *Gastroenterology* 109: 1503; 1995.
62. Kravis L, South M, Rosenlund M. *Clin Pediatr* 21: 713; 1982.
63. Leinbach GE, Rubin CE. *Gastroenterology* 59: 874; 1970.

64. Scudamore HH, Phillips SF, Swedlund HA, Gleich GJ. *J Allergy Clin Immunol* 70: 129; 1982.
65. Ferguson A. *Allergy* 50: 32; 1995.
66. Cavell B, Stenhammar L, Ascher H. *Acta Paediatr* 81: 589; 1992.
67. Holmes G, Prior P, Lane M. *Gut* 30: 333; 1989.
68. Forget PP, Arenda JW. *Eur J Pediatr* 144: 298; 1985.
69. Cavataio F, Iacono G, Montalto G, et al. *Am J Gastroenterol* 91: 1215; 1996.
70. Cavataio F, Iacono G, Montalto G, et al. *Arch Dis Child* 75: 51; 1996.
71. Iacono G, Carroccio A, Cavataio F, et al. *J Allergy Clin Immunol* 97: 822; 1996.
72. Iacono G, Carroccio A, Cavataio F, et al. *J Pediatr* 126: 34; 1995.
73. Iacono G, Cavataio F, Montalto G, et al. *N Engl J Med* 339: 1100; 1998.
74. Zeigler RE, Fomon SJ, Nelson SE, et al. *J Pediatr* 116: 11; 1990.
75. Jakobsson I, Lindberg T. *Pediatrics* 71: 268; 1983.
76. Gerrard JW, MacKenzie JWA, Goluboff N, et al. *Acta Paediatr Scand Suppl* 234: 1; 1973.
77. Lothe L, Lindberg T. *Pediatrics* 83: 262; 1989.
78. Winitz M, Adams RF, Seedman DA, et al. *Am J Clin Nutr* 23: 546; 1970.
79. Teahon K, Smethurst P, Pearson M, et al. *Gastroenterology* 101: 84; 1991.
80. Griffiths AM, Ohlsson A, Sherman PM, Sutherland LR. *Gastroenterology* 108: 1056; 1995.
81. Messori A, Trallori G, D'Albasio G, et al. *Scand J Gastroenterol* 31: 267; 1996.
82. Fernandez-Banares F, Cabre E, Esteve-Comas M, Gassull MA. *J Parent Enteral Nutr* 19: 356; 1995.
83. Dainese R, Galliani EA, DeLazzari F, et al. *Am J Gastroenterol* 94: 1892; 1999.
84. Niec AM, Frankum B, Talley NJ. *Am J Gastroenterol* 93: 2184; 1998.
85. Addolorato G, Gasbarrini G, Marsigli L, Stefanini GF. *Gastroenterology* 111: 833; 1996.
86. Sampson H, Eigenmann PA. In: *Rhinitis: Mechanisms and Management* (Naclerio R, Durham SR, Mygind N, Eds) New York: Marcel Dekker, pg 95, 1999.
87. Raphael G, Raphael M, Kaliner M. *J Allergy Clin Immunol* 83: 110; 1989.
88. James JM, Bernhisel-Broadbent J, Sampson HA. *Am J Respir Crit Care Med* 149: 59; 1994.
89. Bock SA. *Pediatr Allergy Immunol* 3: 188; 1992.
90. Thiel H, Ulmer W. *Chest* 78: 400; 1980.
91. Novembre E, deMartino M, Vierucci A. *J Allergy Clin Immunol* 81: 1059; 1988.
92. Onorato J, Merland N, Terral C. *J Allergy Clin Immunol* 78: 1139; 1986.
93. Heiner DC, Sears JW. *Am J Dis Child* 100: 500; 1960.
94. Joint Task Force on Practice Parameters, American Academy of Allergy, Asthma and Immunology, American College of Allergy, Asthma and Immunology, and the Joint Council of Allergy, Asthma and Immunology, *J Allergy Clin Immunol* 101: S465; 1998.
95. Yocum MW, Khan DA. *Mayo Clin Proc* 69: 16; 1994.
96. Kemp SF, Lockey RF, Wolf BL, Lieberman P. *Arch Intern Med* 155: 1749; 1995.
97. Novembre E, Cianferoni A, Bernardini R, et al. *Pediatrics* 101: E8; 1998.
98. Settipane G. *Allergy Proc* 10: 271; 1989.
99. Bock SA. *J Allergy Clin Immunol* 90: 683; 1992.
100. Romano A, Fonso M, Giuffreda F, et al. *Allergy* 50: 817; 1995.
101. Kidd IJM, Cohen SH, Sosman AJ, Fink JN. *J Allergy Clin Immunol* 71: 407; 1983.
102. Horan RF, Sheffer AL. *Immunol Allergy Clin NA* 11: 757; 1991.
103. Weber RW, Vaughan TR. *Immunol Allergy Clin NA* 11: 831; 1991.
104. Warner JO. *Pediatr Allergy Immunol* 4: 112; 1993.
105. National Institutes of Health Consensus Development Panel *Am J Clin Nutr* 37: 161; 1983.
106. Sicherer SH, Sampson HA. *Immunol Allergy Clin NA* 18: 49; 1998.
107. Sicherer SH, Sampson HA. *J Allergy Clin Immunol* 104: 114S; 1999.
108. Sampson HA, Albergo R. *J Allergy Clin Immunol* 74: 26; 1984.
109. Bock S, Buckley J, Holst A, May C. *Clin Allergy* 8: 559; 1978.
110. Ortolani C, Ispano M, Pastorello EA, et al. *J Allergy Clin Immunol* 83: 683; 1989.
111. Sampson H, Ho D. *J Allergy Clin Immunol* 100: 444; 1997.
112. Crespo JF, Pascual C, Ferrer A, et al. *Allergy Proc* 15: 73; 1994.
113. Sicherer SH, Sampson HA. *Clin Exp Allergy* 29: 507; 1999.
114. Bernhisel-Broadbent J, Taylor S, Sampson HA. *J Allergy Clin Immunol* 84: 701; 1989.

115. Terr AI, Salvaggio JE. In: *Allergy, Asthma, and Immunology from Infancy to Adulthood*. (Pearlman CW, Shapiro DS, Bierman GG, Busse WW, Eds): Philadelphia, W.B. Saunders, 749, 1996.
116. Bock SA, Sampson HA, Atkins FM, et al. *J Allergy Clin Immunol* 82: 986; 1988.
117. AAAAI Board of Directors, American Academy of Allergy, Asthma and Immunology. *J Allergy Clin Immunol* 102: 173; 1998.
118. Bock SA, Atkins FM. *J Allergy Clin Immunol* 83: 900; 1989.
119. Hourihane JO, Dean TP, Warner JO. *Br Med J* 313: 518; 1996.
120. Hourihane JO, Kilburn SA, Dean P, Warner JO. *Clin Exp Allergy* 27: 634; 1997.
121. Hourihane JO, Roberts SA, Warner JO. *Br Med J* 316: 1271; 1998.
122. James JM, Sampson HA. *J Pediatr* 121: 371; 1992.
123. Zeiger RS. In: *Allergy: Principles and Practice*. (Middleton E, Reed C, Ellis E, Adkinson N, Yunginger J, Busse W, Eds) St. Louis: Mosby, 1993, 1137.
124. Zeiger RS. *Pediatr Allergy Immunol* 5: 33; 1994.
125. Hattevig G, Kjellman B, Bjorksten B, Kjellman N. *Clin Exper Allergy* 19: 27; 1989.
126. Sigurs N, Hattevig G, Kjellman B. *Pediatrics* 89: 735; 1992.
127. Zeiger R, Heller S. *J Allergy Clin Immunol* 95: 1179; 1995.
128. Fergusson DM, Horwood LJ, Shannon FT. *Pediatrics* 86: 541; 1990.
129. Fergusson D, Horwood L, Shannon F. *Arch Dis Child 58*: 48; 1983.
130. Kajosaari M, Saarinen UM. *Arch Paediatr Scand* 72: 411; 1983.
131. Kajosaari M. *Adv Exp Med Biol* 310: 453; 1991.
132. Nelson HS, Lahr J, Rule R, et al. *J Allergy Clin Immunol* 99: 744; 1997.
133. Kelso J, Jones R, Tellez R, Yunginge J. *Ann Allergy Asthma Immunol* 74: 391; 1995.
134. Bannon GA, Li X-F, Rabjohn P, et al. *J Allergy Clin Immunol* 99: 141S; 1998.
135. Burks AW, Bannon GA, Sicherer SH, Sampson HA, *Int Arch Allergy Immunol* 119: 165; 1999.
136. Burks AW, King N, Bannon GA. *Int Arch Allergy Immunol* 118: 313; 1999.
137. Rabjohn P, Helm EM, Stanley JS, et al. *J Clin Invest* 103: 535; 1999.
138. Li X, Huang CK, Schofield BH, et al. *J Immunol* 162: 3045; 1999.
139. Roy K, Mao HQ, Huang SK, Leong KW. *Nat Med* 5: 387; 1999.
140. Sampson HA. *J Allergy Clin Immunol* 103: 981; 1999.
141. Sampson HA. *J Allergy Clin Immunol* 78: 212; 1986.
142. Pumphrey RSH, Stanworth SJ. *Clin Exp Allergy* 26: 1364; 1996.
143. Sehgal VN, Rege VL. *Ann Allergy* 31: 279; 1973.
144. Champion R, Roberts S, Carpenter R, Roger J. *Br J Dermatol* 81: 588; 1969.
145. Iacono G, Carroccio A, Cavataio F, et al. *J Allergy Clin Immunol* 97: 822; 1996.
146. Dreborg S, Foucard T. *Allergy* 38: 167; 1983.
147. Ortolani C, Pastorello EA, Farioli L, et al. *Ann Allergy* 71: 470; 1993.
148. Amlot PL, Kemeny DM, Zachary C, et al. *Clin Allergy* 17: 33; 1987.
149. Anderson L, Dreyfuss E, Logan J, et al. *J Allergy Clin Immunol* 45: 310; 1970.
150. Pastorello E, Ortolani C, Farioli L, et al. *J Allergy Clin Immunol* 94: 699; 1994.
151. Walker-Smith JA. *Clin Gastroenterol* 15: 55; 1986.
152. Trier JS. *N Engl J Med* 325: 1709; 1991.

42

Enteral Nutrition

Gail A. Cresci and Robert G. Martindale

Introduction

Historically, enteral feeding can be traced back to ancient Egypt and Greece, where nutrient enemas were used when patients were unable to take oral nutrition. Various combinations of wine, milk, broth, grains, and raw eggs were used with limited success.[1] Rectal delivery of nutrients was continued up until the early 1900s despite lack of supportive benefit. In fact, President James Garfield was given nutrient enemas every 4 hours for 79 days following his attempted assassination until his death.[1]

The first reports of nutrient provision through feeding tubes into the esophagus were in 1598, when an enteral feeding tube was fashioned from eel skin. In 1790 John Hunter initiated the modern era of gastrointestinal (GI) access with his reports of tube feeding the stomach.[1] Up until this time, nutrient mixtures were delivered by gravity force limiting flow rate consistency. The first stomach pump was invented in the 18th century, allowing for consistent enteral nutrient delivery as well as gastric irrigation and emptying.[1] Tubes remained very primitive and uncomfortable until rubber was developed, thus leading to the evolution of the currently available selections. In 1910 Max Einhorn began feeding the duodenum through a rubber tube when gastric access was not feasible, claiming that rectal feeding was unacceptable.[1] The implementation of orojejunal tube feeding in surgical patients implemented by Ravdin and Stengel followed in 1939. In 1950 the use of polyethylene tubes was described with gastric and jejunal tubes 27 inches and 6 feet in length, respectively. With these tubes came the introduction of the feeding pump to deliver the formulation.[1]

Experimentation with the enteral formulations began in the early 1900s with the introduction of the chemically defined or "elemental" diet. The late 1950s through the 1970s marked the space age and the beginning of space diet research. These chemically defined diets were investigated in both animals and healthy humans to produce a low residue diet that would decrease fecal output during space travel. In the late 1960s chemically defined diets were first reported being used in critically ill surgical patients.[1] Since that time, enteral formulations have undergone extensive modification and now exist for nearly every metabolic disease state.

0-8493-2705-9/01/$0.00+$1.50

TABLE 42.1

Immune Benefits of Enteral Feeding

Improved mucosal integrity
Enhanced glycemic control
Normalization of GI flora
Preserved GALT
All epithelial surfaces benefit
common mucosal immune hypothesis
Increased secretory IgA

GI: gastrointestinal; GALT: Gut associated lymphoid tissue

Rationale and Benefits

In most major patient care centers enteral nutrition is the preferred route of nutrient delivery. Parenteral nutrition is substituted only if safe access is unavailable or unsuccessful. Extensive review of the numerous benefits of enteral nutrition is beyond the scope of this section and is only briefly addressed. Available reviews provide more extensive background in these areas.[2-5]

One proposed benefit of enteral nutrition is that it is more physiologic than parenteral nutrition. The gut and the liver process enteral nutrients prior to their release into systemic circulation (first pass). When compared to parenteral nutrition, enteral nutrition positively influences nitrogen balance,[6,7] serum protein levels,[5,8,9] and the metabolic response to stress.[2-5,10,11]

Another benefit of enteral nutrition is its affect on the immune system (Table 42.1). The lack of GI stimulation by enteral nutrients may promote gut mucosal atrophy. This may lead to increased intestinal permeability potentially leaving the gut vulnerable to bacterial translocation. Enteral nutrition provides maintenance of the gut-associated lymphoid tissue,[12,13] maintenance of the normal GI flora,[14-16] and a lowering of infectious complications.[13,17-19]

Enteral nutrition is generally less expensive than parenteral nutrition.[20,21] The lower total cost includes factors such as the cost of enteral formulations, cost of equipment used for formula preparation and administration, and cost of personnel specialists. The delivery of enteral nutrition has been shown to be safe in stable as well as in most critical patients.[17-19,22]

Indications/Contraindications

Enteral nutrition is indicated for patients with access to an adequately functional GI tract and whose oral nutrient intake is insufficient to meet estimated needs. Specific conditions for which enteral nutrition is indicated are found in Table 42.2. Although enteral nutrition is the preferred route of nutrient delivery, it is not innocuous and there are some contraindications to its use (Table 42.3). It is not always clear when enteral nutrition will be tolerated. If the individual's needs are not met enterally, parenteral nutrition may be implemented for either full nutrient provision or concurrently with the enteral delivery to provide the balance of nutrients not tolerated.

Enteral Access

Route of administration and type of access for tube feedings are usually determined by the expected length of therapy (Figure 42.1), risk of aspiration (Table 42.4), and local

TABLE 42.2

Enteral Feeding Indications

Hypermetabolism	*Oncologic Disease*
Postoperative major surgery	Chemotherapy
Trauma	Radiotherapy
Sepsis	Neoplasms
Burns	
Organ Transplantation	
Neurologic Disease	*Psychiatric Disease*
Cerebrovascular accident	Anorexia nervosa
Dysphagia	Severe depression
Head trauma	
Demyelinating disease	*Organ System Failure*
Neoplasm	Respiratory failure (ventilator dependence)
Gastrointestinal Disease	Renal failure
Short bowel syndrome (if remaining bowel has sufficient absorptive capacity ~50-100 cm and intact ileocecal valve)	Cardiac failure (cardiac cachexia)
	Hepatic failure
	Multiple organ system failure
Inflammatory bowel disease	Comatose state
Enterocutaneous fistula (<800 mL output/day)	
Pancreatitis	

TABLE 42.3

Enteral Feeding Contraindications

Bowel obstruction
Persistent intolerance (e.g., emesis, diarrhea)
Hemodynamic instability
Major upper GI bleeds
Ileus
Unable to safely access
Relative Contraindications
Significant bowel wall edema
Nutrient infusion proximal to recent GI anastamosis
High output fistula (>800 mL/day)

expertise. Nasoenteric or oroenteric tubes are generally used when therapy is anticipated to be of short duration (i.e., <4 weeks) or for interim access before the placement of a long-term device. Long-term access requires a percutaneous or surgically placed feeding tube.

Nasoenteric Access

Multiple methods exist for gaining enteral access (Table 42.5), all of which carry various degrees of expertise, risk, and expense. The nasoenteric tube is the most commonly used method of enteral access. It can be inserted into the stomach, duodenum, or jejunum. Since these tubes have low complication rates, are relatively inexpensive, and are easy to place, they are used most often for short-term use. The most common complications are tube malposition and dislodgement.

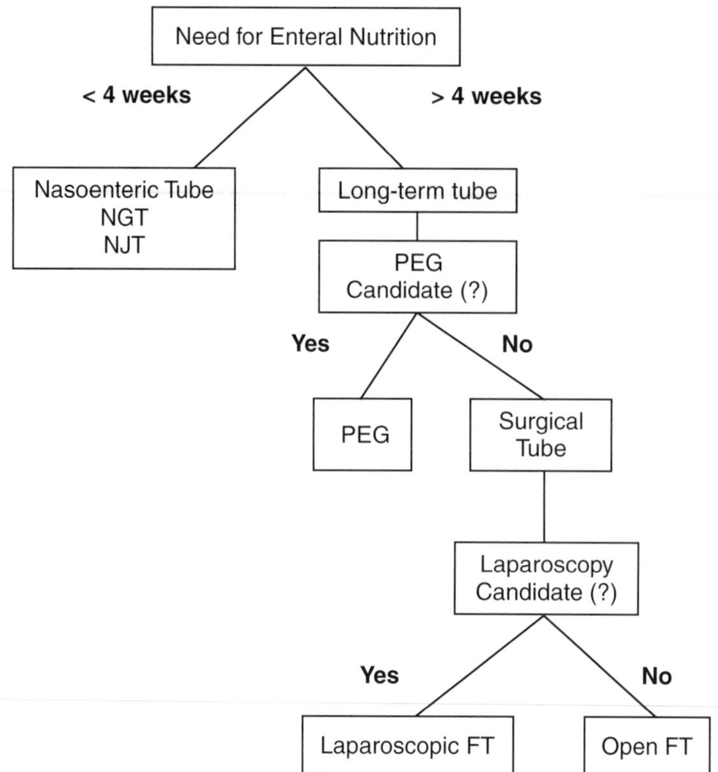

FIGURE 42.1
Enteral access decision tree.

TABLE 42.4
Risk Factors for Aspiration

Altered mental status with inability to protect airway
Swallowing dysfunction
Central (CVA)
Local (vagal disruption, trauma)
History of aspiration
Severe gastroesophageal reflux
Gastric outlet obstruction
Gastroparesis
Patient position restrictions (supine versus semirecumbent)

It is often desirable to place tubes beyond the pylorus in patients with delayed gastric emptying or absent gag reflex to potentially decrease the risk of aspiration. Positioning a nasoenteric tube into the small bowel is much more difficult than positioning into the stomach. Transpyloric tubes can be placed intraoperatively, at bedside, or with endoscopic or fluoroscopic guidance. Intraoperative placement of a nasoenteric tube involves manual manipulation during the surgery; however, this is not common practice, as it requires open laparotomy. Spontaneous placement of a nasoenteric tubes involves advancing the tube into the stomach and allowing it to migrate independently into the small bowel. This technique is not very successful in hospitalized patients, especially the critically ill, due to motility derangements. Several bedside manual methods using special placement techniques, weighted versus non-weighted tubes, pH sensor tubes, prokinetic agents,

TABLE 42.5
Methods of GI Access

Nasoenteric Feeding Tubes	*Percutaneous Feeding Tubes*
Spontaneous Passage	Percutaneous Endoscopic
Bedside — prokinetic agent	Gastric (PEG)
Active Passage	Gastric/Jejunal (PEG/J)
Bedside — assisted	Direct Jejunal (DPEJ)
Endoscopic	*Laparoscopic*
Fluoroscopic	Gastrostomy
Operative	Jejunostomy
	Surgical
	Gastrostomy
	Jejunostomy

magnets, and bioelectrical detection devices have been reported, all with similar success rates (~85%).[23-29]

Do to lack of universal success in manual placement of nasoenteric tubes, fluoroscopic or endoscopic guidance is often sought. If portable equipment is not available, both of these techniques require patient transport to the endoscopy or radiology suite, which may not be feasible for critically ill patients. Fluoroscopic techniques of nasoenteric tube placement involve manipulation of the tube with a long guide wire. Endoscopic techniques include use of a guide wire as well as a "drag" method. In the drag method, a gastrically placed tube is grasped with a snare or biopsy forceps and dragged with the endoscope into the duodenum or farther, and then released. All risks of endoscopy accompany these methods including dental injury, pharyngeal or esophageal injury, gastric bleeding, perforation, and risk of aspiration with the use of intravenous sedation.[30] Both fluoroscopic and endoscopic placement methods are ~85 to 95% successful in obtaining postpyloric feeding tube placement. Although placement of postpyloric feeding tubes using endoscopic, fluoroscopic, and manual techniques may be successful, these tubes are frequently dislodged. Repeated tube insertion increases risk and costs of these access methods. For this reason, patients requiring long-term enteral nutrition should receive more permanent access.

Gastrostomy

Gastrostomy is the most common method for long-term enteral access since it eliminates nasal irritation, psychological stress, and requirement for an infusion pump, as complex formulas may be given as boluses. Gastric tubes, due to their large diameter, can serve many other functions besides feeding, including gastric decompression, gastric pH monitoring, and medication delivery. Insertion can be via laparatomy, laparoscopy, endoscopy, or fluoroscopy.

Permanent gastric placement can be obtained either by surgical procedures (laparotomy or laparoscopically) or by nonoperative procedures. Percutaneous endoscopic gastrostomy (PEG) is the most popular nonoperative procedure for obtaining permanent gastric access. Gauderer et al.[31] first described the procedure in 1980, and despite some modifications, the basic technique used by most endoscopists is similar. Compared to surgically placed tubes, PEGs are less costly, have decreased procedure-related morbidity and mortality, usually do not require general anesthesia, and allow enteral feeding to be initiated

TABLE 42.6

PEG Indications and Contraindications

Indications	*Contraindications*
Long-term access (>4 weeks)	No stomach
Decompression	Unable to scope
Swallowing dysfunction	Hemodynamic instability
Neurologic event precluding swallowing	Coagulation disorders
Tracheoesophageal fistula	Obstruction
	Portal hypertension, esophageal varicies, ascites
	Relative Contraindications
	Peritoneal dialysis
	Prior upper abdominal procedures
	Pregnancy
	Morbid obesity

quickly.[30-36] Indications as well as contraindications for a PEG are described in Table 42.6. Complications of PEGs include dislodgment, bleeding, tube site infection, intra-abdominal leak, site leak, and persistent gastric fistula.[30]

Jejunostomy

The advantage of percutaneous tubes is less apparent when small bowel feeding is required, owing to the high failure rate of PEG tubes with a jejunal extension (PEG/J). While a PEG/J tube is beneficial in the acute care setting when a critically ill patient requiring long-term access is intolerant of gastric feeds, they are not very practical for long-term use. Long-term failure of the jejunal extension is attributed to its small lumen leading to frequent clogging, as well as separation of the inner PEJ tube from the outer gastrostomy tube.[37] For these reasons as well as the expertise required to place the jejunal extension, surgical placement of jejunal tubes is often preferred for long-term jejunal access.

Several choices are available for intraoperative feeding jejunostomy placement. The needle catheter jejunostomy (NCJ) is a quick and easy method that involves inserting a small catheter into the lumen of the jejunum proximal to the ligament of Treitz. The advantage of an NCJ is that nutrients can be administered almost immediately and the catheter can easily be removed when it is no longer needed. Unfortunately, the small lumen of the catheter occludes more readily than larger-bore feeding tubes. Catheters originally designed for other uses have been adapted for jejunal feeding, with the red rubber catheter most frequently used.

Jejunal access has also been obtained by direct percutanous endoscopic jejunostomy placement (DPEJ).[38] This method is similar to PEG placement except that the endoscope is passed through the duodenum, past the ligament of Treitz, into a loop of jejunum adjacent to the abdominal wall. A regular pull-through PEG tube is used for access. This procedure is technically more difficult than a PEG due to the peristaltic action and narrow lumen of the jejunum, but this procedure has many advantages over a PEG/J such as a decrease in clogging due to the use of a larger diameter tube, and decreased migration or kinking. As this is a fairly new procedure, data on long-term complications are lacking.

Enteral Formulas

The increase in the use of enteral over parenteral nutrition in the past few decades has led to a rapid expansion in the number of commercially available enteral nutrition products. These products do not currently require Food and Drug Administration (FDA) approval for their proposed clinical implications, and fall under the category of food supplements. Nearly every major enteral formula company in the United States today carries a similar line of products. These formulas can be categorized as oral supplements, standard tube feedings, high-protein tube feedings, and disease-specific products. Table 42.7 provides an overview of these categories, specifying the types of macronutrients and physical properties of the select formulas. Since these products do not require the rigorous FDA examination prior to their marketing, it is left up to the experienced nutritionist to decipher the product indications. The optimal selection and administration of a formula requires a thorough knowledge of normal and abnormal digestive and absorptive physiology and formula composition. The physical form and quantity of each nutrient may determine the extent of absorption of and tolerance to the formula (e.g., long-chain versus medium-chain triglyceride). The following discussion provides an overview of select macronutrients found in these products, with related supportive research as available.

Macronutrients

Carbohydrate

Among formulas, the two main differences in carbohydrate composition are form and concentration. The form, ranging from starch to simple glucose, contributes to the characteristics of osmolality, sweetness, and digestibility. In general, the larger carbohydrate molecules (e.g., starch) exert less osmotic pressure, taste less sweet, and require more digestion than shorter ones (e.g., maltodextrin, sucrose, corn syrup solids). In the critical care setting, optimal carbohydrate delivery should be at a level to allow maximal protein sparing while minimizing hyperglycemia. Currently 4 to 6 mg/kg/min appears to meet these criteria during states of hypermetabolism.

Fiber

It has been claimed that fiber is beneficial in the control of a myriad of gastrointestinal disorders, as well as treatment of hyperlipidemia and control of blood glucose. Fiber-containing formulas have 5 to 14 gm of total dietary fiber per liter. The form of fiber used is primarily insoluble fiber (e.g., soy fiber), but some formulas also contain extra-soluble fiber (e.g., guars, pectins). The insoluble fiber is beneficial with regard to colonic function and bowel regulation. The soluble fibers may slow gastric emptying and decrease the rise in postprandial blood glucose levels as well as bind bile acids and dietary cholesterol, thus lowering serum cholesterol levels. The soluble fibers are also substrates for bacterial fermentation in the colon, yielding short-chain fatty acids (SCFA), carbon dioxide, methane, hydrogen, and water. SCFAs are known to be the primary fuel for the colonocyte. It is believed that SCFAs are required to maintain optimal colonocyte function. In patients requiring long-term tube feeding, a fiber-containing formula may help to regulate GI motility. Because of the higher viscosity of these formulas, the use of larger bore tubes (10 Fr or greater) or an infusion pump is suggested.

TABLE 42.7

Overview of Select Enteral Formulas

Formula Category	Protein Sources	% Calories from Protein	Carbohydrate Sources	% Calories from Carbohydrate	Fat Sources	% Calories from Fat	Caloric Density (Calories/mL)	NPC:g N	mL for 100% RDI	% Free Water	mOsm/kg Water	Product Names (Select Number)
Oral supplements	Sodium & calcium caseinates, soy protein isolate	14-24	Corn syrup, sugar, sucrose, maltodextrin	47-64	Corn oil, canola oil, soy oil, sunflower oil, safflower oil	21-39	1.0-2.0	78-154:1	946-2000	73-85	480-870	Ensure, Ensure Plus, Sustacal, Sustacal with Fiber, Resource Plus, NuBasics, Sustacal Plus
Standard tube feedings	Sodium & calcium caseinates, soy protein isolates	13-18	Corn syrup, maltodextrin	45-57	Soy oil, corn oil, canola oil, MCT, safflower oil	29-39	1.0-1.5	116-167:1	830-1890	77-85	270-500	Isocal, IsoSource HN, Nutren 1.0, Nutren 1.5, Osmolite, Osmolite HN, Comply
Standard tube feedings with fiber	Sodium & calcium caseinates, soy protein isolate	14-18	Corn syrup, maltodextrin, corn syrup solids, soy fiber, guar gum, oat fiber, FOS	44-57	Canola oil, soybean oil, corn oil, MCT	29-37	1.0-1.2	110-149:1	933-1500	78-85	300-500	Fibersource, Jevity, Jevity Plus, ProBalance, Ultracal, Nutren 1.0 with Fiber
High protein tube feedings	Sodium and calcium caseinates	22-25	Hydrolyzed cornstarch, maltodextrin, sucrose, fructose, oat fiber, soy fiber	38-52	Canola oil, MCT, soybean oil, safflower oil	23-40	1.0-1.5	75-91:1	1000-2000	78-85	300-490	IsoSource VHN, Replete with Fiber, Promote, Protain XL, TraumaCal

Elemental & semi-elemental	Free amino acids, soy hydrolysates, hydrolyzed whey, hydrolyzed casein, hydrolyzed soy	12-25	Hydrolyzed cornstarch, maltodextrin, sucrose, modified cornstarch	36-82	Soybean oil, safflower oil, canola oil, MCT sunflower oil	3-39	1.0-1.5	67-175:1	1150-2000	76-86	270-650	Vivonex T.E.N., Crucial, Peptamen, Perative, Reablin, AlitraQ, Sandosource Peptide, Subdue, Optimental
Pulmonary	Sodium and calcium caseinates	17-20	Hydrolyzed cornstarch, corn syrup, sucrose, maltodextrin, sugar	27-40	Canola oil, soybean oil, MCT, corn oil, safflower oil, sardine oil, borage oil	40-55	1.5	102-125:1	933-1420	76-79	330-650	Nutrivent, Pulmocare, Respalor, Novasource Pulmonary, Oxepa
Renal	Sodium & calcium caseinates, Whey-L-amino acids	7-15	Corn syrup, sucrose, fructose, maltodextrin, sugar	40-58	Corn oil, safflower oil, canola oil, MCT	35-45	2.0	140-340:1	947-1000	70-71	570-700	Nepro, Magnacal Renal, Novasource Renal RenalCal
Diabetic	Sodium & calcium caseinates, beef, milk protein, soy protein isolate	16-24	Maltodextrin, hydrolyzed cornstarch, fructose, sucrose, guar gum, vegetables, fruits, soy fiber	34-40	Sunflower oil, soybean oil, canola oil, MCT, safflower oil	40-49	1.0-1.06	79-125:1	1000-1890 or N/A	85	355-450	Glucerna, Glytrol, Choice dm, DiabetiSource, Resource Diabetic
Immune Modulated	Sodium & calcium caseinates, L-Arginine, L-glutamine, BCAA	22-32	Hydrolyzed cornstarch, maltodextrin, soy fiber	38-53	Canola oil, structured lipids: sunflower oil and menhaden fish oil, MCT	20-40	1.0-1.5	52-71:1	1250-2000	78-86	375-550	Impact, Impact 1.5 ImmunAid, Crucial
Hepatic	L-amino acids, Whey	11-15	Sucrose, maltodextrin, modified cornstarch	57-77	Soybean oil, MCT, canola oil, corn oil, lecithin	12-28	1.2-1.5	148-209:1	N/A-1000	76-82	560-690	NutriHep, Hepatic Aid II

Fructooligosaccharides

Fructooligosaccharides (FOS) are undigestible sugars that occur naturally in food (e.g. onions, blueberries). These sugars consist of a sucrose molecule linked to one, two, or three additional fructose units. Gastric acid or digestive enzymes do not degrade FOS. These oligosaccharides appear to remain intact in the small intestine and pass into the colon unaltered, where they are fermented by colonic microorganisms (e.g., *bifidobacteria*) to lactate and SCFAs. It is suggested that the proliferation of *bifidobacteria* species and the presence of FOS with the consequent production of the fermented byproducts acetate and lactate, produce an environment undesirable for some pathogenic bacteria such as *Clostridium difficile* by lowering the colonic pH.[14,16] A few enteral formulations now contain FOS, but proposed benefits remain to be elucidated.

Fat

The major sources of fat in standard lactose-free formulas are corn, soy, safflower, and canola oils, lecithin, and medium-chain triacylglycerol (MCT). In addition to their importance as a concentrated caloric source (9 kcalories/gm), fat is required for essential fatty acids, and serves as a carrier for the fat-soluble vitamins. Fat also enhances the flavor and palatability of a formula without increasing osmolality. Long-chain triacylglycerol (LCT) is a rich source of essential fatty acids, linoleic and linolenic acid. The estimated daily requirement for essential fatty acids is 3 to 4% of total kcalories. However, due to LCT route of absorption via the lymphatic system, their limited utilization during hypermetabolism, and their immunosuppressive effects when given in large quantities, many formulas now combine LCT with MCT.

MCTs are 6 to 12 carbons long and are prepared from palm kernel or coconut oil. MCT is advantageous because it is more rapidly hydrolyzed and water soluble than LCT, requires little or no pancreatic lipase or bile salts for absorption, and can be transported directly into portal venous circulation where it crosses the mitochondrial membrane and can be oxidized independent of carnitine.[39] MCTs are generally well tolerated by the enteral route but can be associated with some GI symptoms such as nausea, vomiting, and diarrhea. As they produce ketones, they should not be used in patients who are prone to high ketone levels.[39] Since they do not contain essential fatty acids (EFA), most enteral formulas that contain MCT also provide some LCT in order to meet the requirement for EFA.

Recent metabolic research has led to the incorporation of omega-3 fatty acids (linolenic) into enteral formulas. Numerous reports using various *in vivo* and *in vitro* models suggest that the slight structural difference between omega-3 and omega-6 fatty acids strongly favors anti-inflammatory, antithrombotic, antiarrhythmic, hypolipidemic, and antiatherosclerotic effects.[40-42]

Structured lipids are a chemical mixture of LCTs and MCTs incorporated onto the same glycerol molecule. They differ from the more simple random physical mixtures of LCT and MCT. Structured lipids may offer the advantages of both types of fats. Structured lipids have been shown to decrease infection and improve survival by producing less inflammatory and immunosuppressive eicosanoids as compared with conventional triacylglycerols.[39] Enteral formulas, particularly the immune-modulated category, are beginning to include structured lipids as a source of fat.

Protein

Protein contained in enteral formulas may be in the form of intact protein (e.g., lactalbumin, casein, caseinates), partially hydrolyzed protein (e.g., oligopeptides, di- or tripeptides), or crystalline L-amino acids. Intact protein and protein hydrolysates (≥4 amino acid residues) require further luminal digestion by pancreatic or brush border enzymes into peptides (di- or tripeptides) and free amino acids, which are then absorbed primarily in the proximal small bowel. The peptide transport mechanisms are felt to be responsible for absorption of the majority of nitrogen, with the single amino acid carriers playing a minority role in protein absorption. Intact proteins do not add appreciably to the osmolality of the formula, unlike hydrolyzed or crystalline amino acids. The higher the percentage of hydrolyzed protein or free amino acids, the greater the solution osmolality will be. A knowledge of the source and form of protein is essential when prescribing diets for patients with defects in either protein digestion (e.g., pancreatic insufficiency) or absorption (e.g., short bowel syndrome).

Stress and other forms of injury may alter protein metabolism. In times of decreased absorptive surface area, ischemic injury, or malabsorption, provision of enteral formulas containing hydrolyzed protein or free amino acids has been suggested. At present, no clear consistent clinical data support the use of solutions in which protein is in the form of free amino acids or hydrolysates. This may be due to the fact that the small bowel has a very adaptive absorptive mucosa, even when a large percentage of the small bowel mucosa is nonfunctional or resected. Although patients with maldigestion and/or malabsorption may benefit from a peptide-based enteral formula, the higher cost of these formulas and lack of clinical supportive data discourage routine use in patients with normal GI physiology.

Glutamine

Glutamine is the most abundant amino acid in the body and in normal situations is considered a non-essential amino acid. It can be synthesized in many tissues of the body, predominantly skeletal muscle, and is the primary fuel for rapidly dividing tissues such as the small bowel. Glutamine serves many purposes including maintenance of acid-base status as a precursor of urinary ammonia, as a primary fuel source for enterocytes, as a fuel source for lymphocytes and macrophages, and as a precursor for nucleotide synthesis.[43,44] Glutamine is also a precursor for glutathione, an important antioxidant that may be protective in a variety of circumstances. During catabolic illness, glutamine uptake by the small intestine and immunologically active cells may exceed glutamine synthesis and release from skeletal muscle, making glutamine conditionally essential.[43]

Limited human data exist regarding the use of enteral glutamine supplementation. In animal models, supplemental glutamine has been shown to enhance intestinal adaptation after massive small bowel resection, to attenuate intestinal and pancreatic atrophy, and to prevent hepatic steatosis associated with parenteral and elemental enteral feeding.[43] Glutamine appears to maintain GI tract mucosal thickness, maintain DNA and protein content, reduce bacteremia and mortality after chemotherapy, and reduce bacteremia and mortality following sepsis or endotoxemia.[43,44]

In humans with surgical stress, glutamine-supplemented parenteral nutrition appears to maintain nitrogen balance and the intracellular glutamine pool in skeletal muscle.[43] In critically ill patients, glutamine supplementation may attenuate villous atrophy and increased intestinal mucosal permeability associated with parenteral nutrition.[45] Parenteral nutrition supplemented with glutamine has also resulted in fewer infections, improved nitrogen balance, and significantly shorter mean hospital length of stay in bone marrow transplantation patients.[46] Glutamine supplementation may also play a role in protecting the GI tract against chemotherapy-induced toxicity. Oral glutamine supplementation reduced the severity and decreased the duration of stomatitis that occurred during chemotherapy.[47]

While a large volume of animal data supports the beneficial effects of glutamine in a variety of experimental models, the benefit of enteral glutamine supplementation in critically ill human patients is less clear. Well-designed clinical trials with clearly defined endpoints and adequate statistical power are needed to assess whether the animal effects translate into a reduction in hospital stay and mortality rate in humans.

Arginine

Arginine is classified as a nonessential amino acid in normal situations, since the body synthesizes adequate arginine for normal maintenance of tissue metabolism. During injuries such as trauma or stress an increase in urinary nitrogen, excreted largely as urea, represents the end-products of increased tissue catabolism and reprioritized protein synthesis. As the activity of the urea cycle increases, so does the demand for arginine.

Studies indicate that supplemental dietary arginine is beneficial for accelerated wound healing, enhanced immune response, and positive nitrogen balance.[43] The exact mechanism for these benefits is unknown but may in part result from arginine's role as a potent stimulant of growth hormone, glucagon, prolactin, and insulin release.[43] Arginine is also a precursor for nitric oxide, a highly reactive molecule synthesized from arginine by the action of nitric oxide synthase resulting in the formation of nitric oxide and citrulline.[48] Nitric oxide is a ubiquitous molecule with important roles in the maintenance of vascular tone, coagulation, the immune system, and the GI tract, and has been implicated as a factor in disease states as diverse as sepsis, hypertension, and cirrhosis.[48]

In animal models, arginine supplementation has been associated with improved wound healing, with increased wound tensile strength and collagen deposition.[49] Arginine-supplemented rats also had improved thymic function as assessed by thymic weight, the total number of thymic lymphocytes in each thymus, and the mitogenic reactivity of thymic lymphocytes to phytohemagglutinin and concanavalin A.[48] Animal arginine supplementation resulted in improved survival in burns, and with intraperitoneal bacterial challenge.

Multiple human clinical trials have been conducted comparing the use of various enteral formulations that contain arginine as well as other supplemental nutrients (e.g., glutamine, omega-3 fatty acids, nucleotides) to a standard nonsupplemented formula. Results of these trials have found the supplemented formula groups to have various improved outcomes such as decreased number and severity of septic complications,[50-53] decreased antibiotic use,[50] and decreased hospital and intensive care unit stay.[50, 54]

While supplemental arginine has been shown to improve survival in various animal models and to improve a number of *in vitro* measures of immune function, the benefit of arginine supplementation alone in critically ill humans is uncertain.

Other Nutrients

Vitamins and Minerals

Most nutritionally complete commercial formulas contain adequate vitamins and minerals when a sufficient volume of formula to meet energy and macronutrient needs is provided. Some disease-specific formulas are nutritionally incomplete in relation to vitamin and mineral content (e.g., hepatic formulas). Liquid vitamin and mineral supplements may be indicated for patients receiving nutritionally incomplete or diluted formulas for prolonged periods of time. Fat-soluble vitamin supplementation such as vitamin K may be indicated for patients with fat malabsorption or for patients with vitamin K deficiency; most commercial formulas include vitamin K.

Water

A large percentage of all enteral formulas is free water. The quantity of water in enteral formulas is often described as water content or moisture content. The quantity of water is usually reported in milliliters of water either per 1000 mL of formula or per liter of formula. Most enteral formulas contain water in the general range of 690 to 860 mL per 1000 mL of enteral formula. This must be considered when making fluid recommendations.

Physical Properties

Osmolality

Osmolality is the function of size and quantity of ionic and molecular particles (protein, carbohydrate, electrolytes, and minerals) within a given volume. The unit of measure for osmolality is mOsm/kg of water versus the unit of measure for osmolarity, which is mOsm/L. Osmolality is considered the preferred term to use in reference to enteral formulas.

Osmolality is important because of its role in maintaining the balance between intracellular and extracellular fluids. Several factors affect the osmolality of enteral formulas. The primary factor is nutrient hydrolysis. The smaller the chain length of carbohydrates and proteins, the greater will be the formulation's osmolality. Hence, formulas containing increased amounts of simple sugars or free amino acids and/or di- and tripeptides will have a greater osmolality than those containing starch and longer-chain intact proteins. Lipids contribute minimally to the osmolality of an enteral formula with the exception of MCT, owing to their water solubility. Because of dissociation properties and small size, minerals and electrolytes also increase the osmolality.

GI tolerance (e.g., gastric retention, abdominal distention, diarrhea, nausea, and vomiting) is influenced by the osmolality of enteral formulas. Generally, the greater the osmolality, the greater the likelihood of GI intolerance. Administering hypertonic formulas at a slow, continuous rate initially (10 to 20 cc/h) with a gradual titration to the final volume while monitoring for GI complications can reduce the incidence of GI intolerance and allow these formulas to be administered at full strength. What may be more important than the osmolality of the enteral formula is the osmotic contribution from liquid medications either infused with the enteral formula or bolused through the feeding tube. The average osmolality range of commercially prepared liquid medications is reported to be 450 to 10,950 mOsm/kg. The osmolality of enteral formulas ranges from 270 to 700 mOsm/kg.

Hydrogen Ion Concentration (pH)

Gastric motility is reportedly slowed with solutions with a pH lower than 3.5. The pH level of most commercial formulas is >3.5. Feeding tube occlusion can be caused in part by the pH of the enteral formula. Most intact protein formulas coagulate when acidified to a pH of less than 5.0.

kcalorie-Nutrient Density

The kcalorie density of enteral formulas is generally 1.0, 1.5, or 2.0 kcalories per milliliter. This is important as it not only determines how many kcalories, but also the other macro- and micronutrients that the patient receives. As a formula becomes more nutrient dense, it contains less free water.

Caloric density often affects the patient's tolerance for tube feeding. Delayed gastric emptying frequently occurs in patients who are given concentrated formulas. High fat formulas contribute to this, being potent inhibitors of gastric emptying. Since the patient's nutrient needs are met by a decreased volume of this class of formula, free water supplementation should be given to ensure that fluid requirements are met, and to prevent dehydration and constipation. Generally, these products are best tolerated as voluntary oral supplements and not as tube feeding.

Non-Protein Calorie to Gram of Nitrogen Ration (npc:gm N)

In general, the average healthy adult requires a non-protein calorie to gram of nitrogen (npc:gm N) ratio of 150-250:1. In a catabolic state, the body catabolizes lean body mass as a nitrogen and energy source. To minimize this process, it is recommended to provide a npc:gm N of 100-150:1. This protein content of enteral formulas becomes extremely important in patients who require wound healing due to trauma, burns, metabolic stress, infection, and increased wound healing requirements.

Renal Solute Load

Renal solute load refers to the constituents in the formula that must be excreted by the kidneys. Major contributors to renal solute load in enteral formulas are protein, sodium, potassium, and chloride. There is an obligatory water loss for each unit of solute. Therefore, as a formula becomes more concentrated or its renal solute load increases, the patient will require more water.[39] Pediatric and geriatric patients, as well as those with diarrhea, emesis, fistulas, or fevers, should be monitored closely for hydration status.

Disease-Specific Formulations

Most patients can tolerate enteral nutrition safely with a standard enteral formula and do not require specialty enteral formulations. Specialty enteral formulas have an increased cost that often may not be reimbursable; however, factors such as severe hypercatabolism, renal or hepatic failure, pulmonary insufficiency, or malnutrition may alter nutrient metabolism and may thereby warrant an enteral formulation tailored to the specific disease process. Determining the location of enteral nutrient delivery, mode of delivery, and the patient's overall current clinical condition as well as past medical history is necessary for appropriate cost-effective formula selection.

Renal Formulas

The clinical status of patients with renal failure is diverse; therefore, prescribed nutrient intake may vary greatly among patients and should depend on individual nutritional status, catabolic rate, residual glomerular filtration rate, and intensity of dialysis or hemofiltration therapy. Formulas for renal insufficiency do not clearly distinguish the difference between patients with acute failure and those with chronic renal failure.

Renal enteral formulas were first developed as oral supplements; therefore, they tend to be hyperosmolar secondary to their large simple sugar content for flavor enhancement. This hypertonicity often causes GI complications if these formulas are tube fed. The simple sugar content can also be problematic, causing impaired glycemic control in patients who are hypermetabolic, insulin resistant, or diabetic. The goal of feeding patients with renal failure is to provide optimal nutrients without compromising their medical condition through the accumulation of nitrogenous compounds, electrolytes, and fluid. Hence, renal formulas are all calorically rich, providing 2 kcalories per milliliter and containing low-to-moderate amounts of protein, electrolytes, and various minerals. Essential amino acid

(EAA) formulas were developed to decrease urea toxicity. However, previously presumed nonessential amino acids (NEAAs) are probably conditionally essential (e.g., arginine, glutamine, histidine) during metabolic stress. Recent guidelines recommend the use of EAAs and NEAAs for enhanced protein synthesis, correction of low plasma NEAA values, provision of nonspecific nitrogen via NEAAs, and enhanced protein synthesis.[55,56] Nutrients should be provided as needed. The development of fluid and electrolyte disorders or accumulation of metabolic waste products should not be minimized solely by nutrient restriction, but also by adjusting the intensity of dialysis treatment as tolerated.[57] Many patients with stable levels of creatinine, blood urea nitrogen, and electrolytes with or without dialysis can be fed with standard complete enteral formulas.

Pulmonary Formulas

Respiratory insufficiency and ventilator dependence can have a major impact on the feeding of critically ill patients. Often these patients do not receive their full nutritional needs due to the increased work of breathing, carbon dioxide retention, and fluid and electrolyte restrictions. This reduced nutrient intake results in loss of lean body tissue (e.g., intercostals, diaphragm) and malnutrition that in turn leads to fatigue and further difficulty with weaning from the ventilator.

Lipid oxidation is known to produce less carbon dioxide than oxidation of either glucose or protein. This has been the basis for the development of high fat (~45 to 55% of kcalories) and calorically concentrated (1.5 kcalories per milliliter) enteral formulas. Originally these products consisted of 100% long-chain triacylglycerol, which can suppress the immune system as well as cause malabsorption. Pulmonary formulas now contain a variety of lipids including MCT, omega-6 and omega-3 fatty acids, and more recently, γ-linolenic acid (GLA).

Animal research has shown that omega-3 fatty acids produce reduced amounts of proinflammatory eicosanoids relative to animals fed omega-6 fatty acids.[58] In another study, animals fed diets enriched by GLA, as borage oil, were found to have higher inflammatory exudate cellular levels of GLA and dihomogamma-linolenic acid (DGLA) with reduced levels of prostaglandin E_2 (PGE_2) and leukotrienes,[59] suggesting that GLA modulates inflammatory status in a manner similar to that of omega-3 fatty acids. In another animal study, authors concluded that dietary fish oil and fish and borage oil as compared with corn oil may ameliorate endotoxin-induced acute lung injury by suppressing the levels of proinflammatory eicosanoids in bronchoalveolar lavage fluid, and reduce pulmonary neutrophil accumulation.[60] More clinical trials are necessary to determine these claims and patient indications.

Aside from the previously mentioned studies with pulmonary patients, previous research evaluating the use of pulmonary enteral formulas has not demonstrated a clear benefit in providing a high-fat, reduced-carbohydrate nutrient prescription for the patient with compromised pulmonary function.[61] The excessive carbohydrate associated with overfeeding can result in a significant rise in pCO_2 and respiratory quotient that influences respiratory function. Close attention should be made to the avoidance of overfeeding by providing energy intakes from 1.2 to 1.5 times the predicted resting energy expenditure or by measuring energy expenditure via indirect calorimetry.[61]

There are potential detrimental effects in using a high-fat, low-carbohydrate enteral formula. It is well known that high-fat diets can impair gastric emptying.[62] Delayed gastric emptying can result in increased gastric residual volumes and increased risk of aspiration. Carbohydrate is the primary energy source during vigorous muscle exercise, as required during ventilator weaning. During vigorous exercise, depleted muscle glycogen stores may limit muscle endurance and strength. Nutritional support for the pulmonary compromised patient requires a balanced energy mix so that prompt replenishment of respiratory muscle glycogen can occur.[61] Pulmonary formulas, with their low carbohydrate levels, are a potential disadvantage to fully support muscle glycogen repletion during ventilator weaning.

Literature and clinical practice demonstrate that by not calorically overfeeding pulmonary compromised patients, especially if they are septic, nutritional goals may be met with a standard enteral product (~30% kcalories as fat).[56,61]

Diabetic Formulas

Nutrition is an integral component in the management of diabetes mellitus (DM). Whether during critical illness or long-term support, it can be extremely challenging. Over the past several years, enteral formulas have been developed emphasizing glycemic control for patients with DM. These formulations contain high fat- low-carbohydrate nutrient ratios, with actual ingredients varying among the manufacturers (see Table 42.7). The carbohydrate sources include fructose and fiber to assist in glycemic management. Some fat sources have been modified to contain a higher ratio of monounsaturated fatty acids than saturated fatty acids to better meet the 1994 guidelines of the American Diabetes Association.

A few individual outcome studies have been conducted to determine any benefit of providing these formulations to gain optimal glycemic control.[63,64] Overall, the recommendation is to begin by administering a standard, fiber-containing enteral formula with moderate carbohydrate and fat content. Blood glucose levels will vary based on the patient's diabetes history, metabolic stress level, and nutrient delivery method. Blood glucose levels should be monitored closely with appropriate insulin management, especially if feeding regimens are altered or interrupted. If metabolically stable diabetic patients do not exhibit desired glycemic control with a standard formula, then a diabetic enteral formula may be beneficial.

Hepatic Failure Formulas

The specialized formulas for patients with cirrhosis and hepatic failure are designed to correct the abnormal amino acid profile associated with hepatic encephalopathy. In certain instances of hepatic failure, amino acid metabolism is altered, resulting in increased plasma aromatic amino acids (AAA) with a significant change in the branched-chain amino acid (BCAA)-to-AAA ratio. This change results in altered blood-brain barrier transport, with resultant hepatic encephalopathy. Specialized enteral formulas for hepatic enchephalopathy have been designed to reduce the availability of AAAs and decrease their passage through the blood-brain barrier. Therefore, these formulas contain low quantities of AAAs and methionine and high quantities of BCAAs.

In metabolically stressed, malnourished cirrhotic patients with encephalopathy, the effectiveness of the BCAA-enriched formulas may lie in correcting malnutrition by increasing nitrogen intake without aggravating the encephalopathy. However, some life-threatening derangement in liver failure, such as portal hypertension and esophageal varices, are unaffected by nutritional repletion. Therefore, these formulas should be provided only in malnourished patients with liver failure and concomitant encephalopathy who have failed to respond to conventional medical therapy, and in whom a potentially dangerous higher level of nitrogen intake is required to induce anabolism.[56] Due to the incidence of associated fluid and electrolyte abnormalities, these formulas are calorically concentrated and contain minimal amounts of electrolytes, with some formulations failing to provide 100% of the U.S. recommended daily intake. Therefore, patients receiving these formulations should be monitored closely to ensure that no further associated nutrient deficiencies occur.

Immune-Modulated Formulas

Over the past several decades, predominantly animal models have shown that certain individual nutrients demonstrate immune benefits. These nutrients include arginine, glutamine, omega-3 fatty acids, and nucleotides. Because of this, several enteral formula manufacturers have developed immune-modulated enteral formulas to potentially improve clinical outcomes in high-risk or critically ill patients. These products all vary in the amounts of these nutrients they contain. More recently, several human studies have been conducted to determine if critically ill or other immune-compromised individuals experience positive outcomes as a result of receiving these formulations. Results of these studies vary; they have been scrutinized for several variables, including lack of feeding comparisons, lack of homogeneous study population comparisons, and the manner in which the data were analyzed. Outcomes from the studies also vary, with some showing no benefits regarding the immune formulas and others showing reduced rates of infection, antibiotic use, incidence of intra-abdominal abscesses, and reduced intensive care unit and hospital length of stay.[40]

Overall, the literature suggests that these immune-modulated formulas may be beneficial for some patients. In patients who had undergone complicated GI surgery, sustained severe trauma, or had complicated ICU stays, immune formulas were linked with decreased incidence of infections and hospital length of stay, but were not shown to reduce mortality in severely injured and immune-compromised patients.[65] More research is necessary to determine the optimal patient populations and duration of therapy for which these formulas may be appropriate.

Methods of Administration

The method for enteral tube feeding is limited to the type and site of enteral feeding access. The formula delivery method selected for the patient also depends on the patient's hemodynamic stability, gastric emptying rate, GI tolerance to tube feeding, type of formula selected, nutrient needs, patient mobility, and ease of administration. The main methods of tube feeding are by continuous, intermittent, or bolus delivery. Each institution should have an established protocol for the initiation and advancement of enteral feedings.

Bolus Feeding

Bolus feedings involve the delivery of larger amounts of formula over short periods of time, usually five minutes or less. The bolus method should only be used with gastric delivery. The stomach can act as a reservoir to handle relatively large volumes of formula (e.g., 400 mL) over a short time as opposed to the small intestine. The feedings are usually administered via a gastrostomy tube, owing to the large lumen, but they can also be given through a small-bore nasogastric tube. Usually a syringe or bulb is used to push 200 to 500 mL of formula into the feeding tube several times a day. A patient should demonstrate adequate gastric emptying and the ability to protect his/her airway (i.e., an intact gag reflex) prior to initiating bolus feedings, especially in the critical care setting, to decrease the risk of aspiration. The ability to absorb nutrients using this type of feeding depends on the access site and the functional capability of the gut.

Bolus feedings are considered the most physiologic method of administration since the gut can rest between feedings and allow for normal hormonal fluctuations. They are the easiest to administer since a pump is not required. Bolus feedings also allow for increased patient mobility, since they are delivered intermittently and do not require a pump. For these reasons, this method of feeding is most desirable for stable patients who are going home or to an extended care facility with tube feedings.

Intermittent Feedings

This method of feeding requires the formula to be infused over a 20- to 30-minute period. A feeding container and gravity drip is usually used for this method. Intermittent feedings are less likely to cause GI side effects than bolus feeding, since the formula is administered over a longer interval. Depending on the volume delivered, this method may be used for gastric as well as small bowel formula delivery.

Continuous Feedings

Continuous formula delivery is usually the enteral delivery method best tolerated. Continuous feedings are delivered slowly over 12 to 24 hours, typically with an infusion pump. In order to avoid accidental bolus delivery, continuous infusion is preferred over gravity, as a constant infusion rate can be sustained. Postpyloric feedings require continuous infusion. The small bowel does not act as a reservoir for large volumes of fluid within a short time, and GI complications usually arise if feedings are delivered in this manner.

Initiation and progression of continuous feedings should be individualized and based upon the patient's clinical condition and feeding tolerance. Typically, feedings may be initiated at 10 to 50 mL/hour, with the lower range for the critically ill. Progression of tube feedings may range from 10 to 25 mL/hour every 4 to 24 hours, depending on the patient's tolerance, until the desired goal rate is achieved. As a patient is beginning to transition to oral intake, the tube feedings may be cycled to allow for appetite stimulation, or to allow for bowel rest and time away from the pump. The feedings may be administered at night and held during the day to allow for patient mobility and an opportunity to eat.

Enteral Feeding Complications

Although enteral nutrition is the preferred route of nutrient provision in those individuals unable to consume adequate nutrients orally, it is not without complications. Compared to parenteral nutrition, enteral nutrition complications are less serious. Most of the complications with enteral nutrition are minor; however there are a few that may be serious. Most complications can be prevented, or at least made less severe. Appropriate patient assessment for needs and risks, proper feeding route and formula selection, in addition to appropriate monitoring of the enteral nutrition feeding regimen can increase the success of enteral feeding. The most common complications can be categorized as mechanical, metabolic, and gastrointestinal. Table 42.8 lists some of the common complications; their possible causes, and suggested corrective measures.

Monitoring

It is very important to continuously monitor patients for signs of formula intolerance, hydration and electrolyte status, and nutritional status. Physical indicators that should be

TABLE 42.8

Common Complications Associated with Enteral Feeding[66,67]

Complication	Possible Causes	Suggested Corrective Measures
Mechanical		
Obstructed feeding tube	Formula viscosity excessive for feeding tube	Use less viscous formula or larger bore tube
	Obstruction from crushed medications administered through tube	Flush tube before and after feeding
		Give medications as elixir or assure medications are crushed thoroughly
		Flush tube before and after delivering each medication
	Coagulation of formula protein in tube when in contact with acidic medium (medication, flushing solution)	Flush feeding tube only with warm water
		Avoid flushing with sodas, coffee, juices or any other acidic medium
Metabolic		
Hyperglycemia	Metabolic stress, sepsis, trauma	Treat origin of stress and provide insulin as needed
	Diabetes	Avoid excessive carbohydrate delivery
		Give appropriate insulin dose
Elevated or depressed serum electrolytes	Excessive or inadequate electrolytes in the formula	Change formula
	Refeeding syndrome	Monitor electrolytes closely (e.g., potassium, magnesium, phosphorus) and replace as indicated
		Initiate carbohydrate gradually, not increasing amount provided until electrolytes and blood glucose levels stabilized
Dehydration	Osmotic diarrhea caused by rapid infusion of hypertonic formula	Infuse formula slowly
		Change to isotonic formula or dilute with water
	Excessive protein, electrolytes, or both	Reduce protein, electrolytes or increase fluid provision
	Inadequate free water provision	Assure patient receives adequate free water, especially if provided calorically dense formula
Overhydration	Excessive fluid intake	Assess fluid intake; monitor daily fluid intake and output
	Rapid refeeding in malnourished patient	Monitor serum electrolytes, body weight daily; weight change >0.2 kg/d reflects decrease or increase of extracellular fluid
	Increased extracellular mass catabolism causing loss of body cell mass with subsequent potassium loss	
	Cardiac, hepatic, or renal insufficiency	Use calorically dense formula to decrease free water if needed
		Diuretic therapy
Gradual weight loss	Inadequate calories	Assure patient is receiving prescribed amount of calories
		Assure to monitor patient over time as nutrient requirements may change due to metabolic alterations
Excessive weight gain	Excess calories	Decrease calories provided, change formula or decrease volume per day
Visceral protein depletion	Inadequate protein or calories	Increase protein and/or calorie provision

TABLE 42.8 *(Continued)*

Common Complications Associated with Enteral Feeding[66,67]

Complication	Possible Causes	Suggested Corrective Measures
Essential fatty acid (EFA) deficiency	Inadequate EFA intake Prolonged use of low fat formula	Include at least 4% of kcal needs as EFA
Gastrointestinal		
Nausea and vomiting	Improper tube location	Reposition or replace feeding tube
	Excessive formula volume or rate infusion	Decrease rate of infusion or volume infused
	Very cold formula	Administer formula at room temperature
	High osmolality formula infused	Change to isotonic formula or dilute with water prior to infusing
	High fat formula infused	Change to lower fat formula
	Smell of enteral formulas	Add flavorings to formula; use polymeric as have less offensive odor
Diarrhea	Too rapid infusion	Decrease rate of infusion
	Lactose intolerance	Use lactose-free formula
	Bolus feedings into small bowel	Only provide continuous or slow gravity feedings into small bowel
	High osmolality formula infused	Change to isotonic formula or dilute with water prior to infusing
	Hyperosmolar medication delivery	Change medications or dilute with water to make isotonic prior to delivery
	Altered GI anatomy or short gut	Change to hydrolyzed or free amino acid formula with MCT oil
Vomiting and diarrhea	Contamination	Check sanitation of formula and equipment; assure proper handling techniques
Abdominal distention, bloating, cramping, gas	Rapid bolus or intermittent infusion of cold formula	Administer formula at room temperature
	Rapid infusion via syringe	Infuse continuously at low rate and gradually increase to goal
	Nutrient malabsorption	Use hydrolyzed formula, MCT containing, lactose free
	Rapid administration of MCT	Administer MCT gradually as tolerated
Constipation	Lack of fiber	Use fiber containing formula or add stool softener
	Inadequate free water	Increase free water intake
	Fecal impaction, GI obstruction	Rectal exam, digital disimpaction
	Inadequate physical activity	Increase ambulation if able
Aspiration or gastric retention	Altered gastric motility, diabetic gastroparesis, altered gag reflex, altered mental status	Assure post-pyloric nutrient delivery with continuous infusion Add prokinetic agent if changed feeding position does not help
	Head of bed <30 degrees	Elevate head of bed to >30 degrees if possible
	Displaced feeding tube	Verify feeding tube placement and replace as needed
	Ileus or hemodynamic instability	If small bowel feedings not tolerated then hold feedings and initiate TPN for prolonged intolerance
	Medications that may slow gastric motility (e.g., opiates, anticholinergics) Gastric or vagotomy surgery	Evaluate medications and change if feasible

TABLE 42.9

Example Monitoring Protocol for Enteral Feeding

Parameters	During Initiation and Advancement of Feedings Until Stable at Goal Rate	Stable at Goal Rate	Long-term Enteral Support — Stable
Body weight	Daily	1-2 times per week	Monthly
Fluid intake/output	Daily	Daily	Daily
Bowel function			
Glucose	Daily unless abnormal then every 1 to 8 hours until stable	2-3 times per week; unless diabetic, then daily	Every 6 months; unless diabetic, then daily
Electrolytes Blood urea nitrogen Creatinine Magnesium Phosphorus Calcium	Daily	2-3 times per week	Every 3-6 months
Liver function tests Triglyceride	1-2 times per week	1-2 times per month	Every 3-6 months
Visceral proteins (prealbumin, transferrin)	1-2 times per week	Weekly	Every 3-6 months
Gastric residuals (for gastric feeds only)	Every 4-6 hours	If < 200 mL, then discontinue	N/A unless gastroparesis, then every 4-6 hours

From Ideno, K.T. In: *Nutrition Support Dietetics Core Curriculum*, Gottschlich, M.M., Matarese, L.E., Shronts, E.P., Eds., ASPEN, Silver Spring, 1993, 71. With permission.

monitored include incidence of vomiting, stool frequency, diarrhea, abdominal cramps, bloating, signs of edema or dehydration, and weight changes. In addition, several laboratory parameters should be monitored daily with the initiation of enteral feeding and tapered as the patient stabilizes and demonstrates tolerance (Table 42.9).

Summary

Enteral feeding is the preferred method of providing nutrition in those who cannot consume adequate nutrients orally. Enteral feeding has many advantages over parenteral nutrition, including preservation of the structure and function of the GI tract, more efficient nutrient utilization, fewer infections and metabolic complications, greater ease of administration, and lower cost. In order for enteral nutrition to be successful, patient assessment for the optimal access site, appropriate formula selection, nutrient requirements, monitoring, and trouble-shooting complications are required.

References

1. McCamish M, Bounous G, Geraghty M. In: *Clinical Nutrition: Enteral and Tubefeeding* (Rombeau J, Rolandelli R, Eds) WB Saunders, Philadelphia, 1997, 1.
2. King BK, Kudsk KA, Li J, et al. *Ann Surg* 229: 272; 1999.
3. Kudsk KA. *Ann Surg* 215: 503; 1992.
4. Minard G, Kudsk KA. *World J Surg* 22: 213; 1998.
5. Suchner U, Senftleben U, Eckart T. *Nutrition* 12:13; 1996.
6. Hindmarsh JT, Clark RG. *Br J Surg* 60: 589; 1973.
7. Rowlands BJ, Giddings AB, Johnston AB, et al. *Br J Anaesth* 49: 781; 1977.
8. Peterson VM, Moore EE, Jones TN, et al. *Surgery* 104: 199; 1988.
9. Kudsk KA, Minard G, Wojtysiak SL, et al. *Surgery* 116: 516; 1994.
10. McArdle AH, Palmason C, Morency I, et al. *Surgery* 90: 616; 1981.
11. Bennegard K, Lindmark L, Wickstrom I, et al. *Am J Clin Nutr* 40: 752; 1984.
12. Swank GM, Deitch W. *J Surgery* 20: 411; 1996.
13. Kudsk KA. *Nutrition* 14: 541; 1998.
14. Bengmark S. *Curr Opinion Clin Nutr* 2: 83; 1999.
15. Cunningham-Rundles S, Ho Lin D. *Nutrition* 14: 573; 1998.
16. Bengmark S. *J Parent Enter Nutr* 19: 410; 1995.
17. Moore FA, Feliciano DV, Andrassy RJ, et al. *Ann Surg* 216: 172; 1992.
18. Kudsk KA, Croce MA, Fabian TC, et al. *Ann Surg* 215: 503; 1992.
19. Moore FA, Moore EE, Jones TN, et al. *J Trauma* 29: 916; 1989.
20. Trice S, Melnik G, Page C. *Nutr Clin Prac* 12: 114; 1997.
21. Lipman TO. *J Parent Enteral Nutr* 22: 167; 1998.
22. Adams S, Dellinger EP, Wertz MJ, et al. *J Trauma* 26: 882; 1986.
23. Zaloga GP. *Chest* 100: 1643; 1991.
24. Thurlow PM. *J Parent Enteral Nutr* 10: 104; 1986.
25. Heiselman DE, Vidovich RR, Milkovich G, et al. *J Parent Enteral Nutr* 17: 562; 1993.
26. Levenson R, Turner WW, Dyson A, et al. *J Parent Enteral Nutr* 12: 135; 1988.
27. Lord LM, Weiser-Maimone A, Pulhamus M, et al. *J Parent Enteral Nutr* 17: 271; 1993.
28. Kittinger JW, Sandler RS, Heizer WD. *J Parent Enteral Nutr* 11: 33; 1987.
29. Cresci G, Grace M, Park M, et al. *Nutr Clin Pract* 14:101; 1999.
30. Minard G. *Nutr Clin Prac* 9:172; 1994.
31. Gauderer MWL, Ponsky JL, Izant RJ, Jr. *J Pediatr Surg* 15: 872; 1980.
32. Baskin WN. *Gastroenterologist* 4: S40; 1996.
33. Larson DE, Burton DD, Schroeder KW, et al. *Gastroenterol* 93: 48; 1987.
34. Wasiljew BK, Ujiki GT, Beal JM. *Am J Surg* 143: 194; 1982.
35. Ruge J, Vasquez RM. *Surg Gynecol Obstet* 162:13; 1986.
36. Kirby DF, Craig RM, Tsang T, et al. *J Parent Enteral Nutr* 10: 155; 1986.
37. Kaplan DS, Murthy UK, Linscheer WG. *Gastrointest Endosc* 35: 403; 1989.
38. Shike M, Latkany L, Gerdes H, et al. *Nutr Clin Prac* 12: 38S; 1997.
39. Trujilo EB. *In*: *Contemporay Nutrition Support Practice*, Gottschlich MM, Matarese LE, Eds, WB Saunders, Philadelphia, 1998, p. 192.
40. Barton RG. *Nutr Clin Prac* 12: 51; 1997.
41. Blackburn GL. *Soc Exp Biology Med* 200: 183; 1992.
42. Lin E, Kotani J, Lowry S. *Nutrition* 14: 545; 1998.
43. Barton RG, *Nutr Clin Prac* 12: 51; 1997.
44. Heys SD, Ashkanani F. *Br J Surgery* 86: 289; 1999.
45. Van Der Hulst RRW, Van Krell BK, Von Meyenfeldt MF, et al. *Lancet* 341: 1363; 1993.
46. Ziegler TR, Young LS, Benfell K, et al. *Ann Intern Med* 116: 821; 1992.
47. Anderson PM, Schroeder G, Skubitz KM. *Cancer* 83: 1433; 1998.
48. Evoy D, Lieberman MD, Fahey TJ, et al. *Nutrition* 14: 611; 1998.
49. Barbul A, Fishel RS, Shimazu S, et al. *J Surg Res* 38: 328; 1986.

50. Kudsk DA, Minard G, Croce MA, et al. *Ann Surg* 224: 531; 1996.
51. Gottschlich MM, Jenkins M, Warden GD, et al. *J Parent Enter Nutr* 14: 225; 1990.
52. Moore FA, Moore EE, Kudsk KA, et al. *J Trauma* 37: 607; 1994.
53. Braga M, Vignali A, Gianotti L, et al. *Eur J Surg* 162: 105; 1996.
54. Bower RH, Cerra FB, Bershadsky B, et al. *Crit Care Med* 23: 436; 1995.
55. Oldrizzi L, Rugiu C, Maschio G. *Nutr Clin Prac* 9: 3; 1994.
56. ASPEN Board of Directors. *J Parent Enteral Nutr* 17: 1SA; 1993.
57. Kopple JD. *J Parenter Enteral Nutr* 20: 3; 1996.
58. Barton RG, Wells CL, Carlson A, et al. *J Trauma* 31: 768; 1991.
59. Karlstad MD, DeMichele SJ, Leathem WD, et al. *Crit Care Med* 21: 1740; 1993.
60. Mancuso P, Whelan J, DeMichele S, et al. *Crit Care Med* 25: 1198; 1997.
61. Malone AM. *Nutr Clin Prac* 12: 168; 1997.
62. Didery MB, MacDonald IA, Blackshaw PE. *Gut* 35: 186; 1994.
63. Printz H, Reche B, Fehmann HC, Goke B. *Exp Clin Endocrinol Diabetes* 105: 134; 1997.
64. Peters A, Davidson M. *J Parent Enteral Nutr* 16: 69; 1992.
65. Heys SD, Walker LG, Smith I, et al. *Ann Surg* 229: 467; 1999.
66. Stuart S, Melanie S, Unger L. In: *Medical Nutrition and Disease*, Morrison G, Hark L, Eds, Blackwell Science, Cambridge, MA, 1996, p. 339.
67. Ideno KT. In: *Nutrition Support Dietetics Core Curriculum*, Gottschlich MM, Matarese LE, Shronts EP, Eds, ASPEN, Silver Spring, MD, 1993, p. 71.

43

Parenteral Nutrition

Gail A. Cresci and Robert G. Martindale

Introduction

Parenteral nutrition can be considered one of the 20th century's medical breakthroughs. Its discovery and first implementation in the 1960s greatly enhanced clinical medicine by providing a means for complete and safe feeding of patients with nonfunctional gastrointestinal (GI) tracts. Experimentation with intravenous feeding can be traced as far back as the 1600s, when sharpened quills were used to administer a mixture of milk and wine into the veins of dogs.[1] The 1800s brought the administration of saline, and by the 1930s 5% dextrose and protein hydrolysates were being infused intravenously.[2] Several factors limited the safe infusion of nutrients intravenously. One factor was the large volumes that were provided, usually more than 3 liters per day.[2] These volumes were generally not tolerated by patients for long periods of time, and often resulted in pulmonary edema. Another factor was the attempt to deliver hyperosmolar solutions peripherally, which was the common practice in the early years. Dextrose solutions greater than 10% concentration were not tolerated, and resulted in thrombosis. Lastly, volume and the osmolality restrictions resulted in caloric delivery limitations. This all led to experimentation with alternate fuel substrates, alcohol and fat, due to their increased caloric provision of 7 and 9 kcalories per gram, respectively. Research quickly revealed that alcohol was not going to be the answer, as it resulted in hepatoxicity and other side effects when delivered in large amounts.[1] Intravenous fat delivery was an enticing alternative due to its high caloric load and decreased osmolality. Initially, provision of intravenous fat was achieved with cottonseed oil in the 1950s. However, it was removed from the market, as it was associated with jaundice, fever, and bleeding.[3] Research continued in Europe, where emulsions made from soybean oil were successfully administered.[2]

Great advancement came in 1967, when cannulating the subclavian vein was introduced to administer intravenous nutrients. Wilmore and Dudrick[4] first reported successful provision of centrally administered nutrition to an infant with intestinal atresia. In the 1970s advancements continued with the use of crystalline amino acids rather than protein hydrolysates, recommendations for standard amounts of vitamins and minerals, and the reintroduction of lipids in the United States.[1] After the 1970s, the focus turned to fine-tuning the parenteral solutions with the development of specialized amino acid sources

0-8493-2705-9/01/$0.00+$1.50

TABLE 43.1

Development of Total Parenteral Nutrition (TPN) Guidelines

Organization	Year
American Society for Parenteral and Enteral Nutrition	1986, 1993
American College of Physicians	1987, 1989
American Gastroenterology Association	1989
U.S. Dept of Health and Human Services	1990

TABLE 43.2

Indications for TPN[5-8]

Clinical Situation	Consensus
Short bowel syndrome	Inability to absorb adequate nutrients orally <60 cm small bowel may require indefinite use
Severe pancreatitis	Recommended if enteral nutrition causes abdominal pain, ascites, or elevated amylase/lipase Increased fistula output with enteral feedings Intravenous lipids are considered safe if serum triglyceride levels are <400 mg/dl
Enterocutaneous fistula	Fistula that exhibits increased output with enteral nutrition
Intractable diarrhea or vomiting	Recommended for losses greater than 500-1000 ml/day with inability to maintain adequate nutritional status
Bowel obstruction, ileus	With obstruction and malnutrition awaiting surgery >7 days Prolonged ileus >5-7 days with poor nutritional status
Perioperative support	Preoperative support is indicated for severely malnourished patients with expected postoperative NPO status >10 days For those with postoperative complications rendering NPO >10 days
Inflammatory bowel	If enteral nutrition not tolerated or if precluded by GI fistulas
Critical care	Unable to gain enteral access, instability, abdominal distention with prolonged reflux of enteral feedings, expected to remain NPO >7 days
Eating disorders	Severe malnutrition and inability to tolerate enteral feeding for psychological reasons
Pregnancy	Safe in pregnancy; hyperemesis gravidarum

for disease states, approval of total nutrient admixtures by the Food and Drug Administration, and development of new access devices and delivery systems.[1]

Rationale for Use of Parenteral Nutrition

Parenteral nutrition was first developed to provide nutrition to those unable to take complete nutrition via the GI tract due to an inability to digest or absorb nutrients. A nonfunctioning GI tract and failure to tolerate enteral nutrition still remain the primary reasons for parenteral nutrition. Certain accompanying conditions also need consideration, such as a patient being nutritionally at risk, and projected inability to consume anything by mouth for at least 7 to 14 days.[5] Over the past two decades several organizations have developed practice guidelines to identify the appropriate use for parenteral nutrition (Table 43.1). Situations that indicate the need for parenteral nutrition include short bowel syndrome and malabsorption, bowel obstruction, severe pancreatitis, intractable diarrhea or vomiting, prolonged ileus, and high-output GI fistulas (Table 43.2).[5-8]

Comparison of Parenteral and Enteral Nutrition

While parenteral nutrition can be lifesaving when used appropriately, it may also potentiate adverse clinical outcomes. The GI tract not only functions to digest and absorb

TABLE 43.3

Factors that Contribute to Increased Gut Permeability

Absence of enteral stimulation
Broad spectrum antibiotics
H_2-receptor blockers
Decreased GI hormone secretion

nutrients, but also serves as a large immunologic organ in the body by acting as a protective barrier against intraluminal toxins and bacteria. Approximately 50% of the body's immunoglobulin-producing cells line the GI tract, with 80% of the body's manufactured immunoglobulin being secreted across the GI tract.[9] During severe physiologic stress gut ischemia can occur, leading to mucosal damage and disruption of the barrier function and ultimately passage of bacteria and toxins into the bloodstream.[10] In addition, common clinical practices as well as physiologic changes during acute stress can lend to bacterial overgrowth in the proximal GI tract and impact the gut's protective barrier (Table 43.3). Whether or not bacterial translocation occurring in animals and humans during acute stress is clinically significant remains debatable. Animal studies support the statement that enteral rather than parenteral nutrition maintains gut integrity and immune responsiveness, and prevents bacterial translocation.[11-15] However, there was no significant difference in overall outcome in an acute pancreatitis model,[11] but in animals with induced bacterial pneumonia, those that received total parenteral nutrition (TPN) had a higher mortality rate.[15] There is no hard evidence to support the statement that parenteral nutrition results in clinically significant bacterial translocation in humans.[16,17]

Despite this lack of evidence, other disadvantages of parenteral nutrition exist. The metabolic response to intravenous glucose differs from oral glucose. This may be due to the fact that the liver retains a large portion of glucose when provided orally, resulting in less systemic hyperglycemia and hyperinsulinemia.[18] A meta-analysis comparing enteral and parenteral nutrition also concluded that plasma glucose concentrations are lower during enteral than parenteral nutrition.[19] Plasma glucose and insulin concentrations, glucose oxidation, CO_2 production, and minute ventilation increase in proportion to the proportion of kcalories administered in TPN.[20] Prolonged infusion of high rates of glucose (>4 mg/kg/min) results in *de novo* lipogenesis in the majority of critically ill patients.[20] Furthermore, TPN is associated with increased septic morbidity[16,19,21,22] and increased cost[16, 23] when compared with enteral nutrition in trauma patients.

Vascular Access

Peripheral

Prior to initiating parenteral nutrition, vascular access is obtained. Determination of venous access is based upon the duration of therapy, patient limitations, and availability of equipment and facilities. Central or peripheral veins may be used for the provision of parenteral nutrition. Peripheral access with conventional needles uses the small veins of the extremities — typically the hands and forearms. These small veins are easily sclerosed by hypertonic parenteral solutions. Therefore, to minimize phlebitis and thrombosis of the veins, it is recommended that peripheral parenteral solutions (PPN) consist of osmolalities ≤900 mOsm/L.[5] Even with appropriate PPN, intravenous sites may need frequent changing to maintain venous patency.[1] The increased fluid requirement necessary to

TABLE 43.4

Typical PPN Order

Macronutrient	Usual Concentration in PPN Solution	gm/L or mEq/L	Kcal/L	mOsmol/L
Dextrose (6%)	5-10%	60*	240	150
Amino acids (3%)	3-5%	30*	120	300
Lipid (20%)	30-60% (of kcal)	20*	200	300
Sodium		35+	—	70
Potassium		30+	—	60
Magnesium		5+	—	5
Calcium			—	7
Total			560	892

* gm/L; + mEq/L

TABLE 43.5

Indications for Peripheral Parenteral Nutrition

Indication	Example
Patient expected to be NPO 5-7 days	Postoperative ileus
Inadequate GI function expected for 5-7 days	Hyperemesis gravidarum
Transitioning to an oral diet or tube feeding	Patient with Crohn's disease flare
Central venous access is contraindicated	Coagulopathy, sepsis, venous thrombosis
Malnourished patients expected to be NPO for several days	Preoperative small bowel obstruction
Patients with nutrient requirements that can be met with PPN	Obese patient with good venous access, small or elderly people

minimize the PPN solution's osmolality limits nutrient provision as well as the clinical utility of PPN (Table 43.4).

PPN solutions vary considerably among institutions. Some may only use dextrose with electrolytes, vitamins, and minerals while others may include lipids and amino acids to increase the kcalories and minimize catabolism. PPN formulations composed of carbohydrate, amino acids, and lipid generally provide 1000 to 1500 kcal/day . However, PPN may be useful when the long term plan for nutrition is uncertain and the patient requires interim nutrition intervention in which the GI tract is nonfunctional, such as with prolonged ileus or hyperemesis gravidarum (Table 43.5).

Central

Central venous access refers to the large veins in the trunk. The primary indications for central venous access include chemotherapy, antibiotic administration, risk of tissue necrosis with vesicant medications, and provision of TPN due to its pH and increased osmolality. Access is obtained with specialized catheters, with the distal tip placed into the vena cava or right atrial area. The most common venipuncture sites include the subclavian, jugular, femoral, cephalic, and basilic veins (Table 43.6). Several varieties of central venous catheters are available, the most common being polyurethane and silicone (Table 43.7). Most catheters are available in a variety of French sizes, lengths, and number of portals or lumens. Multilumen versions provide for simultaneous infusion of TPN with multiple or incompatible drugs.

Physiologic, functional, psychological, and social factors all need consideration prior to determining the type and location of catheter placement (Table 43.8). If the patient is in the acute care setting and unlikely to be discharged with TPN, the physiologic factors are

TABLE 43.6

Central Venous Catheter Placement[24,25]

Method	Vessels	Description
Percutaneous approach a. Modified Seldinger technique	Subclavian Internal & external jugular Antecubital	a. Venipuncture and passage of a guidewire through the needle followed by removal of the needle and catheter placement over the guidewire
b. Peel-away introducer sheath and tissue dilator		b. Catheter passes through the introducer into the vein and introducer tears longitudinally, leaving the catheter in place
Cutdown	Cephalic External & internal jugular	Surgical dissection, isolation of the vessel, and catheter placement
Tunneled		6 cm catheter segment is tunneled through the subcutaneous tissues between the venipuncture site and the skin exit site
Implanted ports		A reservoir with a silicone disk and attached silicone tube is implanted under the clavicle in a subcutaneous pocket

TABLE 43.7

Central Venous Catheter Characteristics

Material	Description
Silicone elastomer	Known as Silastic (Dow Corning) Biomaterial for longterm indwelling devices Increased elasticity and flexibility for minimal damage to intima Resistant to hydrolytic enzymes; hydrophobic surface resists bacterial adherence Considered chemically inert in blood Guide wire or peel-away introducer needed for insertion due to soft texture
Polyurethane	Increased flexibility and strength; resistance to hydrolytic enzymes Decreased incidence of inflammatory changes and thrombophlebitis with short term use Anticoagulation required with long term use for thrombosis prevention
Polyvinyl chloride	Stiff material Increased rate of thrombogenicity Infrequently used
Polyethylene	High tensile strength Minimal irritation if used for short duration Associated with platelet adherance and fibrous capsule formation with long duration
Polytetrafluoroethylene	Known as Teflon; stable; demonstrates nonadhesive, antifriction properties; resistant to degradative enzymes Smooth and hydrophobic catheter surface Not suitable for long term use due to rigidity which causes irritation and thrombosis formation
Hydrogel	Hydrophilic polymers designed for biological use Absorbs water up to 90% of the catheter's dry weight without dissolving Most inert and nonthrombogenic of biomaterials Material lacks durability unless copolymerized with other monomers
Coated/bonded catheters	Antimicrobial impregnated catheters: catherters with the cationic surfactant tridodecylmethylammonium chloride facilitate bonding of anionic antibiotics to both the internal and external catheter surfaces Antiseptic-coated catheters: polyurethane catheters bonded with silver sulfadiazine and chlorhexidine to the external surface

From Krzywda, E.A. and Edmiston, C.E. *ASPEN Practice Manual*, 1998. With permission.

TABLE 43.8

Patient Factors for Vascular Access Device Selection

Patient Factor	Considerations
Physiologic	Vein physiology
	Hypercoagulable states
	Diabetes
	Clotting abnormalities
	Skin disorders and conditions
	Previous surgical procedures in the thorax or vascular system
	Morbid obesity
	Surgical risk
	Known allergies to vascular materials
Functional	Impaired vision, dexterity
	Developmental disabilities
	Frailty
Psychological	Needle phobia (not ideal candidates for implanted ports)
	Body image issues (implanted port less disturbing than tunneled)
	Previous experience with vascular access devices
Social	Support system for line and catheter care
	Financial implications

From Evans, M. *Nutr. Clin. Prac.* 14: 172; 1999. With permission.

of primary concern. However, if a patient is to receive parenteral nutrition in an alternate care setting, practitioners should consider the other listed factors for optimal patient compliance.[24]

Parenteral Nutrient Components

Parenteral nutrient solutions are complex formulations that usually contain the macronutrients, carbohydrate, protein, and fat for energy provision, as well as electrolytes, trace elements, vitamins, water, and occasionally medications. These components need to be individualized for patients based upon their primary diagnosis, chronic diseases, fluid and electrolyte balance, acid-base status, and specific nutrition goals.[26]

Carbohydrate

Carbohydrate serves as the primary energy source in parenteral solutions. The amount of carbohydrate provided is based upon the patient's individual nutrient requirements and glucose oxidation rate. Although the exact requirement is individualized, guidelines are available. A minimum of 100 gm per day is often used as the obligate need for the central nervous system, white blood cells, red blood cells, and renal medulla.[26] The maximum rate of glucose oxidation in adults is 4 to 7 mg/kg/min,[5] or 400 to 700 gm for a 70-kg person, with the lower range suggested for critically ill patients secondary to endogenous glucose production. Excessive carbohydrate provision is associated with hyperglycemia, excessive carbon dioxide production, and hepatic steatosis.[26]

Carbohydrate is provided almost exclusively as dextrose monohydrate in parenteral solutions. Each gram of hydrated dextrose provides 3.4 kcal/gram. Commercial dextrose preparations are available in concentrations from 5 to 70% (Table 43.9). Dextrose solutions have an acidic pH (3.5 to 5.5) and are stable after autoclave sterilization.[26] Sterilization

TABLE 43.9

Intravenous Dextrose Solutions

Dextrose Concentration %	Carbohydrate (gm/L)	Calories (kcal/L)	Osmolarity (mOsm/L)
5	50	170	250
10	100	340	500
20	200	680	1000
30	300	1020	1500
50	500	1700	2500
70	700	2380	3500

also increases the shelf life of dextrose solutions so that they can be stored for extended periods at room temperature.

Glycerol is a simple organic compound consisting of the elements carbon, hydrogen, and oxygen. Glycerol yields 4.3 kcal/gram when oxidized to carbon dioxide and water, and does not require insulin for cellular uptake. When provided in low concentrations (3%) with amino acids, it has been found to be protein sparing.[27] Because of these advantages, glycerol is used an alternative source of calories in some parenteral formulations, primarily in PPN.

Fat

Since its introduction in Europe in the mid-1960s, intravenous fat emulsions have been extensively used as a nutrient source in parenteral nutrition. The aqueous fat emulsions available in the U.S. as of 1999 consist of long-chain triacylglycerols (TAG) manufactured from soybean and safflower oil. Therefore, the lipid emulsions not only provide a source of kcalories but also essential fatty acids. These products contain egg yolk phospholipid as an emulsifying agent and glycerin, which make the products nearly isotonic. The glycerol raises the caloric concentration of the 10% emulsion to 1.1 kcal/mL and the 20% emulsion to 2.0 kcal/mL. The phospholipid may contribute to the phosphorus intake of patients who receive large amounts of lipids (>500 mL/day). Combinations of long-chain and medium-chain TAG emulsions have been available in Europe for several years.

Most patients tolerate daily infusion of lipids provided as an intermittent or continuous infusion, often as part of a total nutrient admixture (TNA). Continuous delivery with a moderate dose is favored over intermittent infusion due to decreased fluctuations in serum TAG levels and improved fat oxidation.[28] The requirement of a test dose is usually eliminated with continuous delivery, as the administration rate tends to be less than that with the test dose. Patients should still be monitored for fever, chills, headache, and back pain during the first dose of intravenous lipid. Absolute contraindications to intravenous fat emulsions include pathologic hyperlipidemia, lipoid nephrosis, severe egg allergy, and acute pancreatitis associated with severe hypertriglyceridemia.[26] Caution should be taken in delivery to patients with severe liver disease, adult respiratory distress syndrome, or severe metabolic stress. If serum TAG levels are greater than 500 mg/dL, lipids should be held with only the minimal requirements for essential fatty acids (EFA) provided to avoid further metabolic complications.

Lipid requirements are met by providing at least 4% of energy as EFA or approximately 10% of energy as a commercial lipid emulsion from safflower oil[1] to prevent EFA deficiency. Since lipid emulsions vary in their composition of EFA depending on the oil source, the minimum amount provided is based upon the EFA content rather than a percentage of total energy. Recommendations for optimal lipid delivery have evolved over the years. It once was common practice to provide 50 to 70% of energy as lipid due to its concentrated energy source and decreased volume. However, over the years concerns that long-chain triglycerides impair neutraphil function, endotoxin clearance, and complement synthesis have resulted in the recommendation to limit lipid administration to 1 gm/kg per day[29] or 25 to 30% of total energy.[30]

Protein

The primary function of protein in parenteral nutrition is to provide nitrogen to maintain nitrogen balance to help minimize loss of lean body mass and protein degradation for gluconeogenesis. The protein utilized for parenteral nutrition is primarily in the form of crystalline amino acids. Parenteral amino acid products can be divided into standard and modified. Standard amino acid products are suitable for the majority of patients. They contain a balanced or physiologic mixture of essential and nonessential amino acids in which the ratios are based on FAO/WHO recommendations for optimal proportions of essential amino acids. Standard formulations are available in a range of concentrations from 3 to 15%. Most institutions stock 10 and 15% concentrations, since more dilute solutions can be made readily by adding sterile water with an automated compounder.

Modified amino acid solutions are designed for patients with disease- or age-specific amino acid requirements. Formulations are marketed for adults with hepatic failure, renal dysfunction, metabolic stress, and for neonates with special requirements for growth and development. These modified formulations are significantly more costly than the standard formulations and may not always prove as cost-effective; therefore, strict criteria should be established for their use.

Patients with hepatic failure develop multiple metabolic abnormalities including electrolyte disturbances and alterations in amino acid metabolism. In severe liver disease, hepatic encephalopathy can occur which is associated with decreased branched chain amino acid (BCAA) serum levels and elevated aromatic amino acid (AAA) and methionine serum levels. Patients with hepatic disease without encephalopathy may be provided with moderate levels of standard amino acids with close monitoring of their mental status. When hepatic encephalopathy is severe (≥Grade II), a modified hepatic protein formulation may be beneficial. These formulations have high concentrations of BCAA (~45% of protein) and low concentrations of AAA and methionine. Improvement in hepatic encephalopathy and lower mortality have been found in some patients who received this formulation.[31]

Modified formulations are marketed for patients with renal failure. These formulas contain mainly essential amino acids, and were designed on the premise that endogenous urea could be used to synthesize nonessential amino acids. This hypothesis has been challenged, thus questioning the usefulness of these formulas. Prospective, randomized, controlled studies have demonstrated that standard amino acids are as effective as modified amino acids in patients who have renal failure and who require parenteral nutrition.[32,33] Thus, patients with severe renal failure may be given standard amino acids as part of parenteral nutrition in most clinical situations.[24]

A parenteral formulation with an enhanced BCAA formulation is marketed for patients with metabolic stress such as that caused by trauma, burns, and sepsis. Metabolic stress causes an efflux of amino acids from skeletal muscle and the gut to the liver for gluconeogenesis and support of acute phase protein synthesis.[34] Metabolically stressed patients have also been shown to have increased serum levels of AAA and decreased BCAA levels. Therefore, the rationale of using a high BCAA formula in these patients is to provide the preferential fuel to the body and normalize the patient's amino acid patterns. Multiple studies have evaluated the benefits of high BCAA formulations in metabolic stress. Some studies have shown positive benefits when using these formulations, such as nitrogen retention, improved visceral protein levels, and reversal of skin test anergy, but there were no differences in morbidity or mortality.[35-37] Other studies have failed to exhibit significant outcome advantages of BCAAs over standard amino acid formulas in metabolic stress.[38-40] Therefore, since the cost-effectiveness of high BCAA solutions has not been clearly demonstrated, initiation of nutrition support with a standard amino acid solution is recommended in patients with metabolic stress.[5]

Protein requirements are based upon the patient's clinical condition. For normal healthy adults the recommendation is for 0.8 gm/kg per day.[41] In the critically ill population, a range of 1.5 to 2.0 gm/kg/day is appropriate.[5] For patients with renal or hepatic disease, protein recommendations vary according to the disease stage and its intervention. For those with renal disease on peritoneal dialysis, 1.2 to 1.5 gm/kg/day of ideal body weight is recommended for maintenance or repletion. For hemodialysis, 1.1 to 1.4 gm/kg of ideal body weight per day is recommended for maintenance or repletion.[42] For patients with uncomplicated hepatic dysfunction, 0.8 to 1.5 gm/kg dry weight is suggested; for end-stage liver disease with encephalopathy, 0.5 to 0.7 gm/kg; if a high BCAA formula is used, then 0.8 to 1.2 gm/kg/day is suggested.[43]

Electrolytes

Electrolytes are essential nutrients that perform many critical physiologic functions. Electrolytes are added to parenteral solutions based upon individual need. The amount added daily varies based upon the patient's weight, disease state, renal and hepatic function, nutrition status, pharmacotherapy, acid-base status, and overall electrolyte balance. Extrarenal electrolyte losses may be a result of diarrhea, ostomy output, vomiting, fistulas, or nasogastric suctioning. As patients become anabolic during parenteral nutrient delivery they may experience increased requirements for the major intracellular electrolytes (potassium, phosphorus, and magnesium). During refeeding of undernourished patients, these electrolytes should be monitored frequently and replenished accordingly.

Small adjustments in electrolyte intake can affect patient morbidity and mortality and therefore need careful monitoring. General recommendations for electrolyte provision are provided in Table 43.10. Electrolyte products are commercially available (Table 43.11), and the composition of the parenteral solution is dependent upon the compatibility of each electrolyte with the other components of the admixture. For calcium provision, calcium gluconate is the preferred form for parenteral formulations due to its stability in solution and decreased chance of dissociating and forming a precipitate with phosphorus. Whether to provide an electrolyte as a chloride or an acetate salt depends on the patient's acid-base status. Generally, acid-base balance is maintained with providing chloride and acetate

TABLE 43.10

Parenteral Electrolyte Recommendations

Sodium	60-150 mEq/d
Potassium	70-150 mEq/d
Phosphorus	20-30 mmol/d
Magnesium	15-20 mEq/d
Calcium	10-20 mmol
Chloride	Equal to Na+ to prevent acid-base disturbances

From Skipper, A. In: *Contemporary Nutrition Support Practice.* W.B. Saunders, Philadelphia, 1998, p. 227. With permission.

TABLE 43.11

Commercially Available Electrolyte Formulations[25,26]

Sodium chloride	Magnesium sulfate
Sodium acetate	Magnesium chloride
Sodium phosphate	Calcium chloride
Sodium lactate	Calcium gluconate
Potassium chloride	
Potassium acetate	
Potassium phosphate	
Potassium lactate	

in a 1:1 ratio. If a patient has altered acid-base status with skewed electrolyte levels, then the chloride:acetate ratio can be adjusted to facilitate correction. Acetate and chloride are also present in the base amino acid solutions in various amounts, and should be considered when attempting electrolyte homeostasis.

Electrolytes increase the osmolarity of the parenteral solution; however, large amounts can be added to solutions with amino acids and dextrose without affecting the stability. When lipids are added to the parenteral solutions caution is needed when adding electrolytes, as there are limitations and hazards.[1] An insoluble precipitate can form when there are excess cations in the parenteral solutions, as with calcium and phosphate, which may not be visualized in total nutrient admixtures. Crystal formation in the lungs with subsequent death was reported in patients as a result of precipitate formation in TPN solutions.[44] The solubility of calcium and phosphorus varies with the volume of the solution, its pH, the type of calcium preparation, the temperature at which the solutions are stored, and the order of admixture.[1] Solutions can be prepared with a range of calcium and phosphorus contents as long as the product of calcium (in mEq) and phosphorus (in mmols) is less than 200.[45]

Vitamins and Trace Elements

Vitamins are typically added to every parenteral formulation in doses consistent with the American Medical Association Nutrition Advisory Group's recommendations.[46] Guidelines are established for the 12 essential vitamins (Table 43.12). Most institutions use a

TABLE 43.12

AMA Recommendations for Parenteral Vitamin Intake

Vitamin	Amount
Vitamin A	3,300 IU
Vitamin D	200 IU
Vitamin E	10 IU
Vitamin C (ascorbic acid)	100 mg
Folacin	400 μg
Niacin	40 mg
Riboflavin	3.6 mg
Thiamine	3 mg
Vitamin B_6 (pyridoxine)	4 mg
Vitamin B_{12} (cyanocobalamin)	5 μg
Pantothenic acid	15 mg
Biotin	60 μg

Adapted from Multivitamin preparations for parenteral use. A statement by the Nutrition Advisory Group. *J Parenter Enteral Nutr* 3: 258, 1979.

TABLE 43.13

AMA Recommendations for Parenteral Mineral Intake

Element	Amount
Zinc	2.5-4 mg/day
Copper	0.5-1.5 mg/day
Manganese	150-180 μg/day
Chromium	10-15 μg/day
Selenium*	40-80 μg/day

* Suggested intake.

Adapted from Guidelines for essential trace element preparations for parenteral use: A statement by the Nutrition Advisory Group. *J Parenter Enteral Nutr* 3: 263, 1979.

commercially available multiple-entity product which contains 12 essential vitamins for adults. The multivitamin preparations for adults do not contain vitamin K because it antagonizes the effects of warfarin in patients receiving this medication. In adults, vitamin K may be administered by adding 1 to 2 mg/day to the parenteral solution or by giving 5 to 10 mg/week intramuscularly or subcutaneously.[26] Individual vitamin preparations are also available and are used to supplement the multivitamin doses when a deficiency state exists, or with increased needs due to disease or medical condition.

Trace minerals are essential to normal metabolism and growth, and serve as metabolic cofactors essential for the proper functioning of several enzyme systems. Although the requirements are minute, deficiency states can develop rapidly secondary to increased metabolic demands or excessive losses. Most clinicians add these micronutrients daily; however, there are clinical conditions necessitating trace mineral restriction and therefore adjustments in the daily intakes.

The Nutrition Advisory Group of the American Medical Association has also published guidelines for four trace elements known to be important in human nutrition.[47] The suggested amounts of zinc, copper, manganese, and chromium for adults are listed in Table 43.13. Since the original recommendations, it has become more evident that selenium also is essential, and many clinicians add this element to the parenteral solution daily along with the other four.[26] Most institutions use a commercially available multiple-entity product, but there are also single-entity mineral solutions available for use during times of increased requirements or when certain minerals are contraindicated. Zinc requirements are increased during metabolic stress due to increased urinary losses, and with excessive GI losses as with diarrhea and increased ostomy output. Manganese and copper are excreted through the biliary tract, whereas zinc, chromium, and selenium are excreted via the kidney. Therefore, copper and manganese should be restricted or withheld from parenteral nutrition in patients with cholestatic liver disease.[26] Selenium depletion has been found in patients receiving long-term TPN, as well as with thermal injury, acquired immunodeficiency syndrome, liver failure, and critical illness.[26,47]

Other Additives

Many patients receiving TPN are also receiving multiple medications, leading to the desire to add the medications to the TPN solutions. Using TPN as a drug delivery vehicle is very tempting, as it may allow for continuous medication infusion in addition to minimizing fluid volume delivery by eliminating the need for a separate dilutent for each medication

TABLE 43.14

Medications Compatible with Parenteral Solutions

Albumin[a]	Cyanocobalamin	Hydromorphone	Nafcillin
Amikacin	Cyclophosphamide	Imipenem-cilastatin	Neostigmine
Aminophylline[a]	Cytarabine	Insulin, regular[a]	Netilmicin
Azlocillin	Digoxin[a]	Iron dextran	Oxacillin[a]
Caffeine	Dipyridamole	Isoproterenol[a]	Oxytocin
Carbenicillin[a,b]	Dobutamine	Kanamycin[a]	Penicillin G[a]
Cefamandole[a]	Dopamine[a]	Lidocaine[a]	Phenobarbital
Cefazolin[a]	Doxycycline	Meperidine[a]	Phytonadione[a]
Cefoperazone	Erythromycin[a]	Metaraminol	Piperacillin
Cefotaxime	Famotidine[a]	Methicillin[a]	Polymyxin B
Cefoxitin[a]	Fluorouracil[b]	Methotrexate	Ranitidine[a,b]
Ceftazidine	Folic Acid	Methyldopa	Tetracycline
Ceftriazone	Furosemide[a]	Methylprednisolone	Ticarcillin[a,b]
Cephalothin[a,b]	Ganciclovir	Metoclopramide[a]	Tobramycin[a]
Chloramphenicol[a]	Gentamicin[a]	Mezlocillin	Vancomycin
Chlorpromazine	Heparin[a]	Miconazole	
Cimetidine[a]	Hydralazine	Morphine	
Clindamycin[a]	Hydrochloric acid	Moxalactam	

[a] Compatible with total nutrient admixtures (TNA)

[b] Some data suggest incompatibility under certain conditions. Visual compatibility only; tested with parenteral nutrition solution without electrolytes; drug may chelate with divalent cations and cause precipitation.

From Strausburg, K. Parenteral nutrition admixture. *ASPEN Practice Manual,* 1998. With permission.

administered. However, scrutiny is needed prior to adding medications to the TPN solution, as there is potential for drug-drug and drug-nutrient interactions. Issues needing consideration include medication compatibility with TPN constituents, the effect of pH changes on TPN compatibility and drug effectiveness, whether the infusion schedule of the TPN is appropriate to achieve therapeutic levels of the drug, and the potential for interactions among the drugs if more than one is added.[1] The complexity of these issues usually leads to consultation with a pharmacist experienced in TPN compounding and compatibility, reference to the institution's policy and procedure manual, or contact with the drug manufacturers. Medications most frequently added to TPN include albumin, aminophylline, cimetidine, famotidine, ranitidine, heparin, hydrochloric acid, and regular insulin.[1] Table 43.14 list medications compatible with TPN solutions, and Table 43.15 lists those medications which are incompatible with TPN solutions.

Insulin

Even with care to avoid excess carbohydrate delivery, patients receiving TPN often become hyperglycemic. One method of achieving desired blood glucose control with continuous TPN infusions is by adding regular insulin to the TPN solution. A few studies have suggested that absorbance of insulin to glass bottles, polyvinyl chloride bags, and tubing occurs,[49,50] with the greatest loss occurring during the first hour of infusion.[51] So, when adding insulin to TPN solutions to optimize blood glucose control, it is important to remember that the patient may have an increased insulin requirement due to absorbance.

Histamine H_2-Receptor Blockers

Stress ulcer prophylaxis with the addition of H_2-receptor blockers to avoid stress ulcers is common practice with patients on TPN who are not receiving any gastric nutrients.

TABLE 43.15

Medications Incompatible with Parenteral Solutions

Amphotericin B	Methyldopa[a]
Amikacin[a]	Metronidazole (with $NaHCO_3$)
Ampicillin[b]	Phenytoin[a]
Cephradine	Tetracycline[a,c]
Iron dextran[a,d]	

[a] Incompatible with total nutrient admixtures (TNA)
[b] Some visual compatibility data suggest compatibility under certain conditions
[c] Compatible with lipid alone; however, may chelate with divalent cations of TNAs
[d] Visually incompatible with TNAs when reconstituted with 5% dextrose in water; visually compatible when reconstituted with normal saline solution

From Strausberg, K. Parenteral nutrition admixture. *ASPEN Practice Manual*, 1998. With permission.

This may be achieved by adding the H_2-receptor blockers to the TPN solution. Famotidine (20 and 40 mg/L) and ranitidine hydrochloride have been shown to be stable in parenteral nutrition solutions and three-in-one admixtures.[52-56]

Heparin

In order to reduce the complications of catheter occlusion related to fibrin formation around the catheter tip, heparin may be added to the TPN solution. Adding up to 1000 units of heparin per liter reduces the incidence of catheter occlusion without exhibiting anticoagulant effects on serum.[1] Larger amounts of heparin may be used for peripheral parenteral nutrition.

Methods of Administration

Serious complications with TPN may develop if careful initiation and monitoring are not followed. TPN solutions may be infused continuously over a 24-hour period, or cycled over shorter time intervals. If a patient is critically ill or just beginning to receive TPN, it is suggested to infuse it over a 24-hour period until patient tolerance is demonstrated. TPN should not be initiated at goal levels of nutrients, as many patients may not tolerate this prescription. Proportional increases in carbohydrate-dependent electrolytes such as magnesium and phosphorus, in protein-dependent electrolytes such as potassium, and in volume-dependent electrolytes such as sodium should be made as the macronutrients are increased.

For patients with diabetes mellitus, stress hyperglycemia, steroids, or risk for refeeding syndrome, dextrose should be restricted initially to approximately 100 to 150 gm/day. For other patients with normal glucose tolerance, dextrose may be initiated at 200 to 250 gm/day. If after 24 hours serum glucose levels are acceptable, then the dextrose may be advanced to goal over the next 24 to 48 hours as indicated. Capillary glucose measurements should be obtained three to four times daily until the values are normal for two consecutive days. Regular insulin may be administered according to a sliding scale.[1] A continuous intravenous insulin infusion may be substituted for sliding scale if serum glucose levels are consistently elevated beyond suggested levels. Insulin may also be added to the TPN solution; however, one needs to remember that providing insulin in this manner confines the delivery over the time period of the TPN mixture, and if the hyperglycemia resolves then the TPN bag must be discontinued to avoid inadvertent hypoglycemia. For patients requiring insulin prior to TPN institution, approximately half of the established insulin requirement may be included as regular insulin in the initial bag of TPN formula.[1] If blood glucose levels are less than 200 mg/dL, approximately two-thirds of the previous day's subcutaneous insulin dose may be added to the TPN as regular insulin. Regardless of the method of insulin delivery, the goal is to consistently maintain blood glucose levels between 120 and 200 mg/dl.[5]

Lipids may be infused for up to 24 hours, and may reduce the effect of lipids on the reticuloendothelial system.[29] Lipids can be given with the first TPN infusion unless serum triacylglycerol levels are elevated. It is suggested to maintain triacylglycerol levels at ≤400 mg/dL while lipids are being infused.[1] If triacylglycerol levels exceed the recommended level, lipids should be held until levels normalize. As this occurs, patients may be provided with lipids in amounts to prevent essential fatty acid deficiency. For persistent or severe hypertriacylglycerolemia or for patients with egg allergy, oral or topical safflower oil can be administered to alleviate the symptoms of essential fatty acid deficiency.[58] Critically ill patients may also be receiving significant amounts of lipid from lipid-based medications, which may predispose them to hypertriacylglycerolemia prior to TPN infusion. The amount of lipid from medications should be considered in the final TPN formulation to avoid providing excess long-chain triacylglycerol.

Although parenteral nutrition is usually provided over a 24-hour continuous rate, it may also be delivered in a cyclic pattern. Cyclic TPN has been suggested for patients who are stable and receiving TPN for an extended duration. During TPN, circulating insulin levels remain elevated, reducing the amount of carbohydrate that enters the cell, thus favoring hepatic lipogenesis.[1] Cyclic TPN also allows for some time off of the TPN pump, allowing for patient mobility, and therefore it is usually utilized with ambulatory patients. For individuals with limited vascular access, cyclic infusion may be required in order to administer necessary medications or blood products. Conversion from 24-hour continuous infusion to cyclic infusion can be accomplished in two to three days. The largest concern is with the initiation and discontinuation of the carbohydrate infusion and potential for hyperglycemia and rebound hypoglycemia. Another concern is with the increased volume delivery over a shorter time frame. Most stable patients can tolerate cyclic TPN over 8 to 14 hours.

Parenteral Nutrition Discontinuation

Eventually in all patients, the goal is to transition from TPN to enteral nutrition — either tube feeding or oral intake. Prior to discontinuing TPN, assurance that the patient is consuming and absorbing adequate nutrients enterally is imperative. This is usually assessed by diet histories and kcalorie counts. TPN should be decreased as the enteral intake and tolerance improves to avoid overfeeding. TPN may be discontinued once the patient is tolerating approximately 65 to 75% of goal nutrients. For patients who are eating, TPN may be reduced and stopped over a 24- to 48-hour period. If TPN is inadvertently but abruptly discontinued in patients who are not eating, all insulin should be stopped and blood glucose levels should be monitored for 30 minutes after discontinuation of TPN. Based upon the blood glucose levels, appropriate therapy should be implemented.[1] Lastly, if the TPN was used as a vehicle for medication or electrolyte administration, an alternate plan should be made once it is discontinued. Attempting to switch medications to the enteral route is usually employed. Consultation with a pharmacist can help facilitate this transition.

Complications of Parenteral Nutrition

Complications of parenteral nutrition have been widely reported. However, TPN can be safe with minimal complications when it is managed and monitored by a multidisciplinary team of trained professionals. The type of complications that may arise are diverse and include mechanical, infectious, and metabolic.

Mechanical complications of catheter insertion (Table 43.16) include pneumothorax, hydrothorax, and great vessel injury. The catheter malposition may result in venous thrombosis, causing head, neck, or arm swelling, or possibly a pulmonary emobolus. To minimize morbidity, obtaining a chest radiograph before using a new central line for TPN

TABLE 43.16

Mechanical Complications of Parenteral Nutrition

Complication	Possible Cause	Symptoms	Treatment	Prevention
Pneumothorax	Catheter placement by inexperienced personnel	Tachycardia, dyspnea, persistent cough, diaphoresis	Large pneumothorax may require chest tube placement	Experienced personnel to place catheter
Catheter embolization	Pulling catheter back through needle used for insertion	Cardiac arrhythmias	Surgical removal of catheter tip	Avoid withdrawing catheter through insertion needle
Air embolism	Air is inspired while line is interrupted and uncapped	Cyanosis, tachypnea, hypotension, churning heart murmur	Immediately place patient on left side and lower head of bed to keep air in apex of the right ventricle until it is reabsorbed	Experienced personnel to place catheter
Venous thrombosis	Mechanical trauma to vein, hypotension, hyperosmolar solution, hyper-coagulopathy, sepsis	Swelling or pain in one or both arms or shoulders or neck	Anticoagulation therapy with urokinase or streptokinase; catheter removal	Silicone catheter, adding heparin to TPN, low dose warfarin therapy
Catheter occlusion	Hypotension, failure to maintain line patency, formation of fibrin sheath outside the catheter, solution precipitates	Increasing need for greater pressure to maintain continuous infusion rate	Anticoagulation therapy with urokinase or streptokinase	Larger diameter catheter, routine catheter flushing, monitor solution for a precipitate
Phlebitis	Peripheral administration of hypertonic solution	Redness, swelling, pain at peripheral site	Change peripheral line site, begin central TPN if necessary	Maintain osmolarity of peripheral solution $\leq$ 900 mOsm/kg
Catheter-related sepsis	Inappropriate technique of line placement, poor catheter care, contaminated solution	Unexplained fever, chills, red, indurated area around catheter site	Remove catheter and replace at another site	Follow strict protocols for line placement and care

From Skipper, A. In: *Contemporary Nutrition Support Practice.* W.B. Saunders, Philadelphia, 1998: p. 227. With permission.

is important to ensure correct line placement and absence of internal injuries that may have occurred during insertion.

Catheter-related infections can carry a high mortality rate and increased medical costs for a single event. A catheter infection rate of less than 3% is desirable.[5] Appropriate use of aseptic technique by trained personnel is essential to maintain an acceptable catheter infection rate. Nursing protocols should be established for dressing changes and line manipulation. Dressings should be changed every 48 hours and should include local sterilizing ointment and an occlusive dressing. Since gram-positive catheter-related sepsis may be treated with antibiotics, removal of the catheter is not always necessary. Catheter removal is usually necessary with gram-negative organisms.

With close monitoring of TPN, avoidance of metabolic complications (Table 43.17) is possible. Refeeding syndrome may be defined as a constellation of fluid, micronutrient, electrolyte, and vitamin imbalances that occur within the first few days after refeeding a starved patient. Refeeding syndrome may involve hemolytic anemia, respiratory distress, paresthesias, tetany, and cardiac arrythmias.[59] Typical biochemical findings include hypokalemia, hypophosphatemia, and hypomagnesemia. Proposed risk factors for refeeding include alcoholism, anorexia nervosa, marasmus, rapid refeeding, and excessive dextrose infusion. In order to prevent the syndrome from occurring it is suggested to replete serum potassium, phosphorus, and magnesium concentrations prior to beginning TPN; limit initial carbohydrate to 150 gm/day, fluid to 800 mL, and sodium intake to no more than 20 mEq/day in at-risk patients; include adequate amounts of potassium, magnesium, phosphorus, and vitamins in the TPN solution; and increase carbohydrate-dependent minerals in proportion to increases in carbohydrate when TPN is advanced.[59]

Hyperglycemia (nonfasting blood glucose >220 mg/dL) is a common metabolic complication of TPN. Risk factors include metabolic stress, medications, obesity, diabetes, and excess dextrose administration. Careful glucose monitoring, especially in the first few days of TPN administration, can help guide advancement of dextrose to goal. Administration of dextrose in amounts less than the maximum glucose oxidation rate (4 to 7 mg/kg/min) and initiating dextrose in reduced amounts (100 to 150 gm/day) in at-risk patients may help minimize the occurrence of hyperglycemia.[5]

Patients receiving TPN may also experience fluid and electrolyte abnormalities (Table 43.17). The etiology of the abnormalities may be related to several factors including the patient's medical condition and treatment, medications, or excessive or inadequate free water provision. Fluid balance and electrolyte status should be monitored closely (Table 43.18), with corrections in abnormalities made accordingly.

Summary

Parenteral nutrition has been a major medical advancement over the past several decades. Its institution has saved lives of many people who may have otherwise died of malnutrition. The next several decades will most likely bring more advances in the technology and science of parenteral nutrition. With careful selection, implementation, and monitoring, parenteral nutrition is a medical vehicle for nutritional supplementation of numerous diseases.

TABLE 43.17

Metabolic Complications of Parenteral Nutrition

Complication	Possible Cause	Treatment
Hypovolemia	Inadequate fluid provision, overdiuresis	Increase fluid delivery
Hypervolemia	Excess fluid delivery, renal dysfunction, congestive heart failure, hepatic failure	Fluid restriction, diruetics, dialysis
Hypokalemia	Refeeding syndrome, inadequate potassium provision, increased losses	Increase intravenous or parenteral potassium
Hyperkalemia	Renal dysfuntion, too much potassium provision, metabolic acidosis, potassium-sparing drugs	Decrease potassium intake, potassium binders, dialysis in extreme cases
Hyponatremia	Excessive fluid provision, nephritis, adrenal insufficiency, dilutional states	Restrict fluid intake, increase sodium intake as indicated clinically
Hypernatremia	Inadequate free water provision, excessive sodium intake, excessive water losses	Decrease sodium intake, replete free water deficit
Hypoglycemia	Abrupt discontinuation of parenteral nutrition, insulin overdose	Dextrose delivery
Hyperglycemia	Rapid infusion of large dextrose load, sepsis, pancreatitis, steroids, diabetes, elderly	Insulin, reduce dextrose delivery
Hypertriglyceridemia	Inability to clear lipid provision, sepsis, multisystem organ failure, medications altering fat absorption, history of hyperlipidemia	Decrease lipid volume provided, increase infusion time, hold lipids up to 14 days to normalize level
Hypocalcemia	Decrease vitamin D intake, hypoparathyroidism, citrate binding of calcium due to excessive blood transfusion, hypoalbuminemia	Calcium supplementation
Hypercalcemia	Renal failure, tumor lysis syndrome, bone cancer, excess vitamin D delivery, prolonged immobilization, stress hyperparathyroidism	Isotonic saline, inorganic phosphate supplementation, corticosteroids, mithramycin
Hypomagnesemia	Refeeding syndrome, alcoholism, diruetic use, increased losses, medications, diabetic ketoacidosis, chemotherapy	Magnesium supplementation
Hypermagnesemia	Excessive magnesium provision, renal insufficiency	Decrease magnesium provision
Hypophosphatemia	Refeeding syndrome, alcoholism, phophate-binding antacids, dextrose infusion, overfeeding, secondary hyperparathyroidism, insulin therapy	Phosphate supplementation, discontinue phosphate-binding antacids, avoid overfeeding, initiate dextrose delivery cautiously
Hyperphosphatemia	Renal dysfunction, excessive provision	Decrease phosphate delivery, phosphate binders
Prerenal azotemia	Dehydration, excessive protein provision, inadequate nonprotein calorie provision with mobilization of own protein stores	Increase fluid intake, decrease protein delivery, increase non-protein calories
Essential fatty acid deficiency	Inadequate polyunsaturated long-chain fatty acid provision	Lipid administration

From Skipper, A. In: *Contemporary Nutrition Support Practice.* W.B. Saunders, Philadelphia, 1998: p. 227. With permission.

TABLE 43.18

Suggested Monitoring of TPN

Parameter	Baseline Level	Acute Patients	Stable Patients
Electrolytes, BUN, Cr	Yes	Daily	1-2 × week
Chemistry Panel Ca^{2+}, PO^{4-}, Mg^{2+}	Yes	Daily until stable, then 2-3 × week	Weekly
LFTs	Yes	2 × week	Weekly-monthly
Triacylglycerol	Yes	Weekly unless abnormal then 2 × week	Weekly-monthly
Capillary glucose	2-3 × day	3 × day until consistently < 200 mg/dl	2 × day until consistently < 200 mg/dl
Intake and output	Yes	Daily	Daily or by physical exam
Weight	If available	Daily	Monthly
CBC with differential	Yes	Weekly	Weekly
PT, PTT	Yes	Weekly	Weekly

BUN: blood urea nitrogen; PT: prothrombin time;
PTT: partial thromboplastin time; CBC: complete blood count;
LFT: liver function test; Cr: creatinine

References

1. Skipper A In: *Contemporary Nutrition Support Practice.* WB Saunders, Philadelphia, 1998: p. 227.
2. Rhoads JE, Dudrick SJ. In: *Clinical Nutrition: Parenteral Nutrition.* WB Saunders, Philadelphia, 1993, p. 1.
3. Meyer CE, Fancher JA, Schurr PE, Webster HD. *Metabolism* 6: 591; 1957.
4. Wilmore DW, Dudrick SJ. *JAMA* 203: 860; 1968.
5. ASPEN Board of Directors. *J Parent Enteral Nutr* 17(4): 1S; 1993.
6. American College of Physicians. *Ann Intern Med* 107: 252; 1987.
7. Sitzman JV, Pitt HA. *Dig Dis Sci* 34: 489; 1989.
8. Pillar B, Perry S. *Nutrition* 6: 314; 1990.
9. Levine GN, Derin JJ, Steiger E, Zinno R. *Gastroenterology* 67: 975; 1974.
10. Deitch EA. *Arch Surg* 124: 699; 1989.
11. Kotani J, Usami M, Nomura H, et al. *Arch Surg* 134: 287; 1999.
12. Li J, Kudsk D, Gocinski B, et al. *J Trauma* 39: 44; 1995.
13. King BK, Li J, Kudsk KA. *Arch Surg* 132:1303; 1997.
14. DaZhong X, Lu Q, Deitch E. *J Parent Enteral Nutr* 22: 37; 1998.
15. King B, Kudsk K, Li J, et al. *Ann Surg* 229: 272; 1999.
16. Lipman T. *J Parent Enteral Nutr* 22: 167; 1998.
17. Heyland D, MacDonald S, Keefe L, Drover J. *JAMA* 280: 2013; 1998.
18. Vernet O, Christin L, Schultz Y, et al. *Am J Physiol* 250: E47; 1986.
19. Moore FA, Feliciano DV, Andrassy RJ, et al. *Ann Surg* 216: 172; 1992.
20. Tappy L, Schwarz J, Schneiter P, Cayeux C, et al. *Crit Care Med* 26: 860; 1998.
21. Moore FA, Moore EE, Jones TN, et al. *J Trauma* 29: 916; 1989.
22. Kudsk K, Croce M, Fabian T, et al. *Ann Surg* 215: 503; 1992.
23. Trice S, Melnik G, Page C. *Nutr Clin Prac* 12: 114; 1997.
24. Evans M. *Nutr Clin Prac* 14: 172; 1999.
25. Krzywda EA, Edmiston CE. *ASPEN Practice Manual,* 1998.
26. Dickerson R, Brown R, Whithe, K. In: *Clinical Nutrition: Parenteral Nutrition.* WB Saunders, Philadelphia, 1993: p. 310.
27. Freeman JB, Fairfull-Smith R, Rodman G, et al. *Surgery* 156: 625; 1983.
28. Abbott WC, Grakauskas AM, Bistrian BR, et al. *Arch Surg* 119: 1367; 1984.
29. Seidner DL, Mascioli EA, Istfan NW, et al. *J Parent Enteral Nutr* 13: 614; 1989.

30. Jensen GL, Mascioli EA, Deidner DL, et al. *J Parent Enteral Nutr* 14: 467; 1990.
31. Cerra FB, Cheung NK, Fischer JE, et al. *J Parent Enteral Nutr* 9: 288; 1985.
32. Mirtallo JM, Schneider PJ, Mavko K, et al. *J Parent Enteral Nutr* 6: 109; 1982.
33. Feinstein EL, Blumenkrantz MJ, Healy M, et al. *Medicine* 60: 124; 1981.
34. Chiolero R, Revelly J, Tappy L. *Nutrition* 13: 45S; 1997.
35. Cerra FB, Shronts EP, Konstantinides NN, et al. *Surgery* 98: 632; 1985.
36. Cerra FB, Mazuski JE, Chute E, et al. *Ann Surg* 199: 286; 1984.
37. Bower RH, Muggia-Sullum M, Vallgren S, et al. *Ann Surg* 203: 13; 1986.
38. Yu YM, Wagner DA, Walesrewski JC, et al. *Ann Surg* 207: 421; 1988.
39. Freund H, Hoover HC, Atamian S, et al. *Ann Surg* 190: 18; 1979.
40. von Meyenfeldt MF, Soeters PB, Vente JP, et al. *Br J Surg* 77: 924; 1990.
41. Recommended Dietary Allowances, 10th ed, Washington, DC: National Academy Press, 1989, pg 3.
42. Stover J (Ed). *A Clinical Guide to Nutrition Care in End Stage Renal Disease.* Chicago: American Dietetic Association, 1994, pg 28, 43.
43. Shronts E, Fish J. In: *Nutrition Support Dietetics: Core Curriculum,* 2nd ed. Gottschlich M, Matarese L, Shronts E, Eds, ASPEN, Silver Spring, MD, 1993, pg 311.
44. Lumpkin MM, Burlington DB. FDA safety alert: Hazards of precipitation associated with parenteral nutrition. Rockville, MD: U.S. Food and Drug Administration, 1994.
45. Dunham B, Marcuard S, Khazanie PG, et al. *J Parent Enteral Nutr* 15: 608; 1991.
46. American Medical Association Department of Foods and Nutrition. *J Parent Enteral Nutr* 3: 258, 1979.
47. Guidelines for essential trace element preparations for parenteral use: A statement by the Nutrition Advisory Group. *J Parent Enteral Nutr* 3: 263; 1979.
48. Forceville X, Vitoux D, Gauzit R, et al. *Crit Care Med* 26: 1536; 1998.
49. Weber SS, Wood WA, Jackson EA. *Am J Hosp Pharm* 34: 353; 1977.
50. Macuard SP, Dunham B, Hobbs A, Caro JF. *J Parent Enteral Nutr* 14: 262; 1990.
51. Hirsch JJ, Wood JH, Thomas RB. *Am J Hosp Pharm* 38: 995;1981.
52. Bullock L, Fitzgerald JF, Glick MR, et al. *Am J Hosp Pharm* 46: 2321; 1989.
53. Montov JB, Pou L, Salvador P, et al. *Am J Hosp Pharm* 46: 2329; 1989.
54. Williams MF, Hak LJ, Dukes G. *Am J Hosp Pharm* 47: 1547; 1990.
55. Cano SM, Montoro JB, Pastor C, et al. *Am J Hosp Pharm* 45: 1100; 1989.
56. Moore RA, Feldman S, Trenting J, et al. *J Parent Enteral Nutr* 5: 61; 1981.
57. Strausburg K. Parenteral nutrition admixture. *ASPEN Practice Manual,* 1998.
58. Miller DG. *Am J Clin Nutr* 46: 419; 1987.
59. Skipper A, Willikan KW. Parenteral nutrition implementation and management. *ASPEN Practice Manual,* 1998.

44

Sports — Elite Athletes

Michael F. Bergeron

Good nutrition is crucial in any athlete's quest to reach peak performance. At all levels of competition, whether for a local recreational league championship or in preparation for the Olympics, athletes seem to be constantly searching for ways to improve their performance and gain a competitive edge. This often includes trying the latest dietary fad or nutritional supplements. However, dietary strategies for training and competition should address the athlete's need for nutrients as influenced by age, fitness, level of competition and intensity of training, environment, time of competition, duration of play, amount of time between competitions, and type of activity. Moreover, an effective diet for the athlete also includes the same general dietary recommendations as for the non-athlete, and these are intended to promote good health.

Although a healthy diet and body can clearly contribute to better performance, this section will not focus on general nutrition guidelines to eating for good health; this is comprehensively addressed in other sections. This section will review several basic nutrition principles and other current nutrition issues as they relate to athletic performance. The following recommendations are based on established results from research in adults competing in certain sports or participating in exercise activities. While there has been extensive research on nutrition and exercise performance in adults, such studies on children and adolescents are lacking.

Much of the following information and guidelines related to preparing for competition, competition, and recovery are also generally appropriate for training and practice sessions. The unique metabolic demand characteristics and environmental circumstances associated with the myriad activities classified as sports makes it nearly impossible to address all athletes' nutritional concerns for achieving peak performance. Individual preferences also play a role. Therefore, this section focuses on selected general nutritional aspects that are applicable for a variety of athletes, especially those who engage in long-duration, endurance-based events.

A Balanced Diet

The primary dietary concern for all athletes should be to generally avoid the known nutritional risk factors associated with health problems and to follow nutritional guidelines that will help promote good health. A diet that provides excess or deficient energy,

0-8493-2705-9/01/$0.00+$1.50

saturated fat, or alcohol or chronic vitamin and/or mineral deficiencies or excesses should be avoided by anyone interested in good health or good athletic performance. A good diet is one that supports normal growth and development, regulates metabolism, maintains normal menstrual status, and provides adequate energy during training and competition. By following any of the various scientifically based food guides, such as the United States Food Guide Pyramid,[1] athletes, coaches, and parents can achieve appropriate variety, proportions, and balance in their daily dietary planning such that an adequate regular intake of all the essential nutrients is not left to chance.

Carbohydrates

Bread, cereal, rice, pasta, fruits, and vegetables are all good primary sources of carbohydrate that should be regularly included in any athlete's diet. Sport drinks and sport bars are also effective in helping to meet the athlete's carbohydrate needs. It is generally recommended that 55 to 70% of an athlete's daily energy comes from carbohydrates. However, this recommendation may not always be appropriate or practical, particularly if the daily total energy requirement is very high. A better guideline for the athlete in training or during competition would be to ingest at least 7 grams of carbohydrate per kilogram of body weight each day, and up to 10 grams of carbohydrate per kilogram if daily training or competition is intense and lasts for several hours or more.[2,3] This is equivalent to at least 490 grams (or 1960 kcalories) from carbohydrates for a 70-kg person, and would represent roughly 65% of a 3000-calorie daily diet. This relative amount should provide enough dietary carbohydrate to adequately replenish muscle and liver glycogen each day under most circumstances.

Before they are absorbed into the blood, dietary carbohydrates are reduced by digestion to single sugar units (the monosaccharides: glucose, fructose, and galactose). Glucose is the body's primary fuel for energy. Fructose (the very sweet sugar of fruit which is also found in soft drinks and some sport drinks) and galactose (part of lactose or milk sugar) are converted to glucose prior to use as an energy source. Foods that elicit a large and rapid rise in blood glucose are categorized as having a high glycemic index.[4] These foods (Table 44.1) provide a rapid and readily utilizable energy source.[5] Other carbohydrate-rich foods provide glucose at a slower rate due to differences in rates of digestion, absorption, and metabolism. Fructose, for example, is not actively absorbed by the intestine but is absorbed via the less efficient facilitated diffusion. Consumption of large quantities of fructose may slow down fluid absorption and cause a feeling of gastrointestinal distress, particularly during exercise.[6]

Fats

The general recommendation for dietary fat intake is 20 to 30% of total daily energy intake.[7] Further, saturated fats should account for less than 10% of each day's energy supply. Not only is fat needed for many biological functions, fat (as fatty acids) can be an effective metabolic fuel for working trained muscle. Hence, fat provides considerable energy during many sport activities.[2,8,9] Fortunately, most athletes have enough body fat to support their

TABLE 44.1

Glycemic Index (Number in Parentheses) of a Variety of Foods. The index was calculated using glucose as the reference. Average serving size is used; data are from Foster-Powel, K., and Brand Miller, J., *Am. J. Clin. Nutr.* 62: 871S; 1995.

High	Medium	Low
Glucose (100)	Banana (53)	Fructose(23)
Sucrose (65)	Orange juice (57)	Apple, raw (36)
Honey (73)	Potato chips (54)	Soy beans (18)
Bagel (white flour) (72)	White rice (56)	Lentils (29)
Ready-to-eat cereal (70-90)	Spaghetti, white (41)	Peach, raw (28)
Carrots (71)	Bread, mixed grain (45)	Ice Cream, rich (27)
Graham crackers (74)		Skim milk (32)
Potatoes (83)		Yogurt (33)
Raisins (64)		
Jelly beans (80)		
White bread (70)		
Sport drinks, high glucose (70)		

performance energy requirement for fat, and fat intake during or just prior to exercise is not necessary or appropriate.

Some athletes regularly exceed the recommendations for daily fat intake. This may be for convenience or preference, but, for those involved with extensive competition or training that carries a recurring high energy demand, it is often a practical means to help maintain body weight. This practice is fairly common[10-13] among many athletes and has been promoted as being beneficial.[14] As long as the daily energy need is met the athlete is not in chronic positive energy balance, then from a performance point of view, this periodic use of a high-fat diet is appropriate. From a long-term health perspective, the risks associated with such a diet with fit, very active athletes have not yet been studied. Presumably, however, excessive fat intake might adversely affect certain diet-related risk factors for coronary heart disease, even in a fit population.[9,15,16]

Protein

The need for extra protein in an athlete's diet has been a topic of considerable debate. The general recommendation for daily protein intake has been 0.8 grams of high quality protein per kilogram of body weight (about 10 to 15% of daily energy intake).[7] However, a growing body of research[17-20] suggests that many athletes may need more protein than non-athletes.

During and immediately after strenuous exercise, there is an increase in protein breakdown. This is followed by an increase in protein synthesis during the recovery period. This suggests that more dietary protein is needed to maintain body protein mass and/or to support increases in muscle size and muscle energy-producing components. Current thought[17-20] for endurance athletes suggests an intake of 1.2 to 1.8 grams of protein per kilogram of body weight per day. Given the strong endurance component and physiological demands of many competitive sports, athletes involved in extensive regular training and competition may require this much protein each day to maintain protein balance. Body builders and power lifters, for example, could require up to 2.0 grams of protein per kilogram of body weight each day. Such an increase in dietary protein is likely already met by the typical diets that athletes usually consume. Unless an athlete is inappropriately restricting energy, protein supplements are generally not needed — particularly not to the extent that many resistance training athletes ingest regularly.[20-22] There are instances such as when traveling to competition events (especially abroad, where the foods available may be unacceptable to the athlete) and when the travel/competition time is extensive, that sufficient nutrient intake may be challenged or in question. Here, a protein-fortified drink or an energy bar can be a convenient and effective food source to augment the athlete's diet.

Carbohydrate and Fat: Primary Energy Sources

Many factors contribute to the energy expenditure of an athlete during competition or during training. Modestly, 600 to 800 kcalories per hour would not be difficult for many adults to achieve while engaging in sports such as basketball or tennis — and this could readily be much higher with activities such as long distance running or marathon swimming. In fact, large, well-trained athletes might expend up to 10,000 kcal in a single day if the intensity and duration of activity is high.[23]

During continuous endurance activities and other long-duration sports, the metabolic emphasis shifts to utilizing more carbohydrate and proportionately less fat, as the intensity of exercise and overall energy expenditure increase.[2,3] This is necessary because carbohydrate can supply energy for muscle contraction at a much faster rate than fat. However, the intermittent nature of many sports reduces the duration of a continuous high demand for energy within any specific muscle group during and between play. Consequently, even during intense activities such as singles tennis or basketball, fat is used to supply considerable energy throughout the course of the match or game.[24]

Importantly, using fat for energy still requires a continual simultaneous breakdown of glucose. Therefore all athletes, regardless of the intensity of activity, will eventually feel the effects of depleting glycogen stores if the event is long and carbohydrate is not consumed during the activity. Carbohydrate sufficiency can be further challenged in hot environments. As the temperature goes up, the rate of carbohydrate usage can also increase;[27] thus, fatigue can occur more rapidly without regular and adequate carbohydrate intake.

During the latter part of competition, protein could become a more significant contributor in meeting an athlete's energy demands, especially if the pre-event and during-competition dietary carbohydrate intake is inadequate.[20,28] There are ways to reduce potential protein utilization for energy through ensuring sufficient carbohydrate intake and availability. Protein breakdown produces amino acids that in turn are deaminated and used for energy. This, however, puts an additional burden on the body, because the amino group must be converted to urea and excreted.

Effects of Endurance Training on Carbohydrate, Fat, and Protein Utilization

As previously noted, many competitive sports have a significant endurance component. Regularly participating in these sports or other endurance-enhancing exercise or activities (such as bicycling or running) will cause many specific changes in an athlete's body that will positively affect performance.[29,30] A comprehensive discussion of these enhancements is beyond the scope of this section. However, several adaptations relating to the use of nutrients for energy during competition are worth noting.

As a result of regular endurance training and the associated increase in muscle mitochondrial number and activity, there will be an increase in the muscle enzymes that are used for glucose oxidation as well as for glucose conversion to glycogen and for glycogenolysis.[31,32] This, along with other changes that improve the delivery and use of oxygen in the muscles (e.g. an increase in capillary density), permits a more efficient use of carbohydrate for energy.[2] With endurance training there is also an increase in fatty acid uptake and oxidation by the muscle fibers, due to the training-induced increase in mitochondrial number and an induction of the enzymes involved in this process. These are important considerations for an athlete who consequently might not have to rely on blood glucose as much and deplete glycogen stores as readily as a lesser-trained individual — again, fatigue could be delayed, even during high-intensity competition. At the same time, these changes could indirectly defer an undesirable increased reliance on protein for energy as carbohydrate stores are diminished.[28] Some research[34] shows that training results in an enhanced ability and tendency to use protein for energy during exercise. This could supplement the use of glucose and fatty acids as metabolic fuel, and potentially delay fatigue.

Precompetition Nutrition

The nutritional state of the athlete before competition can have a significant impact on performance.[25,35] Many precompetition nutritional strategies are designed to ensure adequate hydration. Appropriate fat, protein, mineral, and vitamin intake are also important, but, because of the metabolic nature of most sports, the other primary precompetition nutritional concern for athletes is adequate carbohydrate intake. How to ensure that carbohydrate stores are maximized prior to competition is the focus of this section.

Ideally, before competition begins, an athlete's carbohydrate stores (muscle and liver glycogen) should be full. The emphasis on precompetition dietary carbohydrates ought to begin at least by the previous evening. The evening meal is typically when the majority of daily energy intake occurs. Moreover, a progressive increase over several days in carbohydrate intake and a concomitant decrease in training duration and intensity just before the start of an event can optimize an athlete's glycogen stores prior to competition.[2]

The immediate precompetition meal is often more of a challenge. Here, the goal is to eat a well-balanced meal with an emphasis on carbohydrate-rich foods and fluids. The recommended energy intake depends, in part, on the competition schedule. In general, the meal size should be moderate. By the time competition begins, the athlete's stomach should be relatively empty, but without feelings of hunger. Prior to competition (three to four hours) a variety of nutritious, easily digestible, nondistress-causing (e.g., low fiber) solid foods can be consumed.[2,36] Based on a person's body weight, a general guideline is to consume approximately 4 to 5 grams of carbohydrate per kilogram of body weight with this meal. This means that a 70-kilogram athlete could consume 280 to 350 grams of carbohydrate. This meal should be low in fat and protein, since too much of either could reduce gastric emptying time. Various fluids (e.g., water, juice, milk, and sport drinks) can be consumed with the precompetition meal, so long as alcohol and excessive caffeine are avoided.

The precompetition meal depends on the time of the competition within the context of the athlete's usual meal pattern. Whatever meal or combination it is, the athlete should not completely skip other regularly scheduled meals. For example, if a game, match, or race is to begin in the early or middle afternoon, a good-sized early breakfast (emphasizing carbohydrates) should be eaten, followed by a smaller precompetition lunch during the late morning or midday. Alternatively, if the competition begins 3 to 4 hours after a precompetition breakfast or lunch, the athlete should eat an additional small (1 to 1.5 grams of carbohydrate per kilogram of body weight), easily digestible carbohydrate snack about 1 to 1.5 hours prior to the start of the event.[2,36] A combination such as 500 ml of a sport drink along with a sport bar or other solid carbohydrate food works well to "top off" carbohydrate stores and body water.

A common problem encountered at some events arises when an early morning competition is scheduled — say, for 8 or 9 a.m. Athletes, parents, and coaches often wonder how to manage breakfast. In this case, it's usually best to have a smaller-than-usual breakfast, again with an emphasis on carbohydrates and easily digestible foods, at least 90 minutes before competition begins. Commercial high-carbohydrate, low-fat liquid meals work well here, because they have less bulk and are easily digested and absorbed. Then, during competition, it will be important to consume a carbohydrate-electrolyte drink throughout, because the body's stored carbohydrate levels will be initially somewhat lower at the outset, and the supplemental carbohydrate will likely have a more readily prominent role in providing energy and deferring hunger.[25]

Whether because of scheduling, preference, or precompetition anxiety, many athletes simply do not consume enough energy before they compete. Inadequate precompetition energy intake and perhaps partially depleted carbohydrate stores can result in premature fatigue.[36]

Another common mistake is to neglect regular fluid and carbohydrate intake during the precompetition warmup session. Such an oversight, especially if it is compounded by a warmup that is too long and consists of excessive exercise, might increase the likelihood that the athlete will begin competition unnecessarily fatigued, dehydrated, and carbohydrate-depleted. Thus, it is important that appropriate rates of fluid and carbohydrate intake be followed during the precompetition warmup as well as during competition. If carbohydrate is not consumed during the warmup period, a small carbohydrate snack after warmup could be sufficient; its content and size depends on how much time is available before competition begins.

Nutrition during Competition

Carbohydrate and fat are the primary energy sources used during sport participation and training activities.[2] Yet, because an athlete's body fat supply is not going to run out in the course of competition, carbohydrate and water are the only principal nutrients that need to be consumed while competing (aside from multi-day or ultra-endurance events).[2,25,37-39] In some situations, salt intake during competition has a more significant role in maintaining fluid balance, but generally it is not a major dietary concern for most athletes while they compete.

Even if an athlete eats well prior to competition, after 60 to 90 minutes of intense exercise, liver and muscle glycogen stores will likely be significantly decreased.[2] Further, the ability to maintain blood glucose and meet the muscles' demand for energy may be seriously challenged. Lack of carbohydrate can be prevented by periodically ingesting carbohydrate during the activity.[25] The amount of supplemental carbohydrate depends on factors such as precompetition dietary status, body weight, environment, and intensity of exercise or play. The body can generally utilize up to 60 grams per hour.[36] This can be provided by a liter of a carbohydrate-electrolyte drink.[25] A number of commercial sport drinks are designed to rapidly deliver carbohydrate and water to maximize performance. Carbohydrate-electrolyte sport drinks can provide energy in the form of carbohydrate. These have been shown to delay the onset of fatigue and perception of effort, increase voluntary fluid intake, and provide electrolytes which help to maintain mineral and fluid balance.[2,25,36,39-42] Moreover, some carbohydrate-electrolyte drinks may be absorbed a little faster than water. Any of these factors can be an important contributor to maintaining performance, especially when competing in a hot environment. In fact, supplemental energy intake may be more readily beneficial during competition in the heat, since glycogen utilization tends to occur more rapidly as body temperature rises.[27] Furthermore, the positive performance effects of carbohydrate and water ingestion during long-term exercise are additive.[43] In other words, appropriate carbohydrate and water consumption (e.g., as a sport drink) during exercise is better than carbohydrate or water consumption alone. Those sport drinks designed for consumption during exercise have a carbohydrate concentration of 5 to 8%. Each liter contains 50 to 80 grams of carbohydrate. Research shows that higher carbohydrate concentrations (i.e., >10%) delay emptying of the stomach, which in turn delays water and carbohydrate from getting into the bloodstream.[40,42]

During the first hour or so of exercise, liver and muscle glycogen often support most of the body's demand for glucose.[2] Thus, from a standpoint of providing energy, the supplemental carbohydrate from a sport drink may not have much of an effect on performance, especially if an athlete's carbohydrate stores are fully replenished at the start of competition. However, it may still be best to drink a carbohydrate-electrolyte drink (perhaps at a diluted concentration at first) from the onset of exercise, even though glycogen stores may not be low. This will help to maintain blood glucose levels and may enhance fluid absorption.[36,39] Moreover, ingesting carbohydrate throughout the early stages of competition might have a sparing effect on some of the body's carbohydrate stores.[36]

Often, athletes drink more than one liter during each hour of exercise in an attempt to offset very high rates of fluid loss from sweating. Exclusive use of a sport drink (even if the carbohydrate content is in the 5 to 8% range) in these situations might not be well tolerated (and may be detrimental) because of the overall excessive amount of carbohydrate that would be ingested. As an alternative, many athletes drink a sport drink and plain water during competition. This combination permits the desired amount of fluid replenishment without taking in too much carbohydrate. At first, the emphasis can be on water consumption. As the competition continues, the athlete can make a progressive transition toward consuming more carbohydrate when he rehydrates.[38] Similarly, eating too large a snack (such as fruit or a sport bar) during competition, while regularly drinking a sport drink at the same time, might also delay stomach emptying and fluid delivery, again, because of the excessive carbohydrate intake. Ingesting a high amount of fructose (liquid or solid) could also cause gastrointestinal distress, since fructose is absorbed more slowly from the intestine compared to other carbohydrates in sport drinks, such as glucose, sucrose, or glucose polymers.[25] However, a small, easily digestible, high-glycemic index snack (e.g., crackers, raisins, jelly beans, etc.) may provide additional needed energy late in the activity.

Postexercise Nutrition

After exercise, an athlete's primary nutritional interest should be the restoration of lost fluid, electrolytes, and carbohydrate.[36,37,39,44] How immediate and aggressive this effort needs to be depends on how much carbohydrate was used (roughly suggested by how intense and long the activity was), how much sweat was lost, and, most importantly, when the next competitive activity will begin.

Sometimes, with sports such as tennis, an athlete must compete more than once on a given day. If the next activity is scheduled to begin shortly after the completion of the first (e.g., within 1 to 2 hours), rehydration and carbohydrate intake (about 50 to 100 grams or 1 to 1.5 grams of carbohydrate per kilogram of body weight) should begin immediately (i.e., within 15 minutes of the end of the match).[2,36] High-carbohydrate sport drinks, along with sport bars, gels, and other carbohydrate-rich foods with a high glycemic index (e.g., bagels, crackers, certain ready-to-eat cereals, white bread, and jelly beans), are good choices. These will facilitate the rapid restoration of muscle glycogen more than high-fructose foods or meals with an emphasis on low glycemic index carbohydrate sources (e.g., flavored yogurt, apples, oranges, pasta, and mixed-grain bread).[5] Notably, some research[45] suggests that a carbohydrate and protein combination might be better than just carbohydrate for rapid glycogen resynthesis. If convenience is a priority, certain commercial high-carbohydrate sport drinks and sport bars are available that could provide appropriate amounts of carbohydrate and protein for this purpose. Otherwise, various combinations of breads, cereals, and dairy products, for example, can provide similar ratios of carbohydrate and protein. During the next activity, regular consumption of carbohydrate may be necessary at an earlier stage to maintain blood glucose, provide energy, and defer hunger, since the short between-activity recovery period may not have been long enough to adequately replenish liver and muscle carbohydrate stores.

When preparing for a second competitive activity that begins four to five hours or more after the completion of the first, athletes should generally follow the precompetition meal guidelines described earlier; however, many athletes would rather not eat a large meal between same-day events, even if there is plenty of time. Thus, if smaller quantities of food are preferred, 50 to 100 grams of carbohydrate, for example, ingested immediately after exercise, and again every two hours, can be an effective method for replenishing (at least partially) one's carbohydrate stores. Having more time to accomplish this task means that an athlete can choose from a wider variety of foods (low, medium, and high glycemic index). However, it is generally a good idea to consume some rapidly absorbed carbohydrates and fluid (i.e., high glycemic index) right after exercise, so that glycogen and hydration status will be more promptly and completely restored for the next activity.[5,39]

If an athlete is not scheduled to compete again until the next day or later, appropriate regularly scheduled meals and snacks (according to the above guidelines) should provide enough of the necessary nutrients to nutritionally recover from the previous exercise and adequately prepare for the next competition.

Nutrition and Fatigue

From a nutritional standpoint, fatigue during sports and exercise occurs when there is an inadequate supply of carbohydrate and/or a diminished ability to use all available sources (i.e., carbohydrate, fat, and protein) to produce energy at a fast enough rate to meet the body's muscular demands. At this point, the fatigued athlete can no longer continue competing at the desired level of intensity.

Following the initiation of exercise, an athlete's blood glucose level tends to increase in response to a variety of hormonal influences (i.e., cortisol and glucagon) designed to mobilize carbohydrate. Without supplemental carbohydrate intake during the rest of the exercise period, a continued high rate of glucose utilization in the muscles will eventually lead to a much greater reliance on blood glucose for energy, which will, in turn, quickly deplete liver glycogen stores. As exercise continues, blood glucose progressively decreases.[2,33,46] Pre-exercise carbohydrate status, of course, plays a role in how readily this occurs. However, with high-intensity competition and repeated long bouts of muscle activity combined with progressive dehydration, the active muscles' use of energy will be accelerated such that carbohydrate will be utilized at an even faster rate. Eventually, carbohydrate availability will be diminished to the point that performance will be severely hindered.[36,38] This is why regular carbohydrate and fluid intake during difficult and long sport and exercise activities is so important, especially in hot environmental conditions. Moreover, if carbohydrate is not consumed during an extended bout of exercise, there may be a significant increase in the conversion of protein to glucose in order to meet the continued demand for energy. This could lead to a lower concentration of the branched-chain amino acids (BCAA) in the blood, which could act as another contributory factor in an athlete's sense of fatigue (see Nutritional Ergogenic Aids in this section).[47,48]

Fluid Balance

When an athlete is involved with any vigorous physical exercise or sport activity, a considerable amount of heat is produced, which will cause body temperature to rise. And although athletes normally have several inherent means for dealing with this (e.g., convection or radiated heat loss), sweating is typically the most effective and utilized method for dissipating heat during exercise, especially in hot weather. However, long-term, extensive sweating can pose a significant fluid balance challenge for athletes.[49]

If fluid balance and thermoregulation are not effectively managed during competition and an athlete progressively dehydrates and becomes overheated, the athlete will fatigue prematurely and possibly lose the race, game, or match. More severely, heat exhaustion, heat cramps, or, at worst, heat stroke may ultimately ensue.[50]

In warm to hot conditions, most adult athletes will lose between 1 and 2.5 liters of sweat during each hour of intense competition or training.[37,39,51,52] Even more impressive, sweat rates over 3.5 liters per hour have been observed with some well-conditioned, world-class athletes competing in very hot and humid climates.[53] During extended competition or training sessions, it would therefore not be difficult for many athletes to lose 10 or more liters of fluid.

The degree to which one sweats depends on a number of factors, including the environmental heat stress (i.e., temperature, humidity, and solar radiation) and the intensity of exercise — as an athlete works harder, sweating rate increases to offset the progressive rise in core body temperature as a result of a higher metabolic rate.[49,54] Acclimatization is another factor. Athletes who have been training and playing in a hot climate for several weeks or more (and thus, are acclimatized to the heat) may sweat more compared to those who are not accustomed to such conditions. The same goes for cardiorespiratory fitness.

Such training can improve sweat gland function and increase plasma volume, which can help to maintain a higher sweating rate.[54] One must keep in mind that a higher sweating rate is a good adaptation, because it gives an athlete a thermoregulatory advantage, although, at the same time, more extensive sweating will be a greater challenge to offset with fluid intake, especially during competition.

Sweat is mostly water, but it also contains a number of other elements found in the blood, including a variety of minerals in varying concentrations. The major mineral ions found in sweat are sodium (Na^+) and chloride (Cl^-), although the concentration varies with a number of factors. For example, well-conditioned athletes who are fully acclimatized to the heat often have sweat sodium concentrations in the range of 5 to 30 mmol per liter (i.e., 115 to 690 mg of sodium per liter of sweat), whereas heat non-acclimatized athletes typically lose much more sodium through sweating (e.g., 40 to 100 mmol or 920 to 2300 mg per liter). Still, some athletes can have a relatively high concentration of sodium in their sweat, no matter how fit or heat acclimatized they are, which again suggests a strong genetic influence. Sweat sodium and chloride concentrations also vary with sweating rate. As sweating rate goes up, the concentration of these minerals in sweat usually increases as well.[55-57]

Without adequate salt replacement, the cumulative effect of such electrolyte losses can bring about a progressive sweat-induced sodium deficit after several days of playing or training in the heat. This can readily lead to incomplete rehydration, poorer performance, and heat-related muscle cramps,[58] and possibly put an athlete at a higher risk for developing heat exhaustion. In contrast, potassium (K^+) and magnesium (Mg^{2+}) sweat losses, for example, are typically much lower.[56] In fact, athletes will generally lose 3 to 10 times as much sodium as potassium during exercise. With regard to calcium and trace minerals such as iron and zinc, their concentrations in sweat are also very low; however, repeated extensive sweating can lead to a deficit of one or more of these elements.[59-61] Such deficits will not have a direct effect on fluid balance per se, but a chronic dietary deficiency of any one of these nutrients (i.e., not enough consumed to offset sweat and other excretory losses) can clearly have a negative impact on overall health and performance.

Unfortunately, it is also a challenge, and often impossible, to keep up with extensive sweating rates over the course of an entire race or match. Therefore, it is critical that athletes prepare and manage as best they can by following a predetermined and comprehensive hydration plan before, during, and after competition.

Heat-related muscle cramps (heat cramps) often occur during prolonged exercise when there have been previous extensive and repeated fluid and sodium losses. Such is often the case in a tennis tournament, for example, especially by the time a player reaches a later round. Drinking plenty of water helps, but to completely restore fluids, the salt lost through sweating must be replenished as well.[62,63] Importantly, any plan for increasing dietary salt intake should be individually designed and include appropriate and adequate fluid intake. For most people with normal blood pressure, however, a slightly excessive salt intake will not likely pose a health threat.[64]

If sufficient carbohydrates and electrolytes are provided by food, then water alone can serve as a primary or sole precompetition beverage. However, other fluids such as milk, juice, and sport drinks can be used as well, and their consumption should be encouraged as part of a well-balanced dietary plan. Alcohol and excessive tea, coffee, and other caffeine-containing beverages should be avoided, as they can accelerate fluid loss.[65,66] An athlete should be able to urinate, and the urine should be fairly clear or light-colored. This can be interpreted as a good indication of adequate precompetition hydration.[67] As previously stated, before competition begins an athlete's carbohydrate (i.e., glycogen) stores should be at or near capacity. Besides providing a readily available source of energy, muscle glycogen also has a fair amount of water stored with it. Thus, by replenishing carbohydrates (even partially), an athlete can improve hydration status as well.

Ideally, athletes should ingest, during competition, enough fluid, electrolytes, and carbohydrate to fully support all circulatory, metabolic, and thermoregulatory requirements, and to offset all fluid losses so that normal body water status (i.e., euhydration) is maintained. But even with relatively short periods of competition (e.g., less than 75 minutes), it is not unusual for some athletes to end up with a significant body water deficit (i.e., a net loss near or greater than 2% of their precompetition body weight).[51,56] In fact, because many athletes often begin competition or training dehydrated to some degree,[51,58] a post-exercise body water deficit may be even worse than is indicated solely by one's pre- and post-exercise body weight difference. Also, because thirst is not a rapidly responding indicator of body water loss, there may not be a sufficient stimulus to consume enough fluid in the exercise or post-exercise period.[68] For some athletes, there could be a fluid deficit of more than 1 liter before thirst is distinctly perceived. During exercise, sweating rates can readily exceed 1.5 liters per hour. Few athletes can comfortably consume this much fluid to replace such a loss. Moreover, it is likely that such a high rate of fluid intake would readily exceed maximal gastric emptying and intestinal absorption rates.[39,42]

After competition, athletes must rehydrate. Plain water alone will rehydrate an athlete to a point, but it also readily prompts increased urine production and potentially a premature elimination of the thirst drive.[63] Excessive water intake for several hours or more can lead to severe problems related to hyponatremia.[69,70] Unless adequate sodium and chloride are replaced, rehydration will remain incomplete. [62,63] Fluid ingestion after prolonged exercise needs to be greater than the volume of fluid that was lost via sweating, because during the rehydration process there is still an obligatory production of urine, whether or not rehydration is complete. [62] Athletes should also keep in mind that alcohol and caffeine can reduce the rate and amount of postexercise plasma volume restoration and net fluid retention.[62,71]

Nutritional Ergogenic Aids

Advocates of today's growing and seemingly endless selection of nutritional ergogenic (work-enhancing) aids promote these products with promises such as enhanced energy, increased strength, power, and lean body mass, more endurance, better performance, and faster recovery. Because many athletes are constantly in search of anything that will provide a competitive advantage, it's understandable why such claims can be so tantalizing. But do the products work? Are the latest supplements just what some athletes need to perform better? To date, very few nutritional ergogenic supplements have lived up to their claims. More importantly, some have been found to actually impede optimal performance. On the other hand, as a result of well-controlled experimental studies, certain products have shown some promise as being effective ergogenic aids. Too often, however, the purported benefits of new supplements are based on unsubstantiated claims or testimonials, poor research or research findings taken out of context, or simply misinformation. Several currently popular and well-studied nutritional ergogenic aids are discussed here, with particular mention of their appropriateness for most sports.

Creatine

Creatine monohydrate has become one of the most popular "performance-enhancing" nutritional supplements in use today, and for good reason. Supportive preliminary evidence associated with creatine supplementation includes increased one-repetition maximum performance (i.e., how much weight a person can lift one time, such as with a bench press or squat) and peak power, as well as enhanced rowing performance and repetitive sprint performance in experimental swimming, running, and cycling bouts of exercise. In addition, many studies have demonstrated increases in body weight.[72]

Does such laboratory data mean that creatine supplementation will enhance performance during sports? Will the same effects be shown with highly trained and conditioned athletes as have been demonstrated with moderately trained or untrained individuals? Is creatine supplementation appropriate for the physiological demands of many sports? Are the observed weight gains actual gains in muscle or mostly fluid retention? And what about the long-term effects and health risks associated with continued supplementation? The answers to these questions are not known at this point.

Creatine is a natural compound made by the body from two amino acids, arginine and glycine. It is also present in fish, meat, and other animal products. During very brief, explosive-type exercise, the muscles' capacity to adequately meet the high demand for energy is largely dependent on the availability of phosphocreatine (PC), a high-energy compound found in muscle. It has been thought that by increasing the amount of creatine in the muscles, more PC will be readily available to provide energy at a faster rate during very high-intensity exercise.

Reports of increased muscle creatine and PC levels, enhanced performance, and desirable changes in body composition have been inconsistent and remain somewhat equivocal. Regarding potential gains in muscle protein, proven and more effective ways exist to gain the necessary lean body mass required for most sports. And, importantly, the long-term consequences and health risks associated with continued creatine supplementation have not yet been comprehensively examined. Potential negative effects on the kidneys, heart, liver, fluid balance, and thermoregulatory capacity, for example, should be carefully studied. Lastly, given the specific loading patterns and metabolic demands on individual muscle groups during many types of sport activities, the muscle creatine and PC levels are probably (without supplementation) already more than adequate in most well-conditioned athletes. At present, creatine supplementation for most athletes does not appear to be justified.

A recent consensus statement written for the American College of Sports Medicine on oral creatine supplementation provides a comprehensive review of the current creatine literature as well as a critical evaluation of its potential health effects and clinical application.[72]

Medium-Chain Tryglycerides

To increase the availability and oxidation of fats during exercise in an attempt to spare carbohydrate and improve performance, several dietary fat supplements have been suggested for athletes.[9] From this category, medium-chain tryglycerides (MCTs) are one of the ergogenic aids used by athletes today because of the professed ability of MCTs to enhance energy levels, fat metabolism, and endurance.[73] Once ingested, MCTs leave the stomach and are absorbed from the intestine in much the same way as are other triglycerides.[48] Thus far, MCTs or other fat-loading techniques have not been shown to affect the rate of carbohydrate oxidation or improve performance. There have also been a number of reports of gastrointestinal complaints and problems associated with MCT ingestion.[48] Therefore, despite the need for fat in an athlete's diet and the important role of fat in providing energy during competition for many sports, fat loading prior to play or fat supplementation during competition are not currently validated or recommended procedures for most athletes.

Sodium Bicarbonate

During very high-intensity exercise, there is an increasing concentration of hydrogen ions (H^+) in the muscle cells as a result of a continuous rapid production of lactic acid. A high level of H^+ will rapidly lead to fatigue. Unless there is something to offset the growing concentration of H^+, there will soon be a decrease in muscle force output, a lower production of energy, and a resultant decrease in performance, even in the presence of adequate carbohydrate supplies. Fortunately, sodium bicarbonate, which is naturally present in the body, buffers a portion of the H^+ associated with the accumulating lactic acid during anaerobic exercise. This helps to delay fatigue. Would augmented sodium bicarbonate levels do a better job in delaying the onset of fatigue during high-intensity exercise by helping to buffer more lactic acid? Probably. Will ingested bicarbonate enhance an athlete's overall performance during all sports? Probably not.[74,75]

The intermittent nature and overall moderate intensity of many sports precludes the necessity for a great reliance on anaerobic carbohydrate metabolism during competition. Consequently, lactic acid production is seldom very high.[46] Thus, sodium bicarbonate supplementation would not be very helpful for such activities, since these athletes do not need to compensate for a large accumulation of H^+. It likely rarely occurs. On the other hand, certain sports that are characterized by high lactic acid production may be better tolerated with an enhanced capacity to neutralize the accompanying decrease in pH within the intracellular environment of the active muscles. Ingestion of buffering agents such as sodium bicarbonate may provide a performance advantage during these activities.[75]

Branched-Chain Amino Acids

When carbohydrate is in short supply, there is a greater reliance on protein for energy. This can lead to lower circulating levels of the branched-chain amino acids (BCAA); i.e., leucine, isoleucine, and valine. Moreover, during prolonged exercise, there is an increase in the concentration of free fatty acids in the blood, which leads to higher levels of free tryptophan (another amino acid). The resultant effect will be a higher free tryptophan:BCAA ratio. This is thought to be an important factor in the development of fatigue, especially during endurance activities. When free tryptophan enters the brain it is converted to serotonin; high amounts of this neurotransmitter may be associated with fatigue.[48,76] Many athletes could conceivably be susceptible to fatigue related to lowered

BCAA levels and increased free tryptophan, particularly during lengthy competitions.[47] Would BCAA supplementation help to alleviate this situation by maintaining higher levels of BCAA in the blood? As one might expect, some researchers have shown improved performance with BCAA supplementation, and others have demonstrated no change in performance.[48,76] Although BCAA might in theory be helpful in delaying the onset of fatigue during long periods of exercise or competition, especially if carbohydrate stores are significantly diminished, adequate carbohydrate intake prior to and during competition could achieve the same effect by reducing the amount of free fatty acids released and minimizing any potential increase in the free tryptophan:BCAA ratio. Furthermore, BCAA supplementation could lead to higher levels of ammonia in the blood, which would accelerate fatigue.[76]

Vitamins and Minerals

Vitamin and mineral supplements are widely used by athletes, often in great excess, not only to maintain health, but also with the hope that performance will be enhanced as well.[77] Likewise, selected mineral supplementation such as increased chromium, vanadium, and boron intake has been purported to increase muscle mass, despite a lack of research evidence.[21]

B-complex vitamin supplements are particularly popular, likely because of their important role as coenzymes in helping carbohydrate and fat to be used for energy. Logically, it seems that B-complex supplementation would be, in theory, helpful in enhancing the utilization of these nutrients during many sports and exercise activities. However, despite the essential role of these and other vitamins in a variety of physiological processes, including energy metabolism, unless an athlete has a vitamin deficiency, vitamin supplementation will not enhance athletic performance. In fact, excessive intake of the fat-soluble vitamins (A, D, E, and K) can have a toxic effect. Although extra water-soluble vitamin (B-complex and C) intake will mostly end up being excreted in urine, excessive intake of these vitamins can have toxic effects as well. Additional vitamin C and E intake, however, might be worth considering. Both of these vitamins have been shown to have beneficial antioxidant and other health-related properties. Moreover, there is evidence that athletes may need more vitamin C compared to those who do not exercise regularly, and additional vitamin E intake may reduce exercise-related muscle tissue damage.[77]

Minerals are necessary for growth, metabolism, and a variety of other physiological processes. Like vitamins, an athlete's mineral requirements generally can be easily met by a well-balanced diet, although certain minerals may need special attention with some people. These typically include calcium and iron, and sometimes zinc. In addition, excessive and repeated sweating may cause a progressive sodium deficit.[55-58] Calcium and iron deficits can be encouraged by inadequate energy intake (which often includes low intake of protein and dairy products), other dietary influences, and excessive sweating. In women, menstrual bleeding can further challenge iron status. But, unless an athlete is restricting energy intake, mineral status is usually not a problem. As a guide, all athletes should regularly eat foods rich in calcium and iron (e.g., meat, chicken, fish, milk, yogurt, dark, leafy green vegetables, whole-grain breads and fortified cereals, etc.); this will likely ensure adequate intake of these and most other minerals. Importantly, arbitrary excessive mineral supplementation can also have deleterious effects on health and can interfere with the absorption of other minerals.[77]

For many athletes, it is sometimes a challenge to maintain a well-balanced diet, especially when traveling and competing.[78] Therefore, to prevent a potential vitamin or mineral deficiency, it is safe and probably prudent to regularly take a one-a-day multi-vitamin/mineral supplement that provides no more than 100% of the Recommended Dietary Allowance (RDA)[7] for any one vitamin or mineral. Slightly higher amounts of vitamins C and E can be supplemented, although it is probably better to obtain these through careful food selection (e.g., fruits, vegetables, legumes).

Summary

Proper nutrition is important in any athlete's quest to reach peak performance. When integrated with proper training and adequate rest, a well-balanced diet, coupled with a dietary strategy that optimizes hydration status and fuel availability in the pre-competition, and recovery periods will greatly enhance an athlete's opportunity to be a regular winner anywhere he or she competes. Table 44.2 summarizes the key performance-related competition points for the elite athlete.

TABLE 44.2
Nutrition-Related Problems and Recommendations for the Elite Athlete

Water

Many athletes begin play or training dehydrated to some degree.
During training or competition, sweat losses can be extensive — 1-2.5 liters per hour or more!
Any water deficit can have a negative effect on an athlete's performance and wellbeing. A progressive water deficit (from sweating and inadequate fluid intake) can cause:
- Increased cardiovascular strain
- Decreased temperature regulation capacity
- Decreased strength, endurance, and mental capacity

Many athletes do not rehydrate adequately after training or competition.

Recommendations

Drink plenty of fluids (e.g., water, juice, milk, sport drinks) throughout the day.
Drink regularly during training and competition — typically, older adolescents and adults can comfortably consume up to 48 ounces (~1.4 liters) per hour.
After training or competition, drink about 150% of any remaining fluid deficit.

Electrolytes

Athletes lose far more sodium and chloride (salt) from sweating than any other electrolyte.
Sodium and chloride losses are greater with higher sweating rates.
Sodium and chloride losses (via sweating) tend to be less when an athlete is acclimatized to the heat.
Sodium deficits can lead to incomplete rehydration and muscle cramps.
To completely rehydrate, an athlete must replace the sodium and chloride that was lost through sweating.
Excessive rapid water consumption, combined with a large sweat-induced sodium deficit, can lead to hyponatremia.

Recommendations

When an athlete competes or trains in a hot environment, adding salt to the diet (or eating high-salt foods) can help to prevent a sodium deficit and maintain/restore hydration. Good sodium and chloride sources include:
- Salt: 1/4 teaspoon (or 1.5 grams) has 590 mg of sodium
- Salted pretzels

TABLE 44.2 *(Continued)*

Nutrition-Related Problems and Recommendations for the Elite Athlete

Tomato juice
Salted sport drinks (or Pedialyte®)
Soup, cheese, tomato sauce, pizza, and many processed foods

Carbohydrates

Adequate carbohydrate intake is crucial to optimal performance in most sports.
Carbohydrate utilization is greater as intensity of exercise increases and when an athlete competes or trains in the heat.
Even if an athlete eats well prior to competition, after 60 to 90 minutes of intense exercise, glycogen stores will likely be significantly decreased and the ability to maintain blood glucose and meet the muscles' demand for energy may be seriously challenged, which could lead to fatigue.

Recommendations

Generally, 7 to 10 grams of carbohydrate per kilogram of body weight (~500 to 700 grams per day for a 155 lb athlete) is appropriate for periods of intense training or competition.
Athletes should consume about 30 to 60 grams of carbohydrate per hour during training and competition.
Foods and sport drinks with a high glycemic index can be particularly effective for providing rapid carbohydrate energy or restoration during and after competition or training.

Lastly, all athletes differ in what foods and which nutritional strategies they can tolerate and that will enhance their performance. New foods, drinks, or other dietary protocols should be experimented with well prior to any important event.

References

1. USDA, Human Nutrition Service, *Food Guide Pyramid: A Guide to Daily Food Choice*, Home and Garden Bulletin No. 252, 1992.
2. Coyle, EF. In: *Perspectives in Exercise Science and Sports Medicine Volume 10: Optimizing Sport Performance*, Lamb, DR, Murray R, Eds. Cooper, Carmel, IN, 1997, ch. 3.
3. Hargreaves, M. *J Sport Sci* 9: 17; 1991.
4. Foster-Powell K, Brand Miller J. *Am J Clin Nut.* 62: 871S; 1995.
5. Walberg Rankin J. Glycemic index and exercise metabolism, *Sport Science Exchange* (Gatorade Sport Science Institute®), 10, 1997.
6. Murray R, Paul GL, Seifert JG, et al. *Med Sci Sports Exerc* 21: 275; 1989.
7. National Research Council, *Recommended dietary allowances, 10th ed.* Washington: National Academy Press, 1989.
8. Bjorntorp P. *J Sports Sci* 9:71; 1991.
9. Sherman WM, Leenders N. *Int J Sport Nutr* 5: 1S; 1995.
10. Chen JD, Wang JF, Li KJ, et al. *Am J Clin Nutr* 49: 1084; 1989.
11. Faber M, Spinnler-Benade S-J, Daubitzer A. *Int J Sports Med* 10: 140; 1990.
12. Grandjean AC. *Am J Clin Nutr* 49: 1070; 1989.
13. Heinemann L, Zerbes H. *Am J Clin Nutr* 49: 1007; 1989.
14. Sears B. *Essential Fatty Acids, Eicosanoids, and Dietary Endocrinology*, Marblehead, MA: Eicotec Foods, 1993.
15. Coggan A, Coleman E, Hopkins W, Spriet L. Dietary fat and physical activity: fueling the controversy, *Sport Science Exchange: Roundtable* (Gatorade Sport Science Institute®), 7, 1996.
16. Muoio DM, Leddy JJ, Horvath PJ, et al. *Med Sci Sports Exerc* 26: 81; 1994.
17. Brouns F. *Nutritional Needs of Athletes*, West Sussex: John Wiley & Sons, 1993.
18. Evans WJ, In: *World Review of Nutrition and Dietetics Vol. 71: Nutrition and Fitness for Athletes*, Simopoulos AP, Pavlou KN, Eds. Basel, Karger, 1993, p. 21.
19. Lemon PWR. *J Sports Sci* 9: 53; 1991.

20. Lemon PWR. *Int J Sport Nutr* 5: 39S; 1995.
21. Clarkson PM, Rawson ES. *Crit Rev Food Sci Nutr* 39: 317; 1999.
22. Durden Beltz S, Doering PL. *Clin Pharm* 12: 900; 1993.
23. Westerterp KR, Saris WHM. *J Sports Sci* 9: 1; 1991.
24. Ferrauti A. In: Second Annual Congress of the European College of Sport Science. Bangsbo J, Saltin B, Bonde H, Hellsten Y, Ibsen B, Kjær M, Sjøgaard G, Eds. *Book of Abstracts II.* Copenhagen, 1997, 920.
25. Hargreaves M. *Sport Science Exchange* (Gatorade Sport Science Institute®), 12, 1999.
26. Maughan RJ, Greenhaff PL, Leiper JB, et al. *J Sports Sci* 15: 265; 1997.
27. Hargreaves M, Angus D, Howlett K, et al. *Med Sci Sports Exerc* 28: 58S; 1996.
28. Tarnopolsky M. In *Perspectives in Exercise Science and Sports Medicine Volume 12: The Metabolic Basis of Performance in Exercise and Sport.* Lamb DR, Murray R, Eds, Cooper, Carmel, IN, 1999, ch. 4.
29. Bassett, Jr, DR, Howley ET. *Med Sci Sports Exerc* 32: 70; 2000.
30. Spriet LL, Howlett RA. In *Perspectives in Exercise Science and Sports Medicine Volume 12: The Metabolic Basis of Performance in Exercise and Sport.* Lamb DR, Murray R, Eds, Cooper, Carmel, IN, 1999, ch. 1.
31. Holloszy JO. *Exerc Sport Sci Rev* 1: 45; 1973.
32. Holloszy JO, Coyle EF. *J Appl Physiol* 56: 831; 1984.
33. Coyle ED, Hodgkinson BJ. In *Perspectives in Exercise Science and Sports Medicine Volume 12: The Metabolic Basis of Performance in Exercise and Sport.* Lamb DR, Murray R, Eds, Cooper, Carmel, IN, 1999, ch. 5.
34. Henriksson J. *J Experimental Biol* 160: 149; 1991.
35. Hawley JA, Schabort EJ, Noakes TD, Dennis SC. *Sports Med* 24: 73; 1997.
36. Hargreaves M. In *Perspectives in Exercise Science and Sports Medicine Volume 12: The Metabolic Basis of Performance in Exercise and Sport*, Lamb DR, Murray R, Eds, Cooper, Carmel, IN, 1999, ch. 3.
37. American College of Sports Medicine, Position stand on exercise and fluid replacement, *Med Sci Sports Exerc* 28: i-vii; 1996.
38. Dennis SC, Noakes TD, Hawley JA. *J Sports Sci* 15: 305; 1997.
39. Maughan RJ. In *Perspectives in Exercise Science and Sports Medicine Volume 10: Optimizing Sport Performance.* Lamb DR, Murray R, Eds, Cooper, Carmel, IN, 1997, ch. 4.
40. Gisolfi CV, Duchman SM. *Med Sci Sports Exerc* 24: 679; 1992.
41. Meyer F, Bar-Or O, MacDougall D, Heigenhauser GJF. *Med Sci Sports Exerc* 27: 882; 1995.
42. Murray R. *Sports Med* 4: 322; 1987.
43. Below P, Mora-Rodriguez R, Gonzalez-Alonso J, Coyle EF. *Med Sci Sports Exerc* 27: 200; 1994.
44. Shirreffs SM, Maughan RJ. *Exerc Sport Sci Rev* 28: 27; 2000.
45. Zawadzki KM, Yaspelkis III, BB, Ivy JL. *J Appl Physiol* 72: 1854; 1992.
46. Bergeron MF, Maresh CM, Kraemer, WJ, et al. *Int J Sports Med* 12: 474; 1991.
47. Strüder HK, Hollman W, Duperly J, Weber K. *Br J Sp Med* 29: 28; 1995.
48. Wagenmakers AJM. In *Perspectives in Exercise Science and Sports Medicine Volume 12: The Metabolic Basis of Performance in Exercise and Sport.* Lamb DR, Murray R, Eds, Cooper, Carmel, IN, 1999, ch. 6.
49. Sawka MN. *Med Sci Sports Exerc* 24: 657; 1992.
50. Armstrong LE, Maresh CM. *Med Exerc Nutr Health* 2: 125; 1993.
51. Bergeron MF, Maresh CM, Armstrong LE, et al. *Int J Sport Nutr* 5: 180; 1995.
52. Sawka MN, Pandolf KB. In *Perspectives in Exercise Science and Sports Medicine Volume 3: Fluid Homeostasis During Exercise.* Gisolfi CV, Lamb DR, Eds, Benchmark, Carmel, IN, 1990, ch. 1.
53. Armstrong LE, Hubbard RW, Jones BH, Daniels JT, *Physician Sportsmed* 14: 73; 1986.
54. Werner J. In *Perspectives in Exercise Science and Sports Medicine Volume 6: Exercise, Heat, and Thermoregulation.* Gisolfi CV, Lamb DR, Nadel ER, Eds, Benchmark, Carmel, IN, 1993, ch. 2.
55. Bergeron MF, Armstrong LE, Maresh CM. *Clin Sports Med* 14, 23, 1995.
56. Maughan RJ, Shirreffs SM. In *Oxford Textbook of Sports Medicine*, 2nd ed., Harries M, Williams C, Stanish WD, Micheli LJ, Eds, Oxford University Press, Oxford, UK, 1998.
57. Wenger CB. In *Human Performance Physiology and Environmental Medicine at Terrestrial Extremes.* Pandolf KB, Sawka MN, Gonzalez RR, Eds, Benchmark, Indianapolis, 1988, ch. 4.

58. Bergeron MF. *Int J Sport Nutr* 6: 62; 1996.
59. Bergeron MF, Volpe SL, Gelinas Y. *Clin. Chem* 44(Suppl.): A167; 1998.
60. Clarkson PM, Haymes EM. *Med Sci Sports Exerc* 27: 831; 1995.
61. Tipton K, Green NR, Haymes EM, Waller M. *Int J Sport Nutr* 3: 261; 1993.
62. Maughan RJ, Leiper JB, Shirreffs SM. *Br J Sports Med* 31: 175; 1997.
63. Nose H, Mack GW, Shi X, Nadel ER. *J Appl Physiol* 65: 325; 1988.
64. Taubes G. *Science* 281: 898; 1998.
65. Wilcox AR. In: *Sport Science Exchange* (Gatorade Sport Science Institute®), 3; 1990.
66. Williams MH. In: *Sport Science Exchange* (Gatorade Sport Science Institute®), 4; 1992.
67. Armstrong LE, Maresh CM, Castellani JW, et al. *Int J Sport Nutr* 4: 265; 1994.
68. Greenleaf JE. *Med Sci Sports Exerc* 24: 645; 1992.
69. Speedy DB, Noakes TD, Rogers IR, et al. *Med Sci Sports Exerc* 31: 809; 1999.
70. Vrijens DM, Rehrer NJ. *J Appl Physiol* 86: 1847; 1999.
71. Wemple RD, Lamb DR, McKeever KH. *Int J Sports Med* 18: 40; 1997.
72. The American College of Sports Medicine Roundtable on the physiological and health effects of oral creatine supplementation, *Med Sci Sports Exerc* 32: 706; 2000.
73. Lambert EV, Hawley JA, Goedecke J, et al. *J Sports Sci* 15: 315; 1997.
74. Heigenhauser GJF, Jones NL. In *Perspectives in Exercise Science and Sports Medicine Volume 4: Ergogenics — Enhancement of Performance in Exercise and Sport*. Lamb DR, Williams MH, Eds, Brown & Benchmark, Carmel, IN, 1991, ch. 5.
75. Horswill CA. *Int J Sport Nutr* 5: 111S; 1995.
76. Davis JM. *Int J Sport Nutr* 5: 29S; 1995.
77. Lukaski HC. In: *Perspectives in Exercise Science and Sports Medicine Volume 12: The Metabolic Basis of Performance in Exercise and Sport*. Lamb, DR, Murray R, Eds, Cooper, Carmel, IN, 1999, ch. 7.
78. Nelson Steen S. *Sport Science Exchange* (Gatorade Sport Science Institute®), 11; 1998.

Part VII

Clinical Nutrition

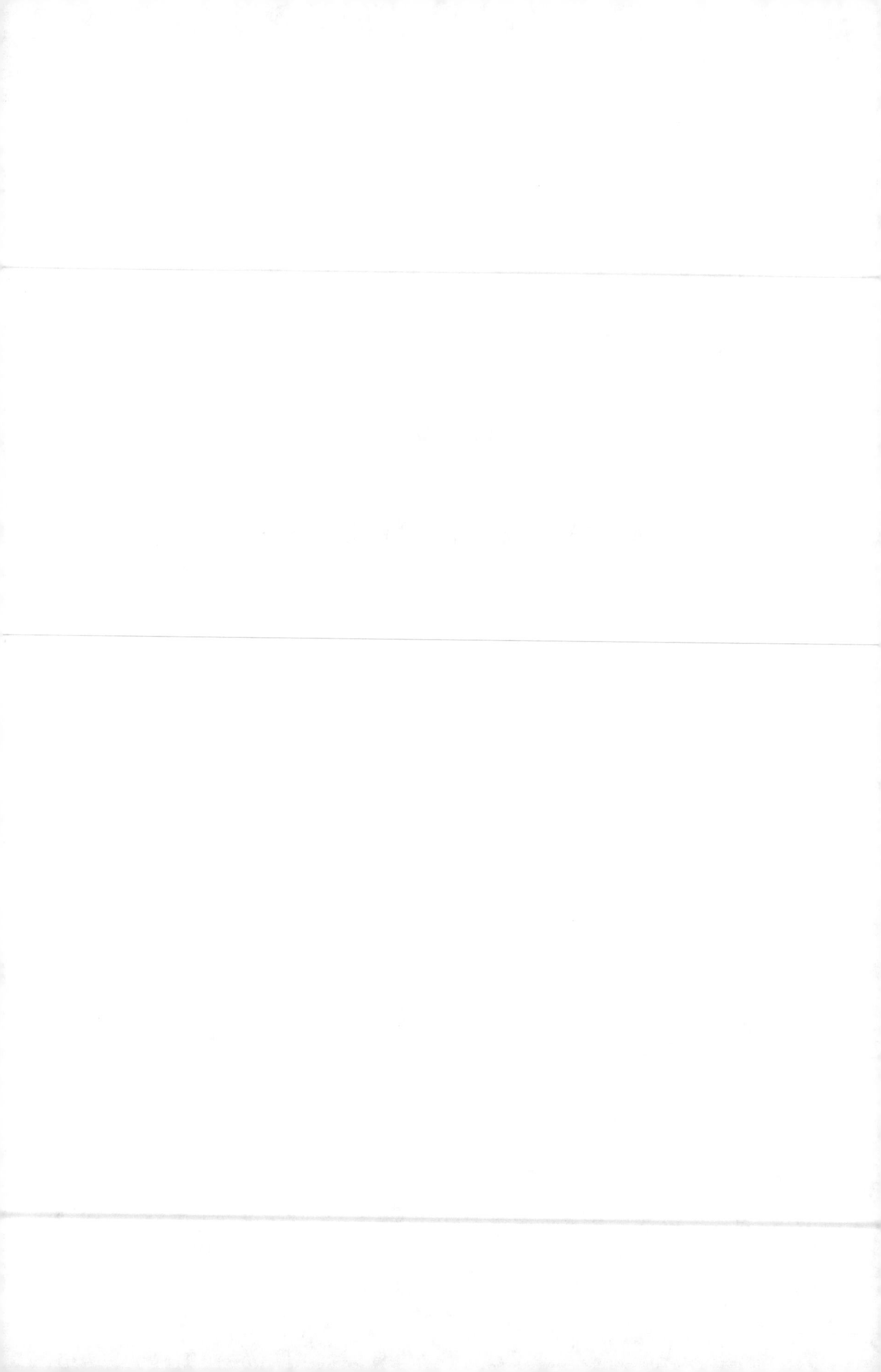

45

Alcohol: Its Metabolism and Interaction with Nutrients

Charles S. Lieber

Respective Role of Alcohol and Nutrition in Organ Damage of the Alcoholic

Ethanol is not only a psychoactive drug. Besides its pharmacologic action, it has a considerable energy value (7.1 kcal/g). Therefore, substantial use of alcohol has profound effects on nutritional status.[1] Such consumption may cause primary malnutrition by displacing other nutrients in the diet because of the high energy content of the alcoholic beverages (Figure 45.1) or because of associated socioeconomic and medical disorders. Secondary malnutrition may result from either maldigestion or malabsorption of nutrients caused by gastrointestinal complications associated with alcoholism, involving especially the pancreas and the small intestine. These effects include malabsorption of thiamine and folate as well as maldigestion and malabsorption secondary to alcohol-induced pancreatic insufficiency and intestinal lactase deficiency.[2] Alcohol also promotes nutrient degradation or impaired activation. Such primary and secondary malnutrition can affect virtually all nutrients (*vide infra*). At the tissue level, alcohol replaces various normal substrates, with the liver being the most seriously affected organ and malnutrition being incriminated as a primary etiologic factor of liver dysfunction.

Theories of the exclusively nutritional origin of alcoholic liver disease were supported by Best, the prominent codiscoverer of insulin who wrote that "there is no more evidence of a specific toxic effect of pure ethyl alcohol upon liver cells than there is for one due to sugar."[3] This notion was based largely on experimental work in rats given ethanol in drinking water.[3] Under these conditions, no liver lesions developed unless the diet was deficient in proteins, methionine, or choline. Deficiency alone sufficed to produce the liver lesions. However, with the technique of alcohol administration in drinking water, ethanol consumption usually does not exceed 10 to 25% of the total energy intake of the animal, because rats have an aversion for alcohol. A comparable amount of alcohol resulted in negligible ethanol concentrations in the blood.[4] Thus, administration of alcohol in drinking water to rodents is not a suitable model for the human disease. When ethanol was incorporated into a totally liquid diet,[4,5] the aversion for alcohol was overcome, because

0-8493-2705-9/01/$0.00+$1.50

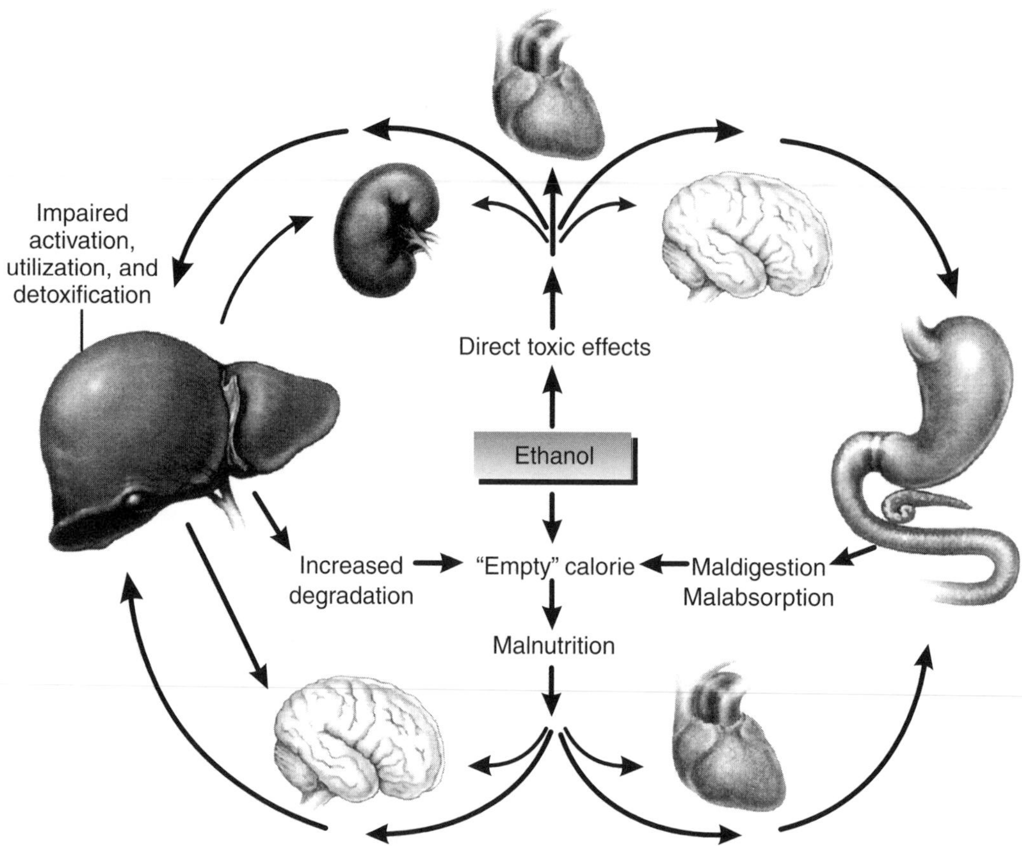

FIGURE 45.1
Organ damage in the alcoholic. Interaction of direct toxicity of ethanol on various organs with malnutrition secondary to dietary deficiencies, maldigestion, and malabsorption, as well as impaired hepatic activation or increased degradation of nutrients. (From Lieber CS, *N Engl J Med* 333: 1058; 1995, with permission.)

in order to eat or drink, the animals had no choice but to take the alcohol along with whatever diet was given. With this technique, the quantity of ethanol consumed was increased to 36% of total energy, an amount relevant to alcohol intake in man. It was found that even with nutritionally adequate diets, isoenergetic replacement of sucrose or other carbohydrates by ethanol consistently produced a 5- to 10-fold increase in hepatic triglycerides.[4-6] Furthermore, isoenergetic replacement of carbohydrate by fat instead of ethanol did not produce steatosis.[4] With this liquid-diet technique, alcohol was also shown to be capable of producing cirrhosis in nonhuman primates, even when there was an adequate diet.[7] In addition, the hepatotoxicity of ethanol was established by controlled clinical investigations which showed that even in the absence of dietary deficiencies, alcohol can produce fatty liver and ultrastructural lesions in humans.[4,5]

Some dietary deficiencies were found to exacerbate the effects of alcohol, and judicious supplementations were shown to have beneficial effects. When protein deficiency is present, the deficiency may potentiate the effect of ethanol. In rats, a combination of ethanol and a diet deficient in both protein and lipotropic factors leads to more pronounced hepatic steatosis than with either factor alone.[8] Indeed, protein deficiency impairs lipoprotein secretion, which can be expected to markedly potentiate hepatic lipid accumulation secondary to the direct effects of alcohol resulting from its metabolism in the liver. However, the effect of protein deficiency has not been clearly delineated in human adults. In children, protein deficiency leads to hepatic steatosis, one of the manifestations of kwashiorkor, but this condition does not progress to cirrhosis. In adolescent baboons, protein restriction to 7% of total energy did not result in conspicuous liver injury (even after 19 months) either by biochemical analysis or by light- and electron-microscopic examination. Significant steatosis was observed only when the protein intake was reduced to 4% of total energy.[9] On the other hand, an excess of protein (25% of total energy or 2.5 times the recommended amount) did not prevent alcohol from producing fat accumulation in human volunteers.[10] Thus, in humans, ethanol is capable of producing striking changes in liver lipids even in the presence of a protein-enriched diet, an effect linked to the metabolism of ethanol.

The hepatocyte contains three main pathways for ethanol metabolism, each located in a different subcellular compartment:

1. The alcohol dehydrogenase (ADH) pathway of the cytosol or the soluble fraction of the cell
2. The microsomal ethanol oxidizing system located in the endoplasmic reticulum
3. Catalase located in the peroxisomes[1]

Each of these pathways produces specific metabolic and toxic disturbance, and all three result in the production of acetaldehyde, a highly toxic metabolite.

The Alcohol Dehydrogenase (ADH) Pathway and Associated Metabolic Disorders of Carbohydrates, Uric Acid, and Lipids

ADH Isozymes

ADH has a broad substrate specificity which includes dehydrogenation of steroids, oxidation of the intermediary alcohols of the shunt pathway of mevalonate metabolism, and ω-oxidation of fatty acids;[11] these processes may act as the "physiologic" substrates for ADH.

Human liver ADH is a zinc metalloenzyme with five classes of multiple molecular forms which arise from the association of eight different types of subunits, $\alpha,\beta1,\beta2,\beta3,\gamma1,\gamma2$, π, and χ, into active dimeric molecules. A genetic model accounts for this multiplicity as products of five gene loci, ADH1 through ADH5.[12] There are three types of subunit, α, β, and γ in class I. Polymorphism occurs at two loci, ADH2 and ADH3, which encode the β and γ subunits. Class II isozymes migrate more anodically than class I isozymes and, unlike the latter, which generally have low K_m values for ethanol, class II (or π) ADH has a relatively high K_m (34 mM) and a relative insensitivity to 4-methylpyrazole inhibition. Class III (χADH) does not participate in the oxidation of ethanol in the liver because of its very low affinity for that substrate. More recently, a new isoenzyme of ADH has been purified from human stomach, so-called σ- or μ-ADH (class IV).

Metabolic Effects of Excessive ADH-Mediated Hepatic NADH Generation

The oxidation of ethanol via the ADH pathway results in the production of acetaldehyde with loss of H which reduces nicotinamide adenine dinucleotide (NAD) to nicotinamide adenine dinucleotide — reduced form (NADH). The large amounts of reducing equivalents generated overwhelm the hepatocyte's ability to maintain redox homeostasis, and a number of metabolic disorders ensue (Figure 45.2),[1] including hypoglycemia and hyperlactacidemia. The latter contributes to the acidosis and also reduces the capacity of the kidney to excrete uric acid, leading to secondary hyperuricemia, which is aggravated by the alcohol-induced ketosis and acetate-mediated enhanced ATP breakdown and purine generation.[13] Hyperuricemia explains, at least in part, the common clinical observation that excessive consumption of alcoholic beverages commonly aggravates or precipitates gouty attacks. The increased NADH also promotes fatty acid synthesis and opposes lipid oxidation with, as a net result, fat accumulation.[14]

The effects of ethanol were reproduced *in vitro* by an alternate NADH-generating system (sorbitol-fructose) and were blocked by an H+ acceptor (methylene blue).[14,15] The preventive effect of methylene blue against ethanol-induced fat accumulation was recently confirmed.[16]

Extrahepatic ADH

The human gastric mucosa possesses several ADH isoenzymes,[17] one of which (class IV ADH or σ-ADH) is not present in the liver. This enzyme has now been purified,[18] its full-length cDNA obtained, the complete amino acid sequence deduced,[19,20] and its gene cloned and localized to chromosome 4.[21] Gastric ADH is responsible for a large portion of ethanol metabolism found in cultured rat[22] and human[23] gastric cells. Its *in vivo* effect is reflected by the first pass metabolism (FPM) of ethanol, namely the fact that for a given dose of ethanol, blood levels are usually higher after IV than after oral administration.[24,25] While the relative contribution of gastric and hepatic ethanol metabolism to FPM is still the subject of debate,[26-28] the role of gastric ethanol metabolism in this FPM has been established experimentally.[29,30] Furthermore, FPM is partly lost in the alcoholic,[31] together with decreased gastric ADH activity. Moreover, FPM disappears after gastrectomy.[32] σ-ADH is also absent or markedly decreased in activity in a large percentage of Japanese subjects,[33] and their FPM is reduced correspondingly[34] in keeping with a predominant role for σ-ADH in human FPM. Thus, the FPM represents some kind of protective barrier against the systemic effects of ethanol, including attenuation of liver damage.[35,36]

Pathogenic Role of ADH Polymorphism

Individual differences in the rate of ethanol metabolism may be genetically controlled. Furthermore, genetic factors influence the severity of alcohol-induced liver disease. Indeed, the frequency of an alcohol dehydrogenase 3 allele has been found to differ in patients with alcohol-related end-organ damage (including cirrhosis) and matched controls, suggesting that genetically determined differences in alcohol metabolism may explain differences in the susceptibility to alcohol-related disease (possibly through the enhanced generation of toxic metabolites),[37] but this hypothesis has been questioned.[38]

Microsomal Ethanol Oxidizing System (MEOS)

This new pathway has been the subject of extensive research, reviewed in detail elsewhere.[39,40] Such a system was demonstrated in liver microsomes *in vitro* and found to be inducible by chronic alcohol feeding *in vivo*,[41] and was named the microsomal ethanol oxidizing system.[41,42]

The key enzyme of the MEOS is the ethanol-inducible cytochrome P4502E1 (CYP2E1) which is increased 4- to 10-fold in liver biopsies of recently drinking subjects,[43] with a corresponding rise in mRNA.[44] This induction contributes to the metabolic tolerance to

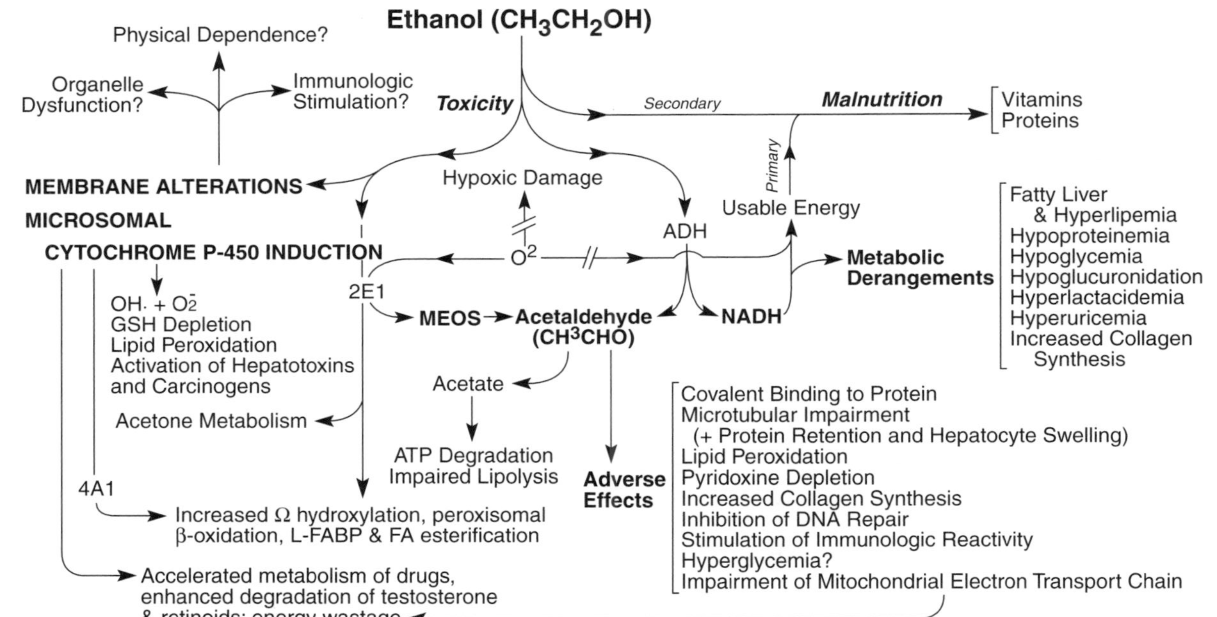

FIGURE 45.2
Hepatic, nutritional, and metabolic abnormalities after ethanol abuse. Malnutrition, whether primary or secondary, can be differentiated from metabolic changes or direct toxicity, resulting partly from ADH-mediated redox changes, effects secondary to microsomal induction, or acetaldehyde production. (From Lieber CS, *J Stud Alcohol* 59: 9; 1998, with permission.)

ethanol that develops in the alcoholic (in addition to the central nervous tolerance), with other cytochromes P450 (CYP1A2, CYP3A4) possibly also involved.[45]

In addition to tolerance to ethanol, alcoholics tend to display tolerance to various other drugs. Indeed, it has been shown that the rate of drug clearance from the blood is enhanced in alcoholics. Of course, this could be caused by a variety of factors other than ethanol, such as the congeners and the use of other drugs so commonly associated with alcoholism. Controlled studies showed, however, that administration of pure ethanol with non-deficient diets either to rats or man (under metabolic ward conditions) resulted in a striking increase in the rate of blood clearance of meprobamate, pentobarbital,[46] and various other drugs.[1] The metabolic tolerance persists several days to weeks after cessation of alcohol abuse, and the duration of recovery varies depending on the drug considered.[47]

Experimentally, this effect of chronic ethanol consumption is modulated, in part, by the dietary content in carbohydrates,[48] lipids,[49] and proteins.[50] It is now recognized that CYP2E1, in addition to its ethanol oxidizing activity, catalyzes fatty acid ω-1 and ω-2 hydroxylations.[51-53] Furthermore, acetone is both an inducer and a substrate of CYP2E1[54-56] (Figure 45.3). Excess ketones and fatty acid commonly accompany diabetes and morbid obesity, conditions associated with non-alcoholic steatohepatitis (NASH). Experimentally, obese, overfed rats also exhibit substantially higher microsomal ethanol oxidation, acetaminophen activation, and p-nitrophenol hydroxylation (monooxygenase activities catalyzed by CYP2E1).[57] These diabetic rats are experimental models relevant to NASH, and indeed the hepatopathology of NASH appears to be due, at least in part, to excess CYP2E1 induction.[58]

Clinically, a most important feature of CYP2E1 is not only ethanol oxidation, but also its extraordinary capacity to convert many xenobiotics to highly toxic metabolites, thereby explaining the increased vulnerability of the alcoholic. These agents include *industrial solvents* (e.g., bromobenzene, vinylidene chloride), *anesthetic agents* (e.g., enflurane,[59] methoxyflurane), commonly used *medications* (e.g., isoniazid, phenylbutazone), illicit drugs (e.g., *cocaine*) and over-the-counter *analgesics* (e.g., acetaminophen),[60] all of which are substrates for, and/or inducers of CYP2E1. The effects of acetaminophen, ethanol, and fasting are synergistic,[61] because all three deplete the level of reduced glutathione (GSH),

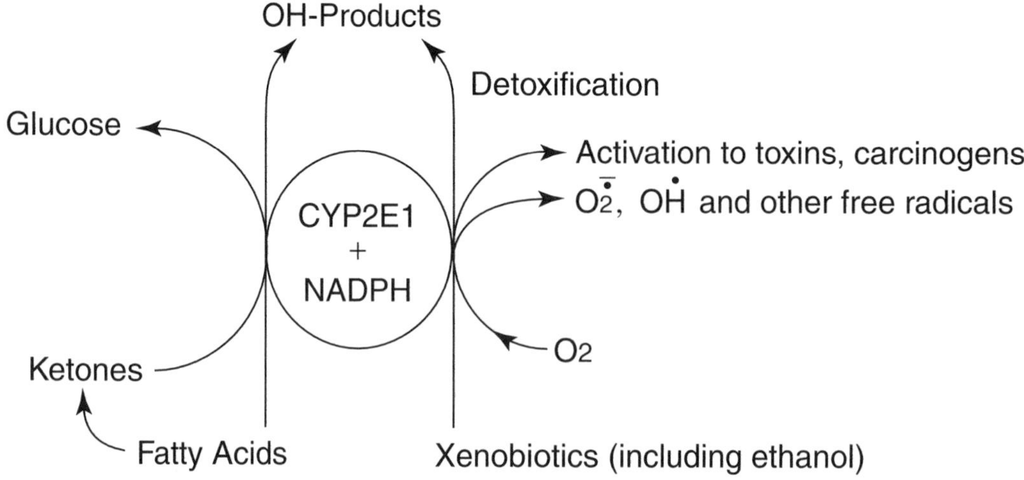

FIGURE 45.3
Physiologic and toxic roles of CYP2E1, the main cytochrome P450 of the microsomal ethanol oxidizing system (MEOS). Many endogenous and xenobiotic compounds are substrates for CYP2E1 and induce its activity through various mechanisms, resulting in an array of beneficial as well as harmful effects. (From Lieber CS, *Alcohol: Clin Exp Res* 23: 991; 1999, with permission.)

a scavenger of toxic free radicals. Rats fed ethanol chronically have increased rates of GSH turnover,[62] and ethanol produces an enhanced loss from the liver.[63] The selective loss of the compound from liver mitochondria[64] contributes to the striking alcohol-induced oxidant stress and impairment of this organelle.

CYP2E1 also generates several species of active oxygen (Figures 45.2, 45.3) which, in concert with a decrease in the level of GSH, promote injury by inactivation of enzymes and peroxidation of lipids. In patients with cirrhosis, hepatic depletion of α-tocopherol,[65] a major antioxidant, potentiates this effect. GSH offers one of the mechanisms for the scavenging of toxic free radicals. Replenishment of GSH can be achieved by administration of precursors of cysteine (one of the amino acids of this tripeptide) such as acetylcysteine or S-adenosyl-L-methionine (SAMe).[66,67] Experimentally, CYP2E1 has also been downregulated by polyenylphosphatidylcholine (PPC),[68] a potentially beneficial therapeutic approach.

Nutritional Status of Alcoholics

Overall Assessment

Alcoholics hospitalized for medical complications of alcohol intoxication (such as states of acute intoxication and withdrawal) have the most severe malnutrition. These alcoholics have inadequate dietary protein,[69] signs of protein malnutrition,[70,71] and anthropometric measurements indicative of impaired nutrition: their height-to-weight ratio is lower,[72] muscle mass estimated by the creatinine-height index is reduced,[71,72] and triceps skin folds are thinner.[71-73] Continued drinking results in weight loss, whereas abstinence results in weight gain[74,75] in patients with and without liver disease.[74]

Many patients who drink to excess are either not malnourished or are less malnourished than the hospitalized group. Women drinking one or more drinks per day weighed on average 2.3 kg less than nondrinkers, and they and their male counterparts continued on a more stable weight over the next ten years than the nondrinkers, whose weight rose.[76] Other surveys, however, found that alcohol intake, especially when accompanied by high fat intake and sedentary behavior,[77] favors truncal obesity, particularly in women.[78] Those with moderate alcohol intake,[79] even those admitted to hospital for alcohol rehabilitation rather than for medical problems,[80] often hardly differ nutritionally from controls (matched for socioeconomic status and health history), except that females have a lower level of thiamin excretion than control patients following a thiamin load test.[80]

The wide range in nutritional status of our alcoholic population surely reflects, in part, differences in what they eat. Moderate alcohol intake, with alcohol accounting for 16% of total kcalories (alcohol included), is associated with slightly increased total energy intake.[81]

Although ethanol is rich in energy (7.1 kcal/g), chronic consumption does not produce the expected gain in body weight.[82] This energy deficit can be attributed, in part, to damaged mitochondria and the resulting poor coupling of oxidation of fat with energy production, as well as to microsomal pathways that oxidize ethanol without conserving chemical energy (Figure 45.2). Thus, perhaps because of these energy considerations, this group with higher total caloric intake has no weight gain, despite physical activity levels comparable to those of the non-alcohol consuming population. This level of alcohol intake, and even slightly higher levels (23%)[83] is associated with a substitution of alcohol for carbohydrate in the diet. In those individuals consuming more than 30% of total kcalories as alcohol, significant decreases in protein and fat intake occur, too, and the consumption of vitamins A, C, and thiamin may descend below the recommended daily allowances.[81] Calcium, iron, and fiber intake are also lowered.[83]

The mechanisms underlying the altered pattern of food intake are under debate. Suppression of appetite has been postulated.[84] Depressed consciousness during inebriation, hangover, and gastroduodenitis due to ethanol, partly explain the decreased food intake. The contribution of subtle nutritional alterations produced by ethanol to the pathogenesis of ethanol-induced or other disease states, including alcoholism, is largely unchartered.

Specific Nutrients

Vitamin C

The vitamin C status of alcoholic patients admitted to a hospital is lower than that of nonalcoholics as measured by serum ascorbic acid, peripheral leukocyte ascorbic acid, or urinary ascorbic acid after an oral challenge.[85] In addition to a lower mean ascorbic acid level, some 25% of patients with Laennec's cirrhosis had serum ascorbic acid levels below the range of healthy controls.[85] Ascorbic acid status is low in alcoholic patients with and without liver disease. When alcohol intake exceeds 30% of total kcalories, vitamin C generally falls below recommended dietary allowances.[86] The clinical significance is unknown for patients who have low ascorbic acid levels but who are not clearly scorbutic.

Vitamin D

Alcoholics have illnesses related to abnormalities of calcium, phosphorus, and vitamin D homeostasis. They have decreases in bone density[87] and bone mass,[88] increased susceptibility to fractures,[89] and increased osteonecrosis.[90] Low blood calcium, phosphorus, magnesium, and low, normal, or high vitamin D_3 levels have been reported, indicating disturbed calcium metabolism.[88] In patients with alcoholic liver disease, vitamin D deficiency probably derives from too little vitamin D substrate, which results from poor dietary intake, malabsorption due to cholestasis or pancreatic insufficiency, and insufficient sunlight.

Vitamin K

Vitamin K deficiency in alcoholism may arise when there is an interruption of fat absorption due to pancreatic insufficiency, biliary obstruction, or intestinal mucosal abnormality secondary to folic acid deficiency. Dietary vitamin K inadequacy is not a likely cause of clinical deficiency unless there is concomitant sterilization of the large gut, a reliable source of the vitamin.

Folic Acid

Alcoholics tend to have low folic acid status when they are drinking heavily and their folic acid intake is reduced. For example, a group of unselected alcoholics showed a 37.5% incidence of low serum folate levels and a 17.6% incidence of low red blood cell folate levels.[74]

In pigs fed ethanol for 11 months, folic acid absorption is normal but jejunal folate hydrolase, an early enzyme of folate polyglutamate breakdown, is decreased.[91,92] *In vitro* preparations of rat intestine absorb folate less well when exposed to a variety of alcohols.[93] Malnourished alcoholics without liver disease also absorb folic acid less well compared to their better-nourished counterparts.[94] Folic acid absorption, usually increased by partial starvation, is less increased in rats when alcohol is ingested.[95] It has not been clearly shown, however, that either protein deficiency or alcohol[94,95] decreases folate absorption *in vivo*.

Thus, it is still unclear what aspects of malnutrition adversely affect folate absorption and under what clinical circumstances alcohol may interfere with folate absorption.

Alcohol accelerates the production of megaloblastic anemia in patients with depleted folate stores[96] and suppresses the hematologic response to folic acid in folic acid-depleted patients.[97] Alcohol also has other effects on folate metabolism but their significance is not clear: alcohol given acutely causes a decrease in serum folate, which is partly explained by increased urinary excretion;[98] alcohol administered chronically to monkeys decreased hepatic folate levels, partly because of the inability of the liver to retain folate,[99] and perhaps partly because of increased urinary and fecal losses.[100]

Vitamin B_{12}

Alcoholics do not commonly have vitamin B_{12} deficiency. Their serum levels are usually normal even when they are deficient in folate, whether they have cirrhosis[101,102] or not.[94,95] This is probably due to large body stores of vitamin B_{12}. Pancreatic insufficiency, however, results in decreased vitamin B_{12} absorption as measured by the Schilling test. In this circumstance there is insufficient luminal protease activity and alkalinity, which normally serve to release vitamin B_{12} from the "r" protein secreted by salivary glands, intestines, and possibly the stomach.[103] Alcohol ingestion has also been shown to decrease vitamin B_{12} absorption in volunteers after several weeks of intake.[104] The alcohol effect may be in the ileum, because co-administration of intrinsic factor or pancreatin does not correct the Schilling test results. It is controversial whether the binding of intrinsic factor-vitamin B_{12} complex to ileal sites is abnormal.[105,106]

Riboflavin

When there is a general lack of B vitamin intake, riboflavin deficiency may be encountered.[107] In one study, deficiency was found in 50% of a small group of patients with medical complications severe enough to warrant hospital admission.[108] Although none of the patients exhibited classic signs of riboflavin deficiency, they had an abnormal activity coefficient (AC) that returned to normal 2 to 7 days after intramuscular replacement with 5 mg riboflavin daily. Activity coefficient is measured as the ratio of erythrocyte glutathione reductase activity upon addition of flavin adenine dinucleotide to the activity with no additions. Riboflavin deficiency could be induced readily by alcohol feeding to the Syrian hamster; the most severe deficiency was seen in animals also restricted in riboflavin intake.[109] Riboflavin and pyridoxine storage in the liver is adversely affected by alcohol, at least in experimental animals.

Vitamin E and Selenium

Vitamin E deficiency is not a recognized complication of alcoholism, although patients with chronic alcoholic pancreatitis have a lower vitamin E-to-total plasma lipid ratio.[110]

When rodents were fed ethanol repeatedly in one study, their hepatic vitamin E levels, measured as α-tocopherol, were low;[111] this was accompanied by increased hepatic lipid peroxidation when alcohol was combined with a low-vitamin E diet.[112] The mechanism of hepatic vitamin E depletion by ethanol is probably enhanced oxidation of α-tocopherol to α-tocopherol quinone in liver microsomes.[112] Alcohol-induced liver injury may be mediated, in part, by stress on cellular antioxidant mechanisms interrelated with vitamin E and selenium. Considering the findings in humans with fat malabsorption or severe cholestasis, and the evidence of vitamin E depletion by chronic alcohol feeding of experimental animals, it would seem that there is great potential for vitamin E deficiency in chronic alcoholics who combine low vitamin E intake with steatorrhea from chronic pancreatitis or prolonged cholestasis.

Magnesium

Acute doses of ethanol cause magnesium loss in the urine,[113] and alcoholism is associated with magnesium deficiency.[114] Alcoholics have low blood magnesium and low body-exchangeable magnesium; symptoms in alcoholics resemble those in patients with magnesium deficiency of other causes; upon withdrawal from alcohol, magnesium balance is positive. Hypocalcemia in alcoholics in the setting of magnesium deficiency has been ascribed, in part, to impaired parathyroid hormone (PTH) secretion as well as renal and skeletal resistance to PTH,[115] and the hypocalcemia may only be responsive to magnesium repletion. Hospitalized alcoholics with normal serum total magnesium had significantly lower serum ionized magnesium.[116]

Iron

There may be either deficiency or excess of iron in the body. Alcoholics may be iron-deficient as a result of the several gastrointestinal lesions to which they are prone and that may bleed.

Hepatic iron content was found to be increased in autopsy studies of most patients with early alcoholic cirrhosis.[117] In most alcoholics, however, the iron content of the liver is normal or only modestly elevated, although there may be stainable iron in reticuloendothelial cells, possibly because of bouts of hemolysis. It is unclear whether increased intestinal absorption of iron because of alcohol[118] or hepatic uptake of iron from plasma in established alcoholic liver disease[119] contributes significantly to increased hepatic iron levels. There is usually little difficulty in distinguishing the hepatic iron increases of alcoholic liver disease from the much higher amounts characteristic of genetic hemochromatosis, using a measure of absolute iron content per gram of liver with upward adjustments for age.[120] The contribution that hepatic iron may make to liver damage via its role in lipid peroxidation[121] (in conjunction with the effects of alcohol) and its possible role in promoting fibrogenesis[122] are of great potential significance.

Zinc

Patients have low plasma zinc,[123] low liver zinc,[124] and increased urinary zinc levels.[124,125] Acute ethanol ingestion, however, does not cause zincuria.[126] The low zinc content of chronic alcoholics with cirrhosis is attributed to decreased intake and absorption as well as increased urinary excretion. Many Americans have a diet marginal in zinc.[127] Alcoholics fall into several of those groups with marginal intake. It is interesting that zinc absorption has been shown to be low in alcoholic cirrhotics but not in patients with cirrhosis of other causes,[128] although cirrhosis of varied etiologies is characterized by low serum zinc.[129] Currently, the therapeutic use of zinc in alcoholism is restricted to the treatment of night blindness not responsive to vitamin A.

Copper

Hepatic copper content is increased in advanced alcoholic cirrhosis.[117] Serum copper content has been reported to be elevated in alcoholics independent of the stage of liver disease,[130] but others have reported normal levels.[131]

Trace Metals

Nickel levels are consistently high in alcoholic liver disease; manganese and chromium are unchanged.[117] Intracellular shifts in trace metals have been described upon acute administration of alcohol.[132] Versieck et al. reported increased serum molybdenum in patients with acute liver disease;[133] increased levels were not seen in those patients with cirrhosis. The clinical significance of trace metal changes is still obscure, except for the cardiotoxicity ascribed to alcoholic beverages with high cobalt content.

Effects of Ethanol on Digestion and Absorption

Diarrhea frequently occurs in alcoholics. In the heavy drinker, diarrhea may occur for a variety of reasons including ethanol-exacerbated lactase deficiency, especially in blacks.[2] Alcohol consumption is also associated with motility changes. In the jejunum, ethanol decreases type I (impeding) waves, while in the ileum it increases type III (propulsive) waves. Another major complication is alcoholic pancreatitis. Intestinal malabsorption may also be secondary to folic acid deficiency (*vide supra*).

Steatorrhea is commonly due to folic acid deficiency and luminal bile salt deficiency. Intraluminal bile salts are decreased by acute ethanol administration.[134] In rodents, long-term ethanol administration delays the half-time excretion of cholic and chenodeoxycholic acids by decreasing the daily excretion and expanding the pool size slightly.[135] Alcoholic cirrhotic patients may have bile low in deoxycholic acid, possibly due to impaired conversion of cholate to deoxycholate by bacteria.[136]

Hospitalized alcoholics were reported to have impaired thiamin absorption compared to control patients when tested by radioactive thiamin excretion,[137] a test also affected by steps not related to absorption. However, folic acid deficiency was not adequately excluded as a cause of thiamin malabsorption in these studies. Refined testing revealed reduced thiamin absorption due to alcohol in a minority of subjects.[138] Jejunal perfusion studies did not show an effect of 5% alcohol on thiamin absorption in man.[139] Thus, whereas human thiamin absorption may not be affected by alcohol, it is clearly impaired in rodents.

Alcohol also interferes with riboflavin absorption in rodents, but this has not been studied in humans. Alcohol impairs folic acid absorption in malnourished humans, but the mechanism is unclear (*vide supra*).

Effect of Alcohol on Nutrient Activation

Thiamine and Pyridoxine

Thiamin deficiency in alcoholics causes Wernicke-Korsakoff syndrome and beriberi heart disease, and probably contributes to polyneuropathy. There has been no confirmation of an inborn error of transketolase affinity for its cofactor thiamine pyrophosphate in Wernicke-Korsakoff syndrome as was once claimed.

Neurologic, hematologic, and dermatologic disorders can be caused in part by pyridoxine deficiency. Pyridoxine deficiency, as measured by low plasma pyridoxal-5′-phosphate (PLP), was reported in over 50% of alcoholics without hematologic findings or abnormal liver function tests.[140,141] Inadequate intake may partly explain low PLP, but increased destruction and reduced formation may also contribute. PLP is more rapidly destroyed in erythrocytes in the presence of acetaldehyde, the product of ethanol oxidation, perhaps by displacement of PLP from protein and consequent exposure to phosphatase.[140,142] Studies showed that chronic ethanol feeding lowered hepatic content of PLP by decreasing net synthesis from pyridoxine.[143-145] The acetaldehyde produced on alcohol oxidation was thought to enhance hydrolysis of PLP by cellular phosphatases.[140]

Methionine and S-Adenosylmethionine (SAMe)

Methionine deficiency has been described and its supplementation has been considered for the treatment of liver diseases, especially the alcoholic variety, but excess methionine was shown to have some adverse effects,[146] including a decrease in hepatic ATP.[147] Furthermore, whereas in some patients with alcoholic liver disease, circulating methionine levels are normal,[148] elevated levels were observed in others.[149-151] Kinsell et al.[152] found a delay in the clearance of plasma methionine after its systemic administration to patients with liver damage. Similarly, Horowitz et al.[153] reported that the blood clearance of methionine after an oral load of this amino acid was slowed. Since about half the methionine is metabolized by the liver, these observations suggested impaired hepatic metabolism of this amino acid in patients with alcoholic liver disease. Indeed, for most of its functions, methionine must be activated to S-adenosylmethionine (SAMe), and in cirrhotic livers Duce et al.[154] reported a decrease in the activity of SAMe synthetase, the enzyme involved, also called methionine adenosyltransferase (Figure 45.4).

Various mechanisms of inactivation of SAMe synthetase have been reviewed recently.[155] One factor that may have contributed to the defect is relative hypoxia, with nitric oxide-mediated inactivation and transcriptional arrest.[156] In addition, long-term alcohol consumption was found to be associated with enhanced methionine utilization and depletion.[157] As a consequence, SAMe depletion as well as its decreased availability could be expected, and indeed, long-term ethanol consumption under controlled conditions by nonhuman primates was associated with a significant depletion of hepatic SAMe.[66] Potentially, such SAMe depletion may have a number of adverse effects. SAMe is the principal methylating agent in various transmethylation reactions which are important to nucleic acid and protein synthesis. Hirata and Axelrod[158] and Hirata et al.[159] also demonstrated the importance of methylation to cell membrane function with regard to membrane fluidity and the transport of metabolites and transmission of signals across membranes. Thus, depletion of SAMe, by impairing methyltransferase activity, may promote the membrane injury which has been documented in alcohol-induced liver damage.[160] Furthermore, SAMe plays a key role in the synthesis of polyamines and provides a source of cysteine for glutathione production (Figure 45.4). Thus, the deficiency in methionine activation and in SAMe production resulting from the decrease in the activity of the corresponding synthetase results in a number of adverse effects, including inadequate cysteine and GSH production, especially when aggravated by associated folate, B_6, or B_{12} deficiencies (Figure 45.4). The consequences of this enzymic defect can be alleviated by providing SAMe, the product of the reaction. SAMe is unstable, but the synthesis of a stable salt allowed for replenishment of SAMe through ingestion of this compound: blood levels of SAMe increased after oral administration in rodents[161] and man.[162] It has been claimed that the liver does not take up SAMe from the bloodstream,[163] but results in baboons[66] clearly showed hepatic uptake of exogenous SAMe. The effective use of SAMe for transmethylation and transsulfuration has also been demonstrated *in vivo*.[164]

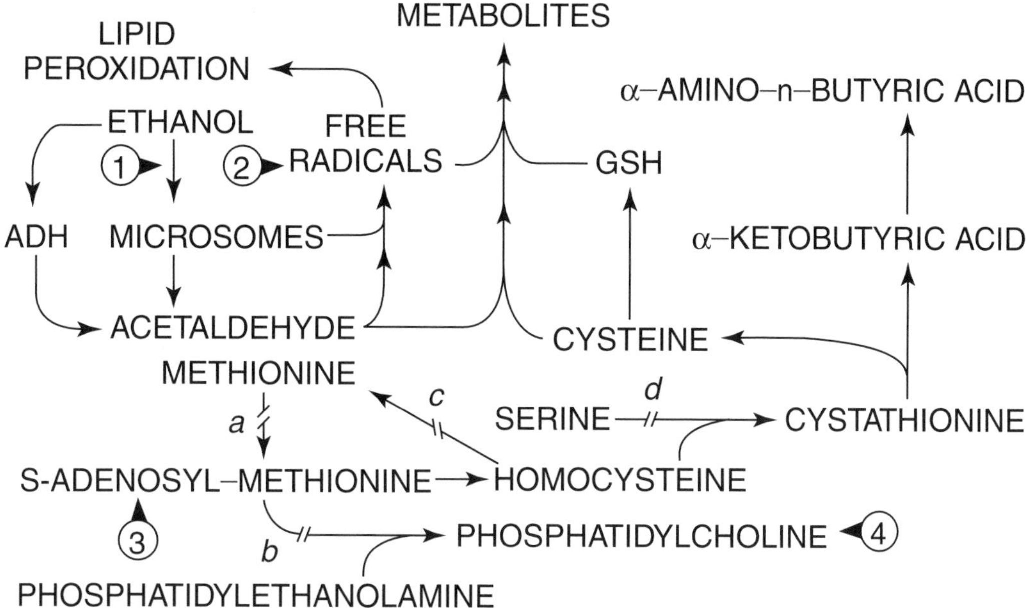

FIGURE 45.4
Lipid peroxidation and other consequences of alcoholic liver disease and/or increased free radical generation and acetaldehyde production by ethanol-induced microsomes, with sites of possible therapeutic interventions. Metabolic blocks caused by liver disease (a,b), folate (c), B_{12} (c) or B_6 (d) deficiencies are illustrated, with corresponding depletions in S-adenosylmethionine, phosphatidylcholine, and glutathione (GSH). New therapeutic approaches include 1) downregulation of microsomal enzyme induction especially of CYP2E1, 2) decrease of free radicals with antioxidants, 3) replenishment of S-adenosylmethionine, and 4) phosphatidylcholine. (From Lieber CS. *J Hepatology*. 32: 113; 2000, with permission.)

Clinical trials revealed that SAMe treatment is beneficial in intrahepatic cholestasis,[165] including recurrent intrahepatic cholestasis and jaundice caused by androgens or estrogens. It was also used successfully in severe cholestasis of pregnancy[166] with few, if any, untoward effects. Oral administration of 1200 mg/day of SAMe for 6 months also resulted in a significant increase of hepatic GSH in patients with alcoholic as well as non-alcoholic liver disease.[167]

The most impressive therapeutic success was achieved in a recent long-term randomized, placebo-controlled, double-blind, multicenter clinical trial of SAMe in patients with alcoholic liver cirrhosis in whom SAMe significantly improved survival or delayed liver transplantation.[168]

Phosphatidylcholine (PC)

In the presence of liver disease, the activity of phosphatidylethanolamine methyltransferase is depressed,[154] with significant pathologic effects. This enzymatic block can again be bypassed through the administration of the product of that reaction, in this case PC[169] (Figure 45.4). This is emerging as potentially important approach to the treatment of liver disease. Indeed, feeding of a mixture rich in polyunsaturated PCs (PPC), especially dilinoleoylphosphatidylcholine (DLPC), which has a high bioavailability, exerted a remarkable protection against alcohol-induced fibrosis and cirrhosis.[170]

PPC contains choline, but in amounts present in PPC, choline had no protective action against the fibrogenic effects of ethanol in the baboon.[171] In primates in general, choline plays a lesser role as a dietary nutrient than in rodents, in part because of lesser choline oxidase activity. In fact, as reviewed elsewhere,[172] choline becomes essential for human nutrition only in severely restricted feeding situations. The decreased phospholipid methyltransferase activity in cirrhotic livers[154] is not simply secondary to the cirrhosis, but may in fact be a primary defect related to alcohol, as suggested by the observation that the enzyme activity is already decreased prior to development of cirrhosis.[169] Another mechanism whereby ethanol may affect phospholipids is increased lipid peroxidation as reflected by increased F_2-isoprostanes,[171] which could explain the associated decrease of arachidonic acid in phospholipids.[173]

One concern was that PPC and DLPC, because of their polyunsaturated nature, may aggravate the oxidative stress, but the opposite was found, both *in vitro* and *in vivo.* In alcohol-fed baboons, PPC not only prevented septal fibrosis and cirrhosis[170] but also resulted in a total protection against oxidative stress, as determined by normalization of 4-hydroxynonenal, F_2-isoprostanes and GSH levels.[174] In patients with hepatitis C, PPC improved the transaminase levels, but the effect on liver fibrosis was not assessed.[175] However, a clinical trial on alcoholic fibrosis is presently ongoing in the U.S.

Toxic Interaction of Alcohol with Nutrients

Adverse Interaction with Retinol

In addition to the classic aspects of vitamin A deficiency due to either poor dietary intake or severe liver disease, direct effects of alcohol on vitamin A metabolism and resulting alterations in hepatic vitamin A levels have been elucidated.[176]

Depletion of Hepatic Vitamin A by Ethanol, its Mechanism and Pathological Consequences

Alcoholic liver disease is associated with severely decreased hepatic vitamin A levels (Figure 45.5), even when liver injury is moderate (fatty liver) and when blood values of vitamin A, retinol binding protein (RBP), and prealbumin are still unaffected.

Malnutrition, when present, can of course contribute to hepatic vitamin A depletion, but the patients with low liver vitamin A in the study of Leo and Lieber[177] appeared well nourished, which suggested a more direct effect of alcohol. Under strictly controlled conditions, chronic ethanol consumption was found to decrease hepatic vitamin A in baboons pair-fed a nutritionally adequate liquid diet containing 50% of total energy either as ethanol or isocaloric carbohydrate. In these baboons, fatty liver developed after 4 months of ethanol feeding, with a 59% decrease in hepatic vitamin A levels, and fibrosis or cirrhosis appeared after 24 to 84 months with a 95% decrease in hepatic vitamin A concentrations.[178] Similarly, hepatic vitamin A levels of rats fed ethanol (36% of total energy) were decreased after 3 weeks (by 42%) and continued to decline up to 9 weeks. In contrast, serum vitamin A and RBP levels were not significantly changed. When dietary vitamin A was increased fivefold, hepatic vitamin A nevertheless decreased in ethanol-fed rats relative to the corresponding controls, and sometimes even compared to the rats given five times less vitamin A (without ethanol).[178] To avoid the confounding effect of dietary vitamin A, it was virtually eliminated in some experiments. Under those conditions, the depletion rate of vitamin A from endogenous hepatic storage was observed to be 2.5 times faster in ethanol-fed rats than in controls.

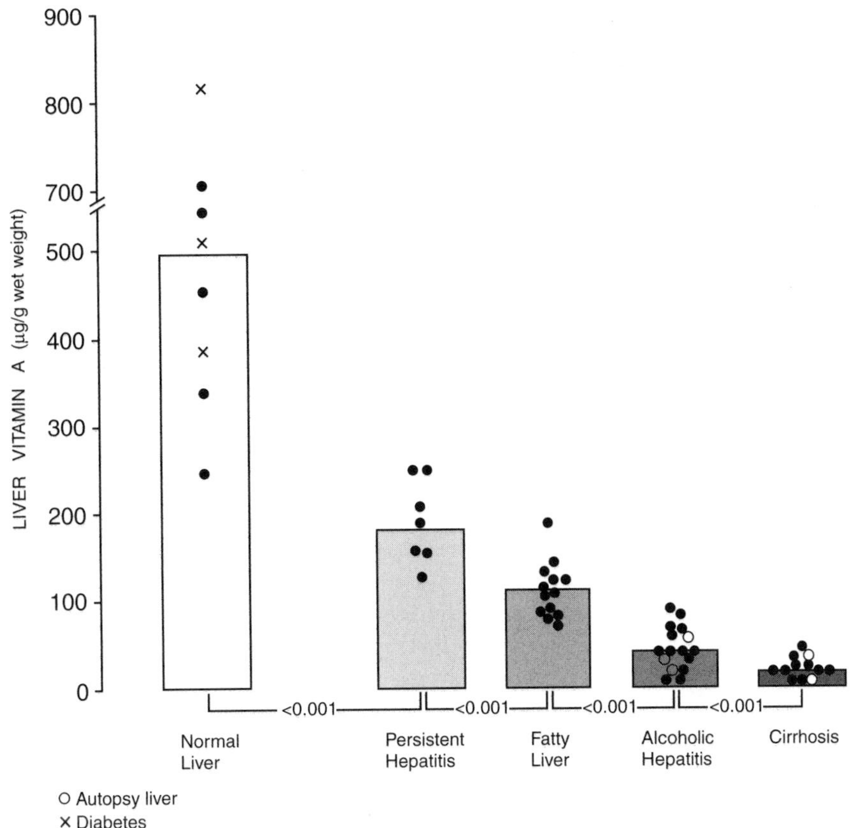

FIGURE 45.5
Hepatic vitamin A levels in subjects with normal livers, chronic persistent hepatitis, and various stages of alcoholic injury (Data from Leo MA, Lieber CS, *N Engl J Med* 307: 597; 1982).

When dietary vitamin A intake was virtually eliminated, the difference in hepatic storage between ethanol-fed rats and controls was much greater than could be accounted for by the total vitamin A intake. Thus, malabsorption was not the only reason for the depletion of hepatic vitamin A. Two possible mechanisms other than malabsorption can be invoked: increased mobilization of vitamin A from the liver, and enhanced catabolism of vitamin A in the liver or in other organs. There is experimental evidence for both.[178-180]

The various pathways involved in hepatic vitamin A metabolism have been reviewed.[181] Drugs that induce the cytochromes P450 in liver microsomes were shown to result in a depletion of hepatic vitamin A.[182] A similar effect was observed after administration of ethanol[177,178] and other xenobiotics that are known to interact with liver microsomes, including carcinogens.[183] The hepatic depletion was strikingly exacerbated when ethanol and drugs were combined,[184] which mimicks a common clinical occurrence.

Retinoic acid has been shown to be degraded in microsomes of hamsters[185] and rats.[180,186] In both species, the reported activity was very low compared to the degree of hepatic vitamin A depletion. These observations prompted the search for alternate pathways of retinol metabolism, and two new pathways of retinol metabolism were described: rat liver microsomes, when fortified with NADPH, converted retinol to polar metabolites, including 4-hydroxyretinol.[186] This activity was also demonstrated in a reconstituted monooxygenase system containing purified forms of rat cytochromes P-450,[187] including P4502B1 (a phenobarbital-inducible isozyme). More recently, it has been shown that other cytochromes (such as P450 CYP 1A1) also catalyze the conversion of retinal to retinoic acid.[188] In addition, a new microsomal NAD^+-dependent retinol dehydrogenase was described.[189] The classic pathway for the conversion of retinol to retinal in the liver involves a cytosolic NAD-dependent retinol dehydrogenase (CRD), believed to be similar, if not identical, to the liver cytosolic alcohol dehydrogenase (ADH, alcohol: NAD^- oxidoreductase, EC 1.1.1.1). The observation that a strain of deermice lacks this enzyme without apparent adverse effects[190] prompted a search for an alternate pathway for the production of retinal, the precursor of retinoic acid. Evidence was obtained for the existence of a NAD-dependent microsomal retinol dehydrogenase (MRD)[189] which can convert retinol to retinal using NAD, and retinal to retinol using NADH as cofactors. The activity of the retinol[189] as well as the retinal[191] dehydrogenases is inducible by chronic alcohol consumption, thereby contributing to hepatic vitamin A depletion. Finally, metabolism of retinol and retinoic acid was also demonstrated with human liver microsomes and purified cytochrome P-4502C8.[191]

In patients with severe as well as moderate depletion of hepatic vitamin A, multivesicular lysosome-like organelles were detected in increased numbers.[192] That a low hepatic vitamin A concentration contributes to these lesions was also verified experimentally in rats.[193]

Hepatic vitamin A depletion plays a key role in hepatic fibrosis, and both hepatocytes and stellate cells are involved. Hepatic stellate cells are the principal storage site of vitamin A. The activation of stellate cells into myofibroblast-like cells, which then synthesize collagen, is associated with a decrease in vitamin A storage in these cells.[194] Retinoic acid, and to a lesser extent retinol, were shown to reduce stellate cell proliferation and collagen production in culture.[194-196] Conversely, lack of retinoids could promote fibrosis in these tissues, especially in the liver, consistent with the associated activation of stellate cells.[194] Paradoxically, however, vitamin A excess may also promote fibrosis (*vide infra).*

Concomitant ethanol consumption and vitamin A deficiency resulted in an increased severity of squamous metaplasia of the trachea.[197,198] This potentiation of vitamin A deficiency by alcohol may predispose the tracheal epithelium to neoplastic transformation.

A relatively high risk of squamous cell carcinoma of the lung was found in a Norwegian population that drank large amounts of alcohol and had a low dietary intake of vitamin A.[199] Furthermore, a positive association of alcohol consumption with lung cancer has been reported in Japanese men in Hawaii.[200] In addition, ethanol-induced vitamin A depletion is associated with decreased detoxification of xenobiotics, including carcinogens such as nitrosodimethylamine,[201] thereby playing a role in chemical carcinogenesis (*vide supra).* Recent data also suggest that functional downregulation of retinoic acid receptors, by inhibiting biosynthesis of retinoic acid and upregulating activator protein-1 (c-Jun and c-Fos) gene expression, may be important mechanisms for causing malignant transformation by ethanol.[202]

In addition to promoting vitamin A depletion, ethanol may interfere more directly with retinoic acid synthesis, since both were shown *in vitro* to serve as substrates for the same enzymes.[203] Specifically, one of the mechanisms by which ethanol induces gastrointestinal cancer may be an inhibition of ADH-catalyzed gastrointestinal retinoic acid synthesis which is needed for epithelial differentiation. Indeed, class I ADH (ADH-I) and class IV ADH (ADH-IV) function as retinol dehydrogenases *in vitro* and are abundantly distributed along the GI tract.[204] Deficiency of retinoic acids can produce birth defects and, as discussed above, ethanol promotes deficiency of retinoids. Duester[203,205] and Pullarkat[206] implicated competitive inhibition by ethanol of the biosynthesis of retinoic acid from retinol, since class I alcohol dehydrogenase (E.C. 1.1.1.1) can contribute to the biosynthesis of retinoic acid from retinol. Indeed, this group identified one human ADH isozyme that exists in the affected embryonic tissues to act as a retinol dehydrogenase catalyzing the synthesis of retinoic acid. Ethanol did, in fact, reduce RA levels in cultured mouse embryos.[207]

However, other results[208] failed to verify, in conceptal tissues, that competitive inhibition of the conversion of retinol to retinoic acid is a significant factor in ethanol-induced embryotoxicity. More recently, Kedishvili et al.[209] characterized an ADH enzyme (ADH-F) that oxidizes all-*trans*-retinol and steroid alcohols in fetal tissues.

Abnormalities Associated with Excess Vitamin A

Vitamin A deficiency promotes carcinogenesis (*vide supra*), but paradoxically, vitamin A excess may have a similar effect: Tuyns et al.[210] and DeCarli et al[211] noted that foods providing large amounts of retinol increase the risk of cancer of the esophagus, and in an epidemiologic study the increased cancer risk associated with the use of cigarettes and alcohol was enhanced upon ingestion of foods containing retinol.[212] Other food constituents could also play a role in that regard.

The teratogenic potential of excessive intake of retinoid has been clearly demonstrated in experimental animals,[213] with corresponding data evolving in humans: teratogenicity of 13-*cis*-retinoic acid, used to treat cystic acne, has been established in epidemiological studies.[214] In addition, among babies born to women who took more than 10,000 IU of preformed vitamin A per day as supplements, about 1 infant in 57 had a malformation.[215] However, some caution in the interpretation of these data is still indicated.[216] Furthermore, acetaldehyde can cross the placenta[217] and may also contribute to the development of the fetal alcohol syndrome, the most prevalent cause of preventable congenital abnormality.[218] Therefore, in addition to potentiating the teratogenicity of vitamin A deficiency, alcohol can be expected to aggravate that of vitamin A excess, and this was indeed verified experimentally.[219]

An excess of vitamin A is also known to be hepatotoxic.[220,221] The smallest daily supplement of vitamin A reported to be associated with liver cirrhosis is 7500 μg RE (25,000 IU) taken for 6 years.[222] These supplements fall well within common therapeutic dosages and amounts used prophylactically with over-the-counter preparations by the population at large.

Potentiation of vitamin A hepatotoxicity by ethanol was first demonstrated in rats fed diets for two months with either normal or fivefold increased vitamin A content, both with and without ethanol.[223] Whereas under these conditions ethanol alone produced only modest changes and vitamin A supplementation at the dose used had no adverse effect, the combination resulted in striking lesions, with giant mitochondria containing paracrystalline filamentous inclusions and depression of oxygen consumption in state 3 respiration with five different substrates. The potentiation of vitamin A toxicity by ethanol was also seen in patients treated with 10,000 IU vitamin A per day for sexual dysfunction attributable to excess alcohol consumption.[224] In addition to giant mitochondria, filamentous or crystalline-like inclusions were seen in the liver mitochondria of patients with hypervitaminosis A.[225,226] The potentiation of vitamin A toxicity by ethanol was most dramatically documented in another study in which rats were given a combination of vitamin A supplementation and ethanol for up to nine months.[227] There was striking hepatic inflammation and necrosis, accompanied by a rise in the serum level of liver enzymes (glutamic dehydrogenase and AST).

Since retinol, retinal, and retinoic acid can be further metabolized by liver microsomes, particularly when the latter system is induced by chronic ethanol consumption,[180,186,187,189] one can postulate that some of these metabolites produced in increased amounts (possibly by some specific forms of cytochrome P-450) might also participate in the enhanced toxicity, but at the present time direct experimental evidence to support such a hypothesis is lacking.

Adverse Interactions of Ethanol with β-Carotene

In contrast with retinoids, carotenoids were not known to produce toxic manifestations, even when ingested chronically in large amounts.[228] Therefore, it made sense to assess whether carotenoids may serve as effective (but less toxic) substitutes for retinol, especially in alcoholic liver injury which has been attributed, in part, to oxidative stress, and since β-carotene is an antioxidant. It was not known, however, whether β-carotene can actually offset alcohol-induced lipid peroxidation.

Effects of Alcohol on β-Carotene Concentrations

Studies in man revealed that for a given β-carotene intake, there is a correlation between alcohol consumption and plasma β-carotene concentration.[229] Thus, whereas in general, alcoholics have low plasma β-carotene levels,[229,230] presumably reflecting low intake, alcohol *per se* might in fact increase blood levels in man.[229] There was also an increase in women with a dose as low as two drinks a day.[231] Furthermore, there was an increase in non-human primates studied under strictly controlled conditions.[232] Indeed, in baboons fed ethanol chronically, liver β-carotene was increased, in contrast with vitamin A, which was depleted. Similarly, plasma β-carotene levels were elevated in these ethanol-fed baboons, with a striking delay in the clearance from the blood after a β-carotene load. Whereas β-carotene administration increased hepatic vitamin A in control baboons, this effect was much less evident in alcohol-fed animals. The combination of an increase in β-carotene and a relative lack of a corresponding rise in vitamin A suggests a blockage in the conversion of β-carotene to vitamin A by ethanol.

β-Carotene, Alcohol, Oxidative Stress, and Liver Injury

In the baboon, the administration of ethanol together with β-carotene resulted in a more striking hepatic injury than with either compound alone,[232] with increased activity of liver enzymes in the plasma, an inflammatory response in the liver and, at the ultrastructural level, striking autophagic vacuoles and alterations of the endoplasmic reticulum and the mitochondria.[233] The ethanol-induced oxidative stress, assessed by an increase in hepatic 4-hydroxynonenal and F_2-isoprostanes (measured by gas chromatography-mass spectrometry), was not improved despite a concomitant rise in hepatic antioxidants (β-carotene and vitamin E).

Extrahepatic Side Effects

Cardiovascular Complications

There was no evidence of lower mortality from cardiovascular disease or other causes following β-carotene supplementation.[234] Similarly, the study of Hennekens et al.[235] ruled out the possibility that there was even a slight reduction in the incidence of mortality from cardiovascular disease with supplementation of 50 mg β-carotene on every other day, for an average of 12 years. Recent results even suggest that β-carotene participates as a pro-oxidant in the oxidative degradation of low density lipoprotein (LDL), and that increased LDL β-carotene may cancel the protective qualities of α-tocopherol.[236]

In the Alpha-Tocopherol, Beta-Carotene and Cancer Prevention (ATBC) Study[237] and the Beta-Carotene and Retinol Efficacy Trial (CARET),[238] it was noted that in smokers, β-carotene supplementation increased death from coronary heart disease.

Interaction with Cancer

Two epidemiologic investigations, namely both the ATBC[237] and the CARET[238] studies, revealed that β-carotene supplementation increases the incidence of pulmonary cancer in smokers. Because heavy smokers are commonly heavy drinkers, we raised the possibility that alcohol abuse was contributory,[239] since alcohol is known to act as a carcinogen and to exacerbate the carcinogenicity of other xenobiotics, especially those of tobacco smoke.[240] Why this should be aggravated by β-carotene is not clear, but β-carotene was found in rat lung to produce a powerful booster effect on phase I carcinogen-bioactivating enzymes, including activators of polycyclic aromatic hydrocarbons (PAHs).[241,242] In addition, since pulmonary cells are exposed to relatively high oxygen pressures, and because β-carotene loses its antioxidant activity and shows an autocatalytic, pro-oxidant effect at these higher pressures,[243] such an interaction is at least plausible and deserves further study, especially since recent studies showed that β-carotene protects against oxidative damage in HT29 cells at low concentrations but rapidly loses this capacity at higher doses,[244] and that β-carotene enhances hydrogen peroxide-induced DNA damage in human hepatocellular HepG2 cells.[245] Furthermore, the more recent publications of the ATBC and CARET studies showed that the increased incidence of pulmonary cancer was related to the amount of alcohol consumed by the participants.[246-248]

Concentrations of carotenoids, retinoids, and tocopherols were also determined in the homogenate of macroscopically normal-appearing oropharygeal mucosa from chronic alcoholics and control patients. All the alcoholics except one had oropharyngeal cancer. No significant difference was found in tissue levels of carotenoids and tocopherols between alcoholics and controls. Furthermore, in 7 of 11 controls, retinol was undetectable in the oropharyngeal mucosa, while in the alcoholics only 2 out of 10 had unmeasurable retinol levels.[249] These results did not support the concept that ethanol-associated oropharyngeal carcinogenesis is due, at least in part, to local deficiencies in retinoids, carotenoids, or α-tocopherol.

Contrasting with the investigations showing a lack of beneficial effects of β-carotene supplementation (reviewed above), β-carotene was found to inhibit rat liver chromosomal aberrations and DNA chain break after a single injection of diethylnitrosamine.[250] Furthermore, a study of nonmelanocytic skin cancer showed that a high intake of vegetables and other β-carotene-containing foods is protective for nonmelanocytic skin cancers.[251] Conversely, Menkes et al.[252] showed an association between low levels of serum β-carotene and the risk of squamous cell carcinoma of the lung. However, the latter two observations do not necessarily prove a causal link, since the beneficial effects may be associated with active nutrients other than β-carotene.

Therapeutic Window of Retinoids and Carotenoids

As already mentioned, vitamin A deficiency aggravates alcohol-induced liver injury, fetal-alcohol syndrome, and carcinogenesis. Vitamin A deficiency results not only from a poor dietary intake, but may also derive from direct effects of ethanol on the breakdown of retinol in the liver. Supplementation of vitamin A in the heavy drinker may thus be indicated, but is complicated by the intrinsic hepatotoxicity of large amounts of vitamin A, which is strikingly potentiated by concomitant alcohol use. β-carotene is a precursor and a nontoxic substitute for retinol, but ethanol interferes with its conversion to vitamin A, and even moderate alcohol intake can result in increased levels of β-carotene when the latter is given in commonly used dosage for supplementation. Side effects observed under these conditions include hepatotoxicity, promotion of pulmonary cancer, and possibly cardiovascular complications. Thus, detrimental effects result from deficiency as well as from excess of retinoids and carotenoids, and paradoxically, both have similar adverse effects in terms of fibrosis, carcinogenesis, and possibly embryotoxicity. Treatment efforts therefore must carefully respect the resulting narrow therapeutic window, especially for drinkers in whom alcohol narrows this therapeutic window even further by promoting the depletion of retinoids and potentiating their toxicity.

Effects of Ethanol on the Metabolism of Proteins

As reviewed elsewhere,[253] ethanol given in single doses causes impaired hepatic amino acid uptake, decreased leucine oxidation,[254] increased serum branched chain amino acids, and impaired synthesis of lipoproteins, albumin,[255-258] and fibrinogen.[254] Given chronically, ethanol causes impaired protein secretion from the liver, probably related to alterations in microtubules and retention of proteins in enlarged hepatocytes.[259] It promotes protein catabolism in the heart[260] and gastrointestinal tract.[261]

Effects of Dietary Factors on Ethanol Metabolism

Low-protein diets reduce hepatic ADH in rats[262] and lower ethanol oxidation rates in rats[262] and man.[263] Prolonged fasting also decreases ethanol oxidation rates as shown in isolated rat liver cells. A mechanism for lowered metabolism of ethanol during fasting is the lack of available metabolites to shuttle reducing equivalents from ethanol oxidation into mitochondria.[264] For a given alcohol intake, malnourished alcoholics may develop higher blood alcohol levels and sustain them longer than normally nourished individuals.[265]

In rats, MEOS activity in the liver showed greater induction by alcohol on a normal than a low-fat diet, although induction of CYP2E1 was the same.[266]

Nutritional Therapy in Alcoholism

Individuals consuming over 30% of total kcalories as alcohol have a high probability of ingesting less than the recommended daily amounts of carbohydrate, protein, fat, vitamins A, C, and B (especially thiamin), and minerals such as calcium and iron (*vide supra*). It is sensible to recommend a complete diet comparable to that of nonalcoholics to forestall deficiency syndromes, although this does not suffice to prevent some organ damage due to the direct toxicity of alcohol (e.g., alcoholic liver disease).

Damage due to lack of thiamin is serious but treatable with a great margin of safety; therefore thiamin deficiency should be presumed and, if not definitely disproved, parenteral therapy with 50 mg of thiamin per day should be given until similar doses can be taken by mouth. Riboflavin and pyridoxine should be routinely administered at the dosages usually contained in standard multivitamin preparations. Adequate folic acid replacement can be accomplished with the usual hospital diet. Additional replacement is optional unless deficiency is severe. Vitamin A replacement should only be given for well-documented deficiency, and to patients whose abstinence from alcohol is assured.

Zinc replacement is indicated only for night blindness unresponsive to vitamin A replacement. Magnesium replacement is recommended for symptomatic patients with low serum magnesium. Iron deficiency that has been clearly diagnosed may be corrected orally.

The nutritional management of acute and chronic liver disease due to alcoholism should include feeding programs to achieve protein replenishment without promoting hepatic encephalopathy, as reviewed elsewhere.[1]

Acute pancreatitis may require withholding oral feeding for prolonged periods, during which time venous alimentation must be given. Chronic pancreatic exocrine insufficiency is treated by dietary manipulation (including decreases in fat) with oral pancreatic enzymes at mealtime. In addition to defining feeding programs to reverse malnutrition, the nutritional management of liver disease due to alcoholism must take into account that, because of the alcohol-induced disease process, some of the nutritional requirements change. This is exemplified by methionine which normally is one of the essential amino acids for humans, but needs to be activated to SAMe, a process impaired by the disease. Thus, SAMe rather than methionine is the compound to be used for supplementation in the presence of significant liver disease, and a resulting prolonged survival has now been documented[16] (*vide supra*). Similarly, because of an impairment in phosphatidylethanolamine methyltransferase activity, supplementation with phosphatidylcholine, particularly the highly bioavailable DLPC, may be useful for prevention and treatment (*vide supra*).

Acknowledgment

Modified from *Annual Review of Nutrition*, Lieber, C.S. 20: 395; 3000 (with permission).

References

1. Lieber CS. *Medical and Nutritional Complications of Alcoholism: Mechanisms and Management.* New York, Plenum Press, 1992, p 579.
2. Perlow W, Baraona E, Lieber CS. *Gastroenterology* 72: 680; 1977.
3. Best CH, Hartroft WS, Lucas CC, Ridout JH. *Br Med J* 2: 1001; 1949.
4. Lieber CS, Jones DP, DeCarli LM. *J Clin Invest* 44: 1009; 1965.
5. Lieber CS, Jones DP, Mendelson J, DeCarli LM. *Trans Assoc Am Phys* 76: 289; 1963.
6. DeCarli LM, Lieber CS. *J Nutr* 91: 331; 1967.
7. Lieber CS, DeCarli LM. *J Med Primatol* 3: 153; 1974.
8. Lieber CS, Spritz N, DeCarli LM. *J Lipid Reds* 10: 283; 1969.
9. Lieber CS, DeCarli LM, Gang H, et al. In: *Medical Primatology,* Part III. Goldsmith EI, Moor-Jankowski J, Eds, Basel: Karger, 1972, p 270.
10. Lieber CS, Rubin E. *Am J Med* 44: 200; 1968.
11. Bjorkhem I. *Eur J Biochem* 30: 441; 1972.
12. Bosron WF, Ehrig T, Li T-K. *Seminars in Liver Disease* 13: 126; 1993.
13. Faller J, Fox IH. *N Engl J Med* 307: 1598; 1982.
14. Lieber CS, Schmid R. *J Clin Invest* 40: 394; 1961.
15. Lieber CS, DeCarli LM, Schmid R. *Biochem Biophys Res Comm* 1: 302; 1959.
16. Galli A, Price D, Crabb D. *Hepatology* 29: 1164; 1999.
17. Hernández-Muñoz R, Caballeria J, Baraona E, et al. *Alcohol: Clin Exp Res* 14: 946; 1990.
18. Stone CL, Thomas HR, Bosron WF, Li T-K. *Alcohol: Clin Exp Res* 17: 911; 1993.
19. Yokoyama H, Baraona E, Lieber CS. *Biochem Biophys Res Comm* 203: 219; 1994.

20. Farrés J, Moreno A, Crosas B, et al. *Eur J Biochem* 224: 549; 1994.
21. Yokoyama H, Baraona E, Lieber CS. *Genomics* 31: 243; 1996.
22. Mirmiran-Yazdy SA, Haber PS, Korsten MA, et al. *Gastroenterology* 108: 737; 1995.
23. Haber PS, Gentry T, Mak KM, et al. *Gastroenterology* 111: 863; 1996.
24. Julkunen RJK, DiPadova C, Lieber CS. *Life Sci* 37: 567; 1985.
25. Julkunen RJK, Tannenbaum L, Baraona E, Lieber CS. *Alcohol* 2: 437; 1985.
26. Levitt MD, Levitt DG. *J Pharmacol Exp Ther* 269: 297; 1993.
27. Lieber CS, Gentry RT, Baraona E. In: *The Biology of Alcohol Problems*, Saunders JB, Whitfield JB, Eds, UK Elsevier Science Publishers, 1996, p 315.
28. Sato N, Kitamura T. *Gastroenterology* 111: 1143; 1996.
29. Caballeria J, Baraona E, Lieber CS. *Life Sci* 41: 1021; 1987.
30. Lim Jr RT, Gentry RT, Ito D, et al. *Alcohol: Clin Exp Res* 17: 1337; 1993.
31. DiPadova C, Worner TM, Julkunen RJK, Lieber CS. *Gastroenterology* 92: 1169; 1987.
32. Caballeria J, Frezza M, Hernández-Muñoz R, et al. *Gastroenterology* 97: 1205; 1989.
33. Baraona E, Yokoyama A, Ishii H, et al. *Life Sci* 49: 1929; 1991.
34. Dohmen K, Baraona E, Ishibadsshi H, et al. *Alcohol: Clin Exp Res* 20: 1569; 1996.
35. Battiston L, Moretti M, Tulissi P, et al. *Life Sci* 56: 241; 1994.
36. Imuro Y, Bradford BU, Forman DT, Thurman RG. *Gastroenterology* 110: 1536; 1996.
37. Day CP, Bashir R, James OF, et al. *Hepatology* 14: 798 and 15: 750; 1991.
38. Poupon RE, Nalpas B, Coutelle C, et al. *Hepatology* 15: 1017; 1992.
39. Lieber CS. *Physiol Rev* 77: 517; 1997.
40. Lieber CS. *Alcohol: Clin Exp Res* 23: 991; 1999.
41. Lieber CS, DeCarli LM. *Science* 162: 917; 1968.
42. Lieber CS, DeCarli LM. *J Biol Chem* 245: 2505; 1970.
43. Tsutsumi M, Lasker JM, Shimizu M, et al. *Hepatology* 10: 437; 1989.
44. Takahashi T, Lasker JM, Rosman AS, Lieber CS. *Hepatology* 17: 236; 1993.
45. Salmela KS, Kessova IG, Tsyrlov IB, Lieber CS. *Alcohol: Clin Exp Res* 22: 2125; 1998.
46. Misra PS, Lefevre A, Ishii H, et al. *Am J Med* 51: 346; 1971.
47. Hetu C, Joly J-G. *Biochem Pharmacol* 34: 1211; 1985.
48. Teschke R, Moreno F, Petrides AS. *Biochem Pharmacol* 30: 45; 1981.
49. Joly J-G, Hetu C. *Biochem Pharmacol* l24: 1475; 1975.
50. Mitchell JR, Mack C, Mezey E, Maddrey WC. *Hepatology* 1: 336; 1981.
51. Laethem RM, Balaxy M, Falck JR, et al. *J Biol Chem* 268: 12912; 1993.
52. Amet Y, Berthou F, Goasduff T, et al. *Biochem Biophys Res Comm* 203: 1168; 1994.
53. Adas F, Betthou F, Picart D. *J Lipid Res* 39: 1210; 1998.
54. Koop DR, Casazza JP. *J Biol Chem* 260: 13607; 1985.
55. Koop DR, Crump BL, Nordblom GD, Coon MJ. *Toxicol Appl Pharmacol* 98: 278; 1989.
56. Yang CS, Yoo J-S, Ishizaki H, Hong J. *Drug Metab Rev* 22: 147; 1990.
57. Raucy JL, Lasker JM, Kramer JC, et al. *Molec Pharmacol* 39: 275; 1991.
58. Weltman MD, Farrell GC, Hall P, et al. *Hepatology* 27: 128; 1998.
59. Tsutsumi M, Leo MA, Kim C, et al. *Alcohol: Clin Exp Res* 14: 174; 1990.
60. Sato C, Nakano M, Lieber CS. *Gastroenterology* 80: 140; 1981.
61. Whitecomb DC, Block GD. *JAMA* 272: 1845; 1994.
62. Morton S, Mitchell MC. *Biochem Pharmacol* 34: 1559; 1985.
63. Speisky H, MacDonald A, Giles G, et al. *Biochem J* 225: 565; 1985.
64. Hirano T, Kaplowitz N, Tsukamoto H, et al. *Hepatology* 6: 1423; 1992.
65. Leo MA, Rosman A, Lieber CS. *Hepatology* 17: 977; 1993.
66. Lieber CS, Casini A, DeCarli LM, et al. *Hepatology* 11: 165; 1990.
67. Lieber CS. J *Hepatology* 30: 1155; 1999.
68. Aleynik MK, Leo MA, Aleynik SI, Lieber CS. *Alcohol: Clin Exp Res* 23: 96; 1999.
69. Patek AJ, Toth EG, Saunders ME, et al. *Arch Intern Med* 135: 1053; 1975.
70. Iber FL. *Nutr Today* 6: 2; 1971.
71. Mendenhall C, Bongiovanni G, Goldberg S, et al. *J Parenter Enteral Nutr* 9: 590; 1985.
72. Morgan MY. *Acta Chir Scand* 507: 81; 1981.
73. Simko V, Connell AM, Banks B. *Am J Clin Nutr* 35: 197; 1982.

74. World MJ, Ryle PR, Jones D, et al. *Alcohol Alcoholism* 19: 281; 1984.
75. World MJ, Ryle PR, Pratt OE, Thompson AD. *Alcohol Alcoholism* 19: 1; 1984.
76. Liu S, Serdula MK, Williamson DF, et al. *Am J Epidemiol* 140: 912; 1994.
77. Armellini F, Zamboni M, Frigo L, et al. *Eur J Clin Nutr* 47: 52; 1993.
78. Tremblay A, Buemann B, Theriault G, Bouchard C. *Eur J Clin Nutr* 49: 824; 1995.
79. Bebb HT, Houser HB, Witschi JC, et al. *Am J Clin Nutr* 24: 1042; 1971.
80. Neville JN, Eagles JA, Samson G, Olson RE. *Am J Clin Nutr* 21: 1329; 1968.
81. Gruchow HW, Sobociaski KA, Barboriak JJ. *JAMA* 253: 1567; 1985.
82. Lieber CS. *Am J Clin Nutr* 54: 976; 1991.
83. Hillers VN, Massey LK. *Am J Clin Nutr* 41: 356; 1985.
84. Westerfeld WW, Schulman MP. *JAMA* 170: 197; 1959.
85. Bonjour JP. *Int J Vitamin Nutr* 49: 434; 1979.
86. Gruchow HW, Sobocinski KA, Barboriak JJ, Scheller JG. *Am J Clin Nutr* 42: 289; 1985.
87. Saville PD. *J Bone Joint Surg [Am]* 47: 492; 1965.
88. Gascon-Barre M. *J Am Coll Nutr* 4: 565; 1985.
89. Nilsson BE. *Acta Chir Scand* 136: 383; 1970.
90. Solomon L. *J Bone Joint Surg [Br]* 55: 246; 1973.
91. Reisenauer AM, Buffington CAT, Villanueva JA, Halsted CH. *Am J Clin Nutr* 50: 1429; 1989.
92. Naughton CA, Chandler CJ, Duplantier RB, Halsted CH. *Am J Clin Nutr* 50: 1436; 1989.
93. Said HM, Strum WB. *Digestion* 35: 129; 1986.
94. Halsted CH, Robles EZ, Mezey E. *N Engl J Med* 285: 701; 1971.
95. Racusen LC, Krawitt EL. *Am J Dig Dis* 22: 915; 1977.
96. Lindenbaum J, Lieber CS. In *Medical Disorders of Alcoholism. Pathogenesis and Treatment.* Vol. 22. Lieber CS, Ed, Philadelphia, W.B. Saunders, 1982, p 313.
97. Sullivan LW, Herbert V. *J Clin Invest* 43: 2048; 1964.
98. Russell RM, Rosenberg IH, Wilson PD, et al. *Am J Clin Nutr* 38: 64; 1983.
99. Tamura T, Romero JJ, Watson JE, et al. *J Lab Clin Med* 97: 654; 1981.
100. Tamura T, Halsted CH. *J Lab Clin Med* 101: 623; 1983.
101. Herbert V, Zalusky R, Davidson CS. *Ann Intern Med* 58: 977; 1963.
102. Klipstein FA, Lindenbaum J. *Blood* 25: 443; 1965.
103. Herzlich B, Herbert V. *Am J Gastroenterol* 81: 678; 1986.
104. Lindenbaum J, Lieber CS. *Ann NY Acad Sci* 252: 228; 1975.
105. Lindenbaum J, Saha JR, Shea N, Lieber CS. *Gastroenterology* 64: 762; 1973.
106. Findlay J, Sellers E, Forstner G. *Can J Physiol Pharmacol* 54: 469; 1976.
107. van der Beek, EJ, Lowik MR, Hulshof KF, Kistemaker C. *J Am Coll Nutr* 13: 383; 1994.
108. Rosenthal WS, Adham NF, Lopez R, Cooperman JM. *Am J Clin Nutr* 26: 858; 1973.
109. Kim C-I, Roe DA. *Drug-Nutr Interact* 3: 99; 1985.
110. Marotta F, Labadarios D, Frazer L, et al. *Dig Dis Sci* 39: 993; 1994.
111. Bjørneboe GE, Bjørneboe A, Hagen BF, et al. *Biochim Biophys Acta* 918: 236; 1987.
112. Kawase T, Kato S, Lieber CS. *Hepatology* 10: 815; 1989.
113. McColister R, Prasad AS, Doe RP. *J Lab Clin Med* 52: 928; 1958.
114. Flink EB. *Alcohol: Clin Exp Res* 10: 590; 1986.
115. Abbott L, Nadler J, Rude RK. *Alcohol: Clin Exp Res* 18: 1076; 1994.
116. Wu C, Kenny MA. *Clin Chem* 42: 625; 1996.
117. Volini F, de la Huerga J, Kent G, et al. In *Laboratory Diagnosis of Liver Disease,* Sunderman FW, Sunderman FW Jr, Eds, St. Louis, W.H. Green, 1968, p 199-206.
118. Chapman RW, Morgan MY, Bell R, Sherlock S. *Gastroenterology* 84: 143; 1983.
119. Chapman RW, Morgan MY, Boss AM, Sherlock S. *Dig Dis Sci* 28: 321; 1983.
120. Olynk J, Hall P, Sallie R, et al. *Hepatology* 12: 26; 1990.
121. Bacon BR, Britton S. *Hepatology* 11: 127; 1990.
122. Chojkier M, Houglum K, Solis-Herruzo J, Brenner DA. *J Biol Chem* 264: 16957; 1989.
123. Vallee BL, Wacker WEC, Bartholomay AF, Robin ED. *N Engl J Med* 255: 403; 1956.
124. Vallee BL, Wacker EC, Bartholomay AF, Hock F. *N Engl J Med* 257: 1055; 1957.
125. Sullivan JF. *Gastroenterology* 42: 439; 1962.
126. Sullivan JF. *QJ Stud Alcohol* 23: 216; 1962.

127. Sandstead HH. *Am J Clin Nutr* 26: 1251; 1973.
128. Valberg LS, Flanagan PR, Ghent CN, Chamberlain MJ. *Dig Dis Sci* 30: 329; 1985.
129. Poo JL, Rosas-Romero R, Rodriguez F, et al. *Dig Dis* 13: 136; 1995.
130. Hartoma TR, Sontaniemi RA, Pelkonen O, Ahlqvist J. *Eur J Clin Pharmacol* 12: 147; 1977.
131. Sullivan JF, Williams RV, Burch RE. *Alcohol: Clin Exp Res* 3: 235; 1979.
132. Szutowski MM, Lipsaka M, Bandolet JP. *Polish J Pharmacol Pharm* 28: 397; 1976.
133. Versieck J, Hoste J, Vanballenberghe L, et al. *J Lab Clin Med* 97: 535; 1981.
134. Marin GA, Ward NL, Fischer R. *Dig Dis* 18: 825; 1973.
135. Lefevre A, DeCarli LM, Lieber CS. *J Lipid Res* 13: 48; 1972.
136. Knodell RG, Kinsey D, Boedeker EC, Collin D. *Gastroenterology* 71: 196; 1976.
137. Thomson AD, Majumdar SK. *Clin Gastroenterol* 10: 263; 1981.
138. Breen KJ, Buttigieg R, Lossifidis S, et al. *Am J Clin Nutr* 42: 121; 1985.
139. Katz D, Metz J, van der Westhuyzen J. *Am J Clin Nutr* 42: 666; 1985.
140. Lumeng L, Li T-K. *J Clin Invest* 53: 693; 1974.
141. Fonda ML, Brown SG, Pendleton MW. *Alcohol: Clin Exp Res* 3: 804; 1989.
142. Lumeng LJ. *J Clin Invest* 62: 286; 1978.
143. Vech RL, Lumeng L, Li TK. *J Clin Invest* 55: 1026; 1975.
144. Parker TH, Marshall JP, Roberts RK, et al. *Am J Clin Nutr* 32: 1246; 1979.
145. Lumeng L, Schenker S, Li T-K, et al. J *Lab Clin Med* 103: 59; 1984.
146. Finkelstein JD, Martin JJ. *J Biol Chem* 261: 1582; 1986.
147. Hardwick DF, Applegarth DA, Cockcroft DM, et al. *Metabolism* 19: 381; 1970.
148. Iob V, Coon WW, Sloan W. *J Surgical Res* 7: 41; 1967.
149. Fischer JE, Yoshimura N, Aguirre A, et al. *Am J Surgery* 127: 40; 1974.
150. Iber FL, Rosen H, Stanley MA, et al. *J Lab Clin Med* 50: 417; 1957.
151. Montanari A, Simoni I, Vallisa D, et al. *Hepatology* 8: 1034; 1988.
152. Kinsell L, Harper HA, Barton HC, et al. *Science* 106: 589; 1947.
153. Horowitz JH, Rypins EB, Henderson JM, et al. *Gastroenterology* 81: 668; 1981.
154. Duce AM, Ortiz P, Cabrero C, Mato JM. *Hepatology* 8: 65; 1988.
155. Lu SC. *Gastroenterology* 114: 403; 1998.
156. Avila MA, Carretero V, Rodriguez N, Mato J. *Gastroenterology* 114: 364; 1998.
157. Finkelstein JD, Cello FP, Kyle WE. *Biochem Biophys Res Commun* 61: 475; 1974.
158. Hirata F, Axelrod J. *Science* 209: 1082; 1980.
159. Hirata F, Viveros OH, Diliberto EJ Jr, Axelrod J. *Proc Natl Acad Sci* 75: 1718; 1978.
160. Yamada S, Mak KM, Lieber CS. *Gastroenterology* 88: 1799; 1985.
161. Stramentinoli G, Gualano M, Galli-Kienle G. *J Pharmacol Exp Ther* 209: 323; 1979.
162. Bornbardieri G, Pappalardo G, Bernardi L, et al. *Int J Clin Pharmacol Therapy Toxicol* 21: 186; 1983.
163. Hoffinan DR, Marion DW, Cornatzer WE, Duerra JA. *J Biol Chem* 255: 10822; 1980.
164. Giulidori P, Stramentinoli G. *Anal Biochem* 137: 217; 1984.
165. Giudici GA, Le Grazie C, Di Padova C. In *Methionine Metabolism: Molecular Mechanism and Clinical Implications,* Mato JM, Lieber CS, Kaplowitz N, Caballero A, Eds, Madrid: CSIC Press 67, 1992.
166. Frezza M, Pozzato G, Chiesa L, et al. *Hepatology* 4: 274; 1984.
167. Vendemiale G, Altomare E, Trizio T. *Scand J Gastroenterol* 24: 407; 1989.
168. Mato JM, Cámara J, Fernández de Paz J, et al. J *Hepatology* 30: 1081; 1999.
169. Lieber CS, Robins SJ, Leo MA. *Alcohol: Clin Exp Res* 18: 592; 1994.
170. Lieber CS, Robins SJ, Li J, et al. *Gastroenterology* 106: 152; 1994.
171. Lieber CS, Leo MA, Mak KM, et al. *Hepatology* 5: 561; 1985.
172. Zeisel S, Busztajn JL. *Annu Rev Nutr* 14: 269; 1994.
173. Arai M, Gordon ER, Lieber CS. *Biochim Biophys Acta* 797: 320; 1984.
174. Lieber CS, Leo MA, Aleynik SI, et al. *Alcohol: Clin Exp Res* 21: 375; 1997.
175. Niederau C, Strohmeyer G, Heinges T, et al. *Hepato Gastroenterol* 45: 797; 1998.
176. Leo MA, Lieber CS. *Amer J Clin Nutr* 69: 1071; 1999.
177. Leo MA, Lieber CS. *N Engl J Med* 307: 597; 1982.
178. Sato M , Lieber CS. *J Nutr* 111: 2015; 1981.
179. Sato M, Lieber CS. *J Nutr* 112: 1188; 1982.

180. Sato M, Lieber CS. *Arch Biochem Biophys* 213: 557; 1982.
181. Duester G. *Biochemistry* 35: 12221; 1996.
182. Leo MA, Lowe N, Lieber CS. *Am J Clin Nutr* 40: 1131; 1984.
183. Reddy TV, Weisburger EK. *Cancer Lett* 10: 39; 1980.
184. Leo MA, Lowe N, Lieber CS. *J Nutr* 117: 70; 1987.
185. Roberts AB, Lamb LC, Spron MB. *Arch Biochem Biophys* 234: 374; 1980.
186. Leo MA, Iida S, Lieber CS. *Arch Biochem Biophys* 234: 305; 1984.
187. Leo MA, Lieber CS. *J Biol Chem* 260: 5228; 1985.
188. Tomita S, Okuyama E, Ohnishi T, Ichikawa Y. *Biochimica Biophys Acta* 1290: 273; 1996.
189. Leo MA, Kim C, Lieber CS. *Arch Biochem Biophys* 259: 241; 1987.
190. Leo MA, Lieber CS. *J Clin Invest* 73: 593; 1984.
191. Leo MA, Lasker JM, Raucy JL, et al. *Arch Biochem Biophys* 269: 305; 1989.
192. Leo MA, Sato M, Lieber CS. *Gastroenterology* 84: 562; 1983.
193. Leo MA, Arai M, Sato M, Lieber CS. In *Biological Approach to Alcoholism: Update.* Research Monograph-11, DHHS Publication No. (ADM) 83-1261, CS Lieber, Ed, Superintendent of Documents, Washington, DC: US Government Printing Office; 1983, p 195.
194. Davis BH, Vucic A. *Hepatology* 8: 788; 1988.
195. Davis BH, Kramer RJ, Davidson NO. *J Clin Invest* 86: 2062; 1990.
196. Friedman SL, Wei S, Blaner W. *Am J Physiol* 264: G947; 1993.
197. Mak KM, Leo MA, Lieber CS. *Gastroenterology* 87: 188; 1984.
198. Mak KM, Leo MA, Lieber CS. *J Natl Cancer Inst* 79: 1001; 1987.
199. Kvale G, Bielke F, Gart JJ. *Intl J Cancer* 31: 397; 1983.
200. Pollack ES, Nomura AMY, Heilbrum L, et al. *N Engl J Med* 310: 617; 1984.
201. Leo MA, Lowe N, Lieber CS. *Biochem Pharmacol* 35: 3949; 1986.
202. Wang X, Liu C, Chung J, et al. *Hepatology* 28: 744; 1998.
203. Duester G. *J Nutr* 128: 459S; 1998.
204. Haselbeck RJ, Duester G. *Alcohol: Clin Exp Res* 21: 1484; 1997.
205. Duester G. *Alcohol: Clin Exp Res* 15: 565; 1991.
206. Pullarkat RK. *Alcohol: Clin Exp Res* 15: 565; 1991.
207. Deltour L, Ang HL, Duester G. *FASEB J* 10: 1050; 1996.
208. Chen H, Namkung J, Juchau MR. *Alcohol: Clin Exp Res* 20: 942; 1996.
209. Kedishvili NY, Gough WH, Chernoff EAG, et al. *J Bio Chem* 272: 7494; 1997.
210. Tuyns AJ, Riboli E, Doornbos G, Pequignot G. *Nutr Cancer* 9: 81; 1987.
211. DeCarli A, Liati P, Negri E, et al. *Nutr Cancer* 10: 29; 1987.
212. Graham S, Marshall J, Haughey B, et al. *Am J Epidemiol* 131: 454; 1990.
213. Soprano DR, Soprano KJ. *Annu Rev Nutr* 111; 1995.
214. Lammer EJ, Chen DT, Hoar RM, *N Engl J Med* 313: 837; 1985.
215. Rothman KJ, Moore LL, Singer MR, et al. *N Engl J Med* 333: 1369; 1995.
216. Oakley GP, Erickson JD. *N Eng J Med* 333: 1414; 1995.
217. Karl PI, Gordon BH, Lieber CS, Fisher SE. *Science* 242: 273; 1988.
218. Abel EL, Sokol RJ. *Alcohol: Clin Exp Res* 15: 514; 1991.
219. Whitby KE, Collins TFX, Welsh JJ, et al. *Fd Chem Toxic* 32: 305; 1994.
220. Russell RM, Boyer JL, Bagheri SA, Hruban Z. *N Engl J Med* 291: 435; 1974.
221. Farrell GC, Bathal PS, Powell LW. *Dig Dis Sci* 22: 724; 1977.
222. Geubel AP, DeGalocsy C, Alves N, et al. *Gastroenterology* 100: 1701; 1991.
223. Leo MA, Arai M, Sato M, Lieber CS. *Gastroenterology* 82: 194; 1982.
224. Worner TM, Gordon G, Leo MA, Lieber CS. *Am J Clin Nutr* 48: 1431; 1988.
225. Minuk GY, Kelly JK, Hwang WS. *Hepatology* 8: 272; 1988.
226. Leo MA, Lieber CS. *Hepatology* 8: 412; 1988.
227. Leo MA, Lieber CS. *Hepatology* 3: 1; 1983.
228. Olson JA. *Am J Clin Nutr* 45: 704; 1987.
229. Ahmed S, Leo MA, Lieber CS. *Am J Clin Nutr* 60: 430; 1994.
230. Ward RJ, Peters TJ. *Alcohol Alcoholism* 27: 359; 1992.
231. Forman MR, Beecher GR, Lanza E, et al. *Am J Clin Nutr* 62: 131; 1995.
232. Leo MA, Kim CI, Lowe N, Lieber CS. *Hepatology* 15: 883; 1992.

233. Leo MA, Aleynik S, Aleynik M, Lieber CS. *Am J Clin Nutr* 66: 1461; 1997.
234. Greenberg ER, Baron JA, Karagas MR, et al. *JAMA* 275: 699; 1996.
235. Hennekens CH, Buring JE, Manson JE. *N Engl J Med* 334: 1145; 1996.
236. Bowen HT, Omaye ST. *J Amer Coll Nutr* 17: 171; 1998.
237. ATBC: α- Tocopherol, β-carotene and Cancer Prevention Study Group. *N Engl J Med* 330: 1029; 1994.
238. Omenn GS, Goodman GE, Thornquist MD, et al. *N Engl J Med* 334: 1150; 1996.
239. Leo MA, Lieber CS. *N Engl J Med* 331: 612; 1994 (letter).
240. Garro AJ, Gordon BHJ, Lieber CS. In *Medical and Nutritional Complications of Alcoholism: Mechanisms and Management,* Lieber CS, ED, New York, Plenum Press, 1992, p 459.
241. Paolini M, Forti GC, Perocco P, et al. *Nature* 398: 760, 1999.
242. Jewell C, O'Brien N. *Br J Nutr* 81: 235; 1999.
243. Burton GW, Ingold KU. *Science* 224: 569; 1984.
244. Lowe GM, Booth LA, Young AJ, Biton RF. *Free Rad Res* 30: 141; 1999.
245. Woods JA, Bilton RF, Young AJ. *FEBS Lett* 449: 255; 1999.
246. Albanes D, Heinonen OP, Taylor PR, et al. *J Natl Cancer Inst* 88: 1560; 1996.
247. Omenn GS, Goodman GE, Thornquist MD, et al. *J Natl Cancer Inst* 88: 155; 1996.
248. Albanes D, Virtamo J, Taylor PR, et al. *Am J Clin Nutr* 66: 366; 1997.
249. Leo MA, Seitz HK, Maier H, Lieber CS. *Alcohol Alcoholism* 30: 163; 1995.
250. Sarkar A, Basak R, Bishayee A, et al. *Br J Cancer* 76;855; 1997.
251. Kune GA, Bannerman S, Field B, et al. *Nutr Cancer* 18: 237; 1992.
252. Menkes MS, Comstock GW, Vuilleumier JP, et al. *N Engl J Med* 315: 1250; 1986.
253. Lieber CS. In *Liver Annual — VI*, Arias IU, Frenkel MS, Wilson JHP, Eds, Amsterdam, Excerpta Medica, 1987, p 163.
254. Klatskin G. *Yale J Biol Med* 34: 124; 1961.
255. Rothschild MA, Oratz M, Mongelli J, Schreiber SS. *J Clin Invest* 50: 1812; 1971.
256. Jeejeebhog KN, Phillips MJ, Bruce-Robertson A, et al. *Biochem J* 126: 1111; 1972.
257. Preedy VR, Marway JS, Siddiq T, et al. *Drug Alcohol Depend* 34: 1; 1993.
258. Preedy VR, Siddiq T, Why H, Richardson PJ. *Alcohol Alcoholism* 29: 141; 1994.
259. Baraona E, Leo M, Borowsky SA, Lieber CS. *Science* 190: 794; 1975.
260. McGhee A, Henderson M, Milikan WJ, et al. *Ann Surg* 197: 288; 1983.
261. Gronbaek M, Deis A, Sørensen TI, et al. *BMJ* 310: 1165; 1995.
262. Bode C, Goebell H, Stahler M. *Z Gesamte Exp Med* 152: 111; 1970.
263. Bode C, Buchwald B, Goebell H. *German Med* 1: 149; 1971.
264. Meijer AJ, Van Woebkon GM, Williamson JR, Tager JM. *Biochem J* 150: 205; 1975.
265. Korsten MA, Matsuzaki S, Feinman L, Lieber CS. *N Engl J Med* 292: 386; 1975.
266. Lieber CS, Lasker JM, DeCarli LM, et al. *J Pharmacol Exp Ther* 1247: 791; 1988.
267. Lieber CS. *N Engl J Med* 333: 1058; 1995.
268. Lieber CS. *J Stud Alcohol* 59: 9; 1998.
269. Lieber CS. 2000. *J Hepatology* 32: 113; 2000.

46

Anemias

Linda K. Hendricks and Abdullah Kutlar

Introduction

Hematopoiesis is the process whereby mature blood cells (red cells, white cells, and platelets) are produced from the pluripotent hematopoietic stem cells in the bone marrow. The process involves the proliferation and differentiation of stem cells into different lineages (megakaryocytic, erythroid, lymphoid, granulocytic/marophage) with the ultimate production of mature blood cells. This process is influenced by many complex factors including the bone marrow microenvironment, an elaborate network of cytokines and hematopoietic growth factors, and an adequate supply of nutrients, vitamins, and some trace elements (Table 46.1). Erythropoiesis refers to the production of red blood cells whose major function is oxygen transport and delivery. A decrease in red blood cell mass and oxygen-carrying capacity results in anemia.

This section will provide an overview of the classification and pathogenesis of anemia, and will primarily focus on a detailed discussion of nutritional deficiencies leading to various types of anemia.

Anemia: Definition and Classification

Anemia is best defined as a reduction in the oxygen-carrying capacity of blood. Since this function is carried out by hemoglobin (Hb) in the red blood cells, measurement of Hb provides an accurate, reproducible means of detecting anemia. The normal values for Hb for different age groups as well as for adult men and women are shown in Table 46.2. Initial laboratory approach to anemia is summarized in Table 46.3.

Anemias can be classified morphologically and functionally. The morphologic classification is based upon the mean corpuscular volume (MCV), average volume of the red cell (Table 46.4). The diameter of a red cell is close to the size of the nucleus of a normal lymphocyte, approximately 7 μm (Color Figure 46.1*). Normal red cells are formed in the shape of two biconcave discs that are flexible and change shape according to a variety of

* Color figures follow page 992.

0-8493-2705-9/01/$0.00+$1.50

TABLE 46.1

Nutrients Important for Normal Red Blood Cell (RBC) Production

Protein/Calories
Vitamin B_{12} (cobalamin)
Folate
Iron
Vitamin B_6 (pyridoxine)
Riboflavin
Nicotinic acid
Ascorbic acid
Vitamin A (retinol)
Vitamin E (α-tocopherol)
Copper

TABLE 46.2

Criteria for Anemia and Normal MCV Values

	Hgb (g/dl)	Hct (%)	MCV (fl)
Infants			
1-3 days	<14.5	<45	95-108
One month	<10	<31	85-104
Two months	<9	<28	77-96
0.5-2 years	<11	<33	70-78
Children			
2-6 years	<11.5	<34	75-81
6-12 years	<11.5	<35	77-86
12-18 yrs			
Female	<12	<36	78-90
Male	<13	<37	78-88
Women	<12	<37	80-90
Men	<14	<40	80-90

MCV = Mean Corpuscular Volume

TABLE 46.3

Initial Laboratory Data in the Evaluation of Anemia

CBC (complete blood count)
White count and differential
Platelet count
Hemoglobin and hematocrit
MCV (mean cell volume)
Reticulocyte count
Red cell morphology on peripheral blood smear

factors. The amount of volume inside the cell membrane is the MCV. The normal MCV of a red cell is 80 to 100 fl. When evaluating either the MCV or the Hb of an individual, it is important to consider the patient's age and sex.

The functional classification takes the pathogenesis of anemia into consideration. Thus, anemias can be hypoproliferative (bone marrow or stem cell defects, decreased stimulation of erythropoiesis), or result from maturation defects (nuclear or cytoplasmic) or from blood loss or destruction (hemorrhage, hemolysis, and sequestration) (Table 46.5).

TABLE 46.4

Classification of Anemias by Morphology

Low MCV (Microcytic)	High MCV (Macrocytic)	Normal MCV (Normocytic)
Fe deficiency	Nonmegaloblastic	Bone marrow failure
Thalassemia	Liver disease	Aplastic anemia
Sideroblastic anemia	Hypothyroidism	Red cell aplasia (acquired and congenital)
Chronic disease	Reticulocytosis	Marrow infiltration
Lead poisoning	Aplastic anemia	Chronic renal failure
Protein deficiency		Endocrine abnormalities
	Megaloblastic	Hypothyroidism
	Vitamin B_{12} deficiency	Adrenal insufficiency
	Folate deficiency	HIV
	Myelodysplastic syndromes	Chronic disease
	Drug Induced	
	Chemotherapeutic agents	
	Nitrous oxide (laughing gas)	

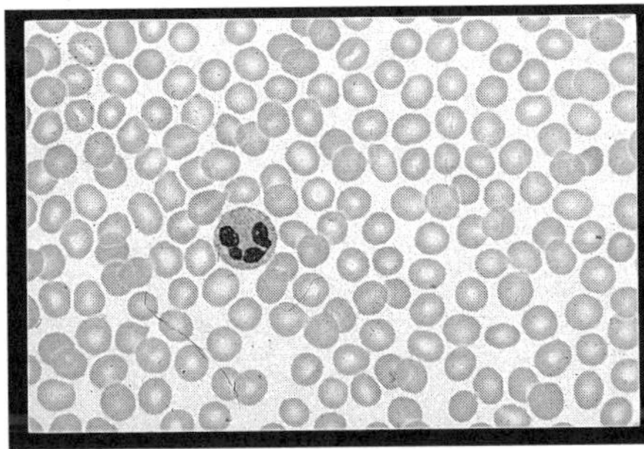

FIGURE 46.1
(See Color Figure 46.1) A normal peripheral blood smear.

Normal Erythropoiesis

A good understanding of normal erythropoiesis will enable one to better understand and appreciate the pathogenesis of different types of anemias (Color Figure 46.2). The earliest red cell precursor, the proerythroblast, is very large (12 to 20 μm) with a large nucleus. The nucleus contains DNA necessary for cell division, and the cytoplasm contains RNA necessary for hemoglobin synthesis. As the cells divide and mature, the nucleus becomes very small and condensed. Eventually the nucleus is extruded and the mature red cell remaining is only the cytoplasm full of hemoglobin. The normal red cell is smaller than the precursor cells and is pink-colored from the hemoglobin.

Perturbations of either the nuclear (DNA) or cytoplasmic (RNA and hemoglobin) maturation leads to anemia. The nucleus of the red cell precursor utilizes cobalamin (vitamin B_{12}) and folate in the synthesis of DNA. When either of these nutrients is sparse the nucleus cannot divide or mature normally, despite normal cytoplasmic development. The red cells formed are large (macrocytic). The bone marrow reveals red cell precursors that are *megaloblastic*, that is, large with fine, sparse nuclear chromatin. Other nucleated bone marrow cells are also affected such as the white cells, resulting in hypersegmented neutrophils in the peripheral blood (Color Figure 46.3).

In the cytoplasm, hemoglobin synthesis proceeds normally as long as both heme and globin are manufactured normally. Defective heme synthesis can occur by two mecha-

TABLE 46.5

Functional Causes of Anemia

- Blood loss
  - Gastrointestinal bleeding
  - Menses/Menorrhagia
  - Internal bleeding
- Decreased production of red blood cells
  - Nutritional deficiencies
  - Primary bone marrow failure
    - (myelodysplastic syndromes, leukemias, infiltrative processes)
  - Secondary bone marrow failure
    - (drugs, toxins, metabolic processes, infections)
- Increased destruction of red blood cells
  - Immune hemolytic anemia
  - Mechanical hemolysis
    - (heart valve, microangiopathic hemolytic anemia, TTP, DIC)
  - Hereditary hemolysis
    - hemoglobinopathies
    - enzyme defects (G6PD, pyruvate kinase)
    - membrane defects
  - Acquired membrane defects
    - paroxysmal nocturnal hemoglobinuria
    - spur cell anemia
  - Infection related hemolysis
    - Clostridia, malaria, babesiosis
- Splenic sequestration
- Increased plasma volume
  - Pregnancy

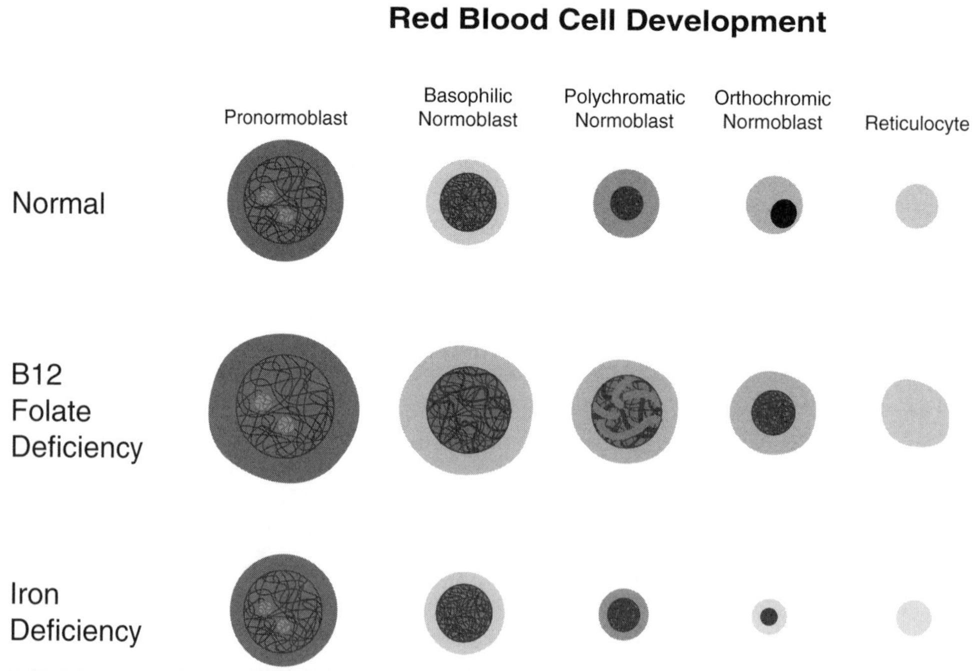

FIGURE 46.2
(See Color Figure 46.2) Erythropoiesis as it is affected by states of iron deficiency and vitamin B_{12} or folate deficiency.

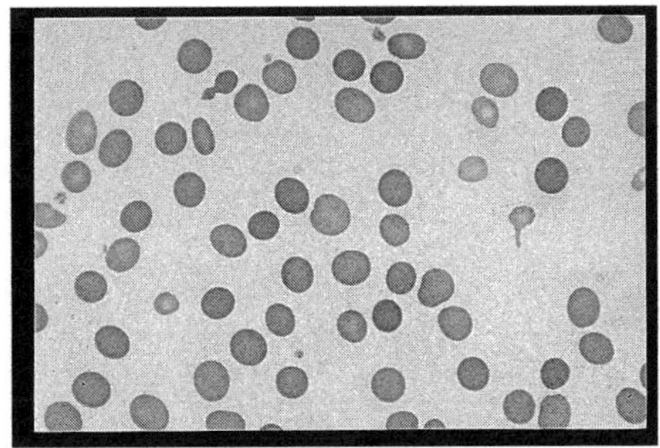

FIGURE 46.3
(See Color Figure 46.3) Macrocytic RBCs. Red blood cells that are larger than normal (macrocytic) and white blood cells that have nuclei with multiple segments (hypersegmented neutrophils) are characteristic of a vitamin B_{12} deficiency anemia.

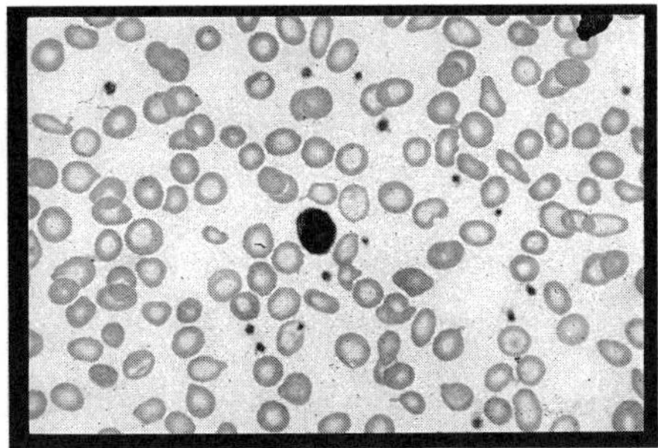

FIGURE 46.4
(See Color Figure 46.4) Microcytic RBCs. Red blood cells that are smaller than normal and have pale features (microcytic and hypochromic) are characteristic of Fe deficiency anemia.

nisms: faulty iron metabolism (iron deficiency anemia) or defective porphyrin metabolism (sideroblastic anemia). A deletion in or defect of the genes encoding globin (thalassemia) causes defective globin synthesis. All of these anemias are characterized by small red cells, *microcytosis*, because the nucleus divides and matures normally (Color Figure 46.4).

The Reticulocyte

The normal red blood cell (RBC) lives about 120 days in the peripheral blood: when the senescent RBC are destroyed they have to be replaced by new RBCs to maintain RBC homeostasis. A newly produced, young RBC still has residual RNA and mitochondria in the cytoplasm and is slightly larger than a normal red cell, appearing a little bluish on the peripheral blood smear. This is called a reticulocyte. A special stain is performed using new methylene blue, which stains the residual RNA, making a reticulocyte easy to identify and count in the blood (Color Figure 46.5). The *reticulocyte count* is the number of reticulocytes counted in 1000 red cells, reported as a percentage. A reticulocyte lives normally two days before it matures into a fully developed RBC. In a normal person with normal red cells and normal bone marrow the reticulocyte count will range from 0.5 to 1.5% (1/120 of RBCs replaced daily). Thus, the reticulocyte count is a sensitive method to detect how rigorous the bone marrow is producing new RBCs. Two corrections need to be made after the reticulocyte percentage is obtained before a conclusion can be drawn about the bone marrow.

One, if a patient has decreased numbers of red cells to begin with, then a reticulocyte count of 0.5 to 1.5% would not be considered an appropriate bone marrow response.

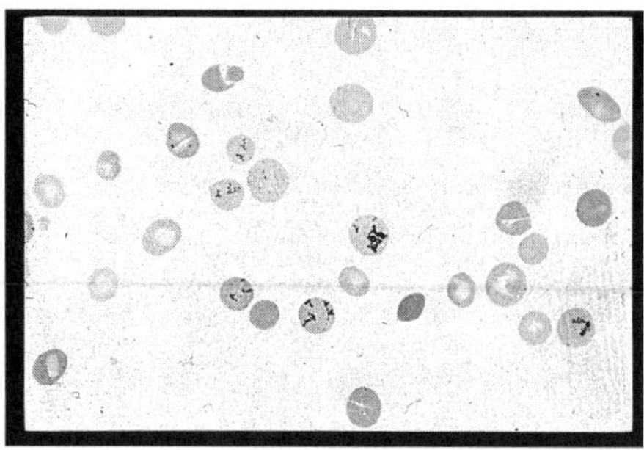

FIGURE 46.5
(See Color Figure 46.5) Reticulocytes. The appearance of young, newly produced red blood cells, reticulocytes, as seen in the peripheral blood smear that has been stained with new methylene blue.

Because of the fewer number of RBCs present, a reticulocyte percentage within that range would actually reflect a much smaller absolute reticulocyte number; i.e., two percent of a hundred cells is less than two percent of a thousand cells. The bone marrow should be producing more reticulocytes in the setting of anemia. Thus, when reticulocytes are counted it is important to take into account the degree of anemia present to avoid a misleading "normal" percentage of reticulocytes. Dividing the patient's hematocrit or hemoglobin by the normal hematocrit or hemoglobin does this. This gives us the fraction of normal red cells the patient has. That fraction is then multiplied by the reticulocyte count giving us the *corrected reticulocyte count*.

Second, the faster the bone marrow is producing reticulocytes, the younger they are when they are released into the peripheral blood. When the reticulocytes are counted on the special stain, both older reticulocytes and younger reticulocytes are counted. Therefore, adjustments for this can be made when calculating a patient's *reticulocyte index* (Color Figure 46.6). The corrected reticulocyte count is divided by the number of days the reticulocyte lives in the peripheral blood. This number, of course, depends on the degree of anemia. The more severely anemic someone is, the earlier the reticulocyte is pushed into the peripheral blood and the longer it stays as a reticulocyte in the blood. (The usual number used in the setting of anemia, however, is two.) After these two corrections have been made to the reticulocyte count, then one has a fair estimate of how well the bone marrow is able to make new RBCs. In the case of nutritionally caused anemias, the reticulocyte index will invariably be low (Table 46.6).

Erythropoietin

Erythropoietin, a glycoprotein hormone produced in the kidney in response to tissue hypoxia, is the major regulator of erythropoiesis. In cases of renal failure the erythropoietin level may be low, causing anemia, usually normocytic. Measuring the erythropoietin level may be a useful step in the evaluation of anemia; however, in cases of nutritionally deficient anemia the level is normal or elevated and is not, therefore, routinely measured.

Symptoms of Anemia

Patients with anemia will often present with similar symptoms regardless of the cause. Low RBCs decrease the oxygen-carrying capacity of the blood, producing generalized symptoms (Table 46.7). The severity of the symptoms, however, is directly related to how rapidly the anemia develops. Anemias that develop rapidly such as in acute bleeding,

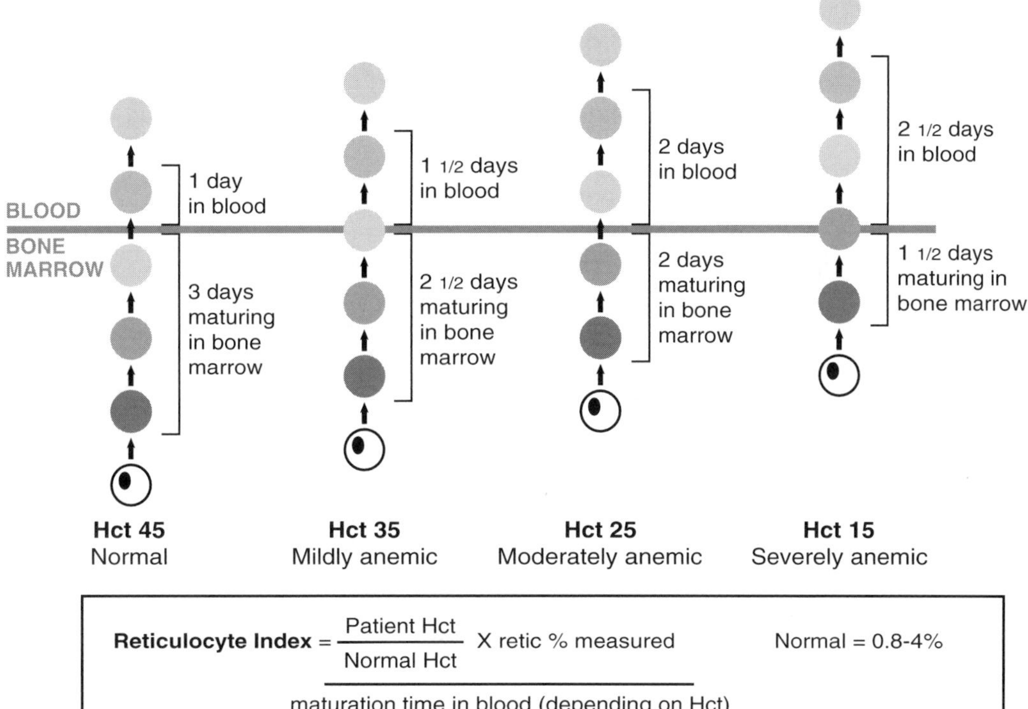

FIGURE 46.6
Understanding the reticulocyte index.

TABLE 46.6
Categorizing Anemias by Reticulocyte Count

Low Reticulocytes	High Reticulocytes
Decreased production:	Acute blood loss
Fe deficiency	Splenic seqestration
B_{12} deficiency	Increased destruction
Folate deficiency	(hemolysis)

TABLE 46.7
Symptoms of Anemia

Symptoms of Anemia
Dyspnea with exertion
Dizziness
Lightheadedness
Throbbing headaches
Tinnitus
Palpitations
Syncope
Fatigue
Disrupted sleep patterns
Decreased libido
Mood disturbances
Difficulty concentrating

TABLE 46.8

Physical Findings in Anemia

Pallor of skin
Pallor of mucous membranes
Mild to moderate tachycardia
Widened pulse pressure
Systolic ejection murmur
Venous hums
Mild peripheral edema

will be more symptomatic than anemias that progress slowly over months to years. The heart must increase the rate of blood flow to the body to compensate for anemia. This may precipitate palpitations, shortness of breath, and throbbing headaches. Syncope occurs with severe anemia due to decreased oxygenation of the brain in the upright position. Often patients with chronic anemia such as those with sickle cell disease will maintain a hemoglobin level much lower than normal and have few symptoms, due to compensation by the body.

Physical Findings

Anemia causes general physical findings independent of the cause of the anemia (Table 46.8). These findings are due to the decrease in hemoglobin; skin and mucous membranes may be pale and the heart rate may be increased. As in symptoms, the physical findings may be influenced by the chronicity of the anemia.

Vitamin B_{12} Deficiency

Mechanism of Anemia

Erythropoiesis depends on proper nuclear (DNA) and cytoplasmic (RNA and hemoglobin) maturation. Vitamin B_{12} (or cobalamin) is important in DNA synthesis. When vitamin B_{12} is not available, the conversion of homocysteine to methionine is impaired. DNA is not synthesized properly and megaloblastic anemia ensues.

Etiology of Vitamin B_{12} Deficiency

The most common cause of vitamin B_{12} deficiency is not the dietary lack of vitamin B_{12} but the inability to absorb the vitamin from food due to a condition known as pernicious anemia. Normally, vitamin B_{12} is released from food in the acidic environment of the stomach and is bound to intrinsic factor formed by the parietal cells of the stomach that allow absorption in the ileum. In pernicious anemia, the stomach does not make intrinsic factor, and the vitamin cannot be absorbed. Pernicious anemia is more commonly seen in people of Northern European descent, but can be seen in all racial groups. Women are affected more than men are. A family history of pernicious anemia may indicate increased risk.

Other causes of vitamin B_{12} deficiency are related to the absorption mechanism (Table 46.9). For example, antibodies to intrinsic factor or to the parietal cells of the stomach may inhibit proper function. Gastrectomy will result in lack of intrinsic factor. Conditions that

TABLE 46.9

Causes of Vitamin B_{12} Deficiency

Pernicious anemia (most common cause)
Gastrectomy
Zollinger Ellison syndrome
Intestinal causes
Ileal resection or disease
Blind loop syndrome
Fish tapeworm
Pancreatic insufficiency
Strict vegetarianism (those who exclude meats, eggs, and milk)

TABLE 46.10

Clinical Features of B_{12} Deficiency

Megaloblastic anemia
Pallor/icterus
Sore tongue or mouth
Gastrointestinal symptoms
Neurologic symptoms
Finger and toe paresthesias
Disturbance of vibration and position sense
Spastic ataxia — subacute combined degeneration
Somnolence, impairment of taste, smell, vision
Dementia, psychosis, "megaloblastic madness"
Well nourished, generally

interfere with the binding of intrinsic factor to the ileum include Crohn's disease, ileal resection, and tropical sprue. The fish tapeworm, Diphyllobothrium latum, competes for vitamin B_{12} and can be a cause of deficiency in infected patients. If pancreatic enzymes are not sufficient to aid in the binding of B_{12} to intrinsic factor, the absorption will be impaired. Only very rarely is dietary deficiency of vitamin B_{12} seen in the United States. Those cases are usually seen in very strict vegans, those who exclude meats, eggs, and milk from their diets. The deficiency develops slowly over many years.

The Clinical Features of B_{12} Deficiency

Full-blown cases of deficiency present with megaloblastic anemia. Sore tongue or mouth and gastrointestinal complaints can occur. Neurologic effects can be devastating (Table 46.10). Demyelination of nerves leads to axonal degeneration and highly variable clinical symptoms. Subacute combined degeneration of the spinal cord and cerebral abnormalities include symptoms of finger and toe paresthesias, disturbance of vibration and position sense, spastic ataxia, impairment of taste, smell, vision, and even psychosis often referred to as "megaloblastic madness." Importantly, the anemia and neurologic effects are not always seen together. A patient could have severe megaloblastic anemia with no neurologic effects, and vice versa. The mechanism of neurologic effects is poorly understood. Unfortunately, treatment with vitamin B_{12} does not always correct the neurologic effects despite correction of the anemia.

The Hematologic Effects of B_{12} Deficiency

The nuclear maturation defect results in a macrocytic anemia (Table 46.11). The mean cell volume is usually greater than 110 fl and can vary depending on the degree of deficiency.

TABLE 46.11

Laboratory Features of B_{12} Deficiency

Hematologic
Megaloblastic anemia (MCV>110)
Leukopenia and thrombocytopenia
Bone marrow
Megaloblastic appearance
Ineffective erythropoiesis
Biochemical
Serum B_{12} level is decreased, i.e., <223 pg/ml
Methylmalonic acid is elevated, i.e., >0.4 µmol/L
Homocysteine is elevated, i.e., >14 µm
Marked increase in LDH, i.e., >3000 units/ml (normal 260 U/ml)
Serum folate levels may be elevated
Schilling Test

In vitamin B_{12} deficiency the red cell precursors in the bone marrow are large with immature nuclei, megaloblastic. Ineffective erythropoiesis (destruction of RBC precursors in the marrow) can be quite significant and is responsible for the elevated indirect bilirubin level and high lactate dehydrogenase (LDH). In fact, up to 90% of the red cells may actually be destroyed in the bone marrow before being released to the peripheral blood as compared to the 10 to 15% seen in normal subjects. Furthermore, the white cell and platelet lineages are affected, and the hematologic picture is often one of pancytopenia.

The Laboratory Diagnosis of B_{12} Deficiency

The serum vitamin B_{12} level reflects the vitamin stores in the body and is the standard method in determining vitamin B_{12} deficiency usually ranging from 200 to 1000 pg/ml. Some conditions such as folic acid deficiency, pregnancy, oral contraceptive use, multiple myeloma, and possibly antibiotic therapy can cause falsely low vitamin B_{12} levels. Because it is important to differentiate true B_{12} deficiency from folic acid deficiency, the serum methylmalonic acid level and serum homocysteine level can be measured (Table 46.12). While the homocysteine level may be elevated in both vitamin B_{12} deficiency and folate deficiency due to interruption of the formation of succinyl CoA, methylmalonic acid will be elevated only in vitamin B_{12} deficiency because it utilizes vitamin B_{12} to form methionine, a process not dependent on folate.

TABLE 46.12

The Laboratory Difference between Negative Nutritional Balance and True Folate and B_{12} Deficiency

Lab Value	Serum Folate	RBC Folate	Serum B_{12}	Serum HCYS	Serum MMA
Condition					
Negative folate balance	⇓	NL	NL	NL	NL
Folate deficiency	⇓	⇓	NL	⇑	NL
Negative B_{12} balance	NL	NL	NL	NL	NL
B_{12} deficiency	NL/⇑	NL/⇓	⇓	⇑	⇑
Combined deficiency	⇓/NL	⇓	⇓	⇑	⇑

HCYS = Homocysteine
MMA = Methylmalonic acid

TABLE 46.13

Treatment of B_{12} Deficiency

Standard dose is 1000 μg intramuscularly
Anemia only: 1000 μg daily for a week, then weekly until Hgb normalizes; maintenance dose is 1000 μg monthly
Neurologic deficits: 1000 μg daily for two weeks, then weekly until Hgb normalizes followed by twice a month for 6 months, then monthly for life
If injections are not an option, oral dose is 1000 μg daily
For the rare case of decreased oral intake from malnutrition, replacement of 50 μg daily is adequate

The Schilling Test

Once vitamin B_{12} deficiency is diagnosed, the cause can be determined by the Schilling Test. The test will differentiate between dietary deficiency, absence of intrinsic factor, and ileal malabsorption. The test consists of two parts: the first part involves administering radiolabeled cobalamin orally to the patient. The urine is collected for 24 hours and radioactivity is measured. If at least 7.5% of the oral dose is excreted in the urine, this means that the patient was able to absorb the vitamin and subsequently excrete the unused amount in the urine. However, if less than 7.5% of radiolabeled cobalamin is excreted in the urine, this means that the vitamin was not absorbed adequately. These patients go on to part two of the test: patients are given the radiolabeled cobalamin orally again. This time they are also given intrinsic factor. The urine collection is repeated. If the excretion is above 7.5% this time, this means that the addition of intrinsic factor corrected the absorption and the patient has pernicious anemia. If the urine excretion is still less than 7.5%, this points to a problem with absorption such as sprue or intrinsic factor receptor abnormalities. Before the test, all patients are given a dose of unlabeled vitamin B_{12} intramuscularly to saturate the cobalamin receptors in the tissues and plasma. This way, the body will absorb and then excrete the unused radiolabeled cobalamin and the test will be valid.

Nutritional Requirements of Vitamin B_{12} and Treatment

The normal total body pool of vitamin B_{12} is 3000 μgs. The daily dietary requirement is approximately 1 μg. The recommended daily allowance is 2 μg, and the average daily diet contains 5 to 15 μg a day (ranging from 1 to 100 μg a day). Thus it is very difficult to become vitamin B_{12} deficient based on poor diet alone. When deficiency is present the treatment requires only 1 μg of B_{12} a day; however, in the setting of neurologic deficiencies, higher doses are often given. The standard maintenance dose is 100 μg intramuscularly each month after an initial loading dose is given (Table 46.13).

Folate Deficiency

Mechanism of Anemia

Like vitamin B_{12}, folate is utilized in the synthesis of DNA in the nucleus. The deficiency of folate causes megaloblastic anemia due to the arrested nuclear maturation. The main function of folate in the biochemistry of hematopoiesis is the transfer of carbon groups to various compounds. The most important compounds formed by this carbon donation are

TABLE 46.14

Causes of Folate Deficiency

Decreased nutritional intake
Poverty
Old age
Alcoholism/ cirrhosis
Children on synthetic diets
Goat's milk anemia
Premature infants
Hemodialysis
Hyperalimentation
Nontropical sprue (gluten-sensitive enteropathy)
Tropical sprue
Congenital folate malabsorption
Other small intestine disease
Pregnancy
Increased cell turnover (chronic hemolysis, exfoliative dermatitis)
Drug induced
Alcohol
Trimethoprim and Pyrimethamine
Methotrexate
Sulfasalazine
Oral contraceptives
Anticonvulsants

the purines, dTMP and methionine. As explained above, methionine formation also requires vitamin B_{12}. Without vitamin B_{12}, methionine is not formed and the prospective folate cannot be recycled, causing a "folate trap." Thus, vitamin B_{12} deficiency can also give a laboratory picture of folate deficiency.

Etiology of Folate Deficiency

Unlike vitamin B_{12} deficiency, nutritional factors play the major role in folate deficiency (Table 46.14). This is seen most commonly in the elderly, the poor, or in alcoholics. Financial reasons, poor nutritional education, and excessive alcohol consumption prohibiting good dietary habits all contribute to the development of folate deficiency. States such as pregnancy or hemolysis, which increase the requirements of folate, will often precipitate a folate deficiency. Drugs can interfere with the recycling of folate by interfering with enzymes necessary to transfer carbon groups to folate. These include methotrexate, some anticonvulsants, and oral contraceptives. Malabsorption of folate, while unusual, is seen in cases of sprue. Bacterial overgrowth in the intestine may utilize the folate before it can be absorbed, such as in blind loop syndrome.

Clinical Features of Folate Deficiency

Unlike patients with vitamin B_{12} deficiency, patients with folate deficiency are more apt to appear malnourished. While the neurologic deficits described above due to vitamin B_{12} deficiency are not seen in folate deficiency, patients with folate deficiency commonly complain of poor sleep, irritability, and depression, and may appear to have a blunted affect (Table 46.15). Folate-deficient patients may also have other nutrient deficiencies such as vitamins A, D, and K, and protein/calorie malnutrition. These concomitant deficiencies may contribute to skin pigmentation changes, sores at the corners of the mouth (angular cheilosis), and pallor such as lemon-tinted skin.

TABLE 46.15

Clinical Features of Folate Deficiency
Blunted affect/ mask-like facies
Depression
Irritability
Forgetfulness
Sleep deprivation
Weight loss from underlying GI disease
Diffuse blotchy brownish skin pigmentation in nail beds/ skin creases
Poor nutritional state
Pallor/icterus from anemia

TABLE 46.16

Laboratory Diagnosis of Folate Deficiency
Red blood cell folate level is reduced
Serum folate level may be reduced but this is not specific; it may also be elevated, depending on the recent folate intake
Serum B_{12} level is normal

The Hematologic Effects of Folate Deficiency

Macrocytosis and megaloblastosis due to folate deficiency are essentially identical to that seen in vitamin B_{12} deficiency.

The Laboratory Diagnosis of Folate Deficiency

The serum folate level reflects only the recent dietary intake of folate and does not provide an accurate assessment of folate stores (Table 46.16). The RBC folate level is low in true folate deficiency. The serum folate level will fall early in dietary restriction, and in true deficiency the red cell folate levels will fall. In vitamin B_{12} deficiency, the folate is trapped in the unconjugated form as described above, leading to a loss of folate in the RBC. Thus, vitamin B_{12} deficiency may give a falsely low RBC folate value, but the serum folate will be normal to increased. Serum homocysteine, the precursor to methionine, will be elevated in folate deficiency as it is in B_{12} deficiency. The methylmalonic acid, however, will be normal in folate deficiency.

Nutritional Requirements of Folate and Treatment

The total body pool of folate stores is 5 to 10 mg. The daily dietary requirement is 50 μg/day and the recommended daily allowance is 200 μg/day for men and 180 μg/day for women. The average daily diet contains 225 μg/day of folate. Foods rich in folate include green leafy vegetables, liver, kidney, fruits, dairy products, and cereals. Because the most common cause of folate deficiency is decreased nutritional intake, treatment is folate supplementation given in one-mg tablets daily (Tables 46.17 and 46.18).

TABLE 46.17

Treatment of Folate Deficiency
Dose is 1-5 mg orally, daily
Pregnancy maintenance dose is 1 mg daily

TABLE 46.18

Causes for Treatment Failure

Wrong diagnosis
Additional vitamin and/or mineral deficiency (concomitant B_{12} and folate, for example)
Additional iron deficiency
Additional hemoglobinopathy (sickle cell disease or thalassemia)
Associated anemia of chronic disease
Hypothyroidism

TABLE 46.19

Who Should Receive Prophylaxis for B_{12} and Folate Deficiency?

Vitamin B_{12}
Infants of mothers with pernicious anemia
Strict vegetarians
Patients who have had total gastrectomy
Folate
ALL women considering pregnancy (0.4 mg/day orally)
Pregnant women
Breastfeeding women
Premature infants
Chronic hemolytic states/ hyperproliferative states
Patients receiving methotrexate for a rheumatologic condition
Certain individuals with hyperhomocysteinemia

Prophylactic Administration of Folate and Vitamin B_{12}

Some patients can be at risk for either folate deficiency or vitamin B_{12} deficiency. These patients should receive supplementation prophylactically (Table 46.19). For vitamin B_{12}, these patients include those with gastrectomy, very strict vegetarians, and infants born to mothers with pernicious anemia, because of the possibility of placental transfer of parietal cell or intrinsic factor antibodies. Folate prophylaxis should be given to pregnant women and women considering pregnancy to prevent neural tube defects. Breastfeeding women and premature infants should also receive folate. Patients with chronic hemolytic states such as sickle cell disease should receive folate as well as patients receiving chronic methotrexate for rheumatologic conditions, as the methotrexate inhibits dihydrofolate reductase, creating a form of "folate trap." Certain individuals with hyperhomocysteinemia may benefit from prophylactic folate administration, because a concomitant folate deficiency would create an exacerbation of the homocysteinemia due to the inhibition of methionine synthesis. Elevated homocysteine levels increase the risk of coronary artery disease.

Iron Deficiency Anemia

Mechanism of Anemia

Every cell in the body requires iron. The cells utilize iron in oxidative metabolism, growth, and cellular proliferation as well as in oxygen transport. The major portion of body iron is found in hemoglobin. Heme is the component of hemoglobin that binds the iron, thus other heme-containing compounds including myoglobin and enzymes also contain iron. Hemoglobin accounts for 85% of all the heme-containing compounds in the body. Iron exists in the body bound to proteins, both in storage and in heme compounds and enzymes (Hb, myoglobin, and cytochrome). Unbound iron is toxic, primarily by generating reactive oxygen species.

Iron is absorbed from the duodenum and transported via transferrin to tissues such as RBC precursors. When not immediately utilized, the iron is stored mostly in the liver in the form of ferritin. During erythropoiesis iron is incorporated in the hemoglobin, where it functions as the transporter of oxygen. When senescent red cells are destroyed in the reticuloendothelial system, macrophages of the spleen and liver take up the iron and recycle it to transferrin to be transported back to the bone marrow.

While vitamin B_{12} and folate are used in DNA synthesis in red cell precursors, iron is utilized in cytoplasmic hemoglobin synthesis. Heme requires adequate iron and porphyrin metabolism for formation. Defective porphyrin metabolism (sideroblastic anemia) sometimes responds to pyridoxine treatment; however, the cause of anemia is not due to a nutritional deficiency of pyridoxine but to inherent enzyme mutations disrupting normal porphyrin metabolism. Thus, sideroblastic anemia is beyond the scope of this section. Deficiency of iron creates a cytoplasmic maturation defect while the nuclear maturation proceeds normally. The result is small (microcytic) cells with poorly hemoglobinized cytoplasm (hypochromia).

Etiology of Iron Deficiency

Iron deficiency is the most common nutritional deficiency in the U.S. In the late 1800s young menstruating females were considered fashionable if they were pale and chlorotic, a state of iron deficiency, though at the time the diagnosis of iron deficiency was not known. The loss of iron through chronic blood loss such as menses in a young female is the classic cause of iron deficiency. Any time iron is removed from the recycling process and lost from the body, iron deficiency can ensue (Table 46.20). Other conditions that remove iron include pregnancy and lactation. Increased iron requirements occur during periods of rapid growth such as in childhood. Adult men or menopausal women who are proven to have iron deficiency must be evaluated for blood loss, such as occurs in occult colon cancer, for example. Dietary causes of iron deficiency are unusual in developed countries except among infants, adolescents, and pregnant women, where the iron requirements are increased and the diet often compromised. The average adult man consumes more than adequate iron daily to make up for the normal iron loss. Therefore, in the U.S., iron deficiency seen in a patient not falling under one of these categories should be thoroughly evaluated for blood loss and not just merely treated.

TABLE 46.20

Causes of Iron Deficiency Anemia
Gastrointestinal bleed
Genitourinary bleed
Menses
Repeated blood donation
Growth
Pregnancy and lactation
Poor diets
Intestinal malabsorption
Hookworm/intestinal parasites
Gastric surgery

TABLE 46.21

Clinical Features of Iron Deficiency

Symptoms of anemia
Pagophagia (heavy ice consumption)
Koilonychia (brittle spoon nails)
Blue sclera
glossitis
Angular stomatitis
Postcricoid esophageal web/stricture (Plummer-Vinson syndrome)
Gastric atrophy
Impaired immunity
Decreased exercise tolerance
Neuropsychological abnormalities

The Clinical Features of Iron Deficiency

Children who develop iron deficiency may demonstrate irritability, memory loss, and learning difficulties. In adults, iron deficiency can develop slowly, and very low levels of hemoglobin may be attained before symptoms of anemia develop (Table 46.21). It is not unusual for a woman to present with hemoglobin of 2 or 3 g/dl with only moderate symptoms of fatigue or shortness of breath. Blood transfusion in these patients can be dangerous and should be performed very carefully, and only with one or two units to avoid congestive heart failure or stroke from rapid increase in intravascular volume and red cell numbers. Iron deficiency anemia may cause brittle "spoon" nails (koilonychia), blue-tinted sclera, and a painful tongue (glossitis). Immunity may be impaired due to the lack of iron needed by white blood cells and the enzymes used in host defense.

Pica is a fascinating manifestation of iron deficiency whereby the appetite is altered and patients crave unusual things to eat. Classic examples include starch, ice, or clay consumption. Pica in most cases is the symptom of iron deficiency and not the cause. However, clay inhibits the absorption of iron and may perpetuate the condition. Furthermore, excessive consumption of these items provides for a poor diet in general, thus exacerbating iron deficiency. In some cultures, pica is practiced as a norm, and in those cases iron deficiency may be the result of and not the cause of pica.

The Hematologic Effects of Iron Deficiency

As mentioned, the perturbation of cytoplasmic maturation during erythropoiesis (decreased Hb synthesis due to Fe deficiency) leads to small, underhemoglobinized red cells (microcytosis and hypochromia). In fact, the MCV can be as low as 50 fl in severe cases. The reticulocyte index is low. Often cells of various shapes and sizes are released from the bone marrow. Platelets may increase in iron deficiency and can even exceed one million (normal being 150 to 400 thousand.) If concurrent folate or vitamin B_{12} deficiency exists, then the red cells may not demonstrate the microcytosis as expected due to the concomitant macrocytosis. However, if folate or vitamin B_{12} is replaced the cells will become small.

The Laboratory Diagnosis of Fe Deficiency

Ferritin is the storage compartment for iron in the body; therefore, serum ferritin levels reflect the state of body Fe stores. A ferritin level of less than 12 μg/dl is diagnostic of

TABLE 46.22

Laboratory Features of Iron Deficiency

Hematologic
Microcytic anemia
Thrombocytosis
Bone marrow
Normal nuclear maturation
Cytoplasmic abnormalities
Absent iron stores on iron stain
Biochemical
Ferritin level is decreased
Total iron binding capacity is elevated
Iron saturation and serum iron are decreased

iron deficiency. Other laboratory features such as the transferrin level (or the iron-binding capacity), the serum iron level, and the transferrin saturation are summarized in Table 46.22. If iron stores are low the iron binding capacity will, of course, be elevated reflecting the vacant binding sites. The transferrin saturation will be decreased. The degree of iron deficiency present and the resultant hematologic effects is an important concept. By the time microcytosis is evident, the red cell hemoglobin content is decreased. Before that stage, however, the body stores of iron will be decreased but the red cell amount of iron will be maintained. This is why a patient may demonstrate a low ferritin, an elevated TIBC, and decreased iron saturation, yet have no evidence of anemia. These patients will develop symptoms of anemia in time if the iron loss is not corrected.

Ferritin is also an acute phase reactant. Thus, conditions such as renal failure, infection, liver disease, acute or chronic inflammatory states will lead to elevated ferritin levels. In these cases it may be necessary to ascertain iron stores directly with a bone marrow aspirate. The bone marrow should demonstrate iron in the interstitium when stained with an iron stain. If no iron is demonstrated in the marrow, the patient definitely has iron depletion. Iron deficiency anemia, however, is only diagnosed by the RBC iron studies.

Nutritional Requirements of Iron and Treatment

Adult men have 50 mg of iron per kilogram of body weight; women have 35 mg/kg. The minimal daily requirement is 1 mg for men and 2 mg for menstruating women. The recommended daily allowance is 12 mg/d for men and 15 mg/d for women. The average daily diet contains 6 mg of iron per 1000 kcal of food consumed (10 to 30 mg/day). Foods rich in iron include red meat. Remember the conditions that increase iron requirements such as pregnancy, childhood, and chronic blood loss. In pregnancy the daily requirement may increase to 5-6 mg. For infants the daily requirement is 0.5 mg, and for children 1 mg.

Oral iron replacement is sufficient in the majority of cases of iron deficiency anemia (Table 46.23). The usual dose is 60 mg of elemental iron administered as 325 mg of iron sulfate three times a day. The best available is in the ferrous form and heme iron as in red meat. The reticulocyte response will peak at day 8 to 10 after initiation of treatment, and the hemoglobin should normalize over 6 to 10 weeks. An improved sense of wellbeing may occur as soon as day 2 or 3 of treatment, however. Often patients complain of gastrointestinal side effects of oral iron (Table 46.24). These include constipation, diarrhea, epigastric discomfort, and nausea. Taking the iron with food can ameliorate the symptoms, though this decreases the absorption as much as 50%. Alternatively, smaller amounts may be given or different preparations tried. Some other iron formulations (iron-sorbitol) may be better tolerated in terms of gastrointestinal side effects. On very rare occasions it may

TABLE 46.23

Treatment of Iron Deficiency

Oral

150-200 mg elemental iron a day given in 3 divided doses on empty stomach
(Children's dose is 3 mg iron/ kilogram body weight per day in 3 divided doses)
Ferrous sulfate is best absorbed and least expensive. One tablet of 325 mg ferrous sulfate contains 60-70 mg of elemental iron. This given 3 times a day is a good standard treatment for adults. Hemoglobin should rise approximately 2 grams/dl every 3 weeks. Treatment should continue for 4-6 months after obtaining normal hemoglobin.

Intravenous

Iron dextran with dose depending on body weight and degree of anemia is the most widely used preparation. This is a one-time dose calculated from a chart included in the product insert. This solution of ferric oxyhydroxide and low-molecular-weight dextran contains 50 mg of elemental iron per ml. An average dose for a 70 kg patient with hemoglobin of 7 g/dl would be 40 ml of iron dextran (2000 mg of elemental iron.)

TABLE 46.24

Possible Side Effects of Iron Therapy

Oral

Constipation
Diarrhea
Nausea
Epigastric discomfort
Vomiting

Intravenous

Anaphylactic reaction (rare)
Fever
Urticaria
Adenopathy
Myalgias
Arthralgias
Phlebitis
Pain at injection site

be necessary to administer intravenous or intramuscular iron. This can be associated with some untoward side effects, but will eliminate the need for oral iron. Oral iron therapy should be continued for six months once the hemoglobin is normalized. Parenteral iron need only be given once. It should be kept in mind that if the cause of the iron deficiency is blood loss and this continues iron deficiency may recur in the future, and chronic iron replacement may be indicated (Table 46.25).

TABLE 46.25

Nutritional Information on B_{12}, Folate, and Iron

	B_{12}	Folate	Iron
Total body pool	3000 μg	5-10 mg	Men: 50 mg/kg Women: 35 mg/kg
Minimal daily adult Requirement (dietary)	0.3-1.2 μg/day	50 μg/day	10-20 mg/day
Recommended dietary allowance (RDA)	2 μg/day	Men: 200 μg/day Women: 180 μg/day	Men: 12 mg/d Women: 15mg/d
Average daily diet	5-15 μg/day (range 1-100 μg/d)	225 μg/day	6 mg/1000 kcal (10-30 mg/d)
Prevalence of deficiency	0.2% of population	8% of men in NA 10-13% of women	2% adult men 8% women
Source foods	Animal origin liver, kidney, mollusks, muscle, eggs, cheese, milk Multivitamins	Green leafy vegs. liver, kidney fruits, breakfast cereals, dairy, tea Multivitamins	Red meat
Time to develop blood signs after abstinence of nutrient	5-6 years	3 weeks	Years

Additional Sources of Information

1. Wintrobe MM. *Clinical Hematology,* Lippincott Williams & Wilkins, Philadelphia, 1999.
2. Israels LG, Israels ED. *Mechanisms in Hematology,* Core Health Services Inc., Ontario, 1998.
3. Hoffman R. *Hematology,* Churchill Livingstone, New York, 1995.
4. Hercberg S, Galan P. Nutritional anemias, *Clinical Haematology,* Vol. 5, Fleming AF, Ed, Bailliere Tindall, London, 1992, pp 143-168.
5. Hughes-Jones NC, Wickramasinghe SN. Lecture Notes on Haematology, Blackwell Science, London, 1996.
6. Foucar K. *Bone Marrow Pathology,* ASCP Press, Chicago, 1995.
7. Jandl JH. *Blood,* Little, Brown, Boston, 1987.
8. Duffy TP. Normochromic, normocytic anemias, *Cecil Textbook of Medicine,* 20th ed, Bennett JC, Plum F, Eds, WB Saunders, Philadelphia, 1996, p 837.
9. Duffy TP. Microcytic and hypochromic anemias, *Cecil Textbook of Medicine,* 20th ed, Bennett JC, Plum F, Eds, WB Saunders, Philadelphia, 1996, p 839.
10. Allen RH, Megaloblastic anemias, *Cecil Textbook of Medicine,* 20th ed, Bennett JC, Plum F, Eds, WB Saunders, Philadelphia, 1996, p 843.

47

Nutritional Treatment of Blood Pressure: Nonpharmacologic Therapy

L. Michael Prisant

Blood pressure is a continuous variable, like temperature and heart rate.[1] The level of blood pressure gradually increases from birth to age 18 years. The dividing line between a normal and an abnormal blood pressure is arbitrary. However, there is a continuous relationship between the level of blood pressure and various cardiovascular events, including myocardial infarction, strokes, congestive heart failure, renal failure, and mortality. An optimal blood pressure is a systolic blood pressure less than 120 mmHg and diastolic blood pressure less than 80 mmHg. Hypertension is defined by the average of multiple measurements with either a systolic blood pressure ≥140 mmHg or a diastolic blood pressure ≥90 mmHg.

The hallmark of hypertension is an elevated systemic vascular resistance. Hypertension may be caused by various adrenal tumors producing cortisol, aldosterone, and norepinephrine, hyperthyroidism, hypothyroidism, hyperparathyroidism with increased parathormone and calcium, acromegaly with increased growth hormone, renal failure, renal artery stenosis resulting in renal ischemia and increased renin, and various drugs that cause salt and water retention, increase renin, or activate the sympathetic nervous system. The majority of patients with arterial hypertension do not have a known cause.

Why the prevalence of essential hypertension increases with aging and what causes it remain an enigma. It is likely that what is called essential hypertension may be the result of diverse causes. Multiple factors alter the level of blood pressure. The sympathetic nervous system is important for modifying the tone of blood vessels. Circulating renin, angiotensin, aldosterone, norepinephrine, and endothelin are vasoconstrictors. The kidney is necessary to regulate sodium excretion and volume. Endothelial damage due to abnormal lipids, glucose intolerance, tobacco use, hyperhomocystinemia, hyperinsulinemia, and circulating vasoconstrictors is less responsive to local endogenous vasodilators such as nitric oxide. Essential hypertension is not a homogenous disease state; it is likely a polygenic trait.

Hypertension affects 24% of the U.S. adult population. Since essential hypertension accounts for 90 to 95% of all causes and the prevalence increases with each decade of life, there is an interest in the role of nutrients and foods for both the etiology and treatment of hypertension. A primary preventive approach is advocated by some epidemiologists and researchers.

0-8493-2705-9/01/$0.00+$1.50

Nutrients and Blood Pressure

Sodium

A large body of data relates salt intake to the level of blood pressure. In a study of chimpanzees that normally eat a fruit and vegetable diet (low sodium and high potassium intake), half had salt (up to 15 g/d) added gradually to their diet over 20 months.[2] Sodium chloride resulted in a blood pressure increase of 33/10 mmHg, which could be reversed within six months of removing sodium chloride from the diet. Similar studies have convinced the medical community that salt may be responsible for the higher prevalence of hypertension in modern society compared to more primitive communities. However, sodium may not be the sole culprit. Studies suggest that the chloride anion with sodium is necessary for an increase in blood pressure, since giving sodium with other anions does not increase blood pressure.[3,4]

The INTERSALT (International Study of Salt and Blood Pressure) Cooperative group examined 10,079 men and women aged 20 to 59 by urine sodium excretion and blood pressure at 52 centers throughout the world.[5] The average intake of sodium was 100 to 200 mmol (6 to 12g NaCl or 2.5 to 5g sodium). The relationship of sodium excretion and systolic blood pressure correlated positively in 33 of 52 centers after correcting for age, gender, body mass index (BMI), alcohol consumption, and urine potassium excretion, but was significant in only eight centers. Negative correlations were observed in 19 centers. For the entire cohort, the adjusted effect of sodium for systolic blood pressure was 2.17 mmHg per 100 mmol 24 hour sodium excretion ($p<0.001$). There was not a significant adjusted effect for diastolic blood pressure. Among the centers with a low BMI (21.8 kg/m^2) and a low sodium intake (26.7 mmol), the mean prevalence of hypertension was 1.7%. For the sites with a low BMI (22.2 kg/m^2) but with a high sodium intake (187.7 mmol), the prevalence of hypertension was 11.9%.[6] Alternatively, the Scottish Heart Health Study of 7354 men and women aged 40 to 59 years reported a weak positive correlation of urinary sodium excretion and either systolic or diastolic blood pressure.[7] The correlation was not significant after adjustment for age, BMI, alcohol consumption, and urinary potassium excretion.

The implication of INTERSALT is that if the population reduces daily sodium intake by 100 mmol or 1 teaspoon of salt per day, systolic blood pressure would decrease 2 to 3 mmHg.[6] This could have the potential to reduce coronary deaths by 4 to 5%, stroke deaths 6 to 8%, and total mortality by 3 to 4%. The impact would be greater over a lifetime for a whole population, reducing total, coronary, and stroke mortality by 13, 16, and 23%, respectively. The public policy sodium intake goal is 6 g per day.[8]

Not every person's blood pressure increases with salt. Salt-sensitivity refers to those individuals whose blood pressure increases with increased salt intake and decreases with reduced salt intake. Up to 50% of hypertensives may be salt sensitive. The blood pressure response to sodium chloride is determined by genetic and environmental factors. African Americans, obese patients, low-renin hypertensives, chronic renal insufficiency patients, and the elderly may benefit more than other groups by reducing sodium intake.

To assess the impact of sodium chloride on blood pressure, trials have been conducted either by restricting or supplementing sodium to the diet. Sodium supplementation trials are conducted less commonly (Table 47.1).[9] In the Study of Sodium and Blood Pressure, normotensive subjects participated in a trial, using a placebo or 96 mEq sodium capsules in 4-week treatment periods separated by a 2-week washout period.[9] Overnight urinary sodium excretion decreased 51 mEq/8 hr from baseline to 9 mEq/8 hr after the low sodium

TABLE 47.1

Randomized Double-Blind Trials of Sodium Supplementation

Author, Year	Study Group	Design	n	Group Differences in Na+ Excretion (mEq/24 hr)	Sodium Effect on Pressure Δ Systolic/Δ Diastolic (mmHg)
Australian National Committee, 1989	Hypertensive	Parallel	103	43	+4.8/+2.8
Dodson, 1989	Hypertensive Type 2 Diabetes	Parallel	9	76	+9.7/+5.1
McCarron, 1997	Hypertensive	Crossover	99	55	+4.9/+2.9
MacGregor, 1982	Hypertensive	Crossover	19	146	+10/+5
MacGregor, 1989	Hypertensive	Crossover	20		
High intake				141	+16/+9
Moderate intake				59	+8/+4
Mascioli, 1991	Normotensive	Crossover	48	60	+3.6/+2.3
Palmer, 1989	Elderly	Crossover	7	—	+11.0/+8.6
Watt, 1983	Hypertensive	Crossover	18	56	+0.5/+0.4

Updated and modified from Mascioli et al., *Hypertension* 17: 121; 1991.

diet run-in period, before treatment periods were initiated. Differences in systolic and diastolic blood pressure between sodium and placebo treatment periods were significant. Sodium excretion increased +20.4 mEq/8 hr ($p < 0.001$). An increase of systolic and diastolic blood pressure with the salt capsules was experienced by 65 and 69% of study participants.

A number of meta-analyses have sought to summarize the impact of sodium restriction on blood pressure.[10-15] One meta-analysis of 2635 subjects with 32 randomized trials on sodium reduction required random allocation, no confounding variables, an objective measure of a change in sodium intake (i.e., urine sodium excretion), and no adolescents,[14] updating an earlier analysis by the same authors.[11] The individual studies are listed in Tables 47.2 and 47.3. The largest meta-analysis of 4294 subjects included 58 trials of hypertensive and 56 trials of normotensive persons.[15] The mean reduction of blood pressure by sodium restriction in hypertensive individuals was –3.9/–1.9 mmHg ($p < 0.001$ for both) and in normotensives was –1.2/–0.26 mmHg ($p < 0.001$ for systolic only). Tables 47.4 and 47.5 provide a comprehensive list of the trials used in that meta-analysis. The authors conclude that the cumulative blood pressure-lowering effect of individual sodium restriction trials in both normotensive and hypertensive populations has been stable since 1985. Future trials are unlikely to change the average treatment effect noted above.

The reduction of sodium intake for primary prevention as well as nonpharmacologic treatment of hypertension has become controversial in recent years.[16-18] In one study, 2937 hypertensive men provided 24-hour urine collections for sodium determination off medication for 3 to 4 weeks.[16] After 3.8 years of average followup, 117 cardiovascular events (including 55 myocardial infarctions) occurred. There was an inverse relationship between baseline urinary sodium excretion and myocardial infarction rate. A recent meta-analysis indicated that renin, aldosterone, norepinephrine, total cholesterol, and low-density lipoprotein cholesterol increases with sodium restriction.[15] Other hazards of moderate sodium restriction suggested include a potential increase in blood pressure in 15% of patients, increased sympathetic activity and sleep disturbances, the potential of simultaneous restriction of grain products, meat, poultry, and fish, and dairy products (which contain 50% of sodium intake), decreased iodine intake, decreased susceptibility of the elderly to respond to blood loss or heat stress, the potential for fetal growth retardation during pregnancy, and unknown effects of alternative food preservatives.[19]

TABLE 47.2

Descriptive Summary of Sodium-Reduction Trials in Normotensive Subjects*

Author , Year	n	Duration (mo)	Blinding	Δ Urinary Na mmol/24 h	(No)¶ Changes in Confounders	Δ Systolic mm Hg	Δ Diastolic mm Hg
Crossover Trials							
Skrabal, 1981	20	0.5	NR	–170	Wt (K)	–2.7	–3.0
Cooper, 1984	113	2	BP obs	–68	Wt, (K)	–0.6	–1.4
Watt, 1985 (H)	35	1	DB	–74	(Wt), K	–1.4	1.2
Watt, 1985 (L)	31	1	DB	–60	(Wt), K	–0.5	1.4
Teow, 1985	9	0.5	BP obs	–210	(Wt), K	–0.6	–2.7
Myers, 1989	172	1	BP obs	–130	(Wt), (K)	–3.5†	–1.9†
Hargreaves, 1989	8	0.5	DB	–106	(Wt), (K)	–6 .0†	–3.0†
Mascioli, 1991	48	1	DB	–20.2/8h	NR	–3.6†	–2.3†
Parallel Trials‡							
Puska , 1983	19, 19‡	0.5	BP obs	–117	Wt, K, Alc, (P:S)	–1.5	–1.1
HPT, 1990	174, 177	36	BP obs (RZ)	–16	(Wt), K	0.1	0.2
Cobiac, 1992	26, 28	1	DB	–71	(Wt), (K)	–1.7	0.8
TOHP, 1992	327, 417	18	BP obs (RZ)	–44	(Wt), (K), (Ca), (mg), (alc), (fat)	–1.7†	–0.9†
Nestel, 993 (Females)	15, 15	6	DB	–94	(Wt), (K)	–6.0†	–2.0†
Nestel, 993 (Males)	17, 19	6	DB	–76	(Wt), (K)	–2.0†	–1.0†

* NR, not reported; Wt, body weight; K, potassium excretion; BP obs, observers blinded; H, high blood pressure; L, low blood pressure; DB, double blind; Alc, alcohol intake; P:S, ratio of polyunsaturated to saturated fat; HPT, Hypertension Prevention Trial; RZ, random zero manometer; TOHP, Trials of Hypertension Prevention Collaborative; Ca, calcium intake; Mg, magnesium intake; fat, fat intake.

† $p < 0.05$.

‡ values are the number of subjects in the sodium-reduction treatment and control groups, respectively.

¶ Parentheses denote controlled factors; no parentheses denotes possible confounders

Modified from Cutler.[11] Reproduced with permission from *Am J Clin Nutr*, 1997; 65(2):643S-651S.

TABLE 47.3

Descriptive Summary of Sodium-Reduction Trials in Hypertensive Subjects*

Author , Year	n	Duration (mo)	Blinding	Δ Urinary Na mmol/24 h	(No)¶ Changes in Confounders	Δ Systolic mm Hg	Δ Diastolic mm Hg
Crossover Trials							
Parijs,1973	15	1	NR	–98	(Wt)	–6.7	3.2
MacGregor, 1982	19	1	DB	–76	Wt, (K)	–10.0†	–5.0†
Watt,1983	18	1	DB	–56	(Wt), (K)	0.5	–0.3
Richards, 1984	12	1–1.5	NR	–105	(Wt), K	–5.2	–1.8
Grobbee, 1987	40	1.5	DB	–72	(Wt), (K)	–0.8	–0.8
MacGregor, 1989	20	1	DB	–82	(Wt), (K)	–8 .0†	–5.0†
Dodson,1989	9	1	DB	–76	(Wt), (K)	9.7†	–5.1
ANHMRC,1989	88	2	DB	–67	(K)	–2.6†	–2.1†
Benetos, 1992	20	1	DB	–78	(Wt), (K), (Ca)	–6.5†	–3.7†
Parallel Trials‡							
Morgan, 1978	31, 31‡	24	BP obs	–27	NR	–1.5†	–6.9†
Morgan,1981	6, 6	2	BP obs	–98	K	NR	–6.02
Morgan, 1981	6, 6	2	BP obs	–78	K	NR	–4.0
Costa, 1981	20, 21	12	NR	NR§	NR	–18.3†	–5.9†
Silman, 1983	10, 15	12	BP obs (RZ)	–53	(Wt), (K)	–8.7	–6.3
Puska, 1983	15, 19	1.5	BP obs	–117	Wt, K, Alc, (P:S)	1.8	0.5
Fagerberg, 1984	15, 15	2.3	NR	–89	(Wt), (K), (Alc)	–13.3†	–6.7†
Maxwell,1984	18, 12	3	NR	–171	Wt	–2.0	2.0
Erwteman,1984	44, 50	6	BP obs (RZ)	–58	NR	–2.7	–3.4†
Chalmers,1986	48, 52	3	NR	–54	(K)	–5.1†	–4.2†
Logan,1986	37, 38	6	BP obs	–32	Wt, (K)	–1.1	–0.2
Dodson, 1989	17, 17	3	BP obs	–59	(Wt). (K)	–13.0†	–1.8
ANHMRC, 1989	50, 53	2	DB	–71	(Alc)	–5.5†	–2.8†
Sciarrone, 1992	46, 45	2	DB	–84	(Wt), (K)	–6 .0†	–1.0
Parker,1990, low EtOH,	16, 15	1	DB	–80	(Wt), (Alc), (K), (Ca), (Mg)	2.2	0.5
Parker ,1990, norm EtOH	15, 13	1	DB	–52	(Wt), (Alc), (K), (Ca), (Mg)	–0.1	0.8

* NR, not reported; Wt, body weight; DB, double blind; K, potassium intake/excretion: ANHMRC, Australian National Health and Medical Research Council; Ca, calcium intake/excretion; BP obs, observers blinded: RZ, random zero manometer; Alc, alcohol intake; P:S, ratio of polyunsaturated to saturated fatty acid; Mg, magnesium excretion.

† $p < 0.05$.

‡ n values given for each study are the number of subjects in the sodium-reduction treatment and control groups, respectively.

§ –23% intracellular Na.

¶ Parentheses denote controlled factors; no parentheses denotes possible confounders

Modified from Cutler.[11] Reproduced with permission from *Am J Clin Nutr*, 1997; 65(2): 643S-651S.

TABLE 47.4

Characteristics of Trials of Sodium Restriction and Blood Pressure in Normotensive Populations*

Author, Year	Design	Dur.	N	Age	NU	SR	Cum SR	Effect SBP	Effect DBP	Cum. SBP	Cum DBP	Z SBP	Z DBP
Sullivan, 1980	Op, CO	4	27	29	1	146	146	–7.1	–1.1	–7.1	–1.1	–2.2	–0.4
Skrabal, 1981	Op, CO	14	20	23	1	150	147	2.7	3.0	–2.7	0.7	–1.0	0.4
Myers, 1982	Op, CO	14	136	39	1	130	133	3.3	2.7	2.4	2.4	1.1	2.2
Puska, 1983	SB, P	72	38	40	3	90	123	1.5	2.1	2.4	2.2	1.1	2.2
Cooper, 1984	SB, CO	24	59	16	1	55	111	1.4	3.4	2.0	3.5	1.6	3.0
Cooper, 1984	SB, CO	24	54	16	1	72	107	–0.3	–0.7	1.3	2.7	1.3	2.6
Skrabal, 1984	Op, CO	14	30	23	1	137	109	–1.4	–0.8	1.2	2.3	1.0	2.2
Skrabal, 1984	Op, CO	14	22	23	1	167	113	7.7	4.6	1.5	2.4	1.9	2.7
Skrabal, 1985	SB, CO	14	34	23	1	144	115	0.1	0.6	0.9	1.9	1.9	2.8
Skrabal, 1985	SB, CO	14	28	23	1	163	118	5.8	3.3	1.4	2.0	3.3	3.9
Watt, 1985	DB, CO	28	31	23	4	60	114	0.5	–1.4	1.3	1.4	3.4	3.3
Watt, 1985	DB, CO	28	35	22	4	75	111	1.4	–1.2	1.3	0.9	3.7	2.8
Teow, 986	Op, CO	14	9	25	1	200	112	0.6	2.7	1.3	0.9	3.6	2.9
Richards, 1986	SB, CO	4	8	36	4	181	114	2.0	–7.0	1.3	0.9	3.5	2.2
Fuchs, 1987	Op, CO	9	6	20	3	99	113	5.8	–3.0	1.3	0.8	3.6	1.9
Fuchs, 1987	Op, CO	9	11	20	3	93	111	1.1	–1.0	1.3	0.8	3.5	1.8
El Ashry, 1987	SB, CO	14	13	24	1	222	111	0.0	4.0	1.3	0.8	3.4	1.9
El Ashry, 1987	SB, CO	14	13	27	1	232	115	0.0	1.0	1.3	0.8	3.3	1.9
Lawton, 1988	Op, CO	6	13	24	1	313	119	2.0	–2.0	1.3	0.8	3.3	1.7
Hargreaves, 1989	DB, CO	14	8	23	2	106	119	6.0	3.0	1.3	0.8	3.4	1.7
Mtabaji, 1990	Op, P	7	30	•	1	272	121	9.0	9.0	1.4	1.0	4.0	2.3
Friberg, 1990	Op, CO	13	10	33	3	117	120	0.0	1.0	1.4	1.0	4.0	2.4
Dimsdale, 1990	Op, CO	5	19	34	2	183	129	–1.4	–4.1	1.2	0.5	3.7	1.6
Dimsdale, 1990	Op, CO	5	23	34	2	178	132	–1.0	–4.4	1.2	0.3	3.6	1.0
HPT, 1990	SB, P	1100	228	40	1	23	125	–0.3	–0.1	1.1	0.3	3.5	0.9
Sharma, 1990	SB, CO	7	15	24	2	192	127	0.9	3.7	1.1	0.3	3.4	1.1
Schmid, 1990	SB, CO	7	9	32	1	190	128	3.0	0.0	1.1	0.3	3.5	1.0
Bruun, 1990	Op, CO	4	10	46	1	341	131	5.0	1.0	1.1	0.3	3.6	1.1
Ruppert, 1991	SB, CO	7	98	35	3	275	179	–0.3	–0.3	1.1	0.3	3.5	1.0
Ruppert, 1991	SB, CO	7	24	36	3	275	190	–6.0	–6.0	0.9	0.1	2.9	0.4
Ruppert, 1991	SB, CO	7	25	46	3	262	198	7.5	7.5	1.0	0.2	3.3	0.9

Sharma, 1991	SB, CO	6	13	25	3	246	198	3.0	–0.5	1.1	0.2	3.6	0.9
Sharma, 1991	SB, CO	6	10	24	3	247	198	6.4	5.9	1.1	0.2	3.7	1.1
Mascioli, 1991	DB, CO	28	48	52	5	70	197	3.6	2.3	1.3	0.4	4.3	1.5
Steegers, 1991	SB, P	140	36	27	5	63	195	–2.0	–2.0	1.3	0.4	4.1	1.4
Cobiac, 1992	DB, P	28	52	66	2	75	194	3.1	2.8	1.3	0.4	4.3	1.8
Cobiac, 1992	DB, P	28	54	67	2	73	192	2.7	–0.6	1.3	0.4	4.4	1.7
TOHP, 1992	SB, P	550	744	43	3	47	135	1.7	0.9	1.4	0.4	4.7	2.0
Burnier, 1993	Op, CO	6	16	29	1	186	136	1.0	–0.5	1.4	0.4	4.7	1.9
Burnier, 1993	Op, CO	6	7	29	1	218	137	1.0	–1.2	1.4	0.4	4.7	1.8
Ruppert, 1993	SB, CO	7	30	46	3	270	146	12.6	5.6	1.4	0.4	5.1	2.3
Ruppert, 1993	SB, CO	7	108	36	3	275	160	1.4	–1.2	1.4	0.4	5.2	2.1
Ruppert, 1993	SB, CO	7	25	35	3	280	165	–5.9	–8.0	1.4	0.3	4.9	1.5
Sharma, 1993	SB, CO	7	16	24	3	224	166	0.8	0.5	1.4	0.3	4.9	1.5
Fliser, 1993	SB, CO	8	8	25	2	190	167	1.3	1.3	1.4	0.3	4.9	1.5
Fliser, 1993	SB, CO	8	8	26	2	181	167	0.6	0.6	1.4	0.3	4.8	1.5
Nestel, 1993	DB, P	42	72	66	4	56	166	2.0	1.0	1.4	0.3	4.9	1.6
Nestel, 1993	DB, P	42	60	65	4	73	165	6.0	2.0	1.4	0.4	5.1	1.7
Donovan, 1993	SB, CO	5	8	36	1	152	164	2.0	–1.0	1.4	0.4	5.1	1.6
Grey, 1996	DB, CO	7	34	23	1	133	164	–1.0	–1.0	1.4	0.3	5.0	1.5
Feldmann, 1996	DB, CO	7	5	27	1	176	164	–5.0	–5.0	1.2	0.2	4.5	1.1
Schorr, 1996	DB, CO	28	16	64	2	61	162	1.0	0.0	1.2	0.2	4.4	1.0
Miller, 1997	Op, CO	7	12	23	2	182	163	1.0	1.0	1.2	0.2	4.5	1.1
Miller, 1997	Op, CO	7	10	•	2	194	163	–1.0	–1.0	1.2	0.2	4.4	1.1
Schorr, 1997	SB, CO	7	27	25	7	208	163	5.6	5.6	1.3	0.3	4.6	1.3
Schorr, 1997	SB, CO	7	76	25	7	208	165	–2.8	–2.8	1.2	0.3	4.5	1.2

* Dur.: duration of intervention, days; Op: open; SB: single blind; DB: double blind; P: parallel; CO: cross–over; N: number of persons in trial; Age: mean age of persons in trial; NU: number of urine collections per person per treatment period; SR: sodium reduction, mmol/24–h; Cum: cumulative; CI: 95% confidence interval of previous column. SBP: systolic blood pressure; DBP: diastolic blood pressure; Z: summary statistic; •: no data.

Personal Communication from NA Graudal of unpublished data from his manuscript.[15]

TABLE 47.5

Characteristics of Trials of Sodium Restriction in Hypertensive Populations*

Author, Year	Design	Dur.	N	Age	NU	SR	Cum SR	Effect SBP	Effect DBP	Cum. SBP	Cum DBP	Z SBP	Z DBP
Parijs, 1973	Op, CO	28	15	41	1	98	98	6.7	–3.2	6.7	–3.2	1.6	–1.2
Mark, 1975	Op, CO	10	6	28	1	305	216	13.1	7.7	9.8	–0.1	2.7	0.4
Morgan, 1978	SB, P	90	62	60	2	23	114	1.0	2.0	6.2	1.2	2.6	0.9
Sullivan, 1980	Op, CO	4	19	27	1	153	121	–1.2	1.2	4.6	1.2	2.2	0.9
Morgan, 1981	SB, P	56	12	38	2	67	106	•	4.0	•	1.9	•	1.1
Morgan, 1981	SB, P	56	12	40	2	92	104	•	8.0	•	3.0	•	1.7
Ambrosioni, 1982	SB, CO	42	25	23	6	60	91	2.2	0.4	3.9	2.6	1.3	1.7
MacGregor, 1982	DB, CO	28	19	49	2	76	89	10.0	5.0	5.4	3.0	2.0	2.2
Beard, 1982	Op, P	84	90	48	3	124	95	5.2	3.4	5.4	3.0	2.2	2.5
Watt, 1983	DB, CO	28	18	52	4	56	92	0.5	0.3	3.6	2.0	2.3	2.5
Silman, 1983	Op, P	90	28	55	4	63	91	–3.5	–0.5	3.5	1.9	2.1	2.4
Puska, 1983	SB, P	72	34	40	3	90	91	–1.8	–0.5	3.3	1.8	2.0	2.3
Koolen, 1984	Op, CO	14	20	41	2	213	97	6.5	4.9	3.4	1.9	2.2	2.5
Richards, 1984	SB, CO	28	12	36	2	100	97	4.0	3.0	3.4	2.0	2.4	2.7
Erwteman, 1984	SB, P	28	94	46	4	58	91	2.7	2.5	3.3	2.0	2.5	2.9
Maxwell, 1984	Op, P	84	30	46	4	161	92	2.0	–2.0	3.3	1.9	2.5	2.8
Fagerberg, 1984	Op, P	63	30	51	4	99	92	3.7	3.1	3.3	2.0	2.6	2.9
Resnick, 1985	Op, CO	5	12	•	1	190	96	3.0	1.0	3.3	1.9	2.7	2.9
Logan, 1986	Op, P	180	86	47	1	43	92	1.1	0.2	3.1	1.9	2.8	2.9
Chalmers, 1986	SB, P	84	100	53	6	70	91	4.8	4.2	3.3	2.3	3.0	3.5
Grobbee, 1987	DB, CO	42	40	24	4	72	88	0.8	0.8	3.1	2.3	3.0	3.5
MacGregor, 1987	DB, CO	30	15	52	2	100	88	13.0	9.0	3.6	2.4	3.6	3.9
Kurtz, 1987	DB, CO	7	5	58	2	217	91	16.0	8.4	4.7	2.6	4.6	4.3
Morgan, 1987	SB, P	60	20	58	5	57	90	6.0	4.0	4.7	2.6	4.5	4.4
Morgan, 1988	SB, CO	14	16	63	1	50	89	3.0	4.0	4.5	2.7	4.7	4.6
Lawton, 1988	Op, CO	6	9	25	1	328	91	1.0	–4.0	4.4	2.6	4.7	4.4
Shore, 1988	SB, CO	5	6	•	5	97	91	9.0	5.6	4.5	2.6	4.8	4.4
ANHMRC, 1989	Op, P	48	103	58	4	63	89	5.5	2.9	4.6	2.7	5.2	4.8
MacGregor, 1989	DB, CO	30	20	57	2	150	91	16.0	9.0	4.8	2.8	5.6	5.2
Dodson, 1989	SB, P	90	34	62	3	44	90	13.0	1.8	4.8	2.8	5.8	5.2
Dimsdale, 1990	Op, CO	5	16	34	2	178	93	6.4	–2.0	4.9	2.7	6.0	5.0

Dimsdale, 1990	Op, CO	5	17	34	2	198	98	0.1	–0.8	4.6	2.6	6.0	4.9
Parker, 1990	DB, P	28	31	50	4	73	97	–1.9	0.1	4.3	2.4	5.8	4.9
Parker, 1990	DB, P	28	28	54	4	49	97	–1.9	–1.8	4.1	2.4	5.6	4.7
Schmid, 1990	SB, CO	7	9	36	1	181	99	6.0	1.9	4.1	2.4	5.7	4.7
Bruun, 1990	Op, CO	4	12	47	1	331	103	8.0	4.0	4.2	2.4	5.8	4.8
Egan, 1991	DB, CO	7	27	39	1	194	106	1.1	1.1	3.9	2.3	5.9	4.8
Carney, 1991	DB, CO	42	11	54	4	102	106	1.0	–1.0	3.9	2.3	5.8	4.8
Singer, 1991	DB, CO	30	21	54	2	91	106	9.0	3.0	4.0	2.3	6.1	4.9
Sciarrone, 1992	DB, P	56	91	54	1	82	104	5.8	0.4	4.0	2.2	6.4	4.9
Benetos, 1992	DB, CO	28	20	42	1	78	103	6.5	3.7	4.1	2.3	6.5	5.1
Del Rio, 1993	DB, CO	14	30	49	1	151	106	1.4	0.5	4.0	2.2	6.5	5.1
Ruilope, 1993	DB, P	21	19	•	1	69	106	4.0	4.0	4.0	2.3	6.4	5.1
Redon-Mas, 1993	Op, P	28	418	55	1	104	105	–1.0	–1.9	3.5	1.6	6.3	4.7
Fotherby, 1993	DB, CO	35	17	73	2	79	105	8.0	0.0	3.6	1.5	6.5	4.7
Buckley, 1994	SB, CO	5	12	49	1	296	106	8.7	8.7	3.7	1.6	6.8	5.0
Jula, 1994	Op, P	365	76	44	3	57	105	6.7	3.8	3.7	1.7	6.9	5.2
Zoccali, 1994	SB, CO	7	15	45	1	163	106	14.0	8.0	3.8	1.7	7.2	5.6
Weir, 1995	SB, CO	14	11	60	5	146	106	9.0	7.0	3.8	1.8	7.2	5.7
Weir, 1995	SB, CO	14	11	60	5	127	106	–4.0	–5.0	3.8	1.7	7.1	5.5
Overlack, 1995	DB, CO	7	11	61	3	240	109	9.9	9.9	3.9	1.8	7.4	5.8
Overlack, 1995	DB, CO	7	27	40	3	249	114	0.8	0.8	3.8	1.8	7.3	5.8
Overlack, 1995	DB, CO	7	8	43	3	234	115	–6.0	–6.0	3.7	1.7	7.1	5.6
Ferri, 1996	DB, CO	14	61	47	2	264	120	7.4	3.5	3.9	1.8	7.6	5.9
Feldmann, 1996	DB, CO	7	8	27	1	178	120	–2.0	–2.0	3.8	1.8	7.4	5.7
Mühlhauser, 1996	DB, P	28	16	36	4	107	120	2.0	0.0	3.8	1.8	7.2	5.5
McCarron, 1997	DB, CO	28	99	52	1	56	119	4.9	2.9	3.8	1.8	7.4	5.7
Cappuccio, 1997	DB, CO	30	47	67	2	83	118	7.3	3.2	3.9	1.9	7.7	6.0

* Dur.: duration of intervention, days; Op: open; SB: single blind; DB: double blind; P: parallel; CO: cross-over; N: number of persons in trial; Age: mean age of persons in trial; NU: number of urine collections per person per treatment period; SR: sodium reduction, mmol/24-h; Cum: cumulative; CI: 95% confidence interval of previous column. SBP: systolic blood pressure; DBP: diastolic blood pressure; Z: summary statistic; •: no data.

Personal Communication from NA Graudal of unpublished data from his manuscript.[15]

Potassium

Intracellular potassium is the major cation responsible for establishing the membrane potential. The blood pressure of normotensives increases with potassium depletion.[20] Observational studies suggest an inverse relationship between potassium intake and blood pressure.[21] Often there is an inverse relationship with dietary potassium and sodium or a positive relationship between urinary Na+/K+ ratio and blood pressure.[5, 21] In the Scottish Heart Health Study, the relationship between blood pressure and the urinary Na+/K+ ratio was stronger than the relationship between excretion of either sodium or potassium individually and blood pressure.[7] After adjusting for age, gender, BMI, ethanol intake, and urinary sodium intake, it was observed in the INTERSALT study that the systolic blood pressure was 2.7 mmHg lower for each 60 mmol/d higher excretion of potassium.[5] Since African Americans have a lower intake of potassium due to decreased consumption of fresh fruits and vegetables, this may explain the higher prevalence of hypertension in blacks compared to whites.[21-24] Potassium supplementation (80 mmol/d) compared to placebo reduced systolic and diastolic blood pressure (–6.9/–2.5 mmHg) significantly in African Americans consuming a diet low in potassium for 21 days.[25] Explanations for the hypotensive effects of potassium include direct vasodilatation, a direct natriuretic effect, altered baroreceptor function, increased urinary kallikrein, or suppression of the renin-angiotensin-aldosterone axis or sympathetic nervous system.[8]

Studies using the Dahl salt-sensitive rat show a protective effect of potassium supplementation, reducing mortality by 93% in the hypertensive rats.[26] In a 12-year prospective population study of 859 older persons, the relative risks of stroke-associated mortality in the lowest tertile of potassium intake, as compared with that in the top two tertiles combined, were 2.6 ($p = 0.16$) in men and 4.8 ($p = 0.01$) in women.[27] A 10-mmol increase in daily potassium decreased stroke-associated mortality by 40% ($p < 0.001$) in a multivariate analysis. In the Health Professionals Follow-up Study, a multivariate analysis demonstrated the greater the potassium intake, the lower the relative risk of stroke ($p = 0.007$) (Figure 47.1).[28] Furthermore, use of potassium supplements, especially among men

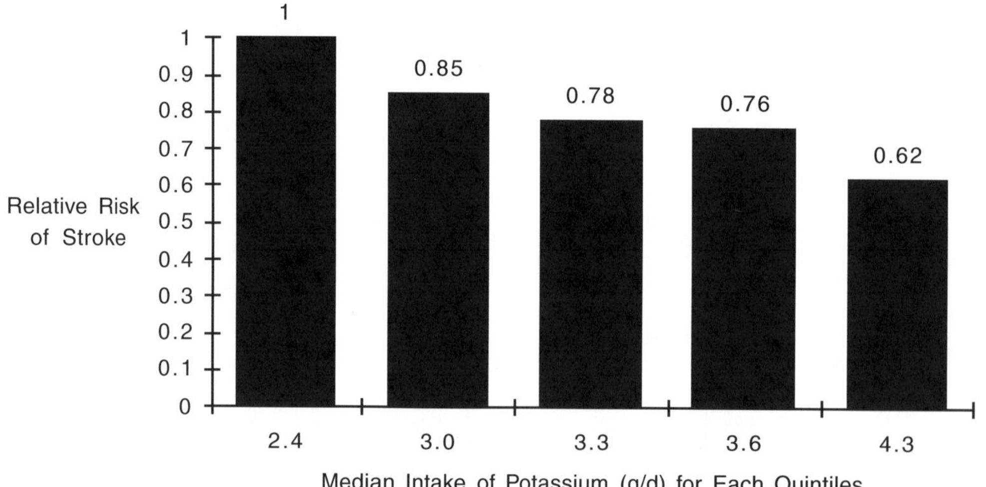

FIGURE 47.1
Multivariate adjusted relative risk of stroke of 43,738 United States men, 40 to 75 years by quintile of potassium intake: adjusted for age, total energy intake, smoking, alcohol consumption, history of hypertension and hypercholesterolemia, family history of premature myocardial infarction, profession, body mass index, and physical activity ($p = 0.007$ for trend). Derived from Ascherio.[28]

taking diuretics, was also inversely related to the risk of stroke. However, after further adjustment for fiber and magnesium intake, the relative risk of stroke was no longer statistically significant.

The largest meta-analysis (see Tables 47.6 and 47.7) observed a significant reduction in both systolic and diastolic blood pressure (–4.44/–2.45 mmHg, $p < 0.01$ for both) for oral potassium supplementation.[29] There was a greater decrease in blood pressure (–4.91/–2.71 mmHg, $p < 0.01$ for both) when trials were examined that achieved a net change in urinary potassium ≥20mmol/d. If trials excluded concomitant antihypertensive drugs, the change in blood pressure was –4.85/–2.71 mmHg, $p < 0.01$ for both). The change in blood pressure was lower for normotensives (–1.8/–1.0 mmHg) compared with hypertensives (–4.4/–2.5 mmHg). The change for systolic blood pressure among black subjects was greater than white subjects (–5.6 mmHg versus –2.0 mmHg, $p = 0.03$); however, the change for diastolic blood pressure was not significant (–3.0 mmHg versus –1.1 mmHg, $p = 0.19$).

Interestingly, there was no overall association between 24-hour urinary potassium excretion and change in systolic or diastolic blood pressure; however, the higher the urinary sodium excretion at followup (see Figure 47.2), the greater the decline in both systolic ($p < 0.001$) and diastolic blood pressure ($p < 0.001$).[29] This explains the lack of benefit seen in a study that combined sodium restriction and potassium supplementation in patients.[30] This randomized, placebo-controlled, double-blind trial of 287 men assessed the effect of 96 mmol of microcrystalline potassium chloride or placebo on a sodium-restricted diet. After the withdrawal of their antihypertensive medication at 12 weeks, there was no significant difference in either systolic or diastolic blood pressure between the two groups at any point in time up to an average of 2.2 years.[30]

Calcium

Most body calcium is found in the skeleton. Calcium is important for its role in smooth muscle relaxation and contraction, especially the vascular smooth muscle that alters peripheral vascular resistance directly. An inverse relationship between water hardness and blood pressure has stimulated an interest in the role of calcium supplementation on blood pressure.[31] Paradoxically, data from the first Health and Nutrition Examination Survey found that daily calcium intake was lower in 1012 hypertensive vs. 8541 normotensive persons (608 mg vs. 722 mg, $p < 0.01$).[32] However, it was not associated with blood pressure when age and BMI were controlled. For 58,218 female nurses with a calcium intake of at least 800 mg/day, the reduction in the risk of hypertension was 22% when compared with an intake of less than 400 mg/day.[33] In men, calcium was inversely associated with baseline blood pressure but not with change in blood pressure; furthermore, intake of calcium in men was not inversely associated with an increased risk of stroke.[28,34] Other observational studies have reported both positive and negative correlations with blood pressure, but many studies did not adjust for weight and alcohol, vitamin D, sodium, and other nutrient intake, and are based on dietary recall.[35] Also, it has been suggested that calcium supplementation is important in African Americans, since intake of dairy products is especially low and the prevalence of hypertension much higher than in caucasians. In addition, sodium excretion and calcium intake interact in salt-sensitive individuals: increased ingested calcium facilitates sodium excretion.[36] Calcium supplementation is associated with controversy because of the association of hyperparathyroidism and hypertension, the pressor effect of hypercalcemia in normotensives, and the direct relationship of calcium and blood pressure.[37] However, responders to calcium supplementation may be a subset of hypertensives with a low renin level, high parathormone level, and low ionized calcium.[36]

TABLE 47.6

Participant and Study Design Characteristics in 33 Potassium Supplementation Trials

Author, Year	No. of Subjects	Age, y Mean	Age, y Range	% Male	% White	% HTN†	AntiHTN Medication	Study Design*	Study Duration, wk
Skrabal, 1981									
(a)	20	...	21-25	100	...	0	No	XO	2
(b)	20	...	21-25	100	...	0	No	XO	2
MacGregor, 1982	23	45	26-66	52	78	100	No	XD	4
Khaw and Thom, 1982	20	...	22-35	100	...	0	No	XD	2
Richards, 1984	12	...	19-52	67	...	100	No	XO	4-6
Smith, 1985	20	53	30-66	55	90	100	No	XD	4
Kaplan, 1985	16	49	35-66	38	19	100	Yes‡	XD	6
Zoccali, 1985	19	38	26-53	53	100	100	No	XD	2
Bulpitt, 1985	33	55	...	45	...	100	Yes‡	PO	12
Matlou, 1986	32	51	34-62	0	0	100	No	XS	6
Barden, 1986	44	32	18-55	0	...	0	No	XD	4
Poulter and Sever ,1986	19	...	18-47	100	0	0	No	XD	2
Chalmers, 1986									
(a)	107	52	...	85	...	100	No	PO	12
(b)	105	52	...	86	...	100	No	PO	12
Grobbee, 1987	40	24	18-28	85	...	100	No	XD	6
Siani, 1987	37	45	21-61	62	...	100	No	PD	15
Svetkey, 1987	101	51	...	74	88	100	No	PD	8
Medical Research Council, 1987	484	...	35-64	56	...	100	Yes‡	PS	24
Grimm, 1988	312	58	45-68	100	...	100	Yes‡	PD	12
Cushman and Langford, 1988	58	54	26-69	100	47	100	No	PD	10
Obell, 1989	48	41	23-56	44	0	100	No	PD	16
Krishna, 1989	10	...	20-40	100	100	0	No	XD	10d
Hypertension Prevention Trial, 1990	391	39	25-49	64	83	0	No	PO	3 y
Mullen and O'Connor, 1990									
(a)	24	25	22-31	100	9	0	No	XD	2
(b)	24	25	22-31	100	92	0	No	XD	2
Patki, 1990	37	50	...	22	...	100	No	XD	8
Valdes, 1991	24	50	...	54		100	No	XD	4
Barden ,1991	37	32	...	0		0	No	XD	4 d
Overlack, 1991	12	37	25-59	67	...	100	No	XS	8
Smith, 1992	22	67	_ 60	57	71	100	No	XD	4 d
Fotherby and Potter, 1992	18	75	66-79	28	...	100	No	XD	4
Whelton, 1995	353	43	30-54	72	86	0	No	PD	24
Brancati, 1996	87	48	27-65	36	0	0	No	PD	3

* XO indicates crossover open; XS, crossover single blind; XD, crossover double blind; PO, parallel open; PS, parallel single blind; PD, parallel double blind; and ellipses, no data.

† HTN indicates hypertensive, BP indicates blood pressure; SBP, systolic BP; and DBP, diastolic BP. Sitting BP was used in the studies by Khaw and Thom, Matlou, Poulter and Sever, Chalmers, Svetkey, Grimm, Hypertension Prevention Trial, Barden, and Overlack.

‡ Study participants were treated with thiazide or thiazide-like diuretics (hydrochlorothiazide [25-75 mg/d] or chlorthalidone [50 mg/d] and in addition, clonidine [0.1 mg twice daily] in 1 subject [Kaplan]; bendrofluazide [2.5-10 mg/d], cyclopenthiazide [25-50 mg/d], hydrochlorothiazide [25 mg/d], furosemide [40-80 mg/d], and chlorthalidone [50-100 mg/d] [Bulpitt]) ; bendrofluazide [5-10 mg/d] [Medical Research Council]; chlorthalidone or hydrochlorothiazide [84%], β-blockers [43%], other medications, e.g., reserpine [6%], hydralazine [6%], and methyldopa [5%] [doses not specified] [Grimm]).

Table Modified from Whelton, PK.[29] Reproduced with permission from May 28, 1997 *JAMA* 277(20):1624-32.

TABLE 47.6

Participant and Study Design Characteristics in 33 Potassium Supplementation Trials

Intervention	Control	Baseline Supine BP, mm Hg† SBP/DBP	Baseline Urinary Electrolytes, mmol/d K+/Na+	Baseline K+ mmol/L
200 mmol K from diet, 200 mmol NaCl	80 mmol KCl, 200 mmol NaCl	...	.../...	4.7
200 mmol K from diet, 50 mmol NaCl	80 mmol KCI,50 mmol NaCl	...	.../...	4.6
64 mmol KCl	Placebo	154/99	68/152	4.0
64 mmol KCl	Placebo	118/74	73/138	...
200 mmol K from diet, 180 mmol NaCl	60 mmol KCI,180 mmol NaCl	140-180/90-105	.../...	3.8
64 mmol KCI, 70 mmol NaCl	Placebo,70 mmol NaCl	163/103	72/68	3.9
60 mmol KCI	Placebo	131/96	46/166	3.0
100 mmol KCI	Placebo	154/96	.../...	3.8
64 mmol KCl	Usual care	150/95	66/...	3.7
65 mmol KCl	Placebo	154/105	62/172	3.8
80 mmol KCl	Placebo	118/71	50/131	...
64 mmol KCl	Placebo	113/69	39/123	...
100 mmol K from diet	Normal diet	150/95	71/155	...
100 mmol K from diet, low Na	Low Na	152/95	68/148	...
72 mmol KCI, low Na	Placebo, low Na	143/78	71/141	3.8
48 mmol KCI	Placebo	145/92	60/190	4.4
120 mmol KCI	Placebo	145/95	.../...	4.4
17-34 mmol KCl	Usual care	161/98	.../...	4.2
96 mmol KCI, low Na	Placebo, low Na	124/80	79/166	4.2
80 mmol KCl	Placebo	150/95	52/176	...
64 mmol KCl	Placebo	174/100	59/171	4.0
90 mmol KCI	10 mmol KCl	120/77	70/164	3.2
100 mmol K from diet, low Na	Low Na	124/82	64/161	...
75 mmol KCI	Placebo	117/69	77/153	4.2
75 mmol K citrate	Placebo	117/69	77/153	4.2
60 mmol KCl	Placebo	155/100	62/196	3.6
64 mmol KCl	Placebo	147/96	57/155	3.8
80 mmol KCl	Placebo	105/63	53/105	...
120 mmol K citrate and bicarbonate	Placebo	150/100	62/169	4.4
120 mmol KCI	Placebo	152/87	70/192	3.9
60 mmol KCI	Placebo	187/96	63/115	4.2
60 mmol KCI	Placebo	122/81	59/153	...
80 mmol KCl	Placebo	125/78	47/147	...

Reproduced with permission from May 28, 1997 *JAMA* 277(20):1624-32. Copyright 1997, American Medical Association.

TABLE 47.7

Urinary Electrolyte Excretion, Body Weight, and Blood Pressure during Followup in 33 Potassium Supplementation Trials*

Author, Year	Mean Net Change in Urinary Electrolytes, mmol/d K+/Na+	Urinary Sodium Excretion during Followup, mmol/d	Mean Net Change in Body Weight, kg	Mean Net Change, in Blood Pressure, mm Hg Systolic/Diastolic
Skrabal, 1981				
(a)	44/-55	155	-0.9	-1.7/-4.5
(b)	107/-12	28	-0.2	0.4/-0.5
MacGregor, 1982	56/29	169	-0.2	-7.0/-4.0
Khaw and Thom, 1982	52/9	164	...	-1.1/-2.4
Richards, 1984	129/5	200	0.8	-1.9/-1.0
Smith, 1985	50/7	80	0.1	-2.0/0
Kaplan, 1985	46/1	168	0.8	-5.6/-5.8
Zoccali, 1985	81/13	195	...	-1.0/-3.0
Bulpitt et at, 1985	40/10	149	1.2	2.3/4.8
Matlou et at, 1986	62/35	165	-0.4	-7.0/-3.0
Barden et at, 1986	68/5	130	...	-1.4/-1.4
Poulter and Sever, 1986	38/1	114	-0.1	-1.2/2.0
Chalmers et at, 1986				
(a)	22/7	150	...	-3.9/-3.1
(b)	12/25	79	...	-1.0/1.6
Grobbee, 1987	57/12	69	0.4	-2.5/-0.6
Siani, 1987	30/6	189	...	-14.0/-10.5
Svetkey, 1987	.../...	...	...	6.3/-2.5
Medical Research Council, 1987	.../...	...	...	0.8/-0.7
Grimm, 1988	80/-9	114	...	0.7/1.4
Cushman and Langford, 1988	36/177	177	...	.../-0.1
Obel, 1989	39/...	172	...	-41.0/-17.0
Krishna, 1989	47/44	144	-0.6	5.5/-7.4
Hypertension Prevention Trial, 1990	0/-6	155	0.2	-1.3/-0.9
Mullen and O'Connor, 1990				
(a)	23/-12	141	-0.1	0/3.0
(b)	34/-15	138	-0.2	-2.0/2.0
Patki, 1990	22/-14	184	...	-12.1/-13.1
Valdes, 1991	68/19	166	-1	-6.3/-3.0
Barden, 1991	72/15	120	...	-1.7/-0.6
Overlack, 1991	105/-13	156	0	2.8/3.0
Smith et at, 1992	109/29	221	0.2	-4.3/-1.7
Fotherby and Potter, 1992	39/13	136	-0.7	-10.0/-6.0
Whelton, 1995	42/6	144	...	-0.3/0.1
Brancati, 1996	70/20	141	-0.1	-6.9/-2.5

* Ellipses indicate no data.

Table Modified from Whelton PK, He J, Cutler JA, et al. Reproduced with permission from May 28, 1997 *JAMA* 277(20):1624-32.

In a randomized, double-blind study of 48 hypertensive persons and 32 normotensive persons, 1000 mg per day of calcium or placebo was given for 8 weeks.[38] Supine blood pressure decreased significantly 3.8/2.3 mmHg in the hypertensive subjects; 25, 23, and 13% of subjects achieved a blood pressure goal of systolic <140 mmHg, diastolic <90 mmHg and both systolic <140 mmHg and diastolic <90 mmHg, respectively. Calcium did not lower blood pressure in the normotensives. 44% of hypertensive and 19% of normotensive subjects lowered their standing systolic blood pressure >10 mmHg. There have been at least 67 randomized trials of calcium supplements in nonpregnant study popula-

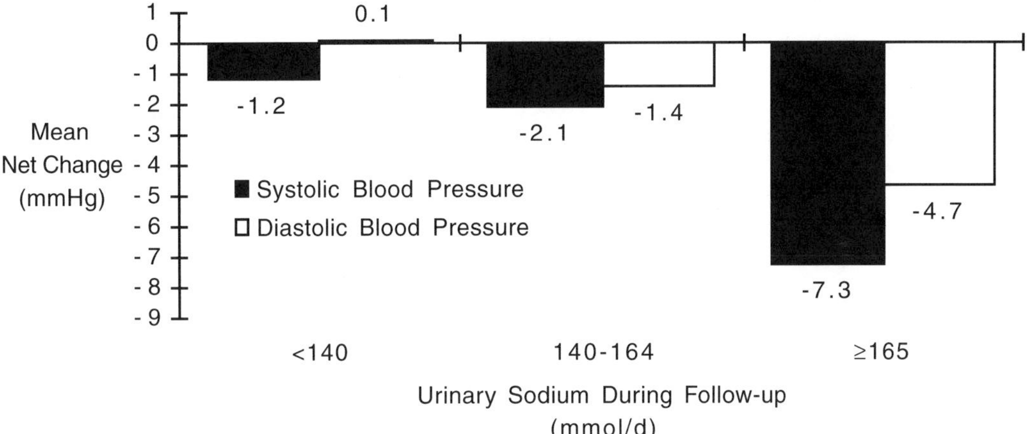

FIGURE 47.2
Effect of potassium supplementation on net blood pressure reduction according to urinary sodium excretion during followup: the greater the sodium excretion, the greater the blood pressure reduction with potassium supplementation (p <0.001 for both systolic and diastolic blood pressure). Derived from Whelton PK, He J, Cutler JA, et al. *JAMA* 277: 1624, 1997. With permission.

tions. There have been several meta-analyses to assess the effect of dietary and nondietary interventions on blood pressure.[35,39-43] A larger effect of calcium supplementation on systolic blood pressure was observed with increasing age and among women.[41] The subgroup of hypertensive subjects had a greater reduction in blood pressure than the normotensives (–4.30/–1.50 mmHg versus –0.27/–0.33 mmHg).[42] The change in systolic and diastolic blood pressure was significant for the hypertensives, but not the normotensives.[42] The largest meta-analysis (see Tables 47.8 and 47.9) shows a reduction of blood pressure of –1.44/–0.84 mmHg (p <0.001 for each).[43] There was no difference in the change in blood pressure comparing 33 nondietary trials (–1.09/–0.87 mmHg) and the 9 dietary trials (–2.01/–1.09 mmHg). The authors concluded that the small reduction in blood pressure of calcium supplements does not merit its use in mild hypertension, and further suggest that the use of calcium must weigh the benefits of reducing cardiovascular disease and increasing bone density versus the risk of nephrolithiasis.

Despite this modest benefit in nonpregnant subjects, a meta-analysis (see Tables 47.10 and 47.11) of calcium supplementation in pregnancy observed a blood pressure reduction of –5.40/–3.44 mmHg and a decrease in the rate of preeclampsia (odds ratio = 0.38 [95% CI: 0.22 to 0.65]).[44] Since the publication of the meta-analysis, the National Institutes of Health sponsored trial, Calcium for Preeclampsia Prevention, has been completed.[45] This placebo-controlled, randomized, multicenter trial assigned 4589 nulliparous women 13 to 21 weeks pregnant to 2 g of calcium carbonate or placebo. There was no benefit in the rate of preeclampsia (6.9 versus 7.3%), the prevalence of gestational hypertension (15.3 versus 17.3%), or pregnancy-associated proteinuria (3.4 versus 3.3%) in the calcium (n = 2295) and placebo (n = 2294) groups.

Magnesium

Magnesium is a divalent intracellular cation. The adult body contains about 25 g distributed between the skeleton (60%) and soft tissues (40%).[46] It serves as a cofactor for many enzyme systems. Intracellular calcium increases and blood pressure rises as magnesium depletion occurs in rats. The hypotensive effect of magnesium is observed best when given

TABLE 47.8

Randomized Controlled Trials Examining the Relationship of Calcium and Blood Pressure

Author, Year, Study Design	No. of Subjects (Intervention/ Control)	Quality Score*	Calcium Formulation	Elemental Calcium (mg/day)	Study Duration (weeks)
Nondietary Interventions					
Belizan, 1983	30/27	4	Calcium gluconate	1000	22
Sunderrajan, 1984[cx]	17/17	0	Calcium carbonate	1000	4
Johnson, 1985	59/56	2	Calcium carbonate	1500	208
McCarron, 1985[cx]	80/80	3	Calcium carbonate	1000	8
Grobbee, 1986	46/44	4	Calcium citrate	1000	12
Nowson, 1986	31/33	3	Calcium carbonate	1600	8
Resnick, 1986[cx, ci]	8/8	0	Calcium carbonate	2000	8
Strazzullo, 1986[cx, ci]	17/17	3	Calcium gluconate	1000	15
Van Berestyn, 1986	29/29	3	Calcium carbonate	1500	6
Cappuccio, 1987[cx]	18/18	4	Calcium gluconate	1600	4
Lyle, 1987	37/38	4	Calcium carbonate	1500	12
Meese, 1987[cx]	19/17	3	Calcium carbonate	800	8
Siani, 1987[cx]	8/8	4	Calcium gluconate	1000	3
Thomsen, 1987	14/14	3	Calcium gluconate	2000	52
Vinson, 1987	4/5	4	Calcium carbonate	500	7
Zoccali, 1987[cx, ci]	11/11	3	Calcium gluconate	1000	2
Siani, 1988[cx]	14/14	5	Calcium gluconate	1000	4
Zoccali, 1988[cx]	21/21	3	Calcium gluconate	1000	8
Orwoll, 1990[ci]	34/28	3	Calcium carbonate	1000	156
Tanji, 1991[cx]	28/28	3	Calcium carbonate	1200	12
Cutler, 1992	237/234	6	Calcium carbonate	1000	26
Lyle, 1992	21/21	3	Calcium carbonate	1500	8
Galloe, 1993[cx]	20/20	4	Calcium gluconate	2000	12
Jespersen, 1993[cx]	7/7	5	Calcium carbonate	1000	8
Pan, 1993[cx]	14/15	1	Calcium citrate and placebo Vitamin D	800	11
Weinberger, 1993[cx]	46/46	4	Calcium carbonate	1500	8
Petersen, 1994[ci]	10/10	1	Calcium gluconate	2000	26
Zhou, 1994	30/27	3	Calcium carbonate	1000	14
Gillman, 1995	51/50	4	Calcium citrate malate	600	12
Sacks, 1995[ci]	34/31	5	Calcium carbonate	1000	26
Lijnen, 1996[ci]	16/16	5	Calcium gluconate	2000	16
Davis, 1997	17/17	3	Calcium gluconate	1500	4
Sanchez, 1997	10/10	4	Calcium gluconate	1500	8
Dietary Interventions					
Margetts, 1986[cx, ci]	39/39	3	Other dietary manipulation	1076	6
Rouse, 1986	18/18	3	Other dietary manipulation	1177	6
Bierenbaum, 1988[cx]	50/50	1	Milk/dairy product suppl	1150	26
Morris, 1988	142/139	4	Other dietary manipulation	1500	12
Hakala, 1989	31/37	3	Other dietary manipulation	1163	52
Van Beresteijn, 1990	28/25	3	Milk/dairy product suppl	1180	6
Kynast-Gales, 1992[cx]	7/7	1	Milk/dairy product suppl	1515	4
McCarron, 1997	274/274	4	Milk/dairy product suppl	1886	10
Appel, 1997	151/154	4	Milk/dairy product suppl	1265	8

[cx], cross-over study; [ci], cointervention.

* A quality score of 6 corresponds to the highest quality level

Adapted from Griffith LE, Guyatt GH, Cook RJ, et al. *Am J Hypertens* 12, 84, 1999. With permission.

TABLE 47.9

Randomized Controlled Trials Studying the Effect of Calcium Supplementation and Blood Pressure

Author, Year	Position of Blood Pressure Measurement	Mean BP at Study End*	Systolic Mean Baseline, mm Hg	Systolic Mean Difference, mmHg (SD)	Diastolic Mean Baseline, mm Hg	Diastolic Mean Difference, mm Hg (SD)
Nondietary Interventions						
Belizan, 1983						
Women	Lateral	1	102	-2.40 (1.03)	68	-4.50 (1.46)
Men	Lateral	1	113	-0.80 (1.05)	71	-6.00 (1.94)
Sunderrajan, 1984						
Normotensive	Sitting	2	NA	1.89 (2.78)	NA	1.89 (2.50)
Hypertensive	Sitting	2	NA	-1.63 (5.93)	NA	-4.13 (2.50)
Johnson, 1985						
Normotensive	Sitting	2	120	0.00 (3.01)	74	0.00 (1.67)
Hypertensive	Sitting	2	141	-13.0 (6.52)	86	0.00 (2.79)
McCarron, 1985						
Normotensive	Standing	2	113	1.30 (2.00)	75	1.00 (2.62)
Hypertensive	Standing	2	144	-5.60 (2.10)	92	-2.30 (1.40)
Grobbee, 1986	Sitting	1	143	-0.40 (2.27)	83	-2.40 (1.90)
Nowson, 1986						
Normotensive	Sitting	1		0.00 (2.97)		0.30 (2.33)
Hypertensive	Sitting	1	157	1.60 (3.83)	92	1.30 (2.90)
Resnick, 1986						
Salt-sensitive	Sitting	1	NA	NA	NA	-8.0 (6.0)
Salt-insensitive	Sitting	1	NA	NA	NA	7.0 (6.0)
Strazzullo, 1986	Standing	2	145	-8.60 (4.98)	98	-1.70 (2.56)
Van Berestevn, 1986	Supine	1	115	-1.36 (1.88)	65	0.79 (1.66)
Cappuccio, 1987	Standing	2	156	2.00 (4.17)	112	0.40 (2.64)
Lyle, 1987						
White	Sitting	1	115	-2.44 (2.00)	75	-1.89 (2.31)
Black	Sitting	1	114	-3.63 (3.85)	71	4.02 (5.67)
Meese, 1987	Sitting	2	143	-5.00 (4.21)	95	-2.00 (2.83)
Siani, 1987	Supine	2	154	5.10 (8.01)	96	1.30 (4.10)
Thomsen, 1987	Supine	2	124	-0.50 (6.10)	76	-1.30 (3.78)
Vinson, 1987	Supine	2	114	7.90 (4.93)	74	2.40 (2.05)
Zoccali, 1987	Sitting	1	141	6.45 (3.35)	88	4.64 (2.21)
Siani, 1988	Supine	2	139	2.20 (4.94)	91	0.70 (3.68)
Zoccali, 1988	Sitting	1	142	-2.80 (2.97)	88	-2.80 (2.47)
Orwoll, 1990	Sitting	1	131	2.60 (3.54)	84	3.08 (2.63)
Tanji, 1991	Sitting	1	146	3.00 (4.20)	95	2.00 (2.40)
Cutler, 1992	Sitting	1	126	-0.46 (0.67)	84	0.20 (0.46)
Lyle, 1992	Sitting	1	133	-5.90 (1.99)	87	-7.20 (1.71)
Galloe, 1993	Sitting	1	168	2.20 (4.49)	97	3.30 (2.75)
Jespersen, 1993	Supine	1	148	-0.57 (7.20)	93	-0.86 (3.88)
Pan, 1993	Sitting	1	136	-7.09 (7.89)	72	-0.87 (3.29)
Weinberger, 1993						
Normotensive	Sitting	2	116	1.00 (3.00)	72	-1.00 (2.64)
Hypertensive	Sitting	2	131	-2.00 (5.68)	87	-1.00 (2.92)
Petersen, 1994	Sitting	2	145	4.50 (13.2)	81	-8.20 (5.10)
Zhou, 1994	Sitting	1	158	-14.6 (4.48)	103	-7.11 (2.43)
Gillman, 1995	Sitting	1	102	-2.20 (11.0)	58	-0.80 (7.16)
Sacks, 1995	Sitting	1	NA	3.70 (2.45)	NA	3.60 (2.32)
Lijnen, 1996	Supine	1	114	-5.70 (2.18)	73	-3.50 (1.79)
Davis, 1997	Mean 24 h ambulatory	1	125	-1.72 (1.20)	91	-0.49 (0.35)
Sanchez, 1997	Sitting	1	166	1.60 (1.60)	99	0.40 (1.21)

TABLE 47.9 *(Continued)*

Randomized Controlled Trials Studying the Effect of Calcium Supplementation and Blood Pressure

Author, Year	Position of Blood Pressure Measurement	Mean BP at Study End*	Systolic Mean Baseline, mm Hg	Systolic Mean Difference, mmHg (SD)	Diastolic Mean Baseline, mm Hg	Diastolic Mean Difference, mm Hg (SD)
Dietary Interventions						
Margetts, 1986	Sitting	1	NA	-3.50 (1.75)	NA	-1.20 (1.00)
Rouse, 1986	Sitting	2	NA	1.90 (2.30)	NA	2.30 (1.40)
Bierenbaum, 1988	Sitting	2	119	-2.00 (2.19)	79	-1.00 (1.33)
Morris, 1988						
Normotensive	Standing	1	113	-1.00 (1.04)	77	-0.90 (0.80)
Hypertensive	Standing	1	145	-3.60 (1.50)	94	-1.20 (0.86)
Hakala, 1989	Sitting	1	129	3.80 (11.9)	84	3.20 (4.53)
Van Beresteijn, 1990	Supine	1	114	-2.82 (1.83)	63	0.43 (1.89)
Kynast-Gales, 1992	Supine	1	136	-8.29 (8.12)	83	-0.14 (6.15)
McCarron, 1997	Sitting	1	134	-1.80 (0.78)	85	-1.20 (0.46)
Appel, 1997	Sitting	1	131	-2.70 (0.83)	84	-1.90 (0.60)

* For mean blood pressure at study end, 1 indicates change and 2 indicates mean.

Modified from Griffith LE, Guyatt GH, Cook RJ, et al. *Am J Hypertens* 12, 84, 1999. With permission.

in preeclampsia and toxemia. Magnesium supplementation in 400 normotensive primigravida women given from 13 to 24 weeks gestation did not lower blood pressure or the incidence of preeclampsia.[47] However, among 2138 hypertensive women admitted in labor, intramuscular magnesium sulfate was superior to phenytoin in preventing eclamptic seizures (0 versus 0.92%, $p = 0.004$).[48]

Magnesium and calcium contribute to water hardness. There is an inverse relationship between water hardness and blood pressure.[49,50] However, epidemiologic studies assessing the role of magnesium and blood pressure often do not control for potential confounders, including caloric, ethanol, sodium, potassium, and calcium intake, and use of antihypertensive medication.[50] Thus, observational studies using 24-hour dietary recall, food records, and food frequency questionnaires have not always shown a consistent correlation, but generally show a negative correlation with both systolic and diastolic blood pressure after adjustment.[50] In the Health Professionals Follow-up Study, the relative risk of a stroke among 43,738 men between the lowest quintile of magnesium intake and highest quintile, after adjustment for age, BMI, various risk factors, family history, profession, and physical activity, was 0.62 ($p < 0.002$).[28] In the Atherosclerosis Risk in Communities Study of four U.S. communities (n = 15,248 participants), an early report suggested that low serum and dietary magnesium may be related to the etiology of hypertension; however, a subsequent report found no association between dietary magnesium intake and incident hypertension.[51,52]

The mechanism most often cited for the apparent antihypertensive effect of magnesium is a calcium antagonist property. Other mechanisms include stimulation of vascular prostacyclin release, renal vasodilation, acceleration of the cell membrane sodium pump, and alterations in vascular responsiveness to vasoactive agents.[53] One 1988 analysis concluded that there were inadequate data from the four randomized, controlled trials to suggest a hypotensive effect.[49] Since that report, there have been a number of trials reported with mixed results (see Table 47.12). It has been suggested that combinations of cations may act in concert; however, in a randomized, double-blind, multicenter trial of 125 participants, there was no hypotensive effect of magnesium in combination with either calcium or potassium.[53] In normotensive women whose reported intake of magnesium was

TABLE 47.10

Randomized Controlled Trials of Calcium Supplementation in Pregnancy

Author, Year	No. of Participants, Calcium Supplementation/ Placebo	Calcium Formulation	Elemental Calcium Equivalent, mg/d	Type of Control	Weeks of Gestation	Treatment Duration, wk	Cointervention	Compliance Assessed	Quality Score†
Trials Providing Data on Treatment Effects of Systolic and Diastolic Blood Pressure									
Belizan, 1983	11/14	Calcium Sandoz	2000	Placebo	15	22	NA*	NA	3
Marya , 1987	188/182	Unknown calcium supplement	375	Placebo	22	18	No	Yes	5
Villar,1987	25/27	Os-Cal tablets	1500	Placebo	26	14	Yes	Yes	0
Lopez-Jaramillo,1989	49/43	Calcium gluconate	2000	Placebo	23	17	No	Yes	1
Repke, 1989	16/18	Os-Cal tablets	1500	Placebo	25	10	No	Yes	4
Lopez-Jaramillo,1990	22/34	Elemental calcium	2000	Placebo	30	10	No	No	4
Belizan, 1991	579/588	Calcium carbonate	2000	Placebo	20	20	No	Yes	2
Felix, 1991	14/11	Elemental calcium	2000	Placebo	20	20	No	Yes	3
Knight, 1992	10/10	Os-Cal tablets	1000	Normal diet	12	20	Yes	Yes	5
Sanchez-Ramos, 1993	36/39	Unknown calcium supplement	NA	Unknown	22	18	No	No	6
Sanchez-Ramos, 1994	29/34	Calcium carbonate	2000	Placebo	25	15	No	Yes	4
Levine, 1997‡	2294/2295	Calcium carbonate	2000	Placebo	17	21	No	Yes	6
Trials Providing Data on Binary Outcomes Exclusively									
Montanaro, 1990	84/86	Calcium carbonate	2000	Placebo	24	16	No	No	1
Villar and Repke 1990	95/95	Os-Cal tablets‡	2000	Placebo	23	20	Yes	Yes	2
Cong, 1993	50/50	Shen gu capsules	Unknown	Placebo	22	18	No	No	0

* NA indicates not applicable.

† Quality scores range from 0 to 6 with 6 indicating the highest quality score

‡ Calcium for the Preeclampsia Prevention Trial (Not in the original meta-analysis)

Modified from Bucher HC. Reproduced with permission from April 10, 1996 *JAMA* 275(14):1113-7. Copyright 1996, American Medical Association.

TABLE 47.11

Change in Blood Pressure in Randomized Controlled Trials of Calcium Supplementation in Pregnancy

Author, Year	Mean Difference In Systolic Blood Pressure, mm Hg	Mean Difference in Diastolic Blood Pressure, mm Hg
Belizan, 1983	-5.10	-5.70
Marya, 1987	-6.90	-3.40
Villar, 1987	-4.10	-4.90
Lopez-Jaramillo, 1989	-8.70	-6.60
Repke, 1989	-2.50	-2.77
Lopez-Jaramillo, 1990	-13.10	-11.80
Belizan 1991	-1.70	-0.90
Felix, 1991	-6.30	-5.80
Knight and Keith, 1992		
Normotensive	-2.70	0.50
Hypertensive	+4.8	0
Sanchez-Ramos, 1993	+4.6	-0.82
Sanchez-Ramos, 1994	-4.08	-3.00
Levine, 1997*	-0.3	+0.3

* Calcium for the Preeclampsia Prevention Trial (not in the original meta-analysis)

Modified from Bucher HC. Reproduced with permission from April 10, 1996 *JAMA* 275(14):1113-7. Copyright 1996, American Medical Association.

between the 10th and 15th percentiles, 16 weeks' daily supplement of magnesium 14 mmol had no significant treatment effect (–0.9/–0.7 mmHg). The administration of magnesium with potassium did not enhance the effect of potassium alone.[54]

ω-3 Polyunsaturated Fatty Acids

ω-3 polyunsaturated fatty acids refer to the fish oil, very long chain fatty acids eicosapentaenoic (EPA) and docosahexaenoic (DHA) acids. ω-3 polyunsaturated fatty acids are thought to lower blood pressure by altering the balance of the vasoconstrictor thromboxane A_2 and the vasodilator prostacyclin prostaglandin I_3, modulating the vasoconstrictor response to pressors, or decreasing blood viscosity.[8]

A meta-analysis by Appel identified 40 studies testing the impact of ω-3 polyunsaturated fatty acids on blood pressure; however, 23 were eliminated because of design, including concurrent antihypertensive medications, no control group, unhealthy study population, concurrent use of ω-3 polyunsaturated fatty acids in the control group, or insufficient data.[55] Most trials used a combined dose of 3 g daily of EPA and DHA, which is equal to 6 to 10 capsules of commercial fish oil supplements or two 100 g servings of fish that are high in ω-3 polyunsaturated fatty acids. The overall change in blood pressure, –1.5/–1.0 mmHg, was significant. For normotensives, the change in blood pressure, –1.0/–0.5 mmHg, was significant for the systolic blood pressure only. However, the decline in blood pressure, –5.5/–3.5 mmHg, for hypertensives was significant for both systolic and diastolic blood pressure ($p < 0.001$). Interestingly, the higher the blood pressure, the greater the reduction ($p < 0.05$); however, this was not a function of the dose of the ω-3 polyunsaturated fatty acids, duration of treatment, type of intervention (food versus oil capsules), or age of participants. Side effects summarized include the unpleasant or fishy taste, gastrointes-

TABLE 47.12

Randomized Trials of Magnesium Supplementation

Author, Year	n	Mean Age, Yr	Men, %	Cohort	BP Meds	Mg Salt, mmol Mg/d	Study Design	Duration, Weeks	Control ΔSBP/ΔDBP	Magnesium ΔSBP/ΔDBP
Itoh, 1997	33	65	33	Mixed	?	Hydroxide, 17-23	DB, PR	4	+1/-1	-5/-2
TOHP, 1992‡	461	43	70	Normotensive	No	Diglycine, 15	DB, PR	24	-2.9/-2.7	-3.0/-2.9
Sacks, 1998	153	39	0	Normotensive	No	Lactate, 14	DB, PR	16	+0.4/+0.2	-0.5/-0.5
de Valk, 1998	50	62.5	56	Diabetes (insulin)	?	Aspartate, 15	DB, PR	12	-10.4/-0.8	-7.7/-0.3
Purvis, 1994	28	53.8	86	Diabetes (no insulin)	?	Chloride, 15.7	DB, CO	6		-7.4/-2.3
Cappuccio, 1985	17	52	53	Hypertensive	No	Aspartate, 15	DB, CO	4	-3/-3	0/-2
Dyckner, 1983	20	65	33	90% Hypertensive	Yes	Aspartate, 15	O,PR	24	-0/-4	-12/-8
Ferrara, 1992	14	47.5	57	Hypertensive	No	Pidolate, 15	DB, PR	24	-17/-4	-7/-7
Henderson, 1986	41	62	?	Hypertensive	Yes	Oxide, 12.5	DB, PR	24	-3/-1	-4/-3
Kawano, 1998	60	58	57	Hypertensive	Some	Oxide, 20	CO	8		-3.7/-1.7
Lind, 1991	71	61	52	Hypertensive	No	Mixed†, 15	DB, PR	24	-2/-4.2	+1/-2
Plum-Wirell, 1994	39	39	62	Hypertensive	No	Aspartate, 15	DB, CO	8	-0.8/-0.4	-2.4/-0.4
Reyes, 1984	21	57	19	Hypertensive	Yes	Chloride, 15.8	DB, PR	3	-13/-4	-11/-7
Sanjuliani, 1996	15	36-65	47	Hypertensive	No	Oxide, 25	DB, CO	3	+1.7/-1.0	-7.6/-3.8
Sibai, 1989	374	18	0	Pregnancy	No	Aspartate, 15	DB, PR	21	+16/+18	+15/+16
Widman, 1993	17	50	88	Hypertensive	No	Hydroxide, 15-40	DB, CO	9	-1/0.0	-7.9/-8.2
Wirell, 1994	39	26-69	77	Hypertensive	Yes	Aspartate, 15	DB, CO	8	+3.2/+2.3	-3.8//-1.7
Witteman, 1994	91	57	0	Hypertensive	No	Aspartate, 20	DB, PR	24	+0.2/+0.1	-3.3/-2.4
Zemel, 1990	13	~49	86	Hypertensive	No	Aspartate, 40	DB, PR	12	-1/+1	+3/+2

† 4.58 mmol Mg lactate + 0.42 Mg Citrate; ‡ TOPH, Trial of Hypertension Prevention (Phase I)

tinal symptoms, eructation, loose stool or diarrhea, and obstipation occurring in 28% of experimental subjects — 13% of the control group ($p < 0.001$).[55]

Another meta-analysis included 31 of 52 studies that included trials with a placebo group and a report of pretreatment and post-treatment blood pressures (see Table 47.13).[56] Like the previous meta-analysis, hypertensives (–3.4/–2.0 mmHg) had greater blood pressure decline than normotensives (–0.4/–0.7 mmHg), but the dose of the fish oils was higher in the hypertensive group (5.6 g/d) than the normotensive group (4.2 g/d). There also was a statistically significant dose-dependent decline in blood pressure: ≤ 3g/d, –1.3/–0.7 mmHg; >3 to 7g/d, –2.9/–1.6 mmHg; and 15g/d, –8.1/–5.8 mmHg. The effect of fish oil on blood pressure is maximally manifested by 3 to 4 weeks.

Since the completion of these meta-analyses, several new studies have supported their conclusions. In a double-blind, placebo-controlled trial of parallel design, 59 overweight, mildly hyperlipidemic men were randomized to 4 g/d of purified EPA, DHA, or olive oil (placebo) capsules and continued their usual diets for 6 weeks. Fifty-six subjects completed the study. Only DHA significantly reduced 24-hour and daytime ambulatory blood pressure ($p < 0.05$).[57] In 63 overweight hypertensives, combining a daily fish meal with a weight-reducing regimen led to additive reduction on ambulatory blood pressure and decreased heart rate.[58]

Dietary Protein

Cross-sectional studies show that dietary protein intake is inversely related to blood pressure, although a direct relationship was considered to exist.[59] Protein intake was thought to increase blood pressure due to adverse effects on renal function in partially nephrectomized rats. The mechanism of action of high dietary protein intake is not clear, but multicollinearity (multiple nutrient intake that correlated with one another) is a problem. Amino acid production (e.g., tryptophan, tyrosine, and arginine) may affect hormones or neurotransmitters that ultimately alter blood pressure. For instance, the sulfonic amino acid taurine given 6 g for 7 days in 19 young hypertensive subjects decreased blood pressure –9.0/–4.1 mm Hg compared with to –2.7/–1.2 mmHg in the placebo-treated subjects in a double-blind, placebo-controlled trial.[60] Perhaps other protein metabolites have natriuretic or diuretic activity.

Human observational studies on protein and blood pressure are displayed in Table 47.14. These studies show in aggregate that increased protein intake, determined by food records or recall or by urine studies of sulfate and urea nitrogen, is associated with decreased blood pressure. The relationship of blood pressure and vegetable protein versus animal protein is unclear. After adjustment for age, BMI, alcohol consumption, urinary sodium excretion, dietary intake, and resident area for each one standard deviation higher level of dietary protein intake (39 g), a 3.55 mmHg lower systolic blood pressure was observed.

Most intervention trials (Table 47.15) have been conducted in normotensive subjects, were not designed to assess the relationship between protein and blood pressure or determine a dose relationship, and were not powered adequately or randomized.[59,61]

Dietary Fiber

Vegetarians and other persons with high fiber intakes have lower average blood pressures than persons with low fiber intakes do. In the Coronary Artery Risk Development in Young Adults (CARDIA) Study, fiber intake predicted insulin levels, weight gain, and other cardiovascular risk factors more potently than did fat consumption.[62] High intake of fiber was associated with lower systolic and diastolic blood pressure in whites but not African-

TABLE 47.13

Characteristics of the 31 Trials used for the Meta-Analysis of Fish Oil and Blood Pressure*

Study, Year	Study Design*	Blinding Subject	Blinding Observer§	Study Length	n, Treatment*	ω-3 Dose (g/d)‡	Gender (Age Range)	Baseline Pressure¶	BP Effect SBP/DBP¶
Health Subjects									
Mortensen, 1983	XO	+	+	4	20 Fish oil 20 Mixed oil	3.3	Men (25-40 y)	120/76	-4.0/-4.0
Bruckner, 1987	PG	+	-	3	10 Fish oil 11 Olive oil	3.9	Men (19-40 y)	119/80	+5.0/+1.0
v Houwelingen, 1987									
Maastricht	PG	-	+	6	19 Fish 20 Meat	4.7	Men (20-45 y)	121/77	+1.1/-0.9
Tromso	PG	-	+	6	11 Fish 12 Meat	4.7	Men (20-45 y)	118/77	+0.1/-0.9
Zeist	PG	-	+	6	10 Fish 10 Meat	4.7	Men (20-45 y)	115/73	-3.7/-3.0
Flaten, 1990	PG	+	+	6	27 Fish oil 29 Olive oil	6.5	Men (35-45 y)	119/80	+1.5/+0.8
Ryu, 1990	PG	NS†	NS	4	10 Fish oil 10 Wheat germ	3	Men (20-39 y)	124/73	-4.3/-2.0
TOHP, 1992	PG	+	+	24	175 Fish oil 175 Olive oil	2.4	Men & Women (30-54y)	123/81	-0.2/-0.6
Hypertensive Subjects									
Norris, 1986	XO	+	+	6	16 Fish oil 16 Placebo	NS	Men & Women (45-74 y)	161/95	-10.0/-2.0
Knapp, 1989	PG	-	-	4	8 Fish oil 8 Saturated mix	3	Men (age NS)	137/94	-2.6/-0.1
Meland, 1989	PG	+	+	6	20 Fish oil 20 Mixed oil	6	Men (26-66 y)	149/101	+1.0/-1.0
Bonaa, 1990	PG	NS	NS	10	78 Fish oil 78 Corn oil	5.1	Men & Women (34-60 y)	144/95	-6.4/-2.8

TABLE 47.13 *(Continued)*

Characteristics of the 31 Trials used for the Meta-Analysis of Fish Oil and Blood Pressure*

Study, Year	Study Design*	Blinding Subject	Blinding Observer§	Study Length	n, Treatment*	ω-3 Dose (g/d)‡	Gender (Age Range)	Baseline Pressure¶	BP Effect SBP/DBP¶
Levinson, 1990	PG	+	+	6	8 Fish oil 8 Saturated mix	15	Men & Women (18-75 y)	147/94	-8.0/-9.0
Wing, 1990	XO	+	+	8	20 Fish oil 20 Olive oil	4.5	Men & Women (32-75 y)	139/81	+0.6/-0.3
Radack, 1991	PG	+	+	12	16 Fish oil 17 Safflower	2	Men & Women (mean, 46 y)	136/95	-7.2/-6.7
Margolin, 1991	PG	+	+	8	22 Fish oil 24 Corn oil	4.7	Men & Women (60-80 y)	164/94	+1.1/+0.1
Morris, 1992	XO	+	+	6	18 Fish oil 18 Olive oil	4.8	Men & Women (32-64 y)	130/87	-2.4/-1.8
Hypercholesterolemic Subjects									
Demke, 1988	PG	+	+	4	13 Fish oil 18 Safflower	1.7	Men & Women (18-60y)	119/74	-3/+1.0
Bach, 1989	PG	+	+	5	30 Total saturated	2.5	Men & Women (mean, 31 y)	130/85	-9.0-4.0
Dart, 1989	XO	NS	NS	8	21 Fish oil 21 Olive oil	6	Men & Women (mean, 46 y)	125/77	-5.3/-2.0
Wilt, 1989	XO	NS	NS	12	38 Fish oil 38 Safflower	6	Men (mean, 42 y)	124/84	-2.7/-1.8
Kestin, 1990	PG	+	+	6	11 Fish oil 11 Linoleic	3.4	Men (mean, 46 y)	124/75	-5.1/0.0
Cobiac, 1991	PG	-	-	5	12 Fish 13 Fish oil 6 Saturated mix	4.5	Men (30-60 y)	128/79	-0.6/+1.3
Davidson, 1986	PG	+	+	4	30 Total olive oil	6	Age, sex: NS†	142/88	-9.8/-3.2

Cardiovascular Disease Subjects									
Mehta, 1988	XO	+	+	4	8 Fish oil 8 Placebo	5.4	Men (52-73 y)	138/80	-10.0/-4.0
Solomon, 1990	PG	+	+	12	5 Fish oil 5 Olive oil	4.6	Men & Women (42-64y)	142/87	-16.8/-9.6
Gans, 1990	PG	+	+	16	16 Fish oil 16 Corn oil	3	Men & Women (mean, 66 y)	148/80	+9.0/+1.0
Diabetic Subjects									
Haines, 1986	PG	-	-	6	19 Fish oil 22 Olive oil	4.6	Men & Women (30-59 y)	136/82	+1.0/+1.7
Jensen, 1989	XO	+	+	8	18 Fish oil 18 Olive oil	4.6	Men & Women (22-47 y)	148/89	-9.0/-4.0
Hendra, 1990	PG	+	+	6	40 Fish oil 40 Olive oil	3	Men & Women (mean, 56 y)	143/83	+0.4/-0.6
Mixed Sample†									
Rogers, 1987	PG	+	+	4	30 Fish oil 30 Olive oil	3.3	Men (22-65 y)	130/76	-3.1/-5.0

* The number of subjects in each treatment period is listed for crossover studies. XO, Crossover, PG, Parallel Group. The number of subjects in each treatment group was not reported for Davidson, 1986 and Bach, 1989. Saturated mix is a mixture of saturated and other oils; mixed oil is a mixture of corn and olive oils.

† NS, not specified. Mixed sample indicates that there were no inclusion criteria for health of the sample.

‡ ω–3 Dose represents eicosapentaenoic acid plus docosahexaenoic acid. The ω–3 dose for Bruckner, 1987, reported as 1.5 g/10 kg body wt, is estimated based on a mean weight of 85 kg.

¶ Average blood pressure at baseline for active and control groups for parallel group studies and blood pressure during the placebo period for crossover studies. SBP, systolic blood pressure; DBP, diastolic blood pressure; NS, not specified. Change in BP attributed to fish oil treatment.

§ Blinded to treatment status.

Tabulated from Tables 2 and 3 from Morris.[56]

TABLE 47.14

Observational Studies on Protein and Blood Pressure*

Study	Number, Age	Protein Measurement	Results
Cross-Sectional Studies			
Yamori, 1981	1120, NS*	Spot urine: sulfate:urea nitrogen ratio	↓ SBP with ↑ animal protein
Kihara, 1984	1120, 30-70+ y	Spot urine: sulfate:urea nitrogen ratio	↓ SBP in men with ↑ animal protein
Reed, 1981	6496 men, NS	Single 24-h recall: g/d	↓ SBP, ↓ DBP with ↑ total protein
Pellum, 1983	61, 22-25 y	3-d food record: g/d	↓ SBP with ↑ total protein
Elliott, 1991	1190, 20-59 y	24-h urine: total nitrogen, urea nitrogen, sulfate	↓ SBP with ↑ total and animal protein
Dyer, 1992	2325, 20-59 y	24-h urine: total nitrogen, urea nitrogen	↓ SBP with ↑ total protein
Stamler, 1992	11342 men, 35-57 y	Four or five 24-h recalls: % energy intake	↓ SBP with ↑ total protein
Eliott, 1992	1922, mean age 39 y	7-d weighed food record: g/d, % energy intake	↓ SBP in women, ↓ DBP in men and women with ↑ total protein
Liu, 1992	3809, 18-30 y	Interviewer-administered food-frequency questionnaire: % energy intake	↓ DBP in white women, black women, and black men with ↑ vegetable protein only
Zhou, 1989	2672, 35-50 y	Three 24-h recalls: percentage energy intake	↓ SBP with ↑ animal protein only
Zhou, 1994	705, 40-59 y	Three 24-h recalls: % energy intake	↓ SBP, ↓ DBP with ↑ animal protein only
Havlik, 1990	402 male twins, 42-56 y	Interviewer-administered food-frequency questionnaire: % energy intake, g/d, g/d adjusted for energy	↑ DBP with ↑ total protein
He, 1995	827 men, mean 31-45 y	Three 24-h recalls: % energy intake	↓ SBP with ↑ total protein
Stamler, 1996	10020, 20-59 y	24-h urine: total nitrogen, urea nitrogen, sulfate	↓ SBP, ↓ DBP with ↑ total protein
Stamler, 1996	11342 men, 35-57 y	Four or five 24-h recalls: % energy intake	↓ DBP with ↑ total protein
Longitudinal Studies			
Liu, 1993	1804 men, 40-56 y	Quantitative diet history: % energy intake	↓ SBP with ↑ vegetable protein only
Liu, 1995†	3809, 18-30 y	Interviewer-administered food-frequency questionnaire: % energy intake	No change, with ↑ total, animal, or vegetable protein

* SBP indicates systolic blood pressure; DBP, diastolic blood pressure; NS, not stated

† Personal communication

TABLE 47.15

Human Intervention Studies on Protein and Blood Pressure*

Study	Number, Age, Cohort	Study Design	Results	Conclusion
Chapman, 1950	8 men, 31-58 y, hypertensive protein	Sequential: (1) control, (2) rice-fruit; (3) rice-fruit + 40 g milk (animal)	↓SBP and ↓DBP, but both NS	Compared with rice-fruit diet, no effect of animal protein on BP
Hatch, 1954	9, 36-66 y, hypertensive	Sequential: (1) low-sodium control; (2) low-sodium + 30-50 g milk and meat protein	↓SBP and ↓DBP, but both NS	No effect of ↑animal protein on BP
Brussaard, 1981	69, 18-30 y, normotensive	Parallel, randomized, each for 4 wk: (1) control; (2) casein protein; (3) soy protein	Casein: ↓SBP and ↑ DBP, but both NS; Soy: ↑ SBP and ↑ DBP, but both NS	No effect of animal or vegetable protein on BP
Sacks , 1981	21, 20-55 y normotensive vegans	Sequential: (1) 2 wk control vegetarian diet; (2) 4 wk 250 g of added beef	↑ SBP ($p<0.05$), ↓DBP (NS)	Animal protein ↑ SBP
Sacks, 1984	18, 22-41 y, normotensive vegans	Crossover, randomized each for 6 wk (1) high protein (58 g soy and wheat protein); (2) low protein (7 g rice protein)	Compared with low protein, high protein: ↑ SBP and ↑ DBP, but both NS	No effect of ↑ vegetable protein on BP
Sacks, 1984	Study 1 — 19, 14-54 y normotensive	Study I — Sequential: (1) 3 wk at baseline (2) 3 mo lactovegetarian diet	Study 1 — Low-fat vegetarian protein diet: ↑ SBP and ↑ DBP, but both NS	Study 1 — No effect of vegetarian diet on BP
	Study 2 — 17, 18-24 y, normotensive vegetarians	Study 2 — Crossover, randomized, each for 3 wk: (1) no eggs; (2) 1 egg/d	Study 2 — 1 egg/d: ↑ SBP and ↑ DBP, but both NS	Study 2 — No effect of eggs on BP
Prescott , 1987	50, 18-60 y, normotensive	Parallel, randomized, each for 12 wk: (1) meat protein (93 g of protein) (2) vegetable protein (84 g protein)	Compared with meat protein diet, vegetable protein: ↓SBP and ↑ DBP, but both NS	No difference in BP between vegetable and animal protein
Sacks, 1988	13, 21-41 y, normotensive vegans	Crossover, randomized, each for 3 wk: (1) 27 g casein protein; (2) 27 g soy protein	Compared with casein protein; soy protein: ↓SBP, and ↓DBP, but both NS	No difference in BP between vegetable and animal protein
Kestin, 1989	26 men, 28-64 y, normotensive	Crossover, randomized, each for 6 wk: (1) lean meat (high animal protein); (2) lactoovovegetarian (high vegetable protein)	Lactoovovegetarian diet: No change in SBP and ↑ DBP, but both NS	No difference in BP between low-fat animal and low-fat vegetable protein diet

* SBP indicates systolic blood pressure; DBP, diastolic blood pressure; BP, blood pressure; and NS, not significant.

Americans. Among 30,681 white male health professionals, only dietary fiber had an independent inverse association with hypertension after four years of follow up.[34] The relative risk of hypertension was 1.57 times greater for men with a fiber intake of less than 12 g/day versus greater than 24 g/day. In the Health Professionals Follow-up Study (43,738 men), high intakes of cereal fiber and magnesium were inversely associated with the risk of all strokes after 8 years.[28] Among 827 Chinese men, a 10 g higher intake of dietary fiber was significantly associated with a reduced systolic and diastolic blood pressure (–2.2/–2.1 mmHg).[63]

The explanation for lower blood pressure with fiber is unclear. Suggestions include an increased intake in dietary potassium and Vitamin C and/or a decreased sodium intake.[64] Among controlled studies the average intake of fiber (primarily cereal) was increased by 14 g, resulting in an average reduction of blood pressure of –1.6/–2.0 mmHg.[65] Better studies need to be conducted to understand the relationship of fiber with blood pressure.

Ascorbic Acid (Vitamin C) and Antioxidant Combinations

Ascorbic acid is an antioxidant and a free radical scavenger. Low vitamin C levels might decrease the production of nitric oxide and increase blood pressure by increasing free radical formation.[66] Other mechanisms include decreased vasodilating prostaglandin formation, modified leukotriene metabolism, altered vascular sodium content, or nutrient multicollinearity.[67] Several studies suggest an inverse relationship between blood pressure or stroke and vitamin C levels. Differences in nutritional consumption between hypertensives and normotensives are shown in Figure 47.3.[68]

It has been observed that a low potassium could also explain this association.[69] In 722 Eastern Finnish men in the Kuopio Ischaemic Heart Disease Risk Factor Study, both plasma ascorbic acid and serum selenium concentrations had independent inverse associations with the blood pressure.[66] However, neither vitamin E nor vitamin C supplements

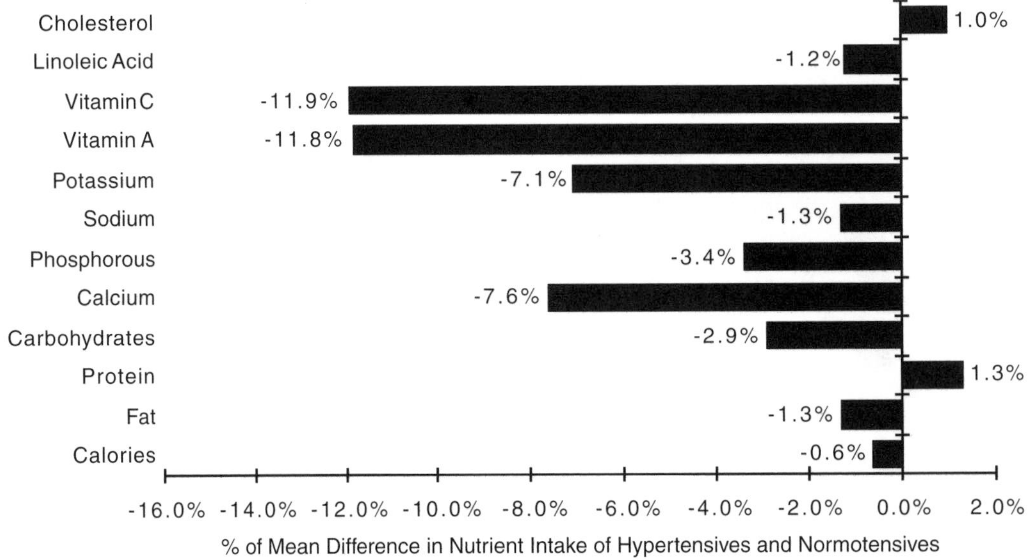

FIGURE 47.3
Health and Nutrition Examination Survey I: % mean difference in average nutritional consumption between hypertensive and normotensive persons, adjusted for age. Derived from McCarron DA, Morris CD, Henry HJ, Stanton JL. *Science* 224(4656), 1392, 1984. With permission.

TABLE 47.16

Trials of Ascorbic Acid and Blood Pressure

Study	Patient Number	Design	Duration	Intervention	Blood Pressure (mm Hg) Systolic/Diastolic
Osilesi O, 1991	20	Crossover	6 wks	1000 mg/d	-6.3 /0.6
Feldman EB, 1992	21	Single Blind	4 wks	1000 mg/d	-4.2/-2.9
Lovat LB, 1993	27	Crossover	4 wks	400 mg/d	--2 to -5·3 /-0.2 to -1.9
Ghosh SK,1994	48	Controlled	6 wks	500 mg/d	-2.5/-1.2
Duffy SJ, 1999	39	Controlled	4 wks	2000 mg bolus 500 mg per day	-11/-6

Table modified from Ness A, Sterne J. *Lancet* 335(9211), 1271, 2000.

reduced the risk of stroke in the Health Professionals Follow-up Study of 43,738 men.[70] In 168 healthy subjects, plasma concentrations of ascorbic acid (but not α-tocopherol, selenium, or taurine) were significantly inversely related to systolic and diastolic blood pressure.[67] Intravenous vitamin C, thiopronine, and glutathione (all antioxidants) individually demonstrated an acute decrease in blood pressure in 20 unmedicated hypertensive and 20 diabetic subjects.[71] Few studies assess the impact of ascorbic acid supplementation alone. Ascorbic acid — 500 mg twice daily in 21 subjects — lowered blood pressure 4.2/2.9 mmHg in a pilot study.[72] In a double-blind randomized crossover study, ascorbic acid 200 mg twice daily or placebo for four weeks was given to 27 elderly hypertensives.[73] No significant treatment effect was observed. Following a 2-week run-in phase, 48 untreated elderly hypertensive subjects in a randomized, double-blind, placebo-controlled six week study received ascorbic acid 250 mg twice daily or placebo.[74] The change in blood pressure in the vitamin C group was –10.3/–5.9 mmHg, and in the placebo group –7.7/–4.7 mmHg (p = nonsignificant). In a controlled trial, 20 subjects received placebo and 19 subjects received a 2 g bolus followed by 500 mg daily of ascorbic acid for 30 days.[75] Systolic blood pressure decreased 13 mmHg ($p < 0.05$); the change in diastolic blood pressure was not significant. Table 47.16 summarizes several trials of vitamin C supplementation and blood pressure.[76] The effect on systolic blood pressure is consistently greater than diastolic blood pressure.

Several studies have combined several antioxidants to assess an effect on blood pressure. In a randomized, placebo-controlled, clinical trial of 297 retired teachers randomly assigned to 2 to 4 months of the combination of 400 IU/day vitamin E, 500 mg/day vitamin C, and 6 mg/day β-carotene or placebo, the antioxidant combination capsule had no significant hypotensive effect.[77] In a randomized, double-blind, crossover design placebo-controlled study of 21 hypertensives and 17 normotensives, participants were assigned to receive either 8 weeks of placebo followed by 2 weeks washout, then 8 weeks antioxidants 200 mg of zinc sulfate, 500 mg of ascorbic acid, 600 mg of α-tocopherol and 30 mg of β-carotene daily, or the opposite sequence. Only systolic blood pressure (–5.3 mmHg) decreased significantly at the end of the antioxidant phase compared with the placebo phase (+3.7 mmHg) in hypertensive subjects ($p < 0.01$).[78]

Garlic (Allium Sativum)

Garlic has been reported to decrease blood pressure and attenuate age-related increased aortic stiffness, which could alter blood pressure rise with aging.[79-83] Allicin is believed to be the component responsible for the medicinal effects of garlic. In rabbits and dogs, garlic elicits a dose-dependent diuretic-natriuretic response.[84,85] In a randomized, placebo-controlled, double-blind trial, 47 subjects with mild hypertension (diastolic blood pressures from 95 to 104 mmHg) took either garlic powder or a placebo of identical appearance for 12 weeks.[79] The supine diastolic blood pressure in the garlic treatment group decreased 13 mmHg after 12 weeks ($p < 0.01$) compared with no significant changes in the placebo group. In a double-blind crossover study of 41 moderately hypercholesterolemic men assessing the effect of aged garlic extract versus placebo on blood lipids, there was a 5.5% decrease in systolic blood pressure and a modest reduction of diastolic blood pressure.[81] Another study of 40 hypercholesterolemic men treated with 900 mg of garlic powder observed a similar finding.[80] In a randomized, double-blind study, 42 healthy adults took either 300 mg three times a day of standardized garlic powder in tablet form, or placebo for 12 weeks.[86] There was no significant change in blood pressure.

A meta-analysis of 8 trials (415 subjects) using dried garlic powder 600 to 900 mg observed a decrease for systolic blood pressure of –7.7 (95% CI –11.0 to –4.3) and diastolic blood pressure of –5.0 (95% CI –7.1 to –2.9) mmHg, which represented the overall pooled difference in the absolute change (baseline to final measurement) in blood pressure relative to placebo (see Table 47.17).[87] The same analysis for hypertensive subjects reported an –11.1/–6.5 mmHg decline in blood pressure. The authors observe that blinding may have been difficult due to the odor of garlic. Furthermore, they emphasize that their quality assessment of the trials was poor because the authors did not state their technique to achieve effective randomization. Side effects appear to be rare. A recent randomized, multicenter, double-blind, placebo-controlled, 12-week parallel treatment study in hypercholesterolemic subjects using garlic powder (Kwai) 300 mg 3 times per day found no benefits in lowering blood pressure.[88] The authors of this paper emphasize that negative studies tend not to be submitted or published, suggesting that the current literature on garlic represents a publication bias.[87,88] Despite the suggested benefit, more trials need to be conducted to assess the benefit in hypertensives.

Ethanol

Alcohol consumption increases the risk of the development of hypertension.[89,90] The risk increases above 28 g of ethanol per day (which is equivalent to 24 oz of beer, 10 oz wine, and 3 oz of distilled spirits).[91] The maximum addition to the prevalence of hypertension of alcohol usage greater than two drinks daily is estimated to be 5 to 7%; however, the 11% risk in men is greater than in women because of greater alcohol intake.[92] In another study, alcohol consumption greater than 20 g per day gradually increases the risk of hypertension among women.[93] The relationship of alcohol intake to blood pressure is graded and continuous with the effect clearer in men than in women and more consistent in whites than in blacks (see Figure 47.4).[94] The effect of alcohol consumption on systolic blood pressure is independent of the effects of age, obesity, cigarette smoking, and physical activity.[95] In the INTERSALT Study (n = 10,079), both BMI and heavy alcohol consumption were significantly and independently correlated with both systolic and diastolic blood pressure ($p < 0.001$).[5] The effect of alcohol consumption on blood pressure is independent of and additive to BMI and urinary excretion of sodium and potassium.[96] The effect of alcohol on change in blood pressure independent of other risk factors is displayed in Figure 47.4.[94] In the Scottish Health Heart Study, alcohol consumption showed a weak positive correlation with blood pressure among 7354 men, but the correlation was greater than for sodium.[7]

Resting plasma concentrations of norepinephrine, epinephrine, renin activity, angiotensin II, aldosterone, and cortisol are similar in drinkers and nondrinkers.[97] In a prospective study of 7735 middle-aged British men, the prevalence of measured hypertension and

TABLE 47.17

Randomized Controlled Trials of Garlic and Blood Pressure*

Reference	Participants	Dose per day (mg)	Control	Blinding	Number of Subjects	Duration	Position	Heart Rate	Analysis
Kandziora, 1988	Hypertensives	600	Reserpine-diuretic	Single	40	12 weeks	Sup/St	UC	ITT
Kandziora, 1988	Hypertensives	600	Placebo	Double	40	12 weeks	Sup/St	UC	ITT
Auer, 1990	Hypertensives	600	Placebo	Double	47	12 weeks	Sup/St	NS	NS
Vorberg, 1990	Hyperlipidemics	900	Placebo	Double	40	16 weeks	Sup	NS	NS
Kiesewetter, 1991	SWISA	800	Placebo	Double	60	4 weeks	NS	NS	NS
Holzgartner, 1992	Hyperlipidemics	900	Bezafibrate	Double	94	12 weeks	NS	UC	ITT
Santos, 1993	NS	900	Placebo	Double	60	6 months	NS	NS	ORT
Jain, 1993	Hyperlipidemics	900	Placebo	Double	42	12 months	NS	NA	NS

* Sup, supine; St, standing; UC, unchanged; ITT intention to treat; NS, not stated; SWISA, subjects with increased spontaneous aggregation; ORT, on randomized treatment; NA. not available. Crossover study.

Modified from Silagy CA, Neil HA. *J Hypertens* 12(4), 463, 1994. With permission.

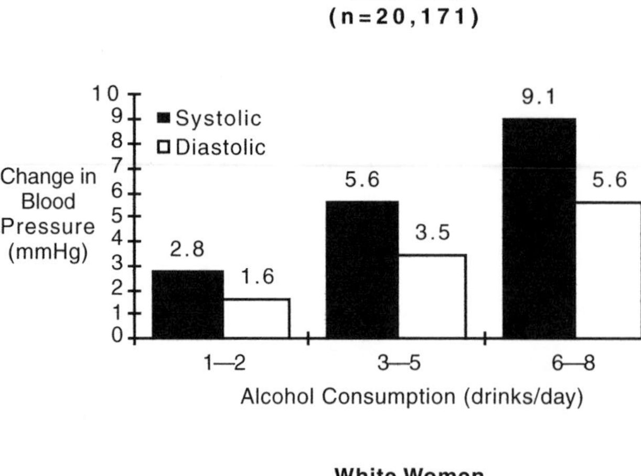

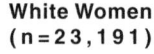

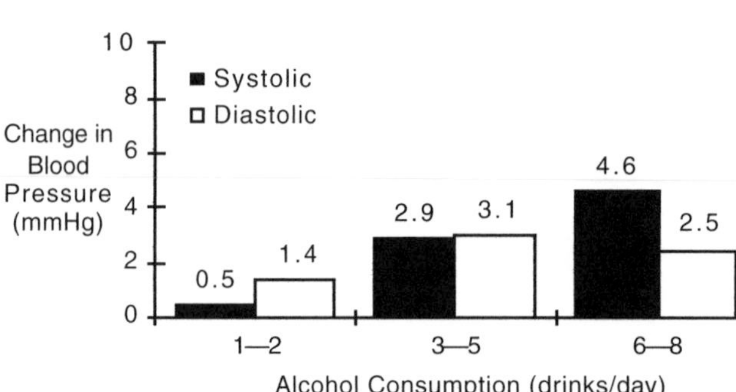

FIGURE 47.4
The effect of ethanol consumption on the change in blood pressure independent of other factors. Graph derived from data of Klatsky AL, Friedman GD, Armstrong MA. *Circulation* 73(4): 628, 1986.

level of blood pressure were significantly higher on Mondays and lower on Fridays than on other weekdays.[98] This suggests a withdrawal effect of weekend ethanol consumption.

Modest alcohol intake has been associated with a protective effect on ischemic heart disease events. Heavy alcohol intake has been associated with an increased rate of hemorrhagic strokes.[99,100] However, mild to moderate consumption in men reduced the risk of ischemic stroke without increasing the risk of hemorrhagic stroke.[101]

Several trials have been conducted to assess the impact of alcohol in moderation on blood pressure. These are listed in Table 47.18. Prevention and Treatment of Hypertension Study (PATHS)[91,102] was designed to assess alcohol intake reduction in nondependent moderate to heavy drinkers. 641 outpatient hypertensive and nonhypertensive veterans with a diastolic blood pressure of 80 to 99 mmHg were randomized to observation or behavioral cognitive intervention. To qualify for enrollment, self-reported alcohol intake had to be ≥294 g/week or ≥21 drinks/week for the preceding six months. The goal of behavioral cognitive intervention was to reduce alcohol intake to less than 50% of baseline intake or 14 drinks per week.

For the entire cohort, the average reduction of alcohol intake at 6 and 24 months between groups was 131 and 124 g/wk ($p < 0.001$ for each). For the 265 hypertensive subjects, the average reduction at 6 and 24 months was 157 and 135 g/wk (each $p < 0.001$). At 6 and 12 months, this translated to a nonsignificant reduction in blood pressure (i.e., treatment

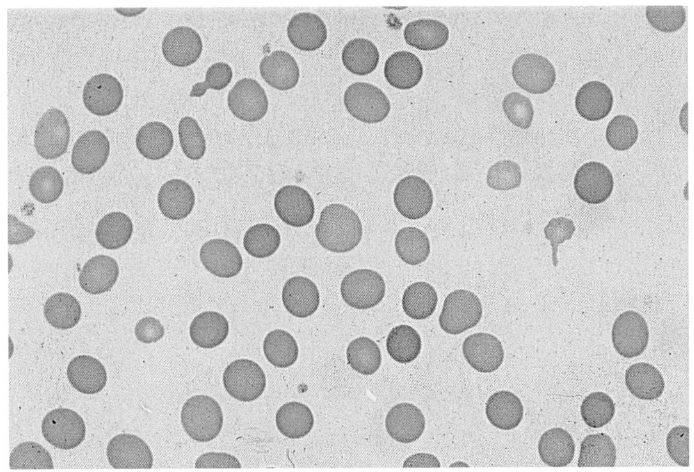

COLOR FIGURE 46.3
Macrocytic RBCs. Red blood cells that are larger than normal (macrocytic) and white blood cells that have nuclei with multiple segments (hypersegmented neutrophils) are characteristic of a vitamin B_{12} deficiency anemia.

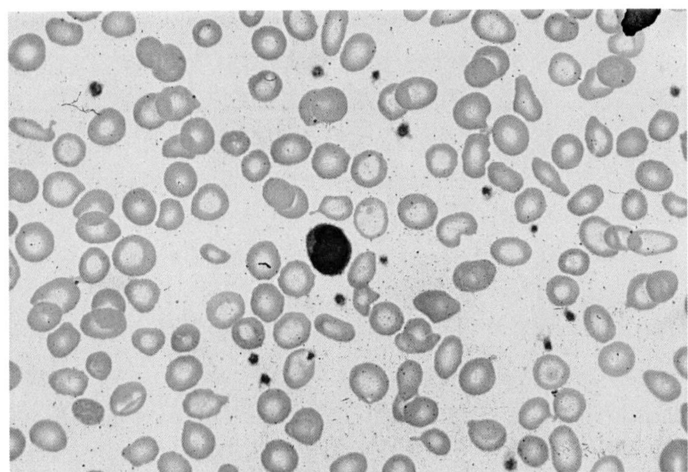

COLOR FIGURE 46.4
Microcytic RBCs. Red blood cells that are smaller than normal and have pale features (microcytic and hypochromic) are characteristic of Fe deficiency anemia.

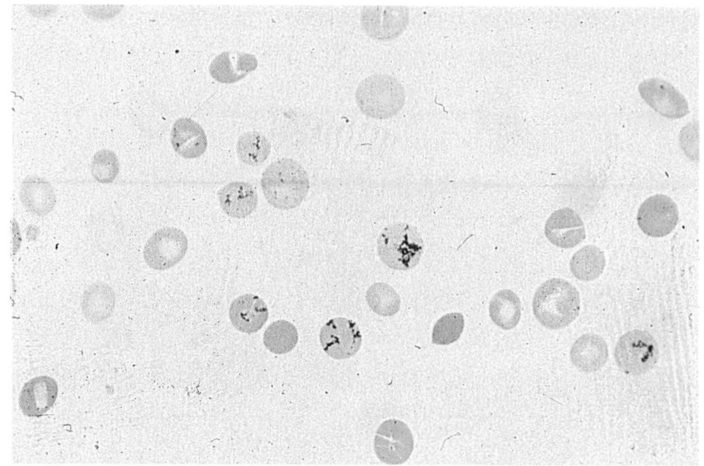

COLOR FIGURE 46.5
Reticulocytes. The appearance of young, newly produced red blood cells, reticulocytes, as seen in the peripheral blood smear that has been stained with new methylene blue.

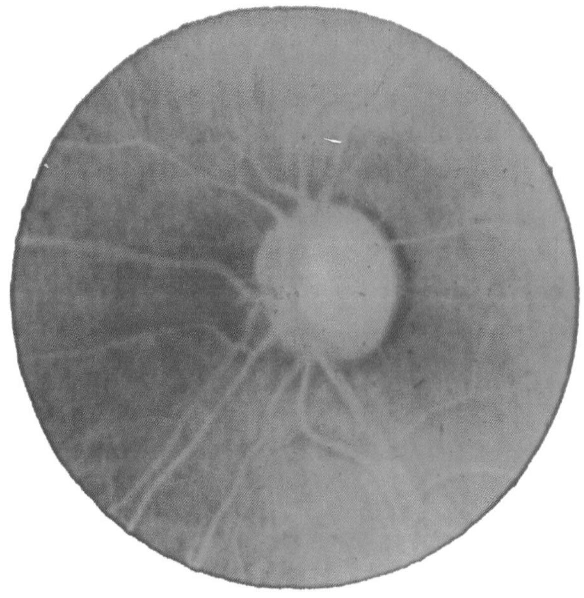

COLOR FIGURE 52.1
Lipemia retinalis visualized in the optical fundus of a patient with chylomicronemia with TAG levels exceeding 3000 mg/dl.

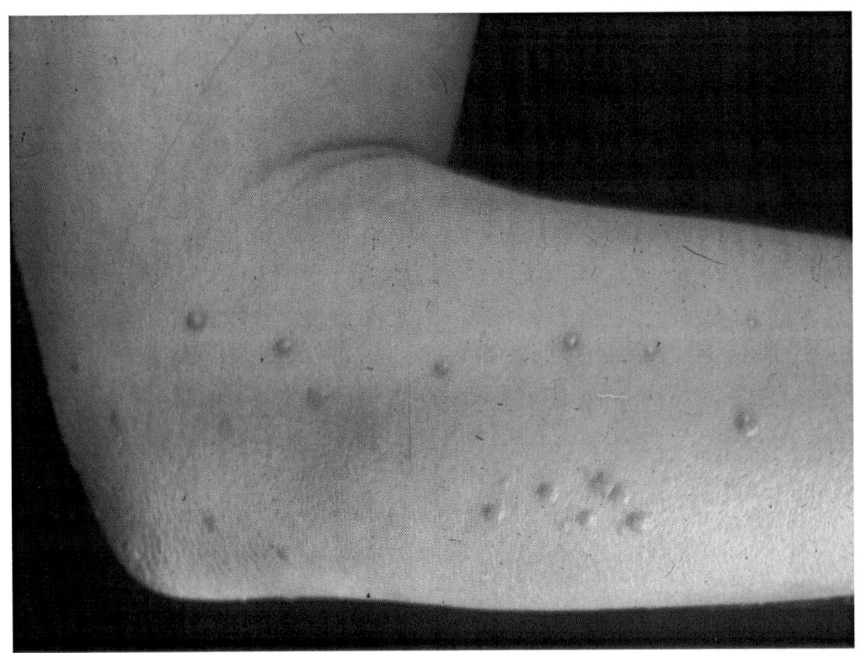

COLOR FIGURE 52.2
Eruptive xanthomas observed in a patient with chylomicronemia.

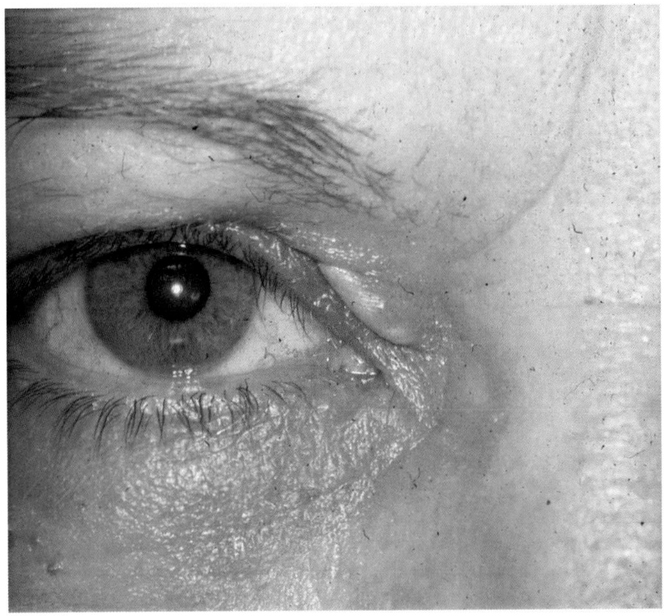

COLOR FIGURE 52.3
Eyelid xanthelasma from a woman with familial hypercholesterolemia.

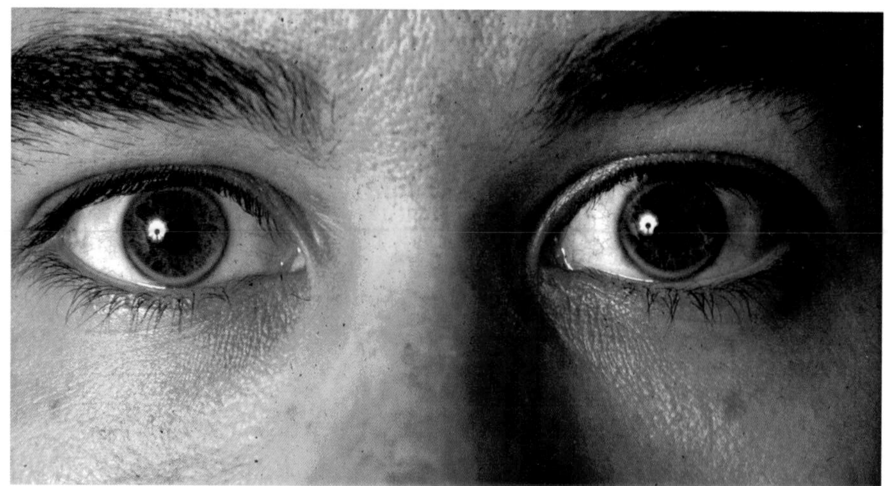

COLOR FIGURE 52.4
Corneal arcus observed in a 31-year-old man with familial hypercholesterolemia.

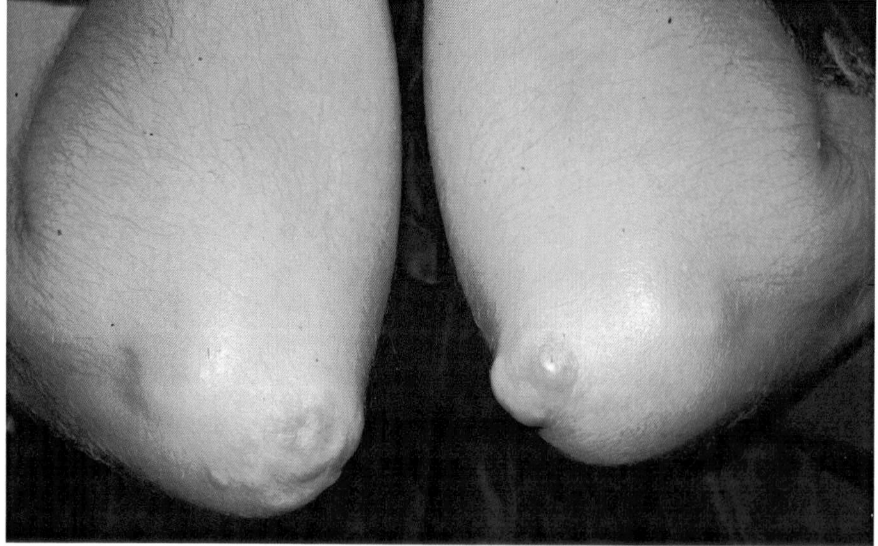

COLOR FIGURE 52.5
Tuberous xanthomas in the skin of the elbows of a teenage girl with familial hypercholesterolemia.

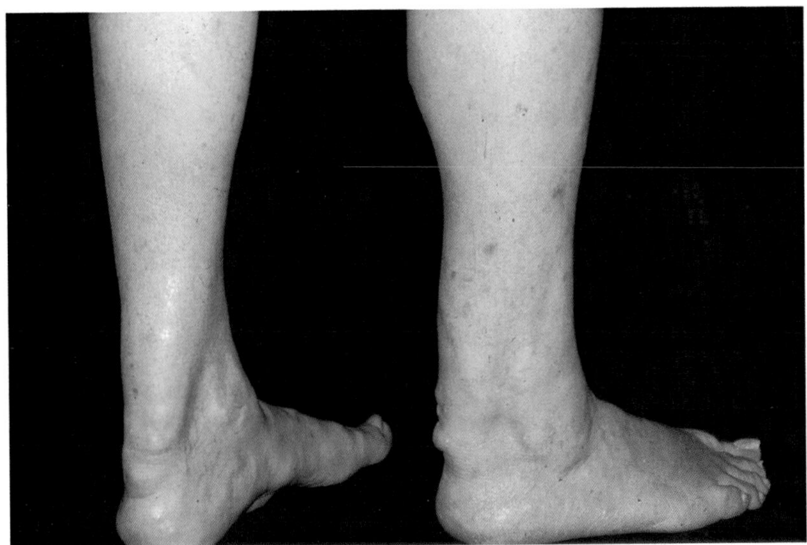

COLOR FIGURE 52.6
Xanthomas of the Achilles tendons of a patient with familial hypercholesterolemia.

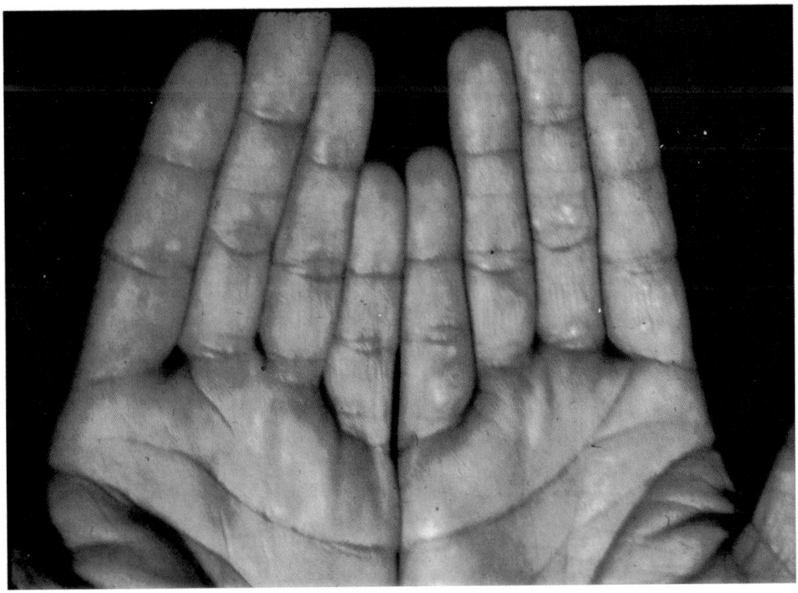

COLOR FIGURE 52.7
Yellow linear deposits in the creases of the fingers and palms of the hands of a 33-year-old man with Type III hyperlipoproteinemia.

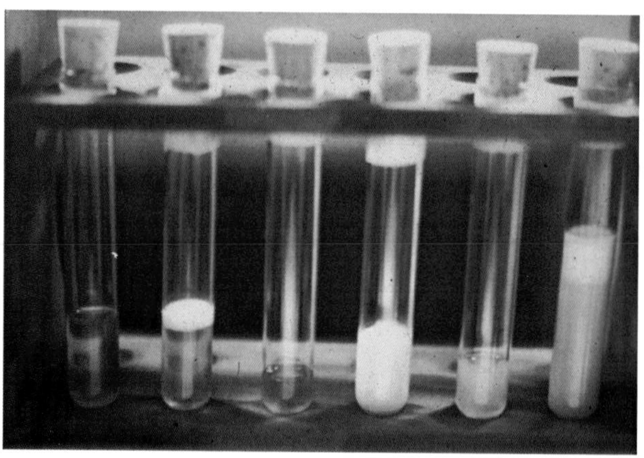

COLOR FIGURE 52.8
The appearance of plasma, refrigerated overnight, from fasting patients. The tubes with plasma samples are taken from (left to right): A subject with normal lipid levels and clear plasma (similar to a patient with Type IIa); a patient with chylomicronemia (Type I) with a creamy top layer above a clear infranatant; a patient with hypercholesterolemia (Type IIa) with clear plasma; a patient with Type III hyperlipoproteinemia with diffusely turbid plasma; a patient with Type IV hyperlipoproteinemia also showing diffuse turbidity; and a patient with Type V hyperlipoproteinemia with plasma exhibiting a creamy top layer over a turbid infranatant.

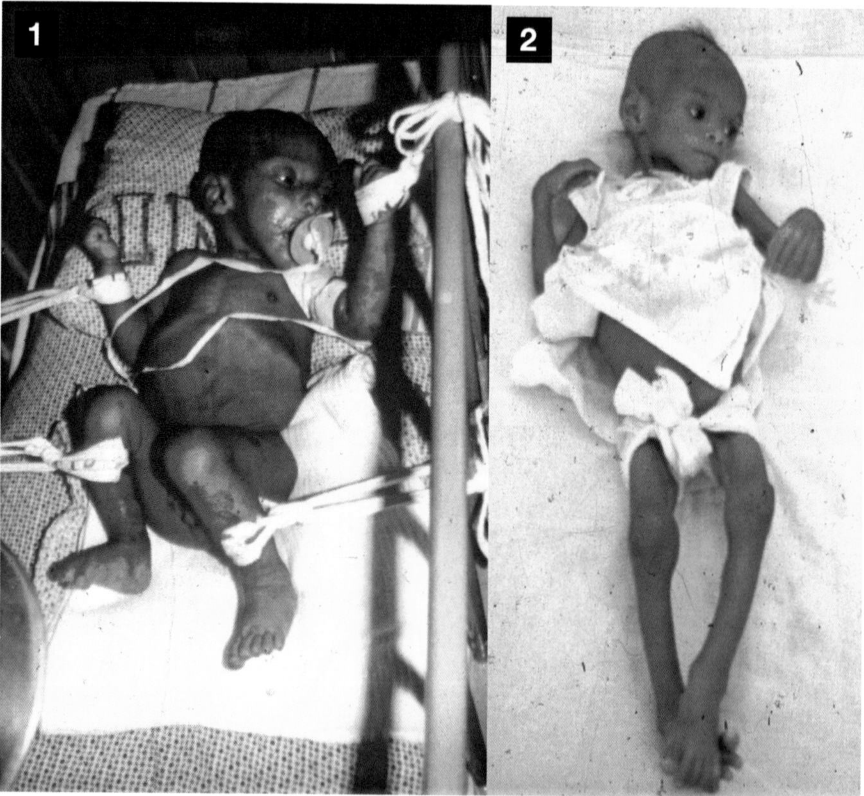

FIGURE 63.1
1. Kwashiorkor in a child. 2. Marasmic infant. (Photos are from Brazil and were provided by Dr. T. Kuske, reproduced from Feldman, E.B., *Essentials of Clinical Nutrition*, Philadelphia, F.A. Davis, 1988, pp. 321-325. With permission.)

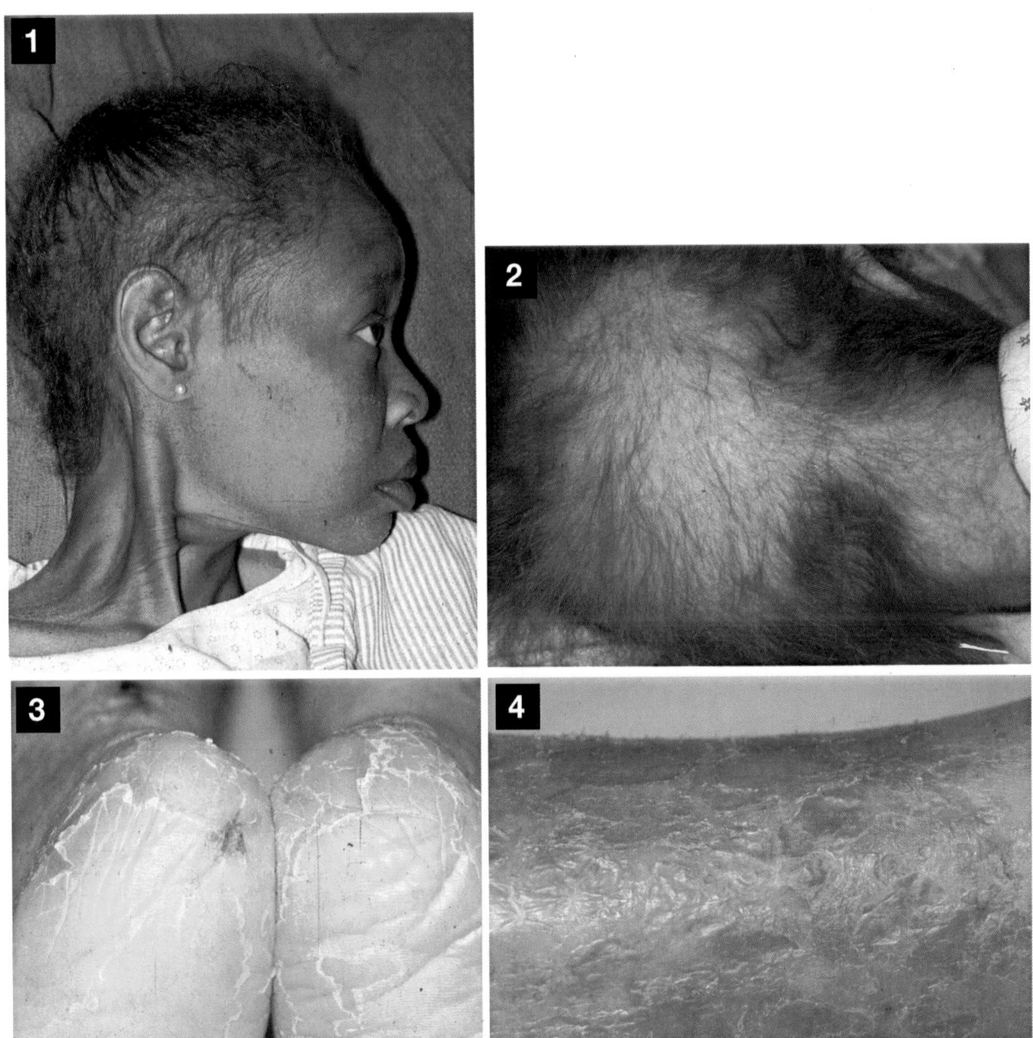

COLOR FIGURE 63.2
Examples of some of the physical findings associated with PEM. (1) Reddish hair, (2) hair loss, (3) flaking skin of the heels and (4) legs. (Photos of patients at the Medical College of Georgia, Augusta, courtesy of Elaine B. Feldman, M.D.)

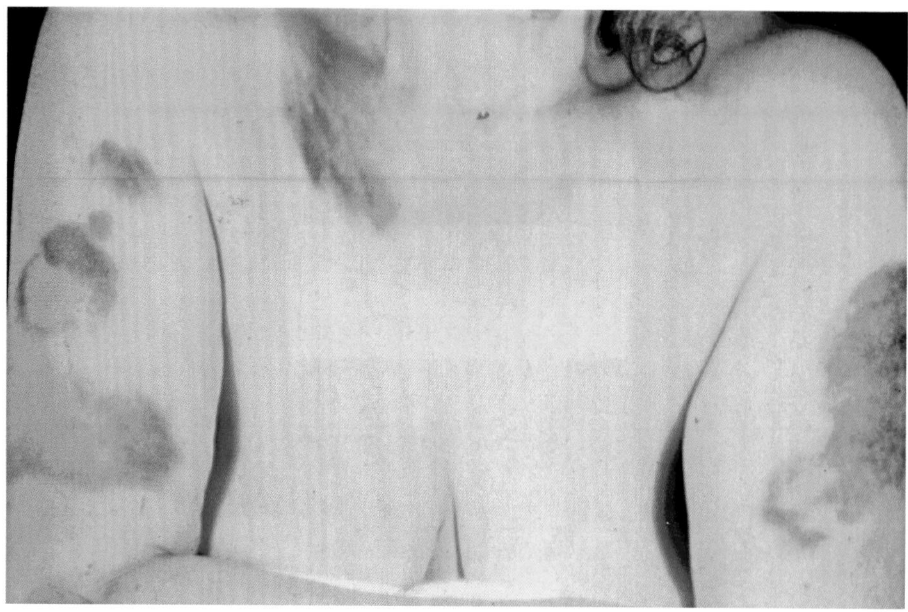

COLOR FIGURE 64.1
Patient with severe vitamin K deficiency, illustrating multiple purpuric areas occurring spontaneously. (Photo courtesy of Elaine B. Feldman, M.D.)

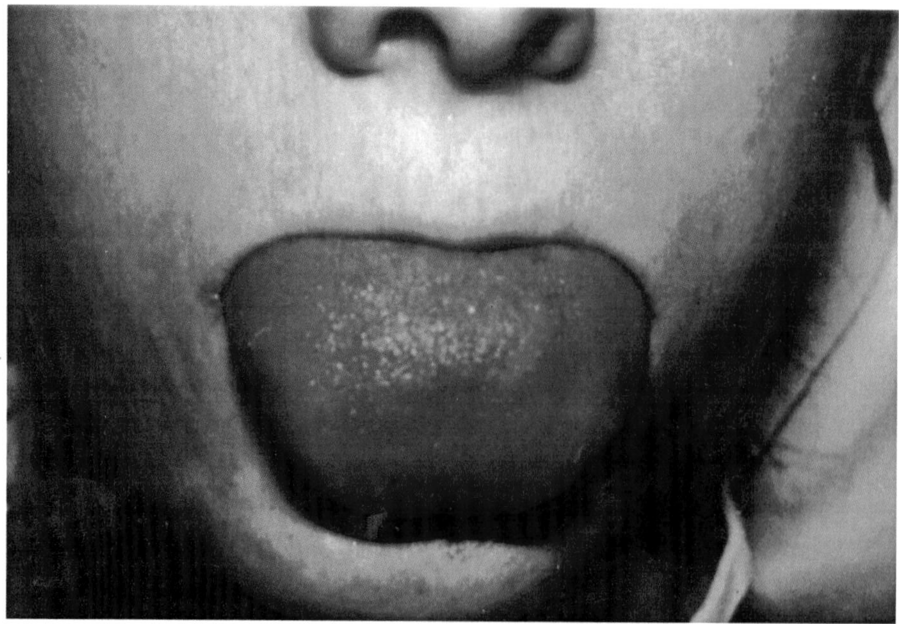

COLOR FIGURE 64.2
Patient with classical riboflavin (vitamin B_2) deficiency illustrating pallor, cheilosis, and a large, red, smooth tongue. (Photo courtesy of Elaine B. Feldman, M.D.)

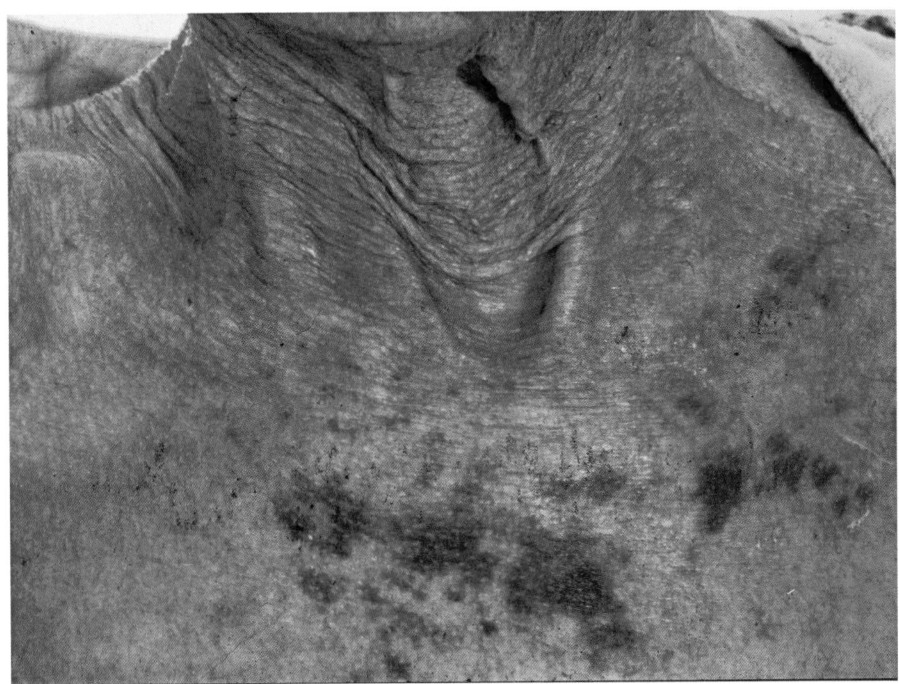

COLOR FIGURE 64.3
Patient with advanced pellagra resulting from niacin deficiency, illustrating a dark, scaly eruption over sun-exposed surfaces. (Photo courtesy of Elaine B. Feldman, M.D.)

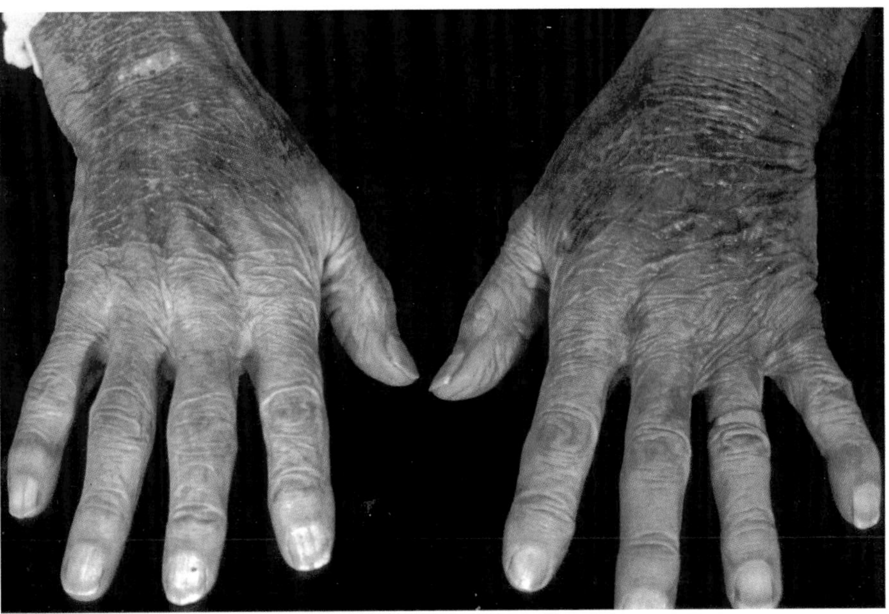

COLOR FIGURE 64.4
Hands of a patient with advanced pellagra, illustrating dark, scaly, thickened lesions. (Photo courtesy of Elaine B. Feldman, M.D.)

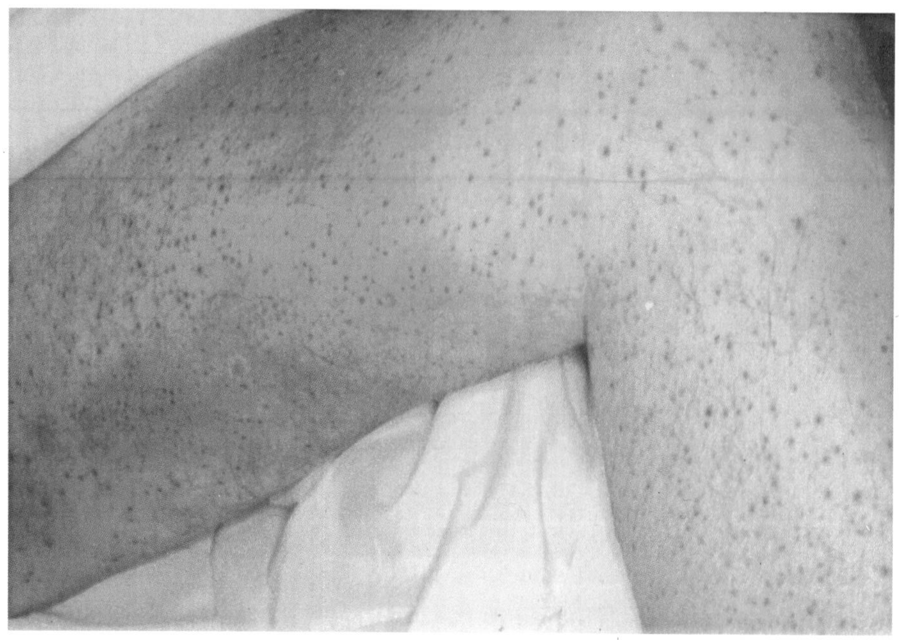

COLOR FIGURE 64.5
Leg of an adult patient with severe scurvy, illustrating multiple perifollicular hemorrhages. Some corkscrew hairs are visible. (Photo courtesy of Elaine B. Feldman, M.D.)

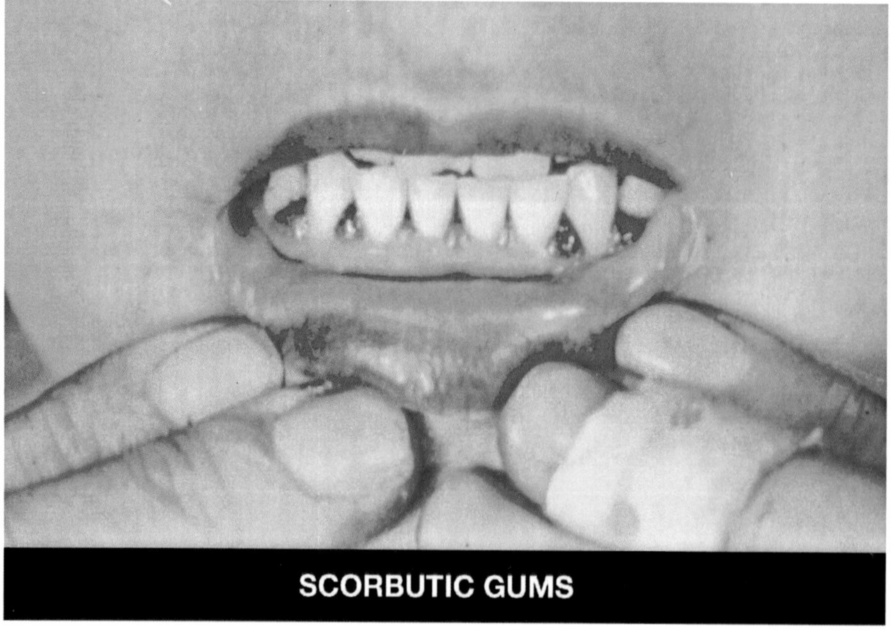

COLOR FIGURE 64.6
Mouth and teeth of a patient with far-advanced scurvy, showing swollen, bleeding gingiva. (Photo courtesy of Elaine B. Feldman, M.D.)

TABLE 47.18

Randomized Controlled Trials of Alcohol Reduction on Blood Pressure

Study, Year	n	Age, Years (Mean ± SD or Range)	Duration, Weeks	Baseline BP, mm Hg	Alcohol Intake Difference, Drinks†/Day	Blood Pressure Reduction, mm Hg	p Value
Puddey, 1985	46	35 ± 8	6	133/76	3.7	3.8/1.4	<.001/<.05
Howes, 1985	10	25-41	0.6	120/66	5.7	8/6	<.025/<.001
Puddey, 1987	44	53 ± 16	6	142/84	4.0	5/3	<.001/<.001
Ueshima, 1987	50	46 ± 7	2	148/93	2.6	5.2/2.2	<.005/NS
Wallace, 1988	641	42 ± 20	52	136/82	1.0	2.1/?	<.05/NS
Parker, 1990	59	52 ± 11	4	138/85	3.8	5.4/3.2	<.01/<.01
Cox, 1990	72	20-45	4	132/73	3.4	4.1/1.6	<.05/<-05
Maheswaran, 1992	41	40s	8	144/90	3.1	Not reported	NS
Puddey, 1992	86	44	18	137/85	3.0	4.8/3.3	<.01/<.01
Ueshima, 1993	54	44 ± 8	3	144/96	1.7	3.6/1.9	<.05/NS
PATHS, 1998‡	641	57 ± 11	104	140/86	1.3	0.9/0.6	0.16/0.10

† A standard drink is defined as 14 g of ethanol and is contained in a 12-oz glass of beer, a 5-oz glass of table wine, or 1.5 oz of distilled spirits.

‡ PATHS is Prevention and Treatment of Hypertension Study.

Modified from report of Cushman WC, Cutler JA, Bingham SF, et al. *Am J Hypertens* 7(9PT1), 814, 1994.

effect) for the entire cohort of –1.0/–0.6 mmHg and –0.9/–0.6 mmHg. For the hypertensive participants, the nonsignificant treatment effect at 6 and 12 months was –1.9/–0.6 and –1.6/–0.4 mmHg. There was no significant difference in the incidence of hypertension at 24 months: 16.6% in the intervention group and 21.8% in the control group. Weight declined more in the intervention group by –0.5 and –1.0 kg at 6 and 24 months.

PATHS was designed to achieve a 2-drink reduction in alcohol between treatments, but only achieved a reduction of 1.3 drinks per day. Furthermore, it was anticipated that 60% of the intervention group and 20% of the control group could reduce baseline alcohol intake to less than 50%; however, at 6 months the level for the control group was 23% and the intervention group was 44%.

Caffeine

Caffeine may increase peripheral vascular resistance by blocking the adenosine receptors. There are few randomized, controlled trials assessing the impact of coffee consumption on blood pressure. A meta-analysis (see Table 47.19) reviewed 36 studies and identified 11 controlled trials with 522 subjects.[103] The median duration of the trials was 56 days. They estimated the overall pooled treatment effect attributable for a median coffee intake of 5 cups/d as +2.4 mmHg (95% CI +1.0 to +3.7) for systolic blood pressure and +1.2 mmHg (95% CI +0.4 to +2.1) for diastolic blood pressure. Only one of the 11 trials included a hypertensive cohort. This meta-analysis did not observe a treatment effect on blood pressure based on treatment duration, the type of coffee (instant or not), whether coffee was filtered, or the type of coffee control (decaffeinated or no coffee). Age, coffee consumption, and sample size were independently associated with both systolic and diastolic blood pressure. The systolic and diastolic blood pressure increased 0.8 and 0.5 mmHg per cup of coffee consumed. A recent study using ambulatory blood pressure monitoring to study nonsmoking men and women older than 50 years reported a +4.8/+3.0 mmHg higher 24-hour systolic and diastolic blood pressure comparing 14 hypertensive coffee drinkers of 5 cups/d for two weeks compared with 13 hypertensive abstainers after a mandatory period of abstention of caffeine-containing foods for two weeks.[104]

TABLE 47.19

Controlled Studies of Coffee Consumption

Author, Year	No. of Subjects	Age, y Mean	Age, y Range	% Male	BP Drugs	Study Design*	Random Study	Study Duration	Baseline BP, mmHg SBP/DBP	Habitual Intake, cups/d	Run-time Time, d	Coffee Method	Coffee Filtered	No Cups of Coffee	Caffeine Content
Ammon, 1983	8	27	20-30	100	No	XO, D	No	28 d	123/82‡	...	7	Instant	No	504	
	...								126/85§						
Burr, 1989	54	35	18-58	65	No	XO, S	Yes	28 d	116/69	...	7	Instant	No	5	...
Bak, 1989a	67	26	18-33	54	No	PG, ...	Yes	63 d	122/71	5.9	21	Boiled	No	5	630
Bak, 1989b	68	26	18-33	54	No	PG, ...	Yes	63 d	122/71	5.5	21	Boiled	Yes	5	670
Van Dusseldorp, 1980	45	38	25-45	49	No	XO, D	Yes	42 d	124/76	..	0	Drip	Yes	5	435
Rosmarin, 1990	21	36	...	100	No	XO, ...	Yes	56 d	115/72	...	0	Drip	Yes	3.6	...
MacDonald, 1991†	52	47	26-67	44	No	XO, D	Yes	14 d	134/87¶	...	0	Instant	No	3	...
Van Dusseldorp, 1992a	43	39	17-57	42	No	PG, D	Yes	79 d	110/69¶	5.5	17	Boiled	No	6	860
Van Dusseldorp, 1992b	42	39	17-57	42	No	PG, D	Yes	79 d	110/70¶	5.5	17	Boiled	Yes	6	887
Eggertsen, 1993	23	56	28-74	57	Yes	XO, D	Yes	14 d	130/80¶	3.5	14	Instant	No	3.5	...
Superko, 1994	99	46	43-48#	100	No	PG, D	Yes	56 d	116/74	4.5	0	Drip	Yes	4.5	584

* BP indicates blood pressure; SBP, systolic blood pressure; DBP, diastolic blood pressure; XO, crossover; D, double-blind; S, single-blind; and PG, parallel group.
† MacDonald (1991): mean ambulatory BID during caffeinated coffee regimen vs caffeine-free diet.
‡ Regular coffee group.
§ Decaffeinated coffee group.
¶ Ambulatory BP measurements.
\# Range of means.

Modified from Jee SH, He J, Whelton PK, et al. *Hypertension* 33(2), 647, 1999.

Weight Reduction (Caloric Deprivation)

The relationship between obesity and hypertension is well documented. All adults with a BMI of 25 kg/m^2 or greater are at risk for hypertension.[105] The impact of weight reduction as a modality for preventing or reducing blood pressure is addressed in the section on major nonpharmacologic trials.

Summary

Table 47.20 summarizes the meta-analyses on nonpharmacologic intervention and blood pressure. The importance of the amount of change in blood pressure varies with the perspective of the clinician vs. that of the epidemiologist.

TABLE 47.20

Meta-Analysis of Results of Studies on Nonpharmacologic Intervention and Blood Pressure

Author, Year	Number of Trials	Nutrient	Systolic Pressure (95% CI)	Diastolic Pressure (95% CI)
Jee, 1999[103]	11	Caffeine	+2.4 (+1.0 to +3.7)	+1.2 (+0.4 to +2.1)
Normotensives	10		+2.4 (+1.0 to +3.8)	+1.2 (+0.4 to +2.1)
Cappuccio, 1989[39]	15	Calcium	-0.13 (-0.46 to +0.19)	+0.03 (-0.17 to +0.22)
Hypertensives	10		+0.06 (-0.59 to +0.72)	+0.03 (-0.21 to +0.27)
Cutler, 1990[35]	19	Calcium	-1.8 (-3.0 to -0.6)	-0.7 (-1.5 to +0.2)
Normotensives	9		-1.3 (-3.2 to +0.8)	-1.3 (-2.6 to -0.1)
Hypertensives	12		-2.1 (-3.6 to -0.6)	-0.1 (-1.3 to +1.0)
Allender, 1996[41]	22	Calcium	-0.89 (-1.74 to -0.05)	-0.18 (-0.75 to +0.40)
Normotensives	13		-0.53 (-1.56 to +0.49)	-0.28 (-0.99 to +0.42)
Hypertensives	16		-1.68 (-3.18 to -0.18)	+0.02 (-0.96 to +1.00)
Buchner, 1996[42]	33	Calcium	-1.27 (-2.25 to -0.29)	-0.24 (-0.92 to +0.44)
Normotensives	33		-0.27 (-1.80 to +1.27)	-0.33 (-1.56 to +0.90)
Hypertensives	6		-4.30 (-6.47 to -2.13)	-1.50 (-2.77 to -0.23)
Griffith, 1999[43]	42	Calcium	-1.44 (-2.20 to -0.68)	-0.84 (-1.44 to -0.24)
He, 1996[65]	20	Fiber	-1.6 (-2.7 to -0.4)	-2.0 (-2.9 to -1.1)
Silagy, 1994[87]	8	Garlic	-7.7 (-11.0 to -4.3)	-5.0 (-7.1 to -2.9)
Hypertensives	2		-11.1 (-17.2 to -5.0)	-6.5 (-9.6 to -3.4)
Appel, 1993[55]	17	ω-3-Fatty Acids	-1.5 (-2.4 to -0.6)	-1.0 (-1.6 to -0.4)
Normotensives	11		-1.0 (-2.0 to 0.0)	-0.5 (-1.2 to +0.20)
Hypertensives	6		-5.5 (-8.1 to -2.9)	-3.5 (-5.0 to -2.1)
Morris, 1993[56]	31	ω-3- Fatty Acids	-3.0 (-4.5 to -1.5)	-1.5 (-2.2 to -0.8)
Normotensives	8		-0.4 (-1.6 to +0.8)	-0.7 (-1.5 to +0.1)
Hypertensives	9		-3.4 (-5.9 to -0.9)	-2.0 (-3.3 to -0.7)
Cappuccio, 1991[106]	18	Potassium	-4.0 (-4.7 to -3.2)	-2.4 (-3.0 to -1.8)
Hypertensives	12		-5.3 (-6.2 to -4.4)	-3.0 (-3.7 to -2.3)
Whelton, 1997[29]	32	Potassium	-3.11 (-4.31 to -1.91)	-1.97 (-3.42 to -0.52)
Normotensives	12		-1.8 (-2.9 to -0.6)	-1.0 (-2.1 to 0.0)
Hypertensives	20		-4.4 (-6.6 to -2.2)	-2.5 (-4.9 to -0.1)
Cutler,1991[11]	23	Sodium	-2.91 (-3.67 to -2.15)	-1.60 (-2.09 to -1.11)
Normotensives	6		-1.70 (-2.68 to -0.72)	-0.97 (-1.62 to -0.32)
Hypertensives	18		-4.92 (-6.19 to -3.65)	-2.64 (-3.46 to -1.82)
Midgley, 1996[13]	56	Sodium	-0.5 (-1.17 to -0.07)	-1.6 (-2.10 to -1.02)
Normotensives	28		-0.1 (-0.76 to +0.63)	-0.5 (-1.16 to +0.14)
Hypertensives	28		-2.0 (-3.57 to -0.49)	-2.7 (-3.77 to -1.58)
Cutler, 1997[14]	32	Sodium	-2.81 (-3.39 to -2.23)	-1.52 (-1.90 to -1.14)
Normotensives	12		-1.90 (-2.62 to -1.18)	-1.09 (-1.57 to -0.61)
Hypertensives	22		-4.83 (-5.87 to -3.79)	-2.45 (-3.13 to -1.77)
Graudal, 1998[15]		Sodium		
Normotensives	56		-1.2 (-1.8 to -0.6)	-0.26 (-0.3 to +0.9)
Hypertensives	58		-3.9 (-4.8 to -3.0)	-1.9 (-2.5 to -1.3)

References

1. Prisant LM. Hypertension. In: *Current Diagnosis* 9. Conn RB, Borer WZ, Snyder JW, Eds. Philadelphia: W. B. Saunders, 1997: p 349.
2. Denton D, Weisinger R, Mundy NI, et al. *Nat Med* 1(10), 1009, 1995.
3. Kurtz TW, Al-Bander HA, Morris RC. *N Engl J Med* 317(17), 1043, 1987.
4. Boegehold MA, Kotchen TA. *Hypertension* 17(1 Suppl), I158, 1991.
5. _________. *Br Med J* 297(6644), 319, 1988.
6. Stamler R. *Hypertension* 17(1 Suppl), I16, 1991.

7. Smith WC, Crombie IK, Tavendale RT, et al. *Br Med J* 297(6644), 329, 1988.
8. ________. *Arch Intern Med* 153(2), 186, 1993.
9. Mascioli S, Grimm R, Jr, Launer C, et al. *Hypertension* 17(1 Suppl), I21, 1991.
10. Grobbee DE, Hofman A. *Br Med J* 293(6538), 27, 1986.
11. Cutler JA, Follmann D, Elliott P, Suh I. *Hypertension* 17(1 Suppl), I27, 1991.
12. Law MR, Frost CD, Wald NJ. *Br Med J* 302(6780), 819, 1991.
13. Midgley JP, Matthew AG, Greenwood CM, Logan AG. *JAMA* 275(20), 1590, 1996.
14. Cutler JA, Follmann D, Allender PS. *Am J Clin Nutr* 65(2 Suppl), 643, 1997.
15. Graudal NA, Galloe AM, Garred P. *JAMA* 279(17), 1383, 1998.
16. Alderman MH, Madhavan S, Cohen H, et al. *Hypertension* 25(6), 1144, 1995.
17. Alderman MH. *Am J Hypertens* 10(5 Pt 1), 584, 1997.
18. Alderman MH, Cohen H, Madhavan S. *Lancet* 351(9105), 781, 1998.
19. Alderman MH, Lamport B. *Am J Hypertens* 3(6 Pt 1), 499, 1990.
20. Krishna GG, Miller E, Kapoor S. *N Engl J Med* 320(18), 1177, 1989.
21. Langford HG. *Ann Intern Med* 98(5 Pt 2), 770, 1983.
22. Grim CE, Luft FC, Miller JZ, et al. *J Chronic Dis* 33(2), 87, 1980.
23. *J Chronic Dis* 40(9), 839, 1987.
24. Adrogue HJ, Wesson DE. *Semin Nephrol* 16(2), 94, 1996.
25. Brancati FL, Appel LJ, Seidler AJ, Whelton PK. *Arch Intern Med* 156(1), 61, 1996.
26. Tobian L, Lange J, Ulm K, et al. *Hypertension* 7(3 Pt 2), I110, 1985.
27. Khaw KT, Barrett-Connor E. *N Engl J Med* 316(5), 235, 1987.
28. Ascherio A, Rimm EB, Hernan MA, et al. *Circulation* 98(12), 1198, 1998.
29. Whelton PK, He J, Cutler JA, et al. *JAMA* 277(20), 1624, 1997.
30. Grimm R, Jr, Neaton JD, Elmer PJ, et al. *N Engl J Med* 322(9), 569, 1990.
31. Stitt FW, Clayton DG, Crawford MD, Morris JN. *Lancet* 1(7795), 122, 1973.
32. Gruchow HW, Sobocinski KA, Barboriak JJ. *JAMA* 253(11), 1567, 1985.
33. Witteman JC, Willett WC, Stampfer M, et al. *Circulation* 80(5), 1320, 1989.
34. Ascherio A, Rimm EB, Giovannucci EL, et al. *Circulation* 86(5), 1475, 1992.
35. Cutler JA, Brittain E. *Am J Hypertens* 3(8 Pt 2), 137, 1990.
36. Resnick LM, *Am J Hypertens* 12(1 Pt 1), 99, 1999.
37. *Hypertension* 8(5), 444, 1986.
38. McCarron DA, Morris CD. *Ann Intern Med* 103(6 (Pt 1)), 825, 1985.
39. Cappuccio FP, Siani A, Strazzullo P. *J Hypertens* 7(12), 941, 1989.
40. Cappuccio FP, Elliott P, Allender PS, et al. *Am J Epidemiol* 142(9), 935, 1995.
41. Allender PS, Cutler JA, Follmann D, et al. *Ann Intern Med* 124(9), 825, 1996.
42. Bucher HC, Cook RJ, Guyatt GH, et al. *JAMA* 275(13), 1016, 1996.
43. Griffith LE, Guyatt GH, Cook RJ, et al. *Am J Hypertens* 12(1 Pt 1), 84, 1999.
44. Bucher HC, Guyatt GH, Cook RJ, et al. *JAMA* 275(14), 1113, 1996.
45. Levine RJ, Hauth JC, Curet LB, et al. *N Engl J Med* 337(2), 69, 1997.
46. Appel LJ. Calcium, magnesium, and blood pressure. In: Izzo JH, Black HR, Eds. *Hypertension Primer. The Essentials of High Blood Pressure.* Dallas: Lippincott Williams &Wilkins, 1999: p 253.
47. Sibai BM, Villar MA, Bray E. *Am J Obstet Gynecol* 161(1), 115, 1989.
48. Lucas MJ, Leveno KJ, Cunningham FG, *N Engl J Med* 333(4), 201, 1995.
49. Whelton PK, Klag MJ. *Am J Cardiol* 63, 26, 1989.
50. Mizushima S, Cappuccio FP, Nichols R, Elliott P. *J Hum Hypertens* 12, 447, 1998.
51. Ma J, Folsom AR, Melnick SL, et al. *J Clin Epidemiol* 48(7), 927, 1995.
52. Peacock JM, Folsom AR, Arnett DK, et al. *Ann Epidemiol* 9(3), 159, 1999.
53. Sacks FM, Brown LE, Appel L, et al. *Hypertension* 26(6 Pt 1), 950, 1995.
54. Sacks FM, Willett WC, Smith A, et al. *Hypertension* 31(1), 131, 1998.
55. Appel LJ, Miller ER, Seidler AJ, Whelton PK. *Arch Intern Med* 153(12), 1429, 1993.
56. Morris MC, Sacks F, Rosner B. *Circulation* 88(2), 523, 1993.
57. Mori TA, Bao DQ, Burke V, et al. *Hypertension* 34(2), 253, 1999.
58. Bao DQ, Mori TA, Burke V, et al. *Hypertension* 32(4), 710, 1998.
59. Obarzanek E, Velletri PA, Cutler JA, *JAMA* 275(20), 1598, 1996.
60. Fujita T, Ando K, Noda H, et al. *Circulation* 75(3), 525, 1987.

61. He J, Whelton PK. *Clin Exp Hypertens* 21(5-6), 785, 1999.
62. Ludwig DS, Pereira MA, Kroenke CH, et al. *JAMA* 282(16), 1539, 1999.
63. He J, Klag MJ, Whelton PK, et al. *J Hypertens* 13(11), 1267, 1995.
64. Singh RB, Rastogi SS, Singh R, et al. *Am J Cardiol* 70(15), 1287, 1992.
65. He J, Whelton PK, Klag MJ. *Am J Hypertens* 9(4 Part 2), 74, 1996.
66. Salonen JT, *Ann Med* 23(3), 295, 1991.
67. Moran JP, Cohen L, Greene JM, et al. *Am J Clin Nutr* 57(2), 213, 1993.
68. McCarron DA, Morris CD, Henry HJ, Stanton JL. *Science* 224(4656), 1392, 1984.
69. Bulpitt CJ. *J Hypertens* 8, 1071, 1990.
70. Ascherio A, Rimm EB, Hernan MA, et al. *Ann Intern Med* 130(12), 963, 1999.
71. Ceriello A, Giugliano D, Quatraro A, Lefebvre PJ. *Clin Sci* 81(6), 739, 1991.
72. Feldman EB, Gold S, Greene J, et al. *Ann N Y Acad Sci* 669, 342, 1992.
73. Lovat LB, Lu Y, Palmer AJ, et al. *J Hum Hypertens* 7(4), 403, 1993.
74. Ghosh SK, Ekpo EB, Shah IU, et al. *Gerontology* 40(5), 268, 1994.
75. Duffy SJ, Gokce N, Holbrook M, et al. *Lancet* 354(9195), 2048, 1999.
76. Ness A, Sterne J. *Lancet* 355(9211), 1271, 2000.
77. Miller E3, Appel LJ, Levander OA, Levine DM. *J Cardiovasc Risk* 4(1), 19, 1997.
78. Galley HF, Thornton J, Howdle PD, et al. *Clin Sci* 92(4), 361, 1997.
79. Auer W, Eiber A, Hertkorn E, et al. *Br J Clin Pract Suppl* 69, 3, 1990.
80. Vorberg G, Schneider B. *Br J Clin Pract Suppl* 69, 7, 1990.
81. Steiner M, Khan AH, Holbert D, Lin RI. *Am J Clin Nutr* 64(6), 866, 1996.
82. Breithaupt-Grogler K, Ling M, Boudoulas H, Belz GG. *Circulation* 96(8), 2649, 1997.
83. Ernst E. *Pharmatherapeutica* 5(2), 83, 1987.
84. Pantoja CV, Chiang LC, Norris BC, Concha JB. *J Ethnopharmacol* 31(3), 325, 1991.
85. Pantoja CV, Norris BC, Contreras CM. *J Ethnopharmacol* 52(2), 101, 1996.
86. Jain AK, Vargas R, Gotzkowsky S, McMahon FG. *Am J Med* 94(6), 632, 1993.
87. Silagy CA, Neil HA. *J Hypertens* 12(4), 463, 1994.
88. Isaacsohn JL, Moser M, Stein EA, et al. *Arch Intern Med* 158(11), 1189, 1998.
89. Klatsky AL, Friedman GD, Siegelaub AB, Gerard MJ. *N Engl J Med* 296(21), 1194, 1977.
90. Beilin LJ. *Ann N Y Acad Sci* 676, 83, 1993.
91. Cushman WC, Cutler JA, Bingham SF, et al. *Am J Hypertens* 7(9 Pt 1), 814, 1994.
92. MacMahon S. *Hypertension* 9(2), 111, 1987.
93. Witteman JC, Willett WC, Stampfer MJ, et al. *Am J Cardiol* 65(9), 633, 1990.
94. Klatsky AL, Friedman GD, Armstrong MA. *Circulation* 73(4), 628, 1986.
95. Arkwright PD, Beilin J, Vandongen R, et al. *Circulation* 66(3), 515, 1982.
96. Marmot MG, Elliott P, Shipley MJ, et al. *BMJ* 308(6939), 1263, 1994.
97. Arkwright PD, Beilin LJ, Rouse I, et al. *Circulation* 66(1), 60, 1982.
98. Wannamethee G, Shaper AG. *J Hum Hypertens* 5(2), 59, 1991.
99. Iso H, Kitamura A, Shimamoto T, et al. *Stroke* 26(5), 767, 1995.
100. Camargo CA. *Stroke* 20(12), 1611, 1989.
101. Berger K, Ajani UA, Kase CS, et al. *N Engl J Med* 341(21), 1557, 1999.
102. Cushman WC, Cutler JA, Hanna E, et al. *Arch Intern Med* 158(11), 1197, 1998.
103. Jee SH, He J, Whelton PK, et al. *Hypertension* 33(2), 647, 1999.
104. Rakic V, Burke V, Beilin LJ. *Hypertension* 33(3), 869, 1999.
105. *Arch Intern Med* 158(17), 1855, 1998.
106. Cappuccio FP, MacGregor GA. *J Hypertens* 9(5), 465, 1991.

48

Nutritional Treatment of Blood Pressure: Major Nonpharmacologic Trials of Prevention or Treatment of Hypertension

L. Michael Prisant

Major Nonpharmacologic Trials of Prevention or Treatment of Hypertension

Primary Prevention Trials

Primary Prevention of Hypertension (PPH) Trial

The purpose of PPH was to determine whether intense lifestyle modifications would reduce the incidence of hypertension and lower blood pressure in the intervention versus the monitored (control) group.[1] "Hypertension-prone" individuals between the ages of 30 to 44 years were screened. Diastolic blood pressure < 90 mmHg was required for enrollment. Greater than 50% above desirable weight, excess alcohol use, diabetes mellitus, and major cardiovascular diseases precluded participation in the trial. Diastolic blood pressure ≥90 mmHg or initiation of antihypertensive drug therapy was the primary endpoint. Interventions by nutrition counselors and physicians included either:

The greater of a 4.5 kg decrease or 5% weight loss in overweight subjects

Decreased sodium intake to ≤1800 mg (4.5g NaCl)

Reduced alcohol intake (≤26g)

Increased physical activity (30 minutes for 3 days per week)

The group that did not receive the intervention was monitored. Baseline characteristics are shown in Table 48.1. The incidence of hypertension was 8.8% of 102 intervention and 19.2% of monitored subjects (p = 0.027) over 5 years. The odds ratio for hypertension development in the control group was 2.4 (90% CI 1.2-4.8, p <0.027).

0-8493-2705-9/01/$0.00+$1.50

TABLE 48.1

Nonpharmacologic Interventions in High Normal Blood Pressure*

Trial	n	Mean Age (Yr)	% Male	% White	Study Duration	Intervention	Initial Blood Pressure	Systolic/ Diastolic Change	Relative Risk of Hypertension*
Primary Prevention of Hypertension[1]	201	38	87	82	5 yr	↓calories & NaCl ↓ethanol ↑physical activity	123/83	-1.3/-1.2	0.46†
Hypertension Prevention Trial[2]	252	38	68	80	3 yr	↓calories	125/83	-2.4/-1.8	0.77
	392	39	62	84	3 yr	↓NaCl	124/83	+0.2/+0.1	0.79
	255	39	62	82	3 yr	↓calories & NaCl	125/83	-1.0/-1.3	0.95
	391	38	63	85	3 yr	↓NaCl & ↑ KCl	124/83	-1.2/-0.7	0.77
Trial of Hypertension Prevention[3] (Phase 1)	564	43	72	79	18 mo	↓calories & ↑physical activity	124/84	-2.9/-2.3	0.49†
	744	43	72	79	18 mo	↓NaCl	125/84	-1.7/-0.9	0.76
	562	43	71	84	18 mo	Manage Stress	125/84	-0.5/-0.8	1.07
	471	43	68	85	6 mo	↑ Calcium	126/84	-0.5/+0.2	0.91
	461	43	68	85	6 mo	↑ Magnesium	125/84	-0.2/-0.1	0.63
	351	43	72	87	6 mo	↑ Potassium	122/81	+0.1/-0.4	0.87
	350	43	70	86	6 mo	↑ Fish Oil	123/81	-0.2/-0.6	1.11
Trial of Hypertension Prevention[4] (Phase 2)	1191	43	66	79	36 mo	↓calories	127/86	-1.3/-0.9	0.81†
	1190	43	67	80	36 mo	↓NaCl	128/86	-1.2/-0.7	0.88
	1193	43	69	79	36 mo	↓calories & NaCl	127/86	-1.1/-0.6	0.84†

* Defined as diastolic blood pressure of ≥90 mmHg or antihypertensive drug therapy during followup.

† $p < 0.05$.

Modified from *Arch Intern Med* 1993;153 January 2 :186-208.[19] Used with permission and Copyright 1993, American Medical Association.

TABLE 48.2
Hypertension Prevention Trial (HPT): Six-Month Change in Interventions

	High BMI				Low BMI		
	Control	Kcalories	Sodium	Sodium/ Calories	Control	Sodium	Sodium/ Potassium
Number of subjects	121	112	109	113	191	173	180
ΔSBP/DBP (mmHg)	-1.8/-2.5	-6.9†/-5.3‡	-3.6/-3.4	-5.8/-4.0	-2.1/-3.0	-3.8/-3.4	-3.4/-3.7
ΔWeight (kg)	+0.18	-5.58†	-0.04	-3.90	+0.27	+0.00*	+0.27
ΔNa+Excretion (mmol/8h)	-4.5	-4.2	-7.8	-8.4	-3.9	-9.4¶	-11.4
ΔK+Excretion (mmol/8h)	0.3	-1.1	0.9	-0.1	-0.1	0.2	1.2

* p = 0.025; † p <0.001; ‡ p <0.01; ¶ p = 0.002.
Derived from Tables 4 and 5 in the report of The Hypertension Prevention Trial, *Arch Intern Med* 150: 153; 1990.

Hypertension Prevention Trial (HPT)

Men and women between the ages of 25 to 49 years with a diastolic blood pressure ≤89 mmHg were randomized.[2] Group and individual dietary counseling was performed. This primary prevention trial allocated subjects (see Table 48.1) on the basis of body mass index (BMI) into several interventions. Low BMI (men <25 kg/m^2 and women <23 kg/m^2 were randomized to either a control group (n = 70), sodium restriction (n = 70) ≤70 mmol/d (≤1610 mg/d) or sodium restriction and potassium augmentation (n = 71) ≥100 mmol/d (3900 mg/d). High BMI individuals were randomized to control (n = 126), caloric restriction (n = 125), sodium restriction (n = 126), sodium and caloric restriction (n = 129), and sodium restriction and potassium augmentation (n = 124).

The mean change in blood pressure for the interventions is displayed for both systolic and diastolic blood pressure at six months in Table 48.2. Caloric restriction reduced blood pressure significantly. Caloric and sodium restriction was a less effective strategy in this cohort. Sodium restriction with or without caloric restriction or potassium supplementation had no effect on blood pressure reduction. After three years, weight reduction was still significant (3.5 kg, p <0.001) and was associated with a significant blood pressure reduction of –2.4/–1.8 mmHg. After three years, the incidence of hypertension was significantly reduced in the low BMI group only (p <0.01), but only marginally so in the high BMI group (p = 0.066) as shown in Figure 48.1.

Trials of Hypertension Prevention (TOHP), Phase I

The TOHP (Phase I) was designed to assess the effect of various nonpharmacologic interventions in nonhypertensive subjects to lower blood pressure, and to determine the long-term impact on preventing the development of hypertension (see Table 48.1).[3] The trial was a multicenter, randomized study that examined three lifestyle interventions — weight reduction (n = 308), sodium restriction (n = 327), and stress management (n = 242) — compared to usual care (n = 589), and various nutritional supplements in two stages with an intervening washout period:

1. 25 mmol or 1g QD of calcium carbonate (n = 237), 15 mmol or 360 mg QD of magnesium diglycine (n = 227), and placebo (n = 234)
2. 6 g of fish oil containing 3g of ω-3 fatty acids (n = 175), 60 mmol or 4.5 g of potassium chloride (n = 178), and placebo (n = 175)

Weight reduction used a combination of caloric reduction, exercise increase, and behavioral self-management. Stress management involved teaching slow breathing, progressive

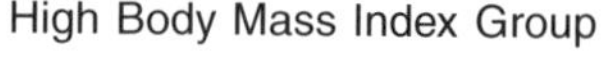

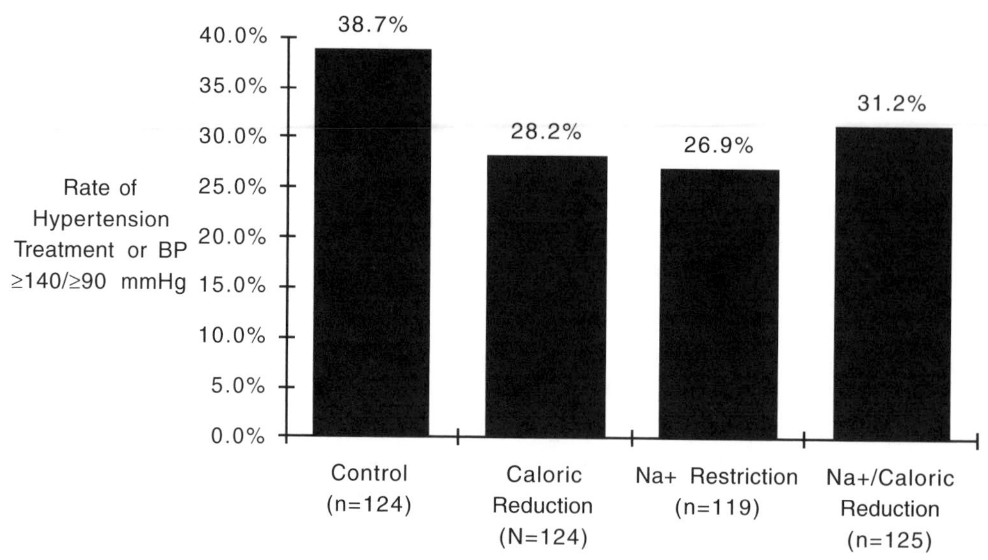

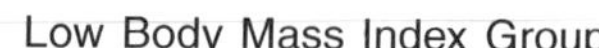

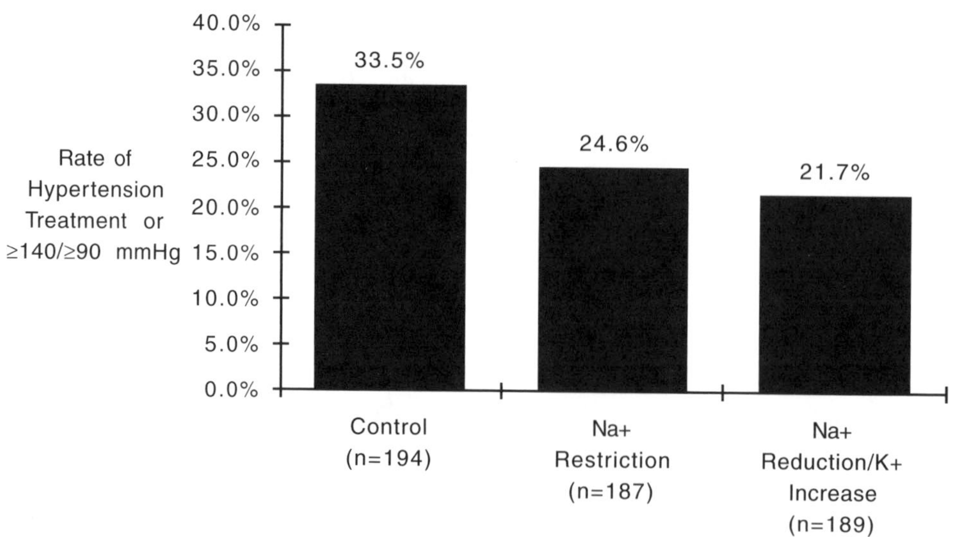

FIGURE 48.1
The Hypertension Prevention Trial: three-year rate of elevated blood pressure or treatment for hypertension, according to BMI and intervention.

muscular relaxation, mental imagery, stretching, and managing stress perceptions, reactions, and situations. The lifestyle modifications lasted 18 months and used blinded measurement of blood pressure as an endpoint. The nutritional supplements were placebo controlled, doubled blinded, and lasted 6 months.

The primary outcomes are displayed in Table 48.3 and Figure 48.2. Only weight reduction significantly lowered blood pressure and reduced the development of hypertension

TABLE 48.3

Intervention Outcome, Treatment Effect, and Blood Pressure Effect (Active – Control) in Trial of Hypertension Prevention, Phase I

Intervention	Outcome Treatment Effect	Blood Pressure Effect
18 Months Maximum Followup		
Sodium excretion (mmol/24h)	-43.86†	-1.69†/-0.85*
Weight change (kg)	-3.90†	-2.90†/-2.28†
Stress score frequency/intensity	+2.35†/-0.01	-0.47/-0.82
6 Months Maximum Followup		
Magnesium excretion (mmol/24h)/serum (mmol/L)	1.31†/+0.04†	-0.20/-0.05
Calcium excretion (mmol/24h)	0.91†	-0.46/+0.20
Potassium excretion (mmol/24h)	42.29†	+0.06/-0.42
% Eicosapentaenoic/Docosahexaenoic fatty acid	2.90†/2.04†	-0.22/-0.62

* p <0.05; † p <0.01.

Derived from Tables 2 and 3 in Trial of Hypertension Prevention, Phase 1, *JAMA* 267: 1213; 1992.

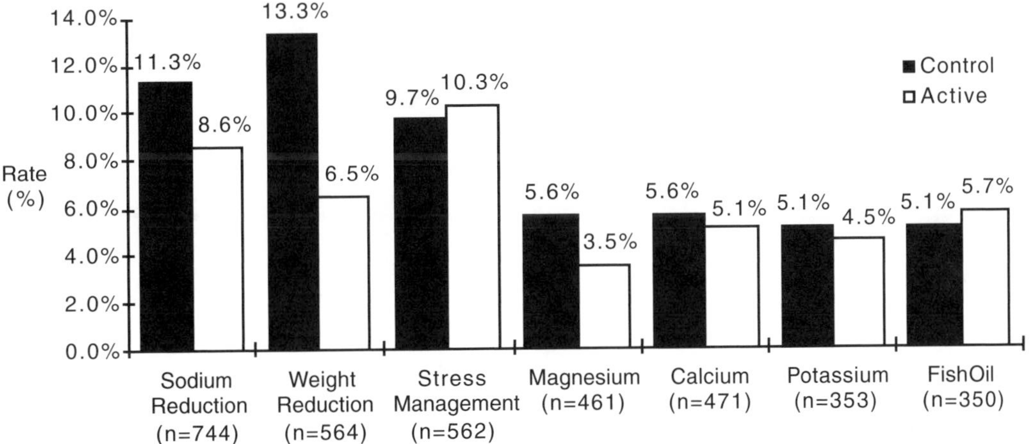

FIGURE 48.2
Trial of Hypertension Prevention, Phase 1. Incidence of hypertension in each lifestyle change and nutritional supplement group. Only weight reduction significantly reduced incidence of hypertension, relative risk = 0.49 (95% CI, 0.29 to 0.83). Derived from corrected table in *JAMA* 1992; 267(17): 2330.

at maximal followup at 18 months. Sodium restriction significantly lowered systolic and diastolic blood pressure, –1.7/–0.9 mmHg, but did not significantly reduce the incidence of hypertension.

The weight loss goal was 4.5 kg for the participants with 115 to 165% of desirable body weight that were enrolled. 45% of men and 26% of women in the intervention group compared with 12% of men and 18% of women in the control group met the weight loss goal at 18 months. The net change in weight at 18 months was 4.7 kg for men and 1.8 kg for women (p <0.01). Rather than being related to gender, the treatment effect was related to the higher baseline weight in males. In fact, the amount of blood pressure change, by gender related more to the quintile of weight change as shown in Table 48.4.

TABLE 48.4

Trial of Hypertension Prevention, Phase 1: Effect of Weight Change on Blood Pressure Reduction at 18 Months by Gender

	Quintile of Weight Change, kg				
	<-9.5	-9.5 to <-4.5	-4.5 to <-2.0	-2.0 to <1.0	≥1.0
Δ Systolic Blood Pressure (mmHg)					
Men	-9.0	-6.6	-4.8	-3.3	-1.6
Women	-5.7	-7.5	-5.0	-0.8	-1.2
Δ Diastolic Blood Pressure (mmHg)					
Men	-9.4	-6.8	-5.5	-4.2	-2.6
Women	-9.1	-7.1	-4.3	-4.9	-4.1

Derived from Figures 3, 4, and 5 in Trial of Hypertension Prevention, Phase 1, *JAMA* 267: 1213; 1992.

TABLE 48.5

Baseline Characteristics and Outcomes of Trials of Hypertension Prevention (Phase II)

	Weight Loss	Sodium Restriction	Combined	Usual Care
Number	595	594	597	596
Age, y	43.4	44.2	43.6	43.2
Male, %	63.0	64.8	68.8	68.3
White, %	78.0	81.1	78.4	79.5
Weight, kg	93.4	94.0	93.6	93.6
Baseline sodium excretion, mmol/d	180.9	186.1	179.3	188.0
Baseline blood pressure, mmHg	127.6/86.0	127.7/86.1	127.4/86.0	127.3/85.8
Six Month Followup				
Weight change, kg	-4.4 p <0.001*	-1.1 p <0.001*	-4.1 p <0.006*	0.1
Sodium excretion change, mmol/d	-18.2 p = 0.48*	-78.0 p <0.001*	-64.3 p = 0.006*	-27.6
Change in blood pressure, mmHg	-6.0/-5.5 p <0.001/<0.001†	-5.1/-4.4 p <0.001/<0.001†	-6.2/-5.6 p <0.001/<0.001†	-2.2/-2.8
Incidence of hypertension, %	4.2 p = 0.02*	4.5 p = 0.04*	2.7 p <0.001*	7.3
36 Month Followup				
Weight change, kg	-0.2 p <0.001*	+1.7 p = 0.92*	-0.3 p <0.001*	+1.8
Sodium excretion change, mmol/d	-9.0 p = 0.79*	-50.9 p <0.001*	-34.1 p <0.001*	-10.5
Change in blood pressure, mmHg	-0.8/-3.2 p = 0.01/0.04†	-0.7/-3.0 p = 0.02/0.10†	-0.5/-3.0 p = 0.05/0.19†	+0.6/-2.4
Incidence of hypertension, %	31.9	34.4	32.8	39.2

* significance vs. usual care group
† significance of systolic and diastolic blood pressure vs. usual group

Derived from Tables 1 through 4 from The Trials of Hypertension Prevention (Phase II) Prevention Collaborative Research Group, *Arch Intern Med* 157: 657; 1997.

Trials of Hypertension Prevention (TOHP II), Phase II

The randomized TOHP II was conducted as a two-by-two factorial design study to assess the effect of weight reduction, sodium restriction, or both compared to usual care in lowering blood pressure and preventing the development of hypertension after three to four years of followup.[4] Diastolic blood pressure was required to be 83 to 89 mmHg at the third screening visit, and weight 110 to 165% of desirable body weight. Intervention goals for the weight reduction group was weight loss ≥4.5 kg, and for the sodium reduction group a decrease in sodium intake ≤80 mmol/d. Blinded observers measured blood pressure. 2382 subjects were recruited.

Baseline and treatment outcomes are displayed in Table 48.5. By 6 months, neither the weight loss nor sodium restriction goals were met by the groups; however, the net blood pressure reduction compared to the usual care group was significant (p <0.001 for each intervention): weight loss, –3.7/–2.7 mmHg; sodium restriction, –2.9/–1.6 mmHg; and the combination, –4.0/–2.8 mmHg. At 36 months, many of the treatment effects were lost. The 38% incidence of hypertension was similar in all treatment groups, compared to 44% in the usual care group, and did not appear additive at 36 months. The relative risk of hypertension (compared with the usual care group) was 0.87 for the weight loss group (p = 0.06), 0.86 for the sodium reduction group (p = 0.04), and 0.85 for the combined intervention group (p = 0.02).[4]

Secondary Prevention Trials

Dietary Intervention Study of Hypertension (DISH)

Participants in DISH were former medicated participants of the Hypertension Detection and Follow-up Program.[5] The cohort (n = 496) was grouped into obese (≥120% of ideal body weight) or nonobese. The obese group was randomized into one of four groups: 1) continue drug therapy or 2) discontinue drug therapy and a) receive no dietary intervention, the control group, b) decrease sodium intake, or c) lose weight. The nonobese group was randomized to 1) continue drug therapy or 2) discontinue drug therapy and a) receive no dietary intervention, the control group, or b) decrease sodium intake.

Demographics and outcomes are shown in Table 48.6. Among overweight persons, 46.3% lost an average of 5% of weight, or greater than 4.5 kg after 56 weeks. The average weight

TABLE 48.6

Dietary Intervention Study in Hypertension: Demographics and Outcome

	Obese Drug Therapy Control	Obese No Drug Control	Obese Sodium Restriction	Obese Weight Reduction	Lean Drug Therapy Control	Lean No Drug Control	Lean Sodium Restriction
Number	48	89	101	87	33	70	68
Age (Yr)	59	57	57	56	58	57	56
% Black	75	70	64	62	58	73	56
% Women	69	64	59	68	52	50	47
BP (mmHg)	131/80	128/80	128/81	128/81	126/80	124/80	127/81
ΔWeight (kg)	-0.46	-0.46	0	-4.0	+0.46	0	+0.46
Δ Urine Na+ (mEq/d)	-13	-10	-59	0	+2	-5	-44
% on *no* BP Drugs	0	35	45	60	0	45	53

Derived from Tables 1, 2, and 3 in article by Langford, H.G., et al. *JAMA* 253: 657; 1985.

TABLE 48.7

Hypertension Control Program: Demographics and Outcome

	No BP Drugs Nutritional Therapy	No BP Drugs No Nutritional Therapy	BP Drugs No Nutritional Therapy
Number	97	44	48
Age (Yr)	57	55	55
% Female	35	39	38
% Black	11	21	15
BP (mmHg)	122/78	118/77	119/79
Δ Weight (kg)*	-1.8‡	+2.0	+2.0
Δ Urinary Na+ (mEq/d)	-60‡	+20	-5
Δ Ethanol (g/d)†	-12.5	-7.1	-10.2
% Without BP Drugs	39%‡	5%	0%

* Among obese subjects only; † Among drinkers only; ‡ p <0.001

Derived from tables and manuscript of Stamler, R. et al. *JAMA* 257: 1484; 1987.

loss in this group was 4.0 kg (p <0.05 versus the no-medication control group). Among obese and nonobese persons who were sodium restricted, the mean decrease in urine sodium output was –59 mEq/24 hr and –44 mEq/24 hr (each p <0.05 versus the no-medication control group) after 56 weeks. The percent not taking antihypertensive medication among obese individuals was 35.3% in the control group, 44.9% in the sodium restricted group, and 59.5% in weight loss group (p = 0.0015 versus control). In the lean group, the percent not taking antihypertensive medication was 45% in the control group and 53.4% in the sodium-restricted group (not significantly different).

The Hypertension Control Program (HCP)

Participants in the HCP were former drug-treated participants of the Hypertension Detection and Follow-up Program. Subjects (n = 189) were randomized to three groups:

1. Discontinue antihypertensive therapy and reduce overweight, excess salt, and alcohol
2. Stop medication without nutritional intervention (the control group)
3. Continue drug treatment with no nutritional program

The primary endpoint was the percentage of subjects remaining hypertensive in the intervention versus the control group.

As shown in Table 48.7, in the nutritional intervention group, weight decreased (p <0.001) and sodium output increased (p <0.001) significantly after four years. 39% of the nutritional therapy group were maintained on no drug therapy compared to only 5% of the control group (p <0.001).

Trial of Antihypertensive Intervention and Management (TAIM)

This multicenter, placebo-controlled trial randomized 787 overweight (110 to 160% ideal body weight) hypertensive (baseline diastolic pressure 90 to 100 mmHg) men and women to one of three drugs (placebo, chlorthalidone 25 mg QD, or atenolol 50 mg QD) and three dietary interventions (usual diet, weight loss, or sodium decrease/potassium increase).[6] The weight loss goal was 10% of baseline weight or 4.54 kg, whichever was greater. Sodium reduction was 52 to 100 mmoles/d and potassium increase 62 to 115 mmoles/d, and depended on weight. Both weight reduction and electrolyte changes required group nutri-

TABLE 48.8

Trial of Antihypertensive Intervention and Management: Change in Blood Pressure from Baseline by Treatment Group at Six Months

	Usual Diet	Weight Loss	Low Na+/High K+
Placebo	-10.34/-7.96 (n = 90)	-11.49/-8.78 (n = 90)	-8.66/-7.91 (n = 79)
Chlorthalidone	-17.41/-10.78 (n = 87)	-21.72/-15.06 (n = 87)	-19.51/-12.18 (n = 89)
Atenolol	-15.06/-12.43 (n = 87)	-18.11/-14.81 (n = 88)	-18.29/-12.76 (n = 90)

Derived from Tables 2 and 3 from Langford, H.G. et al. *Hypertension* 17: 210; 1991.

tional counseling weekly for 10 weeks, and individually thereafter every 6 to 12 weeks. There was no change in the drugs or their dosages during the first six months of the trial unless critical diastolic blood pressures were reached (treatment crossovers). Change in diastolic blood pressure treatment failure (as assessed by the need to increase drug treatment), quality of life, and calculated cardiovascular risk were assessed.

Table 48.8 shows the change in systolic and diastolic blood pressure from baseline to six months by treatment group. In the weight loss group, the average decrease in weight was 4.5 kg after six months. Weight loss was more effective than usual diet ($p = 0.001$) or the low sodium/high potassium diet ($p = 0.019$) in lowering diastolic blood pressure. Weight loss in combination with either a diuretic (–4.3 mmHg, $p = 0.002$), added significantly to blood pressure reduction compared to usual diet with a diuretic. The combination of weight loss with a β-blocker (–2.4 mmHg, $p = 0.07$) did not add to the effect of the drug alone.

45% of the weight loss cohort lost ≥4.5 kg. For patients who were not treatment crossovers, placebo and usual diet (n = 71) was associated with a 7 mmHg decrease in blood pressure and a 0.63 kg change in weight, and was less effective than placebo with >4.5 kg weight loss and diastolic blood pressure decrease of 11.6 mmHg ($p < .01$). There was a graded relationship with the amount of weight reduction and blood pressure decrease: <2.25 kg, –6.9 mmHg; –2.25 to 4.5 kg, –8.9 mmHg; and >4.5 kg, –11.6 mmHg. The change in diastolic blood pressure inversely correlated with the baseline plasma renin indexed to the 24-hour urinary sodium in the weight loss diet group.[7] In fact, the change in diastolic blood pressure with >4.5 kg weight change is comparable to low-dose drug therapy as seen in Table 48.9. After 24 months, there was gradual return of weight toward the baseline.[8] Among the weight-loss diet patients, the least mean change in weight occurred among atenolol-treated subjects. In fact, among atenolol-treated subjects assigned to usual diet or electrolyte modification, there was a mean weight gain. The 5-year incidence of treatment failure was lower in the weight loss group (49.8 per 100 subjects) than in the usual diet group (56.7 per 100 subjects).[9]

TABLE 48.9

Trial of Antihypertensive Intervention and Management: Change in Diastolic Blood Pressure with >4.5 kg Weight Change — Comparable to Low-Dose Drug Therapy

	Usual Diet	≥4.5 kg Weight Loss
Placebo	-7.0 (n = 71)	-11.6 (n = 33)*
Chlorthalidone	-11.1 (n = 80)	-15.3 (n = 53)†
Atenolol	-12.4 (n = 79)	-18.4 (n = 26)‡

* $p < 0.01$, † $p = .002$, and ‡ $p = 0.0005$ compared to usual diet.

Derived from Figures 2 and 3 from Wassertheil-Smoller, S. et al. *Arch Intern Med* 152: 131; 1992.

In the low sodium/high potassium group, the average decrease in urinary sodium was 27.4 mmol/d and the average increase in urinary potassium 10.9 mmol/d. The effect on blood pressure of the low sodium/high potassium diet did not differ from that of the usual diet ($p = 0.347$) on blood pressure. The low sodium/high potassium diet did not further lower diastolic blood pressure, but the baseline urinary sodium excretion was already relatively low (133 mmol/d). However, in the placebo group, when urinary sodium excretion ≤70 mEq/d was achieved, systolic and diastolic blood pressure reduction was greater than in the usual diet group (–23.7/–13.9 mmHg versus –9.6/–7.0 mmHg, each $p < 0.005$).[10]

After 3 years, compared to the usual diet, the net difference of urinary sodium excretion reduction was 30 mmol/d and urinary potassium excretion augmentation was 11 mmol/d.[11] There was a 41% decrease ($p = 0.01$) in the risk of treatment failure for women and 34% decrease ($p = 0.03$) among less obese patients. After 3.5 years among patients assigned to low sodium/high potassium diet, treatment failures occurred in 68% of placebo-, 47% of diuretic-, and 35% of β-blocker-assigned subjects.

Quality of life was improved with weight reduction.[12] Weight reduction significantly reduced symptoms of physical problems, especially sexual problems, and improved satisfaction with physical health. Weight loss improved the erectile dysfunction reported with chlorthalidone and usual diet (12.1 versus 26.2%).[13] Weight reduction reduced symptoms of sexual problems in both men and women significantly. The low sodium/high potassium diet with placebo was associated with greater fatigue (34.3%) than was either usual diet (18.1%, $p = 0.04$) or weight reduction (14.6%, $p = 0.009$). The electrolyte intervention group in combination with chlorthalidone (32.0%, $p = 0.04$) was associated with more sleep disturbances than chlorthalidone versus usual diet (16%). A nonsignificant ($p = 0.07$) similar trend was observed with atenolol.

Overall calculated cardiovascular risk worsened with chlorthalidone therapy in the usual diet group at six months due to the changes in cholesterol and glucose.[14] Those persons treated with atenolol or weight reduction showed the lowest relative risk.

Trial of Nonpharmacologic Interventions in the Elderly

This was a randomized, multicenter, controlled trial of 975 men and women aged 60 to 80 years with blood pressure of <145/<85 mmHg on a single hypertensive drug.[15] Patients were randomized to treatment based on their body habitus. 585 obese patients either received usual care, sodium restriction (a dietary intake of less than 80 mmoles per day as measured by 24-hour urine sodium collection), a weight loss program to achieve a loss of 4.5 kilograms or greater, or a combination of sodium restriction and weight loss. 390 nonobese patients were randomized to either usual care or sodium restriction.

The mean change in blood pressure prior to attempted medication withdrawal for each group was: sodium reduction, –3.4/–1.9 mmHg; weight reduction, –4.0/–1.1 mmHg; combination intervention, –5.3/–3.4 mmHg; and usual care, –0.8/–0.8 mmHg. Sodium reduction, weight reduction, and the combination intervention lower blood pressure significantly more than usual care. After three months of nonpharmacological therapy, antihypertensive medication withdrawal was attempted. After 30 months, 44% of patients in the combined sodium and weight reduction group were free of a primary endpoint (sustained blood pressure of 150/90 mmHg or higher, pharmacologic treatment of hypertension, or occurrence a clinical cardiovascular event). Compared to 16% in the usual care group, 34% of the sodium restriction group and 37% of the weight reduction group did not have a primary endpoint at 30 months. The sodium-restricted group reduced average sodium intake about 40 mmoles per day. In the weight loss group, average body weight decreased by 3.5 kilograms. Sodium restriction was equally effective in the obese and lean subjects; however, the combined intervention was not more effective than either single intervention. Predictors of successful long-term withdrawal of pharmacologic treatment include lower baseline systolic blood pressure, shorter duration of hypertension or drug treatment, and absence of a history of cardiovascular disease.[16]

Dietary Approaches to Stop Hypertension (DASH)

The DASH trial was a multicenter, randomized feeding study that sought to assess the impact of nutrients naturally occurring in food in contrast to nutritional supplements.[17] Subjects were required to have a systolic blood pressure less than 160 mmHg and a diastolic blood pressure 80 to 95 mmHg. Persons consuming greater than 14 alcoholic beverages per week were excluded from the study. After screening, all subjects completed a three-week control diet. The control diet included magnesium, potassium, and calcium at the 25th percentile of consumption, and fiber at the average level of consumption. After the control period, 459 study participants received either a control diet, a fruit and vegetable diet, or combination diet for eight weeks. The fruit and vegetable diet provided magnesium and potassium at the 75th percentile of consumption and was also high in fiber. The combination diet was high in protein and fiber, provided increased calcium, magnesium, and potassium to the 75th percentile of consumption, and reduced intake of total fat, total cholesterol, and saturated fat. The sodium content (~3000 mg per day) was similar for all three diets, and caloric intake was adjusted so that weight gain did not occur in the study.

The average age of the subjects was 44 years; 60% were African Americans and 49% were women. About 14% had a diastolic blood pressure ≥90 mmHg, and 23.5% had a systolic blood pressure ≥140 mmHg. Change in the diastolic blood pressure was the primary outcome. The change in blood pressure in the combination group (corrected for the change in the control group) was –5.5/–3.0 mmHg (p <0.001 for each). The change in blood pressure among hypertensive subjects was larger than in nonhypertensive subjects (–11.4/–5.5 mmHg versus –3.5/–2.1 mmHg), and among minority subjects was larger than nonminority subjects (–6.8/–3.5 mmHg versus –3.0/–2.0 mmHg). The change in blood pressure in the fruit and vegetable group minus the change in the control group was –2.8/–1.1 mmHg (p <0.001 for each). Hypertensive subjects had a greater blood pressure reduction (–7.2/–2.8 mmHg) on the fruit and vegetable diet.

The combination diet demonstrated superiority over the fruits and vegetables in reducing blood pressure significantly an average of –2.5/–1.9 mmHg more. The combination diet lowered systolic blood pressure significantly more in African Americans (6.8 mm Hg) than in whites (3.0 mm Hg), and in hypertensive subjects (11.4 mm Hg) than in nonhypertensive subjects (3.4 mm Hg) (p <0.05 for both).[18]

Since the DASH trial showed a blood pressure-lowering effect for a diet rich in vegetables, fruits, grains, low-fat dairy products, fish, poultry, and nuts, a logical question was whether there was an additional benefit of a low sodium diet. To answer this question, 412 subjects were randomly assigned to either the DASH diet or a control diet.[21] Each person for their assigned diet was rotated in random order at 30-day intervals to a low (50 mmol/d), intermediate (100 mmol/d) or high (150 mmol/d) sodium intake diet. The study population included 57% females, 57% blacks, and 41% hypertensives. Since this was a feeding trial, it was not surprising that urinary excretion of sodium was reduced according to treatment assignment in both the DASH and control diet groups. The change in blood pressure in the control diet group from high to intermediate sodium intake was –2.1/–1.1 mmHg, and from intermediate to low sodium intake –4.6/–2.4 mmHg. The corresponding values for the DASH diet were –1.3/–0.6 mmHg and –1.7/–1.0 mmHg. All of these values are statistically significant except for the change in diastolic blood pressure from high to intermediate sodium intake in the DASH group. The benefit of the DASH diet over the control diet was confirmed by the change in blood pressure in the high (–5.9/–2.9 mmHg), intermediate (–5.0/–2.5 mmHg), and low sodium intake (-2.2/-1.0 mmHg) groups. The greatest benefit was seen in hypertensive subjects, African Americans, and women. There was a less than additive effect of decreased sodium intake and DASH diet, but a greater effect than either intervention individually.

Summary

The primary prevention trials prove that sodium restriction and weight reduction are effective in reducing the rate of development of hypertension. However, the behavioral changes are difficult to sustain over a 36-month period, and the treatment effects are modest. Individual strategies of potassium, calcium, magnesium, or fish oil supplementation are not effective in nonhypertensive subjects in lowering blood pressure or preventing the development of hypertension.

The secondary prevention trials document a clear benefit for sodium restriction and weight reduction in controlling blood pressure. However, the combination of weight reduction and sodium restriction was not additive. Weight loss was additive to diuretic therapy and improved quality of life, including sexual dysfunction. Although individual dietary components of potassium, calcium, magnesium, and fish oil supplementation have not been successful strategies for primary prevention, the DASH feeding study, which reduced intake of total fat, total cholesterol, and saturated fat, and increased protein, fiber, fruit, and vegetable intake, demonstrates the potential that can be achieved with nonpharmacological interventions rich in these individual components.

References

1. Stamler R, Stamler J, Gosch FC, et al. *JAMA*, 262: 1801; 1989.
2. *Arch Intern Med* 150: 153; 1990.
3. *JAMA* 267: 1213; 1992.
4. *Arch Intern Med* 157(6): 657; 1997.
5. Langford HG, Blaufox MD, Oberman A, et al. *JAMA* 253: 657; 1985.
6. Langford HG, Davis BR, Blaufox D, et al. *Hypertension* 17: 210; 1991.
7. Blaufox MD, Lee HB, Davis B, et al. *JAMA* 267: 1221; 1992.
8. Davis BR, Oberman A, Blaufox MD, et al. *Hypertension* 19: 393; 1992.
9. Davis BR, Blaufox MD, Oberman A, et al. *Arch Intern Med* 153: 1773; 1993.
10. Wassertheil-Smoller S, Blaufox MD, Oberman AS, et al. *Arch Intern Med* 152(1): 131, 1992.
11. Davis BR, Oberman A, Blaufox MD, et al. *Am J Hypertens* 7: 926; 1994.
12. Wassertheil-Smoller S, Blaufox MD, Oberman A, et al. *Ann Intern Med* 114: 613; 1991.
13. Wassertheil-Smoller S, Oberman A, Blaufox MD, et al. *Am J Hypertens* 5: 37; 1992.
14. Oberman A, Wassertheil-Smoller S, Langford HG, et al. *Ann Intern Med* 112: 89; 1990.
15. Whelton PK, Appel LJ, Espeland MA, et al. *JAMA* 279: 839; 1998.
16. Espeland MA, Whelton PK, Kostis JB, et al. *Arch Fam Med* 8: 228; 1999.
17. Appel LJ, Moore TJ, Obarzanek E, et al. *N Engl J Med* 336: 1117; 1997.
18. Svetkey LP, Simons-Morton D, Vollmer WM, et al. *Arch Intern Med* 159: 285; 1999.
19. __________ *Arch Intern Med* 153: 186; 1993.
20. Stamler R, Stamler J, Grimm R, et al. *JAMA* 257: 1484; 1987.
21. Sacks FM, Svetkey LP, Vollmer WM, et al. *N Engl J Med* 344: 3; 2001.

49

Chemoprevention of Cancer in Humans by Dietary Means

Elizabeth K. Weisburger and Ritva Butrum

This section will attempt to describe succinctly the basis for prevention of cancer by dietary means. An understanding of the processes involved in carcinogenesis is vital to any efforts in prevention. Reference 1 provides information on the metabolic activation of chemical carcinogens to the ultimate forms, which interact with the genetic material of the cell. In addition, the separate stages in carcinogenesis are described; namely, initiation or the first step, promotion or enhancement of the process, and progression or increased growth and expansion of the cancerous cells. Examples of how the different stages can be inhibited or altered are provided.

Diet or nutrition is an essential part of life, for it furnishes the food elements needed to sustain life, wards off some disease conditions, and helps insure a reasonable level of well being. The choices we make for our diets can have an appreciable impact on our health and vigor. Balanced and varied diets of natural foodstuffs, high in whole-grain products, fruits, and vegetables, are more likely to enhance our health than diets of highly refined foods. For a proper balance, various macronutrients, vitamins, minerals, and even non-nutritive food constituents are necessary, as discussed herewith.

Macronutrients

Carbohydrates

Carbohydrates, either simple sugars or starches, are formed in plants through the process of photosynthesis from carbon dioxide and water, and thus represent the means by which the energy from the sun is converted into food. The simple sugars of dietary carbohydrates are mono- and disaccharides such as glucose, sucrose, and fructose. Oligo and higher polysaccharides, which include both starch and non-starch polysaccharides constitute the major portion of dietary fiber. Starch occurs in cereals, legumes, roots, tubers, plantains, and bananas; it is the energy source for plants, equivalent to liver glycogen in animals.

Starch which is resistant to digestion in the small intestine occurs in whole grains, legumes, and potatoes, for example. This resistant starch is metabolized by the bacteria in the large intestine to compounds which are important for both the growth of endogeneous bacteria and for colonic epithelial cell proliferation. Nonstarch polysaccharides, along with

0-8493-2705-9/01/$0.00+$1.50

lignan from plant cell walls comprise dietary fiber, which plays an important role in regulation of stool bulk and weight. Dietary fiber is considered to have a preventative effect against colorectal cancer, since by increasing stool bulk, it dilutes any toxic material.[2]

Dietary carbohydrates should account for about 40 to 85% of total energy. Diets outside these guidelines may be lacking in other needed constituents.[3] Preferably, dietary carbohydrates should include high fiber sources, since besides decreasing the risk of colorectal cancer, there may be a preventative action for pancreatic and breast cancer. Conversely, high starch diets or those high in refined starch may increase risk for stomach cancer. Thus, the type of dietary carbohydrate can either be beneficial or deleterious with respect to cancer risk.

Fats

Fats, often maligned as relatively undesirable dietary constituents, are nevertheless essential components of food. They are necessary building blocks for biological membranes, have a high nutritive value, are a source of certain essential fatty acids and vitamins, impart a pleasant feel to foods, solubilize or carry many of the flavor components of foods, and serve as an energy storage depot. Chemically, fats are composed chiefly of the triesters of long-chain aliphatic carboxylic acids with glycerol, along with minor amounts of free acids and mono- and diacylglycerols. The composition of fat is affected by the source — animal or vegetable, growth environment, type of food if from an animal, climate, and location.

During the digestive process, fats are hydrolyzed by lipases to the respective acids which serve as an energy source. The major acids from most domestic food animals are stearic, palmitic, and oleic acids, while plant fats yield more of the unsaturated acids such as oleic, linoleic, and linolenic. Fish oils, although containing some palmitic and stearic acids, have varying amounts of other unsaturated fatty acids. As for nomenclature, the double bond position is determined by counting from the methyl end of the aliphatic chain, using the notation Ω (omega). Fatty acids from fish contain large amounts of Ω-3 fatty acids; those from plants contain more of the Ω-6 type. The "shorthand" description of the fatty acid depicts the number of carbon atoms in the chain and the number, positions, and configurations (cis/trans) of the double bonds (see Table 49.1).

The acids derived from fats or oils, besides being energy sources, have a role in enhancing or promoting, and suppressing or inhibiting, the processes involved with carcinogenesis. Generally, oleic acid and the Ω-3 unsaturated acids from fish oils appear to suppress neoplastic effects, both in experimental and epidemiologic studies. Although epidemiologic studies cannot be controlled to the extent of animal studies, they indicate that populations consuming diets richer in olive oil have a lower breast cancer incidence.[4,5] In some cases, higher fish consumption was associated with possibly decreased risk for cancer of the larynx, pharynx, liver, colon, endometrium, and kidney.[6,7] There are many confounding factors in such studies, but the indications are that olive and fish oils are beneficial, while the saturated fats from most meats and some of the Ω-6 unsaturated fats from many oilseeds may enhance the action of exogenous or endogenous carcinogens.

An additional fatty acid with antimutagenic and anticarcinogenic effects in animal systems is conjugated linoleic acid (CLA), a mixture of positional isomers of linoleic acid where the double bonds are in positions 9 and 11 or 10 and 12 along the carbon chain. Since the bonds can be in the cis or trans configuration, eight isomers are possible. CLA was originally identified in grilled ground beef, but it has also been found in meat from other ruminants, and in dairy products such as cheese. In animal experiments, CLA has been effective as an inhibitor of tumors from application of polycyclic aromatic hydrocarbons, in decreasing the action of tumor promoters, decreasing cell proliferation, reducing

TABLE 49.1

Typical Dietary Fatty Acids

Designation	Structure	Name		Melting Point(°C)
		Systematic	Common	
4:0	$H_3C(CH_2)_2COOH$	Butanoic	Butyric acid	-7.9
5:0	$H_3C(CH_2)_3COOH$	Pentanoic	Valeric	-34.5
6:0	$H_3C(CH_2)_4COOH$	Hexanoic	Caproic	-3.9
7:0	$H_3C(CH_2)_5COOH$	Heptanoic	Enanthoic	-7.5
8:0	$H_3C(CH_2)_6COOH$	Octanoic	Caprylic	16.3
9:0	$H_3C(CH_2)_7COOH$	Nonanoic	Pelargonic	12.4
10:0	$H_3C(CH_2)_8COOH$	Decanoic	Capric	31.3
12:0	$H_3C(CH_2)_{10}COOH$	Dodecanoic	Lauric	44.0
14:0	$H_3C(CH_2)_{12}COOH$	Tetradecanoic	Myristic	54.4
15:0	$H_3C(CH_2)_{13}COOH$	Pentadecanoic	Pentadecylic	52.1
16:0	$H_3C(CH_2)_{14}COOH$	Hexadecanoic	Palmitic	62.9
17:0	$H_3C(CH_2)_{15}COOH$	Heptadecanoic	Margaric	61.3
18:0	$H_3C(CH_2)_{16}COOH$	Octadecanoic	Stearic	69.6
20:0	$H_3C(CH_2)_{18}COOH$	Eicosanoic	Arachidic	75.4
22:0	$H_3C(CH_2)_{20}COOH$	Docosanoic	Behenic	80.0
24:0	$H_3C(CH_2)_{22}COOH$	Tetracasonoic	Lignoceric	84.2
26:0	$H_3C(CH_2)_{24}COOH$	Hexacosanoic	Cerotic	87.7
18:1 (9)	$CH_3(CH_2)_7CH{=}CH\text{-}(CH_2)_7COOH$	Oleic		13.4
22:1 (13)	$CH_3(CH_2)_7CH{=}CH\text{-}(CH_2)_{11}COOH$	Erucic		34.7
18:2 (9,12)	$CH_3(CH_2)_4\text{-}(CH{=}CH\text{-}CH_2)_2(CH_2)_6COOH$	Linoleic		-5.0
18:3 (6,9,12)	$CH_3(CH_2)_4\text{-}(CH{=}CH\text{-}CH_2)_3(CH_2)_3COOH$	γ-Linoleic		
20:4 (5,8,11,14)	$CH_3(CH_2)_4\text{-}(CH{=}CH\text{-}CH_2)_4(CH_2)_2COOH$	Arachidonic		-49.5
18:1 (tr 9)	$CH_3(CH_2)_7CH{=}CH(CH_2)_7COOH$	Elaidic		46.0
18:3 (9,12,15)	$CH_3\text{-}CH_2(CH{=}CH\text{-}CH_2)_3(CH_2)_6COOH$	α-Linolenic		-11.0

From *CRC Handbook of Chemistry and Physics*, D.R. Lide, Ed., 80th ed., 1999-2000.

the activation of heterocyclic amine carcinogens for some organ sites but not others, and modulating the action of protein kinase C proteins involved in signal transduction.[8,9] CLA was effective at a dietary level of 0.1%, one-hundredfold less than the level of dietary fish oil needed to inhibit animal tumors. Despite the effectiveness in both animal and cell culture studies, CLA as such has not been investigated in any sizable population studies.

A controversial aspect of the fatty acid situation relates to trans fatty acids. These compounds, where the hydrogens are on opposite sides of the carbons in the double bonds, are linear, akin to the shape of saturated fatty acids. Although trans fatty acids occur in nature in plants and in milk and meat from ruminants, the main source of dietary intake is through partial hydrogenation of vegetable oils, which have been used in margarine, salad oils, shortenings, and cooking fats for most of this century. Animal studies have shown that diets with up to 35% trans fat had no effect on growth or reproduction, but like natural saturated fats, they increased blood cholesterol levels. Epidemiological studies are controversial, but they have not shown untoward effects of trans fatty acids if used prudently.[10,11]

Thus, monounsaturated dietary fatty acids and perhaps the Ω-3 unsaturated acids found in fish oils may have a suppressing action against certain human cancers. Nevertheless, even such advantageous fats should be used prudently.[12,13]

Protein

Proteins are complex molecules comprising combinations of amino acids. They can be of plant or animal origin; for example, about 20 to 35% of legumes is protein, 8 to 25%

of nuts and seeds, 8 to 16% of cereals, 10 to 20% of meat and fish, 15% of eggs, 3.5% of milk, and 13% of vegetables. Proteins are important nutritionally, as they supply the necessary building blocks for protein biosynthesis in specific organisms, contribute to the physical properties of food, and are either part of the flavor of food or are the precursors for flavor components formed during thermal or enzymatic reactions occurring during food processing.

Protein intake usually varies between 10 and 18% of total energy in different countries, and the composition varies depending whether animal or vegetable proteins are consumed.[14] There are no definitive data in humans indicating an association between cancer risk and protein intake, due to the presence of other macroconstituents in protein sources and various micronutrients. Dietary use of soy products has been suggestive for a lower risk of breast and endometrial cancer in Asian women.[15-17] Whether this is due to the soy protein, or more likely, the flavonoids present in soy has not been exactly determined. In animal studies, however, low protein diets tend to inhibit cancer, probably due to slower growth, while a high intake tends to enhance cancer development at various sites.

Proteins themselves are hydrolyzed or split by proteases to the individual amino acids, some of which are essential for mammalian growth and development while others are not (Table 49.2). Proteins from animal sources (animals, birds, fish, shellfish) are considered complete proteins since all the essential amino acids are present. Proteins from plant sources are generally incomplete since one or the other of the essential amino acids is low. However, combinations of plant proteins can usually supply all the essential amino acids; for example, corn and beans or rice and beans.

Chemically, some of the amino acids have nonpolar uncharged side chains; others have uncharged polar side chains, while still others have charged polar side chains (Table 49.2). These side chains are involved in the reactions and configurations of amino acids and the proteins from them.

Of all the amino acids, only methionine appears to be involved in physiological processes which have a chemopreventive action against cancer. As its S-adenosyl derivative or SAM, it is important, in conjunction with folate, in methylation of nucleic acid bases. Under- or hypomethylation of these cell constituents has been associated with cancer in animal studies. In animal experiments, deficiencies of SAM and folate led to tumors in rats and mice. The data for the folate/SAM effect for decreasing colorectal cancer in humans are suggestive but not definitive.[18,19]

Total Energy

Total energy denotes the sum of the kcalories from fats, proteins, and carbohydrates within the diet of an individual. Energy requirements for each person vary with weight, height, age, body mass, and physical activity. Persons involved in strenuous physical activity such as competitive sports or mountain climbing obviously require more kcalories than those with sedentary lifestyles. However, it is excess total energy that becomes a problem, for the caloric matter in excess food is converted to fat and stored as such in the body. Fat, besides being an energy storage depot, also serves as a repository for all lipid-soluble xenobiotics and leads to greater conversion of endogenous steroids to estrogen. Estrogen, in turn, is a risk factor associated with breast and endometrial cancers. Higher body mass index is linked to an increased risk for cancer of the kidney and possibly gallbladder, colon, pancreas, and prostate. Continued physical activity and a body mass index below average tend to a decrease in cancer risk. Thus, continued physical activity tends to decrease cancer risk.[20]

Recommendations on a diet for prevention of cancer emphasize the need to rely on a low-fat diet, since dietary fat contains more kcalories on a weight basis than other macro-

TABLE 49.2
Amino Acids

Name	Formula	Essential	Non-essential	Non-polar, Uncharged Sidechain	Polar, Uncharged Sidechain	Charged Sidechain
Alanine	(Ala) $H_2N\text{-}CH(CH_3)\ COOH$		X	X		
Arginine	(Arg) $H_2N\text{-}C(=NH)\ NH(CH_2)_3\ CH(NH_2)\ COOH$	X				X
Asparagine	(Asn) $H_2N\text{-}CH\ (COOH)\ CH_2\ CONH_2$		X		X	
Aspartic acid	(Asp) $H_2N\text{-}CH\ (COOH)\ CH_2\ COOH$		X			X
Cysteine	(Cys) $H_2N\text{-}CH\ (CH_2SH)\ COOH$		X		X	
Glutamic acid	(Glu) $H_2N\text{-}CH\ (COOH)\ (CH_2)_2\ COOH$		X			X
Glutamine	(Gln) $H_2N\text{-}CH\ (COOH)\ (CH_2)_2\ CONH_2$		X		X	
Glycine	(Gly) $H_2N\text{-}CH_2\ COOH$		X	X		
Histidine	(His) $H_2N\text{-}CH\ (COOH)\ CH_2\ (C_3N_2H_3)$	X (infant)				X
Isoleucine	(Ile) $H_2N\text{-}CH\ (COOH)\ CH(CH_3)\ CH_2\ CH_3$	X		X		
Leucine	(Leu) $H_2N\text{-}CH\ (COOH)\ CH_2\ (CHCH_2CH_3)$	X		X		
Lysine	(Lys) $H_2N\text{-}CH\ (COOH)\ (CH_2)_4NH_2$	X				X
Methionine	(Met) $H_2N\text{-}CH\ (COOH)\ (CH_2)_2\ SCH_3$	X		X		
Phenylalanine	(Phe) $H_2N\ CH\ (COOH)\ CH_2\ C_6H_5$	X		X		
Proline	(Pro) $HN\ (CH_2)_3\ CH\ (COOH)$		X	X		
Serine	(Ser) $H_2N\text{-}CH\ (COOH)\ CH_2\ OH$		X		X	
Threonine	(Thr) $H_2N\text{-}CH\ (COOH)\ CH\ (OH)\ CH_3$	X			X	
Tryptophan	(Try) $H_2N\text{-}CH\ (COOH)\ CH_2\ C_8H_6N$	X		X		
Tyrosine	(Tyr) $H_2N\text{-}CH\ (COOH)\ CH_2\ C_6H_4\ OH$		X		X	
Valine	(Val) $H_2N\text{-}CH\ (COOH)\ CH_2\ CH\ (CH_3)_2$	X		X		

nutrients. However, there is no clear association between dietary fat and cancer in all cases. In one study, a higher risk of prostate cancer was associated with higher energy intake, but there was no clear association between fat intake and the cancer risk.[21] Conversely, in a study of skin cancer patients, reducing the level of dietary fat from 37 to 40% to about 20% led to a significant reduction in the incidence of new actinic keratosis and nonmelanoma skin cancer.[22]

Numerous animal studies have shown an inverse relationship between cancer incidence and lower body weight due to a calorie-restricted diet.[23] Such results may not apply to humans, but it seems that obesity, a sign of excess total energy, should be avoided by matching energy intake with expenditure and increasing physical activity.[24,25]

Vitamins and Minerals

Vitamins

Vitamin A

Vitamin A or retinol is a fat-soluble vitamin with an unsaturated aliphatic chain. It has a role in cell differentiation, in the protein metabolism of cells originating from the ectoderm, and in formation of the chromosphere component of visual cycle chromoproteins. Lack of retinol causes night blindness and thickening of the skin; conversely, excess vitamin A is toxic. Except for the occurrence in milk fat, egg yolk, and liver of mammals, most vitamin A is usually obtained from carotenoids. These precursors to vitamin A occur in vegetables, mostly green, yellow, and dark green leafy vegetables, and many yellow or orange fruits.[26] They are converted to vitamin A in the intestinal tract. Investigations in different animal species have shown that retinol esters and beta-carotene can inhibit the effects of various carcinogens through modulating DNA stability and decreasing lipid peroxidation.[27]

As for humans, there have been many epidemiologic studies of retinol and carotenes, with conflicting results. There were no protective effects against melanoma of the skin, suggestive but insufficient evidence for a decreased risk of bladder cancer with higher dietary retinol, and no consistent protective effect for cancer of the lung, stomach, breast, and cervix. An IARC (International Agency for Research on Cancer) group concluded that there is little evidence that vitamin A intake has a substantial cancer-preventive effect.[28]

The situation differs for dietary carotenoids, where there is evidence for a modest to weak protective action against lung cancer[29-31] and a possible decreased risk for esophageal,[32] stomach, colorectal, breast, and cervical cancers,[33-35] as well as an effect against cancers of the thyroid[36] and salivary gland.[37] Some epidemiologic surveys showed no such protective action.[38-41] Conversely, supplemental beta-carotene or megadose vitamin supplementation did not lead to any benefit.[42]

The controversy about carotenoids was heightened when studies of Finnish smokers receiving supplemental beta-carotene showed a higher death rate from lung cancer in those receiving additional beta-carotene than in those who did not.[43] Likewise, a combination study of beta-carotene with retinol had a similar trend, leading to termination of these studies.[44]

Nevertheless, another carotenoid which is not a vitamin A precursor, namely lycopene, responsible for the color of tomatoes, has shown a protective action against chemical carcinogens in animals.[45] Furthermore, epidemiologic studies have indicated that consumption of tomato products, along with a modest amount of fat to facilitate absorption, has been associated with a lower incidence of prostate[46] and digestive tract cancers.[47]

On balance, although dietary supplements do not seem efficacious, obtaining vitamin A or carotenoids through a diet with high levels of fruits and vegetables seems to afford modest protection against cancer.

Vitamin B

Vitamin B actually consists of several water-soluble compounds without any apparent structural similarity. All are necessary for proper physiological function; the requirements for some are actually filled through synthesis by endogenous intestinal bacteria (Table 49.3). Riboflavin, one of the B vitamins, was shown relatively early to have a chemopreventive action in rats fed a carcinogenic aminoazo dye. In this situation, as part of the enzyme system that reductively split the dye to two non-effective groups, dietary riboflavin definitely was a preventive agent.[48] However, there are no epidemiologic studies that indicate a connection between riboflavin and the prevention of cancer.

The situation differs for the B_6, B_{12}, and B_c vitamins, as these are involved in reactions of amino acids and one–carbon units. Methionine, an essential amino acid, combines with adenosine triphosphate to form S-adenosylmethionine (SAM); in turn, SAM transfers methyl groups to adjacent molecules, thereby regulating expression of genes, preservation of membranes, and the action of various hormones and neurotransmitters. After the transfer of the methyl group, methionine becomes homocysteine, which has toxic effects on the cardiovascular system and the developing fetus. In the presence of B_{12} and B_c, homocysteine is remethylated to methionine, with folate being especially important. Vitamin B_6, in turn, is involved by converting homocysteine to glutathione, another protective body constituent.

Both hypo- and hypermethylation of DNA are markers of the early stages of carcinogenesis. By maintaining a normal methylation pattern, folic acid may aid in decreasing cancer risk. For example, high dietary folate intake was weakly associated with decreased risk of colon cancer.[18,19]

Vitamin C

Vitamin C has been widely studied, both in animal systems and in epidemiologic trials. Vitamin C, or ascorbic acid, is involved in biological hydroxylation reactions and formation of collagen in connective tissues, is important in wound healing, and is necessary for the prevention of scurvy. Most animals, except for primates and guinea pigs, synthesize their daily requirements, but for species which do not, the following foods are excellent sources: citrus fruits, strawberries, currants, cabbages, and potatoes. A great excess of vitamin C is not especially beneficial, as it is metabolized to oxalic acid, which is harmful to the kidneys. The recommended daily intake is 175 to 400 mg.

In many animal experiments, vitamin C had a beneficial action against skin or mammary cancer with dimethylbenz(a)anthracene, benzo(a)pyrene, or against estrogen-induced kidney cancer in hamsters. The most effective action was against formation of N-nitrosamines *in vivo* by combined administration of nitrite and a secondary amine; in this case, ascorbic acid reacts preferentially with nitrite, yielding non-effective compounds. However, in other cases vitamin C had no beneficial action.[49,50]

Epidemiologic trials have been less definitive. Most studies have shown some possible decrease in cancers of many organ systems, but the effects were not dramatic. Thus, the question of whether any protection was due solely to vitamin C or to a combined action with other constituents of the diet cannot be answered definitely.[38,51]

TABLE 49.3
B Vitamins

Vitamin	Name	Function	Dietary Sources	Result of Deficiency
B_1	Thiamine	Component of enzymes catalyzing oxidative decarboxylation reactions in Krebs cycle.	Wheat germ, pork	Beri-beri
B_2	Riboflavin	Occurs in flavin mononucleotides (FMN) and flavin adenine dinucleotide (FAD), prosthetic groups in flavoproteins which are respiratory enzymes.	Yeast , liver, egg yolk, milk, fish, green vegetables	Chellosis (cracking of lips)
B_3	Niacin	Component of nicotinamide adenine dinucleotide (NAD) and its phosphate derivatives (NADP) which are electron carriers in respiratory systems.	Wheat germ, yeast, liver	Pellagra
B_5	Pantothenic Acid	Constituent of coenzyme A, important in many physiological processes such as fatty acid metabolism.	Animal or plant tissue, produced by intestinal bacteria	Deficiency rare
B_6	Pyridoxine	Pyridoxine and derivatives, pyridoxal, pyridoxamines and their phosphates are co-factors for enzymes involved in metabolism of proteins and amino acids	Fish, meat, poultry, grains, legumes, potatoes	Skin lesions, anemia, muscle cramps
B_{12}	Cyanocobalamin	Essential growth factor, component of enzyme involved in reactions of one-carbon units.	Animal tissues, produced by intestinal bacteria	Pernicious anemia
B_C	Folic Acid (pteroylglutamic acid)	Needed for amino acid metabolism and formation of red blood cells; involved in reactions of one-carbon units (methylation)	Yeast extract, green vegetables	Anemia, spina bifida in fetus

Data from Kingston, R., Supplementary benefits, *Chem. Brit.*, 35, 29, 1999.

Vitamin D

Vitamin D, a fat-soluble vitamin (cholecalciferol; D_3), is formed naturally from cholesterol in the skin through photolysis of 7-dehydrocholesterol under the influence of ultraviolet light. The active metabolites are the 1, 25-dihydroxy- and 1-α-hydroxy-forms. These are needed for intestinal resorption of calcium and for its deposition into the organic matrix of the bones, which then triggers the biosynthesis of calcium-binding proteins. Deficiency of vitamin D in children leads to increased excretion of calcium and phosphate, thus impairing bone formation due to inadequate calcification of cartilage and bones — the disease known as rickets. In adults, deficiency leads to softening and weakening of bones, or osteomalacia. Some foods, especially milk, are fortified with vitamin D. Biochemically, vitamin D interacts with the vitamin D receptor, a member of the steroid/thyroid/retinoic acid family of nuclear receptors, which either induce or repress the expression of specific genes. In turn, the protein products of these genes include calcium-binding proteins (calbindins), bone matrix proteins (osteocalcin, osteopontin), digestive enzymes such as alkaline phosphatase, and vitamin D-metabolizing enzymes.[52]

The effect of vitamin D is linked to the level of dietary calcium, while therapeutic use is limited due to the calcemic effect of vitamin D, which causes calcium carbonate or phosphate disorders in various organs.

Although vitamin D inhibits the growth of breast cancer cells *in vitro*, the exact mechanism has not been delineated; induction of apoptosis has been implicated.[53] There is some evidence from population studies that higher serum vitamin D was associated with lower risk of breast cancer; likewise vitamin D may possibly reduce the risk of colorectal and prostate cancer.[53-55] As with other protective factors, the effect of vitamin D alone is relatively small. Animal studies with vitamin D in the chemoprevention of cancer have been few, and the results were positive in some cases, but not in others.[50] However, both animal and human studies lend support to the concept that increased intake of calcium and vitamin D can reduce the risk of colon cancer associated with high dietary fat.[56]

Vitamin E

Vitamin E occurs in vegetable oils, especially the germ oils of cereals as tocopherols; of all these, d-α-tocopherol has the greatest biological activity. Tocopherols are antioxidants, and thus retard the oxidation of lipids or stabilize vitamin A, ubiquinones, hormones, and various enzymes. Vitamin E protects polyunsaturated fatty acids against autooxidation, protects against the immune response, and decreases the adherence of platelets to blood vessel walls.[57] In experiments using the hamster buccal pouch or other animal systems, vitamin E had a protective action against chemical carcinogens, but the effect on colon cancer in model animal systems was inconsistent.[50] In humans, vitamin E possibly protects against cancer of the mouth and pharynx, esophagus, pancreas, stomach, colon and rectum, cervix, and prostate.[58] For breast cancer, the epidemiologic results have been inconclusive.[38,51,59] The mechanism of its action, apart from the antioxidant properties, has not been elucidated.

Minerals

Calcium

Calcium, one of the more abundant essential minerals of the body, has several roles in building and maintaining bones and teeth, in blood clotting, and in muscle contraction. The usual requirement is 500 to 700 mg daily, with more necessary during pregnancy and lactation, or in osteoporosis patients. The main dietary sources are milk and dairy products, although some vegetables (watercress, kale, spinach, broccoli) have reasonable levels. Supplementation of fruit juices with calcium has also become popular.

As for any chemopreventive action against cancer, a number of studies show a beneficial effect, but conflicts remain. A protective association for pancreatic cancer was noted in one study,[60] and for colorectal cancer, the weight of the evidence points toward an inhibitory action, as do some animal tests.[61-65] However, conflicting results were also noted.[54] Higher intake of calcium may reduce breast cancer risks,[51] but the data on prostate cancer and calcium intake levels are conflicting.[55,66]

Thus, for continued good health and body function, sufficient calcium is necessary. Except for breast and colorectal cancer, the epidemiologic studies are not definitive on whether calcium protects against other cancers.

Chromium

Chromium is an essential micronutrient for utilization of glucose, since it activates phosphoglucomutase and increases insulin activity. The daily intake varies depending on the region of the country, with most foods containing some chromium; brown sugar is a good source along with meat and seafood. Average intake is about 80 μg per day.[67] Few, if any, chemopreventive experiments have been done with chromium, since hexavalent chromium has been considered a human carcinogen by the IARC.[68] Animal tests with trivalent chromium were negative, and surveys on chromium levels in diets and cancer incidence are lacking. Nevertheless, a sufficient supply is needed for good health. Although no long-term toxicity studies have been done, the use of chromium picolinate as a dietary supplement has increased recently. Chromium thus represents a paradox — it is needed for proper body function, but it presents a hazard under certain conditions.[69]

Iodine

Iodine is an essential element for the thyroid gland to biosynthesize the hormones thyroxine or tetraiodothyronine and triiodothyronine; the requirement is 100 to 200 μg/day. A deficiency of iodine is associated with goiter or thyroid enlargement, which in turn is associated with a higher risk of cancer. Many epidemiologic studies have confirmed such an effect.[1]

The opposite, excess intake of iodine (18 to 1000 mg/day) can block uptake of iodine by the thyroid, leading to elevated thyroid-stimulating hormone (TSH) levels and an increased risk of thyroid cancer, as confirmed by animal experiments.[1] Thus, a proper balance in iodine uptake is required to maintain thyroid hormone levels and to decrease the risk of thyroid cancer.

Iron

The essential micronutrient iron is mostly present in the body in the hemoglobin of the blood and the myoglobin of muscle tissue. Iron also occurs in various oxidative enzymes such as the P450s, peroxidases, catalases, hydroxylases, and flavine enzymes. The daily requirement is about 1 to 3 mg, but an intake of about 15 to 25 mg is needed due to poor absorption of iron. Good sources of iron are egg yolks, liver, wheat germ, lentils, and spinach.[70]

Deficiency of iron leads to anemia and has been associated with cancer of the esophagus and Plummer-Vinson syndrome.[71] Conversely, the risk of various other types of cancer increases in association with higher body iron stores. High serum ferritin levels were associated with an increased risk of colorectal adenomas or cancer,[72] and a high concentration of iron in the liver was linked to a greater risk of liver cancer.[73] The suggestion has been made that high dietary intakes of iron enhance the generation of free radicals, which are implicated in the initiation or promotion phases of carcinogenesis. As with other essential micronutrients, a balance between a deficiency and an excess of iron is needed to maintain good health.

Selenium

Selenium was recognized only about 30 years ago as an essential micronutrient, with a recommended intake of 75 to 125 μg daily. It is a component of the glutathione peroxidase system and occurs in organ meats, seafood, and in cereals and seeds at levels proportional to those in the soil.[74] An excess of selenium is toxic, resulting in damaged hooves and hair in range animals. A deficiency leads to "white muscle disease" in calves and lambs; thus, a proper balance in selenium levels is needed.

A survey of soil selenium levels in the U.S. versus cancer incidence pointed toward a decreased risk in high selenium areas. Likewise, animal studies with selenium, mostly as the selenite salt, have shown an inhibitory action against tumor development in various organs.[75] In humans, the data are often conflicting. High blood levels of selenium were correlated with esophageal cancer in a Chinese population,[76] while in other studies, high body selenium was protective against stomach cancer. Data for liver and pancreatic cancer are somewhat conflicting, but overall there was some inhibitory effect. Evidence for a protective action against colorectal and breast cancer in humans is limited.

Consumption of high-selenium brewer's yeast did not prevent the appearance of new skin cancers in patients who already had developed basal cell and squamous cell skin cancers, but total cancer incidence and deaths were lower in the selenium-using group.[77] Furthermore, higher body stores of selenium were associated with reduced risk of advanced prostate cancer.[78] Accordingly, although selenium suppresses most types of cancer and has a beneficial action, the toxicity of selenium limits the amount that can be administered, and must be considered.

Zinc

Zinc is an essential trace element, as it is a component of several enzymes, including alcohol, glutamate, lactate, and malate dehydrogenases, carboxypeptidases, and carbonic anhydrase. In addition, several other enzymes are activated by zinc. Zinc deficiency causes serious disorders, but high zinc intake is toxic. A normal diet usually provides the daily requirement of a little over 10 mg (6 to 22 mg).[79]

Many animal experiments have shown that dietary zinc deficiency as well as zinc supplementation can increase the incidence of some carcinogen-induced tumors and decrease the incidence of others.[80] However, there are no definitive epidemiologic studies that associate human cancers with either a deficiency or an excess of zinc.

Nonnutritive Components

Fiber

Of all the nonnutritive food constituents, dietary fiber has been the one most extensively investigated in humans. The evidence is suggestive that high dietary fiber decreases the risk of stomach, pancreatic, and breast cancer, and is protective against colorectal (and possibly endometrial) cancer,[17,3981-83] although contradicting studies are also available.[84] Animal studies showing the preventive effects of fiber against intestinal cancer predated most epidemiologic studies by a decade or more.[34,85-87]

Several possible reasons exist for the beneficial action of dietary fiber. The fiber may physically trap or attach to various deleterious substances ranging from carcinogen metabolites to certain bile acids, and sweep them out of the intestinal tract. Fiber may also trap hormonal constituents and thus help decrease breast cancer. Further, some fiber is eventually fermented by intestinal bacteria to butyric acid, which regulates cell cycles.[88,89]

For continued good health and function of the digestive system, a reasonable level of fiber in the diet is needed. Generally, this can be attained by eating a diet with whole grain products and fruits and vegetables.

Flavonoids, Isoflavones, and Polyphenols

Flavonoids and isoflavones are present in plants and their various parts in combination with sugars (glycosides). The common property of many chemopreventive plant products is the presence of several hydroxyl groups in the molecule; thus the designation as polyphenols is appropriate for a wide range of these substances.

Many polyphenols from foods have demonstrated preventive effects against chemical carcinogens in animal experiments. Examples include ellagic acid,[90] silymarin from the artichoke,[91] quercetin, found in most plant materials,[92] the flavones or epicatechins common in tea,[93] curcumin in tumeric and mustard, caffeic and ferulic acids, resveratrol from grapes, and lignans derived from plant phenolics through bacterial action in the intestinal tract. Further, several plant phenolics can inhibit nitrosamine formation *in vivo* and thus have a chemopreventive action. The beneficial effects of these polyphenols are difficult to delineate separately, since they occur in many fruits and vegetables. Epidemiologic studies definitely associating one or the other dietary polyphenol with a reduction in cancer incidence are lacking or inconclusive.

That is not the case with the soybean compounds genistein and daidzein, examples of isoflavones. Various surveys have indicated a lower risk of breast and possibly endometrial cancer in women who consume soybean products,[15,94] while animal studies have confirmed the chemopreventive action of genistein.[95,96] The mechanism probably resides in the weak estrogenic effect of these compounds which then bind to estrogen receptors, thus blocking the action of the more potent natural estrogens.[16] Plant lignans, which also are beneficial, appear to bind weakly to estrogen receptors. Furthermore, daidzein sulfoconjugates inhibit the enzymes involved in estrogen steroid activation.[97]

An additional benefit of soy, reported recently, was that a soy-based beverage had suppressed an increase in prostate specific antigen (PSA) in prostate cancer patients.[98]

Despite these beneficial aspects of soy consumption, soy should be used in moderation. Soy consumption is associated with a goitrogenic effect, as confirmed by mechanistic studies in animals.[99] Thus, moderation in use is a reasonable policy.

Indole-3-carbinol

Indole-3-carbinol (I3C) was one of the first specific cancer chemopreventive compounds to be isolated from a cruciferous vegetable, namely Brussels sprouts.[100] Many animal studies have shown its ability to suppress the effects of chemical carcinogens, presumably through its induction of detoxifying enzymes.[101] There is a concern that under certain conditions it may act as a promoting agent, and possible application of I3C as a chemopreventive agent in humans should be approached cautiously.[102]

Isothiocyanates

Isothiocyanates occur naturally in the form of their glucosinolate conjugates in a variety of cruciferous vegetables. When the plant cells are damaged by cutting or chewing, the enzyme myrosinase is released, which causes hydrolysis of the glucosinolates followed by a rearrangement which affords the isothiocyanates. These are generally responsible for the sharp taste associated with cruciferous vegetables, mustard, horseradish, and watercress. Animal studies with isothiocyanates have shown definitive and often quite specific inhibition of the action of some carcinogens, largely through suppressing metabolism to an activated intermediate.[103]

Epidemiologic studies focused specifically on isothiocyanates are lacking. However, one trial showed that if confirmed smokers ate watercress, a source of phenethyl isothiocyanate, the oxidative action of 4-(methylnitrosamino)-1-(3-pyridyl)-1-butanone (NNK), a carcinogen present in tobacco smoke, was suppressed and higher urinary levels of a detoxification product of NNK were observed.[104]

Another unique isothiocyanate, sulforaphane or 1-isothiocyanate-4-methylsulfinylbutane, has been isolated from broccoli.[105] Sulforaphorane induces P450 enzymes which tend to detoxify carcinogens.[106] It appears to be still another component of the protective substances present in cruciferous vegetables.

Methods have recently been developed to quantify the metabolic endproducts of isothiocyanates.[107,108] This should expedite the further application of these compounds in both metabolic and epidemiologic studies.[109]

Sulfides

The chemical background for the numerous sulfides and their selenium analogs occurring in "Allium" vegetables has been presented in several reviews. The substances involved are various sulfur derivatives, and in series are: alkyl cysteine-S-oxides, sulfenic acids, and thiosulfinate esters, which in turn afford alkyl and allyl sulfides and the selenium analogs.[110]

Animal tests have shown an inhibitory action of garlic and onion constituents, especially diallyl sulfide, on experimental carcinogenesis of the skin, esophagus, and colon. Epidemiologic studies have noted the same trend — that Allium vegetables protect against stomach and colon cancer — but no such action was noted for breast and lung cancer.[111] In one animal trial, garlic enriched with selenium had a chemopreventive action against the effects of a mammary carcinogen.[112] However, application of these results to the human situation will require much further study.

Terpenoids

The terpenoid substances which occur in foods generally are the monoterpenes; examples include carvone, p-cymene, geraniol, limonene, linalool, nerol, perillyl alcohol, pinene, and thymol, among others. These substances occur in the essential oils of fruits and plants, in citrus and other fruits, cherries, certain grapes, mint, dill, and caraway, and are largely responsible for the pleasant fragrances of the fruits and plants.

The inhibitory action of fruit oil containing a monoterpene on the effect of a potent chemical carcinogen was noted several decades ago. More recent efforts have confirmed

TABLE 49.4

Cancer Preventive Action of Vitamins

Vitamin	Species	Organ/Tissue
A	Mouse	Skin
	Rat	Mammary gland
		Urinary bladder
B (folate)	Mouse	Lung
	Human	Colon (weakly)
C	Mouse	Colon
		Lung
	Rat	Mammary gland
		Colon
		Liver
	Hamster	Kidney
D	Mouse	Skin
	Rat	Colon
	Human	Breast
		Colon/rectum
		Prostate
E	Mouse	Skin
		Colon?
	Rat	Mammary gland
		Stomach
		Colon?
		Ear duct
		Liver
	Hamster	Buccal pouch
	Human	Mouth (possibly)
		Pharynx (possibly)
		Esophagus (possibly)
		Pancreas (possibly)
		Stomach (possibly)
		Colon/rectum (possibly)
		Cervix and prostate (possibly)

that d-limonene, the putative active component of sweet orange oil, has several inhibitory mechanisms.[113] It suppresses the activation of nitrosamines[114] and azoxymethane,[115] induces glutathione-S-transferase, and inhibits oncogene activation by depressing the isoprenylation of oncogene products. The benefits of consuming citrus fruits may lie not only in their vitamin C content, but also in the limonene contained therein. Another monoterpene, perillyl alcohol, also inhibits protein isoprenylation, thus suppressing eventual oncogene activation,[116] even in human-derived cell lines.[117]

Although other monoterpenes have not been investigated, it is gratifying to know that these compounds with a pleasant fragrance are beneficial for health.

The diversity of cancer chemopreventive substances in foods is noteworthy and allows the individual many choices in devising a healthful diet. The aim should be a varied diet with moderation in the amounts of any one constituent. Dietary supplements, in which the active factor has been isolated and administered in a concentrated form, are not as useful as the actual food. However, Tables 49.4 and 49.5 provide results from both animal and human studies with vitamins and nonnutritive food components. In an actual diet, synergism among food constituents may occur with the combination, as in foods, being better than the individual components. All the more incentive to follow a varied moderate diet with plenty of fruits, vegetables, and whole-grain products.

TABLE 49.5

Chemopreventive Action of Nonnutritive Principles of Foods

Substance	Species	Organ/Tissue
Fiber	Human	Stomach
		Pancreas
		Breast
		Colon/rectum
		Endometrium
	Rat	Colon
Flavonoids, isoflavones, polyphenols	Human	Breast
		Endometrium
	Rodents	Mammary gland
		Skin
Indole-3-carbinol	Mouse	Forestomach
	Rat	Mammary gland
Isothiocyanates	Mouse	Lung
		Forestomach
	Rat	Mammary gland
Sulfides	Human	Stomach
		Colon
	Rat	Esophagus
		Lung
		Thyroid
	Mouse	Forestomach
		Lung
		Colon
Terpenoids	Mouse	Forestomach
		Lung
	Rat	Mammary gland

References

1. Food, Nutrition and the Prevention of Cancer: A Global Perspective. World Cancer Research Fund/American Institute for Cancer Research, Washington, DC, 1997.
2. Food, Nutrition and the Prevention of Cancer: A Global Perspective. World Cancer Research Fund/American Institute for Cancer Research, Washington, DC, 1997, p 377.
3. Food, Nutrition and the Prevention of Cancer: A Global Perspective. World Cancer Research Fund/American Institute for Cancer Research, Washington, DC, 1997, p 521.
4. Trichopoulos A, Katsouyanni K, Stuver S, et al. *J Natl Cancer Inst* 87: 110; 1995.
5. LaVecchia C, Negri E, Franeschi S, et al. *Cancer Causes Control* 6: 545; 1995.
6. Caygill CP, Hill MJ, et al. *Eur J Cancer Prev* 4: 329; 1995.
7. Schloss I, Kidd MS, Tichelaar H, et al. *S Afr Med J* 87: 152; 1997.
8. Ip C, Chin SF, Scimeca JA, et al. *Cancer Res* 51: 6118; 1991.
9. Cesano A, Visonneau S, Scimeca JA, et al. *Anticancer Res* 18: 1429; 1998.
10. Leviton A, Shapiro SS, Gans K, et al. *Am J Pub Health* 85: 410; 1995.
11. Kritchevsky D. *Chemistry & Industry* 5: 565; 1996.
12. Cave WT, Jr. In *Nutrition and Cancer Prevention*, Watson RR, Mufti SI, Eds. CRC Press, Boca Raton, 1996, p 84.
13. Reddy BS. In *Nutrition and Cancer Prevention*. Watson RR, Mufti SI, Eds. CRC Press, Boca Raton, 1996, p 105.
14. Food, Nutrition and the Prevention of Cancer: A Global Perspective. World Cancer Research Fund/American Institute for Cancer Research, Washington, DC, 1997, p 395.
15. Wu AH, Ziegler RG, Nomura AM, et al. *Am J Clin Nutr* 68: 1437S; 1998.

16. Nagata C, Kabuto M, Kurisu Y, et al. *Nutr Cancer* 29: 228; 1997.
17. Goodman MT, Wilkens LR, Hankin JH, et al. *Am J Epidemiol* 146: 294; 1997.
18. Slattery ML, Schaffer D, Edwards SL, et al. *Nutr Cancer* 28: 52; 1997.
19. Ma J, Stampfer MJ, Giovannucci E, et al. *Cancer Res* 57: 1098; 1997.
20. Food, Nutrition and the Prevention of Cancer: A Global Perspective. World Cancer Research Fund/American Institute for Cancer Research, Washington, DC, 1997, p 366.
21. Rohan TE, Howe GR, Burch JD, et al, *Cancer Causes Control* 6: 145; 1995.
22. Black HS. *Mutat Res* 422: 185; 1998.
23. Frame LT, Hart RW, Leakey JE. *Environ. Health Perspect* 106: 313S; 1998.
24. Goldin-Long P, Kreuser ED, Zunft HJ. *Rec Results Cancer Res* 142: 163; 1996.
25. Kritchevsky D. In *Nutrition and Cancer Prevention*, Watson RR, Mufti SI, Eds, CRC Press, Boca Raton, 1996, p 91.
26. Yang Y, Huang CY, Peng SS, et al. *Biomed Environ Sci* 9: 386; 1996.
27. Duthie SJ, Collins AR, Duthie GG. *Subcell Biochem* 30: 181; 1998.
28. Vainio H, Rautalahti M. *Cancer Epidemiol Biomarkers Prev* 8: 107; 1999.
29. Nyberg F, Agrenius V, Svartengren K, et al. *Int J Cancer* 78: 430; 1998.
30. Ocke MC, Bueno-de-Mesquita HB, Feskens EJ, et al. *Am J Epidemiol* 145: 358; 1997.
31. Albanes D. *Am J Clin Nutr* 69: 1345S; 1999.
32. Zhang ZF, Kurtz RC, Yu GP, et al. *Nutr Cancer* 27: 298; 1997.
33. Longnecker MP, Newcomb PA, Mittendorf R, et al. *Cancer Epidemiol Biomarkers Prev* 6: 887; 1997.
34. Verhoeven DT, Assen N, Goldbohm RA, et al. *Br J Cancer* 75: 149; 1997.
35. Zhang S, Hunter DJ, Forman MR, et al. *J Natl Cancer Inst* 91: 547; 1999.
36. D'Avanzo B, Ron E, La Vecchia C, et al. *Cancer* 79: 2186; 1997.
37. Horn-Ross PL, Morrow M, Ljung BM. *Am J Epidemiol* 146: 171; 1997.
38. Kushi LH, Fee RM, Sellers TA, et al. *Am J Epidemiol* 144: 165; 1996.
39. MacLennan R, Macrae F, Bain C. *J Natl Cancer Inst* 87: 1733; 1995.
40. Flagg EW, Coates RJ, Greenberg RS. *J Am Coll Nutr* 14: 419; 1995.
41. van Poppel G. *Eur J Clin Nutr* 50(3): S57; 1996.
42. Rose RC. *Med Hypotheses* 51: 239; 1998.
43. Koo LC. *Int J Cancer* 10: 22; 1997.
44. Omenn GS, et al. *N Engl J Med* 334: 1150; 1996.
45. Krinsky NIT. *Proc Soc Exp Biol Med* 218: 95; 1998.
46. Giovannucci E, Clinton SK. *Proc Soc Exp Biol Med* 218: 129; 1998.
47. La Vecchia C. *Proc Soc Exp Biol Med* 218: 125; 1998.
48. Mueller GC, Miller JA. *J Biol Chem* 185: 145; 1950.
49. Mirvish SS. *Eur J Cancer Prev* 5(1): 131S; 1996.
50. Arcos JC, Argus MF, Woo YT, et al. *Chemical Induction of Cancer, Modulation and Combination Effects*, Berkhauser, Table 2, 1995, p 326.
51. Franceshi S. *Eur J Cancer Prev* 6: 535; 1997.
52. Welsh J, Simboli-Campbell M, Narvaez CJ, et al. In *Diet and Cancer*, AICR, Washington, DC, 1995, p 45.
53. Giovannucci E. *Cancer Causes Control* 9: 567; 1998.
54. Pritchard RS, Baron JA, Gerhardsson de Verdier M. *Cancer Epidemiol Biomarkers Prev* 5: 897; 1996.
55. Chan JM, Giovannucci E, Anderson SO, et al. *Cancer Causes Control* 9: 559; 1998.
56. Newmark HL, Lipkin M. *Cancer Res* 52: 2067S; 1992.
57. Weber P, Bendich A, Machlin LJ. *Nutrition* 13: 450; 1997.
58. Moyad MA, Brumfield SK, Pienta KJ. *Semin Urol Oncol* 17: 85; 1999.
59. Kimmick GG, Bell RA, Bostick RM. *Nutr Cancer* 27: 109; 1997.
60. Farrow DC, Davis S. *Am J Epidemiol* 132: 423; 1990.
61. Lipkin M, Newmark H. *J Cell Biochem* 22: 65S; 1995.
62. Holt PR, Atillasoy EO, Gilman J, et al. *J Am Med Assoc* 280: 1095; 1998.
63. Hyman J, Baron JA, Dain BJ, et al. *Cancer Epidemiol. Biomarkers Prev* 7: 291; 1998.
64. Ghadirian P, Lacroix A, Maisonneuve P, et al. *Cancer* 80: 858; 1997.

65. La Vecchia C, Braga C, Negri E. *Int J Cancer* 73: 525; 1997.
66. Vlajinac HD, Marinkovic JM, Ilic MD, et al. *Eur J Cancer* 33: 101; 1997.
67. Belitz HD, Grosch W. *Food Chemistry* Springer-Verlag, Berlin, 1987, p 323.
68. IARC, Monograph on the Evaluation of Carcinogenic Risks to Humans, International Agency for Research on Cancer, *Chromium, Nickel and Welding*, 49: 49; 1990.
69. Salem H, Katz SA. *Sci Total Environ* 86: 1; 1989.
70. Food, Nutrition and the Prevention of Cancer: A Global Perspective. World Cancer Research Fund/American Institute for Cancer Research, Washington, DC, 1997, p 321.
71. Food, Nutrition and the Prevention of Cancer: A Global Perspective. World Cancer Research Fund/American Institute for Cancer Research, Washington, DC, 1997, p 124.
72. Nelson RL, Davis FG, Sutter E. *J Natl Cancer Inst* 86: 455; 1994.
73. Food, Nutrition and the Prevention of Cancer: A Global Perspective. World Cancer Research Fund/American Institute for Cancer Research, Washington, DC, 1997, p 208.
74. Food, Nutrition and the Prevention of Cancer: A Global Perspective. World Cancer Research Fund/American Institute for Cancer Research, Washington, DC, 1997, p 409.
75. Food, Nutrition and the Prevention of Cancer: A Global Perspective. World Cancer Research Fund/American Institute for Cancer Research, Washington, DC, 1997, p 209
76. Food, Nutrition and the Prevention of Cancer: A Global Perspective. World Cancer Research Fund/American Institute for Cancer Research, Washington, DC, 1997, p 124.
77. Clark LC, Combs Jr, GF, Turnbull BW. *JAMA* 276: 1957; 1996.
78. Yoshizawa K, Willett WC, Norris SJ. *J Natl Cancer Inst* 90: 1219; 1998.
79. Belitz HD, Grosch W. *Food Chemistry* Springer-Verlag, Berlin, 1987, p 323.
80. Arcos JC, Argus MF, Woo YT, et al. *Chemical Induction of Cancer, Modulation and Combination Effects*, Berkhauser, 1995, p 348.
81. Food, Nutrition and the Prevention of Cancer: A Global Perspective. World Cancer Research Fund/American Institute for Cancer Research, Washington, DC, 1997, p 151.
82. Bagga D, Ashley JM, Geffrey SP, et al. *Cancer* 76: 2491; 1995.
83. Slattery ML, Potter JD, Coates A, et al. *Cancer Causes Control* 8: 575; 1997.
84. Gerber M. *Eur J Cancer Prev* 7(2): 63S; 1998.
85. Fuchs CS, Giovannucci EL, Colditz GA, et al. *N Engl J Med* 340: 169; 1999.
86. Platz EA, Giovannucci E, Rimm EB, et al. *Cancer Epidemiol Prev* 6: 661; 1997.
87. Alabaster O, Tang Z, Shivapurkar N. *Mutat Res* 350: 185; 1996.
88. Stoll BA. *Br J Cancer* 73: 557; 1996.
89. Goldin BR, Gorbach SL. In *Diet and Breast Cancer*, AICR, Washington, DC, 1994, p 35.
90. Lesca P. *Carcinogenesis* 4: 1651; 1983.
91. Agarwal R, Mukhtar H. In *Dietary Phytochemicals in Cancer Prevention and Treatment*, AICR, Washington, DC, 1996, p 35.
92. Hertog MG, Hollman PC. *Eur J Clin Nutr* 50: 63; 1996.
93. Conney AH, Lou YR, Yie JG, et al. *Proc Soc Exp Biol Med* 216: 234; 1997.
94. Stoll BA. *Ann Oncol* 8: 223; 1997.
95. Zhou JR, Mukherjee P, Gugger ET, et al. *Cancer Res* 58: 5231; 1998.
96. Lamartiniere CA, Zhang JX, Cotroneo MS. *Am J Clin Nutr* 68(6): 1400S; 1998.
97. Wong CK, Keung WM. *Biochem Biophys Res Commun* 233: 579; 1997.
98. Barken I. Proc 3rd Int Symp Soy, Washington, DC, 1999.
99. Divi RL, Chang HC, Doerge DR, *Biochem Pharmacol* 54: 1089; 1997.
100. Wattenberg LW, Loub WD. *Cancer Res* 38: 1410; 1978.
101. Oganesian A, Hendricks JD, Williams DE. *Cancer Lett* 118: 87; 1997.
102. Wong GY, Bradlow L, Sepkovic D, et al. *J Cell Biochem* 28-29: 111S; 1997.
103. Hecht SS. *Environ Health Perspect* 105(4): 955S; 1997.
104. Hecht SS, Chung FL, Richie JP, Jr. *Cancer Epidemiol Biomarkers Prev* 4: 877; 1995.
105. Zhang Y, Talalay P, Chi CG, et al. *Proc Natl Acad Sci USA* 89: 2399; 1992.
106. Barcelo S, Gardiner JM, Gescher A, et al. *Carcinogenesis* 17: 277; 1996.
107. Chung FL, Jiao D, Conaway CC, et al. *J Cell Biochem* 27: 76S; 1997.
108. Chung FL, Jiao D, Getahun SM, et al. *Cancer Epidemiol Biomarkers Prev* 7: 103; 1998.

109. Shapiro TA, Fahey JW, Wade KL, et al. *Cancer Epidemiol Biomarkers Prev* 7: 1091; 1998.
110. Block E. In *Dietary Phytochemicals in Cancer Prevention and Treatment*, AICR, Washington, DC, 1996, p 155.
111. Wargovich MJ, Uda N. In *Dietary Phytochemicals in Cancer Prevention and Treatment*, AICR, Washington, DC, 1996, p 171.
112. Ip C, Lisk DJ. In *Dietary Phytochemicals in Cancer Prevention and Treatment*, AICR, Washington, DC, 1996, p 179.
113. Arcos JC, Argus MF, Woo YT, et al. *Chemical Induction of Cancer, Modulation and Combination Effects*, Berkhauser, 1995, p 106.
114. Wattenberg LW, Coccia JB. *Carcinogenesis* 12: 115; 1991.
115. Kawamori T, Tanaka T, Hirose Y, et al. *Carcinogenesis* 17: 369; 1996.
116. Crowell PL, Ayoubi AS, Burke YD. In *Dietary Phytochemicals in Cancer Prevention and Treatment*, AICR, Washington, DC, 1996, p 131.
117. Hohl RJ. In *Dietary Phytochemicals in Cancer Prevention and Treatment*, AICR, Washington, DC, 1996, p 137.

50

Nutrition and Cancer Treatment

David Heber and Susan Bowerman

Etiology of Malnutrition in the Cancer Patient

Malnutrition is a frequent and serious problem in patients with cancer. Some types of cancers such as lung, prostate, head and neck, and gastric cancer are more frequently affected, but the overall incidence of malnutrition ranges between 30 and 87% of different populations studied.[1,2] The advanced starvation state resulting from decreased food intake and hormonal/metabolic abnormalities characteristic of the interaction between tumor and host has been called cancer cachexia.[3] A retrospective analysis of patient body weight at the beginning of cooperative chemotherapy trials determined that the presence of a 6% weight loss from usual body weight was a significant prognostic factor for survival.[4] The apparent effect of weight loss at the time of diagnosis on median survival for certain common cancers was greater than the impact of chemotherapy. Despite the development of advanced technology and delivery systems for total parenteral nutrition and continuous enteral nutrition, nutrition therapy alone has had little impact on this problem. While nutritional rehabilitation can be demonstrated in selected patients who respond to antineoplastic therapy, the application of parenteral and enteral nutrition as an adjunct to chemotherapy in cancer patients has not resulted in increased survival or predictable weight gain.[5,6] These observations suggest that decreased food intake alone cannot account for the progressive weight loss noted in cancer patients.

Metabolic Abnormalities in the Cancer Patient

Since predictable renutrition of the cancer patient has not been possible, a great deal of research has been conducted concerning specific hormonal and metabolic abnormalities which could interfere with renutrition. Over the last 15 years, research on the basic pathophysiology of cancer cachexia has resulted in the definition of several metabolic and hormonal abnormalities in malnourished cancer patients. These abnormalities are listed in Table 50.1.

Based on these abnormalities, a number of strategies using hormonal and metabolic agents have been tested. These are listed in Table 50.2. None of the above hormonal or metabolic strategies tested resulted in predictable weight gain.

0-8493-2705-9/01/$0.00+$1.50

TABLE 50.1

Metabolic Abnormalities in Cancer Patients

Hypogonadism in male cancer patients[7]
Increased glucose production[8,9]
Increased protein catabolism[10,11]
Increased lipolysis and fatty acid oxidation[12,13]
Insulin resistance[14,15]

TABLE 50.2

Research Strategies to Counter Metabolic Abnormalities

Hydrazine sulfate to inhibit gluconeogenesis[16]
Anabolic androgens to counteract metabolic effects of hypogonadism[17]
Insulin supplementation to counteract apparent insulin resistance[18]

Based on autopsy studies performed in the 1920s[19,20] and animal studies done in the 1950s[21] it was postulated that tumors acted to siphon off needed energy and protein from the host. In the 1970s and 1980s, specific abnormalities of intermediary metabolism were identified in cancer patients that could account for the common observation that such patients lost weight even in the face of apparently adequate nutrition. Studies conducted in a number of laboratories, including our own, have demonstrated that maladaptive metabolic abnormalities occur frequently in patients with cancer. In 1983, we demonstrated that adequate energy and protein administered to six patients with active localized head and neck cancer via forced continuous enteral alimentation under metabolic ward conditions for 29 days failed to lead to significant weight gain.[22] The mean nitrogen balance in these patients is shown in Figure 50.1. The observed failure of these patients to gain weight despite adequate caloric intake under metabolic ward conditions supports the concept that malnourished cancer patients are hypermetabolic.

If metabolic abnormalities promote the development of malnutrition or interfere with renutrition, then there should be some evidence of abnormally increased energy expenditure. A number of investigators have used indirect calorimetry and the abbreviated Weir formula to calculate energy expenditure at rest, and then compared this to the basal energy expenditure (BEE) determined using the Harris-Benedict formulas. Long et al.[23] demonstrated a mean difference of 2% when this comparison was performed in 20 normal controls. In 1980, Bozetti et al.[24] found that 60% of a group of patients with advanced cancer had basal metabolic rates increased 20% above predicted. In 1983, Dempsey et al.[25] studied energy expenditure in a group of 173 malnourished gastrointestinal (GI) cancer patients. Fifty-eight percent had abnormal resting energy expenditure (REE) by indirect calorimetry compared to BEE, but a greater percentage were hypometabolic rather than hypermetabolic (36 versus 22%). Knox et al.[26] studied 200 patients with a variety of cancers and found abnormal energy metabolism in 59%, but found more hypometabolic than hypermetabolic individuals (33 versus 26%). Figure 50.2 shows that while standard formulae accurately predict metabolic rate in normal individuals, the measured metabolic rates in patients with cancer have a much wider distribution.

Lean body mass rather than fat mass correlates with the individual variations observed in measured REE. The hypothesis that the malnourished cancer patient may be hypermetabolic relative to the amount of lean body mass remaining has been examined. Peacock et al.[27] studied resting energy expenditure in non-cachectic patients with sarcomas. These patients had no prior treatment, had large localized sarcomas, and had no weight loss or history of decreased food intake. REE corrected for body cell mass (BCM) determined by total body potassium counting or body surface area was significantly greater in male

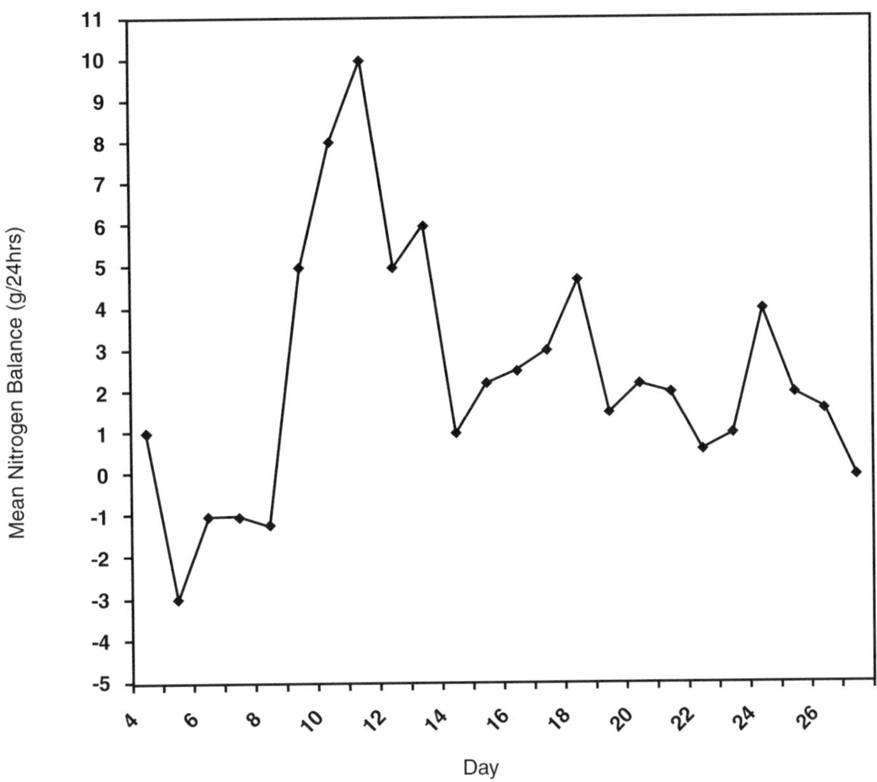

FIGURE 50.1
Mean nitrogen balance in grams per 24 hours in six patients with head and neck cancer receiving 1.25 × BEE kcal for 5 days and 2.25 × BEE for 19 days as a continuous enteral infusion. (From Geber, D., Byerley, L.O., Chi, J., et al. *Cancer* 58: 1867; 1986. With permission.)

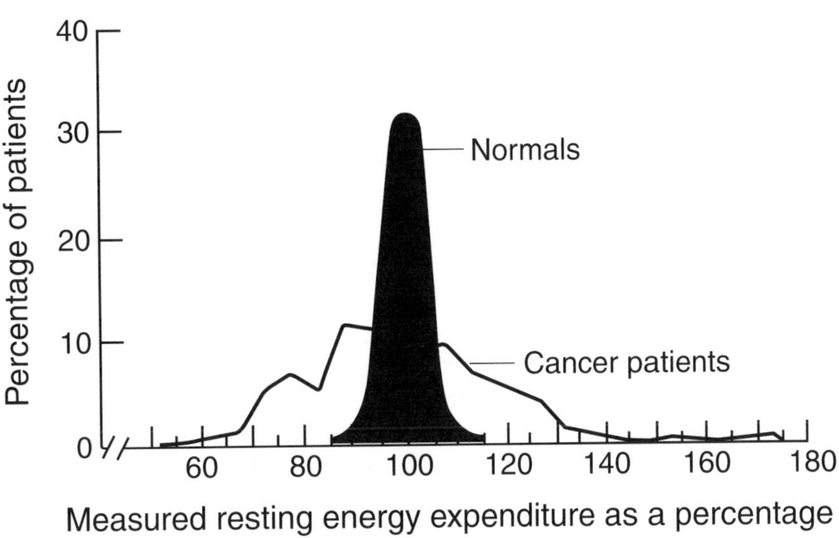

FIGURE 50.2
Measured resting energy expenditure as a percentage of predicted energy expenditure. (From Knox, L.S., Crosby, L.O., Feurer, I.D., et al. *Ann Surg* 197: 152; 1983.

sarcoma patients compared to controls. This difference was due to both a decrease in BCM and an increase in REE in these patients before the onset of weight loss. Tumors have been demonstrated to increase the rate of glucose utilization in a number of tissues.[28] Since there are only 1200 kcal stored in the body as liver and muscle glycogen, blood glucose levels would be expected to fall. This does not occur since there is also an increase in hepatic glucose production in cachectic and anorectic tumor-bearing animals and humans. The regulation of protein metabolism is tightly linked to carbohydrate metabolism, since these processes are critical to the normal adaptation to starvation or underfeeding. During starvation there is a decrease in glucose production, protein synthesis, and protein catabolism. The decrease in glucose production occurs as fat-derived fuels, primarily ketone bodies, are used for energy production. While there are 54,000 kcal of protein stored in the body cell mass, only about half of these are available for energy production. In fact, depletion below 50% of body protein stores is incompatible with life. Whole body protein breakdown is increased in lung cancer patients and has been shown to correlate with the degree of malnutrition such that more malnourished patients have greater elevations of their whole body protein breakdown rates expressed per kg of body weight (Figure 50.3).[11] The results of metabolic studies in lung cancer patients compared

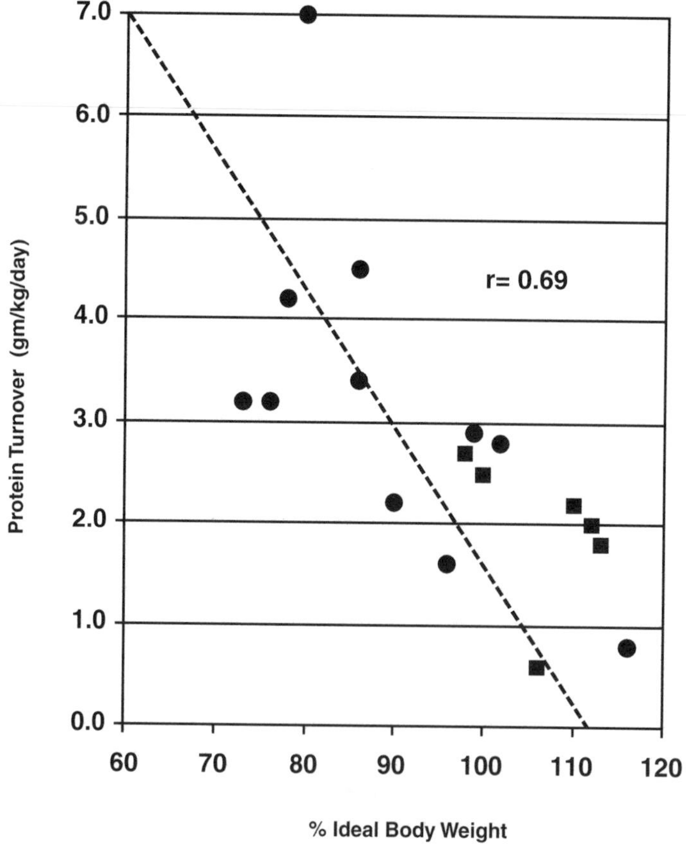

FIGURE 50.3
Whole-body protein turnover determined by [*U*-^{14}C] lysine infusion in the fasting state in g/kg/day versus percentage of ideal body weight for height in non-oat cell lung cancer patients (●) and age-matched healthy controls (■). The correlation coefficient of the linear regression drawn (- - - -) is shown as *r* ($p < 0.05$). (From Heber D, Chlebowski RT, Ishibashi DE, et al. *Cancer Res* 42: 4815, 1982. With permission.)

TABLE 50.3

Total Body Protein Turnover, Glucose Production, and 3-Methylhistidine Excretion in the Fasting State on Day 5 of Constant Nitrogen and Kcalorie Intake in Lung Cancer Patients Compared to Healthy Controls

Group	Protein Turnover (g/kg/day)	Glucose Production (mg/kg/min)	3-Methylhistidine Excretion (μmol/g creatinine/day)
Control	2.12 ± 0.38	2.18 ± 0.06	71 ± 8
Lung Cancer	3.15 ± 0.51[a,b]	2.84 ± 0.16[a]	106 ± 11[a]

[a] $p < 0.05$ versus control subjects.
[b] Mean ± S.D.

to healthy controls are shown in Table 50.3. Muscle catabolism, measured by 3-methylhistidine excretion, was increased in lung cancer patients compared to that of healthy controls. Methylhistidine excretion rates did not correlate with weight loss, percentage of ideal body weight, or age in the lung cancer patients studied. Glucose production rates were markedly increased in lung cancer patients compared with healthy controls, and changes in glucose production rates in the cancer patients studied did not correlate with weight loss, percent of ideal body weight, or age.

Hydrazine sulfate is a non-competitive inhibitor of gluconeogenesis. When this drug is administered to lung cancer patients not only does whole body glucose production decrease as expected, but there is also a decrease in whole body protein breakdown rates.[29] Increases in glucose production are directly and quantitatively linked to increased protein breakdown and changes in the circulating levels of individual glucogenic amino acids. Table 50.4 shows the influence of hydrazine sulfate on lysine flux. At one month, there

TABLE 50.4

Whole Body Lysine Flux in Lung Cancer Patients

	Lysine Flux (μmol/h)	
	Baseline	1 mo
Placebo Group		
1	2172	2812
2	1869	2959
3	2373	2674
4	2772	2269
5	2758	3195
6	3542	3585
Mean (SD)	2580 (580)	2920 (450)[a,b]
Hydrazine Treated		
7	2675	1146
8	2522	2119
9	2666	3129
10	1808	1217
11	2264	1438
12	3114	2006
Mean (SD)	2510 (440)	1840 (750)[b,c]

[a] $p = 0.08$; [b] $p < 0.05$, paired t-tests with baseline; [c] $p < 0.01$ by combined paired t-test both groups

was a significant reduction in the hydrazine group and a nonsignificant increase in the placebo group.

Both anorexia and abnormal metabolic adaptations to starvation play a role in the genesis of cancer cachexia. Anorexia has been given less attention than the metabolic abnormalities of increased glucose production, protein breakdown, and lipolysis. The tumor-bearing host does not adapt to decreased food intake normally, but studies of glucoregulatory and thyroid hormones fail to reveal systematic abnormalities other than insulin resistance which could impair renutrition. The immune response of the host to the tumor results in the local and perhaps systemic release of cytokines with potent metabolic effects. In fact, TNF-α has been shown to cause all of the metabolic abnormalities characteristic of cancer cachexia. It is possible that other cytokines may also participate in the pathogenesis of cancer cachexia. The study of the mechanisms of action of these cytokines and their interactions with cellular and soluble receptors may lead to improved strategies for the treatment of this perplexing clinical problem.

Assessment of the Cancer Patient's Nutritional Status

There are several nutritional assessment factors specific to the cancer patient, and these are listed in Table 50.5. Involuntary weight loss is a key indicator of undernutrition and is often a sign associated with a poorer prognosis and survival. The rate of weight loss is also important. It is accepted that an involuntary weight loss of 10% of the patient's usual body weight over a period of 6 months or less indicates undernutrition in patients with cancer.[30] One complicating factor in cancer patients is the development of edema or ascites; this should be kept in mind when interpreting weight data.

Ideal body weight is the weight associated with optimal survivorship in populations studied by life insurance companies. A commonly used reference is the 1983 Metropolitan Life Insurance Tables. With these tables, ideal weight range is calculated on the basis of height, body frame size, and sex, but no adjustments are made for age. Studies undertaken at the Gerontology Research Center (GRC), however, indicate that age significantly affects ideal body weight, while sex differences are not significant.[31] For a given height, older subjects have a higher ideal body weight range than younger individuals. Importantly, both tables are based on the same database, except that age is introduced as a variable only by the more recent GRC tables. Since cancer affects both the young and the aged, with the majority of patients in the older age groups,[32] it is more appropriate to utilize the age-adjusted tables to calculate ideal body weight range. Serious shortcomings still exist since there is no correction for disease-related changes in height, and no guidelines are provided in these tables for patients 70 years old or older.

Based on these ranges, we determine whether the patient is above, within, or below the ideal weight range. Thus, current weight compared to the expected or ideal body weight

TABLE 50.5

Nutritional Assessment Factors in the Cancer Patient

Nutritional Assessment Factors in the Cancer Patient
Involuntary weight loss
Comparison to usual, pre-illness, or ideal body weight
Anorexia and decreased food intake
Anthropometric measures
Biochemical and cellular biomarkers

range may help us determine the patient's nutritional status. An additional variable for consideration is usual or pre-illness weight. Therefore, both information on percent ideal weight and percent usual or pre-illness weight should be collected on all patients.There are healthy individuals who are below their projected weight for many years. From a clinical standpoint, stable weight and an adequate diet often equate with good nutrition even if the individual is below the ideal body weight range.

Anorexia and decreased food intake have long been recognized as key causes of undernutrition in patients with malignancies.[33,34] Anorexia is a treatable symptom of cancer which, if left untreated, leads to significant patient discomfort in addition to malnutrition.[35]

This information can be obtained by simply questioning the patient about a subjective loss of appetite and decrease in food intake. In order to further quantify these changes, we ask the patient to rate the appetite level from 0 to 7 (0 = no appetite; 1 = very poor; 2 = poor; 3 = fair; 4 = good; 5 = very good; 6 = excellent; 7 = always hungry). We also ask whether the amount eaten is enough to meet the patient's needs (0 = not at all; 1 = less than enough; 2 = enough; 3 = more than enough).

Detailed anthropometric measurements (such as mid-arm circumference and triceps skin fold) have long been utilized to determine skeletal muscle mass and nutritional status.[36] Although the value of these measurements can be limited if done in the hospital setting, serial measurements by the same professional in the outpatient clinic can help assess the patient's ongoing nutritional state. Problems with these measurements include interobserver variability and interference by edema or patient positioning. The decision to do these measurements should be individualized according to the acuteness of the underlying process, the availability of trained personnel, and intervention goals. It should be noted that muscle wasting and loss of adipose tissue reserves seen on physical examination are important but late signs of undernutrition. Ideally, early diagnosis and intervention should be directed at avoiding this advanced stage of undernutrition or cachexia.

The role of laboratory parameters, such as albumin or prealbumin level, transferrin, or total lymphocyte count, are less well defined in patients with cancer. These and other tests can be useful to assess protein depletion, but are difficult to interpret in patients with advanced cancer who often have metastases to visceral sites with organ dysfunction as well as metabolic and immunologic derangements due to cancer therapy.

Routine chemistry panels include albumin levels, which can be a useful indication of nutritional state. Albumin has a half-life in the circulation of about three weeks. Hypoalbuminemia can result from malnutrition but is also associated with liver disease, disseminated malignancies, protein-losing enteropathy, nephrotic syndrome, and conditions leading to expanded plasma volume such as congestive heart failure.

Prealbumin has a half-life of just under two days, and its level may increase with the use of steroid hormones and can be decreased by liver disease, disseminated malignancies, nephrotic syndrome, inflammatory bowel disease, the use of salicylates, or malnutrition.[37,38]

Transferrin can be measured by the transferrin antigen assay; the iron binding capacity provides with roughly equivalent results. Transferrin has a half-life of about one week, and it may increase with storage iron depletion or the use of hormonal agents and decrease with infection, malignancy, inflammation, liver disease, nephrotic syndrome, or malnutrition.[39]

Absolute lymphocyte counts can be reduced by malnutrition as well as a variety of other factors. More sophisticated tests (bioimpedance, total body K, basal metabolic rate [BMR] and others) are clinical research procedures.[40]

In many instances, a brief clinical nutritional assessment based on the degree of weight loss from usual or pre-illness weight, current weight as a percentage of usual and ideal body weight, and dietary history is sufficient to determine the clinical situation and consider potential interventions. We therefore reserve the use of anthropometric and

TABLE 50.6

Patient Characteristics in 644 Consecutive Cancer Patients*

Characteristic	Percent of Patients
Age — Median (range) in Years: 66 (22-91)	
Age <65	45
Age ≥65	55
Sex	
Women	53
Men	47
Type of Cancer	
Breast	16
Colon/rectum	14
Leukemia/lymphoma	13
Lung/non-small cell	14
Prostate	5
Stomach	4
Head/neck squamous	4
Ovary	3
Kidney/urinary bladder	3
Lung/small cell	2
All others	22
Stage of Cancer	
Metastatic	52
Non-metastatic	48

* Seen at Pacific Shores Medical Group and St. Mary Medical Center, Long Beach, California.

laboratory evaluations to specific individual situations. Interpretations of these evaluations should be based on an assessment of the clinical context.

A number of associated conditions are prevalent in older patients and can affect their food intake and nutrition. Mucositis as a side effect of chemotherapy or radiation therapy is common. Oral pain and dryness, poor dentition, periodontal disease, and ill-fitting dentures are also common. Other problems requiring consideration are dysphagia, alteration in taste, fatigue, nausea, vomiting, and diarrhea or constipation. Pain and other symptoms such as dyspnea can also interfere with nutrition. Depression is a well known cause of weight loss, and depression can worsen due to the stress of coping with cancer. Feelings of isolation and actual social isolation are not uncommon, especially in those patients who do not have strong family support. Socioeconomic and living conditions must be taken into account because they may impact food availability and preparation. These can all be very serious problems for patients with cancer, and require a multidisciplinary effort for proper management.

An understanding of the frequency and severity of malnutrition in cancer patients is necessary to better plan preventive, diagnostic, and therapeutic approaches, including the allocation of a variety of resources. To this end and as part of a more comprehensive effort, we studied nutrition-related clinical variables in 644 consecutive oncology patients regardless of type, status, or stage of cancer. The characteristics of these patients is shown in Table 50.6. The majority were seen as outpatients. We divided patients by age (<65 versus ≥65), and we analyzed the entire group as well as the subset of patients who had

TABLE 50.7

Nutritional Variables in 644 Consecutive Cancer Patients*

Variable	All Stages (n = 644)	Patients with Metastases (n = 377)
Decreased appetite	54%	59%
Decreased food intake	61%	67%
Underweight	49%	54%
Normal weight	37%	33%
Overweight	14%	13%
Weight loss		
Any	74%	76%
Up to 5%	15%	15%
>5 to <10%	22%	20%
10-20%	26%	27%
None	26%	24%

* Seen at Pacific Shores Medical Group and St. Mary Medical Center, Long Beach, California.

metastatic disease. Ideal body weight range was calculated using the GRC tables. The vast majority of patients sustained the weight loss shown within a period of six months from cancer diagnosis.

As shown in Table 50.7, the incidence of weight loss is very high in all patients, but particularly in those over the age of 65. Thus, 72% of all patients 65 or older with metastatic cancer had some degree of weight loss; 56% were underweight, 54% had decreased appetite, and 61% reported a decrease in food intake. Thirty-eight percent of patients 65 or older with metastatic disease had weight loss of 10% or more of their usual body weight. These data suggest that undernutrition at various stages is highly prevalent among oncology patients, particularly in the older population. Attention to the nutritional status of patients may afford the clinician opportunities for early diagnosis and intervention.

Nutritional and Adjunctive Pharmacotherapy of Anorexia and Cachexia

Counseling

The benefits of initial and follow-up evaluations and counseling by a registered dietitian, preferably in the context of a team approach, can be enormous, although difficult to quantify.[17] The main benefits relate to patient satisfaction, nutrition improvement or maintenance, compliance with team or institutional management protocols and guidelines, and a judicious use of risky and expensive treatments. The costs of nutritional counseling are modest when compared to other interventions. Table 50.8 shows the benefits, methodology and risks of common nutrition interventions. Nutritional evaluation and counseling, usually undertaken by a registered dietitian, is a first and important step. Ideally, a dietitian should be an integral part of the cancer care team.

In addition to assessing the clinical nutritional parameters previously outlined, it is our practice to first determine, through the dietary history, whether the patient is consuming a "balanced diet." The dietitian obtains a 24- to 72-hour recall diet history either verbally or, preferably, recorded at home. This diet record is then examined to assess the adequacy of kcalories and protein, utilizing food analysis tables compared to estimated energy and protein needs. Usually a weight-maintenance diet depends on the BEE, and is calculated

TABLE 50.8

Benefits, Methodology, and Risks of Nutrition Interventions

	Benefits	Methodology	Risks
1. Counseling	Patient satisfaction Nutrition maintenance Adherence to protocols	1 initial and 2 follow-up visits by dietitian	None
2. Food Supplements a. Home-made b. Commercial	Nutrition maintenance Avoid or delay need for more expensive therapy	a. Three 8-oz servings = 750 kcal/day b. Three 8-oz servings = 750-1080 kcal/day	Limited risks: diarrhea, nausea a. Diarrhea with lactose intolerance b. Patients may not like taste
3. Appetite Stimulants a. Megestrol acetate oral suspension b. Dronabinol c. Prednisone	a. Improved appetite, weight, wellbeing, quality of life b. Improved appetite, no significant weight change c. Short-term (4 weeks) appetite stimulation (see text)	a. 200 mg/d, 1 month supply 400 mg/d, 1 month supply 800 mg/d, 1 month supply b. 2.5 mg/d, 1 month supply 5 mg/d, 1 month supply c. 40 mg/d, 1 month supply	a. Impotence, vaginal bleeding, deep vein thrombosis b. Euphoria, somnolence, dizziness, confusion c. Hypokalemia, muscle weakness, cushingoid features, hyperglycemia, immune suppression
4. Enteral nutrition	Maintenance of nutrition via enteral route when oral route is not possible	Requires nasogastric, gastrostomy, or jejunostomy tube placement	Aspiration, diarrhea, nausea, bloating, infection, bleeding
5. Home parenteral nutrition	Maintenance of nutrition when no other alternative is appropriate; no evidence of improved survival in end-stage cancer	Central catheter surgically placed; parenteral infusion equipment and parenteral formulas: dextrose (20-25% w/w), crystalline amino acids (2-4% w/w), lipid emulsions (500 cc/d → 500 cc/wk)	Catheter-related pneumothorax, sepsis, thrombosis, bleeding; hepatic dysfunction, fluid and electrolyte imbalance

based on the Harris-Benedict formula[15] which, on an average, results in a daily requirement of 20 to 25 kcal per kg of body weight. The minimum recommended protein need is at least 0.8 grams per kg/per day.[16] These values need to be adjusted according to whether weight gain is desirable, and to match the metabolic needs of the patient.

One goal of nutrition education and counseling is to have the patient increase consumption of nutrient-dense foods to correct nutritional imbalances and deficiencies in order to achieve and maintain a desirable weight. Nutrient-dense foods are those with a high content in kcalories, protein, fat, and vitamins relative to their volume. Liquid supplements are the most common types of nutritional supplements, and are readily available for patient consumption. Patients may be anorectic due to illness, or be affected by disabling factors such as difficulty chewing, inability to prepare foods for themselves, visual difficulties, decreased energy level, or poor access to foods. Nutritional supplements may be homemade and are usually milk-based or commercially prepared and packaged. Although somewhat expensive, commercial supplements provide balanced, fortified (vitamin and mineral enriched) nutrition which require little or no preparation.

Not all cancer patients have the same requirements for nutrition. One major difference is whether patients are losing weight or have been treated successfully and are trying to prevent a recurrence through healthful nutrition. In the former case, calorically dense foods including those with low nutrient density can be used to increase the efficiency of kcalorie conversion to body fat stores. One limitation of this approach is that malnourished patients often are limited in their ability to absorb and digest fat due to the effects of malnutrition or enteritis caused by radiation or chemotherapy. Therefore, overprescription of high fat foods can in some cases lead to gastrointestinal distress. Foods containing refined sugar can also be used in these patients, as long as the patient has normal glucose tolerance. Since diabetes is a not uncommon comorbid condition in cancer patients, this is a practical consideration. Table 50.9 lists calorically dense foods and strategies for these types of patients. For patients who have been successfully treated, a preventive diet covered elsewhere in this text should be used.

Food Supplements

Liquid concentrated food supplements provide high kcalorie and protein, low volume nutrients, and are reviewed elsewhere.[17] Instant breakfast and milk provide an inexpensive and usually well-tolerated alternative. Commercial products may be more convenient and better tolerated in those patients with lactose intolerance. Dietitians will help patients select products on the basis of tolerance and palatability. These products are particularly helpful when patients can not maintain an adequate intake through a regular diet but are able to swallow and have a relatively intact GI tract.

Commercially prepared supplements are available in a variety of flavors (including unflavored) and in a variety of nutrient compositions. Most commercially prepared supplements are available in ready-to-drink eight-ounce cans or boxes and are usually lactose free, which for the patients is often more acceptable due to the increased incidence of perceived milk intolerance in this population. When patients have difficulty consuming adequate volumes of enteral supplement, a high-caloric supplement containing 2 kcal/ml (e.g., Isocal HCN [Mead Johnson] or Magnacal [Sherwood Medical]) can be used. Homemade supplements can also be made with commercially available products comprising a dry milk base to which whole milk and flavoring is added for a nutrient-dense

TABLE 50.9

Foods Recommended to Increase Kcalorie and Protein Intake of the Patient with Cancer

Food Group	Recommendations
Fruits and vegetables	Fruit juice added to canned fruit; pureed fruit added to milk, cereals, pudding, ice cream, gelatin; gelatin made with fruit juice to replace water; tender, cooked vegetables (mashed white or sweet potatoes, squash, spinach, carrots); vegetables added to soups and sauces; vegetables in cream or cheese sauces
Grains	Hot cereals prepared with milk instead of water; high protein noodles; noodles or rice in casseroles and soups; breaded and floured meats; bread or rice pudding; dense breads (i.e., bagels) and dense cereals (granolas, mueslis)
Beverages	Milk beverages; shakes made with fruit juices and sherbet when milk is not tolerated
Milk and calcium equivalents	Custards; milkshakes; ice cream; yogurt; cheeses; cheesecake; double-strength milk (1 quart fluid milk mixed with 1 cup nonfat dry milk powder); cottage cheese; flavored milk; pudding; commercial eggnog; cream soups; nonfat dry milk powder added to puddings, soups, sauces and gravies, casseroles and mixed dishes
Meat and protein equivalents	Diced or ground meat; casseroles; smooth peanut butter; cheese; egg and egg dishes; chopped, diced or puréed meats mixed with soups, sauces, and gravies; fish, poultry, and vegetable protein meat substitutes; tuna, meat, or cheese in cream sauces
Fats	Margarine or oil added to vegetables, hot cereals, and casseroles; cream used in place of milk or added to fruits and desserts; sour cream; salad dressings; mayonnaise mixed with tuna, egg, chicken salad
Sweets	Desserts made with dry milk powder, peanut butter, or eggs

beverage. Commercially prepared powdered breakfast drinks (e.g., Ultra Slim-Fast, Instant Breakfast), to which whole milk is added, is an inexpensive effective supplement when lactose intolerance is not an issue. These supplements have vitamin, mineral, kcalorie, fat, carbohydrate, and protein content similar to most commercially prepared supplements.

An eight-ounce supplement varies in nutrient density from 240 to 480 kcals, 7 to 20 grams of protein, 5 to 19 grams of fat and 12 to 25% of the U.S. Recommended Dietary Allowances (USRDA) for vitamins and minerals.

A nutritional supplement is advisable for patients whose GI tract is functional but who are unable to obtain adequate nutrition from a regular diet. The volume and choice of supplement is based on patients' individual nutrient needs and preferences, and GI tolerance. Supplements with fiber, generally soy or oat fiber, are available and may be beneficial to the patient who has diarrhea or constipation. Nutritional supplements are generally well accepted and may offer relief to a patient who has difficulties eating solid food. Tolerability can be enhanced by starting with small quantities and diluting the supplement with water or ice to decrease osmolality. A patient will usually accept one to three 8-ounce supplements per day, but there is great individual variability. Patients who have alterations in taste or nausea may better tolerate an unflavored supplement.

A common concern of patients and families is whether adding vitamins and other micronutrients to the patient's diet is beneficial. An analysis of the dietary record for the recommended number of servings from the Basic Four Food Groups (milk, meat and meat substitutes, vegetable and fruit, and grain) helps establish whether the minimum vitamin and mineral requirements are met. A computerized diet analysis program can help to quickly and accurately assess the nutrient content including vitamins and minerals. When intake is inadequate, we prescribe a daily multivitamin.

Patients should be provided with practical dietary advice about how to improve daily caloric intake, and the following are some simple tips to increase food intake:

- Avoid favorite foods after highly emetogenic chemotherapy to prevent the development of food aversions.
- Patients should be encouraged to consume any foods regardless of foods being labelled "non-nutritious," such as potato chips, nuts, or ice cream.
- Emphasize consumption of "nutrient-dense" foods as part of main meals or snacks, i.e., peanut butter, cheese, whole milk, and yogurt.
- Avoid the "Why don't you eat?" complaint. The patient should not be psychologically punished by the cancer care team and/or the family for not eating, but rather should be supported to overcome anorexia and other problems that lead to decreased food intake.
- Emphasize the pleasurable as well as social aspects of meals. Encourage patients to have their meals in a relaxed, friendly, and familiar atmosphere.
- Moderate alcohol intake is usually compatible with treatments and should be allowed before meals unless contraindicated.
- Avoid odors that can cause nausea. A short walk outside while meals are being prepared is advisable.
- Encourage food supplements and snacks between meals without being concerned that they may affect intake at meal time.

Patients are often deeply interested in the topic of nutrition as an unproven treatement. However, many will not bring up this topic unless encouraged and listened to in a nonjudgmental fashion. Open discussion and patient education may help prevent untoward effects of these diets and introduce nutrition-related issues into the mainstream of oncology care.

Nutrition Options and Alternative Therapies

A number of alternative therapies are being used by cancer patients in addition to standard medical oncology therapy,[41] as listed in Table 50.10. For this section, the nutrition alternatives will be outlined without reference to acupuncture or other non-nutritional therapies. Often patients fail to indicate that they are using these nutritional therapies. A number of potential side effects and concerns, listed in Table 50.11, may arise and need to be addressed.

Up until recently, most uses of vitamins and herbs were thought to be nontoxic. Recent animal studies suggest that antioxidants may affect tumor biology. The ATBC and CARET trials[42] in smokers demonstrated an increased incidence of lung cancer following admin-

TABLE 50.10

Alternative Nutritional Therapies Used by Cancer Patients

Multivitamins and single vitamin supplements
Low fat-, high fiber-, soy protein-supplemented diets
Specific macrobiotic diets
Vegetable and grass juicing
Herbal supplements (green tea extract, antioxidants)
Chinese herbal medicine (mushrooms, teas, roots)

TABLE 50.11

Potential Side Effects and Concerns

Vitamin toxicities (e.g. vitamin A >5000 IU per day)
Possible vitamin effects on tumor biology (apoptosis, proliferation)
Vitamin imbalances and conditioned deficiencies
Drug-nutrient interactions

istration of beta-carotene at a dose of 30 mg per day. There were no cancer-stimulatory effects noted with these doses of beta-carotene in non-smokers in a large heart disease prevention trial. However, there remains real uncertainty as to the safety of vitamin and mineral supplementation during chemotherapy or radiation therapy. For the large numbers of patients diagnosed today with early cancers of the breast and prostate, vitamin supplementation is as safe as in the general population once the treatment has been completed and nutritional intervention may prevent or delay cancer recurrence. However, the possibility of antioxidant effects on tumor biology or the effectiveness of antitumor drugs on radiation therapy requires much more research before general recommendations can be made. At this time, each patient and each oncologist must decide on the advisability of a given regimen for a given cancer patient based on clinical criteria without the benefit of a large scientific basis of controlled trials.

References

1. Nixon DW, Heymsfield SB, Cohen A, et al. *Am J Med* 68: 683; 1980.
2. Shils ME. *Cancer Res* 37: 2366; 1977
3. Brennan MF. *Cancer Res* 58: 1867; 1977
4. DeWys D, Begg C, Lavin PT, et al. *Am J Med* 69: 491; 1980
5. Brennan MF. *New Engl J Med* 305: 375; 1981.
6. Shike M, Russell DM, Detsky AS, et al. *Ann Int Med* 101: 303; 1984.
7. Chlebowski RT, Heber D. *Cancer Res* 42: 2495; 1982.
8. Holroyde CP, Gabuzda T, Putnam R, et al. *Cancer Res* 35: 3710; 1975.
9. Chlebowski RT, Heber D. *Surg Clin North Am* 66: 957; 1986.
10. Burt ME, Stein PT, Schwade JG, Brennan MF. *Cancer* 53: 1246; 1984.
11. Heber D, Chlebowski RT, Ishibashi DE, et al. *Cancer Res* 42: 4815; 1982.
12. Jeevanandam M, Horowitz GD, Lowry SF, Brennan MF, *Metabolism* 35: 304; 1986.
13. Shaw JHF, Wolfe RR. *Ann Surg* 205: 368; 1987.
14. Bennegard K, Lundgren F, Lundholm K. *Clin Physiol* 6: 539; 1986.
15. Byerley LO, Heber D, Bergman RN, et al. *Cancer* 67: 2900; 1991.
16. Chlebowski RT, Heber D, Richardson B, Block JB. *Cancer Res* 44: 857; 1984.
17. Chlebowski RT, Herrold J, Oktay E, et al. *Cancer* 58: 183; 1986.
18. Moley JF, Morrison SD, Norton JA. *Cancer Res* 45: 4925; 1985.
19. Warren S. *Am J Med Sci* 184: 610; 1932.
20. Terepka AR, Waterhouse C. *Am J Med* 20: 225; 1956.
21. Fenninger LD, Mider GB. *Adv Cancer Res* 2: 229; 1954.
22. Heber D, Byerley LO, Chi J, et al. *Cancer* 58: 1867; 1986.
23. Long CL, Schaffel N, Geiger JW, et al. *J Parent Ent Nutr* 5: 366; 1981.
24. Bozzetti F, Pagnoni AM, Del Vecchio M. *Surg Gynecol Obstet* 150: 229; 1980.
25. Dempsey DT, Feurer ID, Knox LS, et al. *Cancer* 53: 1265; 1984.
26. Knox LS, Crosby LO, Feurer ID, et al. *Ann Surg* 197: 152; 1983.
27. Peacock JL, Inculet RI, Corsey R, et al. *Surgery* 102: 465; 1987.
28. Heber D. *Nutrition* 5: 135; 1989.

29. Tayek J, Heber D, Chlebowski RT. *Lancet* 2: 241; 1987.
30. Blackburn G, Bistrian B, Maini B, et al. *J Parent Eenteral Nutr* 1: 11; 1977.
31. Andres R, Elahi D, Tobin JD, et al. *Ann Intern Med* 103: 1030; 1985.
32. Boring C, Squires T, Tong T. *CA: A Cancer Journal of Clinicians* 41: 19; 1991.
33. DeWys W. *Semin Oncol* 12: 452; 1985.
34. Theologides A. *Cancer* 43: 2013; 1979.
35. Tchekmedyian NS, Hickman M, Siau J, et al. *Oncology* 4: 185; 1990.
36. Chumlea WC, Baumgartner RN, *Am J Clin Nutr* 50: 1158; 1989.
37. Henry JB. In: *Clinical Diagnosis and Management by Laboratory Methods, 18th ed.*, WB Saunders, Philadelphia, 1991, p. 316.
38. Sacher RA, McPherson RA, Campos JM. In: *Widmann's Clinical Interpreter of Laboratory Tests, 10th ed.*, FA Davis, Philadelphia, 1991, p. 352.
39. Brittenham GM, In: *Hematology: Basic Principles and Practice*. Ronald Hoffman, Ed., Churchill Livingstone, New York, 1991, p. 334.
40. Harris JA, Benedict FG. Biometric studies of basal metabolism in man. Publication No. 279. Carnegie Institute of Washington, 1919.
41. Wargovich MJ. *Curr Opinion Gastroenterol* 15: 177; 1999.
42. Albanes D, Heinonen OP, Taylor PR, et al. *J Natl Cancer Inst* 88: 1560; 1996.

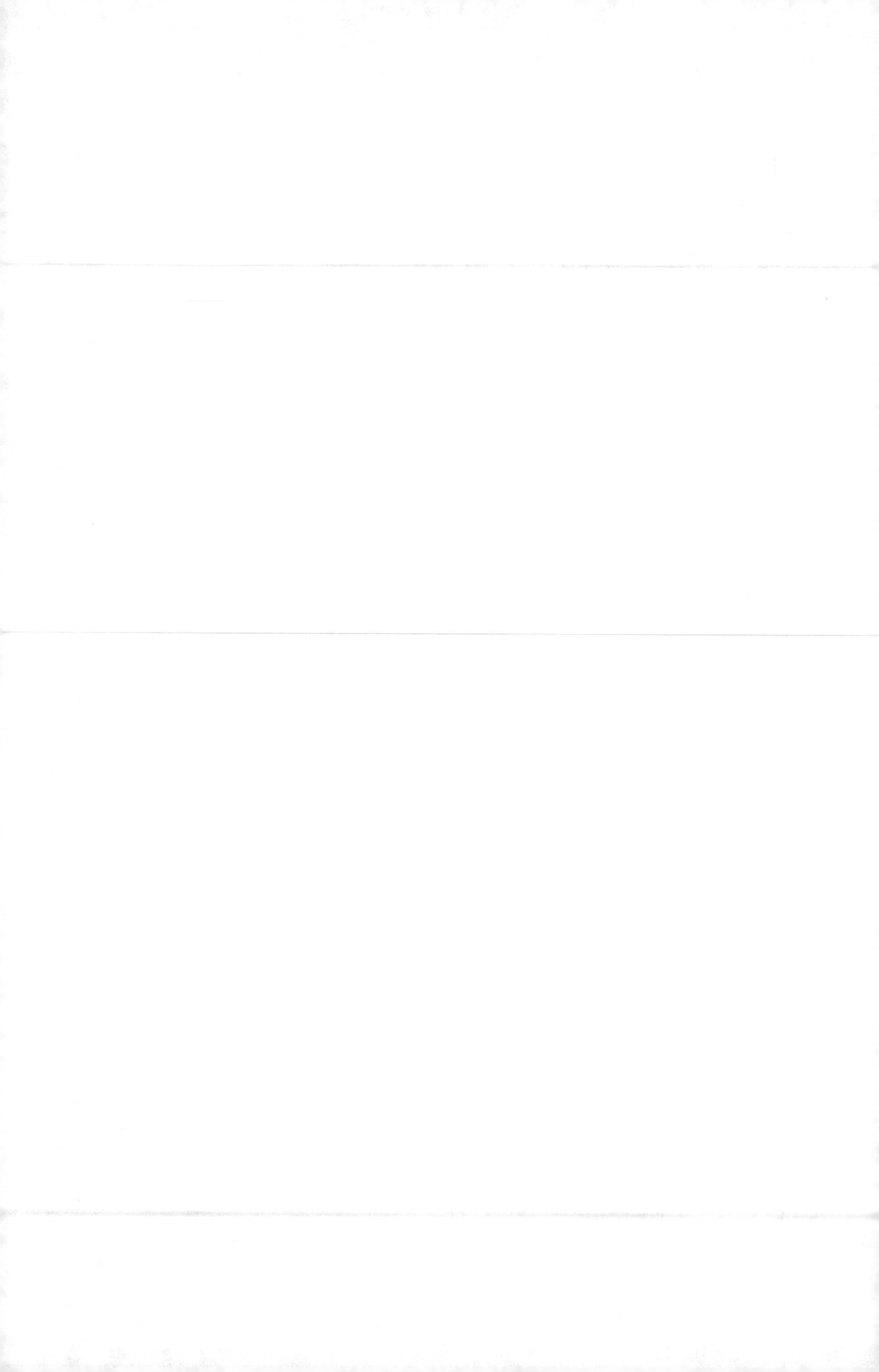

51

Cardiovascular Disease Risk — Prevention by Diet

Elaine B. Feldman

Introduction

Coronary heart disease (CHD) is the leading cause of death in both men and women in developed countries. Mortality rates vary from ~50/100,000 in Japanese women to 436/100,000 in Scottish men.[1] In the U.S. 32% of women and 50% of men will develop CHD, and CHD is the cause of death in 31% of men and 24% of women. The current concepts of the role of the diet in the etiology of cardiovascular disease (CVD) relate components of the diet to the pathogenesis of atherosclerosis. Primarily dietary fats, especially saturated fat and cholesterol, impact on the levels of circulating lipids to raise total and low-density lipoprotein (LDL) cholesterol that increase CHD risk. Dietary factors increase triacylglycerol (TG) levels that also increase the risk of CHD and/or decrease high density lipoprotein (HDL) cholesterol the lipoprotein that lessens CHD risk. Thus, diets that lower LDL cholesterol and/or TG and/or raise (or do not lower) HDL are protective against CHD. Other dietary components such as antioxidants (carotenoids, vitamin C, vitamin E) may lessen the risk of CVD by decreasing oxidized LDL, which is more atherogenic. High blood levels of homocysteine are atherogenic, and the levels of this amino acid are decreased by intake of folate, vitamin B_6 and vitamin B_{12}. This section will review:

- The background for these hypotheses and associations
- The dietary factors that influence circulating lipids and lipoproteins (Table 51.1) and their mechanisms of atherogenesis
- The role of some nutrients in vascular biology
- The diet that may best prevent CHD in those without the disease or in individuals post-myocardial infarction

The Extended Lipid Hypothesis

The fat content and fatty acid composition of the diet were determined to be important factors in the pathogenesis of atherosclerosis as an inference from the decline in cardio-

0-8493-2705-9/01/$0.00+$1.50

TABLE 51.1

Foods and Nutrients that Affect Cholesterol Levels

Cholesterol-Lowering	Cholesterol-Raising
Plant sterols, 3 g/day	Saturated fatty acids
Fruits and vegetables, 5 servings/day	Trans fatty acids
Soy proteins, 25 g/day	Dietary cholesterol
Whole grains	
Soluble fiber, 30 g/day	
Psyllium	
Monounsaturated fatty acids	
The Mediterranean diet	
N-6 polyunsaturated fatty acids	

vascular mortality that was observed during the depression and with World War II.[2] Food was scarce, with a decrease in the consumption of dairy products and eggs, rich sources of saturated fat and cholesterol. The dietary fat–heart hypothesis was proposed by Keys.[3] Epidemiologic studies related CHD rates to the intake of dietary fat, especially saturated fat (Figure 51.1). A high-fat diet, enriched in saturated fats, was also related to the rise in serum cholesterol with age. The related cholesterol hypothesis proposes that increasing serum cholesterol raises the risk of CHD, and that decreasing serum cholesterol levels will reduce risk.[2]

The risk of developing CHD is continuous over the range of serum total cholesterol levels. Cholesterol levels exceeding the 75th percentile are associated with moderate risk of atherosclerosis, and at >90th percentile with high risk.[4] Low-density lipoprotein cholesterol levels similarly can be classified into low, moderate, and high risk.[5] Small, dense LDL particles are associated with a tripling of the risk of myocardial infarction (MI), compared to the larger, more buoyant LDL particle.[6] Elevated lp (a) increases the risk of

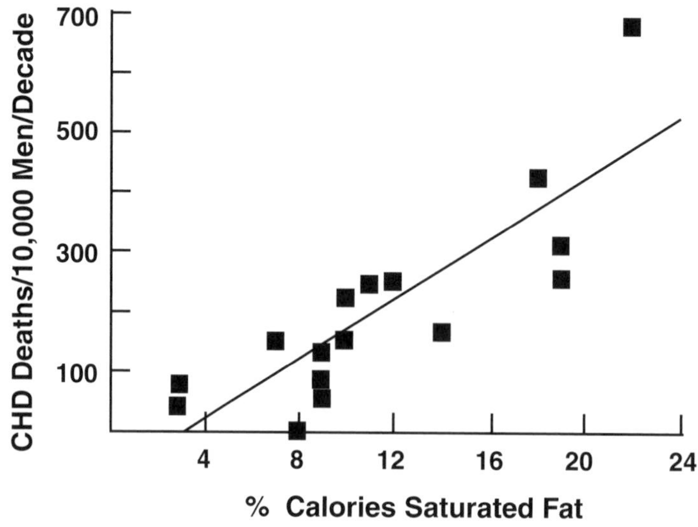

FIGURE 51.1
Death rates from CHD and the intake of saturated fat in the Seven Countries Study. The ordinate represents deaths from coronary heart disease that occurred over a 10-year period per 10,000 men enrolled in the study. The cohorts are from sites in seven countries: the U.S., Japan, Greece, Italy, Yugoslavia, the Netherlands, Finland. The regression equation is y = –83 + 25.1x, r + 0.84. Adapted from Keys A. *Seven Countries Study — A Multivariate Study of Death and Coronary Heart Disease,* Harvard University Press, Cambridge, 1980.)

TABLE 51.2
Factors Affecting HDL Cholesterol Levels

Increased Levels	Decreased Levels
Saturated fats	Polyunsaturated fat, high
Dietary cholesterol	Simple sugars/high carbohydrate diet (short period)
Alcohol <2 drinks/day	Some antihypertensive drugs
Long-term aerobic exercise program	Physical inactivity
Estrogens	Androgens
	Progestogens
	Anabolic steroids
Female gender	Male gender
	Obesity
	Diabetes mellitus
	Cigarette smoking

atherosclerosis,[7] although it is unknown whether decreasing levels with any intervention reduces risk. Elevated lp (a) levels are resistant to treatment other than high doses of niacin. The smaller lp (a) particles are more atherogenic, may act by promoting LDL oxidation, and may decrease endothelial-dependent vasodilatation. This additional risk factor is an indication for more aggressive management of other risk factors. Coronary events are reduced by 2 to 3% for every 1% decrease in LDL cholesterol.[1]

HDL cholesterol levels are inversely related to CVD risk.[8] Risk is appreciably higher in subjects with HDL levels < 0.92 mmol/L (35 mg/dl), and decreases when HDL levels are >1.5 mol/L (60 mg/dl). In addition, the ratio of total cholesterol to HDL cholesterol, or of LDL:HDL cholesterol, or total to non-HDL cholesterol indicate varying degrees of CVD risk. Factors influencing HDL cholesterol levels are listed in Table 51.2. Coronary events are reduced by 3% for every 1% increase in HDL cholesterol.[1]

TG levels in blood are increased by excess energy intake, fats, carbohydrates, and alcohol. Whether TG levels are independent risk factors for CHD has been debated over decades. Recent data have supported the concept that higher TG levels increase risk independent of HDL levels or other confounding factors of the dyslipidemic syndrome such as glucose intolerance, hyperinsulinism, obesity, hypertension, etc.[9] Results from one prospective study in Quebec males followed for up to five years suggest that fasting plasma insulin, apolipoprotein B levels, and LDL particle size may improve risk assessment. Identification of individuals with this cluster of abnormalities may lead to effective diet and exercise interventions.[10] This study supports conclusions from the Physicians' Health Study that elevated TG levels may help identify individuals at high risk because of the associated predominance of small, dense LDL particles.[11] Data from the Framingham Offspring Study indicate that elevated levels of fasting insulin are associated with impaired fibrinolysis and hypercoagulability in individuals with normal or abnormal glucose tolerance. This suggests that the risk factors of hyperinsulinemia and glucose intolerance may be mediated in part by enhanced potential for acute thrombosis.[12]

A meta-analysis of studies of TG levels and CVD showed that a 1 mmol/L increase in TG levels was associated with a 76% increase in CVD risk in women and a 31% increase in men.[13] Current data indicate that TG levels >100 mg/dl raise CVD risk, independent of the usual accompanying low HDL.[14] In the Copenhagen Male Study, fasting hypertriglyceridemia was found to be a stronger predictive risk factor than total cholesterol.[15]

Levels of circulating apoproteins may be useful in predicting the risk of CVD. Absolute levels, or changes in lipoprotein particle size or amino acid composition may be better predictors of CHD than are lipid levels.

A puzzling and as yet unanswered aspect of CHD risk is that the lipid levels of patients with various clinical symptoms or pathologic signs of atherosclerosis often fall within the "normal range." In the most recent National Health and Nutrition Examination Survey (NHANES III) (Table 26.4), the average level of total cholesterol in the U.S. was 225 mg/dl, and the average level of LDL cholesterol was 142 mg/dl.[16] Patients studied with CHD, such as in the Framingham Study, have had total cholesterol levels ranging from 200 to 250 mg/dl and LDL cholesterol ranges of 132 to 156 mg/dl.[8]

Dietary Effects on Serum Lipids and Lipoproteins

Lipids

Diets high in total fat, saturated fat, and cholesterol are atherogenic for many animal species. Long-chain saturated fatty acids (Figure 51.2) in animal or vegetable fats raise plasma cholesterol levels and decrease LDL receptor activity.[17] Paradoxically, these fats also raise HDL cholesterol levels. Predominantly monounsaturated liquid vegetable oils have a cholesterol-lowering effect, lowering LDL cholesterol, but not HDL cholesterol; some monounsaturated oils have shown a TG-lowering effect.[18,19] Polyunsaturated fats of the n-6 series in liquid vegetable oils decrease LDL cholesterol and increased amounts lower HDL cholesterol.[4] The n-3 series of polyunsaturated fatty acids found in fish (especially deep-water ocean fatty fish) and fish oil have variable effects on total LDL, and HDL cholesterol, and lower TG levels.[20] Trans-fatty acids produced from some processes of partial or complete hydrogenation of unsaturated liquid vegetable oils (in the U.S. predominantly soybean oil) raise LDL cholesterol to a somewhat lesser degree than long-chain saturated fats or butter, but in contrast, lower HDL cholesterol.[21] Investigators concluded that vegetable shortening and stick margarine have advantages over butter with respect to LDL cholesterol levels (–5 to 7%), with ingestion of liquid soybean oil or semiliquid margarine resulting in 11 to 12% lowering of LDL cholesterol in comparison

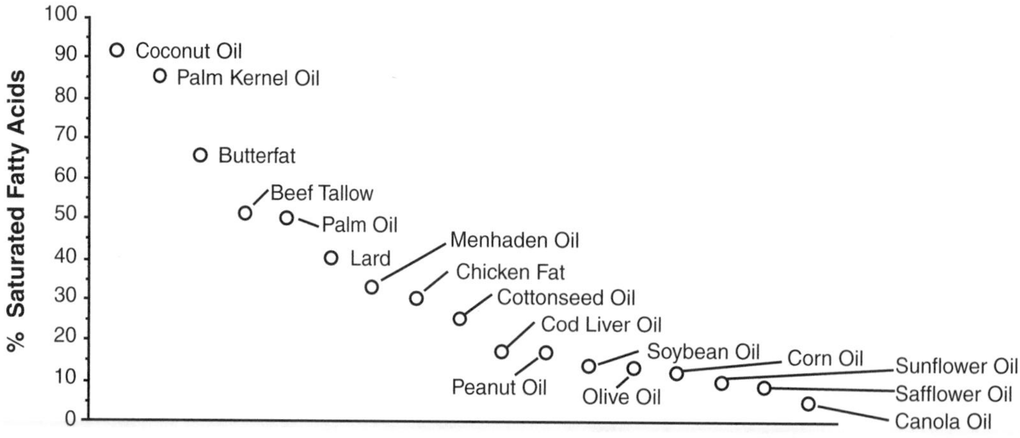

FIGURE 51.2
The saturated fatty acid content of various fats and oils.

to butter. Cholesterol is found in the diet only in animal products and is not present in any plant sources.

Atherosclerosis

Theories of Atherogenesis

Theories of atherogenesis propose that LDL cholesterol is the pathogen, delivering cholesterol to the arterial wall. Endothelial injury initiates proliferation of vascular smooth muscle cells and conversion of monocytes to macrophages (cholesterol ester-laden foam cells) and fibroblasts under the influence of growth factors and cytokines.[22] Oxidized LDL accelerates formation of foam cells, atheroma, and the fibrous plaque.[23] Plaque rupture initiates the events of myocardial infarction. CHD progression is related to levels of total and LDL cholesterol, and decreased levels of HDL cholesterol, especially HDL_2, or the ratio of HDL_2 to LDL cholesterol.[1,2] Levels of TG >2.28 mmol/L (250 mg/dl) also increase the risk of MI and warrant intervention; more recent data suggest lowering this level, perhaps to 0.91 mmol/L (100 mg/dl).[13,14] Regression of atherosclerosis occurs when cholesterol ester is mobilized from the superficial layers of plaque. Cholesterol is removed from plaque when LDL cholesterol levels are reduced to <2.5 mmol/L (95 mg/dl).[2] This level of LDL usually parallels a total cholesterol value <4.6 mmol/L (180 mg/dl).

Current theories of atherogenesis implicate plaque rupture with release of a necrotic lipid core as the precipitating factor for thrombosis at the site and MI.[22] Lipid lowering, especially of LDL cholesterol, stabilizes the plaque and reduces the risk of MI. Lower lipid levels may also decrease local concentrations of modified lipoproteins that have proinflammatory effects.[24] Evaluation of recent cholesterol-lowering clinical trials in the aggregate suggests that with treatment, CVD mortality is decreased by 25% and MI by 50%, and that a drop of 44% in LDL cholesterol halts progression of coronary atherosclerosis. The percent drop in LDL correlates 1:1 with the decrease in coronary events.[25,26]

Atherosclerosis begins in childhood and is strongly associated with LDL cholesterol levels. A lipid-lowering diet applicable to the general population can be recommended for children over the age of two years.[27]

Some mutations that predispose to atherosclerosis by affecting lipid levels and lipoprotein concentrations and composition are listed in Table 51.3.

TABLE 51.3

Mutations that Predispose to Atherosclerosis

Heterozygous LPL gene mutation
(May be associated with pattern B LDL)
LDL subclass pattern B (small dense)
Increased apo C-II, C-III or A-II on TG-rich lipoproteins
(Delays clearance and increases atherogenic remnant particles)
? Subtle polymorphisms in ABC-1 gene contribute to reduction in HDL levels

Risk Factors for Atherosclerotic CVD

In addition to the composition and concentration of serum lipids and lipoproteins that have been associated with risk of CVD, i.e., hypercholesterolemia, high lp (a), other factors modify risk and may interact with the lipids. These risk factors include:[28,29]

TABLE 51.4

National Cholesterol Education Program Guidelines, Adult Treatment Panel III, mg/dl[a]

Factor	Optimal	Near/Above Optimal	Borderline High	High	Very High
LDL cholesterol	<100	100-129	130-159	160-189	>190
Non-HDL cholesterol	<130	<160	<190		
Total cholesterol	***Desirable*** <200		200-239	>240	
HDL cholesterol	***Low*** <40 men <50 women			>60	
Triglycerides	***Normal*** <150		150-199	200-499	>500

[a] Full report available on the NHLBI Web site: http//www.nhlbi.nih.gov/guidelines/cholesterol/index.htm

Adapted from expert panel on detection, evaluation, and treatment of high blood cholesterol in adults. *JAMA* 285: 2486, 2001.

- Cigarette smoking
- Hypertension
- Diabetes mellitus
- Obesity, especially truncal; weight gain 5 kg+ after age 18 (women)
- A sedentary lifestyle (physical inactivity)
- Gender (males at increased risk, females at lower risk)
- Increasing age
- Excessive alcohol
- (Low socioeconomic status)

Obviously, optimal prevention should aim at modifying any or all of these factors that can be manipulated.

NCEP and Dietary Guidelines

The National Cholesterol Education Program Adult Treatment Plan (NCEP ATP) recommends strategies for identifying and managing subjects at risk for CHD, either primary prevention in healthy people, or secondary prevention for those with CHD[5] (Table 51.4). Dietary and lifestyle modification is the first intervention, with lipid-lowering drugs added if target goals are not reached. Diet is more aggressive when lipid levels are higher. The more potent drug intervention is introduced earlier when lipid levels are very high, when there are multiple risk factors, or in patients who already have CVD (MI, unstable angina, stroke).

Diet modifications and the strategies proposed to lessen the risk of CVD and optimize the lipid and lipoprotein risk factors include:

- Lower total fat from the usual 35% in the American diet to 30% (low fat), or to <20% (very low fat)

TABLE 51.5

Selected Foods High in Monounsaturated Fatty Acids

Food	g/30 g Portion
Canola oil	16.4
Olive oil	20.0
High oleic safflower oil	20.4
High oleic sunflower oil	23.4
Hazelnuts	14.7
Macadamia nuts	16.5
Pistachios	10.1
Pecans	11.4

- Emphasize that the decrease in fat content should mainly reduce saturated fat (+trans) intake to <10%, or to <7% (Figure 51.1 shows the saturated fatty acid content of some common fats and oils)
- Decrease saturated fat similarly but not total fat by substituting monounsaturated fat for saturated fat (Mediterranean diet)
- Concentrate on the ratio of saturated, monounsaturated, and polyunsaturated fats to decrease saturates, increase polyunsaturates, and result in a l:l:l proportion of the three types of long-chain fatty acids
- Consume primarily a plant-based diet and limit meat and dairy products
- Increase whole grains and soluble fiber and limit refined sugars and foods with a high glycemic index. Dietary fiber has been estimated to lower LDL cholesterol from 3 to 10%.[1,2] Fiber sources include oats, barley, beans, psyllium, pectin, and guar gum. Gastrointestinal side effects are common. The AHA recommends a total dietary fiber intake of 25 to 30 g/day from food, about double the current intake in the U.S.
- Balance energy intake with energy expenditure to prevent or treat obesity which contributes to the atherogenic lipid pattern

Food sources of saturated fat, monounsaturated fat, and cholesterol are listed in Tables 51.5 through 51.7. The AHA Step 1 and Step 2 diets are described in Table 51.8.

Maximal dietary therapy typically reduced LDL cholesterol by 15 to 25 mg/dL, or about 5 to 10%.[5,30,31] Addition of a vigorous exercise program (10 miles/week of brisk walking or jogging) doubled LDL lowering in contrast to the Step 2 diet while preserving HDL cholesterol levels.[32]

Other proposals emphasize increasing the intake of fish and n-3 oils like flaxseed, in part because of their favorable action on eicosanoids.[33-35] Recently, commercial food products have been developed that add cholesterol-lowering plant sterols or their derivatives (sitosterol, sitostanol) to fats and salad dressings. Studies have shown a reduction in total cholesterol of 6 to 13% and a 9 to 20% reduction of LDL cholesterol with 3 g/day of stanol ester in margarine.[36] Other dietary components that lower cholesterol or reduce oxidized cholesterol include 25 g/day of soy protein, perhaps 35 mg/day of the soy isoflavones,[37] and antioxidant vitamins (E, C, and carotenoids).[38] The amount and type of dietary protein can affect levels of total and LDL cholesterol, i.e., animal proteins are hypercholesterolemic, and plant proteins are cholesterol-lowering. This may be attributable to the content of amino acids lysine and methionine in animal proteins, and arginine in plant proteins.[39] Some additional foods that may favorably influence CV risk and lipid/lipoprotein levels and atherogenicity include garlic (putative lipid lowering) or green tea (antioxidant).[40] In

TABLE 51.6

Dietary Sources of Cholesterol[a]

Food[b]	Cholesterol
Fruits, grains, vegetables	0 mg LOW
Scallops (cooked)	53 mg
Oysters (cooked)	45 mg
Clams (cooked)	65 mg
Fish, lean	65 mg
Chicken, turkey, light meat (without skin)	80 mg
Lobster	85 mg
Beef, lean	90 mg
Chicken, turkey, dark meat (without skin)	95 mg
Crab	100 mg
Shrimp	150 mg
Egg yolk	270 mg
Beef liver	440 mg
Beef kidney	700 mg

[a] From National Heart, Lung, and Blood Institute, NIH Publication No. 85-2606, January 1985.

[b] Seafood, fish, poultry, and meat are cooked, and portion size is about 3 1/2 oz.

TABLE 51.7

Selected Foods High in Saturated Fatty Acids

Food	g/100 g Edible Portion
Beef, roast, chuck, cooked	11.2
Beef, steak, prime rib, cooked	12.8
Ground beef, cooked	9.9
Bologna, beef, regular	13.8
Frankfurter, all beef, Kosher, regular	13.6
Frankfurter, regular, beef and pork	13.7
Salami, hard or dry, pork	16.0
Bacon, regular cut	23.7
Egg, yolk only, cooked	9.6
Cream, half-and-half	32.6
Cream, light, coffee cream	12.0
Parmesan cheese, dry	19.1
American cheese, processed	18.7
Cream cheese, Neufchatel	13.8
Cheddar cheese, natural	21.1
Cheddar cheese, low fat	10.9
Swiss cheese, natural	17.8
Monterey Jack cheese, natural	19.1
Mozzarella cheese, part skim milk	10.9
Brie cheese	15.3
American flavor cheese, low fat	9.8
Coconut oil	86.5
Palm oil	49.3
Palm kernel oil	71.5
Lard	39.2
Butter, regular, salted	50.5
Coconut, fresh	29.7

Adapted from Table A 21-a in *Modern Nutrition in Health and Disease*, Shils M.E., Olson J.A., Shike M., Ross, A.C., Eds, 9th ed, Williams & Wilkins, Baltimore, 1999, p A-121.

TABLE 51.8

Step I and Step II Diets

Nutrient	Step I Recommend	Step II Recommend
Total fat	<30 % of kcalories	<30% of kcalories
Saturated fat	8%-10% of kcalories	<7% of kcalories
Polyunsaturated fat	Up to 10% of kcalories	Up to 10% of kcalories
Monounsaturated fat	Up to 15% of kcalories	Up to 15% of kcalories
Carbohydrate	>55% of kcalories	>55% of kcalories
Protein	~15% of kcalories	~15% of kcalories
Cholesterol	<300 mg/day	<200 mg/day
Kcalories	Achieve, maintain desirable weight	Achieve, maintain desirable weight

addition to effects on blood lipids and LDL oxidation, these nutrients also may influence factors involved in vascular reactivity, such as nitric oxide and thrombus formation.[41] Chinese red yeast rice is another traditional herbal remedy that may be lipid lowering because of its content of statins and precursors.[42]

HDL cholesterol levels are raised by moderate intake of alcoholic beverages;[43] red wine, grapes, and grapeseed oil also may contain favorable antioxidants.[44] Short-term replacement of usual dietary oil with grapeseed oil in subjects with moderate elevations of LDL cholesterol and low HDL cholesterol resulted in a 7% lowering and 8% increment respectively (personal communication, D.T. Nash). Similar antioxidants are found in rice bran oil.[45] Ingestion of rice bran oil has resulted in decreases in LDL and increases in HDL comparable to effects of canola oil. Components of fats and oils that are not the fatty acids, but perhaps the tocotrienols, plant sterols, or flavonoids may be partially responsible for an antiatherogenic effect. As vascular biologists derive more scientific data, foods may influence atherogenesis by mechanisms less dependent on lipid/lipoprotein levels.

Nutritionists debate the importance of limiting dietary cholesterol intake (see Table 51.7 for sources), especially in relation to the established merit of decreased saturated fat. Examples of some menus and foods for lipid-lowering diets are provided in Table 51.9.

Diet Trials

There has been no large scale long-term trial of the effects of diet on serum lipids and lipoproteins, or most importantly on cardiovascular risk (morbidity, mortality). Dietary recommendations are derived by consensus and are modified as new scientific information is obtained, usually from epidemiologic or animal studies.

Some relevant diet and lifestyle trials include the GISSI (Gruppo Italiano per lo Studio della Sopravvivenza nell Infarto [Miocardico]) trial that evaluated dietary supplementation with n-3 polyunsaturated fatty acids and vitamin E in patients after MI.[33] Patients who took 1 g daily of n-3 PUFA (equivalent to about 100 g/day of fatty fish), but not those who took 300 mg/day of vitamin E, had significant benefit attributable to the 20 to 30% decrease in risk for overall and cardiovascular mortality. The fish oil capsule contained 375 mg DHA ethyl ester and 465 mg EPA ethyl ester. All of these study patients in Italy were also ingesting a Mediterranean diet and were taking cardiac medications. The investigators propose the benefit of n-3 PUFA on arrhythmogenesis over the 3 1/2 years of treatment. A similar protective effect of fatty fish in the secondary prevention of CHD (29% reduction in overall mortality) has been reported in the Diet and Reinfarction Trial

TABLE 51.9
Step I AHA — Meal Plan

Food	Total Kcal	Fat (g)	Sat. Fat (g)	Chol. (mg)
		Goals:	<30% Fat <10% Sat. Fat <300 mg Chol.	
Breakfast				
Cantaloupe, pieces, 1 c	56	0.4	0.1	0
Toast, whole wheat, 2 sl	130	2	0.4	0
Margarine, Promise Extra Lite soft, 1 Tb	50	5.6	0.9	0
Milk, 1% Fat, 8 fl. oz	102	2.6	1.6	10
Breakfast subtotal	338	10.6	3	10
Lunch				
Grilled chicken sandwich:				
Chicken breast w/o skin, boneless, 2 oz	95	2.1	0.6	47
Bun, 1	133	2.2	0.2	0
Mayonnaise, light, 1 Tb	50	5	1	0
Lettuce, 1 leaf	2	0	0	0
Carrot, raw, 1 med	31	0.1	0	0
Pretzels, 1 oz	108	1	0.2	0
Apple, raw w/peel, 1 med	81	0.5	0.1	0
Lunch subtotal	500	10.9	2.1	47
Dinner				
Grouper, baked, 4 oz	133	1.4	0.4	52
Rice, 1/2 c cooked	100	0.5	0.1	0
Green peas, 1/2 c	59	0.3	0.1	0
Margarine, Promise Extra Lite, soft, 1 Tb	50	5.6	0.9	0
Dinner roll, 1	85	2.1	0.5	0
Sherbert, 1/2 c	132	1.9	1.1	5
Pineapple, raw, pieces, 1/2 c	37	0.4	0	0
Dinner subtotal	596	12.2	3.1	57
Snacks				
Oatbran muffin, 1 med	154	4.2	0.5	0
Milk, 1%, 8 fl. oz	102	2.6	1.6	10
Snacks subtotal	256	6.8	2.1	10
Daily Total	1690	40.5	10.3	124
		22%	5%	
20% Protein				
58% Carbohydrate				

(DART).[46] The protective effect of fish also was reported in the observational Health Professionals Study[34] and the U.S. Physicians Health Study.[35] Diet recommendations developed and updated by the American Heart Association and the federal government will be modified in 2000.

Since TG levels are raised by diets high in carbohydrate, especially refined sugars, and also are sensitive to alcohol and excess kcalories, TG-lowering diets limit sugars, alcohol, and kcalories, and increase energy expenditure.[47]

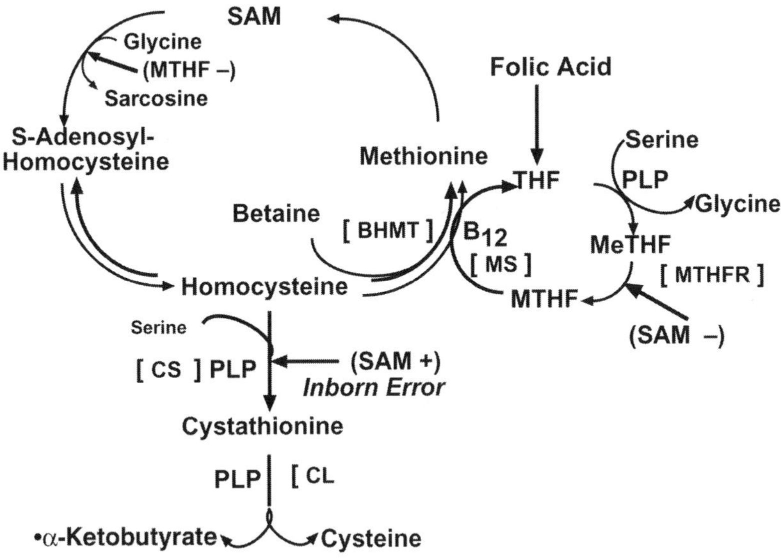

FIGURE 51.3
Homocysteine metabolism is regulated by enzymes dependent on folate and vitamins B_6 and B_{12}. + = activation, – = inhibition. Abbreviations: THF = tetrayhydrofolate; MeTHF = methylene tetrahydrofolate; MTHF = methyltetrahydrofolate; SAM = S-adenosylmethionine; PLP = pyridoxalphosphate (biological active form of vitamin B_6); CS + cystathionine synthase; CL = cystathionine lyase; MS = methionine synthase; MTHFR = methylene tetrahydrofolate reductase; BHMT = betaine homocysteine methyl transferase.

Other Nutritional Factors and CVD Risk

Homocysteine

An important nutritional risk factor for CVD is the blood homocysteine level, which increases in relation to deficient intake or metabolism of folate, and vitamins B_6 and B_{12} (see Figure 51.3). Elevated levels of homocysteine may be due to defects in enzymes catalyzing transsulfuration or remethylation pathways caused by drugs (methotrexate, phenytoin, theophylline, carbamazepine), deficiency of cofactors or cosubstrates (folate, B_{12}, B_6), impaired renal clearance, hypothyroidism, ovarian, pancreatic or breast cancer, or increasing age impairing vitamin absorption.

In recent years evidence has accumulated concerning the efficacy of folate (folic acid) in preventing heart disease. It is arguable whether folate from food sources (polyglutamates) is as effective as folic acid supplements (monoglutamate) in risk reduction. Folate bioavailability from food is 50%, whereas bioavailability from synthetic folic acid approaches 85% (1.7×).

Dietary folate or folic acid supplements may reduce the risk of cardiovascular disease in individuals with hyperhomocysteinemia resulting from genetic disorders of methionine metabolism and/or subclinical deficiencies of the B vitamins folate, B_{12}, and B_6. The genetic disorder is associated with premature cerebral, peripheral, and possibly coronary vascular disease. Homocyst(e)ine has been proposed as a risk factor for atherosclerotic CHD for more than 30 years.[48] Recent studies have concluded that homocyst(e)ine is an independent risk factor for coronary heart disease equivalent in importance to hyperlipidemia and smoking.[49,50] It promotes prothrombotic changes in the vascular environment, arterial narrowing and endothelial cell toxicity, affects platelets and clotting control mechanisms, and stimulates smooth muscle cell proliferation. Investigators have linked hyperhomocysteinemia with premature vascular occlusive diseases: carotid occlusive disease, cerebrovascular disease, CHD, peripheral arterial occlusive disease, and veno-occlusive disease. Homocysteine may be synergistic for thromboembolic disease with other risk factors, e.g., diabetes mellitus, hyperlipidemia, smoking, deficient antithrombin II, protein C, protein S, or Factor V Leiden.

Normal fasting levels are slightly lower in women (6 to 10 μmol/L) than in men (8 to 12 μmol/L). Risk of CVD is significantly increased when homocysteine levels exceed the 95th percentile (~15.8 nmol/ml). There appears to be a graded effect of the homocysteine level on risk of CVD, and homocysteine level is a strong predictor of cardiovascular mortality. Elevated homocysteine may account for 10% of the attributable risk of CHD.

Importantly, elevated blood levels of homocysteine can be normalized with vitamin supplements (0.2 to 1 mg folic acid, with or without 0.4 mg cyanocobalamin, 10 mg pyridoxal), potentially decreasing cardiovascular risk. Results of such intervention have not yet been reported in any prospective large scale randomized placebo-controlled clinical prevention trial. Whether reduction of plasma homocysteine by diet and/or vitamin therapy will reduce CVD risk is not known. Thus, at the present time emphasis should be placed on meeting requirements for folate and vitamins B_6 and B_{12}. Screening for fasting plasma homocysteine may be indicated in patients with premature CVD or with a family history of premature CVD.

Vitamins and Minerals

Other nutrients that have been associated with CVD risk include niacin that is lipid lowering only in pharmacologic doses at minimum 50 times the daily requirement for the vitamin,[51] copper (cholesterol and LDL-lowering),[52] and zinc (increasing cholesterol and LDL).[53] Vitamin D may be atherogenic, and retinoids have been shown to raise TG levels.

The possible role of antioxidant vitamins (beta-carotene and carotenoids, vitamin C, vitamin E) and dietary supplements in reducing CVD risk is under investigation. At present the dose of vitamin E that may be effective and safe, and the minimum duration of treatment for protection are unknown. The Canadian Heart Outcome Prevention Evaluation Study in patients at high risk for CV events found that treatment with 400 IU daily of vitamin E for 4.5 years had no apparent effect on cardiovascular outcomes.[54]

CVD Risk Prevention by Non-Lifestyle Modifications

In recent years successful primary and secondary prevention as well as documented slowing of progression or regression of atherosclerotic lesions have been achieved by a variety of modalities established by sound randomized, often double-blind, intervention trials that have been carried out in the U.S. and abroad.[25] Most trials address the lipid risk factors by use of lipid-lowering medications or ileal bypass. Other modalities include LDL plasmapheresis.[55] Chelation therapy with EDTA is unorthodox therapy that is generally not recognized as effective or safe. Low-dose aspirin has been shown to reduce the risk of MI in men, and oral anticoagulants continue to be proposed to reduce the risk of MI and stroke.[41] Some studies have shown a reduction in the risk of stroke as well as cardiovascular events with the use of statin drugs.[56] Of interest and debate is whether the favorable response is proportional to lowering of cholesterol and LDL, or raising of HDL, or whether a threshold is achieved for optimal prevention. In some trials, favorable results decreasing morbidity and mortality occurred too soon to expect them to be related to the degree of atherosclerosis but were more likely associated with stabilization of plaque. These trials also have demonstrated favorable effects in patients with lipid levels within the normal or average range, which is the level found in many patients with CHD. In fact, 20 to 25% of MIs occur in people with LDL cholesterol levels between 100 and 129 mg/dl.[8,57]

The first effective and safe cholesterol-lowering drugs were the bile acid-binding resins cholestyramine and colestipol. The efficacy of resins and the newer statin drugs (HMG Co A reductase inhibitors) and fibric acid derivatives on lipids and lipoproteins is depicted in Figure 52.9 of the Hyperlipidemia section. High-dose niacin therapy has also been administered for several decades, and is included as well. Often these drugs are used in combination to aggressively treat resistant forms of hyperlipidemia. Adverse effects of lipid-lowering drugs are observed on the gastrointestinal tract, liver, and muscles. The diet modifications initiated prior to drug therapy are usually continued during drug treatment in order to minimize the drug dosage, thereby decreasing adverse events and cost. If the diet, however, has been shown to be ineffective, then emphasis during drug treatment might better be placed on controlling body weight and eating a balanced diet.

Clinical Trials, Lifestyle

The studies of the effects on circulating lipids of changes in the content and composition of the diet are too numerous to cite in this section. Rather, more recent multicenter or large scale diet trials and three randomized controlled lifestyle intervention trials that address disease outcomes and/or angiographic endpoints over five years will be discussed.

The Lifestyle Heart Trial in patients with moderate to severe CHD demonstrated that intensive lifestyle changes lead to regression of coronary atherosclerosis.[58,59] The diet prescribed was a 10% fat, vegetarian diet and moderate aerobic exercise, stress management training, smoking cessation, and group support.

The St. Thomas' Atherosclerosis Regression Study (STARS) in patients with CHD included one arm of a 27% fat, weight reduction diet supervised by dietitians.[60] Dietary change retarded overall progression and induced regression of CHD.

The diet and exercise trial from Heidelberg in high-risk young men included rigorous exercise and a 20% fat diet.[28] A significant slowing of progression of coronary lesions was demonstrated.

Despite the demonstrated benefits of the Ornish regimen, other investigators have reported no benefit in lowering fat some 3 to 5% below the Step 1 diet in hypercholesterolemic men with and without hypertriglyceridemia followed for one year.[61] The Diet Effects on Lipoproteins and Thrombogenic Activity (DELTA) study at four sites included women, minorities, and older subjects in a comparison of eight weeks of the Step 1 diet (6% lower in total fat and saturated fat) and a 3% even lower-fat and saturated fatty acid diet in contrast to the average American diet (34% fat, 15% saturated fat).[31] Confirming other studies, the significant results were that with the Step 1 diet there was a drop in total (5%), LDL and HDL cholesterol (7%), apo B (–3%), and apo A-1 (5%), with a 9% increase in TG and 10% increase in lp (a). Further fat reduction resulted in a significant 4 to 5% fall in total, LDL, and HDL cholesterol and apo A-1, and a 7% increase in lp (a). The increase in negative risk factors lp (a) and TG raised questions about benefit in lowering CHD risk. The degree of lipid lowering with diet was similar to that observed in the earlier diet-lovastatin study[30] and continue to be less than earlier predictions from Keys-Hegsted.[1]

Lessons from Large-Scale Clinical Trials of Lipid-Lowering Therapy[25,26,65]

Many studies using effective lipid-lowering drugs, primarily statins, in primary and secondary prevention of CHD have yielded an overwhelming body of evidence to confirm that significant risk reduction can be achieved in about five years of treatment. Interestingly, the benefit is beyond the change in plaque in angiographic studies, but extends to symptoms of unstable angina and precipitation of acute MI from plaque rupture. Thus, the conclusion is that lesions are stabilized as a result of effective lipid-lowering treatments that may affect a number of inflammatory and thrombotic mechanisms. More aggressive treatment with LDL cholesterol lowered to <100 mg/dl reduces progression still more. The implication is that all patients with CHD should be treated to lower their cholesterol. This recommendation also may apply to individuals with very high LDL (>220 mg/dl) or with LDL levels >160 mg/dl and other risk factors, especially diabetes mellitus.

References

1. Feldman EB. In *Modern Nutriton in Health and Disease,* Shils ME, Olson JA, Shike M, Eds, 8th ed. Lea & Febiger, Philadelphia, 1993, ch 72.
2. Grundy S.M. In *Modern Nutrition in Health and Disease,* Shils ME, Olson JA, Shike M, Ross AC, Eds, 9th ed, Williams & Wilkins, Baltimore, 1999, ch 75.
3. Keys A. *Seven Countries Study — A Multivariate Study of Death and Coronary Heart Disease,* Harvard University Press, Cambridge, 1980.
4. Feldman EB. *Essentials of Clinical Nutrition,* FA Davis, Philadelphia, 1988.
5. National Cholesterol Education Program. *Circulation* 89: 1329; 1994.
6. Austin MA, Breslow JL, Hennekens CH, et al. *JAMA* 260: 1917; 1988.
7. Assmann G, Schulte H, von Eckardstein A. *Am J Cardiol* 77: 1179; 1996.
8. Dawber TR. *The Framingham Study: The Epidemiology of Atherosclerotic Disease,* Harvard University Press, Cambridge, 1980.
9. Austin MA. *Am J Cardiol* 83: 13F; 1999.
10. Lamarche B, Tchernof A, Mauriege P, et al. *JAMA* 279: 1955; 1998.
11. Stampfer MJ, Krauss R, Ma J, et al. *JAMA* 276: 882; 1996.
12. Meigs JB, Mittleman MA, Nathan DM, et al. *JAMA* 283: 221; 2000.
13. Austin MA. *Am J Cardiol* 83: 13F; 1999.
14. Miller M. *Clin Cardiol* 22: II-1; 1999.
15. Jeppeson J, Hein HO, Svadicani DD, Gyntelberg MD. *Circulation* 97: 1029; 1998.
16. NHANES III. *JAMA* 269: 3000; 1993.
17. Dupont J, White PD, Feldman EB. *J Am Coll Nutr* 10: 577; 1991.
18. Kris-Etherton PM. *Circulation* 100: 1253; 1999.
19. Lorgeril M de, Salen P, Martin JL, et al. *Circulation* 99: 779; 1999.
20. Harris WS. *Clin Cardiol* 22: II-40; 1999.
21. Lichtenstein AH, Ausman LM, Jalbert SM, Schaefer EJ. *N Engl J Med* 340: 1933; 1999.
22. Libby P. *Circulation* 91: 2844; 1995.
23. Steinberg D. *Circulation* 95: 1062; 1997.
24. Steinberg D, Gotto AM, Jr. *JAMA* 282: 2041; 1999.

25. Grundy SM. In: *Cholesterol-Lowering Therapy — Evaluation of Clinical Trial Evidence*, Grundy SM, Ed, Marcel Dekker, New York, 2000, ch 1.
26. Ferraro-Borgida M, Waters D. *In: Cholesterol-Lowering Therapy — Evaluation of Clinical Trial Evidence*, Grundy SM, Ed, Marcel Dekker, New York, 2000, p. 221.
27. Fisher EA, Van Horn L, McGill HC, Jr. *Circulation* 95: 2332; 1997.
28. Schuler G, Hambrecht R, Schlierf G, et al. *Circulation* 86: 1; 1992.
29. Willett WC, Manson JE, Stampfer MJ, et al. *JAMA* 273: 461; 1995.
30. Hunninghake DB, Stein EA, Dujovne CA, et al. *N Engl J Med* 328: 1213; 1993.
31. Ginsberg HN, Kris-Etherton P, Dennis B, et al. *Arterioscler Thromb Vasc Biol* 18: 441; 1998.
32. Stefanick ML, Mackey S, Sheehan M, et al. *N Engl J Med* 339: 12; 1998.
33. GISSI-Prevenzione Investigators. *Lancet* 354: 447; 1999.
34. Ascherio A, Rimm EB, Stampfer MJ, et al. *N Engl J Med* 332: 977; 1997.
35. Albert CM, Hennekens CH, O'Donnell CJ, et al. *JAMA* 279: 23; 1998.
36. Hallikainen MA, Uusitupa MIJ. *Am J Clin Nutr* 69: 403; 1999.
37. Anderson JW, Johnstone BM, Cook-Newell ME. *N Engl J Med* 333: 276; 1995.
38. Tribble DL. *Circulation* 99: 591; 1999.
39. Stone NJ, Nicolosi RJ, Kris-Etherton P, et al. *Circulation* 94: 3388; 1996.
40. Neil HAW, Silagy C. *Curr Opin Lipidol* 5: 6; 1994.
41. Anand SS, Yusuf S. *JAMA* 282: 2058; 1999.
42. Heber D, Yip I, Ashley JM, et al. *Am J Clin Nutr* 69: 231; 1999.
43. Pearson TA. *Circulation* 94: 3023; 1996.
44. Weisburger JH. *Food Chem Toxicol* 37: 943; 1999.
45. Seetharamaiah GS, Chandrasekhra N. *Atherosclerosis* 78: 218; 1989.
46. Burr ML, Fehily AM, Gilbert JF, et al. *Lancet* 2: 757a; 1989.
47. Greene JM, Feldman EB. *J Am Coll Nutr* 10: 443; 1991.
48. Graham IM, Daly LE, Refsum HM, et al. *JAMA* 277: 1775; 1997.
49. Malinow MR, Bostom AG, Krauss RM. *Circulation* 99: 178; 1999.
50. Stein JH, McBride PE. *Arch Intern Med* 158: 1301; 1998.
51. Feldman EB. In *Nicotinic Acid,* Altschul R, Ed, CC Thomas, Springfield, 1964.
52. Medeiros DM, Milton A, Brunett E, et al. *Biol Trace Elements Res* 30: 19; 1991.
53. The Heart Outcome Prevention Evaluation Study Investigators. *N Engl J Med* 342: 154; 2000.
54. Keller C. *Atherosclerosis* 86: 1; 1991.
55. Holmes CL, Schulzer M, Mancini GBJ. In *Cholesterol-Lowering Therapy — Evaluation of Clinical Trial Evidence*, Grundy SM, Ed, Marcel Dekker, New York, 2000, p 191.
56. Kannel WB. *Am J Cardiol* 76: 69C; 1995.
57. Gould KL, Ornish D, Kirkeeide R, et al. *Am J Cardiol* 69: 845; 1992.
58. Ornish D, Scherwitz L, Billings JH, et al. *JAMA* 280: 2901; 1998.
59. Watts GF, Lewis B, Brunt JNH, et al. *Lancet* 339: 563; 1992.
60. Knopp RH, Walden CE, Retzleff BM, et al. *JAMA* 278: 1509; 1997.

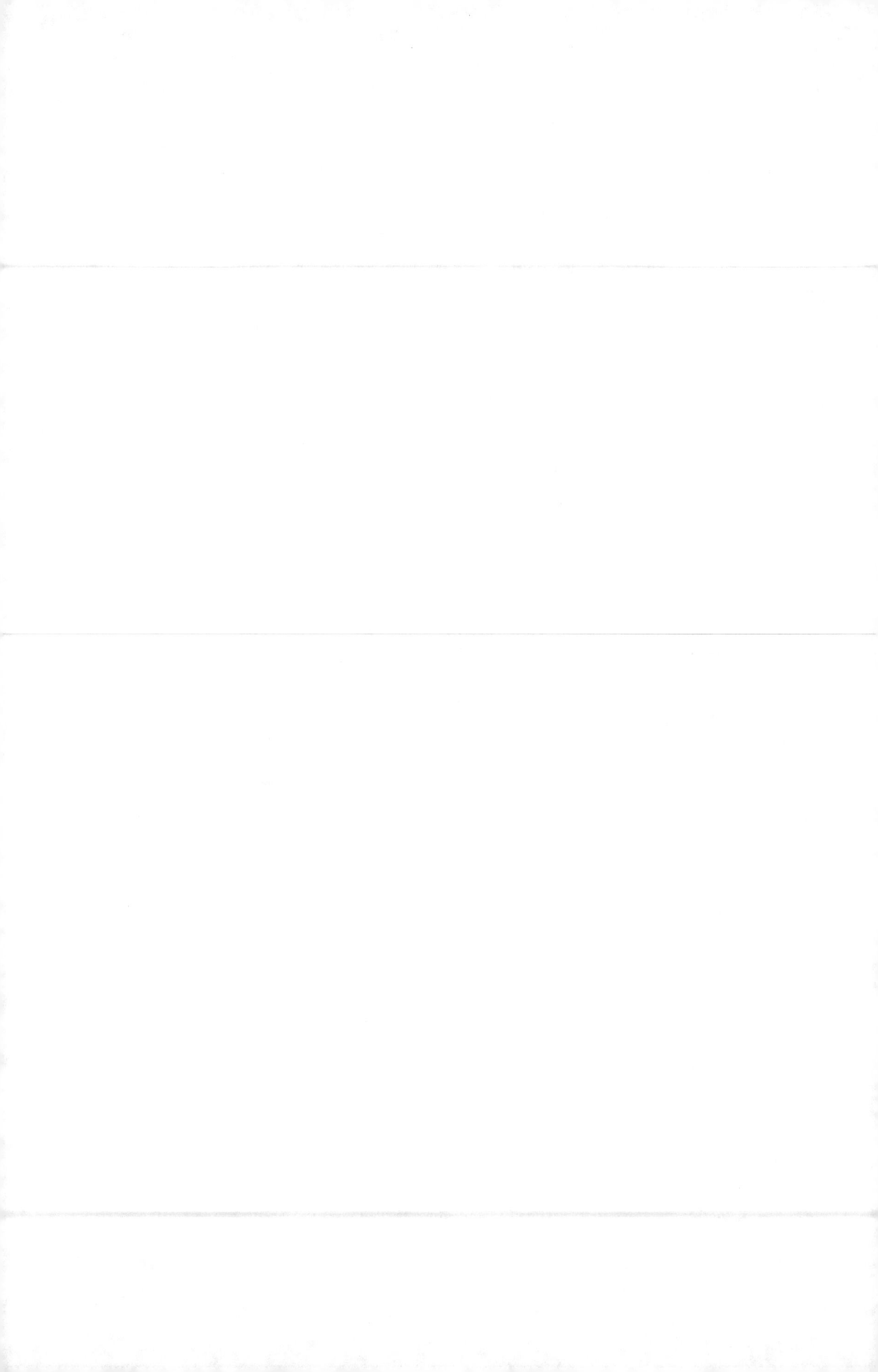

52

Hyperlipidemias and Nutrient-Gene Interactions

Elaine B. Feldman

A variety of factors under genetic control are involved in the production and metabolism of serum lipids and lipoproteins (Table 52.1).[1,2] Nutrients in the diet may affect one or more steps of gene regulation of lipoproteins, resulting in abnormal lipid or lipoprotein levels and predisposition to atherosclerosis. The factors affected are listed in Table 52.1. Examples of effects of diet and lifestyle on genetic mechanisms are included in Table 52.2.[1]

Hyperlipidemias

These lipid disorders reflect abnormal increase in one or another serum lipid component and/or lipoprotein carrier (Tables 52.3, 52.4). The abnormalities often are inherited and are strongly influenced by the diet. Their management requires accurate diagnosis and evaluation, searching for other diseases that may induce secondary hyperlipidemia.[3] The dietary intervention, if unsuccessful, should be followed by appropriate medication that normalizes the lipids and lipoproteins in order to prevent complications of atherosclerotic disease (myocardial infarction, peripheral vascular disease) or pancreatitis.[4]

These subjects have lipid levels generally above the 90th percentile for their age and sex (Table 26.3). Blood samples should be obtained after a 12 to 14-hour fast in individuals ingesting their usual diet. At least three blood samples should be evaluated, two or three weeks apart. The lipid studies may need to be more elaborate than the usual lipid screen or profile (see Section 26). Ultracentrifugation of the plasma often is necessary, usually performed in a specialized lipid laboratory. These lipid disorders can be suspected from the patient's history, family history, and physical examination. First degree relatives should also be investigated in order to detect others with the disorder and to characterize the genetics.

Numerous mutations have been associated with the various types of familial hyperlipoproteinemias (Table 52.4).[5] In the future, nutrient modulation of gene expression may be used as therapy. More than half the variability in serum cholesterol (low density lipoprotein, LDL cholesterol) among individuals is attributable to genetic variation, presumably polygenic. Polymorphisms in apo-E or apo-B are examples. The remaining variability in cholesterol levels may be attributable to the diet, diet-gene interactions, or postulated genes that control variability of response to the environment. The prevalence of hyperlipidemias is increased in patients with premature coronary heart disease (CHD), i.e., <55 years of age.

0-8493-2705-9/02/$0.00+$1.50

TABLE 52.1

Factors Involved in the Formation and Metabolism of Lipoproteins

Type	Action
Apoproteins	
Apo A-I	Anti-atherogenic
Apo A-II	Apo A-II-containing lipoproteins are not effectively metabolized by lipoprotein lipase (defective lipolysis)
Apo B_{100}	Ligand for the LDL receptor
Apo C-I	Blocks apo E binding to receptors
Apo C-II	Activates lipoprotein lipase (LPL)
Apo C-III	Impairs TAG hydrolysis delaying clearance of remnants of chylomicrons; inhibits LPL; decreases LDL binding to receptors; displaces apo E from lipoprotein particles
Apo E	Ligand for the LDL receptor; interacts with the LDL receptor-related protein (LRP); enhances lipolysis
Enzymes	
Lipoprotein lipase (LPL)	Hydrolyzes TAGs to free fatty acids in chylomicrons and VLDL to form chylomicron remnants and IDL. Excess lipoprotein surface components are released to form HDL particles
Hepatic lipase (HL)	Functions as a phospholipase and TAG hydrolase. Important for conversion of IDL to LDL. Increased activity leads to LDL pattern B (small dense) and low HDL
Lecithin:cholesterol acyltransferase (LCAT)	Catalyzes the esterification of free cholesterol to cholesterol ester on plasma lipoproteins
Acyl CoA:cholesterol acyltransferase (ACAT)	Catalyzes cholesterol esterification
Carboxyl ester lipase (CEL)	
Receptors	
LDL receptor	Binds apo B-containing lipoproteins, such as LDL
LDL receptor-related protein (LRP)	Takes up chylomicron remnants
Scavenger receptor A (SR-A)	Binds LDL modified by oxidation
CD-36, a scavenger receptor on macrophages	Binds modified LDL
Scavenger receptor B1 (SR-B1)	Selectively removes cholesterol esters from HDL and apo B-containing lipoproteins
Peroxisome proliferator-activated receptor-α (PPARα)	Putative HDL receptor takes up HDL particles
VLDL receptor	
Transfer Proteins	
Cholesterol ester transfer protein (CETP)	Required for normal clearance of HDL. Transfers cholesterol esters synthesized in HDL to the apo B-containing lipoproteins in exchange for TAG
ATP-binding-cassette transporter 1 (ABC-1)	Actively transports free cholesterol out of cells and into HDL particles transforming lipid-poor A-I particles into nascent HDL particles
Microsomal triglyceride transfer protein (MTP)	Necessary to generate LDL (VLDL)

TABLE 52.2
Effects of Diet and Lifestyle on Gene Regulation of Lipoprotein Expression

Factor	Effect
Cholesterol	Decreases expression of the LDL receptor by suppressing transcription of its gene
	Regulates H:MG CoA reductase expression by controlling the stability of the HMG CoA reductase protein (post-translational level)
Polyunsaturated fatty acids	Block transcription of the fatty acid synthase gene
Fats	Excessive intake induces excessive secretion of apo-B containing lipoproteins by stabilizing the protein (post-translational)
	Affects LDL receptor expression
	Increases expression of LPL activity, inducing adipose tissue LPL activity and suppressing skeletal muscle LPL activity (perhaps via insulin). Post-translational regulation by glycosylation is possible.
Atherogenic diet	Decreases HDL
	Decreases the expression of the gene encoding paraoxonase, an enzyme that protects LDL from oxidation
Exercise	Increases muscle LPL activity pre-translationally
Glucose	Increases fatty acid synthesis by stabilizing the fatty acid synthase mRNA (post-transcriptional)
Other	Subjects with the E_3/E_4 phenotype respond to a low fat, low cholesterol diet intervention with a greater LDL decrease than those with the E_3/E_3 or E_3/E_2 phenotype

TABLE 52.3
Classification (Type) of Hyperlipidemia and the Underlying Lipoprotein Abnormality

Type	Lipoprotein Abnormality
I	Increased exogenous triacylglycerols (TAG) in the form of chylomicrons
IIa	Hypercholesterolemia with increase in LDL and normal TAG levels
Iib	Hypercholesterolemia combined with mild hypertriglyceridemia (increase in LDL and VLDL particle number, overproduction of apo-B)
III	Remnant hyperlipemia; hypercholesterolemia with hypertriglyceridemia and increase in IDL
IV	Mild to moderate endogenous hyperlipemia; increased VLDL with TAG 2.8-7.9 mmol/L or 250-700 mg/dl
V	Mixed hyperlipemia; moderate to severe hypertriglyceridemia (>11.3 mmol/L or 1000 mg/dl) with mixed VLDL and chylomicrons

Types of Hyperlipidemias

Chylomicronemia (Type I Hyperlipoproteinemia)[3-7]

Dietary TAGs that are transported as chylomicrons are increased in Type I. This rare disorder results from a defect in removal of chylomicrons from the blood due to the presence of a recessive gene that results in deficiency of lipoprotein lipase (LPL, Table 52.4).[6] A similar disorder results from the absence or abnormal function of the apo-C II activator of LPL,[7] or from the presence of a circulating inhibitor of LPL. Type I may present in infants and children. It does not usually predispose to vascular disease, but patients are at risk of recurrent severe pancreatitis. Signs of lipemia retinalis (Color Figure 52.1*), eruptive xanthomas (Color Figure 52.2), and hepatosplenomegaly may be present. The plasma shows a chylomicron creamy layer over a clear infranatant. Plasma TAG levels usually exceed 17 mmol/L.

* Color figures follow page 994.

TABLE 52.4

Genetic Basis of Familial Hyperlipidemias

Type	Abnormality	Mutation
Type I	Familial lipoprotein lipase deficiency	40 known missense and nonsense mutations of gene encoding enzyme
	Familial lipoprotein lipase inhibitor	
	Familial apo C-II deficiency	14 defects identified
	Familial hepatic lipase deficiency	
Type II	Familial hypercholesterolemia	400 deletions/point mutations in 5 classes of the LDL gene
	Familial defective apo B_{100}	Apo B 3500 mutation impairs binding to the LDL receptor
	Polygenic hypercholesterolemia	Apo A-I/C-III/A-IV gene clusters
Type Iib	Familial combined hyperlipidemia	Apo A-I/C-III/A-IV
		LCAT
		Mn superoxide dismutase linkage
		Partial LPL deficiency
Type III	Familial dysbetalipoproteinemia	Apo E gene polymorphism affects amino acid coding E_2/E_2 phenotype
Type IV	Familial hypertriglyceridemia (mild)	Apo A-I/C-III/A-IV
		?Hepatic lipase deficiency
Type V	Familial hypertriglyceridemia (severe)	Apo A-I/C-III/A-IV
	Familial lipoprotein lipase deficiency	Apo A-II
	Apo C-II deficiency	

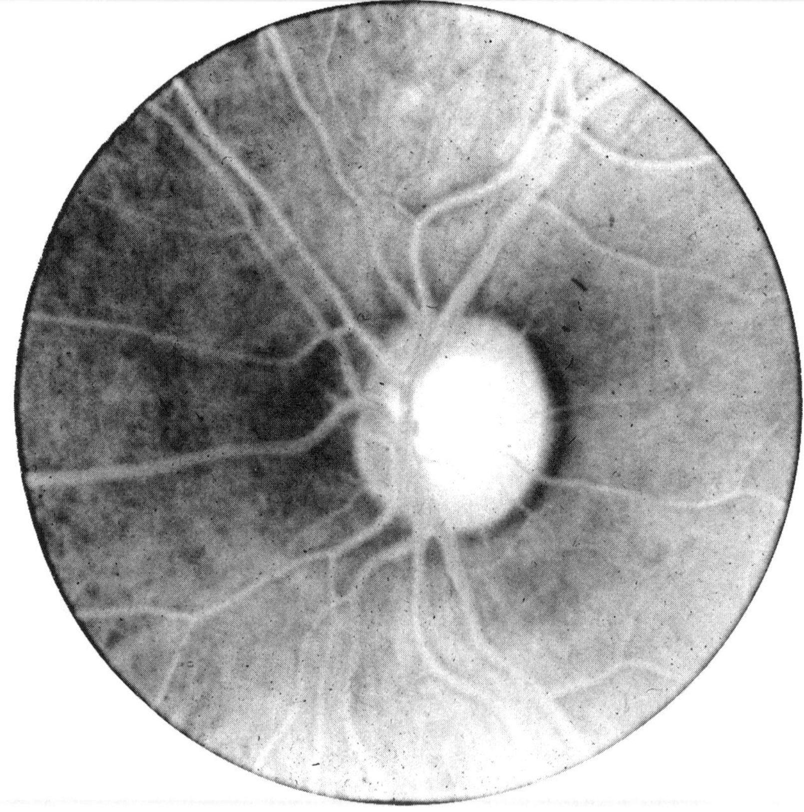

FIGURE 52.1
(See Color Figure 52.1) Lipemia retinalis visualized in the optical fundus of a patient with chylomicronemia with TAG levels exceeding 3000 mg/dl.

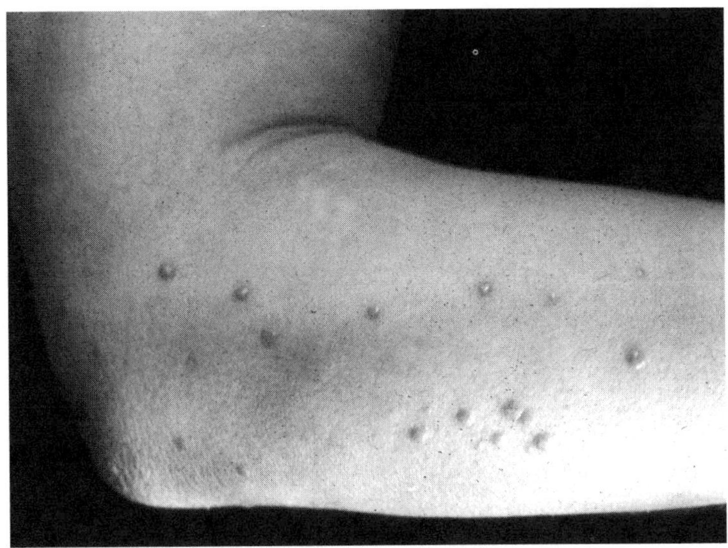

FIGURE 52.2
(See Color Figure 52.2) Eruptive xanthomas observed in a patient with chylomicronemia.

Hypercholesterolemia (Type IIa and Type IIb Hyperlipoproteinemias)[3,4,9]

In Type IIa hypercholesterolemia, increased LDL is present with normal levels of TAGs. Familial hypercholesterolemia (FH) is a single-gene defect of the cell surface receptor that binds circulating LDL and delivers cholesterol to cells.[8] To date, more than 400 mutations have been characterized in five classes.[5,9] In the heterozygote, receptor number or activity is about half normal. LDL cholesterol does not enter the cell and does not suppress the activity of hydroxymethylglutaryl coenzyme A (HMG CoA) reductase, the rate-limiting step in cholesterol synthesis. Cholesterol synthesis continues and esterified cholesterol accumulates in the cell, suppressing LDL receptor synthesis. The LDL cholesterol level in blood doubles (to about 9 mmol/L) and the fractional catabolic rate of LDL is halved. In the FH homozygote with no receptors, LDL production is greatly enhanced and removal severely decreased. LDL cholesterol levels average 19 mmol/L.

Signs of FH include lipid deposits such as eyelid xanthelasma (Color Figure 52.3), corneal arcus (Color Figure 52.4), and tendon and tuberous xanthomas of the skin (Color Figures 52.5, 52.6) that appear in the second or third decade of life. Hypercholesterolemia is present from birth.[10] FH homozygotes may have xanthomas in infancy or early childhood. The incidence of CHD is increased 25-fold in FH patients and occurs prematurely (before age 50). In FH homozygotes, CHD may be present in infancy and early childhood, with death occurring by age 21.

Patients with familial defective apo B (Table 52.4) may exhibit a phenotype identical to FH.[5] In Type IIb, hypercholesterolema is combined with hypertriglyceridemia, with LDL and very low density lipoprotein (VLDL) increased, and overproduction of apo-B. Familial combined hyperlipidemia (FCH) is the most common hyperlipidemic syndrome in patients with premature CHD. In this condition, small, dense LDL is overproduced, with increased levels of apo-B.[11-13]

Type III Hyperlipoproteinemia (Dysbetalipoproteinemia, Broad-beta or Floating-beta Disease)[14]

In this syndrome, hypercholesterolemia is combined with hypertriglyceridemia. Intermediate density lipoprotein (IDL) remnants are increased, at times mixed with chylomicrons.

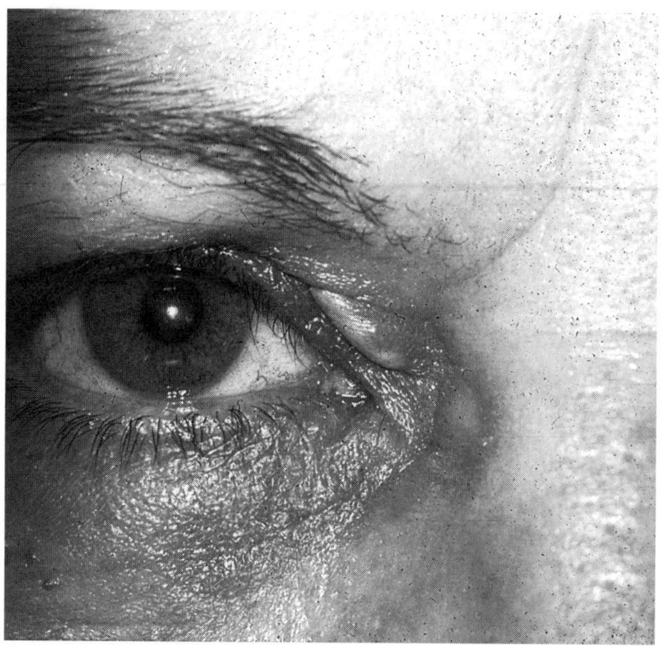

FIGURE 52.3
(See Color Figure 52.3) Eyelid xanthelasma from a woman with familial hypercholesterolemia.

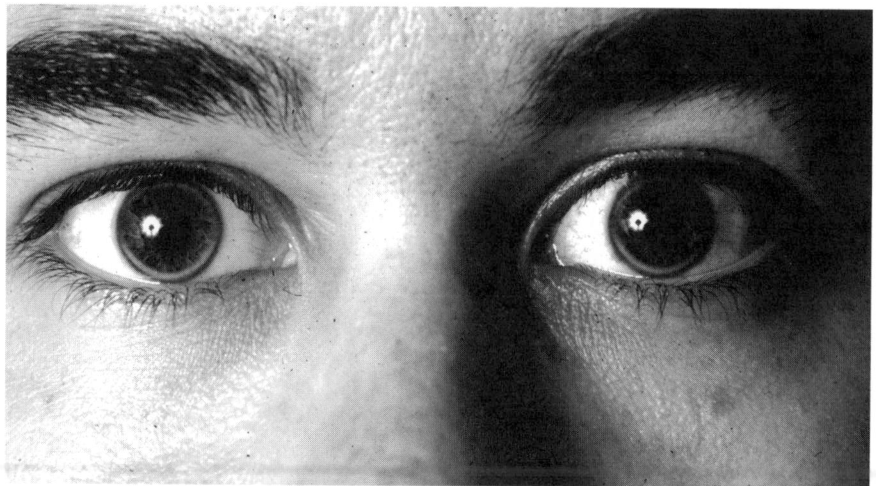

FIGURE 52.4
(See Color Figure 52.4) Corneal arcus observed in a 31-year-old man with familial hypercholesterolemia.

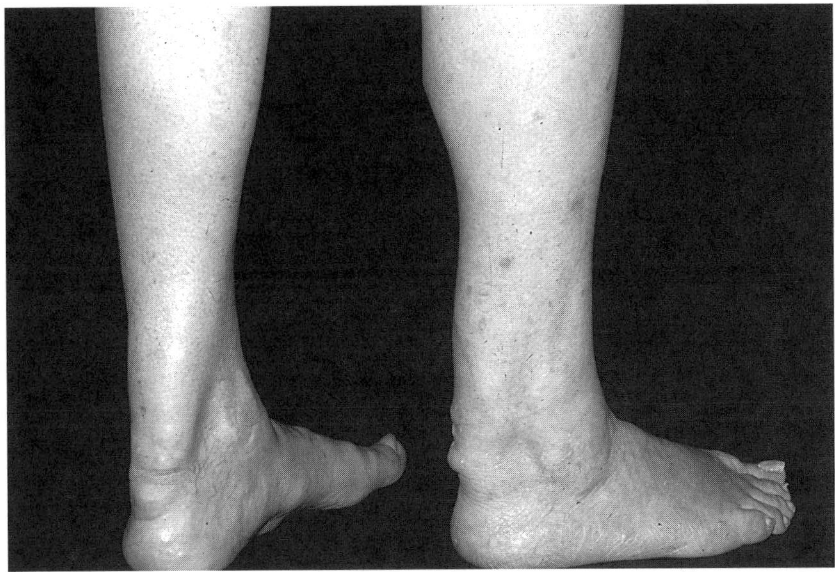

FIGURE 52.5
(See Color Figure 52.5) Xanthomas of the Achilles tendons of a patient with familial hypercholesterolemia.

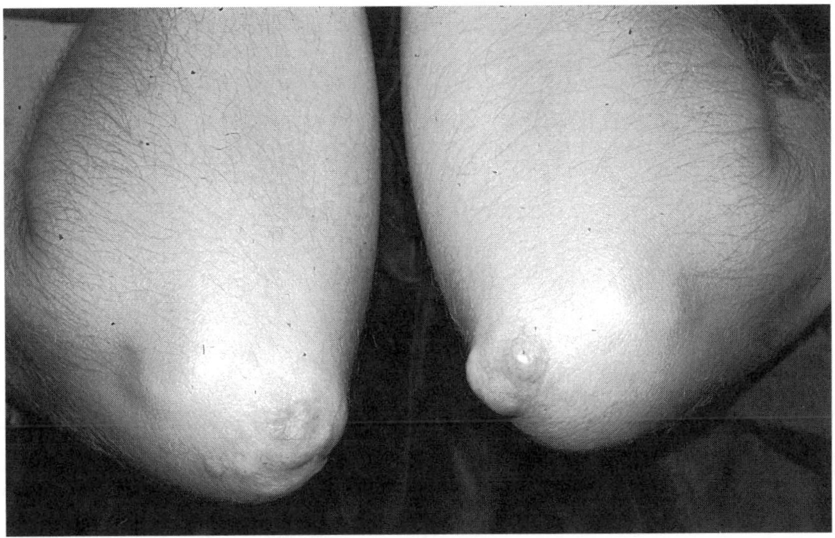

FIGURE 52.6
(See Color Figure 52.6) Tuberous xanthomas in the skin of the elbows of a teenage girl with familial hypercholesterolemia.

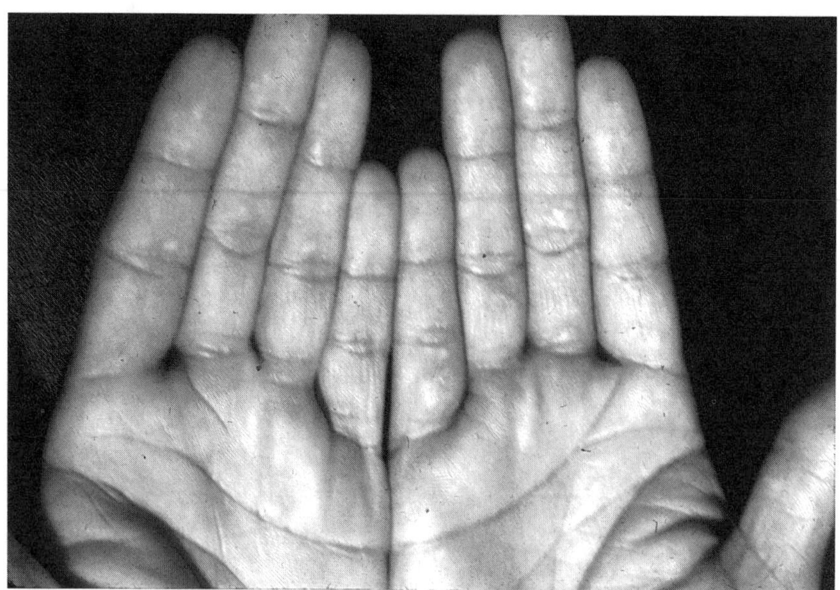

FIGURE 52.7
(See Color Figure 52.7) Yellow linear deposits in the creases of the fingers and palms of the hands of a 33-year-old man with Type III hyperlipoproteinemia.

The disorder is due to a genetic defect in the apo-E isoforms. The normal E_3 is replaced by one or two E_2 proteins that have defective receptor binding. This results in a lesser rate of removal and increases the circulating level of IDL. Preparative ultracentrifugation demonstrates increased cholesterol relative to TAG in the VLDL fraction, with more rapid migration of the lipoprotein on electrophoresis. Apo-E isoforms should be determined (E phenotype). Patients show planar xanthomas of the palms (Color Figure 52.7) and tuberous xanthomas as early as the third decade of life. Patients have premature peripheral vascular disease and CHD.[15]

Type IV Hyperlipoproteinemia[5]

Endogenous hypertriglyceridemia is characterized by mild to moderate increase in TAG levels (3 to 8 mmol/L, 250 to 700 mg/dl), with increase in VLDL.[16,17] Both overproduction and decreased removal of VLDL TAG may be responsible. LDL cholesterol levels are within the normal range. Usually HDL cholesterol is decreased. These subjects may be at increased risk of atherosclerosis, and hypertriglyceridemia per se may be an independent risk factor for cardiovascular disease (CVD).[16,17] Patients often have no signs or symptoms other than the abnormal lipid and lipoprotein values, and may present initially with cardiovascular events. Underlying mechanisms and genetic defects are multiple.[5] See also atherogenic dyslipidemia, below.

Type V Hyperlipoproteinemia

Moderate to severe increases in TAG levels exceeding 11.3 mmol/L or 1000 mg/dl characterize this disorder, often termed the chylomicronemia syndrome.[3,4,6,15] Chylomicrons appear along with increased levels of VLDL. Patients exhibit eruptive xanthomas and lipemia retinalis (TAG levels >34 mmol/L, 3000 mg/dl) (Color Figures 52.1, 52.2). They are at high risk for recurrent episodes of acute pancreatitis, at times resulting in pancreatic insufficiency. Fifty percent or more of these patients have diabetes mellitus that must be

TABLE 52.5

Metabolic Syndrome Risk Factors
Insulin resistance
Elevated Triaglycerides
Increased dense LDL
Low HDL
Hyperinsulinemia
Glucose intolerance
Hypertension
Prothrombotic state
Truncal obesity
Premature CVD

controlled to effectively lower TAG levels. Alcohol intake or estrogen treatment may convert a type IV patient to type V, or worsen type V and precipitate pancreatitis.[3] Underlying mechanisms and genetic defects are a mixture of those of Type I and Type IV (Table 52.4).

Dyslipoproteinemia (Atherogenic Dislipidemia)

Some lipidologists have proposed and prefer a simpler classification into subgroups of hypercholesterolemia, chylomicronemia, or atherogenic dyslipidemia.[4] This metabolic syndrome encompasses hypertriglyceridemia, small dense LDL, low HDL, insulin resistance, abdominal obesity, and hypertension (Table 52.5). These patients are at high risk of atherosclerosis.[1,7]

Evaluation of Patients with Hyperlipidemia

Table 52.6 enumerates the details of the history, physical examination, and laboratory tests used for the evaluation of subjects who may have one of the hyperlipidemic syndromes (Color Figure 52.8).

Dietary Management of Hyperlipidemias

Appropriate diet tailored to the lipid abnormality is the initial intervention. Treatment goals are to normalize lipids, or in patients with vascular disease, to lower these to optimal levels that promote regression of atherosclerotic disease and stabilize plaque. Lipid levels should be monitored at six- to eight-week intervals. After a three- to six-month trial of diet, depending on the response and the severity of the disease, appropriate cholesterol- and/or triglyceride-lowering medication should be added. The diet is continued (unless the response is adverse) so that medication dose can be lower, thereby minimizing side effects and cost. Treatment is lifelong.

Diets to Lower Serum Cholesterol and LDL Cholesterol[3,4]

Cholesterol lowering is achieved by a diet that regulates kcalories to achieve desirable weight, and includes an exercise regimen. Depending on the severity of hypercholesterolemia, total fat should be decreased to 30% or less of energy, with saturated fat reduced to <10% or <7% of kcalories depending on severity and response, and cholesterol intake should be 70 to 100 mg/1000 kcal. Consumption of plant based foods, complex carbohydrates, and dietary fiber should be increased.

TABLE 52.6

Evaluation of Patient for Hyperlipidemia

History of:

Vascular disease, angina, MI, angioplasty, bypass surgery, claudication
Abdominal pain
Diabetes
Thyroid, hepatic, renal, disease, gout
Smoking habits, exercise, medications
Body weight
Family history of vascular disease, diabetes, gout
Diet history: alcohol, supplement use, amount and type of fat and cholesterol, energy, protein, carbohydrate, sucrose intakes (best done by a dietitian)

Physical Examination:

Blood pressure, height, and weight
Corneal arcus, xanthelasma, retinopathy, lipemia retinalis
Xanthomas of skin and/or tendons
Dry skin, hair loss
Bruits, murmurs, absent pulses, arrhythmias
Liver, spleen size

Laboratory:

Blood, after 12-14 hour overnight fast, cholesterol, TAG, HDL cholesterol, glucose
Plasma turbidity
Apoproteins, ultracentrifugation, electrophoresis
Post-heparin lipolytic activity
Tests of renal, hepatic, and thyroid function
Electrocardiogram

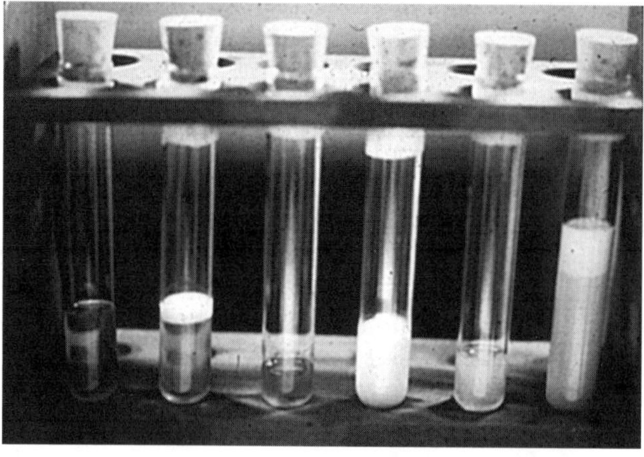

FIGURE 52.8
(See Color Figure 52.8) The appearance of plasma, refrigerated overnight, from fasting patients. The tubes with plasma samples are taken from (left to right): a subject with normal lipid levels and clear plasma (similar to a patient with Type IIa); a patient with chylomicronemia (Type I) with a creamy top layer above a clear infranatant; a patient with hypercholesterolemia (Type IIa) with clear plasma; a patient with Type III hyperlipoproteinemia with diffusely turbid plasma; a patient with Type IV hyperlipoproteinemia also showing diffuse turbidity; and a patient with Type V hyperlipoproteinemia with plasma exhibiting a creamy top layer over a turbid infranatant.

TABLE 52.7

Guidelines of Food Choices and Menu Plans for Patients with Severe Hypercholesterolemia (FH)[a]

Very Low-Fat Diet-Meal Plan	Goal 10-15% Fat Kcals			
Food	Total Kcal	Fat (g)	Sat Fat (g)	Chol (mg)
Breakfast				
Orange juice, fresh, 6 fl. oz	84	0	0	0
Banana slices, 1/2 med	52	0.5	0	0
Shredded wheat, spoon size, 1 c	170	0.5	0	0
Milk, fat-free, 8 fl. oz	86	0.4	0.3	4
Breakfast subtotal	392	1.4	0.3	4
Lunch				
Turkey sandwich:				
Turkey breast, fat-free luncheon meat, 2 oz	52	0.4	0.2	23
Mayonnaise, light, 1 Tb	50	5	1	0
Whole wheat bread, 2 slices	130	2	0.4	0
Sliced tomato, 1/2 med	13	0.2	0	0
Apple, 1 med	81	0.5	0.1	0
Lunch subtotal	326	8.1	0.7	23
Dinner				
Pork tenderloin, marinated, 4 oz	140	4	1.5	65
Baked potato, w/skin, 8 oz	220	0.2	0.1	0
Fat-free sour cream, 2 Tb	35	0	0	5
Margarine, Promise Ultra fat free, 1 Tb	5	0	0	0
Broccoli, steamed, 1 c	44	0.6	0	0
Angel food cake, 1/12	130	0	0	0
Strawberries, fresh, 1/2 c	23	0.6	0	0
Whipped topping, fat-free, 2 Tb	15	0	0	0
Dinner subtotal	612	5.4	1.6	70
Snacks				
Non-fat vanilla yogurt, 8 fl oz	200	0	0	5
Honeydew melon, cubed pieces, 1c	60	0.2	0	0
Snacks subtotal	298	0.7	0	5
Daily Total	1628	15.6	2.6	102
		8.6%	1.4%	
19% Protein				
72% Carbohydrate				

[a] Prepared by Sandra Leonard, M.S., R.D.

See Table 52.7 for food choices and menu plans for patients with Type II hyperlipidemia or FH.[19,20] Compliance with and response to these changes may lower total and LDL cholesterol by 10 to 20%.

Diets to Lower Serum TAG[3,4]

TAG in VLDL are decreased when kcalories are restricted, especially the intake from refined carbohydrates and alcohol. N-3 fatty acids in fish and fish oils lower TAG.[21]

Chylomicron TAG are lowered by limiting fat intake severely to 50 g or less daily, or to less than 20% of kcalories. Patients with Type V who become pregnant may require

TABLE 52.8

Guidelines of Food Choices and Menu Plans for Patients with Severe Hypertriglyceridemia (Type V)[a]

Triglyceride-Lowering Meal Plan	Goals:	<30% Fat <10% Sat Fat low refined sugar low cholesterol		
Food	**Total Kcal**	**Fat (g)**	**Sat Fat (g)**	**Sugar (g)**	**Cholesterol (mg)**
Breakfast					
Cheerios, 1 1/2 c	165	3	0	1.5	0
Milk, 1%, 8 fl. oz	102	2.6	1.6	*N/A	10
Blackberries, fresh, 1/2 c	37	0.3	0	*N/A	0
Orange juice, 1/2 c	56	0.2	0	8	0
Breakfast subtotal	360	6.1	1.6	9.5	10
Lunch					
Ham and cheese sandwich					
Lean ham, 2 oz	69	2.2	0.8	1.8	29
Cheese, cheddar, lowfat, 1 oz	49	2	1.2	0	6
Mustard, 1 Tb	0	0	0	0	0
Whole wheat bread, 2 sl	130	2	0.4	4	0
Peach, fresh, 1 med	37	0.1	0	*N/A	0
Tea, w/sugar substitute	0	0	0	0	0
Lunch subtotal	285	6.3	2.4	5.8	35
Dinner					
Pink salmon, broiled, 6 oz	254	7.6	1.2	0	114
Salad:					
Romaine, 1 c	8	0.2	0	1.2	0
Tomato, 1/2 med	13	0.2	0	1.7	0
Ranch dressing, light, 2 Tb	100	8.0	1.0	1.0	5
Pasta, cooked, 1/2 c	100	0.5	0	0	0
Marinara sauce, 1/4 c	55	2.5	0.8	4.0	0
Asparagus, 6 spears	22	0.3	0.1	1.4	0
Lemon juice	0	0	0	0	0
Cherries, sweet, fresh, 10	49	0.7	0.1	*N/A	0
Dinner subtotal	601	20	3.2	9.3	119
Snacks					
Pear, raw, 1 med	98	0.7	0	*N/A	0
Triscuits, reduced fat, 8 wafers	130	3	0.5	0	0
Snacks subtotal	228	3.7	0.5	0	0
Daily Total	1474	36.1	7.7	24.6	164
		22%	4.7%		
19% Protein					
56% Carbohydrate					

* N/A = Not Available

[a] Provided by Sandra Leonard, M.S., R.D.

placement on diets with the fat content lowered to 20 g/day. Alcohol should be eliminated from the diet, which also controls kcalories and increases exercise to optimize weight. Table 52.8 indicates some food choices and menu plans for TAG lowering in patients with more severe forms of hypertriglyceridemia (Type V). [20] Patients may respond rapidly to withdrawal of dietary fat, with TAG levels falling by 50%/day.

Diet and Lp(a)[22]

The only effects of diet on levels of Lp(a) are the decrease observed with trans-fatty acids. Niacin is the only intervention that lowers Lp(a). Therefore, the advice to individuals with elevated Lp(a) is to aggressively treat any known risk factors for CHD, especially elevated levels of LDL cholesterol.

Drug Management of Hyperlipidemias[4,23-26]

Patients with severe hypercholesterolemia (FH) are unlikely to reach desirable levels in terms of CHD prevention with diet alone. Therefore the trial of diet should be shortened and medication added. The diet trial is worthwhile in order to ascertain whether the subject is diet responsive. Patients with CHD and hypercholesterolemia who are at higher risk also may be placed on medication after a shortened diet trial period. Drug treatment should be monitored for efficacy and safety, and medication needs to be taken throughout life.

Drugs to Lower Cholesterol[23,24]

Drugs that primarily lower total and LDL cholesterol include: the bile acid-binding resins cholestyramine and colestipol, niacin and the statins (lovastatin, pravastatin, simvastatin, atorvastatin, fluvastatin, cerivastatin). Relative efficacy of these classes of drugs is depicted in Figure 52.9. Niacin and statins also increase HDL cholesterol. Side effects with resins (constipation) and niacin (flushing, hepatotoxicity) are more common and serious than those encountered with statins (hepatotoxicity, myositis). Drugs may need to be used in combination in the management of severe hypercholesterolemia. Timing of medication and efficacy in combination with food vary among these drugs, so that the patient must be advised appropriately by health caregiver or pharmacist.

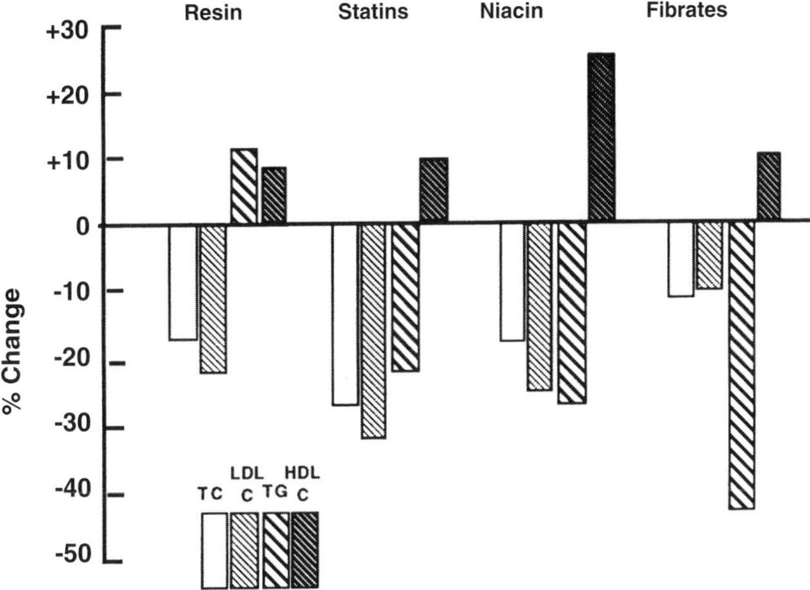

FIGURE 52.9
The efficacy of various lipid-lowering drugs in treating patients with hypercholesterolemia. Data represent the percent change in lipoprotein lipid levels from levels obtained from patients ingesting a baseline lipid-lowering diet.

Plasmapheresis has been used successfully for treating severe forms of FH that are poorly controlled with diet and multiple medications. Liver transplant may improve patients with homozygous FH.

Drugs Affecting TAG Levels[25,26]

Fibric acid derivatives (clofibrate, gemfibrozil, fenofibrate) and niacin are potent TAG-lowering medications that also increase HDL cholesterol. These medications should be added to the diet early in patients with Type V with severe elevations of TAG in order to prevent attacks of acute pancreatitis. At times the LDL levels will increase with fibric acid derivatives as VLDL and chylomicrons decrease, so that a statin may need to be combined with the initial agent. Side effects of fibric acid derivatives include lithogenic bile and gallstones, gastrointestinal distress, and myositis. Oral contraceptives, estrogens, or corticosteroids may raise triglycerides and worsen hypertriglyceridemia. TAG levels should be monitored carefully in patients with Type V using these drugs.

Additional relevant information may be found in Section 26, that addresses the laboratory assessment of lipids and lipoproteins and Section 51, that discusses the role of nutrition in preventing and modifying cardiovascular risk factors.

References

1. Semenkovich CF. In *Modern Nutrition in Health and Disease*, 9th ed, Shils ME, Olson JA, Shike M, Ross AC, Eds, Williams & Wilkins, Baltimore, 1999, ch 74.
2. Havel RJ, Kane JP. In: *The Metabolic and Molecular Bases of Inherited Disease*, 7th ed, Scriver CL, Beaudet AL, Sly WS, Valle D, Eds, McGraw Hill, NY, 1995, ch 56.
3. Feldman EB. In: *Modern Nutrition in Health and Disease*, 8th ed, Shils ME, Olson JA, Shike M, Eds, Lea & Febiger, Philadelphia, 1993, ch 72.
4. Grundy SM. In: *Modern Nutrition in Health and Disease*, 9th ed, (Shils ME, Olson JA, Shike M, Ross AC, Eds, Williams & Wilkins, Baltimore, 1999, ch 75.
5. Humphries SE, Peacock R, Gudnason V. In *Lipoproteins in Health and Disease,* Betteridge DJ, Illingworth DR, Shepherd J, Eds, Oxford University Press, NY, 1999.
6. Brunzell JD. In *The Metabolic and Molecular Bases of Inherited Disease*, 7th ed, Scriver CL, Beaudet AL, Sly WS, Valle D, Eds, McGraw Hill, NY, 1995, ch 59.
7. Santmarina-Fojo S. *Curr Opin Lipidology* 3: 186; 1992.
8. Brown MS, Goldstein JL. *Science* 232: 34; 1986.
9. Goldstein JL, Hobbs HH, Brown MS. In *The Metabolic and Molecular Bases of Inherited Disease*, 7th ed, Scriver CL, Beaudet AL, Sly WS, Valle D, Eds, McGraw Hill, NY, 1995, ch 62.
10. Sohar E, Bossak, ET, Wang CI, Adlersberg D. *Science* 123: 461; 1957.
11. Aouizerat BE, Allayee H, Cantor RM, et al. *Arterioscler Thromb Vasc Biol* 19: 2730; 19XX.
12. Kwiterovich PO, Jr. *Curr Opin Lipidology* 4: 133; 1993.
13. Campos H, Dreon DM, Krauss RM. *J Lipid Res* 34: 397; 1993.
14. Mahley RW, Rall SC, Jr. In *The Metabolic and Molecular Bases of Inherited Disease*, 7th ed, Scriver CL, Beaudet AL, Sly WS, Valle D, Eds, McGraw Hill, NY, 1995, ch 61.
15. Feldman EB. In *Essentials of Clinical Nutrition*. FA Davis, Philadelphia, 1988, ch 19.
16. Brewer HB, Jr. *Am J Cardiol* 83: 3F; 1999.
17. Austin MA, Hokanson HE, Edwards KL, *Am J Cardiol* 82: 7B; 19XX.
18. Grundy SM. *Circulation* 95: 1; 1997.
19. Greene JM, Feldman EB. *J Am Coll Nutr* 10: 443; 1991.
20. Bloch AS, Shils ME. In *Modern Nutrition in Health and Disease*, 9th ed, Shils ME, Olson JA, Shike M, Ross AC, Eds, Williams & Wilkins, Baltimore, 1999, pp A167, 170.
21. Harris WS. *Curr Opin Lipidology* 7: 3; 1996.

22. Nestel P, Noakes M, Belling B, et al. *J Lipid Res* 33: 1029; 1992.
23. Lipid Research Clinics Program. *JAMA* 251: 351; 1984.
24. Jones P, Kalonek S, Laurora I, Hunninghake D. for the CURVES Investigators, *Am J Cardiol* 81: 582; 1998.
25. Knopp RH, Waldaen CE, Rezlaff BM, et al. *JAMA* 278: 1509; 1997.
26. Goldberg AC, Schonfeld G, Feldman EB, et al. *Clin Ther* 11: 69; 1989.

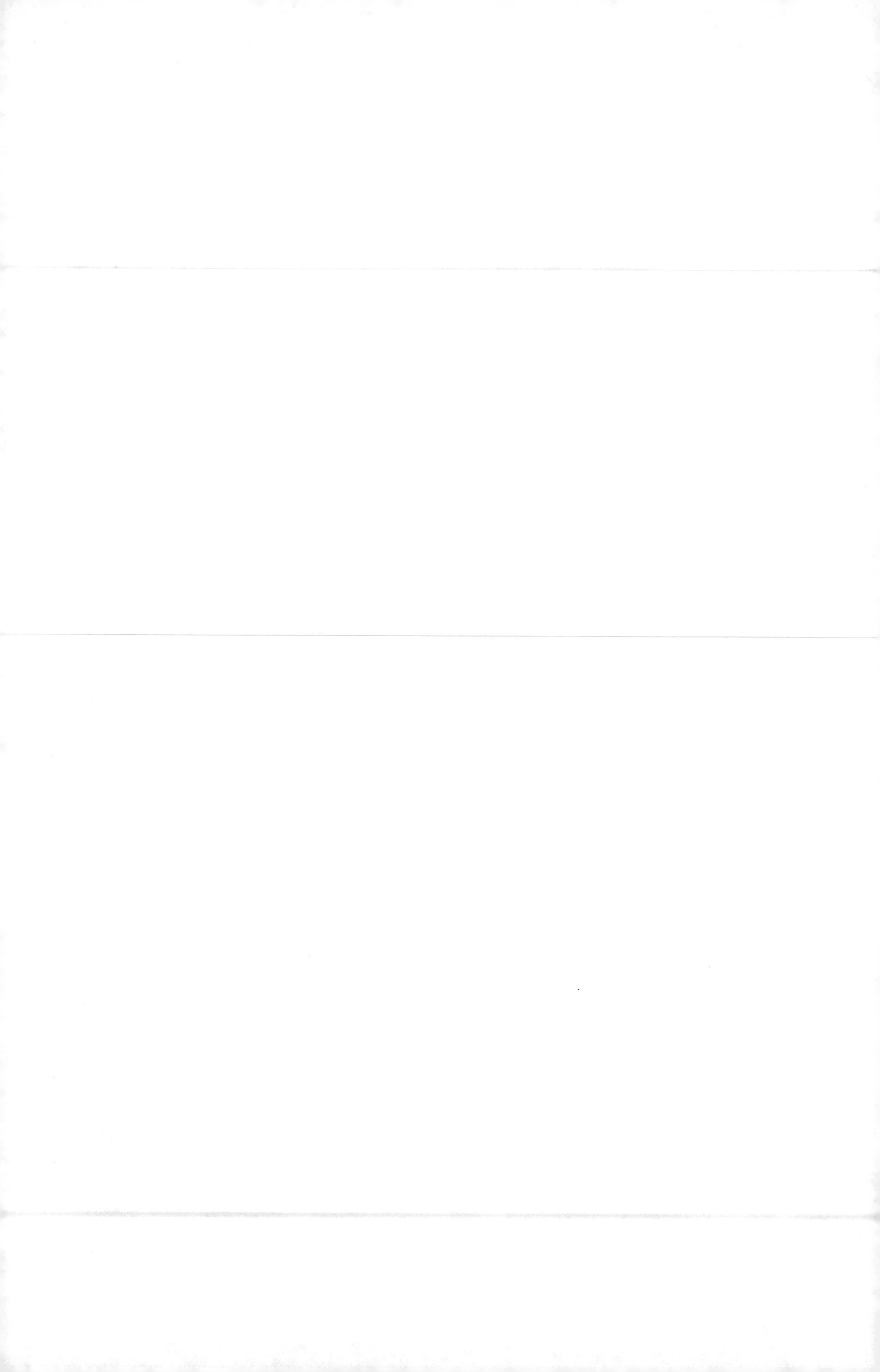

53

Nutrition in Diabetes Mellitus

Maria F. Lopes-Virella, Carolyn H. Jenkins, and Marina Mironova

Introduction

Diabetes mellitus is a common metabolic disorder.[1,2] The hallmark of diabetes is fasting and/or post-prandial hyperglycemia. Hyperglycemia results from insulin deficiency or interference with its action (insulin resistance) or both. Uncontrolled diabetes leads to widespread metabolic derangement. Sixteen million people in the United States have diabetes mellitus. The prevalence of diabetes is increasing at an alarming rate in all age groups, from children to the elderly. The disorder is progressively more common with advancing age. Fifty percent or more of the population after 80 to 90 years of age has glucose intolerance or diabetes. It is the sixth leading cause of death due to disease in the U.S. and decreases the average life expectancy up to 15 years when compared to the population without diabetes. Diabetes has an enormous social impact, mostly due to its chronic microvascular (retinopathy, nephropathy, and neuropathy) and macrovascular complications. Diabetic retinopathy is the leading cause of blindness in the U.S. In people with diabetes, age 20 to 74 years, there are 12,000 to 24,000 new cases of blindness each year. Diabetic nephropathy is responsible for a large number of the patients on renal dialysis and undergoing renal transplantation. In 1996 more than 130,000 people with diabetes underwent either dialysis or kidney transplantation. Diabetic neuropathy is present in 60 to 70% of all patients with diabetes. Besides increasing the risk for sudden death and silent myocardial infarction, diabetic neuropathy leads to impotence, which is experienced by 50% of men with diabetes. Diabetic neuropathy together with peripheral vascular disease is responsible for more than 200,000 cases of foot ulcers and 80,000 limb amputations each year. Finally, diabetes is also responsible for macrovascular complications including peripheral vascular disease, stroke, and cardiovascular disease. Cardiovascular disease is the leading cause of death in diabetes (80% of all patients with diabetes die of cardiovascular disease). Seventy five percent of the cardiovascular mortality in diabetes is from coronary heart disease and 25% is from cerebral or peripheral vascular disease. Coronary heart disease, peripheral vascular disease, and stroke account for nearly one million hospital admissions each year among patients with diabetes. In women, diabetes carries yet another burden since it may lead to problems during pregnancy — mainly congenital malformations in babies born to diabetic mothers. The rate of major

0-8493-2705-9/02/$0.00+$1.50

congenital malformations is 10% compared to 2% in non-diabetic women, and fetal mortality occurs in 3 to 5% of pregnancies.

Classification and Diagnostic Criteria of the Several Subtypes of Diabetes and Intermediate Syndromes

Classification of Diabetes Mellitus

Type 1 Diabetes

Type 1 diabetes is characterized by pancreatic β-cell destruction, usually leading to absolute insulin deficiency.[3,4] Its etiology is likely due to a combination of genetic and environment factors. Most type 1 diabetes is an organ-specific autoimmune disease characterized by T-cell mediated autoimmune destruction of the pancreatic β-cells. In a few cases there is no evidence of an autoimmune process, and these cases are classified as idiopathic.

Type 2 Diabetes

Type 2 diabetes is characterized by insulin resistance and an insulin secretory defect.[3,4] It is the most prevalent type of diabetes, and comprises 90% of the population with diabetes. As with type 1 diabetes, type 2 has both a genetic and an environment component. Type 2 diabetes may range from cases with predominantly insulin resistance and relative insulin deficiency to cases with a predominantly secretory defect and some degree of insulin resistance.

Other Specific Types of Diabetes

Genetic defects in β-cell function or in insulin action as well as several diseases of the exocrine pancreas, endocrinopathies, infections, drugs or chemicals, uncommon forms of immune-mediated diabetes, and other genetic syndromes that may lead to hyperglycemia are included under the definition of other specific types of diabetes. A comprehensive list is included in Table 53.1.

Gestational Diabetes (GDM)

Gestational diabetes is defined by any degree of glucose intolerance that is initially recognized during pregnancy. The type of treatment required to manage glucose intolerance in pregnancy and whether or not the glucose intolerance continues after pregnancy does not affect the diagnosis. Six or more weeks after pregnancy it is necessary to reclassify the patient and determine whether diabetes, impaired glucose tolerance, impaired fasting glucose, or normoglycemia is present. About 4% of all pregnancies are complicated by gestational diabetes, and the diagnosis is commonly made during the third trimester.

At present it is not recommended that all women be screened for gestational diabetes. Screening should, however, be performed in women if they a) are more than 25 years of age, b) are overweight, c) have family history of diabetes, or d) are Hispanic, Asian, Afro-American, or native American. The first test to be performed is a screening test using a 50 g load of glucose. If the screening test is positive, a 100 g diagnostic loading test needs to be performed.

TABLE 53.1

Etiologic Classification of Diabetes Mellitus

- I. Type I diabetes* (β-cell destruction, usually leading to absolute insulin deficiency)
  - A. Immune mediated
  - B. Idiopathic
- II. Type II diabetes* (may range from predominantly insulin resistance with relative insulin deficiency to a predominantly secretory defect)
- III. Other specific types
  - A. Genetic defects of β-cell function
    1. Chromosome 12, HNF-1a (MODY3)
    2. Chromosome 7, glucokinase (MODY2)
    3. Chromosome 20, HNF-4a (MODY1)
    4. Mitochondrial DNA
    5. Others
  - B. Genetic defects in insulin action
    1. Type A insulin resistance
    2. Leprechaunism
    3. Rabson — Mendenhall syndrome
    4. Lipoatrophic diabetes
    5. Others
  - C. Diseases of the exocrine pancreas
    1. Pancreatitis
    2. Trauma/pancreatectomy
    3. Neoplasia
    4. Cystic fibrosis
    5. Hemochromatosis
    6. Fibrocalculous pancreatopathy
    7. Others
  - D. Endocrinopathies
    1. Acromegaly
    2. Cushing's syndrome
    3. Glucagonoma
    4. Pheochromocytoma
    5. Hyperthyroidism
    6. Somatostatinoma
    7. Aldosteronoma
    8. Others
  - E. Drug- or chemical-induced
    1. Vacor
    2. Pentamidine
    3. Nicotinic acid
    4. Glucocorticoids
    5. Thyroid hormone
    6. Diazoxide
    7. β-adrenergic agonists
    8. Thiazides
    9. Dilantin
    10. α-interferon
    11. Others
  - F. Infections
    1. Congenital rubella
    2. Cytomegalovirus
    3. Others
  - G. Uncommon forms of immune-mediated diabetes
    1. "Stiff-man" syndrome
    2. Anti-insulin receptor antibodies
    3. Others
  - H. Other genetic syndromes sometimes associated with diabetes
    1. Down's syndrome

TABLE 53.1 *(Continued)*

Etiologic Classification of Diabetes Mellitus

2. Klinefelter's syndrome
3. Turner's syndrome
4. Wolfram's syndrome
5. Friedreich's ataxia
6. Huntington's chorea
7. Laurence-Moon-Biedl syndrome
8. Myotonic dystrophy
9. Porphyria
10. Prader-Willi syndrome
11. Others

IV. Gestational diabetes mellitus (GDM)

* Patients with any form of diabetes may require insulin treatment at some stage of their disease. Such use of insulin does not, of itself, classify the patient.

Reprinted with authorization from American Diabetes Association (*Diabetes Care* 23(1): 6S; 2000).

Impaired Glucose Tolerance and Impaired Fasting Glucose

These two syndromes are usually associated with an intermediate metabolic stage between normal glucose metabolism and diabetes. Impaired glucose tolerance is associated with levels of plasma glucose ≥140 mg/dl but <200 mg/dl after an oral load of 75 g of glucose. Patients with glucose intolerance are often hyperglycemic if challenged with an oral glucose load, but in normal conditions they may have normal or near-normal plasma glucose levels and hemoglobin A1c. Impaired fasting glucose corresponds to fasting levels of plasma glucose ≥110 mg/dl but <126 mg/dl. Neither of these two syndromes is a disease per se, but they are considered risk factors for the development of macrovascular disease and diabetes. They are considered as risk factors for macrovascular disease because both syndromes can be associated with the insulin resistance syndrome, a metabolic syndrome previously named by Reaven as syndrome X.[5] This syndrome includes visceral obesity, insulin resistance, compensatory hyperinsulinemia, hypertriglyceridemia, low HDL-cholesterol, hypertension, and the presence of dense LDL. The two syndromes can also be observed in the disease processes listed in Table 53.1. Interestingly however, a recent study by Tominaga et al.[6] examining the cumulative survival rates from cardiovascular disease in a Japanese population of 2534 individuals with normal glucose tolerance, impaired glucose tolerance, impaired fasting glucose, or diabetes showed no significant difference between the survival rates from cardiovascular disease in subjects with normal glucose tolerance and subjects with impaired fasting glucose, but a significant decrease in survival in subjects with impaired glucose tolerance and diabetes. They therefore concluded that impaired glucose tolerance was a risk factor for cardiovascular disease, but impaired fasting glucose was not.

Diagnostic Criteria

The diagnostic criteria for diabetes, for type 1, type 2, and other specific types of diabetes, have been modified recently. In the past, the criteria used was that recommended by the National Diabetes Data Group[3] or World Health Organization (WHO);[1] the revised criteria are shown in Table 53.2. For epidemiological studies determining prevalence and/or incidence of diabetes, the first criterion (fasting plasma glucose >126 mg/dl) can be used, but it will lead to slightly lower estimates of prevalence/incidence than the combined use of the fasting plasma glucose and oral glucose tolerance test. That is clearly demonstrated by the data obtained in NHANES III[2] as summarized in Table 53.3. WHO criteria were

TABLE 53.2

Criteria for the Diagnosis of Diabetes Mellitus*

1. Symptoms of diabetes plus casual plasma glucose concentration ≥200 mg/dl (11.1 mmol/l). Casual is defined as any time of day without regard to time since last meal. The classic symptoms of diabetes include polyuria, polydipsia, and unexpected weight loss.

or

2. FPG ≥126 mg/dl (7.0 mmol/l). Fasting is defined as no caloric intake for at least 8 h.

or

3. 2-h PG ≥200 mg/dl (11.1 mmol/l) during an OGTT. The test should be performed as described by WHO (2), using a glucose load containing the equivalent of 75-g anhydrous glucose dissolved in water.

* In the absence of unequivocal hyperglycemia with acute metabolic decompensation, these criteria should be confirmed by repeat testing on a different day. The third measure (OGTT) is not recommended for routine clinical use.

Reprinted with authorization from American Diabetes Association (*Diabetes Care* 23(1): 11S; 2000).

TABLE 53.3

Estimated Prevalence of Diabetes in the U.S. in Individuals 40 to 74 Years of Age using Data from the NHANES III

Diabetes Diagnostic Criteria	Prevalence (%) of Diabetes by Glucose Criteria without a Medical History of Diabetes*	Total Diabetes Prevalence (%)#
Medical history of diabetes	—	7.92
WHO (2) criteria for diabetes:		
FPG ≥140 mg/dl (7.8 mmol/l) or 2-h PG ≥200 mg/dl (11.1 mmol/l)	6.34	14.26
FPG ≥126 mg/dl (7.0 mmol/l)	4.35	12.27

* Diabetes prevalence (by glucose criteria) in those without a medical history of diabetes × (100%-prevalence of diabetes by medical history).

\# First column of data plus 7.92.

Data are from K. Flegal, National Center for Health Statistics, personal communication. Reprinted with authorization from American Diabetes Association (*Diabetes Care* 23(1): 11S; 2000).

based on the fact that the prevalence of retinopathy and nephropathy would rise markedly when the level of glucose 2 h after a standardized glucose load was >200 mg/dl. The revised criteria are based on results of several studies showing that fasting plasma level >126 mg/dl, like a 2-h post glucose load of >200 mg/dl, is associated with a marked rise in the prevalence of vascular complications.[4] In other words, levels of glucose ≥126 mg/dl reflect a serious metabolic disorder associated with the development of serious chronic diabetic complications.

Impaired fasting glucose is defined by glucose levels ≥110 mg/dl and <126 mg/dl after an eight-hour fast. Impaired glucose tolerance is defined by a level of glucose ≥140 mg/dl but <200 mg/dl two hours after a 75 g oral glucose load. The impaired glucose tolerance criteria will identify more people with impaired glucose homeostasis than the criteria of impaired fasting glucose.

Criteria for Screening for Diabetes

Screening for type 1 diabetes is not recommended. Type 1 diabetes is commonly an autoimmune process characterized by a variety of auto-antibodies against intracellular or

TABLE 53.4

Major Risk Factors for Diabetes Mellitus

Family history of diabetes (i.e., parents or siblings with diabetes)
Obesity (i.e., ≥20% over desired body weight or BMI ≥27 kg/m^2)
Race/ethnicity (i.e., African-Americans, Hispanic-Americans, Native Americans, Asian-Americans, Pacific Islanders)
Age ≥45 years
Previously identified IFG or IGT
Hypertension (≥140/90 mm Hg)
HDL cholesterol level ≥35 mg/dl (0.90 mmol/l) and/or a triglyceride level ≥250 mg/dl (2.82/l)
History of GDM or delivery of babies over 9 lb

Reprinted with authorization from American Diabetes Association (*Diabetes Care* 23(1): 21S; 2000).

surface protein epitopes in the β-cell. The markers that may identify patients at risk before development of the disease are many. However, the levels of the markers that would permit the diagnosis of high-risk patients are not well established. Furthermore, the methodology is not easily accessible, and there is no consensus about what to do if high levels of auto-antibodies are observed. Nowadays, there is no effective and safe treatment to prevent the development of type 1 diabetes. A number of ongoing clinical trials testing various ways to prevent the development of type 1 diabetes are being conducted, and it is possible that in the near future, screening for patients at high risk for developing type 1 diabetes will be justifiable. At present the cost effectiveness and clinical relevance of such testing is questionable.

Screening for type 2 diabetes is, however, highly recommended. Undiagnosed type 2 diabetes is very common in the U.S. Approximately 50% of patients with type 2 diabetes are undiagnosed.[7] Some epidemiological studies have shown that retinopathy will start developing seven years prior to making the diagnosis of diabetes.[8] Even more worrisome is the fact that patients with undiagnosed diabetes are at significantly higher risk of developing premature macrovascular disease.[9] The risk of developing type 2 diabetes increases with age, obesity, and lack of physical activity. Furthermore, diabetes is more common in certain racial/ethnic groups (Hispanic, Asian, African-Americans, and native Americans), in women with gestational diabetes, and in individuals with a family history of diabetes, hypertension, or dyslipidemia. The major risk factors for developing diabetes are listed in Table 53.4.

The American Diabetes Association (ADA) recommends screening individuals who have one or more of the risk factors shown in Table 53.4 at three-year intervals. Fasting plasma glucose measurement or oral glucose tolerance test are adequate to perform screening for diabetes. Fasting, as mentioned before, represents a period of at least eight hours without food or beverage other than water. When an oral glucose tolerance test is performed, a load of 75 g of anhydrous glucose is considered the standard load for adult testing. Interpretation of the results is crucial, and should be made according to the criteria shown in Table 53.5. It is important to remember that certain drugs including furosemide, glucocorticosteroids, thiazides, estrogen-containing preparations, β-blockers, and nicotinic acid may induce hyperglycemia. In community screening tests it is sometimes impossible to use a fasting plasma glucose assay; therefore, a fasting capillary whole blood glucose is performed due to its convenience and simplicity of measurement. The levels are not, however, as accurate as those measured in plasma, and they are lower. If the measurement is made in capillary whole blood, individuals with blood glucose ≥110 mg/dl should be referred to a physician for further evaluation and testing. Criteria for diagnosis of gestational diabetes mellitus (GDM) is summarized in Table 53.6.

TABLE 53.5

Criteria for the Diagnosis of Diabetes Mellitus using Glucose Tolerance Results

Normoglycemia	Impaired Glucose Metabolism	DM*
FPG < 110 mg/dl	FPG ≥ 110 mg/dl and < 126 mg/dl	FPG ≥ 126 mg/dl
2-h PG† < 140 mg/dl	2-h PG† ≥ 140 mg/dl and < 200 mg/dl	2-h PG† ≥ 200 mg/dl
		Symptoms of DM and random plasma glucose concentration ≥ 200 mg/dl

* A diagnosis of diabetes must be confirmed on a subsequent day by measurement of FPG, 2-h PG or random plasma glucose (if symptoms are present). The FPG test is greatly preferred because of ease of administration, acceptability to patients, and lower cost. Fasting is defined as no caloric intake for at least 8 h.

† This test requires the use of a glucose load containing 75 g anhydrous glucose dissolved in water.

* DM, diabetes mellitus; 2-h PG, 2-h postload glucose.

Reprinted with authorization from American Diabetes Association (*Diabetes Care* 23(1): 21S; 2000).

TABLE 53.6

Screening and Diagnosis Scheme for Gestational Diabetes Mellitus (GDM)*

Plasma Glucose	75-g Oral Glucose Load	100-g Oral Glucose Load
Fasting	95 mg/dl	95 mg/dl
1-h	180 mg/dl	180 mg/dl
2-h	155 mg/dl	155 mg/dl
3-h	not done	140 mg/dl

* The diagnosis of GDM requires any two or more plasma glucose values obtained during the test to meet or exceed the values shown above.

Reprinted with authorization from American Diabetes Association (*Diabetes Care* 23(1): 78S; 2000).

Diabetic Complications: Microvascular

Retinopathy

Diabetic retinopathy is a specific microvascular complication present in both type 1 and type 2 diabetes, strongly correlated with the duration of diabetes. After 20 years of diabetes, nearly all patients with type 1 diabetes and more than 60% of the patients with type 2 diabetes will have some degree of retinopathy.[10]

Retinopathy can be defined as damage to the retina, a cell layer in the posterior part of the eye that contains the photoreceptors necessary for vision. It can be classified as mild, nonproliferative (also called background retinopathy), or moderate to severe non-proliferative retinopathy, characterized by hard exudates and retinal blot hemorrhages. This type of retinopathy advances to a preproliferative phase when retinal ischemia becomes more severe. Proliferative retinopathy is the most advanced stage of retinopathy, and is characterized by the growth of new blood vessels on the retina and posterior surface of the vitreous. Proliferative retinopathy usually leads to loss of vision due to retinal detachment, and is the leading cause of blindness in persons 30 to 65 years of age. Vision loss may also occur in patients without proliferative retinopathy when vascular leakage (macular edema) and/or occlusion occurs in the area of the macula. Maculopathy is more common in type 2 than type 1 diabetes and is an important cause for decreased visual acuity in this group of patients.

TABLE 53.7

Screening and Followup of Patients with Diabetes for Retinopathy

	Recommended Ophthalmologic Examination*	Recommended Minimum Followup
Type 1 diabetes > 10 years of age	Within 3-5 years after onset of disease	Yearly
Type 2 diabetes	At the time of diagnosis of diabetes	Yearly or more often if retinopathy is progressing
Diabetic patients during pregnancy	Prior to conception if programmed and during the 1st trimester	As often as necessary, according to physician
Patients with macular edema, severe proliferative retinopathy	Immediately after diagnosis of the condition	As often as necessary, according to physician

* The ophthalmologic exam recommended is a dilated and comprehensive exam by an ophthalmologist or optometrist.

Screening

Screening for the presence of retinopathy depends on the rates of progression of diabetic retinopathy and the risk factors that may alter these rates. Most of the available data is based on studies on Caucasian populations, and it is not certain whether these data can be applied to the ethnic groups with the highest incidence of diabetes and complications. The guidelines for screening and followup of patients with diabetic retinopathy are summarized in Table 53.7.

Influence of Glycemic Control and Treatment of Hypertension and Dyslipidemia

Data from the Diabetes Control and Complications Trial Research Group (DCCT) clearly show a definitive and direct relationship between glycemic control and diabetic microvascular complications, including retinopathy.[11] The DCCT shows that intensive insulin therapy for type 1 diabetes reduced or prevented the progression of diabetic retinopathy by 27% when compared with conventional therapy. Similar results were observed in type 2 diabetes as shown by the U.K. Prospective Diabetes Study Group (UKPDS).[12,13] The earlier that intensive control is started in the course of diabetes, the more effective it is in preventing the development of retinopathy. Besides poor glycemic control, proteinuria is also associated with retinopathy. Hypertension is an established risk factor for proteinuria. Thus, it is important to tightly control hypertension. Finally, maculopathy consists of edema and/or lipid exudates; since the lipid exudates observed in cases of maculopathy originate from circulating blood lipids, aggressive treatment of lipid abnormalities is also important in the prevention of retinopathy/maculopathy.

The main reason that screening for diabetic retinopathy is essential is the well known efficacy of laser photocoagulation therapy in patients with proliferative retinopathy and macular edema. The surgery, as well demonstrated in the Early Treatment Diabetic Retinopathy Study and the Diabetic Retinopathy Study, is extremely efficient in preventing loss of vision, but does not have much impact in reversing visual acuity if already diminished. Since proliferative retinopathy and macular edema are quite often asymptomatic, screening is crucial.

Neuropathy

Symptomatic and potentially disabling neuropathy affects nearly 50% of diabetic patients. Neuropathy can be symmetrical or focal, and often involves the autonomic nervous

TABLE 53.8

Classification of Diabetic Neuropathy

Diabetic Polyneuropathies	Diabetic Mononeuropathies
Distal symmetrical	Peripheral
Chronic sensorimotor	Cranial
Autonomic	Radiculopathy
Proximal motor	Isolated nerve lesions
Acute sensory	

TABLE 53.9

Symptoms and Signs of Diabetic Polyneuropathy

	Symptoms	Signs
Polyneuropathy	Pain and paresthesias most common at night	Diminished sensation to touch, temperature, pain, and vibration; loss of reflexes Atrophy of intrinsic hand muscles; sensory impairment

system. The prevalence of symmetrical neuropathy is similar in type 1 and type 2 diabetes, but the focal forms of neuropathy are more common in the older type 2 diabetic patient. The classification of neuropathy is made according to the areas affected due to the relatively poor understanding of the pathogenic mechanisms of this diabetic complication. Table 53.8 includes the most commonly accepted classification of diabetic neuropathic syndromes.

The cause for mononeuropathies is unknown, but they usually have a sudden onset, which suggests a vascular component in their pathogenesis. They usually tend to resolve with time, and although they occur in diabetes they are not the typical neuropathic lesions of diabetes. Diabetic polyneuropathies are the main problem for diabetic patients, and they will be discussed in some detail. To assess diabetic neuropathy, history of clinical symptoms and physical exam, electrodiagnostic studies, quantitative sensory testing, and autonomic function testing should be performed. Table 53.9 summarizes the clinical signs and symptoms of diabetic polyneuropathy, and Table 53.10 summarizes the functional changes associated with autonomic failure. In Table 53.11, adequate diagnostic testing to assess diabetic neuropathy is summarized.

TABLE 53.10

Functional Changes Associated with Autonomic Failure

Systems Involved	Manifestations
Cardiovascular	Resting tachycardia, impaired exercise-induced cardiovascular responses, cardiac denervation, orthostatic hypotension, heat intolerance, impaired vasodilatation, impaired venoarteriolar reflex (dependent edema)
Eye	Decreased diameter of dark-adapted pupil (dark-adapted miosis)
Gastrointestinal	Esophageal enteropathy, gallbladder atony, impaired colonic motility (diarrhea, constipation), anorectal sphincter dysfunction (incontinence)
Genitourinary	Neurogenic vesical dysfunction (decreased bladder sensitivity/incontinence/retention), sexual dysfunction, (male: penile erectile failure and retrograde ejaculation; female: defective lubrication)
Sudomotor	Anhidrosis/hyperhidrosis (heat intolerance), gustatory sweating
Endocrine	Hypoglycemia-associated autonomic failure

Reprinted with authorization from American Diabetes Association (*Diabetes Care* 19(1): 82S; 1996).

TABLE 53.11

Electrodiagnostic Studies, Sensory Testing, and Autonomic Function Testing for the Diagnosis of Diabetic Neuropathy

Sensory Testing	Electrodiagnosis	Autonomic Function Testing
Vibration/touch thresholds Thermal thresholds Pain thresholds	Motor and sensory nerve conduction studies Needle electromyography of extremity and paraspinal muscles	R-R variations, orthostasis, Valsalva Resting heart rate QTc, DAPS, NPT, CMG+BST REPs, QSART, TST Solid phase gastric motility Clamped hypoglycemia Clamped insulin infusion test

Abbreviations: QTc — corrected QT interval on EKG; DAPS — dark-adapted pupil size; NPT — nocturnal penile tumescence, CMG+BST — cystometrogram+Bethanechol supersensivity test; REPs — reflex-evoked potentials; QSART — quantitative sudomotor axon reflex test; TST — thermoregulated sweat test.

TABLE 53.12

Definition of Abnormalities in Albumin Excretion

	24-h Collection	Timed Collection	Spot Collection
Normal	<30 mg/24 h	<20μg/min	<30 mg/g creatinine
Microalbuminuria* (incipient nephropathy)	30-300 mg/24 h	20-200 μg/min	30-300 mg/g creatinine
Nephropathy*	>300 mg/24 h	>200 μg/min	>300 mg/g creatinine

* Two out of three urine specimens collected within a 3 to 6 month period should be abnormal before diagnosing a patient as having incipient nephropathy or nephropathy.

Influence of Glycemic Control

Data from the DCCT and UKPDS clearly show a definitive and direct relationship between glycemic control and diabetic microvascular complications, including neuropathy.[11-13] The DCCT data showed that intensive insulin therapy when compared with conventional therapy reduced or prevented the progression of diabetic neuropathy in patients with type 1 diabetes. The UKPDS showed the same results in patients with type 2 diabetes.

Nephropathy

Diabetic nephropathy is characterized by persistent albumin excretion exceeding 300 mg/24 h, a progressive decline in the glomerular filtration rate, and increased blood pressure.[14] The earliest clinical evidence of nephropathy is the increased excretion of albumin in the urine. This phase of incipient nephropathy is designated as microalbuminuria. The levels of albumin excretion in the microalbuminuria stage of nephropathy range from 30 to 300 mg/24 h. Table 53.12 summarizes the cutoff levels for diagnostic purposes as well as the correspondent values in spot urine collections. Measurement of creatinine and albumin excretion simultaneously in the same urine specimen is necessary when a spot urine is collected, and it is also recommended in timed specimens to ensure that a proper urine collection was obtained. Interpretation of microalbuminuria needs to take into consideration factors such as hyperglycemia, level of exercise preceding the urine collection, uncontrolled hypertension, urinary tract infections, acute febrile illnesses, and heart failure, since all of these conditions may lead to increased albuminuria. Diagnosis of nephropathy needs to be based on data from three urine specimens collected within a three- to six-month period. At least two of the specimens may be concordant to allow establishment of a valid diagnosis.

About 20 to 30% of patients with type 1 or type 2 diabetes develop nephropathy. A high percentage of subjects with type 2 diabetes are found to have microalbuminuria shortly after their initial diagnosis. Two possible reasons are that in many cases diabetes has been present for many years and not diagnosed, and microalbuminuria in type 2 diabetes is less specific of diabetic nephropathy, as shown by renal biopsy studies.

Approximately 80% of individuals with type 1 diabetes who develop sustained microalbuminuria will progress to overt nephropathy over a period of 10 to 15 years. Once overt nephropathy occurs and if there is no therapeutic intervention, 50% of these patients will progress to end-stage renal disease in 10 years, and 75% in 20 years. The progression to overt nephropathy in type 2 diabetes, without therapeutic intervention, is less than in type 1 diabetes (approximately in 20 to 40% of the cases), and only approximately 20% will progress to end-stage renal disease. A marked racial/ethnic variability exists, however, as far as progression to end-stage renal disease in type 2 diabetes. Native Americans, Mexican-Americans and African-Americans have a much higher risk of developing end-stage renal disease than the other populations with type 2 diabetes. In the U.S., diabetic nephropathy is responsible for one third of all cases of end-stage renal disease, and that is a terrible burden in the country's economy. Regardless of the fact that subjects with type 1 diabetes are more prone to progress to end-stage renal disease, half of the patients with diabetes on dialysis have type 2 diabetes due to the higher prevalence of type 2 diabetes in the population.

Two major risk factors that can be easily intervened upon are involved in the progression of nephropathy: hypertension and hyperglycemia. The standards of care for hypertension and hyperglycemia in diabetes will be discussed later in this section.

Influence of Hypertension and Glycemic Control

In type 1 diabetes, hypertension is usually caused by the underlying diabetic nephropathy, and typically is detected at the time microalbuminuria becomes apparent. In type 2 diabetes, hypertension is present at the time diabetes is diagnosed in one third of the patients. The hypertension may be related to the underlying diabetic nephropathy, may be secondary to other diseases, or may be a coexisting disease, "essential hypertension." Commonly, subjects with type 2 diabetes, before being diagnosed as having diabetes, have been found to have an insulin resistance syndrome, which basically comprises a cluster of problems including hypertension, obesity, dyslipidemia, and glucose intolerance. The presence of both systolic and diastolic hypertension contributes to the accelerated development of diabetic nephropathy, and therefore treating hypertension aggressively in patients with diabetes is an essential step that cannot be overemphasized.

Hyperglycemia has been shown in recent trials to have a major impact in the development of microvascular complications, including nephropathy. Intensive treatment of diabetes to obtain near-normal glucose and hemoglobin A1c levels has significantly reduced the risk of development of microalbuminuria and overt nephropathy.[11-13]

Influence of Protein Restriction and Treatment of Lipid Disorders

It is well known that microalbuminuria is a marker for increased cardiovascular mortality and morbidity in patients with either type 1 or type 2 diabetes. In reality, microalbuminuria is considered as an indicator to screen patients for macrovascular complications (see Macrovascular Complications). Interestingly, some preliminary evidence also shows that lowering cholesterol leads to a reduction in the level of proteinuria. More work is needed to adequately validate this observation. Protein restriction has been shown to be of great benefit in animal studies to reduce progression of renal disease, including diabetic nephropathy. However, studies in humans are less clear. Several small studies seem to indicate that patients with overt nephropathy treated with a diet containing protein at 0.7 g/kg of body weight had mild retardation in the fall of the glomerular filtration rate. A recent study of patients with renal disease in which 3% had type 2 diabetes failed to show any benefit of protein restriction. In reality, marked decrease of protein intake in patients with end-stage renal disease on dialysis showed that the main predictive factor of mortality was low albumin due to protein-energy malnutrition.

Diabetic Complications: Macrovascular Disease

General Considerations

Macrovascular disease, which includes coronary artery disease (CAD), cerebrovascular disease, and peripheral vascular disease, is the leading cause of mortality in people with diabetes. Individuals with diabetes have at least a two- to fourfold increased risk of cardiovascular events and stroke, and an eightfold increased likelihood of peripheral vascular disease compared with age-matched subjects without diabetes. The atherosclerotic process in diabetic patients is indistinguishable from that affecting the nondiabetic population, but begins earlier and is more severe. Most deaths in the diabetic population are due to complications of CAD. Although diabetic patients have a higher prevalence of traditional CAD risk factors (i.e., hypertension, dyslipidemia, obesity) compared to people without diabetes, these risk factors account for less than half the excess mortality associated with diabetes. Thus, the diagnosis of diabetes is a major independent risk factor for the development of CAD and adverse outcomes following a myocardial event. Other abnormalities induced by diabetes such as increased levels of small, dense atherogenic LDL, oxidized or glycated LDL, increased platelet aggregation, hyperviscosity, endothelial cell dysfunction, decreased fibrinolysis, and increased clotting factors and fibrinogen are likely responsible for accelerated atherosclerosis in diabetic patients.

Current Treatment and Prevention Strategies

Current treatment of macrovascular complications includes reduction of cardiovascular risk factors (obesity, smoking, sedentary lifestyle), with special emphasis on the treatment of hypertension and dyslipidemia. Diabetic patients with existing or incipient macrovascular disease in general require multiple modifications of lifestyle and diet, as well as a polypharmaceutical approach to address the optimization of lipid level, blood pressure, and other disease risk factors. Glycemic control seems also to contribute to a reduction in macrovascular events both in type 1 and type 2 diabetes, but its impact is much less marked than impact of treatment of cardiovascular risk factors such as dyslipidemia and hypertension.

Treatment of Hypertension

Hypertension accelerates not only atherosclerosis, but also nephropathy and probably retinopathy. Thus in diabetes, it is important to treat even minimal elevations of blood pressure that in nondiabetic patients might be dismissed. The normal nocturnal fall in blood pressure may be lost in diabetic patients, leading to a more sustained hypertension throughout the day. Initially, nonpharmacologic measures such as weight loss, exercise training, and sodium restriction should be implemented (see Section 48). If blood pressure is not lower than 130/85 mmHg, drug therapy is indicated. Among the various therapeutic options, ACE inhibitors offer special advantages, mainly when there is concomitant renal disease. Calcium channel blockers and vasodilators have no adverse metabolic effects, and therefore are good alternatives.

Treatment of Dyslipidemia

Dyslipidemia is common in subjects with diabetes. The more common lipid abnormalities in diabetes are increased triglycerides and low HDL cholesterol levels. Small, cholesterol-poor, dense LDL particles are also common in patients with hypertriglyceridemia and the insulin resistance syndrome. Dense LDL is more readily oxidized and more atherogenic. Aggressive treatment of dyslipoproteinemia is crucial to prevent the development and/or progression of macrovascular complications in diabetes.[15] Recommendations by the ADA concerning goals for therapy of hyperlipidemia as well as guidelines for medical nutrition therapy (MNT), physical activity, and drug treatment have been widely promulgated. Optimal triglyceride levels in diabetes are below 150 mg/dl, as in nondiabetic patients. This level was recommended by the National Cholesterol Education Program Adult Treatment Panel III (NCEP0-ATP III) on the recently released guidelines[15a] and it is lower than the 200 mg/dl previously recommended by both the NCEP-ATP II and the ADA. HDL-cholesterol levels above 45 mg/dl are the target in diabetes. According to ADA guidelines and the NCEP-ATP III guidelines, values below 40 μg/dl for men and above 50 mg/dl are used to define the metabolic syndrome. Levels of HDL-cholesterol below 40 mg/dl instead of 35 mg/dl are considered in the new NCEP guidelines a risk factor for CHD. The AFCAPS-Tex CAPS trial was instrumental in this change since it showed clearly that CHD risk decreases with levels of HDL-cholesterol above 40 mg/dl. Weight loss, increased physical activity, and good glycemic control are important measures to lower triglycerides and increase HDL-cholesterol levels. Increased LDL-cholesterol levels were not considered important in the treatment of diabetic dyslipidemia until recently. However, in the past decade it became apparent that lowering LDL-cholesterol levels in diabetes led to a significant reduction in the risk of a major congestive heart disease (CHD) event. That was clearly shown in several clinical trials including two major secondary prevention trials: Scandinavian Simvastatin Survival Study[16] and CARE trial.[17] The results of these trials were instrumental in the establishment of the guidelines to treat dyslipidemia in diabetes recently published by the ADA, and together with the results of several studies, among them the East West Study,[17a] were behind the change in the NCEP-ATP III guidelines that now considers diabetes as a CHD equivalent. Optimal LDL-cholesterol levels for adults with diabetes are <100 mg/dl, regardless of their risk factor profile or presence or absence of established cardiovascular disease.

Indications for Cardiac Testing

Asymptomatic CAD and silent myocardial infarction (MI) are frequent in subjects with diabetes. Thus, early diagnosis of CAD in patients with diabetes is very important, and allows earlier implementation of preventive programs aimed at reducing the risk of future coronary morbidity and mortality, initiation of treatment with anti-ischemic medications in silent ischemia, and earlier identification of patients in whom revascularization is appropriate. Indications for cardiac testing are summarized in Table 53.13.

Diabetic Complications: Hypoglycemia

It is well established that glycemic control will prevent specific long-term complications of diabetes. However, in order to prevent complications intensive treatment of diabetes is necessary, and unfortunately this may lead to hypoglycemia. It is obvious that even in optimal conditions, hypoglycemia is the limiting factor in the management of patients

TABLE 53.13

Indications for Cardiac Testing in Diabetic Patients

Testing for CAD is warranted in patients with the following:

1. Typical or atypical cardiac symptoms
2. Resting EKG suggestive of ischemia or infarction
3. Peripheral or carotid occlusive arterial disease
4. Sedentary lifestyle, age ≥ 35 years, and plans to begin a vigorous exercise program
5. Two or more of the risk factors listed below (a-e) in addition to diabetes
   a) Total cholesterol ≥ 240 mg/dl, LDL cholesterol ≥ 160 mg/dl, or HDL cholesterol < 35 mg/dl
   b) Blood pressure > 140/90 mm Hg
   c) Smoking
   d) Family history of premature CAD
   e) Positive micro/macroalbuminuria test

Reprinted with authorization from American Diabetes Association (*Diabetes Care* 21: 1551; 1998).

with type 1 diabetes. Hypoglycemia is defined as a blood glucose of ≤60 mg/dl that may occur with or without symptoms.[18] During the course of the DCCT trial and even under optimal conditions, the incidence of severe hypoglycemia was more than three times higher in patients on intensive therapy when compared with patients treated with conventional therapy. The effects of hypoglycemia cannot be ignored, since they can be devastating, particularly on the brain. The first signs of hypoglycemia are shakiness, sweating, tachycardia, hunger, irritability, and dizziness. These symptoms are followed by inability to concentrate, confusion, slurred speech, irrational behavior, blurred vision, and extreme fatigue. Finally, the symptoms of severe hypoglycemia are seizures, unresponsiveness, and loss of consciousness. Symptoms of hypoglycemia may occur at any time, and therefore patients with diabetes should always be prepared to address them.

The level of glucose that leads to symptoms of hypoglycemia may vary from person to person and also varies in the same individual under different circumstances. Hypoglycemia is a much less frequent problem for people with type 2 diabetes except in the elderly, mainly when they have associated diseases that require the use of beta blockers. Hypoglycemia usually occurs gradually, and in general is associated with warning signs, including rapid heart beat, perspiration, shakiness, anxiety, and hunger. However, warning symptoms of hypoglycemia may be absent, causing the clinical syndrome of hypoglycemia unawareness. This syndrome results from excessive insulin in the setting of absent glucagon secretory responses to falling glucose levels. These episodes, in turn, cause reduced autonomic responses and lead to further decrease of the warning symptoms of hypoglycemia. This creates a vicious cycle that can only be broken by avoiding inducing iatrogenic hypoglycemia. The most common causes of hypoglycemia include: a) skipping, delaying, or reducing the size of the meals and snacks; b) increased physical activity without adequately adjusting therapy; c) alcohol intake mainly on an empty stomach; and d) treatment with excessively high levels of insulin or other antidiabetic medications. Hypoglycemia occurs mainly when the patient is being treated with insulin or sulphonylureas. In theory, biguanidines, thiazolidinediones, and α-glucosidase inhibitors would not be expected to induce hypoglycemia, since by themselves they will not increase the level of plasma insulin. However, it is conceivable that any intervention that limits hepatic glucose production, favors glucose utilization, or both may lead to hypoglycemia, since increased hepatic glucose production and limited glucose utilization are mechanisms of defense against a drop in plasma glucose levels. In the elderly, it is not uncommon to have hypoglycemia episodes, and these may be dangerous since these subjects often live alone. A recent study examining the risk of sulphonylurea-induced hypoglycemia in elderly type

2 diabetic patients concluded that therapy with sulphonylureas is well tolerated by the elderly, and that the primary mechanism of protection against hypoglycemia is an increase in epinephrine secretion.[19] That suggests that glucagon secretion in elderly patients is diminished, and supports the concept that treatment of these patients with sulphonylureas or insulin when they are also being treated with β-blockers may be dangerous, and close followup is needed. Oral antidiabetic agents other than sulphonylureas are probably better candidates for the treatment of these patients if their hyperglycemia is relatively modest. Although hypoglycemia during treatment with these agents may also occur, it is likely to be less frequently observed and less severe.

Standards of Medical Care for Diabetic Patients

Standards of medical care for diabetic patients have been markedly influenced by the results of recent major clinical trials. Some of the trials were specifically designed to address the importance of intensive glycemic control in subjects with type 1 or type 2 diabetes (DCCT and UKPDS). Some clinical trials, although not designed to specifically address questions related to diabetic patients, had a sufficiently large number of patients with type 2 diabetes and glucose intolerance to allow drawing conclusions on the effect of lipid-lowering therapy in the development of macrovascular complications (CARE, 4S, AF-CAPS/TEX-CAPS). The data published concerning these trials as well as the technical reviews of the ADA[20] will provide evidence for the standard-of-care measures proposed by the ADA for the treatment of patients with diabetes.

Standards of diabetes care are expected to provide health care providers taking care of patients with diabetes the means to establish treatment goals, assess the quality of the diabetes treatment provided, identify areas where more self management is needed, and define situations when referral to specialists is necessary. Also, the same standards of diabetes care should allow patients with diabetes to assess the quality of medical care that they receive, understand their role in the treatment of their disease, and compare their treatment outcomes with standard goals.

General Principles

It is accepted that lowering blood glucose levels to normal or near-normal levels will reduce:

- The danger of acute decompensation due to diabetic ketoacydosis or hyperosmolar hyperglycemic nonketotic syndrome
- The symptoms of blurred vision and symptoms/signs usually accompanying diabetes (polyuria, polydipsia, weight loss with polyphagia, fatigue) as well as vaginitis or balanitis
- The development or progression of diabetic retinopathy, nephropathy, and neuropathy
- Triglycerides leading to a less atherogenic lipid profile

It is also well accepted that lowering lipid levels will result in a decrease in diabetic macrovascular complications.

Thus, proper standards of diabetes care should include:

- Appropriate frequency of self monitoring of blood glucose
- Adequate medical nutrition therapy
- Regular exercise
- Adequate regimens with insulin and/or oral glucose-lowering agents
- Instructions in the prevention and treatment of hypoglycemia
- Instructions in the prevention and treatment of acute and chronic diabetes complications
- Adequate regimens of lipid-lowering therapy
- Continuing education and reinforcement programs
- Periodic assessment of treatment goals

Specific Goals for Management of Diabetes

An overview of the steps, goals, and treatment needed to obtain optimal care of patients with diabetes is summarized in Table 53.14.

Special Considirations

Pregnancy

To reduce the risk of fetal malformations and maternal and fetal complications, pregnant diabetic women require excellent glycemic control. Followup by a multidisciplinary team including a diabetologist, internist or family physician, obstetrician, and diabetes educator is essential. Other specialists need to be called upon if necessary. Self-management skills essential for glycemic control and preparation for pregnancy include:

- Designing an appropriate meal plan, with timing of meals and snacks and an appropriate physical activity plan
- Self-monitoring blood glucose levels, choosing the time and site for insulin injections, using therapy with glucagon or carbohydrate intake for treatment of hypoglycemia, and self-adjusting insulin dosages
- Reducing stress and coping with denial

Before conception, it is essential to have a good laboratory evaluation including HbA1c, baseline assessment of renal function, thyroid function tests, and lipid profile. Other tests may need to be added according to medical history and physical exam. Conception should be deferred until the initial evaluation is completed and specific goals of therapy, including glucose control and dietary and physical activity adherence, are attained. Since the safety of oral antidiabetic agents is not well established for the fetus, patients need to be switched to insulin therapy. The goals for blood glucose are 70 to 100 mg/dl preprandial and <140 or <120 mg/dl respectively one or two hours postprandial. Hypertension, retinopathy, nephropathy, gastroparesis, and other neuropathies as well as elevated lipid levels need to be stabilized prior to conception. Pregnancy will exacerbate and accelerate acute and long-term complications of diabetes. Continuing care by a team of professionals is essential in the management of pregnant diabetic patients.

Macrovascular Disease

Recommendations listed in Table 53.14 for LDL and HDL cholesterol levels as well as for triglycerides have a goal of reducing the risk for development of coronary heart disease

TABLE 53.14

Recommended Diabetes Management Guidelines

Parameters to Assess	Frequency of Evaluation	Goal	Action Indicated If:	Recommended Treatment
Assessment of Metabolic Control				
HbA1c	Quarterly	≤7%	≥8%	Diet, exercise, oral agents, and/or insulin
Self-monitoring of blood glucose:				
Preprandial	As necessary for glycemic control	80-120mg/dL	>140 mg/dL	Stepped adjustment of medication/diet to obtain adequate glycemic control
Bedtime		100-140 mg/dL	>160mg/dL	
Technique check	Annually	Proficient	Not proficient	Referral for teaching
Hypoglycemic episodes	Each visit	No episodes	Episodes occur	Change in lifestyle, diet, and/or drug treatment
Hyperglycemic episodes/ketonuria	Each visit	No episodes	Episodes occur	Change in lifestyle, diet, and drug treatment
Assessment Macrovascular Complications				
Blood pressure	Each visit	≤ 130/80 mm Hg	> 130/80 mm Hg	ACE Inhibitors and off other antihypertensive medications
Lipid profile:	At least yearly. Quarterly or more frequently if levels are abnormal			Stepped approach to lipid control with lipid lowering medications, diet, and exercise
LDL-Cholesterol		< 100 mg/dL**	>100 mg/dL	Low dosage aspirin for patients with established macrovascular disease or patients with several risk factors for macrovascular disease
HDL-Cholesterol		>45 mg/dL	< 45 mg/dL	
Triglycerides		<150 mg/dL	> 150 mg/dL	
EKG	Annually	Normal	Abnormal	Stress test and/or referral to cardiology
Ankle/brachial ratio	Annually	Normal	Abnormal	Peripheral vascular assessment and/or referral to vascular surgery

TABLE 53.14 *(Continued)*

Recommended Diabetes Management Guidlines

Parameters to Assess	Frequency of Evaluation	Goal	Action Indicated If:	Recommended Treatment
Peripheral pulses	Each visit	Normal	Abnormal	See above
Assessment of Microvascular Complications				
Retinopathy:				
Dilated eye exam by eye care specialist	Annually	Normal	Abnormal	Referral to ophthamology Adequate glycemic control
Nephropathy:				
Microalbumin	Annually or quarterly if abnormal	< 30 mg/24 h or < 30 mg/g of creatinine (spot urine)	≥ 30 mg/24 h or ≥ 30 mg/g of creatinine (spot urine)	Adequate glycemic control Adequate treatment with ACE inhibitors Adequate treatment of hyperlipidemia Referral to nephrology if necessary
Neuropathy:				
Peripheral sensory	Annually	Intact sensation	Abnormal	Protective and preventive education Adequate glycemic control Drug treatment for symptomatic disease
Feet exam	Each visit	No complications	Corns, calluses, ulcers, wounds, infections	Referral to podiatry and/or vascular surgery specialist Adequate control of lipid abnormalities and blood glucose Treatment of infections if present

Assessment of Other Complications				
Oral/periodontal	Each visit Dental visit and hygiene every 6 months	Healthy gums/teeth	If no routine dental visits and hygiene are being performed	Referral for dental hygiene and care Adequate glycemic control*
Other infection	Each visit	Absence of infection	If infection is present	Adequate glycemic control* Appropriate treatment of infection and referral to ID if necessary
Lifestyle Assessment				
Exercise	Each visit	20-45 minutes on most days	< 3 times weekly	Exercise counseling related to type, frequency, duration, and intensity
Smoking, tobacco use	Each visit	No use	Any use	Smoking cessation counseling
Weight	Each visit	Ideal body weight	Patient is over- or underweight	For overweight: diet adjustment for short term-weight lost of 0.2-0.5 kg/week; for long term weight loss as much as needed to attain IBW For underweight: if severe — consult NST If mild — assess the reasons for weight loss and treat accordingly
Nutrition	Each visit Annual in-depth assessment by RD	Healthy eating daily weight control Metabolic control	Poor glucose or lipid control or increased weight	Referral for nutrition counseling In-depth nutrition assessment, plan, and followup by RD
Overall diabetes self-management practices	Each visit Annual in-depth assessment and self-management update	Healthy diabetes management with metabolic control and at least annual diabetes assessment and self-management education update	Early signs of complications and early signs of poor self-management of diabetes	Referral to diabetes educator or formal diabetes education classes for assessment, plan, evaluation, and followup by CDE

Severe gum disease or any local of systemic infection is associated with higher glucose levels. Treatment of infection improves glycemic control.

TABLE 53.15

Treatment Decisions Based on LDL Cholesterol Levels in Adults

	Medical Nutrition Therapy		Drug Therapy	
	Initiation Level	LDL Goal	Initiation Level	LDL Goal
With CAD, PVD, or CVD	>100	≤100	>100	≤100
Without CAD, PVD, or CVD	>100	≤100	≥130	≤100

Data are given in mg/dl.

Reprinted with authorization from American Diabetes Association (*Diabetes Care* 23(1): 58S; 2000).

and to stop progression or cause regression in patients with already established macrovascular disease. The goal for LDL cholesterol levels is 100 mg/dl for all diabetics. Lipid-lowering drug therapy is recommended to be started in patients with established vascular disease (coronary heart disease, peripheral vascular or cerebrovascular disease) if the levels of LDL-cholesterol are above 100 mg/dl. In diabetic patients without established macrovascular disease, lipid-lowering drug therapy is recommended for LDL-cholesterol of 130 mg/dl or above. The recommendations for treatment of elevated LDL-cholesterol are summarized in Table 53.15. Pharmacological therapy should be initiated after behavioral interventions are used. However, in patients with clinical CAD or very high LDL-cholesterol levels (i.e., ≥200 mg/dl), pharmacological therapy should be initiated at the same time that behavioral therapy is started. According to the NCEP-ATP III guidelines, diabetes drug treatment and behavioral modification should be performed simultaneously. The ADA guidelines recommend that diabetic subjects with clinical CAD and an LDL cholesterol level of >100 mg/dl be treated with pharmacological agents. For diabetics without pre-existing CAD, the current ADA recommendations for starting pharmacological therapy are LDL-cholesterol levels ≥130 mg/dl. Recent clinical trial data strongly suggests that these goals may become more stringent soon.

A point to consider in diabetic patients is the method used to measure LDL-cholesterol. Due to the prevalence of dense LDL in these patients, the conventional method to calculate LDL-cholesterol is inappropriate and the levels determined are in general falsely low.

Increased triglyceride levels are also recognized as a target for intervention. The levels of triglycerides considered acceptable are <150 mg/dl, and the HDL-cholesterol levels >45 mg/dl. The initial therapy for hypertriglyceridemia is behavioral modification with weight loss, increased physical activity, and no alcohol consumption. In the case of severe hypertriglyceridemia (≥1,000 mg/dl according to the ADA guidelines and ≥500 mg/dl according to NCEP-ATP III guidelines), severe dietary fat restriction (15 to 20% of kcalories as fat) in addition to pharmacological therapy is necessary to reduce the risk of pancreatitis. These patients are hard to manage, and improving glycemic control rather tightly is a very effective measure for reducing triglyceride levels and should be aggressively used before the introduction of fibric acid derivatives.

Nutritional Recommendations and Principles for the Dietary Treatment of Diabetics

Goals of Nutrition Therapy

The goals of medical nutrition therapy are to optimize health, control diabetes, and prevent or delay complications of diabetes.[21] The goals are summarized in Table 53.16. MNT is

TABLE 53.16

Goals of Medical Nutrition Therapy for Diabetes

- Achieve and maintain near-normal blood glucose goals
- Achieve and/or maintain optimal blood lipid levels
- Achieve and/or maintain normal blood pressure
- Prevent, delay or treat nutrition-related complications
- Provide adequate kcalories for achievement of reasonable body weight
- Provide optimal nutrition for maximizing health and for growth, development, pregnancy, and lactation

individualized for the person with diabetes to integrate the therapy into the daily routine of living. A registered dietitian completes a nutritional assessment and develops the individualized meal plan and behavioral interventions with the person with diabetes and the family.[22] The effectiveness of the dietary interventions in helping the person with diabetes achieve the identified goals should be evaluated routinely until goals are achieved. If goals are not met, changes in the overall management plan are needed. When goals are achieved, reassessment, continuing education, and evaluation should occur at least annually, and more often with changes in lifestyle, to assure optimal control of diabetes and maintenance of health.

Nutrition Therapy for Different Types of Diabetes

Type 1 Diabetes

The person with type 1 diabetes is typically thin or within recommended weight range. Prior to diagnosis the patient may have experienced weight loss, frequent urination (polyuria), thirst and increased fluid intake (polydipsia), and hunger (polyphagia). The initial goals of MNT are to replace fluids, normalize blood glucose and lipids, and provide appropriate kcalories for healthy living. Food, insulin administration, and physical activity need to be well balanced to obtain optimal control. It is essential that the person with diabetes coordinates the eating and exercise patterns with the onset of action and the duration of the insulin. The person with newly diagnosed type 1 diabetes may be overwhelmed with changes in daily routine; thus, initially the focus is on survival skills for managing diabetes (Table 53.17) followed by teaching self-management knowledge and skills which are needed to optimally control diabetes and its complications.[23,24] Dietary changes to optimize health can be made more slowly over time. Figure 53.1 outlines the

TABLE 53.17

Survival Skills for Managing Diabetes

- To acquire an adequate knowledge of:
  - Basic food and meal guidelines (including when eating out)
  - Effect of carbohydrates on blood glucose
  - Amount of carbohydrates taken daily
  - Carbohydrate food groups, portion sizes, and label information
- To coordinate insulin administration with food intake
- To be able to perform self-monitoring of blood glucose
- To schedule exercise according to food intake and glucose control
- To acquire knowledge of how to treat hypoglycemia:
  (in general, 15 grams of carbohydrates should raise blood glucose 50-100 mg/dl in 15 minutes)
- To know that alcohol intake may cause hypoglycemia (by inhibiting gluconeogenesis in liver)
- To know why, when, and how to call the health care provider and/or dietitian
- To have an established plan for recording self-management and returning for continuing care

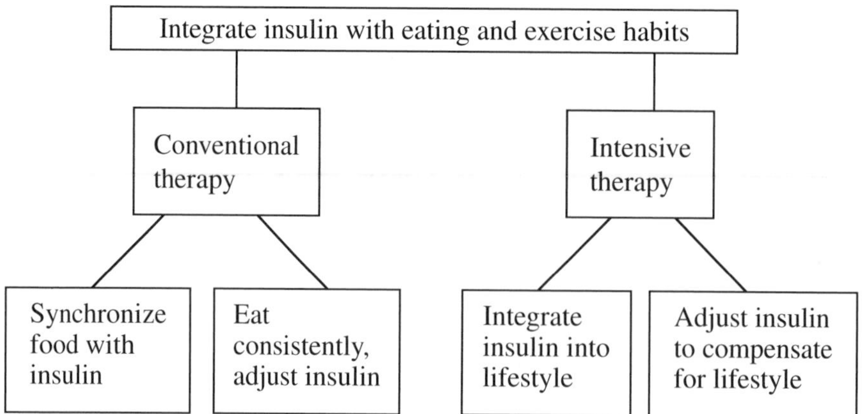

FIGURE 53.1
Nutrition therapy for type 1 diabetes. Reprinted with permission from *Maximizing the Role of Nutrition in Diabetes Management*, American Diabetes Association, Alexandria, 1994.

two approaches to nutrition therapy currently recommended by the ADA.[25] Blood glucose levels need to be monitored and insulin doses and/or food intake to control blood glucose adjusted according to recommended levels (Table 53.14).

Type 2 Diabetes

The person with newly diagnosed type 2 diabetes may have had asymptomatic type 2 diabetes for a number of years prior to diagnosis, and may present with one or more complications. Most are obese or have increased percentage of body fat distributed predominately in the abdominal region. The goals of therapy are to achieve and maintain glucose, lipid, and blood pressure within the recommended range and to achieve a moderate weight loss (5 to 9 pounds) if overweight.[26,27] Methods for attaining these goals are outlined in Figure 53.2. There is no clear answer about which goal should have first priority; however, the UKPDS researchers found that blood pressure control produced the most improved outcomes.[28] The desired outcomes of medical nutrition therapy for persons with type 2 diabetes are outlined in Tables 53.14 and 53.16.

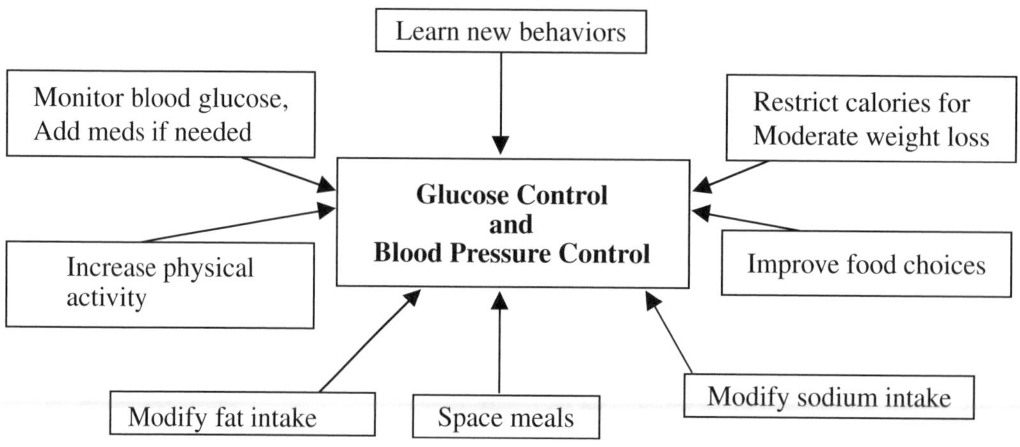

FIGURE 53.2
Nutrition therapy for type 2 diabetes. Adapted with permission from *Maximizing the Role of Nutrition in Diabetes Management*, American Diabetes Association, Alexandria, 1994.

TABLE 53.18

Goals for Medical Nutrition Therapy in GDM

- Optimal nutrition for developing fetus
- Optimal nutrition for mother
- To maintain maternal euglycemia keeping an adequate diet
- Good nutrition patterns taught to the family 'gatekeeper'
- To develop nutritional patterns that prevent or forestall recurrence of GDM and onset of type 2 diabetes mellitus

Reprinted with permission from American Diabetes Association: Thomas-Dobersen, D., et al. *Clinical Diabetes* 1: 172; 1999.

TABLE 53.19

Blood Glucose Goals for Pregnancy

	Preexisting Diabetes Mellitus	Gestational Diabetes
Fasting	70-100 mg/dl	≤105 mg/dl
Premeal	70-100 mg/dl	70-105 mg/dl
Postprandial 1 hour	≤140 mg/dl	≤120 mg/dl
Postprandial 2 hour	≤120 mg/dl	≤120 mg/dl

Adapted with permission from Hoeer, J.H., Green-Pastors, J., *Diabetes Medical Nutrition Therapy,* American Diabetes Association, Alexandria, ch. 8, 1997.

Diabetes in Pregnancy

The goal of nutrition therapy for diabetes in pregnancy is to produce a healthy baby at term and maintain optimal health for the mother. If type 1 or type 2 diabetes is diagnosed prior to pregnancy, counseling is recommended to attain optimal control of diabetes prior to conception and throughout pregnancy. The pregnant woman is defined as having gestational diabetes if first diagnosed during the present pregnancy. GDM does not exclude the possibility that diabetes may have been unrecognized prior to pregnancy; however, GDM typically occurs around the 24th week of pregnancy. Women diagnosed with GDM in a prior pregnancy have a 30 to 65% probability of developing GDM in a subsequent pregnancy. Studies also show that women with GDM have a 22 to 30% probability of developing type 2 diabetes in 7 to 10 years and a 50 to 60% risk of developing diabetes in their lifetime. Additionally, the offspring have an increased risk of obesity and GDM.[29]

The overall goals for medical nutrition therapy are shown in Table 53.18, and blood glucose goals are shown in Table 53.19. To accomplish these goals, meal patterns, nutrient composition, and caloric needs are reviewed in Table 53.20, and a typical meal/snack pattern is shown in Table 53.21.

Nutritional Recommendations

Guidelines for nutrient consumption and other nutrition components such as sweeteners and cholesterol along with technical reviews of the evidence for the guidelines have been published by the ADA,[30-34] and are summarized in Table 53.22. The energy nutrients can be converted into blood glucose, and Table 53.23 summarizes their degree of conversion. Protein and fats have minimal effect on blood glucose except in patients whose diabetes is poorly controlled, since these nutrients may lead to a rapid increase in gluconeogenesis and deteriorated glycemic control.[32] Many persons with diabetes initially think that only sugar can increase blood glucose; thus, diabetes education about the effect of nutrients (especially carbohydrates) is essential to good control.

TABLE 53.20

Summary of Intensive Nutritional Therapy for GDM

Meal Pattern

Three meals plus three or more snacks (2-3 hour intervals)
(breakfast with low carbohydrate content)
ADA exchange pattern individualized

Composition

Nutrition therapy and exercise only (no insulin)
38-45% carbohydrate complex, high fiber, >150 g minimum
(lower level can be used as long as no ketonuria is present)
20-25% protein (1.3 g/kg body weight)
30-40% fat (mono or polyunsaturated emphasized)

Energy Levels

Second trimester, 25-30 kcal/kg IBW prepregnant
Third trimester, 30-35 kcal/kg IBW prepregnant

Weight Gain

Adjust kcalorie level to achieve appropriate weight gain for prepregnancy BMI category:

	Prepregnancy BMI	Total gain
Underweight	<19.8	28-40 lbs. (12.5-18 kg)
Normal weight	19.8-26	25-35 lbs. (11.5-16 kg)
Overweight	>26-29	15-25 lbs. (7-11.5 kg)
Obese	>29	Minimum 15 lbs. (7.1 kg)

Reprinted with permission from American Diabetes Association. Gunderson, E.P., *Diabetes Care* 20: 223; 1997.

TABLE 53.21

Intensive Medical Nutrition Therapy for GDM

Meal or Snack	Total Carbohydrate kcalories (%)	Carbohydrate (g)
Breakfast	10-15	15-30
A.M. snack	10	15-30
Lunch	20-25	30-60
P.M. snack	15	15-45
Dinner	25	45-60
Bedtime snack	15	30 or more
Daily total	100	150-250

Reprinted with permission from American Diabetes Association. Gunderson, E.P., *Diabetes Care* 20: 223; 1997.

Carbohydrate level should vary according to kcalorie prescription and the individual's tolerance for carbohydrate, which worsens as gestation progresses. The restricted levels listed above are characteristic of late gestation.

TABLE 53.22

Medical Nutrition Therapy Recommendations

Nutrient	Recommendation	Comments
Protein Sources: chicken, fish, meat, eggs, milk, tofu, nuts, peanut butter	10-20% of total kcalories should come from protein sources.	Research indicates needs are similar for people with or without diabetes. With onset of nephropathy, limit protein to adult RDA (0.8 g/kg/day). Some research studies suggest vegetable protein may not be as harmful to the kidneys as animal protein.
Carbohydrate Sources: starch (grains, bread, pasta, rice, potato, beans) milk, fruit, vegetables, sugar, honey, jam, molasses, etc.	80-90% of kcalories are divided between carbohydrate and fats based on individual risk factors and needs. Depending on nutritional assessment and medical nutritional therapy goals, this generally equates to 45-60% of total kcalories from carbohydrate.	Total carbohydrate intake has greater impact on blood glucose control than source of carbohydrate, i.e., whether complex carbohydrate or sucrose. Sucrose and sucrose-containing foods should be consumed within the context of a healthful diet. These foods are often high in total carbohydrate and fat and low in vitamins and minerals.
Sugars and Other Sweeteners Sources: sucrose, fructose, corn sweeteners such as corn syrup, fruit juice, or fruit juice concentrate, honey, molasses, dextrose, maltose; sorbitol, mannitol, xylitol (sugar alcohols)	% of kcalories will vary and is individualized based on usual eating habits, glucose and lipid goals. Sucrose and other sugars/sweeteners can be integrated into a healthy eating pattern for persons with diabetes.	Sucrose and sucrose-containing foods should be consumed within the context of a healthful diet. These foods are often high in total carbohydrate and fat and low in vitamins and minerals. Individuals can be taught to substitute sucrose-containing foods for other carbohydrate foods in their meal plans.
Nonnutritive sweeteners such as saccharin, aspartame, acesulfame K, and sucralose	All are approved by the FDA and the FDA determines an acceptable daily intake (ADI) which includes a 100-fold safety factor. Actual intake by persons with diabetes is well below the ADI.	
Fat Sources: monounsaturated: olive and canola oils, avocado, nuts polyunsaturated: safflower, sunflower, corn, and soy oils	60-70% of total kcalories should be divided between monounsaturated fats and carbohydrates. Up to 10% of kcalories should be from polyunsaturated fats.	Individuals with diabetes should limit total fat to 25-35% of total kcalories and <200 mg of dietary cholesterol per day. If obesity and weight management are the primary issues, reduced total fat to reduce total kcalories and increasing exercise should be recommended.

TABLE 53.22 *(Continued)*

Medical Nutrition Therapy Recommendations

Nutrient	Recommendation	Comments
saturated: butter, lard, shortening, animal fats, coconut, and palm oils	Less than 7% of total kcalories should be from saturated fats. Depending on nutritional assessment, total fat intake equates to 25-35% of total kcalories.	Guidelines for reducing cardiovascular risk are emphasized — nobody should exceed 7% of total kcalories from saturated fats. If elevated triglyceride and very low-density lipoprotein cholesterol are the primary concerns, a moderate increase in monounsaturated fat intake, with <7% of total kcalories from saturated fat, and a more moderate (slight decrease) in carbohydrate can be tried. Some studies have shown that a diet with increased total fat from monounsaturated fats can lower plasma triglycerides, glucose, and insulin levels more than a high-carbohydrate diet in some individuals. In individuals with triglycerides >1000, reduction of all types of dietary fats to reduce levels of plasma dietary fat in the form of chylomicrons should be implemented.
Fat replacers		
Typically fall into three categories based on their nutrient content: Carbohydrate-based: includes carrageenan, cellulose gum, corn syrup solids, dextrin, guar gum, hydrolyzed corn starch, maltodextrin, modified food starch, pectin, polydextrose, sugar beet fiber, tapioca dextrin, xanthan gum. Protein-based: includes microparticulated egg white and milk protein (Simplesse, K-Blazer), whey protein concentrate Fat-based: includes caprenin, olestra (Olean), salatrin (Benefat), and others.	Foods with fat replacers can be substituted in an individual's meal plan based on the nutrient profile of the food product.	Food products that contain <20 kcalories or 5 grams of carbohydrate per serving have a negligible effect on metabolic control. Foods containing 20 kcalories per serving should be limited to 3 servings spread throughout the day.

Dietary cholesterol	<200 mg per day	MNT typically reduces LDL Cholesterol 15-25 mg/dl (0.40-0.65 mmol/l)
Fiber	10-25 grams of soluble fiber per day — same recommendation as for individuals without diabetes.*	Research suggests that in the amounts typically consumed, fiber intake has very little impact on blood glucose levels.
Sodium	Same as for general population: <3000 mg per day. If hypertensive, individuals should reduce sodium intake to <2400 mg per day. Food selection guidelines: <400 mg sodium per single serving of food; <800 mg sodium per entree or convenience meal.	There is an association between hypertension and both IDDM and NIDDM, with an increase for people with NIDDM who are obese. There is also evidence that individuals with NIDDM are more salt sensitive.
Alcohol 1 drink = 12 oz. beer, 5 oz. wine, 1 oz. 80-proof liquor	Insulin users: limit to 2 drinks per day and do not cut back on food. Non-insulin users: substitute alcohol for fat.	Abstinence is recommended for those with history of alcohol abuse or alcohol-induced hypertriglyceridemia, and during pregnancy. Drink only with food. Alcohol can lead to hypoglycemia via inhibition of gluconeogenesis. Limit for weight loss and elevated triglycerides.
Micronutrients	The vitamin and mineral needs of people who are healthy appear to be adequately met by the RDAs, which include a generous safety factor.	Individuals at greatest risk for vitamin/mineral deficiency include those on weight loss diets, strict vegetarians, the elderly, pregnant or lactating women, those taking medications known to alter micronutrient metabolism, people with poor glycemic control (i.e., glycosuria), people with malabsorption disorders, and people with congestive heart failure or myocardial infarction.

* Exception in patients with autonomic neuropathy who should not have increased fiber in their diet.

Adapted and expanded from Karlsen, M., Khakpour, D., and Thomson, L.L. *Clinical Diabetes* 14: 54; 1996.

TABLE 53.23

Energy Nutrients and Their Absorption

Nutrient	Kcalories/Gram	% Nutrient Converted to Glucose	Estimated Time for Absorption*
Carbohydrate	4	100%	
Simple			5-30 min
Complex			1-3 h
Protein	4	50-60%	3-6 h
Fat	9	10%	3-8 h

* The absorption time is affected by the nutrient mix. For example, the sugar from a candy bar with high fat content is more slowly absorbed than a piece of candy than contains no fat.

TABLE 53.24

Meal Planning Approaches

Approach	Benefits	Drawbacks
Food guide pyramid	Well known by the general public	Little focus on meal spacing
Health food choices	Mixes guidelines with meal plan	Often perceived as diet
Exchange lists for meal planning	Places emphasis on all nutrient groups	Concept difficult to understand by the lay person
Counting plans	Good approach for specific nutrient intervention	Requires committed learner
Carbohydrate indications	Useful for adequate glucose control	Ignores other nutrients
Protein indications	Address diabetic nephropathy	Ignores other nutrients
Fat indications	Address weight or hyperlipidemia	Ignores other nutrients

Reprinted with permission from American Diabetes Association. Karlsen, M., Khakpour, D., and Thomson, L.L. *Clincal Diabetes,* May/June: 54; 1996.

Food Guides and Planning Food Intake for Persons with Diabetes

Historically, the approaches to planning food intake for persons with diabetes have ranged from starvation diets (during the pre-insulin era) to high-fat, low-carbohydrate diet plans, to our present system of more liberalized food intake. Various food guides and methods for planning food intake have been used. An overview of the meal planning approaches for providing MNT to persons with diabetes is reviewed in Table 53.24. A meal planning approach that provides the desired outcomes (decrease of complications and optimal health and satisfaction) is desirable. Carbohydrate counting is one method that allows maximum flexibility as well as excellent glycemic control. The different ways to count carbohydrates are reviewed in Table 53.25.

Food Labeling

Teaching patients with diabetes how to read a food label is especially important to those who count carbohydrate, fat, or protein in their meal plans. For persons using exchange

TABLE 53.25
Ways to Count Carbohydrates

Method	Description	Ease vs. Accuracy	Premeal or Bolus Dose Calculation*
Counting carbohydrate exchanges (interchanges)	Count each serving of starch, fruit, and milk as one carbohydrate exchange and consider them equal in carbohydrate value	Easiest method but also the least accurate Requires the least math skill	Calculate pre-meal dose units/exchange
Counting food exchanges	Add the carbohydrate values of all exchanges that contain carbohydrate (including vegetables) to obtain the carbohydrate total for a meal	Easy and fairly accurate	Calculate pre-meal dose as units/exchange, counting vegetables as carbohydrates, or calculate the bolus by dividing the total grams of carbohydrate in the meal by the insulin-to-carbohydrate ratio
Carbohydrate gram counting	Add carbohydrate gram values for all foods eaten to obtain the total carbohydrate intake per meal	More time-consuming than methods 1 and 2 but also quite accurate. Requires more math skill to add and divide 2- and 3-digit number	Calculate pre-meal dose by dividing the total grams of carbohydrate in the meal by the insulin-to-carbohydrate ratio
Calculating available glucose	Count grams of carbohydrate for all foods eaten, then calculate the glucose available from protein and add this value to the carbohydrate grams to obtain the meal total	Most difficult; requires the most math skill of all methods	Multiply grams of protein in meal by 0.6 to obtain available glucose, add to grams of carbohydrate; calculate the dose by dividing this total by the insulin-to-carbohydrate ratio

* Short-acting insulin adminstered before meals to control the meal-related glucose rise. The calibration of insulin to food intake is recommended for individuals with type 1 diabetes, especially those following intensive therapy.

lists for meal planning, information about how to use the nutrition information to fit foods into the exchange lists is helpful (and essential for combination foods). The key question for the patient to ask is "how does this food, based on the nutritional information, fit into my food plan for controlling diabetes?"[35]

Diabetes and Physical Activity

Exercise can be used as a therapeutic tool for controlling diabetes, and the person with diabetes needs to incorporate exercise into the lifestyle for healthy living with diabetes.

Patient Evaluation before Exercise

The person with diabetes should undergo a medical evaluation with appropriate diagnostic studies and should be screened for complications that may be worsened by the exercise program.[36] If complications are present, the patient should have an individualized exercise program prescription that specifies the frequency, intensity, and duration of exercise, along with specific precautions for minimizing risks. The benefits of physical activity are many, including cardiovascular fitness and psychological wellbeing. However, the risks of exercise for the person with diabetes are many, including fluctuations in blood glucose control, ketosis, lower-extremity injury, and exacerbation of pre-existing complications.

Exercise Recommendations

For Persons with Cardiovascular Disease

Diabetics at risk or with diagnosed cardiovascular disease should undergo medical evaluation of cardiac status and special evaluation for exercise tolerance before participating in increased physical activities. Supervised cardiovascular risk reduction or rehabilitation programs often provide the patient and his family with increased support for increasing physical activities.

Positive effects of regular exercise on reducing blood pressure have been consistently demonstrated in hyperinsulinemic persons.

For Persons with Peripheral Arterial Disease

Following an evaluation of peripheral arterial disease, the basic treatment is a supervised exercise program and no smoking, carried out under the supervision of a physician. A walking program may improve muscle metabolism and collateral circulation for a person with intermittent claudication. If pain is severe and does not improve, further evaluation and possible limitation of exercises involving the lower extremities may be considered.

For Persons with Retinopathy

Following a dilated eye exam, if proliferative diabetic retinopathy is present, the person with diabetes may need to avoid anaerobic exercise and exercise that involves straining, jarring, or Valsalva maneuvers, and any other activities that increase systolic blood pressure. Medical status dictates the level of risks associated with exercise; however, low-impact cardiovascular conditioning such as swimming, walking, low-impact aerobics, stationary cycling, and endurance exercises are low risk.

For Persons with Nephropathy

Specific exercise recommendations have not been developed for persons with nephropathy, but some patients may self-limit exercise based on a reduced capacity for activity. High-intensity or strenuous exercises should probably be discouraged for persons with overt nephropathy, but other low intensity-physical activities may increase a sense of wellbeing and socialization.

For Persons with Neuropathy

Peripheral

For the person who has loss of protective sensation in the feet on testing, weight-bearing exercises are contraindicated. This includes use of treadmill, prolonged walking, jogging, and step exercises. Recommended exercises include swimming, bicycling, rowing, chair and arm exercises, along with other nonweight-bearing exercises.

Autonomic

Autonomic neuropathy increases the risks of exercise-related problems, and certain precautions need to be taken to tailor the exercise prescription to each individual patient following an in-depth evaluation. Thermoregulation may be difficult, so avoiding exercise in hot or cold environments, and special attention to adequate hydration are most important.

Exercise and Glycemic Control

Regular exercise activities (30 or more minutes on most days) have demonstrated consistent beneficial effects on carbohydrate metabolism and insulin sensitivity, as well as enhanced weight loss.

Exercise for Persons with Type 1 Diabetes

Persons with type 1 diabetes, who do not exhibit some of the limiting complications previously discussed or poor glycemic control, can enjoy all types of exercise.[37] The key is regulating the glycemic response to exercise. The person should avoid exercise if fasting glucose levels are >250 mg/dl with ketosis present or if glucose levels are >300 mg/dl. If glucose levels are <100 mg/dl prior to exercise, additional carbohydrates are recommended. Food adjustments for exercise for persons with type 1 diabetes are shown in Table 53.26. Food and fluids should be readily available for persons with type 1 diabetes

TABLE 53.26

Food Adjustments for Exercise for Persons with Type 1 Diabetes

Types of Exercise and Examples	General Guidelines: If Blood Glucose Is:	General Guidelines: Increase Food Intake By:	Suggestion of Food Exchanges to Use:
Short duration, low-to-moderate intensity (walking a half mile or leisurely bicycling for <30 minutes)	<100 mg/dL	10 to 15 g of CHO	1 Fruit or 1 starch
	≥100 mg/dL	None	
Moderate intensity (1 hour of tennis, swimming, jogging, leisurely bicycling, golfing, etc.)	<100 mg/dL	25 to 50 g CHO before exercise, then 10 to 15 g/h of exercise	1 Meat sandwich with a milk or fruit
	100-180 mg/dL	10 to 15 gm CHO	1 Fruit or 1 starch
	180-300 mg/dL	None	
	>300 mg/dL	Do not begin exercise until blood glucose is under control	
Strenuous (about 1-2 hours of football, hockey, racquetball, or basketball; strenuous bicycling or swimming; shoveling heavy snow)	<100 mg/dL	50 g CHO, monitor blood glucose carefully	1 Meat sandwich (2 slices of bread) with a milk and fruit
	100-180 mg/dL	25 to 50 g CHO depending on intensity and duration	Meat sandwich with a milk and fruit
	180-300 mg/dL	10 to 15 g CHO	1 Fruit or 1 starch
	>300 mg/dL	Do not begin exercise until blood glucose is under better control	

Self-blood glucose monitoring is essential for all persons to determine their carbohydrate needs. Persons with type 2 diabetes usually do not need an exercise snack. During periods of exercise, all individuals need to increase fluid intake.

CHO = carbohydrates.

Adapted with permission from Franz, M.J., and Barry, B., *Diabetes and Exercise*: Guidelines for Safe and Enjoyable Activity, American Diabetes Association, Alexandria, 1996, p. 16.

during exercise. If the duration of exercise is 30 minutes or more during peak action time of insulin and blood glucose is in good control, reduction of insulin is recommended. The reduction of insulin is based on duration and intensity of exercise, and usually ranges from 5 to 60% of daily requirements. After exercise, an extra carabohydrate snack may be necessary. Frequent monitoring of blood glucose and adequate food/fluid intake to prevent hypoglycemia are essential for self-management and maintaining a healthy lifestyle.

Exercise for Persons with Type 2 Diabetes

Many persons with type 2 diabetes may have some of the previously mentioned complications at diagnosis, and also may have been sedentary for many years. Thus, before beginning an exercise program, an in-depth physical examination and recommendations for exercise frequency, intensity, and duration is recommended.[38] Beginning with 5 to 10 minute sessions with gradual increases usually is successful and safe. Unless treated with insulin or glucose-lowering medications, the person with type 2 diabetes does not usually need additional food before, during, or following exercise, except for exercise that is intense or of long duration. Recent attention has focused on the useful role of exercise in preventing or delaying the onset of type 2 diabetes.

Exercise for Older Adults with Diabetes

Exercise for older adults with diabetes is recommended, and may lead to an improved quality of life and less chronic disease. The same precautions should be taken with older adults with and without diabetes.

Hospital Admission Guidelines for Persons with Diabetes

If the standard of care is adequate, seldom will a diabetic patient require hospitalization. According to the guidelines of the ADA, inpatient care may be required in:

- Life-threatening acute metabolic complications of diabetes
- Newly diagnosed diabetes in children and adolescents
- Patients with chronic poor metabolic control that necessitates close monitoring to determine the problem behind the poor control and changes in therapy
- Patients with severe chronic complications that require intensive treatment either of diabetes or of conditions that significantly affect diabetes control and further development of complications
- Uncontrolled or newly discovered insulin-requiring diabetes during pregnancy
- Patients in whom institution of insulin-pump therapy or other intensive insulin regimens are being contemplated

Translation of Medical Nutrition Therapy for Diabetes to Health Care Institutions

Today's recommendations for MNT in health care facilities are based on individualized needs of the patients with diabetes. One of the approaches frequently used is the "con-

TABLE 53.27

Developing a Consistent Carbohydrate Diabetes Meal Plan Menu for Health Care Facilities

1. Establish the desired kcalorie range.
2. Determine the desired percentages of macronutrients (carbohydrate, protein, saturated fat, total fat).
3. Determine the numbers of CHO choices to be given at each meal, and if included, at bedtime snack.
4. Determine how often to include sucrose-containing desserts and the maximum number of CHO choices to be allotted to each dessert.
5. Analyze current fat-modified menus for distribution of macronutrients (% carbohydrate, protein, saturated fat, total fat) to determine if they meet goal ranges of new diabetic menus.
6. Determine how many grams of carbohydrate or CHO choices are in each item in the fat-modified menu (i.e., fruits, salads, starches, casseroles, desserts, milk, juices).
7. For nonselective menus, adjust the fat-modified menus to provide the established number of CHO choices, and include a bedtime snack if desired.
8. For facilities with menu selections, identify the CHO choices for each carbohydrate item, and include instructions on the menu regarding the number of carbohydrate choices to make at each meal.
9. For long-term care facilities that wish to base their diabetic diet (consistent carbohydrate diet) on regular menus, use the same process as for fat-modified menus.

Reprinted with permission from Schafer, R.G. *Practical Diabetology* 16:3, 48; 1997.

sistent carbohydrate diabetes meal plan;" a plan for developing a menu is shown in Table 53.27.

Acute Health Care Facilities

Approximately one out of seven hospital beds is occupied by a person with diabetes. In the acute care facility, many of the patients have complex health problems in addition to diabetes. Thus, the challenge is to maximize health potential and provide foods that are culturally acceptable to the patient. Each acute care facility has a different meal planning system that best meets its needs. The consistent carbohydrate menu plan can be used to improve metabolic control. The ideal meal plan reflects the diabetes nutrition recommendations and does not unnecessarily restrict sucrose.[39]

Long-Term Health Care Facilities

Since the risk of diabetes increases with age, the patient population in long-term care includes many individuals with diabetes. Additionally, malnutrition is a recognized challenge in the older adult population. Food intake should be adequate and not overly restricted. Regular menus, with consistent amounts of carbohydrate at meals and snacks, are the recommended approach. Monitoring of blood glucose and hemoglobin A_{1c} should be used to evaluate glycemic control, with individualized approaches to achieve goals of MNT.

Self-Management Education for Persons with Diabetes

Diabetes self-management education and continuing nutrition care is essential for meeting the goals of MNT and diabetes control.[23,30] The outpatient and home settings are the ideal environments. If the patient is hospitalized with multiple other priorities, usually the concern of the patient and the family is not focused on diabetes self-management education. Learning readiness is the cornerstone for self-management education. At discharge from the inpatient facility, plans are made for continuing education and followup by the health care team.

Education for Health Care Professionals and Administrators

The role of MNT in helping the team and person with diabetes attain the desired treatment goals is cost effective and leads to quality health services. One of the roles of the registered dietitian is to translate nutrition recommendations for the diabetes care team and to integrate these recommendations into the overall care of the person with diabetes. Team members should have access to simplified guidelines for patient nutrition care until a registered dietitian is available.

Third Party Reimbursement for Diabetes Care, Supplies, and Self-Management Education

Currently, 37 states have enacted diabetes reform laws that improve insurance coverage for supplies, equipment, and education for people with diabetes. States that have enacted these laws are listed in Table 53.28.[40] MNT counseling is usually included in diabetes education coverage; however, examination of each state's reform laws is necessary to determine the extent of coverage. New Medicare regulations are expected to be released in 2000, and diabetes advocates and nutrition professionals are working to assure inclusion of MNT in these regulations. Medicaid, a federal–state partnership program for persons unable to afford health care and private third-party insurance, offers coverage for MNT in some states. To determine if your state offers coverage, contact the state's Medicaid program.

The frequency of dietitian contact with the patient and the essential care processes for MNT have not been clearly delineated; yet quality health care today requires consistently applied, evidence-based care that leads to positive outcomes for most patients. In a research study conducted by the Diabetes Care and Education Practice Group of the ADA, use of guidelines resulted in changes in dietitian practices and produced greater improvement in patient blood glucose outcomes at three months compared to usual care.[41] Self-management education is critical to successful diabetes management, and medical treatment without self-management education is regarded as substandard and unethical. Numerous studies have demonstrated that self-management education and MNT improve outcomes for persons with diabetes.

TABLE 53.28

States that have Enacted Diabetes Reform Laws (as of January 2000)[27]

Arizona	Iowa	Nebraska	Rhode Island
Arkansas	Kansas	Nevada	South Carolina
California	Kentucky	New Hampshire	South Dakota
Colorado	Louisiana	New Jersey	Tennessee
Connecticut	Maine	New Mexico	Texas
Florida	Maryland	New York	Vermont
Georgia	Minnesota	North Carolina	Virginia
Illinois	Mississippi	Oklahoma	Washington
Indiana	Missouri	Pennsylvania	West Virginia
			Wisconsin

From Maggio, C.A., Pi-Sunyer, F.X. *Diabetes Care* 20: 1744; 1997.

References

1. World Health Organization: Diabetes Mellitus: Report of a WHO Study Group. Geneva, World Health Org, 1985 (Tech Rep Ser no 727).
2. Harris MI, Flegal KM, Cowie CC, Eberhardt MS, Goldshtein DE, Little RR, Wiedmeyer HM, Byrd-Holt DD. *Diabetes Care* 21: 518; 1998.
3. National Diabetes Data Group. *Diabetes* 28: 1039; 1979.
4. Expert Committee on the Diagnosis and Classification of Diabetes Mellitus, *Diabetes Care* 21(1): 5S; 1998.
5. Reaven GM. *Diabetes* 37: 1595; 1988.
6. Tominaga M, Eguchi H, Manaka H, et al. *Diabetes Care* 22: 920; 1999.
7. Harris MI, Hadden WC, Knowler WC, Bennett PH. *Diabetes* 36: 523; 1987.
8. Harris MI. *Diabetes Care* 16: 642; 1993.
9. Klein R. *Diabetes Care* 18: 258; 1995.
10. Aiello LP, Gardner TW, King GL, et al. *Diabetes Care* 21: 143; 1998.
11. The Diabetes Control and Complications Trial Research Group, *N Engl J Med* 329: 997; 1993.
12. UK Prospective Diabetes Study Group, *Lancet* 352: 837; 1998.
13. UK Prospective Diabetes Study Group, *Lancet* 352: 854; 1998.
14. DeFronzo RA. *Diabetes Reviews* 3: 510; 1995.
15. Haffner SM. *Diabetes Care* 21: 160; 1998.

15a. Expert Panel on Detection, Evaluation, and Treatment of High Blood Cholesterol in Adults. *JAMA* 285: 2486, 2001.

16. Pyorala K, Pederson TR, Kjekshus J, et al. *Diabetes Care* 20: 614; 1997.
17. Sacks FM, Pfeffer MA, Moye LA, et al. *N Engl J Med* 335: 1001; 1996.

17a. Haffner SM, et al. *N Engl J Med* 339, 229, 1998.

18. Cryer PE, Fisher JN, Shamoon H. *Diabetes Care* 17: 734; 1994.
19. Burge MR, Schmitz-Firentino K, Fischett C, et al. *JAMA* 279: 137; 1998.
20. Weir GC, Nathan DM, Singer DE. *Diabetes Care* 17: 1514; 1994.
21. Franz MJ, Horton ES, Bantle JP, et al. *Diabetes Care* 17: 490; 1994.
22. Schafer RG, Bohannon B, Franz M, et al. *Diabetes Care* 20: 96; 1997.
23. Clement S. *Diabetes Care* 18: 1204; 1995.
24. Funnell MM, Haas LB. *Diabetes Care* 18: 100; 1995.
25. American Diabetes Association. *Maximizing the role of nutrition in diabetes management*, American Diabetes Association, Alexandria, 1994, ch 5, 6.
26. Hoeer JH, Green-Pastors J. *Diabetes Medical Nutrition Therapy.* American Diabetes Association, Alexandria, 1997, ch 3.
27. Maggio CA, Pi-Sunyer FX. *Diabetes Care* 20: 1744; 1997.
28. American Diabetes Association. *Diabetes Care* 23(1): 27S; 2000.
29. Thomas-Dobersen D. *Clinical Diabetes* 17: 179; 1999.
30. Franz MJ, Horton ES, Bantle JP, et al. *Diabetes Care* 17: 490; 1994.
31. Karlsen M, Khakpour D, Thomson LL. *Clinical Diabetes* 14: 54; 1996.
32. Henry RR. *Diabetes Care* 17: 1502; 1994.
33. Warshaw H, Franz M, Powers MS. *Diabetes Care* 19: 1294; 1996.
34. Mooradian AD, Failla M, Hoogwerf B, et al. *Diabetes Care* 17: 464; 1994.
35. Wheeler ML, Franz M, Heins J, et al. *Diabetes Care* 17: 489; 1994.
36. American Diabetes Association. *Diabetes Care* 22(1): 50S; 2000.
37. Wasserman DH, Zinman B. *Diabetes Care* 17: 924; 1994.
38. Schneuider SH, Ruderman NB. *Diabetes Care* 13: 785; 1990.
39. American Diabetes Association. *Diabetes Care* 22(1): 47S; 2000.
40. American Diabetes Association. *Diabetes Advocate (Newsletter)* January, 2000.
41. Kulkarni K, Castle G, Gregory R, et al. *J Am Diet Assoc* 98: 62; 1998.

54

Nutrition and Oral Medicine

Dominick P. DePaola, Connie Mobley, and Riva Touger-Decker

Introduction

In the Spring of 2000, the Surgeon General of the United States released the first-ever report on "Oral Health in America." The intent of this landmark report is to alert the American people to the full meaning of oral health and its importance to general health and well being. The report has five major themes:[1]

1. Oral health means much more than healthy teeth.
2. Oral health is integral to general health.
3. Safe and effective disease prevention measures exist that everyone can adopt to improve oral health and prevent disease.
4. General health risk factors, such as tobacco use and poor dietary practices, also affect oral and craniofacial health.
5. There are significant oral health disparities among racial and ethnic minority population cohorts.

The overlying theme is that the etiology and pathogenesis of diseases and disorders affecting the craniofacial structures are complex and multifactional, involving an interplay and interaction among genetic, environmental, and behavioral factors. The major environmental factor in this interplay is diet and nutrition during development of the craniofacial complex, the maintenance of craniofacial structure integrity, and fending off subsequent microbial challenge. In fact, the two classic dental diseases, caries and periodontal disease(s), both have vital nutrition and dietary components. Caries is intimately linked to adequate nutrient intake during development of teeth and salivary glands, and to the frequent ingestion of fermentable carbohydrates post-eruption. Periodontal disease is generally considered to be caused by bacterial plaque residing on the tooth structure, but the inflammatory response can be modulated by adequate systemic nutriture. In terms of craniofacial disorders, cleft lip and palate — among the most common birth defects affecting humans — are linked, in part, to adequate folate nutriture during critical periods in craniofacial development, much the same way that neural tube defects are linked to

0-8493-2705-9/02/$0.00+$1.50

folate nutriture. Importantly, the diet and nutrition relationship to oral, dental, and craniofacial diseases is much more extensive than those classic illustrations. For example, systemic disease resulting from infectious oral microbes is generally recognized to occur in patients with immunological and nutritional deficiencies such that individual host defenses are compromised, allowing oral microbes to gain systemic access.[2] In turn, the oral, dental, and craniofacial tissues are the sites of signs and symptoms of about 120 systemic diseases.[1] Additionally, changing demographics suggest that an aging population will increasingly present medically significant oral problems.[1]

This section reviews the relationship between nutrition and oral, dental, and craniofacial diseases and disorders, the nutrient-tissue interplay, and, where appropriate, prevention, treatment, or intervention strategies using diet and nutrition. The section begins with an illustration of the burden of oral disease and proceeds to discuss chronic oral infectious disease (caries, periodontal disease, others); selected systemic diseases; neoplastic diseases; craniofacial-dental-oral birth defects; and health promotion, health education, and behavioral change.

The Burden of Oral Disease

Dental, oral, and craniofacial diseases and disorders are among the most common of human maladies, with widespread tooth loss due to caries and periodontal disease. Dental caries, in particular, disproportionately affects low socioeconomic populations and some racial/ethnic minorities. Additionally, oral and pharyngeal cancer results in over 12,000 deaths per year and has one of the worst morbidity and mortality rates of any cancer. Birth defects, particularly cleft lip and/or palate, are highly prevalent, as are a variety of chronic and disabling diseases and disorders, the oral complications of systemic diseases, and the oral complications of those interventions and medications consequent to treating systemic disease. Figure 54.1 illustrates the burden of disease according to the most recent NIDCR data.[1,3]

Chronic Oral Infectious Disease

Dental Caries

In spite of a substantial reduction over the last 20 years, dental caries continues to be a major problem for adults and children worldwide. For example, a 1988 to 1991 survey of the U.S. population showed that over 45% of children and adolescents in the 5- to 17-year age group had carious teeth.[4] In adults, over 93% had evidence of caries, with an increasing incidence of root caries with age.[5] The impact of dental caries on pain and suffering remains profound. The Surgeon General's Report estimates that 51 million school hours are lost each year to dental related illness, and in adults more than 164 million work hours are lost each year for dental related illness or treatment.[1]

The etiology of dental caries is well documented and results from the interplay of dental plaque present on the tooth surface with ingested fermentable carbohydrates. Many studies have documented that a demineralization-mineralization equilibrium occurs at the tooth-plaque-saliva interface, where the equilibrium balance favors demineralization

Birth Defect
- Cleft lip/palate births estimated at 1 in 600 for whites and 1 out of 850 for African Americans

Dental Caries
- 5-10% of pre-school age children have early childhood caries; rates are substantially higher in low income families and some racial/ethnic minorities
- 19% of all young children age 2-5 have untreated caries in primary teeth; the rate is 30% for children living in poverty
- 45% of school children and 94% of adults have experienced caries in permanent teeth
- 5x more common than asthma and 7x more common than hay fever

Dental Orthopedics
- 20% of adults and 18% of children have mild to severe malocclusions requiring orthodontic treatment

Candidiasis
- Candidiasis is the most common oral fungal infection in patients with immunodeficiency disorders, such as HIV infection

Edentulism - Total Loss of Teeth
- 11% of adults 25 and older have lost all natural teeth; the rate is 17% for adults living in poverty
- 30% of adults 65 and older are toothless; the rate is 46% for those in poverty

Head and Neck Cancer
- 12,300 deaths and 40,400 new cases per year for oral, pharyngeal and laryngeal cancers combined
- Five years after diagnosis, half of all patients with oral and pharyngeal cancers survive; less than a third of African American male patients survive that long

Osteoporosis & Oral Bone Loss
- Osteoporosis is a major health threat for 28 million Americans, 80% female
- Oral bone loss is also found in patients with osteoporosis

Salivary Gland Dysfunction
- Between 1 and 4 million Americans are estimated to have Sjögren's syndrome
- Cystic fibrosis affects about 30,000 Americans. More than 500 prescription and over-the-counter drugs have xerostomic effects

Trauma
- 19.8 Million emergency room visits are estimated for craniofacial injuries each year
- Motor vehicle crashes are leading cause of unintentional injury deaths in children, with majority resulting from head injuries
- 25% of people age 6-50 show evidence of anterior tooth trauma

Pain
- 22% of adults report some form of orofacial pain in last 6 months
- 6% of adults report pain symptoms commonly associated with temporomandibular joint disorders (TMD)
- Orofacial pain is a major component of Bell's palsy, trigeminal neuralgia, fibromyalgia, and diabetic neuropathy

Periodontal Diseases
- 90% of people 13 and older show evidence of periodontal problems
- Maternal periodontal infection appears associated with increased risk of spontaneous pre-term birth and low birth weight
- Periodontal infection appears to be a risk factor for cardiovascular diseases and stroke

Oral Complications of Cancer Therapy
- Each year an estimated 490,000 patients undergoing cancer therapy suffer from such complications as painful mouth ulcers, mucositis, rampant caries, fungal infections, impaired taste, and salivary gland dysfunction

Older Adults
- About 30% of adults 65 years and older are edentulous
- 23% of 65- to 74-year-olds have severe periodontal disease
- Most older Americans take medications which have oral side effects, especially dry mouth

FIGURE 54.1
The burden of disease. From: NIDCR (www.nih.nidcr.gov) 1999 and Surgeon General's Report, 2000.

Protective Factors	Pathological Factors
Salivary flow and components Proteins, antibacterial components, and agents Fluoride, calcium, and phosphate Dietary components: protective	Reduced salivary function Bacteria: mutans streptococci, lactobacilli Dietary components: frequency carbohydrates

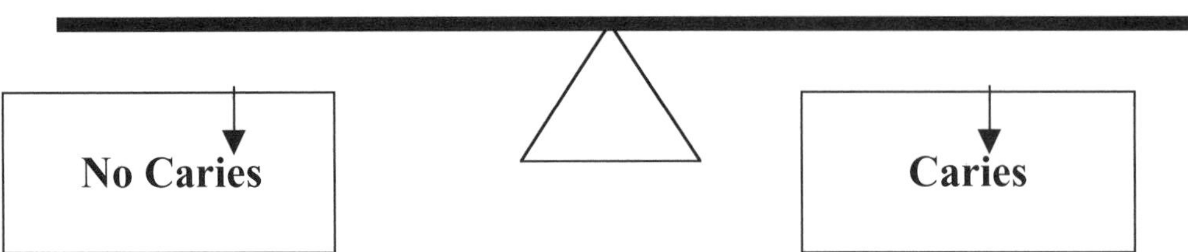

FIGURE 54.2
The caries balance: a schematic diagram of the balance between pathological and protective factors in the caries process. From: Featherstone, J.D.B., *J. Amer. Dent. Assoc.* 131: 887; 2000. With permission.

when the plaque pH drops, such as when carbohydrates (sugars) are fermented by plaque bacteria to form organic acids.[6] Mineral flows back when the pH is neutralized mostly due to the presence of salivary buffers and mineral ions, particularly when supplemented with fluoride.[6] Fluoride, when ingested at optimum amounts during tooth development (about 0.7 to 1.0 ppm), makes the enamel hydroxapatite crystal less soluble. Additionally, individuals with hyposalivation or xerostomia due to use of specific medications, head and neck irradiation, or chronic diseases like Sjögren's syndrome, lack appropriate salivary buffering capacity and thus have increased risk for caries.[7]

In a recent review, Featherstone illustrated that caries balance is dependent on the interaction of protective and pathological factors (Figure 54.2).[6] Dental caries represent an excellent example of how understanding the complex etiological agents of this multifactorial disease can have health promotion, intervention, and treatment consequences that can effect not only the disease itself, but the intricate interactions between health and nutritional status. As shown in Figure 54.3, the balance between health and disease in the oral and craniofacial complex is dependent on food choices and dietary patterns interwoven with nutritional and oral health status. Furthermore, there is a synergy between these two measures of health, (nutriture and oral status) that has a significant impact on general health and thus individual risk for many contemporary chronic and disabling diseases. If dietary intake leads to poor nutritional status, chronic disease is more likely to occur in the presence of additional risk factors that might include other lifestyle, environmental, and genetic factors.

Periodontal Disease(s)

Periodontal disease is an infection with local and systemic inflammatory effects. The initiation and progression of periodontal disease is markedly affected by risk factors. The relationship between nutrition and periodontal disease is multifaceted, where environmental and host risk factors contribute to its pathogenesis. Some of the host factors related to diet and nutrition include presence of other systemic or chronic disease, lifestage (preg-

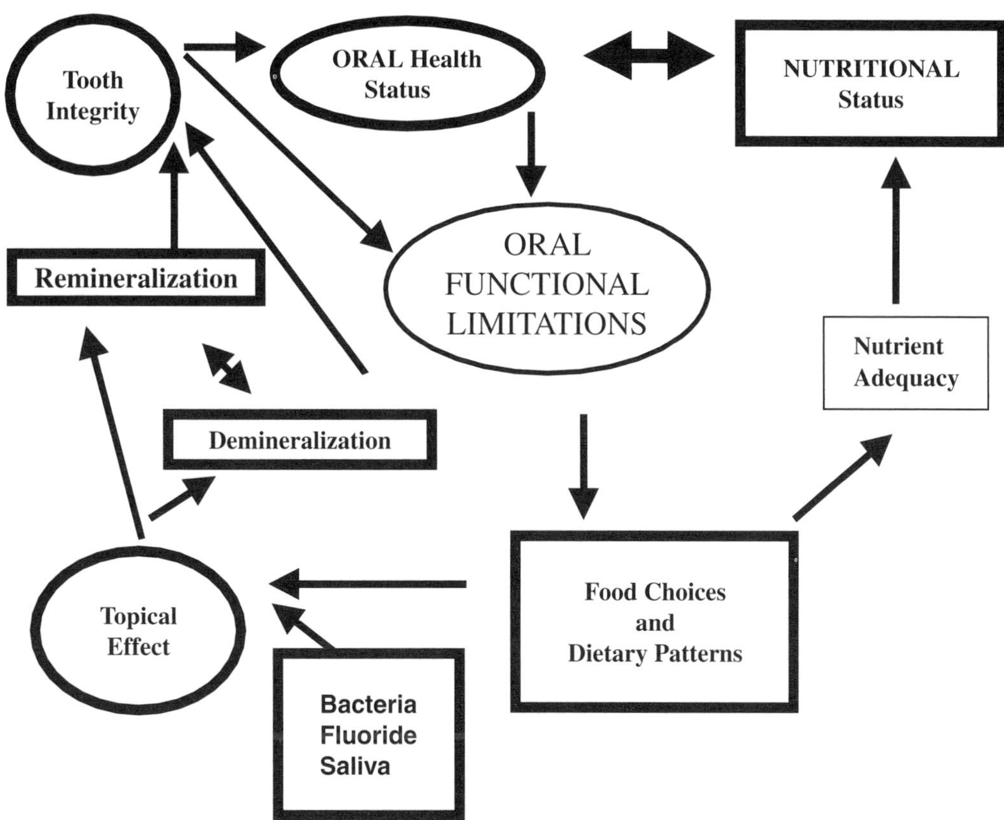

FIGURE 54.3
Diet and dental health.

nancy, menopause, elderly, etc.), osteoporosis, medications, and nutrition status. The current knowledge of nutrition and periodontal disease can be viewed in one of three ways:

1. Known relationships between periodontal disease, nutrition status, and immune response
2. Relationships of periodontal disease with nutrients that have been demonstrated in select populations
3. Unknown and yet to be tested relationships between periodontal disease, individual nutrients, and select host defense and health status variables

Known relationships include the impact of malnutrition on inflammation and infection, and the associations between calcium and periodontal disease. A superb overview of the new paradigm for the pathogenesis of periodontitis was provided recently by Page and Kornman, and is depicted in Figure 54.4.[8]

Nutrient deficiencies can compromise the system's response to inflammation and infection and increase the kcalories and protein needs necessary for adequate wound healing.[9] In this manner, poor nutritional status can impact host response to the inflammatory process and infection imposed by periodontal disease. A balanced diet along with good nutrition status is the appropriate nutrition management strategy for nutritional wellbeing

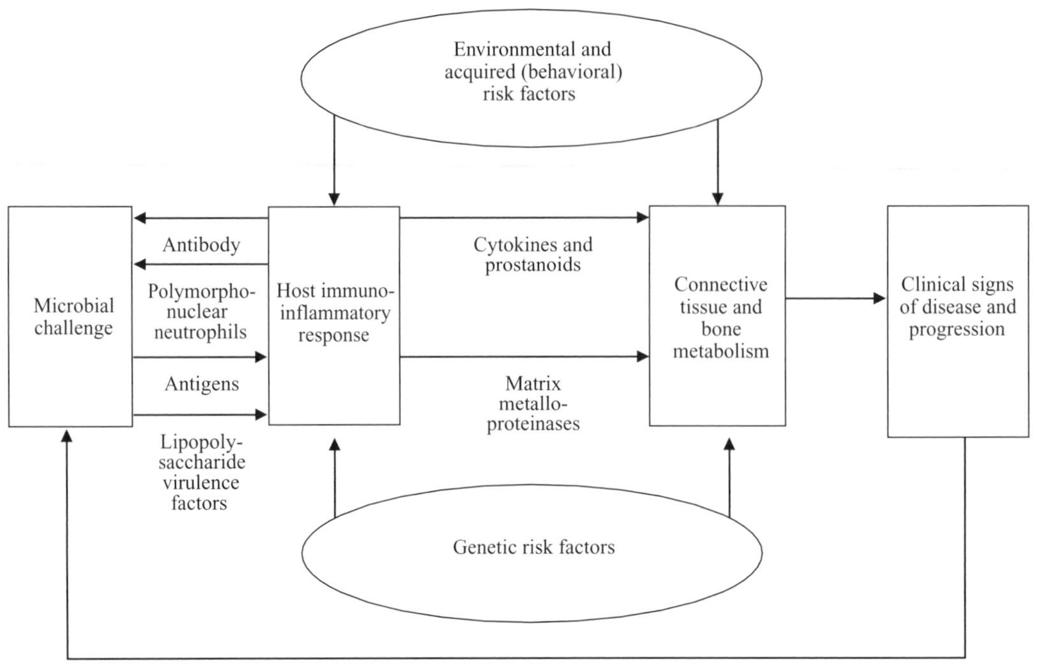

FIGURE 54.4
A new paradigm for the pathobiology of periodontitis. From: Page and Kornman, 1997, Periodontology 2000, 14: 9; 1997, with permission. Reprinted in Surgeon General's Report.

to reduce risk of malnutrition-associated compromises in immune and inflammatory responses and wound healing.

Relationships between periodontal disease, osteoporosis, and calcium intake is presented elsewhere in this section. Krall et al. have demonstrated that osteopenia and bone loss are associated with oral bone loss.[10] Treatments for osteoporosis, including hormone replacement therapy and biphosphanides, are associated with reduced oral bone and tooth loss. The relationship between calcium and vitamin D and incidence of periodontal disease remains to be demonstrated in broader gender- and age-related populations. The need for adequate calcium in the diet (either with foods and/or supplements) is important for prevention and management of osteopenia and osteoporosis as well as for periodontal disease.

The relationship between various antioxidants and periodontal disease is a developing area of research. Nishida et al. demonstrated that low dietary intake of vitamin C was significantly (although "weakly") associated with periodontal disease in individuals who currently smoke or have a history of smoking tobacco.[11] However, vitamin C has not been proven efficacious for improving periodontal health or reducing risk of disease in the general population.[11] Several studies have implicated deficiencies in ascorbate and folate with severity of gingivitis. For example, Leggott demonstrated that depletion of vitamin C was associated with increased gingival bleeding but no other markers of periodontal disease.[12]

The relationship between diabetes and periodontal disease is discussed elsewhere. However, the potential relationship between obesity and periodontal disease is a new area for investigation. In a study of obese, healthy Japanese men undergoing evaluation of periodontal status, there was a positive association between degree of obesity, as measured by body mass index, and incidence of periodontal disease.[13] After adjusting for age, sex, oral hygiene status, and smoking, the relative risk of periodontal disease was 1.3 for each

5% increase in body mass index.[13] Although type 2 diabetes is a recognized risk factor for periodontal disease, there was no association in this study between fasting blood glucose or glycosolated hemoglobin values and periodontal disease.[13] Further research is needed to explore relationships between obesity and periodontal disease, particularly in individuals with diabetes, a disease in which obesity can further compromise metabolic control.

Changes in oral tissues associated with aging can also impact periodontal status. Alveolar bone loses approximately 1% per year after age 30, and tooth mobility occurs more frequently in the elderly.[1] Soft tissue changes include thinning of the surface epithelium of the mucus membranes and gingival recession. Decreased salivary flow, most often secondary to medications or disease, is also common. These changes can also impact on nutrition status and eating ability. If severe, diet intake and nutrition status can suffer. The combined changes in the oral cavity increase the risk for nutrient intake compromise and periodontal disease.

Consumption of a balanced diet consistent with the food guide pyramid and inclusive of fruits, vegetables, grains, and adequate protein will provide sufficient vitamins, minerals, phytochemicals, and protein for overall and oral health. At this point, no published scientifically sound evidence exists to support the notion that individuals with periodontal disease need supplemental doses of any individual nutrients or groups of nutrients.

Environmental Oral Health Promotion: Fluoridation

In the early 1900s, Americans could expect to lose their teeth by middle age. With the discovery of the properties of fluoride and the adjustment of the concentration of fluoride in the supply of drinking water in the 1940s, this trend was reversed. Community water fluoridation remains one of the great achievements of public health and health promotion in the 20th century.[14] It is considered an inexpensive means of improving oral health benefits for all residents of a community. In 1992, 56% of the U.S. population was receiving fluoridated water at levels equal to or greater than 0.7 parts per million, either from natural or fluoridated public water systems. Dental caries prevention is effective at 0.7 to 1.2 part per million.[14] Some foods, beverages, and other dental products provide additional sources of fluoride to individuals.

Since the early days of community water fluoridation, the prevalence of dental caries in the U.S. has declined in communities with and without fluoridated water. This has been largely due to the diffusion of fluoridated water to areas without fluoridated water via food/beverage distribution channels and the widespread use of fluoride toothpaste.[15] Although early studies focused mostly on children, water fluoridation also reduces enamel caries in adults by 20 to 40%, and prevents root surface caries, a condition that particularly affects older adults.[1,16]

Health care providers are agents of health promotion at both individual and community levels. In the absence of a water supply with adequate fluoride to prevent dental caries, health promotion practices that support primary prevention through fluoride supplementation are encouraged. The American Dental Association Council on Scientific Affairs[17] and the American Academy of Pediatrics[18] recommend safe levels of daily fluoride supplementation for children living in unfluoridated communities. Table 54.1 describes the recommended supplementation schedule. Dietary fluoride supplements are available as tablets, drops, or lozenges. Supplementation has not been shown to be beneficial during pregnancy.[19,20] Flouridation is an inexpensive means of improving oral health, and benefits all residents of a community.

TABLE 54.1

Supplemental Fluoride Dosage Schedule (mg/day)[a]

	Concentration of Fluoride in Drinking Water (ppm)		
Age	< 0.3	0.3 to 0.6	>0.6
6 months to 3 years	0.25 mg	0	0
3 to 6 years	0.50 mg	0.25 mg	0
6 to 16 years	1.00 mg	0.50 mg	0

[a] ppm = parts per million; 2.2 mg sodium fluoride contains 1 mg fluoride.

From American Dental Association, *J. Am. Dent. Assoc.* 126: 19S; 1995. With permission.

Systemic Diseases

General Observations

The oral cavity is the gateway to the rest of the body, and at times reflects systemic as well as oral health and disease.[1] The mechanisms by which oral manifestations occur as a result of some systemic diseases are not fully known. Systemic diseases which affect the integrity of the oral cavity, and oral diseases themselves, may impact upon nutrition status, as well as the converse. Any condition affecting the functional capacity of the oral cavity (sensory or motor function) and/or the health and integrity of the soft tissue may impact on diet intake. If the integrity of the oral tissues is compromised due to infection, surgery, trauma, or medications, nutrient needs are increased. Unfortunately, this is often in the face of compromised intake due to pain, dysphagia, or anorexia. In these situations, nutrition status is compromised and the risk of malnutrition is increased. Malnutrition in turn can compromise wound healing and integrity of the immune system, further increasing the risk of oral infectious disease.

Emerging areas of research in dentistry in the 21st century include the relationships between oral infections and systemic diseases, and the oral manifestations and complications of systemic diseases and chronic disabling diseases.[2] It is anticipated that when fully appraised of these oral health–systemic health and nutrition interactions, health care professionals will be able to work collectively to identify dental and nutrition patient management strategies.

It is well documented that nutritional status may influence disease progression and recovery from illness, infection, and surgery. Malnutrition and individual nutrient deficiencies can affect tissue integrity and muscle function. A selected list of chronic diseases with recognized oral manifestations affecting nutrition status, and diseases with associated oral infections are listed in Table 54.2. Nutrition status may be affected via two primary mechanisms, functionally and metabolically, both of which can effect the sense of taste. Additionally, functional integrity of the oral cavity is critical for optimal smell, mastication, and swallowing; negative impacts on any of these functions can influence food and fluid intake, and consequently nutrition status. Metabolic impacts also include altered nutrient metabolism, typically increased catabolism of protein stores for energy, as well as increased protein and kcalorie needs due to infection. The end result of either a functional or metabolic mechanism(s) is often compromised nutrition status, increased risk of secondary infection, and altered response to disease and treatment. Weight loss of 10% or more, which can occur as a result of these diseases, increases morbidity and mortality.

TABLE 54.2

Selected Systemic Diseases with Potential Oral Manifestations Affecting Nutrition Status

Arthropathies	Autoimmune disorders
Cancers	Chronic orofacial pain
Cardiovascular disease	Diabetes
End-stage renal disease	HIV infection/AIDS
Inflammatory bowel disease	Liver disease
Megaloblastic anemia	Oral-facial pain syndromes
Osteoporosis	Pulmonary disease
Vesiculobullous diseases	Herpes Zoster

TABLE 54.3

Medications with Associated Oral Manifestations

Anticonvulsants	Antipsychotics
Antidepressants	Corticosteroids
Diuretics	Immune suppressing agents
Opiates	Serotonin uptake inhibitors
Tricyclic antidepressants	Protease inhibitors
Anti-anxiety agents	

Medications used to treat chronic diseases may also have oral sequellae that in turn compromise food intake and nutrition status. Xerostomia may occur independently, as a consequence of another systemic disease, or as a side effect of medication. More than 400 prescribed and over-the-counter medications are associated with xerostomia.[1] Xerostomia can affect sense of taste and swallowing ability as well as caries risk. Food texture and temperature may need to be modified for individuals with moderate to severe xerostomia. Drugs may also alter appetite and nutrient metabolism. Antidepressant medications and steroids can increase appetite, thus leading to increased risk of weight gain and subsequent obesity. Steroids increase catabolism of protein and carbohydrate, and lead to calcium losses. Individuals on long-term steroids are at risk for type 2 diabetes, and require calcium supplementation and added protein in their diets to reduce risk of osteoporosis and malnutrition, respectively. Classes of medications with oral manifestations are found in Table 54.3. Individual drugs are not listed; practitioners should check the Physicians Desk Reference (PDR) for individual drugs and their associated oral manifestations.

Table 54.4 addresses clinical symptomatology with associated oral clinical and systemic disorders and nutritional implications. Clinical features may represent one or more local and systemic diseases. It is imperative that clinicians look beyond the symptom to discern the actual cause of the symptomatology so as to treat the symptoms and the primary cause or disease. Although select clinical features may have an associated nutritional etiology, all other causes must be considered, and treatment aimed at the root cause and associated symptoms.

HIV-AIDS

As of December 1999, there were 33.6 million individuals with HIV/AIDS.[21] Estimates indicated 5.6 million new cases alone in 1999 and 2.6 million deaths worldwide from AIDS.[21] In the U.S., combination antiretroviral therapies have contributed to a decline in death due to AIDS as well as a reduction in the incidence of complications. Individuals with immunosuppressive diseases including HIV infection and AIDS are at increased risk

TABLE 54.4

Abnormal Oral Findings: Associated Local and Systemic Diseases

Clinical Feature	Associated Finding	Associated Disorders	Nutritional Considerations
Xerostomia	Excessive dental caries, candidiasis, dysphagia, dysgeusia, burning mouth/tongue	Drug-induced xerostomia, head and neck irradiation, Sjögren's syndrome, diabetes	Increase fluids, minimize cariogenic foods, modify food consistency and flavoring, evaluate glucose control in diabetes
Burning mouth/tongue	May be associated with mucosal erythema/atrophy, glossitis	Anemia, diabetes, candidiasis	Determine etiology of anemia (iron, folate, B_{12}), check riboflavin, modify food consistency and flavoring, evaluate glucose control
Angular cheilitis	Dry, cracked, fissured corner of the mouth	Dehydration, anemia, ill-fitting dentures (drooling)	Determine etiology
Candidiasis	White and/or red removable patches on the oral mucosa	Immunodeficiency, diabetes	Determine etiology
Difficulty chewing	Partial or complete edentulism, poor occlusion, ill fitting dentures	Cranial nerve disorders	Determine etiology, referral for medical nutrition therapy

Adapted from Touger-Decker R, Sirois D. *Support Line* 3: 1; 1996.

of oral complications and malnutrition due to the disease and associated metabolic, oral, GI, immune, psychosocial, and pharmacological sequellae. Macronutrient metabolism is often altered; women lose more fat tissue, further contributing to malnutrition, while men tend to lose lean tissue, again contributing to malnutrition and increased needs.[21] The psychological and physiological stress associated with HIV and AIDS contributes to alterations in nutrient intake and subsequent nutrition status.

Poor oral hygiene, malnutrition, and lack of dental care are key factors in the development and severity of oral lesions in this population. Candidiasis occurs in 80 to 100% of HIV patients with AIDS upon onset of the disease.[3] Periodontal disease including necrotizing ulcerative periodontitis (NUP) is common in patients with HIV. Cancers of the oral cavity, Kaposi's sarcoma, and lymphoma may also occur. Thus, oral challenges, combined with common nutrition problems such as wasting syndrome, visceral and somatic protein depletion, maldigestion and malabsorption, altered nutrient and energy needs, polypharmacy, and reduced oral food intake secondary to anorexia, nausea, or compromised oral health status further contribute to the malnutrition observed in this population.

The possible causes of anorexia in this population can be seen in Table 54.5. Medical Nutrition Therapy (MNT) by the Registered Dietician (RD) and physician is warranted to prevent further nutritional depletion, altered taste perception, odynophagia/dysphagia,

TABLE 54.5

Possible Causes of Anorexia in HIV/AIDS

Polypharmacy	Dysgeusia
Odynophagia/dysphagia	Nausea/vomiting
Depression	Weakness/lethargy
Oral infections/lesions	Tooth loss
GI disease	Kaposi's sarcoma

TABLE 54.6

Impact of HIV Infection on Nutrition and Diet in the Upper GI Tract

Location	Problem	Effect	Diet Management
Oral cavity	Candidiasis, KS herpes, stomatitis, apthous ulcers	Pain, infection, lesions, altered ability to eat, saliva; dysgeusia	Increase kcalories & protein Oral supplements Caries risk reduction
	Xerostomia	Caries risk, pain, no moistening power, food sticks, dysgeusia	Moist, soft foods; non-spicy, "smooth," cool/warm, fluids Caries risk reduction
Esophagus	Candidiasis, herpes, KS, Cryptosporidius	Dysphagia, odynophagia	Oral supp 1st, 2nd = NG using silastic feeding tube or PEG
	CMV CMV + ulceration	Dysphagia, food accumulation	Percutaneous endoscopic gastrostomy

nausea/vomiting, psychosocial considerations, weakness/lethargy, and the expanded use of other medications.

Wasting syndrome is characteristic of later stages of HIV and is defined as "a greater than (>)10% unintentional weight loss from usual body weight in the presence of diarrhea or fever for greater than (>) 30 days that is not attributable to other disease processes."[22] Wasting Syndrome is also defined as "a process of decline characterized by pathological alterations in body composition, weight loss, fatigue and loss of strength and a decrease in quality of life."[23] The pathogenesis of wasting can be attributed to several factors including decreased energy intake, anorexia, GI dysfunction, and deranged metabolism including increased insulin sensitivity, altered carbohydrate metabolism, and increased protein turnover. During acute phases of the disease, drugs and medical nutrition therapy are critical to manage the disease and preserve lean body mass. As individuals progress to lifelong drug management with combinations of antiretroviral therapies, nutrition status is challenged by the associated drug side effects. These side effects may include food-drug interactions, oral lesions, and infection as well as alterations in appetite and intake.

Table 54.6 outlines the impact of HIV infection in the GI tract. Common HIV-associated oral infectious disorders include those of fungal, viral, and bacterial origin, detailed in Table 54.7.[24] Oropharyngeal fungal infections may cause a burning, painful mouth and dysphagia. The ulcers found with viral infections such as herpes simplex and cytomega-

TABLE 54.7

Common HIV-Associated Oral Disorders

Infection	
Bacterial	Linear erythematous gingivitis, necrotizing ulcerative periodontitis, syphilis, caries
Fungal	Candida, cryptococcus, histoplasmosis
Viral	Herpes simplex, hairy leukoplakia, human papiloma
Neoplasm	
Fungal	Kaposi's sarcoma
Viral	Non-Hodgkin's lymphoma
Other	
Fungal	Parotid disease, xerostomia, apthous ulcers
Viral	Pain syndromes, necrotizing stomatitis

Adapted with permission from D. Sirois, *Mt. Sinai J. Med.* 65: 322; 1998.

TABLE 54.8

Oral Manifestations of Diabetes

Gingivitis	Altered taste
Periodontal disease	Burning mouth
Reduced saliva (with resultant xerostomia)	Increased thirst
Salivary hyperglycemia	Neuropathies
Increased risk of infectious disorders and complications	
Slowed wound healing	

lovirus cause pain and reduced oral intake. Oral and esophageal candidiasis results in painful chewing, sucking, and swallowing, consequently reducing an already compromised appetite and intake. Kaposi's sarcoma compromises oral intake and increases nutrient needs. The oral disorders found with HIV and AIDS increase nutrient demands on the body for healing, and compromise eating ability. MNT is critical to healing and maintenance of lean body mass. Oral diets with or without nutritional supplements should be tried first, followed by tube feedings if needed. The dental professional should observe patients for changes in intake, weight, and overall nutritional wellbeing, and refer individuals to an RD and/or physician early in the process of disease management.[25,26]

Diabetes

Over 11 million individuals in the U.S. have diabetes; another 13 million have impaired glucose tolerance.[27] Diabetes is the seventh leading cause of death in the U.S. Oral sequellae occurring with diabetes are usually a result of poorly controlled diabetes, or hyperglycemia. Oral cell metabolism, immune surveillance, and vascular integrity as well as salivary chemistry may be altered in individuals with diabetes, particularly when uncontrolled. Over 90% of individuals over age 13 with diabetes have some periodontal problems relative to diabetes.[28] While there is limited evidence that periodontal infection affects glycemic control,[29] any infection can contribute to adverse alterations in glycemic control. Other oral manifestations may occur, impacting diet intake and nutrition status. These can be seen in Table 54.8.

Diabetes, particularly when poorly controlled, is associated with a higher prevalence of all infections including oral infections, as compared to non-diabetics.[28] The susceptibility to periodontal disease in diabetes is likely directly related to impaired defense mechanisms. Micro- and macrovascular circulation are altered, along with wound healing, collagen metabolism, neutrophil chemotaxis, and proteolysis. Pathologic tissue destruction contributes to periodontal tissue destruction. Increased salivary glucose increases bacterial substrate and plaque formation. Microangiopathies, altered vascular permeability, and metabolic alterations may lead to an altered immune response and precipitate periodontal disease progression. The oral complications associated with diabetes are often referred to as the sixth major medical complication of diabetes.

The relationship between oral manifestations in diabetes and diet/nutrition is a complex two-way street. While uncontrolled diabetes is partly due to poor diet management, oral manifestations challenge and ultimately compromise eating ability and consequent dietary intake. Taste in patients with diabetes is often altered due to salivary chemistry, xerostomia, and/or candidiasis. Management of burning mouth/tongue requires a determination of the cause. When due to a nutrient deficiency, augmentation of the diet with the appropriate nutrient(s) or supplements will treat the cause and subsequent symptomatology. When a physical or biochemical abnormality cannot be found, the symptoms of burning mouth can be improved using tricyclic antidepressant medications. However, the unfortunate side effect of tricyclic antidepressants is xerostomia, which may compound any existing alterations in saliva, and increase risk of candidiasis and dental caries.

Diet management is the cornerstone of diabetes care. Proper diet control, in kcalorie and macronutrient distribution throughout the day, is critical to glycemic control, particularly in type 1 diabetes. In both type 1 and type 2 diabetes, a diet consistent with the food guide pyramid consisting of 50% carbohydrate, 20% protein, and 30% fat is recommended with attainment and maintenance of desirable body weight. In most states, MNT by an RD with several follow-up visits is a benefit covered by all third party payers and Medicaid. The oral health professional should work closely with the patient's physician and refer patients, as appropriate, to an RD, reinforce the need to adhere to the diabetic diet, integrate oral hygiene into daily routines, and modify diet consistencies as needed to manage oral conditions and surgeries.

Crohn's Disease

Crohn's disease can present with apthous ulcers, angular stomatitis, and/or glossitis. Oral lesions present on the lips, gingiva, and buccal mucosa may precede gastrointestinal symptoms and have a dramatic impact on oral function. The size of the lesion may not coincide with the intensity of pain reported or degree of compromise in food and fluid intake. Ability to eat may be hampered by pain; topical anesthetic agents (or a 1:1 mixture of Milk of Magnesia and Benadryl as a rinse and spit) prior to meals may temporarily relieve pain and allow more comfort in eating. Pharmacological management is critical; steroids are often needed. The impact of steroids on nutritional wellbeing has been addressed in other sections of this handbook.

Autoimmune Disease

Autoimmune diseases such as Pemphigus Vulgaris (PV) increase nutrition risk by virtue of the oral and facial sequellae of the disease and the medications used to manage it. Steroids are often used in the management of vesiculobullous diseases of the oral cavity including PV. PV can impact diet intake and nutrition status by virtue of the disease process as well as the medications used to manage it. Much like other diseases with oral lesions, PV affects appetite and eating ability due to associated pain. In addition to the medications used for the disease, topical anesthetics, as well as a rinse-and-spit 1:1 mixture of Benadryl and Milk of Magnesia immediately prior to eating, provides a topical coating, allowing more comfort during mealtime. Other autoimmune diseases including Sjögren's Syndrome and rheumatoid arthritis (RA) can affect the oral cavity and subsequent nutrition status. Oral and nutritional implications of select diseases in this category are outlined in Table 54.9. While diet modifications are addressed, particular attention needs to be paid to the individual's stage of disease. During disease exacerbation, eating ability may be severely compromised and a liquid diet using oral supplements (meal replacement formulas) such as Sustacal or Boost (Mead Johnson) or Ensure+ (Ross) may be required to meet energy and protein needs. During remission, individuals may be able to liberalize diets considerably.

Osteoporosis

Osteoporosis is the most common bone disease.[30] Osteoporosis is clinically defined as reduced bone mineral density.[30] The majority of individuals with osteoporosis are women

TABLE 54.9
Autoimmune Disorders with Associated Oral and Nutritional Side Effects

Disease	Oral Manifestation	Nutrition Implications
Rheumatoid arthritis	TMJ ankylosis Limited mandibular opening	Pain upon eating Modify diet consistency
Erythema multiforme	Oral mucosal lesions, often ulcerative	Pain upon eating Increased needs for healing Modify diet, often liquid consistency with straw during exacerbation If treated with steroids: increase calcium, protein
Pemphigus Vulgaris	Oral mucosal lesions	Eating painful and difficult If treated with steroids: increase calcium, protein Modify diet as needed in temperature, consistency
Sjögrens syndrome	Xerostomia; mucosa dry, erythematous; fissures; more susceptible to trauma; increased risk of caries; fissured tongue; periodontal disease; cervical caries	Increased fluids with and between meals, increase fluidity of foods, soft, temperate foods, non-spicy
Systemic lupus erythematosus	Ulcerations of mucosa	Manage side effects of steroids and medications, diet as per Sjögrens

(80%); however it is a risk for up to 28 million Americans, and is often known as a "silent killer."[1] One in two caucasian women will have an osteoporotic fracture in their lifetime.[30] Nonmodifiable and modifiable causes of osteoporosis are listed in Table 54.10. Since dental health care professionals see patients on a regular basis and since alveolar boss loss is associated with osteoporosis, the dental professional is in an ideal situation to access patients at risk for osteoporosis. Simple screening in the dental office can include asking patients about calcium intake in the form of dairy products (milk, cheese, yogurt), functional foods or foods fortified with calcium (orange juice, cereal), and calcium supplements. Other individuals at risk for osteoporosis (see Table 54.10) should be referred for a dexascan to determine risk for or presence of osteopenia or osteoporosis.

Bone loss is a common denominator for both periodontal disease and osteoporosis. The relationship between the two diseases remains to be fully determined.[31] However, an association between periodontal disease and systemic osteopenia and osteoporosis has been documented in adults.[31,32] The relationship between calcium intake and risk of periodontal disease has also been demonstrated; lowered dietary intakes in adults have been found to be associated with increased periodontal disease risk.[11] While a serum calcium level may not be associated with actual calcium intake, decreasing levels of intake below the recommended dietary intakes is associated with increased risk and incidence of osteoporosis.[33] Tezal et al. pose "four possible pathways" for the relationship between osteoporosis and severity of periodontal disease, including systemic loss of bone mineral density, modified local tissue response to infection as a result of "systemic factors of bone remodeling", genetics, and lifestyle factors.[31] The final pathway, lifestyle factor, links the issues of hygiene, diet, and exercise with local and systemic disease. Osteoporosis has also been linked to the development of tooth loss, particularly in post-menopausal women.[10] Please refer to Section 61 for a thorough description of osteoporosis and other bone diseases and disorders.

TABLE 54.10
Risk Factors for Osteoporosis

Nonmodifiable
History of fracture as an adult
Caucasian or Asian race
Advanced age
Female gender
Dementia
Poor health/frailty
Prolonged use of glucocorticoids, phenytoin
Estrogen deficiency:
Menopause/early menopause (<age 45) or bilateral ovariectomy; prolonged premenopausal amenorrhea (>1 year)
Prolonged immobilization, i.e., spinal cord injury
Potentially Modifiable
Current cigarette smoking
Low body weight (<127 lbs)
Low calcium intake (lifelong)
Alcoholism
Impaired eyesight despite adequate correction
Recurrent falls
Inadequate physical activity
Poor health/frailty
End-stage renal disease

From National Osteoporosis Foundation, *Physicians Guide to Prevention and Treatment of Osteoporosis*, 1998. With permission.

Neoplastic Diseases: Oral Cancer

Oral cancer develops from a precancerous lesion most commonly on the tongue, lips, and floor of the mouth. White leukoplakia or reddish erythroplakia are usually induced by tobacco use alone or in combination with alcohol abuse.[34,35] It is the sixth most common cancer in males living in the U.S. Over 90% of oral cancers are squamous cell carcinomas — cancers of the epithelial cells. Tobacco components act as promoters of carcinogenesis, and alcohol may act as a solvent to facilitate penetration of the tobacco carcinogens into oral tissue.[36] Viruses, including the herpes simplex type 1 and human papilloma virus, have both been implicated in oral cancer. Of the known oncogenes, many have been implicated in oral and pharyngeal cancer.[37] Both disarmament of the cell's DNA repair mechanisms and mutation of tumor suppressor genes have been linked to smoking and alcohol use, and play a major role in oral cancer development. Likewise, nicotine stimulates negative changes in immune cells that can promote tumor growth.

Ecologic and case-control studies have suggested that nutrients may play an important role in the prevention and management of early oral cancer and precancerous leukoplakia. Likewise, several studies have shown that smokers have lower plasma levels of vitamin E, C, beta-carotene, and other antioxidants due to both low intake and increased metabolic use.[38] Total fruits and vegetables, fresh fruits, green leafy vegetables, other vegetables, total bread and cereals, and whole grain breads and cereals which are excellent sources of multiple antioxidants have been shown to be associated with decreased risk of oral cancer.[39] More specifically, citrus, dark yellow and other fruits were more consistently associated with decreased risk than were estimated intake of specific nutrients including carotene, vitamin C, fiber, folate, thiamine, riboflavin, niacin, vitamin E, and iron. A case-control study conducted in Italy illustrated that the more a micronutrient, such as vitamin C, carotene, or vitamin E, was correlated to total vegetable and fruit intake, the stronger was its protective effect against oral cancer.[40] Thus, it appears that total fruit and vegetable intake may offer greater risk reduction than singular antioxidant nutrients in supplemental doses. Fioretti et al. reported that even in the absence of tobacco use, if subjects reduced alcohol and saturated fat intake and increased fruit and carrot consumption, there appeared to be a favorable effect on oral cancer risk among subjects who participated in a large case-control study.[41]

Nutritional care of the patient with oral cancer will vary based on treatment modalities and side effects that can include changes in weight, sore mouth or throat, xerostomia, mucositis, dental caries, gingival infection, changes in sense of taste and smell, nausea, vomiting, and fatigue. Nutritional management strategies will require the services of oncology health care professionals.

Craniofacial-Oral-Dental Birth Defects

Nearly two infants in every 1000 live births have some type of craniofacial birth defect.[42] These defects can occur in isolation or as a component of a larger birth defect syndrome caused by genetic influences, environmental disturbances, or the interplay between gene and environment. A number of congenital oral-dental-craniofacial birth defects can be prevented by reducing risk factors associated with human craniofacial malformations. Among the common environmental risk factors are alcohol (associated with fetal alcohol syndrome); smoking (associated with risk of cleft lip with or without cleft palate); anti-convulsant medications, such as phenytoin and other teratogens (associated with a variety of birth defects involving the face, teeth, and jaws); retinoic acid analogues (associated with severe craniofacial and oral clefts and limb defects); and vitamin deficiency, particularly folate (associated with increased risk of cleft lip with or without cleft palate).[42]

Available data from the NIDCR revealed that about 20% of craniofacial-oral-dental birth defects are either genetic or familial.[42] The largest majority are caused by the defined risk factors noted above or unknown causes. From a nutrition perspective, there are a number of important discoveries that could be applied to oral-dental-craniofacial defects. One application relates to the preventive effects of micronutrients. A growing body of evidence strongly suggests that the use of multivitamin supplements and folic acid result in the prevention of cleft lip and/or cleft palate in much the same way that these micronutrients work to prevent neural tube defects such spina bifida. As these studies progress, it will become important to carefully titrate the dose of the micronutrient provided to an expectant woman that will result in a maximum protective effect. This is vital because there is a possibility that excessive amounts of some nutrients, such as vitamin A or retinoic acid, can result in the opposite effect; that is, they could be teratogenic.[42,43] Retinoic acid-induced embryopathy includes defects in craniofacial, skeletal, cardiac, thymic, and central nervous system structures.[42,43]

The protective molecular mechanism for retinoic acid-induced embryopathy relates to the binding of retinoic acid to cognate receptors that, in turn, bind to unique regions within the promoter region of structural and/or regulatory genes.[44] Indeed, the expression of the homeobox gene, Hoxb-1, is highly responsive to vitamin A. Since Hoxb-1 regulates embryonic axial patterning, excess vitamin A induces altered pattern formation with apoptosis.[44] Thus, folic acid and vitamin A represent excellent examples of the exquisite sensitivity of embryogenesis, and the craniofacial complex in particular, to nutrients. A critical message for the oral health practitioner is the necessity to work closely with the nutritionist and physician to educate prospective and expectant parents regarding nutrition and oral health.

Importantly, following the birth of a "cleft" child, depending on the extent and severity of clefting, a series of physiological, psychological, medical, dental, and social issues emerges. The establishment of a craniofacial anomaly or cleft team to manage patients with clefting and/or other craniofacial defects is ideal. This multidisciplinary team assesses the child and his/her various medical, nutritional, social, and psychological needs. Often a nutritionist/dietician is an integral part of such a team, since one of the major issues to overcome for such children is the ability to ingest adequate amounts of food and nutrients consistent with increased nutrient requirements of the early developmental years. These nutrition requirements are exacerbated by multiple surgical interventions and the extent of the defects. Therefore, craniofacial anomalies present two challenges for the health care professional and the nutrition community in particular. One is to identify women at risk for birth defects and use appropriate interventions to prevent craniofacial anomalies. The second is to work closely in an interdisciplinary team to mitigate the effects of the anomaly.

Health Promotion, Health Education, and Behavior Change

Health promotion is a term used to describe not only heath education but also organizational, economic, and environmental channels that provide support for enabling people to increase control over and improvement of their health.[45,46] Dental nutrition is an integral part of general health promotion and disease prevention.

According to health promotion theoretical models, personal health practices and behaviors that enhance lifestyle lead to reduced morbidity and mortality, improved health status, and improved quality of life. Frequently, oral diseases in children are associated with eating difficulty, general health problems, and even lost school time.[47] In aging populations strong associations exist between oral health status and ability to swallow, chew efficiently, and select a variety of foods.[48] Numerous nutrition and dietary practices enhance positive oral health outcomes throughout the life span. Thus, it is imperative that dietary intake provide adequate nutrients to support oral health and function.

Nutrition education programs focused on changing dietary behaviors should include oral health promotion within the Food Guide Pyramid and U.S. Dietary Guidelines messages.[49] Table 54.11 describes global nutrition messages appropriate for inclusion in oral health promotion programs targeting primary and secondary prevention of dental caries. Table 54.12 identifies messages appropriate for early childhood caries (ECC) prevention. Effort has been made to reduce ECC, particularly in high-risk populations that include minority and low socioeconomic groups. Unfortunately, the nutrition focus has been limited to infant feeding practices, promoting early weaning with transition from bottle to cup and the impression that milk sugar (lactose) is the primary culprit. Sucrose, glucose, and fructose found in fruit juices and drinks as well as sweetened solid foods are probably the main sugars associated with ECC.[55] Due to the casein as well as calcium and phosphate

TABLE 54.11

Global Nutrition Messages Addressing Primary and Secondary Prevention of Dental Caries

Message	Rationale
Eat a balanced diet representing moderation and variety	Focus on positive aspects of healthy eating. Fermentable carbohydrates can contribute to dietary intake and be consumed in moderation.
Combine and sequence foods to encourage chewing and saliva production	Combinations of raw and cooked foods can increase saliva flow. Protein-rich foods combined with cooked carbohydrates, and dairy foods combined with fermentable carbohydrates can alter dental plaque pH. (Rugg-Gunn, 1993)[50]
Space the frequency of eating or drinking fermentable carbohydrates at least two hours apart	It may take up to 120 minutes for dental plaque pH to return to neutral after exposure to fermentable carbohydrate. (Edgar, 1996)[51]
Chew sugarless gum after meals and snacks to increase saliva	The Food and Drug Administration authorized the use of sugar alcohol containing foods to be labeled "does not promote," or "useful in not promoting," or "expressly for not promoting" dental caries if the food does not cause a drop in dental plaque pH below 5.7 when a fermentable carbohydrate is present. (U.S. Food and Drug Administration, 1996)[52]
Drink water to satisfy thirst and hydration needs	A review of fermentable carbohydrate consumption in the U.S. identified carbonated beverages as the major contributor to total intake. (Gibney, 1995)[53]

content, milk formulas (with the exception of some soy-based and protein hydrolyzed formulas), bovine milk, and human milk may indeed be cariostatic and not a source of cariogenic substrate in ECC. However, the nursing bottle can effectively block salivary access to tooth surfaces and may increase the caries-promoting potential of any food that remains in the mouth.[56] Reisine and Douglass have suggested that psychosocial and behavioral issues related to elements of the environment may be greater modulators of ECC than the baby bottle.[57]

Numerous opportunities exist for nutrition messages to be included in oral health promotion initiatives. Table 54.13 lists a variety of health topics that impact oral health outcomes and status. With the advent of The Surgeon General's Report on Oral Health, attention has been drawn to the need for health care professionals to address oral health and systemic health as one entity: health![1] This list in Table 54.13 provides insight into the aforementioned synergy between oral and nutritional status, and offers targeted messages for health promotion in public health and private practice.

Better understanding of the role of behavioral variables in health and disease, including the role of prevention, is important in the delivery of messages that promote both nutritional and oral health status. Practices that attempt to translate the scientific discoveries in nutrition and oral health will provide a basis upon which to plan and execute future health promotion activities.

TABLE 54.12

Nutrition Messages to Integrate into Parenting Practices for Primary Prevention of ECC

Message	Rationale
Birth to 6 Months of Age	
Encourage feeding schedules that encourage breast milk and formula consumption on a regular routine basis rather than continuously on-demand.	The American Academy of Pediatrics (AAP) encourages breastfeeding on demand in response to signs of hunger, described as increased alertness or activity, mouthing or rooting. The American Academy of Pediatric Dentistry (AAPD) recommend that infants not be put to sleep with a bottle and that nocturnal breastfeeding should be avoided after the first primary tooth begins to erupt.
Instruct mothers to avoid introduction of food until the infant doubles the birth weight or weighs at least 13 pounds.	The AAP recommends breastfeeding exclusively for about the first six months after birth, after which time iron-enriched solid foods can be added to complement the breast milk diet. Infants will double their birth weight or reach 13 pounds at between 4 and 6 months of age, or approximately 5 months.
Hold the infant when bottle and/or breast feeding.	This will prevent bottle propping, prolonged exposure to caries-promoting substrate, and allowing infants to drink from bottles on a continuing basis.
6 to 12 Months	
Promote weaning from the bottle in combination with the introduction of a cup and spoon.	The AAPD encourages parents to have infants drink from a cup prior to their first birthday and be weaned from the bottle at 12-14 months of age.
Promote introduction of foods to encourage self-feeding and growth and development as well as dental health.	The AAPD recommends implementation of oral hygiene measures by the time of eruption of the first primary tooth.
1 to 16 Years of Age	
Promote snacking habits that support growth and development and dental health.	The AAPD endorses the Dietary Guidelines for Americans that promote variety, a healthy weight, a diet that includes vegetables, fruits, and grains, and use of sugars in moderation for children and adults.
Advocate discontinued bottle and breast feeding practice.	
Stress the value of mealtime and the importance of variety and moderation.	
Encourage the beginning of routine dental visits for the child.	The AAPD recommends an oral evaluation visit within six months of the eruption of the first tooth and no later than twelve months of age.

American Academy of Pediatrics, *Pediatrics* 11: 1035; 1997.

Journal of The American Academy of Pediatric Dentistry Reference Manual 1996-97. *Pediatr. Dent.* 18: 25; 1996.

TABLE 54.13

Nutrition Messages for Targeted Oral Health Promotion Topics

Oral Health Promotion Topics	Nutrition Messages
Hypomineralized or hypoplastic primary teeth and caries risk	Children who are malnourished pre-, peri-, or postnatally and/or low birthweight are more likely to have this condition. (Alvarez 1995, Lai 1998)[58,59]
Craniofacial development	Causes are attributed to genetic defects often working in concert with environmental factors such as alcohol intake and possibly excessive therapeutic vitamin A. Neural tube defects and risks of cleft lip and palate may be reduced in children if women support dietary folic acid intake with additional supplementation to equal 400 μg. (Bonin 1998)[60]
Bone status	Loss of teeth leads to bone atrophy. Localized diseases like periodontal disease and systemic diseases like osteoporosis may further affect alveolar bone loss. Promotion of diets adequate in calcium and vitamin D to target these effects should be discussed in the context of oral health. (Bhaskar 1991)[61]
Oral soft tissue integrity	Nutritional status can enhance the ability of healthy epithelial tissue to prevent penetration of bacterial endotoxins into gingival tissue. Protein, vitamins A, C, and E, as well as the B-compex vitamins and zinc will help to maintain immune system integrity, but there is a paucity of scientific data to support supplemental use of these nutrients. Prevention of diseases of the soft tissue related to diseases like periodontal disease and systemic diabetes may challenge utilization of nutrients and can increase risk of decreased oral soft tissue integrity. (Touger-Decker 2000)[62]
Salivary output	Saliva and salivary glands provide clues to overall health and disease and function in the mucosal immune system to protect oral tissue integrity. Saliva moistens food and lubricates the bolus for swallowing. Fiber intake and frequency of eating can promote salivary output. Xerostomia (dry mouth) associated with disease and drug therapies may require medical nutrition therapy. (Martin 1999)[48]
Edentulous state	Toothless persons or those who wear dentures need to be encouraged to modify food selection habits and method of preparing foods for easier biting and chewing. One can still achieve good nutritional status important to the maintenance of the oral tissue.
Oral cancer prevention	Promoting five or more servings a day of fruits and vegetables from a variety of sources that include both dark green and yellow sources may decrease risk for oral cancer. Weight management strategies for those interested in smoking cessation can possibly enhance success and should be explored when appropriate. (Jones and Mobley 2000)[63]
Dental erosion	Fruit juices, citrus fruits, acid sweet candies and mints, pickles, and cola drinks can cause loss of tooth enamel. Vomiting and regurgitation associated with gastroesophageal reflux and eating disorders can also cause this dental condition. Encourage dietary practices to neutralize the impact of these products and conditions. (Rugg-Gunn 1993)[50]

References

1. U.S. Department of Health and Human Services. *Oral Health in America: A Report of the Surgeon General*. Rockville, MD: U.S. Department of Health and Human Services, National Institute of Dental and Craniofacial Research, National Institutes of Health, 2000.
2. Slavkin H, Baum BJ. *JAMA* 284: 1215; 2000.
3. National Institute of Dental and Craniofacial Research. *Burden of Disease*. www.nidcr.nih.gov/discover/ctfy2001, accessed July 26, 2000.
4. Kaste LM, Selwitz RH, Oldakowski RJ, et al. *J Dent Res* 75: 631; 1996.
5. Winn DM, Brunell JA, Selwitz RH, et al. *J Dent Res* 75: 642; 1996.
6. Feathersone JDB. *J Am Dent Assoc* 131: 887; 2000.
7. Winston AE, Bhaskar SN. *J Am Dent Assoc* 129: 1579; 1998.
8. Page RC, Kornman KS. *Periodontology 2000* 14: 9; 1997.
9. American Dietetic Association. Position of The American Dietetic Association: Oral Health and Nutrition. *J Am Diet Assoc* 96: 184; 1996.
10. Krall EA, Garcia RI, Dawson-Hughes B. *Calcif Tissue Int* 59: 433; 1996.
11. Nishida M, et al. *J Periodontal* 71: 1215; 2000.
12. Leggot PJ, et al. *J Dent Res* 70: 1531; 1991.
13. Saito T, et al. *N Engl J Med* 339: 482; 1998.
14. Achievement in public health, 1900-1999; *MMWR Weekly* 48: 933; 1999.
15. Horowitz HS. *J Public Health Dent* 56: 253; 1996.
16. Newbrun E. *J Public Health Dent* 49: 279; 1989.
17. American Dental Association. *J Am Dent Assoc* 126: 15; 1995.
18. American Academy of Pediatrics. *Pediatrics* 11: 1035; 1997.
19. Leverett DH, Vaughn BW, Adair SM, et al. *J Public Health Dent* 53: 205A; 1993.
20. Clarkson HB, Fejerskov O, Ekstrand et al. In: *Fluorides in Dentistry*. Fejerskov O, Ekstrand J, Burt BA, Eds, 2nd ed. Copenhagen: Munksgaad; 1996, p 347.
21. American Dietetic Association. *J Am Diet Assoc* 100: 708; 2000.
22. Centers for Disease Control. *MMWR* 41: 1; 1992.
23. Kotler D, Tierney AR, et al. *Am J Clin Nutr* 57: 1; 1989.
24. Sirois D. *Mt Sinai J Med* 65: 322; 1998.
25. Touger-Decker R. *Mt Sinai J Med* 65: 355; 1998.
26. Touger-Decker R, Sirois D. *Support Line* 3: 1; 1996.
27. National Institute of Dental and Craniofacial Research. *Workshop on Oral Disease and Diabetes*, December 6-7, 1999.
28. Baron S. Bacterial Infection in Diabetes. *Workshop on Oral Disease and Diabetes*, National Institute of Dental and Craniofacial Research, December 6-7, 1999.
29. Taylor G, Burt B, Becker M, et al. *J Periodontol* 67: 1085; 1996.
30. Osteoporosis Coalition of New Jersey and the New Jersey Department of Health and Senior Services. *Recommended Practice Guidelines for the Diagnosis and Treatment of Osteoporosis*. Washington Crossing PA: Scientific Frontiers Inc, 1998.
31. Tezal M, Wactawski-Wende J, Grossi SG. *J Periodontol* 71: 1492; 2000.
32. Payne JB, Reinhardt RA, et al. *Osteoporosis Int* 10: 34; 1999.
33. National Osteoporosis Foundation, *Physicians Guide to Prevention and Treatment of Osteoporosis*. Washington DC: National Osteoporosis Foundation, 1998.
34. Mashberg A. *J Am Dent Assoc* 96: 615; 1978.
35. Shklar G. *N Engl J Med* 315: 1544; 1986.
36. Blot WJ, McLaughlin JK, Winn DM, et al. *Cancer Res* 48: 3282; 1988.
37. Spandidos DA, Lamothe A, Field JK. *Anticancer Res* 5: 221; 1985.
38. Handelman GJ, Packer L, Cross CE. *Am J Clin Nutr* 63: 559; 1996.
39. Marshall JR, Boyle P. *Cancer Causes Control* 7: 101; 1996.
40. Negri E, Franceschi S, Bosetti C, et al. *Int J Cancer* 86: 122; 2000.
41. Fioretti F, Bosetti C, Tavani A, et al. *Oral Oncology* 35: 375; 1999.

42. Slavkin H. Meeting the Challenge of Craniofacial-Oral-Dental Birth Defects, *J Am Dent Assoc* 127: 681; 1996.
43. Slavkin H. *Prospects for Dental, Science, Education and Practice in the 21st Century.* 2nd Asia Pacific Congress, Japan, May 2000. www.nidcr.nih.gov/discover/slides.
44. Slavkin H. *Nutrients and Micronutrients: Progress is Science-Based Understanding, Insights on Human Health,* NIDCR; 1-11, 1998. www.nih.nidcr.gov.
45. Green LW, Kreuter MW. *Health Promotion Planning: An Educational and Environmental Approach.* 3rd ed. Mountain View CA: Mayfield Publishing Company, 1999.
46. Epp L. Achieving Health of All: A Framework for Health Promotion in Canada. Toronto: Health and Welfare Canada, 1986.
47. Edmunds M, Coye MJ, Eds. *America's Children: Health Insurance and Access to Care.* Committee on Children, Health Insurance and Access to Care, Division of Health Care Services, Institute of Medicine. Washington: National Academy Press, 1998.
48. Martin WE. Oral health in the elderly. In: *Geriatric Nutrition; The Health Professional's Handbook.* 2nd ed. Chernoff R, Ed, Aspen Publishers, Gaithersburg, 1999, p 107.
49. Nutrition and Your Health: Dietary Guidelines for Americans. 5th ed, Washington, DC, U.S. Depts of Agriculture and Health and Human Services, *Home and Garden Bulletin,* No. 232, 2000.
50. Rugg-Gunn AJ. *Nutrition and Dental Health.* Oxford: Oxford University Press, 1993.
51. Edgar WM, O'Mullane DM. *Saliva and Oral Health.* London: British Dental Association, 1996.
52. United States Food and Drug Administration. Health claims: dietary sugar alcohols and dental caries, *Fed Reg,* 43433, August 23, 1996.
53. Gibney M, Sigman-Grant M, Stanton Jr, JL, et al. *Am J Clin Nutr* 62: 178S; 1995.
54. Journal of The American Academy of Pediatric Dentistry Reference Manual 1996-97. *Pediatr Dent* 18: 25; 1996.
55. Seow WK. *Community Dent Oral Epidemiol* 26: 8; 1998.
56. Bowen WH. *Community Dent Oral Epidemiol* 26: 28; 1998.
57. Reisine S, Douglass JM. *Community Dent Oral Epidemiol* 26: 32; 1998.
58. Alvarez JO. *Am J Clin Nutr* 61: 410S; 1995.
59. Lai PY, Seow WK, Tudehope DI, et al. *Pediatr Dent* 19: 42; 1997.
60. Bonin MM, Bretzlaff JA, Therrien SA, et al. Northeastern Ontario Primary Care Research Group, *Arch Fam Med* 7: 438; 1998.
61. Bhaskar SN. In: *Orban's Oral Histology and Embryology.* Bhaskar SN, Ed, St Louis, Mosby Yearbook; 1991, p 239.
62. Touger-Decker R. In: *Krause's Food, Nutrition and Diet Therapy.* 10th ed. Mahan LK, Escott-Stump S, Eds, WB Saunders: Philadelphia, 1999, p 633.
63. Jones DL, Mobley CC. *Tx Dent J* 26; 2000.

55

Foodborne Infections and Infestations

Kumar S. Venkitanarayanan and Michael P. Doyle

Introduction

The microbiological safety of foods is a major concern to consumers and to the food industry. During the last decade, food safety received considerable attention due to the emergence of several new foodborne pathogens, and the involvement of foods that traditionally have been considered safe in many foodborne disease outbreaks. Further, increased globalization of the food supply and consumer demands for preservative-free convenience foods and ready-to-eat meals highlight the relevance of the microbial safety of foods. A recently published study by the U.S. Centers for Disease Control and Prevention reported an estimated 76 million cases of foodborne illness which resulted in 325,000 hospitalizations and 5000 deaths in the United States annually.[1] Besides the public health impact, outbreaks of foodborne illness impose major economic losses to both the food industry and society. The various microbiological hazards associated with foods can be classified as bacterial, viral, fungal, and parasitic.

Bacterial Foodborne Pathogens (Table 55.1)

Bacteria are a major agent of microbial foodborne illnesses. Bacterial foodborne illnesses can be classified into foodborne infections resulting from ingestion of foods containing viable cells of bacterial pathogens, and foodborne intoxications, which result from consumption of foods containing preformed toxins produced by toxigenic bacteria. The various bacterial pathogens associated with foodborne diseases are discussed below.

Escherichia coli O157:H7

Enterohemorrhagic *Escherichia coli* O157:H7 emerged in 1982 as a food-borne pathogen and is now recognized as a major public health concern in the United States. Many food-

0-8493-2705-9/02/$0.00+$1.50

TABLE 55.1

Bacterial Foodborne Pathogens

Microorganism	Biochemical and Growth Characteristics	Sources/ Reservoirs	Vehicles	Estimated No. of Foodborne Cases Annually in USA[1]	Incubation Period, Symptoms and Duration	Detection Methods	Control/Prevention
Escherichia coli O157:H7	Gram negative, facultative anaerobe, nonsporeforming, optimum growth at 37°-40°C, inability to grow at ≥ 44.5°C in presence of selective agents, inability to ferment sorbitol within 24 h, does not produce β-glucuronidase, acid tolerance	Cattle, humans	Raw or undercooked beef, unpasteurized milk and apple juice, lettuce, alfalfa sprouts, water	62,500	3 to 9 days Severe abdominal cramps, watery diarrhea that can become bloody, absence of fever, kidney failure, seizures, coma Duration is days to weeks	Cultural methods followed by confirmatory biochemical tests[102,103] Latex agglutination assay[104, 105] ELISA[106, 107] PCR[108]	Adequate cooking of beef; pasteurization of milk and apple juice; use of potable water for drinking; avoid eating alfalfa and vegetable sprouts; good personal hygiene
Salmonella spp. (non typhoid)	Gram negative, facultative anaerobe, oxidase negative, catalase positive, nonsporeforming, growth at 5°-47°C, optimum growth at 37°C, metabolize nutrients by respiratory and fermentative pathways	Cattle, swine, poultry, humans	Raw or undercooked meat, poultry, eggs, and milk and untreated water	1,340,000	6 to 72 h up to 4 days. Abdominal cramps, diarrhea, fever, chills, headache and vomiting. Duration is few days to one week, occasionally up to 3 weeks.	Cultural methods followed by confirmatory biochemical tests[109, 110] Latex agglutination assay[111] ELISA[112] PCR[113, 114]	Adequate cooking of food; avoid cross-contamination of raw foods of animal origin with cooked or ready to eat foods; avoid eating raw or undercooked foods of animal origin; use of potable water; good personal hygiene
Salmonella enterica serovar Typhi	Gram negative, facultative anaerobe, ferment D-xylose	Humans	Raw milk, shellfish, raw salads, under cooked foods	660 (> 70% of cases acquired abroad)	7 to 28 days Remittent fever with stepwise increments over a period of days, high temperature of 103 to 104°F, abdominal pain, diarrhea, and headache Duration is up to 3 weeks	Biochemical tests[115] Latex test[116] ELISA[117] PCR[118]	Good personal hygiene and food handling practices; proper sewage systems; effective surveillance of known carriers

Campylobacter jejuni and *coli*	Gram negative, microaerophilic, nonsporeforming, optimal growth at 42°C, CO_2 is required for good growth, growth optimal in 3-6% O_2, sensitive to dehydration, survives best at refrigeration temperature	Poultry Swine Cattle Sheep Wild birds	Raw or undercooked chicken, pork, and beef, and unpasteurized milk	1,960,000	1 to 11 days, usually 2 to 5 days Abdominal pain, diarrhea, malaise, headache, fever Duration is up to 10 days	Cultural methods followed by confirmatory biochemical tests[31, 119] Immunoassay[120] PCR[121, 122]	Adequate cooking of meat; avoid cross-contamination of raw foods of animal origin with cooked or ready to eat foods; pasteurization of milk
Shigella spp.	Gram negative, facultative anaerobe, nonspore-forming, does not ferment lactose, growth at 10°-45°C, optimal growth at 37°C	Humans	Raw foods and water contaminated with human feces; prepared salads	89,600	1 to 7 days Severe abdominal and rectal pain, bloody diarrhea with mucus, fever Dehydration Duration is few days to few weeks	Cultural methods followed by confirmatory biochemical tests[123] ELISA[124] PCR[125]	Good personal hygiene, including adequate cooking of food, drinking potable water
Yersinia enterocolitica	Gram negative, facultative anaerobe, nonspore-forming, growth at 0°-44°C, optimal growth at ca. 29°C, growth at pH 4.6-9.0, growth in presence of 5% NaCl but not 7% NaCl	Swine is principal reservoir of pathogenic strains	Undercooked or raw pork, especially tongue	86,700	1 to 11 days, usually 24 to 36 h Severe abdominal pain, nausea, diarrhea, fever, sometimes vomiting Duration is usually 2-3 days but may continue for up to 3 weeks	Cultural methods followed by confirmatory biochemical tests[126] PCR[127]	Adequate cooking of pork, disinfection of drinking water, control of *Y. enterocolitica* in pigs, prevent cross-contamination of pig viscera, feces, and hair with food and water
Vibrio cholerae	Gram negative, facultative anaerobe, nonsporeforming, growth at 18°-42°C with optimal growth at 37°C, growth is stimulated in presence of 3% NaCl, pH range for growth is 6-11	Humans, marine waters, especially brackish water and estuaries	Undercooked or raw seafoods; vegetables fertilized with contaminated human feces or irrigated with contaminated water; water	49	1 to 3 days Profuse watery diarrhea, which can lead to severe dehydration, abdominal pain, vomiting Duration is up to 7 days	Cultural methods followed by confirmatory biochemical tests[128, 129] ELISA[130] PCR[131, 132]	Safe disposal of human sewage, disinfection of drinking water, avoid eating raw seafood, adequate cooking of food
Vibrio parahaemolyticus	Gram negative, facultative anaerobe, nonspore-forming, growth in presence of 8% NaCl, optimal growth at 37°C with rapid generation time (ca. 10 minutes), growth at 10°C, sensitive to storage at refrigeration temperature	Coastal seawater, estuarine brackish waters above 15°C, marine fish, shellfish	Raw or undercooked fish and seafoods	5100	9 to 25 hours, up to 3 days, Profuse watery diarrhea, abdominal pain, vomiting, fever Duration is up to 8 days	Cultural methods followed by confirmatory biochemical tests[128, 129] ELISA[133] PCR[134]	Adequate cooking of seafood, rapid chilling of seafoods, prevent cross-contamination from raw seafoods to other foods and preparation surfaces

TABLE 55.1 *(Continued)*

Bacterial Foodborne Pathogens

Microorganism	Biochemical and Growth Characteristics	Sources/ Reservoirs	Vehicles	Estimated No. of Foodborne Cases Annually in USA[1]	Incubation Period, Symptoms and Duration	Detection Methods	Control/Prevention
Vibrio vulnificus	Gram negative, nonsporeforming, optimal growth at 37°C	Coastal and estuarine waters	Raw seafood, especially raw oysters	47	12 h to 3 days, Profuse diarrhea with blood in feces, fulminating septicemia, hypotension Duration is days to weeks	Cultural methods followed by confirmatory biochemical tests[128,129] ELISA[135] PCR[136]	Avoid eating raw seafood, especially raw oysters when have a history of liver disease or alcoholism
Aeromonas hydrophila	Gram negative, facultative anaerobe, nonsporeforming, oxidase positive, some strains are psychrotrophic (4°C) optimum growth at ca. 28°C	Aquatic environment, freshwater fish (especially Salmonids)	Untreated water	Very few	24 to 48 h Abdominal pain, vomiting, watery stools, mild fever Duration is days to weeks	Cultural methods followed by confirmatory biochemical tests[137, 138, 139] PCR[140, 141]	Avoid consumption of raw seafoods, avoid long-term storage of refrigerated foods, adequate cooking of foods, disinfection of drinking water
Plesiomonas shigelloides	Gram negative, facultative anaerobe, nonsporeforming, oxidase positive, some strains are psychrotrophic	Fresh and estuarine waters, fish, and shellfish	Fish, shellfish, oysters, shrimp and untreated water	Very few	1 to 2 days Abdominal pain, nausea, vomiting, diarrhea, chills, headache Duration is days to weeks	Cultural methods followed by confirmatory biochemical tests[137, 138]	Avoid consumption of raw seafoods, disinfection of drinking water
Listeria monocytogenes	Gram positive, facultative anaerobe, nonsporeforming, growth at 2°-45°C, optimal growth at 30°-35°C, growth in presence of 10% NaCl	Soil, sewage, vegetation, water, and feces of humans and animals	Raw milk, soft cheese, pâte, ready-to-eat cooked meat products (poultry, hot dogs) and cooked seafoods (smoked fish), and raw vegetables	2490	Few days to several weeks Flu-like symptoms such as fever, chills, headache Abdominal pain and diarrhea are present in some cases In pregnant women, spontaneous abortion and stillbirth Duration is days to weeks	Cultural methods followed by confirmatory biochemical tests[142, 143, 144] Immunoassay[145] PCR[146]	Proper sanitation of food processing equipment and environments, adequate cooking of meat and meat products, prevent recontamination of cooked products, proper reheating of cooked food, avoid drinking raw milk, avoid certain high risk foods (e.g., soft cheeses and pâtes) by pregnant women and immunocompromised individuals

Staphylococcus aureus (staphylococcal enterotoxin)	Gram positive, facultative anaerobe, nonsporeforming, coagulase positive, growth at 7°-48°C, optimal growth at ca. 37°C, toxin production at a_w of 0.86, toxin is heat stable (can withstand boiling for 1 h)	Humans (nose, throat and skin) and animals	Ham, chicken and egg salads, cream-filled pastries	185,000	2 to 6 h Abdominal cramps, nausea, vomiting, diarrhea, headache, chills, and dizziness Duration is up to 2 days	Cultural methods followed by confirmatory biochemical tests[147, 148] PCR[149, 150] Detection of toxin by microslide gel double diffusion test[151]	Good personal hygiene in food preparation and handling, adequate cooking of foods, proper refrigeration of cooked foods
Clostridium botulinum (botulinum neurotoxin)	Gram positive, obligate anaerobe, sporeforming, produce seven potent neurotoxins A-G (only A, B, E and rarely F associated with human illness), proteolytic strains grow at 10°-50°C, nonproteolytic strains can grow at 3.3°C, spores are resistant to normal cooking temperatures, and survive freezing and drying	Soil, dust, vegetation, animals, birds, insects, and marine and fresh water sediments and the intestinal tracts of fish (type E)	Beef, pork, fish, vegetables, and honey (infant botulism)	58	12 to 36 h, can range from few h to 8 days Very severe life threatening intoxication, headache, fixed and dilated pupils, vertigo, blurred or double vision, lack of muscle coordination, dry mouth, difficulty in breathing Gastrointestinal symptoms include abdominal pain, nausea, vomiting, constipation Duration is days to months (8 months)	Cultural methods followed by confirmatory biochemical tests[152] PCR[153, 154] Detection of toxin by mouse bioassay[155]	Boiling of foods will destroy toxin, adequate heat processing of home-canned foods, proper refrigeration of vacuum-packaged fresh or lightly cooked/smoked foods, acid-preserved foods should be below pH 4.6, discard swollen cans, avoid feeding honey to infants
Clostridium perfringens	Gram positive, anaerobe, sporeforming, optimum growth at 37°-47°C, grows slowly below 20°C	Soil, sewage, dust, vegetation, feces of humans and animals	Cooked meat and poultry, especially roast beef, turkey and gravies	249,000	8 to 24 h Abdominal pain and diarrhea Duration is 1 to 2 days	Cultural methods followed by confirmatory biochemical tests[68] Latex agglutination test[156] Colony hybridization assay[157] PCR[156]	Adequate cooking of foods; cooked food should be rapidly cooled (<5°C) or held hot (>60°C); proper refrigeration and adequate reheating of stored cooked foods
Bacillus cereus	Gram positive, facultative anaerobe, sporeforming, some strains can grow at 4°-6°C; optimum growth at 28°-37°C	Widely distributed in nature, soil, dust, vegetation	Cereals, fried rice, potatoes, cooked meat products, milk and dairy products, spices, dried foods	27,000	*Diarrheal syndrome* (toxic infection): 8 to 16 h Abdominal pain, watery diarrhea Duration is 24 to 36 h *Emetic syndrome* (preformed, heat stable toxin): 1 to 5 h Nausea, vomiting, malaise, sometimes diarrhea Duration is 24 to 36 h	Cultural methods followed by confirmatory biochemical tests[158] ELISA[159] PCR[160]	Adequate cooking of foods; cooked foods should be rapidly cooled (<5°C) or held hot (60°C); avoid leaving cooked foods at room temperature for long time

TABLE 55.1 *(Continued)*

Bacterial Foodborne Pathogens

Microorganism	Biochemical and Growth Characteristics	Sources/ Reservoirs	Vehicles	Estimated No. of Foodborne Cases Annually in USA[1]	Incubation Period, Symptoms and Duration	Detection Methods	Control/Prevention
Brucella spp.	Gram negative, aerobe, nonsporeforming, optimal growth at 37°C	Cattle, sheep, pig, goat	Raw milk and products made from unpasteurized milk	780	Acute form: 3 to 21 days, infrequently months Pyrexia, profuse sweats, chills, constipation, weakness, malaise, body aches, joint pains, weight loss, anorexia Chronic form: several months Long history of fever, inertia, recurrent depression, sexual impotence, insomnia Duration is weeks	Cultural methods[161] ELISA[162, 163] PCR[163]	Vaccination of livestock against *Brucella* spp., avoid contact with infected animals, eradication of diseased animals; pasteurization of milk; avoid eating unpasteurized dairy products
Helicobacter pylori	Gram negative, microaerophile to anaerobe	Humans, cats	Untreated water, foodborne transmission of disease has not been proven	Unknown	Gastritis, dyspepsia, peptic ulcer, gastric carcinoma	Cultural methods[78] ELISA[76] PCR[77]	Avoid contact with infected animals, use of chlorinated water for cooking and drinking

associated outbreaks are reported each year, with 340 outbreak-associated confirmed cases reported in 1997.[2] A wide variety of foods, including undercooked ground beef, raw milk, roast beef, venison jerky, salami, yogurt, lettuce, unpasteurized apple juice, cantaloupe, alfalfa sprouts, and coleslaw, have been implicated as vehicles of *E. coli* O157:H7 infection.[3] In addition, outbreaks involving person-to-person and waterborne transmission have been reported.[3] Cattle have been identified as an important reservoir of *E. coli* O157:H7,[4,5] with undercooked ground beef being a major vehicle of foodborne outbreaks.[6] A survey performed by the National Animal Monitoring System of the U.S. Department of Agriculture revealed that 1.6% of feedlot cattle shed *E. coli* O157:H7 and 0.4% shed *E. coli* O157 nonmotile bacteria in their feces.[7] This is likely an underestimate of the actual percentage of *E. coli* O157:H7 harbored by cattle. The use of more sensitive isolation procedures will likely identify considerably higher carriage rates. *E. coli* O157:H7 localizes in cattle primarily in the rumen and colon, and is shed in feces.[8] *E. coli* O157:H7 can survive in bovine feces for many months,[9] hence potentially contaminating cattle, food, water, and the environment. During slaughter and subsequent processing operations, contamination of carcasses with *E. coli* O157:H7 from the digesta or feces of cattle can occur. Moreover, fruits and vegetables grown on soil fertilized with cattle manure or irrigated with water contaminated with cattle manure has the potential of being a vehicle of *E. coli* O157:H7.

Acidification is commonly used in food processing to control growth and survival of spoilage-causing and pathogenic microorganisms in foods. The U.S. Food and Drug Administration does not regard foods with pH $\leq$ 4.6 (high-acid foods) to be microbiologically hazardous. However, *E. coli* O157:H7 has been associated with outbreaks attributed to high-acid foods, including apple juice, mayonnaise, fermented sausage, and yogurt,[10] raising concerns about the safety of these foods. Several studies have revealed that many strains of *E. coli* O157:H7 are highly tolerant to acidic conditions, being able to survive for extended periods of time in synthetic gastric juice and in highly acidic foods.[10,11] Further, exposure of *E. coli* O157:H7 to mild or moderate acidic environments can induce an acid tolerance response, which enables the pathogen to survive extreme acidic conditions. For example, acid-adapted cells of *E. coli* O157:H7 survived longer in apple cider, fermented sausage, and hydrochloric acid than non-acid adapted cells.[12,13] However, *E. coli* O157:H7 is not unusually heat resistant[14] or salt tolerant[15] unless cells are preexposed to acid to become acid adapted. Acid-adapted *E. coli* O157:H7 cells have been determined to have increased heat tolerance.

In humans, three important manifestations of illness have been reported in *E. coli* O157:H7 infection. These include hemorrhagic colitis, hemolytic uremic syndrome, and thrombocytopenic purpura.[16] Two important factors attributed to the pathogenesis of *E. coli* O157:H7 include the ability of the pathogen to adhere to the intestinal mucosa of the host, and production of Shiga toxin I and/or Shiga toxin II.[16] Retrospective analysis of foods implicated in outbreaks of *E. coli* O157:H7 infection suggest a low infectious dose of the pathogen, probably less than a hundred cells.[17]

Salmonella Species

Salmonella spp. are facultatively anaerobic, gram-negative, rod-shaped bacteria belonging to the family *Enterobacteriaceae*. Members of the genus *Salmonella* have an optimum growth temperature of 37°C and utilize glucose with the production of acid and gas.[18] *Salmonella* spp. are widely distributed in nature. They colonize the intestinal tracts of humans, animals, birds, and reptiles, and are excreted in feces, which contaminate the environment, water, and foods.[19] Many food products, especially foods having contact with animal feces, including beef, pork, poultry, eggs, milk, fruits, and vegetables, have been associated with outbreaks of salmonellosis.[20] *Salmonella* spp. can be divided into host-adapted serovars and those without any host preferences. Most of the foodborne serovars are in the latter group.

The ability of many strains of *Salmonella* to adapt to extreme environmental conditions emphasizes the potential risk of these microorganisms as foodborne pathogens. Although salmonellae optimally grow at 37°C, the genus *Salmonella* consists of strains which are capable of growth from 5° to 47°C.[21] *Salmonella* spp. can grow at pH values ranging from 4.5 to 7.0, with optimum growth observed near neutral pH.[19] Pre-exposure of *Salmonella* to mild acidic environments (pH 5.5 to 6.0) can induce in some strains an acid tolerance response, which enables the bacteria to survive for extended periods of time exposure to acidic and other adverse environmental conditions such as heat and low water activity.[22,23] However, most *Salmonella* spp. possess no unusual tolerance to salt and heat. A concentration of 3 to 4% NaCl can inhibit the growth of *Salmonella*.[24] Most salmonellae are sensitive to heat, hence ordinary pasteurization and cooking temperatures are capable of killing the pathogen.[25]

The most common species of *Salmonella* that cause foodborne salmonellosis in humans are *S. enterica* serovar Typhimurium and *S. enterica* serovar Enteritiditis.[26] A wide variety of foods, including beef, pork, milk, chicken, and turkey have been associated with outbreaks caused by *S.* Typhimurium. *S.* Enteritidis outbreaks, however, are most frequently associated with consumption of poultry products, especially eggs. During the period from 1985 to 1987, 77% of *S.* Enteritidis outbreaks in the U.S. was associated with Grade A shell eggs or foods containing eggs.[27] One of the major routes of *S.* Enteritidis contamination of intact eggs is through transovarian transmission of the pathogen to the yolk.[28]

S. enterica serovar Typhi is the causative agent of typhoid (enteric fever), a serious human disease. Typhoid fever has a long incubation period of 7 to 28 days, and is characterized by prolonged and spiking fever, abdominal pain, diarrhea, and headache.[18] The disease can be diagnosed by isolation of the pathogen from urine, blood, or stool specimens of affected individuals. *S. typhi* is an uncommon cause of foodborne illness in the U.S.

Campylobacter Species

The genus *Campylobacter* consists of 14 species, however, *C. jejuni* subsp. *jejuni* and *C. coli* are the dominant foodborne pathogens. *C. jejuni* is a slender, rod-shaped, microaerophilic bacterium that requires approximately 3 to 6% oxygen for growth. It can be differentiated from *C. coli* by its ability to hydrolyze hippurate.[29] *C. jejuni* is the most common bacterial agent causing diarrheal disease in humans in the U.S. and many other countries.[30] Many animals including poultry, swine, cattle, sheep, horses, and domestic pets harbor *C. jejuni* in their intestinal tracts, hence serving as reservoirs of human infection. Although a number of vehicles such as beef, pork, eggs, and untreated water have been implicated in outbreaks of campylobacter enteritis, chicken and unpasteurized milk are reported as the most commonly involved foods.[31] The organism does not survive well in the environment, being sensitive to drying, highly acidic conditions, and freezing. It is also readily killed in foods by adequate cooking.[32]

Usually campylobacter enteritis in humans is a self-limiting illness characterized by abdominal cramps, diarrhea, headache, and fever lasting up to four days. However, severe cases, involving bloody diarrhea and abdominal pain mimicking appendicitis, also occur.[29] Guillain-Barré syndrome (GBS) is an infrequent sequela to *Campylobacter* infection in humans. GBS is characterized by acute neuromuscular paralysis[32] and is estimated to occur in approximately one of every 1000 cases of campylobacter enteritis.[33] A few strains of *C. jejuni* reportedly produce a heat-labile enterotoxin similar to that produced by *Vibrio cholerae* and enterotoxigenic *E. coli*.[29] Some strains of *C. jejuni* and *C. coli* also can produce a cytolethal distending toxin, which causes a rapid and specific cell cycle arrest in HeLa and Caco-2 cells.[30]

Shigella Species

The genus *Shigella* is divided into four major groups: *S. dysenteriae* (group A), *S. flexneri* (group B), *S. boydii* (group C), and *S. sonnei* (group D) based on the organism's somatic (O) antigen. Humans are the natural reservoir of *Shigella* spp. The fecal-oral route is the primary mode of transmission of shigellae, and proper personal hygiene and sanitary practices of cooks and food handlers can greatly reduce the occurrence of outbreaks of shigellosis. Most foodborne outbreaks of shigellosis are associated with ingestion of foods such as salads and water contaminated with human feces containing the pathogen. Shigellosis is characterized by diarrhea containing bloody mucus, which lasts one to two weeks. The infectious dose for *Shigella* infection is low. The ID_{50} of *S. flexneri* and *S. sonnei* in humans is approximately 5000 microorganisms, and that of *S. dysenteriae* is a few hundred cells; hence secondary transmission of *Shigella* by person-to-person contact frequently occurs in outbreaks of foodborne illness.

Yersinia enterocolitica

Swine have been identified as an important reservoir of *Yersinia enterocolitica*, in which the pathogen colonizes primarily the buccal cavity.[34] Although pork and pork products are considered to be the primary vehicles of *Y. enterocolitica*, a variety of other foods, including milk, beef, lamb, seafood, and vegetables, has been identified as vehicles of *Y. enterocolitica* infection.[35] One of the largest outbreaks of yersiniosis in the U.S. was associated with milk.[36] Water has also been a vehicle of several outbreaks of *Y. enterocolitica* infection.[36] Surveys have revealed that *Y. enterocolitica* is frequently present in foods, having been isolated from 11% of sandwiches, 15% of chilled foods, and 22% of raw milk in Europe.[37] However, most isolates from foods of non-pork origin are nonpathogenic for humans. Although contaminated foods are a major source of *Y. enterocolitica* infection, contaminated blood used in transfusions has resulted in many cases of *Y. enterocolitica* sepsis.[38] Several serovars of pathogenic *Y. enterocolitica* have been reported, which include O:3, O:5, O:8, and O:9,[39] with serovar 0:8 being common in the U.S.[40]

An unusual characteristic of *Y. enterocolitica* that influences food safety is its ability to grow at low temperatures, even as low as –1°C.[41] Several studies have revealed growth of *Y. enterocolitica* in foods stored at refrigeration temperature. *Y. enterocolitica* grew on pork, chicken, and beef at 0 to 1°C.[42,43] The ability of *Y. enterocolitica* to grow well at refrigeration temperature has been exploited for isolating the pathogen from foods, water, and stool specimens. Such samples are incubated at 4 to 8°C in an enrichment broth for several days to selectively culture *Y. enterocolitica* based on its psychrotrophic nature.

Vibrio Species

The genus *Vibrio* consists of 28 species, of which *V. parahaemolyticus*, *V. vulnificus*, and *V. cholerae* are the most important foodborne pathogens. Vibrios are associated with estuarine and marine waters, and their populations in surface waters and in seafoods are higher during the warm than cold months of the year.[44] *V. parahaemolyticus* is present in coastal waters of the U.S. and the world. A survey by the U.S. Food and Drug Administration revealed that 86% of 635 seafood samples contained *V. parahaemolyticus*, being isolated from clams, oysters, lobsters, scallops, shrimp, fish, and shellfish.[44] An important virulence characteristic of pathogenic strains of *V. parahemolyticus* is their ability to produce a thermostable hemolysin (Kanagawa hemolysin).[45] Studies in humans on the infectious dose of pathogenic *V. parahemolyticus* strains revealed that ingestion of approximately 10^5 to 10^7 organisms can cause gastroenteritis.[44]

V. cholerae serovars O1 and O139, the causative agents of cholera in humans, are a part of the normal estuarine microflora, and foods such as raw fish, mussels, oysters, and clams have been associated with outbreaks of cholera.[46] Infected humans can serve as short-term carriers, shedding the pathogen in feces. Cholera is characterized by profuse diarrhea, potentially fatal in severe cases, and often described as "rice water" diarrhea due to the presence of prolific amounts of mucus in the stools. Gastroenteritis caused by non-O1 and non-O139 serovars of *V. cholerae* is usually mild in nature.

V. vulnificus is the most serious of the vibrios and is responsible for most of the seafood-associated deaths in the U.S., especially in Florida.[44] Although a number of seafoods has been associated with *V. vulnificus* infection, raw oysters are the most common vehicle associated with cases of illness.[47] This pathogen causes a fulminating septicemia with a 40 to 50% mortality rate.

Aeromonas hydrophila

Although *Aeromonas* species have been recognized as pathogens of cold-blooded animals, their potential to cause human infections, especially foodborne illness, received attention only recently. *A. hydrophila* has been isolated from drinking water, fresh and saline waters, and sewage.[48] It also has been isolated from a variety of foods such as fish, oyster, shellfish, raw milk, ground beef, chicken, and pork.[48] Although *A. hydrophila* is sensitive to highly acidic conditions and does not possess any unusual thermal resistance, some strains are psychrotrophic and grow at refrigeration temperature.[49] *A. hydrophila* can grow on a variety of refrigerated foods, including pork, asparagus, cauliflower, and broccoli.[50,51] However, considering the widespread occurrence of *A. hydrophila* in water and food and its relatively infrequent association with human illness, it is likely that most strains of this bacterium are not pathogenic for humans. *A. hydrophila* infection in humans is characterized by watery diarrhea and mild fever. Virulent strains of *A. hydrophila* produce a 52-kDa polypeptide, which possesses enterotoxic, cytotoxic, and hemolytic activities.[52]

Plesiomonas shigelloides

P. shigelloides has been implicated in several cases of sporadic and epidemic gastroenteritis.[53] The pathogen is present in fresh and estuarine waters, and has been isolated from various aquatic animals.[49] Seafoods such as fish, crabs, and oysters have been associated with cases of *P. shigelloides* infection. The most common symptoms of *P. shigelloides* infection include abdominal pain, nausea, chills, fever, and diarrhea. Potential virulence factors of *P. shigelloides* include cytotoxic enterotoxin, invasins, and β-hemolysin.[49]

Listeria monocytogenes

L. monocytogenes has emerged into a highly significant and fatal foodborne pathogen throughout the world, especially in the U.S. There is an estimated approximately 2500 cases of listeriosis annually in the U.S., with a mortality rate of ca. 25%.[1] A large outbreak of listeriosis involving more than 100 cases and associated with eating contaminated turkey frankfurters occurred during 1998-99.[54] During this period of time there were more than 35 recalls of a number of different food products contaminated with listeriae.[54] *L. monocytogenes* is widespread in nature, occurring in soil, vegetation, and untreated water. Humans and a wide variety of farm animals, including cattle, sheep, goat, pig, and poultry, are known sources of *L. monocytogenes*.[55] *L. monocytogenes* also occurs frequently in food processing facilities, especially in moist areas such as floor drains, floors, and processing equipment.[56] *L. monocytogenes* can also grow in biofilms attached to a variety of processing plant surfaces such as stainless steel, glass, and rubber.[57]

A wide spectrum of foods, including milk, cheese, beef, pork, chicken, seafoods, fruits, and vegetables, has been identified as vehicles of *L. monocytogenes*.[55] However, ready-to-eat cooked foods such as low-acid soft cheese, pâtes, and cooked poultry meat which can support the growth of listeriae to large populations (>10^6 cells per gram) when held at refrigeration temperature for several weeks, have been regarded as high-risk foods.[58,59] *L. monocytogenes* possesses several characteristics which enable the pathogen to successfully contaminate, survive, and grow in foods, thereby resulting in outbreaks. These traits include an ability to grow at refrigeration temperature and in a medium with minimal nutrients, ability to survive in acidic conditions, e.g., pH 4.2, ability to tolerate up to 10% sodium chloride, ability to survive incomplete cooking or subminimal pasteurization treatments, and the ability to survive in biofilms on equipment in food processing plants and resist superficial cleaning and disinfection treatments.[54]

Human listeriosis is an uncommon illness with a high mortality rate. Clinical manifestations range from mild influenza-like symptoms to meningitis and meningoencephalitis. Pregnant females infected with the pathogen may not present symptoms of illness or may exhibit only mild influenza-like symptoms. However, spontaneous abortion, premature birth, or stillbirth are frequent sequela to listeriosis in pregnant females.[59] Although the infective dose of *L. monocytogenes* is not known, published reports indicate that it is likely more than 100 CFU per gram of food.[59] However, the infective dose depends on the age, condition of health, and immunological status of the host. Important virulence factors of *L. monocytogenes* include intracellular invasin and production of listeriolysin O.[60]

Staphylococcus aureus

Pre-formed, heat stable enterotoxin that can resist boiling for several minutes is the agent responsible for staphylococcal food poisoning. Humans are the principal reservoir of *S. aureus* strains involved in outbreaks of foodborne illness. Colonized humans can be long-term carriers of *S. aureus*, and thereby contaminate foods and other humans.[61] The organism commonly resides in the throat and nasal cavity, and on the skin, especially in boils and carbuncles.[61] Protein-rich foods such as ham, poultry, fish, dairy products, custards, cream-filled bakery products, and salads containing cooked meat, chicken, and potatoes are the vehicles most frequently associated with *S. aureus* food poisoning.[62] *S. aureus* is usually overgrown by competing bacterial flora in raw foods; hence raw foods are not typical vehicles of staphylococcal food poisoning. Cooking eliminates most of the normal bacterial flora of raw foods, thereby enabling the growth of *S. aureus*, which can be introduced by infected cooks and food handlers into foods after cooking. The incubation period of staphylococcal food poisoning is very short, with symptoms observed within two to six hours after eating toxin-contaminated food. Symptoms include nausea, vomiting, diarrhea, and abdominal pain.

S. aureus can grow within a wide range of pH values from 4 to 9.3, with optimum growth occurring at pH 6 to 7. *S. aureus* has an exceptional tolerance to sodium chloride, being able to grow in foods in the presence of 7 to 10% NaCl, with some strains tolerating up to 20% NaCl.[62] *S. aureus* has the unique ability to grow at a water activity as low as 0.83

to 0.86, which is unusual for a nonhalophilic bacterium.[63] *S. aureus* produces nine different enterotoxins which are quite heat resistant, losing their serological activity at 121°C but not at 100°C for several minutes.[63]

Clostridium botulinum

Foodborne botulism is an intoxication caused by ingestion of foods containing pre-formed botulinal toxin, which is produced by *C. botulinum* under anaerobic conditions. There are seven types of *C. botulinum* (A, B, C, D, E, F, and G) classified on the basis of the antigenic specificity of the neurotoxin they produce.[64] The organism is present in soil, vegetation, and sedimentation under water. Type A strains are proteolytic, whereas type E strains are nonproteolytic.[65] Another classification divides *C. botulinum* into four groups: group 1 (type A strains and proteolytic strains of types B and F), group II (type E strains and nonproteolytic strains of B and F), group III (type C and D strains), and group IV (type G strains). Types A, B, E, and F are associated with botulism in humans. Type A *C. botulinum* occurs frequently in soils of the western U.S., whereas type B strains are more often present in the eastern states and in Europe.[65] Type E strains are largely associated with aquatic environments and fish. Foods most often associated with cases of botulism include fish, meat, honey, and home-canned vegetables.[64] Type A cases of botulism in the U.S. are frequently associated with temperature-abused, home-prepared foods. Proteolytic type A, B, and F strains produce heat-resistant spores, which pose a safety concern in low-acid canned foods. In contrast, nonproteolytic type B, E, and F strains produce heat-labile spores, which are of concern in pasteurized or unheated foods.[65] The minimum pH for growth of group I and group II strains is 4.6 and 5, respectively.[64] Group I strains can grow at a minimum water activity of 0.94, whereas group II strains do not grow below a water activity of 0.97.[66] The proteolytic strains of *C. botulinum* are generally more resistant to heat than nonproteolytic strains.

Clostridium perfringens

C. perfringens strains are grouped into five types: A, B, C, D, and E, based on the type(s) of toxin(s) produced. *C. perfringens* foodborne illness is almost exclusively associated with type A isolates of *C. perfringens. C. perfringens* is commonly present in soil, dust, water, and in the intestinal tracts of humans and animals.[67] It is frequently present in foods; about 50% of raw or frozen meat and poultry contain *C. perfringens*.[68] Spores produced by *C. perfringens* are quite heat resistant, and can survive boiling for up to one hour.[68] *C. perfringens* spores can survive in cooked foods, and if not properly cooled before refrigerated storage, the spores will germinate and vegetative cells can grow to large populations during holding at growth temperatures. Large populations of *C. perfringens* cells ($>10^6$/g) ingested with contaminated food will enter the small intestine, multiply, and sporulate. During sporulation in the small intestine *C. perfringens* enterotoxin is produced, which induces a diarrheal response. Although vegetative cells of *C. perfringens* are sensitive to cold temperature and freezing, spores tolerate cold temperature well and can survive in refrigerated foods.

Bacillus cereus

B. cereus is a spore-forming pathogen present in soil and on vegetation. It is frequently isolated from foods such as meat, spices, vegetables, dairy products, and cereal grains, especially fried rice.[69] There are two types of foodborne illness caused by *B. cereus*, i.e., a diarrheagenic illness and an emetic syndrome.[70] The diarrheal syndrome is usually mild and is characterized by abdominal cramps, nausea, and watery stools. Types of foods implicated in outbreaks of diarrheal syndrome include cereal food products containing corn and corn starch, mashed potatoes, vegetables, milk, and cooked meat products. The emetic syndrome is more severe and acute in nature, characterized by severe vomiting. Refried or rewarmed boiled rice dishes are frequently implicated in outbreaks of emetic syndrome.[71] The dose of *B. cereus* required to produce diarrheal illness is estimated at more than 10^5 cells/g.[72]

Brucella Species

Brucella spp. are pathogens in many animals, causing sterility and abortion. In humans, *Brucella* is the etiologic agent of undulant fever. The genus *Brucella* consists of six species, of which those of principal concern are *B. abortus*, *B. suis*, and *B. melitensis*.[73] *B. abortus* causes disease in cattle, *B. suis* in swine, and *B. melitensis* is the primary pathogen of sheep. *B. melitensis* is the most pathogenic species for humans. Human brucellosis is primarily an occupational disease of veterinarians and meat industry workers. Brucellosis can be transmitted by aerosols and dust. Foodborne brucellosis can be transmitted to humans by consumption of meat and milk products from infected farm animals. The most common food vehicle of brucellosis for humans is unpasteurized milk.[73] Meat is a less common source of foodborne brucellosis because the organisms are destroyed by cooking.

Helicobacter pylori

H. pylori is a human pathogen causing chronic gastritis, gastric ulcer, and gastric carcinoma.[74,75] Although, humans are the primary host of *H. pylori*, the bacterium has been isolated from cats.[58] *H. pylori* does not survive well outside its host, but it has been detected in water and vegetables.[76,77] A study on the effect of environmental and substrate factors on the growth of *H. pylori* indicated that the pathogen likely lacks the ability to grow in most foods.[78] However, *H. pylori* may survive for long periods in low-acid environments under refrigerated conditions. Presently, the mode of transmission of *H. pylori* in human infection has not been elucidated, but contaminated water and food are considered potential vehicles.

Viral Foodborne Pathogens (Table 55.2)

Recent estimates by the Centers for Disease Control and Prevention of the incidence of foodborne illness in the U.S. indicate that viruses are responsible for approximately 67% of the total foodborne illnesses of known etiology annually.[1] Viruses are obligate intracellular microorganisms, and most foodborne viruses contain RNA rather than DNA. Since viruses require a host for multiplication, they cannot grow in foods. Foodborne viruses are generally enteric in nature, causing illness through ingestion of foods and water contaminated with human feces. Viruses disseminated through foods also can be spread by person-to-person contact. Hepatitis A virus, Norwalk-like viruses, and possibly rotavirus are among the most significant of the foodborne viruses.

TABLE 55.2
Viral Foodborne Pathogens

Microorganism	Significant Characteristics	Sources/ Reservoirs	Vehicles	Estimated No. of Foodborne Cases Annually in USA[121]	Incubation Period, Symptoms and Duration	Detection Methods	Control/Prevention
Hepatitis A virus	Single-stranded RNA virus, spherical in shape, remains viable for long periods of time in foods stored at refrigeration temperature, virus multiplies in the gut epitheliums before being carried by blood to the liver. Virus is shed in feces before symptoms of liver damage become apparent	Humans, sewage-polluted waters	Raw or undercooked shellfish and seafoods harvested from sewage-polluted water, ready-to-eat foods such as salads prepared by infected food handler	4170	15 to 45 days, usually ca. 25 days Loss of appetite, nausea, abdominal pain, fever, jaundice, dark urine, pale stools Duration is a few weeks to months	Cultural methods[164, 165] Enzyme immunoassay[166] PCR[167, 168]	Avoid consumption of raw seafoods, disinfection of drinking water, good personal hygiene and food handling practices, vaccination of professional food handlers, safe sewage disposal
Norwalk-like viruses (small round structured viruses; SRSV)	Single-stranded RNA virus, spherical in shape, does not multiply in any known laboratory host	Humans, sewage-polluted waters	Raw or undercooked shellfish and seafoods harvested from sewage polluted water, drinking water	9,200,000	1 to 2 days Loss of appetite, nausea, abdominal pain, diarrhea, vomiting, headache Duration is 2 days	Enzyme immunoassay[169] PCR[168]	Avoid consumption of raw seafoods, disinfection of drinking water, good personal hygiene and food handling practices, hygienic sewage disposal, treatment of wastewater used for irrigation
Rotavirus	Double-stranded RNA virus, icosahedral in shape	Humans	To be determined	39,000	1 to 3 days Vomiting, abdominal pain followed by watery diarrhea Duration is 6 to 8 days	Cultural methods[164, 165] ELISA[170] PCR[171]	Avoid consumption of raw seafoods Avoid drinking of untreated water, Good personal hygiene

Hepatitis A virus

Hepatitis A virus is a member of the family *Picornaviridae* and is transmitted by the fecal-oral route. Raw shellfish harvested from waters contaminated by human sewage is among the foods most frequently associated with outbreaks of hepatitis A virus.[79] Hepatitis A virus is more resistant to heat and drying than other picornaviruses.[79] The incubation period for onset of symptoms of hepatitis A infection ranges from 15 to 45 days, and symptoms include nausea, abdominal pain, jaundice, and fever. The virus is shed in feces by infected humans many days before the onset of symptoms, indicating the importance of good personal hygienic practices of cooks and food handlers who could otherwise contaminate food during the period of asymptomatic fecal shedding.

Norwalk-like viruses

Norwalk-like viruses belong to the family *Calciviridae*, and are often referred to as small, round structured viruses. Viruses of this type are believed to be the most common cause of foodborne viral diseases in the U.S. Raw or undercooked shellfish and other seafoods are common vehicles of Norwalk-like viruses. The incubation period of infection ranges from 24 to 48 h, and symptoms include nausea, vomiting, and diarrhea. Infected humans shed the virus in feces for up to a week after symptoms have subsided. Although little information is available on the stability of these viruses in foods, qualitative studies in human volunteers indicate that the viruses are infective for up to 3 h when exposed to a medium at pH 2.2 at room temperature or for 60 minutes at pH 7 at 60°C.[80]

Rotavirus

Rotavirus is the most common cause of diarrhea in children worldwide, especially in developing countries. In the U.S., there are an estimated 3.9 million cases of rotavirus diarrhea each year; however, only 39,000 cases are estimated to be acquired through contaminated foods.[1] Rotavirus infection has an incubation period of one to three days, and is characterized by fever, vomiting, and diarrhea. The virus is shed in the feces of infected humans and can survive on vegetables at 4° or 20°C for many days.[81] It also has been shown to survive the process of making soft cheese.[81]

Fungal Foodborne Pathogens (Table 55.3)

Molds are widely distributed in nature and are an integral part of the microflora of foods. Although molds are major spoilage agents of many foods, many molds also produce mycotoxins of which some are carcinogenic and mutagenic. Mycotoxins are secondary metabolites produced by molds usually at the end of their exponential phase of growth. Some of the principal species of molds which produce mycotoxins in foods are described here.

Aspergillus Species

A. flavus and *A. parasiticus* are the most important toxigenic foodborne aspergilli. A wide variety of foods such as nuts, corn, oil seeds, and sorghum are potential vehicles of these

TABLE 55.3
Fungal Foodborne Pathogens

Microorganism/ Toxin	Significant Characteristics	Sources/ Reservoirs of Fungi	Vehicles of Toxins	Toxic Effects	Detection Methods	Control/ Prevention
Aspergillus parasiticus and *Aspergillus flavus*/ Aflatoxin	Growth at 10°-43°C, optimal growth at 32°C, produces aflatoxins at 12°-40°C, growth at pH 3 to 11	Environment, soil, vegetation	Corn, peanuts, cottonseed	Effects of aflatoxin in animals: Acute: hemorrhage in the gastrointestinal tract, liver damage, death Chronic: cirrhosis of liver, liver tumors, immunosuppression	Cultural methods[172, 173, 174] ELISA[175] PCR[176]	Proper storage of cereal products, detoxification of mycotoxins in cereal products by treatment with hydrogen peroxide, ammonia
Penicillium expansum/ Patulin; *Penicillium citrinum*/Citrinin	*P. expansum* is psychrotrophic, capable of growth at -2° to -3°C, optimal growth at 25°C	Environment, soil, vegetation	*P. expansum*: Fruits, especially apples and pears *P. citrinum*: Cereals, especially rice, wheat, corn	Effects of patulin: Gastrointestinal, neurological, and immunological effects in animals Citrinin: fatty degeneration and necrosis of kidneys of pigs and dogs; significance in human health is unresolved	Cultural methods[173, 174, 177] Gas chromatography[178]	Avoid consumption of rotten apples and pears, proper storage of cereal products
Fusarium graminearum/ Deoxynivalernol, nivalenol, zearalenone	Growth at 5°C but not at 37°C, optimal growth at 25°C	Environment, soil, vegetation	Cereals, especially wheat, barley and corn	Effects of deoxynivolenol: nausea, vomiting, abdominal pain, diarrhea, headache, fever, chills, throat irritation	Cultural methods followed by morphology[179, 180] PCR[181]	Proper storage of cereal products

aspergilli. *A. flavus* and *A. parasiticus* produce aflatoxins, which are difuranocoumarin derivatives.[82] The common types of aflatoxins produced are B_1, B_2, G_1, and G_2.[83] Aflatoxicosis in animals can be acute or chronic. Acute cases are characterized by severe liver damage, whereas liver cirrhosis, liver cancer, and teratogenesis occur in chronic toxicity. Chronic intake of aflatoxins in animals can lead to poor feed conversion and low weight gain.

Penicillium Species

The genus *Penicillium* consists of more than 150 species, of which nearly 100 produce known toxins. Three important foodborne toxigenic *Penicillium* species include *P. verrucosum, P. expansum,* and *P. citrinum. P. verrucosum* is present on grains grown in temperate zones, and is commonly associated with Scandanavian barley and wheat.[84] *P. verrucosum* produces Ochratoxin A, which has immunosuppressive and potential carcinogenic properties.[84] Ochratoxin A also has been associated with nephritis in pigs in Scandanavia.[85] *P. expansum,* which is frequently associated with fresh fruits, produces patulin, a toxin that produces immunological, neurological, and gastrointestinal toxic effects in animal models. *P. expansum* is commonly present in rotten apples and pears, and to a lesser extent in cereals. An unusual characteristic of *P. expansum* is its ability to grow at low temperature, i.e., –2° to –3°C.[84] *P. citrinin* is a widely occurring mold commonly present on rice, wheat, and corn. *P. citrinin* produces the metabolite citrinin. Although the toxicological effect of citrinin in humans is not known, it has been reported to cause renal toxicity in pigs and cats.[86]

Fusarium graminearum

F. graminearum is a toxigenic mold commonly present in soil and on cereals such as wheat and corn. It produces a number of mycotoxins, including deoxynevalenol and zearalenone.[87] Ingestion of foods containing deoxynevalenol produces illness termed Scabby grain intoxication, which is characterized by anorexia, nausea, vomiting, diarrhea, dizziness, and convulsions. Foods most frequently implicated as vehicles of deoxynevalenol include cereal grains, wheat, barley, and noodles.

Parasitic Foodborne Pathogens (Table 55.4)

Foods can be vehicles of several types of parasites, including protozoa, roundworms, and flatworms. Although foodborne transmission of parasites such as *Trichinella spiralis* and *Taenia solium* has been known for many years, the foodborne disease potential of many protozoan parasites such as *Cryptosporidium* and *Cyclospora* has only recently been recognized. Unlike bacteria, parasites do not multiply in foods. Moreover, parasites need at least one specific host to complete their life cycle. Many of the well-recognized parasites that can be transmitted to humans through foods are listed below.

Giardia lamblia

G. lamblia is a flagellated protozoan parasite that colonizes the intestinal tract of humans and animals. It is commonly present in lakes, rivers, and stagnated waters. The life cycle of *G. lamblia* includes flagellated trophozoites, which become pear-shaped cysts.[88] The

TABLE 55.4
Parasitic Foodborne Pathogens

Parasite	Significant Characteristics	Sources/ Reservoirs	Vehicles	Estimated No. of Foodborne Cases Annually in USA[1]	Incubation Period, Symptoms and Duration	Detection Methods	Control/ Prevention
Giardia lamblia	Flagellate protozoa, produces oval-shaped cysts ranging from 8 to 20 μm in length and 5 to 12 μm in width, cysts contain four nuclei and are resistant to chlorination used to disinfect water	Humans, animals, especially beavers and muskrats, water	Drinking water, raw fruits and vegetables contaminated with cysts, ready-to-eat foods such as salads contaminated by infected food handlers	200,000	4 to 25 days, usually 7 to 10 days Abdominal cramps, nausea, abdominal distension, diarrhea which can be chronic and relapsing, fatigue, weight loss, anorexia Duration is weeks to years	Immuno-fluorescence[182] Immunochromato-graphy[183] PCR[184]	Adequate cooking of foods, filtration of drinking water, good personal hygiene and food handling practices
Entamoeba histolytica	Amoeboid protozoa, anaerobe survives in environment in crypted form, cysts remain viable in feces for several days and in soil for at least 8 days at 30°C and for more than 1 month at 10°C, relatively resistant to chlorine	Humans, dogs, rats	Foods and water contaminated with feces or irrigation water	Unknown	2 to 4 weeks Abdominal pain, fever, vomiting, diarrhea containing blood and mucus, weight loss Duration is weeks to months	Microscopic examination ELISA[185] PCR[185, 186]	Good personal hygiene and food handling practices, adequate cooking of foods, filtration of water, hygienic disposal of sewage water, treatment of irrigation water
Cryptosporidium parvum	Obligate intracellular coccidian parasite, oocysts are spherical to oval in shape with an average size of 4.5 to 5.0 μm, oocysts are resistant to chlorination used to disinfect water	Humans, wild and domestic animals, especially calves	Contaminated drinking and recreational water, raw milk from infected cattle, fresh vegetables and other foods contaminated with feces from infected humans and animals	30,000	2 to 14 days Profuse, watery diarrhea, abdominal pain, nausea, vomiting Duration is few days to 3 weeks	Immunofluorescence assay[187] PCR[188]	Thorough cooking of food, avoid contact with infected animals, filtration of drinking water, good personal hygiene and food handling practices
Cyclospora cayetanesis	Obligate intracellular coccidian parasite, oocysts are spherical in shape with an average size of 8 to 10 μm	Humans	Water, fruits and vegetables contaminated with oocysts	14,600	1 week Watery diarrhea, abdominal pain, nausea, vomiting, anorexia, myalgia, weight loss Duration is a few days to 1 month	Staining and microscopic examination[189] PCR[190]	Good personal hygiene, filtration of drinking water

Toxoplasma gondii	Obligate intracellular coccidian protozoa	Cats, farm animals, transplacental transmission from infected mother to fetus	Raw or undercooked meat, raw goat milk, raw vegetables	112,500	5 to 23 days Fever, rash, headache, muscle pain, swelling of lymph nodes; transplacental infection may cause abortion Duration is variable	Cell culture and mouse inoculation[191] Immunoassay[192] PCR[191]	Prevent environmental contamination with cat feces, avoid consumption of raw meat and milk, safe disposal of cat feces, wash hands after contact with cats
Trichinella spiralis	Nematode with no free living stage in the life cycle, adult female worms are 3 to 4 mm in length, transmissible form is larval cyst which can occur in pork muscle	Wild and domestic animals, especially swine and horses	Raw or undercooked meat of animals containing encysted larvae such as swine or horses	50	Initial symptoms: 24 to 72 h, Systemic symptoms: 8 to 21 days Initial phase: abdominal pain, fever, nausea, vomiting, diarrhea Systemic phase: periorbital oedema, eosinophilia, myalgia, difficulty in breathing, thirst, profuse sweating, chills, weakness, prostration Duration is 2 weeks to 3 months	Microscopic examination ELISA[193] PCR[194]	Adequate cooking of meat, freezing of meat at -15°C for 30 days or at -35°C, preventing trichinosis in pigs by not feeding swine garbage containing infected meat
Anisakis spp.	Nematode, slender threadlike parasite measuring 1.5 to 1.6 cm in length and 0.1 cm in diameter	Sea mammals	Some undercooked salt water fish, sushi, herring, sashimi, ceviche	Unknown	4 to 12 h Epigastric pain, nausea, vomiting, sometimes hematemesis Duration is variable	ELISA[195] PCR[196]	Adequate cooking of saltwater fish, freezing fish at -23°C for 7 days
Taenia solium *Taenia saginata*	Tapeworm, dependent on the digestive system of the host for nutrition	Humans, cattle, swine	Raw or undercooked beef or pork	Unknown	Few days to >10 years Nausea, epigastric pain, nervousness, insomnia, anorexia, weight loss, digestive disturbances, weakness, dizziness Duration is weeks to months	Detection of eggs or proglottids in feces ELISA[197] PCR[198]	Adequate cooking of beef and pork, proper disposal of sewage and human wastes, freezing of meat at -10°C for 2 weeks
Diphyllobothrium latum	Largest human tapeworm	Saltwater fish, humans	Raw or undercooked saltwater fish	Unknown	Epigastric pain, nausea, abdominal pain, diarrhea, weakness, pernicious anemia Duration is months to years	Detection of eggs in feces	Adequate cooking of fish, proper disposal of sewage and human waste

cysts contaminate water or food through feces of infected animals or humans. Following ingestion of cyst-contaminated water or food, the trophozoites reach the small intestine, where they undergo excystation and multiply by binary fission. New trophozoites subsequently become cysts in the distal small intestine, and the encysted trophozoites are shed in the feces. The symptoms of giardiasis include abdominal pain, abdominal distension, nausea, vomiting, and diarrhea. Although water and foods contaminated with cysts are primary vehicles of giardiasis, little is known about the survival characteristics of the cysts in foods. In most cases of foodborne transmission, infected food handlers transfer the cysts to foods they prepare.

Entamoeba histolytica

E. histolytica is a protozoan parasite that causes amoebiasis or amoebic dysentery in humans. Although the parasite survives in the environment and water, humans are the principal source of amoebiasis. In humans, cysts containing the trophozites are released, which in turn multiply and are subsequently excreted in the feces as cysts.[89] Foods and water contaminated with the cysts transmit the disease. Since the fecal-oral route is the principal route of transmission of amoebiasis, personal hygiene of infected food handlers plays a critical role in preventing foodborne amoebiasis. Human amoebiasis can occur in two forms: intestinal amoebiasis and amoebic liver abscess, which is usually a sequela to the intestinal form. Intestinal amoebiasis is characterized by abdominal pain, vomiting, and watery diarrhea containing mucus and blood. Symptoms of the hepatic form of amoebiasis include wasting, painful and enlarged liver, weight loss, and anemia.

Cryptosporidium parvum

C. parvum is a protozoan parasite that infects a wide range of animals and humans. *C. parvum* is monoexenous in its life cycle, requiring only one host for its development.[88] Infected hosts shed in their feces oocysts of the parasite, subsequently contaminating the environment, food, and water. The life cycle of *C. parvum* can be summarized as follows.[88] Upon ingestion of contaminated water or food, or by inhalation of oocysts, sporozoites are released by excystation of oocysts into the gastrointestinal or respiratory tract. The sporozoites enter the epithelial cells and develop into trophozoites, which in turn differentiate into type I and type II meronts. The merozoites from type I meronts invade new tissues and develop into trophozoites to continue the life cycle. The merozoites from type II meronts invade infected cells and undergo sexual multiplication to give rise to male and female gametes. The zygotes resulting from fertilized gametes become infectious by sporulation, and the sporulated oocysts are excreted in feces.

Cryptosporidiosis is a self-limiting disease with an incubation period of one to two weeks, and is characterized by profuse, watery diarrhea, abdominal pain, vomiting, and low-grade fever. Water is the most common source of *C. parvum* for human infections.[58] Oocysts of the pathogen have been detected in fresh vegetables, raw milk, sausage, and apple cider.[58] Infected food handlers can also transfer the oocysts to foods.[90, 91] *C. parvum* oocysts are sensitive to freezing and freeze-drying. The oocysts lose infectivity in distilled water stored at 4°C.[92] However, the oocysts are quite resistant to chlorine; no loss in infectivity was observed in water containing 1 to 3% chlorine for up to 18 hours.[93] However, the oocysts are sensitive to ozone, losing more than 90% infectivity in the presence of 1 ppm ozone for 5 minutes.[94]

Cyclospora cayetanensis

C. cayetanensis is an emerging foodborne, protozoan pathogen, especially in the U.S. The parasite was implicated in several foodborne outbreaks in the U.S. during 1996 and 1997.[95] *C. cayetanensis* is spread through infected feces and is transmitted to humans by the fecal-oral route. Water and foods, especially fruits and vegetables containing oocysts, are common vehicles of human infection. The symptoms of *C. cayetanensis* infection in humans include watery diarrhea, nausea, abdominal pain, vomiting, and weight loss. Presently, very little information is available on the effects of heat, freezing, and disinfection agents on *Cyclospora* oocysts. Preliminary studies revealed that exposure of oocysts to –20°C for 24 h or 60°C for 1 h prevented oocysts from sporulating. Exposing oocysts to 4° or 37°C for 14 days delayed sporulation.[96]

Toxoplasma gondii

T. gondii is an obligate intracellular protozoan parasite for which cats are the definitive hosts. In the intestines of cats, the parasite undergoes sexual reproduction to form oocysts, which are excreted in feces.[97] The oocysts undergo maturation and survive in the environment for months. Toxoplasmosis in humans results following ingestion of food or water contaminated with oocysts. Transmission also occurs from an infected pregnant mother to child by transplacental transmission.[89] Symptoms in healthy adults are usually mild, and include rash, headache, muscle pain, and swelling of lymph nodes. The oocysts are sensitive to both heat and cold;[98] hence the cysts are killed in properly cooked foods.[99]

Trichinella spiralis

T. spiralis is a roundworm that primarily infects wild and domestic animals, especially pigs. Humans contract trichinosis by consumption of raw or undercooked meat containing larvae of the parasite. Pigs are infected by consuming uncooked scraps of infected pork. The encysted larvae upon ingestion are liberated from the cyst in the intestine, where they sexually mature.[100] The mature male and female worms copulate in the lumen of the small intestine, giving rise to a new generation of larvae. The newly born larvae migrate to various tissues in the body. Those larvae that reach the striated muscles penetrate into the sarcolemma of the muscle fibers and develop to maturity as encapsulated cysts.[100] The larvae continue their life cycle when raw or undercooked meat, especially pork containing the larvae, is consumed by humans.

Anisakis Species

Anisakiasis in humans is caused by two foodborne roundworms. These include *A. simplex*, whose definitive host is whales, and *Pseudoterranova decipiens*, which primarily inhabits seals. The eggs of these roundworms are excreted in feces by their respective hosts. The eggs then undergo molting in suitable intermediate hosts and subsequently develop into larvae, which are ingested by fish.[101] Humans contract anisakiasis by consumption of raw or undercooked fish and seafoods containing the larvae. In noninvasive anisakiasis, the worms released from ingested foods migrate to the pharynx, resulting in "tingling throat syndrome."[101] The worms are ultimately expelled by coughing. In the invasive form of anisakiasis, the worms penetrate the intestinal mucosa, causing symptoms that include epigastric pain, nausea, vomiting, and diarrhea.

Taenia Species

The genus *Taenia* includes two meatborne pathogenic flat worms, *T. saginata* (beef tapeworm) and *T. solium* (pork tapeworm). The eggs of *T. saginata* survive in the environment, including on pastures, and are ingested by cattle in which they hatch into embryos.[100] The embryos migrate to skeletal muscles or the heart, and develop into larvae known as cysticercus bovis. Humans become infected by consuming raw or undercooked beef containing the larvae. Larvae that are released into the small intestine develop into mature, adult worms. The symptoms of *T. saginata* infection in humans include decreased appetite, headache, dizziness, diarrhea, and weight loss.

In the normal life cycle of *T. solium*, pigs serve as the intermediate host. Eggs ingested by pigs develop into embryos in the duodenum, penetrate the intestinal wall, migrate through the blood and the lymphatic system, and finally reach the skeletal muscles and myocardium, where they develop into larvae known as cysticercus cellulose. Humans consuming raw or undercooked pork are infected with the larvae, which develop into adult worms in the small intestine. The symptoms of *T. solium* infection in humans include discomfort, hunger pains, anorexia, and nervous disorders. Worms are passed in the feces. In the abnormal life cycle of *T. solium*, humans serve as intermediate hosts in which the larvae develop in striated muscles and in subcutaneous tissue.

Diphyllobothrium latum

D. latum is commonly referred to as the broad tapeworm because it is the largest human tapeworm.[101] Humans contract diphyllobothriasis by consuming raw or undercooked fish containing the larval forms called plerocercoids. Upon ingestion, the larvae develop into mature worms in the intestines. Eggs produced by mature worms are excreted in feces. If feces containing the eggs contaminate water, the eggs develop into free-swimming larvae called coricidia. Coricidia are ingested by crustaceans, where they develop into a juvenile stage known as procercoid. Following ingestion of infected crustaceans by fish, procercoids develop into plerocercoids to continue the life cycle. Diphyllobothriasis in humans is characterized by nausea, abdominal pain, diarrhea, weakness, and pernicious anemia.[101] Cases of diphyllobothriasis have been associated with eating raw salmon and sushi.

References

1. Mead, PS, Slutsker, L, Dietz, W et al. *Emerg Infect Dis* 5: 607; 1999.
2. Centers for Disease Control and Prevention, *Morbid Mortal Weekly Rep* 47: 782; 1997.
3. Meng, J, Doyle, MP. In: *Microbiology of Shiga Toxin-Producing* Escherichia coli *in Foods,* Escherichia coli *O157:H7 and Other Shiga Toxin-Producing* E. coli *Strains,* Kaper, JB, O'Brien, AD, Eds, ASM Press, Washington, DC, 1998, p 92.
4. Faith, NG, Shere, JA, Brosch, R, et al. *Appl Environ Microbiol* 62: 1519; 1996.
5. Zhao, T, Doyle, MP, Shere, J, Gerber, L. *Appl Environ Microbiol* 61: 1290; 1995.
6. Riley, LW, Remis, RS, Helgerson, SD, et al. *N Engl J Med* 308: 681; 1983.
7. Zhao, T, Doyle, MP, Harmon, BG, et al. *J Clin Microbiol* 36: 641; 1998.
8. Brown, CA, Harmon, BG, Zhao, T, Doyle, MP. *Appl Environ Microbiol* 63: 27; 1997.
9. Wang, GT, Zhao, T, Doyle, MP. *Appl Environ Microbiol* 62: 2567; 1998.
10. Uljas, HE, Ingham, SC. *J Food Prot* 61: 939; 1998.
11. Arnold, KW, Kaspar, CW. *Appl Environ Microbiol* 61: 2037; 1995.
12. Buchanan, RL, Edelson, SG. *Appl Environ Microbiol* 62: 4009; 1996.
13. Leyer, GJ, Wang, L, Johnson, EA. *Appl Environ Microbiol* 61: 3152; 1995.

14. Doyle, MP, Schoeni, JL. *Appl Environ Microbiol* 48: 855; 1984.
15. Glass, KA, Loeffelholz, JM, Ford, JP, Doyle, MP. *Appl Environ Microbiol* 58: 2513; 1992.
16. Padhye, NV, Doyle, MP. *J Food Prot* 55: 555; 1992.
17. Doyle, MP, Zhao, T, Meng, J, Zhao, S. In: *Food Microbiology: Fundamentals and Frontiers*, Doyle, MP, Beuchat, LR, Montville, TJ, Eds, ASM Press, Washington, DC, 1997, p 171.
18. D'Aoust, J-Y. In: *Food Microbiology: Fundamentals and Frontiers*, Doyle, MP, Beuchat, LR, Montville, TJ, Eds, ASM Press, Washington, DC, 1997, p 129.
19. Jay, JM. *Modern Food Microbiology*, Aspen Publishers, Gaithersburg, 1998, p 509.
20. Bean, NH, Griffin, PM, Goulding, JS, Ivey, CB. *J Food Prot* 53: 711; 1983.
21. D'Aoust, J-Y. *Int J Food Microbiol* 13: 207; 1991.
22. Leyer, GJ, Johnson, EA. *Appl Environ Microbiol* 59: 1842; 1993.
23. Leyer, GJ, Johnson, EA. *Appl Environ Microbiol* 58: 2075; 1992.
24. D'Aoust, J-Y. In: *Foodborne Bacterial Pathogens*, Doyle, MP, Ed, Marcel Dekker, New York, 1998, p 336.
25. Flowers, RS. *Food Technol* 42: 182; 1988.
26. Millemann, Y, Lesage, MC, Chaslus-Dancla, E, Lafont, JP. *J Clin Microbiol* 33: 173; 1995.
27. Banhart, HM, Dreesen, DW, Bastien, R, Pancorbo, OC. *J Food Prot* 54: 488; 1991.
28. Keller, LH, Benson, CE, Krotec, K, Eckroade, RJ. *Infect Immun* 63: 1134; 1995.
29. Jay, JM. *Modern Food Microbiology*, Aspen Publishers, Gaithersburg, 1998, p 556.
30. Whitehouse, CA, Balbo, PB, Pesci, EC, et al. *Infect Immun* 66: 1934; 1998.
31. Stern, NJ, Kazmi, SU. In: *Foodborne Bacterial Pathogens*, Doyle, MP, Ed, Marcel Dekker, New York, 1989, p 71.
32. Altekruse, SF, Stern, NJ, Fields, PI, Swerdlow, DL. *Emerg Infect Dis* 5: 28; 1999.
33. Allos, BM. *J Infect Dis* 176: 125S; 1997.
34. Robins-Browne, RM. In: *Food Microbiology: Fundamentals and Frontiers*, Doyle, MP, Beuchat, LR, Montville, TJ, Eds, ASM Press, Washington, DC, 1997, p 192.
35. Jay, JM. *Modern Food Microbiology*, Aspen Publishers, Gaithersburg, 1998, p 555.
36. Shiemann, DA. In: *Foodborne Bacterial Pathogens*, Doyle, MP, Ed, Marcel Dekker, New York, 1989, p 631.
37. Greenwood, M. Leatherhead: Leatherhead Food Research Association. 1990.
38. Bottone, EJ. *Clin Microbiol Rev* 10: 257; 1997.
39. Schifield, GM. *J Appl Bacteriol* 72: 267; 1992.
40. Toma, S, Lafleur, L. *Appl Microbiol* 28: 469; 1974.
41. Walker, S. Organisms of emerging significance, *Microbiological and Environmental Health Issues Relevant to the Food and Catering Industries*. Symposium Proceedings, Campden Food and Drink Research Association, Chipping Campden, UK, 1990.
42. Hanna, MO, Stewart, JC, Zink, DL, et al. *J Food Sci* 42: 1180; 1977.
43. Palumbo, SA. *J Food Prot* 49: 1003; 1986.
44. Oliver, JD, Kaper, JB. In: *Food Microbiology: Fundamentals and Frontiers*, Doyle, MP, Beuchat, LR, Montville, TJ, Eds, ASM Press, Washington, DC, 1997, p 228.
45. Miyamato, Y, Obara, Y, Nikkawa, T, et al. *Infect Immun* 28, 567, 1980.
46. Mintz, ED, Popovic, T, Blake, PA. In: *Vibrio cholerae and Cholera: Molecular to Global Perspectives*, ASM Press, Washington, DC, 1994, p 345.
47. Jay, JM. *Modern Food Microbiology*, Aspen Publishers, Gaithersburg, 1998, p 544.
48. Beuchat, LR. *Int J Food Microbiol* 13: 217; 1991.
49. Kirov, SM. In: *Food Microbiology: Fundamentals and Frontiers*, Doyle, MP, Beuchat, LR, Montville, TJ, Eds, ASM Press, Washington, DC, 1997, p 265.
50. Berrang, ME, Brackett, RE, Beuchat, LR. *Appl Environ Microbiol* 55: 2167; 1989.
51. Palumbo, SA. *Int J Food Microbiol* 7: 41; 1988.
52. Jay, JM. *Modern Food Microbiology*, Aspen Publishers, Gaithersburg, 1998, p 620.
53. Holmberg, SD, Wachsmuth, IK, Hickmann-Brenner, FW, et al. *Ann Intern Med* 105: 690; 1986.
54. Nickelson, N. Food Quality, April, 28, 1999.
55. Brackett, RE. *Food Technol* 52: 162; 1998.
56. Cox, LJ, Keiss,T, Cordier, JL, et al. *Food Microbiol* 6: 49; 1989.
57. Jeong, DK, Frank, JF. *J Food Prot* 57: 576; 1994.

58. Meng, J, Doyle, MP. *Annu Rev Nutr* 17: 255; 1997.
59. Rocourt, J, Cossart, P. In: *Food Microbiology: Fundamentals and Frontiers*, Doyle, MP, Beuchat, LR, Montville, TJ, Eds, ASM Press, Washington, DC, 1997, p 337.
60. Jay, JM. *Modern Food Microbiology*, Aspen Publishers, Gaithersburg, 1998, p 490.
61. Jablonski, LM, Bohac, GA. In: *Food Microbiology: Fundamentals and Frontiers*, Doyle, MP, Beuchat, LR, Montville, TJ, Eds, ASM Press, Washington, DC, 1997, p 353.
62. Newsome, RL. *Food Technol* 42: 182; 1988.
63. Bergdoll, ML. In: *Foodborne Bacterial Pathogens*, Doyle, MP, Ed, Marcel Dekker, New York, 1989, p 463.
64. Dodds, KL, Austin, JW. In: *Food Microbiology: Fundamentals and Frontiers*, Doyle, MP, Beuchat, LR, Montville, TJ, Eds, ASM Press, Washington, DC, 1997, p 288.
65. Pierson, MD, Reddy, NR. *Food Technol* 42: 196; 1988.
66. Jay, JM. *Modern Food Microbiology*, Aspen Publishers, Gaithersburg, 1998, p 462.
67. Hobbs, BC. In: *Foodborne Infections and Intoxications*, Riemann, H, Bryan, FL, Eds, Academic Press, New York, 1979, p 131.
68. Labbe, R. In: *Foodborne Bacterial Pathogens*, Doyle, MP, Ed, Marcel Dekker, New York, 1989, p 191.
69. Doyle, MP. *Food Technol* 42: 199; 1988.
70. Kramer, JM, Gilbert, RJ. In: *Foodborne Bacterial Pathogens*, Doyle, MP, Ed, Marcel Dekker, New York, 1989, p 327.
71. Johnson, KM. *J Food Prot* 47: 145; 1984.
72. Hobbs, BC, Gilbert, RJ. Microbiological counts in relation to food poisoning, *Proc IV Intl Cong Food Sci Technol* 3: 159; 1974.
73. Stiles, ME. In: *Foodborne Bacterial Pathogens*, Doyle, MP, Ed, Marcel Dekker, New York, 1989, p 706.
74. Labigne, A, De Reuse, H. *Infect Agents Dis* 5: 191; 1996.
75. McColl, KEL. *J Infect Dis* 34: 7; 1997.
76. Goodman, KJ, Correa, P. *Int J Epidemiol* 24: 875; 1995.
77. Hopkins, RJ, Vial, PA, Ferreccio, C, et al. *J Infect Dis* 168: 222; 1993.
78. Jiang, X, Doyle, MP. *J Food Prot* 61: 929; 1998.
79. Cromeans, T, Nainan, OV, Fields, HA, et al. In: *Foodborne Diseases Handbook, Vol 2, Diseases Caused by Viruses, Parasites, and Fungi*, Hui, YH, Gorham, JR, Murrel, KD, Cliver, DO, Eds, Marcel Dekker, New York, 1994, p 1.
80. Dolin, R, Blacklow, NR, Dupont, H, et al. *Proc Soc Exp Biol Med* 140: 578; 1972.
81. Sattar, SA, Springthorpe, VS, Ansari, SA. In: *Foodborne Diseases Handbook, Vol 2, Diseases Caused by Viruses, Parasites, and Fungi*, Hui, YH, Gorham, JR, Murrel, KD, Cliver, DO, Eds, Marcel Dekker, New York, 1994, p 81.
82. Buchi, G, Rae, ID. In: *Aflatoxins*, Goldbatt, LA, Ed, Academic Press, New York, 1969, p 55.
83. Hocking, AD. In: *Food Microbiology: Fundamentals and Frontiers*, Doyle, MP, Beuchat, LR, Montville, TJ, Eds, ASM Press, Washington, DC, 1997, p 343.
84. Pitt, JI. In: *Food Microbiology: Fundamentals and Frontiers*, Doyle, MP, Beuchat, LR, Montville, TJ, Eds, ASM Press, Washington, DC, 1997, p 406.
85. Krogh, P, Hald, B, Perdersen, EJ. *Acta Pathol Microbiol Scand Sect* B81: 689; 1977.
86. Friis, P, Hasselager, E, Krogh, P. *Acta Pathol Microbiol Scand* 77: 559; 1969.
87. Bullerman, LB. *Food Microbiology: Fundamentals and Frontiers*, Doyle, MP, Beuchat, LR, Montville, TJ, Eds, ASM Press, Washington, DC, 1997, p 419.
88. Smith, J. *J Food Prot* 56: 451; 1993.
89. Speer, CA. In: *Food Microbiology: Fundamentals and Frontiers*, Doyle, MP, Beuchat, LR, Montville, TJ, Eds, ASM Press, Washington, DC, 1997, p 478.
90. Hoskin, JC, Wright, RE. *J Food Prot* 54: 53; 1991.
91. Petersen, C. *Lancet* 345: 1128; 1995.
92. Tzipori, S. *Microbiol Rev* 47: 84; 1983.
93. Reduker, DW, Speer, CA. *J Parasitol* 71: 112; 1985.
94. Korich, DG, Mead, JR, Madore, MS, et al. *Appl Environ Microbiol* 56: 1423; 1990.
95. Sterling, CR, Ortega, YR. *Emerg Infect Dis* 5: 48; 1999.

96. Smith, HV, Paton, CA, Mtambo, MMA, Girdwood, RWA. *Appl Environ Microbiol* 63: 1631; 1997.
97. Casemore, DP. *Lancet* 336: 1427; 1990.
98. Fayer, R, Dubey, JP. *Food Technol* 39: 57; 1985.
99. Fleck, DG. *PHLS Microbiol Digest* 6: 69; 1989.
100. Kim, CW. In: *Food Microbiology: Fundamentals and Frontiers*, Doyle, MP, Beuchat, LR, Montville, TJ, Eds, ASM Press, Washington, DC, 1997, p 449.
101. Hayunga, EG. In: *Food Microbiology: Fundamentals and Frontiers*, Doyle, MP, Beuchat, LR, Montville, TJ, Eds, ASM Press, Washington, DC, 1997, p 463.
102. Kleanthous, H, Fry, NK, Smith, HR, et al. *Epidemiol Infect* 101: 327; 1988.
103. March, SB, Ratnam, S. *J Clin Microbiol* 23: 869; 1986.
104. Doyle, MP, Schoeni, JL. *Appl Environ Microbiol* 53: 2394; 1987.
105. March, SB, Ratnam, S. *J Clin Microbiol* 27: 1675; 1989.
106. Okrend, AJG, Rose, BE, Matner, R. *J Food Prot* 53: 936; 1990.
107. Padhye, NV, Doyle, MP. *Appl Environ Microbiol* 57: 2693; 1991.
108. Pollard, DR, Johnson, WM, Lior, H, et al. *J Clin Microbiol* 28: 540; 1990.
109. Cox, NA, Fung, DYC, Bailey, JS, et al. *Dairy Food Environ Sanitat* 7: 628; 1987.
110. Cox, NA, Fung, DYC, Goldschmidt, MC, et al. *J Food Prot* 47: 74; 1984.
111. Feng, P. *J Food Prot* 55: 927; 1992.
112. Tietjen, M, Fung, DYC. *Crit Rev Microbiol* 21: 53; 1995.
113. Cano, RJ, Rasmussen, SR, Sanchez Fraga, G, Palomers, JC. *J Appl Bacteriol* 75: 247; 1993.
114. Nguyen, AV, Khan, MI, Lu, Z. *Avian Dis* 38: 119; 1994.
115. Le Minor, L, Craige, J, Yen, CH. *Can Publ Health J* 29: 484; 1938.
116. Lim, P, Tam, FCH, Cheong, Y, Jegathesan, M. *J Clin Microbiol* 36: 2271; 1998.
117. Chaicumpa, W, Ruangkunaporn, D, Burr, D, et al. *J Clin Microbiol* 30: 2513; 1992.
118. Hashimoto, Y, Itho, Y, Fujinaga, Y, et al. *J Clin Microbiol* 33: 775; 1995.
119. Park, CE, Smibert, RM, Blaser, MJ, et al. *Compendium of Methods for the Microbiological Examination of Foods*, 2nd ed, Speck, ML, Ed, American Public Health Association, Washington, DC, 1984, p 386.
120. Rice, BE, Lamichhane, C, Joseph, SW, Rollins, DM. *Clin Diagn Lab Immunol* 3: 669; 1996.
121. Linton, D, Lawson, AJ, Owen, RJ, Stanley, J. *J Clin Microbiol* 35: 2568; 1997.
122. Ng, LK, Kingombe, CI, Yan, W, et al. *Appl Environ Microbiol* 63: 4558; 1997.
123. Morris, GK. *Compendium of Methods for the Microbiological Examination of Foods*, 2nd ed, Speck, ML, Ed, American Public Health Association, Washington, DC, 1984, p 343.
124. Pal, T, Al-sweih, N, Herpay, M, Chugh, TD. *J Clin Microbiol* 35: 1757; 1997.
125. Lampel, KA, Jagow, JA, Trucksess, M, Hill, WE. *Appl Environ Microbiol* 56: 1536; 1990.
126. Restaino, L, Grauman, GS, McCall, WA, Hill, WM. *J Food Prot* 42: 120; 1979.
127. Kapperud, G, Vardund, T, Skjerve, E, Michaelsen, TE. *Appl Environ Microbiol* 59: 2938; 1993.
128. Farmer, JJ III, Hickmann-Brenner, FW, Kelly, MT. *Manual of Clinical Microbiology*, 4th ed, Lennette, EH, Balows, A, Hausler, WJ, Jean-Shadomy, H, Eds, American Society for Microbiology, Washington, DC, 1985, p 282.
129. Twedt, RM, Madden, JM, Colwell, RR. *Compendium of Methods for the Microbiological Examination of Foods*, 2nd ed, Speck, ML, Ed, American Public Health Association, Washington, DC, 1984, p 368.
130. Castillo, L, Castillo, D, Silva, W, et al. *Hybridoma* 14: 271; 1995.
131. Miyagi, K, Sano, K, Imura, S, et al. *J Med Microbiol* 48: 883; 1999.
132. Varela, P, Pollevick, GD, Rivas, M, et al. *J Clin Microbiol* 32: 1246; 1994.
133. Honda, T, Yoh, M, Kongmuang, U, Miwatani, T. *J Clin Microbiol* 22: 383; 1985.
134. Kim, YB, Okuda, J, Takahashi, C, et al. *J Clin Microbiol* 37: 1173; 1999.
135. Parker, RW, Lewis, DH. *Appl Environ Microbiol* 61: 476; 1995.
136. Hill, WE, Keasler, SP, Truckess, MW, et al. *App Environ Microbiol* 57: 707; 1991.
137. Janda, JM, Abott, SL, Carnahan, AM. In: *Manual of Clinical Microbiology*, 6th ed, Murray, PR, Baron, EJ, Pfaller, MA, Tenover, FC, Yolken, RH, Eds, American Society for Microbiology, Washington, DC, 1995, p 477.
138. Jeppesen, C. *Int J Food Microbiol* 26: 25; 1995.
139. Joseph, SW, Carnahan, A. *Ann Rev Fish Dis* 4: 315; 1994.

140. Borrel, N, Acinas, SG, Figueras, MJ, Martinez-Murcia, AJ. *J Clin Microbiol* 35: 1671; 1997.
141. Cascon, A, Anguita, J, Hernanz, C, et al. *Appl Environ Microbiol* 62: 1167; 1996.
142. Jones, GL. *Isolation and identification of* Listeria monocytogenes, U.S. Department of Health and Human Services, Public Health Service, Centers for Disease Control, 1989.
143. McClain, D, Lee, WH. *J Assoc Off Anal Chem* 71: 876; 1988.
144. VanNetten, P, Perales, I, van de Moosdijk, A, et al. *Int J Food Microbiol* 8: 299; 1989.
145. Fliss, I, St. Laurent, M, Emond, E, et al. *Appl Environ Microbiol* 59: 2698; 1993.
146. Bubert, A, Hein, I, Rauch, M, et al. *Appl Environ Microbiol* 65: 4688; 1999.
147. Bennett, RW. In: *Foodborne Microorganisms and Their Toxins: Developing Methodology,* Pierson, MD, Stern, NJ, Eds, Marcel Dekker, New York, 1986, p 345.
148. Taitini, SR, Hoover, DG, Lachicha, RVF. In: *Compendium of Methods for the Microbiological Examination of Foods,* 2nd ed, Speck, ML, Ed, American Public Health Association, Washington, DC, 1984, p 411.
149. Tsen, H-Y, Chen, TR. *Appl Microbiol Biotechnol* 37: 685; 1992.
150. Van der Zee, A, Verbakel, H, van Zon, J, et al. *J Clin Microbiol* 37: 342; 1999.
151. Bennett, RW. In: *Bacteriological Analytical Manual,* 6th ed, U.S. Food and Drug Administration, Association of Official Analytical Chemists, Arlington, 1984, 15.01.
152. Dowell, VR, Lombard, GL, Thompson, FS, Armfield, AY. Media for isolation, characterization, and identification of obligate anaerobic bacteria, Center for Disease Control, Atlanta, Georgia, 1981.
153. Aranda, E, Rodriguez, MM, Asenio, MA, Cordoba, JJ. *Lett Appl Microbiol* 25: 186; 1997.
154. Fach, P, Gilbert, M, Griffais, R, et al. *Appl Environ Microbiol* 61: 389; 1995.
155. Kautter, DA, Lynt, RK, Solomon, HM. Clostridium botulinum, *Bacteriological Analytical Manual,* 6th ed, US Food and Drug Administration, Association of Official Analytical Chemists, Arlington, 1984, 18.01.
156. Fach, P, Popoff, MR. *Appl Environ Microbiol* 63: 4232; 1997.
157. Baez, LA, Juneja, VK. *Appl Environ Microbiol* 61: 807; 1995.
158. Harmon, M, Goepfert, JM. *Compendium of Methods for the Microbiological Examination of Foods,* 2nd ed, Speck, ML, Ed, American Public Health Association, Washington, DC, 1984, p 458.
159. Beecher, DJ, Wong, ACL. *Appl Environ Microbiol* 60: 4614; 1994.
160. Mantynen, V, Lindstrom, K. *Appl Environ Microbiol* 64: 1634; 1998.
161. Ruiz, J, Lorente, I, Perez, J, Simarro, E, Martinez-Campos, L. *J Clin Microbiol* 35: 2417; 1997.
162. Luccero, NE, Foglia, L, Ayala, SM, et al. *J Clin Microbiol* 37: 3245; 1999.
163. Romero, C, Pardo, M, Grillo, MJ, et al. *J Clin Microbiol* 33: 3198; 1995.
164. Smith, EM. In: *Methods in Environmental Virology,* Gerba, CP, Goyal, SM, Eds, Marcel Dekker, New York, 1982, p 15.
165. Williams, Jr, FP, Fout, GS. *Environ Sci Technol* 26: 689; 1992.
166. Polish, LB, Robertson, BH, Khanna, B, et al. *J Clin Microbiol* 37: 3615; 1977.
167. Abbaszadegan, M, Stewart, P, LeChavallier, M. *Appl Environ Microbiol* 65: 444; 1999.
168. Atmar, RL, Neill, FH, Romalde, JL, et al. *Appl Environ Microbiol* 61: 3014; 1995.
169. Herrmann, JE, Blacklow, NR, Matsui, SM, et al. *J Clin Microbiol* 33: 2511; 1995.
170. Tsunemitsu, H, Jiang, B, Saif, LJ. *J Clin Microbiol* 30: 2129; 1992.
171. Le Guyader, F, Dubois, E, Menard, D, Pommepuy, M. *Appl Environ Microbiol* 60: 3665; 1994.
172. Pitt, JI, Hocking, AD, Glenn, DR. *J Appl Bacteriol* 54: 109; 1983.
173. Pitt, JI, Hocking, AD. *Fungi and Food Spoilage,* Academic Press, Sydney, 1985.
174. Samson, RA, Hoekstra, ES, Frisvad, JC, Filtenborg, O. *Introduction to Foodborne Fungi,* 4th ed, Centraalbureau voor Schimmelcultures, Baarn, The Netherlands, 1995.
175. Shapira, R, Paster, N, Menasherov, M, et al. *Appl Environ Microbiol* 63: 990; 1997.
176. Shapira, R, Paster, N, Eyal, O, et al. *Appl Environ Microbiol* 62: 3270; 1996.
177. King, AD, Pitt, JI, Beuchat, L, Corry, JEL. *Methods for the Mycological Examination of Food,* Plenum Press, New York, 1986.
178. Matheis, JP, Roberts, RG. *Appl Environ Microbiol* 58: 3170; 1992.
179. Nelson, PE, Tousoun, TA, Marasas, WFO. *Fusarium Species: An Illustrated Manual for Identification,* The Pennsylvania State University Press, University Park, 1983.

180. Trane, U, Filtenborg, O, Frisvad, FC, Lund, F. In: *Modern Methods in Food Microbiology*, Hocking, AD, Pitt, JI, King, AD, Eds, Elsevier Science, New York, 1992, p 285.
181. Hue, F, Huerre, M, Rouffault, M, de Bievre, C. *J Clin Microbiol* 37: 2434; 1999.
182. Deng, MQ, Cliver, DO. *Parasitol Res* 85: 733; 1999.
183. Pillai, DR, Kain, KC. *J Clin Microbiol* 37: 3017; 1999.
184. Mahubhani, MH, Schafer, FW, Jones, DD, Bej, AK. *Curr Microbiol* 36: 107; 1998.
185. Zengzhu, G, Bracha, R, Nuchamowitz, Y, et al. *J Clin Microbiol* 37: 3034; 1999.
186. Haque, R, Ali, K, Akther, S, Petri, WA Jr. *J Clin Microbiol* 36: 449; 1998.
187. Sterling, CR, Arrowood, MJ. *Pediat Infect Dis* 5: 139; 1986.
188. Laxter, MA, Timlin, BK, Patel, RJ. *Am J Trop Med Hyg* 320: 1372; 1989.
189. Eberhard, ML, Pieniazek, NJ, Arrowood, MJ. *Arch Pathol Lab Med* 121: 792; 1997.
190. Jinneman, KC, Wetherington, JH, Hill, WE, et al. *Food Prot* 62: 682; 1999.
191. Hitt, JA, Filice, GA. *J Clin Microbiol* 30: 3181; 1992.
192. Hofgartner, WT, Swanzy, SR, Bacina, RM, et al. *J Clin Microbiol* 35: 3313; 1997.
193. Yopez-Mulia, L, Arriaga, C, Viveros, N, et al. *Vet Parasitol* 81: 57; 1999.
194. Wu, Z, Nagano, I, Pozio, E, Takahashi, Y. *Parasitol*ogy 118: 211; 1999.
195. Yagihashi, A, Sato, N, Takahashi, S, et al. *J Infect Dis* 161: 995; 1990.
196. Zhu, X, Gasser, RB, Podolska, M, Chilton, NB. *Int J Parasitol* 28: 1911; 1998.
197. D'Souza, PE, Hafeez, M. *Vet Res Commun* 23: 293; 1999.
198. Gottstein, B, Deplazes, P, Tanner, I, Skaggs, JS. *Trans R Soc Trop Hyg* 85: 248; 1991.

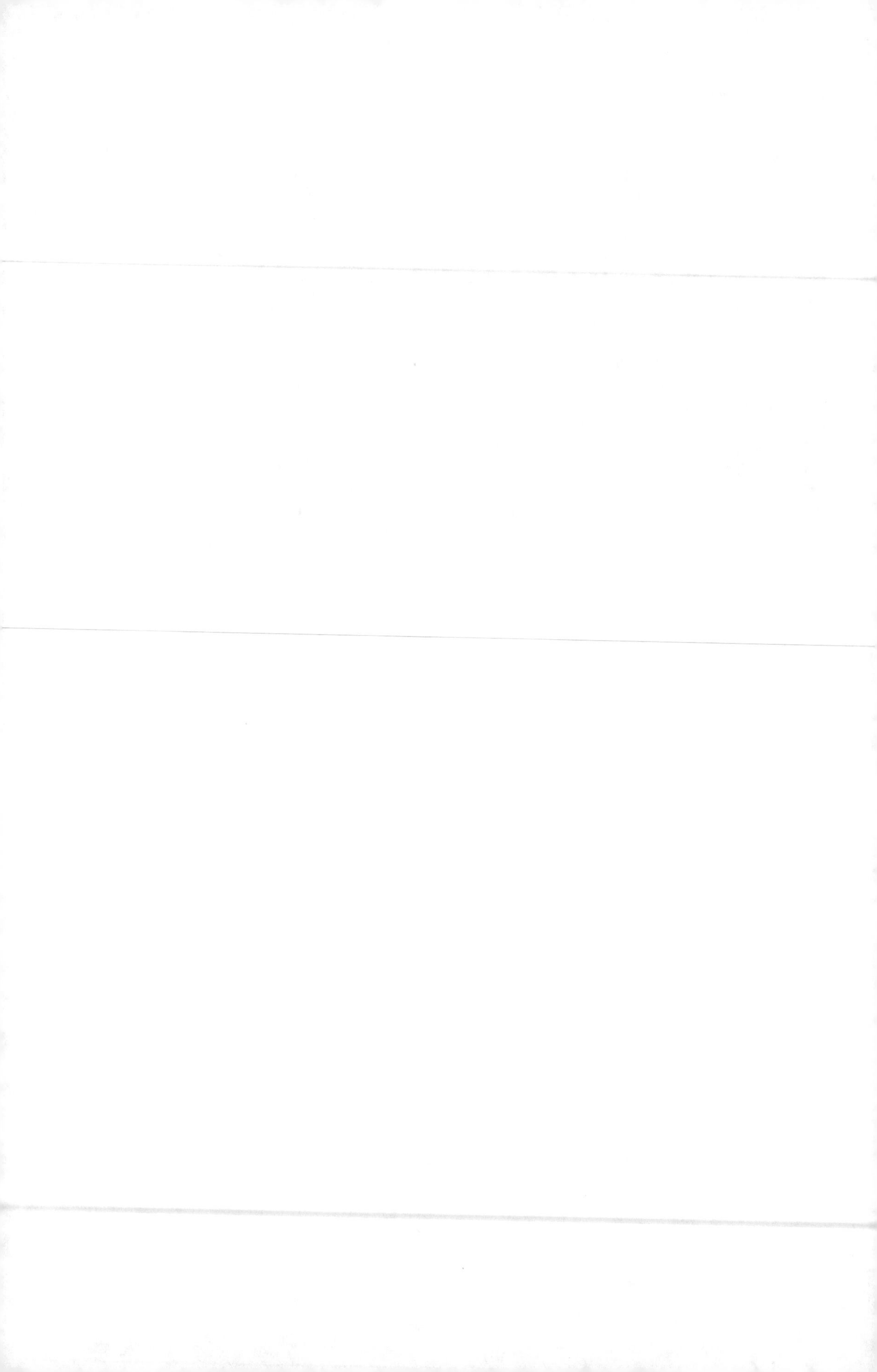

56

Nutrition and Hollow Organs of the Upper Gastrointestinal Tract

Ece A. Mutlu, Gökhan M. Mutlu, and Sohrab Mobarhan

Nutrition is an integral part of the management of gastrointestinal illness. The following two sections will elucidate the basic mechanisms of how the hollow organs of the gastrointestinal (GI) tract handle and digest food, how illnesses of these organs affect nutritional status, and the role of nutrition in the management of these illnesses. The readers are referred to a GI textbook for further details on diseases mentioned in these sections. Neoplasms of the GI tract are not included (see Section 50).

Introduction

The general roles of the various parts of the digestive system are given in Table 56.1. Diseases of these various parts not only cause damage to individual organs but also disrupt the harmonious mechanisms that enable adequate handling and digestion of food.

Food enters through the mouth where it is lubricated and broken down into pieces by mastication. Lubrication serves several purposes including protection of the mouth from damage by food, ease of transfer of food over surfaces of the GI tract and, formation of a liquid medium in which chemical reactions of digestion can occur. Mastication is not only necessary for food breakdown, but also helps to increase the surface area of the food particles to allow reach by digestive enzymes.

Transport of food through the mouth and the pharynx into the esophagus is accomplished by the swallowing reflex. This reflex involves coordinated actions of the tongue, the soft and hard palates, the pharyngeal muscles, the glottis, the epiglottis, and the upper esophageal sphincter. It is extremely rapid with a duration less than a second, and is regulated by both peripheral nerves and a swallowing center in the brain stem.[1] The multiple levels of control of swallowing and the redundancy of the control mechanisms allow compensating for minor problems.

Once swallowing is initiated voluntarily or involuntarily and the content of the mouth is pushed back into the pharynx, the swallowing reflex results in closure of the larynx by the epiglottis and concomitant relaxation of the upper esophageal sphincter (UES) to enable reception of bolus into the esophagus. Subsequently, the esophageal body, which has a short segment of striated muscle proximally but mainly is made up of smooth muscle,

0-8493-2705-9/02/$0.00+$1.50

TABLE 56.1

Parts of the Digestive System and Their Functions

Parts	Functions
Mouth, salivary glands, and pharynx	Breakdown of food into parts for transport to downstream; lubrication of food pieces for transport; initiation of the digestion of carbohydrates in food
Esophagus	Transport and lubrication of food pieces; protection of the airway from food entry
Stomach	Storage and trituration of food into small pieces (<1 mm^3); initiation of the digestion of proteins with acid and proteases; initiation of the digestion of fats
Small intestines	Breakdown of foods into molecules; and absorption of macro- and micronutrients; maintenance of water and electrolyte balance
Colon	Absorption of water and electrolytes; synthesis of certain vitamins and breakdown of carbohydrates to short chain fatty acids by bacteria; excretion of waste

propels the bolus downward with peristaltic motion. As the bolus travels through the distal esophagus, the lower esophageal sphincter (LES) relaxes and food is transported into the stomach for short-term storage and digestion. The integrity of the entire esophageal food transfer mechanism is very important to prevent food entering the airway.

Food goes through two functionally distinct compartments in the stomach. The proximal compartment, consisting of the fundus and upper body, acts as a reservoir. An adequate capacity in this compartment is achieved through receptive relaxation of the stomach wall, mediated by inhibition of vagal pathways and hormones such as secretin, gastric inhibitory peptide, and cholecystokinin (CCK). This relaxation allows for a wide range of storage volumes up to 1 to 2 liters without significant increases in intragastric pressure. At the same time, release of acid and digestive enzymes into the reservoir initiates gastric digestion.

The distal and second compartment of the stomach consists of the lower body and antrum, whose main function is dissolution of food into gastric chyme with particle size <1 to 2 millimeters prior to exit through the pylorus. This process, termed trituration, is achieved by the strong propulsive motor activity of the stomach. After initiation of the electrical signal that is generated by specialized pacemaker cells located in the mid-portion of the greater curvature, the stomach begins to contract from the mid-body, the contraction gradually spreads towards the antrum in a peristaltic fashion, and partial closure of the pyloric channel occurs. The stomach contents are forced backward against the antral walls and a closed pylorus, with passage of only a small amount of well-ground food into the duodenum. The shearing physical forces generated in this repetitive propulsion and retropulsion of gastric contents attain the particle size required of solid foods before passage into the small intestine.

Antral contractions cause emptying of solid food from the stomach. Liquids exit proportional to the pressure gradient between the duodenum and the stomach. This pressure gradient increases after completion of a meal when receptive relaxation fades away and the gastric fundus returns to its normal tone, increasing intragastric pressure. The rate of emptying from the stomach is also determined by the chemical and physical composition of the meal, as well as the way the body reacts to the food via the vagus nerve and the GI hormones. Liquids empty faster than solids; foods with high carbohydrate contents empty faster than foods that contain fat or are high in fiber. Hypo- or hypertonic fluids, highly viscous fluids, acid (pH 3.5), chyme with a high caloric density, polypeptides, oligosaccharides, and fatty acids entering the duodenum, or overdistention of the small intestine inhibit gastric emptying. If nutrients rapidly enter or bypass the jejunum, rapidly reaching the ileum and colon, GI transit time is extended via an ileal "brake." This brake is mediated through neurohumoral mechanisms and GI hormones, the most important of which is peptide YY. These mechanisms assure that food is gradually released into the small intestine, is optimally mixed with pancreatic and biliary secretions, and has adequate contact time with digestive enzymes and the small intestinal absorptive mucosa.

The small intestine is designed to have a large surface area, by arrangement of its cells into villi and crypts. The epithelial cells' lumenal surfaces have fingerlike projections termed microvilli that collectively make up the brush border. Most intestinal secretions come from the crypt cells, whereas the major function of the cells of the villi is digestion and absorption of water and nutrients. The villi, as well as their lining cells, are taller in the jejunum, and the height of both decreases caudally towards the ileum. Intestinal cells also become more specialized towards the ileum, where absorption of bile salts and certain vitamins occurs. Digestion of nutrients is accomplished both by brush border and intraluminal enzymes, especially pancreatic exocrine ones. The different types of nutrients and how they are digested by the various enzymes in the GI tract are shown in Figure 56.1.

After gastric chyme arrives at the small intestine, its acidity is rapidly neutralized by duodenal secretions and bicarbonate released from the pancreas. This neutralization is important for establishing a favorable milieu for optimal enzyme action. Furthermore, large amounts of electrolytes and water are secreted into the jejunal lumen to make chyme isoosmolar, dilute toxins, and enable mucosal defense mechanisms such as secretory IgA. Almost simultaneously, motor activity of the intestines changes: propulsive movement decreases and segmental motor contractility increases. The net effect is stirring of intestinal contents with slow forward motion, which in turn increases contact of nutrients with intestinal cells.

During this process, blood flow and lymphatic drainage of the intestine are tightly regulated. Both flows increase as food, electrolytes, and water are absorbed, rapidly carrying these away to facilitate further diffusion. This rapid circulation ensures meeting intestinal oxygen, salt, and water demands, especially during secretion.

The products of digestion get absorbed, utilizing various mechanisms such as passive diffusion and osmosis, facilitated diffusion, and active transport. The sites of absorption of different nutrients and the mechanism(s) involved in this process are given in Table 56.2. A small amount of macronutrients leaves the small intestine undigested. Undigested portions are larger for complex carbohydrates, vary with fat intake, and are minimal for proteins.

In the colon, bacteria act on the remaining nutrients and fiber, forming short chain fatty acids and a variety of vitamins. These and large amounts of electrolyte and water are avidly absorbed by the colon, resulting in a small amount of feces. Together with the enterohepatic circulation of bile, the absorption of 98% of all GI fluid and electrolytes makes the GI system one of the most efficient parts of the body. The various GI secretions are listed in Table 56.3, along with calculation of the net fluid balance.

Nutrition in Selected Diseases of the Upper Gastrointestinal Tract

Gastroesophageal Reflux Disease (GERD)

Definition and Epidemiology

GERD exists in individuals who have symptoms or histopathological changes related to backflow of gastric contents into the esophagus (see Tables 56.4 and 56.5). There is no gold standard test to diagnose GERD; its incidence is estimated from either the disease symptoms (most frequently heartburn) or from findings of esophageal injury such as

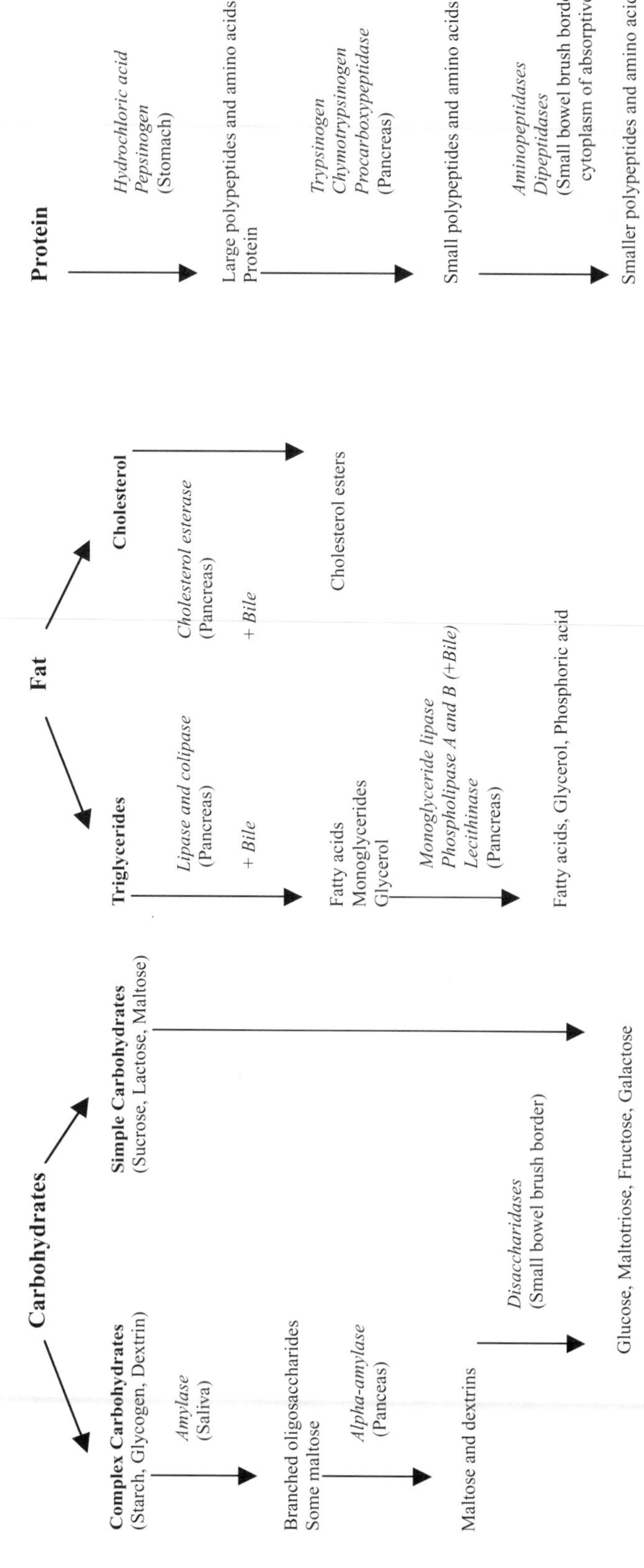

FIGURE 56.1
Digestion of macronutrients.

TABLE 56.2

Overview of Nutrient Absorption

Nutrient	Absorption Site	Mechanism of Absorption
Lipids	Proximal and distal jejunum, colon	Passive diffusion, facilitated diffusion*
Monosaccharides	Proximal and distal jejunum	Na-dependent active transport
Amino acids	Proximal and distal jejunum	Carrier-mediated active transport, simple diffusion
Small peptides	Proximal and distal jejunum	Na-independent tertiary active transport
Bile salts and acids	Distal ileum	Passive absorption, specific active absorption
Vitamin A	Duodenum, mid-jejunum	Passive diffusion**
Vitamin D	Duodenum, mid-jejunum, ileum	Passive diffusion**
Vitamin E	Duodenum, mid-jejunum	Passive diffusion**
Vitamin K_1	Duodenum, mid-jejunum, ileum, colon	Carrier-mediated uptake**
Vitamin K_2	Duodenum, mid-jejunum, ileum, colon	Passive diffusion**
Ascorbic acid	Mid-jejunum, ileum	Na-dependent active transport
Vitamin B_{12}	Ileum	Intrinsic factor binding, specific receptor med
Vitamin B_6	Jejunum	Passive diffusion
Thiamine	Duodenum, mid-jejunum	Na-dependent active transport***
Riboflavin	Duodenum, mid-jejunum	Na-dependent active transport***
Niacin	Duodenum, mid-jejunum	Awaits further study
Pantothenic acid	Mid-jejunum	Na-dependent active transport
Biotin	Duodenum, jejunum, colon	Na-dependent active transport
Folate	Duodenum, mid-jejunum, ileum	Specific carrier mediated Na-dependent active transport pH-sensitive process
Sodium	Colon	Ion-specific channel Carrier mediated coupling sodium and nutrients Antiport carrier
Chloride	Colon	Electrogenic diffusion created by Na absorption Transcellular transport linked to Na via dual antiport Anion exchangers
Potassium	Colon	Active transport by K-ATPase pumps
Calcium	Duodenum, mid-jejunum, ileum colon	Active transcellular process via specific channels, binding to calbindin and Ca-ATPase Passive paracellular diffusive process
Phosphorus	Duodenum, mid-jejunum	Active transport, passive diffusion
Magnesium	Duodenum, mid-jejunum, ileum	Passive paracellular diffusive process Transcellular carrier mediated saturable process
Iron	Duodenum, mid-jejunum	Passive paracellular diffusive process Nonessential fatty acid stimulated pathway Intracellular iron binding proteins
Zinc	Mid-jejunum	Saturable carrier mediated process Nonsaturable diffusion process
Iodine	Stomach	Active transport, passive diffusion†
Selenium	Duodenum	Active transport, passive diffusion†

TABLE 56.2 *(Continued)*

Overview of Nutrient Absorption

Nutrient	Absorption Site	Mechanism of Absorption
Copper	Stomach, duodenum	Unknown[††]
Molybdenum	Stomach, mid-jejunum	Unknown[††]
Chromium	Mid-jejunum	Unknown[††]
Manganese	Mid-jejunum	Unknown[††]
Fluoride	Stomach	Unknown[††]

* linoleic acid uptake occurs by facilitated diffusion
** bile salts are required for solubilization of the vitamins
*** includes hydrolytic acid phosphorilation steps
† some is also transported as amino acid complexes
†† possibly via facilitated diffusion or active diffusion or passive diffusion

TABLE 56.3

Gastrointestinal Secretions

Site	Approximate Volume (in ml)
1. Salivary glands	1500
2. Stomach	2500
3. Liver (as bile)	500
4. Pancreas	1500
5. Small intestine	1000
GI tract secretions(1+2+3+4+5)	+7000
Daily oral intake	+2500
Absorption	–9300
Net excretion in the form of stool	200

TABLE 56.4

Symptoms of GERD

Esophageal	Extraesophageal
Heartburn (pyrosis)	Hypersalivation
Acid regurgitation	Nocturnal choking sensation
Dysphagia	Symptoms related to asthma:
Odynophagia	Wheezing
Chest pain	Shortness of breath
Globus sensation	Chronic cough
Nausea/Vomiting	Other symptoms of asthma
Symptoms of GI bleeding:	Symptoms related to posterior laryngitis:
Coffee ground emesis	Chronic hoarseness/Dysphonia
Melena	Frequent throat clearing
	Chronic cough
	Sore throat
	Other symptoms of laryngitis
	Symptoms related to dental caries

TABLE 56.5

Histopathological Changes Related to GERD

Reflux esophagitis:	Destruction of esophageal epithelium: erosions, ulcers, balloon cells in epithelium
	Neutrophilic or eosinophilic infiltration of the mucosa
	Large basal zone (>15% of the total epithelial thickness)
	Extension of mucosal papillae
	Regenerative changes in the epithelium
Barrett's esophagus:	Metaplastic columnar epithelium replacing normal esophageal mucosa
Adenocarcinoma of the esophagus	
Peptic strictures	
Inflammatory polyps of the esophagus	
Pseudodiverticula	
Esophageal fistulas	

TABLE 56.6

Major Mechanisms Thought to be Involved in the Pathogenesis of GERD

1. Incompetent lower esophageal sphincter (LES)
   a. Increased transient relaxations of LES
   b. Hypotensive LES, i.e., decreased LES tone
   c. High gastroesophageal pressure gradient
2. Irritant effects of the refluxed material (especially gastric acid and pepsin)
3. Abnormal esophageal clearance/ neutralization of the refluxed material
4. Delayed gastric emptying
5. Increased esophageal sensory perception

esophagitis. Heartburn is very common: 36% of the population experience heartburn at least once a month.[2] Esophagitis is estimated to occur in 3 to 5% of the general population.

Mechanisms

Factors and mechanisms important in GERD pathogenesis are listed in Table 56.6. Current dietary management of GERD is based on preventing or counteracting these mechanisms.

Effects on Nutritional Status

Uncomplicated GERD occasionally may lead to malnutrition in infants and children, although this is extremely rare in adults. Scurvy has been reported as a result of long-term avoidance of foods that contain vitamin C.[3] Additionally, megaloblastic anemia has occurred in association with long-term use of a proton pump inhibitor.[4]

In cases of significant malnutrition with GERD symptoms, diseases giving rise to similar symptomatology and complications of GERD need to be sought. Examples include eating disorders and scleroderma, which are easily overlooked. Complications of GERD are given in Table 56.7.

Lifestyle Factors That May Affect GERD

Lifestyle factors that may adversely affect the severity or frequency of GERD-related symptoms are given in Table 56.8.

TABLE 56.7

Major Complications of GERD

1. Acute GI bleeding
2. Chronic GI bleeding with anemia
3. Peptic strictures
4. Esophageal perforation
5. Barrett's esophagus
6. Adenocarcinoma of the esophagus

TABLE 56.8

Lifestyle Factors That May Adversely Affect Severity or Frequency of GERD

1. Obesity
2. Smoking
3. Exercise
4. Alcohol consumption
5. Recumbent body position
6. Tight clothing over abdomen

Obesity

GERD is associated with obesity, and the occurrence of GERD is positively correlated with increasing body mass index (BMI). The frequency and severity of GERD seems to be worse in obese individuals; a significantly higher number of GERD-related hospitalizations occurred among the obese in the NHANES study.[5] Obese individuals also tend to have a higher incidence of hiatal hernia that adversely affects LES function and competence.[6] In some obese individuals, LES pressures are lower than controls,[7] but this is not a consistent mechanism of GERD.[8] It is postulated that the gastroesophageal pressure gradient (difference between the pressures in the esophagus and stomach) may play a more important role. As a result of the mechanical effects of increased intraabdominal fat, this gradient may be high in many obese patients with GERD. This forces gastric contents towards the relatively lower pressure esophageal environment and may promote reflux during any sphincter relaxation. Additionally, obese individuals have a higher incidence of esophageal motility disturbances[8] and cannot clear acid/gastric contents from the esophagus as fast as non-obese controls.[9] Combination of the high gastroesophageal pressure gradient with decreased clearance may explain the frequency and severity of GERD with obesity.

One study among obese GERD patients who are not medication dependent for symptom control showed significant symptomatic improvement with weight loss.[10] The authors have anecdotal evidence that even loss of a few pounds may improve symptoms. However, definitive evidence that relates weight reduction to improvement in GERD is lacking. Some studies show no benefit, although most of these studies have been undertaken in individuals who are medication dependent with severely symptomatic disease. Large amounts of weight loss may be required in the morbidly obese before symptomatic improvement is evident. Nevertheless, most obese individuals should be encouraged to lose weight as first line treatment not only for GERD, but also for other health benefits.

Exercise

Exercise such as rowing, cycling, or jogging may cause GERD in healthy volunteers.[11] Reflux is further potentiated if the exercise is performed after meals.[11-13] There are no definitive studies of GERD patients in this area.

Tight Clothing

Tight clothing worn over the abdomen and stomach has been postulated to elevate the gastroesophageal pressure gradient, especially postprandially.[14] Therefore, loose-fitting clothing has been recommended, although no clinical data support this recommendation.

Food and Diet in GERD

Dietary Habits, Body Position after Meals, and GERD

Gastric distention is a potent stimulus for inappropriate transient LES relaxations. Especially after the first few hours of eating, meal size is the most important determinant of gastric distention. Therefore, GERD patients are advised to eat smaller meals and drink liquids between, as opposed to with, meals.

Recumbent body position and sleep both decrease the clearance of refluxed gastric contents from the esophagus, resulting in prolonged esophageal exposure to acid, pepsin, etc.[15] Such exposure is a major contributor to the severity of esophagitis and stricture formation. Intraesophageal pH recordings in sleeping GERD patients show that elevation of the head of the bed significantly improves nocturnal acid clearance times.[16-18] Combined with H_2 blocker therapy, use of blocks to raise the head of the bed decreases retrosternal chest pain better than medication alone.[19] This effect is especially prominent for smokers and alcohol consumers. Thus, GERD patients are advised not to sleep for at least two hours after eating, to assume an upright body posture while awake, and to elevate the head of their bed using blocks or a foam wedge.

Meal Types and Foods That May Adversely Affect the GERD Patient

A recent study comparing various different meals suggests that more than one component or feature of the meal determines induction of GERD.[20] Use of spices, caloric density, fat content, and alcohol consumption with the meal, alone or in combination, may affect initiation of symptoms.

Various foods that are known to induce GERD, worsen its severity, or adversely affect healing of esophagitis are given in Table 56.9 together with their mechanisms of action. Alcohol's effects on promoting reflux are well documented and may be potentiated in the presence of fatty meals. Different than other alcoholic beverages, wine is very hypertonic, acidic, and has high tyramine content. Tyramine competes with histamine for degradation and may therefore delay the breakdown of the latter, which increases gastric acid secretion. In a survey of 349 individuals with GERD, wine has been reported to cause reflux in 37%.[21]

While there is no evidence that meal consistency (solid vs. liquid) affects reflux, osmolality of food may be important. Hyperosmolar versus isoosmolar foods reproduce esophageal symptoms. Coffee is thought to provoke GERD symptoms because of its high osmolality and irritant effects on the esophageal mucosa[22,23] rather than its effects on LES pressure and transient LES relaxations, which are variable.

The relationship between fat intake and GERD is unclear. Fat may increase GERD by decreasing LES pressure[24] caused by cholecystokinin (CCK) release, and by slowing gastric emptying, which in turn is thought to increase the frequency of transient LES relaxations resulting from a vagovagal reflex originating in stomach mechanoreceptors.[25]

Survey findings show that fatty foods precipitate symptoms of GERD in 38% of normal subjects. Earlier studies show that in healthy volunteers, LES pressures decrease after ingestion of a fatty meal, as opposed to increase with a protein meal. When adjusted for body position, this effect of fat on LES pressure was present only in recumbency in one study,[26] and only in the upright position in another.[27] In a third study, high fat content (50%) compared to low (10%) made no difference.[28] However, nonphysiological fat expo-

TABLE 56.9

Foods That May Worsen GERD

Food	Effect(s)
Methylxanthines (e.g., theophylline in tea)	↓ LES pressure 2° inhibition of phosphodiesterase → increased cAMP and smooth muscle relaxation
Carminatives (e.g., peppermint)	↓ LES pressure ↑ transient LES relaxations
Chocolate	Methylxanthines in it cause ↓ LES pressure High fat content ↓ gastric emptying ↑ transient LES relaxations
Alcohol	↓ or ↑ LES pressure ↓ esophageal peristalsis → ↓ acid clearance Caustic effect on mucosa Adverse effects on protective mucus ↑ gastric acid secretion ↑ number of reflux episodes ↑ nocturnal acid reflux
Citrus juice	Directly irritant to the esophageal mucosa
Tomatoes	Directly irritant to the esophageal mucosa ↑ transient LES relaxations possibly secondary to salicylate content
Capsaicin (found in peppers)	Directly irritant to the esophageal mucosa ↑ gastric acid and pepsin secretion
Spearmint	Directly irritant to the esophageal mucosa
Coffee	Directly irritant to the esophageal mucosa ↑ gastric acid secretion ↓ or ↑ LES pressure (effects worse with concomitant food intake) (effects vary with brand and treatment prior to consumption)
Onions	↑ transient LES relaxations ↑ acid-pepsin injury possibly through inhibition of arachidonic acid metabolism (raw ones create worse symptoms compared to cooked)
Milk	↑ gastric acid secretion

sures (100% fat infused into the duodenum) increased the rate of reflux episodes and the incidence of reflux during transient LES relaxations.[29] The discrepancy in results may be related to variations in composition of the diets used, the small number of patients involved, and the differences in baseline characteristics of the study subjects.

Results are more consistent for GERD patients. In terms of esophageal acid exposure when identical protein content, volume, and kcalories are provided to patients, fat does not seem to matter.[27] Recent work confirms that a high fat meal (52%), compared to 24% fat meal in an isovolumic and isoosmolar balanced one, affects neither the acidity of the esophagus nor resting LES pressures and the rate of transient LES relaxations three hours postprandially in healthy subjects and GERD patients.[30] However, these studies involve small numbers of subjects; findings may not apply to various subgroups of patients, and there may not be enough power to detect significant differences. Nevertheless, based on these results, a low fat diet cannot be recommended for all patients with GERD. For the individual symptomatic patient who cannot tolerate fat, avoidance of fatty meals is reasonable.

The type of fat in a meal may also affect GERD. In preterm infants, medium-chain triglycerides have been shown to significantly increase gastric emptying compared to long-chain triglycerides. One study investigating reflux rates two hours postprandially has found no difference with or without medium-chain triglycerides in pediatric formulas.[31] In healthy adults, new non-digestible fats (e.g., olestra) do not alter esophageal acid exposure or delay gastric emptying.[32]

TABLE 56.10

Summary of Tips for the GERD Patient

1. If overweight, lose weight
2. Try avoiding foods that may worsen GERD (given in Table 56.9)
3. Eat small quantities of food at a time
4. Eat in an upright position
5. Avoid drinking large quantities of liquids with meals
6. Do not recline for at least 2 hours after meals
7. Do not exercise for several hours after meals
8. If night time symptoms are present, try elevating the head of the bed with a wedge
9. If taking proton pump inhibitors, take medication 30 minutes before a meal

Data on other macronutrients and components of diet and GERD are sparse. High protein meals increased LES pressure in volunteers in one study,[24] but a commercially available amino acid solution infused intravenously or given intragastrically did not change reflux episodes or transient LES relaxations.[33] Oral L-Arginine did not promote reflux, despite increasing nitric oxide and lowering LES pressures.[34] High fiber did not cause reflux in 20 patients with suspected GERD.[35]

Gas-containing foods such as carbonated beverages are commonly believed to initiate reflux episodes through belching. Although no definitive data exists, in one study among GERD patients, postprandial gas reflux made up 47% of the reflux episodes versus liquid reflux, which happened 78% of the time. Only 24% of liquid retroflow into the esophagus was preceded by gas reflux, which suggests that most episodes occur without belching.[36] Another reflux-promoting mechanism may be stimulation of gastric acid secretion, as seen with cola beverages.

Do We Really Need a Certain Diet for GERD? Is There Enough Scientific Evidence for a Particular Diet?

There is no scientific evidence for a specific diet for all or most GERD patients. While a combination of lifestyle modifications such as weight loss, bland diet, elevation of the head of the bed, and antacids has been used in the past, the majority of patients with chronic symptoms and complications (about 81% in one study) do not respond, and ultimately require use of medications like H_2 blockers and proton pump inhibitors (PPIs), or surgical therapy. However, this may not apply to numerous individuals with less severe GERD, who may not even present to physicians. Given the high disease prevalence, the potential side effects of medications, and the expense of chronic PPI therapy, studies pertaining to the utility of diet therapies alone or in combination with other lifestyle modifications in patients with less severe disease are needed urgently. In the meantime, the authors assert that all patients should be educated about various aspects of diet and its effects on GERD. Patients should be given a chance to experience and experiment with the nutritional tips for GERD patients given in Table 56.10. Treatment with a diet consisting of avoidance of reflux-promoting foods (as in Table 56.9) should be reserved for the individual patient responding with the most symptomatic relief. The physician should ascertain that such treatment does not impair the patient's quality of life, as effective alternative management exists.

GERD Therapy and Diet

In general, patients with GERD tolerate all foods while on treatment with medications. Patients who do not symptomatically or histologically improve with standard therapy may have allergic eosinophilic esophagitis. Most such patients are children,[37] for whom therapy is withdrawal of the offending protein and feeding an elemental diet.

Surgical treatment of GERD may be complicated with dumping syndrome, dysphagia, and gas-bloat syndrome. Dietary treatment of dumping syndrome is given below. Dietary treatment of dysphagia and gas-bloat syndrome after fundoplication is based on common sense and anecdotal evidence. For dysphagia, authors suggest that patients eat soft foods, eat slowly, and chew food well. For gas-bloat syndrome, the suggestions are the following: 1. to decrease aerophagia: avoid talking and laughing during meals, avoid chewing gum, hard candy, mints, etc., chew foods well, do not rush through meals or eat on the run; 2. to decrease intestinal gas production: avoid gas-forming foods such as legumes, beans, etc., or foods that contain significant amounts of nondigestible materials like sorbitol, olestra, etc.

Nutritional tips for patients with GERD are summarized in Table 56.10.

The Patient on Enteral Nutrition and GERD

Theoretically, GERD may get worse with nasogastric or nasoenteric feedings as well as with gastrostomy placement. However, these interventions usually involve sick patients who may already have GI motility problems as a result of underlying illnesses. Therefore, worsening of GERD in such settings may not be reflective of these interventions.

Aspiration is the number one complication of enteral feeding via tube placement. Nasoenteric tubes can promote transient LES relaxations[38] and therefore may put patients at a higher risk of aspiration compared to gastrostomy tubes. Differences between gastrostomy and jejunostomy tubes have been evaluated in small or poorly designed studies without clear documentation of tube position. The American Gastroenterological Association recommends reservation of jejunostomy to patients with a history of GERD or recurrent aspiration secondary to gastrostomy tubes.[39]

Peptic Ulcer Disease (PUD)

Definition and Epidemiology

Peptic ulcer disease is characterized by defects in the mucosa that extend through the muscularis mucosa (i.e., ulcers) in the presence of acid-peptic injury. PUD is common, with a lifetime prevalence of 5 to 10%. The etiologies for the disease are given in Table 56.11.

Mechanisms

Proposed mechanisms of peptic ulcer pathogenesis are given in Table 56.12. Of these, the most important is the presence of gastric acid. Many studies have shown that when acid is eliminated, ulcers do not form. Therefore, the current treatment of PUD is directed at

TABLE 56.11

Causes of PUD

Common	Uncommon
Helicobacter pylori	Diseases that cause hyperacidity:
Nonsteroidal anti-inflammatory drugs	Zollinger Ellison syndrome (gastrinoma)
Stress-related mucosal damage	Mastocytosis/Basophilic leukemia
	Antral G cell hyperplasia or hyperfunction
	Infections of the gastric mucosa:
	Cytomegalovirus
	Herpes simplex
	Vascular diseases:
	Chronic radiation injury
	Crack cocaine-related injury
	Chemotherapy related injury

TABLE 56.12

Major Mechanisms of Tissue Damage and Repair Involved in the Pathogenesis of PUD

1. Epithelial cell injury resulting from:
   a. Exogenous irritants like NSAIDs and alcohol
   b. Endogenous irritants like acid, pepsin, bile acids, and lysolecithin
   c. Breakdown of epithelial defense mechanisms:
      i. Weak mucus and bicarbonate layer
      ii. Low resistance of the apical cell membrane to acid back diffusion
      iii. Inadequate acid clearance intracellularly because of derangements of the Na^+/H^+ antiporter
      iv. Inadequate acid clearance extracellularly because of altered mucosal blood flow
2. Inadequate repair of epithelial injury:
   a. Inadequate epithelial cell restitution and growth
   b. Inadequate wound healing

decreasing gastric acidity with medications. If *H. pylori* is present, treatment with antibiotics is undertaken to preven recurrence.

Effects on Nutritional Status

PUD may affect nutritional status, especially if complications related to PUD or to the cause of PUD are present. These are given in Table 56.13. *Helicobacter pylori* or medication-induced atrophic gastritis may lead to vitamin B_{12} deficiency. Repeated blood loss from bleeding ulcers may cause iron deficiency anemia. Chronic long-standing gastric outlet obstruction as a result of scarring of the pyloric channel or development of severe dumping syndrome following surgical treatment of ulcers can cause protein and kcalorie malnutrition. These complications are rare in the U.S.

Diet in PUD

The role of diet in PUD occurrence and treatment has changed tremendously as our knowledge about the pathogenesis of PUD increased. In the early 1900s, with the rationale that food buffers stomach acid, Lenhartz[39a] proposed that frequent small meals might be of benefit in PUD treatment. Physicians of the day followed with restrictive dietary treatment programs that advocated small quantities of bland food at frequent intervals, in the hopes that such a feeding regimen would also stimulate less acid secretion and thereby hasten healing. One PUD treatment consisting of milk, cream, and eggs with subsequent addition of soft and "nonirritating" foods, the Sippy diet, was formulated by Sippy and Hurst in 1910.[40] This diet and its modifications prevailed in PUD treatment over eight decades. A 1977 survey by Welsh et al. of 326 hospitals in the U.S. demonstrated that 77% used a bland diet and 55% routinely or usually gave milk to PUD patients.[41] Marked variations were seen in the composition of these supposedly similar diets.

The benefits of restrictive diets, including the Sippy and its modifications, are refuted in numerous studies.[42-45] First, acidity of the stomach following bland diets and freely

TABLE 56.13

Major Complications Related to PUD

1. Atrophic gastritis
2. Gastric carcinoma related to *H. pylori*
3. Obstruction, esp. at gastric outlet
4. Hemorrhage (acute or chronic)
5. Perforation
6. Penetration of ulcers

chosen diets do not differ.[46] More importantly, controlled studies of radiological ulcer healing or resolution of clinical symptoms show no improvement on these diets.[47,48] The same is true for ulcer recurrence, which is not different with or without such diets when patients are followed up to a year or more.[47,49] Instead, these diets in the long-term may be harmful; they can result in nutritional deficiencies such as scurvy.[50] Given this evidence, there is no reason to support the use of a restricted or bland diet for PUD. Further evidence for and against various dietary interventions are given below.

Small Frequent Feedings

Food-related gastric acid stimulation is prolonged in PUD patients, and therefore it is not logical to expect adequate acid buffering with any type of meal.[51,52] Even though peak acid secretion may be higher as a result of gastric distention with larger meals, studies show that mean acid concentration does not differ when patients are fed two-hourly portions as opposed to four-hourly ones.[53]

Increased Use of Milk

Milk had been advocated as part of the early diets for PUD (including the Sippy and its modifications) because of its acid-buffering capacity. However, in a study of a large group of PUD patients, intragastric milk drip did not improve radiological healing of PUD, although pain relief was quicker.[54] In another study of 65 patients taking equal doses of cimetidine, endoscopic ulcer healing or pain relief at four weeks was worse in the group given milk with seasonal fruits as opposed to the group given a regular diet.[55]

Milk increases gastric acid secretion (about 30% in duodenal ulcer patients)[56] and its capability to neutralize acid is short-lived.[57] Whether milk is whole, low-fat, or non-fat does not make a difference.[57] Amino acids released as a result of hydrolysis of milk proteins stimulate gastrin secretion.[56] The relatively high calcium in milk acts as a second messenger for gastrin and acetylcholine stimulated acid release, and ulcer patients are more sensitive to such effects of calcium.[58]

Milk can also be harmful to ulcer patients who consume large amounts of absorbable antacids concomitantly. These PUD patients may develop acute or chronic milk-alkali syndrome leading to alkalosis, renal insufficiency/calculi and hypercalcemia.[59]

Changing the Macronutrient Composition of Diet

Protein stimulates gastric acid more than carbohydrates and fat;[60] however, there is also evidence that high protein may result in lower gastric and duodenal acidity following meals.[61] Whether this effect is due to satiety induced by the high protein is unknown. Thus, no recommendations concerning the protein content of the meal for PUD can be made. Although fat in the small intestine inhibits gastric acid secretion,[62] there is no satisfactory evidence that high-fat diets are beneficial to ulcer patients, either. In fact, many of the bland diets, including the Sippy diet, are high in fat and have been shown to be harmful by increasing the risk of cardiovascular disease among PUD patients.

Alcohol Consumption

Alcohol ingestion can cause acute erosive gastritis with ulcerations and bleeding. Alcohol concentrations of at least 8% were required to break the gastric mucosal barrier in one study,[63] while higher levels of 40% or more were needed in another study.[64] Alcohol as low as 5% stimulates gastric acid secretion both through direct stimulation of parietal cells and through release of antral gastrin, although the effects may vary depending on the type of beverage consumed.[65] Beer, for example, can increase acid independent of its ethanol content. Intake of alcohol with salicylates may contribute to its irritant effects by causing back-diffusion of acid and stimulating pepsin secretion. Furthermore, acute alcohol ingestion can weaken duodenal defenses against ulcer formation by inhibiting basal and secretin-stimulated pancreatic fluid and bicarbonate secretion,[66-68] which is not entirely due to alcohol-induced contraction of the sphincter of Oddi.[69]

Epidemiological studies, however, show no difference in alcohol consumption between high and low PUD areas throughout different parts of the world, and alcohol intake is not independently predictive of PUD prevalence in surveys (although most studies were conducted before testing for *H. pylori* was implemented.) Indeed, in one prospective study, alcohol consumption was lower among PUD patients compared to controls. Alcohol does not adversely affect ulcer healing either. In one study, moderate alcohol consumption (20g/day or less) promoted healing of duodenal ulcers. An author of this study, Sonnenberg, also reported that alcohol in small amounts is protective against NSAID injury, and hypothesized that alcohol may be similar to mild irritants in that low doses may heighten mucosal defenses through stimulation of prostaglandin production.[70]

Caffeine/Coffee/Tea/Carbonated Drinks

Caffeine stimulates both acid and pepsin release, and patients with duodenal ulcer have a greater and longer response. The effects of coffee and tea, however, exceed what their caffeine content induces.[71] Serum gastrin and gastric acidity (especially in ulcer patients) is higher than caffeine, and decaffeination diminishes this acid-secretory potency only minimally.[71] In one study, the addition of milk and sugar to tea lessened this effect.[72] Whether these translate into clinical significance is unknown. Habitual coffee consumption in college students was linked to development of PUD in later life. Conversely, a very large survey of 37,000 subjects failed to show an association between coffee and PUD. Carbonated beverages similarly stimulate acid production, but this may also be unrelated to caffeine.[71]

Salt Intake

A large oral load of salt can be an irritant to the gastric mucosa, leading to gastritis.[73] In epidemiological studies, PUD mortality correlates linearly with increasing salt consumption.[74] Case control studies also show that gastric ulcer patients have a higher level of salt intake compared to healthy controls.[75]

Avoidance of Certain Spices

Application of spices on upper GI mucosa revealed that cinnamon, nutmeg, allspice, thyme, black pepper, cloves, and paprika cause no endoscopic damage, whereas hot pepper, chili powder, and mustard lead to edema, erythema, and mucosal breakdown.[76] The latter spices also lead to epigastric discomfort in patients.[76] Furthermore, peppers induce supramaximal acid output in duodenal ulcer patients, and have been associated with gastritis.[77] In one study using gastric lavage, both red and black pepper caused higher levels of gastric cell exfoliation, acid and pepsin secretion, and microbleeding, although this was not confirmed endoscopically.[78] In several others, gastric aspirates after use of capsaicin (found in red peppers and paprika) and black peppers showed increased DNA fragment levels, indicating mucosal damage.[72] In other studies, peppers increased production of mucus with only minimal acid secretory effects. Duodenal ulcer patients on acid-suppressive therapy eating 3 g of red chili powder had clinical and endoscopic healing rates similar to patients not eating the spice.[42] Authors of this study suggested that direct installation of spices via tubes in a fasting state in previous studies, as opposed to more physiological consumption of the spice, might explain the discrepancy between prior reports of gastric damage and their findings. Concomitant antacid intake may have altered the effects of the spice in this study. It is also unknown whether chronic consumption of potentially irritant spices leads to an adaptation response by stimulating gastric defenses, explaining some of the earlier work showing high levels of mucous production.

Dietary Fiber

Fiber has been postulated to be beneficial for PUD because of its buffering effects, shortening of GI transit leading to decreased acid secretion, and binding of irritant bile acids.[79] The role of dietary fiber in treatment or prevention of PUD is controversial. Reduction in clinical and endoscopic ulcer recurrence with high-fiber diets has been shown,[80,81] although epidemiological studies have found elevated incidence of PUD in areas of the world with high fiber consumption. Low fiber consumption may predispose to PUD, rather than high fiber having protective effects.[82]

Supplementation of fiber in the form of pectin has not affected ulcer recurrence.[83] Guar gum may reduce gastric acid; it has not been shown to normalize it.[84] Therefore, components of the high fiber diet other than fiber itself may be protective.

Fiber given as wheat bran can bind bile acids and may reduce their elevated concentration in gastric ulcer patients;[85] it may be beneficial in biliary reflux-associated ulcerations.

Essential Fatty Acids

Linoleic acid, an essential fatty acid (EFA) and a major substrate for synthesis of prostaglandins that are protective for upper GI tract mucosa, has been shown to be deficient in the diets of duodenal ulcer patients.[86] Additionally, Hollander and Tarnawksi have shown that the declining incidence of PUD parallels a 200% increase in dietary availability of EFAs.[87] They have hypothesized that this association reflects a cause-and-effect relationship and that higher intakes of EFA induce mucosal prostaglandin E synthesis, thereby conferring protection against mucosal irritants and NSAIDs. Although the epidemiological evidence for this hypothesis is strong, direct evidence is lacking.

Many dietary factors may be significant in the pathogenesis and treatment of ulcer disease, but most studies have been conducted before *H. pylori* was implicated in ulcer formation. Therefore, some of the evidence, especially the epidemiological, for or against various interventions may not be applicable to current PUD patients. The available information is summarized in Table 56.14. A summary of nutritional tips for patients with PUD is given in Table 56.15. With the potent antisecretory medications available today, diet

TABLE 56.14

Summary of Evidence on Diet and PUD

Definitely Not Beneficial and Potentially Harmful to PUD Patients
Bland and restrictive diets including the Sippy diet and its modifications
Frequent milk intake
Probably Harmful to PUD Patients
Alcohol
Caffeine
Coffee/Tea
Carbonated beverages
Certain spices
High salt load
Probably Beneficial to PUD Patients
Essential fatty acids
Fiber intake

TABLE 56.15

Summary of Nutritional Tips for PUD Patients

1. Avoid restrictive diets
2. Avoid frequent milk intake
3. Avoid high salt intake
4. Avoid concentrated alcoholic beverages
5. Avoid directly irritant foods and spices such as peppers, chili powder, etc.
6. Take proton pump inhibitors, 30 minutes before a meal

therapy has a limited role in treatment of PUD. Patients with PUD should be allowed to eat as they desire, with few exceptions.

Food and PUD Medications

Proton pump inhibitors frequently used in the treatment of acid-peptic diseases including PUD are expensive medications that irreversibly bind and block the hydrogen pump of the parietal cell. These drugs are rapidly cleared from the bloodstream within a few hours following intake. Therefore, for utmost efficacy, they should be timed so that effective concentrations are in the circulation when acid secretion is maximally stimulated. This usually requires these drugs to be taken about 30 minutes prior to a meal.

Gastroparesis

Abnormally slow emptying of the stomach from causes other than mechanical obstruction is called gastroparesis. The many causes are given in Table 56.16, with diabetes the most common.

The various factors and medications that affect the rate of gastric emptying are given in Table 56.17. The mainstay of the dietary treatment of gastroparesis involves avoidance of the factors that delay emptying (as shown in Table 56.17) while adopting a diet that exits the stomach easily. No one diet has been shown effective.

In general, dietary fiber usually needs to be decreased, as it may result in bezoar formation. Koch promotes six smaller meals in order to decrease symptom severity, and he advocates a three-step nausea and vomiting diet.[88] These recommendations need to be tested to prove their usefulness.

Dietary treatment frequently needs to be combined with prokinetic medications, usually administered before meals. Oral medications should preferably be in liquid formulations that are absorbed faster than capsules and tablets, which may lie in the stomach for hours.

As the disease progresses, dietary and medical treatment may not suffice, and refractory patients may require drainage gastrostomy with jejunal enteral feeding. Although no controlled studies exist, in one retrospective study, enteral feeding via a jejunostomy improved overall health status in diabetic patients.[89] Nutritional tips for the gastroparetic patient are summarized in Table 56.18.

Dumping Syndrome

Dumping syndrome is the collection of symptoms triggered by rapid entry of large boluses of food into the small bowel. The syndrome most often occurs in patients who have had a vagotomy and/or gastrectomy, frequently done in the past for PUD. The two main types of the syndrome, the symptoms, and possible mechanisms are given in Table 56.19.

Dietary treatment of early dumping aims to slow emptying of the stomach and decrease the volume and osmolality of food boluses delivered to the small bowel. For this purpose,

TABLE 56.16

Causes of Gastroparesis

Metabolic and Endocrine:
Diabetes, thyroid disease, uremia, porphyrias, pregnancy, electrolyte imbalance, Addison's disease

Iatrogenic:
Surgical damage to vagal trunk, drugs, radiation damage to stomach

Neurological:
Intracranial/spinal cord lesions, Guillain-Barré syndrome, acute dysautonomic syndrome, Shy-Drager syndrome, Parkinson's disease, seizure disorder, multiple sclerosis, labyrinthitis

Psychogenic:
Anorexia, bulimia, psychological stress

Inflammatory:
Viral gastritis, Chagas disease, Botulinum toxin, celiac sprue

Rheumatologic:
Scleroderma, SLE, PM/DM, amyloidosis
muscular disorders

Paraneoplastic:
Small cell lung cancer, breast cancer

Idiopathic

TABLE 56.17

Factors that Affect the Rate of Gastric Emptying

Factor	Fast Emptying	←→	Slow Emptying
Luminal:			
Consistency of food	Liquid		Solid
Macronutrient composition	Fat	Protein	Carbohydrate
Fiber content of food	Low		High
Osmolality in stomach or duodenum	Low		High (>800 mOsm/L)
Change in temperature of stomach	Hot/Cold		Body temperature
Gastric distention	High		Low
Volume in duodenum	Low		High
pH in duodenum	High		Low
Drugs:	Cholinergic Erythromycin Metoclopropamide Cisapride Domperidone		Anticholinergic
Gastrointestinal hormones:	Gastrin Motilin		Cholecystokinin Glucagon Secretin

patients are advised to avoid consuming liquid and solids simultaneously, stay away from highly osmolar foods, and eat small meals. Dietary treatment of late dumping syndrome aims to decrease rapid entry of large amounts of carbohydrates, especially concentrated simple sugars, into the small intestine. Patients are advised to keep away from concentrated sweets such as candy, honey, syrup, etc. These latter recommendations have not been rigorously tested but are consistent with the pathophysiology of dumping.

TABLE 56.18

Summary of Tips for the Gastroparesis Patient

1. Eat small quantities at a time
2. Eat in upright position
3. Do not recline until several hours after meals
4. Chew every bite of food well
5. Consume a low fat diet
6. Avoid fiber/roughage
7. Eat well-cooked foods
8. Turn foods into liquid/pureed form if unable to tolerate solids
9. Take medications in liquid formulation, 30 minutes before meals

TABLE 56.19

Types of Dumping Syndrome

	Timing Following a Meal	Cause	Mediators	Symptoms*
Early	15-30 min	Rapid fluid shift from intravascular space to small intestinal lumen	Release of vasoactive intestinal hormones (e.g., VIP, neurotensin, motilin, etc.)	Flushing Dizziness Nausea Palpitations Diaphoresis Syncope
Late	2-4 h	Rapid rise of blood glucose	Rapid rise in insulin in response to glucose	

* Symptoms are similar for both early and late dumping.

TABLE 56.20

Summary of Nutritional Tips in Dumping Syndrome

1. Eat small and drink quantities at a time
2. Spread meals throughout the day
3. Avoid drinking liquids with meals, instead drink liquids in between meals
4. Avoid hypertonic foods and concentrated sweets (such as soft drinks, juices, pies, cakes, cookies, candy, etc.)
5. Avoids foods rich in simple carbohydrates, replace with complex carbohydrates
6. Consume high-protein, moderate fat foods
7. Increase fiber intake if tolerated
8. Lie down after meals if possible

Additionally, in order to delay gastric emptying, and especially bind the liquid component of the meal, fiber such as guar gum and pectin has been added to meals. Results with pectin are variable: in small studies it delays gastric emptying in the majority of patients but may also increase it; therefore, doses may need to be individualized to achieve a particular viscosity.[90,91] In one study, muffins that contain 5 g of pectin failed to alter symptoms or gastric emptying.[92] In open-label studies, addition of 5 g of guar gum to meals for four weeks symptomatically benefited 8/16 patients with proximal selective vagotomy-induced dumping, although the effect was minimal in 3 patients.[93] Recent work also suggests that increasing viscosity of the liquid phase of a meal by pectin or guar gum may stimulate more propulsive forces in the stomach, causing a detrimental effect.[94] Most patients with severe dumping do not respond to the commonly used dietary instructions. In these refractory patients, octreotide is useful.[95]

Nutritional tips for patients with dumping syndrome are summarized in Table 56.20.

References

1. Jean A. *Brain Behav Evol* 25:109; 1984.
2. Nebel OT, Fornes MF, Castell, DO. *Am J Dig Dis* 21:953; 1976.
3. Hiebert CA. *Ann Thorac Surg* 24:108; 1977.
4. Bellou A, Aimone-Gastin I, De Korwin JD, et al. *J Intern Med* 240(3):161; 1996.
5. Ruhl CE, Everhart JE. *Ann Epidemiol* 9:424; 1999.
6. Wilson LJ, Ma W, Hirschowitz BI. *Am J Gastroenterol* 94:2840; 1999.
7. O'Brien TF, Jr. *J Clin Gastroenterol* 2:145; 1980.
8. Jaffin BW, Knoepflmacher P, Greenstein R. *Obes Surg* 9:390; 1999.
9. Mercer CD, Rue C, Hanelin L, Hill LD. *Am J Surg* 149:177; 1985.
10. Murray FE, Ennis J, Lennon JR, Crowe JP. *Ir J Med Sci* 160:2; 1991.
11. Yazaki E, Shawdon A, Beasley I, Evans DF. *Aust J Sci Med Sport* 28:93; 1996.
12. Peters HP, Wiersma JW, Koerselman J, et al. *Int J Sports Med* 21:65; 2000.
13. Clark CS, Kraus BB, Sinclair J, Castell DO. *JAMA* 261:3599; 1989.
14. Dent J. *Baillieres Clin Gastroenterol* 1:727; 1987.
15. Demeester TR, Johnson LF, Joseph GJ, et al. *Ann Surg* 184:459; 1976.
16. Johnson LF, DeMeester TR. *Dig Dis Sci* 26:673; 1981.
17. Hamilton JW, Boisen RJ, Yamamoto DT, et al. *Dig Dis Sci* 33:518; 1988.
18. Stanciu C, Bennett JR. *Digestion* 15:104; 1977.
19. Harvey RF, Gordon PC, Hadley N, et al. *Lancet* 2:1200; 1987.
20. Rodriguez S, Miner P, Robinson M, et al. *Dig Dis Sci* 43:485; 1998.
21. Feldman M, Barnett C. *Gastroenterology* 108:125; 1995.
22. Lloyd DA, Borda IT. *Gastroenterology* 80:740; 1981.
23. Price SF, Smithson KW, Castell DO. *Gastroenterology* 75:240; 1978.
24. Nebel OT, Castell DO. *Gastroenterology* 63:778; 1972.
25. Franzi SJ, Martin CJ, Cox MR, Dent J. *Am J Physiol* 259:G380; 1990.
26. Iwakiri K, Kobayashi M, Kotoyori M, et al. *Dig Dis Sci* 41:926; 1996.
27. Becker DJ, Sinclair J, Castell DO, Wu WC. *Am J Gastroenterol* 84:782; 1989.
28. Pehl C, Waizenhoefer A, Wendl B, et al. *Am J Gastroenterol* 94:1192; 1999.
29. Holloway RH, Lyrenas E, Ireland A, Dent J. *Gut* 40:449; 1997.
30. Penagini R, Mangano M, Bianchi PA. *Gut* 42:330; 1998.
31. Sutphen JL, Dillard VL. *J Pediatr Gastroenterol Nutr* 14:38; 1992.
32. Just R, Katz L, Verhille M, et al. *Am J Gastroenterol* 88:1734.
33. Gielkens HA, Lamers CB, Masclee AA. *Dig Dis Sci* 43:840; 1998.
34. Luiking YC, Weusten BL, Portincasa P, et al. *Am J Physiol* 274:G984; 1998.
35. Floren CH, Johnsson F. *J Intern Med* 225:287; 1989.
36. Sifrim D, Silny J, Holloway RH, Janssens JJ. *Gut* 44:47; 1999.
37. Kelly KJ, Lazenby AJ, Rowe PC, et al. *Gastroenterology* 109:1503; 1995.
38. Mittal RK, Stewart WR, Schirmer B. *Gastroenterology* 103:1236; 1992.
39. Kirby DF, Delegge MH, Fleming CR. *Gastroenterology* 108:1282; 1995.

39a. Lawrence JS. *Lancet* 1:482-485, 1952.

40. Sippy BW. Landmark article May 15, 1915. *JAMA* 250:2192; 1983.
41. Welsh JD. *Gastroenterology* 72:740; 1977.
42. Marotta RB, Floch MH. *Med Clin North Am* 75:967.
43. Berstad A. *Scand J Gastroenterol Suppl* 129:228; 1987.
44. Kirsner JB, Palmer WL. *Am J Dig Dis* 1940:85; 1940.
45. Bingle JP, Lennard-Jones JE. *Gut* 1:337; 1960.
46. Lennard-Jones JE, Babouris N. *Gut* 6:113; 1965.
47. Doll R, Friedlander P, Pygott F. *Lancet* 1:5; 1956.
48. Truelove SC. *Br Med J* 2:559; 1960.
49. Buchman E, Kaung DT, Dolan K, Knapp RN. *Gastroenterology* 56:1016; 1969.
50. Zucker GM, Clayman CB. *JAMA* 250:2198; 1983.

51. Fordtran JS, Walsh JH. *J Clin Invest* 52:645; 1973.
52. Malagelada JR, Longstreth GF, Deering TB, et al. *Gastroenterology* 73:989; 1977.
53. Barbouris N, Fletcher J, Lennard-Jones JE. *Gut* 6:118; 1965.
54. Doll R, Price AV, Pygott F. *Lancet* 1:70; 1970.
55. Kumar N, Kumar A, Broor SL, et al. *Br Med J (Clin Res Ed)* 293:666; 1986.
56. Mathewson M, Farnham C. *Crit Care Nurse* 4:75; 1984.
57. Ippoliti AF, Maxwell V, Isenberg JI. *Ann Intern Med* 84:286; 1976.
58. Feldman M. In: *Gastrointestinal and Liver Disease: Pathophysiology, Diagnosis and Management.* Sleisenger MH, Fordtran JS, Eds, 6th ed. Philadelphia, W.B. Saunders, 1998, p 587.
59. Pursan S, Somer T. *Acta Med Scand* 173:435; 1963.
60. Rune SJ. *Scand J Gastroenterol* 8:605; 1973.
61. Lennard-Jones JE, Fletcher J, Shaw DG. *Gut* 9:177; 1968.
62. Christiansen J, Rehfeld JF, Stadil F. *Scand J Gastroenterol* 11:673; 1976.
63. Davenport HW. *Proc Soc Exp Biol Med* 126:657; 1967.
64. Hollander D. *Nutr MD* 14:1; 1988.
65. Lenz HJ, Ferrari-Taylor J, Isenberg JI. *Gastroenterology* 85:1082; 1983.
66. Davis AE, Pirola RC. *Med J Aust* 2:757; 1966.
67. Marin GA, Ward NL, Fischer R. *Am J Dig Dis* 18:825; 1973.
68. Mott C, Sarles H, Tiscornia O, Gullo L. *Am J Dig Dis* 17:902; 1972.
69. Pirola RC, Davis AE. *Gut* 9:557; 1968.
70. Sonnenberg A. *Scand J Gastroenterol Suppl* 155:119; 1988.
71. Cohen S, Booth GH, Jr. *N Engl J Med* 293:897; 1975.
72. Tovey FI, Jayaraj AP, Lewin MR, Clark CG. *Dig Dis* 7:309; 1989.
73. MacDonald WC, Anderson FH, Hashimoto S. *Can Med Assoc J* 96:1521; 1967.
74. Sonnenberg A. *Gut* 27:1138 and 1523; 1986.
75. Stemmermann G, Haenszel W, Locke F. *J Natl Cancer Inst* 58:13; 1977.
76. Schneider MA, De Luca V, Gray SJ. *Am J Gastroenterol* 2:722; 1956.
77. Solanke TF. *J Surg Res* 15:385; 1973.
78. Myers BM, Smith JL, Graham DY. *Am J Gastroenterol* 82:211; 1987.
79. Rydning A, Weberg R, Lange O, Berstad A. *Gastroenterology* 91:56; 1986.
80. Malhotra SL. *Postgrad Med J* 54:6; 1978.
81. Rydning A, Berstad A. *Scand J Gastroenterol Suppl* 110:29; 1985.
82. Baron JH. *Lancet* 2:980; 1982.
83. Kang JY, Tay HH, Guan R, et al. *Scand J Gastroenterol* 23:95; 1988.
84. Harju E. *Am Surg* 50:668; 1984.
85. Rydning A, Berstad A. *Scand J Gastroenterol* 20:801; 1985.
86. Grant HW, Palmer KR, Riermesma RR, Oliver MF. *Gut* 31:997; 1990.
87. Hollander D, Tarnawski A. *Gut* 27:239; 1986.
88. Koch KL. *Dig Dis Sci* 44:1061; 1999.
89. Fontana RJ, Barnett JL. *Am J Gastroenterol* 91:2174; 1996.
90. Leeds AR, Ralphs DN, Ebied F, et al. *Lancet* 1:1075; 1981.
91. Lawaetz O, Blackburn AM, Bloom SR, et al. *Scand J Gastroenterol* 18:327; 1983.
92. Andersen JR, Holtug K, Uhrenholt A. *Acta Chir Scand* 155:39; 1989.
93. Harju E, Makela J. *Am J Gastroenterol* 79:861; 1984.
94. Prather CM, Thomforde GM, Camilleri M. *Gastroenterology* 103:1377; 1992.
95. Scarpignato C. *Digestion* 57:114-8; 1996.

57

Nutrition and Hollow Organs of the Lower Gastrointestinal Tract

Ece A. Mutlu, Gökhan M. Mutlu, and Sohrab Mobarhan

Basic principles of nutrition in diseases of the small and large intestines are covered in this section. Often the disease processes are complex and result in challenges frequently requiring that nutritional treatment be individualized. Thus, consultation with a nutrition specialist is usually necessary and highly recommended.

Celiac Sprue (CS)

Definition and Epidemiology

Celiac sprue (celiac disease, gluten-sensitive enteropathy) is an allergic disease of the small intestine characterized by malabsorption of nutrients, a specific histological appearance on biopsy (Table 57.1), and prompt improvement after withdrawal of gluten (a water-insoluble protein moiety in certain cereal grains) from the diet. The disease is prevalent in almost every population, with higher numbers among people of northern European descent. In Europe, the prevalence is estimated to be 0.05 to 0.2%; however, the disease is underdiagnosed. When U.S. blood donors were screened using antiendomysial antibodies (AEA), which are serological markers with high specificity for CS, 1 in 250 were positive. The classic symptoms of the disease are diarrhea, flatulence, weight loss, and fatigue, although many patients without extensive small bowel damage may not have one or more of these symptoms. In fact, celiac disease patients may also be asymptomatic in terms of any GI manifestations, and may present with extraintestinal or malnutrition-related problems (such as miscarriages, osteoporosis with fractures, skin diseases, etc.) Clinical manifestations of the disease are given in Table 57.2. Patient populations at risk and their disease prevalence are given in Table 57.3.

Mechanisms

Gluten, the main allergen, is a protein found in wheat. The prolamin fraction of gluten is an alcoholic extract rich in proline and glutamine residues. This fraction is also termed gliadin, and certain amino acid sequences occurring in it (proline-serine-glutamine-

0-8493-2705-9/02/$0.00+$1.50

TABLE 57.1

Histological Features of Celiac Sprue (CS)

1. Loss of villi with resultant flat absorptive surface
2. Presence of cuboidal epithelial cells at surface
3. Hyperplasia of crypts, with increased mitotic figures
4. Increased intraepithelial lymphocytes
5. Increased cellularity in lamina propria

TABLE 57.2

Clinical Manifestations/Presentations of Celiac Sprue

Gastrointestinal	Extra-Intestinal
Diarrhea	Dermatitis herpetiformis
Steatorrhea/Weight loss	Amenorrhea/Infertility/Miscarriages
Nausea/Vomiting	Anemia (iron or folate deficiency)
GERD	Osteoporosis/Osteomalacia
Abdominal pain/Dyspepsia	Brittle diabetes
Bloating/Flatulence	Dementia
Occult blood in stool	Depression
Elevated transaminases	Neuropathy
Recurrent pancreatitis	Seizures
	Hyposplenism
	Headaches
	Hypoparathyroidism
	IgA nephropathy
	Malaise/Fatigue

TABLE 57.3

Patient Populations at Risk for CS

At Risk Population	Disease Prevalence
Family members of a patient with CS:	5-20%
Monozygotic twins	70-90%
Siblings with HLA DQW2 or HLA DR5/DR7	40%
First degree relatives	10-20%
Autoimmune thyroid disease	4-5%
Diabetes mellitus type I	2-5%
Ig A deficiency	15%
Sjögren's syndrome	15%
Down's syndrome	4-5%

glutamine and glutamine-glutamine-glutamine-proline) initiate the allergic reaction in CS. Many grains such as rye, barley and wheat also contain similar prolamin fractions, and are therefore toxic to CS patients (Figure 57.1). Taxonomy of common cereal grains and chemical names for their prolamin fractions are given in Figure 57.1.

In genetically predisposed individuals, the prolamin fractions from cereal grains bind a tissue autoantigen called tissue transglutaminase.[1] The bound complex is believed to initiate an autoimmune reaction leading to activation of intraepithelial T lymphocytes and formation of autoantibodies, resulting in destruction of small intestinal epithelial cells and the interstitium that make up the villus.

Tissue transglutaminase is normally found in the cytoplasm of the small intestinal epithelial cell, and its main function is to cross-link glutamine residues. *In vitro*, the enzyme preferentially acts on gluten, 35% of which is made up of glutamine, and renders it more susceptible to uptake and processing by the enterocyte. Tissue transglutaminase can also

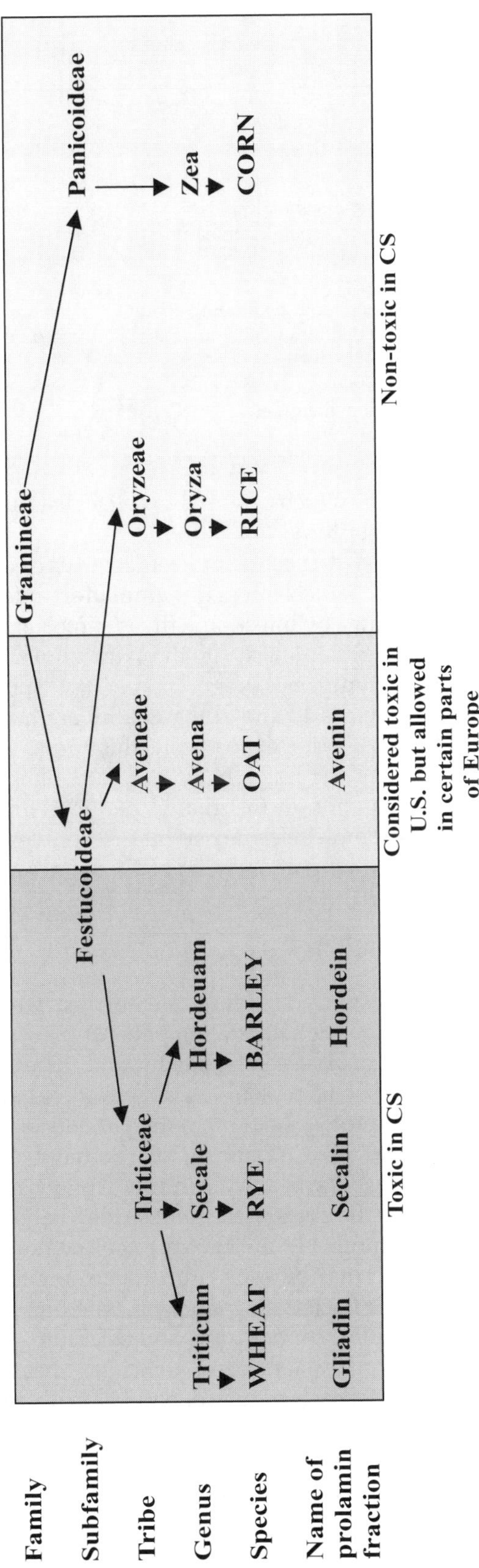

FIGURE 57.1
Taxonomy of grains.

TABLE 57.4

Pathogenetic Factors in Celiac Sprue

1. Dietary gluten
2. Genetic predisposition
   a. Association with HLA-DQw2, B8 and DR3
3. Autoimmunity
   a. Heightened gut permeability to macromolecules
   b. Increased T lymphocytes (esp. $\gamma\Delta$ type) in lamina propria
   c. Increased humoral mucosal immune response
   d. Tissue transglutaminase
      i. Creation of new antigenic epitopes by binding gliadin
      ii. Deamidation of glutamine residues in gliadin, causing increased binding to HLA
4. Acute trigger factors
   a. Infection with viruses
   b. Acute inflammation due to food allergy, etc.
   c. Mechanical stress

deamidate glutamyl donor molecules, which can bind to celiac disease-specific HLA-DQ2 better than their non-deamidated counterparts.

How tissue transglutaminase and gluten come into contact is unclear. Postulated mechanisms include exposure during mechanical stress, inflammation, infection, or apoptosis. For example, instigation of tissue injury by infection with adenovirus 12 has been hypothesized to cause release of tissue transglutaminase into the extracellular environment where it links with gluten. Supporting this hypothesis, Kagnoff et al.[2] have shown that a particular portion of the E1B protein of adenovirus 12 and alpha-gliadin are homologous, and 89% of patients with CS have evidence of prior exposure to this virus. Others propose that gluten is inadequately digested and toxic fractions accumulate. Subsequent sampling of the intestinal milieu leads to presentation of the gliadin peptides on antigen presenting cells within the cleft of the HLA-DQ2 molecules carried by susceptible individuals. Various hypotheses and factors important in the pathogenesis of CS are given in Table 57.4.

Effects on Nutritional Status

CS can profoundly affect nutritional status, leading to steatorrhea, weight loss, and many micronutrient deficiencies, although about half of adult patients present with rather subtle clinical signs of malnutrition, as the disease can be patchy, and the extent of involvement of the small intestine varies from person to person. The degree of malnutrition is positively correlated with the presence of symptoms; asymptomatic patients are less malnourished than symptomatic ones (31 versus 67%).[3] CS patients tend to have lower body fat, bone mass, and lean body mass compared to healthy controls. Total body fat can even be decreased significantly in asymptomatic cases with latent sprue.[4] Laboratory studies show that albumin, triglycerides, and hemoglobin are typically below normal. Anemia is frequent in both overt and latent CS, and may be due to iron, folate, or vitamin B_{12} deficiencies resulting from malabsorption and/or bacterial overgrowth. Micronutrient problems such as low calcium, potassium, magnesium, copper, zinc, and selenium, and vitamin K deficiency have been reported. Additionally, vitamin E deficiency has been linked to the neurological symptoms of CS. Of utmost importance, patients with symptomatic as well as latent CS may have osteomalacia and/or low bone mineral density[5] partly as a result of vitamin D and calcium deficiency, and these need to be supplemented to prevent osteoporosis. There is no correlation between clinical or biochemical abnormalities and bone mineral density, so supplementation with regular screening should be undertaken in all patients.

Diet in Celiac Sprue

The Gluten-Free Diet

CS patients need to avoid foods that contain certain cereal grains. For medical purposes, such a diet is termed a gluten-free diet (GFD). In general, the oryzeae or the tripsaceae such as rice, corn, and maize are safe because the protein fractions of these grains are significantly different from gliadin, due to their different taxonomy, shown in Figure 57.1. Basic principles of the GFD are given in Table 57.5.

Caution should be exercised when the word "gluten" is used to select foods, as it has different meanings to different people. Bakers typically use it to mean the sticky part of grains, whereas chemists only refer to wheat-derived protein fractions, and use the chemical names given in Figure 57.1 for other cereal grains. Therefore, patients are encouraged to ask, "Is this food free of wheat, rye, barley, oats, etc., and ingredients derived from grains?" rather than, "Is this a gluten-free food?."

Unfortunately, many dietary additives exist in processed foods containing hidden ingredients that are derived from cereal grains; therefore, compliance with a truly GFD diet is difficult. A simple watch list for some of these ingredients is given in Table 57.5, Item 3. Chemicals/fillers added to nonfood items such as vitamins and pills may also be sources of gluten. Moreover, food-processing elements, which need not to be reported on food labels, may use grains. Hence, patients are encouraged to consult a dietitian experienced in GFD with questions, as well as to join professional societies such as The Celiac Sprue Association, U.S.A.

Manifestations of the diseases responsive to GFD are given in Table 57.6. Numerous studies show that GFD is not only essential in controlling GI symptoms, but also prevents complications.

Osteopenia and osteoporosis are common, and can result from vitamin D and calcium malabsorption as well as secondary to hypoparathyroidism from hypomagnesaemia.[6] GFD leads to increases in bone mineral density, with the greatest benefit in the first year of treatment,[7-10] but normalization may not occur even on GFD.[10] In a study of 65 patients with CS on GFD, up to 50% had a T score of less than –2 on dual energy x-ray absorptiometry.[11]

There is a two- to threefold relative increase in the risk of cancer among patients with CS.[12,13] Specifically, T-cell lymphomas of the small intestine, adenocarcinoma of the small intestine, cancers of the mouth, nasopharynx, and esophagus are more common in CS.

TABLE 57.5

Principles of the Gluten-Free Diet (GFD)

1. Avoid the following grains: wheat, rye, barley, oat, spelt (dinkel), kamut, buckwheat
2. Avoid the following grain based products: bulgar*, couscous*, wheat starch, wheat germ, semolina*, durum*, bran, oat bran, germ, graham flour
3. Avoid potentially grain based products or additives: malt**, malt flavoring, malt extract, malt syrup, food starch (edible starch)***, icing sugar****, soy sauce*****, filler+, gum base, oat gum, cereal binding, white vinegar*****, hydrolyzed vegetable protein or hydrolyzed plant protein
4. Avoid sauces, salad dressings, and fat substitutes as these may typically contain grain-derived products.
5. Avoid grain-based alcohol such as beer or alcoholic extracts of grains.
6. Corn and rice are the only allowable cereal grains.
7. All fresh vegetables and fruits are allowed.

* derived from wheat
** may be derived from barley
*** may be derived from wheat
**** contains 5% wheat starch
***** may contain wheat or barley
+ found frequently in medications and vitamins

TABLE 57.6

Manifestations of CS Responsive to GFD

1. Gastrointestinal symptoms
   a. Diarrhea
   b. Malbsorption
2. Osteopenia/Osteoporosis
3. Anemia
4. Dermatitis herpetiformis
5. Depression
6. Increased risk of malignancy
7. Amenorrhea/Infertility/Spontaneous abortions

Malignant complications correlate with GFD; in patients who have been on GFD for five years or more, malignancy risk reverts back to that for the general population.[13,14] For those on a reduced gluten or normal diet, the risk for non-Hodgkin's lymphoma and cancers of the mouth, pharynx, and esophagus is 78-fold, and 23-fold higher compared to the general population.[13]

The time to respond to GFD clinically varies, depending on the severity of disease. A prompt improvement in symptoms is expected within days to a few weeks. Patients with milder disease in biopsies tend to respond sooner than those with villus atrophy, in whom resolution of symptoms may take up to several months. Still, normalization of biopsy samples when total villus atrophy is present has been reported incomplete even after two years.[15] Dermatitis herpetiformis takes longer to resolve with GFD than other symptoms (on average two years), and older patients take longer to respond than younger ones.

What to Do in the Patient Who is Unresponsive to a GFD?

From a dietary standpoint, careful review of the patient's diet for hidden sources of gluten is suggested. The most common causes of GI symptoms in such patients are bacterial overgrowth, development of other autoimmune diseases, and a new onset of microscopic/collagenous colitis found in 5% of patients with CS. Treatment of bacterial overgrowth with antibiotics may be beneficial.[16] Complications of CS such as development of T-cell lymphoma, adenocarcinoma, and collagenous sprue should also be investigated.

Exocrine pancreatic insufficiency due to impaired cholecystokinin-pancreozymin release from abnormal mucosa has been reported, suggesting a beneficial role for pancreatic enzyme supplements.[17,18] In fact, mild to moderate pancreatic insufficiency with subnormal levels in one or more pancreatic enzymes was found in 29% of patients with CS in one study, and the presence of insufficiency did not seem to correlate with overall nutritional status.[19] A prospective, double-blind, randomized study of adolescents has shown improvement in anthropometric variables as well as weight gain with enzyme supplementation.[20]

Searches for dietary antigens other than gliadin have shown usefulness to an elimination diet in 77% of patients in one study.[21] This elimination diet excluded foods containing natural salicylates, amines and/or glutamine, food colorings, preservatives, monosodium glutamate, lactose and/or dairy products, soy, and millet-containing foods.

Patients in whom symptoms persists are considered to have "refractory sprue" upon exclusion of other diagnoses. These patients may benefit from corticosteroids,[22] azathioprine,[23] or cyclosporine.[24] Zinc-deficient patients with refractory sprue may respond to zinc supplements,[25] although this issue is controversial.[26]

Is There a Safe Amount of Gluten that CS Patients May Consume?

The amount of gluten required to initiate CS is unknown. One study suggests that at least 10 g-gluten challenge leads to relapse of disease within seven weeks,[27] although there is no consensus in this regard. Diets recommended by professional societies in the U.S. do not allow any gluten, whereas the Codex Alimentarius Commission of the Food and Agricultural Organization of the United Nations (FAO) and the World Health Organization (WHO) permit a gluten-free label on foods that contain up to 0.3% of protein from toxic grains. Most of this protein comes from wheat starch or malt.

Wheat starch (that only contains 0.75 mg/100 g gliadin) is not tolerated well, and its withdrawal from the diet results in marked improvement of intestinal symptoms and dermatitis herpetiformis.[28] In a recent study examining patients who are symptomatic despite the GFD as defined by FAO/WHO standards, conversion to a no-detectable gluten diet resulted in complete resolution or reduction of symptoms in 23 and 45% respectively.[29] Based on these results, there is no safe amount of gluten in the diet.

Can CS Patients Eat Oats?

Evidence that oats may not be harmful to CS patients dates back to the 1970s, when Dissanayake, Truelove, and Whitehead administered 40 to 60 g of oats to four CS patients for one month and showed no damage to the small intestinal mucosa.[30] Several investigators claim that oats, which taxonomically belong to a different subclass in the cereal grains, the aveneae, do not elicit the immune reaction seen with the ones in the triticeae tribe; oats have a lower content of proline, which is abundant in the toxic amino acid sequences (proline-serine-glutamine-glutamine and glutamine-glutamine-glutamine-proline) of prolamin fractions. Also, these sequences occur fewer times per molecule of oat avenin as opposed to wheat prolamin.[31] Whether such lower amounts are enough to elicit the autoimmune reaction of CS or whether there is a certain safe level of oat consumption is unclear. *In vitro* investigations show that antibodies from sera of patients with CS and dermatitis herpetiformis can react against oat avenin, but the significance of this finding is questionable, because similar immunoreactivity against corn has also been demonstrated.[32]

Two small cohort studies with CS and dermatitis herpetiformis patients have shown no rise in antibody titers and no clinical or histological deterioration when oats are given 50 g/day and 62.5 g/day, respectively.[33,34] In the largest randomized placebo-controlled study to date, newly diagnosed European patients and ones in remission on GFD were studied for 12 and 6 months, respectively.[35] The patients were not blinded, although the investigators were. Consumption of 50 g of oats daily did not cause any clinical relapse or histopathological worsening in the established patients with CS, nor did it prevent clinical or histological healing in newly diagnosed cases. The authors concluded that small to moderate amounts of oats can be included in a GFD, and may improve poor compliance with the diet. Despite the well-design of this study, long-term evidence regarding the safety of oats is lacking. Considering crop rotation and lack of specified mills for oats in the U.S., addition of oats to GFD cannot be recommended at this time.

Should CS Patients Also Avoid Lactose?

Lactase, the enzyme needed for digestion of lactose, is located at the very tip of the brush border. As a result of damage to the villi, the levels of lactase are assumed to be lower in most acutely ill patients with CS. Therefore, most professionals advocate a lactose-free diet at the beginning of treatment with a GFD until resolution of symptoms. This is especially true for patients with severe disease, requiring corticosteroids. No controlled studies have been done examining the utility of a lactose-free diet in CS. Long-term avoidance of lactose is not appropriate, considering the high incidence of osteopenia among CS patients.

Does Breastfeeding Prevent Occurrence of CS?

The incidence of CS is increased in the relatives of patients. The relative risks for family members of CS patients are given in Table 57.3. Retrospective studies have shown that

TABLE 57.7

Nutritional Tips for CS Patients

1. Avoid lactose (mainly milk and dairy products) in acute disease
2. Follow a gluten free diet (Table 57.5) at all times:
   a. Read food labels
   b. Ask about grains in foods and medications
   c. Avoid all foods if it is not certain that they do not contain the restricted grains
   d. Select plain meats, fresh fruits, and vegetables when eating outside of the home if not sure
   e. Record weight and symptoms, and keep a food diary until symptoms resolve on the GFD
3. Avoid foods that initiate/exacerbate symptoms as they may contain hidden sources of grains or other food allergens
4. Consult an experienced dietitian with questions
5. Report persistent symptoms promptly
6. Join support groups for people with CS

relative risk of CS development is fourfold less in siblings of Italian children with CS if they are breastfed for over 30 days.[36] Similar findings showing a protective effect of breastfeeding has been confirmed in Tunisian children.[37] This effect may be correlated with duration of breastfeeding, and appears independent of the delays in introduction of wheat and grain products into an infant's diet.[38] Age at gluten introduction seems to be a separate factor. Epidemiological evidence links increasing incidence of CS in Sweden, as opposed to Denmark, to early- and high-level introduction of gluten into infant feedings.[39] However, case control studies have not yet confirmed these results.[40] Presently, this topic needs further study. Nutritional tips for CS are given in Table 57.7.

Inflammatory Bowel Disease (IBD)

Definition and Epidemiology

Inflammatory bowel disease is an idiopathic chronic inflammatory disorder of the gastrointestinal system. The two main forms of the disease are Crohn's disease (CD) and ulcerative colitis (UC). The main differences of these diseases are shown in Table 57.8.

Mechanisms

Various factors and mechanisms important in the pathogenesis of IBD are listed in Table 57.9. Most recently, certain genetic foci associated with IBD have been discovered, and it

TABLE 57.8

Differences between UC and CD

	UC	CD
Clinical	Bloody diarrhea is main symptom	Obstruction, fistulae, perianal disease may be present
Site of involvement	Rectum extending proximally into colon as a continuum	Any part of the GI tract Normal tissue between areas of involvement (i.e., skip areas)
	Small bowel normal	70% small bowel involvement
	Only mucosal involvement	Involvement of the entire bowel wall
Pathological appearance	No granulomas	Presence of granulomas
Prognosis/recurrence	Can be cured with colectomy	Cannot be cured with surgical resection

TABLE 57.9

Factors Important in the Pathogenesis of IBD

1. Genetic predisposition
2. Environmental factors (e.g., smoking, urban lifestyle, etc.)
3. Dietary factors
4. Infectious agents
   a. Mycobacteria
   b. Measles virus
5. Immune reactivity
6. Psychosocial factors and stress

is hypothesized that environmental factors in susceptible individuals ultimately initiate the inflammatory process leading to disease. Environmental factors include diet and dietary antigens as well as the bacterial flora of the intestines.

Effects on Nutritional Status

Malnutrition is common in IBD; however, there is an important difference between CD and UC. CD usually leads to chronic malnutrition that develops insidiously over long periods of time, whereas in most cases, UC causes acute reductions in weight during flareups of disease. Up to 85% of patients hospitalized with IBD and about 23% of outpatients with CD have protein-energy malnutrition.[41] Stable patients with the disease tend to have a normal fat-free mass but low fat stores.

The causes of malnutrition in patients with IBD are multifactorial, and are given in Table 57.10. There is an increase in the resting metabolic rates in active IBD, but mean increases are modest (19% in active UC,[42] 12% in active CD[43]) when compared to the calculated ones from the Harris Benedict Equation, or to controls. Total energy expenditures, however, are comparable to healthy people.[44] Most stable outpatients with IBD do not have increased energy expenditures either.[45] One exception is underweight individuals (body weight <90% of ideal)[45,46] who may represent a special subgroup with specific metabolic abnormalities different than the rest. Interestingly, stable patients with CD who have decreased fat stores but a similar fat-free mass to healthy controls or UC patients, have enhanced utilization of lipids and diet-induced thermogenesis.[47,48] A worse subclinical disease might be the cause in these patients, as increased lipid oxidation is seen with active disease and its level correlates with disease activity.[43]

TABLE 57.10

Causes of Malnutrition in IBD Patients

1. Reduced dietary intake
   a. Anorexia to avoid symptoms
   b. Restricted diets
   c. Drug-induced taste alterations
2. Maldigestion and malabsorption
   a. Inadequate mucosal surface
   b. Bile salt malabsorption from ileal disease
   c. Bacterial overgrowth
   d. Drug induced
3. Increased requirements
   a. Inflammatory catabolism
   b. Drug-induced nutrient wasting
4. Exudative protein losses from inflamed intestine or fistulae

TABLE 57.11

Micronutrient Deficiencies in IBD

Micronutrient	% Prevalance in: UC	CD
Iron	81	39
Folic acid	35	54-67
Vitamin B_{12}	5	48
Potassium		6-20
Calcium		13
Magnesium		14-33
Vitamin A	26-93	11-50
Vitamin D	35	75
Zinc		40-50
Selenium		35-40

Fecal energy and protein losses in IBD are significant in active IBD, but most patients compensate by increased food intake. Generally, patients on corticosteroids are also in positive energy balance, possibly due to the appetite stimulant properties of these drugs.[49] Yet, attention should be paid to the provision of adequate protein to meet increased protein need by the patient with active IBD, especially in malnourished patients who may require as much as 2 g/kg/day of protein.[50]

Food intolerances are twice as common among IBD patients as in the general population.[51] These intolerances are commonly towards corn, wheat, cereals, cruciferous vegetables, and milk, although intolerances to foods such as rice or even tap water have been observed.

In patients without obvious malabsorption, food intolerances together with less hunger, decreased appetite, and fewer sensations of pleasure related to eating lead to significantly reduced food intakes.[52] This is the major cause of weight loss in patients with IBD.[52] In patients without other objective evidence of active inflammation, weight loss should not be attributed to IBD, but rather close attention should be paid to the patient's food intake.

Patients with IBD commonly have many micronutrient deficiencies, as shown in Table 57.11. Low levels of zinc and selenium that are cofactors for oxidant-protective enzymes and low antioxidant vitamins (A, E, and C) have been implicated in worsening of the disease course as well as contributing to the high rate of carcinogenesis among IBD patients.

Osteopenia, a well-recognized complication of IBD, is widespread among both adult and pediatric patients[53] and may occur independent of steroid use. Both osteopenia and osteoporosis have been linked to vitamin D and calcium deficiencies, and supplementation has been beneficial in treatment of these disorders.

Diet in IBD

Diet as a Potential Cause of IBD

Epidemiological evidence suggests that the incidence of Crohn's disease (CD) has been increasing over the last half century, while that of ulcerative colitis (UC) is declining, especially in developed countries. Moreover, migrant populations of Asians into England, or of European Jews into the U.S., have a much greater increase in the incidence of CD compared to their counterparts living in their native countries. Assuming that the migrants and natives have similar genetic pools, the increase has been attributed to environmental factors. Strikingly, a higher incidence of CD in urban areas as opposed to rural ones further suggests environmental factors at play. Among these factors, diet is important.

Pre-Illness Diet Factors and Dietary Habits of Patients with IBD

Many studies on dietary factors in the development of IBD and the roles of many types of food (such as refined sugar, cereals, fiber, and dairy products including milk) have been undertaken.

In general, patients with IBD tend towards higher intake of sugar compared to controls,[54,55] and this trend specifically reaches statistical significance for CD[54,55] in most studies, and for UC in one.[56] Fruit, vegetable, and fiber consumption, on the other hand, was much lower in IBD in these studies. One study in the Japanese population confirmed the lower intakes of vegetables and fruits among IBD patients, and a Westernized diet increased the risk for UC.[57] These findings among IBD patients are not surprising, as they may represent an adaptation to the disease process rather than the cause of IBD.

Realizing this pitfall, in some studies only patients who have recent exacerbation of IBD were questioned about their diets. Such studies also confirmed that there is higher intake of sugars among CD patients but not UC ones.[58-64] In one of these, deleterious effect of increased intake of sugars was only seen with sucrose, but not with lactose or polysaccharides.[58] IBD patients also consume more fat prior to onset of disease.[58] One epidemiological study suggests that IBD is related to increased n-6 polyunsaturated fatty acid and animal protein intake.[65]

Does Milk Cause IBD? Should Patients with IBD Avoid Milk?

The role of milk in initiating or worsening IBD is debatable, and whether lactose intolerance is more common in IBD is controversial. Even among IBD patients who are not lactose malabsorbers, elimination of milk from the diet leads to improvement in diarrhea in 1/5 to 1/4 of the cases with UC, and in 1/3 of the patients with CD.[66,67]

Although no clear-cut explanation for this exists, morphological changes in small intestinal mucosa are well documented in CD and UC.[68,69] The extent to which these changes are related to decreased food intake or starvation as a result of disease symptoms is unknown. Nevertheless, in CD, improvements related to a milk-free diet are not attributable to changes in brush border lactase levels.[70] In UC, measurements of intestinal lactase have shown that deficiencies of lactase are real during active disease, but lactase deficit is not necessarily more frequent in the active phase compared to inactive.[71]

This raises the question of whether milk itself is an allergen. One group of studies has searched for humoral immune responses to milk proteins. Antibodies to milk proteins can be readily detected in sera of IBD patients,[72] but their levels may not be increased[73,74] nor are they particularly common.[75] Some investigators have correlated antibody response against milk to disease activity in CD but not in UC.[76] However, disruptions of the intestinal barrier as a result of inflammation can easily lead to such antibody formation, making it a secondary phenomenon rather than the cause of disease. Other studies have directly looked at the effects of a milk-free diet. In one, elimination of milk from the diet decreased relapses of UC when patients were followed up to one year subsequent to treatment with steroids[77] even though strict statistical comparisons between treatment and control groups were not undertaken. In another small study, 40% of IBD patients without lactose intolerance improved.[66] Allergy to cow milk may play a role in initiating or perpetuating inflammation in IBD in a subset of patients, although no evidence clearly establishes milk as an allergen.

Milk may also modify the intestinal flora, causing harm to individuals genetically susceptible to IBD, or to IBD patients. Supporting this hypothesis, lack of breastfeeding has been an independent risk factor for childhood CD,[78] but not UC.[79]

Is IBD Caused by Allergy to Foods?

In a subset of patients who respond to elimination diets, IBD may be caused by allergy to a specific food item. However, such patients constitute a very small minority and may represent cases with an allergic colitis that is misdiagnosed as IBD. Further studies are needed to answer this question.

Dietary Treatment for IBD

Energy and Protein Requirements in IBD

The Harris Benedict equation is useful in calculating the energy requirements of IBD patients. Active disease may increase calculated requirements up to 20%. Fecal losses of protein are the norm in active disease; therefore, patients should be given or encouraged to consume at least 1.5 g/kg of protein.

Effects of Diet Counseling

Individualized dietary counseling for six months can lead to significant decreases in the CD activity index, the need for medications such as prednisone, days spent in the hospital for acute exacerbations, and number of days lost from work.[80] Counseling can also lead to increased incidence of disease remission, with beneficial effects persisting up to one year, and is useful in both active and inactive disease.

Unproven Diets

High Fiber Diets that Restrict Sugar or Provide Unrefined Carbohydrates

Investigators have studied the impact of a diet with little or no sugar, rich in unrefined carbohydrates and fiber on IBD. In one open-label study of CD patients and matched controls, hospital admissions were significantly fewer and shorter in the treatment group.[64] Subjects were given over 30 g of fiber/day on average, with no adverse effects seen in the patients with strictures. In a larger, better-designed, controlled, multicenter trial with CD, the diet intervention group did not have a clinically different course than the group consuming a low-fiber, unrestricted sugar diet.[81]

Low Residue Diet for Active CD

A study of patients with active nonstenosing CD compared a low-residue diet with an ad-lib diet.[82] There were no differences in the incidence of poor outcomes such as need for surgery, hospitalization, prolonged bedrest, partial obstruction, or new inflammatory mass.

The Simple Carbohydrate Diet

Patients are resorting to diet therapies because of the many side effects of immunosuppressive medications used in treatment of IBD and their lack of effectiveness in a significant number of cases. There is a growing body of anecdotal evidence towards the efficacy of various diets used by patients. One very popular example is the simple carbohydrate diet (SCD) pioneered by Dr. Haas and currently advocated by Elaine Gottschall, whose son has been afflicted with UC.[83] The diet is based on avoidance of all complex sugars and grains, is gluten-free, and is devoid of all additives/preservatives. With a few exceptions, only fresh food is allowed, and it is cooked well to promote easy digestion. The principles of the diet attempt to generate an "elemental carbohydrate diet." Although elemental diets work in IBD, polymeric enteral formulas have been found to be just as effective in one-to-one comparisons. Moreover, many of the elemental formulations do, in fact, contain polymeric carbohydrates, refuting the possibility that taking in only simple carbohydrates will be successful. To date, the SCD diet has not been tested scientifically; therefore it cannot be advocated for general use. If it is proven effective after objective scientific evaluation, this may be based on features other than its "simple carbohydrates." For the patient who wishes to stay on the SCD diet, adequate macro- and micronutrient intake should be supervised by an experienced dietitian.

Elimination Diets

Report of food intolerances by IBD patients have led to investigations into elimination diets as a potential therapy. In an uncontrolled trial, 66% of CD patients were able to find a nutritionally adequate diet after elimination of various foods.[84] More than half of these patients needed elimination of more than one or two foods. The relapse rate was 33% at the end of the first year on the diets, with annual averages of about 14% within the first three years. A controlled trial by the same investigators showed that 7/10 patients in the treatment group remained in remission after three months, as opposed to all patients relapsing in the control group given an unrefined carbohydrate fiber rich diet.[84] Unfortunately, these beneficial results have not been confirmed with better-designed studies to eliminate bias. In fact, in a study of 42 eligible CD patients put into remission with elemental diet, 33% dropped out of the study; 19% did not identify food intolerance, and 48% did.[85] Among this 48%, food sensitivity was confirmed in half, in open-challenge with the item, and this was reproducible in only three patients on double-blind challenge. These findings suggest that elimination diets are of little help in the day-to-day treatment of IBD.

Growth Hormone and High-Protein Diet

The effects of high-protein diet versus glucocorticoids on the course of active CD was considered in a small study of pediatric patients. No significant dissimilarities between the two treatment groups in terms of improvement of pediatric Crohn's Disease activity index (CDAI) or laboratory parameters at two weeks were observed, although the study may not have had adequate power to detect any differences. In a followup of 1.3 years, patients given steroids tended to relapse more than the diet group.[86]

High-protein diet and growth hormone also have been shown to enhance adaptation of the small intestine after massive resection[87] and to improve protein absorption and reduce stool output and requirements for hyperalimentation in short bowel syndrome when used together with glutamine.[88] A pilot study of high-protein diet (protein intake = 2 g/kg/day) in conjunction with growth hormone injections (loading dose 5 mg/day for one week, maintenance 1.5 mg/day for four months) in moderate-to-severe CD patients undergoing conventional treatment has been studied in a double-blind and placebo-controlled fashion. Although the study is limited because of a small number of patients and does not indicate the percentage of patients entering remission, a significantly lower score of CDAI was seen in the treatment group.[89] This effect may be a result of increased amino acid uptake and electrolytes, increased intestinal protein synthesis, and/or decreased intestinal permeability in response to growth hormone. Further studies are needed before this treatment is applicable in clinical practice.

Fish Oils (Omega-3 fatty acids)

Omega-3 fatty acids such as eicosapentaenoic acid and docosahexanoic acid have been shown to inhibit production of leukotriene B_4, a major neutrophil chemo-attractant in IBD. In two trials with active UC patients, oral fish oil decreased steroid requirements and improved histology.[90,91] In another study of patients with moderate UC, decrease in disease activity was seen, although no improvement was noted in histology or leukotriene B_4 levels.[92] In UC, no beneficial effects of fish oil in maintenance of remission were seen.[90,93]

In CD, intravenous administration of eicosapentaenoic acid increases the ratio of leukotriene B_5: leukotriene B_4.[94] A one-year study in CD patients has shown reduced rates of relapse while on high doses of n-3 fatty acids (= 2.7 g/day), given as nine capsules a day. Compliance can be difficult with this regimen because of the large number of pills, and because some patients report a fishy odor at this dosage.

Capsaicin

Capsaicin, found in peppers, worsens colitis in IBD animal models by interfering with sensory neuroimmunomodulation.[95] No data exists in humans.

Short Chain Fatty Acids (SCFAs)

SCFAs are produced in the colon by fermentation of fiber or undigested starch by colonic flora, and represent the primary energy source of colonic cells. Small open-label trials of butyrate, a SCFA, given as an enema to patients with left-sided UC, have shown rates of remission similar to treatments with steroids and mesalamine.[96-99] The expense and the pungent smell of SCFA enemas precludes their clinical use; oral precursors of SCFAs are being developed. In animal studies, pectin increases SCFAs and leads to reduction of inflammation and enhancement of repair.[100]

Gut Microflora/Probiotics/Prebiotics

A large body of research indicates that the intestinal flora may be proinflammatory in IBD. This may explain why antibiotics that alter the flora, such as fluoroquinolones or metronidazole, or diversion of the fecal stream with an ostomy, are utilized in the treatment of IBD. The proinflammatory effect of the flora may be a result of expansion of harmful colonies of normal gut microorganisms in the presence of certain lumenal conditions such as an acidic pH, etc. Therefore, novel probiotic therapies that administer "good colonies (non-inflammatory)" of gut bacteria, which compete with "bad colonies," have been developed for treatment of IBD. One of these, *E. coli* strain *Niessle 1917* most recently has been shown to be as effective as conventional treatment with 5-ASA drugs in the maintenance of remission in UC.[101] Another probiotic preparation containing 5×10^{11} composed of four strains of lactobacilli, three strains of bifidobacteria and one strain of Streptococcus salivarius can prevent recurrence of pouchitis, (inflammation of the ileal pouch anastomosed to the rectum in patients who have undergone colectomy for UC), in a nine month follow-up period.[102] A different approach has been the use of prebiotics, nondigestible food substances that promote only the growth of a defined subset of good bacteria. Certain foodstuffs or their components have been found to be prebiotics (e.g., fructo-oligosaccharides and oats) that can profoundly influence the gut microflora, favoring expansion of good organisms like lactobacillus. Although no controlled studies with these substances exist in humans, a pilot study of patients with IBD has reported increases in favorable intestinal flora as well as SCFA.[103]

Medium-Chain Triglycerides (MCTs)

Foods rich in medium-chain triglycerides are readily absorbed, and enhance kcaloric intakes in malabsorptive states like IBD.

Enteral Nutrition and IBD

Primary Therapy

Many different formulations have been used for enteral nutrition in IBD. Polymeric formulas usually have starches, complex protein, long-chain triglycerides, and MCTs.

Semielemental formulations contain oligosaccharides, peptides, and MCTs. Elemental formulations typically contain predigested nutrients such as amino acids and glucose.

In active CD, comparison of elemental/semielemental diets with corticosteroids have shown equal efficacy in achieving short term remission (≤ 3 months) in the range of 70 to 80% in individual studies,[104-106] but a meta-analysis indicates that steroids may be more effective.[107] Long-term effects of enteral diets are less well known, although percentage of patients in remission at one year ranges from 9 to 56%.[105,106,108] This rate is not significantly different when elemental diets are compared with polymeric or semi-elemental formulations in most studies.[107,109] Elemental diets are poorly tolerated because of their smell/taste, complications such as diarrhea, and high costs. Therefore, polymeric formulations should be favored. Furthermore, relapse rates are generally higher with elemental diets as opposed to conventional therapy;[110] therefore, enteral nutrition as primary therapy should be attempted only in selected cases.

Investigators have found that CD patients with severe disease[111] and/or CDAI >450[112] and patients with colonic disease together with a fever[113] are less likely to respond to enteral nutrition therapy. In one study, the initial response rates were 38 versus 76% for CD patients with moderate disease, as opposed to patients with severe inflammation.[111] Studies with UC reveal no benefit from enteral nutrition for induction of remission.[114]

Comparison of hyperalimentation with enteral nutrition in CD has shown no superiority of parenteral nutrition.[41,109,115] Given the multiple potential side effects of parenteral nutrition, enteral therapy should be used whenever possible.

Parenteral Nutrition and IBD

Preoperative

Parenteral nutrition decreases postoperative complications only in severely malnourished patients with IBD. In one study, therapy duration of at least five days was required to see any beneficial effect.[116]

Primary Therapy

Randomized prospective studies have shown a response rate to parenteral nutrition in the 30 to 50% range in acute UC, but no significant differences over placebo have been demonstrated.[117-120] Furthermore disease-free maintenance rates on total parenteral nutrition (TPN) have been poor, and complications requiring surgery may be higher; therefore, there is no role for TPN as primary therapy of UC.[117-120]

In retrospective and prospective analyses in CD, parenteral nutrition can induce remission in 70 to 100% of patients refractory to conventional treatments,[114,115,117,118] but in at least one prospective study, 60% relapse rate is seen within two years.[121] This rate is four times higher than historical controls treated with surgical resection. Therefore, consideration of parenteral nutrition is recommended only in patients who are malnourished and have extensive disease precluding surgical treatment. Given the many complications of parenteral nutrition, this treatment should be a last resort, after exhaustion of other therapies.

Micronutrients

Antioxidants

Lower levels of antioxidant vitamins such as vitamin A, E, C, and beta-carotene have been shown in both sera and colonic tissue of patients with IBD when compared to healthy controls.[122,123] In one study, vitamin C level also correlated with disease severity.[122] Vitamin C can especially be low in patients with fistulous tracts.

Animal studies suggest that antioxidant supplementation over and above corrections for deficiency states may ameliorate colitis; however, no randomized placebo controlled trials have been performed in humans.

Calcium/Vitamin D

Low levels of vitamin D are found in 75% of patients with CD and 35% of patients with UC.[109] Low levels also correlate with disease activity in undernourished CD patients.[124] Of such patients, 45% have osteoporosis.[125] Therefore, supplementation of vitamin D and calcium is essential for the prevention of osteopenia/osteoporosis in IBD. Smoking also independently increases the rate of osteoporosis, and should be avoided.

Folate

In retrospective analyses, folate supplementation has been shown to reduce incidence of dysplasia and cancer in patients with UC.[126,127] Folate requirements in IBD are increased due to anemia and medications such as azathioprine, 6-mercaptopurine, and sulfasalazine; therefore supplementation is recommended in almost all patients.

Zinc

Zinc deficiency is especially common among patients with fistulous disease, and has been implicated as a cause for poor wound healing in these patients.[128]

Vitamin B_{12}

Deficiency of vitamin B_{12} occurs as a result of ileal involvement or resection as well as bacterial overgrowth in CD. All patients with CD should have supplementation either nasally or as monthly injections, because oral absorption is inadequate. Recently, sublingual administration of two over-the-counter vitamin nuggets (1000 μg/nugget) daily for seven to ten days to a small group of patients with B_{12} deficiency has been reported to be effective in raising blood levels. This latter route requires further study.

Specific Situations

Obstruction

Patients with intermittent obstruction are advised to consume a low-residue diet, although no definite data exists.

Fistulae

Postoperative fistulae may respond to TPN, but CD fistulae are less likely to close and frequently reopen promptly after food intake is resumed.[129,130] Similar results are seen with elemental diet.[111,113,131,132] In the era of effective anti-tumor necrosis factor therapies, TPN cannot be recommended as first-line therapy for fistulae in CD.

Severe Diarrhea and Antidiarrheals/Pectin

Diarrhea can be disabling for patients with IBD, and many require antidiarrheals such as Loperamide or Lomotil. These agents induce their effects by diminishing GI motility by binding opioid receptors in the GI tract, and therefore have been implicated in the pathogenesis of IBD complications such as toxic megacolon. Thus, caution should be exercised when using these, and for severely symptomatic patients without any obstruction, antidiarrheals such as Kaopectate, that bind excess liquid in the lumen, should be tried.

TABLE 57.12

Nutritional Tips for IBD Patients

1. Seek dietary counseling from an experienced dietitian
2. Avoid milk and milk products during active disease
3. Consume 10-20% more kcalories and 50% more protein with active disease
4. Do not avoid fiber, in fact try to increase fiber in diet as long as there is no obstruction in the GI tract
5. Follow a low residue diet if there is partial obstruction in the GI tract, consult with a physician and dietitian before making dietary changes
6. Prefer fish over other dishes (fish with high fat/fish oils such as catfish, salmon, etc., should be selected)
7. Take a multivitamin supplying 100% of RDA of vitamins and minerals, make sure to have monthly vitamin B_{12} injections if having CD
8. During inactive disease, consume foods that are rich in naturally occurring probiotics (such as yogurt containing lactobacillus)

Extraintestinal Manifestations

Unconfirmed reports suggest associations between resolution of pyoderma gangrenosum and uveitis with diet therapy.[133]

Ileal Resection and Kidney Stones

Patients with CD are at increased risk of oxalate kidney stones if their colons are relatively intact and they have had extensive ileal resections. Such patients should be advised to follow a low oxalate diet. Patients with a history of oxalate stones should also be treated with binding resins such as cholestyramine.

Nutritional tips for IBD patients are given in Table 57.12.

Short Bowel Syndrome

Definition and Epidemiology

Short bowel syndrome (SBS) is a malabsorptive state with a distinct group of symptoms and signs that occur as a consequence of major reductions in small intestinal absorptive surface area typically due to intestinal resection(s). Patients usually experience large-volume diarrhea with salient fluid and electrolyte losses as well as weight loss. The most important determinant of SBS is the length of the remaining functional small intestine, and less than 200 cm (6.5 feet) of length invariably is associated with compromised nutritional status. Less than 100 cm (3 to 3.5 feet) usually requires TPN. Small intestinal length is variable from person to person, with a range of 330 to 850 cm; therefore, the length of resected segments is clinically irrelevant. If there is doubt as to the length of the remaining small intestine, this crucial information can be obtained by doing a small bowel followthrough, since surgical and radiographic measurements correlate well.[134]

Although the true incidence and prevalence of SBS is not known, it is estimated that 10 to 20 thousand people in the U.S. require TPN as a result of it. The commonest causes of SBS are Crohn's disease, malignancy, radiation enteritis, and ischemic bowel. Others include jejunoileal bypass operations (used in the past to treat obesity), congenital abnormalities such as intestinal atresia, malrotation of the intestines, aganglionosis, and necrotizing enterocolitis in childhood.

TABLE 57.13

Factors That Affect the Type of Nutrition Required by SBS Patients

Factors	The Effect
Phases of SBS	See Table 57.14
Length of remaining small intestine	Very short lengths (60-100 cm) worsen severity of SBS
The extent of disease in remaining intestine	Impact of even mild disease on nutritional status can be profound. As disease worsens, the length of functioning small intestine decreases
Absence of the stomach	Loss of timed and slow release of gastric chyme decreases contact time between food and digestive/absorptive epithelium, thereby worsening SBS. Lack of stomach acid facilitates bacterial overgrowth aggravating malabsorption
Absence of the ileocecal valve	Leads to bacterial overgrowth enabling passage of colonic bacteria into the small intestine
Absence of the colon	Promotes water and electrolyte losses. Kcaloric losses are more extensive. Lack of gastrocolic reflex results in rapid transit of food, enhancing malabsorption

TABLE 57.14

Phases of SBS with Their Characteristics

Phase	Duration	Main Problems
Postoperative	1-2 weeks	High volume/severe diarrhea Gastric hypersecretion Related fluid and electrolyte imbalances

Transition	1-3 months	Diarrhea with oral intake
		Malabsorption:
		  Increased kcaloric requirements
		  Micronutrient deficiencies
		Social problems
		TPN related problems

Adaptation	3 months to 1-2 years	Dietary restrictions
		Adequacy of oral intake
		Complications:
		  Renal stones
		  Gallstones
		  D-Lactic acidosis

Pathophysiology and Types of SBS

The main factors that affect the type of nutrition required by patients are listed in Table 57.13. The phase of SBS (i.e., the elapsed time after intestinal insult or surgery resulting in SBS) is of utmost importance in the acute management of SBS (Table 57.14). The remaining factors determine how well a patient will handle enteral nutrition in the long run.

In general, jejunal resections are better tolerated than ileal ones for several reasons:

1. Most of the intestinal fluid secretion that balances the osmotic load of gastric chyme entering the small bowel occurs in the jejunum. Subsequently, a large percentage of the proximally secreted water/electrolytes are absorbed distally in the ileum. Therefore, ileal as opposed to jejunal resections/insults result in more voluminous diarrhea, with loss of nutrients in stool.
2. GI transit is faster in patients with ileal resections because of the lack of the ileal brake mechanism, discussed in the first GI section.
3. The ileum has a greater adaptive potential.

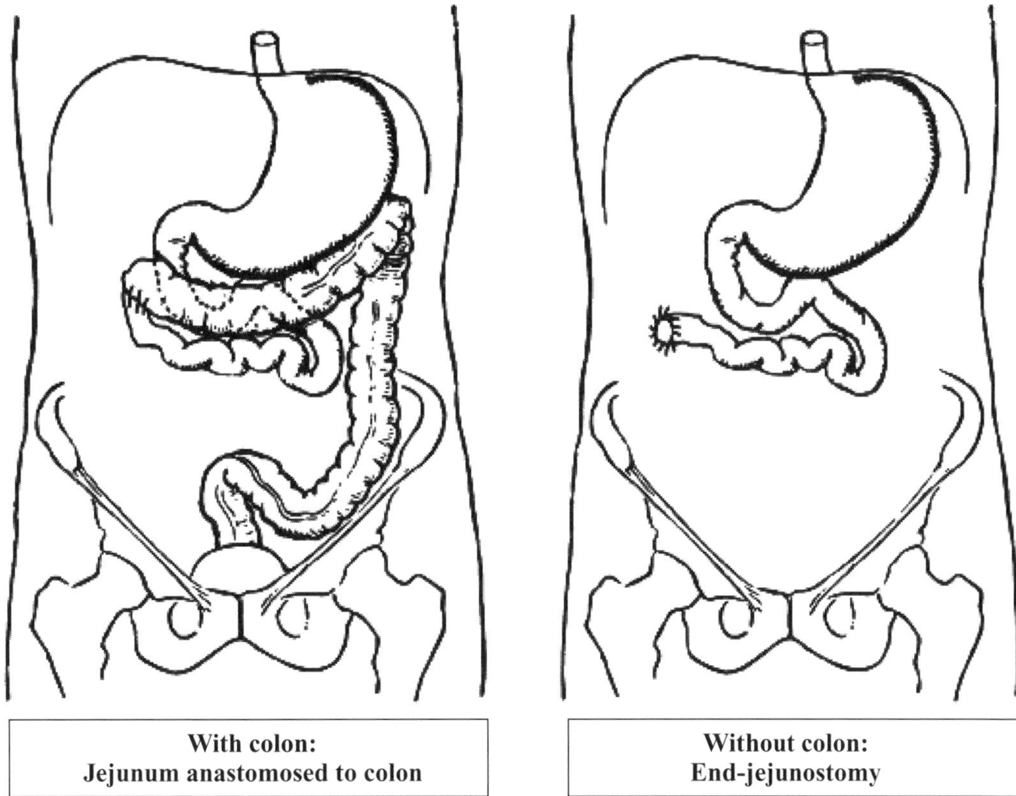

FIGURE 57.2
Anatomic types of short bowel syndrome.

Most patients with SBS fall into two main categories: those with and those without a colon. Patients with a colon usually have the majority of their ileum and some of their jejunum resected, with a resultant jejunocolic anastomosis. Those without a colon usually have end-jejunostomies (see Figure 57.2). Patients with a colon typically do better, especially in maintaining fluid and electrolyte balance, and cases with >50 cm of jejunum remaining may be managed with oral/enteral nutrition instead of TPN.

Diet in SBS

Dietary interventions in SBS should be individualized for each patient, as the needs differ considerably. Some general recommendations are given in the following paragraphs.

Postoperative Phase

No enteral nutrition is given at this phase because of the osmotic effects of food, and all patients require TPN. There are massive losses of fluids and electrolytes, and the amount is highly variable; therefore, careful monitoring of all intake and output as well as daily laboratory tests must be done. Patients should be given back their entire deficit plus an extra estimated 300 to 500 cc/day for insensible losses. Preferably, this type of replacement should be done on an hourly basis and separate from the TPN.

Agents that slow intestinal transit such as parenteral codeine and drugs that reduce the commonly seen gastric hypersecretion are also helpful in reducing the volume of stool output. Gastric hypersecretion is usually comparable to the level seen in duodenal ulcer patients,[135] can lead to significant volume losses, especially within the first six months following surgery,[136] and can contribute to malabsorption by inactivating pancreatic lipase and deconjugating bile salts. Treatment with cimetidine has been shown to improve absorption.[136,137] A study of 13 patients with large-volume ostomy output has shown that omeprazole can increase water absorption in cases with fecal outputs >2.5 kg/day, but does not alter absorption of kcalories, macronutrients, or electrolytes.[138]

Octreotide (50 to 100 μg subcutaneously twice a day) has also been shown useful in patients with end jejunostomies who have >3 L/day of ostomy output.[139] Initial concerns that octreotide may delay adaptation have not been substantiated in animal studies.[140]

Transition Phase and Adaptation Phase

Oral Diet

In the transition phase, TPN is continued while patients are first started on isotonic clear liquids that contain salt and glucose. It is advised to wait until the ostomy output is less than 2 to 3 L/day before commencement of oral intake. The average sodium concentration in the ostomy secretions generally varies between 80 to 100 mEq/L, so the initial hydration solutions should have at least this amount. Alternatively, sodium in the ostomy secretions can be measured to calculate the concentration in the replacement solution. Patients who can tolerate these solutions should also be switched to oral antidiarrheals such as Loperamide, Lomotil, or tincture of opium. The commonly used dosages given in Table 57.15 are typically high.

Subsequently, patients should be transitioned into an oral diet. In general, patients with SBS do not tolerate large amounts of food at one time, foods with concentrated carbohydrates (especially mono and disaccharides) and high lactose, or foods high in oxalate and insoluble fiber. Hypotonic fluids such as water, tea, juices, and alcohol also need to be avoided, especially in patients without a colon, because this type of fluid draws sodium into the jejunal lumen, causing increased salt and water losses. Additionally, patients should be advised not to consume foods or supplements with non-absorbable sugars (such as sorbitol and mannitol) or non-absorbable fat (such as olestra), and to watch out for hidden diarrheal agents (e.g., polyethylene glycol found in certain mints). It is best to try small and frequent amounts of solid food until the patient can consume at least 1200 kcal/day without a significant increase in diarrhea. Once this is achieved, TPN may be gradually cycled to go on only during the night and then on alternate days, together with slow advancement of oral intake.

Enteral Feeding

Patients who are not able to take in adequate kcalories via the oral route should be tried on enteral feedings. There is no consensus on which type of enteral feeding is best for SBS, but isotonic polymeric formulas are recommended over elemental ones, which are expensive and poorly tolerated by patients because of their taste, smell, and high osmolality that increases jejunal secretion.

TABLE 57.15

Dosages for Antidiarrheals in SBS

Antidiarrheal	Typical Dosage
Loperamide	4-6 mg/4-5 times a day
Lomotil	2.5-5 mg/4 times a day
Tincture of opium	5-10 cc every 4 hours
Codeine phosphate	30 mg/3-4 times a day

TABLE 57.16

Selected Complications of TPN in SBS and Their Prevention/Treatment

Complication	Treatment
Line infections	Remove catheter completely if fungal infections or Staph. aureus are the cause (change over a wire is not acceptable) Staph. aureus requires 2-6 weeks of antibiotics Staph. epidermidis may be cured 80% of the time with 7-10 days of iv vancomycin
Bacterial overgrowth	Treat with broad spectrum antibitotics (tetracycline, ciprofloxacin, metronidazole, etc.) Rotate antibiotics every 4-8 weeks
Liver disease	Pursue enteral feedings aggressively Take care to prevent line infections Avoid overfeeding with excessive kcalories Prefer lipid kcalories to high carbohydrate nutrition Treat bacterial overgrowth Screen for cholelithiasis

Parenteral Nutrition

Patients who cannot stop TPN need to be monitored for complications such as feeding catheter infections, liver disease, bacterial overgrowth, and nutritional deficiencies. Some of these, together with their treatments, are given in Table 57.16.

Dietary Requirements and the Composition of the Diet in SBS

Energy

Most patients with SBS only absorb 50 to 60% of total energy, with the highest % malabsorption in fat and carbohydrates.[141] Thus, they need 1.5 to 2 times the amount of food/energy to maintain weight. For patients not able to increase their intake to this level, enteral feedings at night or additional TPN is required.

Carbohydrate versus Fat

In normal individuals, about 20% of all carbohydrates consumed exit the small bowel undigested and are fermented to SCFAs in the colon, where they are absorbed.[142,143] In order to take advantage of this colonic absorption, a well-designed study has compared the use of a high carbohydrate (60:20:20% of kcalories from carbohydrate: fat: protein) versus a high fat diet (20:60:20%) in SBS.[144] Intakes of the various diets did not affect stool or ostomy outputs, but consumption of the high carbohydrate diet by patients with a colon reduced the fecal loss of kcalories by 2 ± 0.2 MJ/day, which may equal up to 20 to 25% of the daily kcaloric intake of an average patient with SBS. Thus, patients with a colon should be advised to consume a high carbohydrate (50 to 60% of kcalories) and lower fat (20 to 30% of kcalories) diet. Diets containing more than 60% of energy as carbohydrates may ultimately overcome the colon's energy salvage capability of 2.2 MJ/day of SCFAs.[145]

In patients without a colon, neither high-fat nor high-carbohydrate diet significantly affects energy or water/electrolyte losses.[144] Furthermore, many patients with very short jejunal segments and high ostomy outputs have been shown not to need or benefit from any particular diet.[146,147] So, restriction of fat in the diet is not recommended, because such restriction limits palatability of food and deprives patients of valuable concentrated energy.

Long-Chain Fatty Acids (LCFAs) versus MCTs

There is a tendency to use MCTs because of their better absorption in the presence of a reduced bile acid pool and/or pancreatic insufficiency. MCTs can help reduce ostomy output[148] in some cases, but they also exert a higher osmotic load in the small intestine and have a lower caloric density compared to LCFAs. Besides, LCFAs are better in inducing intestinal adaptation;[149] thus, a mixture of LCFAs and MCTs seems to be the most logical approach. A recent study compared the effects of a high fat (56% of kcalories as fat) diet in SBS. Patients were given fat in the form of LCFAs or a mixture of MCTs and LCFAs (about 1:1). Only patients with a colon benefited, with an increase in energy absorption from 46 to 58%.[150]

Lactose

Although the concentration of lactase in the intestine of SBS patients is unaltered, there is a reduction in the total quantity of available lactase. Thus, intake of food with high lactose content (e.g., milk) is discouraged, although many patients are able to tolerate small quantities of cheese and yogurt well.

Insoluble Fiber

Insoluble fiber such as bran decreases intestinal transit time and should be avoided by SBS patients.

Micronutrients

Deficiency of divalent cations such as calcium, magnesium, and zinc are typical. Water-soluble vitamin deficiencies are rare because most are absorbed in the proximal jejunum. Vitamin B_{12}, which is absorbed in the terminal ileum, and fat-soluble vitamins A, D, E, and K need to be replaced routinely. A water-soluble form of vitamin A (Aquasol A) may be tried. Monthly injections of 1000 μg vitamin B_{12} are necessary.

Bile Acid Replacement

Although the bile acid pool is reduced in patients with SBS, clinicians do not replace it routinely because of a fear that diarrhea will increase when bile acids are fermented by bacteria, causing secretion of water and electrolytes. A recent case report contradicts this and has demonstrated a 40 g/day increase in fat absorption when the patient was given a natural conjugated bile acid mixture isolated from ox bile or a synthetic bile acid named cholylsarcosine.[151]

Common Problems and Complications in SBS

Hypomagnesemia

Patients with end-jejunostomies tend to have hypomagnesemia more often than those with colons.[152] The condition requires parenteral magnesium frequently but oral 1-α-hydroxycholecalciferol may also be tried.[152] Urinary magnesium levels are a better indicator of deficiency than serum levels, which represent only 4% of the total body pool.[153]

Renal Stones

Risk of oxalate stones is increased, occurring in 25% of all SBS patients with a colon.[154] Calcium, which normally binds to oxalate and causes its excretion with feces, actually binds the malabsorbed fatty acids in the lumen in SBS, leaving oxalate available for absorption in the colon. Unabsorbed bile acids that enter the colon also stimulate absorption of oxalate.

Urinary oxalate excretion should be measured in patients with a colon, and oxalate should be restricted in patients with high levels of excretion. In patients with a history of stones, restriction of fat in the diet may be considered. Additionally, urinary citrate and magnesium, which inhibit stone formation, are low and may need to be supplemented.

Gallstones

There is a two- to threefold increased risk of cholesterol gallstones because of the decreased bile acid pool in SBS. This increased risk is not different for patients with or without a colon, but risk of calcium bilirubinate stones is higher in patients on TPN because of gallbladder stasis and low oral intake. Cholecystokinin injections have been tried in dogs[155] with good success in preventing gallbladder stasis. Some advocate prophylactic cholecystectomy in SBS.[156]

Social Problems

Patients with end-jejunostomies and those dependent on TPN frequently have social problems that require help of psychiatrists and psychologists.

D-Lactic Acidosis

Fermentation of malabsorbed carbohydrates in the colon produces D-lactic acid that cannot be metabolized by humans. Elevated levels cause an anion-gap metabolic acidosis with confusion, ataxia, nystagmus, opthalmoplegia, and dysarthria.[157] The condition is more likely when thiamine deficiency is present, and it is treated with nonabsorbable antibiotics (neomycin or vancomycin) and restriction of carbohydrates (especially mono- and oligosaccharides) in the diet.[158]

In summary, nutritional management of SBS is complex, and patients should best be referred to an experienced multidisciplinary nutrition management team.

Acute Infectious Diarrhea

Acute infectious diarrhea usually does not affect nutritional status, even though it can result in severe water and electrolyte disturbances. Although no specific diet therapy is proven to be effective in this disease, patients should be encouraged to drink plenty of fluids that contain a mixture of glucose and sodium. Absorption of sodium in the intestinal tract is altered in acute diarrhea, but glucose-coupled sodium transport through the SGLT1 transporter is adequate in most cases to sustain hydration. An ideal mixture of glucose and sodium is found in the WHO oral rehydration solution (ORS), which can be made by mixing 20 g glucose, 3.5 g sodium chloride, 2.9 g sodium bicarbonate and 1.5 g potassium chloride in 1 L water. The commonly advocated sports drinks contain far less sodium and much more glucose compared to this ORS solution, and should not replace the latter. Within the last two decades, rice and other cereal-based ORS solutions that take advantage of other apical membrane sodium-dependent solute-transport transporters have been discovered. In these solutions, rice or cereal flour replace glucose found in the original ORS. The rice ORS solution is superior to the glucose-based ORS in decreasing stool output.[159] Most recently, induction of sodium absorption from the colon by short-chain fatty acids was observed.[160] A clinical application of this principle has been tested: 50 g/L amylase-resistant maize starch, which is malabsorbed and fermented to short-chain fatty acids by colonic flora, was added to the original WHO ORS. In adolescents and adults with *Vibrio Cholerae*-induced diarrhea, stool output and duration of diarrhea was less in patients given the maize starch ORS compared to controls given standard ORS.[161] Further studies are needed before the latter is incorporated into common clinical practice.

Although it is rational to advise patients to stay away from hard-to-digest foods such as red meat, high fiber-containing vegetables (e.g., salads, greens, broccoli, etc.), and lactose, because of the increased rate of intestinal transit and concurrent malabsorption that occur in acute diarrhea, there exists no data in this regard. Most recently, an antidiarrheal factor has been found in rice, suggesting that a rice-based diet may be useful.[162] This factor blocks the secretory response of intestinal crypt cells to cyclic adenosine monophosphate and targets the cystic fibrosis transmembrane regulator (CFTR) chloride channel.

Clostridium Difficile Colitis and Probiotics

C. difficile colitis is a major cause of antibiotic-associated diarrhea and acute diarrhea in hospitalized patients. Spores of the bacterium are hard to destroy, and a mean of 20% (range 5 to 66%) of patients have recurrences despite treatment with effective antibiotics. Preliminary results of a trial with yogurt enriched in *Lactobacillus GG* (trial using medicinal microbiotic yogurt = TUMMY) together with standard antibiotic therapy have been promising in prevention of recurrence.[163] Final results are awaited for further recommendations.

Functional Disorders of the Gastrointestinal Tract (FGIDs)

Definition and Epidemiology

Functional gastrointestinal disorders (FGIDs) are the most common diseases of the GI tract, with at least 4.7 million affected individuals in the U.S. They comprise about 20 to 50% of gastroenterology clinic visits and are estimated to cost 8 billion dollars/year to the healthcare system. Definitions for the different types of FGIDs are established, and are known as the Rome II criteria.[164]

Mechanisms

Various factors and mechanisms thought to be important in the pathogenesis of these disorders are listed in Table 57.17. Currently recommended dietary management is based on decreasing food allergies, affecting GI motility and lowering intestinal gas production in an effort to decrease bowel wall distention.

Effects on Nutritional Status

FGIDs usually do not lead to weight loss. If a patient with FGIDs has significant weight loss, other causes should be sought. Although there are no reports of malnutrition, patients with FGIDs have many self-reported food intolerances, resulting in avoidance of various foods. This avoidance may lead to nutritional deficiencies. In one study comparing nutrient intake using 48-hour dietary recall, women with FGID had lower mean consumption of kcalories as well as folate, ascorbic acid, and vitamin A, compared to GERD and IBD patients.[165]

TABLE 57.17

Factors Important in Pathogenesis of FGIDs

1. Cognitive factors
   a. Illness behavior
   b. Illness coping strategies
2. Behavioral/Emotional factors
   a. Psychosocial stress
   b. Physical and/or sexual abuse
   c. Anxiety
   d. Depression
3. Physiological factors
   a. Visceral hyperalgesia
   b. Altered intestinal motility
   c. Altered neuroendocrine response
4. Environmental factors
   a. Dietary allergens
   b. Enteric infections

Diet in FGIDs

There is no particular diet for patients with FGIDs, and there is little evidence for dietary therapies of functional upper digestive tract diseases. Some patients with functional chest pain may improve with diets similar to ones recommended for GERD patients (given in the previous GI section, Table 56.10). Others with functional dyspepsia may benefit from elimination of foods that delay gastric emptying (given in the previous GI section, Table 56.17).

Fiber for Irritable Bowel Syndrome (IBS)

Types of Dietary Fiber

Dietary fiber is defined as endogenous components of plants that are resistant to digestion by human enzymes. Fiber consists either of non-starch polysaccharides (e.g., cellulose, hemicellulose, pectins, and gums) or of non-polysaccharides (e.g., lignins composed of phenylpropane units). Cellulose is a non-digestible glucose polymer found in the cell walls of all vegetation, making it the most abundant organic compound in the world. Hemicellulose fibers are cellulose molecules substituted with other sugars, such as xylan, galactan, mannan, etc. Pectins and gums are composed of arabinose or galactose side chains added on to a galacturonate backbone; they naturally form gels.

Cellulose and hemicellulose are the major components of bran and whole grains. Lignins are commonly found in seeds and stems of vegetation. Pectin is part of apples, citrus fruits, and strawberries, and is widely added to jams and jellies. Gums naturally occur in oats, legumes, guar, and barley. Structural fibers such as celluloses, lignins, and some hemicelluloses are water-insoluble. Gums, pectins, psyllium, oat bran, and beans are water-soluble.

Insoluble fiber mainly adds bulk to stool and increases transit through the colon. Soluble fibers such as guar and pectin delay gastric emptying and transit through the small intestine, but speed transit through the colon and lower intraluminal pressures. Soluble fibers may also bind bile acids and minerals such as calcium and iron.

Bran

Fiber, in the form of bran, for IBS was popularized after Burkitt's initial work in early 1970s demonstrating that it increases stool weight and decreases intestinal transit time.

Others confirmed these findings,[166] and a lack of fiber was implicated for the development of many GI diseases including diverticular disease, colon cancer, and IBS. Consequently, studies in the 1970s undertook bran replacement as therapy for IBS, and the results were positive in some[167] but clearly negative in many others.[168] Most of these studies had methodological flaws, and were usually done with small numbers of patients. Nevertheless, given the lack of other effective therapies for the disease, bran became the standard of care.

Evidence over the last two decades contradicts this, and indicates that patients with IBS consume equal amounts of total fiber but less vegetable fiber compared to healthy controls.[169] Fiber replacement in the form of bran is no more effective than placebo,[170-172] and is poorly tolerated in many subjects. In one study, 55% of patients worsened after bran therapy, with deterioration in bowel habits, abdominal distention, and pain.[173] Improvement was seen in only 10%. These findings are corroborated by data from other studies upon careful review;[174] not only may patients worsen initially and not tolerate bran, but they also may have a high subsequent withdrawal rate.[175]

Soluble Fiber

Soluble fiber replacement seems to be better tolerated and more effective for IBS in comparison with bran.[176] It has also been used in combination with antispasmodics, anxiolytics, and antidepressants, and has a synergistic effect in such combinations[177] in some studies. Soluble fiber (such as psyllium, methylcellulose, or calcium polycarbophil) is most effective for constipation predominant IBS patients, and should be gradually increased over a period of weeks to avoid bloating and flatulence.

High-Fiber Diets

The role of a high-fiber diet for IBS is debatable, given the above controversies regarding bran as treatment for IBS. In an open-label trial, the symptoms that have been shown to benefit most from a high fiber diet are hard stools, constipation, and urgency. In this study, all patients who were able to consume 30 g or more fiber improved symptomatically.[178] In another trial of 14 patients followed for two to three years, 50% improved greatly, whereas 28.5% had worsening of their symptoms.[179] In conclusion, fiber is not ideal therapy for all patients with IBS, but should be tried especially in patients with constipation-predominant symptoms.

Food Allergies and IBS

Patients with IBS have many food intolerances, although a small number of these represent true food allergies. Food intolerances are typically to more than one item and are not specific, suggesting intolerance to food in general exists, rather than true food sensitivity. Problem foods are identified in 6 to 58% of cases, depending on the study.[180] The most common adverse food reactions, confirmed on double-blind challenge, are to milk, wheat, eggs, dairy products, corn, peas, tea, coffee, potatoes, nuts, wine, citrus fruits, tomatoes, chocolate, bananas, tuna fish, celery, and yeast. Some authors believe that these foods represent foods with a high salicylate content.[180] Many adverse reactions to food are not the classical wheal and flare type, a mere 3% are truly anaphylactoid-like and cause rash or swelling of the lips or throat,[181] and only some of the reactions are able to be confirmed by skin prick testing.[182] Most of the true food allergies in IBS are seen in patients with other atopic diseases.[183,184] Furthermore, most true food allergies on testing may not be clinically relevant. In a study of IBS patients, food intolerance was identified in 62.5%; skin prick tests to various foods were positive in 52.3%; but, strikingly, only

13.7% of the patients were symptomatic with foods that they were allergic to on prick tests.[182] These findings argue against undertaking a search for food allergies as part of the clinical evaluation of IBS patients.

A positive response to elimination diets in IBS ranges from 15 to 71%, but most studies have methodological flaws.[180] Supporting the role of food allergy in IBS, equal improvement of symptoms up to 50% has been noted in both study groups in trials with diet versus sodium chromoglycate administration for diarrhea-predominant disease.[185,186] These findings need to be confirmed in well-designed placebo controlled experiments before they can be considered clinically applicable, given a high placebo response rate in IBS.

Recently an *in vivo* colonoscopic allergen provocation (COLAP) test based on wheal and flare reactions in the colonic mucosa has been developed, and has shown positive reactions in 77% of patients with food-related symptoms.[187] The clinical utility of this test in IBS is yet to be determined.

In conclusion, a small subgroup of patients with true food allergies is classified as IBS. These patients tend to have atopy in general, and diarrhea-predominant disease. In selected patients, a symptom and food diary may be useful as an initial investigation for food allergy. Foods that lead to symptoms may then be eliminated and rechallenges may be done. Referral to an allergy specialist may be useful in such cases.

For the majority of cases, however, elimination of certain foods that the individual patient believes to cause symptoms is adequate therapy. Physicians also need to ensure that the patient's self-imposed dietary restrictions do not lead to macro- or micronutrient deficiencies.

Carbohydrates in IBS

Fructose and Sorbitol

A number of studies show that IBS symptoms are exacerbated in patients after ingesting fructose and sorbitol mixtures. Fructose is a natural ingredient of fruits, as is sorbitol. The latter is also a common sweetener in dietetic foods. Ingestion of 10 g of sorbitol, equivalent of 4 to 5 sugar-free mints or two medium pears, can produce moderate to severe abdominal discomfort, bloating, and diarrhea in 27% of healthy volunteers.[188] Symptoms may last up to six hours.

A subset of IBS patients has true malabsorption of fructose and sorbitol as assessed by breath hydrogen production,[189,190] although the level of breath hydrogen produced does not necessarily correlate with the degree of symptoms.[191] Whether fructose and sorbitol malabsorption is more common or more severe among IBS patients compared to healthy controls is uncertain. In one large study, there was no higher incidence or higher level of malabsorption.[192] Among malabsorbers, symptoms cannot be explained by changes in jejunal sensitivity and motor function of the small bowel. At present, avoidance of sorbitol and high intakes of fructose may be considered in selected patients.

Lactose

Subjective lactose intolerance is also increased in IBS, and lactose malabsorption is common. Most lactose malabsorbers among IBS patients are malabsorbers of fructose and sorbitol as well. However, elimination of lactose from the diet does not impact on the disease course or reduce symptoms when assessed objectively in long-term followup.[193] In contrast with these findings, many patients subjectively feel that identification of their lactose malabsorptive state has helped them gain awareness of food-symptom relationships and alleviate their symptoms partially. Treatment with lactase[194] or acidophilus milk have shown no benefit over unaltered milk in IBS patients with and without lactose malabsorption.

Therapies Directed against Gas Production and Enzyme Therapies

Gas in the upper GI tract is a result of swallowed air and the carbon dioxide generated by chemical reactions of acid and alkali substances, whereas in the colon, gas forms as a result of fermentation of nutrients by the bacterial flora. Bloating and gas are common complaints of patients with IBS, even though the total amount of gas in the intestinal tract is not increased.[195] Rather, IBS patients have a hypersensitivity to the presence of gas, resulting in discomfort and pain. Therefore, therapies directed against gas seem reasonable in symptomatic patients.

In order to reduce air in the upper digestive tract, patients may be instructed to eat smaller quantities, avoid eating on the run, not talk during eating, avoid carbonated beverages, chewing gum, smoking, and excessive fluid intake with meals. Additionally, simethicone may be tried despite its questionable efficacy, as it poses no harm to patients other than their pocketbooks.[196]

One small study suggests that pancreatic enzyme supplements (30,000 USP lipase-112,500 USP protease-99,600 USP amylase) may reduce symptomatic bloating, gas, and fullness without significant decreases in breath hydrogen or methane levels in healthy subjects in response to a high-fat meal.[197] It is unknown whether the marginal symptomatic benefit in this study can be translated into patients with functional dyspepsia or IBS.

Activated charcoal has been shown to be partially effective in reducing gas in the lower GI tract.[196,198] A preparation called "Beano," containing the enzyme beanase, has been reported to reduce flatulence and breath hydrogen produced after ingestion of mashed black beans, although no studies exist demonstrating its clinical utility in IBS.[199]

It is commonly recommended that IBS patients avoid known gas-producing foods such as cabbage, legumes, lentils, beans, and certain cruciferous vegetables such as cauliflower and broccoli, although such a diet has not been tested, either. Interestingly, King and colleagues[200] have devised an elimination diet that reduces abnormal colonic fermentation. This diet allows meat and fish except beef, replaces all dairy products with soy products, eliminates all grains except rice, and restricts yeast, citrus, caffeinated drinks, and tap water. A pilot study of diarrhea predominant patients on this elimination diet has demonstrated reduction in median symptom scores, compared to controls. Further studies are needed before such a restrictive diet can be recommended for IBS in general.

Nutritional tips for patients with FGIDs are summarized in Table 57.18.

Diverticular Disease of the Colon

Definition and Epidemiology

Diverticular disease of the colon is common in Western countries. The incidence increases with age, but the true incidence is difficult to determine, since most patients remain asymptomatic. Nonetheless it is rare before age 40, and can be found in up to two-thirds of patients over the age of 80.[201-203] In contrast to Western countries (U.S., Australia, and European countries) diverticula are less common in South America, and extraordinarily rare in Africa and rural Asia. Owing to worldwide geographical variability, diverticular disease of the colon has been termed a disease of Western civilization.

TABLE 57.18

Summary of Nutritional Tips for the IBS Patient

1. If constipation predominant IBS, try soluble fiber supplements
2. If diarrhea predominant disease and atopic patient, keep food diary and seek help from an allergy specialist
3. Avoid only those foods that cause symptoms every time they are consumed
4. Replace consumption of heavily processed foods, containing preservatives, additives, food coloring, etc., with a natural balanced diet
5. Seek help from a dietitian to ensure adequate macro- and micronutrient intake if having to avoid many food items
6. Avoid gas-producing vegetables (e.g., legumes, cruciferous vegetables, etc.)
7. Avoid carbonated and caffeinated beverages

The majority of diverticula are histologically pseudodiverticula, which are herniations of the mucosa and submucosa through the muscular layer of the colon as opposed to true diverticula, which involve all layers. The sigmoid colon is the most frequent location for diverticular disease in the U.S.

Mechanisms

Role of Diet in the Pathogenesis

Dietary fiber deficiency along with the theory of colonic segmentation has been the leading hypothesis for the etiology of diverticular disease of colon. According to the segmentation theory, contraction of the colon at the haustral folds causes the colon to act as a series of "little bladders" instead of a continuous single-chambered lumen.[202] Formation of these segments leads to delayed transport, increased water absorption, and more importantly, a rise in intraluminal pressure, resulting in mucosal herniation.[204]

The incidence of diverticula within a society increases following the adoption of a Western diet that is low in fiber.[205] This is supported by animal data as well as epidemiological studies.[205,206] Compared to patients on a diet high in fiber content, those who consume a low-fiber diet have a threefold increase in the incidence of diverticulosis.[207] Consumption of a low-fiber Westernized diet leads to a lower intake of crude cereal grains, increase in consumption of white flour, refined sugar, conserves, and meat. Lack of "adequate" dietary fiber decreases stool weight, prolongs transit time, and increases the colonic intraluminal pressure, all of which predispose to the diverticula formation in concert with segmentation.[202,208] Additionally, a high meat diet changes bacterial metabolism in the colon, and bacteria may produce a toxic metabolite favoring diverticulosis, which is hypothesized to be a spasmogen, or an agent that weakens the colonic wall.[209]

Diet and Diverticulosis

Diet in Prevention of Diverticulosis

Given the importance of fiber in the pathogenesis of diverticula, it is reasonable to recommend a high-fiber diet in the prevention of diverticular disease. Confirming the importance of high-fiber diet as a prophylactic measure, the Health Professionals Follow-up Study, which included over 50 thousand health professionals, showed an inverse relationship between the amount of dietary fiber intake and the risk of developing symptomatic diverticular disease. Those who consumed more that 32 g/day of fiber had the greatest benefit.[210]

Diet in Treatment of Symptomatic Disease

The beneficial effects of dietary fiber on symptomatic uncomplicated diverticular disease continue to be subject to debate. Two controlled trials that evaluated the impact of fiber supplementation in patients with uncomplicated diverticulosis showed conflicting results.[211,212] However, this disagreement does not preclude the potential benefits from a trial of high-fiber diet, which still seems a reasonable approach. The American Society of Colon and Rectal Surgeons practice guidelines recommend the resumption of a high fiber diet following the resolution of uncomplicated acute diverticulitis.[213] In cases of complicated diverticular disease, the patient should be placed on clear liquid diet or be kept NPO in order to achieve bowel rest, which remains the mainstay of therapy along with the antibiotics. There is neither evidence nor scientific basis for avoidance of nuts, popcorn, or seeds for prevention of symptomatic attacks, even though this recommendation seems to be common.

References

1. Dieterich W, Ehnis T, Bauer M, et al. *Nat Med* 3:797; 1997.
2. Kagnoff MF, Paterson YJ, Kumar PJ, et al. *Gut* 28:995; 1987.
3. Corazza GR, Di Sario A, Sacco G, et al. *J Intern Med* 236:183; 1994.
4. Mazure RM, Vazquez H, Gonzalez D, et al. *Am J Gastroenterol* 91:726; 1996.
5. Mustalahti K, Collin P, Sievanen H, Salmi J, Maki M. *Lancet* 354:744; 1999.
6. Rude RK, Olerich M. *Osteoporos Int* 6:453; 1996.
7. Valdimarsson T, Lofman O, Toss G, Strom M. *Gut* 38:322; 1996.
8. McFarlane XA, Bhalla AK, Robertson DA. *Gut* 39:180; 1996.
9. Mautalen C, Gonzalez D, Mazure R, et al. *Am J Gastroenterol* 92:313 1997.
10. Bai JC, Gonzalez D, Mautalen C, et al. *Aliment Pharmacol Ther* 11:157; 1997.
11. McFarlane XA, Bhalla AK, Reeves DE, et al. *Gut* 36:710; 1995.
12. Logan RF, Rifkind EA, Turner ID, Ferguson A. *Gastroenterology* 97:265; 1989.
13. Holmes GK, Prior P, Lane MR, et al. *Gut* 30:333; 1989.
14. Leonard JN, Tucker WF, Fry JS, et al. *Br Med J (Clin Res Ed)* 286:16; 1983.
15. Grefte JM, Bouman JG, Grond J, et al. *J Clin Pathol* 41:886; 1988.
16. Roufail WM, Ruffin JM. *Am J Dig Dis* 11:587; 1966.
17. Regan PT, DiMagno EP. *Gastroenterology* 78:484; 1980.
18. DiMagno EP, Go WL, Summerskill WH. *Gastroenterology* 63:25; 1972.
19. Carroccio A, Iacono G, Montalto G, et al. *Dig Dis Sci* 39:2235; 1994.
20. Carroccio A, Iacono G, Montalto G, et al. *Dig Dis Sci* 40:2555; 1995.
21. Faulkner-Hogg KB, Selby WS, Loblay RH. *Scand J Gastroenterol* 34:784; 1999.
22. Trier JS, Falchuk ZM, Carey MC, Schreiber DS. *Gastroenterology* 75:307; 1978.
23. Sinclair TS, Kumar JS, Dawson AM. *Gut* 24: A494 1983.
24. Longstreth GF. *Ann Intern Med* 119:1014; 1993 & 120:443; 1994.
25. Love A, Elmes M, Golden M, McMaster D. In: *Perspectives in Celiac Disease*. McNicholl B. MCF, Fottrell PF, Ed, Lancaster, England, MTP, 1978, pg 335.
26. Jones PE, L'Hirondel C, Peters TJ. *Gut* 23:108; 1982.
27. Kumar PJ, O'Donoghue DP, Stenson K, Dawson AM. *Gut* 20:743; 1979.
28. Chartrand LJ, Russo PA, Duhaime AG, Seidman EG. *J Am Diet Assoc* 97:612; 1997.
29. Selby WS, Painter D, Collins A, et al. *Scand J Gastroenterol* 34:909; 1999.
30. Dissanayake AS, Truelove SC, Whitehead R. *Br Med J* 4:189; 1975.
31. de Ritis G, Auricchio S, Jones HW, et al. *Gastroenterology* 94:41; 1988.
32. Vainio E, Varjonen E. *Int Arch Allergy Immunol* 106:134; 1995.
33. Srinivasan U, Leonard N, Jones E, et al. *Br Med J* 313:1300; 1996.
34. Hardman CM, Garioch JJ, Leonard JN, et al. *N Engl J Med* 337:1884; 1997.

35. Janatuinen EK, Pikkarainen PH, Kemppainen TA, et al. *N Engl J Med* 333:1033; 1996.
36. Auricchio S, Follo D, de Ritis G, et al. *J Pediatr Gastroenterol Nutr* 2:428; 1983.
37. Bouguerra F, Hajjem S, Guilloud-Bataille M, et al. *Arch Pediatr* 5:621; 1998.
38. Greco L, Mayer M, Grimaldi M, et al. *J Pediatr Gastroenterol Nutr* 4:52; 1985.
39. Ivarsson A, Persson LA, Nystrom L, et al. *Acta Paediatr* 89:165; 2000.
40. Ascher H, Krantz I, Rydberg L, et al. *Arch Dis Child* 76:;1997.
41. Han PD, Burke A, Baldassano RN, et al. *Gastroenterol Clin North Am* 28:423; 1999.
42. Klein S, Meyers S, O'Sullivan P, et al. *J Clin Gastroenterol* 10:34; 1988.
43. Al-Jaouni R, Hebuterne X, Pouget I, Rampal P. *Nutrition* 16:173; 2000.
44. Stokes MA, Hill GL. *J Parent Enteral Nutr* 17:3; 1993.
45. Kushner RF, Schoeller DA. *Am J Clin Nutr* 53:161; 1982.
46. Barot LR, Rombeau JL, Feurer ID, Mullen JL. *Ann Surg* 195:214; 1982.
47. Capristo E, Mingrone G, Addolorato G, et al. *J Intern Med* 243:339; 1998.
48. Mingrone G, Capristo E, Greco AV, et al. *Am J Clin Nutr* 69:325; 1999.
49. Mingrone G, Benedetti G, Capristo E, et al. *Am J Clin Nutr* 67:118; 1998.
50. Christie PM, Hill GL. *Gastroenterology* 99:730; 1990.
51. Ballegaard M, Bjergstrom A, Brondum S, et al. *Scand J Gastroenterol* 32:569; 1997.
52. Rigaud D, Angel LA, Cerf M, et al. *Am J Clin Nutr* 60:775; 1994.
53. Cowan FJ, Warner JT, Dunstan FD, et al. *Arch Dis Child* 76:325; 1997.
54. Mayberry JF, Rhodes J, Allan R, et al. *Dig Dis Sci* 26:444; 1981.
55. Persson PG, Ahlbom A, Hellers G. *Epidemiology* 3:47; 1992.
56. Panza E, Franceschi S, La Vecchia C, et al. *Ital J Gastro* 19:205; 1987.
57. Dietary and Other Risk Factors of Ulcerative Colitis. A Case-Control Study in Japan. Epidemiology Group of the Research Committee of Inflammatory Bowel Disease in Japan. *J Clin Gastroenterol* 19:166; 1994.
58. Reif S, Klein I, Lubin F, et al. *Gut* 40:754; 1997.
59. Mayberry JF, Rhodes J, Newcombe RG. *Digestion* 20:323; 1980.
60. Jarnerot G, Jarnmark I, Nilsson K. *Scand J Gastroenterol* 18:999; 1983.
61. Thornton JR, Emmett PM, Heaton KW. *Br Med J* 280:293; 1980.
62. Thornton JR, Emmett PM, Heaton KW. *Br Med J (Clin Res Ed)* 290:1786; 1985.
63. Kasper H, Sommer H. *Am J Clin Nutr* 32:1898; 1979.
64. Thornton JR, Emmett PM, Heaton KW. *Br Med J* 2:762; 1979.
65. Shoda R, Matsueda K, Yamato S, Umeda N. *Am J Clin Nutr* 63:741; 1996.
66. Gudmand-Hoyer E, Jarnum S. *Gut* 11:338; 1970.
67. Wright R, Truelove SC. *Br Med J* 250:138; 1965.
68. Salem SN, Truelove SC. *Br Med J* 250:827; 1965.
69. Salem SN, Truelove SC, Richards WCD. *Br Med J* 248:394; 1964.
70. Park RH, Duncan A, Russell RI. *Am J Gastroenterol* 85:708; 1990.
71. Cady AB, Rhodes JB, Littman A, Crane RK. *J Lab Clin Med* 70:279; 1967.
72. Taylor KB, Truelove SC. *Br Med J* 242:924;1961.
73. Dudek B, Spiro HM, Thayer WR. *Gastroenterology* 49:544; 1965.
74. Jewell DP, Truelove SC. *Gut* 13:796; 1972.
75. Sewell P, Cooke WT, Cox EV, Meynell MJ. *Lancet* 2:1132; 1963.
76. Knoflach P, Park BH, Cunningham R, et al. *Gastroenterology* 92:479; 1987.
77. Wright R, Truelove SR. *Am J Dig Dis* 11:847; 1966.
78. Koletzko S, Sherman P, Corey M, et al. *Br Med J* 298:1617; 1989.
79. Koletzko S, Griffiths A, Corey M, et al. *Br Med J* 302:1580; 1991.
80. Imes S, Pinchbeck B, Thomson AB. *Digestion* 39:7; 1988.
81. Ritchie JK, Wadsworth J, Lennard-Jones JE, Rogers E. *Br Med J (Clin Res Ed)* 295:517; 1987.
82. Levenstein S, Prantera C, Luzi C, D'Ubaldi A. *Gut* 26:989; 1985.
83. Gottschall E. Breaking the Vicious Cycle, 1999 ed, Baltimore, Ontario, Kirkton Press Ltd., 1999.
84. Jones VA, Dickinson RJ, Workman E, et al. *Lancet* 2:177; 1985.
85. Pearson M, Teahon K, Levi AJ, Bjarnason I. *Gut* 34:783; 1993.
86. Ruuska T, Savilahti E, Maki M, et al. *J Pediatr Gastroenterol Nutr* 19:175; 1994.
87. Iannoli P, Miller JH, Ryan CK, et al. *Surgery* 122:721 & 728; 1997.

88. Byrne TA, Persinger RL, Young LS, et al. *Ann Surg* 222:243 & 254; 1995.
89. Slonim AE, Bulone L, Damore MB, et al. *N Engl J Med* 342:1633; 2000.
90. Hawthorne AB, Daneshmend TK, Hawkey CJ, et al. *Gut* 33:922; 1992.
91. Stenson WF, Cort D, Rodgers J, et al. *Ann Intern Med* 116:609; 1992.
92. Aslan A, Triadafilopoulos G. *Am J Gastroenterol* 87:432; 1992.
93. Greenfield SM, Green AT, Teare JP, et al. *Aliment Pharmacol Ther* 7:159; 1993.
94. Ikehata A, Hiwatashi N, Kinouchi Y, et al. *Am J Clin Nutr* 56:938; 1992.
95. Eysselein VE, Reinshagen M, Patel A, et al. *Ann N Y Acad Sci* 657:319; 1992.
96. Breuer RI, Buto SK, Christ ML, et al. *Dig Dis Sci* 36:185; 1991.
97. Steinhart AH, Brzezinski A, Baker JP. *Am J Gastroenterol* 89:179; 1994.
98. Patz J, Jacobsohn WZ, Gottschalk-Sabag S, et al. *Am J Gastroenterol* 91:731; 1994.
99. Scheppach W, Sommer H, Kirchner T, et al. *Gastroenterology* 103:51; 1992.
100. Rolandelli RH, Saul SH, Settle RG, et al. *Am J Clin Nutr* 47:715; 1988.
101. Rembacken BJ, Snelling AM, Hawkey PM, et al. *Lancet* 354:635; 1999.
102. Gionchetti P, Rizzello F, Venturi A, et al. *Gastroenterology* 119:305; 2000.
103. Umemoto Y, Tanimura H, Ishimoto K. *Gastroenterology* 114:A1102; 1998.
104. O'Morain C, Segal AW, Levi AJ. *Br Med J (Clin Res Ed)* 288:1859; 1984.
105. Gorard DA, Hunt JB, Payne-James JJ, et al. *Gut* 34:1198; 1993.
106. Seidman EG, Bouthullier L, Weber AM. *Gastroenterology* 90:A1625; 1986.
107. Griffiths AM, Ohlsson A, Sherman PM, Sutherland LR. *Gastroenterology* 108:1056; 1995.
108. Gonzalez-Huix F, de Leon R, Fernandez-Banares F, et al. *Gut* 34:778; 1993.
109. Dieleman LA, Heizer WD. *Gastroenterol Clin North Am* 27:435; 1998.
110. Lochs H, Steinhardt HJ, Klaus-Wentz B, et al. *Gastroenterology* 101:881; 1991.
111. Axelsson C, Jarnum S. *Scand J Gastroenterol* 12:89; 1977.
112. O'Brien CJ, Giaffer MH, Cann PA, Holdsworth CD. *Am J Gastroenterol* 86:1614; 1991.
113. Lochs H, Egger-Schodl M, Schuh R, et al. *Klin Wochenschr* 62:821; 1984.
114. McIntyre PB, Powell-Tuck J, Wood SR, et al. *Gut* 27:481; 1986.
115. Greenberg GR, Fleming CR, Jeejeebhoy KN, et al. *Gut* 29:1309; 1988.
116. Rombeau JL, Barot LR, Williamson CE, Mullen JL. *Am J Surg* 143:139 1982.
117. Dickinson RJ, Ashton MG, Axon AT, et al. *Gastroenterology* 79:1199; 1980.
118. Elson CO, Layden TJ, Nemchausky BA, et al. *Dig Dis Sci* 25:42; 1980.
119. Sitzmann JV, Converse RL, Jr, Bayless TM. *Gastroenterology* 99:1647; 1990.
120. Solomons NW, Rosenberg IH, Sandstead HH, Vo-Khactu KP. *Digestion* 16:87; 1977.
121. Muller JM, Keller HW, Erasmi H, Pichlmaier H. *Br J Surg* 70:40; 1983.
122. Fernandez-Banares F, Abad-Lacruz A, Xiol X, et al. *Am J Gastroenterol* 84:744; 1989.
123. Kuroki F, Iida M, Tominaga M, et al. *Dig Dis Sci* 38:1614; 1993.
124. Harries AD, Brown R, Heatley RV, et al. *Gut* 26:1197; 1985.
125. Vogelsang H, Ferenci P, Woloszczuk W, et al. *Dig Dis Sci* 34:1094; 1989.
126. Lashner BA, Heidenreich PA, Su GL. *Gastroenterology* 97:255; 1989.
127. Lashner BA, Provencher KS, Seidner DL. *Gastroenterology* 112:29; 1997.
128. Kruis W, Rindfleisch GE, Weinzierl M. *Hepatogastroenterology* 32:133; 1985.
129. Ostro MJ, Greenberg GR, Jeejeebhoy KN. *J Parent Enteral Nutr* 9:280; 1985.
130. Hawker PC, Givel JC, Keighley MR, et al. *Gut* 24:284; 1983.
131. Teahon K, Bjarnason I, Pearson M, Levi AJ. *Gut* 31:1133; 1990.
132. Calam J, Crooks PE, Walker RJ. *J Parent Enteral Nutr* 4:4; 1980.
133. Levine JB, Lukawski-Trubish D. *Gastroenterol Clin North Am* 24:633; 1995.
134. Nightingale JM, Bartram CI, Lennard-Jones JE. *Gastrointest Radiol* 16:305; 1991.
135. Fielding JF, Cooke WT, Williams JA. *Lancet* 1:1106; 1971.
136. Murphy JP, Jr., King DR, Dubois A. *N Engl J Med* 300:80; 1979.
137. Cortot A, Fleming CR, Malagelada JR. *N Engl J Med* 300:79; 1979.
138. Jeppesen PB, Staun M, Tjellesen L, Mortensen PB. *Gut* 43:763; 1998.
139. Farthing MJ. *Digestion* 54(Suppl 1):47; 1993.
140. Vanderhoof JA, Kollman KA. *J Pediatr Gastroenterol Nutr* 26:241; 1998.
141. Woolf GM, Miller C, Kurian R, Jeejeebhoy KN. *Dig Dis Sci* 32:8; 1987.
142. Levitt MD. *Gastroenterology* 85:769; 1983.

143. Bond JH, Currier BE, Buchwald H, Levitt MD. *Gastroenterology* 78:444; 1980.
144. Nordgaard I, Hansen BS, Mortensen PB. *Lancet* 343:373; 1994.
145. Mobarhan S. *Nutr Rev* 52:354; 1994.
146. McIntyre PB, Fitchew M, Lennard-Jones JE. *Gastroenterology* 91:25; 1986.
147. Messing B, Pigot F, Rongier M, et al. *Gastroenterology* 100:1502; 1991.
148. Bochenek W, Rodgers JB, Jr., Balint JA. *Ann Intern Med* 72:205; 1970.
149. Vanderhoof JA, Grandjean CJ, Kaufman SS. *J Parent Enteral Nutr* 8:685; 1984.
150. Jeppesen PB, Mortensen PB. *Gut* 43:478; 1998.
151. Gruy-Kapral C, Little KH, Fordtran JS, et al. *Gastroenterology* 116:15; 1999.
152. Selby PL, Peacock M, Bambach CP. *Br J Surg* 71:334; 1984.
153. Fleming CR, George L, Stoner GL, et al. *Mayo Clin Proc* 71:21; 1996.
154. Nightingale JM, Lennard-Jones JE, Gertner DJ. et al. *Gut* 33:1493; 1992.
155. Doty JE, Pitt HA, Porter-Fink V, Denbesten L. *Ann Surg* 201:76; 1985.
156. Thompson JS. *Arch Surg* 131:556 & 559; 1996.
157. Anon. *Lancet* 336:599; 1990.
158. Mayne AJ, Handy DJ, Preece MA, et al. *Arch Dis Child* 65:229; 1990.
159. Pizarro D, Posada G, Sandi L, Moran JR. *N Engl J Med* 324:517; 1991 & 326:488; 1992.
160. Krishnan S, Ramakrishna BS, Binder HJ. *Dig Dis Sci* 44:1924; 1999.
161. Ramakrishna BS, Venkataraman S, Srinivasan P, et al. *N Engl J Med* 342:308; 2000.
162. Mathews CJ, MacLeod RJ, Zheng SX, *Gastroenterology* 116:1342; 1999.
163. Pochapin M. *Am J Gastroenterol* 95:S11; 2000.
164. Drossman DA. *Gut* 45 Suppl 2:II1; 1999.
165. Gee MI, Grace MG, Wensel RH, et al. *J Am Diet Assoc* 85:1591; 1985.
166. Payler DK, Pomare EW, Heaton KW, Harvey RF. *Gut* 16:209; 1975.
167. Manning AP, Heaton KW, Harvey RF. *Lancet* 2:417; 1977.
168. Soltoft J, Krag B, Gudmand-Hoyer E. *Lancet* 1:270; 1974.
169. Hillman LC, Stace NH, Fisher A, Pomare EW. *Am J Clin Nutr* 36:626; 1982.
170. Snook J, Shepherd HA. *Aliment Pharmacol Ther* 8:511; 1994.
171. Lucey MR, Clark ML, Lowndes J, Dawson AM. *Gut* 28:221; 1987.
172. Arffmann S, Andersen JR, Hegnhoj J, et al. *Scand J Gastroenterol* 20:295; 1985.
173. Francis CY, Whorwell PJ. *Lancet* 344:39; 1994.
174. Cann PA, Read NW, Holdsworth CD. *Gut* 25:168; 1984.
175. Kruis W, Weinzierl M, Schussler P, Holl J. *Digestion* 34:196; 1986.
176. Hotz J, Plein K. *Med Klin* 89:645; 1994.
177. Ritchie JA, Truelove SC. *Br Med J* 1:376; 1979.
178. Lambert JP, Brunt PW, Mowat NA, et al. *Eur J Clin Nutr* 45:601; 1991.
179. Hillman LC, Stace NH, Pomare EW. *Am J Gastroenterol* 79:1; 1984.
180. Niec AM, Frankum B, Talley NJ. *Am J Gastroenterol* 93:2184; 1998.
181. Locke GR, 3rd, Zinsmeister AR, Talley NJ, et al. *Am J Gastroenterol* 95:157; 2000.
182. Dainese R, Galliani EA, De Lazzari F, et al. *Am J Gastroenterol* 94:1892; 1999.
183. Bentley SJ, Pearson DJ, Rix KJ. *Lancet* 2:295; 1983.
184. Petitpierre M, Gumowski P, Girard JP. *Ann Allergy* 54:538; 1985.
185. Stefanini GF, Saggioro A, Alvisi V, et al. *Scand J Gastroenterol* 30:535; 1995.
186. Stefanini GF, Prati E, Albini MC, et al. *Am J Gastroenterol* 87:55; 1992.
187. Bischoff SC, Mayer J, Wedemeyer J, et al. *Gut* 40:745; 1997.
188. Jain NK, Rosenberg DB, Ulahannan MJ, et al. *Am J Gastroenterol* 80:678; 1985.
189. Fernandez-Banares F, Esteve-Pardo M, de Leon R, et al. *Am J Gastroenterol* 88:2044; 1993.
190. Rumessen JJ, Gudmand-Hoyer E. *Gastroenterology* 95:694; 1988.
191. Symons P, Jones MP, Kellow JE. *Scand J Gastroenterol* 27:940; 1992.
192. Nelis GF, Vermeeren MA, Jansen W. *Gastroenterology* 99:1016.
193. Tolliver BA, Jackson MS, Jackson KL. *J Clin Gastroenterol* 23:15; 1996.
194. Lisker R, Solomons NW, Perez Briceno R. *Am J Gastroenterol* 84:756; 1989.
195. Lasser RB, Bond JH, Levitt MD. *N Engl J Med* 293:524; 1975.
196. Jain NK, Patel VP, Pitchumoni S. *Ann Intern Med* 105:61; 1986.
197. Suarez F, Levitt MD, Adshead J, Barkin JS. *Dig Dis Sci* 44:1317; 1999.

198. Jain NK, Patel VP, Pitchumoni CS. *Am J Gastroenterol* 81:532; 1986.
199. Friedman G. *Gastroenterol Clin North Am* 20:313; 1991.
200. King TS, Elia M, Hunter JO. *Lancet* 352:1187; 1998.
201. Painter NS, Burkitt DP. *Br Med J* 2:450; 1975.
202. Painter NS, Burkitt DP. *Clin Gastroenterol* 4:3; 1975.
203. Parks TG. *Clin Gastroenterol* 4:53; 1975.
204. Srivastava GS, Smith AN, Painter NS. *Br Med J* 1:315; 1976.
205. Ohi G, Minowa K, Oyama T, et al. *Am J Clin Nutr* 38:115; 1983.
206. Berry CS, Fearn T, Fisher N, et al. *Lancet* 2:294; 1984.
207. Gear JS, Ware A, Fursdon P, et al. *Lancet* 1:511; 1979.
208. Burkitt DP, Walker AR, Painter NS. *JAMA* 229:1068; 1974.
209. Cummings JH, Hill MJ, Jivraj T, et al. *Am J Clin Nutr* 32:2086; 1979.
210. Aldoori WH, Giovannucci EL, Rockett HR. *J Nutr* 128:714; 1998.
211. Brodribb AJ. *Lancet* 1:664; 1977.
212. Ornstein MH, Littlewood ER, Baird IM, *Br Med J (Clin Res Ed)* 282:1353; 1981.
213. Roberts P, Abel M, Rosen L, et al. *Dis. Colon Rectum* 38:125; 1995.

58

Nutrient Metabolism and Support in the Normal and Diseased Liver

Mark T. DeMeo

Introduction

The liver plays a dual role in nutritional wellbeing. First, it contributes to nutrient assimilation through the synthesis of bile acids. At the time of a meal, as the gallbladder contracts, bile acids are released into the gut lumen. These bile acids enable lipids to be absorbed efficiently. Second, the liver plays a major role in substrate metabolism and allocation. It maintains nutrient blood levels at a constant level despite variations in substrate availability. It is therefore not surprising that damage to this vital organ has a tremendous impact on nutritional status.

Role of the Liver in Normal Nutrient Metabolism

Carbohydrates

Certain cells such as neutrophils, erythrocytes, and platelets are obligate utilizers of glucose. Therefore, during periods when glucose is not ingested, such as an overnight fast, glucose requirements continue. Many organs that use glucose during the fed state use fatty acids when supplies of glucose are low. It is estimated that carbohydrates account for 45% of the resting energy expenditure in overnight-fasted humans.[1] In this setting, the liver accounts for about 90% of the glucose released into circulation. Earlier studies suggested that approximately three-quarters of that glucose comes from glycogen, its liver storage form; however, a more recent study determined that glycogen contributes only about one-third to hepatic glucose production during the first 22 hours of fasting.[2] The remaining portion comes from gluconeogenesis.[1,2] *Gluconeogenesis* is the formation of glucose from precursors such as lactate, pyruvate, glycerol, and the gluconeogenic amino acids (mainly alanine, glutamine, and glycine). Gluconeogenesis is regulated by hormones and facilitated by a drop in insulin level and a rise in glucagon secretion, characteristic

0-8493-2705-9/02/$0.00+$1.50

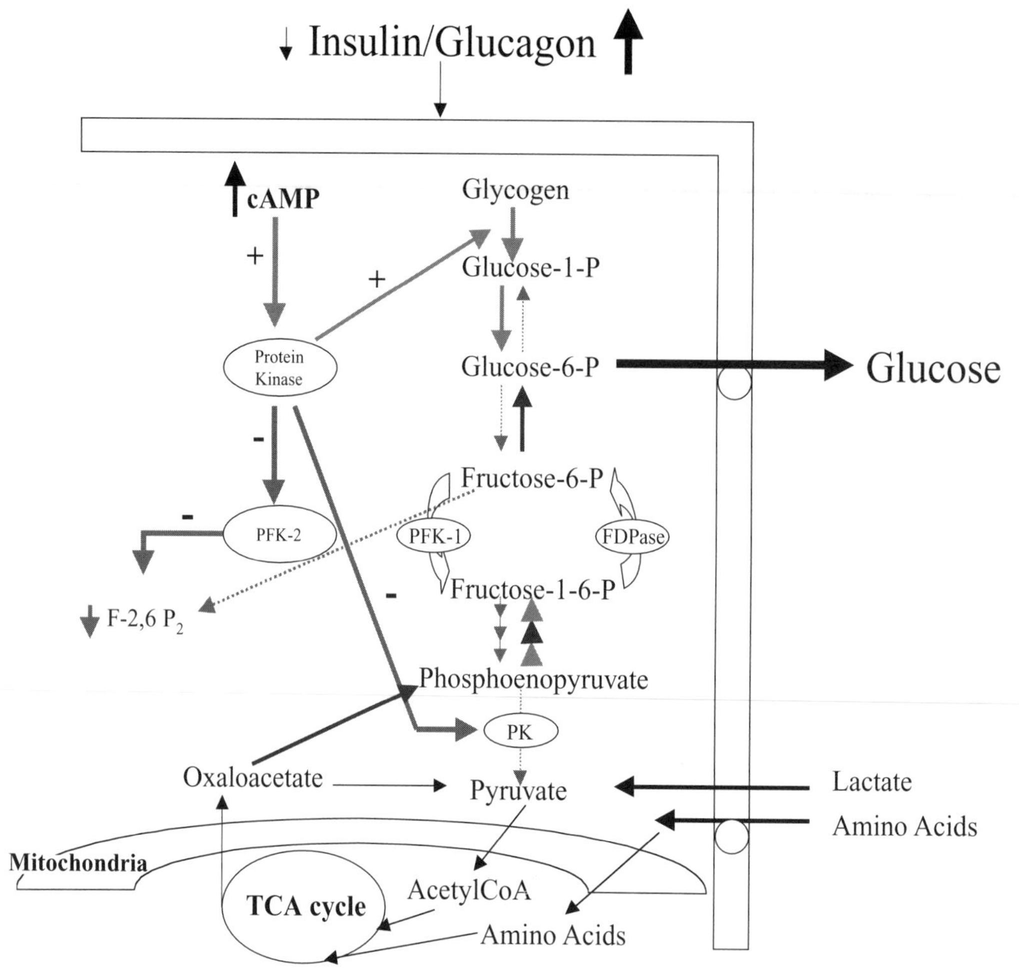

FIGURE 58.1
Hormonal regulation of glucose homeostasis in the liver. During fast, the insulin/glucagon ratio decreases. This stimulates an increase in cAMP in the hepatocyte. cAMP activates cAMP-dependent protein kinase, which activates glycogen phosphorylase. This enzyme leads to the breakdown of glycogen and the formation of glucose-1-phosphate. Protein kinase also inactivates phosphofructokinase-2 (PFK-2). PFK-2 catalyzes the conversion of Fructose-6-Phosphate to fructose-2, 6-bisphosphate (F-2, 6 P_2). F-2, 6 P_2 is an important activator of Phosphofructokinase 1 (PFK-1). The impaired activation of PFK-1 slows glycolysis and favors the conversion of Fructose-1-6-P to Fructose-6-P and ultimately favors the formation of glucose. Protein kinase also interferes with the conversion of Phosphoenopyruvate (PEP) to Pyruvate, by blocking the enzyme pyruvate kinase (PK). This favors the formation of Fructose-1-6-P and ultimately glucose. Glucagon also stimulates gluconeogenesis, in part through carrier mediated uptake of alanine, the major gluconeogenic amino acid. This and other gluconeogenic amino acids enter the TCA cycle with the resultant formation of Oxaloacetate (OAA). OAA is converted to PEP and proceeds toward the formation of Glucose-6-P and ultimately glucose. (Adapted from Brodsky IG. In: *Modern Nutrition in Health and Disease*, 9th ed, Shils ME, Olson JA, Shike M, Ross AC, Eds, Williams and Wilkins, Baltimore, 1999, p. 699.)

of the fasted state. The drop in insulin decreases the activity of pyruvate kinase (Figure 58.1). This "blockage" drives the equation back to Glucose 6-phosphate and ultimately increases hepatic output of glucose.

In the fed state, metabolic and hormonal signals change the liver's response to carbohydrates. It is estimated that between 25 and 45% of an oral glucose load is taken up by the liver. This percentage may increase as the carbohydrate load increases.[1] Glucose taken up by the liver is largely used to replenish the glycogen depleted after an overnight fast.

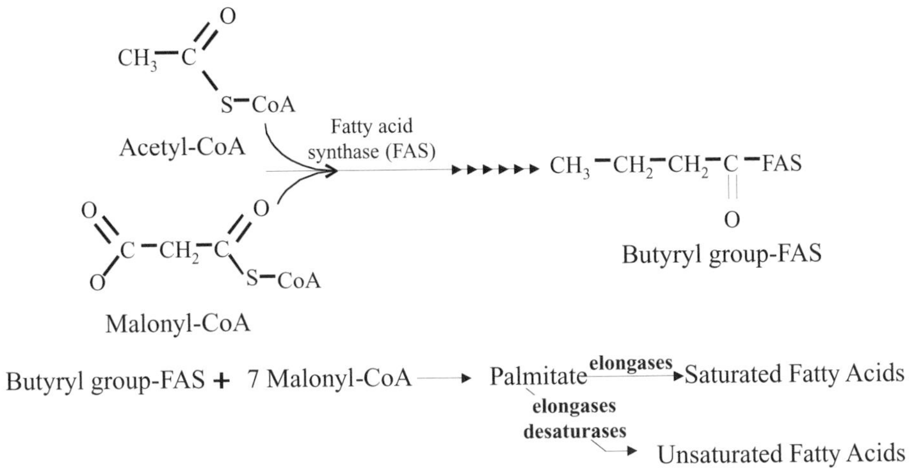

$CH_3-C(=O)-S-CoA$

Acetyl-CoA

Fatty acid synthase (FAS)

$CH_3-CH_2-CH_2-C(=O)-FAS$

Butyryl group-FAS

$^{-}O(O=)C-CH_2-C(=O)-S-CoA$

Malonyl-CoA

Butyryl group-FAS + 7 Malonyl-CoA → Palmitate —elongases→ Saturated Fatty Acids

Palmitate —elongases, desaturases→ Unsaturated Fatty Acids

FIGURE 58.2
Fatty acid synthesis. Acetyl-CoA combines with Malonyl-CoA in the presence of the fatty acid synthase complex. Then through a series of condensation, reduction, dehydration, and translocation steps, a four-carbon, saturated fatty amyl compound is formed. Seven more cycles take place to form plasmatic acid (C16: 0). Other fatty acids, both saturated and unsaturated, can be formed using a series of elongates and desaturases.

High postprandial glucose levels stimulate the pancreas to release insulin. This decreases hepatic glucose production and increases glucose metabolism and storage. Insulin facilitates the synthesis of glycogen by stimulating the enzyme glycogen synthase. However, the liver glycogen concentration also influences synthesis. As the concentration of this storage form of glucose increases, its rate of formation slows. This phenomenon can occur in spite of high insulin levels and glucose concentrations, emphasizing the fact that this is a limited form of energy storage. It should also be noted that glucose is a relatively poor substrate for glycogen synthesis. Only about 50% of "neoglycogens" come from ingested glucose, while the remainder is derived from gluconeogenic precursors. Thus, the amount of carbohydrates presented to the liver could exceed the ability to form glycogen. Insulin also stimulates glucose oxidation by increasing pyruvate dehydrogenase, which converts pyruvate to acetyl-CoA. When the acetyl-CoA generated by glycolysis is not needed for oxidative phosphorylation, it is converted to fatty acids and ultimately to triglycerides[3] (Figure 58.2).

Lipids and Lipoproteins

The liver synthesizes bile acids from cholesterol. The bile acids are secreted in bile and released in response to a meal. When bile acids are released in sufficient quantities, the critical micellar concentration, they will form micelles. Micelles have a hydrophilic or water-soluble surface, and a lipophilic or lipid-soluble core. Most dietary fat is in the form of triglycerides, which are fatty acids esterified to a glycerol backbone. Triglycerides are a major source of both stored and available energy. As pancreatic lipase cleaves the fatty acids from the dietary triglycerides, these water-insoluble molecules are absorbed into the lipophilic core of the micelle. The micelle provides a conduit through the intestinal unstirred water layer to the lipid-soluble membranes of the intestinal enterocyte. The fatty acid diffuses into the lipid-soluble membrane of the enterocyte (Figure 58.3). Medium chain triglycerides can be absorbed directly into the portal vein and do not need this "micellar intermediate" to facilitate absorption. The bile acids are largely taken up by

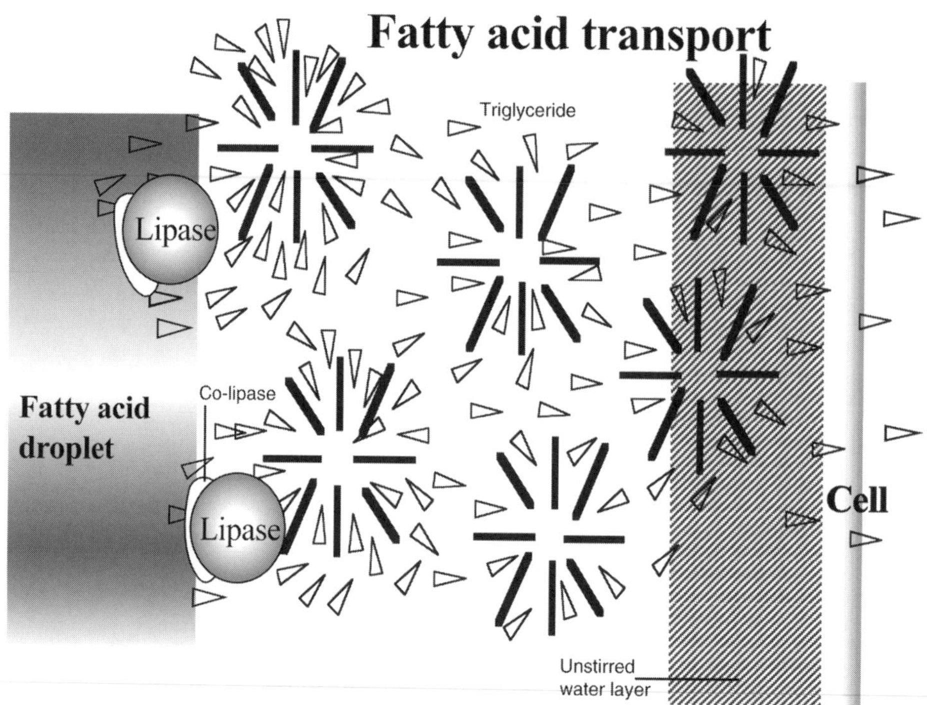

FIGURE 58.3
Fatty acid transport. Co-lipase attaches to the lipid droplet and then binds lipase, the principal enzyme of triglyceride digestion. Lipase then hydrolyzes the ester bonds of the tryglycerides forming free fatty acids. The fatty acids are taken up by the lipophilic inner core of the micelle. The outer core of the micelle is hydrophilic, allowing for this particle to traverse the unstirred water layer of the intestine. The fatty acids in the inner core of the micelle are placed in approximation to the lipid soluble membrane of the enterocyte, allowing for diffusion across the enterocyte membrane. (Adapted from Reference 5.)

receptors in the terminal ileum and transported back to the liver via the enterohepatic circulation. Some unabsorbed bile acids are excreted into the feces.[5]

In the enterocyte, fatty acids are reesterified into triglycerides and packaged into lipoproteins called chylomicrons. Chylomicrons are secreted into the lymphatics, travel through the thoracic duct to the superior vena cava, and are then circulated to target tissues. Chylomicrons are part of the exogenous transport system for lipids. The endogenous system is comprised of three main carriers, VLDL, LDL, and HDL.[5,6] Many of the protein components of these lipoproteins, called apoproteins, are also synthesized in the liver.

The liver can also manufacture triglycerides from fatty acids synthesized by repetitive additions of two carbon fragments, derived from Acetyl-CoA, to malonyl CoA, or from non-esterified fatty acids removed from the blood.[3] Triglycerides synthesized by the liver are transported by the lipoprotein LDL to target tissues. Similarly, cholesterol synthesized in the liver is taken by the LDL carrier to target tissues. Peripheral tissues transport cholesterol back to the liver for excretion by the gallbladder through the action of HDL.

Amino Acids and Proteins

The liver also plays a major role in amino acid homeostasis. Amino acids serve as building blocks of proteins and as precursors to many other important biomolecules, such as purines and pyrimidines. Additionally they can be a source of energy, particularly when they are present in excess of need for visceral or somatic protein synthesis. Amino acids are either essential or non-essential. The distinguishing feature between these two types of amino acids is the ability of the body to synthesize their carbon skeleton. Essential amino acids have a carbon skeleton that cannot be synthesized *de novo* and must be obtained from the diet.

The first step in the catabolic process of most amino acids is the removal of the α-amino group from the carbon skeleton. This occurs via a pathway known as transamination. In the liver, most of α-amino groups derived from ingested protein, muscle protein, or protein from other tissues are separated from the parent carbon skeleton, leaving a ketoacid and an amino group. This amino group is combined with α-ketogluterate to form glutamate. Glutamate then undergoes oxidative deamination in the mitochondria, yielding the protonated form of ammonia (NH_4^+). The NH_4^+ is a co-substrate in forming carbamoyl phosphatase. It then enters the urea cycle. As ammonia is toxic to animals, the urea cycle enzymes, also located largely in the liver, allow excretion of this harmful metabolite (Figure 58.4). Transamination can also occur between other amino acids. The presence of transaminase enzymes in the liver ensures that the liver is able to conserve essential amino acids and interconvert nonessential amino acids. Although most amino acid catabolism occurs in the liver, the three amino acids with branched side chains (leucine, valine, and isoleucine) are particularly noteworthy. They are oxidized as fuels to be used primarily by extrahepatic tissue, particularly muscle, adipose, kidney, and brain. These extrahepatic tissues contain a single aminotransferase not present in the liver. This acts on all three branched chain amino acids (BCAAs) to produce the corresponding α-ketoacid.

Amino acid carbohydrate skeletons can metabolize to pyruvate or intermediates of the tricarboxylic acid cycle. These can be converted into glucose and are called glucogenic amino acids. These precursors contribute to a process known as gluconeogenesis. In humans, gluconeogenesis occurs largely in the liver, and to a much smaller extent in the renal cortex. Since some tissues in the body are obligate glucose utilizers, this pathway is extremely important during periods of relative glucose deficiency. It maintains hepatic glucose output to glucose-utilizing tissues.[8,9]

The liver absorbs amino acids from plasma to be utilized in protein synthesis. The most abundant plasma protein secreted by the liver is albumin. Albumin is the most important regulator of plasma oncotic pressure and is the principal transport protein for many endogenous and exogenous substances. The liver also produces transport proteins for lipids (lipoproteins), iron (transferrin), and copper (caeruloplasmin) as well as steroid hormone-binding proteins, thyroid hormone-binding proteins, and several vitamin-binding proteins. An equally essential role for the liver is the synthesis of many of the coagulation and fibrinolysis proteins. The liver is also the primary site of synthesis of the complement system that plays an important role in host defense against infectious agents. Finally, it is the major site of synthesis of protease inhibitors, inhibitors of coagulation and fibrinolysis, as well as many other proteins involved in immunomodulation, drug binding, and other aspects of the acute phase response.[10]

Impact of Liver Disease on Nutrient Metabolism

Carbohydrates

Damage to the liver can negatively impact glycogen stores. Since the liver is the major source of glucose production in the fasted state, it would be expected that patients with liver disease might have low blood glucose levels after an overnight fast or a prolonged

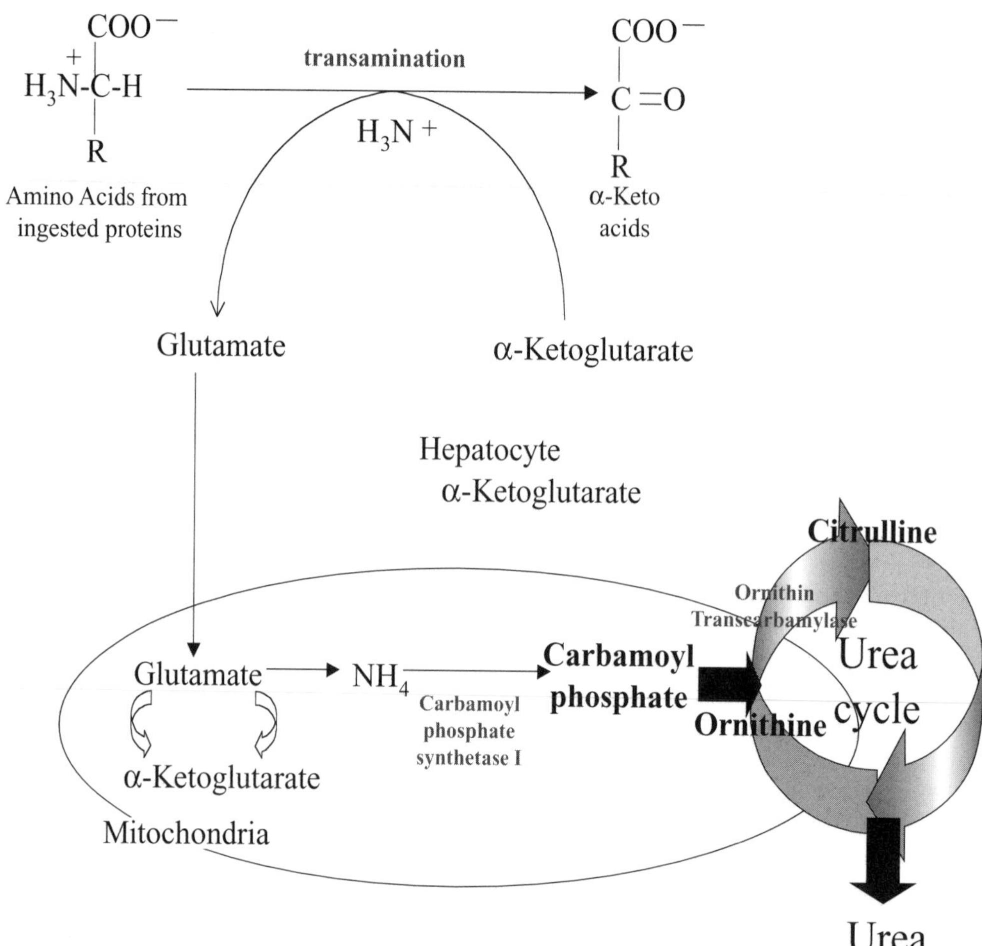

FIGURE 58.4
NH_3 Metabolism. Amino acids from ingested proteins are transaminated to yield NH_3 and α-keto acids. The amino group is then transferred to α-ketogluterate to form glutamate. Glutamate is transported to the hepatocyte mitochondria where α-ketogluterate is reformed with the loss of NH_4. This ammonium group combines with HCO_3 and 2 ATPs to form carbamoyl phosphate. Carbamoyl phosphate enters the urea cycle, is converted to urea after a series of reactions. (Adapted from Nelson DL, Cox MM. In: *Principals of Biochemistry,* 2nd ed, Lehninger AL, Nelson DL, Cox MM, Eds, Worth Publishers, New York, 1993, pg 506.)

absence of oral intake. However, hypoglycemia is rare in liver disease, usually seen only in fulminant hepatic failure or in the terminal stages of chronic hepatic insufficiency. This is probably due to the tremendous reserve capacity of the liver to produce glucose, with approximately 20% of the hepatic mass needed to maintain normal glucose levels in the fasted state.[1]

More commonly, fasting glucose levels in patients with liver disease are normal or high. Despite high levels of glucagon seen in these patients, increased hepatic glucose production does not seem to be a contributing factor. Unless there is coexistent diabetes, studies suggest that hepatic glucose production in liver disease varies from normal to 20-40% lower than normal. However, diabetic cirrhotics with fasting hyperglycemia displayed increased hepatic glucose production, which was not appropriately decreased by insulin.[4]

Since glycogen synthesis is impaired in liver disease and glycogen stores are rapidly depleted in the fasted state, patients with liver disease more rapidly transition to gluconeogeneisis and ketogenesis to fill their glucose and energy needs. It is estimated that gluconeogenesis accounts for about 67% of hepatic glucose production, with the remainder coming from glycogenlysis. The rapid switch to a fatty acid/ketone economy for energy needs is an adaptive response, as it decreases reliance on hepatic glucose production. Glucose production by the damaged liver may be limited due to decreased glycogen stores and potentially diminished delivery of gluconeogenic precursors to the liver.[1]

After glucose ingestion, many patients with liver disease have abnormally elevated blood glucose concentrations.[1] In fact, 60 to 80% of patients with cirrhosis are glucose intolerant, and 10 to 30% eventually develop frank diabetes.[4] In a recent study, non-diabetic cirrhotics given a mixed meal had elevated blood glucose levels in spite of a fivefold increase in blood insulin levels.[12] It appears that in these glucose-intolerant patients, both oxidative and nonoxidative glucose disposal is impaired.[1,4] The oxidative impairment of glucose utilization, the less significant of the two abnormalities, is due in part to the preferential utilization of fatty acids seen in this patient population. The generation of Acetyl-CoA from the metabolism of fatty acids inhibits pyruvate dehydrogenase resulting in a diminution of pyruvate oxidation.[4] The nonoxidative utilization of glucose is essentially the formation of glycogen. In spite of hyperinsulinemia seen in these patients, they demonstrate peripheral insulin resistance. As such, glucose uptake by muscle and stimulation of glycogen synthesis is significantly impaired. This accounts for most of the decreased glucose disposal and consequent glucose intolerance seen in these patients, as hepatic glucose production is still normal in the basal state and normally suppressed by insulin.[1,4] In contrast, liver disease patients with diabetes not only have abnormalities with glucose disposal but also are unable to appropriately suppress hepatic glucose suppression, suggesting a relative lack of insulin. Petrides et al. hypothesized that patients with liver disease become frankly diabetic when the pancreatic β-cells cannot meet the increased demand for insulin secretion due to insulin resistance.[4]

Lipids and Lipoproteins

Since cholesterol is excreted from the body through the biliary tree, the total cholesterol level tends to rise in obstructive jaundice. However, in severe parenchymal disease, cholesterol ester levels tend to fall. This latter sign is the result of reduced activity of lecithin cholesterol acyltransferase (LCAT) activity. LCAT is an enzyme synthesized in the liver that catalyses the transfer of a fatty acid from the 2-position of lecithin to the 3 β-OH group to form cholesterol ester and lysolecithin. It plays a key role in the turnover of cholesterol and lecithin. Low levels of this enzyme also alter the lipid composition of lipoproteins.

Plasma triglycerides are often elevated, both in obstructive, and less often in parenchymal liver disease. Triglycerides are normally cleared by the action of peripheral lipoprotein lipases (LPL) and hepatic triglyceride lipases (HTLP). The latter enzyme levels are reduced in liver disease and may account for triglyceride abnormality.[6]

These changes in lipids may effect membrane lipid content, fluidity, and function. They may, in part, explain the abnormalities associated with liver disease in platelet aggregation and in the morphology of red blood cells.[6] These changes in the lipid content of cell membranes effect all cells in the body. The subsequent effects on membrane fluidity and function have been advanced as a possible contributing factor in the hyporesponsiveness of cirrhotic myocardium to pharmacologic or psychologic stress.[7]

After an overnight fast, cirrhotic patients derive a greater proportion of energy from fat oxidation than do controls. This difference in endogenous energy substrate use has been attributed to diminished glycogen stores. After ingestion of a mixed meal, fat oxidation of cirrhotic patients decreases but still remains elevated compared to controls. The increased reliance on endogenous fat during fasting and the continued high rate of fat oxidation in spite of ingestion of a mixed meal may account for the reduction in body fat stores common in this patient population.[12]

Amino Acids and Proteins

Patients with liver disease often have disturbances in plasma amino acid concentrations, characterized by increased levels of aromatic amino acids and methionine. This is most likely a result of the injured liver's poor utilization of these amino acids as well as portosystemic shunting.[8] Additionally, since the enzymes involved in urea production are largely localized in the liver, urea synthesis, and hence α-amino nitrogen clearance, is lower in cirrhotics compared to controls. In patients with severe decompensated liver disease, the plasma urea level tends to drop and the amount of urea excreted in the urine is reduced. In patients with well-compensated cirrhosis, urea production rates remains stable under basal conditions but maximal urea production capacity is significantly reduced in response to a protein or amino acid load.[8,11]

Chronic alcohol consumption actually increases the synthesis of albumin and constituent hepatic proteins but is also associated with a reduced secretion of these proteins from the liver.[10] However, as liver damage increases, there is a decrease in synthesis of albumin with an apparent significant correlation between its synthesis rate and Childs score (a scoring system based on clinical and laboratory values that is used to demonstrate the severity of the underlying liver disease).[10] Although the albumin is used in many different prognostic scoring systems, it should be remembered that the plasma concentration of albumin is not only dependent on synthesis but also is reliant on the rate of degradation. Additionally, newly synthesized albumin is secreted into the lymph and ascitic fluid, when present, which increases the distribution volume and can contribute to hypoalbuminemia. Therefore, in the acute setting, the serum level of albumin does not purely reflect decreases in hepatic synthesis.

The liver is also important in maintaining homeostasis. All clotting proteins, coagulation factors, and inhibitors, and most of the components of the fibrinolytic system are synthesized by hepatocytes except for von Willebrand factor, which is produced by endothelial cells, and megakaryocytes. Liver damage can lead to decreased levels of the clotting factors produced in the liver. It is unusual for fibrinogen to be reduced significantly unless there is concomitant disseminated intravascular coagulation. Overall, liver impairment favors bleeding due to impaired synthesis of coagulation factors and increased fibrinolytic activity. However, it also increases susceptibility to intravascular coagulation resulting from impaired clearance of procoagulant material.[13]

Nutritional Evaluation in Liver Disease

Energy Expenditure in Liver Disease

There is significant controversy about the ability to accurately predict metabolic rates in cirrhotic patients. This is partly because hypermetabolism occurs only when a measured value (indirect or direct calorimetry) is compared to a predicted value. Thus, depending on the methods of standardization and comparison, (i.e., formula equations versus estimates of lean body tissue), the baseline for comparison differs. Common formula equations that use age, weight, and height are standardized for normal proportioned individuals. They do not make allowances for differences in body compartments that may occur in liver disease. For example, if there is depletion of body fat, a common occurrence in cirrhotics, there is a relative overrepresentation of metabolically active tissue per unit mass. If this were the case, formula equations may predict a lower energy expenditure relative to a measured value. One method to address this potential discrepancy is to correct for lean body mass by using creatinine secretion. Since the secretion of creatinine roughly correlates with the presence of lean body tissue, standardization to this value should help account for discrepancies in somatic protein/fat composition. However, it should be kept in mind that creatine, the precursor of creatinine, is synthesized in the liver. Thus, significant liver disease can compromise the urinary recovery of creatinine and result in an underestimation of the amount of metabolically active tissue. This could subsequently result in an underestimation of lean body tissue and an overestimation of metabolic rate when a measured value is compared to a predicted value corrected for fat-free mass.[14]

Alternatively, fluid retention tends to increase weight or body surface area; formulas that standardize energy expenditure on these values overestimate the predicted metabolic rate compared to a measured value.[15] More recently, researchers have attempted to measure fat-free mass, since this a more accurate indicator of metabolically active tissue. They use this variable in predictive formulas for resting energy expenditure. However, even with these more complicated formulas, only 50 to 60% of the observed variation between measured and predicted values can be accounted for.

Most studies have failed to show significant differences in energy expenditure between cirrhotics and control patients.[14,16,17] However, others, such as in a study by Madden, have demonstrated that the mean measured resting energy expenditure in patients with cirrhosis is significantly higher than in controls when adjusted for body weight. Overall, using multiple predictive formulae, 12% of the patients were considered hypometabolic while 30% were determined to be hypermetabolic. A recent comprehensive study by Müller found a similar proportion of hypermetabolic patients (33.8%). Unfortunately, neither author could identify the hypermetabolic patients on the basis of demographic or clinical variables.[18,19] A possible exception to this is primary biliary cirrhosis patients, in whom worsening disease was associated with increased resting energy expenditure and prolonged diet-induced thermogenesis after a meal.[20]

Müller also demonstrated that increased levels of catecholamines in hypermetabolic patients could be a contributing factor in increased metabolic rate. He further determined that for these patients, a propranolol infusion resulted in a pronounced decrease in energy expenditure.[19]

Clinically, determining hypermetabolism is important for these patients, as they are more likely to present malnourished, and this clinical status may be further complicated by difficulty in nutrient assimilation. Thus, hypermetabolism may further negatively impact outcome. A study assessing preoperative risk factors in patients undergoing liver transplantation associated hypermetabolism and diminished body cell mass (<35% of body weight) with reduced survival after liver transplantation.[21] Given the clinical implications of determining an accurate metabolic rate in cirrhotic patients and the fact that this rate cannot be accurately determined from formulas and clinical variables, many authors are advocating that the metabolic rate should be measured in cirrhotic individuals to accurately determine this value.[18,19]

Prevalence of Malnutrition in Liver Disease

Protein-calorie malnutrition (PCM) is common in advanced liver disease. A summary of five studies using a total of 550 subjects demonstrated a range of PCM from 10 to 100%, depending in part on the criteria used to determine PCM.[22] In the Veterans Administration Cooperative study on alcoholic hepatitis, malnutrition was a ubiquitous finding and correlated with dietary intake and severity of liver dysfunction.[23,24] In hospitalized patients with less severe alcoholic and nonalcoholic liver disease, the prevalence of PCM ranged from 30 to 40%. It should be noted that much of the data on malnutrition is derived from the alcoholic liver disease population. However, a recent study by Sarin et al.[24] demonstrated that malnutrition in patients with alcoholic and nonalcoholic cirrhosis is very common, and present to the same degree. The patterns of malnutrition appear to be different depending on the underlying liver disease. Patients with nonalcoholic cirrhosis demonstrated decreases in both fat and muscle mass, while those with alcoholic liver disease demonstrated a greater decrease in muscle mass but relative sparing of fat stores. The authors of the accompanying editorial hypothesize that this discrepancy may be due to the "precirrhotic nutritional status" of the patient or to toxic effects of alcohol on meal-stimulated protein secretion. They also speculated that alcohol might lead to changes in intestinal permeability, which could potentially lead to transmigration of intestinal bacteria or toxins with resultant release of proteolytic cytokines.[25] The authors determined that the dietary intake of both groups was reduced to a similar degree.[24]

Nutritional Assessment

The presence of liver disease may affect many of the traditional modalities used to evaluate the nutritional status of patients. Visceral protein stores can be greatly influenced by acute and/or extensive damage to the liver. Liver injury can result in decreases in visceral markers that may be unrelated to the nutritional status of the patient, and may therefore not improve significantly with nutritional intervention. In fact, serum visceral protein appears to correlate better with the degree of liver damage than with the nutritional status of the patient. Chronic liver disease can also cause alterations in cellular immunity and total lymphocyte count independent of protein malnutrition.[22] Furthermore, abnormal immunologic reactivity, again independent of nutritional status, is a prominent feature of chronic autoimmune hepatitis, primary biliary cirrhosis, and possibly viral hepatitis.[27] From a clinical standpoint, a thorough nutritional evaluation should be performed and repeated serially. A bedside assessment of somatic protein stores and subcutaneous fat stores usually provides a reliable nutritional assessment.[26] Other important aspects of this subjective global assessment tool adapted for liver patients included the presence of encephalopathy, edema, weight change, renal insufficiency, constipation, satiety, and difficulty chewing. Anthropometric data, specifically the assessment of fat stores by tricep or subscapular skinfold thickness and the assessment of somatic stores by midarm muscle circumference or body weight to height, can yield valuable information. Assessments should be performed by a skilled person, as there can be problems with reproducibility. Additionally, apparent or subclinical edema can lead to a potential underestimation of the severity of protein and fat losses.[27] The creatinine height index is generally a good indicator of lean body mass in patients with liver disease. However, it, too, has shortcomings, as there is frequently associated renal dysfunction which could impair collection. Furthermore, with severe liver disease there can be a decrease in creatinine formation, as its substrate creatine is synthesized in the liver. Both of these circumstances could result in underestimation of lean body tissue.

In summary, given the numerous limitations of standard nutritional parameters in patients with liver disorders, it is preferable to rely on collective information generated from the use of several parameters used simultaneously and on a serial basis.[27]

Nutritional Intervention in Liver Disease

Background Data

It is well known that patients with chronic liver disease are usually malnourished, and that frequently the degree of malnutrition parallels the severity of the liver disease. Reasons for malnutrition include altered metabolism, malabsorption/maldigestion, anorexia, iatrogenic restrictions, and poor dietary intake. Though there appears to be a correlation between the severity of malnutrition and subsequent morbidity and mortality from liver disease, it is intuitive, though less clear, that nutritional intervention can have an impact. An article by Patek et al., published in 1948, was one of the earliest to evidence that nutritional intervention could impact the course of liver disease. In this study, 124 patients (89% of whom had "significant weight loss") were admitted to the hospital with "hepatic failure." These patients were given a diet of approximately 3500 kcals with 140 gms of protein, supplemented with a vitamin B complex preparation. The supplemented group was compared to historic controls. Although the patients' ability to achieve dietary goals was not mentioned, 49% were described as "clinically improved." This improvement was characterized by 1) a disappearance of ascites, jaundice, and edema, 2) weight gain and strength, and 3) improvement in liver function test results. Furthermore, there appeared to be significant differences in survival between the treated group and historical controls at one and five years.[30] This positive study provided the basis for subsequent studies assessing the impact of enteral, parenteral, and oral supplementation in patients with liver disease.

Many recent studies have focused on nutritional intervention in alcoholic liver disease. Acute alcoholic hepatitis is a potentially reversible condition, but is associated with high mortality. The majority of patients with alcoholic liver disease who require hospitalization for their disease are moderately to severely malnourished. Malnutrition can contribute to delayed wound healing, increased risk of infection, increased toxicity of alcohol to the liver, reduced protein synthesis, and impaired regenerative capacity of the injured liver.[28,31] Additionally, both human and animal data suggest that poor nutrition combined with alcohol is more injurious to the liver than alcohol alone.[3,31] These factors imply that nutritional intervention may be beneficial in this disease.[28,31] In an early and much-cited trial by Galambos, 28 days of peripheral amino acid infusion resulted in significant improvement in albumin and bilirubin levels in the supplemented group compared to controls. The supplemented group also showed a trend toward improved survival.[33,34]

Mendenhall authored a series of landmark articles on alcoholic hepatitis. A nutritional investigation of patients with alcoholic hepatitis was part of a larger multicentered VA cooperative study of the effects of steroid therapy in the treatment of this disease. In an early study, the patients were categorized into mild, moderate, and severe protein calorie malnutriton (PCM) based on eight parameters that included tests to assess somatic protein stores, visceral protein stores, and delayed cutaneous hypersensitivity. The investigators were able to demonstrate that 30-day and 6-month mortality rates correlated with nutritional category. Perhaps equally important was that patients who moved from one nutritional category to another assumed the mortality associated with their new category.[35] However, it should be noted that this early observation on nutrition and outcome was a secondary endpoint.

The same researchers subsequently designed a study to intercede with nutritional supplements while providing patients with anabolic steroids (oxandrolone). Oxandrolone was used in this population because the researchers believed it would increase anabolism and liver regeneration. In a group of patients defined as having moderate PCM yet adequate caloric intake (>2500 kcals), oxandralone significantly decreased mortality compared to the placebo group. In addition, patients defined as having severe PCM yet adequate caloric intake had significantly lower 6-month mortality regardless of the use of oxandrolone. Finally, caloric intake during the first month demonstrated a significant inverse correlation, with mortality at six months. It should be noted, however, that as the severity of the liver disease increased, the caloric intake decreased.[29] Unfortunately, it is unclear from this study whether nutritional supplementation, even if the patient accepts and is compliant with this supplementation, will improve the "nutritional category." It is possible that other changes in underlying liver disease also have to occur before nutritional repletion is realized. However, the authors mentioned that there was a "marginally significant correlation" between percent of basal energy expenditure consumed and the improvement in PCM during hospitalization.

These authors published another followup article focused solely on the nutritional indices in this same cohort of patients. The authors were able to identify four nutritional parameters that seem to effect six-month mortality. They included creatinine height index, total lymphocyte count, handgrip strength, and prealbumin levels. The authors suggested that surviving patients tend to improve in most of their measured nutritional parameters, but it is again unclear that either adequate protein or energy intake significantly influences these four variables. Nevertheless, the authors conclude that nutritional therapy improves both prognosis and overall nutritional status. They qualify this statement, however, by stating that the degree of improvement is dependent on the severity of the PCM.[39]

A recent study by Cabre et al. assessed the effects of total enteral nutrition and prednisolone in the treatment of patients with alcoholic hepatitis. Patients were randomized to receive either TEN (2000 kcal/d and 72 g protein via a nasoenteral tube) or prednisolone. The latter group was encouraged to eat a standard hospital diet of approximately 2000 kcals and 1 g/kg of protein. Although no difference was seen in short term or one-year survival, differences in the time to death and cause of death were noted. Deaths occurred earlier in the TEN group (median of seven days). In the prednisolone-treated group, most of the deaths occurred in the immediate six weeks after the end of the treatment period and were largely due to infectious complications. The authors speculate that most of the early mortality may have been caused by inflammatory mediators (thus the early benefit of steroids). The latter mortality may have been caused by changes in the intestinal barrier (supporting the importance of enteral nutrition in maintaining the integrity of the gut barrier). The author suggests that there might be a synergistic effect realized in using both modes of therapy.[41]

The positive effects of nutritional supplementation are not, however, limited to patients with alcoholic hepatitis. In an earlier study, Cabre et al. looked at enteral nutrition in hospitalized cirrhotic patients. The treatment group was given an enteral formula containing 2115 kcal/d with 71 g protein via nasoenteral tube. The control group was offered a standard low-sodium hospital diet supplying 2200 kcals and 70 to 80 g protein. The etiology of the cirrhosis was varied (though largely alcoholic) and there were no differences in Child's scores. All patients in both groups had severe protein energy malnutrition. Although the incidence of major complications was similar in both groups, the Child score improved and mortality fell (47 versus 12%) only in the TEN group. The authors were unable to explain the discrepancy. They suggested that the GI tract stimulation may have decreased the catabolic effect of the injury or resulted in decreased bacterial/endotoxin translocation.[42]

In summary, multiple studies using oral, enteral, and parenteral supplementation have demonstrated only modest improvements in liver function tests and nutritional parameters. A decrease in mortality in nutritionally supplemented patients has not been a consistent or overwhelming finding,[34,40,43-45] though other important facts have emerged. These patients appear to tolerate the protein supplementation, including those with hepatic encephalopathy. Fluid retention has not been a major problem.[34] It should also be noted that there is no published study demonstrating an adverse effect of nutritional supplementation. These studies point out that nutritional supplementation, though very important, is only one of several factors likely to determine the ultimate outcome in liver disease patients. As this is a factor that can be influenced, at least to some degree, and there do not seem to be untoward effects when used appropriately, attention to nutrition, with supplementation when indicated, should be considered a mainstay in the therapy for these patients.

The use of branched chain amino acids (BCAA) has been advocated in the treatment of liver disease. It has been suggested that 50 to 60% of patients with chronic liver failure will tolerate 60 to 80 g/d of a standard amino acid mixture as part of a parenteral nutrition regimen. The remainder, in particular those with grade III or IV hepatic encephalopathy, seem to respond better to with modified solutions containing BCAA.[54] One rationale for their use in hepatic encephalopathy concerns the high aromatic amino acid (AA)-to-BCAA ratio in the blood of patients with decompensated liver disease. This is primarily due to poor metabolism of AAs by the failing/injured liver. Conversely, BCAAs are deaminated mainly by skeletal muscle, and so have an alternate pathway for their metabolism. Since both of these amino acids compete for the same transmembrane transport system in order to cross the blood brain barrier, the increase in AA/BCAA in the blood favors the transport of AAs. In the central nervous system these AAs can be metabolized to false neurotransmitters (octopamine and phenylethanolamine) and thus contribute to hepatic encephalopathy. Additionally, infusion of BCAAs has been shown to reduce blood ammonia levels.[46] The branch chain amino acids have also been reported to augment protein synthesis in humans. Leucine, or more specifically, its deamination product, βα-keto-isocaprioic acid, is thought to have an important role in stimulating protein synthesis and inhibiting protein degradation.[46,47] Thus, it would seem that a BCAA mixture would be an ideal mode of therapy in patients with liver disease.

Several studies have looked at the use of BCAA in the treatment of hepatic encephalopathy. The largest study was by Cerra et al., who concluded that the BCAA-enriched formula resulted in more rapid and complete recovery from encephalopathy as compared to the standard treatment of neomycin. The treatment group also showed improvements in nitrogen balance and survival. Interestingly, the control group was not given any protein, and their sole source of kcalories was a 25% dextrose solution. Both the BCAA and dextrose solutions were started at 1.5 liters and advanced to a maximum of 3 liters over the ensuing days.[48] Unfortunately, the lack of protein in the control group challenges the validity of the nitrogen balance data and perhaps the mortality differences in these populations.

Overall, studies regarding the use of BCAA in encephalopathy have yielded mixed results.[47,69] A recent meta-analysis by Naylor et al. suggests that BCAA solutions have a significant and beneficial effect on recovery from hepatic encephalopathy, though the authors state that analysis is difficult, given the diversity of the studies involved. The same authors were unable to verify an advantage of BCAA solutions on mortality.[54] Another extensive analysis by Eriksson et al. presented a much more skeptical view of the benefits of BCAA solutions in either acute or chronic encephalopathy. The authors proposed that problems with data analysis, biased assignment of patients to groups in regard to etiology of the encephalopathy, and study design disallowed any firm conclusion that BCAA or their keto analogues were beneficial.[55] Thus, though the use of BCAA-enriched supplements may lead to mild improvement in encephalopathy compared to standard therapy, other positive effects are not consistently demonstrated. The benefits do not seem to justify routine use of this enriched formula at the present time.

An exception to this may be the patient with chronic encephalopathy who is intolerant to increases in protein or standard amino acid solutions. Eriksson's analysis did concede that in the setting of chronic encephalopathy in which increases in standard protein supplements worsened or precipitated encepahalopathy, BCAA mixtures were better tolerated. A study by Egberts et al. of this population demonstrated significant improvements in psychomotor function, attention, and practical intelligence when stable patients were supplemented with a BCAA-enriched mixture.[50] However, the clinical applicability of these improvements in psychomotor testing has been called into question.[55]

In vitro studies of isolated hepatocytes suggest that the keto acid analogues of BCAAs augment protein synthesis.[51] However, when the effects of these BCAA solutions were evaluated in cirrhotic patients, no such augmentation was seen.[46,52] In an editorial accompanying this paper, Charlton speculated that because the BCAA-enriched infusate lacked sufficient AAs for protein synthesis, the expected protein synthetic response may have been dampened. Alternately, he suggests that relative hyperglucagonemia may shunt amino acids toward gluconeogenesis and thus render them unavailable for protein synthesis. He concluded that these abnormalities may account for the less-than-convincing "improved outcomes" with BCAA-enriched formulas for patients with liver disease.

Nutritional Recommendations

In multiple diverse populations, malnutrition can negatively impact infection, wound healing, and organ function. The great majority of patients who present for liver disease are malnourished, and the severity of their malnutrition has prognostic implications. However, when studies on nutritional intervention in liver disease are considered, it is difficult to ascertain whether nutritional intervention can positively impact the course of the disease. A similar conclusion can be arrived at in most disease states, both acute and chronic, in which nutritional intervention has been critically assessed. This does not necessarily mean that nutritional intervention is not important in the individual patient. The diverse baseline nutritional status in patients (both from a macronutrient as well as a micronutrient perspective), the differences in insult severity, and the myriad of therapies and approaches given to the individual patient, explain why there does not appear to be a guiding light for nutritional intervention. In spite of this, some general recommendations can be made with regard to energy and protein requirements.

Energy Needs

As discussed previously, difficulties in estimating energy expenditure in cirrhotics have been attributed to fluid retention, relative changes in body compartments, and other variables related to metabolic abnormalities in patients with liver disease. Nonetheless, in stable cirrhotics, various studies have measured energy expenditures ranging from approximately 1500 to 2100 kcals/d.[16,18,19] Thus, though the controversy over whether these patients are hypermetabolic compared to controls remains unanswered, the absolute energy requirements in these patients do not appear to be excessive. Furthermore, in the acute setting, increases in the metabolic rate are influenced by many variables including the severity of the insult, the presence of infection, and medications that the patient may be receiving. These latter variables further complicate accurate extrapolation of energy needs from formula equations. REE, or resting energy expenditure, is measurement of the body's daily energy expenditure, not involving activity or caloric intake. REE with indirect calorimetry remains the most accurate and practical way of estimating total caloric needs. In the absence of indirect calorimetry, the simplest and most accurate predictive formula is the Schofield formula. This formula, referenced by Madden et al.,[18] varies significantly by age. In men between the ages of 30 to 60 it is as follows:

$$(11.48 \times \text{wt}) - (2.63 \times \text{ht}) + 877.57$$

Most interventional studies have used a caloric intake of 2000 to 3000 kcals. In the VA cooperative study, a level of 2500 kcalories and above was considered adequate therapy. Alternately, values ranging from 25 kcals/kg/d (stable cirrhotic) to 45 kcals/kg/d (post-operative cirrhotic) have been proposed.[22] Excessive caloric delivery is not beneficial, as it can create metabolic and respiratory stresses. High caloric delivery may also involve increasing the fluids given to these usually fluid-restricted patients. Additionally, nutritional repletion is not usually accomplished during hospitalization in the current medical climate. Energy goals should thus be directed at maintenance without causing metabolic abnormalities.

Perhaps more important than delivery of a caloric load is the mixture of the kcalories provided. In an interesting study by Chanda and Mehendale, rats subjected to a hepatotoxin demonstrated a decrease in hepatocellular regeneration and tissue repair when given 15% glucose in drinking water.[56] Conversely, in a similar experiment, rats given palmitic acid and L-carnitine were protected against similar doses of that hepatotoxin. The authors suggest that the regenerating liver uses fatty acids as the main source of cellular energy. The increased demand for cellular energy in the form of ATP needed to support hepatocellular division is essentially derived from fatty acid oxidation.[57]

It is also interesting to note that the two outwardly "negative studies" doing BCAA supplementation in a test group were compared to a control group on a lipid-based formula. It is possibile that the lack of efficacy in these studies was due to the lipids conveying some advantage to the control group, thus decreasing by comparison the effectiveness of the BCAA solution in the treatment group.

Other interesting animal data suggests that lipids, specifically saturated fatty acids, may offer protection against alcoholic liver injury. Nanji et al. found that diets enriched with saturated fatty acids (palm oil) reverse the pathological changes induced by ethanol. Conversely, omega-3 fatty acids (fish oil) do not improve the severity of alcohol-induced injury. The authors suggest that the protective effects may be explained in part by differences in lipid peroxidation. Dietary fat helps to modify the expression of cytochrome p450 2E1, which contributes to NADPH-dependant lipid peroxidation. The animals fed the diets rich in saturated fatty acids demonstrated less induction of the CYP2E1 enzyme system.[58] Alternately, the protective effect may be through positive changes in eicosanoid metabolism manifested as an increase in the prostacycline-to-thromboxane B_2 ratio. In previous studies, these authors found that decreases in this ratio preceded the production of pathologic liver disease.

Saturated fats are probably not the only nutrients that may have a protective effect against liver disease. Lieber found that baboons maintained on a chronic ethanol-enriched diet supplemented with polyunsaturated phospholipids (55 to 60% of which was polyunsaturated phosphatidylcholine [PPC]) were protected against alcohol-induced fibrosis. In a similar study, the animals were given a purer extract, comprising 94 to 96% phosphatidylcholine. The researchers found that these baboons given ethanol for up to eight years did not develop cirrhosis or septal fibrosis when fed this supplemented diet. Leiber proposed that the phosphatidylcholine directly affects collagen metabolism and opposes oxidative stress.[3,59,60] Unfortunately, supplementing fat does not appear to be the entire answer. In a rat model, Lieber also found that in the setting of chronic alcohol consumption, increased triglycerides in the diet results in increased fat accumulation in the liver.[3] Extrapolating from animal data, it would therefore seem that in the setting of alcoholic liver disease, 25 to 35% of the total kcalories should be derived from a mixture of these lipids. Thus, it would appear that the type as well as amount of fat are important considerations in supplementing patients with liver disease.

Protein supplementation in the patient with acute liver injury is probably the most controversial aspect of macronutreint nutritional supplementation. These patients usually demonstrate somatic protein wasting and decreases in muscle strength, immune reactivity, and protein synthesis. These deficiencies may in part be due to diminished protein stores. Also, repair of injury, extrapolated from other clinical settings, requires adequate protein. Finally, it has been assumed that liver regeneration is delayed when there is insufficient protein.[3]

In their studies of nutritional intervention in patients with alcoholic liver disease, Mendenhall et al. have stated that all patients with alcoholic hepatitis achieved positive nitrogen balance with 1.2 g/kg of protein. Additionally, this intake of protein was well tolerated in spite of severe liver disease. Encephalopathy was observed in 20% of patients, but its occurrence did not correlate with protein intake.[39] In patients with chronic liver disease, Lieber states that positive nitrogen balance can be attained with a protein intake of 0.74 g/kg. Thus it appears that the stringent protein restrictions often imposed on hospitalized patients with liver disease can be eased. Protein provisions in the range of 0.6 to 0.8 g/kg can usually be safely given during the acute setting, increasing protein delivery as tolerated to at least 1.2 g/kg. It should be noted that the protein supplemented in Mendenhall's study, and the basis of his recommendations, was enriched with BCAA. Although there have been no definitive studies comparing tolerability of standard amino acid mixtures to BCAA, it is possible that an individual patient with acute liver injury may tolerate a larger quantity of protein if supplemented with BCAA supplementation. Thus, clinical surveillance is important when increasing protein load in these patients.

Finally, the remainder of patients' energy needs should be met with carbohydrates. As discussed previously, insulin resistance is common in patients with cirrhosis, and this intolerance is further exacerbated in the setting of acute injury. Therefore, providing carbohydrates to the point of inducing metabolic aberrations is not advisable. Cirrhotics may further benefit from complex carbohydrates to reduce insulin requirements. Complex carbohydrates may also be advantageous in the setting of encephalopathy, as they tend to decrease transit time and and lower colonic pH, both of which serve to decrease ammonia absorption from the gastrointestinal tract.[3]

Nutritional Supplements

S-Adenosylmethionine

S-Adenosylmethionine (SAMe) is synthesized by the transfer of an adenosyl group from ATP to the essential amino acid methionine. SAMe serves primarily as a methyl donor. These SAMe-dependent methylations are essential for the biosynthesis of a variety of cellular components including carnitine, phospholipids, proteins, DNA, and RNA, as well as polyamines needed for cell regeneration.[31,61] In addition, it serves as one source of csyteine for glutathione production (Figure 58.5). Furthermore, it has been shown that methionine metabolism is impaired in patients with liver disease and that the activity of SAMe synthase is decreased in human cirrhotic livers.[31,62,63]

The administration of exogenous SAMe should be effective in liver disease. In baboons, correction of ethanol-induced hepatic SAMe depletion with oral SAMe supplementation resulted in a corresponding attenuation of ethanol-induced liver injury.[32,64] Thus, supplementation with SAMe dampens the depletion of hepatic glutathione (GSH) stores. Without supplementation, depletion of GSH leads to inactivation of SAMe synthetase, which would tend to further reduce GSH stores, thereby predisposing to hepatic injury.[32] The studies that have evaluated SAMe supplementation have demonstrated significant improvements in subjective symptoms, serum markers of cholestasis, and hepatic GSH levels.[32,65,66] More recently, Mato et al. demonstrated that SAMe supplementation could improve survival or delay time to transplantation compared to controls. These results demonstrated a positive

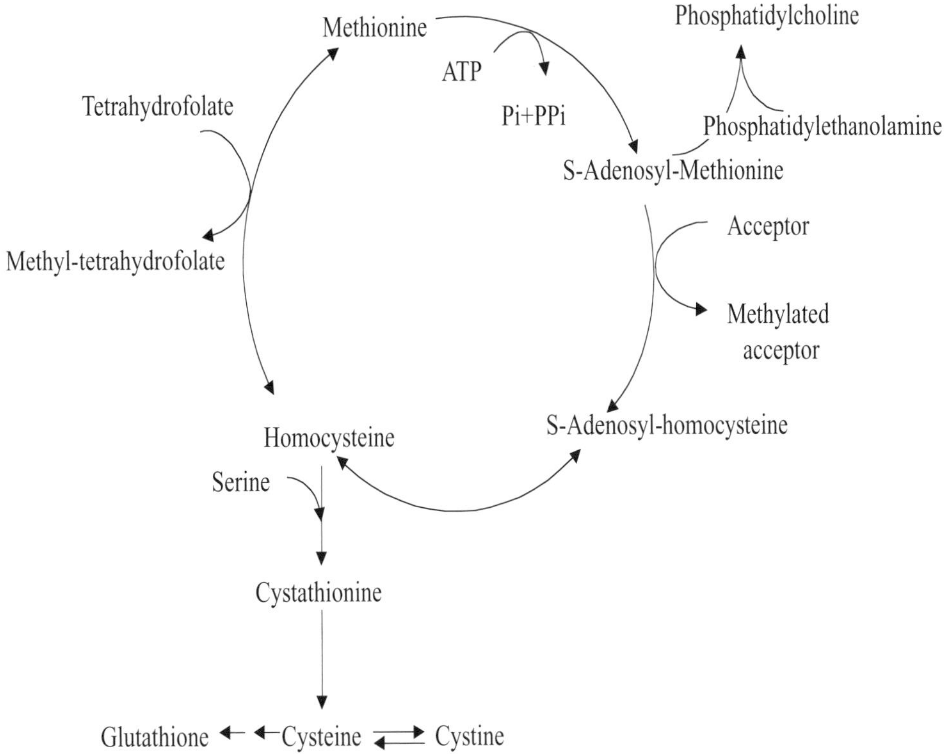

FIGURE 58.5
SAMe synthase. S-Adenosyl-L-Methionine (SAMe) is formed in an irreversible reaction that transfers an adenosyl group from methionine. SAMe is an important donor of methyl groups, and is active in the conversion of creatine to creatinine and of phosphatidylethanolamine to phosphatidylcholine. SAMe is converted to S-adenosyl-homocysteine and then to homocysteine. Homocysteine can combine with serine to form csytathionine which can ultimately be converted to glutathione. (Adapted from Kruszynska YT. In: *Oxford Textbook of Clinical Hepatology*, 2nd ed, Bircher J, Benhamou J, McIntyre N, Rizzetto M, Rodes J, Eds, Oxford University Press, Oxford, 1999, p. 257 and Lieber CS. In: *Modern Nutrition in Health and Disease*, 9th ed, Shils ME, Olson JA, Shike M, Ross AC, Eds, Williams and Wilkins, Baltimore 1999, pg 1177.)

trend in favor of the supplemented group, but achieved significance only when patients with advanced cirrhotic liver disease (Child C) patients were excluded.[31,67]

Supplementation with SAMe shows significant promise in the treatment of liver disease and will undoubtedly be investigated with larger studies in the future.

Zinc

Zinc (Zn) is the most abundant intracellular trace element. It is involved in a multitude of diverse catalytic, structural, and regulatory functions. Many physiologic functions require zinc, including protein metabolism, normal immune functioning and wound healing, neurosensory function such as cognition and taste, and membrane stability.[68,69] Hypozincemia is common in various types of liver disease.[69] The deficiency is multifactorial and is believed to involve poor dietary intake and impaired intestinal absorption (possibly due to a cytokine-induced intestinal metallothionein, which dampens zinc absorption). Additionally, there is decreased affinity of albumin for zinc in cirrhotics, which might influence bioavailability and lead to increased urinary losses of zinc. Finally, increased cytokine or hormonal concentrations may lead to altered zinc metabolism.[69]

Zinc deficiency may play a role in increasing plasma ammonia levels. Zinc deficiency was shown to decrease activity of glutamate dehydrogenase and ornithine transcarbamylase (OTC), enzymes important in normal nitrogen metabolism (Figure 58.4). Urea synthetic capacity is believed to be reduced in zinc-deficient patients due to reduced OTC activity, as zinc acts as a cofactor in the activity of this enzyme. Zinc supplementation speeds up the kinetics of nitrogen conversion from amino acids into urea in cirrhotics.[11] Zinc deficiency also increases muscle glutamine synthetase and adenosine monophosphate deaminase, enzymes that increase ammonia production from aspartate.[70]

Although zinc deficiency may play a role in some of the altered taste sensations seen in liver disease, it is unlikely to be a major cause of anorexia in liver disease. It is much more likely that the anorexia seen in this disease is cytokine mediated.[69] Conversely, zinc deficiency, at least in part, does appear to play a role in immune dysfunction and perhaps in delayed wound healing. The latter may occur through the effect of zinc on insulin-like growth factor.[69] In regard to protein synthesis, a recent study showed lower serum albumin levels in children undergoing liver transplantation than in other transplant patients in whom serum zinc levels were normal. This correlates with the findings by Bates and McClain, which demonstrated improvement or normalization of serum transport proteins in zinc-deficient patients on parenteral nutrition when supplemented with zinc.[71,72]

Selenium

There are at least eleven selenoproteins; the most well known class is the glutathione peroxidases. These proteins are important participants in the body's antioxidant defenses. Selenium concentrations have been reported to be lower in patients with cirrhosis compared to healthy controls. Selenium deficiency could therefore contribute to the morbidity of cirrhosis. This deficiency could be easily addressed with supplementation. However, a recent study by Burk et al. reported that, though plasma selenium is indeed depressed in patients with cirrhosis, the changes noted in plasma selenoproteins of cirrhotics are not the same as those found in selenium-deficient subjects without liver disease. Functionally, these patients had an increase in the plasma gluatathione concentration, arguing against a true selenium deficiency.[73,74]

Carnitine

Fatty acids are the preferred fuel for patients with cirrhosis. Since carnitine is essential for the mitochondrial use of long-chain fatty acids for energy production, decreased availability of this quaternary amine may lead to energy deficiency in cirrhotics. Deficiency can arise from poor dietary intake or disruption of carnitine biosynthesis, the last step occurring almost exclusively in the liver. Measured levels of carnitine in patients with chronic liver disease can be reduced or increased. The literature suggests that plasma and tissue carnitine levels can be altered in patients with chronic liver disease, depending on both its cause and progression.[75,76]

A recent study by Krahenbuhl and Reichen found that patients with chronic liver disease are normally not carnitine deficient. They also concluded that carnitine metabolism can be disturbed in subgroups of patients with liver disease. For example, patients with alcoholic cirrhosis demonstrated increased plasma concentrations. Patients with primary biliary cirrhosis were able to maintain normal plasma levels of carnitine, but demonstrated increased renal excretion.[76]

Conclusion

It is clear that the relationship between nutrition and the liver is intricate and interdependent. Liver disease can result in anorexia, malabsorption, and abnormalities in nutrient metabolism leading to a compromise in the nutritional status of the host. This impaired nutritional status can impact negatively on immune function, compromise the ability of the liver to limit the extent of hepatic insults, and retard an appropriate response to injury. Nutritional deficiencies in patients with liver disease can range from subtle abnormalities to advanced protein calorie malnutrition. Some degree of nutritional compromise is invariably present. In treating patients with liver disease, the recognition and aggressive treatment of these deficiencies is paramount. In milder forms of liver disease, this intervention may take the form of nutrient and vitamin supplementation. In more advanced liver disease, aggressive nutritional support, preferably in the form of enteral access and feeding, may be the "controllable" factor that leads to an improved outcome.

References

1. Kruszynska YT. In: *Oxford Textbook of Clinical Hepatology* 2nd ed, Bircher J, Benhamou J, McIntyre N, Rizzetto M, Rodes J, Eds, Oxford University Press, Oxford, 1999, p 257.
2. Rothman DL, Magnusson I, Katz LD, et al. *Science* 254: 573; 1991.
3. Lieber CS. In: *Modern Nutrition in Health and Disease* 9th ed, Shils ME, Olson JA, Shike M, Ross AC, Eds, Williams and Wilkins, Baltimore, 1999, pg 1177.
4. Petrides AS, Vogt C, Schulze-Berge D, et al. *Hepatology* 19: 616; 1994.
5. Jones PJH, Kubnow S, In: *Modern Nutrition in Health and Disease* 9th ed, Shils ME, Olson JA, Shike M, Ross AC, Eds, Williams and Wilkins, Baltimore, 1999, pg 67.
6. Harry DS, McIntyre N. In: *Oxford Textbook of Clinical Hepatology* 2nd ed, Bircher J, Benhamou J, McIntyre N, Rizzetto M, Rodes J, Eds, Oxford University Press, Oxford, 1999, pg 287.
7. Ma Z, Lee SS. *Hepatology* 24: 451; 1996.
8. Kruszynska YT, McIntyre N. In: *Oxford Textbook of Clinical Hepatology* 2nd ed, Bircher J, Benhamou J, McIntyre N, Rizzetto M, Rodes J, Eds, Oxford University Press, Oxford, 1999, pg 303.
9. Nelson DL, Cox MM. In: *Principals of Biochemistry* 2nd ed, Lehninger, Nelson, Cox, Worth Publisher, New York, 1993, pg 506.
10. Gerok W, Gross V. In: *Oxford Textbook of Clinical Hepatology* 2nd ed, Bircher J, Benhamou J, McIntyre N, Rizzetto M, Rodes J, Eds, Oxford University Press, Oxford, 1999, pg 346.
11. Haussinger D. In: *Oxford Textbook of Clinical Hepatology* 2nd ed, Bircher J, Benhamou J, McIntyre N, Rizzetto M, Rodes J, Eds, Oxford University Press, Oxford, 1999, pg 325.
12. Riggio O, Merli M, Romiti A, et al. *JPEN* 16: 445; 1992.
13. Denninger M. In: *Oxford Textbook of Clinical Hepatology* 2nd ed, Bircher J, Benhamou J, McIntyre N, Rizzetto M, Rodes J, Eds, Oxford University Press, Oxford, 1999, pg 367.
14. Schneeweiss B, Graninger W, Ferenci P, et al. *Hepatology* 11: 387; 1990.
15. Heymsfield SB, Waki M, Reinus J. *Hepatology* 11: 502; 1990.
16. McCullough AJ, Raguso C. *Am J Clin Nutr* 69: 1066; 1999.
17. Merli M, Riggio O, Romiti A. *Hepatology* 12: 106; 1990.
18. Madden AM, Morgan MY. *Hepatology* 30: 655; 1999.
19. Müller MJ, Böttcher J, Selberg O, et al. *Am J Clin Nutr* 69: 1194; 1999.
20. Green JH, Bramley PN, Losowwsky MS. *Hepatology* 14: 464; 1991.
21. Selberg O, Böttcher J, Tusch G, et al. *Hepatology* 25: 652; 1997.
22. McCullough AJ, Mullen KD, Smanik EJ. *Gastro Clin N Am* 18: 619; 1989.
23. Mendenhall CL, Anderson S, Weesner RE, et al. *Am J Med* 76: 211; 1984.
24. Sarin SK, Dhingra N, Bansal A, et al. *Am J Gastro* 92: 777; 1997.
25. McCullough AJ, Bugianesi E. *Am J Gastro* 92: 734; 1997.
26. Hasse J, Strong S, Gorman MA, et al. *Nutrition* 9: 339; 1993.
27. Munoz SJ. *Sem in Liver Dis* 11: 278; 1991.
28. McCullough AJ, Tavill AS. *Sem Liver Dis* 11: 265; 1991.
29. Mendenhall CL, Moritz TE, Roselle GA. *Hepatology* 17: 564; 1993.
30. Patek AJ, Ratnoff OD, Mankin H, et al. *JAMA* 138: 543; 1948.

31. Schenker S, Halff GA. *Sem in Liver Dis* 13: 196; 1993.
32. Lieber CS. *J Hepatol* 32(1): 113S; 2000.
33. Nasrallah SM, Galambos JT. *Lancet* ii: 1276; 1980.
34. Nompleggi DJ, Bonkovsky H. *Hepatology* 19: 518; 1994.
35. Mendenhall CL, Tosch T, Weesner RE. *Am J Clin Nutr* 43: 213; 1986.
36. Mendenhall CL, Anderson S, Weesner RE, et al. *Am J Med* 76: 211; 1983.
37. Silk DBA, O'Keefe SJD, Wicks C. *Gut* 29S; 1991.
38. Achord JL. *Am J of Gastro* 82: 1; 1987.
39. Mendenhall CL, Moritz TE, Roselle GA. *JPEN* 19: 258; 1995.
40. Bonkovsky HL, Fiellin DA, Smith GS. *Am J of Gastro* 86: 1200; 1991.
41. Cabre E, Rodriguez-Iglesias P, Caballeria J. *Hepatology* 32: 36; 2000.
42. Cabre E, Gonzalez-Huix F, Abad-Lacruz A, et al. *Gastroenterology* 98: 715; 1990.
43. Bonkovsky HL, Singh RH, Jafri IH, et al. *Am J Gastro* 86: 1209; 1991.
44. Kearns PJ, Young H, Garcia G, et al. *Gastroenterology* 102: 200; 1992.
45. Morgan TR. *Sem Liver Dis* 13: 384; 1993.
46. Weber FL, Bagby BS, Licate L, et al. *Hepatology* 11: 942; 1990.
47. Buse MG, Reid SS. *J Clin Invest* 56: 1250; 1975.
48. Cerra FB, Cheung NK, Fischer JE. *JPEN* 9: 88; 1985.
49. Fischer JE. *JPEN* 14: 249S; 1990.
50. Egberts EH, Schomerus H, Hamster W, et al. *Gastroenterology* 88: 887; 1985.
51. Base W, Barsigian C, Schaeffer A, et al. *Hepatology* 7: 324; 1987.
52. Tessari P, Zanetti M, Barazzoni R, et al. *Gastrology* 111: 127; 1996.
53. Charlton MR, Branched Chains Revisited *Gastroenterology* 111: 252; 1996.
54. Naylor CD, O'Rourke K, Detsky AS, et al. *Gastroenterology* 97: 1033; 1989.
55. Eriksson LS, Conn HO. *Hepatology* 10: 228; 1989.
56. Chanda S, Mehendale HM. *FASEB J* 9: 240; 1995.
57. Chanda S, Mehendale HM. *Toxicology* 111: 163; 1996.
58. Nanji AA, Sadrzadeh SMH, Yang EK, et al. *Gastroenterology* 109: 547; 1995.
59. Lieber CS, DeCarli LM, Mak KM, et al. *Hepatology* 12: 1390; 1990.
60. Lieber CS, Robins SJ, Li J, et al. *Gastroenterology* 106: 152; 1994.
61. Stipanuk MH. In: *Modern Nutrition in Health and Disease* 9th ed, Shils ME, Olson JA, Shike M, Ross AC, Eds, Williams and Wilkins, Baltimore, 1999, pg 543.
62. Horowitz JH, Rypins EB, Henderson JM, et al. *Gastroenterology* 81: 668; 1981.
63. Duce AM, Ortiz P, Cabrero C, et al. *Hepatology* 8: 65; 1988.
64. Lieber CS, Casini A, Decarli LM, et al. *Hepatology* 11: 165; 1990.
65. Frezza M, Surrenti C, Manzillo G, et al. *Gastroenterology* 99: 211; 1990.
66. Vendemiale G, Altomare E, Trizio T, et al. *Scan J Gastro* 24: 407; 1989.
67. Mato JM, Camara J, Fernendez de Paz J, et al. *J Hepatol* 30: 1081; 1999.
68. King JC, Keen CL. In: *Modern Nutrition in Health and Disease* 9th ed, Shils ME, Olson JA, Shike M, Ross AC, Eds, Williams and Wilkins, Baltimore, 1999, pg 223.
69. McClain CJ, Marsano L, Burk RF, et al. *Sem in Liv Dis* 11: 321; 1991.
70. Mullen KD, Weber FL. *Sem in Liv Dis* 11: 292; 1991.
71. Narkewicz MR, Krebs N, Karrer F. *Hepatology* 29: 830; 1999.
72. Bates J, McClain CJ. *Am J Clin Nutr* 34: 1655; 1981.
73. Burk RF, Levander OA. In: *Modern Nutrition in Health and Disease* 9th ed, Shils ME, Olson JA, Shike M, Ross AC, Eds, Williams and Wilkins, Baltimore, 1999, pg 256.
74. Burk RF, Early DS, Hill KE, et al. *Hepatology* 27: 794; 1998.
75. Rebouche CJ. In: *Modern Nutrition in Health and Disease* 9th ed, Shils ME, Olson JA, Shike M, Ross AC, Eds, Williams and Wilkins, Baltimore, 1999, pg 505.
76. Krahenbuhl S, Reichen J. *Hepatology* 25: 148; 1996.
77. Brodsky IG. In: *Modern Nutrition in Health and Disease* 9th ed, Shils ME, Olson JA, Shike M, Ross AC, Eds, Williams and Wilkins, Baltimore, 1999, pg 699.
78. Nelson DL, Cox MM. In: *Principals of Biochemistry* 2nd ed, Lehninger AL, Nelson DL, Cox MM, Eds, Worth Publishers, New York, 1993, pg 506.

59

Nutrition and the Pancreas: Physiology and Interventional Strategies

Mark T. De Meo

Introduction

The pancreas plays a major role in nutrient digestion as well as in the control of intermediate metabolism. Patients with pancreatic disease will likely have their nutritional homeostasis compromised with both macronutrient and micronutrient deficiencies. This section will explore the effects of a diseased pancreas on nutritional health and nutritional interventions that may be beneficial to patients with a diseased or inflamed pancreas.

Normal Pancreatic Function

The exocrine pancreas delivers two main products to the lumen of the duodenum during the digestive process — digestive enzymes and bicarbonate. The digestive enzymes secreted by the pancreas are key to the breakdown of ingested macronutrients (carbohydrates, proteins, and fats). Table 59.1 demonstrates the various enzymes and their functions. The bicarbonate secreted in pancreatic juice neutralizes the acidic chyme entering the duodenum from the stomach, and in so doing, increases duodenal pH. This alkaline environment in the duodenum in turn allows for optimal functioning of the pancreatic digestive enzymes.

Carbohydrate Digestion

Dietary carbohydrates are an important component of daily caloric intake in adults. Ingested carbohydrates take three major forms: *monosaccarides* such as fructose; *disaccharides* such as lactose and sucrose; and *polysaccharides*, of which starch is the predominant form. Monosaccharides are absorbed directly by the normal small bowel mucosa. Disaccharides require the action of enzymes called disaccharidases, found in the brush border

0-8493-2705-9/02/$0.00+$1.50

TABLE 59.1

Digestive Enzymes Secreted by the Pancreas

Amylase	Splits alpha 1-4 glycosidic linkages of dietary polysaccharides
Trypsin	Cleaves internal bonds with a preference for positively charged amino acids
Chymotrypsin	Cleaves internal bonds with a preference for amino acids with aromatic side groups
Elastase	Cleaves internal bonds with a preference for amino acids with aliphatic side chains
Carboxypeptidase A	Cleaves carboxy-terminal amino acids
Carboxypeptidase B	Cleaves carboxy-terminal amino acids with a preference for peptide bonds after arginine or lysine residues
Lipase	Preferentially hydrolyzes the 1 & 3 position of dietary triglycerides
Colipase	Binds to the lipid/aqueous interface between the emulsion and the unstirred water layer and also binds to lipase; this allows for the approximation of lipase to dietary triglycerides and facilitates digestion
Phospholipase A_2	Cleaves the phospholipid at the 2 position to yield a lysophosphoglyceride and a fatty acid
Cholesterol esterase	Cleaves esterfied fatty acid from cholesterol moiety

From Lowe, M.E. In *Physiology of the Gastrointestinal Tract,* 3rd ed., Johnson, L.R. et al., Eds., Raven Press, New York, 1994, p. 1531, with permission.

of mucosal cells lining the small bowel. The disaccharidases break down these small carbohydrates into their component sugars prior to absorption. Starches are much larger molecules of repeating glucose molecules joined by either a C1-4 or C1-6 linkage (Figure 59.1). Starches require digestion prior to absorption.

Digestion of starch begins with the release of salivary amylase in the mouth. However, salivary amylase becomes neutralized quickly by gastric acid. Starch then passes to the duodenum where α-amylase, secreted by the pancreas, continues the digestive process.

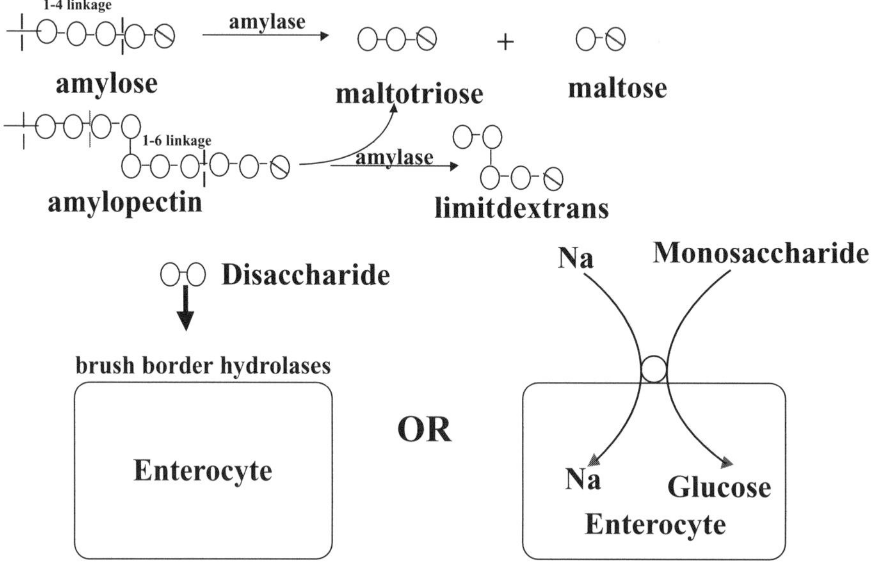

FIGURE 59.1
Mechanism of monosaccharide absorption. Monosaccharides can be absorbed directly by the small bowel mucosa. Disaccharides are futher metabolized by brush border disaccharidases. Polysaccharides are cleaved by amylase at the 1-4 but not the 1-6 linkages forming oligosaccharides. These oligosaccharides are cleaved by brush border enzymes to their constituent monosaccharides.

Pancreatic amylase cleaves the 1-4 glucose linkages but not the 1-6 linkages or the 1-4 linkages juxtaposed to the 1-6 links. This hydrolysis results in the formation of large oligosaccharides, with an average chain length of about eight glucose units with one or more 1-6 linkages. These oligosaccharides are hydrolyzed by intestinal brush border enzymes into their constituent monosaccharides. The resultant monosaccharides are transported into the mucosal epithelial cell.[1,2]

Protein Digestion

Protein digestion begins in the stomach with the nonspecific actions of pepsin and hydrochloric acid. Enzymes secreted from the pancreas also play a major role in protein digestion. These enzymes are released in the form of zymogens or inactivated enzymes. Trypsinogen is activated by enterokinase, which is released from the intestinal mucosa. The active enzyme, trypsin, then activates the proenzyme forms of chymotrypsin, elastase, and carboxypeptidase A and B. Trypsin, chymotrypsin, and elastase are called endopeptidases, as they cleave internal bonds. Interluminal digestion of protein results in the generation of free amino acids and oligopeptides. Oligopeptides are further hydrolyzed by the membrane-bound oligopeptidases of the enterocyte brush border.[3]

Lipid Digestion

Lipid digestion begins in the oral cavity with the secretion of lingual lipase and the mechanical effects of mastication. In the stomach, gastric lipase is released and mixes with lingual lipase. In addition, gastric contractions cause a mechanical grinding of the ingested fat, resulting in the formation of an emulsion. An *emulsion* is a suspension of enzymatically partially digested and mechanically disrupted fat droplets in liquid. The emulsion acquires a coating comprised of phospholipids, bile acids, and triglycerides which serves to stabilize the fat globule. This stabilized emulsion ultimately passes into the duodenum.

Pancreatic lipase, the principal enzyme of triglyceride digestion, hydrolyzes ester bonds at the 1 and 3 positions of the glycerol moiety. However, in the presence of bile acids, this enzymatic process is inefficient. Another enzyme secreted by the pancreas, colipase, avidly binds to the triglyceride/aqueous interface of the emulsion and also has a binding site for lipase. Colipase thus ensures the adhesion of lipase to the lipid droplet and increases the efficiency of the latter enzyme in the digestion of triglycerides. Phospholipase A2 is also secreted by the pancreas and acts upon ingested phospholipids to yield a fatty acid and a lysophosphatidylcholine (Figure 59.2). Finally, cholesterol esterase hydrolyzes an esterafied fatty acid from the parent cholesterol molecule.

Once hydrolyzed, lipid products have to traverse the unstirred water layer of the gut prior to being absorbed by the mucosal absorptive cell. However, since fat is not water soluble, fat digestion products have difficulty crossing this water layer. Bile acids, secreted by the liver, greatly facilitate this diffusion. Bile acids are effective because they have a hydrophilic (water-soluble) end and one hydrophobic or lipophilic end (water-insoluble or, conversely, lipid-soluble). These bile acids, when secreted in sufficient quantity, form micelles, which are small spheres with an outward hydrophilic projection and an inner lipophilic core. The products of fat digestion pass into the fat-soluble core while the outer layer remains soluble in the unstirred water layer. This lipid-rich conduit is able to traverse the unstirred water layer and bring the inner lipid core into proximity with the mucosal absorptive cell membrane, which is largely comprised of lipids. Once in contact with the lipid membrane, the micelle core lipids diffuse into the endothelial absorptive cell. This

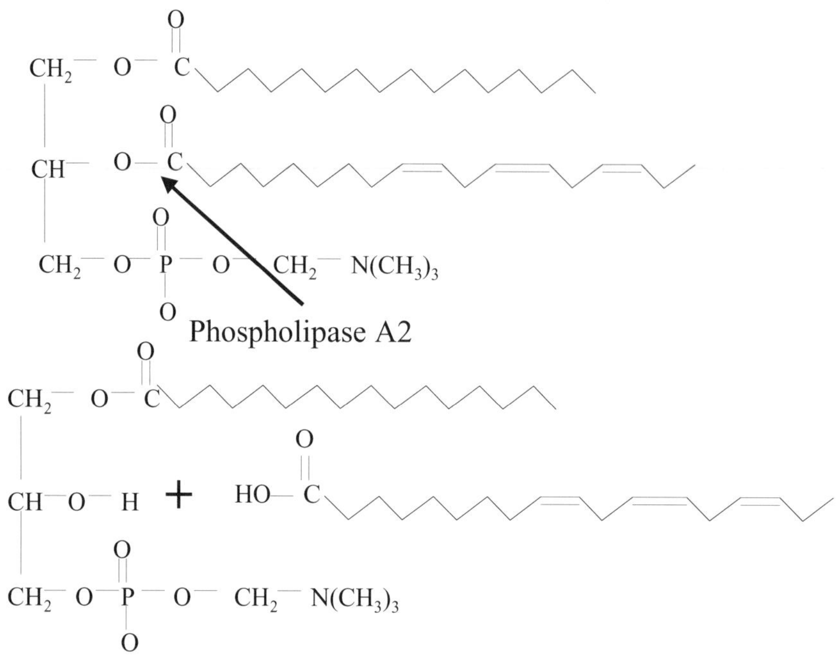

FIGURE 59.2
Phospholipase A_2 action. Phospholipase A_2 hydrolyzes the phospholipid at position 2 to yield a fatty acid, and a lysophospatidylcholine and a fatty acid. (Adapted from Linscheer WG, Vergroesen AJ. In: *Modern Nutrition in Health and Disease* 8th ed, Shils ME, Olson JA, Shike M, Ross AC, Eds, Williams and Wilkins, Baltimore, 1999, pg. 47.)

"shuttling of lipids" from the lumen, where digestion takes place, to the absorptive enterocyte membrane, greatly facilitates lipid absorption.[4,5]

Nutritional Implications and Ramifications in Pancreatic Disease

The nutritional status of patients with pancreatitis is in part dependent on the duration of the disease, the severity of the acute exacerbation, and the underlying etiology of the pancreatitis.

The two most common etiologies of acute pancreatitis in the Western world are alcohol and biliary tract disease. The nutritional status of the patient at the time of acute episode may impact on the clinical course. In a recent study of 99 consecutive patients with acute pancreatitis, 64% of whom had alcohol as an etiology of their disease, only 15% were considered underweight (BMI<19) according to their body mass index (BMI) (weight in kg/height in m^2).[6] Obesity as opposed to malnutrition appears to be a risk factor for severe disease, particularly in alcoholics.[6,7] Still, a severe acute episode could lead to protracted inability to take nutrition by mouth, and relative hypermetabolism.[8] This can lead to depletion of nutritional reserves and, depending on the patient's nutritional status prior to the acute event, may predispose the patient to infection and compromise his ability to survive the acute episode. Thus, although obesity may increase the severity of the presenting episode, it is unclear if a patient whose nutritional reserves are compromised will have a more complicated hospital course.

Alternately, chronic pancreatic patients are generally characterized by an asthenic body type and a low BMI. The causes for a compromised nutritional status are multifactorial but mainly include decreased food intake, maldigestion, and malabsorption.

Decreased Food Intake

Many patients with chronic pancreatitis experience abdominal pain, frequently with accompanying nausea and anorexia. As these symptoms are usually meal related, they often severely limit oral intake.

Maldigestion

Decreases in enzyme and bicarbonate secretion parallel progressive injury to the pancreas. Preliminary studies in patients with pancreatic insufficiency suggest that 5 to 10% of normal postprandial enzyme output by the pancreas is sufficient to maintain normal digestion.[9,10] Maldigestion does not proceed equally among the three macronutrients.

Fat maldigestion is invariably the first to become clinically manifest as nonpancreatic mechanisms do not perform well in lipid digestion. However, there is some compensation for fat digestion, such as to the action of small amounts of lingual or gastric lipases. Given these compensatory mechanisms, an estimated 50% of dietary fat is absorbed.[11] The synthesis and secretion of pancreatic lipase is also more impaired in the damaged pancreas compared to other enzymes. Additionally, lipase is much more sensitive to inactivation in an acidic milieu. Thus, a corresponding decrease in the production of bicarbonate by the damaged gland results in a greater deactivation of lipase. Finally, lipase, once secreted, is more rapidly degraded in the intestinal lumen than the other pancreatic enzymes.

When fat malabsorption is present, the standard for the diagnosis is the finding of greater than 7 g of fat per day in stool collected over a three-day period. Prior to obtaining the specimen, the patient should consume 100 g fat/day for three days and continue on this diet during the three days of collection.[12]

Malabsorption

Malabsorption occurs secondary to the effects of chronic pancreatitis on micelle formation. The failure of the damaged pancreas to secrete sufficient bicarbonate to neutralize the stomach's acidic chyme causes precipitation of bile acids. This impairs micelle formation, which leads to decreased solubility and absorption of ingested fat. A diminished secretion of pancreatic enzymes lessens the bactericidal effect of these enzymes and can result in bacterial overgrowth. The bacteria deconjugate bile acids, which leads to impaired micelle formation, again resulting in malabsorption. Finally, associated complications such as diabetes and cirrhosis can also impair absorption. The former promotes bacterial overgrowth and the latter impairs synthesis of bile acids. Additionally, when diabetes complicates pancreatitis, the nutrient wasting and relatively high glucagon-to-insulin ratio promote malnutrition.

Many patients with chronic pancreatitis have low serum albumin and cholesterol. The latter is in part due to a malabsorption of bile acids which causes increased demand to form bile acids from cholesterol. Other contributing factors include a decrease in the consumption of cholesterol-containing food and malabsorption of luminal cholesterol. Blood fatty acid profiles are also abnormal and can lead to several of the abnormalities that are seen in this disease. Specifically, the blood levels of linoleic acid and arachidonic acid are elevated, while those of eicosapentanoic acid and docosahexanoic acid are increased. There is also a compensatory increase in palmitoleic acid. Polyunsaturated fatty acids play an important role in vascular endothelial cells and platelets in coagulation and thrombus formation. Thus, abnormalities in the levels of these lipids may impact on hemostasis. Finally, the serum concentration of fat-soluble vitamins is low due to poor intake and malabsorption.[13]

A recent study found a slightly greater metabolic rate in patients with chronic pancreatitis compared to a malnourished control group, even when corrected for fat-free mass. There was also a difference within the chronic pancreatis group between those who were normally nourished and those who were undernourished, with the latter group being more "hypercatabolic." This increased resting energy expenditure was seen in over 60% of the stable population with chronic pancreatitis. The authors concluded that the differences were not readily explained by infection, alcohol use, or nicotine use. They suggested that this unexplained metabolic status might contribute to the malnutrition seen in this disease.[14]

Patients with pancreatic cancer are at particularly high risk for nutritional problems. They have the highest incidence of weight loss of any group of patients with cancer, with approximately 80 to 90% losing weight during the course of their illness.[15,16] The development of cachexia and weight loss, which are poor prognostic variables in this disease,[16] is due in part to damage to an organ that is crucial to nutrient digestion as well as constitutional symptoms such as nausea, depression, and anorexia associated with advancing disease. Cytokines released by the tumor or by host cells in response to the tumor lead to anorexia and metabolic dysregulation.

Nutritional Intervention in Pancreatic Disease

Nutritional Intervention in Acute Pancreatitis

Nutritional intervention during an acute episode of pancreatitis is largely determined by the severity of the initial inflammatory event, the estimated period of time that the patient will remain without adequate oral intake, and the patient's underlying nutritional status. The inflammatory response evoked during an acute episode of pancreatitis is largely mediated through the release of cytokines and counterregulatory hormones. This response is teleologically advantageous to the host. Collectively, the acute phase response serves to clear bacteria from the bloodstream, sequester potentially virulent substances, and limit "innocent bystander" oxidative damage. Cytokines also stimulate immune cells and signal them to the appropriate point of engagement, regulating the inflammatory response up or down as needed. This response has been adapted over time to alert, enforce, and aid the immune response as well as limit damage to the host in a response directed against an offending agent. This response, however, can deplete the body's nutrient resources. The greater the insult, the greater the use of endogenous substrate. In spite of exogenous attempts to provide nutritional resources, "autocannibalism" continues, largely unabated. It is therefore plausible, though unproven, that in the setting of poor endogenous resources, a prolonged inflammatory state can overwhelm the body's ability to bring forth an inflammatory response and can contribute to the demise of the host. Unfortunately, there is no simple gauge with which to assess the body's ability to respond appropriately to the challenge.

Ranson Criteria	APACHE-II
At admission	Temperature (rectal)
Age >55	Mean arterial pressure
WBC count >16,000/mm^3	Heart rate
Glucose > 200 mg/dl	Respiratory rate
Lactate dehydrogenase (LDH) > 350 IU/L	Oxygenation
Aspartate transaminase (AST) > 250 U/L	Arterial pH
	Serum sodium
During initial 48 hours	Serum potassium
Hematocrit decrease of > 10 mg/dl	Serum creatinine
Blood urea nitrogen (BUN) increase of > 5 mg/dl	Hematocrit
Calcium < 8 mg/dl	WBC count
PaO_2 < 60 mm Hg	Glasgow coma score
Base deficit > 4 mEq/L	
Fluid sequestration > 6 L	Age points
	Chronic health points

FIGURE 59.3
Ranson criteria and APACHE II severity of pancreatitis. Ranson criteria and the APACHE II severity of disease classification system are two scoring systems used to judge the severity of acute pancreatitis. In the APACHE II system, points were given for each of twelve variables (in box) based on the severity of those variables. Points were also awarded for increasing age, a history of organ dysfunction, immunocompetence, and surgical interventions. Three or more Ranson criteria or eight or more APACHE II points are considered significant disease.

The inflammatory challenge also brings with it a state of substrate intolerance, particularly to carbohydrates and less so to lipids, which makes imprudent use of nutritional support potentially harmful. Additionally, visceral proteins such as albumin, which often are used as nutritional parameters in epidemiological studies, are affected by the inflammatory response and lose value as predictors of substrate exhaustion. Perhaps in the future we will be guided by readily available tests of immune function that will allow us to discern when the immune response is faltering from lack of available substrate. However, currently, we must estimate the severity and duration of the inflammatory response as well as the underlying nutritional status of the host to determine whether nutritional intervention will be of benefit.

Approximately 80% of patients admitted to the hospital with acute pancreatitis have mild disease. These patients are expected to be able to ingest kcalories orally in five to seven days. From a nutritional perspective, unless there is severe underlying malnutrition antedating the episode of pancreatitis, there is little need to intervene.

Severe pancreatitis occurs in about 20% of patients, and with prolonged absence of oral intake nutritional intervention may be necessary. The diagnosis of severe pancreatitis is suspected on the basis of clinical and laboratory evaluations and can be modified by imaging criteria. Several criteria, including Ranson and APACHE II scores, have been established and validated as indicators of severity in acute pancreatitis[17-19] (Figure 59.3).

There is one reason for providing nutrition in acute pancreatitis accompanied by a mitigating circumstance. Nutrition is provided to support the underlying nutritional status of the host while the patient is beseiged by mediators of the inflammatory process. If there is a deficiency in endogenous substrate, artificial nutrition will furnish the needed building blocks to survive the insult. The mitigating circumstance is whether the treatment itself does more harm, as the therapy may stimulate the inflamed pancreas and aggravate the underlying problem. Additionally, metabolic aberrations potentially caused by the therapy may complicate the clinical picture.

Several studies in animals (with and without pancreatitis), healthy humans, and humans with stable pancreatic fistulas demonstrate little convincing evidence that parenteral nutrition or enteral feeding delivered to the jejunum produce significant pancreatic stimulation. The more convincing data come from human trials in patients with pancreatitis, in whom there is no increased rate of pancreas-related complications using either modality.[20,21]

Unfortunately, only a few randomized controlled studies exist on the benefit of nutritional intervention. In a study by Sax et al., patients with mild pancreatitis (average Ranson criteria 1 to 2) were randomized to receive either standard hydration or parenteral nutrition.[22] The authors found no advantage to using parenteral nutrition with respect to hospital days or number of pancreatic complications. The authors did find a greater risk of line infections in this group than in patients with other diseases requiring parenteral nutrition who were cared for concurrently using the same central line care. The importance of parenteral nutrition in this study may have been understated, as all the patients had mild disease.

Another study by Kalfarentzos et al. examined parenteral nutrition in patients with more severe disease (Ranson criteria 3 or greater). The study was retrospective, and the groups were divided on the basis of whether patients began parenteral nutrition within the first 72 hours. The authors stated that the initiation of parenteral nutrition was based on clinical grounds, but it is not clear what factors initiated the use of TPN and why the authors chose 72 hours as a reference point. In spite of these potential biases, the authors showed a statistically significant reduction in local complications and mortality. The authors also reconfirmed the apparent increased risk of catheter-related complications in this group of patients (again, compared to concurrent, nonpancreatic disease patients who were receiving parenteral nutrition).[23] Thus, the interpretation of this one prospective study and several retrospective studies is that parenteral nutrition does not worsen pancreatitis and may be of benefit in severe disease, though the data are not convincing.

McClave et al. compared enteral jejunal feedings to parenteral nutrition in patients with mild pancreatitis, generally of alcoholic etiology. The authors found that the enteral route was safe and there were no differences in clinical or biochemical resolution of pancreatitis in their study patients. However, the cost of nutritional intervention in the enteral group was significantly lower than the parenteral group.[24] Kalfarentzos and colleagues also performed a randomized prospective trial of enteral versus parenteral feeding in severe acute pancreatitis (APACHE II score 8 to 15). They not only showed that enteral feeding was safe, they also showed that these patients had a significantly lower septic complication rate than the parenteral nutrition group. Other morbidities, including the incidence of infectious pancreatic or peripancreatic necrosis, were also lower in the enteral nutrition group but did not reach statistical significance, probably because of the small numbers of patients in the groups.[25]

Jejunal feeding in patients with pancreatitis is not only safe but also as effective as parenteral nutrition in supporting the patient. An additional question is whether the enteral route, by stimulating trophic factors which can potentially maintain the integrity of the gut as a barrier against bacterial translocation, is beneficial to patient care in ways that are not realized with parenteral nutrition. The issue of translocation in other predisposing states such as trauma and sepsis has been more readily proven in animal models than in humans.[26,27] The proof that this process is clinically significant in humans is less established.[28] The causative bacteria in infected pancreatic necrosis are often of gut origin, and translocation of bacteria and/or endotoxin can contribute to the inflammatory process.[29-31] Enteral nutrition in pancreatitis appears to be safe from the available clinical studies, and it offers cost savings and fewer septic complications. It should be considered strongly as the treatment of choice in these patients. If it also decreases the incidence of infected pancreatic necrosis, which is associated with a significantly increased morbidity and mortality, it moves out of the realm of purely nutritional support and into the realm of a therapeutic intervention.

A recent study examined the immunoinflammatory response and its relationship to nutritional outcome with enteral feeding. In addition to finding that enteral nutrition was associated with decreases in sepsis and multiorgan failure (though not significant), the authors reported significant decreases in the APACHE II scores for enterally fed patients (11 to 2) versus parenterally fed patients (12 to 10). They also reported moderate decreases in c-reactive protein (CRP). Parenterally fed patients had significant increases in IgM antiendotoxin response, while these levels remained unchanged in enterally fed patients. These data support enteral feeding as an intervention that will improve disease severity and clinical outcome by modifying the acute phase response. Moreover, these findings lend support to the concept that enteral feeding maintains the integrity of the gut as a barrier against translocation, which can be a contributor to the inflammatory response seen in this disease.[32]

As more evidence shows that enteral nutrition is safe and beneficial, it should begin to supplant parenteral nutrition in the management of pancreatitis. In reality, although these studies are promising, they are still small in number and the practice of enteral nutrition is not widespread.

In severe acute disease, the predominant treatment in most hospitals and medical centers is parenteral nutrition. Knowledge of the appropriate use and the individual components of the parenteral solution becomes a mainstay in treating patients with severe disease.

Parenteral Nutrition Issues

Which Patients are Candidates for Parenteral Nutrition

Candidates are those who have severe disease (as assessed by severity scores), those who are malnourished upon admission to the hospital, and those who have complications of their disease.

Delivery Volume; Total Kcalories; Individual Macronutrients, Micronutrients, and other Additives

Fluid volume: pancreatitis has been compared to an internal burn, with tremendous shifts in fluid. Recent data suggest that the level of hemoconcentration seen at presentation may have prognostic significance in acute pancreatitis. This not only suggests that relative hypovolemia may contribute to pancreatic damage, but also underscores the importance of fluid resuscitation. However, since renal, lung, and cardiac dysfunction can accompany severe pancreatic insult, vigorous or inadequate use of fluids can be detrimental to the patient. Though fluid resuscitation is important, total volume replacement is not an essential goal of parenteral nutrition in a severe, acute setting. At our institution, the volume of solution is based on providing 20 to 35 cc of fluid per kilogram estimated dry weight of the patient. Additionally, adjustments are made for the presence of heart or renal failure, or conversely for the presence of increased fluid loss or sequestration. Usually only one liter of the solution is infused the first day to determine the patient's metabolic response to the infused nutrients. Care should be taken to ensure against metabolic aberrations. Additional volume for resuscitation can be delivered through peripheral intravenous fluids.

Kcalories: when estimating the total kcalories provided to the patient, consider that a significant percentage of patients with pancreatitis are hypermetabolic. However, the same factor, the inflammatory response, that increases the metabolic rate in these patients also introduces an element of substrate intolerance. This intolerance, which is mainly to carbohydrates but is also to a lesser degree to lipids, is not specific to pancreatitis but is a feature of any significant inflammatory response. Similarly, if renal failure or encephalopathy are present, the provision of protein also needs careful monitoring. Additionally, the hypermetabolism seen with an acute insult should be considered dynamic and can decrease or increase during the hospitalization, roughly paralleling the patient's clinical course.

The most reliable indicator of kcaloric needs in the hospital setting is indirect calorimetry. If this is not available, then formula equations can be used to estimate needs, although formula equations are less reliable. These equations were developed in healthy individuals and are secondarily extrapolated to the severely ill. There may be a significant under- or overestimation of metabolic needs in the individual patient. The first tenet in treating these patients is to do no harm. Therefore, although targets for estimating needs may be logically derived or measured, pushing macronutrient delivery to hyperglycemia or hyperlipidemia, especially in the setting of pancreatitis, is clearly not in the patient's best interest.

Protein: though amino acids may be the most important macronutrient provided, there is little data to support an optimal amount. In studies of parenteral nutrition in pancreatitis, the protein provided ranged from 1 to 2.5 g/kg.[22-25,32] In the setting of renal impairment or encephalopathy, the protein load needs to be conservative and monitored closely. Conversely, if protein losses seem very high, protein should move toward the higher end of the range provided there are no intolerances. Initiate a more conservative amount of protein and advance only after the patient demonstrates stability to the initial protein load.

It is controversial whether protein kcalories should be considered as part of total kcalories. Parenterally-provided protein is not intended to be a kcaloric source; yet there is partial metabolism. Thus, including protein in the kcaloric goal will likely result in an underestimation of kcalories, whereas the opposite will result if protein is calculated separately. However, as the kcaloric content of the provided protein is usually modest and since more harm, in the form of metabolic intolerances, is likely from providing too many kcalories, protein kcalories should be included in total kcalories.

Fat: has been used reluctantly in acute pancreatitis. This stems in part from animal and human experimental studies which show conflicting evidence of the ability of intravenous fat to stimulate the pancreas.[34] Additionally, hyperlipidemia with triglyceride levels of greater than 1000 mg/ml appear to be etiologic in some causes of pancreatitis.[35] Furthermore, in 12 to 15% of cases of acute pancreatitis, there appears to be an associated hypertriglyceridemia.[39] In a retrospective study of lipid infusion in acute pancreatitis, no untoward effect occured as a result of lipid infusion. This was noted in spite of two patients who survived the acute attack and had triglyceride levels in the low to mid-300 mg/ml range. In that study, patients who did not survive had significantly higher plasma triglyceride levels than those who survived. Additionally, lipid oxidation was apparently not affected despite elevated triglyceride levels. It therefore seems that lipids can be safely infused in patients with acute pancreatitis that is not secondary to hyperlipidemia. In the setting of hypertriglyceridemia secondary to pancreatitis, continued lipid infusion was safe in spite of at least one patient with a pre-TPN triglyceride level of 880 mg/dl. During TPN the level decreased to the mid- to low- 400 range.[33-38] It is prudent to monitor triglyceride levels closely and avoid the use of parenteral lipids until levels are below 400 mg/ml. Several studies suggest that parenteral fat can be utilized in the absence of high triglyceride levels, though no large prospective study has specifically addressed this issue.[34]

This finding is of particular importance given the increased incidence of glucose intolerance in acute pancreatitis. Thus, in this setting the use of parenteral fat at 1 to 2 g/kg, not to exceed 40% of the nonprotein kcalories, appears to be safe.

Carbohydrates: early studies of the delivery of carbohydrates to stressed patients suggest that amounts greater than 5 mg/kg/min are associated with an increased respiratory quotient (RQ).[40] In other words, carbohydrates delivered above this infusion rate resulted in lipogenesis with a high CO_2 production to O_2 consumption ratio, thus elevating the RQ. As carbohydrates are provided to the patient for oxidative utilization, lipogenesis represents inappropriate carbohydrate utilization. Thus, 5 mg/kg/day should represent the ceiling of carbohydrate utilization. Hyperglycemia should also be taken into consideration in determining the maximal rate of carbohydrate delivered. Hyperglycemia implies impaired clearance or oxidative utilization of the provided glucose and should be avoided. This metabolic abnormality can further lead to fluid and electrolyte problems and has been implicated in immune dysfunction, potentially complicating the underlying clinical situation.

Nutritional Intervention in Pancreatic Insufficiency

Pancreatic insufficiency occurs when enzyme secretion from the pancreas falls below 10% of normal values. Insufficiency becomes clinically manifest in the form of fat malabsorption, steatorrhea, and to a lesser extent, protein malabsorption or azotorrhea. The treatment of pancreatic insufficiency involves the use of exogenous pancreatic enzymes. Fat is the most predominant malabsorbed macronutrient in pancreatic insufficiency. Synthesis of lipase is compromised to a greater degree than synthesis of other pancreatic enzymes, there is less extrapancreatic compensation for fat absorption, and lipase inactivation is greater than inactivation in the other enzymes.[41] Replacement therapy is usually based on providing at least 28,000 IU of lipase per meal, but much higher doses are often needed.[36,37] Since preparations vary in their enzyme amounts, particular attention should be given to the lipase activity (Table 59.2). In spite of providing oral replacement of pancreatic enzymes in various forms, total abolition of steatorrhea is seldom achieved.

There are multiple reasons that replacement enzymes do not normalize fat malabsorption. The most important is the sensitivity of lipase to inactivation by gastric acid. This factor leads to the coadministration of the initial conventional preparations with bicarbonate, and later, acid suppressive agents. This maneuver further improved but did not completely abolish steatorrhea. In a continuing effort to improve the efficacy of these preparations, the enzymes were packed into enteric coated microspheres 1 to 2 mm in size to protect the enzymes from inactivation by gastric acid. The enzymes were liberated at an alkaline pH. Additionally, the size of the particles was engineered to optimize emptying from the stomach. Granules greater than 2 mm may not empty from the stomach at the same time as the meal, and therefore not result in optimal mixing of enzyme with food. In spite of these apparent technologic advances, steatorrhea persisted. One proposed problem was continued poor mixing of enzymes with their intended substrate. This could occur secondary to poor emptying of enzyme from the stomach or a discrepancy between emptying of food and enzyme from the stomach.[42,43]

A contributing reason for poor substrate/enzyme mixing was recently reported by Guarner et al., who found increased amounts of lipase in the ileum. The authors hypothesized that this was due to poor alkalization of the proximal bowel in patients with diseased pancreas, and hence diminished bicarbonate secretion. The enzymes were not liberated until the more distal bowel, thus potentially diminishing their interaction with

TABLE 59.2

Pancreatic Replacement Enzymes and Strengths of Major Constituents

Recommendations are to start with lowest dose that controls symptoms and adjust upward as indicated.

Enzyme Preparation	Description	Lipase	Protease	Amylase	Starting Dosage
Viokase	noncoated	8,000	30,000	30,000	1-3 tabs w/meals
Cotazym	noncoated	8,000	30,000	30,000	1-2 tabs w/meals
Donnazyme	gastric soluble/pancreatin	1,000	12,500	12,500	2 tabs w/meals
Zymase	enteric coated (EC) spheres	12,000	24,000	24,000	1-2 tabs w/meals
Creon	EC minimicrospheres				
5		5,000	18,750	16,600	2-4 tabs w/meals
10		10,000	37,500	33,200	1-2 tabs w/meal
20		20,000	75,000	66,400	1 tab/wmeal
Pancrease	EC microtablets				
4		4,000	12,000	12,000	400 units of lipase
10		10,000	30,000	30,000	per kg per meal
16		16,000	48,000	48,000	per kg per meal
20		20,000	44,000	56,000	per kg per meal
Ultrase	EC minitablets				
12		12,000	39,00	39,000	1-2 tabs w/meals
18		18,000	58,500	58,500	
20		20,000	65,000	65,000	

nutrients.[44] Additionally, because of the acidification seen in the proximal small bowels of patients with chronic pancreatitis, there may be precipitation of bile acids. This serves to decrease effective micelle formation, hence retarding fat absorption.

Usually patients should take two to seven enteric-coated capsules or five to eight non-enteric coated tablets of an enzyme preparation with meals. Some patients using conventional preparations may need adjuvant acid suppressive therapy (see above). A favorable response to therapy is evidenced by a decrease in steatorrhea, relief of diarrhea, and weight gain. If the patient does not respond to this intervention, either a lower fat diet (not to exceed 60 g fat per day) or evaluation of other potential contributing causes of steatorrhea, such as bacterial overgrowth, need to be considered. Of interest, generic brands of enteric enzymes may not contain bioequivalent amounts of enzymes as the name brand.[42]

Nutritional Intervention in Pancreatic Cancer

Nutritional intervention in patients with pancreatic cancer is often frustrating as these patients proceed down the pathway of progressive malnutrition. In this disease, it is estimated that 89% of patients have experienced weight loss at the time of diagnosis.[45] Ultimately, their demise is as much a function of their nutritional status as their underlying malignancy. The ability to provide effective nutrition should improve the quality of life for these patients. The reasons for weight loss are attributed to anorexia, with secondary decreased food intake, abnormal metabolism, and malabsorption. One study suggested that malabsorption is the most important cause of weight loss in this patient population.[45]

Even when intake can be increased in cancer patients, nutritional gains are minimal. A study by Ovesen et al. assessed the role of frequent nutritional counseling on oral intake, anthropometrics, response to chemotherapy, survival, and quality of life in patients with pancreatic and other malignancies. Though counseling effectively increased energy and protein intake, there were no significant gains in weight or lean body mass during the five-month protocol. Additionally, overall survival, quality of life, and tumor response rate was not significantly different.[46]

Cytokines may play an important role in weight loss and, equally important, the inability to accrue lost lean body tissue in the presence of artificial nutrition. A recent study examined the presence of an acute phase response as an indicator of the effects of pro-inflammatory cytokines in patients with pancreatic cancer. Patients with an acute phase protein response (defined as a C-reactive protein level of greater than 10 mg/l) had a substantial reduction in food intake (approximately 29%). The group with the higher acute phase protein response was also mildly more hypermetabolic than the group that did not exhibit this response. These factors seemed to contribute to accelerated wasting in these patients.[47] Furthermore, the ongoing utilization of amino acids for the acute phase response, as well as for other hepatic export proteins such as albumin, may have a significant effect on whole-body nitrogen economy and could contribute to the loss of lean body tissue. Pro-inflammatory cytokine activity therefore appears to be associated not only with altered host energy metabolism, but also with reduced appetite, thereby contributing to the accelerated weight loss observed with cachexia.[47]

A further study by Falconer of weight-losing patients with pancreatic cancer demonstrated that approximately half of the patients had evidence of an acute phase protein response, and in that subset of patients the resting energy expenditure (REE) was significantly elevated. However, in that study, patients who did not demonstrate an acute phase response also had a higher REE than similar weight-matched controls, and both subgroups of patients lost weight. The differences in weight loss between the groups were not significant. Nevertheless, the authors concluded that an inflammatory response might contribute to the hypermetabolism seen in some patients with pancreatic cancer.[48]

The acute phase protein response also was associated with a significant decline in clinical status. The authors proposed that C-reactive protein, an indicator of the acute phase response, could be used as a variable for stratifying patients into prognostic categories. The higher the level of CRP, the poorer the prognosis.[49] The authors postulated that since the association was so strong, this response might be a useful target for metabolic intervention in the weight-losing patient with cancer.[49]

These preliminary observations led to a study of Megace (an appetite stimulant) and ibuprofen in weight-losing cancer patients. These authors had previously performed a similar six-week study in the same population using only Megace. In that study the authors reported a 1.7 kg weight loss during the study period. The ibuprofen was added to blunt the acute phase protein response, and in so doing the authors reported a 1.3 kg weight gain over the same time period. The authors proposed that the addition of the NSAID and the blunting of the acute phase reaction was the only differentiating factor between the two studies, and thus supported a role for these cytokines in cancer cachexia. Unfortunately, the weight gain appeared to largely be confined to adipose tissue.[50]

It has been demonstrated that a diet high in fish, specifically eicosapentaenoic acid (EPA) and docosahexaenoic acid (DHA) decreases proinflammatory cytokines (IL-1, Il-6, TNF).[51] To study how inflammatory cytokines contribute to the weight loss and cachexia in patients with pancreatic cancer, Barber and colleagues investigated the role of a nutritional supplement enriched with EPA/DHA in patients with inoperable pancreatic cancer. Performance status, appetite, and weight gain all significantly increased. The increase in weight did not seem to be due to an increase in body water or fat. There was no change in the acute phase protein response (APPR), but the authors commented that in the supplemented group they did not find the usual increase in the APPR. Median survival was 4.1 months, which was noted to be at the upper limit of survival in chemotherapy trials in patients of similar disease severity, without the concomitant side effects.[52]

Another area of interesting nutritional intervention in pancreatic cancer is retinoid supplementation. *In vitro,* retinoid treatment of human pancreatic cancer cells results in inhibition of growth, induction of cellular differention, and decreased adhesion to basement membranes (decreased ability to metastasize). In addition, two-thirds of patients with unresectable pancreatic cancer treated with 13-cis retinoic acid and interferon demonstrated stable disease with a mean duration of five months.[53,54]

Although, these results are still preliminary and await randomized controlled studies, they may add hope in the nutritionally abysmal outlook of patients with pancreatic cancer.

The Role of Antioxidants in Pancreatic Disease

The similarity between the changes seen in pancreatic tissue in acute pancreatitis and damage in other tissue known to occur as a result of oxygen radical production led researchers to postulate a role of electrophiles in the pathogenesis of acute pancreatitis. Oxygen radicals, once generated, react with all biologic substances, most readily with polyunsaturated fatty acids (PUFA). Since PUFA are present in high concentrations in cellular membranes, free radical attack will invariably lead to cell membrane disruption and ultimately to cell death.[5] In addition to direct tissue damage, these radicals also signal the accumulation of neutrophils. Neutrophils release various enzymes and other mediators which can damage tissue as well as adhere to endothelium, potentially resulting in vascular plugging and further adding to the microcirculatory derangements observed in the inflammatory stage of this disease.[56] Additionally, they also release oxygen radicals, the "respiratory burst," further damaging tissue and recruiting neutrophils. This cascade can continue to upregulate, resulting in extensive tissue damage. Because of the effects of these reactive oxygen species, these substances can be viewed as triggers of various inflammatory processes. The theory of oxygen-free radicals significantly contributing to the pathophysiology of acute pancreatitis was tested in animals. Most animal studies suggest the presence of these radicals in the early stages of pancreatic injury.[57] It was thus theorized that pretreatment with oxygen-free radical scavengers would lessen pancreatic damage.[58-60] Though the results were mixed, it appears that pretreatment helps in some forms of pancreatic damage. However, if pancreatic injury develops too rapidly, other pathomechanisms seem to cause tissue injury, making enhanced generation of reactive oxygen metabolites ineffective. Fewer animal studies are available for treatment with scavengers after the injury, but they demonstrate that treatment after injury helps to minimize the tissue damage.

In early human studies Braganza, Guyan, and Schoenberg demonstrated increased amounts of lipid peroxidation products. This indirectly demonstrated oxygen-free radical attack on cellular lipids in the serum, bile, duodenal juice, and tissue of patients suffering from acute and/or recurrent pancreatitis.[61] Another study observed several antioxidant deficiencies in patients with pancreatitis, though it is not clear whether the deficiencies facilitated damage or merely were an end result of the damage.[62]

Sandilands et al. were the first to propose that antioxidants may also play a role in the pain management of chronic pancreatitis. They described four patients with significant and recurrent pain from pancreatitis in spite of both medical and surgical intervention. The researchers postulated that ongoing damage to the gland might be caused by free oxidant generation. They further suspected that endogenous stores of these antioxidants might be deficient. The patients were given an antioxidant supplement, selenium ACE (containing 1000 mg of selenium, 1500 IU vitamin A, 90 mg vitamin C, and 45 IU of vitamin E per tablet) varying from one to six tablets per day. Three of these patients also received methionine (2 to 4 g/d). All patients became pain free and have remained without recurrent attacks for a follow-up period of five years.[63] Similar dramatic responses were reported in three patients with familial lipoprotein lipase deficiency and consequent recurrent attacks of acute pancreatitis. Lipoprotein lipase removes triglycerides from circulating lipoproteins. Absence of this enzyme leads to extremely elevated triglyceride levels. As such, many patients with this disorder are prone to recurrent pancreatitis. In a report by Heaney, three patients with lipoprotein lipase deficiency were treated with antioxidant therapy (selenium, β-carotene, vitamins C and E, and methionine). Prior to initiating antioxidant therapy, these patients had failed repeated medical and surgical interventions. After initiation of antioxidant therapy, two patients had no further episodes of pancreatitis in the next 4 to 6 years of observation (previously having between three to six episodes per year). The third patient had a dramatic reduction in pain episodes, going from ten or greater the previous four years to an average of one episode per year over the next three years.[64]

These are exciting examples of how nutritional intervention may not only alleviate the effects of pancreatic disease, but also may have an impact on the disease itself.

References

1. Levin RJ. In: *Modern Nutrition in Health and Disease* 9th ed, Shils ME, Olson JA, Shike M, Ross AC, Eds, Williams and Wilkins, Baltimore, 1999, pg 49.
2. Metzger A, DiMagno EP. In: *The Pancreas* 1st ed, Berger HG, Warshaw AL, Buchler MW, Carr-Locke DL, Neoptolemos JP, Russel C, Sarr MG, Eds, Blackwell Science, Cambridge, England 1998, pg 147.
3. Lowe ME. In: *Physiology of the Gastrointestinal Tract* 3rd ed, Johnson LR, Alpers DH, Christensen J, Jacobson ED, Walsh JH, Eds, Raven Press, New York, 1994, pg 1531.
4. Tso P. In: *Physiology of the Gastrointestinal Tract* 3rd ed, Johnson LR, Alpers DH, Christensen J, Jacobson ED, Walsh JH, Eds, Raven Press, New York, 1994, pg 1867.
5. Jones PJH, Kubow S. In: *Modern Nutrition in Health and Disease* 9th ed, Shils ME, Olson JA, Shike M, Ross AC, Eds, Williams and Wilkins, Baltimore, 1999, pg 67.
6. Funnell IC, Bornman PC, Weakley SP, et al. *Br J Surg* 80: 484; 1993.
7. Martinez J, Sanchez-Paya J, Palazon JM, et al. *Pancreas* 19: 15; 1999.
8. Dickerson RN, Vehe KL, Mullen JL, et al. *Crit Care Med* 19: 484; 1991.
9. Grendell JH. *Clin Gastroenterol* 12: 551; 1983.
10. DiMagno EP, Malagelada JR, Go VL, et al. *N Engl J Med* 296: 1318; 1977.
11. Twersky Y, Bank S. *Gastroenterol Clinc N Am* 18: 543; 1989.
12. DiMagno EP, Go VLW, Summerskill WHJ. *NEJOM* 288: 813; 1973.
13. Nakamura T, Takeuchi T. *Pancreas* 14: 323; 1997.
14. Hebuterne X, Hastier P, Peroux J, et al. *Dig Dis Sci* 41: 533; 1996.
15. DeWys WD. In: *Nutritional Support for the Cancer Patient* 1st ed, Calman KC, Fearon KCH, Eds, London, Balliere Tindall, 1986, pg 251.
16. Falconer JS, Fearon KC, Ross JA. *Cancer* 75: 2077; 1994.
17. Ranson JHC, Rifkind KM, Roses DF, et al. *Surg Gyn Obst* 139: 69; 1974.
18. Knaus WA, Draper EA, Wagner DP, et al. *Crit Care Med* 13: 818-829, 1985.
19. Balthazar EJ, Robinson DL, Megibow AJ, et al. *Radiology* 174: 331; 1990.
20. Havala T, Shronts E, Cerra F. *Gastroenterol Clin N Am* 18: 525; 1989.
21. Corcoy R, Sanchez JM, Domingo P, et al. *Nutrition* 4: 269; 1988.
22. Sax HC, Warner BW, Talamini M, et al. *Am J Surg* 153: 117; 1987.
23. Kalfarentzos FE, Karavias DD, Karatzas TM, et al. *J Am Col Nut* 10: 156; 1991.
24. McClave SA, Greene LM, Snider HL, et al. *J Parent Ent Nutr* 21: 14; 1997.

25. Kalfarentzos F, Kehagias J, Mead N, et al. *Brit J Surg* 84: 1665; 1997.
26. Alverdy J. *Sem Resp Infect* 9: 248; 1994.
27. Gianotti L, Alexander JW, Nelson JL, et al. *Crit Care Med* 22: 265; 1994.
28. Sedman PC, Macfie J, Sagar P, et al. *Gastroenterology* 107: 64; 1994.
29. Luiten EJT, Hop WCJ, Lange JF, et al. *Clin Infect Dis* 25: 811; 1997.
30. Ryan C, Schmidt J, Lewandrowski K. *Gastroenterology* 104: 890; 1993.
31. Fong Y, Marano MA, Barber A, et al. *Ann Surg* 210: 449; 1989.
32. Windsor ACJ, Kanwar S, Li ACK, et al. *Gut* 42: 431; 1998.
33. Van Gossum A, Lemoyne M, Greig PD, et al. *J Parent Ent Nutr* 12: 250; 1988.
34. Leibowitz AB, O'Sullivan P, Iberti TJ. *Mount Sinai J of Med* 59: 38; 1992.
35. Amann ST, Toskes PP. In: *The Pancreas* 1st ed, Berger HG, Warshaw AL, Buchler MW, Carr-Locke DL, Neoptolemos JP, Russel C, Sarr MG, Eds, Blackwell Science, Cambridge, England, 1998, pg 311.
36. McClave SA, Spain DA, Snider HL. *Gastro Clin N Am* 27: 421; 1998.
37. Scolapio JS, Malhi-Chowla N, Ukleja A. *Gastrol Clin N Am* 28: 695; 1999.
38. Silberman H, Dixon NP, Eisenberg D. *Am J Gastro* 77: 494; 1982.
39. McClave SA, Snider H, Owens N, et al. *Dig Dis Sci* 42: 2035; 1997.
40. Burke JF, Wolfe RR, Mullany CJ. *Ann Surg* 190: 74; 1979.
41. Layer P, Holtman G. *Int J Pancreatology* 15: 1; 1994.
42. Greenberger NJ. *Gastro Clin N Am* 28: 687; 1999.
43. Grendell JH. *Clin Gastro* 12: 551; 1983.
44. Guarner L, Rodriguez R, Guarner F, et al. *Gut* 34: 708; 1993.
45. Perez MM, Newcomer AD, Mortel CG, et al. *Cancer* 52: 346; 1983.
46. Ovesen L, Allingstrup L, Hannibal J, et al. *J Clin Oncol* 11: 2043; 1993.
47. Fearon KCH, Barber MD, Falconer JS, et al. *World J Surg* 23: 584; 1999.
48. Falconer JS, Fearon KCH, Plester CE. *Ann Surg* 219: 325; 1994.
49. Falconer JS, Fearon KC, Ross JA. *Cancer* 75: 2077; 1994.
50. McMillan DC, Gorman PO, Fearon KCH, et al. *Br J Surg* 76: 788; 1997.
51. Meydani SN, Lichtenstein AH, Cornwall S, et al. *J Clin Invest* 92: 105; 1993.
52. Barber MD, Ross JA, Voss AC. *Br J Cancer* 81: 80; 1999.
53. Riecken EO, Rosewicz S. *Ann Onc* 10: 197S; 1999.
54. Rosewicz S, Wollbergs K, Von Lampe B, et al. *Gastroenterology* 112: 532; 1997.
55. Schoenberg MH, Buchler M, Helfen M, et al. *Eur Surg Res* 24: 74S; 1992.
56. Schoenberg MH, Birk D, Beger HG. *Am J Clin Nutr* 62: 1306S; 1995.
57. Schoenberg MH, Buchler M, Beger HG. *Free Rad Biol Med* 12: 515; 1992.
58. Schoenberg MH, Buchler M, Younes M, et al. *Dig Dis Sci* 39: 1034; 1994.
59. Furukawa M, Kimura T, Yamaguchi H, et al. *Pancreas* 9: 67; 1994.
60. Nonaka A, Manabe T, Kyogoku T, et al. *Dig Dis Sci* 37: 274; 1992.
61. Schoenberg MH, Birk D. In: *The Pancreas* 1st ed, Berger HG, Warshaw AL, Buchler MW, Carr-Locke DL, Neoptolemos JP, Russel C, Sarr MG, Eds, Blackwell Science, Cambridge, England, 1998, pg 702.
62. Gossum AV, Closset P, Noel E, et al. *Dig Dis Sci* 41: 1225; 1996.
63. Sandilands D, Jeffery IJM, Haboubi NY, et al. *Gastroenterology* 98: 766; 1990.
64. Heanney AP, Sharer N, Rameh B, et al. *J Clin Endocrinol Metab* 84: 1203; 1999.
65. Linscheer WG, Vergroesen AJ. In: *Modern Nutrition in Health and Disease* 8th ed, Shils ME, Olson JA, Shike M, Ross AC, Eds, Williams and Wilkins, Baltimore, 1999, pg 47.

60

Renal Nutrition

Jane M. Greene and Lynn Thomas

Introduction

The kidneys play a vital role in the maintenance of normal blood volume/pressure and regulation of acid-base balance. Approximately one-fourth of the cardiac output is filtered through the kidneys each minute. Urinary excretion is the pathway for removal of the waste products of absorption and metabolism. These include ammonia, urea, creatinine, phosphorus, water, sodium, and potassium. Normal bone health is facilitated by activation of vitamin D and regulation of calcium and phosphorus. The kidney produces the hormone erythropoietin. Deficiency of this hormone results in profound anemia.

A decrease in kidney function greatly affects metabolism and nutritional status. These patients are at risk for protein energy malnutrition. Common manifestations include edema, uremia, hypertension, anemia, and metabolic acidosis. The medical nutrition therapy for kidney failure becomes increasingly complex as the renal disease advances. The diet prescription is matched to the stage of renal failure in order to keep the diet as liberal as possible. Table 60.1[1] defines the terms used in this section.

Nutritional Assessment in the Renal Patient

It is a recommended standard of practice that all renal patients are considered at risk for nutritional compromise. Protein energy malnutrition is a common finding among these patients. Acute and chronic renal failure patients should receive baseline assessments as soon as they are identified or admitted to the hospital. New dialysis patients should receive an assessment within thirty days of the initial treatment. Reassessments should be done at least annually. Short-term updates are required monthly by most dialysis clinics. Any significant changes in weight, laboratory values, or medical status should trigger an in-depth investigation. The goal of the assessment is to develop a diet prescription tailored to the patient's individual needs. The diet should be as liberal as possible and include the patients favorite foods. The patient should be provided with written materials covering

0-8493-2705-9/02/$0.00+$1.50

TABLE 60.1

Explanation of Terms Used in this Section

Term	Explanation
Acute renal failure	Sudden onset secondary to shock, trauma, hypertension, exposure to nephrotoxic substances or bacteria; reversible in many cases.
Azotemia	Elevated concentrations of nitrogenous wastes in blood serum.
Chronic renal failure (CRF) or insufficiency (CRI)	Gradual progression terminating with end stage renal disease requiring dialysis or transplant. Causes include obstructive disease of the urinary tract such as congenital birth defects, systemic diseases such as diabetes mellitus or systemic lupus erythematosis, glomerular disease, and overdosing on analgesic medications. Patients follow an increasingly restricted diet as renal failure progresses.
Hemodialysis	Removal from blood of the waste products of metabolism by use of a semipermeable membrane and a dialysis treatment machine. This process takes 3-6 hours three times per week in an outpatient clinic or hospital. Some patients, with appropriate training and assistance, can dialyze at home. Hemodialysis patients follow a diet restricted in sodium, potassium, phosphorus, and fluids.
Nephrotic syndrome	Failure of the glomerular basement membrane to filter waste products appropriately. Large amounts of protein are found in the urine. Patients frequently have edema secondary to hypoalbumenemia.
Peritoneal dialysis	Removal of the waste products of metabolism by perfusion of a sterile dialysate solution throughout the peritoneal cavity. This method of dialysis is done at home. Dialysate exchanges are performed several times per day or continuously at night with the aid of a peritoneal dialysis machine. Peritoneal dialysis patients follow a liberalized diet since dialysis is daily. The diet is normally a low sodium diet with diabetes mellitus restrictions as necessary.
Uremia	A toxic systemic syndrome caused by retention of high levels of urea.

the major points. The diet is modified on a regular basis as indicated. Tables 60.2[2-6] and 60.3[7-9] provide guidelines for various components of the nutrition assessment.

Stages of Renal Failure

The method of treatment and the nutrition recommendations vary as the patient progresses through the various stages of renal failure. The normal kidney removes excess fluid and waste products from the body and maintains acid-base balance. The kidney also regulates blood pressure, stimulates red blood cell production, and regulates the metabolism of calcium and phosphorus. Nephrotic syndrome is a dysfunction of the glomerular capillaries. Symptoms include urine losses of plasma proteins, low serum albumin, edema, and elevated blood lipids. In acute renal failure the nephrons lose function or the glomerular filtration rate (GFR) drops suddenly. Symptoms include increased blood urea nitrogen, catabolism, negative nitrogen balance, elevated electrolytes, acidosis, increased blood pressure, and fluid overload. Nephrotic syndrome and acute renal failure are usually reversible conditions. In chronic renal failure the GFR declines gradually. In early stages, compensation occurs by enlarging the remaining nephrons.

Symptoms similar to those in acute renal failure appear when the kidney is at 75% of normal function. When the GFR is 10% or less of the normal rate the patient is considered to be in end-stage renal disease. Dialysis is started to replace diminished kidney function. Electrolytes, fluids, anemia, and diet are monitored monthly by a registered dietitian. Some patients in end-stage renal failure receive kidney transplants. This restores kidney function and the patient is able to return to a more liberal diet.

TABLE 60.2

Components of the Nutrition Assessment[a]

Component	Approach
Medical history and physical exam	One way to organize findings is to use a review of systems approach. Note any medical problems or surgical procedures that could impact on nutritional status. Look for recent changes in weight and potential drug-nutrient interactions. Measure the patient's height, weight, and other anthropometric measurements. Check for edema and signs of muscle wasting. Activity levels and urine output are helpful in determining energy needs and fluid restriction.
Laboratory values	Look for laboratory values within expected ranges according to the patient's stage of disease. Consider causes for abnormal findings and corrective actions to take.
Food intake assessment	A diet history should be taken using a 24-hour recall and/or food frequency questionnaire. It is important to determine if the recall is typical and if there have been any changes in appetite. Also ask about use of dietary or nutritional supplements. Determine if the patient practices pica (ingestion of nonfood substances such as ice, cornstarch, or clay). Consider if the current intake is adequate and if not, how can the problem be corrected.
Environmental factors	Determine if the patient has an understanding about the necessity for changes in the diet. Investigate psychological and socioeconomic status. Is there someone who helps the patient follow the diet at home? Who does the grocery shopping and cooking? What is the educational level of the patient?

[a] Rating forms for doing a Subjective Global Assessment (SGA) are readily available. This assessment technique looks at weight and weight change, dietary intake, gastrointestinal symptoms, functional capacity, physical examination, and comorbidities. Use of the SGA rating form gives an overall SGA rating that ranges from severely malnourished to well nourished.

TABLE 60.3

Interpretation of Laboratory Results for Hemodialysis and Peritoneal Dialysis Patients

Test	Range in Renal Disease	Reference Range	Comments
Albumin g/L (depends on method of analysis)	35-50	35-55 Infant: 29-55 <3 yrs.: 38-54	Higher values are more desirable; mortality is 50% higher when albumin is <39
Alkaline phosphatase μkat/L	WNL	M 0.317-1.23 F 0.200-1.05 Infant: 1.667-5.50 Child: 1.5-3.83 Teen: 1.667-4.17	High in bone disease
BUN mmol/L	21.43-42.84	1.43-7.85 Infant: 2.86-9.99 Peds: 3.57-7.14	Varies with protein intake and dialysis adequacy
Calcium mmol/L	2.1-2.87	2.1-2.87	Low with insufficient vitamin D; high with excess
Cholesterol mmol/L	<5.52	<5.52	High with nephrotic syndrome, or hereditary disorders of lipid metabolism
HDL-C mmol/L	>1.56	>1.56	
Triglycerides mmol/L	<1.7	<1.7	
Creatinine μmol/L	34.2-256.5	11.97-25.65 Infant: 6.84-20.52 <4 yrs.: 1.71-11.97 4-10 yrs.: 0.34-15.39 10-16 yrs.: 5.13-18.81	Low in extreme muscle wasting
Ferritin mmol/L	2.21-17.7	0.26-6.63 <6 mo.: 0.55-4.42 6 mo.-15 yrs. 0.15-3.09	High in inflammatory states
Glucose mmol/L	3.9-6.1	3.90-6.1	Monthly clinic labs usually are non-fasting

TABLE 60.3 *(Continued)*

Interpretation of Laboratory Results for Hemodialysis and Peritoneal Dialysis Patients

Test	Range in Renal Disease	Reference Range	Comments
Hematocrit	33-36%	M 39-51% F 36-45% Newborn: 40-70% Infant: 30-49% Child: 30-42% Teen: 34-44%	Target for EPO: 30%
Hemogloblin mmol/L	6.84-7.46	7.46-10.57 Newborn: 8.7-14.93 Infant: 6.22-9.33 Child: 6.84-9.95 Teen: 7.46-10.57	
Iron µmol/L	4.48-35.8	10.74-31.32 Infant: 17.9-35.8 4 mo.–2 yrs. 7.2-17.9 Child: 15.2-26.85	Day-to-day variations common
Phosphorus mmol/L	1.48-2.14	0.82-1.55 Newborn: 1.32-2.96 Infant: 1.51-2.20 Child: 1.32-1.97	High serum levels common — binders & low PO4 diet are used for control
Potassium mmol/L	3.5-6.0	3.5-6.0	High serum levels common; low K diet used for control
Sodium mmol/L	WNL	136-145	Varies with fluid status

Acute Renal Failure: Daily Nutrient and Fluid Needs

Table 60.4[10-12] outlines basic nutritional requirements for children who have acute renal failure. Guidelines are adjusted depending on stress level, acute phase, and dialysis treatments. Table 60.5[13-16] outlines basic nutritional requirements for adults who have acute renal failure. Guidelines are adjusted for individuals depending on the stress level, phase of disease, and dialysis treatments.

TABLE 60.4

Daily Nutrient and Fluid Needs for Pediatric Patients with Acute Renal Failure

Age	Energy	Protein
Birth to 1 year	> 100 kcal/kg	1.0-2.0 g/kg
1-3 years	> 100 kcal/kg	1.5-1.8 g/kg
4-10 years	70-90 kcal/kg	1.0-1.5 g/kg
11-18 years	55 kcal/kg	0.8-1.5 g/kg

Nutrient	Recommendations
Sodium	Monitor and adjust as needed
Potassium	Monitor and adjust as needed
Fluids	Individualized
Calcium	Monitor and adjust as needed
Phosphorus	Monitor and adjust as needed
Vitamins and minerals	Follow daily RDA/DRI[45,46] or therapeutic levels depending on needs

Note: Fluids and electrolytes and micronutrients either are unrestricted or individualized by patient rather than age.

TABLE 60.5

Daily Nutrient and Fluid Needs for Adults with Acute Renal Failure

Nutrient	Recommendations
Energy	30-35 kcal/kg
Protein[a]	0.6-0.8 g/kg
Sodium[b]	2 g/day
Potassium[b]	2 g/day
Fluids	Output plus 500 cc
Calcium	Keep serum values within normal limits
Phosphorus	Keep serum values within normal limits
Vitamins and minerals	Follow daily RDA/DRI[45,46] or therapeutic levels (depending on needs)

[a] Increase as renal function improves or if dialysis is started.
[b] Replace in diuretic phase of disease.

TABLE 60.6

Daily Nutrient and Fluid Needs for Pediatric Patients with Chronic Renal Failure

Age	Energy	Protein
Birth-6 months	> 100 kcal/kg	2.2 g/kg
6 months-1 year	~ 100 kcal/kg	1.6 g/kg
1-3 years	~ 100 kcal/kg	1.2 g/kg
4-10 years	70-90 kcal/kg	1.0-1.2 g/kg
11-18 years[a]	> 40-50 kcal/kg	0.9-1.0 g/kg
Nutrient	**Recommendations**	
Sodium	Monitor and adjust with level of renal function	
Potassium	Monitor and adjust with level of renal function	
Fluids	Individualized	
Calcium	Supplement as needed to DRI	
Phosphorus	Restrict if high serum levels	
Vitamins and minerals	Follow daily RDA/DRI[45,46] or therapeutic levels depending on needs	

Note: Fluids, electrolytes, and micronutrients are either unrestricted or individualized by patient rather than age.

[a] Females typically require fewer kcal.

Chronic Renal Failure: Daily Nutrient and Fluid Needs

Table 60.6[10-12] outlines basic nutritional requirements for children who have chronic renal failure. Guidelines are adjusted depending on comorbidity. Table 60.7[13,15,17-20] outlines basic nutritional requirements for adults who have renal insufficiency, but have not yet started dialysis. Guidelines can be adjusted for comorbidities and advanced age.

Post Kidney Transplant: Daily Nutrient and Fluid Needs

Table 60.8[11,12,21] outlines basic nutritional requirements for children who have received renal transplants. Guidelines can be adjusted for comorbidity. Table 60.9[15,18,22-24] outlines basic nutritional requirements for adults who have received kidney transplants. Guidelines can be adjusted for comorbidities and advanced age. As post-transplant patients are at

TABLE 60.7

Daily Nutrient and Fluid Needs for Adults with Chronic Renal Failure

Nutrient	Recommendations
Energy	30-35 kcal/kg
Protein[a]	0.6-0.8 g/kg
Sodium[b]	2-4 g
Potassium[c]	Unrestricted
Fluids	Unrestricted
Calcium	1.0-1.5 g
Phosphorus	10-12 mg/g protein
Vitamins and minerals	Follow daily RDA/DRI[45,46] for B, C, D, iron, & zinc, no supplements for vitamin A or magnesium

[a] 0.8-1.0 g/kg in nephrotic syndrome, do not adjust for urine protein losses.
[b] Possible restriction when gomerular filtration rate <10 ml/minute or when serum values become elevated.
[c] Start restriction when urine output diminishes.

TABLE 60.8

Daily Nutrient and Fluid Needs for Pediatric Patients Post Kidney Transplant

Age	Energy	Protein <3 Months Post Transplant	Protein >3 Months Post Transplant
Birth-5 months	≥ 108 kcal/kg	3.0 g/kg	2.2 g/kg
5 months-1 year	≥ 100 kcal/kg	3.0 g/kg	1.6 g/kg
1-3 years	102 kcal/kg	2.0-3.0 g/kg	1.3 g/kg
4-6 years	90 kcal/kg	2.0-3.0 g/kg	1.2 g/kg
7-10 years	70 kcal/kg	2.0-3.0 g/kg	1.0 g/kg
11-14 years (girls)	47 kcal/kg	1.5-2.0 g/kg	1.0 g/kg
15-18 years (girls)	40 kcal/kg	1.5-2.0 g/kg	0.9 g/kg
11-14 years (boys)	55 kcal/kg	1.5-2.0 g/kg	1.0 g/kg
15-18 years (boys)	45 kcal/kg	1.5-2.0 g/kg	0.9 g/kg

Nutrient	Recommendations
Sodium	1-3 g postoperative, then as tolerated
Potassium	As tolerated
Fluids	Unrestricted
Calcium	Supplement as needed
Phosphorus	Unrestricted
Vitamins and minerals	Supplement as needed

Note: Fluids and electrolytes and micronutrients either are unrestricted or individualized by patient rather than age.

TABLE 60.9

Daily Nutrient and Fluid Needs for Adults Post Kidney Transplant

Nutrient	Recommendations
Energy	25-35 kcal/kg
Protein[a]	1.0-1.5 g/kg
Sodium	2-4 g/day
Potassium	Unrestricted
Fluids	Unrestricted
Calcium	1.0-1.5 g
Phosphorus	Unrestricted
Vitamins and minerals	Follow daily RDA/DRI[45,46]

[a] Higher end for postoperative recovery, 1.0 g/kg for maintenance.

TABLE 60.10

Daily Nutrient and Fluid Needs for Pediatric Patients Undergoing Peritoneal Dialysis

Age	Energy	Protein	Calcium
Birth to 5 months	≥ 108 kcal/kg	2.5-4.0 g/kg	400 mg
5 months — 1 year	≥ 100 kcal/kg	2.0-2.5 g/kg	600 mg
1-3 years	102 kcal/kg	2.0-2.5 g/kg	800 mg
4-6 years	90 kcal/kg	2.0-2.5 g/kg	800 mg
7-10 years	70 kcal/kg	2.0-2.5 g/kg	800 mg
11-14 years (girls)	47 kcal/kg	1.5 g/kg	1200 mg
15-18 years (girls)	40 kcal/kg	1.5 g/kg	1200 mg
11-14 years (boys)	55 kcal/kg	1.5 g/kg	1200 mg
15-18 years (boys)	45 kcal/kg	1.5 g/kg	1200 mg

Nutrient	Recommendations
Sodium	As tolerated
Potassium	As tolerated
Fluids	Usually unrestricted
Phosphorus	As tolerated
Vitamins and minerals	
Infants and toddlers	1 ml multivitamin drops, 1 mg folic acid, vitamin D as needed
Children	1 mg folic acid, 10 mg pyridoxine, 60 mg vitamin C, 5 mg pantothenic acid, 1.0 mg thiamin, 1.2 mg riboflavin, 6 μg B_{12}, 300 μg biotin, 15 mg niacin, vitamin D as needed
Adolescents	1 mg folic acid, 10 mg pyridoxine, 60 mg vitamin C, 10 mg pantothenic acid, 1.5 mg thiamin, 1.7 mg riboflavin, 6 μg B_{12}, 300 μg biotin, 20 mg niacin, vitamin D as needed

Note: Fluids and electrolytes and micronutrients either are unrestricted or individualized by patient rather than age.

increased risk for hyperlipidemia, the diet should incorporate the principles for a Step One Heart Healthy Diet (American Heart Association).

Peritoneal Dialysis: Daily Nutrient and Fluid Needs

Table 60.10[10-12] outlines basic nutritional requirements for children undergoing daily peritoneal dialysis. Guidelines can be adjusted for comorbidity. Table 60.11[15,17,25-27] outlines basic nutritional requirements for adults undergoing daily peritoneal dialysis. Guidelines can be adjusted for comorbidities and advanced age.

Hemodialysis: Daily Nutrient and Fluid Needs

Table 60.12[10-12] outlines basic nutritional assessment parameters for children undergoing hemodialysis at least three times per week. Guidelines can be adjusted for comorbidity. Table 60.13[15,28-30] outlines basic nutritional requirements for adults undergoing hemodialysis three times per week. Guidelines can be adjusted for comorbidities and advanced age.

TABLE 60.11

Daily Nutrient and Fluid Needs for Adults Undergoing Peritoneal Dialysis

Nutrient	Recommendations
Energy[a]	25-35 kcal/kg
Protein	1.2-1.5 g/kg
Sodium	2-4 g
Potassium	3-4 g
Fluids	As tolerated
Calcium	1.0-1.5 g
Phosphorus	12-15 mg/g/protein
Ascorbic acid	60-100 mg
Pyridoxine	5-10 mg
B_{12}	3 μg
Folic acid	0.8-1.0 mg
No A or K	
Zinc	15 mg
Riboflavin	1.8-2.0 mg
Niacin	20 mg
Thiamin	1.5-2.0 mg
Biotin	200-300 μg
Vitamin E	10-15 IU
Pantothenic acid	10 mg
Iron and active vitamin D	Individualized

[a] Includes kcal from dialysate (3.4 kcal/g).

TABLE 60.12

Daily Nutrient and Fluid Needs for Pediatric Patients Undergoing Hemodialysis

Age	Energy	Protein	Calcium
Birth-5 months	≥ 108 kcal/kg	3.3 g/kg	400 mg
5 months-1 year	≥ 100 kcal/kg	2.4 g/kg	600 mg
1-3 years	102 kcal/kg	1.8 g/kg	800 mg
4-6 years	90 kcal/kg	1.8 g/kg	800 mg
7-10 years	70 kcal/kg	1.5 g/kg	800 mg
11-14 years (girls)	47 kcal/kg	1.3-1.5 g/kg	1200 mg
15-18 years (girls)	40 kcal/kg	1.3-1.5 g/kg	1200 mg
11-14 years (boys)	55 kcal/kg	1.3-1.5 g/kg	1200 mg
15-18 years (boys)	45 kcal/kg	1.3-1.5 g/kg	1200 mg

Nutrient	Recommendations
Sodium	As tolerated
Potassium	1-3 mEq/kg
Fluids	Replace urine output and insensible losses
Phosphorus	Supplement PRN
Vitamins and minerals	
Infants & toddlers	1 ml Multivitamin drops, 1 mg folic acid, vitamin D PRN
Children & adolescents	1 mg folic acid, 10 mg pyridoxine, 60 mg vitamin C, 10 mg pantothenic acid, 1.5 mg thiamin, 1.7 mg riboflavin, 6 μg B_{12}, 300 μg biotin, 15 mg niacin, vitamin D PRN

Note: Fluids and electrolytes and micronutrients either are unrestricted or individualized by patient rather than age.

TABLE 60.13

Daily Nutrient and Fluid Needs for Adults Undergoing Hemodialysis

Nutrient	Recommendations
Energy	30-35 kcal/kg
Protein	1.2-1.4 g/kg
Sodium	2-3 g
Potassium	2-3 g
Fluids	Urine output plus 1000 cc
Calcium	1.0-1.5 g
Phosphorus	12-15 mg/g/protein
Ascorbic acid	60-100 mg
Pyridoxine	5-10 mg
B_{12}	3 μg
Folic acid	0.8-1.0 mg
No A or K	
Zinc	15 mg
Riboflavin	1.8-2.0 mg
Niacin	20 mg
Thiamin	1.5-2.0 mg
Biotin	200-300 μg
Vitamin E	10-15 IU
Pantothenic acid	10 mg
Iron and active vitamin D	Individualized

Special Nutrition Focus

According to the 1999 United States Renal Data Systems (USRDS) Renal Data Report, the number of dialysis patients is approaching 200,000. Many practitioners will encounter dialysis patients who have medical nutrition therapy needs beyond the average patient. These patients require intense nutritional management to improve and then maintain good nutritional status either for the short term as in pregnancy, or for the long term as in patients with diabetes or acquired immunodeficiency disease (AIDS).

Pregnant Hemodialysis Patients

The frequency of pregnancy in female dialysis patients is approximately 1.5%. Of these women, 52% will carry to term. Dialysis frequency usually is increased to an average of 24 hours per week. Predialysis BUN is best kept below 60 mg/dl. Table 60.14[31-34] lists the recommendations for nutrients for pregnant women undergoing hemodialysis.

Adult Dialysis Patients with Diabetes Mellitus

Carbohydrate and fat are individualized for diabetic patients with renal disease. New guidelines from the National Cholesterol Education Program state that diabetes is regarded as a cardiovascular disease risk equivalent. Dietary guidelines generally follow the NCEP step II diet. Most sources of fat should be monounsaturated. Plant stanols/sterols can be used in renal patients to enhance LDL lowering. New desirable lipid targets are the same as for the general population; i.e., total cholesterol <5.2 mmol/L, LDL-

TABLE 60.14

Pregnant Hemodialysis Patients

Nutrient	Recommended Amount
Energy	25-45 kcal/kg +250 kcal
Protein	1.0-1.5 g/kg + 10 g
Sodium	Individualize
Potassium	Individualize
Fluids	Individualize
Calcium	1200-1600 mg/day
Phosphorus	Balance of diet/binders
Vitamins and minerals	Consider increased dose of renal vitamins B & C plus zinc, 1,25(OH)2D3 PRN, fat-soluble vitamins A, E, and K are not usually supplemented

TABLE 60.15

Special Nutrition Focus: Adult Patients with Diabetes Mellitus

Nutrient	Recommended Amount		
	Pre-Dialysis	Hemodialysis	Peritoneal Dialysis
Energy	25-35 kcal/kg	30-35 kcal/kg	25-35 kcal/kg[a]
Protein	0.8-1.0 g/kg	1.2-1.4 g/kg	1.5-2.0 g/kg
Sodium	2-4 g	2 g	2-4 g
Potassium	Not restricted	2-3 g	Individualize supplement as needed
Fluids	Not restricted	Urine output plus 1000 cc	Urine output plus 2000 cc
Calcium	1.0-1.5 g	1.0-1.5 g	1.0-1.5 g
Phosphorus	10-12 mg/g/protein	12-15 mg/g/protein	12-15 mg/g/protein
Vitamins & other minerals	Daily RDA/DRI[45,46] for most vitamins and minerals (fat soluble vitamins and magnesium are not supplemented)		

[a] Includes kcal from dialysate (3.4 kcal/g). Many patients will require adjustment of insulin regimens.

cholesterol <2.6 mmol/L, HDL-cholesterol >1.56 mmol/L, triglycerides <1.7 mmol/L. Table 60.15[7,35-39] lists recommendations for nutrients for diabetic patients with renal failure pre-dialysis or undergoing hemo or peritoneal dialysis.

Dialysis Patients with AIDS Nephropathy

Intestinal malabsorption and diarrhea occur in most AIDS patients. It is therefore not uncommon for the patient to be very malnourished when AIDS nephropathy leads to dialysis. Improving and maintaining nutrition status is a special challenge in this population. Table 60.16[40-44] lists the nutrient recommendations for dialysis patients with AIDS.

Medications

Calcium Supplement/Binders

Calcium supplements are used to supplement therapeutic diets that are low in calcium due to the restriction of dairy products and many other foods high in calcium. Calcium products used for supplementation are taken between meals. Calcium products are also used to bind dietary phosphorus in order to change the route of elimination from urine to stool. Products used for phosphate binding are taken within 30 minutes of meals or

TABLE 60.16

Special Nutrition Focus: Dialysis Patients with AIDS Nephropathy

Nutrient	Recommended Amount	
	Hemodialysis	Peritoneal Dialysis
Energy	45-50 kcal/kg	45-50 kcal/kg[a]
Protein	1.4-2.0 g/kg	1.5-2.0 g/kg
Sodium	2-3 g	2-4 g
Potassium	1 meq/kg	Individualize supplement as needed
Fluids	Urine output plus 1000-1200 cc	Urine output plus 2000 cc
Calcium	1.0-1.5 g	1.0-1.5 g
Phosphorus[b]	12-15 mg/g/protein	12-15 mg/g/protein
Vitamins and minerals	Same as non-AIDS patients	

[a] Includes kcal from dialysate (3.4 kcal/g).

[b] Lift restriction if PO intake poor.

TABLE 60.17

List of Products to Provide Suitable Source of Calcium for Patients with Renal Disease[a]

Generic Name	Name Brand	Elemental Ca^{++}	Source
Calcium acetate	PhosLo	169 mg	Braintree Laboratories
	Calphron	169 mg	NephroTech
Calcium carbonate[b]	Calci-chew	500 mg	R&D Laboratories
	Caltrate 600	600 mg	Whitehall Robins Healthcare
	Maalox Quick Dissolve (regular strength)	222 mg	Novartis Consumer Health, Inc.
	Nephro-Calci	600 mg	R&D Laboratories
	Oscal 500	500 mg	SmithKline Beecham
	Rolaids EX	400 mg	Warner Lambert
	TUMS EX	600 mg	SmithKline Beecham
	Viactiv	500 mg	Mead Johnson
Calcium citrate[c]	Citracal	200 mg	Mission Pharmacal

[a] Manufacturer's information.

[b] Efficacy of different brands of calcium carbonate varies due to ability to dissolve. A tablet of calcium carbonate placed in 6 oz. of vinegar at room temperature and stirred frequently should disintegrate within 30 minutes.

[c] Not generally recommended for renal patients secondary to enhanced aluminum absorption.

snacks. Iron supplements should not be taken with calcium supplements. End-stage renal patients do not need to take calcium products with added vitamin D. When vitamin D supplementation is needed it will be prescribed as an activated form. Table 60.17 lists sources of calcium supplementation.

Phosphate Binders (Non-Calcium Based)

Renagel is a polymetric phosphate binder which contains no calcium. Aluminum-containing products are still used to bind dietary phosphorus when calcium supplements are not effective or not medically appropriate. Magnesium binders in combination with calcium acetate are also an alternative in certain situations. The information in Table 60.18 is a sampling of current products.

Vitamin and Mineral Supplements

Vitamin and mineral supplements for renal patients are generally limited to water-soluble vitamins and essential amounts of minerals. Table 60.19 gives recommended supplemen-

TABLE 60.18

Phosphate Binders (Non-Calcium Based)[a]

Active Ingredient	Unit	Aluminum/Unit	Brand Name	Manufacturer
Aluminum Based Binders				
Aluminum carbonate	5 ml	142 mg	Basaljel	Wyeth-Ayerst Laboratories
Aluminum hydroxide	5 ml	208 mg	AlternaGEL suspension	Johnson & Johnson
	5 ml	111 mg	Amphojel suspension	Wyeth-Ayerst Laboratories
	300/600 mg	104/208 mg	Amphojel tablets	Wyeth-Ayerst Laboratories
	1 capsule	134 mg	Dialume	Rhone-Poulenc Rorer
Active Ingredient	**Unit**	**MG/CA++ Per Unit**	**Brand Name**	**Manufacturer**
Magnesium/Calcium Based Binders				
Magnesium carbonate/ calcium acetate	1 Tablet	57 mg MG/ 113 mg CA++	MagneBind™ 200	Nephro-Tech
	1 Tablet	85 mg MG/ 76 mg CA++	MagneBind™ 300	Nephro-Tech
Active Ingredient	**Unit**	**Sevelamer Hydrochloride**	**Brand Name**	**Manufacturer**
Polymetric Binder				
Sevelamer hydrochloride	1 Capsule	403 mg/800 mg	Renagel	Genzyme Pharmaceuticals

[a] Manufacturer's information.

TABLE 60.19

Vitamin and Mineral Supplementation

Vitamin	Recommended Amount	Vitamin	Recommended Amount
Vitamin C	40-100 mg	Thiamin(B_1)	1.5 mg
Riboflavin(B_2)	1.7 mg	Niacin	20 mg
Pyroxdine(B_6)	10 mg	Cobalamin (B_{12})	6 μg
Folic acid	0.8-1.0 mg	Pantothenic acid	5-10 mg
Biotin	150-300 μg	Active vitamin D	Oral or IV-based on need

Sample Vitamin/Mineral Supplement Product List

Product	Manufacturer
Vitamins	
Nephro-Vite	R&D Laboratories
Neprho-Vite RX	R&D Laboratories
Nephrocaps	Flemming
Berocca	Roche Laboratories
Albee with C	Whitehall Robins Healthcare
Multivitamin B+C with Zinc	Vitaline Formulas
Vitamins with Iron	
Nephron FA	Nephro-Tech
Nephro-Vite + FE	R&D Laboratories
Active Vitamin D	
Rocaltrol	Roche Laboratories
Calcijex (Calcitriol Injection)	Abbott Laboratories
Zemplar (Paracalcitol Injection)	Abbott Laboratories

TABLE 60.20

Iron Supplements[a]

Source of Iron	Elemental Iron	Brand Name	Form
Ferric gluconate	62.5 mg/5ml	Ferrlecit	IV
Ferrous gluconate	35 mg	Fergon	PO
Ferrous fumarate	66 mg	Chromagen	PO
	106 mg	Hemocyte	PO
	115 mg	Nephro-Fer	PO
Ferrous sulfate	65 mg	Feosol	PO
	50 mg	SlowFe	PO
Iron dextran	50 mg/ml	InFed	IV
	50 mg/ml	Dexferrin	IV
Iron polysaccharide	150 mg	Niferex	PO
	150 mg	Nulron	PO

[a] Manufacturer's information.

tation level for selected vitamins and minerals for adults. Supplements for children need to be individualized depending on requirements for growth. Oral iron supplements are routinely used in conjunction with intravenous Epoetin alfa (EPO) therapy to control anemia in dialysis patients. EPO is an amino acid glycoprotein manufactured by recombinant DNA technology. It has the same biological effects as endogenous erythropoietin in stimulating red blood cell production. Intravenous supplements need to be given as a test dose before actual therapy to access the potential for allergic reaction. Oral supplements can have gastrointestinal side effects such as nausea, vomiting, and constipation. Table 60.20 lists some of the available iron supplements for use with renal patients.

Enteral Nutrition Supplements for the Renal Patient

Nutritional supplements are frequently used to provide nutrients for persons who, even after liberalization of the diet, cannot consume adequate oral nutrition or to supply a complete source of nutrition for patients who are nourished through an enteral feeding tube. There are many products from which to choose that will meet the nutrition requirements for most types of medical nutrition therapy. In addition to a variety of normal nutrition products, there are specialty products available for persons with acute or chronic renal failure including end-stage disease. Table 60.21 offers a partial listing of these products. Choosing the appropriate product can be a challenge since there is such a wide variety from which to choose and since many renal patients are successfully managed with normal supplements, which tend to be less expensive than the specialty formulas. In choosing a formula, the following points should be considered:

1. Goal of therapy: more protein, more kcalories or both
2. How much of the patient's needs are being met by the diet
3. How much of the patient's fluid restriction can be spared for the supplement
4. Which products are affordable and available in the patient's area

For the patient who must be tube fed, the location of the tube must be considered in making the formula selection. The feedings must be timed in order to allow time for dialysis without compromising the nutrition therapy.

TABLE 60.21A

Enteral Nutrition Supplements for Renal Patients[a]

Product	Kcal/cc	CHO g/L	PRO g/L	FAT g/L	K mg/L	PO4 mg/L	%H_2O/L
Novasource renal (Novartis)	2	200	74	100	810	650	70
Magnacal Renal (Mead Johnson)	2	200	75	101	1270	800	71
Nepro (Ross)	2	222	70	95.6	1060	685	70
Suplena (Ross)	2	255	30	95.6	1120	730	71

TABLE 60.21B

Enteral Nutrition Supplements for Renal Patients[a]

Product	Unit	Kcal	CHO	PRO	FAT	K	PO4
EggPro (Nutra/Balance)	1 T (7.5g)	30	0.6 g	6 g	0 g	84 mg	8 mg
ProMod (Ross)	1 scoop (6.6 g)	28	0.67 g	5 g	0.60 g	45 mg	33 mg
Essential ProPlus (NutriSOY International, Inc.)	1 scoop (25 g)	68.5	6.4 g	16.3 g	0.2 g	112.5 mg	187 mg
Re/Neph cookies (Nutra/Balance)	2 oz. cookie	210	29 g	9 g	7 g	125 mg	64 mg
Re/Neph HP/HC (Nutra/Balance)	4 fl. oz.	250	32 g	8 g	10 g	10 mg	24 mg

[a] Manufacturer's information.

Practical Application of the Diet

Food Choices to Control Potassium and Phosphorus

Potassium is widely distributed in foods. As the kidneys primarily excrete this nutrient, dietary intake of potassium is an important aspect of the diet of patients with end-stage renal disease. The diet should initially be individualized for each patient based on food likes and dislikes, and modified if indicated. Although the potassium content of foods varies greatly, most foods can be incorporated into the diet of the hemodialysis patient by limiting quantities and/or by altering method of preparation. Dietary potassium is usually not a problem with peritoneal dialysis, as the patients are dialyzed daily. Some foods very high in potassium are listed in Table 60.22. Phosphorus level is almost impossible to control in end-stage renal disease by diet alone. Phosphate binders are necessary to maintain acceptable blood levels. It is also important that the patient limit the intake of dietary phosphorus. Dietary restrictions should be individualized for each patient depending on food preferences and compliance with binders. Table 60.23 lists some foods very high in phosphorus.

Suggested Meal Plans and Sample Menus

Listed in Table 60.24 are suggested meal plans for four different kcalorie levels of the diet for patients with end-stage renal disease. Additional modifications may be indicated when other disease states are also present. For diabetics, emphasis should be placed on complex carbohydrates. It is difficult to achieve energy and protein goals using complex carbohydrate sources exclusively, due to foods that must be limited due to potassium, phosphorus,

TABLE 60.22

Some Foods Very High in Potassium

Food	Portion	Amount of Potassium
Orange juice, fresh	1 cup	496 mg
Banana	medium	451 mg
Cantaloupe	1 c pieces	494 mg
Honeydew melon	1 c pieces	461 mg
Prunes, dried, cooked	1/2 cup	354 mg
Peanuts, oil roasted	1/2 cup	573 mg
Potato with skin, baked	1 large (202 g)	844 mg
Black-eyed peas, fresh-cooked	1/2 cup	347 mg
Sweet potato, baked	1 medium (114 g)	397 mg
Spinach, cooked from raw	1/2 cup	419 mg

Source: Pennington JAT. *Bowes and Church's Food Values of Portions Commonly Used,* 17th ed, Lippincott Williams and Wilkins, Philadelphia, 1997. With permission.

TABLE 60.23

Some Foods Very High in Phosphorus

Food	Portion	Amount of Phosphorus
Bran cereal, 100%	1/2 cup	344 mg
Milk, 2%	1 cup	232 mg
Whole wheat bread	1 slice	65 mg
Cheese, cheddar	1 oz	145 mg
Black-eyed peas, frozen, boiled	1 cup	208 mg
Peanuts, oil roasted	1 oz	145 mg
Peanut butter, creamy smooth	2 tbsp	103 mg
Lima beans, boiled	1 cup	208 mg
Yogurt, low-fat fruit flavor	8 oz	247 mg
Cocoa, dry unsweetened	2 T	74 mg

Source: Pennington JAT. *Bowes and Church's Food Values of Portions Commonly Used,* 17th ed, Lippincott Williams and Wilkins, Philadelphia, 1997. With permission.

and sodium content. Carbohydrates should be included with meals, rather than as snacks, to help slow absorption. Emphasis should also be placed on consistent meal content, especially of carbohydrate, and timing of meals and snacks to facilitate glycemic control. Fat should be from unsaturated sources, preferably monounsaturated. The percentage of kcalories provided by fat will most likely need to be higher than the recommended 30%. Hyperlipidemia, especially elevated triglycerides, is often present in renal disease. Because of the high risk for cardiovascular disease in renal patients, a diet high in complex carbohydrates and containing less than 30% of kcalories from fat may be appropriate. In view of other restrictions, this may not be a top priority. In order to provide adequate kcalories it may be necessary to provide more than 30% of kcalories from fat. Providing fat kcalories from monounsaturated and polyunsaturated sources can reduce saturated fat and cholesterol.

Emergency Shopping List

End-stage renal disease patients are dependent on dialysis to sustain life. Emergencies such as earthquakes, hurricanes, tornadoes, or floods may limit access to dialysis in a specific area. The patient must then use a diet restricted in fluids, protein, and electrolytes to survive until dialysis is once again available. Table 60.25 lists some guidelines for use in the event of a disaster or emergency.

TABLE 60.24
Sample Menus

1800 kcal[a]	2000 kcal[b]	2200 kcal[c]	2400 kcal[d]
Breakfast			
1/2 cup grits	1/2 cup grits	1 cup grits	1 cup grits
1 piece toast	1 piece toast	1 piece toast	1 piece toast
1/2 c grape juice	1/2 c apple juice	1/2 c apple juice	1/2 c apple juice
1/2 c 2% milk	1/2 c 2% milk	1/2 c 2% milk	1/2 c 2% milk
1 t margarine	1 t margarine	1 t margarine	1 t margarine
Lunch			
1 c rice	1 c rice	1 c rice	1 c rice
1 slice bread	1 slice bread	1 slice bread	1 slice bread
1 c garden salad	1 c garden salad	1 c garden salad	1 c garden salad
	1/2 c pears	1/2 c corn	1/2 c pears
			1/2 c corn
3 oz. skinless chicken breast	3 oz. skinless chicken breast	3 oz. skinless chicken breast	3 oz. skinless chicken breast
1 t margarine	1 t margarine	1 t margarine	1 t margarine
1 T salad dressing	1 T salad dressing	1 T salad dressing	1 T salad dressing
Afternoon Snack			
10 thin pretzels	2 slices bread	6 2 1/2″ graham crackers	6 2 1/2″ graham crackers
	1 oz. lean ham	1/2 c pears	1/2 c pears
1/2 c cottage cheese	1 t mayonnaise	1/2 c cottage cheese	1/2 c cottage cheese
Dinner			
1/2 c mashed potatoes	1/2 c mashed potatoes	1/2 c mashed potatoes	1/2 c mashed potatoes
1 roll	1 roll	1 roll	2 rolls
1 c greens	1 c greens	1 c greens	1 c greens
1/2 c fruit cocktail	1/2 c fruit cocktail	1/2 c fruit cocktail	1/2 c fruit cocktail
3 oz. lean beef	3 oz. lean beef	3 oz. lean beef	3 oz. lean beef
1 t margarine	1 t margarine	1 t margarine	2 t margarine
2 sugar cookies	2 sugar cookies	2 sugar cookies	2 sugar cookies
Bedtime Snack			
3-2 1/2″ square graham crackers	5 vanilla wafers	1 slice bread	2 slices bread
		1 t mayonnaise	1 t mayonnaise
1/2 cup pears	1/2 c pineapple	1 c strawberries	1/2 c peaches
		1 oz. turkey breast	1 oz. turkey breast

[a] 80 g protein, <2000 mg sodium, <2000 mg potassium, <1200 mg phosphorus.
[b] 80 g protein, <2000 mg sodium, <3000 mg potassium, <1200 mg phosphorus.
[c] 90 g protein, <3000 mg sodium, <3000 mg potassium, <1200 mg phosphorus.
[d] 100 g protein, <3000 mg sodium, <3000 mg potassium, <1300 mg phosphorus.

TABLE 60.25

Emergency Shopping List for the Dialysis Patient (Food for 2 to 3 days)

Bottled water: allow 2-3 quarts
(~2-3 liters) for hygiene purposes plus usual fluid restriction
Loaf of white bread
Dry cereal: corn flakes, rice krispies, cheerios, puffed wheat and rice, or shredded wheat
Box of vanilla wafers or other plain cookies
Box of graham crackers
Box of unsalted crackers
Small jars of mayonnaise (open one each day)
Small cans of chicken and/or tuna (open, eat, then throw away leftovers; do not try to save without refrigeration)
Can of lemonade or Kool-Aid mix
Granulated sugar
Peanut butter
Lemon candy
Hard candy in different flavors
Powdered milk or boxed milk
Small cans of evaporated milk
Canned fruit: peaches, fruit cocktail, pears, and applesauce
Fresh apples, lemons, carrots, if available
Jelly: apple, grape, strawberry, blueberry, blackberry
Marshmallows
Boxed juices
Plastic dinnerware and utensils
Paper towels and napkins

Note: Food stored in the refrigerator and/or freezer should be used first. Limit fluid intake as much as possible.

Summary

Patients with acute or chronic renal disease are susceptible to the development of profound malnutrition. Protein energy imbalances worsen prognosis regardless of disease stage. A complete nutrition assessment plus frequent monitoring can help identify malnutrition before there is significant depletion in visceral protein stores and weight loss. Important treatment objectives are to communicate with the patient, monitor appropriate laboratory indices, and plan the appropriate nutritional therapy.

References

1. Mitch WE, Klahr S, Eds. *Handbook of Nutrition and the Kidney* Lippincott-Raven, Philadelphia, 1998, pg 25.
2. Blackburn G, Bistrian B, Mainai B, et al. *J Parent Enteral Nutr* 11: 1; 1977.
3. Kopple JD, Massry SG, Eds. *Nutritional Management of Renal Disease* Williams and Wilkins, Baltimore, 1997, pg 203.
4. McCann L, Nelson P, Spinozzi N, Eds. *Pocket Guide to Nutrition Assessment of the Renal Patient,* 2nd ed, National Kidney Foundation, New York, 1997, chap. 1.
5. Mitch WE, Klahr S, Eds. *Handbook of Nutrition and the Kidney* Lippincott-Raven, Philadelphia, 1998, pg 45.
6. Stover J, Ed. *A Clinical Guide to Nutrition Care in End Stage Renal Disease* American Dietetics Association, Chicago, 5: 222; 1994.

7. American Diabetes Association Standards of Medical Care for Patients With Diabetes Mellitus *Clinical Diabetes* January/February, 22, 1997.
8. McCann L, Nelson P, Spinozzi N, Eds. *Pocket Guide to Nutrition Assessment of the Renal Patient,* 2nd ed, National Kidney Foundation, New York, NY, 1997, chap. 2.
9. Mitch WE, Klahr S, Eds. *Handbook of Nutrition and the Kidney* Lippincott-Raven, Philadelphia, 1998, pg 213-236.
10. Kopple JD, Massry SG, Eds. *Nutritional Management of Renal Disease* Williams and Wilkins, Baltimore, 1997, pg 687-712.
11. McCann L, Nelson P, Spinozzi N, Ed. *Pocket Guide to Nutrition Assessment of the Renal Patient,* 2nd ed, National Kidney Foundation, New York, 1997, chap. 11.
12. Stover J, Ed. *A Clinical Guide to Nutrition Care in End-Stage Renal Disease* The American Dietetic Association, Chicago, 1994, pg 79-98.
13. Klahr S, Levey AS, Beck GJ, et al. *N Engl J Med* 330: 877; 1994.
14. Kopple JD, Massry SG, Eds. *Nutritional Management of Renal Disease* Williams and Wilkins, 1997, pg 713-754.
15. McCann L, Nelson P, Spinozzi N, Eds. *Pocket Guide to Nutrition Assessment of the Renal Patient,* 2nd ed, National Kidney Foundation, New York, 1997, chap. 3.
16. Stover J, Ed. *A Clinical Guide to Nutrition Care in End Stage Renal Disease* American Dietetics Association, Chicago, 1994, pg 99-110.
17. Beto J. *J Am Diet Assoc* 95: 898; 1995.
18. Fouque D, Laville M, Boissel et al. *Br Med J* 304: 216; 1992.
19. Kopple JD, Massry SG, Ed. *Nutritional Management of Renal Disease* Williams and Wilkins, 1997, pg 317-340.
20. Mitch WE, Klahr S, Eds. *Handbook of Nutrition and the Kidney* Lippincott-Raven, Philadelphia, 1998, pg 237-252.
21. Mahan L, Escott-Stump S, Eds. *Krause's Food, Nutrition, and Diet Therapy,* 9th ed, Saunders, Philadelphia, 1996, pg 771-804.
22. Kopple JD, Massry SG, Eds. *Nutritional Management of Renal Disease* Williams and Wilkins, 1997, pg 669-686.
23. Mitch WE, Klahr S, Eds. *Handbook of Nutrition and the Kidney* Lippincott-Raven, Philadelphia, 1998, pg 294-315.
24. Pagenkemper JJ, Foulks CJ. *J Renal Nutr* 1: 119; 1991.
25. Kopple JD, Massry SG, Eds. *Nutritional Management of Renal Disease* Williams and Wilkins, Baltimore, 1997, pg 619-668.
26. Mitch WE, Klahr S, Eds. *Handbook of Nutrition and the Kidney* Lippincott-Raven, Philadelphia, 1998, pg 269-293.
27. Stover J, Ed. *A Clinical Guide to Nutrition Care in End Stage Renal Disease* American Dietetics Association, Chicago, 1994, pg 37-56.
28. Kopple JD, Massry SG, Eds. *Nutritional Management of Renal Disease* Williams and Wilkins, Baltimore, 1997, pg 563-600.
29. Mitch WE, Klahr S, Eds. *Handbook of Nutrition and the Kidney* Lippincott-Raven, Philadelphia, 1998, pg 253-268.
30. Stover J, Ed. *A Clinical Guide to Nutrition Care in End Stage Renal Disease* American Dietetics Association, Chicago, 1994, pg 25-36.
31. Grossman SD, Hou S, Moretti M, Saran M. *J Renal Nutr* 3: 5; 1993.
32. Henderson N. *J Renal Nutr* 6: 222; 1996.
33. Hou SH. *Am J Kidney Dis* 23: 60; 1994.
34. Stover J, Ed. *A Clinical Guide to Nutrition Care in End Stage Renal Disease* American Dietetics Association, Chicago, 1994, pg 199-206.
35. Third Report of the National Cholesterol Education Program Expert Panel on Detection, Evaluation and Treatment of High Blood Cholesterol in Adults Executive Summary, May 2001, pg 1-40.
36. Kopple JD, Massry SG, Ed. *Nutritional Management of Renal Disease* Williams and Wilkins, 1997, pg 63-77.

37. McCann L, Nelson P, Spinozzi N, Ed. *Pocket Guide to Nutrition Assessment of the Renal Patient*, 2nd ed, National Kidney Foundation, New York, 1997, chap. 4.
38. Renal Dietetians Dietetic Practice Group, *National Renal Diet: Professional Guide*, American Dietetics Association, 1993.
39. Stover J, Ed. *A Clinical Guide to Nutrition Care in End Stage Renal Disease* American Dietetics Association, Chicago, 1994, pg 69-78.
40. Kopple JD, Massry SG, Ed. *Nutritional Management of Renal Disease* Williams and Wilkins, 1997, pg 257-276.
41. McCann L, Nelson P, Spinozzi N, Eds. *Pocket Guide to Nutrition Assessment of the Renal Patient*, 2nd ed, National Kidney Foundation, New York, NY, 1997.
42. Mitch WE, Klahr S, Eds. *Handbook of Nutrition and the Kidney* Lippincott-Raven, Philadelphia, 1998, pg 45-86.
43. Plourd D. *J Renal Nutr* 5: 182; 1995.
44. Stover J, Ed. *A Clinical Guide to Nutrition Care in End Stage Renal Disease* American Dietetics Association, Chicago, 1994, pg 187-189.
45. *Recommended Dietary Allowances,* 10th ed, National Academy of Sciences, National Academy Press, Washington, DC, 1989.
46. Committee on Dietary Reference Intakes, Dietary Reference Intakes for Calcium, Phosphorus, Magnesium, Vitamin D, and Fluoride, National Academy Press, Washington, DC, 1997.
47. Pennington JAT. *Bowes and Church's Food Values of Portions Commonly Used,* 17th ed, Lippincott Williams and Wilkins, Philadelphia, 1997.

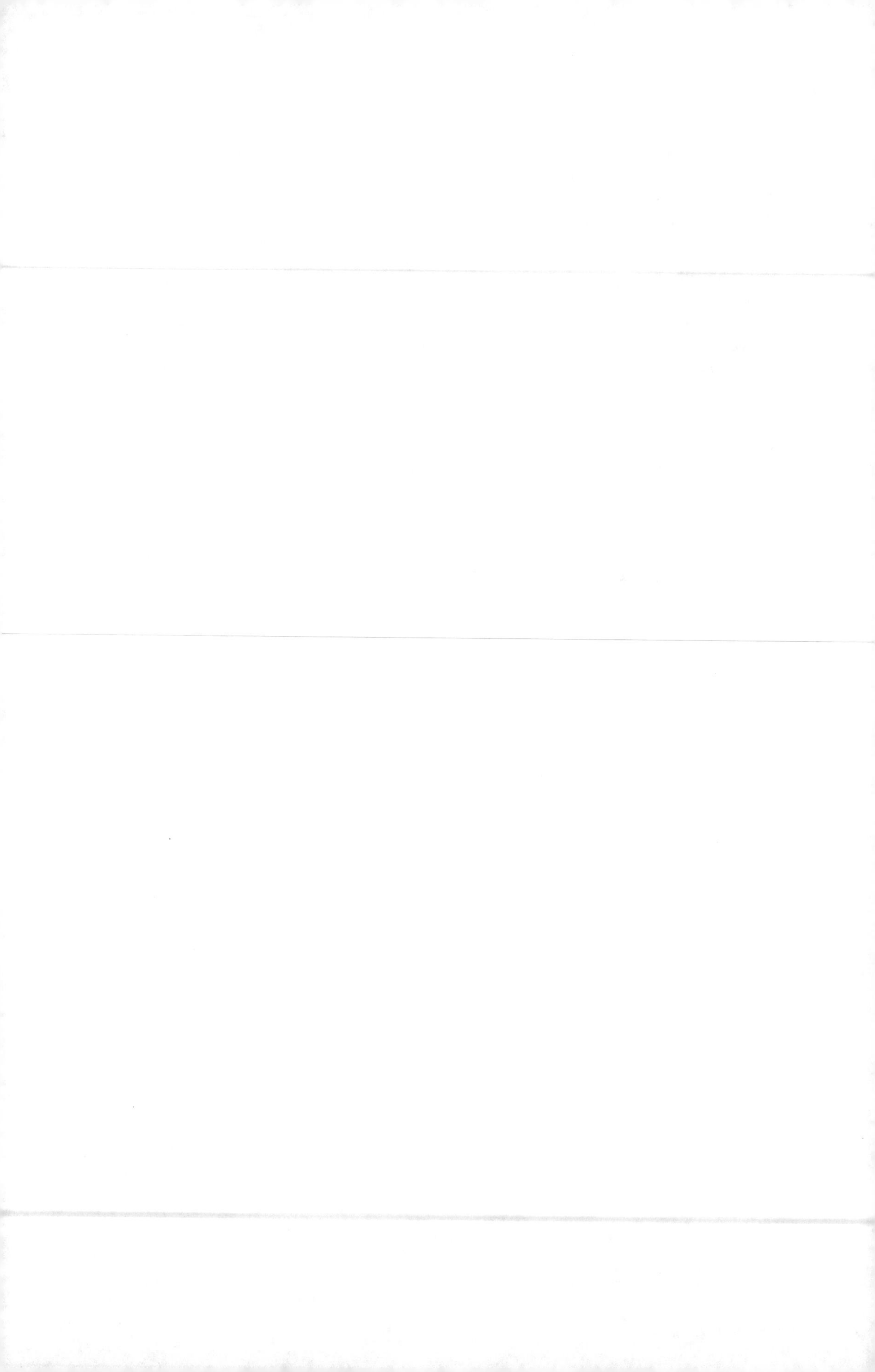

61

Disorders of the Skeleton and Kidney Stones

Stanley Wallach

Introduction

The skeleton is a complex, metabolically active tissue that serves multiple physiologic functions. However, its most important purpose is to maintain normal posture and locomotion by virtue of its hardness. This quality is conferred by a unique arrangement of plates of a calcium/phosphorus-containing mineral called hydroxyapatite [$Ca_{10}(PO_4)_6(OH)_2$] interspaced within the interstices of a protein matrix composed predominately of type 1 collagen (90+%). The matrix also contains a large number of noncollagenous proteins, some of which are unique to bone (Table 61.1). This structure confers extreme hardness, but also sufficient flexibility during strain to minimize brittleness.

The human skeleton matures during growth and development by a process called modeling, during which the enlarging skeleton is repetitively resorbed via osteoclastic activity, and then reformed on a larger template by osteoblastic action. Once growth is complete, these same two opposed processes continue to operate in a coupled manner, so that areas of bone that have undergone microdamage due to the repetitive strain incurred by activities of daily living (plus work-related and athletic activities), can be continually replaced by new, healthy bone. This process, which predominates in the adult, is known as remodeling, and when the two opposing processes of resorption of defunct bone followed by reformation of healthy bone are qualitatively and quantitatively coupled, the skeleton retains normal strength and hardness.

Metabolic Bone Diseases

The term metabolic bone disease refers to an aberration in this orderly cascade which disturbs normal skeletal modeling and/or remodeling. In addition, bone mineralization, which follows reformation of the matrix, also an osteoblastic controlled function, can be involved. Table 61.2 gives examples of the more common disturbances leading to metabolic bone diseases. However, there are literally hundreds of rare, genetically related metabolic bone diseases as well; some examples are given in Table 61.3.

0-8493-2705-9/02/$0.00+$1.50

TABLE 61.1

Skeletal Composition

Comprises 8% of body weight	
35% Organic	Type 1 collagen (90+%)
(FFDW[a])	Non-collagenous proteins: glycosaminoglycans, proteoglycans, glycoproteins, osteocalcin, osteonectin, osteopontin, bone sialoprotein, alkaline phosphatase, etc.
	Growth factors and cytokines
65% Inorganic	Hydroxyapatite: $Ca_{10}(PO_4)_6(OH)_2$
(FFDW[a])	Magnesium, sodium, potassium
	Carbonate-containing salts
	Fluorine
	Deposited "heavy metals"
	Trace elements
Miscellaneous	Water
	Lipids
	Deposited molecules: tetracyclines, etc.

[a] Fat-free dry weight.

TABLE 61.2

Metabolic Bone Diseases

Disturbances in Orderly Sequence of Skeletal Turnover: Resorption-Formation-Mineralization

Examples:
- ↓ resorption: osteopetrosis
- ↓ formation: osteogenesis imperfecta
- ↓ mineralization: osteomalacia
- ↑ resorption: skeletal hyperparathyroidism
- ↑ resorption, ↑ formation: Paget's disease
- ↑ resorption, ↓ formation: osteoporosis

TABLE 61.3

Examples of Genetic Mutations Causing Metabolic Bone Diseases

Enzyme Defects
- Carbonic anhydrase II: Osteopetrosis
- 1-hydroxylase (25-OH-D): Vitamin D dependent rickets

Receptor Defects
- PTH-PTH related protein receptor: Jensen's metaphyseal chondrodysplasia
- Fibroblast growth factor 3 receptor: Achondroplasia
- Calcium sensing receptor: Familial hypocalciuric hypercalcemia (inactivating)
- Calcium sensing receptor: Autosomal dominant hypoparathyroidism (activating)
- Vitamin D receptor: Vitamin D resistance syndromes

Signaling Mechanism Defects
- Gs protein excess: McCune-Albright syndrome
- Gs protein deficiency: Pseudohypoparathyroidism

Structural Gene Defects
- Type I collagen genes: Osteogenesis imperfecta
- Bone morphogenetic protein 4: Fibrodysplasia ossificans progressiva (activating)

The coupling of bone resorption, formation, and mineralization is normally orchestrated and modulated by a large repertoire of hormones, growth factors, resorptive cytokines, and miscellaneous risk factors (Tables 61.4, 61.5) that determine ultimate bone mass and anatomy, and resistance to fracture during casual trauma. Nutritional status is key to

TABLE 61.4

Hormone, Growth Factor, and Cytokine Effects on Bone

Hormones:	Parathyroid Hormone: biphasic effects
	Low dose: ↑↑ trabecular bone formation
	↑ cortical bone formation
	High dose: ↑↑ cortical bone resorption
	↑ trabecular bone resorption
	Vitamin D metabolites: promote calcium absorption and bone mineralization, can also increase bone resorption (high doses)
	Calcitonin: inhibits bone resorption, stimulates bone formation
	Corticosteroids: inhibit bone formation, secondarily stimulate bone resorption
	Gonadal steroids: inhibit bone resorption, ? stimulate bone formation
	Thyroid hormones: increase bone turnover, primarily by stimulating bone resorption
	Growth hormones: stimulate bone formation; stimulate bone resorption (high doses)
	Insulin: stimulates bone formation
	Prolactin: inhibits bone formation
Growth factors:	IGF-1[a] (somatomedin) and IGF-2[a]: stimulate bone formation, inhibit bone resorption
	Transforming growth factor-β: stimulates bone formation, inhibits bone resorption
	Bone morphogenetic proteins: stimulate bone formation
	Fibroblast growth factor — increases bone formation
	Platelet-derived growth factor: stimulates bone formation, inhibits bone resorption
	Interleukin-1 receptor antagonist: opposes interleukin-1 induced bone resorption
	Other interleukin inhibitors: oppose interleukin induced bone resorption
	Prostate carcinoma factor: theoretic stimulator of bone formation
	Prostaglandins: biphasic effects to stimulate both bone formation and resorption
Cytokines:	Interleukins 1, 4, 6, 11: stimulate bone resorption
	Tumor necrosis factor: stimulates bone resorption
	Lymphotoxin: stimulates bone resorption
	Granulocyte/macrophage-CSF[b] and other CSF's[b]: stimulate bone resorption
	Prostaglandins: biphasic effects to stimulate both bone formation and resorption

[a] Insulin-like growth factor.
[b] Colony stimulating factor.

normal interactions among these factors; in the evaluation of individuals in whom skeletal integrity is a clinical issue, consideration of dietary status should take primacy, since all other interactions will be adversely affected by uncorrected dietary deficiencies. Table 61.1 also contains a concise list of macro- and micronutrients present in the skeleton which are considered to have a role in skeletal modeling and remodeling. Many of the micronutrients listed have been shown to exert skeletal effects only in experimental systems, and do not as yet have a proven role in human skeletal metabolism.

Calcium and Vitamin D

Obviously, calcium leads any list of macronutrients, since it is most abundant in bone; the skeleton accounts for greater than 90% of body calcium content. The gastrointestinal (GI) absorption of calcium is affected by a large number of factors such as transit time, mucosal competence, and calcium binding by phosphates, oxalate, and fiber, among others. However, vitamin D is the dominant factor influencing calcium absorption since its active metabolite, 1,25-dihydroxy-vitamin D (calcitriol) stimulates production of a specific calcium-binding protein in mucosal cells, which facilitates transcellular transport of calcium through the GI mucosa. The metabolic cascade involved in vitamin D activation is shown in Figure 61.1 and brings out the point that inadequate vitamin D precursors from the diet,

TABLE 61.5

Risk Factors For Bone Loss

Genetic:	Female sex
	Caucasian/Asian ethnicity
	Family history of osteoporosis
Life Style:	Low calcium intake
	Excessive alcohol use
	Cigarette smoking
	Excessive caffeine use
	Extreme or insufficient athletism
	Excessive acid ash diet (high protein/soft drink intake)
Medical:	Early menopause
	Gonadal hormone deficiency
	Eating disorders
	Chronic liver/kidney disease
	Malabsorption syndromes
Iatrogenic:	Corticosteroids
	Excessive thyroid hormone
	Chronic heparin therapy
	Radiotherapy to skeleton
	Long-term anticonvulsants
	Loop diuretics

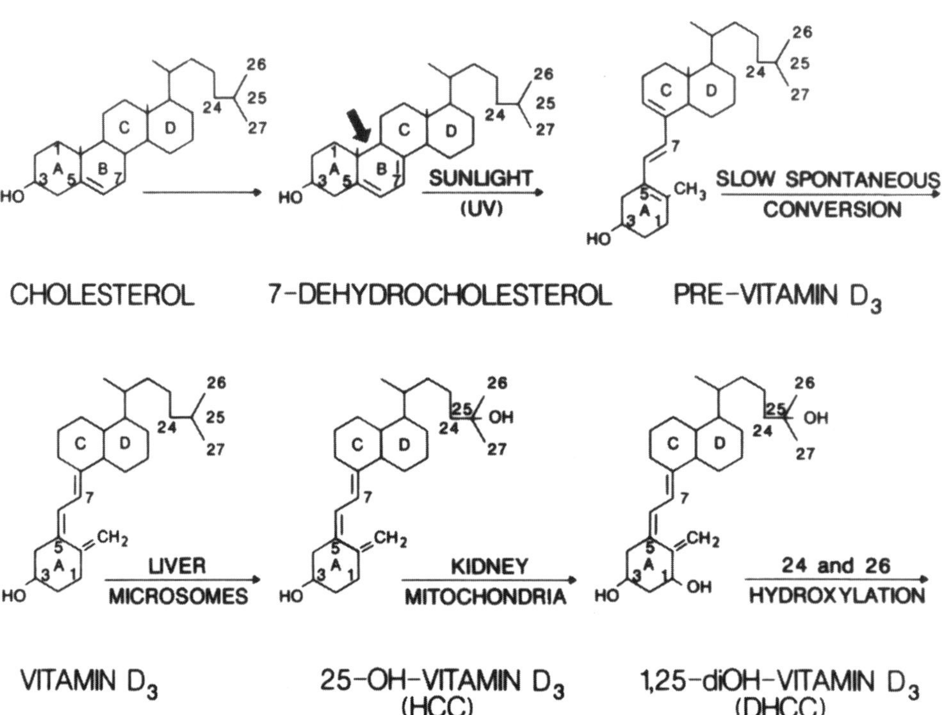

FIGURE 61.1
Conversion cascade for the synthesis of the active metabolite of vitamin D, 1,25-dihydroxy-cholecalciferol (DHCC) from cholesterol. The first three steps take place in the dermis, after which hydroxylations occur in the liver and kidney, respectively. Ingested vitamins D_2 and D_3 enter the cascade as per the lower portion of the figure.

TABLE 61.6

Vitamin D Deficits in Older Patients

Reduced oral intake	Less dairy intake, lactose intolerance
Reduced dermal production	Less sunlight exposure, pollution, sunscreens, intrinsic defect in 7-dehydrocholesterol conversion
Reduced hydroxylation (25 and 1∝)	Age-related declines in hepatic and renal function
Other factors	Anticonvulsants, renal insufficiency, Billroth II surgery, etc.

TABLE 61.7

Revised Recommended Daily Calcium and Vitamin D Intakes

Age	Amount of Calcium (mg)	Vitamin D (units)
Infants		
Birth-6 months	400	200
6 months-1 year	600	400
Children-young adults		
1-10 years	800-1200	400
11-24 years	1200-1500	400
Adult women		
Pregnant and lactating		
Under age 24	1200-1500	400
Over age 24	1200	400
25-49 years (premenopausal)	1000	400
50-64 years (postmenopausal taking estrogen)	1000	600-800
50-64 years (postmenopausal not taking estrogen)	1500	600-800
65+ years	1500	600-800
Adult men		
25-64 years	1000	400
65+ years	1500	600-800

inadequate actinic stimulation of skin precursors of vitamin D, and/or deficits in mucosal, hepatic, or renal handling of vitamin D metabolism can strongly alter vitamin D economy and in turn lead to calcium deficiency. This is especially true for older persons in whom several age-related deficits in vitamin D metabolism and action are common (Table 61.6). Table 61.7 gives the recommended daily intakes of calcium and vitamin D in normal individuals of various ages. Since the average non-dairy diet contains only 300 to 500 mg of calcium, the intentional use of calcium-rich foods daily (Table 61.8) is necessary to meet requirements. Alternately, dietary supplements containing calcium are required. Vitamin D is in even shorter supply, since the only adequate food source is fortified milk (100 IU per 8 oz). Therefore, direct sunlight, which does not have the ultraviolet spectrum screened out, and/or a large milk intake are required. Since this is rarely the case in adults, supplements containing vitamin D should be advocated. In individuals with GI, hepatic, and / or renal deficits, calcium and vitamin D nutrition may have to be further augmented and monitored by measurements of calcium, vitamin D metabolite, and parathyroid hormone levels. When significant hepatic and/or renal disease are present, it may be necessary to substitute vitamin D metabolites such as 25, hydroxy-vitamin D (calcifidiol) or 1,25-dihydroxy vitamin D (calcitriol) for vitamin D. These are prescription drugs and require physician participation in the patient's care. The essentials of adjusting the average patient's intakes of calcium and vitamin D are given in Table 61.9. Vitamin D can be in the form of

TABLE 61.8

Calcium-Rich Foods

Food	Calcium Content (mg)
Skim milk, 1/2 pint (8 oz)	300
Calcium enriched orange juice (6 oz)	260
Ice cream, 1 cup soft serve	240
Calcium enriched juice, 1 glass (8 oz)	225
Fruit yogurt, low fat 8 oz cup	340
Frozen yogurt, 8 oz cup	200
Mozzarella cheese, 1 oz	210
Cheddar cheese, 1 oz	200
Cottage cheese, 2% fat, 4 oz serving	75
Tofu, 4 oz serving	110
Salmon, canned, with bones, 3 oz	170
Sardines, canned, with bones, 3 oz	370
Bok choy, raw, 1 cup	75
Broccoli, raw, 1 cup	140
Collards, 1 cup	370
Kale, frozen, cooked, 1 cup	180

TABLE 61.9

Essentials of Adjusting Calcium and Vitamin D Intakes

Quantitate patient's Ca and vitamin D intakes from the patient's food sources
Determine difference between patient's requirements and actual food source intake
Prescribe daily multivitamin or vitamin D capsule, containing 400 IU
Prescribe $CaCO_3$ or Ca citrate in needed amount but use products that also contain vitamin D
Calculate total intakes of Ca and vitamin D from all sources to verify amount to be taken

either cholecalciferol (D_3) or ergocalciferol (D_2). Another issue is whether to use carbonate- or citrate-based calcium supplements. Both types offer sufficient calcium absorption to be recommended, but in selected patients, one or the other may be preferred (Table 61.10).

Other Macronutrients

Other macronutrients critical to the skeleton include phosphorus (phosphate), magnesium, protein, and lipids. The average American who is not a vegetarian uses meat, dairy products, and phosphoric acid-containing beverages so that phosphorus intake is sufficient, and no additional supplements are required. In fact, excess phosphorus should be avoided since it may increase bone resorption by stimulating excess PTH secretion. Calcium phosphate supplements as a calcium source are not desirable, not only because of a possible stimulatory effect on PTH, but the excess phosphate may excessively bind calcium in the GI tract. Excess phosphate may also combine with calcium internally, and facilitate its removal from the circulation by deposition within soft tissues and on bone surfaces. The latter does not necessarily contribute to bone integrity, except in undermineralized bone (osteomalacia) in which a high phosphorus intake is often beneficial.

The value of magnesium (Mg) in enhancing and/or maintaining skeletal vitality is controversial. *In vitro* and in animal models, Mg exerts the actions indicated in Table 61.11. However, in humans, insufficient studies exist to date to verify comparable actions under

TABLE 61.10

Comparison of Carbonate and Citrate-Based Calcium Supplements

	$CaCO_3$	Ca Citrate
Calcium content per pill	250-600 mg	250-315 mg
Vitamin D content per pill	Up to 200 IU	Up to 200 IU
Pill size	Medium	Large
Average Ca absorption	25-30%	30-40%
Solubility	Requires gastric HCl[a] (take with meals)	Does not require gastric HCl[a]
Special problems	Fe deficiency may occur ($FeCO_3$ insolubility) Constipation Extreme achlorhydria, H_2 blockers, proton pump inhibitors may make Ca absorption uncertain	Pill may be difficult to swallow[b] May require more than 2 pills per day

[a] Hydrochloric acid.
[b] Disintegrates in tap water.

TABLE 61.11

Magnesium Effects on the Skeleton

Promotes matrix formation
Increases mineral content
Increases trabecular bone
Increases mechanical strength
Bone crystal destabilization (in excess)

clinical conditions. Since the U.S. population on the whole has only borderline Mg sufficiency, because of its relatively low concentration in common foodstuffs (Table 61.12), there is some justification in ensuring an adequate Mg intake by the use of supplements (MgO, $MgCl_2$, or Mg-amino/acids salts). However, a superphysiologic amount of magnesium has no scientific basis.

The need for adequate protein of high biologic value to ensure adequate production of bone collagen and noncollagenous bone proteins is obvious. Patients with eating disorders and protein-calorie malnutrition uniformly have deficient skeletons. Perhaps less appreciated is emerging information as to the role of lipids in skeletal metabolism, as summarized in Table 61.13. Most of these basic findings have not been translated into human investigations.

TABLE 61.12

Magnesium Rich Foods

Food	Quantity	Content (mg)
Amaranth, buckwheat	1 cup	300-500
Nuts	1 cup	350-420
Brown rice, unrefined corn products	1 cup	50-320
Other whole grains	1 cup	50-160
Beans (including soy beans)	1 cup	50-150
Tofu	1/2 cup	120
Fish and seafood	3.5 oz	30-150
Avocado	1	70-105
Dark green vegetables	1 cup	25-150
Animal milk products (including yogurt)	1 cup	25-70
Dried fruits	100 g	50

TABLE 61.13
Lipid Effects on the Skeleton

Endogenous	
Prostaglandins	Biphasic effects Low dose: stimulates bone formation High dose: inhibits bone formation, stimulates bone resorption
Leukotrienes	Stimulate bone resorption
Exogenous	
N-3 fatty acids	Stimulate bone formation
Conjugated linoleic acid	Inhibits bone formation
Saturated fats	Increase bone formation, but also increase cortical porosity

Micronutrients

Several nutrients that are variable components of the human diet can have important influences on the skeleton, affecting calcium metabolism or the skeleton directly (Table 61.14). Excess fiber, caffeine, acid-containing foods and beverages all have negative effects, whereas the isoflavones and related compounds present in various foods are "weak estrogens" and exert a positive effect. Alcohol is technically not a nutrient, but is so ubiquitous in the human diet as to be considered so. It has multiple adverse actions, as noted.

Aside from vitamin D, four other vitamins have been shown to have an influence on the skeleton (Table 61.14). Vitamin A in excess and its more powerful retinoic acid derivatives (used to treat acne, other dermatologic conditions, and certain neoplasms) are powerful stimulators of the osteoclast, can cause bone loss and even hypercalcemia. Vitamin C, on the other hand, is an osteoblast promoter, and severe deficiency sufficient to cause borderline scurvy is accompanied by bony lesions. Vitamin E also increases experimental bone formation, but its clinical significance has not been established. Vitamin K, as a co-factor for gamma-hydroxylation, is responsible for the production of osteocalcin, a noncollagenous matrix protein. Although low vitamin K levels have been reported in some osteoporotics, an etiologic connection, if any, is unproven.

A large number of trace elements have either positive or negative effects on the skeleton but the majority are of interest in experimental systems and have no proven benefits or dangers to patients (Table 61.14). Strontium supplementation has been studied in osteoporotics and has been shown to enhance bone density. Lithium, used in the treatment of bipolar disorder, can stimulate the parathyroid glands to excessive activity with increased bone resorption and hypercalcemia. Aluminum overload can occur in chronic renal failure through the use of aluminum containing antacids and other oral sources or the use of aluminum-contaminated renal dialysis fluid. Aluminium toxicity impairs bone formation and mineralization as well as stimulating bone resorption, and is usually manifested in chronic renal failure patients as a resistant osteomalacia, or so-called aplastic bone disease. Iron overload, as occurs in hemochromatosis of both primary and secondary etiologies, hemolytic anemias, and some cases of chronic renal failure, uniformly decreases bone formation and mineralization with measureable bone loss, which can be severe enough to cause osteoporosis. In some cases increased bone resorption has been observed, and in chronic renal failure, iron overload can simulate aluminum toxicity. Cadmium

TABLE 61.14

Nutrient, Vitamin, and Trace Element Effects on the Skeleton

Other Nutrients	
Fiber[a]	Impairs calcium, lipid, and fat soluble vitamin absorption
Caffeine[a]	Decreases bone formation, increases urinary calcium loss
Acid-containing foods and beverages[a]	Increase bone resorption
Alcohol[a]	Decreases bone formation, prevents calcium absorption, increases urinary calcium loss
Isoflavonoids	Decrease bone resorption, through estrogen-like properties
Vitamins	
A[a]	Increases bone resorption when in excess
C	Promotes bone formation
E	Increases bone formation
K	Promotes bone mineralization
Beneficial Trace Elements	
Boron	May enhance estrogen effects on bone
Zinc	Growth factor for the skeleton
Copper	Stimulates cross links in bone, adds strength
Silicon	Enhances skeletal mineralization
Vanadium	Enhances skeletal mineralization
Selenium	Cofactor for maturation of cartilage
Manganese	Promotes skeletal growth
Strontium[a]	Stimulates bone formation
Fluoride[a]	Stimulates bone formation but can increase brittleness if in excess
Detrimental Trace Elements	
Lithium	Causes hyperparathyroidism-related bone resorption
Aluminum	Impairs bone formation and mineralization, increases bone resorption
Iron	Decreases bone formation and mineralization, increases bone resorption
Molybdenum	Causes skeletal deformities
Cadmium	Decreases bone formation and mineralization, increases bone resorption
Tin	Impairs modeling sequence
Lead	Decreases bone formation and mineralization, increases bone resorption

[a] Beneficial nutrients known to be deleterious to the skeleton if taken in excess amounts.

toxicity, which occurs mainly in individuals with industrial exposure, has similar manifestations to iron overload but tends to present itself as defective mineralization, with predominant osteomalacia. Lead toxicity has similar effects to iron and cadmium but rarely shows skeletal manifestations comparable to its CNS, hematologic, and other soft tissue toxicity.

Nutritional Recommendations in Metabolic Bone Diseases

Osteoporosis

Bone loss sufficient to place patients at immediate risk for fracture should always be treated with an FDA-approved drug in addition to a number of nonpharmacologic

TABLE 61.15

Nonpharmacologic Approaches to the Prevention and Treatment of Osteoporosis

Nutrition	Calcium: 1000-1500 mg/day Permits normal growth and development of the skeleton Maximizes peak bone mass Maintains adult bone mass Minimizes age related bone loss Enhances benefits of pharmacologic therapy Vitamin D: 600-1200 IU/day Intake of calcium/vitamin D should be maintained throughout life starting before adolescence. Increase awareness in children and adolescents of needed behavioral/nutritional measures Magnesium: 450-500 mg/day (if tolerated)
Exercise	
Fall prevention	
Other lifestyle modifications (risk factor reduction — see Table 61.5)	

approaches outlined in Table 61.15. The need to achieve an ideal calcium intake cannot be overstated. Opinions vary as to the ideal vitamin D intake, but it is probable that intakes as high as 1200 IU per day would not prove toxic. However, higher vitamin intakes should be avoided. There are also discrepancies in the recommendations for magnesium, but the recommended daily intake of 400 to 500 mg can be taken if there is no tendency to frequent or loose bowel movements. In fact, a high magnesium intake may help to relieve the constipating effects of calcium carbonate preparations. The procedures to ascertain the amount of magnesium supplementation to prescribe are similar to those for calcium in Table 61.9. During nutrition counseling for osteoporosis, the other nonpharmacologic approaches listed in Table 61.15 should be monitored. Falls are particularly serious cofactors in fractures, and are mostly preventable. Adequate protein-kcalorie nutrition promotes muscular strength and agility, and therefore helps prevent falls.

Although these recommendations are intended for primary types of osteoporosis, they are also applicable, with modifications, in secondary forms of osteoporosis. For example, calcium and vitamin D intakes should be carefully monitored by serum and urine calcium measurements in hyperparathyroidism, and idiopathic hypercalciuria, and if urine calcium rises unduly, a thiazide diuretic should be added to reduce urine calcium excretion. In corticosteroid-induced osteoporosis, if the prednisone equivalent dose is 5 mg per day or higher, the vitamin D intake should be drastically increased to the range of 5000 to 7000 IU per day. This can be done most conveniently by prescribing a high-dose vitamin D preparation containing 50,000 IU once a week. The nonpharmacologic approaches in Table 61.15 are equally applicable to patients with lesser degrees of bone loss, or osteopenia. Advanced states of osteopenia may also qualify for a modified drug program.

Osteomalacia

There are many causes of osteomalacia, and most relate to defects in the vitamin D cascade (Figure 61.1), or an endorgan resistance to active vitamin metabolites, either genetic or acquired. Uncomplicated nutritional deficiencies (of calcium and/or vitamin D) are rare but do occur in the financially and socially stressed, and in the institutionalized elderly. A general approach to nutritional therapy of osteomalacia is outlined in Table 61.16, which also indicates modifications to be made in various types of osteomalacia. The reason for advocating a combination of precursor vitamin D and the active metabolite calcitriol is because there is a theoretic possibility that other active metabolites of vitamin D might appear which might have direct stimulatory effects on the mineralization process itself.

TABLE 61.16

Treatment of Osteomalacia

Type	Calcium Intake qd	Vitamin D Intake qd	Other Nutrients	Other Agents
Nutritional (incl. post gastrectomy)	Up to 2000 mg	400-1000 IU		
Malabsorption	Same	Up to 50,000 IU	Other lost nutrients	Gluten-free diet, pancreatic enzymes
Dependent rickets	Same	400-1000 IU plus Calcitriol, up to 0.25 μg qid	Same	
Familial hypophosphatemic rickets	Same	Up to 150,000 IU and/or Calcitriol, up to 0.25 μg qid	Phosphorus (neutral), up to 3000 mg qd	
Oncogenic osteomalacia	Same	Same		Locate and excise mesenchymal tumor
Anticonvulsant-induced osteomalacia	Same	Up to 5000 IU		

TABLE 61.17

Treatment Options for Renal Osteodystrophy

Optimize renal function and dialysis procedures
Consider renal transplantation
Remove excess skeletal aluminum and iron, if present (chelators such as desferrioxamine)
Calcium carbonate supplements (phosphate binder), 500 mg Ca qid[a]
Reduce phosphorus, magnesium, protein, and acid ash in diet
Calcitriol (to tolerance), 0.25 mcg, up to qid[a]
Parathyroidectomy (in selected cases)
Calciomimetic agents (when available)
Calcitonin (in selected cases with a significant osteoporotic component)

[a] Four times a day.

Renal Osteodystrophy

This term refers to the skeletal complications of chronic renal failure and represents a variable combination of secondary hyperparathyroidism, osteomalacia, osteoporosis, and osteosclerosis. Nutritional therapy is an important aspect of treatment (Table 61.17), although pharmacologic and/or surgical approaches may also be necessary in particularly advanced cases. The aim is to suppress the secondary hyperparathyroidism and correct undermineralization by using maximally tolerated doses of the active metabolite of vitamin D, calcitriol (1,25-dihydroxy-vitamin D) and calcium. Calcium carbonate is preferred to calcium citrate, although both have the ability to bind phosphorus in the GI tract and thereby reduce the hyperphosphatemia, a major factor in the genesis of the renal osteodystrophy.

Primary Hyperparathyroidism

Previously, calcium restriction was advocated to lessen the impact of the hypercalcemia characteristic of the condition. However, the availability of bone density measurements has revealed that this results in greater bone loss and worsens the skeletal complications.

Presently, adequate calcium and vitamin D intakes are advocated, preferably as food sources with a minimal use of supplements. The condition is best treated by surgery, although new pharmacologic agents, called calciomimetic agents, are currently under development.

Paget's Disease

Although both bone resorption and formation are increased, their quantitative relationship is variable, so that either positive calcium balance (with hypocalciuria) or negative calcium balance (with hypercalciuria) may be present at any given time during the prolonged course of the condition. In any case, the imbalance rarely disturbs the serum calcium level and does not cause serious bone loss in pagetic lesions. Therefore, normal calcium and vitamin D intakes are the best approach, as having Paget's disease does not protect against osteoporosis in non-pagetic areas. Since the bisphosphonates currently in use can occasionally cause transient mild hypocalcemia, some authorities recommend an increased calcium intake during bisphosphonate treatment. On the other hand, calcium should not be supplemented if there is a history of calcium-containing kidney stones. Another type of stone that can occur in Paget's disease is the uric acid stone, as some pagetic patients also have a concomitant gouty diathesis.

Other Rarer Conditions

Nutritional therapy does not generally play an important role, but may sometimes be useful depending on the features of individual subjects.

Renal Stone Disease

The four major types of kidney stones are outlined in Table 61.18. Although they tend to occur under different clinical conditions, the key to successful categorization and treatment, which is largely a matter of nutritional manipulation, is stone recovery and physicochemical (crystallographic) analysis. When this is not feasible, other clues such as radiographic appearance, clinical data obtained from the patient, and biochemical testing can be used to design a nutritional program.

Calcium Oxalate/Phosphate

This stone type accounts for 80% of renal stones, and approximately 50% of these are idiopathic in that there is no discernible metabolic defect, and both urinary calcium and oxalate levels are normal. In the remainder, either urinary calcium or oxalate is increased; the former may or may not be associated with hypercalcemia. Oxaluria may be a primary genetic condition, may be due to excessive intake of foods that yield oxalate during digestion or metabolism, or may be secondary to the increased oxalate absorption present in inflammatory bowel disease and in some malabsorption syndromes. In the GI-related cases, intestinal calcium becomes bound to unabsorbed fats instead of luminal oxalate, allowing the latter to be absorbed and then excreted, followed by precipitation with

TABLE 61.18

Additional Sources of Information

Calcium and Vitamin D

Heaney RP. *Nutr Rev* 54(4 Pt 2): 3S; 1996.
Reid DM, New SA. *Proceedings of the Nutr Soc* 56: 977; 1997.
Lewis RD, Modlesky CM. *Int J Sport Nutr* 8: 250; 1998.
Bronner F, Pansu D. *J Nutr* 129: 9; 1999.
_______________, Optimal Calcium Intake, NIH Consensus Statement *Nutrition* 12: 1; 1994.
Compston JE. *BMJ* 317: 1466; 1998.

Magnesium

Wallach S. In: *Magnesium and Trace Elements* 10: 281; 1992.
Martini LA. *Nutr Rev* 57: 227; 1999.

Osteoporosis

Nordin BE, Need AG, Steurer TA, Morris HA, Chatterton BE, Horowitz M. *Ann NY Acad Sci* 854: 336; 1998.
Lau EM, Woo J. Nutrition and Osteoporosis *Current Opinion in Rheumatology* 10: 368; 1998.
Raisz LG. *J Bone Min Metab* 17: 79; 1999.
Anderson JJ, Rondano P, Holmes A. *Scand J Rheumatol* 103: 65S; 1996.

Osteomalacia

Francis RM, Selby PL. Osteomalacia *Baillieres Clin Endocrinol Metab* 11: 145; 1997.
Bell NH, Key LL, Jr. Acquired Osteomalacia *Curr Ther Endocrinol Metab* 6: 530; 1997.
Klein GL. *Nutrition* 14: 149; 1998.
Nightingale JM. *Nutrition* 15: 633; 1999.

Renal Osteodystrophy

Sakhaee K, Gonzalez GB. *Am J Med Sci* 317: 251; 1999.
Kurokawa K, Fukagawa M. *Am J Med Sci* 317: 355; 1999.
Slatopolsky E. *Nephrol Dialysis, Transplantation* 13: 3S; 1998.

Trace Elements

D'Haese PC, Couttenye MM, De Broe ME. *Nephrol Dialysis, Transplantation* 11: 3S; 1996.
Wallach S, Chausmer AB. In: *Trace Metals and Fluoride in Bones and Teeth,* Priest ND, Van De Vyver FL, Eds, CRC Press, Boca Raton, 1990, chap. 10.
Chausmer AB, Wallach S. In: *Trace Metals and Fluoride in Bones and Teeth* Priest ND, Van De Vyver FL, Eds, CRC Press, Boca Raton, 1990, chap. 11.

Paget's Disease

Delmas PD, Meunier PJ. *N Engl J Med* 336: 558; 1997.

Renal Stone Disease

Coe FL, Parks JH. Nephrolithiasis In: *Primer on the Metabolic Bone Diseases and Disorders of Mineral Metabolism,* 4th ed, Favus MJ, Ed, Lippincott Williams and Wilkins, Philadelphia, 1999, chap. 81.

calcium in the urinary tract. Calcium stones are difficult to treat, in the sense of preventing or reducing their rate of recurrence, because of their great insolubility. Successful treatment of an underlying medical condition, if present, is the most effective maneuver and should be combined with dietary changes consisting of manipulating calcium intake, limiting vitamins A and D and oxalate intakes, and maintaining maximal hydration compatible with cardiovascular competence. In GI-related oxaluria, an increased calcium intake may allow more oxalate complexation in the GI tract and actually lessen calcium oxalate stone formation. In the case of idiopathic hypercalciuria, an extreme reduction in calcium intake will have an adverse effect on bone density and increase the predisposition to osteoporosis/osteopenia.

$MgNH_4PO_4$

In urinary tract infections with urea-splitting organisms, both urine NH_4 levels and pH rise, and the NH_4 can combine with urinary Mg and PO_4 to precipitate in the alkaline medium. Lowering substrate excretion by dietary restriction and lowering pH with an acid ash diet will retard precipitation, but so long as the infection persists, NH_4 generation will limit the effectiveness of the dietary manipulation. Unfortunately, these infections are difficult to eradicate in the presence of the disturbed anatomy of the renal calyces and pelvis caused by the large, irregularly shaped stones, which sometimes approach the size of staghorn calculi. Dietary manipulations are best instituted before chronic UTIs with urea-splitting organisms begin to generate stones.

Cystine

These are the rarest of kidney stones, since they occur only in an inborn genetic condition, cystinuria. Although organic in composition, they are radio-opaque due to the dense packing of the cystine molecules. In mild cases, urinary alkalinization is successful, but when the stone disease is more aggressive, alkalinization must be combined with agents that can chelate the excess cystine.

Uric Acid (Ureate)

This is the only major radiolucent stone, and its presence may need specialized imaging procedures. Patients with manifest gouty arthritis (acute or tophaceous) are particularly susceptible because of a combination of uricosuria and an intrinsic defect in urinary NH_3 production from purine precursors, which forces the kidney to excrete metabolically derived acids as titratable acidity, a condition under which uric acid is insoluble and can precipitate. A subset of patients exist in whom the urinary defect in NH_3 production is not accompanied by other features of the gouty diathesis, and these patients are easily treated with alkali supplements alone. A simple technique to detect these patients and monitor alkali treatment is to have the patient record the urinary pH of each voided specimen by placing pH-sensitive strips in the urinary stream. In normal individuals, pH will vary from 5.0 or less to 6.5 or higher (the "alkaline tide"), but patients with the defect will show persistent values of 5.0 or less throughout the 24 hours. With successful alkalinization, pH should remain at 6.0 or higher. Excessive purine intake should be curtailed, but not at the expense of causing protein deficiency. Conditions associated with high catabolic states, such as burns, extensive trauma, and certain neoplasms, especially with the use of antineoplastic agents, can cause acute and severe hyperuricosuria which may not only cause stone formation but may clog the renal tubules, causing a "gouty nephropathy." Expectant treatment with alkali and forced hydration is required to forestall this serious complication. Paget's disease patients may also form uric acid stones because of the frequent tendency to a comorbid gouty diathesis, and should also receive careful alkalinization if this is a problem.

Mixed Stones

These represent a challenge in terms of diagnosis and treatment. Since treatment for one component may be deleterious for another component, a full understanding of the qualitative and quantitative nature of the metabolic defects present should be sought before instituting cautious treatment.

Bladder Stones

Stones that form in the urinary bladder and have not migrated from the renal calyces or pelvis are generally not related to metabolic defects, but to stasis. Their composition is quite variable, and is often a mixture of components. They are treated by correcting disturbed anatomy rather than dietary therapy.

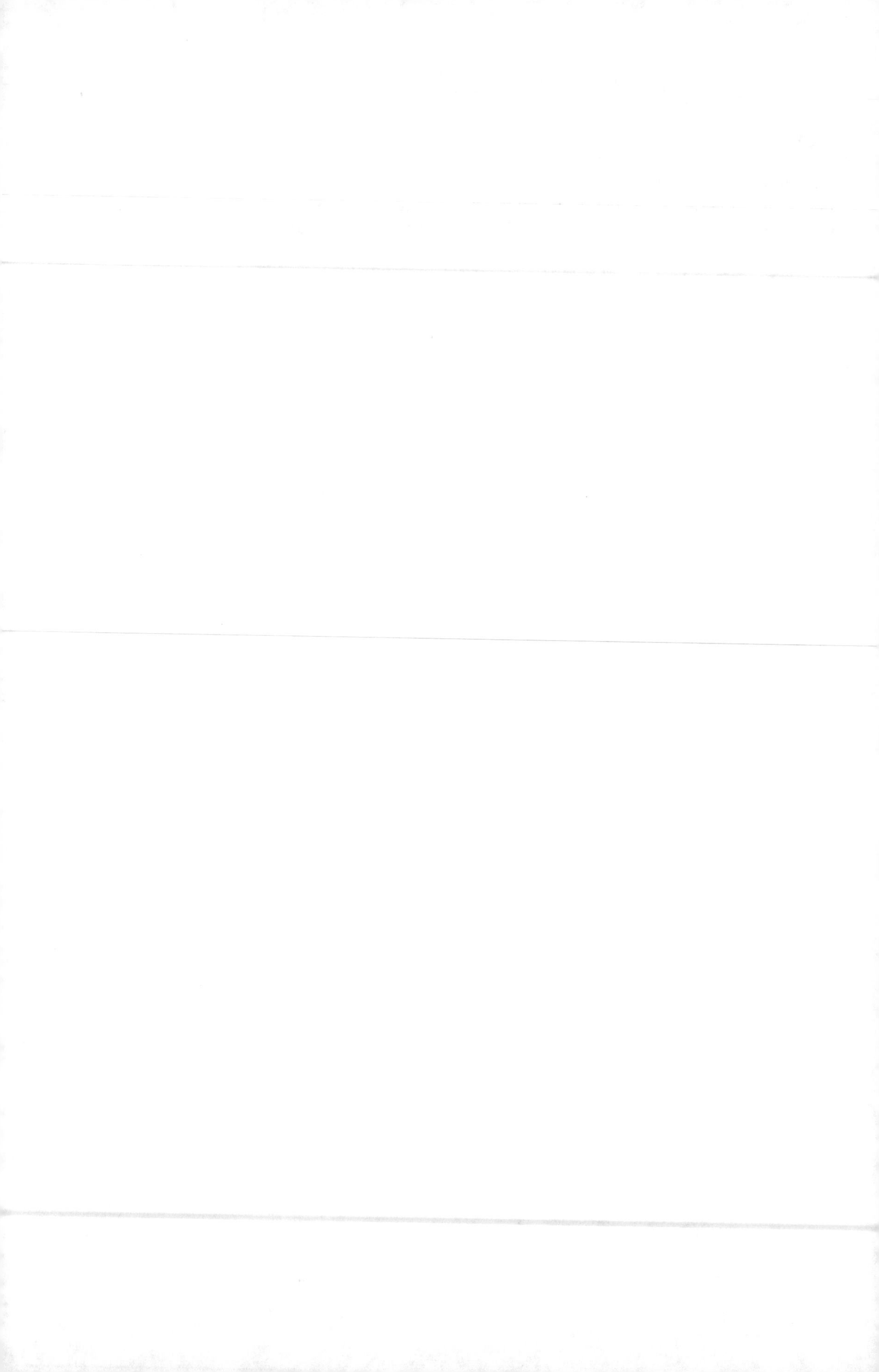

62

Nutrients and Eye Disease

Allen M. Perelson and Leon Ellenbogen

Introduction

Age-related cataract and age-related macular degeneration (AMD) are two of the leading causes of visual impairment in older Americans. Cataracts cloud the lens and impair the entry of light into the eye. AMD results in the loss of central vision due to impingement on the macula, which is responsible for absorption of short wavelengths of light. (See Figure 62.1 for anatomy of the eye.) Studies in animal models indicate a possible role for oxidative mechanisms in the development of both cataract and AMD. Available epidemiological data are derived primarily from observational studies and generally suggest small to moderate benefits for antioxidant nutrients in reducing the risks of cataract and AMD.

Antioxidant Nutrients and Cataract Prevention

There is increasingly strong evidence that the antioxidant nutrients vitamin C, vitamin E, and beta-carotene may help protect against cataracts. Vitamin C is 60 times more concentrated in the lens of the eye than in blood plasma, and other antioxidants, including lutein and other carotenoids, are also found in disproportionately high levels in the eye.

Taylor was among one of the first to suggest that adequate provision of antioxidants from multivitamins might help delay the development of cataracts.[1] This hypothesis was quickly verified by Sperduto et al. in the Linxian cataract studies[2] which showed that vitamin/mineral supplements, particularly niacin and riboflavin, may decrease the risk of nuclear cataract in an undernourished Chinese population. These were the first double-blind, randomized, well-controlled, long-term nutritional intervention studies using multivitamin/mineral supplementation to determine their effect on the prevalence of nuclear, cortical, and posterior subcapsular cataracts. Findings from the Sperduto studies suggested that vitamin/mineral supplements, especially the riboflavin and niacin components, may decrease the risk of nuclear cataract.

0-8493-2705-9/02/$0.00+$1.50

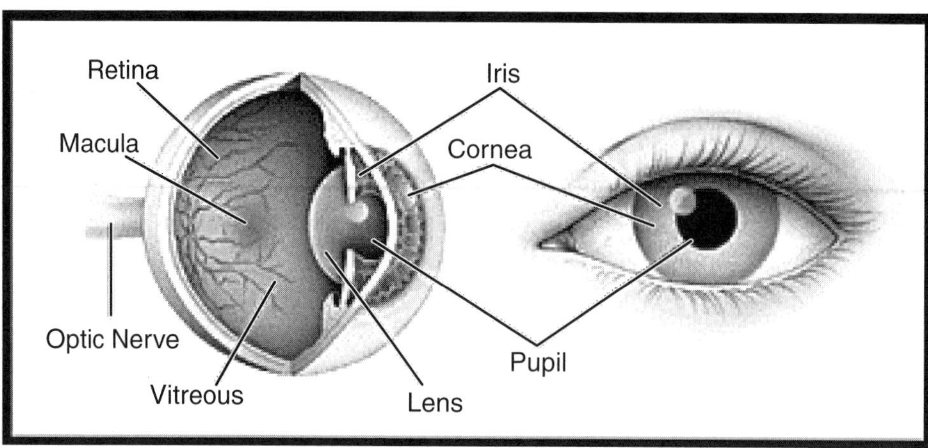

FIGURE 62.1
Anatomy of the eye.

TABLE 62.1
Vitamin E Intake or Plasma Concentration with Reduced Cataract Risk

Reference and Type of Study	Population (Duration)	Endpoint	Risk and Associated Intake or Plasma Concentration of Vitamin E
Jacques (1988)[7]	112 subjects	Plasma levels of vitamins E, C, and carotenoids	High plasma levels of at least two of the three antioxidants were associated with a reduced risk of cataract
Knekt (1992)[8]	47 patients with cataract and 94 controls	Plasma vitamin E and beta-carotene levels	Odds ratio for senile cataract risk was 2.6 for patients in lowest third of serum vitamin E and beta-carotene levels
Rouhaiinen (1996)[5]	410 males	Plasma vitamin E levels	Plasma vitamin E levels in the lowest quartile were associated with a 3.7-fold increased risk of progression of early lens opacities
Robertson (1989)[9]	175 individuals with cataract and 175 individuals without cataract	Vitamin E supplementation	There was a 56% decrease in cataract risk in subjects who took vitamin E supplements
Leske (1998)[6]	764 participants	Vitamin E supplement use and plasma levels	Risk of nuclear cataract was decreased by approximately 50% with regular vitamin E use and in subjects with higher plasma vitamin E levels
Lyle (1999)[10]	400 subjects	Serum carotenoids and tocopherol levels	Nuclear cataract may be linked inversely to vitamin E status but not with carotenoid status

Results of at least two large prospective cohort studies are consistent with a possible benefit of antioxidants in cataract. In the Physicians' Health Study, researchers found that users of multivitamins had a 27% lower risk of developing a cataract and a 21% lower risk of having a cataract operation, compared to non-users.[3] In the Nurses' Health Study, women in the highest quintile for total carotene intake had a 27% reduced risk of cataract.[4]

TABLE 62.2
Vitamin C Intake or Plasma Concentration with Reduced Cataract Risk

Reference and Type of Study	Population (Duration)	Endpoint	Risk and Associated Intake or Plasma Concentration of Vitamin C
Dietary Intake			
Robertson (1989)[9] Case-control	175 Cases, 175 controls	Cataract	>300 mg/d supplement: ↓ risk by 70%
Jacques and Chylack (1991)[11] Case-control	77 Cases, 35 controls	Cataract	>490 compared with <125 mg/d: ↓ risk by 75%
Hankinson (1992)[4] Prospective cohort	50828 Women (8 y)	Cataract (493 extractions)	705 compared with 70 mg/d: no ↓ risk; supplements for >10 y: ↓ risk by 45%
Vitale (1993)[12] Longitudinal	660 Men and women (6 y)	Cataract	>261 compared with <115 mg/d: no ↓ risk
Sperduto (1993)[2] Trial	3249 Chinese men and women (5 y)	Cataract	120 mg/d supplement: ↓ risk by 22% (NS) (+ 30 μg Mo/d cosupplement)
Jacques (1997)[13] Cross-sectional	247 Women (10 y)	Cataract	>359 compared with <93 mg/d: no ↓ risk; supplements for >10 y: ↓ risk by 77–83%
Plasma Concentration			
Jacques and Chylack (1991)[11] Case-control	77 Cases, 35 controls	Cataract	>90 compared with <40 μmol/L: ↓ risk by 71% (>400 compared with 80 mg/d)
Vitale (1993)[12] Longitudinal	660 Men and women (6 y)	Cataract	>80 compared with <60 μmol/L: no ↓ risk (>400 compared with 150 mg/d)

Adapted from Carr, AC, Frei, B. *Am J Clin Nutr* 69: 1086; 1999.

Data from two smaller cohort studies also support the association between antioxidant use and a reduced incidence of cataract. In a study of Finnish men with elevated cholesterol levels, those in the highest quartile of vitamin E intake had a three- to fourfold decreased risk of progression of early cortical lens opacities.[5] In the Longitudinal Study of Cataract, risk of nuclear cataract was reduced by one-third in regular users of multivitamins and by one-half in regular users of vitamin E supplements.[6]

Evidence is also accumulating to assist in characterizing the effect of individual antioxidant nutrients and their contribution to reducing the incidence of cataracts or slowing their progression. A number of epidemiologic studies have suggested an association between cataract incidence and blood levels of vitamin E or intake of vitamin E. These are listed in Table 62.1.

Several epidemiologic studies have investigated the association of vitamin C intake or plasma levels of vitamin C with the incidence of cataract. These are summarized in Table 62.2.

Exciting information concerning lutein and cataract risk has recently been reported from one observational study in men[14] and one in women.[15] Intakes of lutein and zeaxanthin were found to be inversely related to the risk of cataracts severe enough to require extraction. The role of lutein in the prevention of cataracts is discussed in an excellent review by Mares-Perlman.[16]

More research is needed on the impact that nutrient supplementation has on the risk of developing cataracts. Ongoing trials are listed at the end of this section along with

TABLE 62.3

Antioxidant Levels and Intakes and Risk of AMD

Reference	Study Size	Findings
West (1994)[19]	976	Plasma vitamin E levels in lowest quartile associated with two-fold risk of AMD
Smith (1999)[20]	3654	No association between antioxidant intake and risk of AMD
Tsang (1992)[21]	166	No association between vitamin E intake and risk of AMD
Mares-Perlman (1995)[22]	334	Plasma lycopene levels in lowest quintile associated with twofold risk of AMD
Seddon (1994)[23]	876	Carotenoid intake in the highest quintile was associated with a 43% decreased risk of AMD
Eye Disease Case-Control Study Group (1993)[18]	1036	High serum carotenoid levels are associated with a 2/3 risk reduction in AMD

trials examining the role of nutrients in age-related macular degeneration, which is discussed below.

Carotenoids and Acute Macular Degeneration

The macula is the part of the retina responsible for central vision and visual acuity. In primates, including humans, the central area of the macula is yellow due to presence of the "macular pigment," a high concentration of the carotenoids lutein and zeaxanthin. AMD occurs in about 20% of the population, is irreversible, and is the leading cause of visual impairment in the United States.

Supplementation with lutein has been found to increase serum levels of this nutrient, and also to increase macular pigmentation.[17] The Eye Disease Case-Control Study analyzed blood levels of antioxidant nutrients in 421 patients with AMD and in 615 controls. People with medium or high blood carotenoid levels had one-half and one-third the risk of AMD, respectively, compared to people with low carotenoid levels. Carotenoids analyzed were lutein, zeaxanthin, beta-carotene, alpha-carotene, cryptoxanthin, and lycopene. There was no significant protective effect of vitamin C, vitamin E, or selenium.[18]

Table 62.3 summarizes epidemiological studies of antioxidant intakes and plasma levels in association with the risk of AMD.

Recent data from cohort epidemiological studies show zinc to be weakly protective against the development of some forms of early AMD,[24] although this effect is not proven.[20] Newsome et al.[25] undertook the first prospective intervention study using daily doses of zinc 100 mg to determine its effect on visual acuity in subjects with drusen or AMD. Although some eyes in the zinc-treated group lost vision, this group had significantly less visual loss than the placebo group after a followup of 12 to 24 months.

Ongoing Trials

While the majority of evidence suggests a beneficial effect of antioxidants against the development and progression of cataracts and AMD, controlled intervention trials are

TABLE 62.4

Ongoing Trials Investigating Antioxidant Vitamins and Their Effect on Age-Related Cataract and AMD[26]

Trial	Study Population	Agents Tested
Age-Related Eye Disease Study	4753 men and women ages 55-80 with no AMD to relatively severe AMD	High-dose antioxidants (beta-carotene, vitamin C, vitamin E and zinc)
Physicians Health Study II	Approximately 15,000 healthy U.S. male physicians ages 55 and older	Beta-carotene 50 mg on alternate days Vitamin C 500 mg daily Vitamin E 400 IU on alternate days Multivitamin daily
Women's Health Study	39,876 healthy U.S. female health professionals ages 45 and older	Vitamin E 600 IU on alternate days
Collaborative Italian-American Clinical Trial of Nutritional Supplements and Age-Related Cataracts (CTNS)	1020 men and women with no or early cataract at entry	Daily multivitamin/multimineral supplement

Adapted from Christen, WG. *Proc Assoc Am Phys* 111: 16; 1999.

needed to more precisely define the protective role of antioxidants in preserving vision. Table 62.4 lists some ongoing trials.

References

1. Taylor A. *Ann NY Acad Sci* 669: 111; 1992.
2. Sperduto RD, Hu TS, Milton RC, et al. *Arch Ophthalmol* 111: 1246; 1993.
3. Seddon JM, Christen WG, Manson JE, et al. *Am J Public Health* 84: 788; 1994.
4. Hankinson SE, Stampfer MJ, Seddon JM, et al. *BMJ* 305: 335; 1992.
5. Rouhaiinen P, Rouhaiinen H, Salonen JT. *Am J Epidemiol* 144: 496; 1996.
6. Leske MC, Chylack LT, He Q, et al. *Ophthalmology* 105: 831; 1998.
7. Jacques PF, Chylack LT Jr, McGandy RB, et al. *Arch Ophthalmol* 106: 337; 1998.
8. Knekt P, Heliovaara M, Rissanen A, et al. *BMJ* 305: 1392; 1992.
9. Robertson J McD, Donner AP, Trevithick JR. *Ann NY Acad Sci* 570: 372; 1989.
10. Lyle BJ, Mares-Perlman JA, Klein BEK. *Am J Clin Nutr* 69: 272; 1999.
11. Jacques PF, Chylack LT. *Am J Clin Nutr* 53: 352S; 1991.
12. Vitale S, West S, Hallfrisch J, et al. *Epidemiology* 4: 195; 1993.
13. Jacques PF, Taylor A, Hankinson SE, et al. *Am J Clin Nutr* 66: 911; 1997.
14. Brown L, Rimm EB, Seddon JM, et al. *Am J Clin Nutr* 70: 517; 1999.
15. Chasan-Taber L, Willett WC, Seddon JM, et al. *Am J Clin Nutr* 70: 509; 1999.
16. Mares-Perlman JA. *Am J Clin Nutr* 70: 431; 1999.
17. Landrum JT, Bone RA, Kilburn MD. *Adv Pharmacol* 38: 537; 1997.
18. Eye Disease Case-Control Study Group. *Arch Ophthalmol* 111: 104; 1993.
19. West S, Vitale S, Hallfrisch J, et al. *Arch Ophthalmol* 112: 222; 1994.
20. Smith W, Mitchell P, Webb K, et al. *Ophthalmology* 106: 761; 1999.
21. Tsang NCK, Penfold PL, Snitch PF, et al. *Doc Ophthalmol* 81: 387; 1992.
22. Mares-Perlman JA, Brady WE, Klein R, et al. *Arch Ophthalmol* 113: 1518; 1995.
23. Seddon JM, Ajani UA, Sperduto RD, et al. *JAMA* 272: 1413; 1994.
24. Mares-Perlman JA, Klein R, Klein BE, et al. *Arch Ophthalmol* 114: 991; 1996.
25. Newsome DA, Swartz M, Leone NC, et al. *Arch Ophthalmol* 106: 192; 1988.
26. Christen WG. *Proc Assoc Am Phys* 111: 16; 1999.

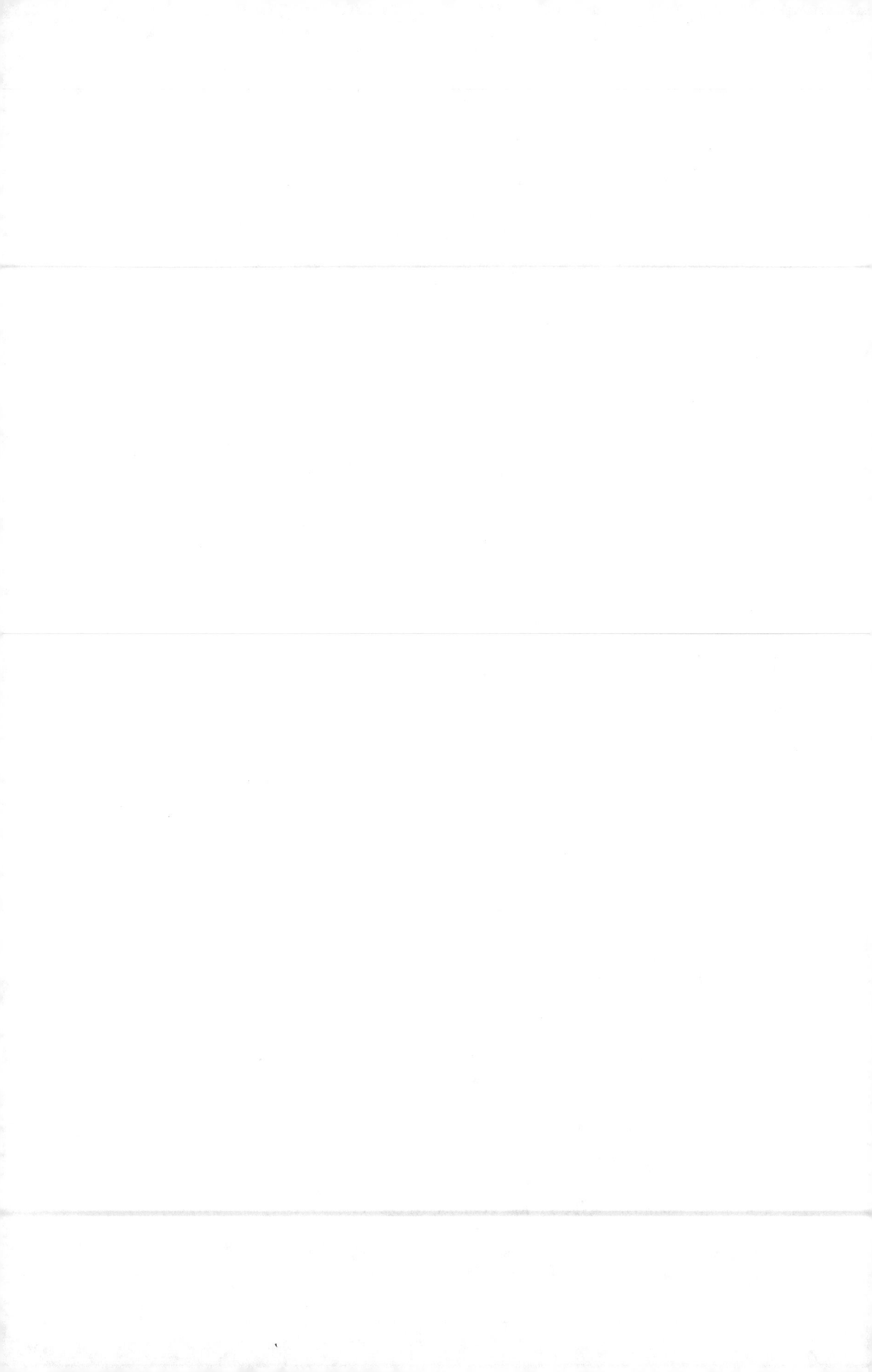

63

Protein-Energy Malnutrition

Naomi K. Fukagawa

Introduction

Protein-energy malnutrition (PEM) is not limited to the severe cases seen in developing countries. Individuals with varying degrees of malnutrition are seen in both inpatient and outpatient settings in the U.S., and all ages may be affected. By definition, PEM results from inadequate intakes of protein, energy fuels, or both. Deficiencies of protein and energy usually occur together but when one predominates and the deficit is severe, kwashiorkor (primarily protein deficiency) or marasmus (predominantly energy deficiency) ensues (Color Figure 63.1*). However, in many cases, it is difficult to recognize which deficit predominates.

Marasmus means wasting. Marasmus results from an overall deficiency of both protein and kcalories, and is characterized by emaciation. Kwashiorkor, a term first used by Williams in 1933,[1] refers to an inadequate protein intake with a fair or normal intake of energy. The classic finding in kwashiorkor is edema, which often masks the degree of wasting. However, because individuals often present with a mixed picture of marasmus and kwashiorkor, the term protein calorie malnutrition was suggested by Jelliffe to include the entire spectrum of undernutrition.[2] In 1973, the World Health Organization (WHO) renamed it PEM.[3] Table 63.1 summarizes the classification of PEM based on standard measures. The best anthropometric measure in children is based on measurements of weight and height or length, and records of age to calculate the two indices: weight for height as an index of current nutritional status, and height for age as an index of past nutritional history. The body mass index (BMI, or Quetelet's index), defined as weight in kg divided by the square of height in meters, is often used for adolescents and adults. Women have more body fat than men at all three cutoff points, but this is an intrinsic biological phenomenon so the same BMI cutoffs may be used for both sexes.

Weight loss is the main feature of mild and moderate PEM, with a decrease in subcutaneous fat. Physical activity and energy expenditure also decline.[4,5] Other functional indicators such as immunocompetence, gastrointestinal function, or behavior may be altered.[6,7] In adults, capacity for prolonged physical work is reduced, but this is usually apparent only in those engaged in intense, energy-demanding jobs. Malnourished women have a higher probability of giving birth to low birth-weight infants.[8] The diagnosis of

* Color figures follow page 992.

0-8493-2705-9/02/$0.00+$1.50

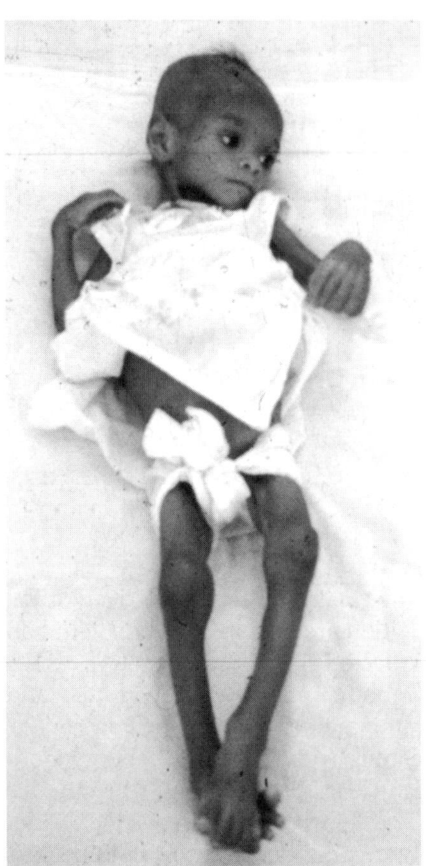

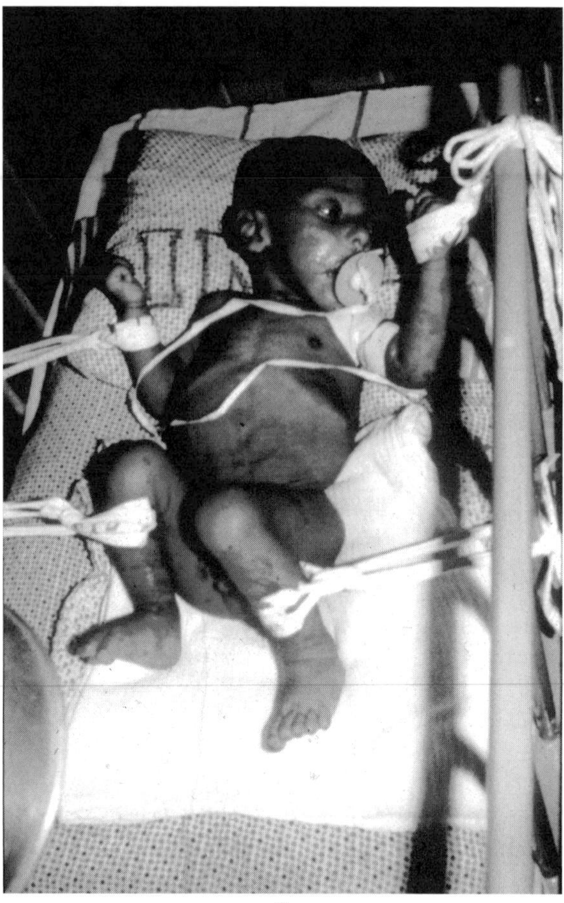

FIGURE 63.1
(See Color Figure 63.1) 1. Kwashiorkor in a child. 2. Marasmic infant. Photographs are from Brazil and were provided by Dr. T. Kuske, reproduced from Feldman, E.B., *Essentials of Clinical Nutrition*, Philadelphia, F.A. Davis, 1988, pp. 321-325. With permission.

TABLE 63.1
Classification of Protein-Energy Malnutrition (PEM)

	Mild	Moderate	Severe
Children			
Weight for height[a] (deficit = wasting)	80-89	70-79	<70 or with edema
Height for age[a] (deficit = stunting)	90-94	85-89	<85
Adults			
Weight:height[b], % of std	90-95	80-90	<80
Triceps skinfold[c], % of std	60-90	40-60	<40
Body Mass Index[d] (wt/ht^2, kg/m^2)	17.0-18.4	16.0-16.9	<16.0

[a] % relative to modern NCHS standards.[47]
[b] Midrange of medium-frame values of the 1959 Metropolitan Life Insurance Tables.
[c] Men 12.5 mm, Women 16.5 mm.
[d] James WP, Ferro-Luzzi A, Waterlow JC. *Eur J Clin Nutr* 42: 969-981; 1988.

severe PEM is principally based on dietary history and clinical features, described later and in the section on Nutritional Assessment.

Etiology and Epidemiology

Causes of PEM may be primary, i.e., as a result of inadequate food intake, or secondary when it is the result of other diseases which lead to limited food intake, poor nutrient absorption or utilization, and/or increased nutrient requirements or losses. Factors that may modify the expression of PEM include age of the patient, cause of the deficiency, and association with other nutritional defects or infectious disease. PEM is the most important nutritional disease in developing countries, especially because of its impact on childhood mortality, growth, and development. In more developed countries, PEM is often seen in chronically ill patients, the elderly, and hospitalized individuals. PEM often develops gradually and is characterized by a series of metabolic and behavioral responses in an attempt to adapt to the reduced food intake. Some of the causes of PEM are listed in Table 63.2.

The global magnitude of PEM is difficult to estimate because mild cases are often not recorded, and many of those afflicted do not receive medical attention. It is estimated that there are about 800 million undernourished people in the world. Most malnourished persons live in developing countries (Africa, Southern and Eastern Asia, Latin America, and the Caribbean). PEM primarily affects infants and preschool children, making it the main cause of growth retardation. About 31% of children under five years of age in developing countries are moderately to severely underweight, 39% are stunted, and 11% are wasted based on a deficit of more than two standard deviations below the WHO/National Center for Health Statistics (NCHS) reference values.[9] There has been a gradual decrease in the prevalence of childhood malnutrition, provided the countries have not been ravaged by natural or manmade disasters such as war, drought, economic crisis, etc. However, the total number of malnourished children worldwide has not decreased because of the rise in populations in countries where malnutrition is prevalent.

TABLE 63.2

Causes of PEM

Primary
Insufficient food intake
Ingestion of proteins of poor nutritional quality
Associated with poverty, ignorance, infectious disease, low food supply
Biologic Factors
Maternal malnutrition prior to and/or during pregnancy
Infectious diseases
Environmental
Overcrowded and/or unsanitary life conditions
Agricultural, climatic, man-made catastrophe (war or forced migration)
Poor food storage

TABLE 63.3

Characteristics of Patients at High Risk for Developing PEM

Gross underweight (<80% weight for height)
Gross overweight (because requirements often overlooked)
Recent weight loss of >10% body weight
Alcoholism
NPO orders >10 days on 5% dextrose in water solution intravenously
Protracted nutrient losses (gut, fistulas, dialysis, extensive exudative or exfoliative cutaneous lesions, or deep decubitus ulcerations)
Increased metabolic needs
Catabolic, anorexogenic, or antinutrient therapies (steroids, chemotherapy, immunosuppression)
Elderly, with polypharmacy and concurrent illness
Infections, especially in those with marginal nutritional status

In industrialized countries, primary PEM is seen among young children of the lower socioeconomic groups, the elderly living alone, adults addicted to alcohol and drugs, or individuals with chronic diseases who have limited food intake. Of interest, in the U.S., 1% of children under five are considered moderately to severely underweight, 1% are wasted, and 2% are stunted.[9] Kwashiorkor has been reported in the U.S. due to peculiar dietary habits imposed upon children by their parents (e.g., unbalanced vegetarian diets), almost total removal of protein in diets of children considered (often incorrectly) to have cow's milk sensitivity, and replacement of milk by low-protein non-dairy creamers. The prevalence of PEM in adults in developed countries is high when considering those who are hospitalized, suffer from chronic diseases, or are disabled. In a recently published study on 369 patients at least 70 years old admitted to a general medical service, 24% were moderately malnourished and 16% severely malnourished.[10] Malnutrition in these patients was associated with greater mortality, delayed functional recovery, and higher rates of nursing home use. These findings emphasize the importance of recognizing and treating PEM if we are to have any impact on the health and well-being of the world population. Some of the characteristics that place patients in the hospital at high risk for PEM are listed in Table 63.3.

Diagnosis

The classical feature of mild to moderate PEM is weight loss (≥5% in 1 month or ≥10% in 6 months in adults; weight for height <80% standard in children). A reduction in subcutaneous adipose tissue is apparent as well as in lean tissue, particularly skeletal muscle, resulting in a marked reduction in upper arm circumference, temporal muscle, and generalized muscle wasting. In infancy and early childhood, poor weight gain is the earliest and most consistent finding with PEM, followed by slowing of linear growth. Some of the physical findings suggestive of PEM are listed in Table 63.4 and illustrated in Color Figure 63.2.

Biochemical information is often not consistent in mild and moderate PEM. Laboratory data related to low protein intake may include low urinary excretion of urea nitrogen and creatinine, altered plasma amino acid patterns (decreased branched-chain amino acids), decreased serum concentrations of albumin and transferrin, and reduced total lymphocyte counts. Severe PEM may be characterized by biochemical changes such as a decline in transport proteins (e.g., transferrin, ceruloplasmin, retinol-, cortisol-, and thyroxine-bind-

TABLE 63.4

Physical Findings Associated with PEM

Area	Findings
General	Poor growth
	Decreased subcutaneous tissue
	Muscle wasting
	Edema
Skin	Dry, scaling, flaking dermatitis
	Altered skin pigmentation
Hair	Dull, altered texture, depigmented, or reddish
	Alopecia
Nails	Transverse ridging, fissuring
Lips	Cheilosis
Tongue	Atrophic lingual papillae
Abdomen	Distention, hepatomegaly

ing proteins, α-, and β- lipoprotein), and decreased enzyme concentrations (e.g., amylase, pseudocholinesterase, alkaline phosphatase). In addition, serum or plasma transaminase concentrations may be increased while the urea cycle or other enzymes associated with degradation (e.g., xanthine oxidase, glycolic acid oxidase, cholinesterase) may be lower. Enzymes utilized in amino acid synthesis may be increased in both forms of PEM.

PEM develops over weeks or months, allowing for a series of metabolic and behavioral adjustments which decrease nutrient demands, and results in a nutritional equilibrium compatible with a lower level of nutrient availability for the cells. Some of the adaptive responses are shown in Table 63.5.[11,12] Many are directed at preserving body protein and essential protein-dependent functions. Energy deficits are initially responded to by a decrease in energy expenditure.[13,14] When compensation fails, fat is mobilized to produce fuel for energy production.[15] This may be followed by protein catabolism, with visceral protein preserved longer.[16] The adaptive response is also characterized by endocrine changes aimed at regulating fuel availability and utilization.[17] As in acute fasting, weight loss early in semistarvation is rapid, but gradually slows even if there is no change in the starvation diet. The reduction in total energy expenditure helps to bring the starving individual back to energy equilibrium, which is further maintained by a reduction in lean tissue mass.

Successful adaptation involves the process of controlled protein loss, which should stop when just enough has been sacrificed to permit energy balance. Since the rate of lean tissue loss is roughly proportional to the amount of lean mass, it automatically slows as the mass of lean tissue decreases.[18] Simultaneously, there is increased efficiency of dietary protein retention until a new state of protein equilibrium is reached.[11] An inverse relationship exists between the amount of lean tissue and the efficiency of retention of protein in the diet. This relationship is affected by the concentration of protein in the diet. As starvation progresses and the lean tissue store diminishes, the rate of protein depletion slows as the amount of protein retained from each meal increases. A new equilibrium is established, and lean tissue loss ceases when a line depicting the relationship between the amount of lean tissue and the rate at which it is depleted crosses over the line which describes the relationship between the amount of lean tissue and the efficiency of retention of protein in the diet. The "price" paid to achieve this physiologic adaptation is the reduction in lean tissue stores. This analytical approach illustrates that a high protein diet may permit protein equilibrium only after moderate lean tissue wasting and that a low-protein diet may also be compatible with protein equilibrium, but the cost, in terms of protein wasting, will be greater.[11]

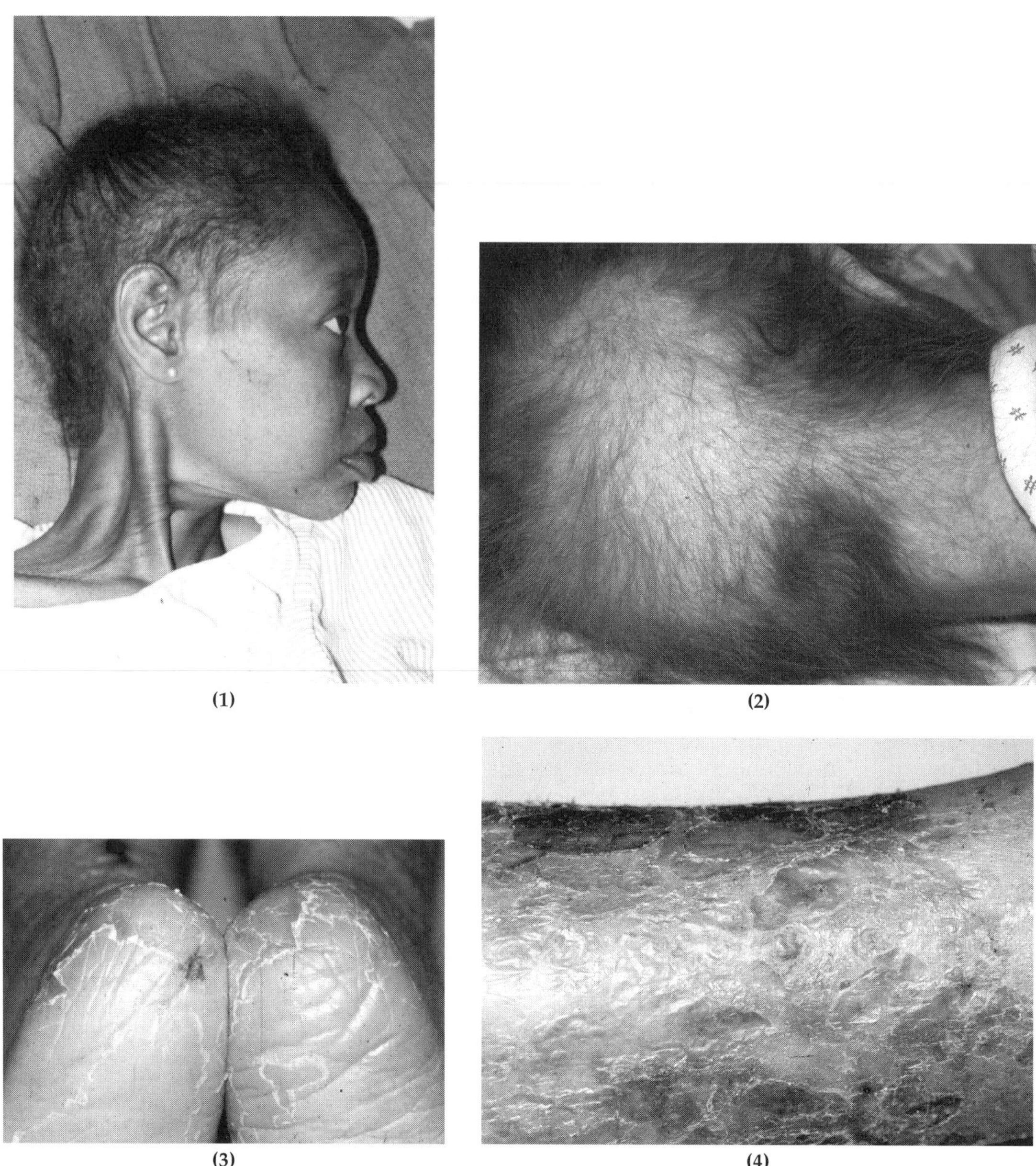

(1) (2) (3) (4)

FIGURE 63.2
(See Color Figure 63.2) Examples of some of the physical findings associated with PEM. (1) Reddish hair, (2) hair loss, (3) flaking skin of the heels, and (4) legs. (Photos of patients at the Medical College of Georgia, Augusta courtesy of Elaine B. Feldman, M.D.)

TABLE 63.5

Adaptive Responses to Protein-Energy Starvation

Hypometabolism (↓ energy expenditure, ↓ physical activity, ↓ protein turnover)
Endocrine changes (↓ serum T_3, ↓ insulin, ↑↓ catecholamines, ↓ IGF-1)
Cardiovascular and renal function (↓ cardiac output, ↓ heart rate, ↓ blood pressure, ↓ renal plasma flow, ↓ glomerular filtration)
Immune system (lymphocyte depletion, ↓ complement components, alterations in monokines or cytokines)

The intimate relationship between dietary energy and the maintenance of body protein should be underscored. Many studies have shown that energy intake influences nitrogen (N) balance at a constant protein intake.[19] The effect of energy is most potent in the modestly submaintenance range of protein and energy intake.[11,20] The amount of dietary energy in surplus or in deficit after energy expenditure is accounted for will influence N balance, making the assessment of energy balance important in managing therapy.[11,20]

Management

Mild to Moderate PEM

If semistarvation is the principal cause for the development of PEM, the patient's response to complete nutrition support is excellent. The response is characterized by marked efficiency of protein utilization when protein intakes increase from the Recommended Daily Allowances (RDA) (0.8 g/kg) to high (1.5 g/kg) and when energy intakes are increased from maintenance to surfeit. In the case of mild to moderate PEM, treating the precipitating event and increasing protein and energy on the basis of the actual height in children and ideal weight in adults may be sufficient. Specific supplementation of individual nutrients is indicated by the presence of signs of specific nutrient deficiency. Table 63.6 outlines the general approach to the treatment of mild to moderate PEM. In children, treatment of mild and moderate PEM corrects the acute signs of the disease, but catch-up growth in height takes a long time or might never be achieved. Weight for height can be restored early but the child may remain stunted. Many severely malnourished children appear to have residual behavioral and mental problems, but the causal role of PEM and poor living conditions are difficult to dissociate.

Severe PEM

Mortality rates in severe PEM can be as high as 40%, with the immediate cause of death being infection. Treatment strategies of severe PEM can be divided into three stages: 1) resolving the life-threatening conditions, 2) restoring nutritional status without disrupting homeostasis, and 3) ensuring nutritional rehabilitation. The most frequent life-threatening conditions associated with severe PEM are described in Table 63.7.

Assessing dehydration in severe PEM is not easy, because the classic signs (sunken eyeballs, decreased skin turgor) may also be found in well-hydrated malnourished

TABLE 63.6

Approach to Treatment of Mild and Moderate PEM

Setting	Ambulatory setting preferred
Foods	Home diet supplemented with easily digested foods containing proteins of high biologic value, high energy density, and adequate micronutrients
Intake Goals	At least twice the protein and 1.5 times the energy requirement (e.g., pre-school child — 2-2.5 g protein and 500-625 KJ (120-150 kcal)/kg body weight)
Food Facts	Appetizing, ready-made or easy to prepare, little commercial value outside the home to avoid sale of items for cash
Special Attention	Avoid a decrease in breastfeeding for infants, ensure adequate vitamins and minerals, perhaps with the use of fortified foods

TABLE 63.7

Life-Threatening Conditions Associated with Severe PEM

Fluid and electrolyte disturbances
Hypoosmolarity with moderate hyponatremia (but intracellular Na excess)
Intracellular K^+ depletion without hypokalemia
Mild to moderate metabolic acidosis
Hypocalcemia
Decreased body magnesium with or without hypomagnesemia
Severe vitamin A deficiency
Infections
Hemodynamic alterations
Cardiac failure secondary to intravenous fluids or after introduction of high-protein and high energy feeding or a diet with high Na^+ content
Pulmonary edema
Severe anemia
Treat only if hemoglobin <4g/dL
Hypothermia
Hypoglycemia

TABLE 63.8

General Approaches to Therapy

Fluid repletion	Allow diuresis of at least 200 ml/24 hrs in children; 500 ml in adults
	Oral or nasogastric rehydration preferred
Electrolytes (if urinating)	~6 mEq K
	2-3 mEq Na
	2-3 mEq Ca^{+2}
Antibiotics	Not used prophylactically
	Choice depends on suspected etiology
Anemia	Treat only in severe cases (hemoglobin <4 g/dL)
Vitamin A deficiency	50,000-100,000 IU for infants and children on day 1
	100,000-200,000 IU for older children and adults on day 1
	Followed by 5000 IU orally each day for the duration of treatment

patients. Furthermore, hypovolemia may coexist with subcutaneous edema. Because of the peculiarities of water and electrolyte disturbances in severe PEM (Table 63.7), the therapeutic approach differs from that used in well-nourished individuals (Table 63.8). Fluid repletion should allow a diuresis of at least 200 ml per 24 hours in children, and 500 ml in adults.[21] Whenever possible, oral or nasogastric rehydration should be used. Although many use the oral rehydration solution (ORS) promoted by the WHO, it is preferable to use solutions that provide more potassium and magnesium, and less sodium (especially for edematous PEM).[22]

Table 63.9 shows the composition of a mineral mix which can complement the diet or be combined with WHO's regular ORS and sucrose to prepare a modified ORS. This modified ORS would be prepared by diluting one standard WHO ORS packet and two 3.12 g packets or 40 mL of concentrated mineral mix and 50 g sucrose in two liters of water. This modified ORS would contain the following: glucose (125 mmol/L), sodium (45 mmol/L), potassium (40 mmol/L), chloride (70 mmol/L), citrate (7 mmol/L), magnesium (3 mmol/L), zinc (0.3 mmol/L), copper (0.04 mmol/L). The osmolarity of this solution would be 300 mOsm/L. The modified ORS solution will have magnesium to begin replenishing the body stores and help potassium retention as well as replace other mineral deficiencies in severe PEM. An approach for rehydration in cases of severe PEM is outlined in Table 63.10.

TABLE 63.9

Mineral Mix for Oral Dehydration Salt Solution and to Complement Liquid Foods

Salt	Amount (g)	mmol in 1 g	mmol in 3.71 g
Potassium chloride	89.5	6.47 K	24 K
Tripotassium chloride	32.4	1.62 K	6 K
Magnesium chloride · $6H_2O$	30.5	0.81 Mg^{2+}	3 Mg
Zinc acetate · $2H_2O$	3.3	0.081 Zn^{2+}	0.300 Zn
Copper sulfate · $7H_2O$	0.56	0.011 Cu^{2+}	0.040 Cu
Total	156.26[a]		

Note: 1 mmol K = 39.1 mg; 1 mmol Mg = 24.3 mg; 1 mmol Zn = 65.4 mg; 1 mmol Cu = 63.5 mg.

[a] Add water to make 1000 mL concentrated mineral mix that can be stored at room temperature or prepare packets with 3.12 g of dry mineral mix. Add 20 mL of concentrated solution or 1 packet to each liter of oral rehydration solution (ORS) or liquid food.

Based on WHO recommendations.

Taken from Torun B, Chew F. Protein-energy malnutrition, *Modern Nutrition in Health and Disease* 9th ed, Shils ME, Olson JA, Shike M, Ross AC. Williams and Wilkins, Baltimore, 1999, pg 963-988. With permission.

TABLE 63.10

Approach to Oral Rehydration for Severe PEM

Initiation	Small sips to provide 70-100 mL/kg body weight over 12 hours (10 ml/kg/hr during first 2 hours for mild to moderate dehydration; up to 30 ml/kg/hr for severe dehydration)
Compensation for ongoing losses	50-100 ml after each loose stool or vomiting for those under 2 years of age; 100-200 ml for older children Continue breast feeding
Evaluation	Monitor every hour; as soon as improvement is seen (usually 4-6 hrs after initiation), small amounts of liquid dietary formula with potassium, calcium, magnesium and other electrolytes may be offered every 2-3 hours
Persistent dehydration	Continue ORS for another 12 hours If signs of overhydration (puffy eyelids, ↑ edema, distended jugular veins, ↑ respiratory rate), use breast milk or liquid diet instead of ORS

Nasogastric tubes may be used in children who vomit constantly or cannot be fed orally. Small portions are key, but if hydration is not improved after four hours, intravenous rehydration may be used. Hypoosmolar solutions (200 to 280 mOsm/L) must be used, and sodium should not be >3 mmol/kg per day. Potassium (not >6 mmol/kg per day) may be added when urination is established. Glucose should provide approximately 63-126 kJ (15 to 30 kcal)/kg/day. The approach to intravenous rehydration is described in Table 63.11.[12]

Hypocalcemia may occur secondary to magnesium deficiency. If magnesium levels cannot be determined, it is necessary to give both calcium and magnesium. Intramuscular or oral magnesium should follow initial parenteral magnesium until repletion with magnesium is complete. A general guideline is intravenous magnesium as a 50% solution of magnesium sulfate in doses of 0.5, 1, and 1.5 mL for patients who weigh less than 7, between 7 and 10, and more than 10 kg, respectively. This may be repeated every 12 hours until there is no recurrence of hypocalcemic symptoms. Calcium replacement may be

TABLE 63.11

Suggested Intravenous Rehydration Regimen

Solutions
1:1 mixture of 10% dextrose with isotonic saline or Ringer's lactated solution (=5% glucose in 0.5 N saline)
Rate
10-30 mL/kg for the first hour followed by 5% dextrose in 0.2 N saline at 5-10 ml/kg/hr
Add K^+ when patient is urinating
Patients with severe hypoproteinemia (<30 g/L), anemia and signs of impending circulatory collapse should be given 10 mL plasma per kg in 1-2 hours followed by 20 mL/kg/hr of a mixture of 2 parts 5% dextrose and one part isotomic saline for 1-2 hours. If diuresis does not improve, the dose of plasma may be repeated 2 hours later.

discontinued when the symptoms disappear or serum Ca^{+2} levels rise to normal. Oral magnesium supplementation of 0.25 to 0.5 mmol magnesium (0.5 to 1 mEq)/kg/day can be given later as described for maintenance therapy.

Infections are frequently the immediate cause of death in severe PEM, and when suspected, appropriate antibiotic therapy should be started immediately. The choice depends on the suspected etiology, patterns of drug resistance, and severity of the disease. Prophylactic antibiotics are not recommended but may be used if close monitoring for signs of infection by experienced personnel is not available. Clinicians should be aware that PEM may alter drug metabolism and that detoxification mechanisms may be compromised.[21] Delayed absorption, abnormal intestinal permeability, reduced protein binding, changes in volume of distribution, decreased hepatic conjugation or oxidation, and decreased renal clearance may all occur. Treatment for intestinal parasites should be deferred until nutritional rehabilitation is under way, because this is rarely urgent. Vaccination against measles for every child over six months should be carried out with a second dose after discharge, because seroconversion may be impaired.

Hemodynamic alterations may occur in severe PEM, especially in the presence of severe anemia, during or after administration of intravenous fluids or shortly after the introduction of high protein and high energy feeding, or a diet with high sodium content. Diuretics such as furosemide (10 mg intravenously or intramuscularly, repeated as necessary) may be given, and other supportive measures taken. The use of diuretics merely to accelerate the disappearance of edema in kwashiorkor, however, is contraindicated. Routine use of blood transfusions for anemia endangers the patients; therefore, it should be given only to those with severe anemia with hemoglobin of <4g/dL, <12% packed cell volume (hematocrit), clinical signs of hypoxia, or impending cardiac failure. In countries with a high prevalence of infection with human immunodeficiency virus (HIV) and few or no resources for screening the blood supply, the risk of transmission of HIV is significant. Therefore, use of blood transfusions should be restricted except in life-threatening situations. Whole blood (10 mL/kg) can be used in marasmic patients, but it is better to use packed red blood cells (6 mL/kg) in edematous PEM. Transfusions must be given slowly, over 2 to 3 hours, and may be repeated as necessary after 12 to 24 hours. At signs of heart failure, 2.5 mL blood/kg should be withdrawn before the transfusion is started and at hourly intervals until the total volume of blood transfusion equals volume of anemic blood removed.

Hypothermia, defined as body temperature below 35.5°C and hypoglycemia, defined as plasma glucose concentrations below 3.3 mmol/L (or 60 mg/dL), may be due to impaired thermoregulation, reduced fuel substrate availability, or severe infection. Asymptomatic hypoglycemia is usually treated by feeding the small volumes of glucose- or sucrose-containing diets described above, whereas severe symptomatic hypoglycemia must be treated with intravenous 50% glucose solution followed by oral or nasogastric administration of 10% glucose solutions at two-hour intervals. Low body temperature will usually rise with frequent feedings of glucose-containing diets or solutions, but patients must be closely monitored when external heat sources are used to reduce the loss of body heat, because they may become rapidly hypothermic when the heat source is removed.

Vitamin A deficiency is usually associated with severe PEM, and therefore a large dose of vitamin A should be given on admission. Water miscible vitamin A as retinol should be given orally or intramuscularly on the first day at a dose of 52 to 105 μmol (15,000 to 30,000 μg or 50,000 to 100,000 IU) for infants and preschool children, or 105 to 210 μmol (30,000 to 60,000 μg or 100,000 to 200,000 IU) for older children and adults, followed by 5.2 μmol (1500 μg or 5000 IU) orally each day for the duration of treatment. Corneal ulceration should be treated with ophthalmic drops of 1% atropine solution and antibiotic ointments or drops until the ulcerations heal.[12]

The refeeding syndrome may develop in severely wasted patients during the first week of nutritional repletion.[23-25] The hyperinsulinemia stimulated by increased carbohydrate consumption results in an antinatriuretic effect.[26] Increased body sodium also results from increased sodium intake. In addition, hypophosphatemia and hypocalemia as well as hypomagnesemia can occur as a result of a stimulation of glycogen synthesis with the refeeding of carbohydrate. Close monitoring is therefore necessary to avoid acute deficiencies, especially of phosphorous and potassium.

Following the attention to life-threatening conditions as described above, the next objective of therapy is to restore nutritional status as rapidly and safely as possible. This may be done with liquid formula diets fed orally or by nasogastric tube, and for older children and adults with good appetites, the liquid formula can be substituted with solid foods that have a high density of high quality and easily digested nutrients. The marasmic patient may require larger amounts of dietary energy after one or two weeks of dietary treatment, which can be provided by adding vegetable oil to increase the energy density of the diet. Intravenous alimentation is not justified in primary PEM, and can actually increase mortality.[27] The protein source in all foods must be of high biologic value and easily digested. Cow's milk protein is frequently available, and although there is concern about lactose malabsorption, cow's milk is usually well tolerated. Eggs, meat, fish, soy isolates, and some vegetable protein mixtures are also good sources of high quality protein. Vitamin and mineral supplements should be included at doses slightly higher than the RDA, and can be accomplished by adding the appropriate amounts of the mineral mix outlined in Table 63.9. Older children and adults should have their diets tailored to their age and general food availability. Initial maintenance treatment should provide average energy and protein requirements followed by a gradual increase to about 1.5 times the energy and 3 to 4 times the protein requirements by the end of the first week. Marasmic patients may need to have further increase in dietary energy intake. Initially, responses to the diet may be no change in weight or a decrease because of the loss of edema and a large diuresis. After 5 to 15 days, there is usually a period of rapid weight gain or "catch-up," but this is usually slower in marasmic patients than kwashiorkor patients.

The final step is ensuring nutritional rehabilitation in patients treated for PEM and usually begins two to three weeks after admission. Traditional foods should be introduced into the dietary regimen, and for the malnourished child, emotional and physical stimulation are important. Adult patients should exercise regularly, with gradual increases in their cardiorespiratory workload. Although the major emphasis of this section appears to be for infants and children, the same physiologic changes and principles apply to adolescents and adults with severe PEM. A brief summary of the approach is provided in Table 63.12. Because adults and adolescents often do not want to eat anything other than habitual foods and resist the intake of formula diets, added sugar and oil may be used to increase the energy density of the traditional diet. Liquid diets with vitamins and minerals can be given between meals and at night.

TABLE 63.12

Dietary Treatment of Adolescents and Adults with Severe PEM

Initial
Energy and protein appropriate for age (45 kcal and 0.75 g protein/kg/day for adolescents; 40 kcal and 0.6 g protein/kg/day for adults)
Rehabilitation
Gradual increase to 1.5 times the energy and 3 to 4 times the protein requirements
RDA for minerals and vitamins
Vitamin A — single dose of 210 μmol (60 mg or 200,000 IU) retinol should be given for all except pregnant women
Monitoring
Supplementary feeding should continue until BMI exceeds 15, 16.5, and 18.5 kg/m^2 for adolescents 11 to 13 years old, 14 to 17 years old, and adults respectively

Monitoring

Monitoring the individual's response to initial therapy encompasses the same principles used to monitor the treatment of life-threatening conditions. Table 63.13 lists the characteristics associated with poor prognosis in patients with PEM. Treatment until full recovery from PEM should not be in the hospital. Ideally, the patient should be followed in a nutrition clinic or rehabilitation center to continue treatment until after all life-threatening conditions have been controlled and the appetite is good, edema and skin lesions have resolved, and the patient appears content and interacts with the staff and other patients. The caretaker of the individual must understand the importance of continuing a high-energy, high-protein diet until full recovery has taken place. An increase in plasma protein or albumin concentration indicates a good response but not full recovery. The most practical criterion for recovery is weight gain, and almost all fully recovered patients should reach the weight expected for their height. Weight for height measures do not necessarily indicate protein repletion, and therefore it is good to use these measures in conjunction with other body composition indices such as creatinine-height index (CHI).[28-31] Table 63.14 summarizes guidelines for CHI and N balance.[31] Premature termination of treatment increases possibility of the recurrence of malnutrition. If body composition cannot be assessed, dietary therapy must continue for a month after the patient admitted with edematous PEM reaches an adequate weight for height without edema and clinical and overall performances are adequate, or for 15 days after the marasmic patient reaches that

TABLE 63.13

Characteristics Associated with Poor Prognosis in Patients with PEM

Age ≤6 months or ≥ 65 years
Significant deficits in weight for age >40% or weight for height >30%
Infections, especially bronchopneumonia or measles, septicemia
Total serum proteins ≤ 3 g/dL
Severe anemia with signs of hypoxia
Hypoglycemia
Hypothermia
Circulatory collapse or signs of heart failure, respiratory distress
Coma, stupor, or other changes in awareness
Severe dehydration or electrolyte disturbance

TABLE 63.14

Guidelines for Creatinine-Height Index and Nitrogen Balance

Creatinine-Height Index (CHI)[31]
  CHI = observed creatinine excretion/expected creatinine excretion x patient ideal weight for height, where expected = 18 mg/kg (women) or 23 mg/kg (men)
  60-80% = moderate muscle mass depletion
  <60% = severe muscle mass depletion
Nitrogen Balance
  Dietary nitrogen (g protein/6.25) – (urinary urea N + 4 g)
Catabolic Index (CI)
  Urinary urea N – (0.5 dietary N intake + 3 g)
  CI = 0, no significant stress
  CI = 1 to 5, mild stress
  CI = >5, moderate to severe stress

weight.[12] The minimum normal limits should be 92% for weight expected for height, or one standard deviation below the reference mean. For children, assuring continual growth at a normal rate with no functional impairments is important.

Nitrogen balance (Table 63.14) is useful for estimating the degree of catabolism and monitoring the response to treatment. N balance is the difference between the quantity of dietary N ingested and the amount of N lost. Because dietary protein is assumed to have an average N content of 16%, protein intake is multiplied by 0.16 or divided by 6.25 to convert protein to N. Since most N is lost in urine as urea, total N excretion may be estimated by adding a correction factor of 4 g to measured urea N: 2 g N for fecal and cutaneous losses, and 2 g for nonurea nitrogenous compounds. One g of N represents approximately 30 g of lean tissue. The catabolic index (CI) (Table 63.14) may be used as an estimate of the degree of stress in an individual. In this case, the amount by which the measured value exceeds the estimated amount is an indicator of the level of stress.[32]

The goal is complete nutritional recovery within three to four months. In children, clearly measurable laboratory changes may be seen within two to three weeks, and anthropomorphic changes from three weeks onwards. Changes in adults are slower unless the PEM was acute and of short duration. Comprehensive programs of nutrition education, psychosocial stimulation, and progressive increments in physical activity must be undertaken.

Impact on Prognosis, Morbidity, and Mortality for Other Illnesses, Especially in the Elderly

PEM is also common in hospitalized patients and individuals with chronic diseases. This has been known since the early 1970s.[33] PEM is an inevitable consequence of chronic liver disease, and reversal of malnutrition is one of the key aims of liver transplantation.[34] Some of the factors contributing to PEM in end-stage liver disease are listed in Table 63.15. Patients with renal disease requiring dialysis are also at significant risk for PEM.[35,36] One of the challenges is to provide adequate nutrition to dialysis patients. Approaches often include dietary supplements, enteral tube feeding, intradialytic parenteral nutrition, and total parenteral nutrition. Appetite stimulants (e.g., megestrol acetate) and growth factors (e.g., anabolic steroids, recombinant growth hormone, or insulin-like growth factor-1) have been used.[37] Another prevalent disease with high incidence of PEM is HIV/acute immunodeficiency disease syndrome (AIDS). PEM is one of the more common findings in AIDS.

TABLE 63.15

Factors Contributing to PEM in End-Stage Liver Disease

Factors Contributing to PEM in End-Stage Liver Disease
Reduced energy intake
Vomiting
Fat malabsorption
Abnormal carbohydrate and protein metabolism
Increased energy requirements
Vitamin and mineral deficiencies

TABLE 63.16

SCALES: Rapid Screen for Risk of PEM

S:	Sadness
C:	Cholesterol < 4.14 mmol/l (160 mg/dl)
A:	Albumin < 40 g/l (4 g/dl)
L:	Loss of weight
E:	Eating problems (cognitive or physical)
S:	Shopping problems or inability to prepare a meal

From Morley JE. *Proc Nutr Soc* 57: 587; 1998. With permission.

Chronic inflammatory bowel disease (e.g., Crohn's disease), anorexia nervosa, or other eating disorders are also commonly associated with PEM.

An important complication of PEM is its impact on wound healing and the development of pressure sores or decubitus ulcers. The majority of studies have looked at the relationship between nutritional factors and the development of pressure ulcers in hospitalized and nursing home patients, most of whom were elderly. Nutritional factors associated with the development of decubitus ulcers include inadequate energy and protein intake, making it one of the many risk factors that is potentially reversible.[38] Providing a diet that is complete in nutrient requirements results in the optimum environment for recovery and healing. A reasonable provision of protein is 1.0 to 1.5 g/kg per day and caloric intake ranging from 30 to 35 kcal/kg per day. Two other nutrients important for wound healing are vitamin C and zinc. Studies have shown that supplements of specific nutrients in patients who are not clinically deficient has little effect on the healing of pressure ulcers.[38] However, since the diagnosis of a subclinical deficiency status is difficult to make, physiologic replacement of dietary deficiencies is prudent when the diet is obviously lacking in sources of vitamins and minerals.

The group at greatest risk for PEM is the elderly, either with or without underlying diseases. Severe PEM occurs in 10 to 38% of older outpatients,[39-41] 5 to 12% of homebound patients,[42] and 5 to 85% of institutionalized older individuals.[43-45] As discussed earlier, a significant number of older hospitalized patients are also at risk for PEM.[10] Unfortunately, the presence of PEM is rarely recognized by physicians, and even when recognized is rarely treated.[41] A number of screening tests for malnutrition risk have been developed, but the SCALES (Table 63.16) was developed to use as a screening tool in the clinic. It has been cross-validated with the Mini Nutritional Assessment (MNA), developed for older subjects.[46] SCALES appears to have superior ability to the MNA to identify subsequent nutritionally associated problems, but has the disadvantage of requiring blood tests. Weight loss remains one of the most sensitive indicators of malnutrition. A useful mnemonic for causes of weight loss, especially in the elderly is shown in Table 63.17. These tables and statistics, however, cannot replace the astute physician or health care provider who remains sensitive to the needs of the elderly and cognizant of this commonly overlooked problem — PEM. Table 63.18 provides a simple checklist which may be useful in the prevention and treatment of PEM in any hospitalized patient.

TABLE 63.17

"Meals on Wheels" Mnemonic for the Causes of Weight Loss

M:	Medications
E:	Emotional (depression)
A:	Alcoholism, anorexia tardive[a], or abuse of elders
L:	Late-life paranoia
S:	Swallowing problems (dysphagia)
O:	Oral problems
N:	No money (poverty)
W:	Wandering and other dementia-related problems
H:	Hyperthyroidism, pheochromocytoma
E:	Enteric problems (malabsorption)
E:	Eating problems
L:	Low-salt low-cholesterol diet
S:	Stones

[a] New onset of food refusal related to a desire to maintain a thin body habitus.[48]

From Morley JE. *Proc Nutr Soc* 57: 587; 1998. With permission.

TABLE 63.18

Checklist of Procedures to Prevent and Treat PEM

1. Accurate record of admission height and weight and weekly follow-up weights.
2. Write specific diet orders; monitor ability to eat and maintain weight.
3. Consult dietician to assess follow-up. Collaborate on oral- and tube-feeding regimens.
4. Regularly check to be sure nutrition composition is sufficient to cover basal and stress-related needs.
5. Know your standard nutrition diets and supplements available.
6. Do not wait >3-5 days before adding protein, kcalories, and other nutrients. Avoid prolonged use of 5% dextrose in water and saline solutions.
7. Use anthropometric measures and available laboratory data to assess and monitor nutritional status.
8. Be cognizant that "hospital food," withholding meals for tests, and anorexia from medications and illness can contribute to malnutrition.
9. Consult Nutrition Support Service when in doubt.
10. Be especially cognizant of patients at high risk (see Tables 63.3 and 63.15).

Adapted from Marliss EB. Protein Calorie Malnutrition, *Cecil Textbook of Medicine* 17th ed, Wyngaarden JB, Smith LH, Jr, Eds, WB Saunders, 1985.

References

1. Williams CD. *Arch Dis Childhood* 8: 423; 1933.
2. Jelliffe DB. *J Pediatr* 54: 227; 1959.
3. Waterlow JC. *Br Med J* 3: 566; 1972.
4. Shetty PS, Kurpad AV. *Eur J Clin Nutr* 44: 47; 1990.
5. Minghelli G, Schutz Y, Charbonnier A, et al. *Am J Clin Nutr* 51: 563; 1990.
6. Chandra RK. *Am J Clin Nutr* 53: 1087; 1991.
7. *The Malnourished Child,* Raven Press, New York, 1990.
8. Habricht JP, Lechtig A, Yarborough C. In: *Size at Birth,* Elliott K, Knight J, Eds, Elsevier, New York, 1974.
9. UNICEF, *The State of the World's Children 2000,* United Nations Publications, New York, 2000.
10. Covinsky KE, Martin GE, Beyth RJ, et al. *J Am Geriatr Soc* 47: 532; 1999.

11. Hoffer LJ. In: *Modern Nutrition in Health and Disease,* 9th ed, Shils ME, Olson JA, Shike M, Ross AC, Eds, Williams and Wilkins, Baltimore, 1999, chap. 41.
12. Torun B, Chew F. In: *Modern Nutrition in Health and Disease,* 9th ed, Shils ME, Olson JA, Shike M, Ross AC, Eds, Williams and Wilkins, Baltimore, 1999, chap. 59.
13. Torun B. *International Dietary Energy Consultancy Group,* 335; 1990.
14. Viteri FE, Torun B. *Bol of Saint Panam* 78: 54; 1975.
15. Torun B, Viteri FE. *United Nations Univ Food Nutr Bull,* 229; 1981.
16. Bistrian BR. In: *Nutritional Assessment,* Wright RA, Heymsfield S, Eds, Blackwell Science Publications, Boston, 1984.
17. Becker DJ. *Ann Rev Nutr* 3: 187; 1983.
18. Grande F. In: *Handbook of Physiology: Adaptation to the Environment,* Dill DB, Ed, APS, Washington, D.C., 1964.
19. Elwyn DH, Gump FE, Munro HN, et al. *Am J Clin Nutr* 32: 1597; 1979.
20. Calloway DH. In: *Protein Quality in Humans: Assessment and In Vitro Estimation,* Bodwell CE, Adkins JS, Hopkins DT, Eds, AVI Pub Co, Westport, CT, 1981.
21. Mehta S. In: *The Malnourished Child,* Suskind RM, Lewinter-Suskind L, Eds, Raven Press, New York, 1990.
22. World Health Organization, *Management of Severe Malnutrition,* WHO Publications, Albany, New York, 1999.
23. McMahon MM, Farnell MB, Murray, MJ. *Mayo Clin Proc* 68: 911; 1993.
24. Graham GG. *N Engl J Med* 328: 1058; 1993.
25. Solomon SM, Kirby DF. *J Parent Enteral Nutr* 14: 90; 1990.
26. Barac-Nieto M, Spurr GG, Lotero H, et al. *Am J Clin Nutr* 32: 981; 1979.
27. Janssen F, Bouton JM, Vuye A, Vis HL. *J Parent Enteral Nutr* 7: 26; 1983.
28. McMahon MM, Bistrian BR. *Disease-A-Month* 36: 373; 1990.
29. Walser M. *J Parenl Enteral Nutr* 11: 73S; 1987.
30. Viteri FE, Alvarado J. *Pediatrics* 46: 696; 1970.
31. Bistrian BR, Blackburn GL, Sherman M, Scrimshaw NS. *Surg Gynecol Obstet* 141: 512; 1975.
32. Bistrian BR. *Surg Gynecol Obstet* 148: 675; 1979.
33. Bistrian BR, Blackburn GL, Vitale J, et al. *JAMA* 235: 1567; 1976.
34. Protheroe SM, Kelly DA. *Baillieres Clin Gastroenterol* 12: 823; 1998.
35. Kopple JD. *J Nutr* 129: 247S; 1999.
36. Bistrian BR, McCowen KC, Chan S. *Am J Kidney Dis* 33: 172; 1999.
37. Kopple JD. *Am J Kidney Dis* 33: 180; 1999.
38. Thomas DR. *Clin Geriatr Med* 13: 497; 1997.
39. Miller DK, Morley JE, Rubenstein LZ, et al. *J Am Geriatr Soc* 38: 645; 1990.
40. Wallace JI, Schwartz RS, LaCroix AZ, et al. *J Am Geriatr Soc* 43: 329; 1995.
41. Wilson MM, Vaswani S, Liu D, et al. *Am J Med* 104: 56; 1998.
42. Morley JE. *Proc Nutr Soc* 57: 587; 1998.
43. Sandman PO, Adolfsson R, Nygren C, et al. *J Am Geriatr Soc* 35: 31; 1987.
44. Silver AJ, Morley JE, Strome LS, et al. *J Am Geriatr Soc* 36: 487; 1988.
45. Morley JE, Silver AJ. *Ann Intern Med* 123: 850; 1995.
46. Guigoz Y, Vellas RJ, Garry PJ. *Facts Res Gerontol* 4: 15; 1994.
47. Waterlow JC. In: *Nutrition in Preventive Medicine,* Beaton GH, Bengod JM, Eds, World Health Organization, Geneva, 1976.
48. Miller DK, Morley JE, Rubenstein LZ, Pietreszka FM. *J Am Geriatr Soc* 39: 462; 1991.

64

Vitamin Deficiencies

Richard S. Rivlin

General Comments on Vitamin Deficiencies

Vitamin deficiencies arise when the diet is inadequate in its content of one or more nutrients or when the body is unable to utilize dietary nutrients adequately. Single nutrient deficiencies are rare these days, because a diet that is suboptimal in one vitamin is nearly always suboptimal in others. Thus, a poor diet tends to have multiple inadequacies. Furthermore, some vitamins are involved in the metabolism of other vitamins, and therefore deficiencies may be interconnected.

A number of factors may serve to intensify the biological effects of a poor diet. For example, exogenous alcohol has specific and selective effects upon vitamin metabolism, interfering with the absorption of some vitamins (e.g., thiamin, riboflavin) and accelerating the metabolic degradation of another (B_6). In addition, a number of medications may affect vitamin metabolism, and at multiple sites. From a practical point of view, laxatives and diuretics, often used for prolonged periods by vulnerable elderly patients with minimal indications, are probably the most common causes of drug-induced vitamin deficiencies.

The concept of risk factors, utilized effectively in the evaluation and prevention of heart disease, needs to be applied to the area of vitamin deficiency. Thus, a patient with alcohol abuse who takes several chronic medications and suffers from malabsorption will have a much enhanced risk of becoming grossly vitamin deficient with a poor diet, and of developing overt deficiency that otherwise might be marginal or subclinical.

A great unknown is the effect of herbal products and so-called alternative/complementary therapies upon vitamin metabolism and on the actions of prescription drugs that, in turn, may affect vitamin metabolism. With large numbers of people consuming a wide variety of products about which there is little information or understanding, a potential exists for developing new forms of malnutrition. We urgently need more information on drug-herbal interactions and their implications for vitamin metabolism.

Several points about the patterns of vitamin deficiency currently emerging in the United States are summarized in Table 64.1.

While the effects of fullblown vitamin deficiencies are well known and have been thoroughly described, the effects of lesser or marginal deficiencies are not as well defined.

0-8493-2705-9/02/$0.00+$1.50

TABLE 64.1

Features of Vitamin Deficiencies

1. Dietary vitamin deficiencies tend to be multiple, not single.
2. Clinical evidence of vitamin deficiencies develops gradually, and early symptoms such as fatigue and weakness may be vague, ill-defined, and non-specific.
3. The physical examination cannot be relied upon to make a diagnosis of early vitamin deficiency; classic features such as the "corkscrew hairs" of scurvy are only detectable after profound deficiency has been attained.
4. The rate of development of vitamin deficiencies is highly variable. Water-soluble vitamins may be depleted within several weeks; longer periods are needed for significant depletion of fat-soluble vitamins. Several years are required for clinical manifestations of vitamin B_{12} deficiency unless there are complicating factors, such as ileal resection or inflammatory bowel disease involving the ileum.
5. The impact of dietary deficiencies of vitamins is greatly augmented by the long-term chronic use of certain medications that may affect absorption, utilization, or excretion of vitamins. Chief among these are laxatives and diuretics. These considerations are particularly relevant to older individuals who use the largest number of drugs, use them for the longest duration, and may have marginal diets to begin with.
6. The concept of "risk factors" may be helpful in assessing the factors such as drugs and alcohol that contribute to determining the clinical significance of a given dietary deficiency.

Within recent years, scientists and the general public have been paying more attention to marginal deficiency in attempting to gain the maximal benefits from diet for health. Recent findings suggest that the concept of so-called "normal" needs to be re-evaluated, inasmuch as there may be different risks for disease within the range considered "normal." For example, individuals with serum folic acid levels in the lower part of the normal range have been shown to have significantly elevated serum concentrations of homocysteine compared to those whose folic acid concentrations are in the upper range of normal. With elevated serum homocysteine concentrations emerging as a risk factor for heart disease, these observations suggest that perhaps we should set higher standards and expectations for the normal range.

In the prevention and treatment of vitamin deficiencies, one must approach the patient in a logical fashion and proceed in an orderly direction. Long-term compliance with an appropriate diet and the use of supplements, if indicated, is the goal, but may be difficult to achieve. Some of the points about correction of vitamin deficiencies are summarized in Table 64.2.

TABLE 64.2

Some Considerations in Correction of Vitamin Deficiencies

1. Approach the patient as a whole; ask yourself, how did a vitamin deficiency develop in the first place? What can be done to prevent a recurrence? Are there complicating factors in addition to the diet?
2. Unless there are specific indications of a single nutrient deficiency, such as vitamin B_{12} in pernicious anemia, most malnourished patients will require rehabilitation with multiple nutrients, primarily with diet, and additionally with supplementation, if necessary.
3. Simple steps can often improve a diet significantly, such as discarding old produce, avoiding "fast food" meals on a regular basis, and increasing the intake of fresh fruits and vegetables. In modern nutrition, one speaks of "junk diets" rather than single "junk foods," and the necessity to have moderation and variety.
4. Learn how to read a label from a nutritional supplement bottle so that you can properly instruct your patients. The array of choices of nutritional supplements is bewildering, and patients must learn that more is not necessarily better.
5. Remember that vitamins may behave like drugs and have a defined toxic:therapeutic ratio. Some vitamins, such as vitamins A and D, have a real potential for causing toxicity. B vitamins may also cause problems, as exemplified by the sensory neuropathy resulting from large doses of vitamin B_6.

Vitamin A

Functions

Vitamin A has a wide variety of functions, including specific roles in vision, embryogenesis, cellular differentiation, growth and reproduction, immune status, and taste sensations.

Deficiency

Deficiency of vitamin A is of crucial importance as a worldwide nutritional problem, because the resultant xerophthalmia is a cause of blindness in approximately half a million preschool children each year in the developing countries. In these areas, the diet is composed primarily of such items as rice, wheat, maize, and tubers that contain far from adequate amounts of vitamin A precursors. The World Health Organization and other groups have made great efforts to plan programs that identify people at risk and to institute appropriate preventive measures on a broad scale.

Clinical deficiency of vitamin A may be overt or subclinical. One of the earliest signs of vitamin A deficiency is night blindness, observed in both children and adults. A characteristic sign that is observed later is Bitot's spots, collections of degenerated cells in the outer aspects of the conjunctivae that appear white in color. The development of xerophthalmia follows a defined sequence, leading eventually to keratomalacia, in which perforation of the cornea occurs. This disorder in its end stages is irreversible, but if ocular abnormalities are detected early and treated vigorously, they may be potentially preventable.

Vitamin A deficiency also causes skin disorders in the form of follicular hyperkeratosis. Although characteristic skin changes occur in response to a deficiency of vitamin A, in practical terms one should remember that skin lesions may be caused by other nutrient deficiencies such as zinc, biotin, niacin, and riboflavin.

Children significantly deficient in vitamin A manifest increased incidence of serious and life-threatening infections and elevated mortality rates. It has been recognized that deficient Vitamin A status is a risk factor for the maternal-to-fetal transmission of human immunodeficiency virus; the relative risk of transmission of the virus is fourfold greater in vitamin A-deficient than vitamin A-sufficient mothers.

Vitamin A deficiency in the U.S. is identified largely with certain risk groups: the urban poor, elderly persons (particularly those living alone), abusers of alcohol, patients with malabsorption disorders, and other persons with a poor diet. Vitamin A deficiency is generally found in a setting in which there are multiple vitamin and mineral deficiencies. Special attention must be paid to deficiency of zinc, a frequent finding in alcoholism, as depletion of zinc interferes with the mobilization of vitamin A from its storage sites in liver. This effect is achieved by blocking the release of holo-retinol-binding protein from the liver.

The physician must keep in mind that deficiency of vitamin A in the U.S. may also develop after the long-term use of several medications. Drug-induced nutritional deficiencies in general, particularly those involving vitamin A, occur most frequently among elderly persons, because they use medications in the largest number and for the most prolonged duration, and may have borderline nutritional status to begin with. Among the drugs most relevant to compromising vitamin A status are mineral oil, which dissolves this nutrient; other laxatives, which accelerate intestinal transit and may diminish the magnitude of vitamin A absorption; cholestyramine and colestipol, which bind vitamin

A; and, under certain conditions, neomycin and colchicine. Patients who are consuming olestra, which may possibly interfere with absorption of a number of vitamins, including A, have been advised to take a multivitamin supplement regularly.

Laboratory Diagnosis of Deficiency

The laboratory diagnosis of vitamin A deficiency is based upon the finding of a low plasma retinol; levels below 10 μg/dl signify severe or advanced deficiency. Interpretation of plasma retinol concentrations may be confounded, however, by a number of other factors such as generalized malnutrition and weight loss. Some authorities have preferred to utilize a form of retinol tolerance test, measuring the increment in serum vitamin A levels over five hours following an oral load of vitamin A.

Prevention

Deficiency of vitamin A can be prevented by a diet high in carotenes, which serve as precursors to vitamin A. The carotenes, particularly beta-carotene, are derived exclusively from plant sources, the richest of which are palm oil, carrots, sweet potatoes, dark green, leafy vegetables, cantaloupe, oranges, and papaya. Vitamin A itself (preformed vitamin A) is derived only from animal sources such as dairy products, meat, and fish. The commercial preparations of fish oils are rich, sometimes too rich, as sources of preformed vitamin A.

The nutritional value of dietary sources of vitamin A may be compromised when the food items are subject to oxidation, particularly in the presence of light and heat. Antioxidants, such as vitamin E, may prevent the loss of vitamin A activity under these conditions.

Treatment

Vitamin A deficiency has been treated worldwide with single intramuscular injections of massive amounts (100,000 to 200,000 IU) of vitamin A, repeated at intervals of approximately six months to one year. Such doses have been effective and are associated with remarkably little toxicity, perhaps because body stores are so depleted at the time of therapy. These doses, however, may produce acute toxic symptoms in well-nourished persons.

Clinical vitamin A deficiency in the U.S. can be treated with either beta-carotene, if there is normal body conversion to vitamin A, or vitamin A itself. Daily doses in the range of 25,000 IU of beta-carotene are being consumed by many healthy individuals. The yellowish discoloration of the skin associated with prolonged use of beta-carotene is not believed to be harmful. Vitamin A, in contrast, is quite toxic when ingested in amounts considerably higher than the Recommended Daily Allowances (RDA), especially for prolonged periods. It is probably advisable not to exceed two to three times the RDA for vitamin A in planning a domestic treatment program involving vitamin A administration.

Congenital malformations, a particularly disturbing consequence of vitamin A overdosage, have been reported in women consuming 25,000 to 50,000 IU daily during pregnancy. The lowest dose of vitamin A that would be completely safe as a supplement for pregnant women is not known definitely. Therefore, it is not a good idea for pregnant women to take supplementary vitamin A unless there are specific indications, such as malabsorption, or proven deficiency. Many advisory groups caution that the maximal intake of preformed vitamin A consumed during pregnancy should not exceed 10,000 IU.

At present, there is widespread interest in other therapeutic applications of vitamin A and its derivatives. Large doses of vitamin A have been found to reduce morbidity and mortality rates among children suffering from severe cases of measles. Certain forms of leukemia have been found to respond to derivatives of vitamin A. The therapeutic potential of this vitamin is being expanded greatly in studies of the chemoprevention and treatment of cancer. The toxicity of large doses of vitamin A places important limits on its feasibility in cancer prevention. Attention has turned to beta-carotene and related agents, which in addition to their role as precursors of vitamin A, have strong antioxidant activity and other effects as well. Beta-carotene, however, may possibly pose a risk in heavy smokers in that two studies in this population have shown an actual increase in prevalence of lung cancer when beta-carotene was administered for several years.

Diminished prevalence of certain cancers has been found among people whose intake of fruits and vegetables is high; this finding has been attributable at least in part to the high content of carotenoids in the diet. Many phytochemicals have been found in fruits and vegetables that have potential health benefits. Some data show that a combination of antioxidants (i.e., vitamin E, vitamin C, and beta-carotene) may be more effective than any of these single agents, providing more evidence in favor of moderation and variety in the diet.

Vitamin D

See Section 65 on calcium and Section 61 on calcium and vitamin D in bone health.

Vitamin E

Functions

A generally accepted role for vitamin E is as a scavenger of free radicals, and in this capacity it protects cell membranes from damage. The role of vitamin E as an antioxidant in health and disease has attracted wide interest. It has many other properties as well. Vitamin E is essential for the immune system, particularly T lymphocytes, and has a role in DNA repair. Interest is growing in the effect of vitamin E on inhibiting oxidation of low-density lipoprotein (LDL); oxidized LDL is quite atherogenic. The neuromuscular system and the retina also require vitamin E for optimal function.

Vitamin E may have additional cellular protective effects. There is evidence that this vitamin may protect sulfhydryl groups in enzymes and other proteins. Similarly, stores of vitamin E may be conserved by the glutathione s-transferase system, which utilizes reduced glutathione and serves similar antioxidant functions.

Deficiency

Dietary vitamin E deficiency is relatively unusual in the U.S. under ordinary circumstances, as sources of vitamin E are widely available from the food supply. The recognizable cases of vitamin E deficiency tend to arise in debilitated patients who have had severe and prolonged periods of fat malabsorption, because vitamin E is incorporated into chylomicrons with other products of fat absorption. Any process that interferes with fat digestion and absorption may also impair absorption of vitamin E. Disorders in which symptomatic vitamin E deficiency may develop include cystic fibrosis, celiac disease, cholestatic liver disease, and short-bowel syndrome of any cause.

Major abnormalities of neurologic function are observed in a severe and prolonged vitamin E deficiency state. Patients display areflexia, ophthalmoplegia, and disturbances of gait, proprioception, and vibration. In premature infants, vitamin E deficiency results in hemolytic anemia, thrombocytosis, edema, and intraventricular hemorrhage. There is increased risk of retrolental fibroplasia and bronchopulmonary dysplasia.

In hemolytic anemia, such as that caused by glucose-6-phosphate dehydrogenase deficiency and sickle cell anemia, vitamin E levels in blood tend to be decreased. Inborn errors of vitamin E metabolism have been identified, but are rare. There are severe neurologic abnormalities in this category. In abetalipoproteinemia, there is a defect in the serum transport of vitamin E. A hallmark of this disease is the finding of an extremely low serum cholesterol level together with a very low serum level of vitamin E.

Laboratory Diagnosis of Deficiency

Ideally, the diagnosis of vitamin E deficiency should be made by detailed chromatographic analysis of the various E isomers. In practice, such a procedure is not realistic, and the clinical evaluation usually depends upon a measurement of plasma E alone. Plasma concentrations of vitamin E below 0.50 μg/ml are generally regarded as indicative of deficiency. It has been observed that despite a wide range of dietary intake, the serum variations in vitamin E levels tend to be more limited.

It is important to keep in mind that vitamin E is transported in blood bound to lipoproteins, particularly LDL. In any condition in which the serum cholesterol is abnormally high or low, the vitamin E level will vary accordingly. Therefore, before concluding that anyone is vitamin E-deficient, the plasma level of this vitamin should be evaluated in relation to the prevailing cholesterol concentrations. In addition, an alpha-tocopherol transport protein has been identified recently.

Prevention

Deficiency of vitamin E can be avoided by regular consumption of the many sources of this vitamin in the food supply. The richest sources of vitamin E in the U.S. diet are vegetable oils, including corn, cottonseed, safflower and soybean oils, and the margarines and other products made from these oils. Green, leafy vegetables are also good sources of vitamin E. In evaluating the adequacy of any given dietary regimen, one should keep in mind that losses of the vitamin occur during storage, cooking, and food processing, particularly with exposure to high temperatures and oxygen.

Because vitamin E deficiency frequently occurs as a result of severe intestinal malabsorption, it is essential to identify this condition early and avoid measures that may intensify the degree of malabsorption. For example, cholestyramine (Questran) and colestipol (Colestid), resins used in the treatment of hypercholesterolemia, by binding to the vitamin, may cause some degree of malabsorption of vitamin E and other fat soluble vitamins. Specific supplementation with vitamin E may be needed. The usual vitamin supplement containing 400 IU should be adequate for this purpose.

Treatment

Vitamin E deficiency can be treated satisfactorily. There is a wide margin of safety in the therapeutic administration of the vitamin. Daily doses of vitamin E in the range of 100 to

800 IU can be given safely to nearly all deficient patients. This dosage is higher than that usually found in multivitamin supplements. This dose range can be used appropriately in those patients with vitamin E deficiency diagnosed in association with celiac disease, inflammatory bowel disease, or other chronic and prolonged forms of intestinal malabsorption. In such instances, many other nutrient deficiencies are likely to be found in association with that of vitamin E, and they, too, necessitate treatment.

In the genetic disorders of vitamin E metabolism, such as isolated vitamin E deficiency, doses in the range of 800 to 1000 IU or higher, must be taken. Large doses of vitamin E given therapeutically under these conditions appear to be generally safe. Some investigators have suggested that pharmacologic doses of vitamin E may interfere with the intestinal absorption of vitamins A and K, but there are few data with which to evaluate this potential risk. In addition, there are suggestive reports that doses of vitamin E in excess of 1200 IU per day may possibly interfere with the action of vitamin K and intensify the actions of anticoagulant drugs. Further information is needed on this subject.

Vitamin K

Functions

The best known role for vitamin K is as cofactor for a post-translational modification in a diverse group of calcium-binding proteins, whereby selective glutamic (Glu) residues are transformed into gamma-carboxyglutamic acid (Gla). The best characterized vitamin K-dependent proteins include the four classic vitamin procoagulants (factors II, VII, IX, and X) and two feedback anticoagulants (proteins C and S), all synthesized by the liver.

Gla proteins also occur in several other tissues. Osteocalcin, which contains three Gla residues, is synthesized by the osteoblasts of bone. It is one of the ten most abundant proteins in the body and may play a role in regulating bone turnover. A second protein isolated from bone that is related structurally to osteocalcin is matrix Gla protein. This protein is more widely distributed, and there is now good evidence that this protein is an important inhibitor of calcification of arteries and cartilage. Gla residues provide efficient chelating sites for calcium ions that enable vitamin K-dependent proteins to bind to other surfaces (e.g., procoagulants to platelet and vessel wall phospholipids, and osteocalcin to the hydroxyapatite matrix of bone). The carboxylation reaction is catalyzed by a microsomal vitamin K-dependent gamma-glutamyl carboxylase, which requires the dietary quinone form of vitamin K to be first reduced to the active cofactor vitamin K hydroquinone, vitamin KH2.

In bone, vitamin K achieves gamma-carboxylation of osteocalcin. In addition, vitamin K regulates interleukin-6 production, synthesis of prostaglandin E2, and urinary excretion of calcium. It is not surprising, therefore, that in patients with low dietary intake of vitamin K long-term, the risk for hip fractures is increased.

Deficiency

Isolated deficiency of vitamin K due entirely to inadequate dietary intake tends to be unusual in adults in the U.S., because this vitamin is widely distributed in the food supply. Overt deficiency of vitamin K is more likely to be observed in conditions in which there are significant complicating factors, such as long-term use of broad spectrum antibiotics, and illnesses and drugs associated with fat malabsorption. It is essential to recognize that vitamin K is synthesized by intestinal bacteria and that this source may provide a significant contribution to the supply of the vitamin. Antibiotic treatment will largely eliminate

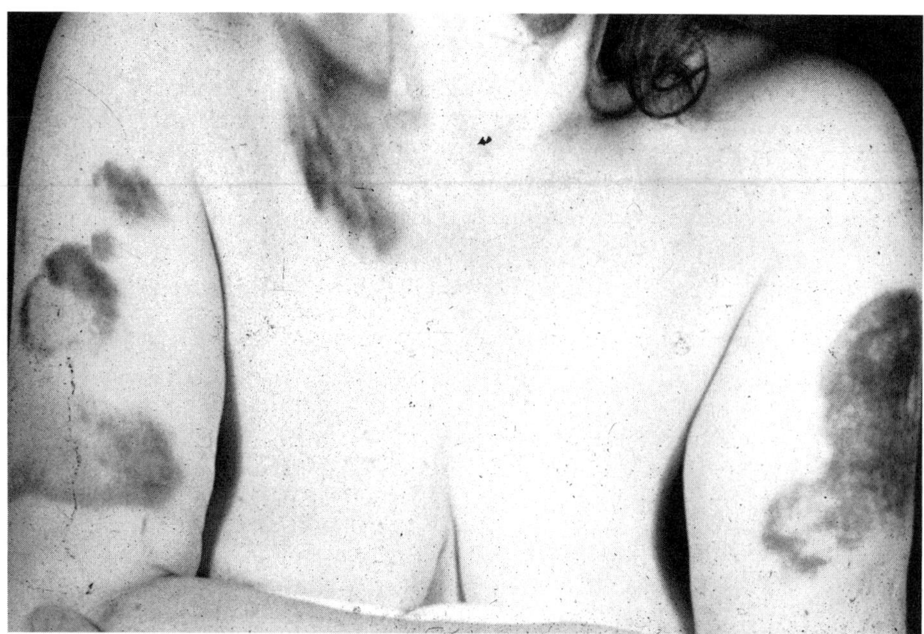

FIGURE 64.1
(See Color Figure 64.1) Patient with severe vitamin K deficiency, illustrating multiple purpuric areas occurring spontaneously. (Photo courtesy of Elaine B. Feldman, M.D.)

these bacterial sources of vitamin K and may have a clinical impact, particularly when treatment is prolonged. One class of antibiotics, the cephalosporins, cause vitamin K deficiency by an entirely different mechanism, namely by inhibiting the vitamin K-dependent hydroxylase.

Severe fat malabsorption is regularly observed as a feature of severe regional enteritis, nontropical sprue, cystic fibrosis, ulcerative colitis, and a number of other disorders. Following extensive intestinal resection, patients are left with a short bowel syndrome, in which fat malabsorption is prominent because of the reduction in intestinal surface area available for absorption and transport.

Vitamin K deficiency with the most serious consequences is that associated with the hemorrhagic disease of the newborn. The pathogenesis of this syndrome derives from (a) the poor placental transport of vitamin K combined with (b) lack of fetal production of vitamin K by intestinal bacteria since the intestinal tract is sterile, and (c) diminished synthesis by an immature liver of prothrombin and its precursors. In adults with vitamin K deficiency, multiple purpuric lesions may be noted (Color Figure 64.1*).

As noted above, dietary sources of vitamin K are widespread in the food supply in the U.S. The highest amounts are found in green leafy vegetables, such as broccoli, Brussels sprouts, spinach, turnip greens, and lettuce. Interestingly, the risk of hip fracture is reported as highest in women who have the lowest consumption of lettuce, which contributes significantly to vitamin K nutrition. Some vitamin K at lower amounts can be found in meat, dairy products, coffee, and certain teas.

Laboratory Diagnosis of Deficiency

Vitamin K in body fluids and in foods can be measured by biological and chemical methods. The vitamin is light sensitive and must be shielded from light during storage

* See color figures following page 992.

and analysis. In practice, functional vitamin K status is assessed indirectly by measurements of serum prothrombin. Clinical vitamin K deficiency should be suspected wherever there is an unusual hemorrhagic tendency.

Prevention

For healthy individuals, dietary vitamin K deficiency should be preventable by maintaining a diet high in green, leafy vegetables. When antibiotics are prescribed long-term, they should be kept to the minimal time period and doses necessary. Efforts should be initiated early to recolonize the gastrointestinal tract through providing live culture yogurt or other sources of normal flora. Similar guidelines should be followed in cases in which drugs causing malabsorption of vitamin K are required. A vitamin supplement containing vitamin K may be advisable. Effective treatment of an underlying disorder of the gastrointestinal tract should be undertaken in a specific fashion where possible, such as a gluten-free diet for nontropical sprue. All of these measures should help to prevent vitamin K deficiency.

Treatment

Treatment of vitamin K deficiency can be accomplished by oral administration of the purified vitamin, consumption of vitamin K-rich foods, or parenteral injection. Water-soluble preparations of vitamin K are available. An oral dose of approximately 500 µg/day should correct vitamin K deficiency, as assessed most simply by measuring serum prothrombin. A poor or inadequate improvement of prothrombin time after vitamin K administration is generally indicative of severe underlying liver disease.

Thiamin (Vitamin B_1)

Functions

The major function of dietary thiamin is to serve as the precursor for the coenzyme, thiamin pyrophosphate, which by the process of oxidative decarboxylation converts alpha-keto-acids to aldehydes. These reactions are an important source of generating energy, and are widely distributed throughout intermediary metabolism. Thiamin pyrophosphate is also the coenzyme for transketolase, which converts xylulose-5-$P0_4$ and ribose-5-$P0_4$ to sedoheptulose-7-$P0_4$ and glyceraldehyde. More recent evidence suggests that thiamin has a role beyond that of a coenzyme in regulating transmission of impulses in peripheral nerves.

Deficiency

The initial clinical presentation of thiamin deficiency is often subtle and nonspecific, comprising anorexia, general malaise, and weight loss. The symptoms, as they progress, are often followed by more intense weakness, peripheral neuropathy, headache, and tachycardia. When thiamin deficiency is advanced, the patient usually exhibits prominent cardiovascular and neurological features.

Cardiac findings include an enlarged heart, tachycardia, edema, and ST-segment and T-wave changes. There is high output failure due, at least in part, to the peripheral vasodilatation. The clinical syndrome has a number of similarities to apathetic hyperthyroidism, with which it is often confused.

The central nervous system findings are those of the Wernicke-Korsakoff syndrome, with vomiting, horizontal nystagmus, ataxia, weakness of the extraocular muscles, mental impairment, memory loss, and confabulation. There may be significant peripheral neuropathy as well.

Laboratory Diagnosis of Deficiency

The diagnosis of thiamin deficiency is based upon the analysis of this vitamin in blood by bioassay or by microbiological, chemical, and functional assays. In practice, urinary thiamin excretion and the erythrocyte transketolase are the most widely utilized assays. Urinary thiamin excretion reflects recent intake, and may be increased after the use of diuretics. The transketolase assay relies upon an indirect measurement of the extent to which the apoenzyme is saturated with its coenzyme, thiamin pyrophosphate. When thiamin stores are depleted, the addition of thiamin pyrophosphate *in vitro* to an erythrocyte lysate produces a large increase in activity. When the percentage increase in activity (activity coefficient) exceeds 15 to 20%, significant thiamin deficiency is diagnosed. Well-nourished individuals have much smaller activity coefficients when tested.

Prevention

Thiamin deficiency can best be prevented by a diet consistently high in meat, grains, peas, beans, and nuts. Treatment of vegetables with baking soda, which is alkaline, a practice often used to enable the bright green colors to be preserved, inactivates thiamin, as does heat.

Intestinal absorption of dietary thiamin is very sensitive to alcohol. A person who drinks alcoholic beverages all day long, but never appears to be intoxicated, is nevertheless at risk for the development of thiamin deficiency. Thiaminases and antithiamin factors in raw fish, seafood, and other food items, significantly break down dietary thiamin and may serve to intensify the effects of a dietary deficiency.

Treatment

Large doses of thiamin (50 to 100 mg) may be administered safely by the parenteral route in the acute syndrome, and the results are often dramatic, with rapid resolution of the nystagmus. Following several days of treatment with doses at this level, treatment with 5 to 10 mg/day is then appropriate. There is little, if any, toxicity when thiamin is given at levels of several times the RDA.

Riboflavin (Vitamin B_2)

Functions

Dietary riboflavin must be converted to its flavin coenzymes, flavin mononucleotide (riboflavin-5′-phosphate, FMN) and flavin adenine dinucleotide (FAD), to fulfill its metabolic functions. Several percent of tissue flavins are bound covalently to proteins, such as monoamine oxidase, and sarcosine and succinate dehydrogenase. The flavin coenzymes catalyze many different types of reactions, particularly oxidation-reduction reactions, dehydrogenations, and oxidative decarboxylations. Flavin coenzymes are involved in the respiratory chain, lipid metabolism, the cytochrome P-450 system, and drug metabolism.

Riboflavin has antioxidant activity in its role as precursor to FAD, the coenzyme required by glutathione reductase. The glutathione redox cycle provides major protection against lipid peroxides. Glutathione reductase generates reduced glutathione (GSH) from glutathione (GSSG), which is the substrate required by glutathione peroxidase to inactivate hydrogen peroxide and other lipid peroxides. Thus, increased lipid peroxidation is a feature of riboflavin deficiency, and one that is not widely appreciated.

Deficiency

The evolution of dietary riboflavin deficiency may be intensified by diseases, drugs, and endocrine disorders that block riboflavin utilization. The conditions in which such effects are observed include thyroid and adrenal insufficiency, treatment with the psychotropic drugs, chlorpromazine, imipramine and amitriptyline, the antimalarial, quinacrine, and the cancer chemotherapeutic drug, adriamycin. Alcohol ingestion may be a significant cause of riboflavin deficiency by interfering with both intestinal absorption and digestion from food sources.

Clinically, patients with riboflavin deficiency exhibit seborrheic dermatitis, burning and itching of the eyes, abnormal vascularization of the cornea, cheilosis, angular stomatitis, anemia, and neuropathy. A smooth red tongue is classically observed in riboflavin deficiency (Color Figure 64.2), but is not pathognomonic.

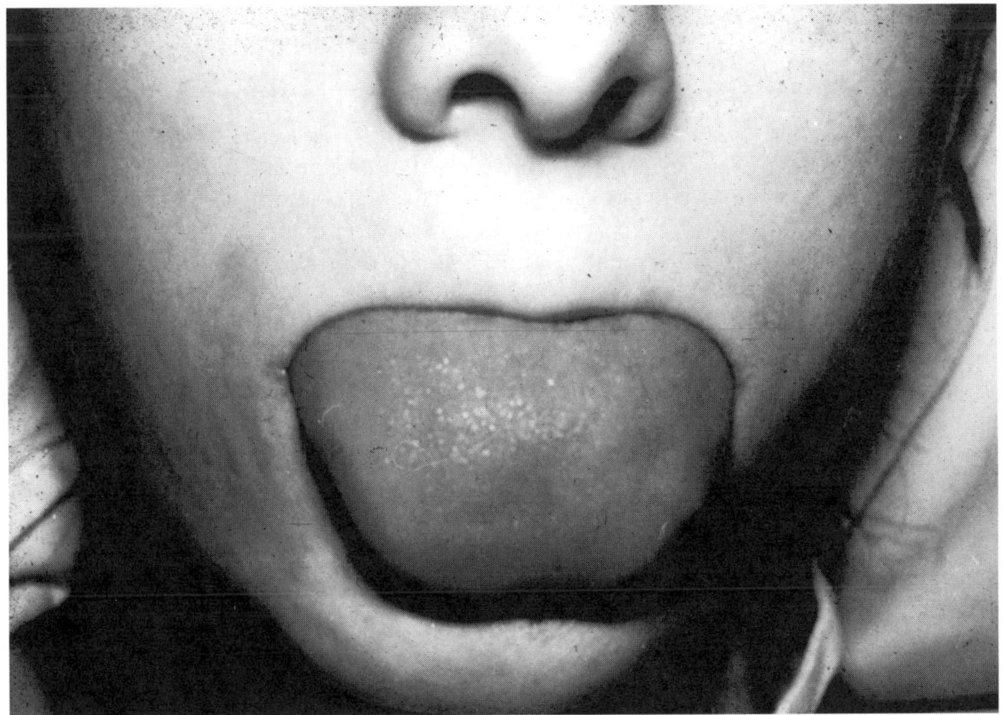

FIGURE 64.2
(See Color Figure 64.2) Patient with classical riboflavin (vitamin B_2) deficiency illustrating pallor, cheilosis and a large, red, smooth tongue. (Photo courtesy of Elaine B. Feldman, M.D.)

Riboflavin deficiency seldom occurs as an isolated entity, and is nearly always detected in association with deficiencies of other B-vitamins.

Laboratory Diagnosis of Deficiency

Riboflavin and its derivatives can be analyzed precisely by high performance liquid chromatography (HPLC) and other techniques which are not generally utilized in clinical practice. Urinary riboflavin excretion is reduced with long-term dietary deficiency, but may be increased acutely after recent intake of the vitamin. Collections have to be made carefully in subdued light and stored in dark bottles because of the light-sensitivity of the vitamin.

A functional test, the erythrocyte glutathione reductase activity coefficiency (EGRAC), measures saturation of the enzyme with its coenzyme (FAD) by the same principle as that used to assess thiamin status with transketolase. An activity coefficient greater than 1.2 to 1.3 indicates some degree of deficiency, with higher levels reflecting more severe deficiency.

Prevention

Riboflavin deficiency can be prevented by maintaining a diet high in meat and dairy products, the major sources of the vitamin in the U.S. Certain green vegetables, including broccoli, asparagus, and spinach, also contain significant quantities of riboflavin, as do fortified cereals. In developing countries, vegetables constitute the major sources of riboflavin.

It should be recalled that because of its heat- and light-sensitivity, considerable amounts of the vitamin can be lost when liquids are stored in clear bottles, when fruits and vegetables are sun-dried, and when baking soda is added to fresh vegetables to maintain color and texture. Under the latter conditions, riboflavin loss is accelerated by photodegradation.

Treatment

Treatment of clinical deficiency can be accomplished by oral intake of the vitamin. Levels greater than 25 mg cannot be completely absorbed as a single dose. This dose level is certainly safe to administer. The parenteral administration of riboflavin is limited by its low solubility. Riboflavin 5′phosphate is more soluble than riboflavin but is not usually available for clinical use.

A theoretical risk involved in treatment with riboflavin is that the vitamin has photosensitizing properties. *In vitro*, phototherapy results in DNA degradation and an increased formation of lipid peroxides. Riboflavin forms an adduct with tryptophan and accelerates its photodegradation. The extent to which these observations have implications for conditions prevailing *in vivo* in humans needs to be elucidated.

Niacin

Functions

The main function of niacin, sometimes referred to as vitamin B_3, is to serve as a precursor of the two coenzymes, nicotinamide adenine dinucleotide (NAD) and nicotinamide adenine dinucleotide phosphate (NADP). Both coenzymes catalyze oxidation-reduction reactions, and are involved in a wide variety of reactions in intermediary metabolism. These reactions include glycolysis, lipid, amino acid, and protein metabolism.

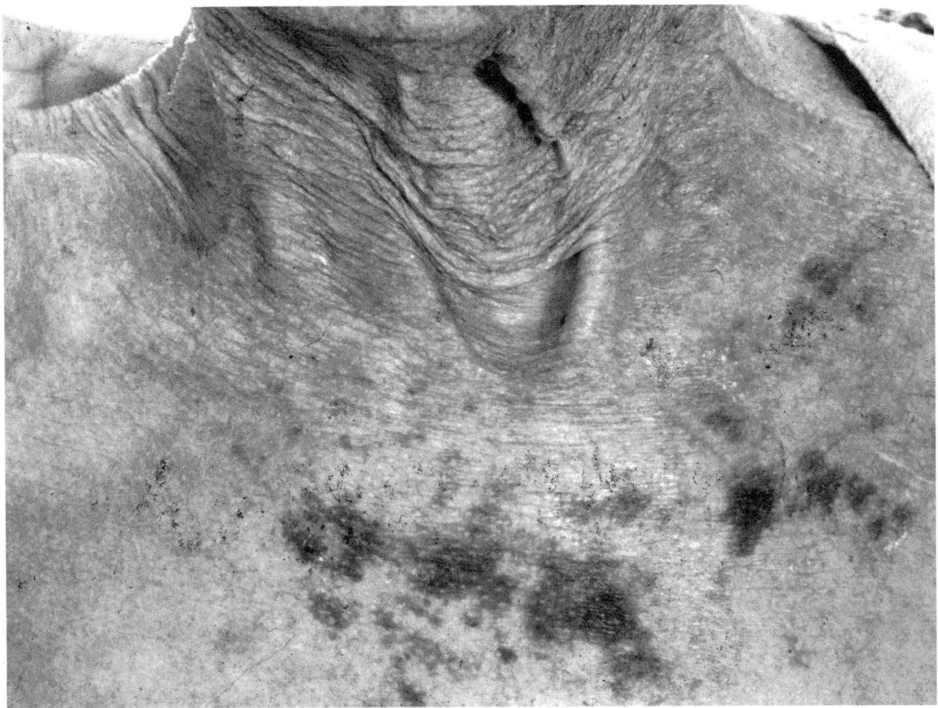

FIGURE 64.3
(See Color Figure 64.3) Patient with advanced pellagra resulting from niacin deficiency, illustrating a dark, scaly eruption over sun-exposed surfaces. (Photo courtesy of Elaine B. Feldman, M.D.)

Deficiency

Dietary deficiency of niacin generally occurs in the presence of other vitamin deficiencies as well. A unique aspect of niacin metabolism is that it is formed from dietary tryptophan. Thus, high quality protein sources tend to protect against niacin deficiency, and poor protein sources that are inadequate in tryptophan, such as corn, tend to accelerate niacin deficiency. Alcoholism may result in niacin deficiency, as will drugs, such as isonicotinic acid hydrazide (isoniazid INH), which interfere with niacin metabolism. The anti-cancer agent, 6-mercoptopurine, may produce severe niacin deficiency. One may also find niacin deficiency in the rare inborn error Hartnup's Disease, and in the malignant carcinoid syndrome in which dietary tryptophan is diverted to the synthesis of serotonin at the expense of niacin.

Early manifestations of niacin deficiency (pellagra) are generally non-specific, with anorexia, weight loss, weakness, and irritability. In later stages of deficiency, the patient may develop glossitis, stomatitis, characteristic scaling, and skin lesions, as shown in Color Figures 64.3 and 64.4. In advanced disease, one may encounter "the four Ds": dermatitis, diarrhea, dementia, and death.

Laboratory Diagnosis and Deficiency

In practice, the diagnosis of niacin deficiency can be established by assay of the urinary excretion of niacin metabolites, specifically N-methylnicotinamide, and less commonly, 2-pyridone. Accurate determinations can be made by HPLC.

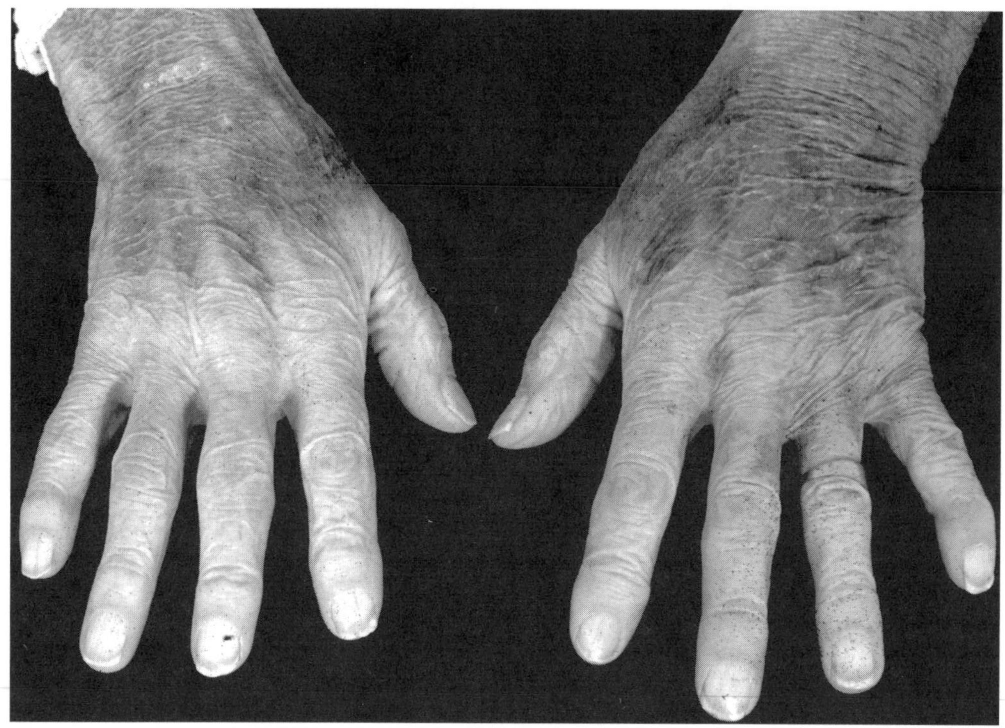

FIGURE 64.4
(See Color Figure 64.4) Hands of a patient with advanced pellagra, illustrating dark, scaly, thickened lesions. (Photo courtesy of Elaine B. Feldman, M.D.)

Prevention

As noted above, the diet needs to be adequate in protein of high biological value that contains tryptophan. Intake of meat and dairy products tends to assure adequate intake of tryptophan. A vegetarian diet may contain adequate amounts of niacin if it is sufficiently balanced and varied.

Treatment

The syndrome of niacin deficiency can be treated with oral administration of the vitamin. Doses in the range of 50 to 150 mg/day of nicotinamide may be recommended to treat severe deficiency, and need to be maintained initially. Improvement is usually noted clinically after only a few days of treatment.

Niacin in the form of nicotinic acid as a drug is a first-line agent for the management of an abnormal serum lipid profile when doses in the range of 1.5 to 6.0 grams are administered daily. Niacin may be effective alone and in combination with other agents in lowering LDL-cholesterol, raising HDL-cholesterol, and reducing serum triacylglycerols (triglycerides). There may, however, be significant side effects noted at this dose range, including worsening of diabetes, abnormalities in liver function tests, elevation of the serum uric acid, and ocular abnormalities. Flushing may be troublesome to the patient, but is often transient. In most instances, the flushing can be minimized by taking a tablet of aspirin shortly before the niacin.

The form of niacin selected is crucial. Nicotinic acid is the form which is effective. Often patients choose niacinamide on their own because it does not cause a flush. Unfortunately, it also will not benefit elevated serum lipid concentrations.

Pyridoxine (Vitamin B_6)

Functions

The role of vitamin B_6 is primarily that of a precursor to pyridoxal phosphate, the coenzyme which participates in a large number of reactions, particularly involving transamination and decarboxylation. In addition, pyridoxal phosphate is involved in side chain cleavage, dehydratase activity, and racemization of amino acids. These reactions relate to gluconeogenesis, lipid metabolism, immune function, cerebral metabolism, nucleic acid synthesis, and endocrine function in relation to steroid hormone action. B_6 deficiency can lead to secondary deficiencies of other vitamins because it plays a role in the pathway leading to synthesis of niacin from tryptophan. B_6, together with B_{12}, folic acid, and possibly B_2, are involved in homocysteine synthetic and degradative pathways.

Although some B_6 is present in the diet in the form of pyridoxal, the majority is in other forms. In plants, B_6 is present largely as pyridoxine, whereas animal sources comprise pyridoxamine as well as pyridoxal phosphate, and other forms.

Deficiency

Like other B vitamins, isolated pyridoxine deficiency entirely on a dietary basis is hardly ever found. In some instances, however, a marginal diet may result in overt deficiency if there are other complicating factors, such as the long-term use of specific pyridoxine antagonists. Two common examples of this are isoniazid and cycloserine, used to treat tuberculosis and generally prescribed for an extended period in order to eradicate the organism. In some individuals a genetic trait may manifest itself, leading to delay in inactivating isoniazid, resulting in their becoming unusually susceptible to developing B_6 deficiency from this drug.

Pyridoxine deficiency is a common feature of chronic alcoholism, found in association with overall malnutrition and inadequate intake of many other vitamins and minerals. An unusual feature of the pathogenesis of B_6 deficiency in alcoholism is that a major effect of alcohol is to accelerate the degradation of pyridoxal into inactive metabolites, particularly pyridoxic acid.

B_6 deficiency is not recognizable as a distinct clinical syndrome. Patients may develop dermatitis, glossitis, cheilosis, and weakness. In more severe deficiency, patients may have dizziness, depression, peripheral neuropathy, and seizures. The risk of kidney stones is increased due to hyperoxaluria. In children, B_6 deficiency may be an important cause of anemia and seizures. Deficiency of B_6 causes a hypochromic, microcytic anemia that resembles the anemia due to iron deficiency.

In a group of rare disorders, called pyridoxine dependency syndromes, large doses of B_6 are required for control. Among these disorders are pyridoxine-dependent convulsions, cystathioninuria, and xanthurenicaciduria.

Laboratory Diagnosis of Deficiency

Vitamin B_6 can be measured directly in blood, with levels less than 50 ng/ml generally considered to represent deficiency. The measurement needs to be interpreted in the light of the patient's diet, as high protein intake depresses plasma pyridoxal phosphate levels, probably because of increased utilization of the coenzyme in protein metabolism.

Urinary tests measure the excretion of metabolites of pyridoxine, most commonly 4-pyridoxic acid. Indirect assessments of vitamin B_6 deficiency can be made using functional assays of the enzymes aspartate or alanine aminotransferase with and without the addition of the cofactor *in vitro*. The principle of this assay is similar to that discussed above for thiamin and riboflavin deficiency. An activity coefficient greater than 1.2 for alanine aminotransferase and 1.5 for aspartate aminotransferase is generally considered to represent vitamin deficiency.

At one time, a specific diagnosis of B_6 deficiency was made by measuring xanthurenic acid after a tryptophan load, inasmuch as B_6 is the coenzyme involved in the transformation. This procedure, although theoretically sound, is somewhat laborious and has largely been abandoned.

Prevention

Vitamin B_6 is widely available in the food supply and is found in vegetables, beans, (especially soy beans), meat, nuts, seeds, and cereals. A diet that is adequate and diversified in these dietary items will generally prevent vitamin B_6 deficiency. It is evident that this kind of diet will prevent deficiencies of the other B vitamins as well. Certain kinds of food processing, particularly heat sterilization, can result in significant losses and reduction of activity of vitamin B_6.

Treatment

Once vitamin B_6 deficiency is diagnosed, it can be satisfactorily managed at a level of 2 to 10 mg/day, which represent doses several times those of the RDA. Vitamin B_6 deficiency during pregnancy should be treated with higher doses in the 10 to 20 mg range because of the increased requirement.

Vitamin B_6 is routinely advised during prolonged treatment with isoniazid, which is a pyridoxine antagonist. In doses of 50 to 100 mg/day, vitamin B_6 has been noted to reduce peripheral neuropathy without apparently lessening efficacy of INH against tuberculosis. In patients with Parkinson's Disease receiving treatment with L-DOPA, too much pyridoxine will interfere with drug action; therefore, these large doses should not be taken as a general rule.

It is important not to exceed certain limits in therapeutic administration of vitamin B_6. Cases of sensory neuropathy have been occasionally noted in patients taking 1 to 2 g per day, but rarely noted when taking only 500 mg/day. The B_6-dependency syndromes can be managed on doses of 100 to 200 mg/day and do not require these megadoses.

Folic Acid and Vitamin B_{12}

See discussion in Section 46.

Vitamin C (Ascorbic Acid)

Functions

Although commonly perceived as a so-called antioxidant, in reality, ascorbic acid serves in both oxidation and reduction reactions, depending upon the prevailing environmental conditions. An important function is that of preventing oxidation of tetrahydrofolate.

Ascorbic acid is involved in collagen biosynthesis, wound healing, immune function, and drug metabolism. It enhances the intestinal absorption of non-heme iron. The vitamin is involved in the biosynthesis of neurotransmitters and carnitine.

Deficiency

Dietary deficiency develops when the diet does not contain adequate amounts of citrus fruits, vegetables, and tomatoes, most commonly among the elderly and the urban poor. Vitamin C deficiency may also arise when there is food faddism or very limited food choices, behaviors that are observed with increased frequency. The classical "tea and toast" diet of the elderly is particularly deficient in vitamin C. The macrobiotic diet may lead to scurvy because of poor sources and the practice of pressure-cooking, which destroys ascorbic acid.

In infancy and childhood, a diet exclusively of unsupplemented cow's milk is deficient in vitamin C and may lead to scurvy. Chronic alcoholism at any age is associated with poor ascorbic acid intake, and if prolonged will greatly increase the risk for scurvy.

The clinical symptoms of vitamin C deficiency develop very slowly, and as with other vitamins are often vague and nonspecific. Patients complain of weakness and fatigue, progressing to dyspnea and lethargy. The characteristic features of scurvy are not observed until the deficiency syndrome is well advanced. Bone and joint pain may occur due to hemorrhages in the subperiosteum. Perifollicular hemorrhages, especially in relation to hair follicles, are observed, as shown in Color Figure 64.5. The hairs may show a corkscrew pattern. Swollen, bleeding gums are observed in advanced deficiency, as shown in Color Figure 64.6. Pallor may be due to the bleeding and the reduction in hematopoiesis. Scurvy results in poor wound healing and secondary breakdown of wounds that had healed previously.

Laboratory Diagnosis

Ascorbic acid can be measured directly in the blood serum or plasma by a variety of chemical methods, most commonly spectrophotometric or fluorometric. Levels of 0.1 mg/dl or lower are generally indicative of vitamin C deficiency. Serum levels may be reduced in many chronic disorders, in smokers, and in some women taking oral contraceptive drugs.

Blood levels tend to segregate in a relatively narrow range in the face of very large differences in dietary intake. Megadoses of ascorbic acid remain almost entirely unabsorbed, and what is absorbed is rapidly metabolized by an efficient hepatic drug-metabolizing enzyme system and, with its low renal threshold, excreted rapidly in the urine.

Prevention

Vitamin C deficiency can be prevented simply by consuming a diet adequate in citrus fruits and vegetables. Consuming orange juice with meals may be a healthy habit that

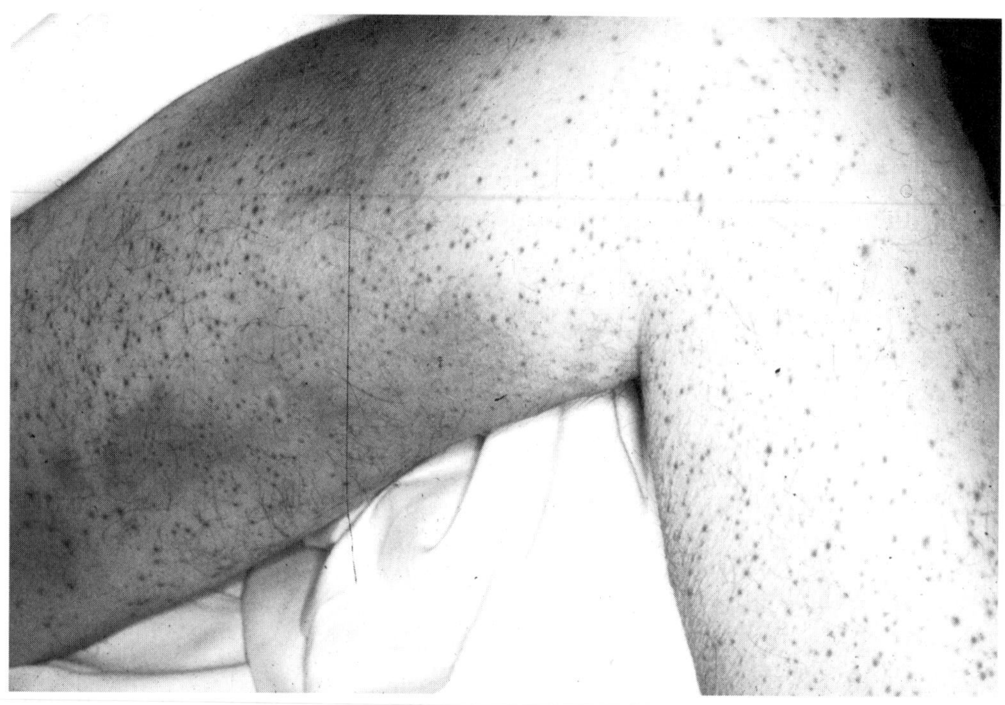

FIGURE 64.5
(See Color Figure 64.5) Leg of an adult patient with severe scurvy, illustrating multiple perifollicular hemorrhages. Some corkscrew hairs are visible. (Photo courtesy of Elaine B. Feldman, M.D.)

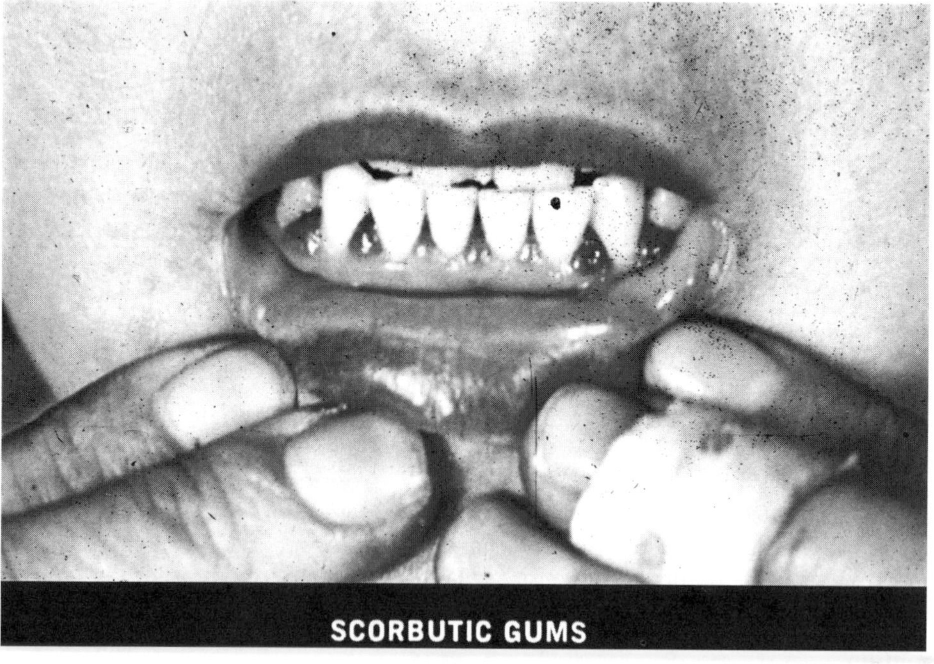

FIGURE 64.6
(See Color Figure 64.6) Mouth and teeth of a patient with far-advanced scurvy showing swollen, bleeding gingiva. (Photo courtesy of Elaine B. Feldman, M.D.)

increases the intestinal absorption of non-heme iron several-fold. Avoiding heating or prolonged storage of foods containing vitamin C can also help maintain adequate stores. Educating people about the potential hazards of a macrobiotic diet, food faddism, and sharply limited food choices should also help to prevent scurvy.

The prevention of scurvy may be accomplished by ingestion of very small amounts of ascorbic acid. Some authorities believe that doses as low as 10 mg/day may be effective. The maintenance of adequate vitamin C status has generally been considered to be in the 40 to 60 mg range, as reflected in the RDA. Recent studies examining the pharmacokinetics of vitamin C and the saturation of tissue stores raise the possibility that larger doses of approximately 200 mg may be optimal.

Treatment

As noted above, doses of ascorbic acid as low as 10 mg/day may prevent scurvy and could achieve benefit in treatment. In advanced cases, a dose range of 100 to 200 mg/day orally may be administered safely and effectively, with a therapeutic benefit evident within a few days. Meat sources containing heme iron are more bioavailable than the non-heme iron present in vegetables. As noted above, efficacy of absorption of non-heme iron can be greatly improved by simultaneous consumption of orange juice.

Megadoses of vitamin C have been given to patients with advanced cancer, and their anticancer efficacy is unproven. Vitamin C has also been advocated to prevent cancer, since its content in fruits and vegetables may be part of the reason that cancer prevalence is reduced in patients who consume several servings a day. There is also a suggestion from some *in vitro* studies that large amounts of vitamin C may not be advisable in terms of possibly accelerating tumor metabolism.

There is some risk for toxicity in doses greater than 1 to 2 g per day in a highly individual fashion. Gastrointestinal upset may occur. Inasmuch as oxalic acid is a direct metabolite of ascorbic acid, the risk of kidney stones theoretically should be increased. The exact prevalence of symptomatic stone formation after ingestion of low doses of vitamin C is not known.

Caution in administering vitamin C should be followed when giving it to individuals with hemochromatosis or those at risk for this disorder, as the intestinal absorption and tissue storage of iron may be increased excessively. Since the gene for hemochromatosis is one of the most common genetic abnormalities known, there may be a risk associated with indiscriminate use of megadoses of ascorbic acid supplements by the general population.

Sources of Additional Information

1. Huttunen JK. Health effects of supplemental use of antioxidant vitamins. Experiences from the alpha-tocopherol beta-carotene (ATBC) cancer prevention study. *Scand J Nutr/Naringsforskning* 39: 103-104; 1995.
2. Goodman GE, Thornquist M, Kestin M, Metch B, et al. The association between participant characteristics and serum concentrations of beta-carotene, retinol, retinyl palmitate, and alpha-tocopherol among participants in the Carotene and Retinol Efficacy Trial (CARET) for prevention of lung cancer. *Cancer Epid Biomark Prevent* 5: 815-821; 1996.
3. Yong LC, Brown CC, Schatzkin A, Dresser CM, et al. Intake of vitamins E, C, and A and risk of lung cancer. *Am J Epid* 146: 231-243; 1997.
4. Rivlin RS. Vitamin deficiency. In: *Conn's Current Therapy* 50th Anniversary Issue, Rakel RE, Ed, Philadelphia, W.B. Saunders, 1998, pg 579-587.

5. Rivlin RS. Riboflavin. In: *Present Knowledge in Nutrition* Ziegler EE, Filer LJ, Jr, Eds, Washington DC, ILSI Press, 1996, pg 167-173.
6. Rivlin RS. Vitamin metabolism in thyrotoxicosis; Vitamin metabolism in hypothyroidism. In: *The Thyroid,* 7th ed, Braverman LE, Utiger R, Eds, Philadelphia, Lippincott, 1996, pg 693-695; pg 863-865.
7. Agus DB, Vera JC, Golde DW. Stromal cell oxidation: A mechanism by which tumors obtain vitamin C. *Cancer Res* 59: 4555-4558; 1999.
8. Vera JC, Reyes AM, Carcamo JG, Velasquez FV, et al. Genistein is a natural inhibitor of hexose and dehydroascorbic acid transport through the glucose transporter, GLUT1. *J Biol Chem* 271: 8719-8724; 1996.
9. Weber P. The role of vitamins in the prevention of osteoporosis — a brief status report. *Int J Vitamin Nutr Res* 69: 194-197; 1999.
10. Rivlin RS. Disorders of vitamin metabolism: Deficiencies, metabolic abnormalities and excesses. In: *Cecil Textbook of Medicine,* 19th ed, Wyngaarden JH, Smith LH, Jr, Bennett JC, Plum F, Eds, Philadelphia, WB Saunders, pg 1170-1183, 1991.
11. Carr A, Frei B. Does vitamin C act as a pro-oxidant under physiological condition? *The FASEB J* 13: 1007-1024; 1999.
12. Subcommittee on the Tenth Edition of the RDAs, National Research Council. Recommended Dietary Allowances, 10th ed, Washington, DC, National Academy Press, 1989.
13. Nichols HK, TK Basu. Thiamin status of the elderly: dietary intake and thiamin pyrophosphate response. *J Am Coll Nutr* 13: 57-61; 1994.
14. Meydani SN, Barklund MP, Liu S, et al. Vitamin E supplementation enhances cell-mediated immunity in healthy elderly subjects. *Am J Clin Nutr* 52: 557-563; 1990.
15. Stephens NG, Parsons A, Schofield PM, et al. Randomised controlled trial of vitamin E in patients with coronary disease: Cambridge heart antioxidant study (CHAOS). *Lancet* 347: 781-786; 1996.
16. Vermeer C, Knapen MHJ, Jie K-SG, Grobbee DE. Physiological importance of extrahepatic vitamin K-dependent carboxylation reactions *Ann NY Acad Sci* 669: 21-33; 1992.

65

Rationale for Use of Vitamin and Mineral Supplements

Allen M. Perelson and Leon Ellenbogen

Introduction

Current research indicates that health benefits which go beyond the repletion of potential deficiency states can be derived from vitamins and minerals. In most instances, these benefits may be conveyed by intakes either at or above recommended daily allowances. For some of these health benefits the scientific evidence base is convincing, while for others, support for potential benefits is just emerging. In many cases the association between a particular vitamin or mineral and its beneficial effect is derived from nutritional epidemiological studies. Intervention studies are needed in many promising areas in order to demonstrate a conclusive nutrient-benefit link. Additionally, in the case of multivitamin supplementation, further investigation is needed in order to determine and characterize the nutrient or nutrient interactions which produce a particular beneficial effect. What follows describes the emerging benefits of vitamins and minerals, and the scientific support for each.

As the increasing importance of nutrients and their health benefits become known, various health agencies and organizations have recognized the need to issue recommendations for vitamin and mineral supplementation and/or fortification of food. These include the U.S. Public Health Department, Centers for Disease Control, Department of Health and Human Services, the National Osteoporosis Foundation, and many international health organizations and boards of health.

Vitamin A

Dietary antioxidants, including carotenoids and vitamin A, are hypothesized to decrease the risk of age-related cataracts by preventing oxidation of proteins or lipids within the lens.[1,2] Information on the role of vitamins in eye disease is discussed in Section 62.

Vitamin A deficiency appears to be common in individuals with HIV infection. Low levels of vitamin A are associated with greater disease severity.[3,4] Transmission of the virus

0-8493-2705-9/02/$0.00+$1.50

TABLE 65.1

Vitamin A — Established Benefits

Important for normal growth in children
Necessary for wound repair
Involved in RNA synthesis
Helps to form and maintain healthy skin, eyes, teeth, gums, hair, mucous membrane, and various glands
Involved in fat metabolism
Important for resisting infectious diseases
Necessary for night and color vision

TABLE 65.2

Vitamin A — Emerging Benefits

Use	Findings	Reference
Age-related cataracts	Vitamin A use not related to decreased risk of cataract	2
HIV	High doses may be protective	3, 4, 5
Measles	High doses decrease morbidity and mortality	6, 7
Acne	High doses may be helpful	8
Crohn's disease	Variable response to high doses	9, 10, 11

from a pregnant mother deficient in vitamin A to her infant has been reported.[5] However, there have been no intervention studies to determine whether vitamin A supplementation is helpful.

The potential benefit of vitamin A therapy for measles was first reported in 1932,[6] and a recent study in South African children under 13 years of age showed that large doses (400,000 IU) of vitamin A resulted in lower complication rates and mortality. Low vitamin A levels have been noted in young children with measles, and are associated with the highest mortality.[7] WHO, UNICEF, and the American Academy of Pediatrics recommend that children with measles be examined for vitamin A deficiency.

Large quantities of analogs of vitamin A, on the order of 300,000 IU per day for females and 400 to 500,000 IU per day for males, have been used successfully to treat a severe type of acne known as cystic acne.[8] However, such high doses of vitamin A are potentially toxic, and topical retinol therapy is more appropriate.

Vitamin A is needed for the growth and repair of cells that line both the small and large intestines. Over the years, reports have appeared of individuals with Crohn's disease responding to vitamin A therapy at a dose of 50,000 IU per day.[9,10,11] See Tables 65.1 and 65.2 for the established and emerging benefits of vitamin A.

Beta-Carotene

Based on the unanimous recommendation by health professionals that diets rich in fruits and vegetables may help reduce the risk of cancer and heart disease, scientists have started to identify the components in these foods which are responsible for the health benefits. Because beta-carotene is one of the more abundant carotenoids in fruits and vegetables, it dominated the research on carotenoids in the 1980s following the report published in *Nature* by Dr. Richard Peto et al., entitled "Can dietary beta-carotene materially reduce cancer rates."[12] See Table 65.3 for the established benefits of beta-carotene.

TABLE 65.3

Beta-Carotene — Established Benefits

Beta-Carotene — Established Benefits
Supplies vitamin A
Antioxidant function
Supports the immune system

TABLE 65.4

Important Beta-Carotene Cancer Trials

Study	Subjects	Intervention	Results
Alpha-Tocopherol, Beta-Carotene Cancer Prevention Study[14] (ATBC Study) — also called the Finnish study	29,133 male smokers, 50-69 years of age	50 mg vitamin E 20 mg beta-carotene or both for 5-8 years	No evidence of prevention of lung and other cancers. Beta-carotene group had a 16% greater incidence of lung cancer in smokers
Beta-Carotene and Retinol Efficacy Trial[15] (CARET)	18,314 men and women smokers and former smokers	25,000 IU vitamin A 30 mg beta-carotene	Increase of 28% in lung cancer and 17% in cancer mortality
Physicians' Health Study[16] (PHS)	22,071 males, mainly non-smokers	50 mg beta-carotene every other day for 12 years	No effect on cancer rates for prostate, bowel or lung or for overall incidence of cancer or mortality

In addition to extensive epidemiological data, beta-carotene showed strong promise in laboratory studies with cancer cells and animals (see Albanes and Hartman, *Antioxidants and Cancer*,[13] for the long list of epidemiological studies). The results of three major double-blind, randomized, placebo-controlled clinical studies, however, were surprising (see Table 65.4).

The conclusions demonstrating a potentially adverse effect of beta-carotene in smokers were questioned because of the evidence from epidemiological and basic biochemical studies whose results were contrary. It has been suggested that the very high doses of beta-carotene used in the above studies might have interfered with the absorption of carotenoids other than beta-carotene.

Several ongoing intervention studies may help clarify the inconsistency of these findings. The Chinese Cancer Prevention Study[17] evaluated beta-carotene (15 mg), vitamin E (30 mg), and selenium (50 μg) and found a non-significant 10% decrease in cerebrovascular mortality in a group receiving treatment compared to that of an untreated group. There was a 13% reduction of borderline significance in total cancer mortality in the treated group and a 21% reduction in gastric cancer, which was significant. Because beta-carotene was evaluated in combination with other nutrients, it is not possible to isolate the effect attributable to beta-carotene alone. Other nutrients may have had an effect in the poorly nourished group included as study subjects, and results may not be applicable to well-nourished individuals.

Several smaller studies of beta-carotene and premalignant lesions have shown interesting preliminary results. A 66% reduction in the frequency of pre-malignant buccal micronuclei was observed after supplementation of 26 mg of beta-carotene for nine weeks.[18] A 71% reduction was observed in patients with oral leukoplakia after a six-month intake of 30 mg per day of beta-carotene.[19]

Apart from cancer prevention, beta-carotene has been studied for its effect in coronary heart disease and cataract. A subgroup of the Physicians' Health Study (PHS) which included 333 physicians with unstable angina or a prior coronary revascularization pro-

TABLE 65.5

Beta-Carotene — Emerging Benefits

Cancer — lung, cervix, oral, colorectal, pancreas, prostate
Cardiovascular disease
Cataracts
Restenosis after angioplasty

TABLE 65.6

Important Beta-Carotene Cardiovascular Trials

Agent	Highest Daily Intake Quintile	Lowest Daily Intake Quintile	Relative Risk	P Value
Nurses Health Study[21]				
Antioxidant Vitamins and Risk of Coronary Heart Disease				
Beta-carotene	>1404 IU	<3850 IU	0.78	.02
Vitamin E	>21.6 mg	<3.5 mg	0.66	<.001
Vitamin C	>359 mg	<93 mg	0.80	.15
Health Professionals Follow-up Study[22]				
Antioxidant Vitamin Intake and Risk of Coronary Heart Disease				
Beta-carotene			0.71	.03
Vitamin E			0.60	.01
Vitamin C			1.25	.98
Massachusetts Elderly Cohort Study[23]				
Beta-Carotene Intake and Risk of Cardiovascular Disease				
Endpoint				
CVD death			0.57	.02
Fatal MI			0.32	.02

cedure had a 20 to 30% reduction in vascular disease. High dietary intakes of beta-carotene were found to be associated with a decreased risk of myocardial infarction in the Rotterdam study, which investigated the dietary intakes of 4802 elderly men and women over the course of four years.[20] A similar effect was not seen for either vitamin C or E. See Table 65.5 for emerging benefits of beta-carotene. The results of several additional important prospective studies are included in Table 65.6.

People with low blood levels of antioxidants and those who eat few antioxidant-rich fruits and vegetables are at high risk for cataracts.[24,25] See information in Section 62 on eye disease.

Lycopene is an antioxidant carotenoid found commonly in tomatoes. Although not a vitamin per se, nor a provitamin (for vitamin A), specific benefits of lycopene are beginning to be elucidated, particularly with respect to certain cancers. Of particular note is an observational finding that high intakes of lycopene are associated with lower rates of prostate cancer. An excellent overview by Giovannucci[26] covers lycopene and the epidemiological evidence supporting its currently known health benefits.

In conclusion, basic metabolic research as well as animal and epidemiological studies all suggest major benefits from carotenoids. These benefits, however, have yet to be confirmed in double-blind intervention studies.

TABLE 65.7

Riboflavin — Established Benefits

Essential for building and maintaining body tissues
Necessary for healthy skin
Prevents sensitivity of the eyes to light
Necessary for protein, fat, and carbohydrate metabolism
Important for the proper function of the nervous system

TABLE 65.8

Riboflavin — Emerging Benefits

Use	Findings	Reference
Age-related cataract	Riboflavin deficiency associated with higher incidence of cataract	27-30
Exercise	Aerobic exercise may deplete riboflavin	31-34
	Supplementation with riboflavin does not appear to increase performance	
Pregnancy and exercise	Riboflavin may be helpful	35
Migraine	High doses in a limited trial produced beneficial results	36

Riboflavin

Deficiency of riboflavin, a precursor of flavin adenine dinucleotide, has been believed by some to be associated with cataract formation,[27,28] Lenticular reduced glutathione, diminished in all forms of human cataract, requires flavin adenine dinucleotide as a coenzyme for glutathione reductase. Despite this putative connection with riboflavin, clinical results of studies in this area are equivocal, and the degree of riboflavin deficiency encountered in the general population would not be considered to be cataractogenic. Clinically, lower intakes of riboflavin are not found to be a risk factor for cataract.[29,30] See Section 62 on eye disease for further discussion of this topic.

Review of riboflavin requirements associated with exercise in several different study groups yields equivocal results. Aerobic exercise may deplete riboflavin as well as other B-vitamins.[31] However, riboflavin status, assessed using erythrocyte glutathione reductase activity coefficient, shows that while riboflavin requirements of women increase with exercise training, additional riboflavin intake does not enhance or result in improvements in endurance.[32,33] Additionally, riboflavin depletion is not related to the rate or composition of weight loss in overweight women.[34] Interestingly, in a cohort of pregnant women who exercised and took vitamin-mineral supplements, participation in a walking program slightly improved aerobic capacity without affecting riboflavin or thiamin status.[35]

Minimal data are available from one study of high doses (400 mg per day) of riboflavin that successfully treated migraine patients.[36] Further work in this area is needed. See Tables 65.7 and 65.8 for established and emerging benefits of riboflavin.

Niacin

The body uses niacin in the process of releasing energy from carbohydrates, to form fat from carbohydrates, and to metabolize alcohol. Niacin comes in two basic forms: niacin

TABLE 65.9

Niacin — Established Benefits

Helps prevent pellagra
Helps cells release energy from food
Aids the nervous system
Helps prevent loss of appetite

TABLE 65.10

Niacin — Emerging Benefits

Use	Findings	Reference
Hypercholesterolemia	Lowers elevated cholesterol levels	37-40
Hypertriglyceridemia	Lowers elevated triacylglcerol levels	37

(also called nicotinic acid) and niacinamide (also called nicotinamide). High levels of niacin — usually several grams per day — lower cholesterol, triglyceride, and triacylglycerol levels and raise HDL cholesterol levels.[37] The niacinamide form, commonly found in multivitamin preparations, does not decrease elevated cholesterol. See Tables 65.9 and 65.10 for established and emerging benefits of niacin.

A variation of niacin, called inositol hexaniacinate, has also been used and has not been linked with the flushing seen with high doses of niacin. It is sometimes prescribed by physicians in Europe to help lower cholesterol. Dosages used are 500 to 1000 mg taken three times per day.[38,39] This form of niacin lowers serum cholesterol but appears to have fewer side effects.[40]

Vitamin B_6

Vitamin B_6 has a significant role to play, along with folate and vitamin B_{12}, in the reduction of elevated homocysteine levels associated with increased risk of cardiovascular disease — specifically, coronary artery disease and stroke. This topic is covered in the section on folate.

Vitamin B_6 also plays a significant role in the immune function of the elderly. *In vitro* indices of cell-mediated immunity in healthy elderly adults indicate that deficiency of vitamin B_6 is associated with impairment of immune function. This impairment appears to be reversible with vitamin B_6 repletion.[41] The levels of vitamin B_6 absorption, phosphorylation, and excretion appear not to be affected by age.[42]

Vitamin B_6 has been shown to reduce the effects of estrogen in animals. Since excess estrogen may be responsible in part for premenstrual symptoms (PMS), a number of studies in humans have demonstrated that 200 to 400 mg of vitamin B_6 per day for several months can relieve symptoms of PMS.[42-46] In other studies, however, the amount of vitamin B_6 used may be too low,[47] or the length of the trial too short,[48] and other studies have not found vitamin B_6 helpful.[49,50]

Many diabetics have low blood levels of vitamin B_6.[51,52] Levels of vitamin B_6 are even lower in diabetics with nerve damage.[53] Vitamin B_6 supplements has been demonstrated to improve glucose tolerance in women with diabetes associated with pregnancy.[54,55] Vitamin B_6 is also partially effective for glucose intolerance induced by birth control pills.[56] For some individuals with diabetes, a form of vitamin B_6 — pyridoxine alpha-ketoglutarate — improves glucose tolerance dramatically.[57] Vitamin B_6 (cyanocobalamin) has been found to help in some,[58] but not all, studies.[59]

TABLE 65.11

Vitamin B_6 — Established Benefits

Important in protein absorption and metabolism
Necessary for red blood cell formation
Necessary for the proper function of the nervous and immune systems
Helps maintain healthy teeth and gums
Needed for serotonin and melatonin production

TABLE 65.12

Vitamin B_6 — Emerging Benefits

Use	Findings	Reference
Immune function	Improves immune function in the elderly	41, 42
Premenstrual symptoms	High doses administered long-term may be helpful	43-50
Diabetes	Low levels are associated with diabetes	51-59
Carpal tunnel syndrome	Inconsistent results	60-68
HIV	Deficiency frequently found and associated with decreased immune function	69

It appears that many people with carpal tunnel syndrome (CTS) have vitamin B_6 deficiencies.[60] Some studies show that people with CTS are helped when given 100 mg of vitamin B_6 three times per day.[61,62] Although a few researchers have found benefits with lesser amounts,[63,64,65] the results have not been consistent.[66,67,68]

Lastly, it is worth noting that vitamin B_6 deficiency was found in more than one-third of HIV-positive men, and a deficiency of this vitamin is associated with decreased immune function.[69] See Tables 65.11 and 65.12 for established and emerging benefits of vitamin B_6.

Vitamin B_{12}

Higher blood levels of vitamins B_6, B_{12}, and folic acid are associated with low levels of homocysteine,[70] and supplementing with these vitamins helps to lower homocysteine levels.[71,72] Preliminary evidence indicates that vitamin B_{12} may be beneficial when included in supplements or in a food-fortification regimen together with folic acid. This topic is discussed further in the section on folate.

The addition of vitamin B_{12} enhances the homocysteine-lowering potential of a folic acid supplement. In one study, female volunteers were given folic acid alone or folic acid combined with one of two supplements containing different doses of vitamin B_{12}. Significant reductions in plasma homocysteine were observed in all groups receiving vitamin treatment. The combination of folic acid 400 μg plus 400 μg of vitamin B_{12} resulted in an 18% decrease in homocysteine levels. This was significantly larger than that obtained with a supplement containing folic acid alone (homocysteine decrease of 11%). Folic acid in combination with a low vitamin B_{12} dose (6 μg) affected homocysteine as well (decrease of 15%). These results suggest that the addition of vitamin B_{12} to folic acid supplements or enriched foods helps maximize the reduction of homocysteine and may thus increase the benefits achieved with the use of folic acid in the prevention of vascular disease.[73]

Lastly, vitamin B_{12} has a role in preventing vitamin B_{12} deficiency in the presence of folate use, especially in light of the increased fortification of foods with folic acid. (See rationale by Oakley.[74]) See Tables 65.13 and 65.14 for established and emerging benefits of vitamin B_{12}.

TABLE 65.13

Vitamin B_{12} — Established Benefits

Necessary for DNA synthesis
Helps prevent pernicious anemia
Helps to form red blood cells
Enhances utilization of nickel

TABLE 65.14

Vitamin B_{12} — Emerging Benefits

Use	Findings	Reference
Hyperhomocysteinemia	Alone and together with folate reduces homocysteine levels	70-73
Folate-induced vitamin B_{12} deficiency	Administration helps unmask vitamin B_{12} deficiency associated with folate use	74

Folic Acid

For the last 40 years, folic acid has almost exclusively been used to treat megaloblastic macrocytic anemia. There is now significant evidence that folate deficiency is associated with increased risk of several diseases. The most convincing is the association of folic acid deficiency with neural tube defects (NTDs) such as spina bifida and anencephaly, a predisposition to occlusive vascular disease associated with hyperhomocysteinemia, and several neoplastic or preneoplastic diseases. In addition, preliminary evidence suggests some association of folate deficiency with neuropsychiatric diseases.

Studies on folate and NTDs were conducted by the British Medical Research Council in 1991.[75] These demonstrated that high-dose folic acid supplements (4.0 mg per day) used by women who had a prior NTD-affected pregnancy reduced the risk of having a subsequent NTD-affected pregnancy by 70%. A conclusive trial conducted in Hungary showed that a multivitamin containing 0.8 mg folic acid protected against a first occurrence of NTD.[76]

In 1992 the Centers for Disease Control in the U.S. issued a recommendation that all women of childbearing age who are capable of becoming pregnant should consume 0.4 mg of folic acid per day to help prevent NTDs.[77] The U.K. Expert Advisory Group and other countries in Europe made similar recommendations.[78] The U.S. Food and Drug Administration has recently authorized a health claim on food labels and dietary supplements that folic acid contained in these products may help reduce the risk of NTD.[79] This is the only health claim currently permitted for a vitamin in the U.S.

A large body of evidence reveals that elevated blood homocysteine is a risk factor for cardiovascular disease, including atherosclerotic coronary heart disease and thromboembolic stroke. There is abundant evidence that folate deficiency and/or a genetic defect in the enzymes involved in homocysteine metabolism give rise to hyperhomocysteinemia. In addition to folate deficiency, vitamin B_6 and B_{12} deficiency has also been associated with elevated homocysteine levels. Patients with higher blood levels of these vitamins are at lower risk for occlusive vascular disease.[80]

Many studies show that folic acid alone or in combination with vitamins B_6 and B_{12} can reduce blood homocysteine levels.[81-90] Observational studies have shown that people who consume multivitamins and/or cereal fortified with folic acid also have reduced homocysteine levels.[91-95] Levels of supplemental folic acid as low as 0.4 mg appear to be effective. A meta-analysis of 12 randomized trials confirms that folic acid has the dominant blood homocysteine-lowering effect.[90] The fortification of enriched grain with folic acid has been shown to increase folate plasma levels and decrease homocysteine levels in middle-aged and older adults.[94] While folic acid fortification was undertaken primarily to reduce the risk of NTDs, it may also have a beneficial effect on vascular disease.

Based on a meta-analysis of 27 studies relating homocysteine to vascular disease and 11 studies of folic acid effects on homocysteine levels, Boushey and Beresford[81] concluded that an increase of 350 μg/day of folate intake by men and 280 μg/day increase by women could potentially prevent 30,500 and 19,000 vascular deaths annually in men and women, respectively. Recent reports show that a small percentage of children, with or without a positive family history of cardiovascular disease,[96-98] have elevated homocysteine levels. Hyperhomocysteinemia may also be a risk factor for ischemic stroke in children. The data on children suggest that tracking of homocysteine levels from childhood on may be helpful in the planning and evaluation of future initiatives aimed at the prevention of cardiovascular disease.

While it has been shown that higher intake of folate may reduce homocysteine levels and that lower homocysteine levels are associated with reduced cardiovascular mortality, clinical intervention trials are needed to prove unequivocally that higher intakes of folate will help reduce the risk of cardiovascular disease. An excellent review of prospective cohort and case-control studies as well as cross-sectional and retrospective case-control studies concerning the association between homocysteine and cardiovascular risk has recently been published by Hankey and Eikelboom.[99]

In a preliminary report, a vitamin mixture of 2.5 mg of folic acid, 25 mg vitamin B_6, and 250 μg vitamin B_{12} stopped the progression of carotid plaques; some regression was also observed.[100] Excellent detailed reviews on homocysteine and vascular disease have been published.[101-105]

Several reports suggest an increased risk of colon, tracheobronchial tree, and cervical cancer, and preneoplastic dysplasia associated with folate deficiency.[106,107] Supplemental folic acid has been shown to partially reverse some cervical dysplasia.[106,108] In some instances, poor folate status may not by itself be carcinogenic, but it may predispose to the carcinogenicity of other agents.[109,110]

Lashner and Heidenreich[110] reported that the rate of colon cancer was 62% lower in patients with ulcerative colitis who were supplemented with folic acid. Giovannucci and Stampfer[111] examined the relationship between the intake of folate, both from supplements and food, and the risk for colon cancer in women in the Nurses Health Study. The results indicate that the use of multivitamin supplements for 15 or more years may decrease the risk for colon cancer by about 75%. The data are consistent with the hypothesis that folate intake is the principal nutritional factor associated with risk reduction. These findings support several recent studies, including the Health Professional Follow-Up Study, which have found a higher risk for colon cancer among persons with low folate. In the Giovannucci report, the association between colon cancer and folate was stronger with supplemental than with dietary folate. This is probably due to the fact that food folate is less bioavailable that supplemental folate. More recently, Zhang and Hunter[112] reported that the excess risk of breast cancer associated with moderate alcohol consumption may be reduced by folate. Alcohol is a known folate antagonist, and this could increase the requirement for folate.

Blount et al.[113] presented data on the possible mechanism by which folate deficiency enhances cancer risk. Folate deficiency results in abnormal DNA synthesis due to misin-

TABLE 65.15

Folic Acid — Established Benefits

Necessary for DNA synthesis
Important for cell formation
Prevents certain types of anemias
Helps maintain the function of the intestinal tract

TABLE 65.16

Folic Acid — Emerging Benefits

Use	Findings	Reference
Neural tube defects	0.4 mg per day prevents neural tube defects	75 -79
Hyperhomocysteinemia	Lowers homocysteine levels	80-104
Cancer	Deficiency is associated with an increased risk of colon, lung, cervical cancer	105-112
Cognitive function	Low levels are associated with Alzheimer's disease	113-115

corporation of uracil into DNA, leading to chromosome breakage. This breakage contributes to the risk of colon cancer.

Data to help elucidate the role of folate in Alzheimer's disease and depression are sparse and just emerging. Low blood levels of folate and vitamin B_{12} are often found in individuals with Alzheimer's disease.[114] The role of elevated homocysteine levels has been reported and needs to be expanded further.[115] Low folate blood levels may be associated with the weaker responses of depressed patients to antidepressants.[116] Factors contributing to low serum levels among depressed patients, as well as the circumstances under which folate may have a role in antidepressant therapy, must be further clarified. See Tables 65.15 and 65.16 for the established and emerging benefits of folate.

Vitamin C

Vitamin C has many functions in the body, including serving as an antioxidant and as a cofactor for several enzymes involved with biosynthesis.[117] The relationship between vitamin C and total serum cholesterol has been investigated in several studies.[118-123] In one intervention study, consumption of 1000 mg of vitamin C per day for four weeks resulted in a reduction in total serum cholesterol.[120] In another study, supplementation with 60 mg per day for two weeks had no effect.[118] Two observational studies found an inverse relationship between vitamin C status and total serum cholesterol concentrations.[122,123]

Low concentrations of plasma vitamin C have been associated with hypertension.[122,124-127] Several studies have reported beneficial effects of the administration of high doses of vitamin C on vasodilation.[128-131] One study found a 128% increase in brachial artery dilation in coronary artery disease patients, while a second found a nonsignificant increase of 27% in chronic heart failure patients.[131] Infusion of 10 mg of vitamin C per minute was observed to effect a 100% reversal of epicardial artery vasoconstriction in coronary spastic angina patients.[132]

Vitamin C may protect against cancer through several mechanisms, including inhibition of DNA oxidation. One potential mechanism is chemoprotection against mutagenic compounds such as nitrosamines.[133,134] In addition, vitamin C may reduce carcinogenesis through stimulation of the immune system, via a beneficial effect on phagocyte functions,

TABLE 65.17

Vitamin C — Established Benefits

Prevents scurvy
Maintains health of teeth, gums, and blood vessels
Necessary for wound repair
Important for collagen formation
Enhances iron absorption

such as chemotaxis,[135-138] or on the activity of natural killer cells and the proliferation of lymphocytes.[139-141] See Table 65.17 for the established benefits of vitamin C.

Table 65.18 (adapted from Carr[142]) lists prospective cohort studies of vitamin C intake associated with reduced cardiovascular disease risk.

TABLE 65.18

Vitamin C Intake Associated with Reduced Cardiovascular Disease Risk (Prospective Cohort Studies)

Reference	Population (Duration)	Endpoint (Events)	Risk and Associated Dietary Intake of Vitamin C
Enstrom[143]	3119 Men and women (10 y)	CVD (127 deaths)	>250 compared with < 250 mg/d: no ↓ risk
Enstrom[144] and Enstrom[145]	4479 Men (10 y) 6809 Women (10 y)	CVD (558 deaths) CVD (371 deaths)	>50 mg/d + vitamin supplement: ↓ risk by 42% >50 mg/d + vitamin supplement: ↓ risk by 25%
Manson[146] and Manson[147]	87,245 Female nurses (8 y)	CAD (552 cases) Stroke (183 cases)	>359 compared with <93 mg/d: ↓ risk by 20% (NS) >359 compared with <93 mg/d: ↓ risk by 24%
Rimm[148]	39,910 Male health professionals (4 y)	CAD (667 cases)	392 compared with 92 mg/d median: no ↓ risk
Fehily[149]	2512 Men (5 y)	CVD (148 cases)	>67 compared with < 35 mg/d: ↓ risk 37% (NS)
Knekt[150]	2748 Finnish men (14 y) 2385 Finnish women (14 y)	CAD (186 deaths) CAD (58 deaths)	>85 compared with < 60 mg/d: no ↓ risk >91 compared with < 61 mg/d: ↓ risk by 51%
Gale[151]	730 UK elderly men and women (20 y)	Stroke (125 deaths) CAD (182 deaths)	>45 compared with < 28 mg/d: ↓ risk by 50% >45 compared with < 28 mg/d: ↓ risk by 20% (NS)
Kritchevsky[152]	4989 Men (3 y) 6318 Women (3 y)	Carotid atherosclerosis Carotid atherosclerosis	>982 compared with < 56 mg/d: ↓ intima thickness >728 compared with < 64 mg/d: ↓ intima thickness
Pandey[153]	1556 Men (24 y)	CAD (231 deaths)	>113 compared with < 82 mg/d: ↓ risk by 25%
Kushi[154]	34,486 Women (7 y)	CAD (242 deaths)	>391 compared with < 112 mg/d (total)2 : no ↓ risk, >196 compared with < 87 mg/d (dietary): no ↓ risk, regular supplement compared with no supplement: no ↓ risk
Losconczy[155]	11,178 Elderly men and women (6 y)	CAD (1101 deaths)	Regular supplement compared with no supplement: no ↓ risk
Sahyoun[156]	725 Elderly men and women (10 y)	CVD (101 deaths)	>388 compared with <90 mg/d: ↓ risk by 62% (NS)
Mark[157]	29,584 Chinese men (5 y)	Stroke	180 mg/d supplement: no ↓ risk (+ 30 μg Mo/d cosupplement)

Note: CVD = Cardiovascular disease; CAD = Coronary artery disease.

Adapted from Carr AC, Frei B. *Am J Clin Nutr* 69: 1086; 1999.

Table 65.19 (adapted from Carr[142]) lists important prospective studies of vitamin C intake associated with reduced cancer risk.

Several epidemiologic studies that have investigated the association of vitamin C intake with the incidence of cataract are discussed in Section 62.

Vitamin D

Vitamin D is an essential element in the maintenance of healthy bones because it helps optimize calcium absorption and prevents increased parathyroid hormone (PTH) secretion.[168] High PTH levels stimulate resorption of bone, which may result in a gradual weakening of bones (osteomalacia) leading to an increase in the incidence of fractures.

Increasing evidence suggests that vitamin D is deficient in a large portion of the elderly population.[169] Vitamin D deficiency in the elderly may be caused by low exposure to sunlight, a reduced ability of the skin to synthesize cholecalciferol, and decreased dietary intakes.[170] This deficiency leads to hyperparathyroidism, bone loss, and increased incidence of fractures.[171] Vitamin D is synthesized in the skin by the action of ultraviolet light.[1] Vitamin D deficiency was found to be common in the elderly due to lack of mobility, which prevents adequate sun exposure.[172] Various studies have also demonstrated that hypovitaminosis D appears prevalent in the winter months due to a reduction in the number of hours spent outside coupled with the use of more protective clothing.[168,171-176]

The effect of age on vitamin D synthesis in the skin may be due to an age-related decline in the dermal production of 7-dehydrocholesterol, the precursor of previtamin D_3.[177] MacLaughlin and Holick compared the amount of previtamin D_3 produced by the skin of young subjects (8 and 18 years old) to the amount produced by the skin of elderly subjects (77 to 82 years).[178] This study revealed that aging appears to produce a greater than twofold reduction in previtamin D_3 production in subjects over 77 years of age.

Vitamin D deficiency, which can cause osteomalacia, is also important in the pathogenesis of age-related osteoporosis.[170] In a study of 3270 elderly women (mean age 84), 800 IU of vitamin D was given in combination with 1.2 g of elemental calcium to 1634 women, and 1636 women received a placebo. The number of hip fractures was reduced by 43% in the group treated with the combination of vitamin D and calcium after 18 months.[173,179] Treatment of the elderly with vitamin D may be a cost-effective method of maintaining bone density and reducing the incidence of osteoporotic fractures.[180]

Vitamin D as 1,25 dihydroxycholecalciferol appears to be potentially useful for people with psoriasis.[181] Topical application has worked well in some,[182-185] but not all, studies.[186,187] Use of vitamin D in psoriatic patients may work by helping skin cells replicate normally.

High doses of calcium combined with vitamin D have also been useful in treating cases of migraine[188,189] at a dose of 400 IU of vitamin D combined with 800 mg of calcium per day.

From epidemiological data, Giovannucci[190] reported that high circulating levels of $1,25(OH)_2$ vitamin D, the biologically active form, may decrease the risk of developing prostate cancer, and that diets high in calcium, phosphorus, and sulfur-containing amino acids from animal protein tend to decrease $1,25(OH)_2$ vitamin D. This effect of vitamin D on prostate cancer may be mediated via vitamin D receptors found on prostate cancer cells, and may be genotype specific.[191]

Animal models suggest that low vitamin D and calcium intake, as commonly found in Western-style diets, may be associated with an increased risk of both colon[192] and breast cancer,[193] although a long-term study of serum vitamin D levels and the incidence of breast

TABLE 65.19

Vitamin C Intake Associated with Reduced Cancer Risk (Prospective Cohort Studies)

Reference	Population (Duration)	Cancer Site (Events)	Risk and Associated Dietary Intake of Vitamin C
Shekelle[158]	1954 Men (19 y)	Lung (33 cases)	101 mg/d in noncases compared with 92 mg/d in cases (NS)
Enstrom[143]	3119 Men and women (10 y)	All cancers (68 deaths)	>250 compared with <250 mg/d no ↓ risk
Kromhout[159]	870 Dutch men (25 y)	Lung (63 deaths)	83–103 compared with <63 mg/d: ↓ risk by 64%
Knekt[160]	4538 Finnish men (20 y)	Lung (117 cases)	83 mg/d in noncases compared with 81 mg/d in cases (NS)
Enstrom[144]	4479 Men (10 y) 6869 Women (10 y)	All cancers (228 deaths) All cancers (169 deaths)	>50 mg/d + regular supplement: ↓ risk by 21% >50 mg/d + regular supplement: no ↓ risk
Shibata[161]	4277 Men (7 y) 7300 Women (7 y)	All cancers (645 cases) All cancers (690 cases)	>210 compared with <145 mg/d: no ↓ risk, 500 mg/d supplement compared with no supplement: no ↓ risk >225 compared with <155 mg/d: ↓ risk by 24%, 500 mg/d supplement compared with no supplement: no ↓ risk
Graham[162]	18,586 Women (7 y)	Breast (344 cases)	>79 compared with <34 mg/d: no ↓ risk
Hunter[163]	89,494 US female nurses (8 y)	Breast (1439 cases)	59 compared with <93 mg/d (total): no ↓ risk, regular supplement compared with no supplement: no ↓ risk, supplement >10 y compared with no supplement: no ↓ risk
Bostick[164]	35,215 Women (5 y)	Colon (212 cases)	>392 compared with <112 mg/d (total) : ↓ risk (NS), >201 compared with <91 mg/d (diet): no ↓ risk, >60 mg/d supplement compared with no supplement: ↓risk by 33%
Blot[165]	29,584 Chinese men and women (5 y)	Esophageal-stomach	120 mg/d supplement: no ↓ risk (+ 30 μg Mo/d cosupplement)
Pandey[153]	1556 Men (24 y)	All cancers (155 deaths)	>113 compared with <82 mg/d: ↓ risk by 39%
Losconczy[155]	11,178 Elderly men and women (6 y)	All cancers (761 deaths)	Regular supplement compared with no supplement: no ↓ risk
Sahyoun[156]	<725 Elderly men and women (10 y)	All cancers (57 deaths)	>388 compared with <90 mg/d: no ↓ risk
Kushi[166]	34,387 Women (5 y)	Breast (879 cases)	>392 compared with <112 mg/d (total): no ↓ risk, >198 compared with <87 mg/d (diet): no ↓ risk, regular supplement compared with no supplement: no ↓ risk
Yong[167]	3968 Men and women (19 y)	6100 Lung (248)	82 mg/d in noncases compared with 64 mg/d in cases

Adapted from Carr AC, Frei B. *Am J Clin Nutr* 69: 1086; 1999.

TABLE 65.20

Vitamin D — Established Benefits

Necessary for the proper formation of bones and teeth
Important for calcium absorption
Aids in the deposition of calcium and phosphorus into bones

TABLE 65.21

Vitamin D — Emerging Benefits

Use	Findings	Reference
Osteoporosis	Reduces the incidence of osteoporosis-related fracture	168-180
Psoriasis	Useful in topical application	181-187
Migraine	May be useful	188, 189
Cancer	May reduce the risk of prostate cancer	190-194
	Low intake is associated with an increased risk of colon and breast cancer	

cancer in humans did not reveal a direct association.[194] See Tables 65.20 and 65.21 for the established and emerging benefits of vitamin D.

Vitamin E

The emerging health benefits for vitamin E are extensive, and include reduction in cardiovascular risk, protection against certain forms of cancer, enhanced immunity, and a potential role in the treatment of certain neurological diseases. See Table 65.22 for the established benefits of vitamin E.

Early research identified that antioxidant scavengers such as vitamin E may reduce oxidative stress that can affect lipid metabolism, thereby producing oxidized low density lipoprotein (LDL) which is more atherogenic than the unoxidized form.[195,196] Because of this action, vitamin E was investigated to determine its efficacy in reducing the risk of cardiovascular disease.

Epidemiological studies found a significant inverse correlation between LDL levels, vitamin E concentration, and degree of coronary artery stenosis,[197] or mortality from ischemic heart disease.[198] The Cholesterol Lowering Atherosclerosis Study demonstrated that supplementary vitamin E intake greater than 100 IU per day was associated with a significant reduction in the progression of atherosclerosis in subjects not treated with lipid-lowering drugs.[199]

Two major epidemiological studies offer the most compelling evidence that vitamin E can reduce the incidence and mortality from coronary heart disease. Data from Stampfer et al.[200] and Rimm et al.[201] lend support to the growing body of evidence which suggests that antioxidants, especially fat-soluble antioxidants such as vitamin E, may protect against

TABLE 65.22

Vitamin E — Established Benefits

Essential for the formation of red blood cells, muscle, and other tissues
Necessary for the proper function of the nervous system
Protects the fat in tissues from oxidation

TABLE 65.23
Vitamin E and Coronary Heart Disease — Epidemiological Trials

Stampfer et al.[200]	87,000 Female nurses aged between 34-59 years	8 year follow-up	Vitamin E supplements for short periods had little apparent benefit, but those who took them for more than 2 years had a 41% reduction in the risk of major coronary artery disease
Rimm et al.[201]	40,000 US male health professionals aged between 40-75 years	4 year follow-up	Men consuming > 60 IU per day of vitamin E had a 36% decreased risk of CHD Men consuming > 100 IU per day for at least two years had a 37% reduced risk of CHD
HOPES Study[203]	2545 Women and 6996 men 55 years of age or older at risk for cardiovascular events	4.5 years	Vitamin E 400IU daily had no apparent effect on cardiovascular outcomes in patients at high risk for cardiovascular disease
GISSI-Prevenzione Study[204]	11,324 Men and women who survived recent myocardial infarction	3.5 years	Treatment with n-3 polyunsaturated fatty acids (PUFA) but not vitamin E 300 mg daily significantly lowered the risk of a fatal cardiovascular event

atherosclerosis by reducing the generation of oxidized LDL. Details of the two studies are listed in Table 65.23.

These data provide evidence of an association between a high intake of vitamin E and a lower risk of coronary heart disease in men. This was further corroborated by the Cambridge Heart Antioxidant Study (CHAOS)[202] wherein the investigators concluded that in patients with angiographically proven symptomatic coronary atherosclerosis, treatment with vitamin E substantially reduces the rate of non-fatal myocardial infarction, with beneficial effects apparent after one year of treatment. Recently, the results from two additional studies appear to contradict the benefit of vitamin E in cardiovascular disease.[203,204] These are also included in Table 65.23.

Although the effect of vitamin E in reducing cardiovascular mortality requires further corroboration, a number of other studies,[205-207] which investigated vitamin E along with other antioxidant vitamins, suggest that antioxidant vitamins reduce the risk of cardiovascular disease, with the clearest effect shown for vitamin E. In a related study, patients randomized after successful percutaneous transluminal coronary angioplasty to receive vitamin E 1200 IU per day for four months were found to have a 35.5% restenosis rate versus a 47.5% restenosis rate in patients receiving a placebo.[208]

Data from a number of epidemiologic studies have shown that individuals with higher intakes of vitamin E have lower risk of cancer. These data are summarized in Table 65.24.

Vitamin E is the major lipid-soluble antioxidant in humans, and its key function is to inhibit lipid peroxidation. Vitamin E deficiency is associated with decreased deep tendon reflexes, decreased proprioception, degeneration of neuronal axons, muscle weakness, and ataxia. Additionally, there is preferential central nervous system transport of vitamin E. These data suggest that vitamin E has a key role as a neurological antioxidant.

It has been hypothesized that Parkinson's patients may lack sufficient antioxidant protection and are susceptible to increased attack by free radicals.[228] A small, open trial of patients with early symptoms of Parkinson's disease was conducted in 1989 in which

TABLE 65.24
Vitamin E Levels and Cancer Incidence

Reference	Cancer Site	Sample Size	Location of Study	Correlation
Stahelin (1984)[207]	Lung, stomach, colon	4224	Switzerland	Vitamin E levels low in colon and stomach cancer cases
Wald (1984)[208]	Breast	5004	U.K.	Five time greater cancer risk for women with lowest vitamin E level
Salonen (1985)[209]	All sites	12,000	Finland	Risk 11.4 times higher with low vitamin E and selenium levels
Menkes (1986)[210]	Lung	25,802	U.S.	Risk 2.5 times higher with low vitamin E levels
Kok (1987)[211]	Lung, other sites	10,532	Holland	Risk 4.4 times higher for those with low vitamin E levels
Miyamoto (1987)[212]	Lung	55 Cancer cases	Japan	Higher cancer risk with low vitamin E levels
Wald (1987)[213]	All sites	22,000	U.K.	Vitamin E levels lower only in newly diagnosed cancer patients
Knekt (1988)[214]	All sites	21,172	Finland	Lower cancer risk with higher vitamin E levels
Knekt (1988)[215]	Gastrointestinal	36,265	Finland	Higher cancer risk with lower vitamin E levels
Knekt (1988)[216]	Reproductive organs	15,093	Finland	Cancer risk 1.6 times greater with lower vitamin E levels
Verreault (1989)[217]	Cervix	189 Cancer cases	U.S.	Lower risk of cervical cancer associated with higher vitamin E intake
LeGardeur (1990)[218]	Lung	59 Cancer cases	U.S.	Lung cancer patients have lower serum vitamin E levels
Buiatti (1990)[219]	Stomach	1016 Cancer cases	Italy	Risk 5 times higher with high vitamin E and C intake vs. low
Gridley (1990)[220]	Oropharynx	190 Cancer cases	U.S.	Lower risk associated with increased intake of vitamin E in men
Palan (1991)[221]	Cervix	116 Cancer cases	U.S.	Serum vitamin E levels lower in cervical cancer cases
Comstock (1991)[222]	Nine sites	25,802	U.S.	Vitamin E protective against lung cancer
Harris (1991)[223]	Lung, skin	96 Cancer cases	U.K.	Vitamin E levels lower in cancer patients
Knekt (1991)[224]	Lung	117 Cancer cases	Finland	Risk in nonsmokers associated with lower vitamin C and E intakes
Gridley (1992)[225]	Oropharynx	1103 Cancer cases	U.S.	Use of vitamin E supplements associated with reduced risk

individuals were given 400 to 3200 IU of vitamin E per day for up to seven years. Treated individuals were found to have an increased ability to carry out activities of daily living as compared to age-matched, unsupplemented controls.[229] A larger trial involved 160 patients with early symptoms of Parkinson's disease given 3200 IU of vitamin E and 3000 mg of vitamin C per day for an extended time. Using these two antioxidants prolonged the time to when treatment with levodopa was needed.[230]

The Deprenyl and Tocopherol Antioxidant Therapy of Parkinsonism (DATATOP) study[231,232] was a double-blind, placebo-controlled, multicenter trial involving 800 patients with early Parkinson's disease given deprenyl, (a monoamine oxidase inhibitor), and/or 2000 IU of vitamin E per day. The study showed that deprenyl alone increased the ability to perform activities of daily living after nine months of treatment; however, there was no effect seen from vitamin E alone or in combination with the deprenyl. An analysis of the results of this trial revealed that the type of vitamin E used was synthetic as opposed to natural vitamin E, which is much more lipid-soluble. This difference in vitamin E may have explained why more positive results were not seen in the antioxidant supplementation group.

The Rotterdam study was a nutritional epidemiological study of 5342 free-living individuals between the ages of 55 and 95, including 31 individuals with pre-existing Parkinson's disease. In examining dietary intakes, there was a significant correlation between the level of daily dietary intake of vitamin E, beta-carotene, and vitamin C and protection against development of Parkinson's disease.[233]

Large intakes of vitamin E are associated with slowing the progression of Alzheimer's disease, according to research from the Alzheimer's Disease Cooperative Study. A two-year study of 341 individuals with Alzheimer's disease of moderate severity found that 2000 IU per day of vitamin E extended the time patients were able to care for themselves compared to that of those taking a placebo.[234]

Vitamin K

Vitamin K is the collective name for a group of compounds all of which contain the 2-methyl-1,4-naphthoquinone moiety. Human tissue contains phylloquinone (vitamin K_1), several menaquinones (types of vitamin K_2), as well as menadione (vitamin K_3).[235] Phytonadione is the name given to common pharmaceutical preparations.[236]

Compounds with vitamin K activity are essential for the formation of prothrombin and at least five other proteins involved in the regulation of blood clotting including Factors VII, IX, and X, as well as protein C and protein S. Although vitamin K is also required for the biosynthesis of several other proteins found in the plasma, bone, and kidney, defective coagulation of the blood is the only major known sign observed in vitamin K deficiency states.[235,237] Vitamin K deficiency in adults is frequently associated with fat malabsorption syndromes.

Although a wide variation exists, decreased vitamin K levels are generally associated with a decrease in the proportion and absolute amount of carboxylated osteocalcin. Osteocalcin is a vitamin K-dependent protein found in bone matrix, and its levels are a reflection of osteoblastic activity. It has therefore been hypothesized that decreased vitamin K levels might be related to an increased risk for osteoporosis.[238,239,240]

Vitamin K deficiency has been shown to be associated with decreased bone mass in post-menopausal women with aortic atherosclerosis, but not in a similar group without

TABLE 65.25

Vitamin K — Established Benefits

Necessary for normal blood clotting
Calcium metabolism

TABLE 65.26

Vitamin K — Emerging Benefits

Use	Findings	Reference
Osteocalcin formation	Decreased levels are associated with decreased osteocalcin	236-239
Osteoporosis	Possible effect in improving bone mass	240, 241

atherosclerosis. This may be due to the fact that gamma-carboxyglutamate, an amino acid formed by vitamin K action, is known to be involved with regulation of calcification in both bone tissue and atherosclerotic vessel walls, and that abdominal calcification is known to be associated with decreased vitamin K status.[241] Patients treated with warfarin appear to have structural alterations in circulating osteocalcin, which suggests the pathophysiological implication of an association of the use of warfarin with osteoporosis.[242]

Low vitamin K intake is known to be associated with an increased risk of hip fracture in women.[242] Vitamin K supplementation in a group of 20 postmenopausal women with osteoporotic fractures resulted in improved carboxylation of osteocalcin.[243] In summary, these studies suggest a possible link between vitamin K deficiency and osteoporosis. Administration of vitamin K appears to improve a key biochemical parameter that has been associated with decreased bone mass; namely, carboxylated osteocalcin. It is unclear whether the administration of vitamin K has beneficial effects in improving bone mass or preventing osteoporosis or osteoporosis-related fractures. See Tables 65.25 and 65.26 for established and emerging benefits of vitamin K.

Calcium

There is an abundance of evidence that adequate dietary calcium intake minimizes bone loss in postmenopausal women[244-248] and reduces the increased risk of fracture associated with osteoporosis.[249-252] Additionally, calcium supplementation has been demonstrated to augment the bone-preserving effect of estrogen replacement therapy in postmenopausal women.[253,254] The U.S. Food and Drug Administration permits a claim for calcium in the prevention and treatment of osteoporosis.

Use of vitamin D in combination with calcium supplementation is particularly important in preventing loss of bone in women who are borderline deficient[255] and reducing the incidence of fractures in the advanced elderly.[256,257,258] Vitamin D is an essential element in the maintenance of healthy bones because it helps optimize calcium absorption and prevents increased parathyroid (PTH) secretion.[259] High PTH levels stimulate resorption of bone that may result in a gradual weakening of bones leading to an increase in the incidence of fractures.

Calcium supplementation has recently been shown to help prevent colorectal adenomas,[260,261] which are precursors of colon cancer (see also Mobarhan[262] and Lipkin et al.[263] for an excellent review of this subject, and a separate review by Lipkin and Newmark[264]

TABLE 65.27

Calcium — Established Benefits

Regulates heart beat
Involved in muscle contraction and nerve transmissions
Assists in blood clotting
Required for bone formation

TABLE 65.28

Calcium — Emerging Benefits

Use	Findings	Reference
Osteoporosis and osteoporotic fracture	Increased bone mass, decreased risk of fracture	242-257
Colon cancer, breast cancer	Reduces the incidence of colorectal adenomas	258-262
Premenstrual syndrome	Reduces severity of PMS symptoms	263
Improved hormone replacement therapy	Permits lower dose of HRT to be used	264
Hypertension	May lower high blood pressure in individuals with calcium-poor diet	265, 266

on vitamin D, calcium, and breast cancer) and to effectively reduce premenstrual symptoms associated with the luteal phase.[265] The administration of 1000 mg of calcium in the presence of normal blood levels of vitamin D has also been demonstrated to permit a lower dose of hormone replacement therapy (HRT) to increase bone density and provide a bone-sparing effect in elderly women similar to or better than that provided by higher-dose HRT without calcium and vitamin D supplementation.[266]

The value of calcium in control of blood pressure is debatable. Despite conflicting data, meta-analysis of a large number of observational and randomized controlled clinical trials indicates that calcium intake has an impact in reducing blood pressure, particularly in persons regularly consuming low levels of dietary calcium.[267,268] Additional work in this area remains to be done. See Tables 65.27 and 65.28 for established and emerging benefits of calcium.

Magnesium

Magnesium appears to be directly involved in bone metabolism, helping in the formation of bone and indirectly interfacing with hormones regulating bone metabolism. Tranquilli et al. demonstrated that both daily intake and bone mineral content of calcium, phosphorus, and magnesium were significantly reduced in a group of postmenopausal women with osteoporosis compared to non-osteoporotic controls.[269] Additionally, supplementation with magnesium has been shown to help increase bone density in postmenopausal osteoporosis.[270]

Magnesium supplements — typically 350 to 500 mg per day — lower blood pressure,[272] but these findings are inconsistent.[273,274] Results appear to be particularly effective in people who are taking diuretics.[275]

Women with PMS are often deficient in magnesium.[276,277] Supplementation with magnesium may help reduce symptoms.[278,279]

Magnesium can increase blood supply by acting as a vasodilator. At least one trial has found that magnesium supplementation of 250 mg per day increases walking distance for

TABLE 65.29

Magnesium — Established Benefits

Regulates heart beat, muscle contractions, and nerve transmissions
Aids in calcium absorption and the deposition of calcium and phosphorus into bones

TABLE 65.30

Magnesium — Emerging Benefits

Use	Findings	Reference
Osteoporosis	Helps increase bone mass	267, 268
Hypertension	May help lower blood pressure, especially where magnesium has been depleted	269-273
PMS symptoms	Deficiency is associated with PMS symptoms	274-277
Intermittent claudication	May respond to magnesium	278

people with intermittent claudication.[280] See Tables 65.29 and 65.30 for established and emerging benefits of magnesium.

Zinc

Zinc supplementation may be helpful in promoting wound healing in individuals who are zinc deficient. A dose of 220 mg of zinc sulfate (equivalent to 50 mg of elemental zinc) given three times a day for seven to eight weeks has been shown to improve wound healing in zinc-deficient patients.[281,282] There is no evidence that zinc supplementation benefits wound healing in individuals whose zinc nutriture is adequate.

Although popular in some countries, the role of zinc supplementation in improving male sexual function is unproven. Studies have shown that zinc is involved in the reproductive process for humans as well as animals. In humans, zinc is thought to be necessary for the formation and maturation of sperm, for ovulation, and for fertilization. High levels of zinc are found in most male reproductive organs, with the highest concentrations located in the prostate. In animal studies, the normal male testis and prostate contain a high concentration of zinc, and zinc deficiency has been shown to lead to defects in sperm along with a depletion of testosterone.[283-286] For men with low testosterone levels, zinc supplementation raises testosterone and increases fertility.[287] For men with low semen zinc levels, zinc supplements may increase both sperm counts and fertility.[288] Most published studies involve infertile men who have taken zinc supplements for at least several months.

Zinc deficiency in humans has been shown to cause retarded growth and slowed skeletal development.[289] Yamaguchi demonstrated that reduced bone growth is sometimes found in conditions associated with zinc deficiency. Additionally, he demonstrated that zinc has a stimulatory effect on bone growth.[290] Other studies have demonstrated a significant correlation between zinc content and bone strength.[291,292] Zinc has an important role in osteogenesis and bone metabolism, although the exact mechanism remains unknown.[289]

Studies have examined the role of zinc in the treatment of anorexia nervosa and in lozenge form to help decrease the duration of symptoms of the common cold. More research is needed to fully characterize the possible benefits of zinc in these conditions. Recent data from cohort epidemiological studies show zinc to be weakly protective against

TABLE 65.31

Zinc — Established Benefits

Involved in protein metabolism
Necessary for insulin synthesis
Important for night vision

TABLE 65.32

Zinc — Emerging Benefits

Use	Findings	Reference
Aids in wound repair	Useful in cases of deficiency	279, 280
Male infertility	No proven benefit	281-286
Osteoporosis	May help increase bone strength	287-290
Age-related macular degeneration	Possibly protective	291-292
Immunity	Increases immune response	293-297

the development of some forms of early age-related macular degeneration (AMD),[293] although this effect is not proven.[294] (See Section 62.)

Zinc also helps support immune function. An older comprehensive review of the literature by Good et al.[295] as well as information from Chandra and McBean[296] and Prasad et al.[297] suggest that inadequate diet, defective absorption of zinc, disturbances in zinc metabolism, or abnormally increased losses of zinc may be associated with deficits in immune function. Low-dose supplementation of zinc (20 mg) and selenium (100 μg) has been shown to provide significant improvement in elderly patients by increasing humoral response after vaccination.[298] Improved cell-mediated immune response was seen following the administration of zinc 25 mg in an institutionalized elderly population.[299] In this study, a similar effect was not seen for vitamin A 800 μg. See Tables 65.31 and 65.32 for established and emerging benefits of zinc.

Selenium

An epidemiological association between increased selenium intakes and reduced cancer risk, as well as the antioxidant role of selenium in glutathione peroxidase, have provided a basis for research on the potential anticarcinogenic effects of selenium. While the exact mechanism by which selenium exerts its preventative effect against certain types of cancer in humans is unknown, selenium supplementation in animal experiments has been shown to result in enhanced primary immune response in mice, as measured by the plaque-forming cell test and hemagglutination.[300] The addition of supplemental amounts of selenium to the diet has been demonstrated to increase humoral antibody production in swine in response to an antigenic challenge with sheep red blood cells.[301] Selenium deficiency is also known to cause impaired mitogen response in cultures of murine spleen cells.[302]

Two clinical intervention trials published to date have demonstrated that selenium, in combination with other nutrients, may reduce cancer risk. In one study,[303] daily administration of 50 μg of selenium in combination with vitamin E and beta-carotene resulted in a moderate reduction in the risk of total mortality, total cancer mortality and stomach cancer mortality. More recently, Clark et al.[304] showed that treatment with 200 μg of

TABLE 65.33

Selenium — Established and Emerging Benefits

Established
Needed for proper immune system response
Helps prevent Keshan disease (a cardiomyopathy)
Antioxidant via glutathione peroxidase
Emerging
Prevents certain types of cancer

selenium per day significantly decreased total mortality and mortality from lung cancer, as well as the incidence of colorectal and prostate cancer.

To test whether supplemental dietary selenium is associated with changes in the incidence of prostate cancer, in another study by Clark, a total of 1312 men with a history of either basal cell or squamous cell carcinoma were randomized to a daily supplement of 200 μg of selenium or a placebo.[305] Patients were treated for a mean of 4.5 years and followed for a mean of 6.4 years. There was no significant change in incidence for the primary endpoints of basal and squamous cell carcinoma of the skin; however, selenium treatment was associated with a significant reduction (63%) in the secondary endpoint of prostate cancer incidence. There were also significant health benefits for other secondary endpoints of total cancer mortality and the incidence of total, lung, and colorectal cancer.

In another study,[306] patients with histories of basal/squamous cell carcinomas of the skin were assigned randomly to either daily oral supplements of selenium-enriched yeast (200 μg Se/day) or a placebo. The results of this study indicate that supplemental selenium intake did not significantly affect the incidence of recurrent basal/squamous cell carcinomas of the skin; however, selenium treatment was associated with reductions in total mortality, mortality from all cancers combined, and the incidence of all cancers combined, lung cancer, colorectal cancer, and prostate cancer.

The consistency of these findings over time strongly suggests that there is an anticancer benefit to selenium supplementation, particularly in reducing the incidence of prostate cancer. An excellent review of selenium and prostate cancer prevention[307] and a review of the mechanisms of the chemopreventive effects of selenium[308,309] have been published. See Table 65.33 for the established and emerging benefits of selenium.

Chromium

Chromium is an essential trace element that is a constituent of glucose tolerance factor and is required for effective insulin action in humans. Data in the literature are equivocal, suggesting a positive benefit of chromium supplementation on glycemic control in diabetes, but a consistent beneficial effect of chromium supplementation remains unproven.

The American Diabetes Association (ADA) does not currently recommend supplementation with chromium for individuals with diabetes. The ADA position statement, "Nutrition Recommendations and Principles for People with Diabetes Mellitus,"[310] states:

> The only known circumstance in which chromium replacement has any beneficial effect on glycemic control is for people who are chromium deficient as a result of long-term chromium-deficient parenteral nutrition. However, it appears that most people with diabetes are not chromium deficient and, therefore, chromium supplementation has no known benefit.

TABLE 65.34
Chromium — Established and Emerging Benefits

Established
Necessary for DNA synthesis
Important for cell formation
Prevents certain types of anemias
Helps maintain the function of the intestinal tract
Emerging
Hyperglycemic control
Increased bone mass
Control of hypertension
Improved lipid profiles

Further studies to assess the effects of dietary chromium supplementation on insulin sensitivity, as well as on other processes such as increased bone mass, improved blood pressure, and lipid profiles in humans are needed.

For further information on this topic the reader is referred to an excellent review by Schmidt Finney[311] as well as an extensive bibliography of material on this subject.[312-329] See Table 65.34 for the established and emerging benefits of chromium.

References

1. Olson JA., In: *Modern Nutrition in Health and Disease*, 8th ed. Shils ME, Olson JA, Shike M. Eds. Philadelphia, Lea and Febiger, 1994, chap. 16.
2. Brown L, Rimm EB, Seddon JM et al. *Am J Clin Nutr* 70: 517; 1999.
3. Tang AM, Graham NMH, Kirby AJ et al. *J Acq Immune Def Syn* 6: 949; 1993.
4. Semba RD. *Arch Int Med* 153: 2149; 1993.
5. Semba RD, Miotti PG, Chiphangwi JD. *Lancet* 343: 1593; 1994.
6. Hussey GD, Klein M. *N Engl J Med* 323: 160; 1990.
7. Committee on Infectious Diseases. *Pediatrics* 91: 1014; 1993.
8. Kligman AM et al. *Int J Dermatol* 20: 278; 1981.
9. Dvorak AM. *Lancet* 1: 1303; 1980.
10. Rachet AJ, Busson A. *Paris Medical* 1: 308; 1935.
11. Skogh M, Sundquist T, Tagesson C. *Lancet* 1: 766; 1980.
12. Peto R, Doll R, Buckley JD et al. *Nature* 290: 201; 1981.
13. Albanes D, Hartman TJ. In: *Antioxidant Status, Diet, Nutrition and Health* (Papas AM Ed) CRC Press, Boca Raton, 1998, pg 497.
14. The α-Tocopherol, β-Carotene Cancer Prevention Study Group. *N Engl J Med* 330: 1029; 1994.
15. Omenn GS, Goodman GE, Thornquist MD et al. *N Engl J Med* 334: 1150; 1996.
16. Hennekens CH, Buring JE, Manson JE et al. *N Engl J Med* 334: 1145; 1996.
17. Blot WJ, Li JY, Taylor PR. *J Natl Cancer Inst* 85: 1483; 1993.
18. Stich HF, Rosin MP, Vallejera MO. *Lancet* 1: 1204; 1984.
19. Garewal HS, Meyske DL, Killen D. *J Clin Oncol* 8: 1715; 1990.
20. Klipstein-Grobusch K, Geleijnse JM, den Breeijen JH et al. *Am J Clin Nutr* 69: 261; 1999.
21. Stampfer MJ, Hennekens CH, Manson JE et al. *N Engl J Med* 328: 1444; 1993.
22. Rimm EB, Stampfer MJ, Ascherio A et al. *N Engl J Med* 328: 1450; 1993.
23. Gaziano JM, Manson JE. *Ann Epidemiol* 5: 255; 1995.
24. Knekt P, Heliovaara M, Rissanen A, et al. *Br Med J* 305: 1392; 1992.
25. Taylor A, Jacques PF, Nadler D, et al. *Curr Eye Res* 10: 751; 1991.
26. Giovannucci E. *J Natl Cancer Inst* 91: 317; 1999.
27. Bhat KS. *Nutr Rep Int* 36: 685; 1987.

28. Parchal JT, Conrad ME, Skalka HW. *Lancet* 1: 12; 1978.
29. Skalka, HW, Prchal JT. *Am J Clin Nutr* 34: 861; 1981.
30. Jacques PF, Hartz SC, Chylack Jr. LT et al. *Am J Clin Nutr* 48: 152; 1988.
31. Keith R, Alt L. *Nutr Res* 11: 727; 1991.
32. Winters, LR, Yoon JS, Kalkwarf HJ et al. *Am J Clin Nutr* 56: 526; 1992.
33. Belko AZ, Obarzanek E, Kalkwarf HJ et al. *Am J Clin Nutr* 37: 509; 1983.
34. Belko AZ, Obarzanek E, Roach R et al. *Am J Clin Nutr* 40: 553; 1984.
35. Lewis RD, Yates CY, and Driskell JA. *Am J Clin Nutr* 48: 110; 1988.
36. Schoenen J, Lenaerts M, Bastings E. *Cephalalgia* 14: 328; 1994.
37. Brown WV. *Postgrad Med* 98: 185; 1995.
38. Head KA. *Alt Med Rev* 1: 176; 1996.
39. Murray M. *Am J Nat Med* 2: 9; 1995.
40. Dorner Von G, Fisher FW. *Arzneimittel Forschung* 11: 110; 1961.
41. Meydani, SN, Ribaya-Mercado JD, Russell RM et al. *Am J Clin Nutr* 53: 1275; 1991.
42. Kant AK, Moser-Veillon PB, and Reynolds RD. *Am J Clin Nutr* 48: 1284; 1988.
43. Barr W. *Practitioner* 228: 425; 1984.
44. Gunn ADG. *Int J Vit Nutr Res* 27: 213S; 1985.
45. Kleijnen J, Riet GT, Knipshcild P. *Brit J Obstet Gynaecol* 97: 847; 1990.
46. Williams MJ, Harris RI, Deand BC. *J Int Med Res* 13: 174; 1985.
47. Brush MG, Perry M. *Lancet* 1: 1399; 1985.
48. Dorsey JL, Debruyne LK, Rady SJ. *Fed Proc* 42: 556; 1983.
49. Malgren R, Collings A, Nilsson CG. *Acta Obstet Gynecol Scand* 64: 667; 1985.
50. Collin C. *Rev Med Brux* 3: 605; 1982.
51. Wilson RG, Davis RE. *Pathology* 9: 95; 1977.
52. Davis RE, Calder JS, Curnow DH. *Pathol* 8: 151; 1976.
53. McCann VJ, Davis RE. *Austral NZ Med* 8: 259; 1978.
54. Spellacy WN, Buhi WC, Birk SA. *Am J Obstet Gynecol* 127: 599; 1977.
55. Coelingh HJT, Schreurs WHP. *Br Med J* 3: 13; 1975.
56. Spellacy WN, Buhi WC, Birk SA. *Contraception* 6: 265; 1972.
57. Passariello N, Fici F, Giugliano D et al. *Internat J Clin Pharmacol Ther Toxicol* 21: 252; 1983.
58. Solomon LR, Cohen K. *Diabetes* 38: 881; 1989.
59. Rao RH, Vigg BL, Rao KSJ. *J Clin Endocrinol Metabol* 50: 198; 1980.
60. Fuhr JF, Farrow A, Nelson HS. *Arch Surg* 124: 1329; 1989.
61. Ellis JM, Azuma J, Watanbe T et al. *Res Comm Chem Path Pharm* 17: 165; 1977.
62. Ellis JM. *Res Comm Chem Path Pharm* 13: 743; 1976.
63. D'Souza M. *Lancet* 1: 1104; 1985.
64. Driskell JA, Wesley RL, Hess IE. *Nutr Rep Internat* 34: 1031; 1986.
65. Ellis JM. *Southern Med J* 80: 882; 1987.
66. Smith GP. *Ann Neurol* 15: 104; 1984.
67. Amadio PC. *J Hand Surg* 10A, 237; 1985.
68. Stransky M. *Southern Med J* 82: 841; 1989.
69. Baum MK. *J Acq Immuno Syn* 4: 1122; 1991.
70. Selhub J, Jacques PF, Wilson PW et al. *JAMA* 270: 2693; 1993.
71. Ubbink JB, Hayward WJ, van der Merwe A et al. *J Nutr* 124: 927; 1994.
72. Manson JB, Miller JW. *Ann NY Acad Sci* 669: 197; 1992.
73. Bronstrup A, Hages M, Prinz-Langenohl R et al. *Am J Clin Nutr* 68: 1104; 1998.
74. Oakley GP. *Am J Clin Nutr* 65: 1889; 1997.
75. Wald N. *Lancet* 338: 131; 1991.
76. Czeizel AE, Dudas I. *N Engl J Med* 327: 1832; 1992.
77. Centers for Disease Control. *Morbidity and Mortality Weekly Report* 41: 5; 1992.
78. deBree A, van Dusseldorp M. *Eur J Clin Nutr* 51: 643; 1997.
79. Food Labeling: Health Claims and Label Statements, Folate and Neural Tube Defects, Proposed Rule and Final Rule 2 CFR part 101. *Federal Register* 61: 8752; 1996.
80. Rimm EB, Willett WC. *JAMA* 279: 359; 1998.
81. Boushey CJ, Beresford SAA. *JAMA* 274: 1049; 1995.

82. Brattstrom LE, Israelsson B. *Scand J Clin Lab Invest* 48: 215; 1988.
83. Brattstrom LE, Israelsson B. *Atherosclerosis* 81: 51; 1990.
84. Jacob RA, Wu Ml. *J Nutr* 124: 1072; 1994.
85. Naurath HJ, Joosten E. *Lancet* 346: 85; 1995.
86. O'Keefe CA, Bailey LB. *J Nutr* 125: 2717; 1995.
87. Ubbink JB, Vermaak WJH. *J Nutr* 124: 1927; 1994.
88. Guttormsen AB, Ueland PM. *J Clin Invest* 98: 2174; 1996.
89. Bostom AG, Shemin D. *Kidney Int* 49: 147; 1996.
90. Homocysteine Lowering Trialists' Collaboration. *Br Med J* 316: 894; 1998.
91. Lobo A, Naso A. *Am J Cardiol* 83: 821; 1999.
92. Brouwer IA, Dusseldorp MJ. *Am J Clin Nutr* 69: 99; 1999.
93. Malinow MR, Nieto FJ. *Arterioscle Thromb Vasc Biol* 17: 1157; 1997.
94. Malinow MR, Duell PB. *N Engl J Med* 338: 1009; 1998.
95. Jacques PF, Selhub J. *N Engl J Med* 340: 1449; 1999.
96. Osdganian J, Stampfer MJ. *JAMA* 281: 1189; 1999.
97. Greenlund KJ, Srinivasan SR. *Circulation* 99: 2144; 1999.
98. Van Beynum IM, Smeitink JAM. *Circulation* 59: 2070; 1999.
99. Hankey GJ, Eikelboom JW. *Lancet* 354: 407; 1999.
100. Peterson JC, Spence JD. *Lancet* 351: 263; 1998.
101. Malinow MR, Bostom AG. *Circulation* 99: 178; 1999.
102. Green R, Miller JW. *Sem Hematol* 36: 47; 1999.
103. Refsum H, Ueland PM. *Ann Rev Med* 49: 31; 1998.
104. Selhub J, D'Angelo A. *Am J Med Sci* 31: 129; 1998.
105. Welch GN, Loscalzo J. *N Engl J Med* 338: 1042; 1998.
106. Mason J. *Nutr Rev* 47: 314; 1989.
107. Butteworth CE. In: *Micronutrients In Health and Disease* Bendich A, Butteworth CE: Eds. New York: Marcel Dekker Inc. 1991, pg 165.
108. Butteworth CE, Hatch KD. *JAMA* 267: 528; 1992.
109. Heimburger DC, Alexander CB. *JAMA* 259: 1525; 1998.
110. Lashner BA, Heidenreich PA. *Gastroenterology* 97: 255; 1989.
111. Giovannucci E, Stampfer MJ. *Ann Int Med* 129: 517; 1998.
112. Zhang S, Hunter DJ. *JAMA* 281: 1632; 1999.
113. Blount BC, Mack MM. *Proc Natl Acad Sci USA* 94: 3290; 1997.
114. Smith CR, Jobst KA. *Arch Neurol* 55: 1449; 1998.
115. McCaddon A, Davies G. *Int J Geriatric Psych* 13: 235; 1998.
116. Alpert JE, Fava M. *Nutr Rev* 55: 145; 1997.
117. Burri BJ, Jacob RA. In: *Vitamin C in Health and Disease,* Packer L, Fuchs J, Eds. New York, Marcel Dekker Inc, 1997, pg 341.
118. Anderson D, Phillips B, Yu T et al. *Environ Mol Mutagen* 30: 161; 1997.
119. Simon JA. *J Am Coll Nutr* 11: 107; 1992.
120. Gatto LM, Hallen GK, Brown AJ et al. *J Am Coll Nutr* 15: 154; 1996.
121. Ness AR, Khaw KT, Bingham S et al. *Eur J Clin Nutr* 50: 724; 1996.
122. Toohey L, Harris MA, Allen KG et al. *J Nutr* 126: 121; 1996.
123. Simon JA, Hudes ES. *J Am Coll Nutr* 17: 250; 1998.
124. Jacques PF. *J Am Coll Nutr* 11: 139; 1992.
125. Moran JP, Cohen L, Greene JM et al. *Am J Clin Nutr* 57: 213; 1993.
126. Jacques PF. *Int J Vitam Nutr Res* 62: 252; 1992.
127. Ness AR, Khaw KT, Bingham S et al. *J Hypertens* 14: 503; 1996.
128. Gokce N, Keaney JF Jr, Frei B et al. *Circulation* (in press).
129. Levine GL, Frei B, Koulouris SN et al. *Circulation* 93: 1107; 1996.
130. Hornig B, Arakawa N, Kohler C et al. *Circulation* 97: 363; 1998.
131. Ito K, Akita H, Kanazawa K et al. *Am J Cardiol* 82: 762; 1998.
132. Kugiyama K, Motoyama T, Hirashima O et al. *J Am Coll Cardiol* 32: 103; 1998.
133. Hecht SS. *Proc Soc Exp Biol Med* 216: 181; 1997.
134. Tannenbaum SR, Wishnok JS. *Ann NY Acad Sci* 498: 354; 1987.

135. Vohra K, Khan AJ, Telang V et al. *J Perinatol* 10: 134; 1990.
136. Johnston CS, Martin LJ, Cai X. *J Am Coll Nutr* 11: 172; 1992.
137. Levy R, Shriker O, Porath A et al. *J Infect Dis* 173: 1502; 1996.
138. Maderazo EG, Woronick CL, Hickingbotham N et al. *J Trauma* 31: 1142; 1991.
139. Hemila H. In: *Vitamin C in health and disease,* Packer L, Fuchs J, Eds., Marcel Dekker Inc, New York, 1997, pg 471.
140. Heuser G, Vojdani A. *Immunopharmacol Immunotoxicol* 19: 291; 1997.
141. Smit MJ, Anderson R. *Agents Actions* 30: 338; 1991.
142. Carr AC, Frei B. *Am J Clin Nutr* 69: 1086; 1999.
143. Enstrom JE, Kanim LE, Breslow L. *Am J Publ Health* 76: 1124; 1986.
144. Enstrom JE, Kanim LE, Klein MA. *Epidemiology* 3: 194; 1992.
145. Enstrom JE. *Nutr Today* 28: 28; 1993.
146. Manson JE, Stampfer MJ, Willett WC et al. *Circulation* 85: 865; 1992.
147. Manson JE, Stampfer MJ, Willett WC et al. *Circulation* 87: 678; 1993.
148. Rimm EB, Stampfer MJ, Asherio A et al. *N Engl J Med* 328: 1450; 1993.
149. Fehily AM, Yarnell JWG, Sweetnam PM et al. *Br J Nutr* 69: 303; 1993.
150. Knekt P, Reunanen A, Jarvinen R et al. *Am J Epidemiol* 139: 1180; 1994.
151. Gale CR, Martyn CN, Winter PD et al. *Br Med J* 310: 1563; 1995.
152. Kritchevsky SB, Shimakawa T, Tell GS et al. *Circulation* 92: 2142; 1995.
153. Pandey DK, Shekelle R, Selwyn BJ et al. *Am J Epidemiol* 142: 1269; 1995.
154. Kushi LH, Folsom AR, Prineas RJ et al. *N Engl J Med* 334: 1156; 1996.
155. Losonczy KG, Harris TB, Havlik RJ. *Am J Clin Nutr* 64: 190; 1996.
156. Sahyoun NR, Jacques PF, Russell RM. *Am J Epidemiol* 144: 501; 1996.
157. Mark SD, Wang W, Fraumeni JF et al. *Epidemiology* 9: 9; 1998.
158. Shekelle RB, Liu S, Raynor WJ et al. *Lancet* 28: 1185; 1981.
159. Kromhout D. *Am J Clin Nutr* 45: 1361; 1987.
160. Knekt P, Jarvinen R, Seppanen R et al. *Am J Epidemiol* 134: 471; 1991.
161. Shibata A, Paganini-Hill A, Ross RK et al. *Br J Cancer* 66: 673; 1992.
162. Graham S, Zielezny M, Marshall J et al. *Am J Epidemiol* 136: 1327; 1992.
163. Hunter DJ, Manson JE, Colditz GA et al. *N Engl J Med* 329: 234; 1993.
164. Bostick RM, Potter JD, McKenzie DR et al. *Cancer Res* 53: 4230; 1993.
165. Blot WJ, Li JY, Taylor PR et al. *J Natl Cancer Inst* 85: 1483; 1993.
166. Kushi LH, Fee RM, Sellers TA et al. *Am J Epidemiol* 144: 165; 1996.
167. Yong L, Brown CC, Schatzkin A et al. *Am J Epidemiol* 146: 231; 1997.
168. Kessenich CR, Rosen CJ. *Orthopaedic Nursing* 15: 67; 1996.
169. Holick MF. *Am J Clin Nutr* 60: 619; 1994.
170. Kinyamu HK, Gallagher JC, Balhorn KE et al. *Am J Clin Nutr* 65: 790; 1997.
171. Goldray D, Mizrahi-Sasson E, Merdler C et al. *J Am Geriatr Soc* 37: 589; 1989.
172. Pogue SJ. *Dermatology Nursing* 7: 103; 1995.
173. Meunier P. *Scan J Rheum* 103: 75S; 1996.
174. McAuley KA, Jones S, Lewis-Barned NJ et al. *NZ Med J* 110: 275; 1997.
175. Compston JE. *Clin Endocrin* 43: 393; 1995.
176. McKenna MJ. *Am J Med* 93: 69; 1992.
177. Ooms ME, Roos JC, Bezemer PD et al. *J Clin Endocrin Metab* 80: 1052; 1995.
178. MacLaughlin J, Holick MF. *J Clin Invest* 76: 1536; 1985.
179. Chapuy MC, Arlot ME, Duboeuf F et al. *N Engl J Med* 327: 1637; 1992.
180. Torgerson DJ, Kanis JA. *QJM* 88: 135; 1995.
181. Morimoto S, Yoshikawa K, Kozuka T et al. *Brit J Dermatol* 115: 421; 1986.
182. Morimoto S, Yoshikawa K. *Arch Dermatol* 125: 231; 1989.
183. Kragballe K. *Arch Dermatol* 125: 1647; 1989.
184. Smith EL, Pincus SH, Donovan L et al. *J Am Acad Dermatol* 19: 516; 1988.
185. Kragballe K, Beck HI, Sogaard H. *Brit J Dermatol* 119: 223; 1988.
186. Henderson CA, Papworth-Smith J, Cunliffe WJ et al. *Brit J Dermatol* 121: 493; 1989.
187. Van de Kerkhof PCM, Van Bokhoven M, Zultak M et al. *Brit J Dermatol* 120: 661; 1989.
188. Thys-Jacobs S. *Headache* 34: 544; 1994.

189. Thys-Jacobs S. *Headache* 34: 590; 1994.
190. Giovannucci E. *Cancer Causes & Control* 9: 567; 1998.
191. Ma J, Stampfer MJ, Gann PH et al. *Cancer Epidemiol, Biomark & Prevent* 7: 385; 1998.
192. Lipkin M, Reddy B, Newmark H et al. *Annu Rev Nutr* 19: 545; 1999.
193. Xue L, Newmark H, Yang K et al. *Nutrition & Cancer* 26: 281; 1996.
194. Hiatt RA, Krieger N, Lobaugh B et al. *J Natl Cancer Inst* 90: 6; 1998.
195. Martindale, The Extra Pharmacopoeia. 32nd Edition, Reynolds JE, Ed., Pharmaceutical Press, London, 1998.
196. Porkkala-Sarataho E, Nyyssonen K, Salonen JT et al. *Atherosclerosis* 124: 83; 1996.
197. Regnstrom J, Nilsson J, Moldeus P et al. *Am J Clin Nutr* 63: 377; 1996.
198. Azen S. *J Am Heart Assoc* 2369; 1996.
199. Gey KF, Puska P, Jordan P et al. *Am J Clin Nutr* 53: 326S; 1991.
200. Stampfer MJ, Hennekens CH, Manson JE et al. *N Engl J Med* 328: 1444; 1993.
201. Rimm EB, Stampfer MJ, Ascherio A et al. *N Engl J Med* 328: 1450; 1993.
202. Stephens NG, Parsons A, Schofield PM et al. *Lancet* 347: 781; 1996.
203. The Heart Outcomes Prevention Evaluation Study Investigators. *N Engl J Med* 342: 154; 2000.
204. GISSI-Prevenzione Investigators. *Lancet* 354: 447; 1999.
205. Losonczy KG, Harris TB, Havlik RJ. *Am J Clin Nutr* 64: 190; 1996.
206. Kushi LH, Folsom AR, Prineas RJ et al. *N Engl J Med* 334: 1156; 1996.
207. Jha P, Flather M, Lonn E et al. *Ann Int Med* 123: 860; 1995.
208. DeMaio SJ, King SB, Lembo NJ et al. *J Am Coll Nutr* 11: 68; 1992.
209. Stahelin HB, Rosel F, Buess E et al. *J Natl Cancer Inst* 73: 1463; 1984.
210. Wald NJ, Boreham J Hayward JL et al. *Br J Cancer* 49: 321; 1984.
211. Salonen JT, Salonen R, Lappetelainen R et al. *Br Med J* 290: 417; 1985.
212. Menkes MS, Comstock GWS, Vuilieumier JP et al. *N Engl J Med* 315: 1250; 1986.
213. Kok FJ, van Duijn CM, Hofman A et al. *N Engl J Med* 316: 1416; 1987.
214. Miyamoto H, Araya Y, Ito M et al. *Cancer* 60: 1159; 1987.
215. Wald NJ, Thompson SG, Densem JW et al. *Br J Cancer* 56: 69; 1987.
216. Knekt P, Aromaa A, Maatela J et al. *Am J Epidemiol* 127: 28; 1988.
217. Knekt P, Aromaa A, Maatela J et al. *Int J Cancer* 42: 846; 1988.
218. Knekt P. *Int J Epidemiol* 17: 281; 1988.
219. Verreault RA, Chu J, Mandelson M et al. *Int J Cancer* 43: 1050; 1989.
220. LeGardeur BY, Lopez A, Johnson WD et al. *Nutr Cancer* 14: 133; 1990.
221. Buiatti E, Palli D, Decarli A et al. *Int J Cancer* 45: 896; 1990.
222. Gridley G, McLaughlin JK, Block G et al. *Nutr Cancer* 14: 219; 1990.
223. Palan PR, Mikhail MS, Basu J et al. *Nutr Cancer* 15: 13; 1991.
224. Comstock GW, Helzlsover KJ, Bush TL. *Am J Clin Nutr* 53: 260S, 1991.
225. Harris RW, Key TJ, Sikocks PB et al. *Nutr Cancer* 15: 63; 1991.
226. Knekt P, Jarvinene R, Seppanen R et al. *Am J Epidemiol* 134: 471; 1991.
227. Gridley G, McLaughlin JK, Block G et al. *Am J Epidemiol* 135: 1083; 1992.
228. Grimes JD, Hassan MN, Thakar JH. *Prog Neuro-Psychopharmacol Biol Psych* 12: 165; 1988.
229. Factor SA, Weiner WJ. *Ann NY Acad Sci* 570: 441; 1989.
230. Fahn S. *Am J Clin Nutr* 53: 380S, 1991.
231. Parkinson Study Group. *N Engl J Med* 328: 176; 1993.
232. Parksinson Study Group. *Ann Neurol* 39: 29; 1996.
233. de Rijk MC, Breteler MM, den Breeijen JH et al. *Arch Neurol* 54: 762; 1997.
234. Sano M, Ernesto C, Thomas RG et al. *N Engl J Med* 336: 1216; 1997.
235. Suttie JW, In: *The Fat Soluble Vitamins,* Diplock AT Ed. William Heinemann Ltd., London, 1985, pg 225.
236. USPDI, Drug Information for the Health Care Professional, Volume 1, The United States Pharmacopoeial Convention, Rockville MD, 1997, pg 2995.
237. Olson RE. *Ann Rev Nutr* 4: 281; 1984.
238. Jie KG, Bots ML, Vermeer C et al. *Calcif Tissue Int* 59: 352; 1996.
239. Vermeer C, Gijsbers BIL, Craciun AM et al. *J Nutr* 126: 187S, 1996.
240. Knapen MH, Hamulyak K, Vermeer C. *Ann Intern Med* 111: 1001; 1989.

241. Menon RK, Gill DS, Thomas M et al. *J Clin Endocrinol Metab* 64: 59; 1987.
242. Feskanich D, Wever P, Willett WC et al. *Am J Clin Nutr* 69: 74; 1999.
243. Douglas AS, Robins SP, Hutchison JD et al. *Bone* 17: 15; 1995.
244. Prince RL, Smith M, Dick IM et al. *N Engl J Med* 325: 1189; 1991.
245. Aloia JF, Vaswani A, Yeh JK et al. *Ann Int Med* 120: 97; 1994.
246. Dawson-Hughes B, Dallal GE, Krall EA et al. *N Engl J Med* 323: 878; 1990.
247. Skaer TL. *P & T* 20: 88; 1995.
248. Riggs BL, Jowsey J, Kelly PJ et al. *J Clin Endo Metab* 42: 1139; 1976.
249. Riggs BL, Seeman E, Hodgson SF et al. *N Engl J Med* 306: 446; 1982.
250. Birge SJ. *Clinics Geri Med* 9: 69; 1993.
251. Lau EM, Cooper C. *Osteoporosis Internat* 3: 23; 1993.
252. NIH Concensus Development Panel on Optimal Calcium Intake. *JAMA* 272: 1942; 1994.
253. Riis BJ, Christiansen C. *Maturitas* 6: 65; 1984.
254. Aloia JF, Vaswani A, Yeh JK et al. *Ann Int Med* 120: 97; 1994.
255. Dawson-Hughes B, Dallal GE, Krall EA et al. *Ann Int Med* 115: 505; 1991.
256. Chapuy MC, Chapuy P, Meunier PF. *Am J Clin Nutr* 46: 324; 1987.
257. Chapuy MC, Arlot MC, DuBoeuf F et al. *N Engl J Med* 327: 1637; 1992.
258. Sankaran SK. *Drugs and Aging* 9: 1; 1996.
259. Kessenich CR, Rosen CJ. *Orthopaedic Nursing* 15: 67; 1996.
260. Baron JA, Beach M, Mandel JS et al. *N Engl J Med* 340: 101; 1999.
261. Whelan RL, Horvath KD, Gleason NR et al. *Dis Colon Rectum* 42: 212; 1999.
262. Mobarhan S. *Nutr Rev* 57: 124; 1999.
263. Lipkin M, Bandaru R, Newmark H et al. *Ann Rev Nutr* 19: 545; 1999.
264. Lipkin M, Newmark HL. *J Am Coll Nutr* 18: 392S, 1999.
265. Thys-Jacobs S, Starkey P, Bernstein D et al. *Am J Obstet Gynecol* 179: 444; 1998.
266. Recker RR, Davies KM, Dowd RM et al. *Ann Intern Med* 130: 897; 1999.
267. McCarron DA, Reusser ME. *J Am Coll Nutr* 18: 398S, 1999.
268. McCarron DA, Metz JA, Hatton DC. *Am J Clin Nutr* 68: 517; 1998.
269. Tranquilli AL, Lucino E, Garzetti GG et al. *Gynecol Endocrinol* 8: 55; 1994.
270. Stendig-Lindberg G, Tepper R, Leichter I. *Magnesium Res* 6: 155; 1993.
271. Motoyama T, Sano H, Fukuzaki H et al. *Hypertens* 13: 227; 1989.
272. Itoh K, Kawasaka T, Nakamura M. *Br J Nutr* 78: 737; 1997.
273. Patki PS, Singh J, Gokhale SV et al. *Br Med J* 301: 521; 1990.
274. Sacks FM, Willett WC, Smith A et al. *Hypertension* 31: 131; 1998.
275. Dyckner T, Wester PO. *Br Med J* 286: 1847; 1983.
276. Abraham GE, Lubran MM. *Am J Clin Nutr* 34: 2364; 1981.
277. Sherwood RA, Rocks BF, Stewart A et al. *Ann Clin Biochem* 23: 667; 1986.
278. Nicholas A. In: *First International Symposium on Magnesium Deficit in Human Pathology*, J Durlach Ed., Springer-Verlag, Paris, 1973; pg 261.
279. Facchinetti F, Borella P, Sances G et al. *Obstet Gynecol* 78: 177; 1991.
280. Neglen P. *VASA* 14: 285; 1985.
281. Greaves MW. *Lancet* 2: 889; 1970.
282. Serjeant GR. *Lancet* 2: 891; 1970.
283. Favier AE. *Biolog Trace Element Res* 32: 363; 1992.
284. Bedwal RS, Bahuguna A. *Experientia* 50: 626; 1994.
285. Apgar J. *J Nutr Biochem* 3: 266; 1992.
286. Hunt CD, Johnson PE, Herbel JL et al. *Am J Clin Nutr* 56: 148; 1992.
287. Netter A, Hartoma R, Nahoul K. *Arch Androl* 7: 69; 1981.
288. Marmar JL. *Fertil Steril* 26: 1057; 1975.
289. Calhoun NR, Smith JC Jr, Becker KL. *Clinical Orthopaedics & Related Research* 1: 212; 1974.
290. Yamaguchi M. *Journal of Nutritional Science & Vitaminology* special no. 522, 1992.
291. Alhava EM, Olkkonen H, Puittinen J et al. *Acta Orthopaedica Scandinavica* 48: 1; 1997.
292. Saltman PD, Strause LG. *J Am Coll Nutr* 12: 384; 1993.
293. Mares-Perlman JA, Klein R, Klein BE et al. *Arch Ophthal* 114: 991; 1996.
294. Smith W, Mitchell P, Webb K et al. *Ophthalmology* 106: 761; 1999.

295. Good RA, Fernandes G, Garofalo JA et al. In: *Clinical, Biochemical and Nutritional Aspects of Trace Elements* Alan R Liss, NY, 1982, pg 189.
296. Chandra RK, McBean LD. *Nutrition* 10: 79; 1994.
297. Prasad AS, Fitzgerald JT, Hess JW et al. *Nutrition* 9: 218; 1993.
298. Girodon F, Galan P, Monget AL. *Arch Int Med* 159: 748; 1999.
299. Fortes C, Forastiere F, Agabiti N et al. *J Am Geriatr Soc* 46: 19; 1998.
300. Spallholz, JE. In: *Diet and Resistance to Disease,* Phillips M, Baetz A, Eds., Plenum, New York, 1981, pg 43.
301. Peplowski MA, Mahan DC, Murray FA et al. *J An Sci* 51: 344; 1980.
302. Mulhern SA, Taylor GL, Magruder LE et al. *Nutr Res* 5: 201; 1985.
303. Blot WJ, Lie JY, Taylor PR et al. *J Natl Can Inst* 85: 1483; 1993.
304. Clark LC, Combs GF, Turnbull BW et al. *JAMA* 276: 1957; 1996.
305. Clark LC, Dalkin B, Krongrad A. *Br J Urol* 81: 730; 1998.
306. Combs GF Jr, Clark LC, Turnbull BW. *Medizinische Klinik* 92: 42S; 1997.
307. Nelson MA, Porterfield BW, Jacobs ET et al. *Sem Urologic Oncol* 17: 91; 1999.
308. Combs GF Jr, Gray WP. *Pharmacol Ther* 79: 179; 1998.
309. Ip C. *J Nutr* 128: 1845; 1998.
310. American Diabetes Association. *Diabetes Care* 19: 16S; 1996.
311. Schmidt Finney L, Gonzalez-Campoy, JM. *Clinical Diabetes* 15: 1; 1997.
312. Anderson, RA. *J Am Coll Nutr* 16: 404; 1997.
313. Anderson RA, Cheng N, Bryden NA et al. *Diabetes* 46: 1786; 1997.
314. Cunningham JJ. *J Am Coll Nutr* 17: 7; 1998.
315. Davies S, McLaren HJ, Hunnisett A et al. *Metabolism* 46: 469; 1997.
316. Davis CM, Vincent JB. *Biochem* 36: 4382; 1997.
317. Fox GN, Sabovic Z. *J Fam Pract* 46: 83; 1998.
318. Hahdi GS. *Diabet Med* 13: 389; 1996.
319. Heller RF. *Med Hypotheses* 45: 325; 1995.
320. Jovanovic-Peterson L, Peterson CM. *J Am Coll Nutr* 15: 14; 1996.
321. Lee NA, Reasner CA. *Diabetes Care* 17: 1449; 1994.
322. Linday LA. *Med Hypotheses* 49: 47; 1997.
323. Littlefield D. *J Am Diet Assoc* 94: 1368; 1994.
324. McCarty MF. *Med Hypotheses* 49: 143; 1997.
325. Porter-Field LM. *RN* 59: 71; 1996.
326. Preuss HG. *J Am Coll Nutr* 16: 397; 1997.
327. Romero RA, Salgado O, Rodriguez-Iturbe B et al. *Transplant Proc* 28: 3382; 1996.
328. Sampson MJ, Griffith VS, Drury PL. *Diabet Med* 11: 150; 1994.
329. Yurkow EJ, Kim G. *Mol Pharmacol* 47: 686; 1995.

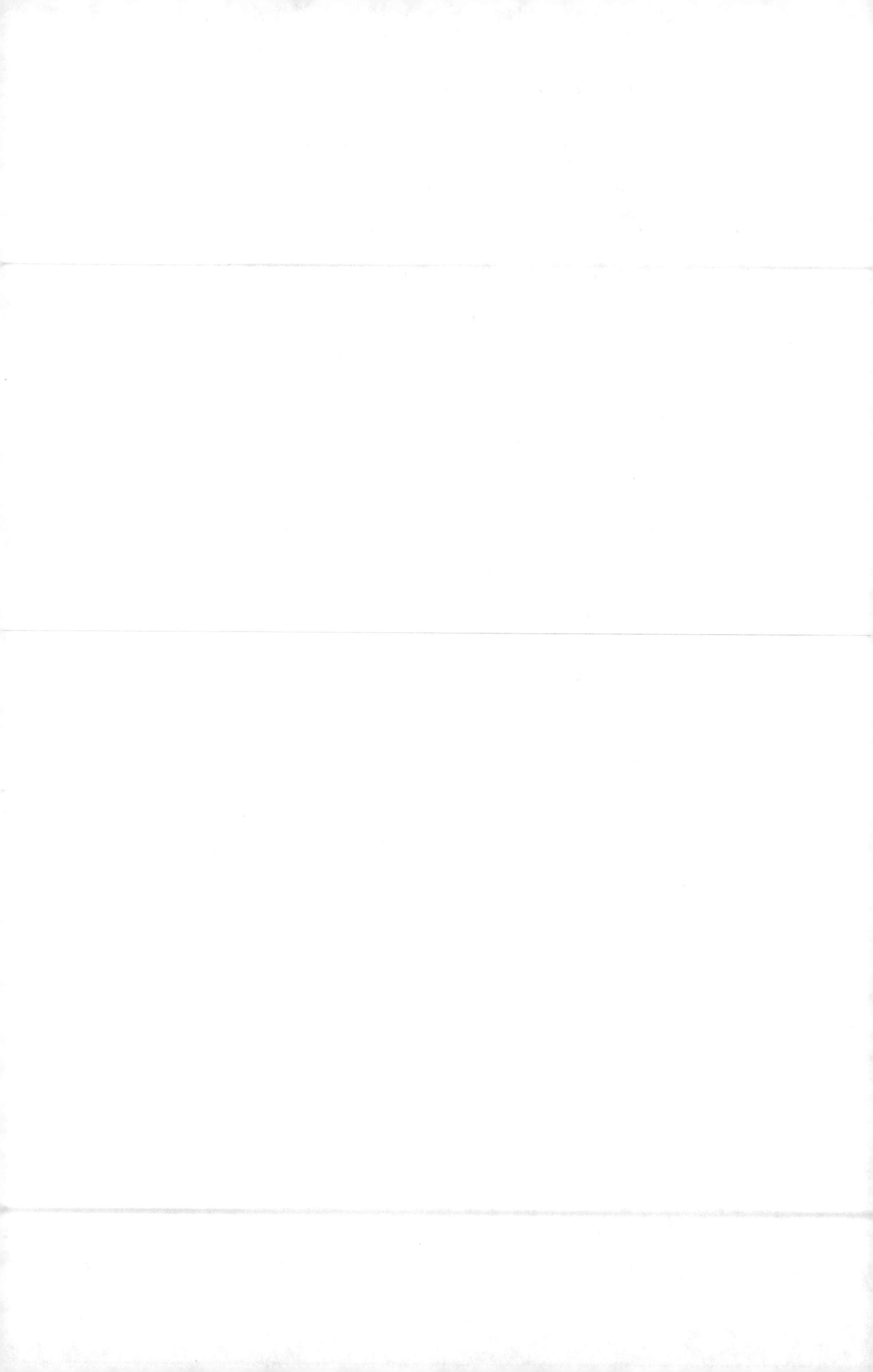

66

Nutrition in Critical Illness

Gail A. Cresci and Robert G. Martindale

Introduction

The human body constantly strives to maintain homeostasis even when challenged by internal and external physical, biological, chemical, or psychological forces. Hospitalized patients are routinely exposed to factors that cause metabolic stress. These include semi-starvation, infection, trauma, surgery, and tissue ischemia. Malnutrition occurs in hospitalized patients mainly through starvation or metabolic stress.[1] These two pathways resulting in malnutrition exhibit very different metabolic alterations (Table 66.1). The development of malnutrition in critically ill patients can occur very rapidly secondary to the hormonal and nonhormonal mediators that result in the complex metabolic alterations.

Metabolic Response to Stress

The metabolic response to injury and sepsis has been well studied after the pioneering work of Kinney.[2] Stressed patients undergo several metabolic phases as a series of ebb and flow states reflecting a patient's response to the severity of the stress (Table 66.2). The earliest, or ebb, state is usually manifested by decreased oxygen consumption, fluid imbalances, inadequate tissue perfusion, and cellular shock. These changes decrease metabolic needs and provide a brief protective environment. The flow state is a hyperdynamic phase in which substrates are mobilized for energy production while increased cellular activity and hormonal stimulation is noted. Subsequently, most patients will enter a third phase of recovery, or anabolism, which is characterized by normalization of vital signs, increased diuresis, improved appetite, and positive nitrogen balance. There is an energy expenditure distinction for each phase, making the goals of nutrition therapy variable depending on the stage in question. As long as the patient is in a hyperdynamic catabolic state, optimal nutrition support can only at best approach zero nitrogen balance in attempts to minimize further protein wasting. Once the patient enters the anabolic phase, it is then realistic to anticipate a positive nitrogen balance and repletion of lean body mass through optimal

0-8493-2705-9/02/$0.00+$1.50

TABLE 66.1

Metabolic Comparisons between Starvation and Stress

	Starvation	Stress
Resting energy expenditure	↓	↑↑
Respiratory quotient	↓	↑
Primary fuels	Fat	Mixed
Glucagon	↑	↑
Insulin	↓	↑
Gluconeogenesis	↓	↑↑↑
Plasma glucose	↓	↑
Ketogenesis	↑↑	↓
Plasma lipids	↑	↑↑
Proteolysis	↑	↑↑↑
Hepatic protein synthesis	↑	↑↑
Urinary nitrogen loss	↑	↑↑↑

TABLE 66.2

Stress Phase Alterations

Phase	Hormonal/Nonhormonal	Metabolic	Clinical Outcomes
Ebb phase	↑ Glucagon ↑ Adrenocorticotropic hormone (ACTH)	Circulatory insufficiency (↑ Heart rate, vascular constriction) ↓ Digestive enzyme production ↓ Urine production	Hemodynamic instability
Flow phase	↑ Counterregulatory hormones (epinephrine, norepinephrine, glucagon, cortisol) ↑ Insulin ↑ Catecholamines ↑ Cytokines (TNF, IL-1,-2, and -6)	Hyperglycemia ↓ Protein synthesis ↑ amino acid efflux ↑ Gluconeogenesis ↑ Glycogenolysis ↑ Lipolysis ↑ Urea nitrogen excretion/ net (-) nitrogen balance	Fluid and electrolyte imbalances Mild metabolic acidosis ↑ Resting energy expenditure
Anabolic phase	↑ Insulin ↓ Counterregulatory hormones ↓ Cytokines	↑ Protein synthesis ↓ Urea nitrogen excretion/ net (+) nitrogen balance ↓ Gluconeogenesis ↓ Lipolysis	↓ Resting energy expenditure ↑ Lean body mass

nutrition intervention. Therefore, early nutrition intervention in critical illness, is primarily geared towards sustaining vital organ structure and immune function, ameliorating the catabolic effects of critical illness and promoting recovery without causing further metabolic derangements.

The high-risk patient usually remains in the catabolic phase for a prolonged period. In order to meet tissue demands for increased oxygen consumption following acute injury, there is an increase in oxygen delivery. This is accomplished by a systemic response that includes increases in heart rate, minute ventilation and myocardial contractility, and decreases in peripheral vascular resistance so that the cardiac index may exceed 4.5 L/min/m.[2,3] Other systemic responses include hypermetabolism yielding increased proteolysis and nitrogen loss, accelerated gluconeogenesis, hyperglycemia and increased glucose utilization, and retention of salt and water. When patients become critically ill, they rapidly shift from an anabolic state of storing protein, fat, and glycogen to a catabolic state by mobilizing these nutrients for energy utilization.[4] There is a direct correlation between the severity of the injury and the degree of substrate mobilization. The mobilization of protein, fat, and glycogen is mediated through the release of cytokines such as tumor necrosis factor, interleukins-1,-2 and -6, and the counterregulatory hormones such as epinephrine, norepinephrine, glucagon, and cortisol.[5] These hormones are labeled counterregulatory because they counter the anabolic effects of insulin and other anabolic hormones. Circulating levels of insulin are elevated in most metabolically stressed patients, but the responsiveness of tissues to insulin, especially skeletal muscle, is severely blunted. This relative insulin resistance is believed to be due to the effects of the counterregulatory hormones. The hormonal milieu normalizes only after the injury or metabolic stress has resolved.

During the hypermetabolic response of critical illness energy expenditure is increased, resulting in an increase in nutrient substrates in an attempt to meet these needs. This is exhibited by an elevated respiratory quotient (RQ) of 0.80 to 0.85 reflecting mixed fuel oxidation, as opposed to a non-stressed starved state where the RQ is in the range of 0.60 to 0.70, reflecting the oxidation of fat as the primary fuel source. Under the influence of the counterregulatory hormones, cytokines, and catecholamines, hepatic glucose production increases through glycogenolysis and gluconeogenesis.[4] The increased endogenous glucose production is poorly suppressed even with exogenous glucose or insulin administration. In stress metabolism, glycogen stores are depleted with 12 to 24 hours of a major catabolic insult, leaving only protein and adipose tissue as potential energy substrates. Gluconeogenic substrates include lactate, alanine, glutamine, glycine, serine, and glycerol. Accompanying the increased glucose production is an increase in flow to and uptake of glucose in the peripheral tissues. Hyperglycemia commonly results due to an increased glucagon/insulin ratio and insulin resistance in peripheral tissues.

Alterations in hormone levels also affect lipid metabolism. Elevations of epinephrine, growth hormone, glucagon, and beta-adrenergic stimulation induce lipolysis and increase glycerol and free fatty acid (FFA) levels which are then used as a fuel source.[5] Despite elevation in lipolysis, a proportionate increase in lipid oxidation is not observed. This is believed to be due to the elevated insulin levels. Therefore, even though lipid stores are abundant in most cases, they are poorly utilized.

With depleted glycogen stores and diminished ability to utilize fat stores, the body shifts to catabolizing and using lean body mass as a main energy source and substrate for gluconeogenesis. Although protein synthesis is higher relative to non-stress starvation, it is overall significantly reduced from the normal state due to the rate of protein catabolism. Increased nitrogen excretion is observed and is proportional to the severity of injury or infection. The major mediators of protein catabolism and the accelerated movement of amino acids from the skeletal muscle to the liver are the glucocorticoids.[4] Amino acids reaching the liver are used to produce glucose and acute-phase proteins such as fibrinogen, haptoglobin, C-reactive protein, ceruloplasmin, and alpha-2 macroglobulin.[5] Alanine is the primary amino acid used for gluconeogenesis, while glutamine supplies the necessary nitrogen to the kidneys for the synthesis of ammonia. Ammonia acts as a neutralizing substrate for the excess acid byproducts produced by the increased protein degradation that occurs during stress. The utilization of amino acids for an energy source results in increased ureagenesis and urinary nitrogen losses which may exceed 15 to 20 g/day.[2]

Nutritional Intervention in Critical Illness

The goals of nutrition intervention in critically ill patients are to minimize lean body tissue loss and support the body's immune system. Nutrient delivery is designed to maintain lean body mass without causing further metabolic complications. Achieving these goals involves accurate and continued nutrition assessment, optimal and timely nutrient delivery, and continuous systematic monitoring of metabolic status.

Determination of Energy Requirements

Regardless of the metabolic state, energy requirements must be met in attempts to minimize the utilization of stored energy reserves. Although the protein-sparing effect of an adequate caloric intake is well recognized in the setting of adaptive starvation, it is equally clear in the setting of stress hypermetabolism that despite adequate caloric provision, protein catabolism continues despite delivery of adequate nutrients.[3]

Determination of energy requirements in the critically ill is often challenging. Critical illness and its treatment can profoundly alter metabolism and significantly increase or decrease energy expenditure.[6] Therefore, accurate determination of resting energy expenditure (REE) is necessary to ensure that energy needs are provided without over- or underfeeding. Overfeeding is associated with numerous metabolic complications. It is usually a result of excessive administration of carbohydrate or fat and can result in hepatic steatosis, hyperglycemia, and pulmonary compromise. Underfeeding leads to poor wound healing, impaired organ function, and altered immunologic status.

There are multiple methods for assessing energy requirements in the critically ill. Some methods actually measure energy expenditure, such as indirect calorimetry, and some predict caloric requirements with various equations, such as the Harris-Benedict Equation (Table 66.3). Each method of determination carries advantages as well as disadvantages. Indirect calorimetry currently remains the gold standard, and is the preferred method for assessment of energy requirements in critically ill patients. However, it is expensive to perform routinely, and many facilities do not have the equipment or trained personnel to conduct the studies. Also, indirect calorimetry can be inaccurate under a variety of circumstances that commonly affect critically ill patients, such as patients receiving greater than 70% FiO_2, or in those with malfunctioning chest tubes or endotracheal tubes in which the expired gas is not completely captured. Therefore, many clinicians rely upon predictive equations for determining energy needs. It is important to know the flaws of these equations to optimally interpret the results. The final estimate of energy needs assumes that the patients demonstrate a predictable metabolic response to their illness. The equations may overestimate the caloric needs of patients who are mechanically ventilated and sedated. Chemical neuromuscular paralysis, which is commonly used as an adjunct to the management of ventilated patients, can decrease the energy requirements of the critically ill patient by as much as 30%.[3] The calculated results are only as accurate as the variables used in the equation. Obesity and resuscitative water weight complicate the use of these equations and lead to a tendency for overfeeding.[7] However, when considering all forms and phases of critical illness, energy requirements can generally range from 20 to 40 kcal/kg lean body mass/day. Patients with extensive burns or head injury may fall at the higher end. In most cases, 20 to 30 kcal/kg per day is a reasonable initial estimate of energy requirements in critically ill adult patients (see Table 66.4). Most clinicians will use an ideal or estimated lean body mass for those individuals who are obese, to avoid overfeeding. For marasmic patients, it is important to use actual body weight to avoid overfeeding when calculating initial energy requirements.

Protein Requirements

Protein metabolism during metabolic stress is characterized by a net proteolysis. In addition to muscle proteolysis, increased ureagenesis, increased hepatic synthesis of acute

TABLE 66.3

Selected Methods for Estimating Energy Requirements

Harris-Benedict Equation — Estimates Basal Energy Expenditure (BEE)

Male: 13.75 (W) + 5 (H) – 6.76 (A) + 66.47
Female: 9.56 (W) + 1.85 (H) – 4.68 (A) + 655.1

W: weight in kilograms; H: height in centimeters; A: age in years
Note: to predict total energy expenditure (TEE) add an injury/activity factor of 1.2 to 1.8 depending on the severity and nature of illness

Ireton-Jones Energy Expenditure Equations (EEE)

Obesity
EEE = (606 × S) + (9 × W) – (12 × A) + (400 × V) + 1444

Spontaneously Breathing Patients
EEE (s) = 629 – 11 (A) + 25 (W) – 609 (O)

Ventilator Dependent Patients
EEE (v) = 1925 – 10 (A) + 5 (W) + 281 (S) + 292 (T) + 851 (B)

Where EEE = kcal/day, v = ventilator dependent, s= spontaneously breathing
A: age in years
W: body weight in kilograms
S: sex (male = 1, female = 0)
V: ventilator support (present = 1, absent = 0)
T: diagnosis of trauma (present = 1, absent = 0)
B: diagnosis of burn (present = 1, absent = 0)
O: obesity > 30% above IBW from 1959 Metropolitan Life Insurance tables (present = 1, absent = 0)

Curreri Burn Formula (EEE: Estimated Energy Expenditure)

EEE for 18-59 years old = (25 kcal × Wt) + (40 × % TBSA burn)
EEE for > 60 years old = BEE + (65 × % TBSA burn)
EEE = kcal/day; Wt: weight in kilograms; TBSA: total body surface area burn

TABLE 66.4

Energy and Substrate Recommendations

Kcalories	20-30 kcal/kg per day
Protein[a]	1.5-2.0 g/kg per day or 20-25% of total kcal
Carbohydrate[b]	≤ 4-5 mg/kg/min per day or 50-60% of total kcal
Fat[c]	15-30% of total kcal
Fluids	1 mL/kcal; maintain optimal urine output
Electrolytes	Maintain normal levels, especially Mg^{2+}, PO^{4-}, K^{+}
Vitamins/minerals	Recommended Daily Allowance; add vitamin K

[a] Adjust protein delivery for renal and hepatic dysfunction.
[b] Adjust glucose administration to maintain serum glucose levels ≤150 gm/dl.
[c] Adjust lipid delivery based on serum triglyceride levels.

phase proteins, increased urinary nitrogen losses, and the increased use of amino acids as oxidative substrate for energy production are also noted. Therefore, the protein needs of critically ill patients are significantly increased compared to those patients with simple starvation. Although the high catabolic rate is not reversed by provision of glucose and protein,[8] the protein synthetic rate is responsive to amino acid infusions, and nitrogen balance is attained through the support of protein synthesis.[9,10] Current recommendations for stressed patients is for 20 to 25% of the total nutrient intake to be provided as protein. This equates to roughly 1.5 to 2.0 g/kg/day, providing the higher range to promote nitrogen equilibrium or at least minimize nitrogen deficit. Excess protein administration has not been shown to be beneficial, and in fact can cause azotemia.[11]

Carbohydrate Requirements

Glucose is the main fuel for the central nervous system (CNS), bone marrow, and injured tissue. A minimum of about 100 g per day is necessary to maintain CNS function. In the metabolically stressed adult, the maximum rate of glucose oxidation is 4 to 7 mg/kg/minute,[12] roughly equivalent to 400 to 700 g/day in a 70-kg person. Provision of glucose greater than this rate usually results in lipogenesis[13] and hyperglycemia. In the hypermetabolic patient, part of the oxidized glucose will be derived from endogenous amino acid substrates via gluconeogenesis. In the severely stressed patient, up to 2 mg/kg/min of glucose may be provided via gluconeogenesis and this endogenous production is poorly suppressed by exogenous glucose administration.[11] In fact, providing additional glucose in these situations can lead to severe hyperglycemia. Exogenous insulin delivery tends to be ineffective with increasing cellular glucose uptake in critically ill patients, since the rate of glucose oxidation is already maximized and because endogenous insulin concentrations are already elevated. Complications of excess glucose administration include hyperglycemia, hyperosmolar states, excess carbon dioxide production, and hepatic steatosis.[11,13] Therefore, it is recommended that glucose be provided at a rate ≤5 mg/kg/min or approximately 50 to 60% of total energy requirements in critically ill patients, and that they be monitored closely for metabolic complications as described above.

Lipid Requirements

Lipids become an important substrate in critically ill patients as they can facilitate protein sparing, decrease the risk of excess carbohydrate, limit volume delivery by their high caloric density, and provide essential fatty acids. Endogenous triglyceride breakdown continues in hypermetabolic patients despite increased plasma levels of glucose and insulin.[14] Daily fat can be provided without adverse effect, as critically ill patients efficiently metabolize exogenous lipids.[15] Fat may comprise 10 to 30% of total energy requirements, with a minimum of 2 to 4% as essential fatty acids to prevent deficiency. Hypermetabolic patients should be monitored for tolerance of lipid delivery, especially if high levels are provided, as it may cause metabolic complications.

These include hyperlipidemia, impaired immune function, and hypoxemia resulting from impaired diffusing capacity and ventilation/perfusion abnormalities. These complications are associated with intravenous infusions and are not only due to the quantity of lipids provided, but also result from the rate of delivery. The rate of infusion should not exceed 0.1 g/kg/hr. Complications may be minimized by infusing lipids continuously over 18 to 24 hours while monitoring serum triglyceride levels and liver function tests to assure tolerance.

The current intravenous lipids available in the U.S. are composed of nearly 100% long-chain triglyceride (LCT) as omega-6 fatty acids, whereas enteral formulations contain mixtures of LCT and medium-chain triglycerides (MCT). In the past several years research has shown that high levels of omega-6 fatty acids provided in critically ill patients can be immunosuppressive.[16] Large and rapid infusions of LCTs favor the production of arachidonic acid and its proinflammatory metabolites such as prostaglandin E_2 (PGE_2), leukotrienes of the 4 series, and thromboxanes.[16-18] Also, LCTs are dependent upon carnitine for

TABLE 66.5

Electrolyte Recommendations for Critically Ill Patients

Electrolyte	Daily Needs (mEq/day)	Reasons for Increased Needs	Reasons for Decreased Needs
Sodium	70-100	Loop diuretics, cerebral salt wasting	Hypertension, fluid overload
Potassium	70-100	Refeeding syndrome, diuretic therapy, amphotericin wasting	Renal failure
Chloride	80-120	Prolonged gastric losses	Acid-base balance
Phosphorus	10-30 mmol/day	Refeeding syndrome	Renal failure
Magnesium	8-24	Refeeding syndrome, diruetic therapy, ↑ GI losses	—
Calcium	5-20	↑ Blood products	—

transfer from cytosol to the mitochondria to undergo beta-oxidation. It has been postulated that critically ill patients have a relative carnitine deficiency[19] due to an increased excretion, thus limiting the oxidation of LCT. MCTs, on the other hand, do not require carnitine for transport and are rapidly and efficiently oxidized to carbon dioxide and water within 24 hours. When MCT is delivered enterally, a significant portion is absorbed into the portal system, thereby bypassing the GI lymphatic LCT absorptive system. MCTs have been shown to be better tolerated in many situations, as they require minimal biliary and pancreatic secretion for absorption. The ideal ratio of LCT:MCT for critically ill patients is currently not known.

Fluid and Electrolytes

Critical illness disrupts normal fluid and electrolyte homeostasis. Sepsis, systemic inflammatory response syndrome (SIRS), gastrointestinal losses, delivery of medications, and acid-base disturbances contribute to the imbalances. Electrolyte deficiencies usually reflect shifts in concentrations between intravascular and extravascular as well as intracellular and extracellular spaces rather than total body depletion. Wound healing and anabolism have been shown to increase requirements of phosphorus, magnesium, and potassium. Altered electrolyte levels can impair organ function and are usually manifested by cardiac dysrhythmias, ileus, and impaired mentation. Fluid and electrolytes should be provided to maintain adequate urine output and normal serum electrolytes, with emphasis on the intracellular electrolytes, potassium, phosphorus, and magnesium. These are required for protein synthesis and the attainment of nitrogen balance. Once nutrition support is initiated, these electrolytes should be monitored closely, as they may deplete rapidly once adequate protein and kcalories have been provided and the patient shifts from catabolism to anabolism. Electrolytes can be safely provided in doses specified in Table 66.5.

Vitamins, Trace Elements, and Minerals

Currently there are no specific guidelines regarding vitamin and mineral requirements in the critically ill. It is presumed that needs are increased during stress and sepsis due to increased metabolic demands; however objective data to support supplementation is lacking. The antioxidant vitamins and minerals have received the most recent attention. Oxygen-free radicals and other reactive oxygen metabolites are believed to be generated during critical illness (trauma, surgery, reperfusion injury, acute respiratory distress syndrome, infection, burns). This response is most likely mediated by release of cytokines and initiation of an acute phase response and redistribution of hepatic protein synthesis.[20] Along

TABLE 66.6

Recommended Vitamin and Mineral Supplementation in the Critically Ill

	Enteral	Parenteral
Vitamin A	800-1000 μg RE	660 μg RE
Vitamin D	5-10 μg	5 μg
Vitamin E	8-10 mg TE	10 mg TE
Vitamin C	60-100 mg	100 mg
Vitamin K	70-140 μg	0.7-2.0 mg
Folate	200 μg	400 μg
Niacin	13-19 mg NE	40 mg NE
Riboflavin	1.2-1.6 mg	3.6 mg
Thiamine	1.0-1.5 mg	3 mg
Pyridoxine	1.8-2.2 mg	4 mg
Cyanocobalamin	2.0 μg	5.0 μg
Pantothenic acid	4.7 mg	15 mg
Biotin	30-100 μg	60 μg
Potassium	1875-5625 mg	60-100 mEq
Sodium	1100-3300 mg	60-100 mEq
Chloride	1700-5100 mg	—
Fluoride	1.5-4.0 mg	—
Calcium	800-1200 mg	600 mg
Phosphorus	800-1200 mg	600 mg
Magnesium	300-400 mg	10-20 mEq
Iron	10-15 mg	1-7 mg
Zinc*	12-15 mg	2.5-4.0* mg
Iodine	150 μg	70-140 μg
Copper	1.5-3 mg	300-500 μg
Manganese	2-5 mg	0.15-0.8 mg
Chromium	0.05-0.2 mg	10-20 μg
Selenium	0.05-0.2 mg	40-80 μg
Molybdenum	75-250 μg	100-200 μg

* Additional 2 mg in acute catabolic states.

with increased levels of free radicals, decreased levels of circulating vitamins C and E have been found after surgery, trauma, burns, sepsis, and long-term parenteral nutrition.[21-25]

Supplementation of large doses of antioxidants in critical illness has not consistently been shown to be beneficial. Current studies in progress are addressing supplementation at various levels and combinations. Apparently, providing more than therapeutic doses of single vitamins or minerals can be harmful by potentially upsetting the balance of metabolic pathways. Current recommendations are to provide the recommended dietary allowance for vitamins and minerals in the critically ill. Enteral formulations contain this recommended level when they are provided at specified volumes. If those volumes are not tolerated, patients should be supplemented intravenously.

Route of Nutrient Delivery

Parenteral vs. Enteral Nutrition

Despite nutrition intervention, critically ill patients undergo an obligatory loss of lean body tissue secondary to the hypercatabolic response of stress as previously described. If

TABLE 66.7

Indications for Parenteral Nutrition

Short bowel syndrome
Malabsorption
Intractable emesis or diarrhea
Severe pancreatitis
Bowel obstruction
Prolonged ileus
High output GI fistula
Unsuccessful enteral access

patients lose greater than 40% of their lean body mass, irreversible changes occur which make survival unlikely. This can occur as soon as 30 days after a serious metabolic insult if the patient is not nutritionally supported. Protein-calorie malnutrition, as a result of hypermetabolic stress, also leads to decreased immune function with subsequent increased infection risk. Impaired wound healing also becomes significant. Therefore, as stated previously, the primary goals of nutrition support in the critically ill are to preserve lean body mass, avoid metabolic complications, and preserve the body's immune function.

The ideal route of nutrition intervention in the critically ill has been well studied. Although total parenteral nutrition (TPN) has been lifesaving and has been successful in reversing malnutrition in many disease states (Table 66.7), several recent studies have found it to have potentially profound negative side effects. It has become more apparent that parenteral formulations currently available in the U.S. may in fact be systemically immunosuppressive, deliver imbalanced nutrient solutions, and alter nutrient uptake and utilization (Table 66.8).[26-28] TPN allows for more rapid achievement of nutrient requirements than enteral nutrition, but also allows for increased nitrogen excretion.[29] TPN has also been associated with a higher rate of hyperglycemia, adding to patient immunocompromise with decreased neutrophil chemotaxis, phagocytosis, oxidative burst, and superoxide production.[30,31] In animal models, TPN is associated with increasing the metabolic stress response, allowing atrophy of the gut mucosa, systemic immunocompromise, and altering gut flora when compared with enteral nutrition.[32-37] More recently, clinical research trials have suggested that TPN therapy may in fact be harmful. Prospective clinical trials

TABLE 66.8

Enteral vs. Parenteral Nutrition

Advantages	Disadvantages
Enteral	
Increased mucosal blood flow	Often difficult to access
Decreased septic morbidity	Aspiration risk
Preservation of gut flora and integrity	GI intolerance
Maintenance of GI hormone axis	Interruptions common
Balanced nutrient delivery	
Parenteral	
Ease of delivery	Overfeeding
Precise nutrient delivery	Exaggerated cytokine response
	Intestinal mucosal atrophy
	Decreased GALT and secretory IgA
	Decreased systemic immunity
	Increased cost

evaluating perioperative TPN have shown that subjects receiving TPN had greater postoperative infectious morbidity rates than those receiving no nutrition intervention.[38-40]

One of the more clinically relevant effects of enteral feeding is the incidence of septic complications.[41] This is most likely related to maintenance of the gut associated lymphoid tissue (GALT) and mucosal integrity. In review of the immunoglobulin-producing cells in the body, the bone marrow, spleen, and extra-GI tract lymph nodes together comprise about 2.5×10^{10} cells; the GI tract from mouth to anus comprises about 8.5×10^{10} immunoglobulin-producing cells. So, clearly 60% of the body's immunoglobulin-producing ability lies in the GI tract. When not utilizing the GI tract, a significant alteration in immune function can be expected. In review of the literature comparing parenteral to enteral nutrition, the gut has become recognized as a metabolically active, immunologically important, and bacteriologically decisive organ in critically ill patients.[42-44]

Low Flow States

Although research supports providing enteral nutrition in critically ill patients, it is often difficult to provide full energy requirements due to patient intolerance. Approximately 20% of the critically ill patient population is intolerant of enteral feeding. The etiology of this intolerance is often multifactorial. One clinically significant factor is low intestinal blood flow. Intestinal ischemia and reperfusion is an important determinant of the subsequent development of the posttraumatic proinflammatory state and multiple organ failure (MOF). Although the gut is able to increase its oxygen extraction up to tenfold in a normal state, it remains extremely vulnerable to ischemic injury during low flow states. Low flow not only exhibits negative effects on mucosal oxygenation and barrier maintenance,[45-47] but also has adverse effects on motility. It is now known that sepsis, endotoxemia, and low flow states have significant negative effects on GI tract motility, with the colon being the most affected, followed by the stomach and small intestine, respectively.[48] Low flow states also cause decreases in nutrient absorption, with protein absorption believed to be significantly altered; carbohydrate and lipid absorption are also altered, but to a lesser degree.[49]

A number of patient populations are at high risk for low flow states. These include those with sepsis, necrotizing enterocolitis, multiple trauma, intra-aortic balloon pump, coronary artery bypass pump, and those who undergo thoracoabdominal aortic aneurysm repair with cross-clamping of the mesenteric vessels.[50,51]

Gut perfusion can be indirectly assessed using tonometric techniques to measure the gastric intramucosal pH (pHi).[52] Trauma patients with a pHi <7.32 and otherwise adequate central hemodynamics and oxygen transport 24 hours after ICU admission showed a higher rate of MOF and mortality compared to a group of patients with adequate central and intestinal perfusion.[53] Several other investigators have attempted to improve the pH in critically ill patients by improving global perfusion, but they were not successful in decreasing mortality or MOF.[54,55] A drawback to this approach has been the inability to selectively improve gut perfusion in the setting of otherwise adequate systemic perfusion. The question remains whether enteral nutrient delivery during low flow states increases potential gut ischemia or whether increased blood flow associated with enteral feeding protects the mucosa. Several investigators using animal models have found that enteral nutrient delivery at low rates will enhance visceral blood flow during low flow states.[56-60]

After trauma or major metabolic insult, ileus commonly results, lasting 24 to 48 hours in the stomach and about 48 to 72 hours in the large intestine. In the small intestine, gut motility returns to near normal 12 to 24 hours after the insult. Several hemodynamic factors can affect the duration of ileus, such as elevated intracranial pressure and significant hyperglycemia. Generally, if small bowel access is available, critically ill patients may be fed enterally as soon as eight hours after insult. Three recent studies have attempted to address the question of how much nutrient delivered into the GI tract is required to yield the immune benefits.[61-63] From these studies it can be estimated that only 15 to 30% of caloric requirements delivered enterally is needed to provide the immune benefits. In other words, full measured or estimated nutrient requirements are not required to be delivered enterally in order to obtain the immunologic and mucosal protective effects. In fact, attempting to obtain 100% of nutrient requirements in critically ill patients often results in intolerance of early enteral feeding. Therefore, a clinically rational approach to enteral feeding in critically ill populations is to initiate and maintain feedings at a low rate (10 to 20 ml/h) until tolerance is demonstrated. Signs of intolerance include abdominal distention and pain, hypermotility, significant ileus, pneumatosis intestinalis, significant increase in nasogastric tube output, and uncontrollable diarrhea. Enteral feeding should only be advanced according to patient tolerance, and decreased or discontinued if any of the above symptoms are present. Most critically ill patients will tolerate full enteral feeds within five to seven days, but if goal tube feedings are not tolerated after five to seven days of injury, then it is appropriate to start parenteral nutrition to either provide the balance of the nutrient requirements or provide full nutrition support as clinically indicated.

Nutrition Support in Trauma and Burns

Trauma and burn patients exhibit similar metabolic alterations as described earlier in critical illness, except that the metabolic alterations often occur to a much greater extent. Few traumatic injuries result in a hypermetabolic state comparable to that of a major burn. As the skin functions to maintain body temperature and fluid balance, loss of this protective barrier leads to excessive fluid, electrolyte, heat, and protein losses.[64] Thermal injury induces hypermetabolism of varying intensity and duration depending on the extent and depth of the body surface affected, the presence of infection, and the efficacy of early treatment.[65] Energy requirements peak at approximately postburn day 12, and typically slowly normalize as the percentage of open wound decreases with reepithelialization or skin grafting.[64] Although still debated, there is no single agent that is entirely responsible for the dramatic rise in metabolic needs observed during the flow phase of burn injury.[66] Rather, the etiology of hypermetabolism appears to be multifactorial (Table 66.9). As

TABLE 66.9

Factors Known to Affect Metabolic Rate in Burn Patients

Activity	Other trauma or injuries
Age	Pain
Ambient temperature and humidity	Physical Therapy
Anxiety	Preexisting medical conditions
Body surface area	Sepsis
Convalescence	Sleep deprivation
Dressing changes	Surgery
Drugs and anesthesia	Treatments rendered
Evaporative heat loss	Type and severity of injury
Gender	
Hormonal and non-hormonal influences	
Lean body mass	
Metabolic cost of various nutrients when digested and absorbed	

Adapted from Mayes T, Gottschlich M. In: *Contemporary Nutrition Support Practice* W.B. Saunders, Philadelphia, 1998: pg 590-607.

TABLE 66.10

Select Nutrients and Their Immune Effect During Critical Illness

Nutrient	Immune Effect
Carbohydrate	↓ (if provision results in blood glucose levels > 200 mg/dL)
Protein	
Glutamine	↑
Arginine	↑
Fat	
n-6 fatty acids	↓ (in large amounts)
n-3 fatty acids	↑
Micronutrients	
Vitamin A	↑ (in burns)
Vitamin C	↑ (in burns)
Vitamin E	??
Zinc	↑ (in burns)
Selenium	↑

previously discussed with critical illness, the goal of acute management in trauma and burns is to stabilize these system-wide effects. Optimal nutrition intervention is an important component in improving immunocompetence, attenuating the hypermetabolic response, and minimizing losses in lean body mass. As in critical illness, enteral feeding is preferred to parenteral. A few select nutrients have been shown to have an impact on the immune system in critical illness (Table 66.10).

Estimating Nutrient Requirements

Energy

Burn patients require individualized nutrition plans to provide optimal energy and protein to accelerate muscle and protein synthesis and minimize proteolysis.[67] There are numerous predictive equations to estimate energy needs in burn patients (Table 66.3).

Several studies have reviewed the accuracy of predictive equations in determining energy requirements in burn patients.[68-70] The consensus appears to be that predictive equations tend to overestimate energy expenditure, and the preferred method of determining energy requirements is by using indirect calorimetry. If indirect calorimetry is not available in the clinical situation, it is suggested that REE can be estimated as 50 to 60% above the Harris-Benedict equation for burns >20% of total body surface area.[71]

Protein

Trauma and sepsis initiate a cascade of events that leads to accelerated protein degradation, decreased rates of synthesis of selected proteins, and increased amino acid catabolism and nitrogen loss. Clinical consequences of these metabolic alterations may increase morbidity and mortality of patients, causing serious organ dysfunction and impaired host defenses. Therefore, trauma and burn patients require increased amounts of protein in attempts to minimize endogenous proteolysis as well as support the large losses from wound exudate. In a landmark study, Alexander et al. found that providing 23% of energy as protein in burned patients resulted in fewer systemic infections and a lower mortality rate when compared to providing 16.5% of energy as protein.[72] Results of another study recommended that burn patients receive 1.5 to 3.0 g/kg/d protein with a nonprotein kcalorie to gram nitrogen ratio of 100:1.[73] More recent studies have questioned these high amounts of protein, as they may cause excessive urea production[74] and protein depletion that is related to altered muscle amino acid transport[67] and/or activation of the ubiquitin-proteasome pathway.[75] Overall recommendations are to provide 1.5 to 2.0, rarely up to 3.0, g protein per kilogram body weight per day in attempts to minimize protein losses. Providing these higher levels of protein requires continuous monitoring of fluid status, blood urea nitrogen, and serum creatinine because of the high renal solute load.

In addition to the quantity of protein provided, the protein quality is also significant. The use of high-biologic value protein, such as whey or casein rather than soy, is preferred for burn patients. Whey protein has been further endorsed over casein due to its beneficial effects on burned children, improvement in tube feeding tolerance, enhanced solubility at low gastric pH, greater digestibility, and improved nitrogen retention.[66] Pharmacologic doses of the single amino acids, arginine and glutamine, have also been explored as to their benefit in critical illness and burns.

Glutamine

Glutamine is known to be a major fuel source for rapidly dividing cells such as enterocytes, reticulocytes, and lymphocytes. In normal metabolic states, glutamine is a non-essential amino acid. However during times of metabolic stress, glutamine is implicated as being conditionally essential as it has been shown to be needed for maintenance of gut metabolism, structure, and function.[76-78] Despite the accelerated skeletal muscle release of amino acids, blood glutamine levels are not increased after burns.[79] In fact, decreased plasma glutamine levels have been reported after severe burns, multiple trauma, or multiple organ failure.[65]

A number of studies have shown beneficial effects with supplemental glutamine, its precursors (ornithine α-ketoglutarate and α-ketoglutarate),[80] or glutamine dipeptides (alanine-glutamine, glycine-glutamine).[81] These studies deliver glutamine in pharmacologic doses of 25 to 35% of the dietary protein.[82] Supplemental glutamine has been shown to have multiple benefits to include increased nitrogen retention and muscle mass,[83] maintenance of the GI mucosa,[84] permeability,[85] preserved immune function,[86] reduced infections,[87] as well as preserved organ glutathione levels (Table 66.11).[88] These protective effects of glutamine supplementation could have significant effects on morbidity and mortality in trauma and burn patients. Safety and cost effectiveness of glutamine supplementation in trauma and burns continues to be researched.

TABLE 66.11

Benefits of Human Glutamine Supplementation

Benefits of Human Glutamine Supplementation
↑ Nitrogen balance
Enhanced gut barrier function
↓ Systemic infections
↓ Ventilator days
↓ Hospital stay
↓ Hospital expense
↓ Sepsis, bacteremia
↑ Survival
Maintenance of tissue glutathione levels

Arginine

Arginine, like glutamine, has gained recent attention in critical care nutrition, and like glutamine is considered a conditionally essential amino acid. Arginine is the specific precursor for nitric oxide production as well as a potent secretagogue for anabolic hormones such as insulin, prolactin, and growth hormone. Under normal circumstances, arginine is considered a non-essential amino acid since it is adequately synthesized endogenously via the urea cycle. However, research suggests that during times of metabolic stress, optimal amounts of arginine are not synthesized to promote tissue regeneration or positive nitrogen balance.[66]

Studies in animal and humans have investigated the effects of supplemental arginine in various injury models. Positive outcomes from supplementation include improved nitrogen balance,[89,90] wound healing,[91-94] immune function,[91-96] and increased anabolic hormones, insulin, and growth hormone.[97] The outcomes are of special interest in the post-trauma and burn patient during the flow phase, when enhancement of these processes would yield the greatest advantage.

However, despite these positive effects, caution with excessive arginine supplementation is warranted in burn patients due to its potential effects on nitric oxide production. The possibility that increased nitric oxide production from arginine supplementation may affect septic patients has not been addressed. Recently it has been shown that marked deregulation of arteriolar tone in patients with endotoxemia septic shock and increased permeability to bacteria in critically ill patients are induced by nitric oxide.[98] Although arginine supplementation for non-septic burn and trauma patients in amounts sufficient to normalize serum and intracellular levels (~2% of kcalories) appears safe and beneficial, the effects of arginine supplementation on nitric oxide production in septic burn patients should be carefully evaluated.[65]

Lipid

Lipid is an important component of a trauma or burn patient's diet for many reasons, as it is an isoosmotic concentrated energy source at 9 kcalories per gram. Carbohydrate and protein provide half as many kcalories as fat and can significantly contribute to the osmolality of the enteral or parenteral formulations. Dietary lipid is also a carrier for fat-soluble vitamins as well as a provider of essential fatty acids, linoleic, and linolenic acids. These essential fatty acids should comprise a minimum of 4% of kcalories in the diet to prevent deficiencies. This often equates to ~10% of total kcalories as fat, since most sources do not solely contain essential fatty acid.

Even though lipids are required in critical illness, excess lipid can be detrimental. Excessive lipid administration has been associated with hyperlipidemia, fatty liver immune suppression, and impaired clotting ability.[99] All of the long-chain fatty acids share the same enzyme systems, as they are elongated and desaturated with each pathway competitive, based upon substrate availability. Dietary fatty acids modulate the phospholipid cell membrane composition and the type and quantities of eicosanoids produced (Figure 66.1). Prostaglandins of the 3 series (PGE3) and series 5 leukotrienes have proven to be anti-inflammatory and immune-enhancing agents.[100,101] Also, PGE3 is a potent vasodilator.[102] These concepts have received considerable attention for the potential of n-3 fatty acids ability to enhance immune function and reduce acute and chronic inflammation.

In most standard enteral formulations, the fat source is predominantly n-6 fatty acids, with a portion coming from medium-chain triglycerides. Formulations supplemented with fish oil, a rich source of n-3 fatty acids (eicosapentenoic [EPA] and docosahexanoic acids [DHA]), and canola oil (alpha-linolenic acid) are now available. Clinical trials utilizing

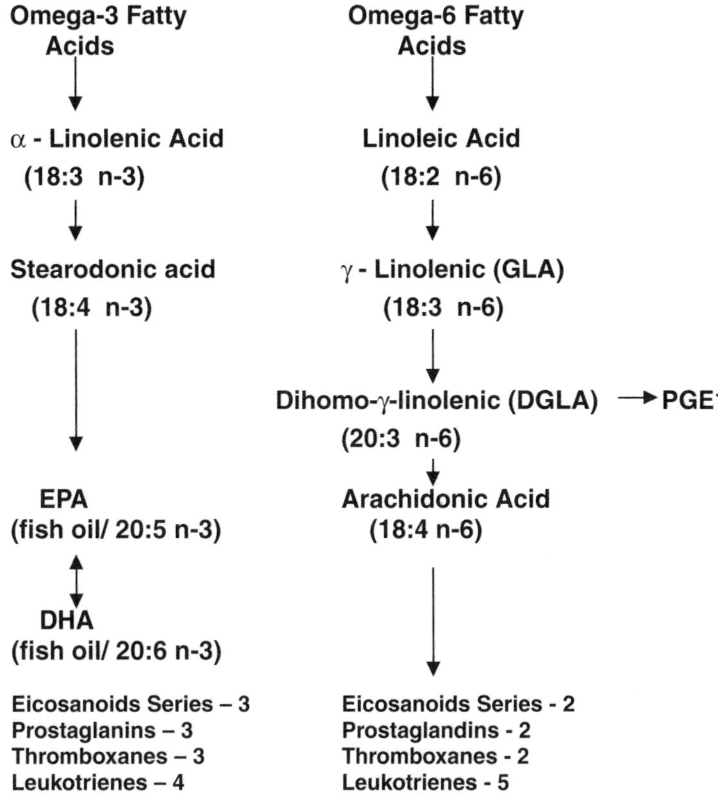

FIGURE 66.1
Metabolism of dietary long-chain fatty acids. EPA — eicosapentenoic acid, DHA — docosahexanoic acid.

these formulations have shown positive benefits in patients with psoriasis,[103] rheumatoid arthritis,[104] burns,[105,106] sepsis,[107,108] and trauma.[109] These benefits are thought to be due to alterations in eicosanoid and leukotriene production, with decreased arachidonic acid metabolites (e.g, PGE2), as well as increased production of the less biologically active trienoic prostaglandins and pentaenoic leukotrienes.[110]

For burn and multiple trauma patients, the recommended amount of total fat delivery is 12 to 15% of total kcalories, with at least 4% coming from essential fatty acids.[65] Provision of formulations with n-3 fatty acids, especially EPA and DHA, is of particular interest for the potential anti-inflammatory and immune-enhancing benefits as described above. Many enteral formulations do not contain these exact proportions of fat and typically have greater amounts, often leading to modular modification. Current parenteral formulations available in the U.S. (Jan. 2000) contain nearly 100% n-6 fatty acids and should not comprise ≥15 to 25% of the total kcalories as fat when delivered to the burn or severely traumatized patient.

Micronutrients

Micronutrients function as coenzymes and cofactors in metabolic pathways at the cellular level. With the increased energy and protein demands associated with traumatic and burn injury, one would expect increased need for vitamins and minerals. In addition, increased nutrient losses from open wounds and altered metabolism, absorption, and excretion, would also be anticipated to have requirements beyond the Recommended Dietary Allow-

TABLE 66.12

Nutrient Recommendations for Burn Patients[a]

Protein	20-25% of total kcalories
Fat	10-15% of total kcalories
Carbohydrate	60-70% of total kcalories (5 mg/kg/min per day)
Vitamins and minerals	Multivitamin and mineral *AND* *Vitamin C*: 500 mg twice daily *Vitamin A*: 5000 IU per 1000 kcalories of enteral nutrition *Zinc*: 220 mg of zinc sulfate (or other compound to provide 45 mg elemental zinc/d)

[a] Patients >40 pounds.

Adapted from Mayes T, Gottschlich M. In: *Contemporary Nutrition Support Practice* W.B. Saunders, Philadelphia, 1998: pg 590-607.

ances. Various vitamins and minerals have also been found to aid with wound healing, immune function, and other biologic functions. Unfortunately, few data are available to support exact requirements during these hypermetabolic states. However, a few studies[111,112] support recommendations in burn patients for vitamin A, vitamin C, and zinc (Table 66.12).

References

1. McWhirter JP, Pennington CR. *Br Med J* 308:945; 1994.
2. Kinney J. *Crit Care Clin* 11:569; 1995.
3. Barton RG. *Nutr Clin Prac* 9:127; 1994.
4. Chiolero R, Revelly JP, Tappy L. *Nutrition* 13:45S; 1997.
5. Gabay C, Kushner I. *N Engl J Med* 340:448; 1999.
6. Flancbaum L, Choban PS, Sambucco S, Verducci J, Burge J. *Am J Clin Nutr* 69:461; 1999.
7. Cutts ME, Dowdy RP, Ellersieck MR, Edes TE. *Am J Clin Nutr* 66:1250; 1997.
8. Elwyn DH. *Crit Care Med* 8:9; 1980.
9. Cerra FB, Siegel JH, Coleman B, et al. *Ann Surg* 192:570; 1980.
10. Shaw JHF, Wildbore M, Wolfe RR. *Ann Surg* 205:288; 1987.
11. Cerra FB. *Surgery* 101:1; 1987.
12. Wolfe R, Allsop J, Burke J. *Metabolism* 28:210; 1979.
13. Burke J, Wolfe R, Mullany C, et al. *Ann Surg* 190:279; 1979.
14. Shaw J, Wolfe R. *Ann Surg* 209:63; 1989.
15. Nordenstrom J, Carpentier YA, Askanazi J, et al. *Ann Surg* 198:725; 1983.
16. Meydani SN, Dinarello CA. *Nutr Clin Prac* 8:65; 1993.
17. Alexander J. *Nutrition* 14:627; 1998.
18. Drumi W, Fischer M, Ratheiser K. *J Parent Enteral Nutr* 22:217; 1998.
19. Brenner J. *Physiol Rev* 63:1420; 1983.
20. Goode HF, Webster NR. Clin Intensive Care 4:265; 1993.
21. Goode HF, Cowley HC, Walker BE, et al. *Crit Care Med* 23:646; 1995.
22. Boosalis MG, Edlund D, Moudry B, et al. *Nutrition* 4:431; 1988.
23. Louw JA, Werbeck A, Louw ME, et al. *Crit Care Med* 20:934; 1992.
24. Downing C, Piripitsi A, Bodenham A, Schorah CJ. *Proc Nutr Soc* 52:314A; 1993.
25. Lemoyne M, Van Gossum A, Kurian R, Jeejeebhoy KN. *Am J Clin Nutr* 48:1310; 1988.
26. McQuiggan MM, Marvin RG, McKinley BA, Moore FA. *New Horizons* 7:131; 1999.
27. Piccone VA, LeVeen HH, Glass P. *Surgery* 87:263; 1980.
28. Enrione EB, Gelfand MJ, Morgan D, et al. *J Surg Res* 40:320; 1986.
29. Moore FA, Feliciano DV, Andrassy RJ, et al. *Ann Surg* 216:62; 1992.

30. Moore FA, Moore EE, Jones TN, et al. *J Trauma* 29:916; 1989.
31. McArdle AH, Palmason C, Morency I, et al. *Surgery* 90:616; 1981.
32. Mochizuki H, Trocki O, Dominioni L, et al. *Ann Surg* 200:297; 1984.
33. Alverdy J, Chi HS, Sheldon GF. *Ann Surg* 202:681; 1985.
34. Kudsk KA, Carpenter G, Peterson SR, et al. *J Surg Res* 31:105; 1981.
35. Birkhan RH, Renk CM *Am J Clin Nutr* 39:45; 1984.
36. Meyer J, Yurt RW, Dehaney R. *Surg Gyn Ob* 167:50; 1988.
37. Lowry SF. *J Trauma* 330:20S; 1990.
38. Sandstrom R, Drott C, Hyltander A, et al. *Ann Surg* 217:183; 1993.
39. Veterans Affair Total Parenteral Cooperative Study Group. *N Engl J Med* 325:525; 1991.
40. Brennan MF, Pisters PWT, Posner M, et al. *Ann Surg* 220:436; 1994.
41. Kudsk KA, Croce MA, Fabian TC, et al. *Ann Surg* 215:503; 1992.
42. Wilmore DW, Smith RJ, O'Dwyer ST, et al. *Surgery* 104:917; 1988.
43. Page CP. *Am J Surg* 158:485; 1989.
44. Border JR, Hassett J, LaDuca J, et al. *Ann Surg* 206:427; 1987.
45. Ohri SK, Somasundaram S, Koak Y, et al. *Gastroenterology* 106:318; 1994.
46. Fink MP. *Crit Care Med* 21:54; 1993.
47. Flynn MP. *Crit Care Med* 19:627; 1991.
48. Singh G, Harkema JM, Mayberry AJ, et al. *J Trauma* 36:803; 1994.
49. Gardiner K, Barbul A. *JPEN* 17:277; 1993.
50. VanLanschott, Mealy K, Wilmore DW, et al. *Ann Surg* 212:663; 1990.
51. Tokyay R, Loick HM, Traber DL, et al. *Surg Gynecol Obstet* 174:125; 1992.
52. Chang M. *New Horizons* 7:35; 1999.
53. Chang MC, Cheatham MC, Nelson LD, et al. *J Trauma* 37:488; 1994.
54. Ivatury RR, Simon RJ, Islam S, et al. *J Am Coll Surg* 183:145; 1996.
55. Gutierrez G, Palizas F, Doglio G. *Lancet* 339:195; 1992.
56. Fiddian-Green RG, Baker S. *Crit Care Med* 15:153; 1987.
57. Gosche JR, Garrison RN, Harris PD, et al. *Arch Surg* 125:1573; 1990.
58. Flynn WJ, Gosche JR, Garrison RN. *J Surg Res* 52:499; 1992.
59. Purcell PN, Davis R, Branson RD, Johnson DJ. *Am J Surg* 165:188; 1993.
60. Kazamias P, Kotzampass K, Koufogiannis D, et al. *W J Surg* 22:6; 1998.
61. Shou J, Lappin J, Minard EA, Daly JM. *Am J Surg* 167:145; 1994.
62. Sax SC, Illig KA, Ryan CK, et al. *Am J Surg* 171:587; 1996.
63. Okada Y, Klein N, Vansaene HKF, et al. *J Ped Surg* 33:16; 1998.
64. Rutan RL. In: *Burn Care and Therapy.* Mosby, Inc., St. Louis, 1998.
65. De-Souza DA, Greene LJ. *J Nutr* 128:797; 1998.
66. Mayes T, Gottschlich M. In: *Contemporary Nutrition Support Practice* W.B. Saunders Co., Philadelphia, 1998: pg 590.
67. Wolfe RR. *Am J Clin Nutr* 64:800; 1996.
68. Saffle JR, Medina E, Raymond J, et al. *J Trauma* 25:32; 1985.
69. Curreri PW, Richmond D, Marvin J, Baxter CR. *J Am Diet Assoc* 65:415; 1974.
70. Turner WW, Ireton CS, Hunt JL, Baxter CR. *J Trauma* 25:11; 1985.
71. Khorram-Sefat R, Behrendt W, Heiden A, Hettich R. *W J Surgery* 23:115; 1999.
72. Alexander JW, MacMillan BG, Stinnett JD, et al. *Ann Surg* 192:505; 1980.
73. Gottschlich MM, Jenkins M, Warden GD, et al. *J Parent Enteral Nutr* 14:225; 1990.
74. Patterson BW, Nguyen T, Pierre, et al. *Metabolism* 46:573; 1997.
75. Mitch WE, Goldberg AL. *N Engl J Med* 335:1897; 1996.
76. Souba WW, Smith RJ, Wilmore DW. *J Parent Enteral Nutr* 9:608; 1985.
77. Souba WW, Smith RJ, Wilmore DW. *J Surg Res* 42:117; 1987.
78. Souba WW, Wilmore DW. *Arch Surg* 120:66; 1985.
79. Gore DC, Jahoor F. *Arch Surg* 129:1318; 1994.
80. Cynober L. *Nutrition* 7:313, 1991.
81. Furst P, Albers S, Stehle P. *J Parent Enteral Nutr* 14S4:118S; 1990.
82. Wilmore DW. *Gastroenterology* 107:1885; 1994.
83. Stehle P, Wurste N, Puchestein C, et al. *Lancet* 1:231; 1989.

84. Scheppach W, Loges C, Bartran P, et al. *Gastroenterology* 107:429; 1994.
85. Van der Hulst RR, van Kreel BK, von Meyernfeldt MF, et al. *Lancet* 341:1363; 1993.
86. Calder PC. *Clin Nutr* 13:2; 1994.
87. Ziegler TR, Young LS, Benfell K, et al. *Ann Int Med* 116:821; 1992.
88. Furst P. *Proc Nutr Soc* 55:945; 1996.
89. Barbul A, Sisto DA, Wasserkrug HL, et al. *Curr Surg* 40:114; 1963.
90. Sitren HS, Fisher H. *Br J Nutr* 37:195; 1977.
91. Barbul A, Rettura G, Levenson SM, Seifter E. *Am J Clin Nutr* 37:786; 1983.
92. Barbul A, Rettura G, Levenson SM, Seifter E. *Surg Forum* 28:101; 1977.
93. Barbul A, Fishel RS, Shimazu, et al. *J Surg Res* 38:328; 1985.
94. Barbul A, Lazarow SA, Efron DT, et al. *Surgery* 108:331; 1990.
95. Daly JM, Reynolds J, Thom A, et al. *Ann Surg* 208:512; 1988.
96. Saito H, Trocki O, Wang S, et al. *Arch Surg* 122:784; 1987.
97. Barbul A, Wasserkrug HL, Sisto DA, et al. *J Parent Enteral Nutr* 4:446; 1980.
98. Gomez-Jimenez J, Salgado A, Mourelle M, et al. *Crit Care Med* 23:253; 1995.
99. Moore FD. *J Parent Enteral Nutr* 4:228; 1980.
100. Ninneman JL, Stockland AE. *J Trauma* 24:201; 1984.
101. Moncada S. *Stroke* 14:157; 1983.
102. Bittiner SB, Tucker WF, Cartwright I, et al. *Lance*t 1:378; 1988.
103. Kremer JM, Jubiz W, Michalek, et al. *Ann Intern Med* 106:497; 1987.
104. Alexander JW, Saito H, Trocki O, et al. *Ann Surg* 204:1; 1986.
105. Trocki O, Heyd TJ, Waymack JP, et al. *J Parent Enteral Nutr* 11:521; 1986.
106. Barton RG, Wells CL, Carlson A, et al. *J Trauma* 31Z:768; 1991.
107. Peck MD, Ogle CK, Alexander JW. *Ann Surg* 214:74; 1991.
108. Kenler AS, Swails WS, Driscoll DF, et al. *Ann Surg* 223:316; 1996.
109. Barton RG. *Nutr Clin Prac* 12:51; 1997.
110. Gottschlich MM, Warden GD. *J Burn Care Rehabil* 11:275; 1990.
111. Gamliel Z, DeBiase MA, Demling RH. *J Burn Care Rehabil* 17:264; 1996.

67

Nutritional Therapies for Neurological and Psychiatric Disorders

G. Franklin Carl

The major neurological and psychiatric disorders are classified into five general categories (Table 67.1) based primarily on the etiology of the disorder. The epilepsies are resistant to etiological classification. Epilepsies may be genetic, developmental, metabolic, or neurodegenerative. Rather than add epilepsy to each of these categories, the epilepsies are treated separately. However, where a specific metabolic cause for the seizures can be identified, or where the seizures are not the major symptom of the disorder, the disorder will be included in the appropriate other category. For example, biotinidase deficiency causes seizures, but the genetic abnormality is easily identified and treatable with high dose biotin, so for the purposes of this section it will be treated separately under Inborn Errors of Metabolism.

Epilepsies

Epilepsy is a neurological disorder characterized by paroxysmal depolarization of cortical neurons causing the external phenomenon known as a seizure. Epilepsy has many causes, but most seizures stem from a cortical focus in which the depolarization of neurons is uncontrolled. The depolarization may remain confined to a specific area of the cortex or it may generalize from the focus to involve much of the brain. Some forms of epilepsy are nonfocal, initiating with a generalized seizure. The preferred treatment for recurrent seizures is pharmacological.

Antiepileptic drugs are the primary therapy for idiopathic seizures. Phenobarbital, phenytoin, primidone, and ethosuximide were the first line of drugs used to treat seizures in the post-bromide years. They were joined by valproate and carbamazepine in the 1970s. Recently a number of new drugs have been added to the neurologist's pharmacopeia for the treatment of seizures. The newer drugs are being developed to improve efficacy and safety. Side effects include interactions of phenytoin, phenobarbital, and primidone with nutrients including folic acid, carnitine, vitamin D, and vitamin K[1-4] (Table 67.2). Carbamazepine causes increased plasma homocysteine,[5] and valproate has been linked to birth defects.[6] Interestingly, valproate inhibits the folate-dependent glycine cleavage system.[7] It has also been shown to cause carnitine depletion[8] (Table 67.2).

0-8493-2705-9/02/$0.00+$1.50

TABLE 67.1

Classification of the Major Neurological and Psychiatric Disorders and the Potential Response of Each to Nutritional Therapy

Category / Disease or Disease Group / Specific Diseases	Defining Characteristics of the Disease	Response to Nutritional Therapy	Therapy	References
Epilepsies	A diverse group of idiopathic disorders characterized by spontaneous seizures resulting from recurrent paroxysmal cerebral neuronal firing	++++	Ketogenic diet	10,12-14
Neurodegenerative Diseases				
Parkinson's disease	Degeneration of the nigrostriatal tract leading to tremor, muscular rigidity, bradykinesia, and unstable posture	+++	MAOI + MAOI diet	16,18
		+++++	L-DOPA + low protein diet	19-21
Alzheimer's disease	Progressive loss of cognitive function associated with the appearance of amyloid plaques and neurofibrillary tangles in the brain	+++	MAOI + MAOI diet	18,24
		+++	Adequate protein and energy intake + supplements with vitamins E, B_1 & B_{12}	25
Multiple sclerosis	Chronic central demyelinating disease of uncertain cause; may have infectious, autoimmune and genetic components	+	Vitamin D	27
		++	Essential fatty acids	28
Amyotrophic lateral sclerosis	Chronic degeneration of motor neuron function; linked to genetic abnormality of Cu/Zn superoxide dismutase	?	? Vitamin E	30
Guam/ALS/Parkinsons/Dementia	Food-induced, chronic degeneration of cells in PNS and CNS	0		32,33
Tardive dyskinesia	Chronic parkinsonian-like syndrome caused by neuroleptics	+++	Choline supplementation	35
		?	?Vitamin E	34
Neurodevelopmental Diseases				
Neural tube defects	Abnormal development of the neural tube in utero	prevention	Folate supplementation periconceptionally	36
Schizophrenia	Psychoses associated with structural abnormalities in the brain	++	Increased requirements for vitamin C essential fats	42
				43

Affective disorders				
Bipolar disorder	Alternating states of mania and depression	++	Choline supplementation	35
		++	n-3 Polyunsaturated fatty acids	48
Endogenous depression	Depression of mood	+++	Low salt diet	44
		++++	S-adenosylmethionine	45,46
		+++	Folic acid	47
		++	n-3 Polyunsaturated fatty acids	48
Hyperactivity	Attention deficit with hyperactivity Disrupts learning	?	Nutritional treatments controversial	
Metabolic Diseases				
Encephalopathies	Metabolic disturbances that affect CNS			
Wernicke-Korsakoff	Thiamine deficiency often induced by alcohol	++++	Thiamine early in disease process	52
Hepatic encephalopathy	Failure of liver to remove neurotoxins from blood	++++	Lactulose and lactitol	51,54
Neuropathies	Metabolic disturbances that affect PNS			
Pyridoxine toxicity	Sensory polyneuropathy	0	Cease vitamin B_6 megadoses	55
Diabetic neuropathy	Slowly progressing, sensorimotor, autonomic polyneuropathy	prevention	Control of blood glucose	57
Vitamin B_{12} deficiency	Dysmyelination leading to parasthesias and weakness	prevention	Vitamin B_{12} early before dysmyelination	56
Pantothenic acid deficiency	Demyelination leading to parasthesias	prevention	Pantothenic acid early before demyelination	56
Inborn Errors (Genetic Diseases)				
Peroxisomal diseases				
Adrenoleukodystrophy	Progressive central demyelination with retardation and death	+++	Lorenzo's oil + polyunsaturated fatty acids	63 64
Refsum's disease	Dysmyelination leading to a polyneuropathy	+++	Lorenzo's oil + polyunsaturated fatty acids	57 64
Maple syrup urine diseases	Defects of branched chain amino acid catabolism leading to accumulation of organic acids causing lethargy, seizures, retardation, coma	++++	Defined amino acid diet	66
		++++	Thiamine, biotin, B_{12} in some patients	67
Functional biotin deficiency	Increased plasma organic acids, psychomotor retardation, seizures, ataxia	+++++	High dose biotin, early	66

TABLE 67.1 *(Continued)*

Classification of the Major Neurological and Psychiatric Disorders and the Potential Response of Each to Nutritional Therapy

Category / Disease or Disease Group / Specific Diseases	Defining Characteristics of the Disease	Response to Nutritional Therapy	Therapy	References
Glucose Transporter Deficiency	Infantile seizures and developmental delay Low CSF glucose and low to normal CSF lactate	++++	Ketogenic diet	67
Diseases of glycogen recall and gluconeogenesis	CNS symptoms of hypoglycemia between meals with rapid onset	+++++	Frequent small meals	68
Deficiencies of fatty acid beta-oxidation	CNS symptoms of hypoglycemia with starvation or fasting	+++++	Avoid depletion of glycogen stores	68
Pyruvate dehydrogenase deficiency	Lactic acidosis	++	Ketogenic diet	68
			Thiamine, lipoic acid with partially active enzyme	68
Defects in respiratory chain proteins	Muscle weakness, ataxia, pyramidal symptoms	++	Vitamins C and K sometimes partially successful	68
Phenylketonuria	Standard genetic screen Failure to treat causes retardation	+++++	Restricted phenylalanine intake	66,69,70
Homocystinuria	High urinary and plasma homocysteine	++++	Betaine, po	66
	Retardation, psychiatric disorders, vascular damage	+++++	Vitamin B_6, po	
		+++	Vitamin B_{12}, im	
Urea cycle defects	Hyperammonemia causes lethargy and coma in neonates accompanied by high blood glutamine and alanine	++++	Sodium benzoate, po	66
		++++	Phenyl acetate, po	
		+++	Arginine, Citrulline	
Glutamate decarboxylase deficiency	Seizures, prenatal, and neonatal	+++	Pyridoxine, iv	66
Wilson's disease	Copper toxicity causes myriad symptoms including tremor, dysarthria, dysphagia, psychiatric disorders	+++++	Penicillamine	72
		+++++	Trientine	
		++++	Zinc, not with chelators	

Treatment ratings:
0 = No known treatment
+ = Suggested or hypothetical treatment
++ = Anecdotal evidence for positive effect
+++ = Treatment shown to have positive effect
++++ = Preferred treatment in some cases
+++++ = Primary treatment

TABLE 67.2

Known Interactions between Antiepileptic Drugs and Nutrients

Drug	Nutrient	Interaction	Treatment	References
Phenytoin	Folic acid	Can cause folate deficiency; high dose folate treatment can decrease plasma phenytoin	Patients receiving phenytoin should be given folate supplement (1-5 mg/d)	1
	Vitamin D	Appears to induce enzymes that cause increased catabolism of vitamin D	Patients need 500-1200 IU/d of vitamin D	2
	Vitamin K	Appears to induce enzymes that cause increased catabolism of vitamin K	Risk in newborn of epileptic mother taking phenytoin	3
			Prophylactic treatment of mother with vitamin K	4
Phenobarbital	Folic acid	Causes decrease in plasma folate concentration	see Phenytoin	1
	Vitamin D	Appears to induce enzymes that cause increased catabolism of vitamin D	see Phenytoin	2
	Vitamin K	Appears to induce enzymes that cause increased catabolism of vitamin K	see Phenytoin	3 4
Primidone	Folic acid	Converted to phenobarbital by the liver; has same effect on folic acid as phenobarbital	see Phenytoin	1
	Vitamn D	Converted to phenobarbital by the liver; has same effect on vitamin D as phenobarbital	see Phenytoin	2
	Vitamin K	Converted to phenobarbital by the liver; has same effect on vitamin K as phenobarbital	see Phenytoin	3 4
Carbamazepine	Folic acid?	Causes increase in plasma homocysteine	?	5
Valproate	Folic acid	Linked to birth defects probably via inhibition of the glycine cleavage system	Suggest betaine or choline (5-10 g/d, po) (personal recommendation)	6,7
	Carnitine	Causes plasma carnitine deficiency by a mechanism not yet understood	Oral carnitine prevents hyperammonemia caused by valproate in patients at risk for carnitine deficiency	8

For seizures unresponsive to drug therapy surgery is often the only option, but some patients are not viable candidates for surgery, and for others surgery doesn't work. The ketogenic diet has proven effective in a portion of the intractable epilepsies.[9,10] The ketogenic diet was first proposed by Wilder[11] in response to his observation that fasting often decreased seizure frequency. Before the advent of effective pharmacotherapy, it was the method of choice for the treatment of epilepsy.[10] High fat with low carbohydrate and low protein intake are used to generate ketone bodies as the main energy source to the brain, reducing the concentration of circulating carbohydrate. In addition, the diet lowers the pH of the blood. Some believe that the lowered pH is responsible for the antiseizure effectiveness of the diet. The ketogenic diet has recently been reviewed from a neurologist's perspective[12] and placed in the context of other treatments for epilepsy.[13]

Ketogenic diets are difficult to maintain because of the blandness and monotony of the high fat foods, but support groups are available through a Stanford University web site (http://www.stanford.edu/group/ketodiet), and a set of palatable diets and acceptable substitutes has been generated by Carroll and Koenigsberger[14] (Tables 67.3 through 67.8).

TABLE 67.3

Sample Menus for the Ketogenic Diet on a 3-Day Rotating Meal Plan (Exchanges for menu items can be picked from Tables 67.4-67.8. Quantities listed are for children ages 1-3. Portions can be increased for older children and adults.)

	Day 1	Day 2	Day 3	Appropriate Exchanges in	Foods and Seasonings That Can Be Used Freely	
Breakfast	1/4 cup corn flakes + 4 2/3 Tbsp heavy cream	1/4 cup cooked oatmeal + 4 2/3 Tbsp heavy cream	1/2 slice wheat bread + 2 1/4 Tbsp margarine	Table 7, starches	Boullion (dilute 1/2 strength) Sugar-free drinks Celery	Basil Cocoa Chives
	2 oz whole milk + 3 1/2 Tbsp heavy cream	2 oz whole milk + 3 1/2 Tbsp heavy cream	1 oz American cheese + 3 Tbsp heavy cream	Table 8, dairy products	Cucumber Iceberg lettuce Endive Pickles (dill)	Cinnamon Curry Dill Garlic powder
Lunch	1 oz cooked chicken + 2 2/3 Tbsp mayonnaise (chicken salad)	1 hardboiled egg + 2 Tbsp mayonnaise (egg salad)	1 Tbsp natural peanut butter + 1 2/3 Tbsp margarine (double butter delight)	Table 5, meats/meat substitutes	Sugar-free gelatin Mustard Vinegar Saccharine, aspartame	Garlic (fresh) Lemon Lemon pepper Lime
	lettuce leaf + 1/4 avocado, sliced + 1 1/2 tsp oil/vingar	1/4 cup cooked carrots, cold + 2 1/2 tsp oil/ vinegar	2 oz tomato juice + 2 Tbsp heavy cream	Table 4, vegetables	Limited extracts of vanilla almond walnut lemon	Onion powder Oregano Paprika Pepper Salt
	1/4 cup pears (water packed) + 3 1/4 Tbsp heavy cream	1/4 cup grapes + 2 2/3 Tbsp heavy cream	1/4 banana + 2 1/2 Tbsp heavy cream (add ice, vanilla, water to make shake)	Table 6, fruits		
			4 celery sticks	Free use vegetable	Conversions	
Dinner	1/2 beef frank + 1/2 tsp margarine	1 oz cooked hamburger + 1 1/3 Tbsp margarine	1 oz fried bologna + 1/2 Tbsp margarine	Table 5, meat/meat substitutes	1 Tbsp margarine = 11.0 g fat 1 Tbsp oil = 15 g fat 1 Tbsp heavy cream = 5.6 g fat 1 Tbsp mayonnaise = 11.2 g fat	
	1/4 cup cooked carrots + 1 Tbsp margarine	1/4 cup broccoli + 1 Tbsp margarine	1/2 cup chopped asparagus + 1 1/2 Tbsp margarine (cooked)	Table 4, vegetables	1 Tbsp margarine = 3/4 Tbsp oil = 2 Tbsp heavy cream = 1 Tbsp mayonnaise	
	1 dill pickle			Free use vegetable	1 g protein = 4 kcal 1 g carbohydrate = 4 kcal 1 g fat = 9 kcal	

Reference: Carroll J, Koenigsberger D. The ketogenic diet: a practical guide for caregivers.

TABLE 67.4

Ketogenic Food Exchange for Vegetables[a]

Vegetable	Amount	Fat (Tbsp), Choose One Margarine	Oil	Heavy Cream
Carrots (cooked)	1/4 cup	1	5/6	2
Cauliflower (cooked)	1/2 cup	1 1/4	11/12	2 1/2
Spinach (cooked)	1/4 cup	1	5/6	2
Broccoli (cooked)	1/4 cup	1	5/6	2
Asparagus (cooked)	1/2 cup	1 1/2	1 1/6	2
Green beans (cooked)	1/4 cup	1	5/6	2
Eggplant (raw, chopped)	1/2 cup	1 1/6	1	2 1/2
Sliced beets (cooked)	1/2 cup	1	5/6	2
Collard greens (cooked)	1/4 cup	1 1/4	11/12	2 1/2
Sauerkraut (cooked)	1/4 cup	1 1/4	5/6	2 1/2
Mushrooms (fresh, small)	5 ea	1 1/4	11/12	2 1/2
Avocado (fresh, small)	1/4	3/4	1/2	1 1/4
Pepper (raw, chopped)	1/2 cup	1 1/6	1	2 1/2
Onions (fresh, chopped)	1/4 cup	1 1/4	11/12	2 1/2
Infant carrots (pureed)	1 1/2 oz	1 1/2	1 1/6	2 1/2
Infant green beans (pureed)	1 1/2 oz	1 1/2	1 1/6	2 1/2
Infant spinach (pureed)	1 1/2 oz	1 1/2	1 1/6	2 1/2
Infant squash (pureed)	1 1/2 oz	1 1/2	1 1/6	2 1/2
Infant sweet potato (pureed)	1 oz	2	1 7/12	3 1/2
Tomato juice	2 oz	1	5/6	2

[a] Each row yields 143 kcal with 0.9 g protein, 2.7 g carbohydrate, 14.5 g fat.

Reference: Carroll J, Koenigsberger D. The ketogenic diet: a practical guide for caregivers. Copyright by The American Dietetic Association. Modified with permission from *JADA* 98: 316-321; 1998.

The caloric intake in these diets is designed for young children (one to three years), but the portions can be increased to meet energy needs as the child grows. The diets can be used for adults, with appropriate adjustment of portions. Initiation of the ketogenic diet requires 12 to 38 hours of fasting to generate ketosis to begin the diet. Once in ketosis, the high fat ketogenic diet will maintain ketosis. Patients should be started on the diet gradually, consuming about half of a high fat meal for the first two meals before ingesting whole meals. Carroll and Koenigsberger[14] have found that small amounts of starch will be tolerated by most children, but some are sensitive to starch. Fluids should not be limited, but should not contain sugar.

Neurodegenerative Diseases

Parkinson's Disease (PD)

PD is caused by the usually slow, irreversible degeneration of the dopaminergic nigrostriatal neurons. This destruction may result from any number of pathological circumstances but is often accelerated by the generation of free radicals. Unfortunately, by the time symptoms appear, most of the dopaminergic function in the nigrostriatal pathway has deteriorated. L-3,4-dihydroxyphenylalanine (L-DOPA), the precursor for dopamine, is the primary treatment for PD, but L-DOPA itself has significant toxicity, and its use should be postponed as long as possible.[15] More efficient use of the endogenous dopamine

TABLE 67.5

Ketogenic Food Exchange for Meats/Meat Substitutes[a]

Meat/Meat Substitute	Amount	Fat (Tbsp), Choose One		
		Margarine	Oil	Heavy Cream
Beef frank	1/2 frank	1/2	5/12	1
Bologna	1 oz	1/2	5/12	1
Cooked steak	1 oz	1 2/3	1 5/12	3 1/2
Cooked hamburger (chuck)	1 oz	1 2/3	1 5/12	3 1/2
Chicken (dark meat, cooked)	1 oz	2 2/3	2	5 1/4
Veal cutlet (cooked)	1 oz	2 1/4	1 2/3	4 1/2
Bacon (use all fat)	3 slices	—	—	—
Ham	1 oz	2	1 1/2	3 2/3
Tuna (in oil)	3/4 oz	1 2/3	1 5/12	3 1/2
Flounder (other fin fish, cooked)	3/4 oz	2	1 1/3	3 1/2
Salami	1/2 oz	1	3/4	2
Pork sausage (cooked)	1/2 link	2	1 1/2	3 2/3
Shrimp (cooked)	3/4 oz	2	1 1/3	3 1/2
Infant beef (strained)	2 oz	1 1/4	1	2 1/2
Infant chicken (strained)	2 oz	1 1/4	1	2 1/2
Infant veal (strained)	2 oz	1 1/4	1	2 1/2
Infant turkey (strained)	2 oz	1 1/4	1	2 1/2
Egg (large)	1	2	1 1/2	3 2/3
Peanut butter (natural)	1 tbsp	1 2/3	1 1/3	3 1/2
Macadamia nut (dry/oil roasted)	1 oz	1/2	1/12	1/4

[a] Each row yields 245 kcal with 6.0 g protein, 24.3 g fat.

Reference: Carroll J, Koenigsberger D. The ketogenic diet: a practical guide for caregivers.

TABLE 67.6

Ketogenic Food Exchange for Fruits[a]

Fruit	Amount	Fat (Tbsp), Choose one		
		Margarine	Oil	Heavy Cream
Applesauce (unsweetened)	1/4 cup	2 1/2	1 5/6	4 2/3
Apricot halves (water packed)	2 halves	1	3/4	2
Fresh blueberries	1/8 cup	1 1/4	1	2 1/2
Fresh cherries	3	1	3/4	2
Banana (small, 6 inches)	1/4	1 7/12	1 1/4	3
Fresh strawberries	1/4 cup	1	3/4	2
Fresh cantaloupe	1/8 cup	1 1/2	1 1/6	2 2/3
Peaches (water packed)	1/4 cup	1 1/2	1 1/6	2 2/3
Fresh grapes	1/4 cup	1 1/2	1 1/6	2 2/3
Pears (water packed)	1/4 cup	1 2/3	1 1/4	3 1/4
Pineapple (water packed)	1/4 cup	1 2/3	1 1/4	3 1/4
Fresh raspberries	1/4 cup	1 1/2	1 1/6	2 2/3
Fresh, small plum	1/2 plum	1 1/2	1 1/6	2 2/3
Infant apple (pureed)	1 oz	1 1/4	1	2 1/4
Infant apple/pineapple (pureed)	1 oz	1 1/4	1	2 1/4
Infant apricots (pureed)	1 oz	1 1/4	1	2 1/4
Infant peaches (pureed)	1 oz	2	1 7/12	4 1/4
Infant pears (pureed)	1 oz	2	1 7/12	4 1/4

[a] Each row yields 168 kcal with 4.2 g carbohydrate, 17 g fat. If fruit packed in fruit juices, soak in water for 1 hour.

Reference: Carroll J, Koenigsberger D. The ketogenic diet: a practical guide for caregivers.

TABLE 67.7

Ketogenic Food Exchange for Starches[a]

Food	Amount	Fat (Tbsp), Choose One Margarine	Oil	Heavy Cream
Cereals				
Corn flakes	1/4 cup	2 1/2	1 2/3	4 2/3
Infant dry cereal (oat, barley or rice)	2 tbsp	1 1/2	1 1/6	3 1/4
Cold rice cereal	1/4 cup	2 1/2	1 5/6	4 2/3
Toasted oat cereal	1/4 cup	1 3/4	1 1/4	3 1/4
Cooked oatmeal (regular)[b]	1/4 cup	3	2	5 1/6
Cooked wheat cereal[b]	1/8 cup	1 1/2	1 1/6	3 1/4
Cooked grits[b]	1 oz	1 1/2	1 1/6	3 1/4
Cooked farina[b]	1/4 cup	2 1/2	1 5/6	4 2/3
Bread/Crackers				
Medium bagel (half)	1/4	1 3/4	1 1/3	3 1/3
Bread stick (0.28 oz)	1 1/2	1 3/4	1 1/3	3 1/3
English muffin	1/4	2 3/4	2	5 1/3
Wheat bread (sliced)	1/2	2 1/2	1 5/6	4 3/4
White bread (sliced)	1/2	2 1/2	1 5/6	4 3/4
Frozen waffle	1/3	2 1/4	11/12	4 1/4
Crackers/arrowroot cookies	1	1 3/4	1 1/3	3 1/3
Rice cakes	1/2	1 1/2	1 1/12	2 3/4
Ritz crackers[c]	2	1 7/12	1 1/6	3 1/4
Saltines	2	1 3/4	1 1/3	3 1/3
Triscuits[c]	2	2 1/4	1 7/12	4 1/4
Wheat Thins[c]	4	1 3/4	1 1/3	3 1/3
Zwieback	1	2 1/4	1 7/12	4 1/4
Starchy Vegetables				
Yellow cooked corn (frozen)	1/8 cup	1 3/4	1 1/3	3 1/3
Peas (frozen in butter sauce)	1/8 cup	1 1/2	1 1/12	2 5/6
Cooked potato (mashed)	1/8 cup	1 3/4	1 1/3	3 1/3
Cooked macaroni	1/8 cup	2 1/4	1 7/12	4 1/4

[a] Each row yields 226 kcal with 4.9 g carbohydrate, 0.75 g protein, 22.6 g fat.
[b] Cereal should be cooked in water only.
[c] Trademark of Nabisco, East Hanover, NJ.

Reference: Carroll J, Koenigsberger D. The ketogenic diet: a practical guide for caregivers. Copyright by The American Dietetic Association. Modified with permission from *JADA* 98: 316-321; 1998.

can accomplish this by inhibiting the dopamine catabolizing enzymes, particularly monoamine oxidase, or by protecting the dopamine with antioxidants. Monoamine oxidase itself generates free radicals as a consequence of its catalytic mechanism in the oxidation of dopamine. Of the two monoamine oxidases in the brain, MAO B is the primary catabolizing enzyme for dopamine. Shoulson and the Parkinson Study Group[16] have shown that L-DOPA use can be postponed by the specific MAO B inhibitor, deprenyl (5 mg, bid). However, alpha-tocopherol treatment did not extend the time between diagnosis and the introduction of L-DOPA treatment for Parkinsonian symptoms in the same study. In an uncontrolled study, a combination of alpha-tocopherol (3200 units/d) and vitamin C (3 g/d) was reported to postpone the need to administer L-DOPA.[17] These levels are so high that the investigator gradually increased the daily dose to reach the levels indicated, but found no significant toxicity.

TABLE 67.8

Ketogenic Food Exchange for Dairy Products[a]

Dairy Product	Amount	Fat (Tbsp), Choose One		
		Margarine	Oil	Heavy Cream
Cheese Products (Measure by Weight)				
Cheddar	3/4 oz	1 1/2	1 1/6	2 1/2
Swiss	3/4 oz	2	1 7/12	3 2/3
Cream cheese	2 tbsp	1/6	1/12	1
American	1 oz	1 1/2	1 1/6	3
Feta	1 oz	1 1/4	1	2 1/2
Mozzarella (whole milk)	1 oz	1 1/2	1 1/6	3
Brie	1 oz	1 1/2	1 1/6	3
Cottage cheese	1 Tbsp	1 1/2	1 1/6	3
Parmesan	1 Tbsp	1/2	1/2	1 1/2
American cheese spread	1 Tbsp	2	1 7/12	4
Milk Products				
Milk (whole)	2 oz	1 2/3	1 1/4	3 1/2
Sour cream	2 Tbsp	1/2	1/6	3
Yogurt (plain)	1/4 cup	2 1/2	1 5/6	5

[a] Each row yields 216 kcal with 0.5 g carbohydrate, 4.7 g protein, 21.7 g fat.

Reference: Carroll J, Koenigsberger D. The ketogenic diet: a practical guide for caregivers. Copyright by The American Dietetic Association. Modified with permission from *JADA* 98: 316-321; 1998.

During the treatment of PD patients with a MAO inhibitor, it is essential that their diet be limited in the content of tyramine. Gardner et al.[18] have analyzed many foods for tyramine content and have proposed a "user-friendly MAOI diet" that is not as restrictive as many other MAOI diets. It appears that any foods that have been processed with microorganisms, whether purposefully or by neglect, are likely to contain high concentrations of tyramine. Such foods include matured or aged cheeses, fermented or dry sausages, foods that have not been properly stored, beverages made by fermentation, certain yeast extracts (Marmite), and sauerkraut. All cheeses except cottage cheese, cream cheese, ricotta cheese, and processed cheese slices should be considered aged or matured cheeses. Pizzas, lasagnas, and many casseroles are made with aged cheeses and should not be eaten when taking MAO inhibitors. Other fresh milk products that have not been allowed to grow fermenting organisms should not contain high levels of tyramine. Fermented or dry meats that have high tyramine levels include pepperoni, salami, mortadella, and summer sausage, among others. Food storage is important in the production of tyramine. Since purposely fermenting foods produces tyramine, neglectful fermenting (poor storage) can also produce tyramine. Foods that have had an opportunity to grow organisms, whether left out at room temperature or stored too long in the refrigerator, should not be consumed by patients taking MAO inhibitors. Meats (all meats) are more likely to produce the tyramine when improperly stored because of the higher protein content of meats. Cooking will destroy the organisms but not the tyramine, so do not assume that cooking will make the meat fit for consumption for the patient. Beer and wine are produced by fermentation processes. Tap beers have high tyramine levels and should be totally avoided, but bottled (canned) beers and wines can be consumed in moderation (no more than two drinks/day; 16 oz. of beer/d, 8 oz. of wine/d). Other foods to avoid are fava, broad bean pods (not the beans), banana peels (not the banana pulp), and soy condiments (not soy milk). Other

TABLE 67.9

Protein Content in Common Foods

Food	Protein Content
Eggs	3.5 g/oz
Milk	8.0 g/cup
Cheeses	7.0 g/oz
Meats, lean beef, poultry, pork, fish	6.9 g/oz
Fruits (apples, figs, plums, and grapes are low in protein)	0.5-1.4 g/cup
Fruit juices	1.0-1.4 g/cup
Breads	2.0 g/slice
Cereal	2.0-4.0 g/cup
Pasta	4.0 g/cup
Rice, cooked	4.0 g/cup
Fats, butter, oils, mayonnaise	trace
Vegetables	2.0-3.4 g/cup
celery	4.0 g/cup
Low protein calorie supplements	
porridge, low protein	0.13 g/cup
noodles, low protein anellini, ragatoni, tagliatelle	0.2 g/cup
bread, low protein	0.1 g/slice
cranberry sauce	0.4 g/cup
honey	0.07 g/tsp
jelly	0.05 g/Tbsp
jam	0.03 g/Tbsp
mints	trace
jelly beans	0.1 g/oz
hard candy	0.1 g/oz
table syrup	0.05 g/Tbsp
marshmallows	0.03 g ea
cranberry juice	0.01 g/oz
Hi-C	0.01 g/oz
Sodas	0.01 g/oz
Dessert topping	0.3-0.6 g/cup

Reference: Burtis G, Davis J, Martin S. *Applied Nutrition and Diet Therapy* W.B. Saunders, Philadelphia, 1988, pp. 784-787.

than those items identified here as tyramine containing or potentially tyramine containing, most foods are allowed on the "user-friendly MAOI diet."

Once treatment with L-DOPA starts, it is necessary to rearrange the protein in the diet of PD patients to maximize the effect of the L-DOPA.[19-21] Because many of the amino acids (the large neutral group) will compete with L-DOPA for uptake into the brain, it is best to ingest the protein when the amino acid competition will have the least detrimental effect. Protein is essential, but if good quality protein is ingested (eggs, milk) the requirement can be reduced to 45 g/d for the average size adult. If the majority of the dietary protein (>80%) is consumed in the evening, the effects of the competition between the amino acids and L-DOPA will be minimized because the decreased L-DOPA uptake into the brain will occur during the night when the patient is asleep and when, presumably, the increase in involuntary movements will be least disruptive. Protein contents of common foods are shown in Table 67.9.

Because constipation is a problem in PD patients, it is recommended that adequate amounts of fiber and fluid be ingested.[22] Ingestion of low protein grains, vegetables, and fruits during the day with at least 64 oz. of water or other non-protein containing drink should accomplish this goal.

Alzheimer's Disease

Alzheimer's disease is characterized by progressive cognitive loss. Early effects appear to involve cholinergic projections from the basal forebrain. Later disease seems to affect many different cell populations, involving several of the neurotransmitters. A diagnosis of Alzheimer's disease is confirmed postmortem by the identification of the typical neurofibrillary tangles and senile plaques. Free radical damage is suspected as a mechanism of cell loss in Alzheimer's, but confirmation is elusive. However, work with Down's syndrome patients and results from the Nun study[23] indicate that mechanisms leading to Alzheimer's may be operative well before cognitive symptoms appear. There is no cure for Alzheimer's or even a moderately effective treatment. It is possible, however, to ameliorate the symptoms and prolong life in these patients with appropriate treatment and diet. As with PD patients, inhibition of the MAO-B (5 mg deprenyl, bid) appears to be effective in conserving transmitter function and prolonging cognitive function.[24] Therefore, Alzheimer's patients treated with MAO-B inhibitors should not eat the tyramine-rich foods discussed in the section on Parkinson's disease. However, unlike PD patients, alpha-tocopherol (1000 IU, bid) is effective in slowing the progress of the Alzheimer's disease,[24] indicating that free radical damage may be a continuing problem in the progression of the disease.

Whether from a chronically poor diet or from an increased need for nutrients, Alzheimer's patients often suffer from protein malnutrition and other nutritional deficiencies that improve the status of the patient when corrected.[25] Whether any of the vitamins has a specific relationship to Alzheimer's is unknown, but vitamin E, thiamine, and vitamin B_{12} have been associated with improvement of symptoms when blood levels are corrected to normal.[25] Vitamin E may help by slowing the rate of free radical-induced tissue damage. Thiamine may help to produce acetylcholine through its participation in the reaction catalyzed by pyruvate dehydrogenase, the rate-limiting step in the synthesis of acetylCoA, a precursor to acetylcholine, the neurotransmitter most closely associated with Alzheimer's symptoms. Vitamin B_{12} is required for the generation of methyl groups that are involved in either the synthesis or the conservation of choline, the other component of acetylcholine. High dose acetyl-L-carnitine (1000 mg with breakfast, 1000 mg with lunch) has also been reported to slow the progression of Alzheimer's disease.[26] Adequate nutriture is essential to preserve as much function as possible.

Multiple Sclerosis (MS)

MS appears to be an autoimmune disease that involves demyelination in the central nervous system. The symptomatology generally progresses slowly and intermittently, but the disease can be fatal. Interestingly, a consistent observation with respect to the etiology of MS is that MS occurs more frequently at higher latitudes. Risk for MS is apparently acquired early in life because one carries the risk associated with the place in which one spends his/her first 15 years. Several hypotheses have been proposed to relate the risk to the disease.

Hayes et al.[27] have hypothesized that the relationship to latitude is a function of the amount of sunlight to which one is exposed. The sunlight activates vitamin D, forming vitamin D_3 which is involved in the regulation of the immune system. Inadequate exposure to sunlight at higher latitudes would create a deficiency in activated vitamin D that translates into an increased risk for development of autoimmune disorders. It has been shown that vitamin D_3 can prevent experimental autoimmune encephalomyelitis (EAE) in mice. EAE is an animal model for MS. Hayes and Ebers are currently examining this hypothesis in a large population at risk for MS (personal communication).

Several studies (see Bates et al.[28] for review) have indicated that treatment of MS patients with essential fatty acids early in the disease ameliorates the symptoms and slows the progression of the disease. However, these studies make no attempt to explain the geographical differences in the incidence of MS, and the oils used to administer the essential fatty acids to the patients will very likely contain significant quantities of the fat-soluble vitamin D.

To affect the disease process with either essential fatty acids or vitamin D, it is necessary to intervene early in the disease process.

Amyotrophic Lateral Sclerosis (ALS)

ALS is a neurodegenerative disease affecting the motor neurons in the spinal cord, brainstem, and motor cortex. It is linked to genetic abnormalities of Cu/Zn superoxide dismutase (SOD1). Lipid peroxidation has been shown to be higher in ALS patients than in controls.[29] Transgenic mice expressing the mutant human SOD1 exhibit the symptoms of ALS.[30] Dietary supplementation of these mice with vitamin E delayed the onset of symptoms and slowed the progress of the disease but did not prolong survival time. Putative inhibitors of the glutamatergic system increased survival time, indicating that excitotoxicity is a factor in the progression of the disease. However, the glutamatergic inhibitors did not delay the onset of the disease, indicating that different mechanisms are involved in disease induction and disease progression. Nutritionally it would seem advisable to maintain adequate levels of antioxidants in patients and in the population at risk for ALS. In this population, adequate levels may be in excess of the RDA. Periodic assessment of antioxidant levels is indicated in this population.

Because of the loss of motor function in ALS patients, they usually develop severe dysphagia, and they often become malnourished from inadequate intake.[31] In addition, impaired respiratory function often demands more energy. Therefore, in end stage treatment, supplying sufficient energy to these patients to maximize life quality is the primary goal.

Guam/ALS/Parkinsons/Dementia (GAPD)

GAPD is a very slowly progressing neurotoxicity apparently induced by diet. The disease, once common in the Chamorro natives of the South Pacific, seems to be disappearing.[32] Cycad seeds, which were part of the Chamorron diet and medicine, appear to contain a neurotoxin that exhibits its effects over decades. Indeed, a very similar disease can be produced in monkeys by feeding them the seeds.[33]

Tardive Dyskinesia (TD)

TD is characterized by choreoform movements, particularly of the tongue, lips, and limbs. It is caused by the chronic use of neuroleptic drugs in the treatment of schizophrenia. Neuroleptic activity is generally exhibited through binding to dopamine receptors. That TD is caused by destruction of susceptible dopaminergic neurons has yet to be shown, but the symptoms produced are very similar to those seen in Parkinson's disease. Treatment with L-DOPA is contraindicated in schizophrenics because it is likely to exacerbate the psychosis. Vitamin E has been used to treat TD in schizophrenic patients, but there is disagreement on whether or not it has an effect.[34] Choline (150-200 mg/kg/d) has been used successfully as a therapy for TD.[35] Administration of the choline as lecithin will prevent the fishy odor associated with the ingestion of high-dose choline.

Neurodevelopmental Diseases

Neural Tube Defects (NTDs)

NTDs are the result of abnormal fetal development in which the neural tube fails to mature normally. NTDs range widely in severity from a very mild spina bifida that may escape notice until adulthood to anencephaly, a fatal birth defect in which the brain fails to grow in utero. Since NTDs are structural defects, most treatments of nonfatal NTDs involve surgery.

NTDs have many causes including diet, drugs, smoking, and genetic susceptibility. Use of several drugs, including the anticonvulsants discussed above, has been associated with increased incidence of NTDs in babies born to mothers taking these drugs, particularly during the formation and closure of the neural tube (16 to 26 days post fertilization). Drugs that interfere with folate absorption or metabolism are particular risks. Diets limited in folate are also known to increase susceptibility to NTDs. This subject is thoroughly reviewed by Lewis et al.[36]

The Center for Disease Control in the United States requested the Food and Drug Administration to mandate that all flour sold in the U.S. be supplemented with folic acid as a mechanism for preventing NTDs. That supplementation has been implemented; data are expected soon to determine the success of this endeavor in decreasing NTDs. Data on hand indicate that folate intake and folate status have already improved.[37]

Schizophrenia

The inclusion of schizophrenia under neurodevelopmental diseases may be controversial. Schizophrenia is still a catchall for a number of diseases that likely have different etiologies.[38,39] However, genetic and structural studies indicate that both genetic and developmental processes are involved in the disease process.[38] Despite significant effort to identify the genetic correlates of schizophrenia, the search has so far been unsuccessful. Moreover, dysmorphology of neurons in the frontal and temporal lobes of the cortex of schizophrenics[38] and the increased incidence of birth of schizophrenics in the winter/spring (environmental factors[39]), indicate that abnormal development (probably in utero) is involved in the formation of the prepsychotic brain. However, whether schizophrenia, or more appropriately, the schizophrenias are caused by disordered developmental processes remains to be proven. Nevertheless, for now it appears most likely that some (or most) are neurodevelopmentally-caused disorders.

Schizophrenia is most often treated with neuroleptics, which can cause tardive dyskinesia (see above) but also are associated with weight gain in the patients. The weight gain correlates with symptom improvement,[40] an observation that can be interpreted in various ways. Neuroleptics also seem to have a negative effect on plasma indicators of nutritional status,[41] indicating that neuroleptics have effects on nutrient absorption or metabolism that should be evaluated periodically. In another study it was shown that schizophrenics consistently had lower plasma vitamin C levels than other hospitalized controls.[42] Whether this is a drug/nutrient interaction or an increased requirement by schizophrenics for vitamin C is unknown, but in either case schizophrenics should be given more vitamin C to attain normal plasma levels.

As in several other neurological disorders, treatment with n-6 and n-3 fatty acids improves symptoms in schizophrenia. Apparently overactivity of phospholipase A_2 causes a vulnerability of these fatty acids to oxidation, resulting in a relative depletion.[43] Dietary replacement ameliorates symptoms by restoring function. Schizophrenics apparently have an increased need for the essential fats, but replacing them, while it improves the symptoms, should not be considered a treatment of the disease, but a nutritional requirement in this population.

Affective Disorders

The primary affective disorders are depression and bipolar disorder. Depression is often divided into endogenous and reactive depression. Reactive depression is a depression of mood in response to an adverse life event. Endogenous depression often has the same symptoms as reactive depression in the absence of any specific adverse life event. Bipolar disorder is characterized by periods of depression interspersed with periods of mania often occurring in a regularly cycling pattern.

The preferred treatment for bipolar disorder is lithium carbonate. Lithium is successful in ameliorating symptoms of both the mania and the depression in most patients with bipolar disorder. It is thought that the mechanism by which this occurs is related to the dampening effect that lithium has on the phosphoinositide cascade.[38]

Lithium is sometimes an effective treatment for unipolar depression as well. However, depression is more commonly treated with tricyclic antidepressants, and more recently with specific serotonin reuptake inhibitors. These drugs are the successors to the monoamine oxidase inhibitors that were used as the first round of effective antidepressants. While monoamine oxidase inhibitors are little used as antidepressants anymore, their use is associated with the potential for toxicity by amines (particularly tyramine) found in some foods.[18] These foods are discussed in the "user friendly MAOI diet" in the section on Parkinson's disease.

Lithium absorption in the gut is inhibited by high salt concentration in the diet,[44] so effective treatment of bipolar disorder is facilitated by a low-salt diet. Care must be taken to balance the dietary salt and the lithium dose, because lithium overdose can cause permanent neurological damage, and the therapeutic window for lithium is relatively narrow.

S-adenosylmethionine, the naturally occurring condensation product of ATP and methionine and the universal methyl donor, has been shown to be an effective antidepressant,[45] just as effective as the tricyclic antidepressants, and with fewer side effects. Indeed, clinical improvement in depressed patients is correlated with plasma levels of S-adenosylmethionine regardless of whether the patients were treated with S-adenosylmethionine or a tricyclic antidepressant.[46] Even though S-adenosylmethionine is a naturally occurring chemical that is found in all foods, it is doubtful that the treatment of depression with S-adenosylmethionine should be considered nutritional therapy, because the doses used (400 mg, tid, PO) are pharmacological. The mechanism by which S-adenosylmethionine improves the symptoms of depression are not yet understood, but it is thought that the methylation process is involved. In support of this hypothesis is the repeated observation that folate deficiency is common in depressed patients and that symptoms improve with folate supplementation whether concomitant with pharmacotherapy or using folate alone.[47] Therefore, it is recommended that folate supplementation be a standard adjunct to pharmacotherapy of depressed patients.

Depression is also characterized by low levels of n-3 polyunsaturated fatty acids (PUFA) in both erythrocyte membranes and plasma. Rather than being a simple deficiency of n-3 PUFA, the ratio of n-6 PUFA/n-3 PUFA may be a problem in depressed patients.[48] This observation may correlate with the action of lithium on the phosphoinositide cascade. In the phosphoinositide cascade the fatty acid substituted in the two position of the phosphoinositide is often a PUFA. If the cascade is poorly controlled in depression or mania, then a deficiency of n-3 fatty acids or an abnormal ratio of n-6/n-3 might be induced by the lack of control. Since the n-3 fatty acids are much more limited in Western diets, a relative deficiency of the n-3 fatty acid would be expected. An increased intake of n-3 PUFA might then ameliorate the symptoms of depression or bipolar disorder. As with schizophrenia, it may be better to consider the increased need for n-3 PUFA in patients with affective disorder a dietary requirement in this patient population rather than a treatment for the disorder.

Tryptophan appears to be a moderately effective treatment for mild depression but does not seem to be effective against severe depression.[35] Tryptophan does seem to be an effective soporific.[35] Small studies indicate that tryptophan is antimanic, but large controlled studies have not been done.[35] Tyrosine may have antidepressant actions in some cases of "dopamine dependent" depression and it may be anxiolytic in stressful situations. These observations have not been established in a large controlled study, but significant differences have been found in small studies.[35] Finally, another nutrient, lecithin (probably the choline portion), has been credited as a significant treatment for mania,[35] but more data are needed.

Hyperactivity

Attention Deficit Hyperactive Disorder (ADHD), a growing problem in children, is either being more frequently or more efficiently diagnosed or the disorder is increasing in frequency in the population. Feingold[49] was convinced that either the salicylates in foods or food additives (colors or flavors) were responsible for the hyperkinesis in children. However, little evidence has been generated to support this hypothesis, even though foods have been shown to have an effect on hyperkinesis in children.[50] Whether the effect is caused by one of Feingold's food components, a nutrient deficiency or food allergy, or a combination of these factors is still an open question. Because of the difficulty in doing research with children, the difficulty in diagnosing the disorder, and the widespread use of methylphenidate to treat the disorder, good research on the causes of hyperactivity is difficult to find. At this time it is difficult to make any solid recommendations for treatment of hyperactivity with the exception that most children would benefit from a more balanced diet with more fresh fruits and vegetables and less fast-food fare.

Metabolic Diseases

Encephalopathies

Encephalopathies are characterized by a gradual decrease in neurological function as toxicity resulting from failure of the liver to remove toxins from the blood progresses.[51] Initial symptoms include slowed reactions, confusion, and changes in mood. As the toxicity becomes more serious the patient becomes drowsy and his/her behavior deteriorates.

The third stage, according to the West Haven criteria, is the induction of a stuporous state with marked confusion and slurred speech. This can be followed by a lapse into coma in which the patient is totally unresponsive. Two common types of encephalopathy are the Wernicke-Korsakoff Syndrome and hepatic encephalopathy.

Wernicke-Korsakoff Syndrome (WKS)

WKS results from thiamine deficiency usually secondary to alcoholism, but can result from other diseases as well, e.g., AIDS or gastrointestinal disease leading to poor absorption of thiamine. WKS exhibits a strictly central nervous system (CNS) pathology.[52] Beriberi, which also results from thiamine deficiency but is rarely seen in Western Society, exhibits peripheral neuropathology. Treatment of WKS is a challenge because it is difficult to recognize the disease in time to prevent permanent damage. However, early treatment will arrest the progress of the disease.[52]

The Wernicke phase of the disease is an acute phase characterized by staggering gait and paralysis of eye movements, and is reversible by thiamine therapy (50 mg/d for 3 days, iv). The chronic Korsakoff phase, a debilitating loss of working memory, is generally not reversible by thiamine.[53]

Hepatic Encephalopathy

Hepatic encephalopathies have a variety of causes that result in failure by the liver to remove toxins from the blood, causing a depression of CNS function. The biochemical mechanism that causes the decreased speed of neurological function is unknown, but most encephalopathies are characterized by increased plasma ammonia concentrations. Traditionally, these encephalopathies have been treated by partial or complete dietary protein withdrawal. This is no longer recommended. Vegetable protein is tolerated better by these patients than is animal protein because of the higher branched chain amino acid component of vegetable protein, and plasma levels of branched chain amino acids are generally lower in patients with hepatic encephalopathy. Non-absorbable disaccharides (lactulose or lactitol) are often used because they inhibit the uptake of toxins sometimes produced by enteric flora and they may alter the absorption of ammonia produced in the gut by the enteric flora.[51,54] The decreased uptake of ammonia in the presence of disaccharides is probably due to acidification of the gut by the metabolism of these disaccharides to organic acids by the gut flora.

Neuropathies

Neuropathies are characterized by the failure of the peripheral nervous system (PNS). Neuropathies may result from a slowed conduction in the PNS, from the absence of sensory input or motor output through specific peripheral nerves, or from diseases leading to the degeneration of specific peripheral nerves. Neuropathies are related to the encephalopathies in that they are generally caused by toxins acting on the peripheral nervous system. These toxins may be caused by genetic defects that allow the accumulation of toxins, by ingestion of toxic substances, or by failure of the body's metabolic control to limit the amounts of potentially toxic metabolites. Genetic neuropathies are discussed under Inborn Errors below. In this section only those neuropathies that have a nutritional component, either cause or treatment, are listed.

Pyridoxine Toxicity

Pyridoxine toxicity generally results from self medication with large doses of vitamin B_6.[55] Pyridoxine binds to proteins in the endoneurium of the PNS axons and blocks normal neuronal function, yielding a sensory polyneuropathy. Ironically, pyridoxine deficiency also contributes to the polyneuropathy of B-complex deficiency.[56] Treatment depends on the cause. Toxicity is treated with cessation of the megadoses of vitamin B_6, and B-complex deficiency is treated with supplements of the B vitamins.

Diabetic Neuropathy

Diabetic neuropathy normally presents as a slowly progressing, mixed sensorimotor, autonomic polyneuropathy. It is probably secondary to diabetes-induced vascular disease. As with other diabetic-induced medical problems, the best treatment is prevention by maintaining control of plasma glucose levels.[57]

Vitamin B_{12} Deficiency

B_{12} deficiency can result in combined system disease characterized by parasthesias, spastic weakness, and malaise. Often these neurological abnormalities are irreversible by the time symptoms are obvious.[56] Vitamin B_{12} deficiency also causes megaloblastic anemia which, in the past, was used as a signal to check plasma B_{12} levels. However, the recent decision to supplement flour with folic acid to prevent birth defects may mask vitamin B_{12} deficiency possibly until the neurological damage is irreversible. Greater care must now be taken to monitor plasma vitamin B_{12} states, especially in vegans. The safest treatment for suspected vitamin B_{12} deficiency is injection of 5 to 15 μg hydroxycobalamin, im. However, injections are expensive, and high dose vitamin B_{12} (150 to 500 μg/d, po) is usually adequate even in cases of pernicious anemia (absence of intrinsic factor).[58] However, to be safe in cases of pernicious anemia, monthly injections of vitamin B_{12} (50 to 150 μg) may be necessary. In the absence of pernicious anemia it is recommended that patients receive 5 to 25 μg/d, po after their plasma levels have been increased to normal range by injection or by the high dose regimen.

Pantothenic Acid Deficiency

Pantothenic acid deficiency leads to parasthesias involving demyelination of peripheral nerves.[56] Pantothenate is a component of coenzyme A which is essential in the synthesis of acetylcholine, the generation of energy in the Krebs cycle, and the synthesis of a number of other metabolic intermediates. Its involvement in the synthesis of fats is probably responsible for the demyelinating effect of its deficiency. Because pantothenic acid is so widely available in the diet, its deficiency normally occurs only in the context of B-complex deficiency. Pantothenic acid deficiency is therefore treated with the daily ingestion of a B-complex vitamin containing at least 10 mg of pantothenic acid.[59]

Inborn Errors (Genetic Diseases)

Peroxisomal Diseases

Peroxisomal diseases are characterized by dysmyelination, hypotonia, retardation, and visual and auditory effects. Peroxisomes are responsible for the oxidative catabolism of a myriad of metabolic products which, if allowed to accumulate, might be toxic to cellular processes. Peroxisomal diseases are a result of either the failure of peroxisome biogenesis in the patient or a defect in one of the proteins essential to the normal function of peroxisomes. Significant advances have been made recently in understanding the genetic causes of these disorders.[60,61] Sixteen separable disorders have been identified, 12 of which cause severe neurological damage.[62] Two groups of these disorders are addressed here.

Adrenoleukodystrophy (ALD) and Adrenomyeloneuropathy (AMN)

ALD and AMN are X-linked genetic disorders characterized by the accumulation of very long chain fatty acids (24:0 and 26:0). The same genetic defect has been identified in both phenotypes. The mutant protein is a peroxisome membrane protein involved in the transport of very long chain fatty acids into the peroxisome for degradation. By a mechanism not yet understood, this deficiency leads to demyelination and progressive loss of neural function. The accumulation of very long chain fatty acids also affects the function of the adrenal gland, and ALD and AMN patients often suffer from primary adrenal insufficiency prior to the onset of neurological symptoms. Dietary restriction of very long chain fatty acids and dietary administration of Lorenzo's oil (glyceryltrioleate + glyceryltrierucate) lower the plasma levels of the primary very long chain fatty acids, but once neurological symptoms have appeared, this treatment does little to reverse the progress of the disease.[63] However, it appears to slow the progress of the disease if it is administered prior to the onset of neurological symptoms.[63] This treatment apparently causes a deficiency of the essential polyunsaturated fatty acids so that supplementation with docosahexaenoic acid and arachadonic acid may be necessary.[64] The treatment of choice at this time is a bone marrow transplant if a suitable donor can be found.

Refsum's Disease — Zellweger's Syndrome

Refsum's disease, Zellweger's syndrome, and neonatal adrenoleukodystrophy are all part of a continuum of diseases that are genetically related.[60,65] They are autosomal recessive defects in the assembly of the peroxisomal system for the oxidation of unusual fatty acids. The inability to catabolize branched chain or very long chain fatty acids leads to the incorporation of the accumulated metabolites into myelin, which then does not function normally. Decreasing the amount of the unusual fats (e.g., phytanic acid or 24:0 and 26:0) in the diet improves the polyneuropathy.[57] Phytanic acid is found in animal fat, especially dairy products. Diets low in animal fat and dairy products relieve some of the symptoms. These peroxisomal disorders can also be treated with Lorenzo's oil, and, as with the ALD and AMN, the plasma levels of n-6 and n-3 polyunsaturated fatty acids should be monitored and supplemented as necessary.[64] Arachidonic and docosahexaenoic acids are the primary representatives of the n-6 and n-3 fatty acids, respectively, in the plasma. Because arachidonic acid is widely available in the diet, the n-3 fatty acids are the most likely to be deficient. The n-3 fatty acids are present in fish oils or in fish, and supplements of both arachidonic acid (n-6) and either docosahexaenoic or eicosapentaenoic acids (n-3) are available as dietary supplements.

Maple Syrup Urine Diseases

There are as many forms of maple syrup urine disease as there are enzymes that catabolize the branched chain amino acids. The disorders present as acidemias or acidurias. Accumulation of many of the metabolites of the branched chain amino acids is toxic. Symptoms commonly include vomiting, lethargy, metabolic acidosis, ketonuria, seizures, mental retardation, and coma. The symptoms typically present during the first few months of life, but milder forms of the genetic defects may not appear until the fourth or fifth year. There are forms of maple syrup urine disease that are responsive to thiamine. These are genetic variants of the branched chain dehydrogenase complex that do not bind thiamine as tightly as the wild type.[56] Some forms of maple syrup urine disease are also responsive to diets restricted in branched chain amino acids. However, the only way to insure adequate intake of the essential amino acids while restricting the branched chain amino acids is to feed the patient a defined amino acid diet.[66] There are several known enzyme defects in the processing of the organic acids formed in the catabolism of the branched chain amino acids. Most of these benefit from a restricted protein diet and some from high dose biotin (10 to 40 mg/d).[66] Those suffering from methylmalonic acidemia may also benefit from high dose (1 to 2 mg/d) vitamin B_{12} therapy.[66]

Functional Biotin Deficiency

Biotin is involved in the carboxylation of organic acids. It is essential for the initiation of gluconeogenesis (carboxylation of pyruvate), the initiation of fatty acid synthesis (carboxylation of acetylCoA), the catabolism of leucine (carboxylation of methylcrotonyl CoA), and the catabolism of propionate from odd chain fatty acids and several amino acids (carboxylation of propionylCoA). Biotin is attached covalently to each of these carboxylases by holocarboxylase synthetase. It is conserved when the carboxylase is degraded by the enzyme biotinidase, which cleaves the covalent attachment. Deficiency of either of these enzymes can cause neurological problems. Both deficiencies are characterized by high plasma levels of organic acids, but the effects of the holocarboxylase synthetase deficiency are more serious and more immediate, because it causes a decreased blood pH. Untreated, the deficiencies will result in psychomotor retardation, seizures, cerebellar signs, and peripheral symptoms at three to six months for biotinidase deficiency, and earlier for holocarboxylase synthetase deficiency. Prompt treatment with pharmacological doses of biotin (10 to 40 mg/d, orally) improves outcome considerably.[66]

Glucose Transporter Deficiency

The brain uses glucose almost exclusively as an energy source. The transport of glucose into the brain by facilitated diffusion is normally not rate-limiting to energy use. However, a relatively newly identified defect in the glucose transporter causes a limited energy supply to the brain.[67] The incidence of this defect in the population is not yet known, but it is suspected that some cases of cerebral palsy and sudden infant death syndrome may be caused by this defect. Symptoms include infantile seizures and developmental delay. It can be diagnosed by hypoglycorrhachia and low to low normal cerebrospinal fluid lactate levels. It can be treated effectively using the ketogenic diet (Tables 67.3 through 67.8). Ketone bodies provide an alternate energy source to the brain, but are not present in significant quantities in the blood unless induced by a high fat, low carbohydrate, low protein diet.

Glycogen Storage Diseases

Fructose-1,6-biphosphatase deficiency, glucose-6-phosphatase deficiency, or deficiency of the glucose-6-phosphate translocation system causes the lack of glucose availability between meals and leads to hepatomegaly, bleeding diathesis, neutropenia, and neurological symptoms from the hypoglycemia. Treatment consists of frequent small meals which may include nocturnal intragastric feeding.[68]

Deficiencies of Fatty Acid Beta-Oxidation

There are several enzymes involved in the oxidation of fatty acids as a source of energy. Carnitine is also needed to transport the fatty acids into the mitochondrion for oxidation. Defects in these processes can cause neurological symptoms including drowsiness, stupor, and coma during acute metabolic crises probably caused by diet-induced hypoglycemia accompanied by a hypoketonemia due to the lack of fatty acid oxidation. The hypoketonemia prevents the brain from receiving the energy it needs to function in the absence of glucose. The treatment is to avoid hypoglycemic states where fatty acids would need to be used for energy.[68] Glycogen is available for immediate energy needs, so that hypoglycemia does not develop as quickly as in glycogen storage diseases. Prolonged fasting or extended exercise, however, deplete the glycogen stores and lead to neurological symptoms and potential neurological damage.

Pyruvate Dehydrogenase Deficiency

As expected from its central position in intermediary metabolism, pyruvate dehydrogenase deficiency is complex. Symptoms range from a mild encephalopathy with retardation to death.[68] It is sex-linked so that males are more often affected. Depending on the defect, the problem may be treatable, especially when it appears in females. Treatment with thiamine, lipoic acid, or ketogenic diets is sometimes partially successful.[68] Treatment with thiamine (25 to 100 mg, po) or lipoic acid (5 to 10 mg, po) requires a partially functional enzyme that responds to pharmacological doses of these vitamins. The use of a ketogenic diet (see Tables 67.3 through 67.8) is an attempt to bypass energy production from carbohydrates, a process which is completely dependent on the activity of pyruvate dehydrogenase.

Defects in the Respiratory Chain Proteins

Abnormalities in the mitochondrial respiratory chain are characterized by both muscle and central nervous system symptoms. Central symptoms include ataxia, pyramidal signs, and dementia, but the course is varied, attributable to the number of proteins involved and the potential for considerable differences in vulnerability. Since the respiratory chain is a process of electron transfer, some redox vitamins can substitute, although very inefficiently, for the abnormal proteins. Vitamin C and vitamin K have been used successfully in this way.[68] Doses differ between patients, but because neither vitamin C nor vitamin K_1 exhibit significant toxicity when taken orally, the doses of both vitamins can be titrated to each patient.

Phenylketonuria (PKU)

There are many genetic forms of PKU. Usually the defect is in the gene for the enzyme phenylalanine hydroxylase. Some of these defects cause a complete loss of enzyme activity, while others cause only partial losses. Because of this variation in activity, some patients are more tolerant to phenylalanine in their diets than are others. The neurological effects of this disease — mental retardation and progressive motor dysfunction — are apparently due to the high blood phenylalanine levels and not to the high plasma levels of phenylalanine metabolites.[66] It is essential that the defect be identified early and treated as soon as possible. PKU at any age is treated using a diet that decreases the amount of phenylalanine ingested. Phenylalanine is so common in high protein foods that it is impossible to ingest sufficient protein to satisfy other amino acid requirements and still maintain the plasma concentration of phenylalanine between 120 and 360 μM in patients with little or no phenylalanine hydroxylase activity. Therefore, high protein foods (see Table 67.9) are usually completely restricted, and a casein hydrolysate stripped of phenylalanine is substituted. Because high protein foods are generally responsible for a significant portion of the vitamins and minerals in the diet, the hydrolysate is usually fortified with vitamins and minerals to ensure that the patients using the hydrolysate as a primary amino acid source do not become deficient in vitamins and minerals. There are several commercial sources of the fortified hydrolysate. It is advisable, particularly in PKU patients with no hydroxylase activity, to continue treatment of the disease with the fortified hydrolysate through the teen years and at least into adulthood.[69,70] Monitoring phenylalanine levels in the plasma is the measure of success in treating the disease. Plasma phenylalanine levels should be maintained between 120 and 360 μM. Because of the expense of the fortified hydrolysate, attempts have been made to restrict dietary phenylalanine without the aid of the fortified hydrolysate. This is difficult at best, often resulting in either a deficiency of essential amino acid intake, a deficiency in one or more of the vitamins, or a deficit in energy intake. Each of these has serious consequences to the patient. Early detection and successful treatment of PKU can lead to a normal independent life.

Phenylketonuria can also be caused by a defect in the metabolism of biopterin, a cofactor in the hydroxylation of phenylalanine. This defect cannot be treated solely by restricting phenylalanine, because it causes a lack of hydroxylation of tyrosine and tryptophan as well. The hydroxylated products of tyrosine and tryptophan are precursors of the neurotransmitters dopamine and serotonin, and consequently, lack of these hydroxylations also has neurological effects. The prognosis for a defect in biopterin metabolism is not as positive as that for a defect in phenylalanine hydroxylase.

Homocystinuria

Homocystinuria can be the result of any one of a series of genetic defects in the transsulfuration pathway. These defects can be either in the enzymes of transsulfuration or in the metabolism of the vitamins that act as cofactors in the pathway. Symptoms are variable but usually include mental retardation, and often include psychiatric disorders, and sometimes seizures. Vascular damage is evident in those who survive into the third decade. Treatment is sometimes successful. High-dose vitamin B_6 (250 to 500 mg/d) works in some cases of cystathionine-beta-synthetase deficiency, depending on the effect of the genetic defect on the capacity of the enzyme to bind B_6. Betaine (6 to 12 g/d) usually helps to remethylate the homocysteine. Defects in the metabolism of folate can also be treated with betaine, while defects in the metabolism of vitamin B_{12} are generally best treated with injections of hydroxycobalamin.[66]

Urea Cycle Defects

There are several enzymes or transporters that can cause the typical hyperammonemia of urea cycle defects. In addition to hyperammonemia, these defects are generally characterized by high serum concentrations of one of the urea cycle intermediates. Glutamine and alanine are usually high, and arginine is low. Orotic acid is often high, especially in ornithine transcarbamylase deficiency, but is normal or low in carbamylphosphate synthetase deficiency. Urea cycle defects are often fatal in the neonatal period, so therapy should start immediately. Patients can be maintained on a low protein diet with adjunct therapy with sodium benzoate (250 mg/kg/d) and phenyl acetate (250 mg/kg/d).[71] These aromatics react with glycine and glutamine, respectively, and are excreted as conjugates of these amino acids, thus excreting ammonia in an alternate form. Arginine can be used as an adjunct to treatment in citrullinemia and arginosuccinic acidemia because it can stimulate the excretion of ammonia as citrulline and arginosuccinate. Arginine is given as a dietary supplement in sufficient quantities to yield a normal plasma level of arginine. The amount of the arginine supplement will depend on the genetic defect, but starting with 700 mg/kg/d is recommended with subsequent titration to normal plasma levels.[71] Lysinuric protein intolerance, a failure of the proximal tubule to reabsorb the dibasic amino acids lysine and ornithine, can be treated by oral citrulline, which is reabsorbed and can act as a source of ornithine for the mitochondrial initiation of the urea cycle.[66] Citrulline is given as a dietary supplement at a rate that allows the plasma ornithine to be normalized.

Glutamate Decarboxylase Deficiency

Glutamate decarboxylase is the enzyme responsible for the synthesis of gamma-aminobutyric acid (GABA), an important inhibitory neurotransmitter. Defective glutamate decarboxylase activity causes a severe seizure disorder, which may begin in utero. Depending on the specific genetic defect, the enzyme can sometimes be stimulated by high dose pyridoxine (10 to 100 mg/d) given parenterally.[66]

Wilson's Disease (WD) or Hepatolenticular Degeneration

WD is caused by copper toxicosis. Copper concentrations in the plasma are normally controlled by an enterohepatic mechanism that causes the excretion of excess copper in the stool. The genetic defect causing WD has been localized to chromosome 13. The defective protein is not ceruloplasmin, since the gene for ceruloplasmin has been localized to chromosome 3. Dietary restriction of copper may delay the onset of symptoms, but it is not preventive. The toxicity of the copper appears to be induced oxidation that damages tissues, particularly nervous tissue, leading to a myriad of symptoms including tremors, rigidity, dysarthria, dysphagia, and psychiatric disorders. The preferred treatment of Wilson's disease is penicillamine (1 g/d, at least 30 min before or 2 hr after meals), a chelator that binds copper and is excreted by the kidney. Trientine at the same dose also works in the same way for patients who have reactions to penicillamine. Zinc supplements (150 mg/d, before meals) can replace copper and are sometimes used, but care must be taken not to give zinc and either of the chelators at the same time, because they can neutralize each other.[72]

References

1. Burtis G, Davis J, Martin S. In: *Applied Nutrition and Diet Therapy.* WB Saunders, Philadelphia, 1988, p.760.
2. Borowitz D. In: *Essentials of Clinical Nutrition.* Feldman EB, Ed., FA Davis, Philadelphia, 1988, p. 172-232.

3. Astedt B. *Seminars in Thrombosis and Hemostasis* 21:364; 1995.
4. Thorp JA, Gaston L, Caspers DR, Pal ML. *Drugs* 49:376; 1995.
5. Schwaninger M, Ringleb P, Winter R, et al. *Epilepsia* 40:345; 1999.
6. Samren EB, van Duijn CM, Koch S, et al. *Epilepsia* 38:981; 1997.
7. Mortensen PB, Kolvraa S, Christensen E. *Epilepsia* 21:563; 1980.
8. Coulter DL. *J. Child Neurol* 10 2:32S; 1995.
9. Tallian KB, Nahata MC, Tsao CY. *Ann Pharmacotherapy* 32:349; 1998.
10. Prasad AN, Stafstrom CF, Holmes GL. *Epilepsia* 37 1:81S; 1996.
11. Wilder RM. *Mayo Clinic Proc* 2:307; 1921.
12. Nordli DR Jr, De Vivo DC. *Epilepsia* 38:743; 1997.
13. Bazil CW Pedley TA. *Ann Rev Med* 49:135; 1998.
14. Carroll J, Koenigsberger D. *J Am Dietetic Assoc* 98:316; 1998.
15. Melamed E, Offen D, Shirvan S, et al. *Ann Neurol* 44:149S; 1998.
16. Shoulson I. *Ann Neurol* 44:160S; 1998.
17. Fahn S. *Ann NY Acad Sci* 570:186; 1989.
18. Gardner DM, Shulman KI, Walker SE, Tailor SA. *J Clin Psychiat* 57:99; 1996.
19. Karstaedt PJ, Pincus JH. *Arch Neurol* 49:149; 1992.
20. Bracco F, Malesani R, Saladini M, Battistin L. *Eur J Neurol* 31:68; 1991.
21. Pincus JH, Barry K. *Arch Neurol* 44:270; 1987.
22. Pandarinath G, Lenhart A. *NC Med J* 58:186; 1997.
23. Snowden DA. *JAMA* 275:528; 1996.
24. Sano M, Ernesto C, Thomas RG, et al. *N Engl J Med* 336:1216; 1997.
25. Folstein M. *Nutr Rev* 55:23; 1997.
26. Spagnoli A, Lucca U, Menasce G, et al. *Neurology* 41:1726; 1991.
27. Hayes CE, Cantorna MT, DeLuca HF. *Proc Soc Exp Biol Med* 216:21; 1997.
28. Bates D, Cartlidge NEF, French JM, et al. *J Neurol Neurosurg Psychiat* 52:18; 1989.
29. Oteiza PI, Uchitel OD, Carrasquedo F, et al. *Neurochem Res* 22:535; 1997.
30. Gurney ME, Cutting FB, Zhai P, et al. *Ann Neurol* 39:147; 1996.
31. Silani V, Kasarskis EJ, Yanagisawa N. *J Neurol* 245 Suppl 2:13S; 1998.
32. Spencer PS. *Can J Neurol Sci* 14:347; 1987.
33. Steele JC, Guzman T. *Can J Neurol Sci* 14:358; 1987.
34. Adler LA, Edson R, Lavori P, et al. *Biol Psychiat* 43:868; 1998.
35. Young SN. *Neurosci Biobehavior Rev* 20:313; 1996.
36. Lewis DP, Van Dyke DC, Stumbo PJ, Berg MJ. *Ann Pharmacother* 32:802; 1998.
37. Jacqes PF, Selhub J, Bostom AG, Wilson PWF, Rosenberg IH. *N Engl J Med* 340:1449; 1999.
38. Barchas JD, Faull KF, Quinn B, Elliot GR. In: *Basic Neurochemistry: Molecular, Cellular and Medical Aspects.* Siegel GJ, Agranoff BW, Albers RW, Molinoff PB, Eds, 5th ed, Raven Press, New York, 1994, pp. 959-977.
39. Franzek E, Beckmann H. *Psychopathology* 29:14; 1996.
40. Lawson WB, Karson CN. *J Neuropsychiat Clin Neurosci* 6:187; 1994.
41. Martinez JA, Velasco JJ, Urbistondo MD. *J Am Coll Nutr* 13:192; 1994.
42. Suboticanec K, Folnegovic-Smalc V, Korbar M, Mestrovic B, Buzina R. *Biol Psychiat* 28:959; 1990.
43. Laugharne JDE, Mellor JE, Peet M. *Lipids* 31:163S; 1996.
44. Yamreudeewong W, Henann NE, Fazio A, Lower DL, Cassidy TG. *J Fam Pract* 40:376; 1995.
45. Bressa GM. *Acta Neurol Scand* 154:7S; 1994.
46. Bell KM, Potkin SG, Carreon D, Plon L. *Acta Neurologica Scandinavica* 154:15S; 1994.
47. Alpert JE, Fava M. *Nutr Rev* 55:145; 1997.
48. Adams PB, Lawson S, Sanigorski A, Sinclair AJ. *Lipids* 31:157S, 1996.
49. Feingold BF. *Ecol Dis* 1:153; 1982.
50. Breakey J. *J Paediatr Child Health* 33:190; 1997.
51. Seery JP, Aspinall RJ, Taylor-Robinson SD. *Hosp Med* 59:200, 1998.
52. Kril JJ. *Metabol Brain Dis* 11:9; 1996.
53. Feldman EB. In: *Essentials of Clinical Nutrition.* Feldman EB, Ed, FA Davis, Philadelphia, 1988, pp. 333-376.
54. Shetty AK, Schmidt-Sommerfeld E, Udall JN, Jr. *Nutrition* 15:727, 1999.

55. Xu Y, Sladky J, Brown MJ. *Neurology* 39:1077; 1989.
56. Blass JP. In: *Basic Neurochemistry: Molecular, Cellular, and Medical Aspects.* Siegel GJ, Agranoff BW, Albers RW, Molinoff PB, Eds, 5th ed, Raven Press, New York, 1994, pp. 749-760.
57. Pleasure DE. In: *Basic Neurochemistry: Molecular, Cellular, and Medical Aspects.* Siegel GJ, Agranoff BW, Albers RW, Molinoff PB, Eds, 5th ed, Raven Press, New York, 1994, pp. 761-770.
58. Burtis G, Davis J, Martin S. In: *Applied Nutrition and Diet Therapy.* WB Saunders, Philadelphia, 1988, pp. 666-679.
59. Burtis G, Davis J, Martin S. In: *Applied Nutrition and Diet Therapy.* WB Saunders, Philadelphia, 1988, pp. 174-193.
60. Powers JM, Moser HW. *Brain Pathol* 8:101; 1998.
61. Wanders RJ. *Neurochem Res* 24:565; 1999.
62. Moser HW. *Sem Pediatr Neurol* 3:298; 1996.
63. Moser AB, Kreiter N, Bezman L, et al. *Ann Neurol* 45:100; 1999.
64. Moser AB, Jones DS, Raymond GV, Moser HW. *Neurochem Res* 24:187; 1999.
65. Geisbrecht BV, Collins CS, Reuber BE, Gould SJ. *Proc Natl Acad Sci* 95:8630; 1998.
66. Yudkoff M. In: *Basic Neurochemistry: Molecular, Cellular, and Medical Aspects.* Siegel GJ, Agranoff BW, Albers RW, Molinoff PB, Eds, 5th ed, Raven Press, New York, 1994, pp. 813-839.
67. De Vivo DC, Trifiletti RR, Jacobson RI, et al. *N Engl J Med* 325:703; 1991.
68. DiMauro S, De Vivo DC. Diseases of carbohydrate, fatty acid, and mitochondrial metabolism. *Basic Neurochemistry: Molecular, Cellular, and Medical Aspects.* Siegel GJ, Agranoff BW, Albers RW, Molinoff PB, Eds, 5th ed, Raven Press, New York, 1994, pp. 723-748.
69. Koch R, Moseley K, Ning J, Romstad A, Guldberg P, Guttler F. *Molec Genetics Metab* 67:148; 1999.
70. Smith I. *Acta Paediatr* 407:60S; 1994.
71. Maestri NE, Hauser ER, Bartholomew D, Brusilow SW. *J Pediatr* 119:923; 1991.
72. Scheinberg IH, Sternlieb I. *Am J Clin Nutr* 63:842S; 1996.

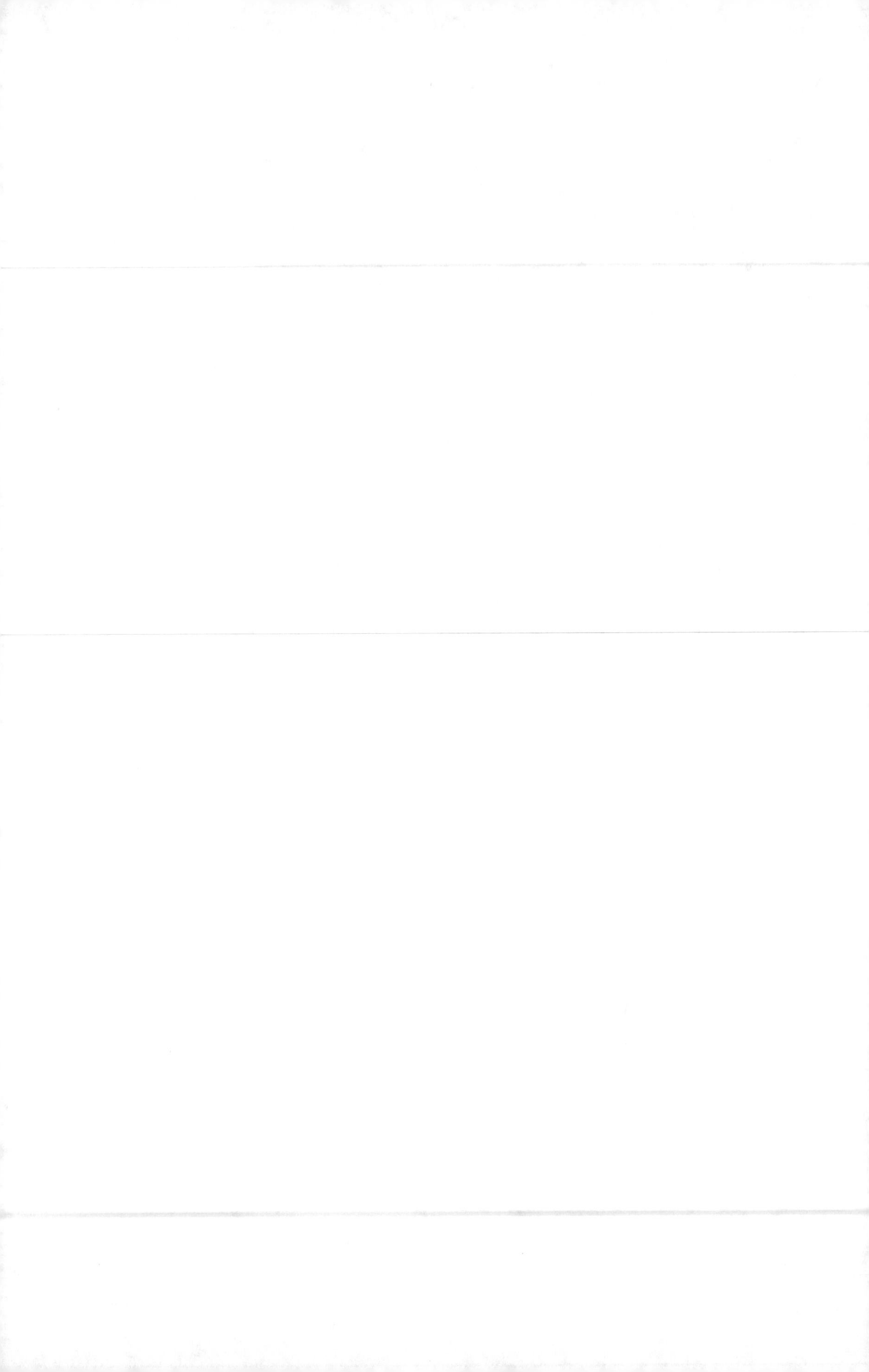

68

Eating Disorders (Anorexia Nervosa, Bulimia Nervosa, Binge Eating Disorder)

Diane K. Smith and Christian R. Lemmon

Introduction

The pursuit of thinness among adolescent and young adult females may leave some of them quickly threatening their physiological and psychological wellbeing as the fear of weight gain and possible obesity drives them into maladaptive eating and dieting habits. The intense preoccupation with dieting and weight control among this segment of the population has become so commonplace that it is often viewed as normal behavior and revered by peers who consider themselves less successful at being able to control their weight and shape. Unfortunately, and sometimes tragically, these maladaptive behaviors may inevitably manifest themselves in the form of eating disorders.

Despite the attention afforded to the eating disorders by medicine and the media, anorexia nervosa (AN), bulimia nervosa (BN) and related feeding disturbances remain difficult psychiatric diagnoses to treat. The American Psychiatric Association[1] recently revised their practice guidelines for the treatment of patients with eating disorders, but practitioners who treat these patients, including psychiatrists and other physicians, psychologists, social workers, counselors, dietitians and other health personnel continue to approach these problems from a wide array of treatment perspectives. Part of this lack of consensus concerning the treatment of eating disorders is attributable to the abundance of theories regarding their etiology. As reported by Yager,[2] "theories regarding the etiology and pathogenesis of the eating disorders have implicated virtually every level of biopsychosocial organization." AN, BN, and related feeding disturbances challenge those who are devoted to their treatment.

Diagnostic Criteria

Eating disorders occur over a continuum of increasingly pathological behavior. Excessive self-evaluation and a preoccupation with weight, shape, and size characterize both AN and BN. Other common characteristics include an intense fear of weight gain and a

0-8493-2705-9/02/$0.00+$1.50

relationship with food that borders on obsession. However, there are distinct differences between the two disorders. Following are the diagnostic criteria for the recognized eating disorders AN and BN. A third eating disorder, Binge Eating Disorder (BED), is currently considered a proposed diagnosis for inclusion in the next revision of the Diagnostic and Statistical Manual, Version IV (DSM-IV) that standardizes psychiatric diagnosis. Other diagnoses and feeding disturbances, including Eating Disorder, Not Otherwise Specified (NOS), will be discussed below.

Anorexia Nervosa (AN)

Although AN often starts with only small reductions in total food intake, patients eventually reduce their energy and fat intake to a point where they are consuming only a limited number of foods in a highly ritualistic fashion. The disorder is characterized by severe, self-induced starvation (300 to 600 kcalories/day). However, an actual loss of appetite is quite rare. Individuals with AN refuse to maintain a minimally normal, healthy body weight, show an intense fear of gaining weight or becoming fat, exhibit a disturbance in their perception of their body weight or shape, and experience abnormal menses. Two subtypes of AN exist, with about 50% classified as the restricting type, and the others exhibiting behaviors indicative of binge-eating and purging. (AN and BN are not mutually exclusive diagnoses.) Further distinctions can be made between AN patients who binge eat and purge and those who purge normal meals or snacks but do not engage in binge-eating episodes. DSM-IV criteria for AN are outlined in Table 68.1.

TABLE 68.1

DSM-IV Criteria for Anorexia Nervosa, including Subtypes[a]

Refusal to maintain body weight at or above 85% of expected for height and age
Intense fear of gaining weight or accumulation of body fat despite underweight status
Body image disturbance which may include the denial or lack of appreciation for the seriousness of one's currently low weight, self-evaluation largely determined by one's shape or weight, or claiming to "feel fat" even though terribly underweight
In females, primary or secondary amenorrhea
Subtypes
Restricting type — person has not regularly engaged in binge eating or various purging behaviors
Binge eating/purging type — person regularly engages in binge eating or various purging behaviors

[a] Adapted from American Psychiatric Association, *Diagnostic and Statistical Manual of Mental Disorders*, 4th ed., American Psychiatric Association, Washington, DC, 1994.

Bulimia Nervosa (BN)

BN is characterized by recurrent episodes of eating unusually large quantities of food in a finite period of time, often until the food is gone or the person is uncomfortably or painfully full. Efforts to purge the excess (3000 to 10,000 kcalories) by some compensatory or purging behavior such as vomiting, laxative or diuretic abuse, excessive exercise, and/or restrictive dieting or fasting occur subsequent to the binge eating episode. These behaviors are associated with a sense of loss of control and typically shame, guilt, and embarrassment are associated with the binge eating and purging process. Nevertheless, patients often report that the purging behaviors diminish the intensity of aversive emotions and provide them with a sense of control. Similar to the diagnosis of AN, patients are classified as either the purging type or nonpurging type. DSM-IV criteria for BN are outlined in Table 68.2.

TABLE 68.2

DSM-IV Criteria for Bulimia Nervosa, including Subtypes[a]

Recurrent episodes (a minimum average of twice per week for at least 3 months) of binge eating, defined as eating abnormally large amounts of food within a 2-hour period, that are associated with a sense of lack of control over the eating process during the episode
Use of compensatory or purging behavior such as self-induced vomiting, laxative/enema or diuretic abuse, restrictive dieting, fasting, or excessive exercise
Self-evaluation largely determined by one's shape and weight
Bulimic behavior does not occur exclusively as a manifestation of anorexia nervosa

Subtypes

Purging type — person regularly uses purging strategies including self-induced vomiting, laxatives, diuretics, or enemas
Nonpurging type — person regularly uses other purging strategies including fasting, restrictive dieting or excessive exercise, but not currently using strategies listed above

[a] Adapted from American Psychiatric Association, *Diagnostic and Statistical Manual of Mental Disorders,* 4th ed., American Psychiatric Association, Washington, DC, 1994.

Binge Eating Disorder

BED is more nebulous, and is characterized by recurrent binge-eating episodes without a compensatory effort to eliminate caloric excess. Although described in the classic paper of Stunkard,[4] it has only recently been widely recognized. In fact, diagnostic criteria for BED were included in the DSM-IV only for research purposes, as it is not yet an approved diagnosis. Although persons diagnosed with BED are seen with a wide range of weights, most are obese. DSM-IV criteria for BED are outlined in Table 68.3.

TABLE 68.3

DSM-IV Proposed Criteria for Binge Eating Disorder[a]

Recurrent episodes (a minimum average of twice per week for at least 6 months) of binge eating, defined as eating an abnormally large amount of food within a 2-hour period, that are associated with a sense of lack of control over the eating process during the episode
At least 3 of the following characteristics are present during binge eating:
- Eating much more rapidly than usual
- Eating until uncomfortably full
- Eating large amounts of food despite not feeling physically hungry
- Eating alone because of embarrassment over quantity of food consumed
- Feeling disgusted, depressed, guilty, or ashamed after the binge

Experience of significant distress about the presence of binge eating
Absence of compensatory behaviors such as self-induced vomiting, laxative or diuretic abuse, restrictive dieting, fasting, or excessive exercise
Binge eating episodes do not occur exclusively as a manifestation of anorexia nervosa or bulimia nervosa.

[a] Adapted from American Psychiatric Association, *Diagnostic and Statistical Manual of Mental Disorders,* 4th ed., American Psychiatric Association, Washington, DC, 1994.

Other Eating Disorders (BED)

Many patients diagnosed with eating disorders do not satisfy criteria for a formal diagnosis of AN or BN. For example, they may not binge and purge often enough to meet the required minimum average occurrence of such behavior. Similarly, a patient's weight may remain in an acceptable or healthy range despite exhibiting all of the other symptoms of AN. Some patients may display all of the characteristics of AN, but continue to menstruate normally. Others may repeatedly chew their food and spit it out in an effort to avoid the ingestion of unwanted energy. Patients who exhibit these and other similar presentations are classified as Eating Disorder, NOS.[3] However, the failure to meet formal criteria for AN or BN does not mean that such an individual does not have a serious disorder or does not require treatment. Many individuals engage in intermittent maladaptive dieting behaviors such as meal skipping, crash dieting, the avoidance of specific foods, excessive exercise, and abuse of drugs (especially appetite suppressants, caffeine, and other stimulants).

Compulsive overeating and night eating have not been formally accepted as eating disorders, but are other maladaptive eating patterns. Compulsive overeating reflects frequent meals and snacks, or continuous eating or "grazing" without the presence of purging behaviors. Usually these individuals become overweight. Night eating is especially common in morbidly obese subjects. It is characterized by delaying the first meal of the day, eating more food after dinner than during that meal, and eating more than half of the day's food after dinner. The eating is often associated with aversive emotions and stress, and the pattern has persisted for at least two months. Nocturnal sleep-related eating is a sleep disorder. Sufferers are in a state somewhere between sleep and wakefulness and do not have recollection of the eating episodes. Another disorder often confused with BN is psychogenic vomiting, which is involuntary postprandial regurgitation in the absence of the core symptoms of fear of weight gain, binge eating, and body image disturbance.

Epidemiology

Eating disorders occur primarily in adolescent and young adult caucasian women, but the onset can be prior to menarche or later in life. Males and non-caucasians are much less frequently afflicted, but recent research suggests an increasing incidence in non-caucasians and persons across the spectrum of socioeconomic class. About 95% of cases of AN are female, and about 90% of cases of BN are female. However, the prevalence in males may be underestimated because of the wide perception that these are "teenage girl" diseases. Bulimic males are typically less likely to seek treatment than bulimic females. Another common misconception is that eating disorders in males signal probable homosexuality. About 20% of males with eating disorders are homosexual.[5] The presentation of males with eating disorders is remarkably similar to that of females. Similar methods of weight control are used by both males and females, and there are comparable rates of psychiatric comorbidity and body image dissatisfaction.[6] A greater percentage of males were overweight before developing their eating disorders.[5] For BED, there is less gender difference.[7]

Estimates of incidence often vary significantly due to variations in the diagnostic criteria utilized and problems with the underreporting of these disorders that are accompanied by denial and secrecy. Reasonable estimates for lifetime prevalence of AN among females in Western countries approach 1% with a range of 0.5 to 3.7%.[1] The lifetime prevalence for BN among women has yielded higher numbers, with a range of 1.1 to 4.2%.[1] Prevalence rates for more broadly defined forms of eating disorder and Eating Disorder, NOS may be substantially higher. Estimates for BED are 2.0% of the general population,[1] with a 3:2 female to male ratio.[8] The incidence of BED increases to about 30% of patients who seek treatment for obesity and about 70% of participants in Overeaters Anonymous.[9] There is no significant racial bias for BED.[9]

Individuals at high risk for the development of eating disorders include dancers, gymnasts, long-distance runners, figure skaters, models, wrestlers, bodybuilders, jockeys, cheerleaders, entertainers, and participants in any other occupations or activities that place a pronounced emphasis on optimal body weight and shape. Patients with certain medical conditions are at risk for developing eating disorders, and may misuse their prescribed treatments or physical conditions to facilitate weight loss and other purging strategies (Table 68.4).[10]

TABLE 68.4

Medical Conditions and Weight Loss Methods[a]

Medical Condition	Weight Loss Method
Diabetes	Misuse of insulin or low fat/low carbohydrate diet
Hypothyroidism	Misuse of thyroid hormones
Hyperthyroidism	Noncompliance with antithyroid medications
Cystic fibrosis	Failure to follow prescribed diet or take pancreatic enzymes
Crohn's disease	Noncompliance with sulfazalazine
Pregnancy	Use of pregnancy-related side effects (nausea, vomiting) to facilitate weight control

[a] Adapted from Powers PS. In: *Handbook of Treatment for Eating Disorders,* 2nd ed., Garner DM, Garfinkel PE, Eds, The Guilford Press, New York, 1997, pg 424.

Etiology

At present no universally accepted theory establishes the etiology of the eating disorders; complex and unique interactions of variables may occur in the affected individual. Disturbances in these interactions may represent primary or secondary phenomena. The current trend is to conceptualize the disorders from a biopsychosocial perspective of multiple converging physiological, psychological, and environmental factors. Table 68.5 summarizes the more accepted etiologic theories.

TABLE 68.5

Etiological Theories of the Eating Disorders

Biological
Genetic
Psychological
Feminist/Social/Cultural
Familial

Numerous biologic theories have been proposed to explain the etiology of the eating disorders; however, no single biologic abnormality unequivocally accounts for the eating disorders. For underweight subjects, most aberrations appear to be the result rather than the cause of the weight loss or malnutrition, and most abate after healthy weight and adequate nutrition are restored.[11] The primary structure controlling ingestive behavior is the hypothalamus of the brain, which also regulates metabolism and end organ function. Other brain structures involved include the limbic system, amygdala, orbitofrontal cortex, and multiple brain stem nuclei. Neuroimaging methods have detected nonspecific abnormalities outside of the secondary changes that accompany malnutrition and hormonal changes.[12] Multiple alterations in neurotransmitters and neuroendocrine axes have been observed in both AN and BN.[13-15] For example, abnormal results have been found in eating disorder patients for levels of luteinizing hormone, follicle-stimulating hormone, gonadotropin, growth hormone, and cortisol and activity of cholecystokinin, opioids, norepinephrine, and serotonin.[11] Once an eating disorder is established, secondary changes in brain chemistry may perpetuate the disease. The fact that amenorrhea is often found in normal-weight bulimics and anorexics before the profound weight loss also suggests some sort of biologic deficit to explain the eating disorders.

Another widely considered theory suggests that the eating disorders, especially BN, are a form of mood disorder.[2] The sufferer of an eating disorder may be using food to self-medicate negative emotions via alterations in brain chemicals. This theory is supported by the high comorbidity of mood disorders found among eating disorder patients, the positive response of patients to antidepressant medications, and the increased prevalence of mood disorders in relatives of eating disorder patients. These findings further emphasize the importance of proper assessment and treatment of depressive symptoms among the eating disorder population.

A genetic predisposition for eating disorders has been suggested. Co-twins of twins with AN were at higher risk for eating disorders.[16] Woodside[17] demonstrated a 45% concordance rate for AN in identical twins, but only a 6.7% concordance in fraternal twins. While the concordance is higher in monozygotic than in dizygotic twins (47.3 versus 31.5%) for BN, the differences were not statistically significant.[17] In a very complete review of the genetic literature, Lilenfeld and Kaye[18] suggested that certain familial tendencies or "vulnerability factors," such as impulsivity, restraint, affective instability, and obsessionality contribute to the development of eating disorders. Others have suggested that a genetically determined vulnerability within the hypothalamic system might contribute to eating disorders.

Many psychological theories have been developed to explain the etiology of eating disorders. Bruch[19] suggested that eating disorders result from disturbances in body image, limited self-esteem, and problems in interoceptive awareness. Another popular theory, especially for AN, relates to conflicts that may develop during adolescence and the sexual maturation process. It has been hypothesized that the physical and emotional regressions that take place in the development of AN are the result of problems encountered during the struggle with independence, the formation of an adult identity, and the realization of sexual urges and sometimes competing parental, personal, and peer pressures.

Learning theorists view eating disorders as evolving out of classical or operant conditioning such that maladaptive learned responses are formed by efforts to reduce anxiety and other aversive emotions. Unwanted emotions and stress are reduced by engaging in restrictive dieting or binge-eating behavior. The guilt, shame, and other feelings that result from binge eating are then reduced by the use of some form of compensatory behavior. Negative reinforcement influences eating disorder behaviors to a large extent. Conditioning principles also may be used to explain the development of weight and body image concerns, specific food avoidance, ritualistic eating behaviors, trauma, and feelings of being out of control. Patients with eating disorders typically struggle with cognitive distortions (dichotomous thinking, overgeneralization, personalization, etc.) that develop in response to low self-esteem, anxiety about one's physical appearance, and other negative core beliefs.

Because of the great gender disparity in the incidence of eating disorders, several feminist explanations for the etiology of the eating disorders have been developed that emphasize the role of various social and cultural influences (e.g., diet, fitness, food, fashion, entertainment, cosmetic, and advertising industries). These influences exert strong pressure on women, especially at the onset of puberty, to be thin at all cost. Other common transitions, such as a new school or job, moves, going off to college, death, marriage, or divorce may trigger eating disorders. Concern about body weight and dieting is manifested among girls as early as the preschool years. Women are uniquely vulnerable to our culture's youth and thinness obsession because they are, more than men, judged and valued based largely on appearance. Bulimic women reveal a greater acceptance of attitudes and beliefs about the relationships between thinness, attractiveness, and success than non-bulimic women.[20] The Westernization of many countries, including Japan, China, and Fiji is believed to have contributed to the increasing prevalence of eating disorders. Western society's similar preoccupation with dieting, exercise, cosmetics, and cosmetic surgery also appears to contribute to the maladaptive behaviors exhibited by patients with eating disorders. When normal individuals are subjected to semistarvation, behavior becomes increasingly and obsessively focused on food.[21]

Another sociocultural variable is the societal expectation that women should be caretakers and nurturers while being self-sacrificing and other-oriented.[22] Schwartz and Barrett[23] suggested that the processes of starvation and purging behavior cause a "numbing effect" that helps the person to deny their feelings, needs, desires, and hunger so that others can be served and satisfied. They also hypothesized that eating disorders have given women a sense of power and control in their lives while they struggle to satisfy society's recommendation to be passive and dependent.

It is also helpful to consider the family system as a whole rather than focusing on the individual patient.[24-25] Whether the dysfunctional family patterns have caused the eating disorders or the individuals with the eating disorders have contributed to the pathology seen in the family remains unclear. Minuchin, Rosman, and Baker[24] reported a number of characteristics of eating disorder families that contribute to the onset and maintenance of the disorder, including enmeshment, overprotectiveness, rigidity, lack of conflict resolution/conflict avoidance, and a pattern by which the symptomatic child diverts marital conflict. Selvini-Palazzoli and Viaro[25] reported that families of AN patients follow a six-stage process by which the patient, usually a daughter, plays out a covert game of switching coalitions between herself and her parents throughout the developmental process, which ultimately results in the daughter perceiving power through her illness and a return to the privileged and overindulged status of her childhood. Other researchers[26-27] have reported unhealthy coalitions formed between the AN patient and a parent, with the eating disorder patient being placed in the role of a parentified child. Root, Fallon, and Friedrich[28] have theorized that the normal adolescent processes of separation and individuation and the establishment of autonomy are adversely affected in bulimic families. They suggested that three different kinds of bulimic families (perfect, overprotective, and chaotic) exist that are different across a number of dimensions, including boundary problems, difficulties with affective expression, parental control or lack thereof, trust issues, enmeshment or isolation, and the function of the eating disorder symptoms within the family system. There is a strong emphasis on weight and appearance in these families.

Comorbid Psychiatric Conditions

Eating disorders are commonly associated with many other psychiatric conditions, with mood, anxiety, and personality disorders appearing to be the most common forms of comorbidity (Table 68.6). AN patients tend to develop eating disorders first and then develop comorbidity, whereas patients with BN tend to manifest mood disorders or anxiety disorders prior to the onset of the eating disorder. It is unclear whether psychiatric comorbidity preceeds or follows the onset of BED.

TABLE 68.6
Common Comorbid Psychiatric Conditions Found in Patients with Eating Disorders

Mood Disorders
Major depressive disorder
Dysthymic disorder
Mood disorder due to general medical condition
Anxiety Disorders
Posttraumatic stress disorder
Obsessive-compulsive disorder
Generalized anxiety disorder
Social phobia
Panic disorder
Personality Disorders
Cluster B (borderline, histrionic, narcissistic)
Cluster C (dependent, passive-aggressive, avoidant, obsessive-compulsive)
Substance Abuse and Dependence
Adjustment Disorders

Other Identified Problems in Patients with Eating Disorders

Other common problems typically found among patients with eating disorders are listed in Table 68.7. They should be evaluated and targeted during treatment, as they may contribute to the development and maintenance of the eating disorder. Many patients experience the struggle between being the model child or conforming to others' rules and expectations and wanting to act out in an irresponsible or oppositional manner. AN patients may strive for and attain high academic achievement, while others, particularly BN patients, may experience academic difficulties. Patients may have a wide range of feelings and attitudes about their sexuality and sexual behavior, including anxiety (AN) or sexual promiscuity (BN).

TABLE 68.7
Other Identified Problems Commonly Found among Patients with Eating Disorders

Perfectionism	Maturity fears
Family dysfunction	Low self-esteem
Low self-efficacy	Control issues
Alexithymia	Poor interoceptive awareness
Cognitive distortions	Self-harming behavior
Relationship problems	Feelings of detachment
Social avoidance and distress	Fear of negative evaluation
Interpersonal distrust and conflict	Mood swings/irritability
Self-destructive anger	Shame and guilt
Emotional, physical, or sexual abuse	Unwanted sexual experience

Bio-Psychosocial Assessment (Table 68.8)

Interview with Referral Source

Most patients are identified by concerned parents, a spouse, relatives, friends, or a primary care physician. Interviewing a referral source is a first step. The practitioner may be better able to communicate understanding, concern, and empathy, and develop better trust with a new or prospective patient if this information is used appropriately. This process will be discussed later in this section.

TABLE 68.8

Bio-Psychosocial Assessment of the Eating Disorders
Interview with referral source
Assessment of the patient's motivation for treatment
Medical evaluation
Nutritional assessment
Clinical interview
Psychological testing
Behavioral assessment
Body image assessment
Interview with family members/significant others

Assessment of the Patient's Motivation for Treatment

The patient's motivation for seeking treatment and her probable stage of readiness for change[29-30] should be considered. A patient may be in the precontemplation, contemplation, preparation, or action stage of change. It is important for the patient, especially the AN patient, to feel that she has some control over the treatment process, although compulsory treatment for AN appears equally effective (in terms of amount of weight gain) when compared to voluntary treatment. The weight gain may take longer in patients receiving compulsory treatment, and their mortality rate is higher.[31]

Medical Evaluation

Nonpsychiatric physicians, especially pediatricians, family physicians, gynecologists, internists, and gastroenterologists play a valuable role in the prevention, early detection, and management of patients suspected of eating disorders.[2] The patient should receive a comprehensive medical evaluation. This evaluation should include a complete history and physical exam, laboratory tests (electrolytes, complete blood count with differential, urinalysis, BUN, creatinine, glucose, albumin, prealbumin, and thyroid function tests), and an electrocardiogram. Consideration also should be given to determining cholesterol, magnesium, calcium, amylase, liver enzymes, muscle enzymes, and performing bone densitometry and a drug screen.

Symptoms and Signs of Anorexia Nervosa

Most of the physical signs and symptoms of AN reflect adaptation to semistarvation. Growth arrest may occur if starvation preceeds epiphyseal closure. Decreases in catecholamine, thyroid, and insulin levels are responsible for the reductions in metabolic rate, pulse rate, blood pressure, respiratory rate, oxygen consumption, carbon dioxide production, cardiac output, hypothermia, cold intolerance, dry skin, dry hair, hypercarotenemia, hypercholesterolemia, prolongation of ankle reflexes, slowed gastric motility, and constipation. Along with emaciation, brain and myocardial atrophy may be present. The latter may produce mitral valve prolapse, which is reversible with weight gain. The QT interval on the electrocardiogram may be prolonged. Cardiac arrest may occur in 5 to 15% of cases. Neurologic signs include peripheral neuropathy, apathy, withdrawal, irritability, impaired cognition, and obsessive thinking about food. Volume deficits in gray matter may persist in spite of weight restoration. The hypothalamic-gonadal axis response to energy deprivation decreases gonodotropic hormones (LH, FSH), testosterone, and estrogen resulting in lanugo hair, anovulation, amenorrhea, infertility, reduced libido, and decreased bone density. Other signs of diffuse hypothalamic dysfunction are altered fluid balance (edema, dehydration, dizziness, syncope) and abnormal thermoregulation (hypothermia, defective shivering, inadequate response to heat and cold exposure). Nonspecific findings include abdominal distress, bloating, delayed gastric emptying, slowed gastrointestinal transit time, anemia, and kidney dysfunction. Osteoporosis and stress fractures may result from both malnutrition and estrogen deficiency. Signs of micronutrient deficiencies such as Wernicke's syndrome, night blindness, scurvy, etc., may develop in occasional patients. Laboratory abnormalities include anemia, leukopenia, thrombocytopenia, hypo- or hypernatremia, hypo- or hyperkalemia, ketoacidosis, abnormal liver functions, and elevated amylase. If the patient participates in purging behavior, signs and symptoms similar to those of bulimia may also be present. Even in the absence of vomiting there may be significant dental disease (decalcification, enamel erosion, tooth decay, gum disease) because the saliva is deficient in buffers and many of the low-calorie foods and soft drinks that AN patients favor provide an acid load.

Symptoms and Signs of Bulimia Nervosa

Body weight may range from underweight to any degree of obesity; significant weight fluctuations are common. Menses may become irregular. Binge eating may induce pancreatitis, disruption of the myenteric plexus, and rupture of the stomach. Subjects who are prone to reactive hypoglycemia may experience symptoms following binges.

The method of purging determines many of the signs. Fluid and electrolyte disturbances may result from any purging method, whereas signs and symptoms of vomiting include swelling of salivary glands, sore throat, dental erosions and caries, calluses of knuckles, tearing of the esophagus, esophagitis, hematemesis, muscle weakness (including cardiac) secondary to ipecac toxicity, alkalosis, and hypokalemia.

Laxative abuse may produce disruption of bowel function leading to laxative dependence, cathartic colon, hyperchloremic metabolic acidosis, hypokalemia, and loss of protective mucus that may increase vulnerability to infection. Diuretic abuse may cause symptomatic hypokalemia with cardiac arrhythmias, palpitations, muscle spasms, myalgia, and weakness.

Laboratory signs include electrolyte imbalance (hypo- or hypernatremia, hypo- or hyperkalemia, hyperchloremia, acidosis, alkalosis), elevated amylase (salivary or pancreatic origin), and elevated creatine phosphokinase.

To the extent that semistarvation is a feature in bulimia, signs and symptoms are similar to those seen in AN.

Symptoms and Signs of Binge Eating Disorder (BED)

The major complications associated with BED are those associated with obesity, including hypertension, diabetes, and dyslipidemia.

Nutritional Assessment

The nutritional assessment (Table 68.9) should include weight and diet history, nutritional knowledge, feelings and thoughts after consuming various foods, medication regimen, and the frequency and severity of various potential purging strategies. Signs and symptoms of macro- and micronutrient deficiencies should be sought (see above). The patient's level of nutritional knowledge should be assessed; while many patients will be able to recite exact fat and calorie contents of many foods, they may not have knowledge of what constitutes a healthy diet or understand nutritional requirements. A food diary (time, place, type and amount of food eaten, mood, level of hunger) will provide additional useful information.

TABLE 68.9

Comprehensive Nutritional Assessment
Growth and weight history (current, maximum, minimum, premorbid, and ideal weights)
Dieting history
24-hr recall of foods consumed (typical vs. atypical)
Binge eating behavior (frequency, types and amounts of food, precipitating factors)
Other behaviors (harsh/restrictive dieting, fasting, tasting, diet pills, overeating, snacking)
Method, frequency, and severity of purging behavior (including ipecac use)
Physical activity patterns and exercise
Review of laboratory results (serum electrolytes, serum glucose, CBC, albumin, prealbumin)
Review of medications and supplements
Completion of baseline food diary
Food surveys
Nutritional knowledge
Food portion size estimation
Physical findings
Interview with family members/significant others

Clinical Interview

The clinical interview (Table 68.10) should include a detailed assessment of the disordered eating behavior as well as comorbid conditions, family dysfunction, and other pathology. In addition to the nutrition assessment, the patient's body image is extremely important (image dissatisfaction, image distortion, image goals, ratings of satisfaction with various body parts, comparisons between current self and ideal self, and thoughts and feelings about weight, shape, and size).

TABLE 68.10

Comprehensive Clinical Interview of Patient with an Eating Disorder
Nutritional assessment (see above)
Body image (overall, specific body parts and areas, dissatisfaction, distortion)
Substance use and abuse
Sleep patterns
Sexual maturation/menstrual history
Mental status exam
Presence of comorbid diagnoses
Other identified problems commonly found among patients with eating disorders
Suicidal ideation/self-harming behavior
History of unwanted/traumatic sexual experiences
Complete developmental history
Medical complications associated with eating disorders
Medical history and family medical history
Psychiatric history (include details about past treatment) and family psychiatric history
Academic and occupational history
Assessment of relationships with family members, peers, significant others

Psychological Testing

A number of psychological tests are designed specifically for the assessment of eating disorders and related problems, and have been validated. A battery of psychological tests designed to assess the presence of other psychiatric diagnoses is also desirable. This includes objective measurements of depression, personality, and other diagnostic categories.

Behavioral Assessment

Completion of a food diary is important not only to assess the patient's baseline level of food intake, but also to determine various factors that may influence the restrictive dieting, binge eating, and purging processes. Direct observation of the consumption of a meal helps the assessment process. Attention should be paid to the types of food selections, the presence of finicky eating behaviors, bite sizes, rate of chewing and swallowing, the duration of the meal, the amount of food and liquid consumed, and the patient's thoughts and feelings present during the meal. Ratings before, during and after the meal concerning hunger level, fear of weight gain, anxiety level, fullness/bloatedness, urge to binge, and urge to purge are helpful. Finally, pulse and blood pressure readings before, during, and after the meal might provide valuable information, given their correlation with one's anxiety level.

Interview with Family Members/Significant Others

Patients with eating disorders are not likely to seek treatment on their own and may falsify and conceal information about their food intake. Therefore, talking to family members or a significant other with permission from the patient can provide valuable information about the extent of disordered eating and purging patterns, the amount of weight loss, the patient's premorbid level of functioning, comorbid symptoms, the patient's family environment, and other potential contributing factors. It also is important to assess the family as a system. Table 68.11 provides a brief outline of family factors to consider.

Treatment

There is no single treatment regimen; optimal treatment must be tailored for the individual. Hospitalization is indicated in the presence of life-threatening malnutrition, severe psychiatric impairment, and overwhelming comorbidity. Less severe illness may be treated with partial hospitalization, outpatient therapy, or in rare cases, with a healthy peer or self-help program. A multidisciplinary approach involving a treatment team with a minimum of a psychologist, psychiatrist, and nutritionist is highly recommended.

A number of factors should be considered in determining the most appropriate setting (Table 68.12) and form of treatment.[1] Inpatient treatment in a medical/psychiatric setting or an eating disorders specialty unit will increase the chances of recovery when compared to general inpatient psychiatric settings whose staffs lack the training and experience typically necessary to treat eating disorder patients.[32]

Refeeding is an absolute requirement of the recovery process. Garner and Needleman[33] and LaVia et al.[34] have provided excellent guides for the development of a treatment plan, within various settings, that is determined by a number of patient characteristics and the

TABLE 68.11

Assessment of the Family of Eating Disorder Patients

General functioning
Emphasis on appearance and thinness
Influence of social and cultural factors
History of eating disorders or obesity among other family members
History of psychopathology among other family members
Physical illness among other family members
Poor relations between parents; divorce, separation
Impact of the eating disorder on the family system and its members
Impaired interactions/communication patterns between family members
Enmeshment, triangulation, and unhealthy alliances or coalitions
Overindulgence of the patient
Overprotectiveness of the patient
Separation/individuation and autonomy issues
Independence/dependence conflict
Poor affective expression
Diffusion of boundaries
Parentification of the patient
Rigidity
Chaotic environment
Conflict avoidance or poor conflict resolution

TABLE 68.12

Determining the Most Appropriate Eating Disorder Treatment Setting[a]

Medical Factors
Orthostatic hypotension
Bradycardia
Tachycardia
Inability to sustain core body temperature
Prior experience with patient at weight required medical intervention
Behavioral/Nutritional Factors
Rapid or persistent decrease in oral food intake and inability to consume adequate diet
Continued decline in weight despite outpatient and partial hospitalization intervention
Failure to abide by reasonable minimum weight contract
Psychiatric Factors
Presence of additional stressors that contribute to patient's inability to consume adequate diet
Significant comorbid diagnoses that warrant intervention on inpatient basis (suicidality)

[a] Adapted from American Psychiatric Association, *Am J Psych* 157:1; 2000.

severity of the illness. Hospitalization alone will probably not be enough for most patients, but is an important and often necessary first step in the treatment process which will need to include outpatient followup and possibly day treatment.

All treatment plans should include the goal of reestablishing a healthy weight (i.e., return of menses and ovulation in females, healthy physical growth, sexual maturation and development in children and adolescents). Efforts should be made to increase patient motivation and commitment to the therapeutic process and facilitate ownership of a goal of "wellness." Nutritional education and counseling also is a necessary component of the treatment regimen. Efforts should be made to modify core thoughts, feelings, and attitudes related to the eating disorder symptomatology, and associated comorbidity and other maladaptive behaviors should be targeted for change. Inclusion of the patient's family or a significant other in the therapeutic process is strongly recommended and is necessary when working with patients who remain in the family home. Treatment should only be considered complete after a period of extensive followup that is designed to enhance relapse prevention. For a thorough review of treatment methods, see Garner and Garfinkel.[35]

Medical Stabilization and Nutritional Rehabilitation, Education, and Counseling

The primary goal of inpatient treatment is medical stabilization with followup care provided within a partial hospitalization or outpatient setting. Fluid and electrolyte abnormalites should be corrected before implementation of refeeding, since these abnormalites will be exacerbated by the refeeding. Dehydration, hypo- or hypernatremia, and hypokalemia are common with any purging method, whereas alkalosis and acidosis accompany vomiting and laxative abuse, respectively. The refeeding syndrome is characterized by glucose and fluid intolerance, hypokalemia, hypophosphatemia, hypomagnesemia, thiamin deficency, and cardiac insufficiency.[36] These electrolyte abnormalites may not be present prior to the initiation of feeding and may develop precipitously. In the face of malnutrition, cells are depleted in potassium, phosphate, and magnesium, and overloaded with sodium. As energy substrate becomes more available, the sodium pump rapidly restores the intracellular electrolyte levels at the expense of extracellular pools.

Standard medical therapy should be provided for pancreatitis and gastrointestinal bleeding. Symptoms related to gastrointestinal dysmotility improve significantly with refeeding.[37] Prokinetic agents improve gastric emptying,[38] but it remains to be determined if they affect outcome of the eating disorder. Osteoporosis is not rapidly reversed by weight gain or resumption of menses; the efficacy of estrogen and/or calcium supplementation remains to be determined. Patients should be referred to a dentist to repair damage and minimize future problems. Parotid swelling may persist for years after recovery[39] but is benign and does not require treatment.

The general principles of nutritional treatment include:

- Education about the physical and psychological consequences of starvation and binge eating
- Encouragement to begin eating a healthy diet
- Interruption of fasting, binge eating, and purging behaviors
- Initial weight stabilization with gradual restitution of a healthy body weight
- Being comfortable with and eventually including all foods in the patient's diet
- Recognition of appropriate weight and body fat proportions of a healthy body

Education also should include information concerning the body's needs for various macronutrients, sources of nutrients, RDAs, and other pertinent information. Patients should learn about the food pyramid, food portion size estimation, food labeling, grocery shopping, and cooking techniques.

Eating disorders are heterogenous; different approaches are needed with different patients. The clinician must be open to whatever treatment approach works best with the particular patient. Regular contact with a nutritionist is warranted, especially in the early stages of treatment.

For AN, encouraging large portions and high-energy snacks is often counterproductive. Due to the low body weight and hypometabolic state, "average" portions of food will begin the weight restoration process. A minimum of 1200 kcal per day is suggested.

Opinions differ regarding the rate of weight gain and appropriate techniques. Increases in energy intake should be gradual to prevent refeeding syndrome (see above). Energy requirements during the weight gain phase may vary widely. In forced feeding (parenteral nutrition) studies, the excess calories required per kilogram of weight gain ranged between 5569 and 15619 kcal, with a mean of 9768 kcal.[40] Subjects who were normal weight prior to the onset of anorexia gain less rapidly and increase their metabolic rate after a glucose challenge more dramatically than subjects who were obese prior to the onset of anorexia.[41] The thermic effect of glucose is greater in AN than in controls.[41] In subjects who have experienced growth arrest, energy intake should be sufficient to support catch-up growth. Exercise should not be severely restricted, so that muscle mass can be restored.

In the inpatient setting, meals and subsequent bathroom access are usually supervised initially. Programs vary in their flexibility regarding refusal to eat certain foods and the use of liquid supplements to replace food not eaten at regular meals. Ultimately, the meal plan should be well-balanced, consist of conventional foods, and be individualized to patient needs. Multiple small meals may be better tolerated than three main meals. Efforts should be made to help patients to eat during three designated meal times, as this meal pattern will probably allow the patient to generalize her behavior to the home environment more easily. "Fattening" and "forbidden foods" should be gradually introduced into the diet. Aversion to fat persists in the recovered state.[42] Educating the patient on a meal plan based on the exchange system rather than counting kcalories is preferred to prevent obsession with the energy content of food. Weight should be tracked, but not overemphasized. Enteral or parenteral nutritional support may be required for life-threatening protein energy malnutrition (i.e., body weight <70% of ideal weight). Therapists disagree about the appropriateness of forced feeding, as control is such an important issue in most AN patients. It should be borne in mind, however, that severe malnutrition may impair cognition. If possible, patients should be allowed approximately 24 h to do as they please with their meals, after which time a supplemental regimen might be considered to ensure adequate energy intake. This will promote autonomy over the eating process for the patient. Refeeding should be done with extreme caution to avoid electrolyte abnormalites (see above), edema, and fatal cardiac arrhythmias.

Since the initial energy intake recommendations in early phases of treatment are likely to be low, a multiple vitamin and mineral supplement is appropriate. If signs and symptoms of micronutrient deficiency syndromes are present, the specific micronutrient should be prescribed.

For BN and BED, initial therapy focuses on regularity in eating habits and stabilization in weight. Bulimic subjects tend to eat more fat and simple carbohydrate and less protein and complex carbohydrate than subjects without eating disorders.[43-44] Normalized eating with adequate protein and complex carbohydrate intake will reduce the risk of a binge being induced by excessive hunger. The energy content of a patient's meal plan should be determined by the Harris-Benedict equation. Patients have been known to respond better to meals if they are allowed to exclude certain high-risk binge foods from their diet early in the course of treatment. Following achievement of appropriate eating behavior, a healthy diet to achieve gradual weight loss can be implemented if appropriate. However, setting strict limitations on fat consumption only perpetuates the notion of "bad" foods, and may trigger bingeing.

Pharmacotherapy

Pharmacologic treatment shoud be considered as an adjunct, especially in the management of comorbid behavior, e.g., depression, obsessive-compulsive behavior, and anxiety. For

BN and BED patients, a selective sertonin reuptake inhibitor (SSRI, e.g., fluoxetine) is usually the drug of choice. SSRIs suppress symptoms of disordered eating independent of their antidepressant effects. Tricyclic antidepressants, mirtazapine and olanzapine, often cause weight gain as a side effect, and thus would be more suitable of AN patients. For overweight BN and BED patients, sibutramine (inhibits reuptake of serotonin and norepinephine) might be helpful.

Individual Therapy

It is important to establish trust and communicate empathy, support, encouragement, and understanding while also setting specific behavioral limitations. Once a therapeutic alliance has been established, the therapist must work toward moving the focus of therapy sessions away from discussions about the amount of food to be consumed, weight, and other specific symptoms, and toward underlying issues related to family dysfunction, relationship problems, low self-esteem, body image concerns, the patient's struggle for autonomy, identity issues, and other identified problems previously outlined. Therapists also should consider exploration of the developmental and cultural factors as well as the family dynamics that may have contributed to the development and maintenance of the eating disorder symptoms. Many forms of individual therapy have been employed in the treatment of the eating disorders, including cognitive-behavioral therapy (CBT), behavioral therapy (BT), interpersonal therapy (IPT), feminist treatment, and various psychodynamically-oriented therapies. Although each of these approaches may prove successful with eating disorder patients, a combination of therapies may prove most helpful, especially as one considers the comorbid disorders that accompany the eating disorders.

CBT, designed to challenge the patient's irrational, distorted, and negative automatic thinking patterns and the negative core belief system, has become the standard of treatment for the eating disorders.[33] CBT is at least comparable, and often superior to, all other types of therapy for eating disorders, especially BN and BED.[45] CBT emphasizes the self-monitoring of food intake and the identification of antecedent stimuli that elicit periods of restrictive dieting and/or binge eating and purging.[46,47] Patients are taught to identify stressful situations and the accompanying aversive thoughts and emotions. Ways to cope (problem-solving skills, cognitive restructuring, and other coping strategies) are emphasized. CBT also targets normalized eating patterns, meal planning, goal setting, cognitive restructuring, education about the eating disorders and related medical complications, and prevention of relapse. CBT appears to be superior to the use of medication alone in reducing bulimic symptoms. The combination of CBT and medication may prove even more beneficial, especially if the medication is indicated after consideration of any comorbidity.[45]

BT utilizes combinations of reinforcers (empathic praise and encouragement, access to exercise, visitation, social activities, and other privileges) contingent upon weight gain, appropriate food consumption, decreased purging behavior, and a general movement toward the display of "well" behavior. BT may prove helpful during the initial stages of inpatient treatment for AN. BT also may include meal monitoring, post-meal observations, exposure with response prevention, and temptation exposure with response prevention procedures. Specifically, patients are exposed to meals or binge foods and guided in their efforts to refrain from vomiting after food consumption. Results are equivocal.[1] The addition of behavior therapy to aid in the weight loss process in BED patients has been shown to contribute to decreases in binge eating and weight loss.[45]

In the last decade, increasing attention has been paid to the use of IPT in the treatment of eating disorders. IPT[48] does not focus directly on the eating disorder symptoms, but rather on the interpersonal difficulties the patient is experiencing. It is believed that problems in relationships with family members, friends, and significant others contribute to the onset and maintenance of eating disorders, and that resolving these interpersonal difficulties will help to eliminate the eating disorder symptoms. Working through issues of grief, interpersonal role disputes, role transitions, and interpersonal deficits are important aspects of this treatment. IPT may be less effective than CBT at the end of treatment for BN. After a one-year follow-up period, CBT and IPT appeared equally effective.[47,49] Similarly, CBT and IPT have proved equally effective in the treatment of BED.[50]

Psychodynamic therapies have been employed in the treatment of eating disorders since Bruch[19] first introduced her etiological theories for the eating disorders. Although numerous case studies have suggested that these approaches may prove helpful, no controlled studies of the effectiveness of these therapies compared to other forms of treatment have been published.[33] Psychodynamic therapies incorporated into the types of therapy described above may be warranted in the treatment of patients who fail to respond.[33]

Scant data exist regarding the efficacy of utilizing a feminist treatment paradigm in the treatment of the eating disorders. Many therapists who specialize in the treatment of eating disorders believe emphasis should be placed on helping the female patient to identify the sociocultural factors that may have contributed to her struggle with body image concerns and maladaptive dieting patterns. It is important to consider the distribution of power in the therapeutic relationship and to encourage the empowerment of the patient through cooperative treatment planning.[51] Russo[52] has provided a detailed outline of principles to consider in treating patients from a feminist perspective. Feminist treatment emphasizes the importance of considering issues such as various forms of victimization, role conflicts and confusion, sexual abuse, the struggle for power and control, and general interpersonal relationships.[33]

Family Therapy

Family therapy is a necessary component of the treatment regimen when working with a child or adolescent or an adult who is still living with his/her family of origin. The primary goal of family therapy is to facilitate the remission of the eating disorder symptomatology and begin a therapeutic process of change within the family. Other goals include changing the status or role of the identified patient within the family, attempting to translate the eating disorder symptoms into a problem of interpersonal communication and family relationships, expanding the problem and taking emphasis off of the eating disorder, and identifying other maladaptive communication patterns. Attempts are made to disengage the patient's parents from using the eating disorder symptoms in a way that leads to further conflict avoidance, overprotectiveness, overindulgence, patient dependence, enmeshment, diffusion of boundaries, and unhealthy coalitions. Family members are taught how to more effectively express and tolerate strong emotions, and the patient's struggle for independence or need for increased dependence is acknowledged and addressed in family therapy. A comprehensive review of family therapy for eating disorders has recently been published by Lemmon and Josephson.[53]

Group Therapy

Oesterheld and colleagues[54] conducted a meta-analysis of 40 group treatment studies, and concluded that group therapy is moderately effective in the treatment of eating disorders. Group therapies prove most helpful when utilized in combination with individual therapies and nutritional education and counseling. Group therapies have merit, since the group experience helps patients reduce the tremendous shame, guilt, and isolation often seen among these patients. Similarly, patients may benefit from the feedback and support provided to them by peers who will typically present with varying degrees of progress in treatment.[1] Group therapy may take the form of a process-oriented group that emphasizes working through difficulties in relationships through the interactions patients experience with their peers, or a more psychoeducational approach that emphasizes the acquisition and practice of new skills. Groups also may be designed to include therapies that closely resemble the types of individual treatment outlined above. Others may emphasize specific problems encountered by patients, such as body image problems, stress management deficits, and other specific skill deficits. A combination of these approaches will probably prove most helpful.

Although little research has investigated the efficacy of treatment programs that follow an addiction model, participation in Overeater's Anonymous has clearly helped some patients. Overeaters Anonymous is a 12-step self-help program, adapted from Alcoholics Anonymous, for people trying to overcome compulsive eating. Groups offer unconditional acceptance and support based on principles grounded in spirituality. Major drawbacks include lack of nutrition education, sometimes the restriction of specific foods (especially sugar and white flour), and lack of data supporting effectiveness.

Participation in group occupational therapy also may prove beneficial, as this type of treatment may help to reduce perfectionism and enhance a patient's self-esteem and self-efficacy.[1]

Physical Therapy

The basic goal of physical therapy is to develop regular moderate physical activity as part of a new lifestyle for the purposes of improving health, stress management, and weight management. Sedentary patients should be counseled about starting an exercise regimen, determining physical activity interests, picking an exercise regimen that will fit into one's daily schedule, setting realistic goals, addressing safety issues, methods of self-reinforcement, and anticipating and refraining from noncompliance. Other important topics include emphasizing improved health rather than weight loss, determining one's resting heart rate, maximum heart rate, and a training-sensitive zone, and the importance of finding an exercise partner.

For BN patients who use excessive exercise as a purging method and for most AN patients, emphasis should be placed on decreasing (but not eliminating) physical activity.

Environmental Exposure

A treatment method often not considered involves exposing patients in graduated steps to environmental situations that they are likely to encounter outside of treatment. This would include activities such as taking more responsibility for refraining from purging behavior by operating without a post-meal observation period, and accepting more responsibility for adequate nutrition by going to the cafeteria and making one's own food selections prior to discharge from the hospital. Other activities might include grocery shopping, eating at a fast-food restaurant or the food court at the mall, eating with one's family, trying on clothes in a store, and any other behaviors the patient has avoided because of his eating disorder. Patients are guided through this process with the help of a therapist, and taught how to use cognitive therapy techniques, self-reinforcement, self-soothing statements, relaxation responses, etc.

Prognosis

Accurate statistics are difficult to determine, but the mortality rate for AN is estimated to be 4 to 6%. Long-term followup shows persistant psychiatric and weight disturbances in the majority of patients.The prognosis is worse for males than females. It is estimated that 50% of BN patients fully recover. The outcome for BED patients is unknown.

Additional Sources of Information

Organizations

AABA — American Anorexia/Bulimia Assoc., 165 West 46th St. #1108, New York, NY 10036, (212) 575-6200, www.aabainc.org

AED — Academy for Eating Disorders, Degnon Associates, Inc., 6728 Old McLean Village Dr., McLean, VA 22101-3906, (703) 556-8729, www.acadeatdis.org

ANAD — Anorexia Nervosa and Associated Disorders, Box 7, Highland Park, IL 60035, (708) 831-3438, www.anad.org

ANRED — Anorexia Nervosa and Related Eating Disorders, P.O. Box 5102, Eugene, OR, 97405, (541) 344-1144, www.anred.com

EDAP — Eating Disorders Awareness and Prevention, 603 Stewart St., Suite 803, Seattle,WA 98101, (206) 382-3587, www.edap.org

IAEDP — International Assoc. of Eating Disorders Professionals, 427 CenterPointe Circle #1819, Altamonte Springs, FL 32701, (800) 800-8126, www.iaedp.com

Overeaters Anonymous Headquarters, World Services Office, 6075 Zenith Ct. NE, Rio Rancho, NM 87124, (505) 891-2664, www.overeatersanonymous.org

Bibliographies

Professional Resources about Eating Disorders (complied by USDA Dec. 1995). www.nal.usda.gov/fnic/pubs/bibs/gen/anorhpbr.htm

EDAP Reading List Resources for the Prevention of Eating Disorders (prepared winter 1999). www.edap.org/reading.html

Online Resources

www.mentalhelp.net
www.something-fishy.com
www.closetoyou.org/eatingdisorders
www.caringonline.com
www.gurze.com

References

1. American Psychiatric Association, *Am J Psych* 157:1; 2000.
2. Yager J. In: *Clinical Psychiatry for Medical Students,* Stoudemire A, Ed, J. B. Lippincott, Philadelphia, PA, 1994, pg 355.

3. American Psychiatric Association. *Diagnostic and Statistical Manual of Mental Disorders*, 4th ed, American Psychiatric Association, Washington, DC, 1994.
4. Stunkard, AJ. *Psychiatr Q* 33:284; 1959.
5. Andersen AE. *Eating Disorders Rev* 4(5):1; 1993.
6. Olivardia R, Pope HG, Mangweth B, Hudson JI. *Am J Psych* 152:1279; 1995.
7. Yanovski SZ, Nelson JE, Dubbert BK, Spitzer RL. *Am J Psych* 150:1472; 1993.
8. National Institutes of Health. *Binge eating disorder*, U.S. Government Printing Office, Washington, DC, 1993, pg 1.
9. Yanovski SZ. *Obesity Res* 1:306; 1993.
10. Powers PS. In *Handbook of Treatment for Eating Disorders*, 2nd ed, Garner DM, Garfinkel PE, Eds, The Guilford Press, New York, 1997, pg 424.
11. Fava M, Copeland P, Schweiger U, Herzog D. *Am J Psych* 146:963; 1989.
12. Herholz K. *Psych Res* 62:105; 1996.
13. Lucas A. *Mayo Clin Proc* 56:254; 1981.
14. Casper RC. *Psych Clin N Am* 7:201; 1984.
15. Goldbloom DS, Kennedy SH. In: *Medical Issues and the Eating Disorders*, Kaplan AS, Garfinkel PE, Eds, Brunner/Mazel, New York, 1993, pg 123.
16. Walters EE, Kendler KS. *Am J Psych* 152:64; 1995.
17. Woodside DB. In: *Medical Issues and the Eating Disorders*, Kaplan AS, Garfinkel PE, Eds, Brunner/Mazel, New York, 1993, pg 193.
18. Lilenfeld LR, Kaye WH. In: *Neurobiology in the Treatment of Eating Disorders* Hoek HW, Treasure JL, Katzman MA, Eds, Wiley, New York, 1998, pg 169.
19. Bruch H. *Eating Disorders: Obesity, Anorexia Nervosa, and the Person Within*, New York, Basic Books, 1973, pg 1.
20. Striegel-Moore RH, Silberstein LR, Rodin J. *Am Psychol* 41:246; 1986.
21. Keys A, Brozek J, Henschel A, et al. *The Biology of Human Starvation*, University of Minnesota Press, Minneapolis, 1950, pg 1.
22. Killian K. *Fam Relations* 43:311; 1994.
23. Schwartz RC, Barrett MJJ. *Psychother Fam* 3:131; 1988.
24. Minuchin S, Rosman BL, Baker L. *Psychosomatic Families: Anorexia Nervosa in Context*, Harvard University Press, Cambridge, MA, 1978, pg 1.
25. Selvini-Palazzoli M, Viaro M. *Fam Proc* 27:129; 1988.
26. Yager J. In: *Family Therapy and Major Psychopathology*, Lansky MR, Ed, Grune and Stratton, New York, NY, 1981, pg 249.
27. Stierlin H, Weber G. *Unlocking the Family Door: A Systemic Approach to the Understanding and Treatment of Anorexia Nervosa*, Brunner/Mazel, New York, 1989, pg 1.
28. Root MPP, Fallon P, Friedrich WN. Bulimia: *A Systems Approach to Treatment*, Norton, NY, 1986, pg 1.
29. Prochaska JO, DiClemente CC, Norcross JC. *Am Psychol* 47:1102; 1992.
30. Vitousek K, Watson S, Wilson GT. *Clin Psych Rev* 18:391; 1998.
31. Ramsay R, Ward A, Treasure J, Russell GFM. *Brit J Psych* 175:147; 1999.
32. Palmer RL, Treasure J. *Brit J Psych* 175:306; 1999.
33. Garner DM, Needleman LD. In: *Handbook of Treatment for Eating Disorders*, 2nd ed, Garner DM, Garfinkel PE, Ed, The Guilford Press, New York, 1997, pg 50.
34. LaVia M, Kaye WH, Andersen A, et al. *Am J Psych* 157:1; 2000.
35. Garner DM, Garfinkel PE, Eds. *Handbook of Treatment for Eating Disorders*, 2nd ed, The Guilford Press, New York, 1997.
36. Solomon SM, Kirby DF. *JPEN* 14:90; 1990.
37. Waldholtz BD, Andersen AE. *Gastroenterology* 98:1415; 1990.
38. Stacher G, Bergmann H, Wiesnagrotzki S, et al. *Gastroenterology* 92:1000; 1987.
39. Hasler JF. *Oral Surg* 52:567; 1982.
40. Dempsey DT, Crosby LO, Pertschuck MJ, et al. *Am J Clin Nutr* 39:236; 1984.
41. Stordy BJ, Marks V, Kalucy RS, Crisp AH, *Am J Clin Nutr* 30:138; 1977.
42. Sunday SR, Einhorn A, Halmi KA. *Am J Clin Nutr* 55:362; 1992.
43. Van der Ster Wallin G, Norring C, Lennernas MAC, Holmgren S. *J Am Coll Nutr* 14:271; 1995.

44. Hetherington MH, Altemus M, Nelson ML, et al. *Am J Clin Nutr* 60:864; 1994.
45. Peterson CB, Mitchell JE. *JCLP/In Session: Psychotherapy in Practice* 55:685; 1999.
46. Fairburn CG. *Psychol Med* 141:631; 1981.
47. Fairburn CG, Marcus MD, Wilson GW. In: *Binge Eating: Nature, Assessment and Treatment* Fairburn CG, Wilson GW, Eds, The Guilford Press, New York, 1993, pg 361.
48. Fairburn CG. In: *Handbook of Treatment for Eating Disorders,* 2nd ed, Garner DM, Garfinkel PE. Eds, The Guilford Press, New York, 1997, pg 278.
49. Fairburn CG, Jones R, Peveler RC, et al. *Arch Gen Psych* 48:463; 1991.
50. Wilfley DE, Agras WS, Telch CF, et al. *J Consulting Clin Psychol* 61:296; 1993.
51. Sesan R. In: *Feminist Perspectives on Eating Disorders* Fallon P, Katzman M, Wooley S, Eds, Guilford Press, New York, NY, 1994, pg 1.
52. Russo D. *Newsletter of the American Psychological Association of Graduate Students* 9:3; 1997.
53. Lemmon CR, Josephson AM. In: *Child and Adolescent Psychiatric Clinics of North America: Current Perspectives on Family Therapy,* Josephson, A, Ed, WB Saunders, Philadelphia, 2001, pg. 519.
54. Oesterheld JR, McKenna MS, Gould NB. *Int J Group Psychotherapy* 37:163; 1987.

69

Adult Obesity

Diane K. Smith and Sandra B. Leonard

Introduction

Obesity is a multifactorial disease that is growing in epidemic proportions. It is associated with significant medical risks that may be ameliorated by modest weight loss. Exercise and behavioral modification of diet are the cornerstones of treatment; pharmacotherapy and surgery may be useful adjuncts.

Etiology

It is estimated that 40 to 70% of the variation in obesity within populations is heritable;[1] however, this predisposition can be overridden by environmental cues and behavior (physical activity and nutrient choices). Less common are secondary causes of obesity (Table 69.1).

Genetic Causes

Genetic background strongly influences the risk of obesity, as demonstrated by adoption studies, where adoptees more closely resembled their biologic parents than their adoptive parents,[2] and twin studies that showed a concordance rate in identical twins twice that of fraternal twins.[3] Both positive and negative energy balance studies in twins show greater variations between pairs than within pairs.[4] Although most forms of monogenetic obesity (Table 69.2) are rare to extremely rare, frame shift mutations of the melanocortin-4 (MC4) receptor have been described in 2 to 7% of populations.

More commonly, polygenetic influences are involved. Although extensively studied, candidate genes remain to be identified.[1] These genes may influence food intake, metabolism, energy expenditure, and hormones (Table 69.3).

0-8493-2705-9/02/$0.00+$1.50

TABLE 69.1
Etiology of Obesity

Primary
Genetic
Nutritional
Environmental
Secondary
Neural
hypothalamic lesions
amygdala lesions
temporal lobe lesions
Endocrine
oophorectomy
insulinoma, insulin therapy
Cushing's syndrome, corticoid therapy
Pharmacologic
Viral?

TABLE 69.2
Monogenetic Human Obesity

Prader-Willi syndrome
Laurence-Moon-Biedl syndrome
Cohen's syndrome
Kleinfelter's syndrome
Leptin deficiency
Truncated leptin receptor
Proopiomelanocortin deficiency
Melanocortin-4 receptor

Environmental Causes

Nutritional

The role of nutrient intake in promoting obesity is quantitative, qualitative, and temporal. The increasing availability of food, often in excessive serving sizes, promotes hyperphagia. The intake of dietary fat is significantly related to adiposity. Dietary fat is converted to body fat with approximately 25% greater efficiency than carbohydrate. Dietary fat may be less satiating than protein and complex carbohydrates, although foods with a high glycemic index (i.e., rapidly converted to glucose) may stimulate hunger and lead to more frequent eating. The long-chain fatty acid composition of dietary fat influences energy utilization; low ratios of polyunsaturated to saturated fat are associated with lower respiratory quotients (RQ; moles of carbon dioxide produced per mole of oxygen consumed).[5] Low protein diets are utilized less efficiently than high protein diets. The pattern of food intake may play a role in the development of obesity. Widely spaced meals are used less efficiently because of the energy cost of storage. Compared to immediate oxidation, the energy cost of converting glucose into glycogen is 5%, and into fat is 28%.

Inactivity

Physical inactivity is increasing as a result of decreased manual labor, the use of labor-saving devices, and a shift in leisure preferences (television, computers, spectator sports).

TABLE 69.3

Obesity-Related Factors Thought to be Genetically Modulated

Diet Related
Dietary fat preferences
Appetite regulation
Amount and rate of eating
Metabolism/Nutrient Partitioning
Adipose tissue distribution
Adipose tissue lipolysis
Adipose tissue and muscle lipoprotein lipase (LPL) activity
Muscle composition and oxidative potential
Free fatty acid and β-receptor activities in adipose tissue
Capacities for fat and carbohydrate oxidation
Energy Expenditure
Metabolic rate
Dietary induced thermogenesis
Nutrient partitioning
Propensity for physical activity/inactivity
Hormonal
Insulin sensitivity/resistance
Growth hormone status
Leptin action

Psychosocial Factors

A cause-and-effect relationship between low socioeconomic status and obesity has been demonstrated.[6] Societal ideals of desirable weight have various ethnic, cultural, and gender determinants. Emotional distress may promote overeating. The hormonal response to stress has been suggested to promote visceral adiposity.[7]

Secondary Obesity

Endocrine changes secondary to obesity (insulin resistance, decreased growth hormone secretion, blunted prolactin responsiveness, hyperparathyroidism, decreased serum testosterone in men) may make it difficult to determine whether obesity is primary or secondary. Secondary obesity may result from hypothyroidism, Cushing's syndrome, insulinoma, hypogonadism, Frolich syndrome, hypothalamic tumors, head injury, or drugs (Table 69.4). There are several known animal models of viral-induced obesity. Antibodies to human adenovirus AD-36 (capable of producing obesity in chickens and mice) have been observed in some obese humans.[8]

Energy Balance

Within groups, there is not a correlation between energy intake and body weight; for the individual, intake does correlate with weight. Therefore, obesity can be viewed as a

TABLE 69.4

Drugs That May Promote Weight Gain

Tricyclic antidepressants
Lithium
Sulfonylureas
Thiazolidinediones
β-adrenergic blockers
Some steroid contraceptives
Corticosteriods
Insulin
Cyproheptadine
Sodium valproate
Neuroleptics

disorder of energy homeostasis. This variability may be either innate or acquired, and may be the result of hyperphagia, energy partitioning, intermediary metabolism, the efficiency of the coupling of electron transport to ATP generation, the efficiency of ATPases, degree of physical activity, the magnitude of adaptive thermogenesis, hormonal influences on energy expenditure, and physiological demands (growth, pregnancy, lactation).

Appetite Regulation

The major loci in the central nervous system that regulate feeding behavior are the dorsomedial, paraventricular, arcuate, and lateral nuclei of the hypothalamus, the prefrontal cortex, the amygdala, the nucleus accumbens, and the nucleus of the solitary tract. These sites respond to a variety of stimuli including deprivation, intracellular glucose concentration, intracellular fat oxidation, food choice, meal timing, desire, mood, stress, metabolic rate, fidgeting, fat stores (via leptin), and ingestive behavior. These areas communicate via complex interactions of neuromodulators that either suppress or stimulate feeding (Table 69.5). Many of these peptides are found in the gut as well as the brain.

Appetite regulation can also be viewed as several interacting feedback loops. The glucostat theory involves glucose-sensitive neurons that stimulate appetite under conditions of low glucose levels, and glucoreceptors in the liver that provide the afferent signal via the vagus nerve. Leptin, a protein produced by adipocytes, appears to drive the adipostat, which is thought to measure the adequacy of fat stores. Thermogenesis in brown adipose tissue has been proposed as a thermostatic regulator of food intake.[9]

Energy Partitioning

Genetic, hormonal, nutritional, and physical activity factors influence the partitioning of energy between fat and fat-free mass, as well as preference for carbohydrate versus fat oxidation to meet energy needs. A high RQ has been shown to predict future weight gain.[10,11] Obese subjects have an attenuation of both basal- and epinephrine-stimulated rates of lipolysis[12] that may in part result from hyperinsulinemia. Dietary fat intake may also influence substrate utilization, with low ratios of polyunsaturated to saturated fats resulting in lower RQs.[13]

A propensity to excessive fat stores may result from increased LPL activity and peroxisome proliferator-activating receptor (PPAR) abnormalities. Lipoprotein lipase activity is increased in obesity, although it is unclear if this increase is a cause or result of obesity. Adipose tissue LPL activity increases during caloric restriction and may lead to rapid weight

TABLE 69.5

Neuromodulators of Appetite Regulation

Stimulatory
Norepinephrine (α-2)
Endogenous opioids
Dopamine (physiologic levels)
Neuropeptide Y
Peptide YY
Orexins
Galanin
Agouti-related protein
Melanin-concentrating hormone
Inhibitory
Norepinephrine (β)
Epinephrine (β)
Dopamine (supraphysiologic)
Serotonin
Cholecystokinin
Somatostatin
Glucagon, glucagon-like protein (GLP-1)
Urocortin
Corticotropin-releasing hormone (CRH)
Melanocortin agonists (e.g., proopiomelanocortin, melanocyte-stimulating hormone)
Cocaine/amphetamine regulated transcript
Leptin

regain when caloric restriction is abandoned. PPARs promote differentiation of preadipocytes. Mutations in gamma-2 PPAR have been described in some severely obese humans.[14]

Energy Expenditure

Basal metabolic rate (BMR) is the rate of energy expenditure upon awakening, before any physical activity and 12 to 18 hours after the last meal. More commonly assessed is resting energy expenditure (REE), which is obtained in the resting state several hours after the last meal. The difference between BMR and REE is small. This energy component is expended for maintenance of body functions and homeostasis (primarily proton pumping and protein turnover) and accounts for 60 to 75% of total energy expenditure in sedentary individuals. Subjects with low REE gain more weight than persons with normal or elevated REE.[15] The REE is increased in obesity, related to the individual's increase in lean body mass. REE increases with overfeeding. With caloric restriction, REE is decreased by both the caloric deficit and the resultant loss in lean tissue. Exercise may help minimize REE decrease. Physical training, i.e., being in the "trained state," can also increase REE independent of body composition or the residual effects of the last bout of exercise.[16]

Energy expenditure on physical activity is the most variable, and is the only component of energy balance that is under volitional control. It includes shivering and fidgeting, as well as physical work. It may range from less than 100 kcal/day in sedentary individuals to greater than 1000 kcal/day with strenuous exericise or labor. Exercise efficiency (energy expenditure/unit work) is not altered by obesity, but because of carrying excess weight, more energy will be expended during weight-bearing activities. In general, the obese are less physically active than the lean. The influence of physical activity on obesity, independent of genotype, has been examined in twins, where discordance for obesity was associated with discordance in activity level.[17]

The thermic effect of food (TEF), also known as diet-induced thermogenesis, is the energy cost of food digestion, absorption, metabolism, and storage, as well as a component resulting from sympathetic nervous system activity. It is lowest for fat and highest for excess carbohydrate stored as fat and protein. It may account for up to 10% of daily energy expenditure and consists of both obiligatory and facultative components. The latter may be decreased in obesity. Weight loss does not normalize TEF and may contribute to weight regain.[18-19] However, longitudinal studies have demonstrated declines in glucose-induced thermogenesis with the evolution of obesity.[20] With caloric restriction, the TEF declines.

Exercise may potentiate TEF, especially in insulin-sensitive subjects. Although study results are inconsistent, at least some obese individuals have lesser magnitudes of energy expenditure than their lean counterparts.

Adaptive thermogenesis is influenced by both genetic and environmental (ambient temperature, food intake, emotional stress) factors and usually accounts for 10 to 15% of total energy expenditure. Mechanisms include changes in the efficiency of oxidative phosphorylation, rates of protein turnover, Na pump activity and futile cycles, and activity/inactivity of brown fat (nonshivering thermogenesis). Examples of futile cycles which waste ATP are:

- Glucose to pyruvate to glucose
- Cyclic lipolysis and reesterification of triglycerides
- Glucose to lactate to glucose (Cori cycle)
- Glucose to glucose-6-phosphate to glucose
- Fructose-6-phosphate to fructose-di-phosphate to fructose-6-phosphate
- Pyruvate to phosphoenolpyruvate to pyruvate

Wastage of ATP may also result directly by phosphatases converting ATP to ADP.

Non-shivering thermogenesis as a mechanism of heat production is well established in hibernating animals and infants of various species, although its contribution to adult human obesity is controversial. This thermogenesis occurs in mitochondria of brown adipose tissue, where an uncoupling protein (uncoupling protein-1, or UCP-1) facilitates a proton leak, and thus fat oxidation is dissociated from oxidative phosphorylation. Recently, additional UCPs have been discovered (currently, five are known). Several of the UCPs have genetic linkage to human obesity, but the importance in obesity remains to be delineated. A polymorphism in the UCP-3 gene has been associated with altered REE.[21]

Prevalence of Obesity

Overweight and obesity are increasing dramatically globally. There has been a greater than 25% increase in the U.S. in the past three decades.[22] The CDC reports an astounding 49% increase in obesity in young adults from 1991 to 1998.[23] For U.S. adults, 42% of men and 28% of women are overweight (body mass index [BMI] ≥25 to 29.9); and 21% of men and 27% of women are obese (BMI ≥30).[22] African- and Hispanic-Americans have a higher prevalence of obesity than Anglo-Americans.

Assessment

Assessment of the patient should include the BMI, waist circumference (measured at the level of the iliac crest), and overall medical risk. Bioimpedance analysis is a simple noninvasive technique that measures total body water and total fat, and calculates lean body mass. Other methods of assessment (underwater weighing, doublely labeled water, calorimetry, dual-energy x-ray absorptiometry [DEXA], computerized tomography [CT] scan, and magnetic resonance imaging [MRI]), are expensive and inaccessible to most practitioners. Although skinfold measurements are inexpensive, they have poor reproducibility, especially with increasing obesity.

Body Mass Index

The BMI is highly correlated with fatness, and minimizes the effect of height. It is calculated as:

$$\text{BMI} = \text{wt (in kg)}/\text{ht}^2 \text{ (in meters) or} \qquad \text{(Eq. 69.1)}$$
$$\text{BMI} = \text{wt (in lb)} \times 703/\text{ht}^2 \text{ (in inches)}$$

As an index of mass, it does not distinguish between fat and fat-free mass. Consequently, it is possible to be overweight without having excess adiposity (very muscular individuals) as well as obese without being overweight (sarcopenic individuals). Table 69.6 presents classification for BMI.

Fat Distribution

In addition to total adiposity, distribution of body fat has medical implications (Table 69.7), with abdominal (visceral) fat presenting a greater health risk than gluteal-femoral fat.[24] A waist circumference >40 inches in men or >35 inches in women reflects excess abdominal fat. Gluteal-femoral fat, which is thought to be estrogen dependent, serves as an energy store for lactation and increases during each pregnancy. Following menopause, this fat depot decreases, while intraabdominal fat increases.

Insulin Resistance

Given the key role of hyperinsulinemia on the medical risks of obesity (see below) assessment of insulin resistance is desirable. Most sensitive is the insulin suppression test, although its performance is not practical in the usual care setting. Fasting plasma insulin levels, although less sensitive, are a useful guide.

TABLE 69.6

Classification for BMI

BMI	Weight Classification
18.5-24.9	Normal weight
25.0-29.9	Overweight
30.0-34.9	Class 1 obesity
35.0-39.9	Class 2 obesity
≥40	Class 3 obesity

TABLE 69.7

Metabolic Consequences of Upper Body Obesity

Increased insulin secretion
Decreased hepatic clearance of insulin
Insulin resistance
Increased lipolysis
Increased circulating free fatty acids
Increased free fatty acid oxidation
Increased gluconeogenesis and decreased glucose utilization
Effects of hyperinsulinemia (see Table 69.8)
Increased free testosterone and free androstenedione levels associated with decreased sex hormone-binding globulin in women
Decreased progesterone levels in women
Decreased testosterone levels in men
Increased cortisol production

Medical Risks of Obesity (Comorbidities)

The medical consequences of obesity may result from hyperinsulinemia, mechanical effects of excess weight, and alterations in sex hormones. Especially damaging is hyperinsulinemia (Table 69.8). Increased insulin secretion is related to total body fat; however, decreased hepatic insulin clearance is related specifically to the amount of abdominal fat (may be related to increased androgen effects on the liver). Exhaustion of pancreatic reserves may lead to impaired glucose tolerance. Glucose intolerance relates to increased intra-abdominal visceral fat as opposed to subcutaneous abdominal fat.[25] Other comorbidities associated with hyperinsulinemia include hypertension, hyperlipidemia, atherosclerotic disease, stroke, and polycystic ovarian syndrome.

Mechanical consequences of obesity include congestive heart failure, sleep apnea, restrictive lung disease, surgery risks (pneumonia, wound infection), high risk pregnancy, cellulitis, degenerative arthritis, and steatohepatitis. Alterations in sex hormones contribute to decreased fertility, menorrhagia, oligomenorrhea, and certain cancers (breast, uterus).

Comorbidities are present in approximately two-thirds of subjects with a BMI >27. Hypertension is the most common obesity-related health risk and its prevalence increases markedly with increasing levels of obesity, as does the incidence of type 2 diabetes, gallbladder disease, and osteoarthritis. Hypercholesterolemia, while more common in the overweight and obese than in normal weight individuals, does not show an increase with increasing levels of obesity. However, the risk of coronary heart disease in women does increase with increasing level of obesity.[22,26] The risk for death from cardiovascular disease, cancer, or other diseases increases with increasing degrees of obesity.[27,28] For more extensive detail, the reader is referred to the NIH Clinical Guidelines[29] or the WHO Consultation on Obesity Report.[30] A modest (5 to 15% of initial weight) sustained weight loss will improve many of the health complications of obesity.[31-36]

Treatment

The most effective weight-loss programs combine diet, exercise, behavior modification, and social support. The patient's motivation can be assessed using the Diet Readiness

TABLE 69.8

Effects of Hyperinsulinemia

Renal
Uric acid — increased production, decreased clearance
Decreased potassium and sodium excretion
Lipid Metabolism
Increased VLDL
Decreased HDL
Decreased clearance of chylomicron remnants and IDL
Increased postprandial lipemia
Increased small, dense LDL
Increased "oxidizabilty" of LDL
Decreased lipolytic activity
Glucose Metabolism
Glucose intolerance
Nervous System
Increased sympathetic activity
Cardiovascular
Increased heart rate
Hypertension
Increased plaque formation
Decreased plaque regression
Smooth muscle and connective tissue proliferation
Enhanced LDL receptor activity
Hemostasis
Increased PAI-1
Increased fibrinogen
Increased von Willebrand factor
Increased factor X
Increased adhesion of mononuclear cells to endothelium
Gonadal
Polycystic ovaries

Questionnaire.[37] For descriptions of popular weight loss programs, see *Weighing the Options*,[38] pg 66-80.

Goals

Practitioners should help patients to set realistic goals to help prevent the patient from being overwhelmed or relapsing. Without guidance, most patients choose goals based on cosmetic criteria, that are usually unachievable. A reasonable or healthy weight loss goal needs to take into account health risks, genetic predisposition to obesity, and whether the patient has hyperplastic (excess fat cell number) versus hypertrophic (excess fat cell size) obesity. When fat cells hypertrophy, they develop insulin resistance, resulting in increased medical risk. When adipocytes reach some maximum size (approximately double optimal

TABLE 69.9

NIH Guidelines for Choosing a Weight-Loss Program

The diet should be safe and include all the Recommended Dietary Allowances for vitamins, minerals, and protein
The program should be directed towards a slow, steady weight loss unless a more rapid weight loss is medically indicated
A doctor should evaluate health status if the client's weight-loss goal is greater than 15 to 20 lb, if the client has any health problems, or if the client takes medication on a regular basis
The program should include plans for weight maintenance
The program should give the prospective client a detailed list of fees and costs of additional items

size), there is a stimulus to proliferate. Hyperplastic obesity is common in patients with childhood/adolescent-onset obesity, morbid obesity, and in some cases of excessive weight gain during pregnancy. Because it is impossible to reduce the number of adipocytes, an appropriate goal for the patient with hyperplastic obesity is to reduce excess fat by approximately one-half.

For patients with a BMI >30, a 10% weight loss over six months (i.e., 1 to 2 lb or 0.5 to 1.0 kg/wk) is a reasonable goal. Slower weight loss is appropriate for those with lesser degrees of obesity. For overweight subjects who are not motivated to lose weight, the goal should be prevention of further weight gain.

Criteria for Choosing a Weight Loss Program

Guidelines for choosing a weight loss program have been developed by the NIH (Table 69.9) and The Institute of Medicine.[38]

Diet

Diets should be individually planned to help create a deficit of 500 to 1000 kcal/day. Succcessful weight reduction is more likely to occur when consideration is given to a patient's food preferences in tailoring a particular diet. The dietitian should ensure that all of the recommended dietary allowances are met; this may necessitate the use of a dietary or vitamin supplement. The diet should also be realistic, i.e., based on dietary modification and practical changes in eating habits. The nutritional recommendations should be based on the patient's current eating habits, lifestyle, ethnicity and culture, other coexisting medical conditions, and potential nutrient-drug interactions.

The diet should be prescribed by the physician and implemented by the dietitian. The active involvement of the physician in such cases is essential, while the role of the dietitian can be invaluable, since caloric intake should be evaluated monthly. Food records should be completed by the patient to assess the relationship of caloric intake to weight loss. However, changes in body weight may not reflect changes in body fat if the patient has edema or has been adding muscle tissue due to an aggressive exercise program. The rate of weight loss can be expected to decline as the patient's energy requirements decline.

Low Calorie Diets (LCD)

Caloric restriction is an integral component of weight loss regimens. The restriction can be moderate to severe; however, compliance decreases with unrealistic restrictions. In general, a 500 to 1000 kcal reduction from maintenance caloric requirements is recommended. Maintenance requirements may be determined by the resting energy equation (REE) recommended by Mifflin et al.[39]

$$\text{REE} = (9.99 \times \text{wt in kg}) + (6.25 \times \text{ht in cm}) - (4.92 \times \text{age in yr}) + (166 \times \text{sex [male = 1; female = 0]}) - 161 \quad \text{(Eq. 69.2)}$$

Multiply the REE by an activity factor (1.5 for women; 1.6 for men) to determinine maintenance requirements.[40]

The Harris-Benedict equation can also be used to calculate REE or basal metabolic rate (BMR); however, this equation overpredicts REE by 5 to 24%.[39] The Harris-Benedict equations are:[40]

$$\text{BMR for males} = 66 + 13.8\ (\text{wt in kg}) + 5\ (\text{ht in cm}) - 6.8\ (\text{age in yr}) \quad \text{(Eq. 69.3)}$$

$$\text{BMR for females} = 655 + 9.6\ (\text{wt in kg}) + 1.8\ (\text{ht in cm}) - 4.7\ (\text{age in yr}) \quad \text{(Eq. 69.4)}$$

Subtract 500 to 1000 kcal to determine the caloric intake needed to achieve a weight loss of approximately 1 to 2 pounds per week.[38]

Implementation of Diet

The dietitian usually uses the exchange system, or the Food Guide Pyramid, to prescribe a specified number of exchanges (or servings) of foods from each food group, and a defined portion size for each food. Thus, weighing and measuring foods is an important requirement in terms of patient compliance. The subject can choose a variety of foods within each food group, and some higher calorie foods can be built in, occasionally. Once caloric needs have been determined, Table 69.10 can be used as a guide for various caloric levels. A sample meal plan for a 1500-calorie exchange diet is shown in Table 69.11.

Because overweight individuals need to lose weight over a period of time, it is imperative that the diet be acceptable. The diet must fit the taste preferences and habits of the individual and be flexible enough to allow eating outside the home as well. Dietary education is necessary to assist in the adaptation to an LCD and should address the topics[29] listed in Table 69.12.

Low Calorie, High Fiber Diets

Reducing dietary fat, along with an increase in dietary fiber and a decrease in refined sugars, is a sound program for weight loss as well as weight maintenance, especially when consuming the recommended number of servings from the Food Guide Pyramid. Consuming ample fruits, vegetables, and whole grains can aid in weight loss because increased fiber intake can increase satiety. The National Research Council and the American Heart Association recommend consuming 25 to 35 grams of fiber each day. A fat intake of 20 to 30% of total kcalories is appropriate, as long as total kcalories from refined sugars are not

TABLE 69.10

Food Group Exchanges for Various Caloric Levels

Calorie Level, kcal	1200	1500	1800
Starch group exchanges	5	6	8
Fruit group exchanges	2	3	4
Vegetable group exchanges	3	4	5
Milk group exchanges	2	2	2
Meat group exchanges	5 oz	6 oz	7 oz
Fat group exchanges	≤3	≤4	≤5
Sweets	use sparingly	use sparingly	use sparingly

TABLE 69.11

Sample Meal Plan for 1500 Calories

Food	Calories (kcal)
Breakfast	
Whole wheat toast, 2 slices	140
Banana, 1 small	60
Milk, fat-free, 8 fl. oz	90
Margarine, 2 tsp	90
Coffee/tea	0
Lunch	
Turkey sandwich	
Turkey breast, 2 oz	70
Bread, 2 slices	140
Mayonnaise, fat-free, 1 Tb	10
Lettuce, 1 leaf	0
Mini carrots, raw, 1 cup	25
Yogurt, fat-free, vanilla, 1 cup	200
Coffee/tea	0
Supper	
Fish, baked, 4 oz	140
Potato, baked, 1 med (6 oz)	160
Sour cream, light, 2 Tb	40
Broccoli, steamed, 1 cup	50
Margarine, 1 tsp	45
Strawberries, fresh, 1 1/4 cup	60
Whipped topping, fat-free, 2 tb	15
Coffee/tea	0
Snack	
Popcorn, air-popped, 6 cups	180
Total calories	1515

TABLE 69.12

Educational Topics for Weight Loss Counseling

Energy value of different foods
Food composition — fats, carbohydrates (including dietary fiber), and proteins
Evaluation of nutrition labels to determine caloric content and food composition
New habits of purchasing — give preference to low-calorie foods
Food preparation — avoid adding high-calorie ingredients during cooking (e.g., fats and oils)
Avoid overconsumption of high-calorie foods (both high-fat and high-carbohydrate foods)
Maintain adequate water intake
Reduction of portion sizes
Limiting alcohol consumption

excessive. Reducing the percentage of dietary fat alone will not produce weight loss unless total kcalories are also reduced.[29] Although lower-fat diets without targeted caloric reduction help promote weight loss by producing a reduced kcalorie intake, lower-fat diets with targeted caloric restriction promote greater weight loss than lower-fat diets alone.[29]

TABLE 69.13

Sample Meal Plan for Low-Fat, High-Fiber Diet

Food	Calories (kcal)	Fat (g)	Fiber (g)
Breakfast			
Orange juice, 1/2 cup	56	0	0.5
Fiber One cereal, 1/4 cup	30	0.5	6.5
Fruit 'n Fiber cereal, 1/2 cup	105	1.5	3
Banana, 1/2 med	52	0.2	1.3
Milk, fat-free, 8 fl oz	86	0.4	0
Whole wheat toast, 1 slice	65	2	2
Margarine, light, 1 tsp	17	2.7	0
Coffee/tea	0	0	0
Lunch			
Split pea soup, 1 cup	133	1.6	3.7
Triscuit crackers, reduced fat, 8	130	3	4
Chicken breast, grilled, skin removed, 2 oz	95	2.1	0
Hamburger bun, 1	123	2.2	1.2
Honey mustard, 1 Tb	25	0	0
Sliced tomato, 1/2 med	13	0.2	0.7
Lettuce, 1 leaf	2	0	0.3
Pear, 1 med	98	0.7	4
Coffee/tea	0	0	0
Supper			
Spinach salad, 1 cup	12	0.2	1.6
Salad dressing, light, 2 Tb	100	8	0
Grouper, baked, 4 oz	133	1.4	0
Brown rice, 1/2 cup	108	0.9	1.8
Asparagus, steamed, 6 spears	22	0.3	1.4
Whole wheat roll, 1	75	1.3	2.1
Margarine, light, 2 tsp	34	5.4	0
Yogurt, fat-free, vanilla, 1 cup	200	0	0
Strawberries, 1 cup	45	0.6	3.4
Coffee/tea	0	0	0
Totals	1759	35.2[a]	37.5

[a] Fat calories provide 18% of total kcalories.

Implementation of Diet

The dietitian should prescribe a caloric level appropriate for a weight loss of one-half to one pound per week. The dietitian should also recommend the fat intake (20 to 30%) and the fiber goal (25 to 35 g). Advising the patient to gradually increase fiber in the diet will help avoid gastrointestinal side effects such as gas, cramps, and bloating. Increasing fluid intake while increasing fiber intake will prevent constipation. Educating the patient on high-fiber cereals, eating the peels on apples and potatoes, and eating the whole fruit rather than just drinking the juice will help fulfill the requirement for fiber. Beans are also an excellent low-fat source of fiber. Patients should be encouraged to keep food records of total kcalories, fat, and fiber to monitor compliance. Recommendations of references for counting calories, fat, and fiber should be given to the patient along with sample meal plans. A sample meal plan is shown in Table 69.13.

TABLE 69.14

Contraindications to Very Low Calorie Diets (VLCDs)
Recent myocardial infarction
Cerebrovascular disease
Chronic renal failure
Hepatic disease
Type I diabetes mellitus
Severe psychiatric disorders
Alcoholism
Cancer
Infection
Acute substance abuse
Human immunodeficiency virus infection

Very Low Calorie Diets (VLCDs)

A very low calorie diet (VLCD) is defined as one that provides <800 kcalories per day. Such diets may severely restrict carbohydrates and induce ketosis (ketogenic diets) or may simply restrict all macronutrients, and can be either a liquid formulation or a food diet.[41] The following discussion will refer to ketogenic VLCDs. Ketosis produces anorexia and thus improves dietary compliance. This diet is appropriate only when a patient has a major health risk(s) and the physician has determined that the diet can be used safely. Indications for patients for VLCDs are a BMI ≥35, or a BMI ≥30, in association with comorbid conditions. The natriuresis associated with ketosis and the rapid reduction in insulin resistance make the diet especially useful in patients with fluid overload and diabetes, respectively. Candidates for VLCDs should have failed prior weight-loss attempts and should demonstrate motivation to adhere to the VLCD. Additionally, the patient should understand that this is a temporary method for weight loss, and that transitioning to a more balanced eating pattern will be necessary for further weight loss and weight maintenance. Patients should not follow this diet for more than 12 to 16 weeks. Contraindications for use of VLCDs are listed in Table 69.14.

VLCDs are not recommended for weight-loss therapy for most patients because they require special monitoring and supplementation.[42] Specialized practitioners experienced in the use of VLCDs are preferable for screening and supervising patients for this diet. Medical monitoring will help the physician detect any patients who may react adversely to the VLCD. Potential complications include excessive loss of lean body mass, orthostatic hypotension, constipation (inadequate fiber in diet), gout (ketones compete with uric acid for excretion), and a likelihood for recidivism. Diuretics should be discontinued to minimize the increased risk of electrolyte imbalance,[43] and diabetic drugs will need to be reduced or discontinued. Clinical trials show that LCDs are as effective as VLCDs in producing sustained weight loss after one year.[44] As with any type of weight loss program, including behavioral therapy and physical activity along with the VLCD seems to improve maintenance of weight loss.[42,45]

Implementation of Diet

The VLCD should provide 1.2 to 1.5 g protein/kg of desirable body weight per day. This protein must be of high biologic value in order to maximize preservation of lean body mass. Lean meat, fish, poultry, and egg whites are recommended. The dietitian determines the protein needs of the patient and converts grams of protein to ounces of meat (7 g protein = 1 oz meat). The meat is divided into three meals per day, and the patient is encouraged not to skip meals. The patient is given the following directions:

TABLE 69.15

VLCD Sample Meal Plan

Breakfast
Lean ham, 4 oz
Coffee, 8 fluid oz
Lunch
Lean ground beef, 5 oz
Carrots, raw, 2 whole
Soda, diet, 12 fluid oz
Supper
Baked chicken breast, skinless, boneless, 6 oz
Green beans, $^1/_2$ cup cooked
Tea, sugar substitute, 12 fl oz
Drink other fluids throughout the day

- Choose only lean meats
- Prepare meats without adding fats, breading, or sauces
- Weigh meat after cooking to comply with prescribed amount
- Include two servings non-starchy vegetables per day
- Drink at least two quarts of non-caloric fluids per day
- Take one multiple vitamin-mineral supplement per day
- Take a calcium supplement providing 1000 to 1500 mg elemental calcium per day
- Test urine for ketones one time per day with KetoStix (available over the counter)

A sample meal plan is shown in Table 69.15 for a VLCD providing 15 oz meat per day. In the case of liquid diets, the protein should be from dairy sources, soy, or albumin. Most liquid formulations provide between 0.8 and 1.5 g protein/kg of desirable body weight, up to 100 g carbohydrate, the minimum of essential fatty acids, and the recommended allowances of vitamins and minerals.

Refeeding, the process of gradual weaning from the VLCD back to a balanced diet, generally takes three to six weeks. The dietitian should follow the patient closely at this time and gradually increase the daily caloric intake, because the decline in resting metabolic rate usually continues for about three months after the VLCD has been discontinued.[43] Patients should be informed that some water weight will most likely be regained when they return to a balanced diet (reversal of the natriuresis associated with ketosis).

High-Protein, Low-Carbohydrate Diets

Diet books such as *Dr. Atkins New Diet Revolution, Protein Power, The Carbohydrate Addict's LifeSpan Program, Sugar Busters,* and *The Zone* all emphasize protein and/or limit carbohydrates or sugar. These diets are similar in some respects to the VLCDs, but typically are not medically supervised. Many of these diets allow/encourage excessive fat and protein, and the authors often suggest that these diets can be followed indefinitely. The diets are based on the idea that carbohydrates are bad, and that many people are insulin-resistant and therefore gain weight when they eat carbohydrates. Proponents espouse severely limiting carbohydrates to force the body to use the fat it already has in storage for energy instead of adding to those fat stores. The authors of these books usually conflict with most mainstream nutritional professionals who recommend ample servings of carbohydrates, especially complex carbohydrates in the form of whole grains, vegetables, and fruit. The authors of these diet books are quick to point out that because of excessive carbohydrate consumption, people are heavier than ever before. However, they don't address the real reason people are overweight — that they are eating more total kcalories and are more sedentary.

Consequences of Dieting

Caloric restriction produces a natriuresis and diuresis that is reversed with resumption of higher kcalorie levels. This may lead to discouragement and abandonment of dietary efforts. With severe caloric restriction, adaptation to starvation produces hypometabolism. Loss of lean tissue will also reduce the REE. Weight loss also produces a reduced capacity for fat oxidation.[46] However, the evidence thus far does not support adverse effects of weight cycling on REE, body composition, or body fat distribution.[47]

Temporary consequences of weight loss include secondary amenorrhea and hair loss. Gallstones may develop during weight loss; a large percentage of these dissolve spontaneously.

Exercise

Adding exercise to a calorie-restricted diet marginally increases weight loss but minimizes the decline in the REE due to the caloric deficit. The major benefits of exercise are its effects on health, mood, and maintenance of weight loss (Table 69.16). The slightly greater proportion of fat used with low-intensity aerobic exercise is offset by the greater total energy

TABLE 69.16

Proposed Mechanisms Linking Exercise with Successful Weight Maintenance

Mechanism
Increased energy expenditure
Improved body composition
Fat loss
Preservation of lean body mass
Reduction of visceral fat depot
Increased capacity for fat mobilization and oxidation
Control of food intake
Short-term reduction of appetite
Reduction of fat intake
Stimulation of thermogenic response
RMR
Diet-induced thermogenesis
Change in muscle morphology and biochemical capacity
Increased insulin sensitivity
Improved plasma lipid and lipoprotein profile
Reduced blood pressure
Better aerobic fitness
Positive psychological effects
Improved mood
Improved self-esteem
Increased adherence to diet

TABLE 69.17

Behavior Modification Techniques

Behavior Modification Techniques
Self monitoring — using food and exercise diaries
Stimulus control — keeping food out of sight
Stress management
Social support
Eating management — eating slower
Behavior substitution — exercising instead of eating
Rewards
Relapse prevention
Cognitive restructuring — positive self-talk
Environmental engineering — eating only at the table
Covert sensitization — imagining unpleasant consequences

expended by high-intensity aerobic exercise. Physical training increases oxidation of fatty acids. By increasing muscle mass, resistance exercise is also beneficial.

Behavior Modification

Behavior modification refers to tools or skills used to improve compliance with diet and exercise regimens. Table 69.17 outlines several approaches. Behavioral therapy is an essential component of any adequate obesity treatment program.

Surgery

Surgical options for the treatment of obesity have been reviewed by Kral.[48] The most common are gastroplasty (creation of a small gastric pouch with restricted outlet along the lesser curvature of the stomach) and gastric bypass (construction of a proximal gastric pouch whose outlet is a Roux-en-Y limb of small intestine). Both procedures produce a >50% reduction of excess weight in the majority of patients, with the bypass having superior results. Additional procedures include gastric banding (adjustable band creating a proximal gastric pouch) and biliopancreatic diversion. Jejunoileal bypasses, which have produced severe complications, are not recommended. Candidates for surgical treatment are those with severe obesity (BMI >35 with comorbidities or >40 without comorbidity) who are well informed and highly motivated, but have failed prior dietary attempts.

Drugs

To be considered for pharmacotherapy, subjects should have a BMI ≥30 without risk factors, or a BMI of ≥27 with obesity-related comorbidities. Centrally acting noradrenergic agents are approved for short-term use, whereas both sibutramine and orlistat are approved for long-term use (Table 69.18). Common side effects of noradrenergic agents are headache, insomnia, nervousness, irritability, and increased blood pressure and pulse. In addition to these effects, sibutramine may cause dry mouth. Side effects of lipase inhibitors are a consequence fat malabsorption and may include abdominal pain, diarrhea, oily stools, fecal incontinence, and malabsorption of fat-soluble vitamins.

The likelihood of long-term effectiveness can be predicted by weight loss during the first month of therapy. Weight loss drugs are not a substitute for a healthy diet and regular exercise, nor are they a cure for obesity. They can, however, promote modest weight loss sufficient to improve health risks.

TABLE 69.18

Weight Loss Agents

Drug	Usual Dose per Day
Noradrenergic Agents	
Phendimetrazine	105 mg
Phentermine	15-37.5 mg
Mazindol	1-3 mg
Diethylproprion	75 mg
Adrenergic/Serotonergic Reuptake Inhibitors	
Sibutramine	5-15 mg
Gastrointestinal lipase inhibitors	
Orlistat	120 mg tid

Outcomes

Treatment outcomes have been reviewed by Brownell and Wadden.[49] Predictors of weight loss and weight maintenance are listed in Tables 69.19 and 69.20, respectively.

TABLE 69.19

Predictors of Weight Loss

Positive Predictors

Personal Factors

High initial body weight or BMI
High REE
High self-management skills

Process Factors

Attendance at program
Weight loss early in program

Treatment Factors

Increased length of treatment
Having social support
Engaging in physical activity
Incorporation of behavior modification techniques
  Self-monitoring
  Goal setting
  Slowing rate of eating

Negative Predictors

Repeated attempts at weight loss
Experiencing perceived stress
(Others include the opposites of the positive indicators)

Nonpredictors

Total body fat, fat distribution, and body composition
Personality/psychopathology test results
Dietary restraint
Binge eating

TABLE 69.20

Predictors of Maintenance of Weight Loss

Positive Predictors
Physical activity
Self-monitoring
Positive coping style
Continued contact
Normalization of eating
Reduction of comorbidities
Negative Predictors
Negative life events
Family dysfunction

References

1. Comuzzie AG, Allison DB. *Science* 280: 1374; 1998.
2. Stunkard AJ, Sorensen TI, Hanis C, et al. *N Engl J Med* 314: 193; 1986.
3. Stunkard AJ, Foch TT, Hrubec Z. *JAMA* 256: 51; 1986.
4. Poehlman ET, Tremblay A, Depres J, et al. *Am J Clin Nutr* 43: 723; 1986.
5. Jones PJH, Schoeller DA. *Metabolism* 37: 145; 1992.
6. Sobal J, Stunkard AJ. *Psychol Bull* 105: 260; 1989.
7. Bjorntorp P. *Obesity Res* 1: 206; 1993.
8. Dhurandhar NV, Augustus A, Atkinson RL. *FASEB J* 11: A230; 1997.
9. Himms-Hagen J. *Obesity Res* 3: 361; 1995.
10. Zurlo F, Lillioja S, Esposito-Del Puente A, et al. *Am J Physiol* 259: E650; 1990.
11. Eckel RH. *Lancet* 340: 1452; 1992.
12. Wolfe RR, Peters EJ, Klein S, et al. *Am J Physiol* 252: E189; 1987.
13. Jones PJH, Schoeller DA. *Metabolism* 37: 145; 1992.
14. Ristow M, Muller-Wieland D, Pfeiffer A, et al. *N Engl J Med* 339: 93; 2990.
15. Ravussin E, Lillioja S, Knowler WC, et al. *N Engl J Med* 318: 462; 1988.
16. Poehlman ET, Horton ES. *Nutr Rev* 47: 129; 1989.
17. Samaras K, Kelly PJ, Chiano MN, et al. *Ann Intern Med* 130: 873; 1999.
18. Golay A, Schutz Y, Felber JP, et al. *Int J Obesity* 13: 767; 1989.
19. Astrup A, Andersen T, Christensen NJ, et al. *Am J Clin Nutr* 51: 331; 1990.
20. Golay A, Jallut D, Schutz Y, et al. *Int J Obesity* 15: 601; 1990.
21. Argyropoulos G, Brown AM, Willi SM, et al. *J Clin Invest* 102: 1345; 1998.
22. Must A, Spadano J, Coakley EH, et al. *JAMA* 282: 1523; 1999.
23. Mokdad AH, Serdula MK, Dietz WH, et al. *JAMA* 282: 1519; 1999.
24. Bjorntorp P. In: *Handbook of Eating Disorders: Physiology, Psychology and Treatment of Obesity, Anorexia, and Bulimia,* Brownell KD, Foreyt JP, Eds, Basic Books, New York, 1986, pg 88.
25. Fujioka S, Matsuzawa Y, Tokunaga K, Tarui S. *Metabolism* 36: 54; 1987.
26. Manson JE, Colditz GA, Stampfer MJ, et al. *N Engl J Med* 322: 882; 1990.
27. Calle EE, Thun MJ, Petrelli JM, et al. *N Engl J Med* 341: 1097; 1999.
28. Lee I-M, Manson JE, Hennekens CH, Paffenbarger RS. *JAMA* 270: 2823; 1993.
29. National Institutes of Health, National Heart, Lung and Blood Institute, *Obesity Res* 6: 51S; 1998.
30. World Health Organization, *Obesity, Preventing and Managing the Global Epidemic,* World Health Organization, Geneva, 1998, pg 1.
31. Wing RR, Koeske R, Epstein LH, et al. *Arch Intern Med* 147: 1749; 1987.
32. Woo PD, Stefanick MI, Dreon DM, et al. *N Engl J Med* 319: 1173; 1988.

33. Hypertension Prevention Trial Research Group, *Arch Intern Med* 150: 153; 1990.
34. Goldstein D. *Int J Obesity* 16: 397; 1992.
35. Van Gaal LF, Wauters MA, De Leeuw IH. *Int J Obesity* 21: 5S; 1997.
36. Bosello O, Armellini F, Zamboni M, Fitchet M. *Int J Obesity* 21: 10S; 1997.
37. Brownell KD. *The LEARN Program for Weight Control,* 7th ed, American Health Publishing Company, Dallas, 1998.
38. Thomas PR. *Weighing the Options, Criteria for Evaluating Weight-Management Programs,* National Academy Press, Washington, DC, 1995; pg 91.
39. Mifflin MD, St Jeor ST, Hill LA, et al. *Am J Clin Nutr* 51: 241; 1990.
40. Frankenfield DC, Muth ER, Rowe WA. *J Am Diet Assoc* 98: 442; 1998.
41. Life Sciences Research Office, *Management of Obesity by Severe Caloric Restriction,* Federation of American Societies for Experimental Biology, Washington, DC, 1979.
42. National Task Force on the Prevention and Treatment of Obesity, National Institutes of Health, *JAMA* 270: 967; 1993.
43. Prasad N. *Postgrad Med* 13: 39; 1990.
44. Wadden TA, Foster GD, Letizia KA. *J Consult Clin Psychol* 62: 165; 1994.
45. Perri MG, McAdoo WG, McAllister DA, et al. *J Consult Clin Psychol* 55: 615; 1987.
46. Wyatt HR, Grunwald GK, Seagle HM, et al. *Am J Clin Nutr* 69: 1189; 1999.
47. Wing R. *Ann Behav Med* 14: 113; 1992.
48. Kral JG. In: *Treatment of the Seriously Obese Patient* Wadden TA, VanItallie TB, Eds, Guilford Press, New York, 1992, pg 496.
49. Brownell KD, Wadden TA. *J Consulting Clin Psychol* 60: 505; 1992.

Sources of Information

Aggregate Database for Investigations on Publications in Obesity and Sequelae (ADIPOS), www.adipos.com

American Council on Exercise, 5820 Oberlin Dr., Suite 102, San Diego, CA 92121, (800) 825-3636, www.acefitness.org

American Dietetic Association, 216 West Jackson Blvd., Chicago, IL 60606, (800) 887-1600, www.eatright.org

American Heart Association, 7272 Greenville Ave., Dallas, TX 75231, (800) AHA-USA1, www.americanheart.org

American Obesity Association, 1250 24th St. NW, Suite 300, Washington, DC 20037, (800) 98-OBESE, www.obesity.org

Center for Nutrition Policy and Promotion, 1120 20th St. NW, Washington, DC 20036, (202) 418-2312, www.usda.gov/cnpp

International Food Information Council, 1100 Connecticut Ave. NW, Suite 430, Washington, DC 20036, (202) 296-6540, www.ific.health.org

Shape Up America, 901 31st St. NW, Washington, DC 20007, (202) 333-7400, www.shapeupamerica.org

Weight-Control Information Network (WIN), 1 Win Way, Bethesda, MD 20892-3665. 1-800-WIN-8098. www.niddk.nih.gov/health/nutrit/win.htm

70

Childhood Obesity and Exercise

Scott Owens, Bernard Gutin, and Paule Barbeau

Introduction

Childhood obesity is the most prevalent nutritional problem among children and adolescents in the United States.[1] Data from the third National Health and Nutrition Examination Survey (NHANES III) suggest that 22% of children and adolescents are overweight, and 11% are obese.[2] Table 70.1 shows the unadjusted prevalence of overweight by body mass index (BMI) for ages 6 to 17 from NHANES III and sex, age, and race-specific 85th and 95th percentile cutoff points from the second and third National Health Examination Surveys (NHES II and NHES III).[2] As shown in Table 70.2, the age-adjusted prevalence of childhood overweight has increased among all sex and ethnic groups since the mid-1960s.[2] Thus, an ever-increasing number of young people are experiencing the host of undesirable social, emotional, and medical implications of obesity.

Definition and Clinical Evaluation of Childhood Obesity

Defining childhood obesity is difficult, and no generally accepted definition has yet emerged.[2] Table 70.3 shows commonly encountered anthropometric definitions of childhood obesity.[2-5] Use of BMI has been recommended for most clinical settings due to its high reliability and ease of measurement.[6-7] A clinical decision about whether a child with a given BMI is truly overfat may require additional information, such as skinfold thickness measurements, comorbidity, family history, and recent health history.[8] A careful family history and physical examination can readily diagnose most of the hormonal causes and genetic syndromes associated with childhood obesity.[1] Table 70.4 lists common hormonal and genetic causes of childhood obesity, and Table 70.5 provides a differential diagnosis of childhood obesity. Although genetic and hormonal disorders are responsible for less than 10% of childhood obesity, they must be ruled out, as they require different modes of therapy.[3]

Age, Gender, Ethnicity, and Socioeconomic Status

Tables 70.6 and 70.7 provide age-, sex-, and race-specific percentiles for BMI and triceps skinfold thickness for ages 6 to 18.[4] NHANES III data (Table 70.8) indicate that lower

0-8493-2705-9/02/$0.00+$1.50

TABLE 70.1

Unadjusted Prevalence of Overweight for NHANES III, from Sex- and Age-Specific 85th and 95th Percentile Cutoff Points of NHES II and NHES III[a]

Category	No.	Percentile	
		85th	95th
Sex and Age, Y			
Both sexes	2920	22.0 ± 1.1	10.9 ± 0.8
6-11	1817	22.3 ± 1.5	11.0 ± 1.0
12-17	1103	21.7 ± 1.9	10.8 ± 1.3
Boys			
6-8	442	21.3 ± 4.3	11.7 ± 3.6
9-11	467	22.7 ± 2.7	10.9 ± 2.3
12-14	253	23.5 ± 3.3	12.0 ± 2.6
15-17	289	20.7 ± 2.9	13.5 ± 2.8
Girls			
6-8	450	24.2 ± 3.6	13.7 ± 2.7
9-11	458	21.4 ± 4.1	8.2 ± 2.1
12-14	288	21.5 ± 2.8	8.5 ± 2.0
15-17	273	21.4 ± 3.1	9.0 ± 1.4
Sex, Age, Y, Race			
Boys age 6 to 11			
Total[b]	909	21.9 ± 2.4	11.3 ± 1.8
Non-Hispanic white	267	20.5 ± 2.8	10.4 ± 2.4
Non-Hispanic black	257	26.5 ± 2.7	13.4 ± 2.3
Mexican American	350	33.3 ± 3.0	17.7 ± 2.3
Boys age 12 to 17			
Total[b]	542	22.0 ± 2.2	12.8 ± 1.9
Non-Hispanic white	155	23.1 ± 3.1	14.4 ± 2.7
Non-Hispanic black	163	21.1 ± 3.7	9.3 ± 2.4
Mexican American	203	26.7 ± 4.6	12.8 ± 3.2
Girls age 6 to 11			
Total[b]	908	22.7 ± 2.4	10.6 ± 1.3
Non-Hispanic white	270	21.5 ± 3.7	9.8 ± 2.0
Non-Hispanic black	224	31.4 ± 4.0	16.9 ± 2.8
Mexican American	389	29.0 ± 2.1	14.3 ± 1.7
Girls age 12 to 17			
Total[b]	561	21.4 ± 2.7	8.8 ± 1.4
Non-Hispanic white	191	20.3 ± 3.5	8.3 ± 1.6
Non-Hispanic black	147	29.9 ± 4.5	14.4 ± 3.1
Mexican American	198	23.4 ± 3.0	8.7 ± 2.5

[a] Values are prevalences ± SEMs. NHANES indicates National Health and Nutrition Examination Survey; NHES, National Health Examination Survey.

[b] Includes data for race-ethnicity groups not shown separately.

From Troiano RP, Flegal KM, Kuczmarski RJ, Campbell M, Johnson CL. *Arch Pediatr Adolesc Med* 149: 1085-1089; 1995. With permission.

TABLE 70.2

Age-Adjusted Prevalence[a] of Overweight from National Surveys (1963 to 1991) by Two Percentile Cutoff Point Definitions

Population Group	Boys 85th Percentile	Boys 95th Percentile	Girls 85th Percentile	Girls 95th Percentile
Ages 6 to 11 y				
All Races[b]				
NHES	15.2	5.2	15.2	5.2
NHANES I	18.2	6.5	13.9	4.3
NHANES II	19.9	7.9	15.8	7.0
NHANES III	22.3	10.8	22.7	10.7
White				
NHES	16.0	5.6	15.7	5.1
NHANES I	19.5	6.7	13.4	4.5
NHANES II	20.8	7.9	15.4	6.4
NHANES III	22.3	10.4	22.0	10.2
Black				
NHES	10.3	2.0	12.1	5.3
NHANES I	12.3	5.6	16.8	3.5
NHANES II	15.1	7.9	18.4	11.3
NHANES III	27.2	13.4	30.7	16.2
Ages 12 to 17 y				
All races[b]				
NHES	15.1	5.2	15.2	5.2
NHANES I	14.9	5.3	19.7	7.2
NHANES II	16.3	5.4	15.5	6.0
NHANES III	21.7	12.8	21.2	8.8
White				
NHES	15.8	5.4	15.0	5.0
NHANES I	15.3	5.5	19.7	6.6
NHANES II	16.6	5.4	15.2	5.3
NHANES III	22.6	14.4	20.3	8.4
Black				
NHES	10.4	3.7	16.5	6.6
NHANES I	12.3	4.3	20.8	11.2
NHANES II	14.5	6.3	18.2	10.4
NHANES III	23.3	9.4	29.9	14.4

[a] Based on sex- and age-specific percentile cutoffs derived from NHES II and III. NHES indicates National Health Examination Survey; 1963 to 1965 for ages 6 to 11 years, and 1966 to 1970 for ages 12 to 17 years for III; NHANES, National Health and Nutrition Examination Survey; 1971 to 1974 for I, 1976 to 1980 for II, and 1988 to 1991 for III.

[b] Includes data for race groups not shown separately.

From Troiano RP, Flegal KM, Kuczmarski RJ, Campbell M, Johnson CL. *Arch Pediatr Adolesc Med* 149: 1085-1089, 1995. With permission.

TABLE 70.3

Anthropometric Definitions of Childhood Overweight/Obesity

Definition	Ref.
Body weight >120% of the value predicted from height	3
Body mass index (BMI) >85% percentile	2
Body mass index (BMI) >95% percentile	2
Triceps skinfold thickness >85% percentile	4
Triceps skinfold thickness >95% percentile	4
Body fat >25% for boys and 30% for girls as estimated from sum of subscapular and triceps skinfolds	5

TABLE 70.4

Hormonal and Genetic Causes of Childhood Obesity

Hormonal Causes	Diagnostic Clues
Hypothyroidism	Increased TSH, decreased thyroxine (T_4) levels
Hypercortisolism	Abnormal dexamethasone test; increased 24-hour free urinary cortisol level
Primary hyperinsulinism	Increased plasma insulin, increased C-peptide levels
Pseudohypoparathyroidism	Hypocalcemia, hyperphosphatemia, increased PTH level
Acquired hypothalamic	Presence of hypothalamic tumor, infection, syndrome trauma, vascular lesion
Genetic Syndromes	**Associated Characteristics**
Prader-Willi	Obesity, unsatiable appetite, mental retardation, hypogonadism
Laurence-Moon-Biedel	Obesity, mental retardation, spastic paraplegia
Alstrom	Obesity, retinitis pigmentosa, deafness, diabetes mellitus
Cohen	Truncal obesity, mental retardation, hypotonia
Turner's	Short stature, undifferentiated gonads, cardiac abnormalities, obesity, X genotype
Weaver	Infant overgrowth syndrome, accelerated skeletal maturation

Adapted from Moran R. Evaluation and treatment of childhood obesity, *Am Fam Phys* 59: 861; 1999. With permission.

TABLE 70.5

Differential Diagnosis of Childhood Obesity

	Hormonal/Genetic	Idiopathic
Family	Obesity not common	Obesity common in family
Height	Short child	Tall child (>50%)
IQ	IQ often low	Normal IQ
Bone age	Bone age retarded	Normal bone age
Physical	Defects common	Normal physical exam

Adapted from Williams CL, Campanaro LA, Squillace M, Bollella M. *Ann NY Acad Sci* 817: 225; 1997. With permission.

TABLE 70.6

Smoothed 85th and 95th Percentiles of Body Mass Index from NHANES I[a] Male Subjects 6 to 18 Years

	Whites						Blacks						Population					
Age	n	5th	15th	50th	85th	95th	n	5th	15th	50th	85th	95th	n	5th	15th	50th	85th	95th
Males																		
6	117	12.93	13.46	14.62	16.52	17.75	47	12.68	13.66	14.49	16.83	18.58	165	12.86	13.43	14.54	16.64	18.02
7	122	13.30	13.88	15.15	17.31	18.98	40	13.11	14.03	14.98	17.29	19.56	164	13.24	13.85	15.07	17.37	19.18
8	117	13.67	14.31	15.70	18.10	20.22	30	13.54	14.41	15.49	17.76	20.51	149	13.63	14.28	15.62	18.11	20.33
9	121	14.04	14.75	16.24	18.88	21.45	55	13.98	14.81	16.00	18.26	21.45	177	14.03	14.71	16.17	18.85	21.47
10	146	14.42	15.19	16.79	19.67	22.66	29	14.41	15.21	16.53	18.78	22.41	177	14.42	15.15	16.72	19.60	22.60
11	122	14.81	15.64	17.35	20.47	23.87	44	14.86	15.62	17.06	19.32	23.42	169	14.83	15.59	17.28	20.35	23.73
12	153	15.21	16.11	17.93	21.28	25.01	50	15.36	16.06	17.61	19.85	24.39	204	15.24	16.06	17.87	21.12	24.89
13	134	15.69	16.65	18.57	22.12	26.06	42	15.89	16.64	18.28	20.62	25.26	177	15.73	16.62	18.53	21.93	25.93
14	131	16.16	17.22	19.25	22.97	27.02	42	16.43	17.22	18.94	21.54	26.13	173	16.18	17.20	19.22	22.77	26.93
15	128	16.57	17.79	19.94	23.82	27.86	43	16.97	17.79	19.56	22.50	27.05	175	16.59	17.76	19.92	23.63	27.76
16	131	17.00	18.35	20.63	24.63	28.69	40	17.51	18.37	20.19	23.45	27.95	172	17.01	18.32	20.63	24.45	28.53
17	133	17.29	18.72	21.13	25.44	29.50	33	17.86	18.77	20.70	24.41	28.89	167	17.31	18.68	21.12	25.28	29.32
18	91	17.50	18.95	21.46	26.08	29.89	28	18.05	19.03	21.09	25.06	29.35	120	17.54	18.89	21.45	25.92	30.02
Females																		
6	118	12.81	13.37	14.33	16.14	17.49	42	12.52	13.40	13.83	16.24	18.58	161	12.83	13.37	14.31	16.17	17.49
7	126	13.18	13.82	15.00	17.16	18.93	47	12.88	13.79	14.55	17.36	19.56	174	13.17	13.79	14.98	17.17	18.93
8	118	13.57	14.27	15.68	18.19	20.36	35	13.25	14.17	15.26	18.49	20.51	153	13.51	14.22	15.66	18.18	20.36
9	125	13.96	14.72	16.35	19.21	21.78	47	13.63	14.57	15.98	19.64	21.45	173	13.87	14.66	16.33	19.19	21.78
10	152	14.36	15.18	17.02	20.23	23.20	41	14.02	14.96	16.69	20.79	22.41	194	14.23	15.09	17.00	20.19	23.20
11	117	14.76	15.64	17.69	21.24	24.59	43	14.41	15.36	17.39	21.96	23.42	163	14.60	15.53	17.67	21.18	24.59
12	129	15.17	16.11	18.36	22.25	25.95	47	14.83	15.77	18.11	23.15	24.39	177	14.98	15.98	18.35	22.17	25.95
13	151	15.59	16.55	18.91	23.13	27.07	47	15.33	16.23	18.78	24.41	25.26	199	15.36	16.43	18.95	23.08	27.07
14	141	15.89	16.89	19.29	23.87	27.97	49	15.77	16.66	19.24	25.46	26.13	192	15.67	16.79	19.32	23.88	27.97
15	117	16.21	17.23	19.69	24.28	28.51	47	16.20	17.07	19.67	26.04	27.05	164	16.01	17.16	19.69	24.29	28.51
16	142	16.55	17.59	20.11	24.68	29.10	30	16.65	17.48	20.11	26.68	27.95	173	16.37	17.54	20.09	24.74	29.10
17	114	16.76	17.84	20.39	25.07	29.72	44	16.92	17.81	20.45	27.38	28.89	159	16.59	17.81	20.36	25.23	29.72
18	109	16.87	18.01	20.58	25.34	30.22	29	17.04	18.06	20.78	27.92	29.35	140	16.71	17.99	20.57	25.56	30.22

[a] NHANES is National Health and Nutrition Examination Survey.

From Must A, Dallal G, Dietz W. *Am J Clin Nutr* 53: 839; 1991. With permission.

TABLE 70.7

Smoothed 85th and 95th Percentiles of Triceps Skinfold Thickness from NHANES I[a] Male Subjects 6 to 18 Years

	Whites						Blacks						Population					
Age	n	5th	15th	50th	85th	95th	n	5th	15th	50th	85th	95th	n	5th	15th	50th	85th	95th
Males																		
6	117	5.26	6.09	8.74	11.63	14.47	47	4.01	4.86	6.85	9.35	12.86	165	5.04	6.19	8.36	11.10	14.12
7	122	5.28	6.12	8.94	12.78	15.95	40	4.01	4.88	6.85	10.09	14.11	164	5.01	6.14	8.59	12.38	15.61
8	117	5.28	6.15	9.12	13.95	17.51	30	4.00	4.88	6.84	10.76	15.35	149	4.96	6.08	8.79	13.66	17.18
9	121	5.27	6.17	9.27	15.10	19.11	55	3.99	4.88	6.83	11.37	16.50	177	4.91	6.02	8.96	14.93	18.81
10	146	5.24	6.18	9.40	16.29	20.96	29	3.98	4.88	6.81	11.52	17.79	177	4.84	5.95	9.10	16.02	20.68
11	122	5.20	6.20	9.51	17.32	22.53	44	3.97	4.89	6.81	11.31	18.68	169	4.78	5.88	9.23	16.87	22.20
12	153	5.15	6.23	9.59	17.79	23.53	50	3.97	4.91	6.80	10.79	18.74	204	4.69	5.79	9.35	17.26	23.25
13	134	5.01	6.21	9.42	17.63	23.87	42	3.94	4.88	6.72	10.23	18.67	177	4.56	5.65	9.17	17.12	23.71
14	131	4.91	6.15	9.26	16.88	23.42	42	3.86	4.84	6.66	9.92	18.58	173	4.47	5.60	8.93	16.35	23.46
15	128	4.81	6.10	9.12	16.11	22.42	43	3.81	4.80	6.62	9.96	18.99	175	4.40	5.59	8.70	15.75	22.34
16	131	4.69	6.05	8.95	15.81	22.05	40	3.76	4.77	6.58	10.30	20.18	172	4.33	5.55	8.45	15.75	21.53
17	133	4.61	6.02	8.92	15.95	21.99	33	3.69	4.72	6.63	10.73	21.12	167	4.29	5.58	8.38	15.95	21.51
18	91	4.53	6.01	9.02	16.69	22.28	28	3.60	4.64	6.79	11.34	21.95	120	4.25	5.63	8.53	16.59	21.83
Females																		
6	118	5.65	6.96	10.19	13.48	15.47	42	4.90	6.10	7.99	13.71	14.94	161	6.00	6.76	10.01	13.44	15.57
7	126	6.09	7.42	10.89	14.93	18.08	47	5.09	6.33	8.60	15.27	17.20	174	6.24	7.17	10.68	14.94	17.89
8	118	6.52	7.86	11.60	16.35	20.60	35	5.29	6.57	9.22	16.82	19.41	153	6.47	7.58	11.36	16.41	20.18
9	125	6.94	8.31	12.31	17.74	23.07	47	5.51	6.83	9.85	18.40	21.65	173	6.71	8.01	12.05	17.85	22.47
10	152	7.37	8.77	13.02	18.84	24.84	41	5.73	7.09	10.47	19.63	23.76	194	6.95	8.44	12.74	19.01	24.38
11	117	7.80	9.23	13.74	19.82	26.23	43	5.96	7.36	11.08	20.72	25.84	163	7.20	8.87	13.43	20.13	26.15
12	129	8.17	9.68	14.44	20.97	27.73	47	6.21	7.62	11.68	21.58	27.53	177	7.45	9.31	14.13	21.25	27.98
13	151	8.49	10.19	15.14	22.00	29.08	47	6.50	8.05	12.22	21.86	29.17	199	7.78	9.84	14.87	22.25	29.51
14	141	8.78	10.76	15.77	22.99	30.22	49	6.81	8.53	12.56	21.71	30.48	192	8.15	10.37	15.47	23.27	30.86
15	117	9.06	11.29	16.39	24.08	31.48	47	7.11	8.94	12.95	21.77	30.54	164	8.46	10.85	16.03	24.32	32.22
16	142	9.34	11.83	17.03	24.85	32.35	30	7.41	9.35	13.36	22.06	30.07	173	8.78	11.34	16.62	25.12	33.22
17	114	9.55	12.18	17.45	25.48	32.95	44	7.67	9.70	13.75	23.03	30.46	159	9.03	11.66	17.02	25.80	33.83
18	109	9.66	12.29	17.67	26.22	33.51	29	7.87	10.03	14.19	24.94	31.42	140	9.21	11.79	17.24	26.51	34.26

[a] NHANES is National Health and Nutrition Examination Survey.

From Must A, Dallal G, Dietz W. *Am J Clin Nutr* 53: 839; 1991. With permission.

TABLE 70.8

Regression Coefficients (β) and p Values from Linear Models for Body Mass Index (BMI) in Black, Mexican-American, and White Youths Age 6 to 24 Years, Third National Health and Nutrition Examination Survey (NHANES III), 1988 to 1994

	β (SE)	P
Girls		
Main Effects		
Ethnicity		
Black	1.20 (0.26)	<0.001
Mexican-American	0.85 (0.33)	0.01
SES[a]	–0.23 (0.06)	<0.001
Age	0.46 (0.04)	<0.001
Boys		
Main Effects		
Ethnicity		
Black	–0.10 (0.21)	0.66
Mexican-American	0.48 (0.25)	0.06
SES[a]	–0.13 (0.09)	0.15
Age	0.44 (0.04)	<0.001

[a] Socioeconomic status as measured by years of education of head of household

Adapted from Winkleby MA, Robinson TN, Sundquist J, Kraemer HC. *JAMA* 281: 1006; 1999.

TABLE 70.9

Visceral Adipose Tissue in White and African-American Youth

Age	Boys	Girls	Boys	Girls	Significant Effects[a]	Ref.
4-10 y	27 ± 16 cm² (n = 16)	54 ± 27 cm² (n = 20)	22 ± 17 cm² (n = 27)	28 ± 17 cm² (n = 38)	race × sex	10[b]
13-16 y	433 ± 105 cm³ (n = 10)	355 ± 151 cm³ (n = 15)	279 ± 107 cm³ (n = 16)	263 ± 109 cm³ (n = 38)	race	11[c]

[a] Significant effects by two-way ANOVA, $p < 0.05$.

[b] Visceral adipose tissue measured as single-slice computed tomography scan at the level of the umbilicus and expressed in cm².

[c] Visceral adipose tissue measured as the sum of five abdominal MRI scans and expressed in cm³.

Source: Goran MI, Nagy TR, Treuth MS, et al. *Am J Clin Nutr* 65: 1703; 1997. With permission.

socioeconomic status is predictive of greater BMI in girls but not boys.[9] White children appear to accumulate greater quantities of deleterious visceral adipose tissue than do African-American children (Table 70.9).[10-11]

Health Risks of Childhood Obesity

Although obesity-related health problems such as coronary artery disease, hypertension, and diabetes tend to present their clinical manifestations in adulthood, these disorders

TABLE 70.10

Health-Related Risk Factors Associated with Childhood Obesity

Risk Factor	References
Elevated triglycerides	13,14
Elevated LDL cholesterol	15
Reduced HDL cholesterol	13,5
Elevated blood pressure	17
Elevated insulin	14,15
Elevated left ventricular mass	18
Endothelial dysfunction	19
Orthopedic abnormalities (e.g., Blount's disease)	20,21
Gallstone formation	22,23
Asthma and reduced pulmonary function	24,25
Sleep disorders	26,27

TABLE 70.11

Visceral Adiposity and Increased Health Risk in Childhood Obesity

Health Risk	References
Elevated LDL cholesterol and triglycerides associated with visceral but not subcutaneous fat in obese children	28
Elevated triglycerides and insulin and lowered HDL cholesterol associated with visceral fat in obese but not in non-obese adolescents	29
Visceral fat, but not subcutaneous or total body fat, explained significant proportions of the variance in triglycerides, HDL cholesterol, and LDL particle size in obese children	30

have their beginnings in childhood,[12] with obese children tending to have a poorer risk profile than their normal-weight counterparts. A variety of additional health problems occur at significantly greater frequencies in obese children (Table 70.10).[13-27] Children with increased visceral adiposity may be at especially high risk (Table 70.11).[28-30]

Etiology of Childhood Obesity

Heredity

Feeding studies with identical twins have helped to elucidate the role of genetic background in determining obesity. When groups of identical twins are exposed to overfeeding, significantly more variance occurs in the response between pairs of twins than within pairs for the changes in body weight, suggesting a genetic component for susceptibility to weight gain.[31] Still, results from family studies suggest that the maximal heritability of obesity phenotypes ranges from about 30 to 50%,[32] indicating that non-genetic factors also play an important role. Quantifying the influence of the non-genetic factors has proven difficult, however.

Diet

Definitive data on the relationship between free-living energy intake and childhood obesity are lacking. Interestingly, as the prevalence of childhood obesity has increased over the past two decades, the reported mean energy intakes of 6- to 11-year-olds showed a

TABLE 70.12

Mean Energy Intake by Age, 1976-1980 and 1988-1991

	NHANES II (1976-1980)		NHANES III (1988-1991)		
Age	n	Energy kj (kcal)	n	Energy kj (kcal)	Percent Change
1-2 y	1417	5385 (1287)	1231	5393 (1289)	<1
3-5 y	2345	6565 (1569)	1547	6657 (1591)	1
6-11 y	1725	8201 (1960)	1745	7937 (1897)	–3

Adapted from Briefel RR, McDowell MA, Alaimo K, Caughman CR, Bischof AL, Carroll MD, Johnson CL. *Am J Clin Nutr* 62: 1072S; 1995.

slight decline from NHANES II (1976-1980) to NHANES III (1988-1991) (Table 70.12).[33] With respect to fat intake, most,[34-38] but not all, juvenile studies[39,40] support the idea that diets high in fat are associated with body fatness or gain in weight. As early as age three, children of obese parents demonstrate an increased preference for high-fat foods.[41] Data also suggest that food preferences developed in childhood tend to track into aduldhood.[42]

Resting Metabolism

Some studies that measured resting metabolic rate in children utilizing 30-minute measures of oxygen consumption support the notion that a lower than normal resting metabolism contributes to childhood obesity.[43,44] On the other hand, two recent reviews of the isotope dilution (doubly-labeled water) method for measuring energy expenditure concluded that low levels of resting energy expenditure are probably not responsible for obesity in most children.[45,46]

Physical Inactivity

Several lines of evidence suggest the importance of physical inactivity in childhood obesity. Preschoolers who were classified as inactive were 3.8 times as likely as active children to have increasing triceps skinfold slopes during the average 2.5 years of followup.[47] An analysis of doubly-labeled water studies concluded that low levels of physical activity were associated with higher levels of body fatness.[45] Time–motion studies have shown that inactive children are more fat than active children,[48,49] even while ingesting less energy.[50]

Treatment of Childhood Obesity

Family Involvement

Studies that have examined successful five-year[51] and ten-year[52] outcomes for childhood obesity interventions emphasize the importance of family involvement in the weight loss process and recommend a treatment model that integrates improved dietary habits, increased physical activity, and behavior modification. Active parental participation is a crucial component of the model, given that parenting styles not only influence the development of food preferences but establish the type of family environment that may be conducive to overeating or a sedentary lifestyle. Parents also function as role models and reinforcers for eating and exercise behaviors. Family-based behavioral interventions for childhood obesity typically include an initial, short-term (8 to 16 weeks) treatment phase followed by a longer-term (1 year) maintenance or continued improvement phase.[53] During initial treatment, children typically meet in group settings once per week for 45 to 90 minutes.[51,54] Follow-up sessions usually occur once or twice per month for up to one year.[54,55] Facilitators for treatment sessions may be pediatricians, child psychologists, or nutritionists.[53]

Dietary Intervention

A variety of dietary approaches have been utilized in family-based childhood obesity interventions; some focus on healthy eating habits rather than energy restriction, while others prescribe significant caloric reduction. From a behavior change perspective, the specific content of the diet may be less important than how it is presented. The diet should be simple, explicit, and unambiguous, so that it is easy to implement and monitor, and not subject to confusion or easy rationalization of exceptions.[56] A trained nutritionist can assist the family in evaluating their cooking and eating patterns and by making suggestions relative to the purchasing and preparing of foods. The nutritionist should also help the family understand the concepts of portion size, nutritional contents of foods, and the use of food exchange lists such as the *Exchange Lists for Weight Management*.[57] It is recommended that obese children practice maintaining a food diary. Although in most cases the diary will be inaccurate in figuring total energy intake, it can prove useful for reviewing problem foods and eating patterns.[1,58] Dietary fiber is also useful in the treatment of childhood obesity, as it increases satiety and often displaces fat in the diet.[3,59] The recommended daily dietary intake of fiber for children aged 3 to 20 years is equivalent to their age in years plus 5 g per day, as the minimum, and increases to age in years plus 10 g per day as the maximum.[60] The "age + 10" upper level of fiber intake is the recommended goal for the obese child.[3] Table 70.13 summarizes the dietary component from several successful family-based behavioral interventions for childhood obesity. By way of note, The Traffic Light Diet was designed to maximize healthy food choices, decrease energy intake, and encourage individual control over the diet.[55] Foods are categorized as red, yellow, or green on the basis of their kcalorie and nutrient content. Green foods (primarily vegetables) are very low in kcalories. Yellow foods (skim milk, apple) are higher in

TABLE 70.13

Selected Family-Based Interventions for Childhood Obesity

Ages	n	Diet	Exercise	Outcome	Ref
12-16	36	Nutrition education, emphasis on low sugar, salt, and fat	Increasing physical activity encouraged	(1 y) % Overweight declined by 10.7%	54
7-17	4	Hypocaloric diets (600 kcal/d for 10 wk); 1200 kcal/d next 42 wk	Gradual increase in physical activity using aerobic points system	(1 y) % Overweight declined by 20%	61
8-12	18	Traffic Light Diet, target of 1000-1200 kcal/d	Children reinforced for decreasing sedentary activities	(1 y) % Body fat (electrical impedance) declined 4.7%	55
7-16	60	Nutrition education, emphasis on healthy eating rather than eating less	Moderate intensity exercise for 30 min/d, lifestyle changes to increase activity	(1 y) % Overweight declined by 11%	63
8-16	12	Modified Traffic Light Diet	Moderate intensity exercise for up to 45 min/d, 5-7 d/wk	(5 y) % Overweight declined by 23%	51

TABLE 70.14

Two Studies of After-School Exercise (without Dietary Intervention) in the Treatment of Childhood Obesity

Subjects (n)	Obesity Status[a]	Exercise Program	Results	Ref.
7-11 y girls (n = 25)	Ex = 42.8% fat C = 43.3% fat	Ex = aerobics, 5 d/wk, 12 wk C = lifestyle education only	-1.4% fat[b] + 0.4% fat[c]	68
7-11 y boys and girls (n = 74)	Ex = 44.5% fat C = 44.1% fat	Ex = aerobics, 5 d/wk, 17 wk C = maintain normal activities	-2.2% fat[b] no change	69

[a] Ex is exercise group, C is control group. % Fat is percentage of body fat measured with dual-energy x-ray absorptiometry.
[b] Significant change ($p<0.05$) from pre-test.
[c] Non-significant change ($p>0.05$) from pre-test.

kcalories and include the dietary staples needed for a balanced diet. Red foods (potato chips, candy) are foods higher in kcalories, with low nutrient density.

Exercise

Although energy restriction can result in significant short-term weight loss in obese children, it tends to reduce fat-free mass and resting metabolic rate,[64] thus setting the stage for regain of the lost fat when the dieting stops.[65] Recent data suggest that exercise (walking 2 to 3 miles per day, 5 days per week) offers metabolic benefits to obese children during diet-induced weight loss by reversing the potentially adverse changes in protein turnover consequent to the hypocaloric diet.[66] Data also suggest that adding exercise to a diet restriction regimen can result in a total daily energy expenditure above that predicted by the addition of the exercise.[67] Within the context of after-school physical activity programs, two recent studies demonstrated the efficacy of exercise alone (no dietary intervention) in reducing childhood obesity (Table 70.14).[68,69] The study by Owens et al.[69] also showed the efficacy of exercise alone in attenuating the increase in visceral adipose tissue in obese children.

Optimal Exercise Dose

Little is known about the optimal dose of exercise for the treatment of childhood obesity. The National Association for Sport and Physical Education recommends that children obtain at least one to two hours of exercise each day.[70] Examination of Tables 70.15 and 70.16 suggests that the exercise component of successful obesity treatment programs can vary widely and may fall short of the recommended one to two hours of daily exercise. For the obese child, increasing the level of physical activity gradually may be an important consideration, so that failure and discouragement do not sabotage both exercise and dietary resolve.[3] Adding 20 to 30 minutes per day of moderate physical activity to the obese child's routine would appear to be a reasonable initial goal. Exercise programs should be designed to increase the interaction between parents and children or with other children.[1] Behavioral research also suggests that obese children are more likely to continue being physically active over time if they perceive themselves as having choice and control over being more physically active, rather than attributing control to their parents.[55]

TABLE 70.15

Behavior Modification Components for Treatment of Childhood Obesity

Component	Comment
Self-monitoring	Utilize food and physical activity log books; monitor body weight changes (usually daily or weekly)
Stimulus control	Limit amount of high-kcalorie foods kept in house; establish set routines for meals and snacks; model physically active lifestyle
Reinforcement	Reward targeted behaviors by child with verbal praise by parents; include predetermined (with input from child) tangible rewards that encourage further physical activity (sporting equipment, trips to recreational areas) or healthy eating habits (favorite fruits)
Eating behavior	Avoid second helpings, take smaller bites, put down fork between bites, leave food on plate at meal's end, avoid TV watching while eating
Goal setting and contracting	Parent and child establish realistic goals for physical activity, weight loss, and eating behaviors; use contracts to help maintain focus and provide structure for rewarding desired changes
Managing high-risk situations	Pre-plan management strategies for holidays, birthdays, parties, and eating in restaurants; practice using role playing

Behavior Modification

The work of Epstein et al.[52,71] represents the current state of the art in behavioral treatment of childhood obesity. They have systematically studied a progression of behavioral methods and demonstrated beneficial long-term effects on weight control.[56] Table 70.15 summarizes components of behavior modification commonly utilized in the treatment of childhood obesity.

Resources on Childhood Obesity

Table 70.16 provides a topical list of sources of information on childhood obesity.

TABLE 70.16

Selected Resources on Childhood Obesity

Topic	Resource
Recent review articles on childhood obesity	References 1, 3, 53, 56, 58,
Recent books on childhood obesity	1. Smith, J.C., *Understanding Childhood Obesity,* University Press of Mississippi, 1999 2. Williams, C.L. (ed), *Prevention and Treatment of Childhood Obesity,* New York Academy of Sciences, 1993 3. Krasnegor, N.A., *Childhood Obesity: A Biobehavioral Perspective,* The Telford Press, 1990
Obesity-related professional journals	1. *International Journal of Obesity and Related Metabolic Disorders* 2. *Obesity Research*
Obesity-related research organizations	1. Center for Child and Adolescent Obesity (University of California, San Francisco) 2. Weight Control Information Network (National Institutes of Health, Bethesda, MD) 3. The National Institute of Child Health and Human Development (National Institutes of Health, Bethesda, MD) 4. European Childhood Obesity Group (Lyon, France)
Childhood exercise and fitness	1. *Pediatric Exercise Science* 2. American College of Sports Medicine (Indianapolis, IN) 3. American Alliance for Health, Physical Education, Recreation and Dance (Reston, VA) 4. President's Council on Physical Fitness and Sports (Washington, D.C.)
Childhood nutrition	1. The American Dietetic Association (Chicago, IL) 2. Food and Nutrition Information Center, U.S. Department of Agriculture 3. American Academy of Pediatrics

References

1. Strauss R. *Curr Prob Pediatr* 29: 5; 1999.
2. Troiano RP, Flegal KM, Kuczmarski RJ, et al. *Arch Pediatr Adolesc Med* 149: 1085; 1995.
3. Williams CL, Campanaro LA, Squillace M, Bollella M. *Ann NY Acad Sci* 817: 225; 1997.
4. Must A, Dallal G, Dietz W. *Am J Clin Nutr* 53: 839; 1991.
5. Williams D, Going S, Lohman T, et al. *Am J Pub Health* 82: 358; 1992.
6. Power C, Lake JK, Cole TJ. *Int J Obes Relat Metab Disord* 21: 507; 1997.
7. Himes JH, Dietz WH. *Am J Clin Nutr* 59: 307; 1994.
8. Bellizzi MC, Dietz WH. *Am J Clin Nutr* 70: 173S; 1999.
9. Winkleby MA, Robinson TN, Sundquist J, Kraemer HC. *JAMA* 281: 1006; 1999.
10. Goran MI, Nagy TR, Treuth MS, et al. *Am J Clin Nutr* 65: 1703; 1997.
11. Owens S, Gutin B, Barbeau P, et al. *Obes Res* [in press].
12. Berenson GS, Srinivasan SR, Bao W. *Ann NY Acad Sci* 817: 189; 1997.
13. Gidding SS, Bao W, Srinivasan SR, Berenson GS. *J Pediatr* 127: 868; 1995.
14. Gutin B, Islam S, Manos T, et al. *J Pediatr* 125: 847; 1994.
15. Kikuchi DA, Srinivasan SR, Harsha DW, et al. *Prev Med* 21: 177; 1992.
16. Gutin B, Owens S, Treiber F, et al. *Arch Pediatr Adolesc Med* 151: 462; 1997.
17. Lauer RM, Burns TL, Clarke WR, Mahoney LT. *Hypertension* 18: I74S; 1991.
18. Gutin B, Treiber F, Owens S, Mensah G. *J Pediatr* 132: 1023; 1998.
19. Treiber F, Papavassiliou D, Gutin B, et al. *Psychosom Med* 59: 376; 1997.
20. Loder RT, Aronson DD, Greenfield ML. *J Bone Joint Surg* 75: 1141; 1993.
21. Dietz WH, Gross WL, Kirkpatrick JA. *J Pediatr* 101: 735; 1982.

22. Friesen CA, Roberts CC. *Clin Pediatr* 7: 294; 1989.
23. Honore LH. *Arch Surg* 115: 62; 1980.
24. Unger R, Kreeger L, Christoffel KK. *Clin Pediatr* 29: 368; 1990.
25. Kaplan TA, Montana E. *Clin Pediatr* 32: 220; 1993.
26. Mallory GB, Fiser DH, Jackson R. *J Pediatr* 115: 892; 1989.
27. Marcus CL, Curtis S, Koerner CB, et al. *Pediatr Pulmonol* 21: 176; 1996.
28. Brambilla P, Manzoni P, Sironi S, et al. *Int J Obes Relat Metab Disord* 18: 795; 1994.
29. Caprio S, Hyman LD, McCarthy S, et al. *Am J Clin Nutr* 64: 12; 1996.
30. Owens S, Gutin B, Ferguson M, et al. *J Pediatr* 133: 41; 1998.
31. Bouchard C, Tremblay A, Despres JP, et al. *N Engl J Med* 322: 1477; 1990.
32. Perusse L, Bouchard C. *Ann Med* 31: 19; 1999.
33. Briefel RR, McDowell MA, Alaimo K, et al. *Am J Clin Nutr* 62: 1072S; 1995.
34. Eck LH, Kleges RC, Hanson CL, Slawson D. *Int J Obes Relat Metab Disord* 16: 71; 1992.
35. Gazzaniga JM, Burns T. *Am J Clin Nutr* 58: 21; 1993.
36. Maffeis C, Schutz Y. *Int J Obes Relat Metab Disord* 20: 170; 1996.
37. Nguyen VT, Larson DE, Johnson RK, Goran MI. *Am J Clin Nutr* 63: 507; 1996.
38. Tucker LA, Seljaas GT, Hager RL. *J Am Dietetic Assn* 97: 981; 1997.
39. Davies PSW, Wells JCK, Fieldhouse CA, Day JME, Lucas A. *Am J Clin Nurtr* 61: 1026; 1995.
40. Muecke L, Simons-Morton B, Huang IE, Parcel G. *J School Health* 62: 19; 1992.
41. Fisher JO, Birch LL. *J Am Diet Assoc* 95: 759; 1995.
42. Kelder SH, Perry CL, Klepp KI, Lytlle LL. *Am J Pub Health* 84: 1121; 1994.
43. Kaplan AS, Zemel BS, Stallings VA. *J Pediatr* 129: 643; 1996.
44. Morrison JA, Alfaro MP, Khoury P, et al. *J Pediatr* 129: 637; 1996.
45. DeLany JP. *Am J Clin Nurtr* 68: 950S; 1998.
46. Goran MI, Sun M. *Am J Clin Nutr* 68: 944S; 1998.
47. Moore LL, Nguyen UDT, Rothman KJ, et al. *Am J Epidemiol* 142: 982; 1995.
48. Goran MI, Hunter G, Nagy TR, Johnson R. *Int J Obes Relat Metab Disord* 21: 171; 1997.
49. Maffeis C, Zaffanello M, Schutz Y. *J Pediatr* 131: 288; 1997.
50. Deheeger M, Rolland-Cachera MF, Fontvielle AM. *Int J Obes Relat Metab Disord* 21: 372; 1997.
51. Johnson WG, Hinkle LK, Carr RE, et al. *Obes Res* 5: 257; 1997.
52. Epstein LH, Valoski A, Wing RR, McCurley J. *Health Psychol* 13: 373; 1994.
53. Owens S, Gutin B. In: *Lifestyle Medicine* Rippe, JM, Ed, Blackwell Science, Malden, MA, 1999; ch 50.
54. Brownell KD, Kelman JH, Strunkard AJ. *Pediatrics* 71: 515; 1983.
55. Epstein LH, Valoski AM, Vara LS, et al. *Health Psychol* 14: 109; 1995.
56. Robinson TN. *Int J Obes Relat Metab Disord* 23: 52S; 1999.
57. American Dietetic Association and American Diabetes Association, *Exchange Lists for Weight Management*, Revised ed, Chicago, 1995.
58. Moran R. *Am Fam Phys* 59: 861; 1999.
59. Kelsay JL, Behall KM, Prather ES. *Am J Clin Nutr* 31: 1149; 1978.
60. Williams CL. *Pediatrics* 5: 985S; 1995.
61. Figueroa-Colon R, Almen K, Franklin F, et al. *Am J Dis Child* 147: 160; 1993.
62. Epstein LH, Valoski AM, Vara LS, et al. *Health Psychol* 14: 109; 1995.
63. Braet C, van Winckel M, van Leeuwen K. *Acta Paediatr* 86: 397; 1997.
64. Maffeis C, Schutz Y, Pinelli L. *Int J Obes Relat Metab Disord* 16: 41; 1992.
65. Schwingshandl J, Borkenstein M. *Int J Obes Relat Metab Disord* 19: 752; 1995.
66. Ebbeling CB, Rodriguez NR. *Med Sci Sports Exerc* 31: 378; 1999.
67. Blaak EE, Westerterp KR, Bar-Or O, et al. *Am J Clin Nutr* 55: 777; 1992.
68. Gutin B, Cucuzzo N, Islam S, et al. *Obes Res* 3: 305; 1995.
69. Owens S, Gutin B, Allison J, et al. *Med Sci Sports Exerc* 31: 143; 1999.
70. National Association for Sport and Physical Education (NASPE), Physical activity guidelines for pre-adolescent children, 1998.
71. Epstein LH, Valoski A, Wing RR, McCurley J. *JAMA* 264: 2519; 1990.

71

Trace Mineral Deficiencies

Forrest H. Nielsen

Introduction

By 1940 the concept of essential nutrients was well established; they were defined as chemical substances found in food that could not be synthesized by the body to perform functions necessary for life. In the 1960s and 1970s, the standard for essentiality was liberalized for mineral elements that could not be fed at dietary concentrations low enough to cause death or interrupt the life cycle (interfere with growth, development, or maturation such that procreation is prevented). Thus, an essential element during this time period was defined as one whose dietary deficiency consistently and adversely changed a biological function from optimal, and this change was preventable or reversible by physiological amounts of the element. This definition of essentiality became less acceptable when a large number of elements was suggested to be essential based on small changes in physiological or biochemical variables. Many of these changes were questioned as to whether they were necessarily the result of a suboptimal function, and sometimes were suggested to be the consequence of a pharmacologic or toxic action in the body, including an effect on intestinal microorganisms. As a result, if the lack of an element cannot be shown to cause death or to interrupt the life cycle, many scientists, perhaps a majority, now do not consider an element essential unless it has a defined biochemical function. However, there are still scientists who base essentiality on older criteria. Thus, no universally accepted list of essential trace elements exists. Nonetheless, it is hoped that most of the mineral elements that are essential, possibly essential, or beneficial have been included in this section.

Biological Roles of Mineral Elements

Trace elements have at least five roles in living organisms. In close association with enzymes, some trace elements are integral parts of catalytic centers at which the reactions necessary for life occur. Working in concert with a protein, and frequently with other

0-8493-2705-9/02/$0.00+$1.50

organic coenzymes, trace elements are involved in attracting substrate molecules and converting them to specific end products. Some trace elements donate or accept electrons in reactions of reduction or oxidation. In addition to the generation and utilization of metabolic energy, redox reactions frequently involve the chemical transformation of molecules. One trace element, iron, is involved in binding, transporting, and releasing oxygen in the body. Some trace elements have structural roles; that is, imparting stability and three-dimensional structure to important biological molecules. Some trace elements have regulatory roles. They control important biological processes through such actions as inhibiting enzymatic reactions, facilitating the binding of molecules to receptor sites on cell membranes, altering the structure or ionic nature of membranes to prevent or allow specific molecules to enter a cell, and inducing genes to express themselves resulting in the formation of proteins involved in life processes.

Homeostatic Regulation of Mineral Elements

Homeostasis is a term used to describe the ability of the body to maintain the content of a specific substance within a certain range despite varying intakes. Homeostasis involves the processes of absorption, storage, and excretion. The relative importance of these three processes varies among the trace elements. The amount absorbed from the gastrointestinal tract often is a primary controlling factor for trace elements needed in the cationic state such as copper, iron, and zinc. Trace elements absorbed as negatively charged anions, such as boron and selenium, are usually absorbed freely and completely from the gastrointestinal tract. Excretion through the urine, bile, sweat, and breath is, therefore, the primary mechanism for controlling the amount of these trace elements in an organism. By being stored in inactive sites, some trace elements are prevented from causing adverse reactions when present in high quantities. An example of this homeostatic process is the storage of iron in the form of ferritin. Release of a trace element from a storage site also can be important in preventing deficiency.

Factors Affecting the Manifestation of Deficiency Signs

Although trace elements play key roles in a variety of processes necessary for life, except for iodine and iron, the occurrence of overt, simple, or uncomplicated deficiency of any trace element in humans is not common. The reasons for this are the powerful homeostatic mechanisms for trace elements described above, and the consumption of diets with different types of foods from different sources. However, reductions in health and wellbeing because of suboptimal status in some trace elements probably are not uncommon because of other factors affecting their metabolism or utilization. For example, genetic errors and diseases that affect absorption, retention, or excretion of a trace element can result in deficiency pathology even though intake may meet dietary guidelines. In other words, most important in making trace elements of nutritional concern is that their metabolism or utilization can be impaired or their need can be increased by nutritional, metabolic, hormonal, or physiological stressors. This is exemplified by selenium, for which it is difficult to produce signs of pathology caused by a simple deficiency in animals or humans.

A stressor such as vitamin E deficiency or viral infection is needed to obtain marked pathology such as that seen with Keshan disease, a cardiomyopathy that primarily affects children and women of childbearing age in some areas of China.

Treatment of Trace Mineral Deficiencies

Because most mineral elements can have adverse effects if taken orally in excess of the Recommended Dietary Allowance (RDA), Estimated Safe and Adequate Daily Dietary Intake (ESADDI), or Adequate Intake (AI), deficiencies of mineral elements are best treated by giving supplements that supply one or two times these amounts. Higher amounts may be indicated if a deficiency is caused by a factor resulting in malabsorption or excessive excretion; these amounts need to be adjusted until indicators of deficiency have been abated and normal status is maintained. The response to treatment of a trace mineral deficiency is best monitored by determining that desirable changes are occurring in indicators of deficiency or status. Once indicators are within normal ranges, intakes near the RDA, ESADDI, or AI that maintain these normal values should be maintained. A diet providing the needed intakes is preferable over supplements.

Mineral Elements Essential for Humans

Essential Trace Elements

Trace elements essential for life generally occur in the body in microgram per gram of tissue, and are usually required by humans in amounts of milligrams per day; these elements are copper, iron, manganese, and zinc. The evidence for essentiality for humans is substantial and noncontroversial for these elements. Specific biochemical functions have been defined for all of them. Another element, boron, has recently joined the list of those accepted as essential; it has been found to be required to complete the life cycle of fish[1] and frogs.[2,3] Because magnesium has many characteristics of a trace element, it also will be included in this grouping.

Boron

Knowledge about the role and clinical aspects of boron in nutrition is just emerging. The biological function of boron has not been defined, but boron apparently has a role that influences the metabolism and utilization of several other nutrients. Thus, described deficiency signs and the pathological consequences of inadequate boron intake, because they can be affected by the intake of several other dietary substances, are numerous and variable. As a result, providing sound factual descriptions in each of the categories in Table 71.1 is not possible, and the information provided could be changed quickly by new research findings. Indicators of boron status are still being established. However, a plasma boron concentration below 25 ng/mL might be indicative of a low boron status. Changes in biochemical indices affected by physiological amounts of boron (shown in Table 71.1) with boron supplementation also may be an indicator of a low boron status. Most of the information in Table 71.1 can be found in reviews by Nielsen,[4-6] Hunt,[7] and Penland.[8]

TABLE 71.1

Biochemical, Clinical, and Nutritional Aspects of Boron

Biological Function:

Established — None
Hypothesized — 1. A role in cell membrane function that influences the response to hormone action, transmembrane signaling, or transmembrane movement of regulatory cations or anions.
2. A metabolic regulator through complexing with a variety of substrate or reactant compounds in which there are hydroxyl groups in favorable positions. Regulation is mainly negative.

Signs of Deficiency:

Biochemical — Because boron apparently affects calcium metabolism and hormone action, low dietary boron has a variety of effects in humans. These include:
Calcium indicators — Decreased serum 25-hydroxycholecalciferol; increased serum calcitonin
Energy metabolism — Increased serum glucose; decreased serum triglycerides
Nitrogen metabolism — Increased blood urea; increased serum creatinine; decreased urinary hydroxyproline excretion
Reactive oxygen metabolism — Decreased erythrocyte superoxide dismutase; decreased ceruloplasmin
Response to estrogen — Decreased serum 17β-estradiol; decreased plasma copper
Physiological — Because boron can cause a variety of biochemical responses depending upon other dietary factors, it is not surprising that boron deprivation also has a variety of physiological effects. These include:
Altered electroencephalograms such that they suggest impaired behavior activation (e.g., more drowsiness) and mental alertness
Impaired psychomotor skills
Impaired cognitive processes of attention and memory
Increased platelet and erythrocyte numbers; decreased white blood cells

A number of physiological signs of deficiency have been found in animals that may eventually have some counterparts in humans. Reported signs [1-3, 9] include:

Frog — Increased necrotic eggs; high frequency of abnormal gastrulation in embryo; abnormal development of the gut, craniofacial region, and eye, visceral edema, and kinking of the tail during organogenesis; delayed tail absorption during metamorphosis
Zebrafish — Embryo death during the zygote and cleavage periods before the formation of a blastula during embryo development; photophobia characterized by photoreceptor dystrophy in adults
Rat — Exacerbation of distortion of marrow sprouts and delay in the initiation of cartilage calcification in bones during marginal vitamin D deficiency; decreased circulating concentrations of natural killer cells and $CD8a^+/CD4^-$ cells during antigen-induced arthritis

Pathological Consequences of Deficiency:

Established — None
Hypothesized — Increased susceptibility to osteoporosis and arthritis
Impaired cognitive and psychomotor function
Predisposing factors for deficiency: stressors affecting calcium metabolism and utilization especially low dietary intakes of vitamin D or calcium; stressors affecting cell membrane function or signal transduction including low dietary intakes of magnesium, potassium or copper

Recommended Intakes:

Prevention of deficiency — Suggested to be 1.0 mg/day
Therapeutic or beneficial — Luxuriant intakes (e.g., 3 mg/day) *may* be beneficial when stressors are present that lead to osteoporotic or arthritic changes

Food Sources:

Food and drink of plant origin, especially noncitrus fruits, leafy vegetables, nuts, pulses, legumes, wine, cider

Copper

Although copper is a well-established essential trace element, its practical nutritional importance, and thus its dietary requirement, remain debatable. Well-established consequences of copper deprivation in humans have come mainly from findings with premature infants and infants with the genetic disorder Menkes' disease; other consequences have been projected from epidemiological, animal, and short-term human copper depletion findings. Most of the information found in Table 71.2 has been obtained from reviews by Harris,[10] Klevay and Medeiros,[11] Milne,[12] Cordano,[13] and Uauy et al.[14]

Iron

Among the mineral nutrients, iron has the longest and best described history. Despite long and effective intervention activities, iron deficiency is the primary mineral deficiency in the U.S. and the world. Recently, it has been suggested that high intakes of iron also may be a health concern. Table 71.3 only briefly outlines some important aspects of iron nutrition, using information from reviews by Beard and Dawson[28] and Baynes and Stipanuk.[29]

Magnesium

Magnesium is the fourth most abundant cation in the body and is second only to potassium in its intracellular concentration. This concentration reflects that magnesium is critical for a great number of cellular functions including oxidative phosphorylation, glycolysis, DNA transcription, fatty acid degradation, and protein synthesis. Surprisingly, although it is such a critically important element, reported descriptions of signs and symptoms of magnesium deficiency in humans through dietary restriction alone are very limited. Described cases of clinical magnesium deficiency have generally been conditioned deficiencies where factors interfering with absorption or promoting excretion were present (see Table 71.4). Table 71.4 briefly outlines some of the important aspects of magnesium nutrition using information from reviews by Rude[40] and Shils.[41]

Manganese

The essentiality of manganese for animals has been known for over 50 years. Deficiency causes testicular degeneration (rats), slipped tendons (chicks), osteodystrophy, severe glucose intolerance (guinea pigs), ataxia (mice, mink), depigmentation of hair, and seizures. However, only one description of an unequivocal case of human manganese deficiency has been reported. A child with a postoperative short bowel receiving over 90% of her nutrition parenterally, which was low in manganese, developed short stature and brittle bones. Because manganese deficiency has been so difficult to identify in humans, manganese is considered not of nutritional concern. Most of the information in Table 71.5 has been obtained from reviews by Leach and Harris,[49] Nielsen,[50] and Freeland-Graves and Llanes.[51]

Zinc

Signs of zinc deficiency in humans were first described in the 1960s. However, the prevalence of zinc deficiency is controversial because of the lack of satisfactory indicators of zinc status. Nonetheless, unquestionable zinc deficiency has been induced often by providing zinc-deficient total parenteral nutrition (TPN), and by feeding cow's milk to infants who have a genetic inability to absorb zinc from such a source. The information in Table 71.6 primarily comes from reviews by Chesters,[60] Prasad,[61] and Sandstead.[62]

TABLE 71.2

Biochemical, Clinical, and Nutritional Aspects of Copper

Biological Function:

Copper is a cofactor for a number of oxidase enzymes and has roles in angiogenesis, neurohormone release, oxygen transport, and the regulation of genetic expression. Copper enzymes are involved in the generation of oxidative energy, oxidation of ferrous iron, synthesis of neurotransmitters, bestowment of pigment to hair and skin, provision of strength to bones and arteries, assurance of competence of the immune system, and stabilization of the matrices of connective tissues. These enzymes include: lysyl oxidase, ferroxidase (ceruloplasmin), dopamine B-monooxygenase, tyrosinase, alpha-amidating monooxygenase, cytochrome c oxidase, and superoxide dismutase.

Signs of Deficiency:

Biochemical — Although not consistently seen, the following have been reported to be the result of copper deprivation in humans: decreased erythrocyte superoxide dismutase; decreased enzymatic and immunoreactive ceruloplasmin and ratio; decreased platelet and mononuclear white cell cytochrome c oxidase; increased plasma LDL and total cholesterol; increased plasma glutathione; decreased platelet and plasma copper; decreased plasma HDL cholesterol and interleukin-2.

Physiological — Premature and malnourished infants: hematologic changes characterized by hypochromic, normocytic or macrocytic anemia accompanied by reduced reticulocyte count, neutropenia and thrombocytopenia; bone abnormalities which mimic scurvy by showing osteoporosis, fractures of the long bones and ribs, epiphyseal separation, fraying and cupping of the metaphyses with spur formation, and subperiostal new bone formation; hypopigmentation of hair; impaired growth; impaired immunity.

Adults (reported experimentally induced): abnormal electrocardiograms; impaired glucose tolerance; increased blood pressure with exercise.

Pathological Consequences of Deficiency:

Established — Premature and malnourished infants: anemia; osteoporosis and bone fractures; increased incidence of infections; poor growth; Menkes' disease; "kinky-type" steely hair; progressive neurologic disorder; death.

Hypothesized — Fetus and children: impaired brain development; [15,16] teratogenesis. [17, 18] Adults: osteoporosis,[19] ischemic heart disease,[20-22] increased susceptibility to infections[14, 23] and cancer,[25] accelerated aging.[26]

Predisposing Factors for Deficiency:

Factors causing impaired absorption including high intakes of iron and zinc, celiac disease, short bowel syndrome, cystic fibrosis, tropical and nontropical sprue, diarrhea, and jejunoileal bypass surgery; and factors causing excessive copper loss including ambulatory peritoneal dialysis, burn trauma, penicillamine therapy, dexamethasone treatment, and excessive use of antacids.

Recommended Intakes:

Prevention of deficiency — The estimated safe and adequate daily dietary intakes (in mg/day) are: infants age 0-0.5 years, 0.4-0.6 and age 0.5-1 year, 0.6-0.7; children and adolescents age 1-3 years, 0.7-1.0, age 4-6, 1.0 1.5, age 7-10 years, 1.0-2.0, and age 11+ years, 1.5-2.5; adults, 1.5-3.0.[27] The lack of a recommended dietary allowance for copper indicates that the amount needed to prevent deficiency is a debatable issue.

Therapeutic or beneficial — Increased intakes of copper (e.g., 3 mg/day) *may* be beneficial in preventing osteoporosis, overcoming the adverse effects of high zinc intake, and more quickly overcoming the consequences of copper deficiency.

Food Sources:

Legumes, whole grains, nuts, organ meats (e.g., liver), seafood (e.g., oysters, crab), peanut butter, chocolate, mushrooms, ready-to-eat cereals.

TABLE 71.3

Biochemical, Clinical, and Nutritional Aspects of Iron

Biological Function:

Iron is involved in oxygen transport and storage, electron transport, and in numerous enzymatic reactions involving substrate oxidation and reduction. The classes of enzymes dependent on iron for activity include the oxidoreductases exemplified by xanthine oxidase/dehydrogenase, monooxygenases exemplified by the amino acid oxidases and cytochrome P450, dioxygenases exemplified by amino acid or amine dioxygenases, lipoxygenases, peroxidases, fatty acid desaturases and NO synthases, and miscellaneous enzymes such as aconitase.

Signs of Deficiency:

Biochemical — Decreased tissue and blood iron enzymes, myoglobin, hemoglobin, ferritin, transferrin saturation, and iron; increased erythrocyte protoporphyrin

Physiological — Anemia, glossitis, angular stomatitis, spoon nails (koilonychia), blue sclera, lethargy, apathy, listlessness, and fatigue

Pathological Consequences of Deficiency:

Established — Impaired thermoregulation, immune function, mental function, and physical performance; complications in pregnancy including increased risk of premature delivery, low birth weight, and infant morbidity

Hypothesized — Osteoporosis,[30] abnormal brain development[31]

Predisposing Factors for Deficiency:

Blood loss including that through menstruation; vegetarian diets

Recommended Intakes:

Prevention of deficiency — The recommended dietary allowances (RDA) for iron (in mg/day) are: infants age 0-0.5 years, 6, and age 0.5-1 year, 10; children 1-10 years, 10; males age 11-18 years, 12, age 19+ years, 10; females age 11-50, 15, and age 50+, 10; pregnant females, 30; lactating females, 15. [27]

Therapeutic or beneficial — Higher doses than the above can be given to more quickly overcome iron deficiency, usually caused by blood loss; doses used include 50-60 mg/day or 120 mg/week.[30-34] However, caution is in order because high intakes of iron have been associated with cardiovascular disease,[35, 36] cancer,[37,38] and neurodegenerative disorders. [39]

Food Sources:

Red meat, organ meats (e.g., liver), seafood (e.g., oysters, shrimp), fortified cereals, potatoes with skin, tofu; some whole grains and vegetables (e.g., spinach) are high in iron, but the bioavailability of this iron may be low

TABLE 71.4

Biochemical, Clinical, and Nutritional Aspects of Magnesium

Biological Function:

Magnesium is a cofactor for more than 300 enzymes in the body. This cofactor role is either as a direct allosteric activator of enzymes or as a part of enzyme substrates for some enzyme reactions (e.g., MgATP and MgGTP). Magnesium also has functions that affect membrane properties and thus influence potassium and calcium channels and nerve conduction.

Signs of Deficiency:

Biochemical — Low blood potassium, calcium, and magnesium; decreased intracellular potassium; excessive renal potassium excretion; impaired parathyroid hormone excretion and vitamin D function; renal and skeletal resistance to parathyroid hormone

Physiological — Neuromuscular signs (e.g., positive Trousseau's sign, tremors, fasciculations, gross muscle spasms, muscle cramps and weakness, seizures, dizziness, disequilibrium); electrocardiographic abnormalities; cardiac arrhythmias (e.g., rapid heart rate, ventricular premature discharges, atrial and ventricular fibrillation)

Pathological Consequences of Deficiency:

Established — Conditioned deficiencies result in cardiac disorders, seizures, cramps, depression, and psychosis

Hypothesized — Numerous epidemiological findings and magnesium supplementation trials show that low magnesium status is associated with numerous disorders including coronary heart disease,[42,43] hypertension,[44] migraine headaches,[45] sleep disorders,[46] mood disturbances,[46] and osteoporosis[47]

Predisposing Factors for Deficiency:

Factors interfering with absorption or promoting excretion including alcoholism, cirrhosis, kidney failure, malabsorption syndromes, extensive bowel resection, gastroileal bypass, severe or prolonged diarrhea, protein-calorie malnutrition, acute pancreatitis, hyperaldosteronism, diabetes mellitus, thyroid gland disease, parathyroid gland disease, vitamin D-resistant rickets, pellagra, malignant osteolytic disease, burns and diuretic therapy

Recommended Intakes:

Prevention of deficiency — The recommended dietary allowances (RDA) for magnesium (in mg/day) are: children age 1-3 years, 80, age 4-8 years, 130, and age 9-13 years, 240; male adults age 14-18 years, 410, age 19-30 years, 400, and age 31+ years, 420; female adults age 14-18 years, 360, age 19-30 years, 310, and age 31+ years, 320; pregnant females, +40. Adequate intakes have been indicated for infants; they are for age 0 0.5 years, 30, and age 0.5-1 years, 75. [48]

Therapeutic or beneficial — Although the infusion of magnesium has been suggested as a therapeutic measure to reduce the frequency of arrhythmias and mortality in cases of suspected acute myocardial infarction, this has not been confirmed in large trials.

Food Sources:

Whole grains, nuts, legumes, green leafy vegetables

TABLE 71.5

Biochemical, Clinical, and Nutritional Aspects of Manganese

Biological Function:

Manganese is a cofactor for enzymes involved in protein and energy metabolism, antioxidant action, and mucopolysaccharide synthesis. These enzymes include the metalloenzymes manganese-dependent superoxide dismutase, pyruvate carboxylase and arginase, and the manganese-activated enzymes phosphoenolpyruvate carboxykinase, glycosyl transferases, glutamine synthetase, and farnesyl pyrophosphate synthetase.

Signs of Deficiency:

Biochemical — Possible signs include hypocholesterolemia, and increased serum calcium, phosphorus and alkaline phosphatase activity
Physiological — Impaired growth and brittle bones; another possible sign is a fleeting dermatitis

Pathological Consequences of Deficiency:

Established — Osteoporosis (one case report in a child)[52]
Hypothetical — Low dietary manganese or low blood and tissue manganese has been associated with osteoporosis,[53] epilepsy,[54] atherosclerosis,[55] impaired wound healing,[56] and increased susceptibility to cancer[57,58]
Predisposing factors for deficiency: High dietary intakes of calcium, phosphorus, iron, fiber, phytaes and polyphenolic compounds

Recommended Intakes:

Prevention of deficiency — The estimated safe and adequate daily dietary intakes for manganese (in mg/day) are: infants age 0-0.5 years, 0.3-0.6, and age 0.5-1 year, 0.6-1.0; children and adolescents age 1-3 years, 1.0 1.5, age 4-6 years, 1.5-2.0, age 7-10 years, 2.0-3.0, and age 11+ years, 2.0-5.0; adults, 2.0-5.0. [27]
Therapeutic or beneficial — High intakes of manganese are ill-advised because of potential neurotoxicological effects, [59] especially in people with compromised homeostatic mechanisms, or infants whose homeostatic control of manganese is not fully developed.

Food Sources

Unrefined grains, nuts, green leafy vegetables, and tea

TABLE 71.6

Biochemical, Clinical, and Nutritional Aspects of Zinc

Biological Function:

Zinc is unique in that it is the only trace element with essential actions in all six enzyme classes. Over 50 zinc metalloenzymes have been identified. Another function of zinc is as a component of transcription factors also known as zinc finger proteins that bind to DNA and activate transcription of a message. Zinc also imparts stability to cell membranes.

Signs of Deficiency:

Biochemical — Decreased plasma and leukocyte zinc, plasma metallothionein, thymulin and alkaline phosphatase, and extracellular superoxide dismutase; increased plasma 5′-nucleotidase and platelet amyloid precursor protein[60-63]

Physiological — Depressed growth; anorexia; parakeratotic skin lesions; diarrhea; impaired testicular development, immune function, and cognitive function

Pathological Consequences of Deficiency:

Established — Dwarfism, delayed puberty, failure to thrive (acrodermatitis enteropathica infants), impaired wound healing, and increased susceptibility to infectious disease

Hypothesized — Osteoporosis,[69] infertility,[61] teratogenesis,[18] increased susceptibility to diabetes,[65] and rheumatic disease, especially rheumatoid arthritis[66]

Predisposing Factors for Deficiency:

Factors affecting absorption including phytate intake, vegetarianism, intestinal infestation by bacteria, protozoa and helminths, gastric and intestinal resection, inflammatory bowel disease, exocrine pancreatic insufficiency, biliary obstruction, and high intakes of copper and iron; factors increasing loss including protein losing enteropathies, renal failure, renal dialysis, diuretic therapy, chronic blood loss (e.g., sickle cell disease), exfoliative dermatoses; factors increasing utilization including rapid tissue synthesis and postcatabolic convalescence.

Recommended Intakes:

Prevention of deficiency — The recommended dietary allowances (RDA) for zinc (in mg/day) are: infants age 0-1.0 year, 5; children age 1-10 years, 10; males age 11-51+ years, 15; females age 11-51+ years, 12; pregnant females, 15; lactating females, first 6 months, 19, second 6 months, 16.[27]

Therapeutic or beneficial — High zinc intakes have been used for the alleviation and prevention of colds, treatment of macular degeneration, acute diarrhea and Wilson's disease; doses have ranged from 20 mg day for children with diarrhea to 150 mg/day for treatment of Wilson's disease.[61,67]

Food Sources:

Red meats, organ meats (e.g., liver), shellfish, nuts, legumes

Essential Ultra Trace Elements

In 1980, the term ultra trace elements began to appear in the nutritional literature; the definition for this term was an element required by animals in amounts of 50 nanograms or less per gram of diet. For humans, the term has been used recently to indicate elements with established or estimated requirements quantified by micrograms per day.[50] Five elements fit in this category. The evidence of essentiality for humans is substantial and noncontroversial for cobalt, iodine, molybdenum, and selenium; specific biochemical functions have been identified for all of them. Another element, chromium, has recently joined the list of ultra trace elements accepted as essential because a defined biochemical function has been identified for it.

Chromium

Many nutritionists have considered chromium as essential for humans since 1977, when a subject on long-term TPN apparently containing a low amount of chromium developed impaired glucose tolerance and insulin resistance that were reversed by an infusion of chromium.[68] However, not until 1997 did evidence come forth which conclusively showed that chromium was essential; then a biochemical function was identified for chromium.[69] Nonetheless, since 1966 numerous reports have described beneficial effects from chromium supplements in subjects with degrees of glucose intolerance ranging from hypoglycemia to insulin-dependent diabetes.[70,71] The information in Table 71.7 comes primarily from reviews by Anderson,[70] Nielsen,[72] and Lukaski.[73]

Cobalt

Ionic cobalt is not an essential nutrient for humans; however, vitamin B_{12}, in which cobalt is an integral component, is an essential nutrient for humans. In the 19th century, a megaloblastic anemia was described that was called pernicious anemia because it was invariably fatal. The first effective treatment for this disease was one pound of raw liver daily. In 1948, the anti-pernicious anemia factor in liver was isolated and named vitamin B_{12}, and was found to contain 4% cobalt. Vitamin B_{12} deficiency is rarely caused by a dietary insufficiency and most commonly arises from a defect in vitamin B_{12} absorption. People with low vitamin B_{12} status (e.g., vegetarians) can also display signs of deficiency if stressed with a substance such as nitrous oxide (used in dentistry), which inhibits vitamin B_{12} activity. Most of the information in Table 71.8 was obtained from reviews by Herbert,[74] Smith,[75] Shane,[76] and Nilsson-Ehle.[77]

Iodine

The consequences of iodine deficiency, which is common, are so profound that it is one of the largest public health problems in the world today. Recognition that iodine was nutritionally important began in the 1920s when it was found that iodine prevented goiter, and increased iodine intake was associated with decreased endemic cretinism. Most of the information in Table 71.9 has been obtained from reviews by Freake,[79] and Hetzel and Wellby.[80]

Molybdenum

Because molybdenum is a cofactor for some enzymes, its essentiality is well established. However, molybdenum deficiency has not been unequivocally identified in humans other than in an individual nourished by TPN and in individuals with a genetic disease that

TABLE 71.7

Biochemical, Clinical, and Nutritional Aspects of Chromium

Biological Function:

A naturally occurring biologically active form of chromium named Low-Molecular-Weight Chromium-Binding Substance (LMWCr) has been identified that has a role in carbohydrate and lipid metabolism as part of a novel insulin-amplification mechanism. LMWCr is an oligopeptide of about 1500 Da that binds four chromic ions and potentiates the ability of insulin to stimulate the conversion of glucose into lipids and carbon dioxide by isolated rat adipocytes.

Signs of Deficiency:

Biochemical — Elevated serum glucose, cholesterol, triglycerides and insulin; glycosuria; decreased insulin binding and insulin receptor number
Physiological — Impaired glucose tolerance

Pathological Consequences of Deficiency:

Established — Impaired glucose tolerance
Hypothesized — Diabetes, atherosclerosis, impaired immune function, increased susceptibility to osteoporosis

Predisposing Factors for Deficiency:

Factors promoting urinary excretion including acute exercise, physical trauma, lactation, and high dietary simple sugars; and factors inhibiting absorption including phytate and drugs that reduce stomach acidity (e.g., antacids) or alter gastrointestinal prostaglandins (e.g., dimethylprostaglandin)

Recommended Intakes:

Prevention of deficiency — The estimated safe and adequate daily dietary intakes for chromium (in µg/day) are: infants age 0 to 0.5 years, 10-40, and age 0.5-1 year, 20-60; children and adolescents age 1-3 years, 20-80, age 4-6 years, 30-120, and age 7 years and older, 50-200; adults, 50-200. [27]
Therapeutic or beneficial — Doses of 200-1000 µg/day of chromium have been shown to potentiate the action of low amounts of insulin or improve the efficacy of insulin such that the need for exogenous sources is reduced or eliminated for some type II diabetics.

Food Sources:

Whole grains, pulses (e.g., dried beans), some vegetables (including broccoli and mushrooms), liver, processed meats, ready-to-eat cereals, spices

TABLE 71.8

Biochemical, Clinical, and Nutritional Aspects of Cobalt

Biological Function:

Vitamin B_{12} is a cofactor for two enzymes, methionine synthase which methylates homocysteine to form methionine, and methylmalonyl CoA mutase which converts L-methylmalonyl CoA, formed by the oxidation of odd-chain fatty acids, to succinyl CoA.

Signs of Deficiency:

Biochemical — Decreased erythrocyte and plasma folate, and plasma vitamin B_{12}; increased plasma homocysteine and urinary formiminoglutamate and methylmalonate
Physiological — Megaloblastic anemia; spinal cord demyelination and peripheral neuropathy

Pathological Consequences of Deficiency:

Established — Pernicious anemia, memory loss, dementia, irreversible neurological disease called subacute degeneration of the spinal cord, death
Hypothesized — Cardiovascular disease associated with elevated plasma homocysteine

Predisposing Factors for Deficiency:

Factors resulting in malabsorption including Type A atrophic gastritis, *Helicobacter pylori* infection, GI bacteria overgrowth caused by achlorhydria and intestinal blind loops, total gastrectomy leading to loss of intrinsic factor excretion, pancreatic insufficiency and coeliac disease; drugs affecting utilization such as histamine H_2 receptor antagonists and proton pump inhibitors, and oral biguanides used in the treatment of type II diabetes; vegetarian diets; nitrous oxide anesthesia.

Recommended Intakes:

Prevention of deficiency — The recommended dietary allowances (RDA) for vitamin B_{12} (in µg/day) are: infants age 0-0.5 year, 0.3 and age 0.5-1 year, 0.6; children age 1-3 years, 1.0; age 4-6 years, 1.1; and age 7-10 years, 1.4; males age 11-14 years, 1.7, and age 14 years and older, 2.0; females age 11-14 years, 1.4, age 15-18 years, 1.5, and age 19 years and older, 1.6; pregnant females, 2.2; lactating females 2.1.[78]
Therapeutic or beneficial — Milligram doses are used to treat vitamin B_{12} malabsorption deficiency syndromes; a common dose is 1 mg/day of oral vitamin B_{12} or monthly injections of a minimum of 100 µg of vitamin B_{12}.

Food Sources:

Meat, dairy products, some seafoods, fortified cereals

TABLE 71.9

Biochemical, Clinical, and Nutritional Aspects of Iodine

Biological Function:

Iodine has only one function; it is a component of thyroid hormones. However, thyroid hormones have an impact on a wide range of metabolic and developmental functions.

Signs of Deficiency:

Biochemical — Decreased plasma or serum thyroxine (T_4) and triiodothyronine (T_3), and urinary iodine; increased plasma or serum thyroid-stimulating hormone (TSH) and cholesterol

Physiological — Decreased basal metabolic rate; decreased heart rate, size, stroke volume, and output; reduced muscle mass and delayed skeletal maturation; abnormal production of glial cells and myelinogenesis

Pathological Consequences of Deficiency:

Established — The spectrum of iodine deficiency disorders is large and includes fetal congenital anomalies and perinatal mortality; neurological cretinism characterized by mental deficiency, deaf mutism, spastic diplegia, and squint; psychomotor defects; goiter; fatigue, slowing of bodily and mental functions, weight increase and cold intolerance caused by slowing of the metabolic rate

Predisposing Factors for Deficiency:

Residence in an area with low soil iodine, lithium treatment, and possibly selenium deprivation

Recommended Intakes:

Prevention of deficiency — The recommended dietary allowances (RDA) for iodine (in µg/day) are: infants age 0-0.5 years, 40, and age 0.5-1 year, 50; children age 1-3 years, 70, age 4-6 years, 90, and age 7-10 years, 120; males and females age 11+, 150; pregnant females, 175; lactating females, 200.[27]

Therapeutic or beneficial — Iodized oil, in which the fatty acids are chemically modified by iodination, slowly releases iodine over a period of months or years in the body. In populations with a high prevalence of severe iodine deficiency disorders(goiter incidence 30% or more), 1 ml of iodized oil containing 480 mg of iodine administered orally or by injection is a therapeutic measure for long term protection against iodine deficiency. An oral iodide dose of 30 mg monthly, or 8 mg biweekly has been found to be an effective prophylaxis for iodine deficiency.[81]

Food Sources:

Iodized salt has been the major method for assuring adequate iodine intake since the 1920s. Other sources are seafoods and foods from plants grown on high-iodine soils.

results in a sulfite oxidase (a molybdoenzyme) deficiency. The information in Table 71.10 has been obtained primarily from reviews by Nielsen.[50,72]

Selenium

Although selenium was first suggested to be essential in 1957, this was not firmly established until a biochemical role was identified in 1972. The first report of human selenium deficiency appeared in 1979; the subject resided in a low-selenium area and was receiving TPN after surgery. The practical nutritional importance of selenium is still being established, but findings of selenium-responsive disorders in certain populations (e.g., Keshan disease in China), and selenium supplementation resulting in reduced incidence of certain cancers suggest that it is quite important. The information in Table 71.11 primarily comes from reviews by Sunde,[84,85] and Levander and Burk.[86]

TABLE 71.10

Biochemical, Clinical, and Nutritional Aspects of Molybdenum

Biological Function:

In humans, three molybdoenzymes have been identified; these are aldehyde oxidase, xanthine oxidase/dehydrogenase, and sulfite oxidase in which molybdenum exists as a small nonprotein factor containing a pterin nucleus. Molybdoenzymes oxidize and detoxify various pyrimidines, purines, and pteridines; catalyze the transformation of hypoxanthine to xanthine and xanthine to uric acid; and catalyze the conversion of sulfite to sulfate.

Signs of Deficiency:

Biochemical — TPN patient: hypermethioninemia, hypouricemia, hyperoxypurinemia, hypouricosuria, low urinary sulfate excretion

Genetic sulfite oxidase deficiency patients: increased plasma and urine sulfite, sulfate, thiosulfate, S-sulfocysteine, taurine

Physiological — TPN patient: mental disturbances progressing to coma. Genetic sulfite oxidase deficiency patients: seizures, brain atrophy/lesions

Pathological Consequences of Deficiency:

Established — Genetic sulfite oxidase deficiency patients: mental retardation, dislocated lenses, death at early age

Hypothesized — Increased susceptibility to cancer[82]

Predisposing Factors for Deficiency:

None known; high sulfur amino acid intake possibly could increase the need for molybdenum

Recommended Intakes:

Prevention of deficiency — The estimated safe and adequate daily dietary intakes for molybdenum (in μg/day) are: infants age 0-0.5 years, 15-30, age 0.5-1 year, 20-40; children and adolescents age 1-3 years, 25-50, age 4-6 years, 30-75; age 7-10 years, 50-150, age 11+ years, 75-250; adults, 75-250.[27] Recent findings suggest that an intake of 25 μg/day would be sufficient to prevent deficiency signs.[83]

Therapeutic or beneficial — None have been proposed.

Food Sources:

Milk and milk products, dried legumes, pulses, organ meats (e.g., liver and kidney), cereals, baked goods

TABLE 71.11

Biochemical, Clinical, and Nutritional Aspects of Selenium

Biological Function:

Selenium is a component of enzymes that catalyze redox reactions; these enzymes include various types of glutathione peroxidases and iodothyronine 5′-deiodinases, and thioredoxin reductase.

Signs of Deficiency:

Biochemical — Decreased plasma and erythrocyte selenium, plasma selenoprotein P and erythrocyte glutathione peroxidase

Physiological — Bilateral muscular discomfort, muscle pain and wasting, cardiomyopathy

Pathological Consequences of Deficiency:

Established — In the presence of other contributing factors, Keshan disease, a multiple focal myocardial necrosis resulting in acute or chronic heart function insufficiency, heart enlargement, arrhythmia, pulmonary edema, and death; other consequences include mood disturbances[87] impaired immune function, and increased susceptibility to viral infections[88]

Hypothesized — Increased susceptibility to certain types of cancer;[89] Kashin-Beck disease, an endemic osteoarthritis

Predisposing Factors for Deficiency:

Conditions that increase oxidative stress including vitamin E deficiency and coxsackievirus B3 infection

Recommended Intakes:

Prevention of deficiency — The recommended dietary allowances (RDA) for selenium (in µg/day) are: infants age 0-0.5 years, 10, and age 0.5-1 year, 15; children age 1-6 years, 20, and age 7-10 years, 30; males age 11-14 years, 40, age 15-18 years, 50, and age 19 years and over, 70; females age 11-14 years, 45, age 15-18 years, 50, and age 19 years and over, 55; pregnant females, 65; lactating females, 75.[27]

Therapeutic or beneficial — A supplement of 200 µg/day of selenium was found to have cancer protective effects.[90, 91]

Food Sources:

Fish, eggs and meat from animals fed luxuriant selenium, grains grown on high-selenium soil

Possibly Essential Ultra Trace Elements

Circumstantial evidence often is used to contend that an element is essential. This evidence generally fits into four categories. These are:

1. A dietary deprivation in some animal model consistently results in a changed biological function, body structure, or tissue composition that is preventable or reversible by an intake of an apparent physiological amount of the element in question.
2. The element fills the need at physiological concentrations for a known *in vivo* biochemical action to proceed *in vitro*.
3. The element is a component of known biologically important molecules in some life form.
4. The element has an essential function in lower forms of life.

An element is considered to have strong circumstantial support for essentiality if all four types of evidence exist for it. There is strong circumstantial evidence for the essentiality of arsenic, nickel, silicon, and vanadium; thus, they are considered possibly essential ultra trace elements.

Arsenic

In addition to the information in Table 71.12, other findings supporting arsenic essentiality are that arsenic can activate some enzymes *in vitro,* enhance DNA synthesis in unsensitized

TABLE 71.12

Arsenic. Biological Function in Lower Forms of Life, Deficiency Signs in Animals, and Speculated Importance and Postulated Adequate Intake for Humans

Biological Function in Lower Forms of Life:

A biochemical function for arsenic has not been identified in lower forms of life, although a bacterium *Chrysiogenes arsenatis* reduces As^{5+} to As^{3+} to gain energy for growth.[96] However, there are enzymes in higher animals and humans that methylate arsenic with S-adenosylmethionine as the methyl donor. Arsenite methytransferase methylates arsenite to monomethylarsenic acid, which is methylated by monomethylarsenic acid methyltransferase to yield dimethylarsinic acid, the major form of arsenic in urine.[97]

Possible Biological Function in Humans:

Arsenic might have a function that affects the formation and utilization of labile methyl groups arising from methionine. Through this effect on methyl group metabolism, arsenic possibly affects the methylation of important molecules such as DNA.

Deficiency Signs in Experimental Animals:

Chick — Depressed growth
Goat — Depressed growth and serum triglycerides; abnormal reproduction characterized by impaired fertility and elevated perinatal mortality; death during lactation with myocardial damage
Hamster — Depressed plasma taurine and hepatic S-adenosylmethionine; elevated hepatic S-adenosylhomocysteine
Pig — Depressed growth; abnormal reproduction characterized by impaired fertility and elevated perinatal mortality
Rat — Depressed growth and hepatic putrescine, spermidine, spermine and S-adenosylmethionine; elevated hepatic S-adenosylhomocysteine; abnormal reproduction

Speculated Importance for Humans:

Decreased serum arsenic concentrations in patients undergoing hemodialysis correlated with injuries to the central nervous system, vascular diseases, and cancer

Predisposing Factors for Deficiency:

Stressors that affect sulfur amino acid or labile methyl group metabolism including high dietary arginine and selenium, low dietary methionine, zinc, selenium and choline, and taurine and guanidoacetic acid supplementation

Postulated Adequate Intake for Humans:

Based on the possible requirements for experimental animals, a possible arsenic requirement of 12 to 25 μg/day has been suggested for humans.

Food Sources:

Shellfish, fish, grains, cereal products

human lymphocytes and in those stimulated by phytohemagglutinin, and induce the isolated production of certain proteins known as heat shock or stress proteins. The control of production of these proteins is apparently at the transcriptional level, and may involve changes in methylation of core histones. Arsenic can increase the methylation of the p53 promoter in human lung cells. Interestingly, although arsenic is commonly thought to be carcinogenic, it has recently been found to be effective in the treatment of some forms of leukemia.[92,93] The information in Table 71.12 primarily comes from reviews by Nielsen.[50,94,95]

Nickel

By 1984, extensive signs of nickel deprivation had been reported for six animal species. Unfortunately, many of the reported signs may have been misinterpretations of pharmacologic actions because nickel was provided in relatively high amounts to supplemented controls in some experiments. Thus, many of the early reported nickel deprivation findings are not shown in Table 71.13. The information in Table 71.13 primarily comes from reviews by Nielsen,[50,72,95,98] and Eder and Kirchgessner.[99]

Silicon

In addition to the information in Table 71.14, other findings supporting silicon essentiality include its localization in the active growth areas, or osteoid layer, and within the osteoblasts in young bone of mice and rats; its consistent presence in collagen and glycosaminoglycan fractions in several types of connective tissue; and its requirement for maximal bone prolylhydroxylase activity in bone tissue culture. Also, silicon nutriture can affect the response to other dietary manipulations; for example, silicon supplementation can prevent the accumulation of aluminum in the brains of rats fed a diet low in silicon and calcium and high in aluminum. The information in Table 71.14 primarily comes from reviews by Nielsen[50,94,95,98] and Carlisle.[100]

Vanadium

In addition to the information in Table 71.15, other findings supporting vanadium essentiality have come from *in vitro* studies with cells and pharmacologic studies with animals. These studies have shown that vanadium has insulin-mimetic properties, stimulates cell proliferation and differentiation, affects cell phosphorylation-dephosphorylation, and affects oxidation-reduction processes. The information in Table 71.15 primarily comes from reviews by Nielsen[50,72,94,95,98,101,102] and Willsky et al.[103]

Other Elements with Beneficial or Biological Actions

If an element has only one or two types of circumstantial evidence to support essentiality, it generally does not get widespread support for being a possibly essential element. However, some of these elements have beneficial pharmacological actions (fluoride and lithium), and others may eventually be found to be of some importance from the nutritional point of view. Elements that fit into this category include aluminum, bromine,

TABLE 71.13

Nickel. Biological Function in Lower Forms of Life, Deficiency Signs in Animals, and Speculated Importance and Postulated Adequate Intake for Humans

Biological Function in Lower Forms of Life:

Component of urease from bacteria, mycoplasma, fungi, yeast, algae, higher plants, and invertebrates; present in hydrogenases from over 35 species of bacteria, may be a common constituent of hydrogenases that function physiologically to oxidize rather than evolve H_2; component of carbon monoxide; (acceptor) oxidoreductase found in acetogenic, methanogenic, phototrophic, and sulfate-reducing anaerobic bacteria; component of a tetrapyrrole known as factor F_{430} found in methyl-S-coenzyme-M reductase that converts CO_2 to methane in methanogenic bacteria; required for the hydrogenase gene to be expressed in *Bradyrhizobium japonicum.*

Possible Functions in Humans:

Cofactor in enzymes involved in hydrolysis or redox reactions; stabilization of a biological molecule; regulation of gene expression; regulation of a cellular calcium channel

Deficiency Signs in Experimental Animals:

Chick — Depressed hematocrits; ultrastructural abnormalities in the liver
Cow — Depressed ruminal urease activity, serum urea nitrogen, growth
Goat — Depressed growth, hematocrits, reproductive performance
Pig — Depressed growth; altered distribution and proper functioning of zinc and calcium
Rat — Depressed growth, hematocrits, plasma glucose; altered distribution and proper functioning of other nutrients including iron, sulfur amino acids, vitamin B_{12}, pyridoxine, and folic acid
Sheep — Depressed growth, total serum protein, erythrocyte counts, ruminal urease activity, total hepatic lipids, cholesterol; altered tissue distribution of copper and iron

Speculated Importance for Humans:

Because nickel can affect sulfur amino acid, vitamin B_{12}, pyridoxine, and folic acid metabolism in animals; nickel nutriture might have an affect on the association between homocysteine and cardiovascular disease in humans

Predisposing Factors for Deficiency:

Low dietary protein, inadequate dietary iron, high dietary simple sugars, and stressors that alter sulfur amino acid or labile methyl metabolism including vitamin B_{12}, vitamin B_6 and folic acid deficiency, and homocysteine supplementation

Postulated Adequate Intake for Humans:

Based on animal studies, should be less than 100 μg/day; a nickel requirement of 25-35 μg/day has been suggested

Food Sources:

Nuts, leguminous seeds (e.g., beans, peas), pulses, grains, chocolate

TABLE 71.14

Silicon. Biological Function in Lower Forms of Life, Deficiency Signs in Animals, and Speculated Importance and Postulated Adequate Intake for Humans

Biological Function in Lower Forms of Life:

Silicon is a component of body structure in some primitive classes of organisms including diatoms (unicellular plants), radiolarians, and some sponges; affects gene expression in diatoms.

Possible Biological Function in Humans:

Structural or other function that influences bone cartilage composition and ultimately calcification; needed for proper collagen formation

Deficiency Signs in Experimental Animals:

Chick — Skull structure abnormalities associated with depressed collagen content; long bone abnormalities characterized by small, poorly formed joints; defective endochondral bone growth associated with depressed contents of articular cartilage, water, hexosamine, and collagen

Rat — Increased humerus hexose; decreased humerus hydroxyproline, femur alkaline and acid phosphatase, and plasma ornithine aminotransferase activity (a key enzyme in collagen synthesis); altered plasma and amino acid and bone mineral composition

Speculated Importance for Humans:

Needed for the initiation of bone calcification and thus proper bone growth and remodeling; needed for proper wound healing

Predisposing Factors for Deficiency:

Inadequate dietary calcium and excessive dietary aluminum

Postulated Adequate Intake for Humans:

On the basis of animal data, the human requirement, if silicon is highly available, would be about 2 to 5 mg/day. However, on the basis of balance data, a silicon intake of 30 to 35 mg/day was suggested for athletes, which was 5 to 10 mg higher than that suggested for nonathletes.

Food Sources:

Unrefined grains of high fiber content and cereal products

TABLE 71.15

Vanadium. Biological Function in Lower Forms of Life, Deficiency Signs in Animals, and Speculated Importance and Postulated Adequate Intake for Humans

Biological Function in Lower Forms of Life:

Vanadium is an essential cofactor for some nitrogenases which reduce nitrogen gas to ammonia in bacteria, and for bromoperoxidase, iodoperoxidase and chloroperoxidase in algae, lichens, and fungi, respectively. The haloperoxidases catalyze the oxidation of halide ions by hydrogen peroxide, thus facilitating the formation of a carbon-halogen bond.[104]

Possible Biological Function in Humans:

Vanadium may have a role in optimal thyroid hormone function.

Deficiency Signs in Experimental Animals:

Goat — Depressed milk production and life span; increased rate of spontaneous abortion; death, sometimes preceded by convulsions, between ages 7 and 91 days; skeletal deformities in the forelegs; thickened forefoot tarsal joints

Rat — Increased thyroid weight and thyroid weight/body weight ratio; decreased erythrocyte glucose-6-phosphate dehydrogenase and cecal total carbonic anhydrase; altered response to high and low dietary iodide

Speculated Importance for Humans:

Identification of a specific biochemical function for vanadium is necessary to disentangle pharmacologic from nutritional findings. Otherwise, the possible nutritional importance of vanadium is unclear. Because vanadium is so pharmacologically active, a beneficial pharmaceutical role for this element might be found; this includes as a treatment for diabetes[105,106] and as an anti-tumorgenic substance.[103]

Predisposing Factors for Deficiency:

Stressors that change thyroid status or iodine metabolism; factors reducing absorption including high iron, aluminum hydroxide, and chromium

Postulated Adequate Intake for Humans:

Based on animal data, a daily dietary intake of 10 μg probably would meet the postulated human requirement for vanadium. To date, pharmacologic doses used to experimentally treat diabetes, e.g., 100 mg/day of vanadyl sulfate, 125 mg/day of sodium orthovanadate, and 50 mg vanadium/day as vanadyl sulfate, have not been established as safe or nontoxic.

Food Sources:

Shellfish, mushrooms, prepared foods, whole grains

cadmium, fluorine, germanium, lead, lithium, rubidium, and tin. The information in Table 71.16 comes from reviews by Nielsen.[72,95,98,108]

Summary

It is likely that not all the essential mineral elements for humans have been identified. Biochemical functions have not been established for some mineral elements. Except for iodine and iron, the full extent of the pathological consequences of marginal or deficient intakes of the trace and ultratrace elements has not been established, which makes it

TABLE 71.16

Reported Deficiency Signs in Experimental Animals and Usual Dietary Intakes of Elements with Beneficial or Biological Actions

Element	Deficiency Signs (Experimental Animals)	Usual Daily Dietary Intakes	Food Sources
Aluminum	Chick — Depressed growth Goat — Depressed growth and life expectancy, increased spontaneous abortions, incoordination and weakness in hind legs	2-10 mg	Baked goods prepared with chemical leavening agents, grains, vegetables, tea
Bromine	Goat — Depressed growth, fertility, milk fat production, hematocrit, hemoglobin, and liefe expectancy; increased spontaneous abortions	2-8 mg	Grains, nuts, fish
Cadmium	Goat — Depressed growth Rat — Depressed growth	10-20 μg	Shellfish, grains, leafy vegetables
Fluorine	Goat — Depressed growth and life span; histological changes in kidney and endocrine organs Rat — Depressed growth; altered incisor pigmentation	Fluoridated water areas 1-3 mg; Nonfluoridated water areas 0.3-0.6 mg	Fish, tea, fluoridated water
Germanium	Rat — Decreased tibial DNA; altered bone and liver mineral composition	0.4-3.4 mg	Vegetables, wheat bran, leguminous seeds
Lead	Pig — Depressed growth; elevated serum cholesterol, phospholipids, and bile acids Rat — Depressed growth, liver glucose, triglycerides, LDL-cholesterol, phospholipids, glutamic-oxalacetic transaminase activity, and glutamic-pyruvate transaminase activity, and blood catalase; increased liver cholesterol and alkaline phosphatase activity and serum ceruloplasmin; anemia	15-100 μg	Seafood, food from plants grown under high-lead conditions
Lithium	Goat — Depressed fertility, birth weight, lifespan, liver monoamine oxidase activity, and serum isocitrate dehydrogenase, malate dehydrogenase, aldolase, and glutamine dehydrogenase activities; increased serum creatine kinase activity	200-600 μg	Meat, eggs, fish, milk, milk products, processed meats, potatoes, vegetables (content varies with geological origin)
Rubidium	Goat — Depressed growth, food intake, and life expectancy; increased spontaneous abortions	1-5 mg	Fruits, poultry, fish, vegetables (especially asparagus), coffee, tea
Tin	Rat — Depressed growth, feed efficiency, and response to sound; altered mineral composition of heart, tibia, muscle, spleen, kidney, and lung		Canned foods

difficult to tabulate deficiency signs and symptoms for humans. Some mineral elements, in addition to fluoride and lithium, are being found to have therapeutic value against disease. Thus, the tables in this section are works in progress and can rapidly change because of ongoing research. This research suggests that the mineral elements are of more practical nutritional concern than currently acknowledged.

References

1. Eckhert, CD, and Rowe, RI. *J Trace Elem Exp Med* 12: 213; 1999.
2. Fort, DJ, Propst, TL, Stover, EL, et al. *J Trace Elem Exp Med* 12: 175; 1999.
3. Fort, DJ, Stover, EL, Strong, PL, Murray, FJ. *J Trace Elem Exp Med* 12: 187; 1999.
4. Nielsen, FH. *J Trace Elem Exp Med* 9: 215; 1996.
5. Nielsen, FH. *Plant Soil* 193: 199; 1997.
6. Nielsen, FH. *Biol Trace Elem Res* 66: 319; 1998.
7. Hunt, CD. *J Trace Elem Exp Med* 9: 185; 1996.
8. Penland, JG. *Biol Trace Elem Res* 66: 299; 1998.
9. Hunt, CD, Idso, JP. *J Trace Elem Exp Med* 12: 221; 1999.
10. Harris, ED. In: *Handbook of Nutritionally Essential Mineral Elements*, O'Dell, BL, Sunde, RA, Eds, Marcel Dekker, New York, 1997, ch 8.
11. Klevay, LM, Medeiros, DM. *J Nutr* 126: 2419S; 1996.
12. Milne, DB. *Am J Clin Nutr* 67: 1041S; 1998.
13. Cordano, A. *Am J Clin Nutr* 67: 1012S; 1998.
14. Uauy, R, Olivares, M, Gonzalez, M. *Am J Clin Nutr* 67: 952S; 1998.
15. Prohaska, JR, Hoffman, RG. *J Nutr* 126: 618; 1996.
16. Hunt, CD, Idso, JP. *J Nutr* 125: 2700; 1995.
17. Keen, CL, Uriu-Hare, JY, Hawk, SN, et al. *Am J Clin Nutr* 67: 1003S; 1998.
18. Keen, CL. In: *Toxicology of Metals*, Chang, LW, Ed, CRC Press, 1996, ch 63.
19. Strain, JJ. In: *Copper and Zinc in Inflammatory and Degenerative Diseases*, Rainsford, KD, Milanino, R, Sorenson, JRJ, Velo, GP, Eds, Kluwer, Dordrecht, 1998, ch 12.
20. Klevay, LM. In: *Role of Copper in Lipid Metabolism*, Lei, KY, Carr, TP, Eds, CRC Press, Boca Raton, 1990, pg 233.
21. Strain, JJ. In: *Role of Trace Elements for Health Promotion and Disease Prevention, Bibl Nutr Dieta*, Sandstrom, B, Walter, P, Eds, Karger, Basel, 1998, pg 127.
22. Medeiros, DM, Wildman, REC. *Proc Soc Exp Biol Med* 215: 299; 1997.
23. Percival, SS. *Am J Clin Nutr* 67: 1064S; 1998.
24. Milanino, R, Marrella, M, Velo, GP, et al. In: *Copper and Zinc in Inflammatory and Degenerative Diseases*, Rainsford, KD, Milanino, R, Sorenson, JRJ, Velo, GP, Eds, Kluwer, London, 1998, ch 10.
25. Davis, CD, Feng, Y. *J Nutr* 129: 1060; 1999.
26. Saari, J. *Can J Physiol Pharmacol* 78: 848; 2000.
27. Food and Nutrition Board, National Research Council, *Recommended Dietary Allowances, 10th Ed.*, National Academy Press, Washington, DC.
28. Beard, JL, Dawson, HD. In: *Handbook of Nutritionally Essential Mineral Elements*, O'Dell, BL, Sunde, RA, Eds, Marcel Dekker, New York, 1997, ch 9.
29. Baynes, RD, Stipanuk, MH. In: *Biochemical and Physiological Aspects of Human Nutrition*, Stipanuk, MA, Ed, Saunders, Philadelphia, 2000, ch 31.
30. Kipp, DE, Pinero, D, Beard, JL. *FASEB J* 12: A508; 1998.
31. Felt, BT, Lozoff, B. *J Nutr* 126: 693; 1996.
32. Cook, JD, Reddy, MB. *Am J Clin Nutr* 62: 117; 1995.
33. Viteri, FE. *Am J Clin Nutr* 63: 610; 1996.
34. Ridwan, E, Schultink, W, Dillon, D, Gross, R. *Am J Clin Nutr* 63: 884; 1996.
35. Salonen, JT. In: *Role of Trace Elements for Health Promotion and Disease Prevention, Bibl Nutr Dieta*, Sandstrom, B, Walter, P, Eds, Karger, Basel, 1998, pg 112.
36. Klipstein-Grobusch, K, Koster, JF, Grobbee, DE, et al. *Am J Clin Nutr* 69: 1231; 1999.
37. Selby, JV, Friedman, GD. *Int J Cancer* 41: 67; 1988.
38. Stevens, RG, Jones, DY, Micozzi, MS, Taylor, PR. *N Engl J Med* 316: 1047; 1988.
39. Youdin, M, Benshachar, D, Riederer, P. *Movement Disord* 8: 1; 1993.
40. Rude, RK. In: *Biochemical and Physiological Aspects of Human Nutrition*, Stipanuk, MH, Ed, Saunders, Philadelphia, 2000, ch 29.

41. Shils, ME. In: *Handbook of Nutritionally Essential Mineral Elements*, O'Dell, BL, Sunde, RA, Eds, Marcel Dekker, New York, 1997, ch 5.
42. Seelig, M. *Am J Cardiol* 63: 4G; 1989.
43. Altura, BM, Altura, BT. In: *Magnesium: Current Status and New Developments*, Theophanides, T, Anastassopoulou, J, Eds, Kluwer, Dordrecht, 1997, pg 383.
44. Mizushima, S, Cappuccio, FP, Nichols, R, Elliott, P. *J Hum Hyperten* 12: 7; 447, 1998.
45. Yasui, M, Ota, K, Murphy, VA. In: *Mineral and Metal Neurotoxicology*, Yasui, M, Strong, MJ, Ota, K, Verity, MA, Eds, CRC Press, Boca Raton, 1997, ch 22.
46. Depoortere, H, Francon, D, Llopis, J. *Neuropsychobiology* 27: 237; 1993.
47. Rude, RK. In: *Principles of Bone Biology*, Bilezikian, JP, Raisz, LG, Rodan, GA, Eds, Academic Press, San Diego, 1996, ch 21.
48. Food and Nutrition Board, Institute of Medicine, *Dietary Reference Intakes for Calcium, Phosphorus, Magnesium, Vitamin D, and Fluoride*, National Academy Press, Washington, DC, 1997.
49. Leach, RM, Jr, Harris, ED. In: *Handbook of Nutritionally Essential Mineral Elements*, O'Dell, BL, Sunde, RA, Eds, Marcel Dekker, New York, 1997, ch 10.
50. Nielsen, FH. In: *Modern Nutrition in Health and Disease*, 9th ed, Shils, ME, Olson, JA, Shike, M, Ross, AC, Eds, Williams and Wilkins, Baltimore, 1999, ch 16.
51. Freeland-Graves, J, Llanes, C. In: *Manganese in Health and Disease*, Klimis-Tavantzis, DJ, Ed, CRC Press, Boca Raton, 1994, ch 3.
52. Norose, N, Terai, M, Norose, K. *J Trace Elem Exp Med* 5: 100; 1992.
53. Wolinsky, I, Klimis-Tavantzis, DJ, Richards, LJ. In: *Manganese in Health and Disease*, Klimis-Tavantzis, DJ, Ed, CRC Press, Boca Raton, 1994, ch 6.
54. Carl, GF, Gallagher BB. In: *Manganese in Health and Disease*, Klimis-Tavantzis, DJ, Ed, CRC Press, Boca Raton, 1994, ch 8.
55. Klimis-Tavantzis, DJ, Taylor, PN, Wolinsky, I. In: *Manganese in Health and Disease*, Klimis-Tavantzis, DJ, Ed, CRC Press, Boca Raton, 1994, ch 4.
56. Shetlar, MR, Shetlar, CL. In: *Manganese in Health and Disease*, Klimis-Tavantzis, DJ, Ed, CRC Press, Boca Raton, 1994, ch 9.
57. Kuratko, CN. *Food Chem Toxicol* 36: 819; 1998.
58. Robinson, BH. *J Inher Metab Dis* 21: 598; 1998.
59. Aschner, M. In: *Metals and Oxidative Damage in Neurological Disorders*, Connor, J, Ed, Plenum Press, New York, 1997, ch 5.
60. Chesters, JK. In: *Handbook of Nutritionally Essential Mineral Elements*, O'Dell, BL, Sunde, RA, Eds, Marcel Dekker, New York, 1997, ch 7.
61. Prasad, AS. *J Trace Elem Exp Med* 11: 63; 1998.
62. Sandstead, HH. In: *Risk Assessment of Essential Elements*, Mertz, W, Abernathy, CO, Olin, SS, Eds, ILSI Press, Washington, DC, 1994, pg 91.
63. Davis, CD, Milne, DB, Nielsen, FH. *Am J Clin Nutr* 71: 781; 2000.
64. Yamaguchi, M. *J Trace Elem Exp Med* 11: 119; 1998.
65. Hadrzynski, C. *J Trace Elem Exp Med* 12: 367; 1999.
66. Fernandez-Madrid, F. In: *Copper and Zinc in Inflammatory and Degenerative Diseases*, Rainsford, KD, Milanino, R, Sorenson, JRJ, Velo, GP, Eds, Kluwer, London, 1998, ch 8.
67. Olson, RJ, DeBry, P. *J Trace Elem Exp Med* 11: 137; 1998.
68. Jeejeebhoy, KN. *J Trace Elem Exp Med* 12: 85; 1999.
69. Davis, CM, Vincent, JB. *JIBC* 2: 675; 1997.
70. Anderson, RA. In: *Essential and Toxic Trace Elements in Human Health and Disease: An Update*, Prasad, AS, Ed, Wiley-Liss, New York, 1993, pg 221.
71. Anderson, RA, Cheng, N, Bryden, NA, et al. *Diabetes* 46: 1786; 1997.
72. Nielsen, FH. In: *Biochemical and Physiological Aspects of Human Nutrition*, Stipanuk, MH, Ed, WB Saunders, Philadelphia, 2000, ch 36.
73. Lukaski, HC. *Ann Rev Nutr* 19: 279; 1999.
74. Herbert, V. In: *Present Knowledge in Nutrition*, 7th ed, Ziegler, EE, Filer, LJ, Jr, Eds, ILSI Press, Washington, DC, 1996, ch 20.
75. Smith, RM. In: *Handbook of Nutritionally Essential Mineral Elements*, O'Dell, BL, Sunde, RA, Eds, Marcel Dekker, New York, 1997, ch 11.

76. Shane, B. In: *Biochemical and Physiological Aspects of Human Nutrition*, Stipanuk, MH, Ed, WB Saunders, Philadelphia, 2000, ch 21.
77. Nilsson-Ehle, H. *Drugs Aging* 12: 277; 1998.
78. Food and Nutrition Board, Institute of Medicine, *Dietary Reference Intakes: Thiamin, Riboflavin, Niacin, Vitamin* B_6*, Folate, Vitamin* B_{12}*, Pantothenic Acid, Biotin, and Choline*, National Academy Press, Washington, DC, 1998.
79. Freake, HC. In: *Biochemical and Physiological Aspects of Human Nutrition*, Stipanuk, MH, Ed, WB Saunders, Philadelphia, 2000, ch 33.
80. Hetzel, BS, Wellby, ML. In: *Handbook of Nutritionally Essential Mineral Elements*, O'Dell, BL, Sunde, RA, Eds, Marcel Dekker, New York, 1997, ch 19.
81. Todd, CH, Dunn, JT. *Am J Clin Nutr* 67: 1279; 1998.
82. Seaborn, CD, Yang, SP. *Biol Trace Elem Res* 39: 245; 1993.
83. Turnland, JR, Keyes, WR, Peiffer, GL, Chiang, G. *Am J Clin Nutr* 61: 1102; 1995.
84. Sunde, RA. In: *Handbook of Nutritionally Essential Mineral Elements*, O'Dell, BL, Sunde, RA, Eds, Marcel Dekker, New York, 1997, ch 18.
85. Sunde, RA. In *Biochemical and Physiological Aspects of Human Nutrition*, Stipanuk, MH, Ed, WB Saunders, Philadelphia, 2000, ch 34.
86. Levander, OA, Burk, RF. In: *Present Knowledge in Nutrition,* 7th ed, Ziegler, EE, Filer, LF, Jr, Eds, ILSI Press, Washington, DC, 1996, ch 31.
87. Finley, JW, Penland, JG. *J Trace Elem Exp Med* 11: 11; 1998.
88. Beck, MA. *J Nutr* 127: 966S; 1997.
89. Ip, C. *J Nutr* 128: 1845; 1998.
90. Clark, LC, Combs, GF, Jr, Turnbull, BW, et al. *JAMA* 276: 1957; 1996.
91. Clark, LC, Dalkin, B, Krongrad, A, et al. *Brit J Urol* 81: 730; 1998.
92. Quignon, F, Chen, Z, de The, H. *Biochim Biophys Acta* 1333: M53; 1997.
93. Wang, Z-G, Rivi, R, Delva, L, et al. *Blood* 92: 1497; 1998.
94. Nielsen, FH. *FASEB J* 5: 2661; 1991.
95. Nielsen, FH. *J Trace Elem Exp Med* 11: 251; 1998.
96. Kraft, T, Macy, M. *Eur J Biochem* 255: 647; 1998.
97. Healy, SM, Wildfang, E, Zakharyan, RA, Aposhian, HV. *Biol Trace Elem Res* 68: 249; 1999.
98. Nielsen, FH. *J Nutr* 126: 2377S; 1996.
99. Eder, K, Kirchgessner, M. In: *Handbook of Nutritionally Essential Mineral Elements*, O'Dell, BL, Sunde, RA, Eds, Marcel Dekker, New York, 1997, ch 14.
100. Carlisle, EM. In: *Handbook of Nutritionally Essential Mineral Elements*, O'Dell, BL, Sunde, RA, Eds, Marcel Dekker, New York, 1997, ch 21.
101. Nielsen, FH. In: *Handbook of Nutritionally Essential Mineral Elements*, O'Dell, BL, Sunde, RA, Eds, Marcel Dekker, New York, 1997, ch 22.
102. Nielsen, FH. In: *Vanadium Compounds: Chemistry, Biochemistry, and Therapeutic Applications, ACS Series 711*, Tracey, AS, Crans, DC, Eds, American Chemical Society, Washington, DC, 1998, ch 23.
103. Willsky, GR, Goldfine, AB, Kostyniak, PJ. In: *Vanadium Compounds: Chemistry, Biochemistry, and Therapeutic Applications, ACS Series 711*, Tracey, AS, Crans, DC, Eds, American Chemical Society, Washington, DC, 1998, ch 22.
104. Butler, A. *Curr Opin Chem Biol* 2: 279; 1998.
105. Thompson, KH, McNeill, JH, Orvig, C. *Chem Rev* 99: 2561; 1999.
106. Sakurai, H, Tsuji, A. In: *Vanadium in the Environment Part 2: Health Effects*, Nriagu, J, Ed, John Wiley & Sons, New York, 1998, ch 15.
107. Morinville, A, Maysinger, D, Shaver, A. *TIPS* 19: 452; 1998.
108. Nielsen, FH. In: *Trace Elements in Human and Animal Nutrition, Vol. 2*, Mertz, W, Ed, Academic Press, Orlando, 1986, ch 10.

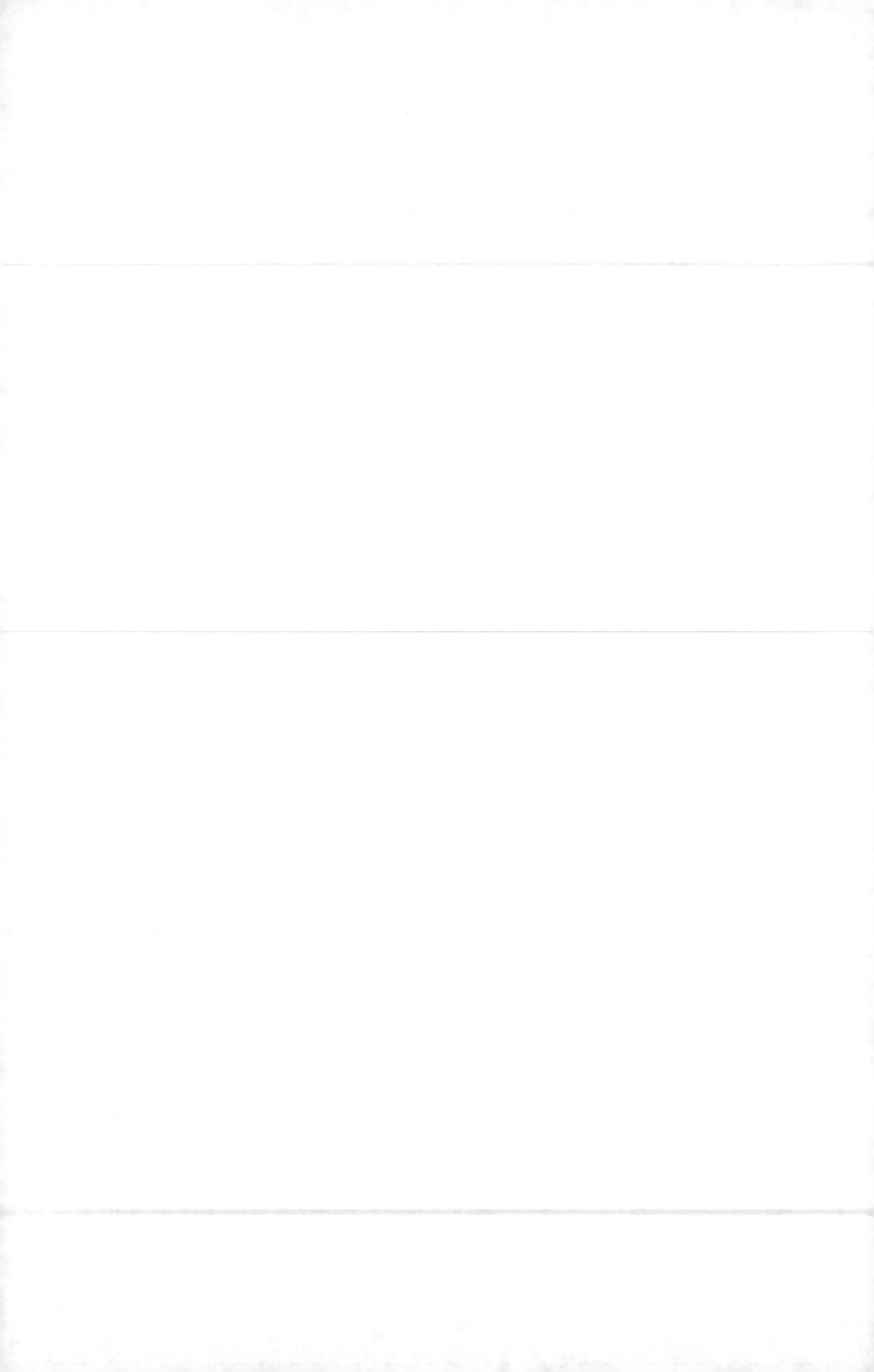

72

Questionable Practices in Foods and Nutrition: Definitions and Descriptions

Stephen Barrett and Victor Herbert

The past decade has seen an enormous increase in the promotion and use of questionable health practices, many of which are nutrition-related. The main factors have been the propaganda associated with "complementary" and "alternative" medicine (CAM) and the ease of acquiring misinformation through the Internet. As a result, alternative medicine has become the politically correct term for questionable practices formerly labeled as quack and/or fraudulent.

In recent years, most media reports have featured the views of proponents and their satisfied clients. Confusion has been accelerated by the erosion of standards that normally signify scientific legitimacy. Accreditation, once a reliable indicator of quality, has been granted to acupuncture, naturopathic, and chiropractic schools that teach unscientific methods. Many medical institutions and professional organizations are sponsoring CAM coursework and/or services that include senseless methods. Many medical journals have published poorly reasoned articles, and a few journals specializing in CAM misinformation are now indexed in *Index Medicus.* As a result, CAM-related literature searches are likely to include low-quality articles. Several government, voluntary, and professional organizations have added to the problem by withdrawing previously published position papers that accurately characterized certain practices as "quack" and/or by publishing "balanced" information that describes these methods without evaluating them. Consumer protection laws have also been weakened.

Pertinent Definitions

The alternative movement is part of a general societal trend toward rejection of science as a method of determining truths. This movement embraces the postmodernist doctrine that science is not necessarily more valid than pseudoscience.[1] In line with this philosophy, alternative proponents assert that scientific medicine (which they mislabel as allopathic, conventional, or traditional medicine) is but one of a vast array of health-care options. Alternative promoters often gain public sympathy by portraying themselves as a beleaguered minority fighting a self-serving, monolithic "Establishment."

0-8493-2705-9/02/$0.00+$1.50

To avoid confusion, alternative methods should be classified as genuine, experimental, or questionable. *Genuine* alternatives are comparable methods that have met science-based criteria for safety and effectiveness. Under the rules of science, proponents who make health claims bear the burden of proof. It is their responsibility to conduct suitable studies and report them in sufficient detail to permit evaluation and confirmation by others. Detailed standards for reporting and evaluating studies have been published.[2]

Experimental alternatives are unproven but have a scientifically plausible rationale and are undergoing responsible investigation. The most noteworthy is the use of a 10%-fat diet for treating coronary heart disease. *Questionable* alternatives are groundless because they lack plausibility or have been disproved. The archetype is homeopathy, which claims that "remedies" so dilute that they contain no active ingredient can exert powerful therapeutic effects. When the three types of alternatives are lumped together, promoters of questionable methods can argue that because some have merit, the rest deserve equal consideration and respect. This section uses the word alternative in the questionable sense.

Proponents describe "complementary medicine" as a synthesis of standard and alternative methods that uses the best of both. However, no data have been reported in peer-reviewed scientific journals that compare standard methods with alternative ones. There is no indication of the extent to which the practitioners actually use proven versus unproven methods. These practitioners typically claim credit for any improvement experienced by the patient, and blame standard treatments for any negative effects. The result may be to undermine the patient's confidence in standard care, reducing compliance or causing the patient to abandon it altogether.

The best way to avoid confusion is to sort methods into three groups: (1) those that work, (2) those that don't work, and (3) those we are not sure about. Most methods described as alternative fall into the second group. A 1998 editorial in the *Journal of the American Medical Association* made this point in another way:

> There is no alternative medicine. There is only scientifically proven, evidence-based medicine supported by solid data or unproven medicine, for which scientific evidence is lacking. Whether a therapeutic practice is "Eastern" or "Western," is unconventional or mainstream, or involves mind-body techniques or molecular genetics is largely irrelevant except for historical purposes and cultural interest. We recognize that there are vastly different types of practitioners and proponents of the various forms of alternative medicine and conventional medicine, and that there are vast differences in the skills, capabilities, and beliefs of individuals within them and the nature of their actual practices. Moreover, the economic and political forces in these fields are large and increasingly complex and have the capability for being highly contentious. Nonetheless, as believers in science and evidence, we must focus on fundamental issues — namely, the patient, the target disease or condition, the proposed or practiced treatment, and the need for convincing data on safety and therapeutic efficacy.[3]

Under the rules of science, people who make the claims bear the burden of proof. It is their responsibility to conduct suitable studies and report them in sufficient detail to permit evaluation and confirmation by others. Instead of subjecting their work to scientific standards, promoters of questionable alternatives would like to change the rules by which they are judged and regulated. Alternative promoters may give lip service to these standards. However, they regard personal experience, subjective judgment, and emotional satisfaction as preferable to objectivity and hard evidence. Instead of conducting scientific studies, they use anecdotes and testimonials to promote their practices and political maneuvering to keep regulatory agencies at bay.

When someone feels better after using a product or procedure, it is natural to credit whatever was done. This can mislead, however, because most ailments resolve spontaneously, and those that persist can have symptoms that wax and wane. Even serious conditions can have sufficient month-to-month variation to enable spurious methods to gain large followings. In addition, taking action often temporarily relieves symptoms via the placebo effect. This effect is a beneficial change in a person's condition that occurs in relation to a treatment but is not due to the pharmacologic or physical aspects of the treatment. Belief in the treatment is not essential, but the placebo effect may be enhanced by such factors as faith, sympathetic attention, sensational claims, testimonials, and the use of scientific-looking charts, devices, and terminology. Another drawback of individual success stories is that they don't indicate how many failures might occur for each success. (In other words, no score is kept.) People unaware of these facts often give undeserved credit to alternative methods. Failure to keep score is the hallmark of quack therapies.

Each of the approaches listed below has one or more of the following characteristics: (a) its rationale or underlying theory has no scientific basis; (b) it has not been demonstrated safe and/or effective by well-designed studies; (c) it is deceptively promoted; or (d) its practitioners are not qualified to make appropriate diagnoses.

Treatment Systems

Many alternative approaches involve nutrition. Special diets and dietary supplements enable people to take an active role in their treatment and feel more in control of their fate. Their proponents typically claim that: (a) nutrient deficiency is widespread and causes a multitude of diseases; (b) various foods or nutrients have special ability to cure specific diseases; (c) certain foods are harmful and should be eliminated from the diet; and (d) "organically grown" and "natural" foods are best.

Some alternative approaches are rooted in vitalism, the concept that bodily functions are due to a vital principle or "life force" distinct from the physical forces explainable by the laws of physics and chemistry. Vitalistic methods are claimed to "stimulate the body's ability to heal itself" rather than treating symptoms. Homeopaths, for example, claim that illness is due to a disturbance of the body's "vital force," which they can correct with special remedies, while many acupuncturists claim that disease is due to imbalance in the flow of "life energy" (chi or Qi), which they can balance by twirling needles in the skin. Many chiropractors claim to assist the body's "innate intelligence" by adjusting the patient's spine. Naturopaths speak of vis medicatrix naturae. Ayurvedic physicians refer to prana. Some vitalists assert that food can be "dead" or "living" and that "live" foods contain a dormant or primitive life force that humans can assimilate. The "energies" postulated by vitalists cannot be measured by scientific methods. Although vitalists often pretend to be scientific, they really reject the scientific method with its basic assumptions of material reality, mechanisms of cause and effect, and testability of hypotheses. They regard personal experience, subjective judgment, and emotional satisfaction as preferable to objectivity and hard evidence.

Chinese Medicine

Traditional Chinese medicine (TCM), also called Oriental medicine, is based on metaphysical beliefs. Its advocates state that the body's vital energy (Chi or Qi) circulates through channels called meridians that have branches connected to bodily organs and functions. They attribute illness to imbalance or interruption of Chi and claim that acupuncture, herbs, and various other modalities can restore balance. Many TCM practitioners are nonphysicians who are licensed as acupuncturists and permitted to prescribe dietary supplements and herbs. The diagnostic process they use may include questioning (medical history, lifestyle), observations (skin, tongue, color), listening (breath sounds), and pulse-taking. Medical science recognizes only one pulse, corresponding to the heartbeat, which can be felt in the wrist, neck, feet, and various other places throughout the body. TCM practitioners check six alleged pulses at each wrist and identify more than 25 alleged pulse qualities such as "sinking, slippery, soggy, tight, and wiry." TCM's pulses supposedly reflect the type of imbalance, the condition of each organ system, and the status of the patient's Chi. The herbs they prescribe are not regulated for safety, potency, or effectiveness. Although some cases of adverse effects from herbs have been reported, no systematic assessment of this problem has been published. A National Council Against Health Fraud task force concluded that (a) acupuncture has not been proven effective for the treatment of any disease; (b) the greater the benefit claimed in a research report, the worse the experimental design; and (c) the best designed experiments — those with the highest number of controls on variables — found no difference between acupuncture and control groups.[4] An NIH Consensus Conference reported more favorably but was dominated by acupuncture proponents.[5]

Macrobiotic Diets

Macrobiotics is a quasireligious philosophical system founded by the late George Ohsawa and popularized by Michio Kushi. (Macrobiotic means "way of long life.") The system advocates a semivegetarian diet in which foods of animal origin are used as condiments rather than as full-fledged menu items. The optimal diet is achieved by balancing "yin" and "yang" foods. The yin/yang classification is based largely on sensory characteristics and is unrelated to nutrient composition. Macrobiotic practitioners may base their recommendations on pulse diagnosis and other unscientific procedures related to TCM.

Ohsawa outlined a ten-stage Zen macrobiotic diet in which each stage was progressively more restrictive. Current proponents espouse a diet that is less restrictive but still can be nutritionally inadequate. They recommend whole grains (50 to 60% of each meal), vegetables (25 to 30% of each meal), whole beans or soybean-based products (5 to 10% of daily food), nuts and seeds (small amounts as snacks), miso soup, herbal teas, and small amounts of white meat or seafood once or twice a week. Kushi Institute publications recommend chewing food at least 50 times per mouthful (or until it becomes liquid), not wearing synthetic or woolen clothing next to the skin, avoiding long hot baths or showers (unless you have been consuming too much salt or animal food), having large green plants in your house to enrich the oxygen content of the air, and singing a happy song every day.

Proponents claim that macrobiotic eating can help prevent cancer and many other diseases. They also present case histories of people whose cancers have supposedly disappeared after they adopted the macrobiotic diet. However, there is no scientific evidence of benefit, and the diet itself can cause cancer patients to undergo serious weight loss.[6]

Maharishi Ayur-Ved

Proponents state that ayurvedic medicine originated in ancient times but was reconstituted in the early 1980s by the Maharishi Mahesh Yogi, who also popularized transcendental meditation (TM). As popularized today, its basic theory attributes the regulation of body functions to three "irreducible physiologic principles" called doshas, whose Sanskrit names are *vata*, *pitta*, and *kapha*. These terms are used to designate body types as well as the physical and mental characteristics of each constitutional type. Through various combinations of vata, pitta, and kapha, 10 body types are possible. However, one's doshas (and therefore one's body type) can vary from hour to hour and season to season.

Ayurvedic proponents state that the symptoms of disease are always related to balance of the doshas, which can be determined by feeling the patient's wrist pulse or completing a questionnaire. Balance is supposedly achieved through "pacifying" diets, "purification" (to remove "impurities due to faulty diet and behavioral patterns"), TM, and a long list of procedures and ayurvedic products, many of which are said to be formulated for specific body types. Most of these cost several hundred dollars, but some cost thousands and require the services of a practitioner.

Naturopathy

Naturopathy, sometimes referred to as natural medicine, is a largely pseudoscientific approach said to assist nature, support the body's own innate capacity to achieve optimal health, and facilitate the body's inherent healing mechanisms. Naturopaths assert that diseases are the body's effort to purify itself, and that cures result from increasing the patient's vital force. They claim to stimulate the body's natural healing processes by ridding it of waste products and toxins which are questionable and are not measurable in a lab.

Naturopaths offer treatment at their offices and at spas where patients may reside for several weeks. Their offerings include fasting, "natural food" diets, vitamins, herbs, tissue minerals, homeopathic remedies, cell salts, manipulation, massage, exercise, colonic enemas, acupuncture, Chinese medicine, natural childbirth, minor surgery, and applications of water, heat, cold, air, sunlight, and electricity. Radiation may be used for diagnosis, but not for treatment. They claim that many of these methods rid the body of unnamed toxins.

Naturopaths are licensed as independent practitioners in eleven states and may legally practice in a few others. The total number of practitioners is unknown but includes chiropractors and acupuncturists who practice naturopathy. Many naturopaths espouse nutrition and lifestyle measures that coincide with current medical recommendations. However, this advice is often accompanied by nonstandard advice that is irrational. Although naturopaths claim to emphasize prevention, most oppose or are overly critical of immunization.

Most naturopaths allege that virtually all diseases are within their scope. The most comprehensive naturopathic publications, *A Textbook of Natural Medicine*[7] (for students and professionals) and *Encyclopedia of Natural Medicine*[8] (for laypersons), recommend special diets, vitamins, minerals, and/or herbs for more than 70 health problems ranging from acne to AIDS. For many of these conditions, daily administration of ten or more products is recommended — some in dosages high enough to cause toxicity.

Natural Hygiene

Natural Hygiene, an offshoot of naturopathy, is a philosophy of health and natural living that advocates a raw food diet of vegetables, fruits, and nuts. It also advocates periodic fasting and food combining (avoiding food combinations it considers detrimental).[18] Natural hygienists oppose immunization, fluoridation, and food irradiation, and eschew most forms of medical treatment.

Iridology

Iridology (iris diagnosis) claims that each area of the body is represented by a corresponding area in the iris of the eye (the colored area around the pupil) and that the body's state of health and disease can be diagnosed from the color, texture, and location of pigment flecks in the eye. The leading proponent, Bernard Jensen, D.C., has written that "Nature has provided us with a miniature television screen showing the most remote portions of the body by way of nerve reflex responses." Iridology practitioners claim to diagnose "imbalances" that can be treated with vitamins, minerals, herbs, and similar products. Some also claim that the eye markings can reveal a complete history of past illnesses as well as previous treatment. Some iridologists use computers to help them analyze eye photographs and select the products they recommend. Two well-designed studies have found that iridology practitioners who examined the same patients (or photographs of their eyes) disagreed among themselves and were unable to state what was medically wrong with the patients.[9,10]

Metabolic Therapy

Proponents of metabolic therapy claim to diagnose abnormalities at the cellular level and correct them by normalizing the patient's metabolism. They regard cancer, arthritis, multiple sclerosis, and other degenerative diseases as the result of metabolic imbalance caused by a buildup of toxic substances in the body. They claim that scientific practitioners merely treat the symptoms of the disease, while they treat the cause by removing toxins and strengthening the immune system so the body can heal itself. The toxins are neither defined nor objectively measurable. Metabolic treatment regimens vary from practitioner to practitioner and may include a "natural food" diet, coffee enemas, vitamins, minerals, glandulars, enzymes, laetrile, and various other nostrums that are not legally marketable in the United States. No controlled study has shown that any of its components has any value against cancer or any other chronic disease. However, many people find its concepts appealing because they do not seem far removed from scientific medicine's concerns with diet, lifestyle, and the relationship between emotions and bodily responses.

Orthomolecular Therapy

Proponents define orthomolecular therapy as "the treatment of disease by varying the concentrations of substances normally present in the human body." They claim that many diseases are caused by molecular imbalances that are correctable by administration of the right nutrient molecules at the right time. (Ortho is Greek for "right.") Linus Pauling coined the term orthomolecular therapy in 1968, but the approach actually dates back to the early 1950s when a few psychiatrists began adding massive doses of nutrients to their treatment of severe mental problems. The original substance was vitamin B_3 (nicotinic acid or nicotinamide), and the therapy was termed megavitamin therapy. Later the treatment regimen was expanded to include other vitamins, minerals, hormones, and diets, any of which may be combined with conventional drug therapy and electroshock treatments.

Pauling postulated that people's nutrient needs vary markedly and that to maintain good health, many people need amounts much greater than the RDAs. In 1970, he announced in *Vitamin C and the Common Cold* that taking 1000 mg of vitamin C daily will reduce the incidence of colds by 45% for most people, but that some people need much larger amounts. A 1976 expansion of the book suggested even higher dosages, and a third book, *Vitamin C and Cancer* (1979) claimed that high doses of vitamin C might be effective against cancer. Yet another book, *How to Feel Better and Live Longer* (1986) stated that megadoses of vitamins "can improve your general health … to increase your enjoyment of life and can help in controlling heart disease, cancer, and other diseases and in slowing down the process of aging."

At least 16 well-designed, double-blind studies have shown that supplementation with vitamin C does not prevent colds and at best may slightly reduce the symptoms of a cold. Slight symptom reduction may occur as the result of an antihistamine-like effect, but whether this has practical value is a matter of dispute. Pauling's views are based on the same studies considered by other scientists, but his analyses are flawed.

The largest clinical trials, involving thousands of volunteers, were directed by Dr. Terence Anderson, professor of epidemiology at the University of Toronto. Taken together, his studies suggest that extra vitamin C may slightly reduce the severity of colds, but it is not necessary to take the high doses suggested by Pauling to achieve this result. Nor is there anything to be gained by taking vitamin C supplements year-round in the hope of preventing colds.

Another important study was reported in 1975 by scientists at the National Institutes of Health who compared vitamin C pills with a placebo before and during colds. Although the experiment was supposed to be double-blind, half the subjects were able to guess which pill they were getting. When the results were tabulated with all subjects lumped together, the vitamin group reported fewer colds per person over a nine-month period. But among the half who hadn't guessed which pill they had been taking, no difference in the incidence or severity was found. This illustrates how people who think they are doing something effective (such as taking a vitamin) can report a favorable result even when none exists.

In 1976, Pauling and Dr. Ewan Cameron, a Scottish physician, reported that a majority of 100 terminal cancer patients treated with 10,000 mg of vitamin C daily survived three to four times longer than similar patients who did not receive vitamin C supplements. However, Dr. William DeWys, chief of clinical investigations at the National Cancer Institute, found that the study was poorly designed because the patient groups were not comparable. The vitamin C patients were Cameron's, while the other patients were under the care of other physicians. Cameron's patients were started on vitamin C when he labeled them untreatable by other methods, and their subsequent survival was compared to the survival of the control patients after they were labeled untreatable by their doctors. DeWys reasoned that if the two groups were comparable, the lengths of time from entry into the hospital to being labeled untreatable should be equivalent in both groups. However, he found that Cameron's patients were labeled untreatable much earlier in the course of their disease — which means that they entered the hospital before they were as sick as the other doctors' patients, and would naturally be expected to live longer.

Nevertheless, to test whether Pauling might be correct, the Mayo Clinic conducted three double-blind studies involving a total of 367 patients with advanced cancer. The studies, reported in 1979, 1983, and 1985, found that patients given 10,000 mg of vitamin C daily did no better than those given a placebo.

Several expert teams have concluded that the claims of orthomolecular psychiatry are unsubstantiated. In the early 1970s, a special American Psychiatric Association task force investigated the claims of psychiatrists who espoused the orthomolecular approach. The task force noted that these practitioners used unconventional methods not only in treatment but also for diagnosis.[11] Claims that megavitamins and megaminerals are effective against psychosis, learning disorders, and mental retardation in children were debunked in reports by the nutrition committees of the American Academy of Pediatrics in 1976 and 1981 and the Canadian Academy of Pediatrics in 1990.[12] Both groups warned that there was no proven benefit in any of these conditions, and that megadoses can have serious toxic effects. The 1976 report concluded that a "cult" had developed among followers of megavitamin therapy.[13]

In 1991, Dutch researchers reported their evaluation of controlled trials of the effects of niacin, vitamin B_6, and multivitamins on mental functions. They concluded that for hyperactive children, children with Down's syndrome, IQ changes in healthy schoolchildren, schizophrenia, psychological functions in healthy adults, and geriatric patients, there was no adequate support from controlled trials in favor of vitamin supplementation.[14] A subsequent review of 12 studies of B_6 and magnesium for autism concluded that although the majority of studies were favorable, most were poorly designed, were reported by researchers who were closely associated, and involved unsafe dosages of B_6.[15] A recent randomized double-blind study published in 1999 found no evidence that regulating the vitamin levels of adult schizophrenics influenced the clinical status of these subjects. The experimental group received amounts of megavitamins based on their individual serum vitamin levels plus dietary restriction-based on radioallergosorbent (RAST) tests. The control group received 25 mg vitamin C and were prescribed substances considered allergenic from the RAST test. After five months, there were marked differences in serum levels of vitamins but no consistent symptomatic or behavioral differences between the groups.[16]

A few situations exist in which high doses of vitamins are known to be beneficial, but they must still be used with caution because of potential toxicity. Orthomolecular practitioners go far beyond this, however, by prescribing large amounts of supplements to all or most of the patients who consult them. This approach can result in great harm — particularly to psychiatric patients — when used instead of effective medications.

Chiropractic Nutrition

Chiropractic is based on the faulty notion that most ailments are related to spinal problems. Although some aspects of scientific nutrition are taught in chiropractic schools, many chiropractors use methods that clash with what is known about the anatomy and physiology of the body.

Applied kinesiology (AK), for example, is based on the notion that every organ dysfunction is accompanied by a specific muscle weakness, which enables health problems to be diagnosed through muscle-testing procedures. Testing is typically carried out by pulling on the patient's outstretched arm after placing the test substance (such as a vitamin or food extract) in the patient's mouth until salivation occurs. However, some practitioners place the test material in the patient's hand or touch it to other parts of the body. If a weak muscle becomes stronger when a nutrient (or a food high in the nutrient) is tested, that supposedly indicates "a deficiency normally associated with that muscle." Treatment may include special diets, food supplements, acupressure, and spinal manipulation.

Contact Reflex Analysis (CRA) proponents claim that over a thousand health problems can be diagnosed with a muscle test during which the chiropractor's finger or hand is placed on one of 75 "reflex points" on the patient's body. If the patient's arm can be pulled downward, a condition corresponding to the "reflex" is considered present, and dietary supplements (typically made from freeze-dried vegetables or animal organs) are prescribed. CRA's chief proponent teaches that 80% of disease is due to allergy, the two main causes of disease are gallbladder disease and staph infections, and obesity is commonly caused by parasites.

The Morter Health System is claimed to be "a complete alternative healthcare system" that can correct physical (biomagnetic), nutritional, and emotional stresses. Its followers postulate that an imbalance in the patient's electromagnetic field causes unequal leg length, which the chiropractor can instantly correct by applying his own electromagnetic energy to points on the body. Supposedly, two fingers on each of the chiropractor's hands are North poles, two are South poles, and the thumbs are electromagnetically neutral. When imbalance is detected, the hands are held for a few seconds at "contact points" on the patient's body until the patient's legs test equally long. Proponents recommend testing early in infancy and at least monthly throughout life. The "nutritional" component is based on the belief that "patients can maintain life and vitality by consuming four times as much alkaline-forming as acid-forming foods." Proponents claim that saliva pH testing can determine whether to use nutritional supplementation and/or spinal manipulation. The recommended supplements include a barley juice formula said to be the best "overall body alkalizer."

NutraBalance is one of several systems in which the results of legitimate blood and urine tests are fed into a computer which determines alleged "metabolic types," lists supposed problem areas, and recommends dietary changes and food supplements from a manufacturer chosen by the chiropractor. Neither the existence of the types nor the recommended nutritional strategies have been scientifically substantiated.

At least 50 companies are marketing irrationally formulated supplement products exclusively or primarily through chiropractors. Some of these companies (or their distributors) sponsor seminars at which chiropractors are taught pseudoscientific nutrition concepts — including the use of supplements to treat disease. These seminars enable manufacturers and distributors to provide information on alleged therapeutic uses that would not be legal to place on product labels. Most chiropractors who recommend supplements sell them to their patients at two to three times their wholesale cost.

Fad Diagnoses

Many practitioners label patients with diagnoses not recognized by the scientific community. Some apply one or more of these diagnoses to almost every patient they see.

Years ago, many people who were tired or nervous were said to have "adrenal insufficiency." The vast majority of these people were not only misdiagnosed but were also treated with adrenal gland extract, a substance that the FDA later banned because it was too weak to treat the actual disease. "Low thyroid" (hypothyroidism) was likewise unjustifiably diagnosed in many cases of fatigue and/or obesity. Today's fad diagnoses used to explain various common symptoms are chronic fatigue syndrome, hypoglycemia, food allergies, parasites, environmental illness, candidiasis hypersensitivity, Wilson's Syndrome, leaky gut syndrome, and mercury amalgam toxicity. The first four on this list are legitimate conditions that unscientific practitioners overdiagnose. The rest lack scientific recognition.

Only a small percentage of people troubled by fatigue have chronic fatigue syndrome (CFS). The U.S. Centers for Disease Control and Prevention states that CFS should never be diagnosed unless fatigue persists or recurs for at least six months and is severe enough to reduce the patient's activity level by more than half. In addition, the fatigue should be accompanied by several other symptoms, such as severe headaches, low-grade fever, joint or muscle pain, general muscle weakness, sleep disturbance, and various psychological symptoms.

Real cases of hypoglycemia exist but are rare. The diagnosis should be reserved for patients who get symptoms two to four hours after eating, develop blood glucose levels below 45 mg per 100 ml whenever symptoms occur, and are immediately relieved of symptoms when blood sugar is raised. Low blood sugar levels without symptoms have no diagnostic significance because they occur commonly in normal individuals fed large amounts of sugar.

Doctors who overdiagnose hypothyroidism typically base their diagnosis on low temperature readings determined by placing the thermometer under the armpit. Proper diagnosis requires blood tests that measure hormone levels. Wilson's Syndrome was coined in 1990 by E. Denis Wilson, M.D. Its supposed manifestations include fatigue, headaches, PMS, hair loss, irritability, fluid retention, depression, decreased memory, low sex drive, unhealthy nails, easy weight gain, and about 60 other symptoms. However, Wilson claims that his "syndrome" can cause "virtually every symptom known to man." He also claims that it is "the most common of all chronic" ailments and "probably takes a greater toll on society than any other medical condition." Wilson claims to have discovered a type of low thyroid function in which routine blood tests of thyroid are often normal and the main diagnostic sign is body temperature that averages less than 98.6°F (oral). In 1992, the Florida Board of Medicine fined him $10,000, suspended his license for six months, and ordered him to undergo psychological testing. He has not reinstated his license. (Note: "Wilson's Syndrome" is not Wilson's disease, a rare condition caused by a defect in the body's ability to metabolize copper.)

Multiple chemical sensitivity is based on the notion that when the "total load" of physical and psychological stresses exceeds what a person can tolerate, the immune system goes haywire and hypersensitivity to tiny amounts of common foods and chemicals can trigger a wide range of symptoms. Doctors advocating this notion call themselves clinical ecologists or specialists in environmental medicine. Their treatment approach involves elimination of exposure to foods and environmental substances to which they consider the patient hypersensitive. Extreme restrictions can involve staying at home for months or living in a trailer designed to prevent exposure to airborne pollutants and synthetic substances. In many cases, the patient's life becomes centered around the treatment. In 1986, the American Academy of Allergy, Asthma and Immunology, the nation's largest professional organization of allergists, warned that, "Although the idea that the environment is responsible for a multitude of health problems is very appealing, to present such ideas as facts, conclusions, or even likely mechanisms without adequate support is poor medical practice."[17] In 1997, it reviewed the evidence again and reached similar conclusions.[18]

Clinical ecologists base their diagnoses primarily on "provocation" and "neutralization" tests in which patients report symptoms that occur soon after suspected substances are administered under the tongue or injected into the skin. If any symptoms occur, the test is considered positive, and lower concentrations are given until a dose is found that "neutralizes" the symptoms. Researchers at the University of California have demonstrated that these procedures are not valid. In a double-blind study, eighteen patients each received three injections of suspected food extracts and nine of normal saline over a three-hour period. The tests were conducted in the offices of clinical ecologists who had been treating them. In nonblinded tests, these patients had consistently reported symptoms when exposed to food extracts and no symptoms when given injections of saline (dilute salt water). But during the experiment, they reported as many symptoms following saline injections as they did after food-extract injections, indicating that their symptoms were nothing more than placebo reactions.[19]

Candidiasis hypersensitivity is another alleged diagnosis with multiple symptoms that include fatigue, depression, inability to concentrate, hyperactivity, headaches, skin problems (including hives), abdominal pain and bloating, constipation, diarrhea, respiratory symptoms, and problems of the urinary and reproductive organs. The main proponent claims that, "If a careful checkup doesn't reveal the cause for your symptoms, and your medical history [as described in his book] is typical, it's possible or even probable that your health problems are yeast-connected." The recommended treatment includes antifungal drugs, vitamin and mineral supplements, and diets that avoid refined carbohydrates, processed foods, and (initially) fruits and milk. The American Academy of Allergy, Asthma and Immunology regards the concept of candidiasis hypersensitivity as "speculative and unproven," and notes that everyone has some of its supposed symptoms from time to time.[20] The Academy has warned that some patients who take the inappropriately prescribed antifungal drugs will suffer side effects and that overuse of these drugs could lead to the development of drug-resistant microorganisms that endanger everyone.

Some unscientific practitioners claim that food allergies can cause virtually any symptom. Some measure the responses of white blood cells exposed to food extracts. Others measure the blood levels of various immune complexes. Some practitioners use muscle testing (described below) to diagnose allergies. The test results are then used to explain the patient's symptoms and dietary modification and supplements are recommended. Neither the tests nor the supplement regimens have a scientifically plausible rationale.

Another popular diagnosis among supplement promoters is "parasites," which may be treated with laxatives and other intestinal cleansers, colonic irrigation, plant enzymes, dietary measures, and homeopathic remedies. Yet another, "leaky gut syndrome," is described by proponents as a condition in which the intestinal lining becomes irritated and porous so that unwanted food particles, "toxins," bacteria, parasites, and "Candida" enter the bloodstream and result in "a weakened immune system, digestive disorders, and eventually chronic and autoimmune disease." Treatment of this alleged condition can include dietary changes (such as not eating protein and starch at the same meal); "cleansing" with herbal products; "reestablishing good balance" of intestinal bacteria; and supplemental concoctions claimed to strengthen and repair the intestinal lining.

Several hundred dentists, physicians, and various other holistic advocates claim that mercury-amalgam (silver) fillings are toxic and cause a wide range of health problems including multiple sclerosis, arthritis, headaches, Parkinson's disease, and emotional stress. They recommend that mercury fillings be replaced with either gold or plastic ones and that vitamin supplements be taken to prevent trouble during and after the process. Scientific testing has shown that the amount of mercury absorbed from fillings is only a tiny fraction of the average daily intake from food and is insignificant.[21] In 1996, the leading antiamalgamist, Hal A. Huggins, D.D.S., of Colorado Springs, Colorado, had his licensed revoked. During the revocation proceedings the administrative law judge concluded that Huggins had diagnosed "mercury toxicity" in all patients who consulted him in his office, even some without mercury fillings.

Dubious Tests

Many unscientific practitioners use nonstandard tests as gimmicks for recommending supplements. The most widely used include hair analysis, muscle-testing, live-cell analysis, Functional Intracellular Analysis, EAV testing, and symptom-based questionnaires.

Hair analysis is performed by obtaining a sample of hair, usually from the back of the neck, and sending it to a laboratory for analysis. The customer and the referring source usually receive a computerized printout that supposedly indicates deficiencies or excesses of minerals. Some also report supposed deficiencies of vitamins. Medical authorities agree that hair analysis is not appropriate for assessing the body's nutritional state but has very limited usefulness as a screening procedure for detecting toxic levels of lead or other heavy metals. Nor can it identify mineral deficiencies, because the lower limits of normal have not been scientifically established. Moreover, the mineral composition of hair can be affected by a person's age, natural hair color, and rate of hair growth, as well as the use of hair dyes, bleaches, and shampoos.[22]

When 52 hair samples from two healthy teenagers were sent under assumed names to 13 commercial hair analysis laboratories, the reported levels of minerals varied considerably between identical samples sent to the same lab and from lab to lab. The labs also disagreed about what was normal or usual for many of the minerals. Most reports contained computerized interpretations that were voluminous, bizarre, and potentially frightening to patients. Six labs recommended food supplements, but the types and amounts varied widely from report to report. Literature from most of the labs suggested falsely that their reports were useful against a wide variety of diseases and supposed nutrient imbalances.[23] The study demonstrated that even if the minerals can be accurately measured, the data have little or no practical value. A recent 2-year study of students exposed to fumes from metal welding found that hair analysis did not consistently reflect blood levels of 11 heavy metals.[24]

Muscle testing is part of a pseudoscientific system of diagnosis and treatment called applied kinesiology (AK). AK is based on the notion that every organ dysfunction is accompanied by a specific muscle weakness, which enables diseases to be diagnosed through muscle-testing procedures. Its practitioners, most of whom are chiropractors, also claim that nutritional deficiencies, allergies, and other adverse reactions to food substances can be detected by placing substances in the mouth so that the patient salivates. "Good" substances will make specific muscles stronger, whereas "bad" substances will cause specific weaknesses. Treatment may include special diets, food supplements, acupressure, and spinal manipulation. Applied kinesiology should be distinguished from kinesiology (biomechanics), which is the scientific study of movement. The concepts of applied kinesiology do not conform to scientific facts about the causes of disease. Controlled studies have found no difference between the results with test substances and with placebos.[25] Differences from one test to another may be due to suggestibility, variations in the amount of force or leverage involved, and/or muscle fatigue.

Live-cell analysis is carried out by placing a drop of blood from the patient's fingertip on a microscope slide under a glass coverslip to slow down the process of drying out. The slide is then viewed with a dark-field microscope to which a television monitor has been attached. Both practitioner and patient can see the blood cells, which appear as dark bodies outlined in white. The practitioner may also take Polaroid photographs of the television screen or make a videotape for himself and the patient. Proponents of live-cell analysis claim that it is useful for diagnosing vitamin and mineral deficiencies, enzyme deficiencies, tendencies toward allergic reactions, liver weakness, and many other health problems.

Dark-field microscopy is a valid scientific tool in which special lighting is used to examine specimens of cells and tissues. Connecting a television monitor to a microscope for diagnostic purposes is also a legitimate practice. However, experts believe that live-cell analysis is useless in diagnosing most of the conditions that its practitioners claim to detect.[26] Many of the reported observations are the result of cell changes that occur as the preparation begins to dry out.

Functional Intracellular Analysis (FIA) is claimed to precisely measure an individual's nutrient status. Its marketers have claimed that most Americans have nutrient deficiencies, and that "intracellular nutrient deficiencies" even occur in over 40% of the more than 100 million Americans taking multivitamins as "insurance." During the test, lymphocytes from the patient's blood are placed into petri dishes containing various concentrations of nutrients. A growth stimulant is added and, a few days later, technicians identify the dishes in which greatest cell growth takes place, which supposedly points to a deficiency. Properly performed lymphocyte cultures have a legitimate role in medical practice, but they are not appropriate for general screening or for diagnosing nutrient deficiencies in the manner used by FIA. The test merely measures the amounts of nutrients stored in the lymphocytes at the time of the test and not whether the body has a shortage.[27]

Some practitioners operate devices they claim can detect diseases, food allergies, and/or nutrient deficiencies by measuring "imbalances in the flow of electromagnetic energy along acupuncture meridians." The procedure is called electroacupuncture of Voll (EAV) or electrodermal testing. The devices are fancy galvanometers that measure electrical resistance of the patient's skin when touched by a probe. One wire from the device goes to a brass cylinder covered by moist gauze, which the patient holds in one hand. A second wire is connected to a probe that the operator touches to the patient's other hand or a foot. This completes a low-voltage circuit, and the device registers the flow of current. The information is then relayed to a gauge or computer screen that provides a numerical readout. However, the size of the number actually depends on how hard the probe is pressed against the patient's skin. The findings are then used to prescribe homeopathic remedies, acupuncture, dietary change, and/or vitamin supplements. These devices cannot be legally marketed in the U.S. for diagnostic or treatment purposes, but state and federal agencies have done little to curtail their use.

Some practitioners and retailers use questionnaires to help decide what supplements to recommend. The tests usually involve completion of questionnaires about diet, other lifestyle factors, and symptoms that supposedly signify deficiency. Some tests are scored by hand, and others are scored by a computer. Tests of this type are also available online. Questionnaires or computer programs used by supplement sellers invariably recommend supplements for everyone.

Herbal Treatment

Americans spend billions of dollars per year for capsules, tablets, bulk herbs, and herbal teas used for supposed medicinal qualities. Most are purchased over the counter, but some are prescribed by practitioners. Many herbs contain hundreds or even thousands of chemicals that have not been completely catalogued. While some may ultimately prove useful as therapeutic agents, others could well prove toxic. Most herbal products sold in the U.S. are not standardized. This means that determining the exact amounts of their active ingredients can be difficult to impossible. Moreover, many herbal practitioners are non-physicians who are not qualified to make appropriate diagnoses or to determine how herbs compare to proven drugs.

The Dietary Supplement Health and Education Act of 1994 includes herbal products in its definition of dietary supplements, even though herbs have little or no nutritional value. Since herbs are not regulated as drugs, no legal standards exist for their processing, harvesting, or packaging. In many cases, particularly for products with expensive raw ingredients, contents and potency are not accurately disclosed on the label. Many products marked as herbs contain no useful ingredients, and some even lack the principal ingredient for which people buy them. Some manufacturers are trying to develop industrywide quality-assurance standards, but possible solutions to the problem of product identification and standardization are a long way off.

Herbal advocates like to point out that about half of today's medicines were derived from plants. (Digitalis, for example, was originally derived from leaves of the foxglove plant.) This statement is true but misleading. Drug products contain specified amounts of active ingredients. Herbs in their natural state can vary greatly from batch to batch and often contain chemicals that cause side effects but provide no benefit. Surveys have found that the ingredients and doses of similar products vary considerably from brand to brand and even between lots of the same product. For example, researchers at the University of

Arkansas tested 20 supplement products containing ephedra (ma huang) and found that half the products exhibited discrepancies of 20% or more between the label claim and the actual content, and one product contained no ephedra alkaloids.[28] Ephedra products are marketed as "energy boosters" and/or "thermogenic" diet aids, even though no published clinical trials substantiate that they are safe or effective for these purposes. The researchers also noted that hundreds of such products are marketed, and that their number exceeds that of conventional prescription and nonprescription ephedra products, which are FDA-approved as decongestants. Products that combine ephedra with caffeine or a high-caffeine herb such as guarana or kola nut have harmed many users.

To make a rational decision about an herbal product, it would be necessary to know what it contains, whether it is safe, and whether it has been demonstrated to be as good or better than pharmaceutical products available for the same purpose. For most herbal ingredients this information is incomplete or unavailable. However, more than 60 natural remedies have been implicated in reactions that were fatal or potentially fatal.[29]

Even when a botanical product has some effectiveness, it may not be practical to use. For example, allicin, which is present in whole garlic cloves, has been demonstrated to moderately lower high blood pressure and high blood cholesterol. However, prescription drugs are more potent and predictable for this purpose. Some garlic supplement products contain no allicin, and some studies of these garlic products have found no beneficial effects. Allicin also has anticoagulant properties, which means that it may enhance the anticoagulant effects of such commonly used products as vitamin E, ginkgo, fish oil, aspirin, and prescription anticoagulants.

The best source of information about herbs is the *Natural Medicines Comprehensive Database,* which is available online (http://www.naturaldatabase.com) and in print[30] for $92 per year (or $132 for both versions). The online version is updated daily, while the print version is updated several times a year. The 1999 book covered 964 herbs and dietary supplements, of which only 15% had been proven safe and 11% had been proven effective.[31] Another excellent resource is the *Professional's Handbook of Complementary and Alternative Medicines,* which provides practical advice for over 300 herbs.[32] The widely touted Commission E report and its derivative, the *PDR for Herbal Medicine,* are not as reliable or practical.[33]

The recent entry of drug companies into the herbal marketplace may result in standardization of dosage for some products; and recent public and professional interest in herbs is likely to stimulate more research. However, with safe and effective medicines available, treatment with herbs rarely makes sense; and many of the conditions for which herbs are recommended are not suitable for self-treatment.

Other Questionable Methods

Chelation Therapy

Chelation therapy is a series of intravenous infusions containing EDTA, vitamins, and various other substances. It is claimed to be effective against kidney and heart disease, arthritis, Parkinson's disease, emphysema, multiple sclerosis, gangrene, psoriasis, and many other serious conditions. However, no well-designed research has shown that chelation therapy can help these conditions, and manufacturers of EDTA do not list them as appropriate for EDTA treatment. A course of treatment consisting of 20 to 50 intravenous infusions costs several thousand dollars.

Chelation therapy is heavily promoted as an alternative to coronary bypass surgery. It is sometimes claimed to be a "chemical Roto-Rooter" that can clean out atherosclerotic plaque from the body's arteries. However, there is no scientific evidence to support this claim. Lifestyle modification, which includes stress reduction, caffeine avoidance, alcohol limitation, smoking cessation, exercise, and nutritional counseling, is encouraged as part of the complete therapeutic program and may be responsible for some of the reported improvements.

The primary organization promoting chelation therapy is the American College for Advancement in Medicine (ACAM), which conducts courses, sponsors a journal, and administers a "board certification" program not recognized by the scientific community. ACAM's chelation protocol calls for intravenous infusion of 500 to 1000 ml of a solution containing 50 mg of disodium EDTA per kg of body weight, plus heparin, magnesium chloride, a local anesthetic (to prevent pain at the infusion site), several B-vitamins, and 4 to 20 g of vitamin C. This solution is infused slowly over 3.5 to 4 hours, one to three times a week. Additional vitamins, minerals, and other substances — prescribed orally — "vary according to preferences of both patients and physicians."

Chelation therapy is one of several legitimate methods for treating cases of heavy metal poisoning, but the chelating substance is calcium EDTA and the frequency of visits is different. Some chelation therapists submit fraudulent insurance reports claiming to have treated lead poisoning or another alleged toxic state. Lead poisoning in adults is uncommon and occurs primarily through (a) occupational exposure or (b) failing to take proper precautions when repainting an old house that had been painted with lead paint. If lead poisoning actually exists, whether discontinuation of exposure is sufficient treatment or chelation therapy should be administered depends on the blood lead concentration, the severity of clinical symptoms, the biochemical and blood abnormalities, and the nature of the exposure. The appropriate test for lead poisoning is a blood lead level, but some chelation therapists test urine and/or hair, which is unreliable to worthless.

In 1998, the Federal Trade Commission (FTC) secured a consent agreement barring ACAM from making unsubstantiated claims that chelation therapy is effective against atherosclerosis or any other disease of the circulatory system. Although the FTC could act against individual doctors who advertise falsely, it usually leaves that up to the state licensing boards. A few chelation therapists have had their licenses revoked, but most practice without government interference.

Colonic Irrigation

Some chiropractors and naturopaths advocate colonic irrigation as part of their treatment system. In this procedure, a rubber tube is passed into the rectum for a distance of up to 20 or 30 inches, and warm water is pumped in and out, a few pints at a time, typically using 20 or more gallons. Some practitioners add herbs, coffee, or other substances to the water. The procedure is said to "detoxify" the body. Its advocates claim that as a result of intestinal stasis, intestinal contents putrefy and toxins are formed and absorbed, which causes chronic poisoning of the body.

This "autointoxication" theory was popular around the turn of the century but was abandoned by the scientific community during the 1930s. No toxins have ever been identified, and careful observations have shown that individuals in good health can vary greatly in bowel habits. Proponents may also suggest that fecal material collects on the lining of the intestine and causes trouble unless removed by laxatives, colonic irrigation, special diets, and/or various herbs or food supplements that "cleanse" the body. The falsity of this notion is obvious to doctors who perform intestinal surgery or peer within the large intestine with a diagnostic instrument. Fecal material does not adhere to the intestinal lining, which is continuously desquamated as part of every stool.

Colonic irrigation is not only therapeutically worthless but can cause fatal electrolyte imbalance. Cases of death due to intestinal perforation and infection (from contaminated equipment) have also been reported.[34]

The Feingold Diet

In 1973, Benjamin Feingold, M.D., a pediatric allergist from California, proposed that salicylates, artificial colors, and artificial flavors caused hyperactivity in children. (Hyperactivity is now medically classified as an attention deficit disorder [ADD] or attention deficit-hyperactivity disorder [ADHD]). To treat or prevent this condition, Feingold suggested a diet free of such chemicals. Feingold's followers now claim that asthma, bed wetting, ear infections, eye-muscle disorders, seizures, sleep disorders, stomach aches, and a long list of other symptoms may respond to the Feingold program and that sensitivity to synthetic additives and/or salicylates may be a factor in antisocial traits, compulsive aggression, self-mutilation, difficulty in reasoning, stuttering, and exceptional clumsiness. The "Symptom Checklist" of the Feingold Association of the United States (FAUS) includes many additional problems.

Adherence to the Feingold diet requires a change in family lifestyle and eating patterns, particularly for families who prepare many meals from scratch. Feingold strongly recommends that the hyperactive child help prepare the special foods, and encourages the entire family to participate in the dietary program. Parents are also advised to avoid certain over-the-counter and prescription drugs and to limit their purchases of mouthwash, toothpaste, cough drops, perfume, and various other nonfood products to those published in FAUS's annual "Food List and Shopping Guide."

Current recommendations advise a two-stage plan that begins by eliminating artificial colors and flavors, the antioxidants BGA, BHT, and TBHQ; aspirin-containing products, and foods containing natural salicylates. If improvement occurs for four to six weeks, certain foods can be carefully reintroduced, one at a time. However, the *Feingold Cookbook* (published in 1979 but still in print) warns that, "A successful response to the diet depends on 100 percent compliance. The slightest infraction can lead to failure: a single bite or drink can cause an undesirable response that may persist for 72 hours or more."

Many parents who have followed Feingold's recommendations have reported improvement in their children's behavior, but carefully designed experiments fail to support the idea that additives are responsible for such symptoms in the vast majority of children.[35-37] Most improvement, if any occurs, appears related to changes in family dynamics, such as paying more attention to the children. Sugar and aspartame have also been blamed for hyperactivity, but well-designed studies have found no evidence supporting such claims.[38-40]

Questionable Cancer Methods

Cancer quackery is as old as recorded history and presumably has existed since cancer was recognized as a disease. Thousands of worthless folk remedies, diets, drugs, devices, and procedures have been promoted for cancer management. Questionable methods can be defined as diagnostic tests, or alleged therapeutic modalities that are (a) promoted for general use for cancer prevention, diagnosis, or treatment; (b) unsubstantiated; and (c) lack a scientifically plausible rationale. They include corrosive agents, plant products, diets and dietary supplements, herbs, drugs, correction of "imbalances," biologic methods,

TABLE 72.1

Signs of Quackery

When talking about nutrients, they tell only part of the story
They claim that most Americans are poorly nourished
They recommend "nutrition insurance" for everyone
They say that most diseases are due to faulty diet and can be treated with "nutritional" methods
They allege that modern processing methods and storage remove all nutritive value from our food
They claim that diet is a major factor in behavior
They claim that fluoridation is dangerous
They claim that soil depletion and the use of pesticides and "chemical" fertilizers result in food that is less safe and less nourishing
They claim you are in danger of being "poisoned" by ordinary food additives and preservatives
They charge that the Recommended Dietary Allowances (RDAs) have been set too low
They claim that under everyday stress your need for nutrients is increased
They recommend "supplements" and "health foods" for everyone
They claim that "natural" vitamins are better than "synthetic" ones
They suggest that a questionnaire can be used to indicate whether you need dietary supplements
They say it is easy to lose weight
They promise quick, dramatic, miraculous results
They routinely sell vitamins and other "dietary supplements" as part of their practice
They use disclaimers couched in pseudomedical jargon
They use anecdotes and testimonials to support their claims
They claim that sugar is a deadly poison
They display credentials not recognized by responsible scientists or educators
They offer to determine your body's nutritional state with a laboratory test or a questionnaire
They claim they are being persecuted by orthodox medicine and that their work is being suppressed because it's controversial
They warn you not to trust your doctor
They encourage patients to lend political support to their treatment methods

Note: Quackery can be defined as the promotion of unsubstantiated health methods for profit. Profit includes personal aggrandizement as well as monetary gain. The above are 25 ways to spot nutrition quacks.

devices, psychologic approaches, and worthless diagnostic tests. Many promoters combine methods to make themselves more marketable.

Promoters typically explain their approach in commonsense terms and appear to offer patients an active role in their care. They claim that:

- Cancer is a symptom, not a disease
- Symptoms are caused by diet, stress, or environment
- Proper fitness, nutrition, and mental attitude allow biologic and mental defense against cancer
- Conventional therapy weakens the body's reserves, treats the symptoms rather than the disease

Questionable therapies are portrayed as natural and nontoxic, while standard (responsible) therapies are portrayed as highly dangerous. Nutrition-related methods are compatible with each of these selling points. Most include self-care components that enable patients to feel more in control of their destiny. Many are claimed to cure by strengthening the immune system, even though cancer does not represent a failure of the immune system.[41] Cures attributed to questionable methods usually fall into one or more of five categories:

1. The patient never had cancer
2. A cancer was cured or put into remission by proven therapy, but questionable therapy was also used and erroneously credited for the beneficial result

TABLE 72.2

More Ploys That Can Fool You

"We really care about you!"
"We treat the whole patient."
"We attack the cause of disease."
"Out treatments have no side effects."
"We treat medicine's failures."
"Think positive!"
"Jump on the bandwagon."
"Our methods are time-tested"
"Backed by scientific studies"
"Take charge of your health!"
"Think for yourself."
"What have you got to lose?"
"If only you had come earlier."
"Science doesn't have all the answers."
"Don't be afraid to experiment."

Note: "Alternative" promoters offer solutions for virtually every health problem, including some they have invented. To those in pain, they promise relief. To the incurable, they offer hope. To gain a patient's allegiance it is not necessary to persuade the patient that all of the statements above are true. Just one may be enough.

3. The cancer is progressing but is erroneously represented as slowed or cured
4. The patient has died as a result of the cancer (or is lost to followup) but is represented as cured
5. The patient had a spontaneous remission (very rare) or slow-growing cancer that is publicized as a cure

Maintaining adequate nutrition is important for the general health of cancer patients, as it is with all patients, and diet plays a role in preventing certain cancers. However, no diet or dietary supplement product has been proven to improve the outcome of an established cancer. Detailed information on today's questionable cancer methods is available on the Quackwatch web site.[42]

Consumer Protection Laws

The Food, Drug, and Cosmetic Act defines drug as any article (except devices) "intended for use in the diagnosis, cure, mitigation, treatment, or prevention of disease" and "articles (other than food) intended to affect the structure or function of the body." These words permit the FDA to stop the marketing of products with unsubstantiated drug claims on their labels. The Dietary Supplement Health and Education Act (DSHEA) of 1994 undermined this situation by increasing the amount of misinformation that can be transmitted to prospective customers through third-party literature.[43] It also expanded the types of products that could be marketed as supplements. The most logical definition of dietary supplement would be something that supplies one or more essential nutrients missing from the diet. DSHEA went far beyond this to include vitamins, minerals, herbs or other botanicals, amino acids, other dietary substances to supplement the diet by increasing dietary intake, and any concentrate, metabolite, constituent, extract, or combination of

TABLE 72.3

Recipe for a New Fad Disease

Pick any symptoms — the more common the better
Pick any disease — real or invented (Real diseases have more potential for confusion because their existence can't be denied)
Assign lots of symptoms to the disease
Say that millions of undiagnosed people suffer from it
Pick a few treatments — Including supplements which will enable health food stores and chiropractors to get in on the action
Promote your theories through books and talk shows
Don't compete with other fad diseases; say that yours predisposes people to the rest or vice versa
Claim that the medical establishment, the drug companies, and the chemical industry are against you
State that the medical profession is afraid of your competition or trying to protect its turf
If challenged to prove your claims, say that you lack the money for research, that you are too busy getting sick people well, and that your clinical results speak for themselves

such ingredients. Although many such products (particularly herbs) are marketed for their alleged preventive or therapeutic effects, the 1994 law has made it difficult or impossible for the FDA to regulate them as drugs. Since its passage, even hormones such as dehydroepiandrosterone (DHEA, a steroid hormone intermediate) and melatonin are being hawked as supplements.

DSHEA also weakened the FDA's ability to regulate product safety by permitting it to restrict only substances that pose "significant and unreasonable risk" under ordinary conditions of use. However, the agency does not have sufficient resources to evaluate the safety of thousands of individual products. Because manufacturers are not required to submit safety information before marketing dietary supplements, the FDA must rely on adverse event reports, product sampling, information in the scientific literature, and other sources of evidence of danger. In addition, there is no practical way to ensure that the ingredients listed on product labels are actually in the products. Thus, the public is virtually unprotected against unsafe supplement and herbal products.

Consumer protection laws face further erosion. Within the past few years, several states have passed "Medical Freedom of Choice" bills that make it difficult for licensing boards to discipline alternative practitioners who mistreat their patients. The federal *Access to Medical Treatment Act* has been introduced to prevent the FDA from protecting the public against the sale and distribution of questionable drugs and devices. These measures reflect the "law of the jungle," under which the strong are free to feed upon the weak.

References

1. Sampson, W. In: *The Flight from Science and Reason* (Gross, PR, Levitt, N, Lewis, MW, Eds) *NY Acad Sci* 1996, pg 188.
2. Standards of Reporting Trials Group. *JAMA* 272: 1926; 1994.
3. Fonterosa, PB, Lundberg, GD. *JAMA* 280: 1618; 1998.
4. Sampson, W et al. *Clin J Pain* 7: 162; 1991.
5. Sampson, W. *Sci Rev Alt Med* 2: 54; 1998.
6. Dwyer, J. *Nutr Forum* 7: 9; 1990.
7. Pizzorno, JE, Jr, Murray, MT, Eds, *Textbook of Natural Medicine* 2nd Edition, WB Saunders, Philadelphia, 1999.
8. Pizzorno, JE, Jr, Murray, MT. *Encyclopedia of Natural Medicine* 2nd Edition, Prima Publishing & Communications, Rocklin, CA 1998.

9. Simon, A et al. *JAMA* 242: 1385; 1979.
10. Knipschild, P. *Br Med J* 297: 1578; 1988.
11. Lipton, M et al. *Task Force Report on Megavitamin and Orthomolecular Therapy in Psychiatry* American Psychiatric Association, Washington, DC, 1973.
12. Nutrition Comm. Can. Ped. Soc. *Can Med Assoc J* 143: 1009; 1990.
13. Committee on Nutrition, Am. Acad. Ped. *Pediatrics* 58: 910; 1976.
14. Kleijnen, J, Knipschild, P. *Biol Psychiatry* 29: 931; 1991.
15. Pfeiffer, SI et al. *J Autism Dev Disor* 25: 481; 1995.
16. Vaughan, K, McConaghy, M. *Austral N/Professional's Z J Psychiatry* 33: 84; 1999.
17. Anderson, JA et al. *J Allergy Clin Immunol* 78: 269; 1986.
18. Terr AI, Bardana EJ, Altman LC. *J Allergy Clin Immunol* 103: 36; 1999.
19. Jewett, DL, Fein, G, Greenberg, MH. *N Engl J Med* 323: 429; 1990.
20. Anderson, JA et al. *J Allergy Clin Immunol* 78: 273; 1986.
21. Mackert, JR, Jr, Berglund, A. *Crit Rev Oral Biol Med* 8: 410; 1997.
22. Hambidge, KM. *Am J Clin Nutr* 36: 943; 1982.
23. Barrett, S. *JAMA* 253: 1041; 1985.
24. Teresa, M, Vasconcelos, SD, Tavares, HM. *Sci Total Environ* 205: 189; 1997.
25. Kenny, JJ, Clemens, R, Forsythe, KD. *J Am Diet Assoc* 88: 698; 1988.
26. Lowell, J. *Nutr Forum* 3: 81; 1986.
27. Barrett, S, Herbert, V. *The Vitamin Pushers: How the Health-Food Industry is Selling America a Bill of Goods.* Prometheus, Amherst, NY, 1994.
28. Gurley, BJ et al. *Am J Health-System Pharm* 57: 963; 2000.
29. Marty, T. *Am Fam Physician* 59: 116; 1999.
30. Jellin, JM, Batz, F, Hitchens K, Eds, *Natural Medicines Comprehensive Database,* Therapeutic Research Faculty, Stockton, CA, 1999.
31. Marty, AT. *JAMA* 283: 2992; 2000.
32. Fetrow, CW, Avila, JR. *Professional's Handbook of Complementary and Alternative Medicines*, 2nd Edition, Springer, Springhouse, PA, 2001.
33. Marty, AT. *JAMA* 282: 1852; 1999.
34. Istre, GR et al. *N Engl J Med* 307: 339; 1982.
35. Wender, EH, Lipton, MA. *The National Advisory Committee Report on Hyperkinesis and Food Additives — Final Report to the Nutrition Foundation.* Nutrition Foundation, Washington, DC, 1980.
36. Lipton, MA, Mayo, JP. *J Am Diet Assoc* 83: 132; 1983.
37. Rowe, KS. *Aust Paediatr J* 24: 143; 1988.
38. Wolraich, ML et al. *N Engl J Med* 330: 301; 1994.
39. Wolraich, ML et al. *JAMA* 274: 1621; 1995.
40. Krummel, DA et al. *Sci Crit Rev Food Nutr* 36: 31; 1996.
41. Green, S. *Biomed Res* 1: 17; 1999.
42. Barrett, S. http://www.quackwatch.com/00AboutQuackwatch/altseek.html.
43. Barrett, S. http://www.quackwatch.com/02ConsumerProtection/dshea.html, 2000.

Index

A

B

C

D

E

F

G

H

I

J

K

L

M

N

O

P

Q

R

S

T

U

V

W

X

Y

Z